The ESC Textbook of
Heart Failure

European Society of Cardiology publications portfolio

The ESC Textbook of Cardiovascular Medicine (Third Edition)
Edited by A. John Camm, Thomas F. Lüscher, Gerald Maurer, and Patrick W. Serruys

The ESC Textbook of Preventive Cardiology
Edited by Stephan Gielen, Guy De Backer, Massimo Piepoli, and David Wood

The EHRA Book of Pacemaker, ICD, and CRT Troubleshooting: *Case-based learning with multiple choice questions*
Edited by Haran Burri, Carsten Israel, and Jean-Claude Deharo

The EACVI Echo Handbook
Edited by Patrizio Lancellotti and Bernard Cosyns

The ESC Handbook of Preventive Cardiology: *Putting prevention into practice*
Edited by Catriona Jennings, Ian Graham, and Stephan Gielen

The EACVI Textbook of Echocardiography (Second Edition)
Edited by Patrizio Lancellotti, José Luis Zamorano, Gilbert Habib, and Luigi Badano

The EHRA Book of Interventional Electrophysiology: *Case-based learning with multiple choice questions*
Edited by Hein Heidbuchel, Mattias Duytschaever, and Haran Burri

The ESC Textbook of Vascular Biology
Edited by Robert Krams and Magnus Bäck

The ESC Textbook of Cardiovascular Development
Edited by José Maria Pérez-Pomares and Robert Kelly

The EACVI Textbook of Cardiovascular Magnetic Resonance
Edited by Massimo Lombardi, Sven Plein, Steffen Petersen, Chiara Bucciarelli-Ducci, Emanuela Valsangiacomo Buechel, Cristina Basso, and Victor Ferrari

The ESC Textbook of Sports Cardiology
Edited by Antonio Pelliccia, Hein Heidbuchel, Domenico Corrado, Mats Borjesson, and Sanjay Sharma

The ESC Handbook of Cardiac Rehabilitation: *A practical clinical guide*
Edited by Ana Abreu, Jean-Paul Schmid, and Massimo Piepoli

The ESC Textbook of Intensive and Acute Cardiovascular Care (Third Edition)
Edited by Marco Tubaro, Pascal Vranckx, Susanna Price, Christiaan Vrints, and Eric Bonnefoy

The ESC Textbook of Cardiovascular Imaging (Third Edition)
Edited by José Luis Zamorano, Jeroen J. Bax, Juhani Knuuti, Patrizio Lancellotti, Fausto J. Pinto, Bogdan A. Popescu, and Udo Sechtem

The ESC Textbook of Cardiovascular Nursing
Edited by Catriona Jennings, Felicity Astin, Donna Fitzsimons, Ekaterini Lambrinou, Lis Neubeck, and David R. Thompson

The EHRA Book of Pacemaker, ICD, and CRT Troubleshooting Vol. 2: *Case-based learning with multiple choice questions*
Edited by Haran Burri, Jens Brock Johansen, Nicholas J. Linker, and Dominic Theuns

The EACVI Handbook of Cardiovascular CT
Edited by Oliver Gaemperli, Pál Maurovich-Horvat, Koen Nieman, Gianluca Pontone, and Francesca Pugliese

The ESC Textbook of Thrombosis
Edited by Raffaele De Caterina, David J. Moliterno, and Steen Dalby Kristensen

The ESC Textbook of
Heart Failure

Edited by

Petar M. Seferović
Serbian Academy of Sciences and Arts, University Medical Center Belgrade, Belgrade, Serbia

Andrew J.S. Coats
Heart Research Institute, Sydney, Australia

Gerasimos Filippatos
Attikon University Hospital, Athens, Greece

Stefan D. Anker
Charité University Hospital, Berlin, Germany

Johann Bauersachs
Hannover Medical School, Hannover, Germany

Giuseppe Rosano
St Georges Medical School, London, UK

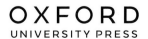

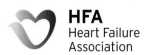

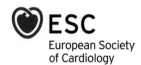

OXFORD UNIVERSITY PRESS

HFA Heart Failure Association

ESC European Society of Cardiology

OXFORD
UNIVERSITY PRESS

Great Clarendon Street, Oxford, OX2 6DP,
United Kingdom

Oxford University Press is a department of the University of Oxford.
It furthers the University's objective of excellence in research, scholarship,
and education by publishing worldwide. Oxford is a registered trade mark of
Oxford University Press in the UK and in certain other countries

Published in the United States of America by Oxford University Press
198 Madison Avenue, New York, NY 10016, United States of America

British Library Cataloguing in Publication Data
Data available

Library of Congress Control Number: 2023937963

ISBN 978–0–19–889162–8

DOI: 10.1093/med/9780198891628.001.0001

Printed in the UK by
Bell & Bain Ltd., Glasgow

Oxford University Press makes no representation, express or implied, that the
drug dosages in this book are correct. Readers must therefore always check
the product information and clinical procedures with the most up-to-date
published product information and data sheets provided by the manufacturers
and the most recent codes of conduct and safety regulations. The authors and
the publishers do not accept responsibility or legal liability for any errors in the
text or for the misuse or misapplication of material in this work. Except where
otherwise stated, drug dosages and recommendations are for the non-pregnant
adult who is not breast-feeding

Links to third party websites are provided by Oxford in good faith and
for information only. Oxford disclaims any responsibility for the materials
contained in any third party website referenced in this work.

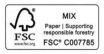

Contents

† Author deceased.

Contributors

Magdy Abdelhamid
Department of Cardiology, Kasr Al Ainy, Faculty of Medicine, Cairo University, Egypt

William T Abraham
Division of Cardiovascular Medicine, The Ohio State University, Columbus, Ohio, USA

Stephan Achenbach
Department of Cardiology, Friedrich-Alexander-Universität Erlangen-Nürnberg, Erlangen, Germany

Marianna Adamo
Institute of Cardiology, ASST Spedali Civili di Brescia and Department of Medical and Surgical Specialties, Radiological Sciences and Public Health, University of Brescia, Brescia, Italy

Stamatis Adamopoulos
Heart Failure and Transplant Unit, Onassis Cardiac Surgery Centre, Athens, Greece

Yehuda Adler
Leviev Heart Centre, Chaim Sheba Medical Centre, Sackler School of Medicine, Tel Aviv University, Tel Aviv, Israel

Stefan Agewall
Oslo University Hospital Institute of Clinical Medicine, University of Oslo, Norway; Karolinska Institute, Danderyd Hospital, Sweden

Piergiuseppe Agostoni
Centro Cardiologico Monzino, IRCCS, Milan; Department of Clinical Sciences and Community Health, University of Milan, Milan, Italy

Alberto Aimo
Interdisciplinary Center for Health Sciences, Sant'Anna School of Advanced Studies, Pisa; Cardiology Division, Fondazione Toscana Gabriele Monasterio, Pisa, Italy

Aris Anastasakis
Onassis Cardiac Surgery Center, Athens, Greece

Stefan D Anker
Department of Cardiology of German Heart Center Charité; Institute of Health Center for Regenerative Therapies (BCRT), German Centre for Cardiovascular Research (DZHK) partner Site Berlin, Charité Universitätsmedizin, Berlin, Germany

Carlo Arnò
Insubria University, Italy

Mattia Arrigo
Department of Internal Medicine, Stadtspital Zurich, Zurich, Switzerland

Birgit Assmus
Department of Internal Medicine, Cardiology and Angiology, Cardio-Pulmonary Institute (CPI), Justus-Liebig University, Giessen, Germany

Johannes Backs
Institute of Experimental Cardiology, Heidelberg University, Heidelberg; and DZHK (German Centre for Cardiovascular Research), Partner Site Heidelberg/Mannheim, Heidelberg, Germany

Lina Badimon
Cardiovascular Program-ICCC, IR-Hospital de la Santa Creu i Sant Pau, IIBSantPau, CiberCV, National Scientific Research Council (CSIC), Autonomous University of Barcelona, Barcelona, Spain

Anna Baritussio
Department of Cardiac, Thoracic, Vascular Sciences and Public Health, Padua University Hospital, Padua, Italy

Cristina Basso
Cardiovascular Pathology Unit, Department of Cardiac, Thoracic, Vascular Sciences and Public Health, University of Padua, Padua, Italy

Johann Bauersachs
Department of Cardiology and Angiology, Medical School Hannover, Hannover, Germany

Helmut Baumgartner
Department of Cardiology III: Adult Congenital and
Valvular Heart Disease, University Hospital Münster,
Münster, Germany

Udo Bavendiek
Department of Cardiology and Angiology, Medical School
Hannover, Hannover, Germany

Jeroen J Bax
Department of Cardiology, Leiden University Medical Centre,
Leiden, the Netherlands

Antoni Bayes-Genis
Heart Institute, Hospital Universitari Germans Trias i Pujol,
Badalona; Universitat Autonoma de Barcelona,
Barcelona, Spain

Tarek Bekfani
Department of Internal Medicine and Cardiology, University
Hospital Magdeburg, Magdeburg, Germany

Yuri Belenkov
Department of Hospital Therapy, I.M. Sechenov First Moscow
State Medical University, Moscow, Russian Federation

Tuvia Ben Gal
Heart Failure Unit, Cardiology Department, Rabin Medical
Center, Sackler Faculty of Medicine, Tel Aviv University,
Tel Aviv, Israel

Edoardo Bertero
Comprehensive Heart Failure Center (CHFC),
University Clinic Würzburg, Würzburg, Germany;
Department of Internal Medicine and Specialties,
University of Genova, Genova, Italy

Jan Biegus
Institute of Heart Diseases, Wroclaw Medical University,
Poland

Rudolf A de Boer
Department of Cardiology, Erasmus MC, Rotterdam,
the Netherlands

Michael Böhm
Klinik für Innere Medizin III, Universitätsklinikum des
Saarlandes, Saarland University, Homburg/Saar, Germany

Barry A Borlaug
Department of Cardiovascular Medicine, Mayo Clinic,
Rochester, Minnesota, USA

Biykem Bozkurt
Winters Center for Heart Failure, Cardiology, Baylor College of
Medicine and Michael E. DeBakey VA Medical Center, Houston,
Texas, USA

Hans-Peter Brunner-La-Rocca
Department of Cardiology, School for Cardiovascular Diseases
CARIM, Maastricht University and Maastricht University
Medical Centre, Maastricht, the Netherlands

Chiara Bucciarelli-Ducci
Royal Brompton and Harefield Hospitals, Guys and St Thomas
NHS Trust and School of Biomedical Engineering and Imaging
Sciences, Faculty of Life Sciences and Medicine, King's College
London, London, UK

Werner Budts
Congenital and Structural Cardiology, University Hospitals
Leuven; Department of Cardiovascular Sciences, Catholic
University of Leuven, Leuven, Belgium

Javed Butler
Baylor Scott and White Research Institute, Dallas, Texas
and University of Mississippi Medical Center, Jackson,
Mississippi, USA

Alida LP Caforio
Cardiology, Department of Cardiac, Thoracic, Vascular Sciences
and Public Health, University of Padova, Padova, Italy

Hugh Calkins
Cardiology Division, Department of Medicine, Johns Hopkins
Institutions, Baltimore, Maryland, USA

Daniela Cardinale
Cardioncology Unit, Division of Cardioncology and Second
Opinion, European Institute of Oncology, IRCCS, Milan, Italy

Ovidiu Chioncel
Emergency Institute for Cardiovascular Diseases 'Prof. C.C.
Iliescu', Bucharest, Romania and University of Medicine Carol
Davila, Bucharest, Romania

Dong-Ju Choi
Department of Cardiology, Cardiovascular Center, Seoul
National University Bundang Hospital and Division of
Cardiology, Department of Internal Medicine, College of
Medicine, Seoul National University, Seoul, South Korea

Andrew JS Coats
Heart Research Institute, Sydney, Australia

Alain Cohen-Solal
Université Paris Cité, IMRS 942 MASCOT, Department of
Cardiology, Hopital Lariboisiere, AP-HP, Paris, France

Sean Collins
Department of Emergency Medicine, Vanderbilt University
Medical Center, Veterans Affairs Tennessee Valley Healthcare
System, Geriatric Research, Education and Clinical Center
(GRECC), Nashville, Tennessee, USA

Gianluigi Condorelli
Department of Cardiovascular Medicine, IRCCS-Humanitas Research Hospital, Rozzano (MI) and Department of Biomedical Sciences, Humanitas University, Pieve Emanuele (MI), Italy

Domenico Corrado
Department of Cardiac, Thoracic and Vascular Sciences, University of Padova Medical School, Padova, Italy

Francesco Cosentino
Cardiology Unit, Department of Medicine Solna, Karolinska Institutet and Heart and Vascular Theme, Karolinska University Hospital, Stockholm, Sweden

Maria-Rosa Costanzo
Heart Failure Program, Midwest Cardiovascular Institute, Naperville, Illinois, USA

Martin R Cowie
Royal Brompton Hospital, London; School of Cardiovascular Medicine, Faculty of Medicine and Life Sciences, King's College London, London, UK

Filippo Crea
Department of Cardiovascular Sciences, Fondazione Policlinico Universitario A. Gemelli IRCCS, Rome and Department of Cardiovascular and Pulmonary Sciences, Catholic University of the Sacred Heart, Rome, Italy

Lorenzo Dagna
Unit of Immunology, Rheumatology, Allergy and Rare Diseases, IRCCS San Raffaele Hospital, Milan, and School of Medicine, Vita-Salute San Raffaele University, Milan, Italy

Kevin Damman
Department of Cardiology, University Medical Center Groningen, University of Groningen, Groningen, the Netherlands

Jeroen Dauw
Department of Cardiology, AZ Sint-Lucas, Ghent and Hasselt University, Diepenbeek, Belgium

Philippe Debonnaire
Department of Cardiology, Sint-Jan Hospital Bruges, Bruges, Belgium

Victoria Delgado
Department of Cardiology, Hospital University Germans Trias i Pujol, Badalona, Spain

Giacomo De Luca
Vita-Salute San Raffaele University, Milan; IRCCS San Raffaele Hospital - Unit of Immunology, Rheumatology, Allergy and Rare Diseases, Milan, Italy

Paul Dendale
Faculty of Medicine and Life Sciences, Hasselt University and Jessa Hospital, Hasselt, Belgium

Kenneth Dickstein
Stavanger University Hospital, University of Bergen, Stavanger, Norway

Javier Díez
Department of Cardiovascular Diseases, Center of Applied Medical Research and School of Medicine, University of Navarra, Pamplona, Spain

Wolfram Doehner
BIH Center for Regenerative Therapies, Charité-Universitätsmedizin Berlin, Berlin; Department of Cardiology, Virchow Campus; German Centre for Cardiovascular Research (DZHK), Partner Site Berlin; and Center for Stroke Research Berlin, Charité Universitätsmedizin Berlin, Germany

Thor Edvardsen
Department of Cardiology, Oslo University Hospital, Oslo and Institute for Clinical Medicine, University of Oslo, Oslo, Norway

Perry Elliott
Institute of Cardiovascular Science, University College London; Barts Heart Centre, Inherited Cardiovascular Disease, St Bartholomew's Hospital, London, UK

Volkmar Falk
Department of Cardiothoracic and Vascular Surgery, Deutsches Herzzentrum der Charité, Berlin; Charité – Universitätsmedizin Berlin, corporate member of Freie Universität Berlin, Humboldt-Universität zu Berlin, and Berlin Institute of Health; DZHK (German Centre for Cardiovascular Research), Partner Site Berlin, Germany; Department of Health Sciences and Technology, ETH Zürich, Zürich, Switzerland

Dimitrios Farmakis
Second Department of Cardiology, Athens University Hospital Attikon, National and Kapodistrian University of Athens Medical School, Athens, Greece

Roberto Ferrari
Centro Cardiologico Universitario di Ferrara, University of Ferrara, Ferrara, Italy

João Pedro Ferreira
Unidade de Investigaçao Cardiovascular-UnIC, Faculdade de Medicina Universidade do Porto, Porto, Portugal and Centre d'Investigations Cliniques Plurithématique 1433 and Inserm U1116, CHRU, FCRIN INI-CRCT (Cardiovascular and Renal Clinical Trialists), Université de Lorraine, Nancy, France

Gerasimos Filippatos
Attikon University Hospital, Department of Cardiology, National and Kapodistrian University of Athens, School of Medicine, Athens, Greece

Donna Fitzsimons
School of Nursing and Midwifery, Queen's University, Belfast, Northern Ireland, UK

Katerina Fountoulaki
2nd Department of Cardiology, National and Kapodistrian University of Athens Medical School, Athens, Greece

Nikolaos G Frangogiannis
Department of Medicine, Albert Einstein College of Medicine, Bronx, New York, USA

Stefan Frantz
University Hospital of Würzburg, Department of Internal Medicine I, Würzburg, Germany

Michael A Gatzoulis
Adult Congenital Heart Centre and National Centre for Pulmonary Hypertension, Royal Brompton and Harefield Hospitals, Guys & St Thomas's NHS Trust and Imperial College, London, UK

Antonello Gavazzi
FROM Research Foundation, Papa Giovanni XXIII Hospital, Bergamo, Italy

Isabelle C van Gelder
University of Groningen, University Medical Center Groningen, Groningen, the Netherlands

Alessia Gimelli
Fondazione Toscana Gabriele Monasterio, Imaging Department, Pisa, Italy

Eva Goncalvesova
National Cardiovascular Institute, Bratislava, Slovakia

Thomas M Gorter
Department of Cardiology, University Medical Centre Groningen, University of Groningen, Groningen, the Netherlands

Stephen Gottlieb
University of Maryland School of Medicine and Baltimore VAMC, Baltimore, Maryland, USA

Amy Groenewegen
Julius Center for Health Sciences and Primary Care, University Medical Center Utrecht, Utrecht, the Netherlands

Gabriele Guardigli
Centro Cardiologico Universitario di Ferrara, University of Ferrara, Ferrara, Italy

Finn Gustafsson
Rigshospitalet – Copenhagen University Hospital, Copenhagen, Denmark

Stephan von Haehling
Department of Cardiology and Pneumology, Heart Center, University of Göttingen Medical Center, Georg-August-University, Göttingen and German Center for Cardiovascular Research, Partner Site Göttingen, Göttingen, Germany

Brian P Halliday
Royal Brompton and Harefield Hospitals, Heart Division, Imperial College, National Heart and Lung Institute, King's College, London, UK

Christian W Hamm
Department of Internal Medicine, Cardiology and Angiology, Cardio-Pulmonary Institute (CPI), Justus-Liebig University, Giessen; Department of Cardiology, Kerckhoff-Klinik, Bad Nauheim, Germany

Tina Hansen
Department of Cardiology, Zealand University Hospital, Denmark

Veli-Pekka Harjola
Emergency Medicine, University of Helsinki and Department of Emergency Medicine and Services, Helsinki University Hospital, Helsinki, Finland

Stephane Heymans
Department of Cardiovascular Sciences, Center for Vascular and Molecular Biology, KU Leuven, Leuven, Belgium and Department of Cardiology, CARIM School for Cardiovascular Diseases, Maastricht University Medical Center, Maastricht, the Netherlands

Denise Hilfiker-Kleiner
Department of Cardiology and Angiology, Hannover Medical School, Hannover and Institute of Cardiovascular Complications in Pregnancy and in Oncologic Therapies, Comprehensive Cancer Centre, Philipps-Universität Marburg, Germany

Loreena Hill
School of Nursing and Midwifery, Queen's University, Belfast, Northern Ireland, UK

Lisa Hjelmfors
Department of Health, Medicine and Caring Sciences, Linkoping University, Linkoping, Sweden

Arno W Hoes
University Medical Center Utrecht, Utrecht, the Netherlands

Ulrich Hofmann
University Hospital of Würzburg, Department of Internal Medicine I, Würzburg, Germany

Martin Huelsmann
Department of Cardiology, University of Vienna, Vienna, Austria

Ferdinando Iellamo
Department of Clinical Science and Translational Medicine – University Tor Vergata, Rome, Italy

Massimo Imazio
Cardiology and Cardiothoracic Department, University Hospital 'Santa Maria della Misericordia', ASUFC, Udine; Department of Medicine, University of Udine, Udine, Italy

Tiny Jaarsma
Department of Health, Medicine and Caring Sciences, Linkoping University, Sweden and Julius Center for Health Sciences and Primary Care, University Medical Center Utrecht, the Netherlands

Ewa A Jankowska
Institute of Heart Diseases, Wroclaw Medical University and University Hospital in Wroclaw, Wroclaw, Poland

James L Januzzi
Cardiology Division, Massachusetts General Hospital and Harvard Medical School, Boston, Massachusetts, USA

Mariell Jessup
University of Pennsylvania, Philadelphia; American Heart Association, Dallas, Texas, USA

Andre Keren
Cardiology Division, Hadassah Hebrew University Hospital, Jerusalem and Heart Failure Center, Clalit Health Services, Jerusalem, Israel

Paulus Kirchhof
Department of Cardiology, University Heart and Vascular Center Hamburg; German Center for Cardiovascular Research (DZHK), partner Site Hamburg/Kiel/Lübeck, Germany and Institute of Cardiovascular Sciences, University of Birmingham, Birmingham, UK

Friedrich Köhler
Centre for Cardiovascular Telemedicine, Deutsches Herzzentrum der Charité, Berlin, and Charité – Universitätsmedizin Berlin, corporate member of Freie Universität Berlin and Humboldt-Universität zu Berlin, Berlin, Germany

Michel Komajda
Department of Cardiology, Groupe Hospitalier Paris Saint Joseph and Sorbonne University, Paris, France

Dipak Kotecha
Institute of Cardiovascular Sciences, University of Birmingham, Birmingham; UK Health Data Research UK Midlands, Queen Elizabeth Hospital Birmingham, University Hospitals Birmingham NHS Foundation Trust, Birmingham, UK

Deni Kukavica
University of Pavia, Pavia; Istituti Clinici Scientifici Maugeri, IRCCS, Maugeri, Italy; and Centro Nacional de Investigaciones Cardiovasculares (CNIC), Madrid, Spain

Carolyn SP Lam
National Heart Centre Singapore; Duke-National University of Singapore, Singapore

Ekaterini Lambrinou
Department of Nursing, School of Health Sciences, Cyprus University of Technology, Limassol, Cyprus

Irene Marthe Lang
Division of Cardiology, Department of Internal Medicine II, Vienna General Hospital, Medical University of Vienna, Vienna, Austria

Alessia Chiara Latini
Humanitas University, Italy

Davide Lazzeroni
Prevention and Rehabilitation Unit, IRCCS Fondazione Don Carlo Gnocchi ONLUS, Florence, Italy

Cecilia Linde
Department of Medicine, Karolinska Institutet; Heart and Vascular Theme, Karolinska University Hospital, Stockholm, Sweden

Ales Linhart
General University Hospital and First Faculty of Medicine, Charles University in Prague, Czech Republic

Yuri Lopatin
Department of Cardiology, Volgograd State Medical University, Volgograd, Russian Federation

Teresa López-Fernández
Cardio-oncology Unit, Cardiology Department, La Paz University Hospital, IdiPAZ Research Institute, Spain

Lars H Lund
Department of Medicine, Karolinska Institutet and Heart and Vascular Theme, Karolinska University Hospital, Stockholm, Sweden

Thomas F Lüscher
Royal Brompton and Harefield Hospitals, Heart Division, Imperial College, National Heart and Lung Institute, King's College London, UK and Center for Molecular Cardiology, University of Zurich, Switzerland

Alexander R Lyon
Royal Brompton Hospital, London, UK

Christoph Maack
Comprehensive Heart Failure Center (CHFC), University Clinic Würzburg, Würzburg, Germany

Mamas A Mamas
Keele Cardiovascular Research Group, Centre for Prognosis Research, Institute for Primary Care and Health Sciences, Keele University, UK

Athanasios Manolis
Cardiology Department, Metropolitan Hospital, Piraeus, Greece

Renzo Marcolongo
Cardiology, Department of Cardiac Thoracic Vascular Sciences and Public Health, University of Padova, Padova, Italy

Pieter Martens
Ziekenhuis Oost Limburg, Genk, - University Hasselt, Hasselt, Belgium and Kaufman Center for Heart Failure Treatment and Recovery, Department of Cardiovascular Medicine, Heart, Vascular and Thoracic Institute, Cleveland Clinic, Cleveland, Ohio, USA

Josep Masip
Research Direction, Consorci Sanitari Integral, University of Barcelona, Barcelona, Spain

Maria Benedetta Matrone
Cardiac Unit, Guglielmo da Saliceto Hospital, Piacenza, Italy

Marco Matucci-Cerinic
Unit of Immunology, Rheumatology, Allergy and Rare Diseases, IRCCS San Raffaele Hospital, Milan; Department of Experimental and Clinical Medicine, University of Florence; and Division of Rheumatology AOUC, Florence, Italy

Andrea Mazzanti
University of Pavia, Pavia; Istituti Clinici Scientifici Maugeri, IRCCS, Maugeri, Italy; and Centro Nacional de Investigaciones Cardiovasculares (CNIC), Madrid, Spain

Katherine McCreary
Cardiovascular Department, Belfast Health and Social Care Trust, Belfast, Northern Ireland, UK

Alexandre Mebazaa
Department of Anaesthesiology and Intensive Care, Hôpitaux Universitaires Saint Louis – Lariboisière, Paris, France

Mandeep R Mehra
Center for Advanced Heart Disease, Brigham and Women's Hospital and Harvard Medical School, Boston, Massachusetts, USA

Marco Metra
Institute of Cardiology, ASST Spedali Civili di Brescia and Department of Medical and Surgical Specialties, Radiological Sciences and Public Health, University of Brescia, Brescia, Italy

Andreas Metzner
Department of Cardiology, University Heart and Vascular Center Hamburg and German Center for Cardiovascular Research (DZHK), partner Site Hamburg/Kiel/Lübeck, Germany

Davor Miličić
University of Zagreb School of Medicine, Department of Cardiovascular Diseases, University Hospital Center Zagreb, Zagreb, Croatia

Ivan Milinković
Faculty of Medicine, Belgrade University, Belgrade and University Clinical Center of Serbia, Department of Cardiology, Belgrade, Serbia

Dimitris Miliopoulos
Heart Failure and Transplant Units, Onassis Cardiac Surgery Centre, Kallithea, Greece

Veselin Mitrović
Department Administration Forschung und Lehre, Kerckhoff-Klinik, Bad Nauheim, Germany

Luca Moderato
Heart Failure Unit, Cardiology, Guglielmo da Saliceto Hospital, Piacenza, Italy

Rocco A Montone
Department of Cardiovascular Sciences, Fondazione Policlinico Universitario A. Gemelli IRCCS, Rome, Italy

Luca Moroni
Unit of Immunology, Rheumatology, Allergy and Rare Diseases, IRCCS San Raffaele Hospital, Milan, Italy

Fabian Moser
Department of Cardiology, University Heart and Vascular Center Hamburg, Germany

Arend Mosterd
Meander Medical Center, Department of Cardiology, Amersfoort, the Netherlands

Brenda Moura
Cardiology Department, Porto Armed Forces Hospital and CINTESIS-Center for Health Technology and Services Research, Porto, Portugal

Wilfried Mullens
Department of Cardiology, Ziekenhuis Oost Limburg Genk, and Faculty of Medicine and Life Sciences, University Hasselt, Belgium

Danilo Neglia
Department of Cardiology, Fondazione Toscana Gabriele Monasterio, Pisa, Italy

Franz-Josef Neumann
Department of Cardiology and Angiology, University Heart Centre Freiburg-Bad Krozingen, Bad Krozingen, Germany

Maria Nikolaou
Cardiology Department, Sismanoglio General Hospital, Athens, Greece

Michael Noutsias
Department of Cardiology, Hospital of Brilon, Brilon and Faculty of Medicine, Martin-Luther-University Halle-Wittenberg, Halle (Saale), Germany

Maria Carmo Nunes
Hospital das Clinicas, School of Medicine, Federal University of Minas Gerais, Belo Horizonte, Minas Gerais, Brazil

Stefan Orwat
Department of Cardiology III: Adult Congenital and
Valvular Heart Disease, University Hospital Münster,
Münster, Germany

Ana Pardo Sanz
Department of Cardiology, Ciber CV, University Hospital
Ramón y Cajal, Madrid, Spain

John T Parissis
University Clinic of Emergency Medicine, Attikon General
Hospital, University of Athens, Athens, Greece

Massimo Francesco Piepoli
Clinical Cardiology, IRCCS Policlinico San Donato,
Milan, Italy; Department of Biomedical Sciences for Health,
University of Milan, Milan, Italy and Department of Preventive
Cardiology, Wroclaw Medical University, Wroclaw, Poland

Burkert Pieske
Department of Internal Medicine and Cardiology, Charité,
Universitätsmedizin Berlin; Campus Virchow Klinikum; and
German Center for Cardiovascular Research (DZHK), Berlin,
Partner Site, Berlin, Germany

Ileana L Piña
Thomas Jefferson University, Philadelphia; Central Michigan
University, Midlands, Michigan, USA

Fausto Pinto
Cardiology Department, Heart and Vascular Department,
University Hospital, Lisbon, Portugal

Bertram Pitt
School of Medicine, University of Michigan, Ann Arbor,
Michigan, USA

Sven Plein
Multidisciplinary Cardiovascular Research Centre and
Biomedical Imaging Science Department, Leeds Institute of
Cardiovascular and Metabolic Medicine, University of Leeds,
Leeds and School of Biomedical Engineering and Imaging
Sciences, Faculty of Life Sciences and Medicine, King's College
London, UK

Marija Polovina
Faculty of Medicine, Belgrade University, Belgrade and
Department of Cardiology, University Clinical Centre of Serbia,
Belgrade, Serbia

Eftihia Polyzogopoulou
Emergency Medicine, Attikon General Hospital, University of
Athens, Athens, Greece

Piotr P Ponikowski
Institute of Heart Diseases, Wroclaw Medical
University, Poland

Bogdan A Popescu
Department of Cardiology, University of Medicine and Pharmacy
'Carol Davila'-Euroecolab, Emergency Institute for Cardiovascular
Diseases 'Prof. Dr. C. C. Iliescu', Bucharest, Romania

Karina Portillo
Pneumology Department, Hospital Universitari Germans
Trias i Pujol, Fundació Institut d'Investigació en Ciències de la
Salut Germans Trias i Pujol, Badalona, Barcelona, Universitat
Autònoma de Barcelona, Spain

Susanna Price
Royal Brompton and Harefield Hospitals, Heart Division,
Imperial College, National Heart and Lung Institute, King's
College London, UK

Silvia G Priori
University of Pavia, Pavia; Istituti Clinici Scientifici Maugeri,
IRCCS, Maugeri, Italy; and Centro Nacional de Investigaciones
Cardiovasculares (CNIC), Madrid, Spain

Amina G Rakisheva
Department of Cardiology, Scientific Institution of Cardiology
and Internal Diseases, Almaty; Oonaev City Hospital, Almaty
Region, Kazakhstan

Claudio Rapezzi[†]
Cardiologic Centre, University of Ferrara and Maria Cecilia
Hospital, GVM Care and Research, Cotignola (Ravenna), Italy

Anneline te Riele
Division of Cardiology, Department of Heart and Lungs,
University Medical Centre Utrecht, Utrecht; Netherlands Heart
Institute, Utrecht, the Netherlands

Arsen D Ristić
Department of Cardiology, University Clinical Centre of Serbia,
Faculty of Medicine, University of Belgrade, Belgrade, Serbia

Jolien W Roos-Hesselink
Department of Cardiology, Erasmus Medical Center, Rotterdam,
the Netherlands

Giuseppe Rosano
IRCCS San Raffaele and San Raffaele University, Roma, Italy

Stephan Rosenkranz
Heart Center at the University of Cologne, Cologne, Germany

Patrick Rossignol
Université de Lorraine, INSERM, Centre d'Investigations
Cliniques 1433, CHRU de Nancy, Inserm 1116 and INI-
CRCT (Cardiovascular and Renal Clinical Trialists) F-CRIN
Network, Nancy, France; and Medical specialties – Nephrology
Hemodialysis Departments, Princess Grace Hospital Monaco,
and Monaco Private Hemodialysis centre, Monaco, Monaco

† Author deceased.

Laura Rottner
Department of Cardiology, University Heart and Vascular
Center Hamburg and German Center for Cardiovascular
Research (DZHK), partner Site Hamburg/Kiel/Lübeck, Germany

Frans H Rutten
Julius Center for Health Sciences and Primary Care, University
Medical Center Utrecht, Utrecht, the Netherlands

Elisabetta Salvioni
Centro Cardiologico Monzino, IRCCS, Milan, Italy

Gianluigi Savarese
Division of Cardiology, Department of Medicine, Karolinska
Institutet; Heart, Vascular and Neuro Theme, Karolinska
University Hospital, Stockholm, Sweden

Irina Savelieva
Molecular and Clinical Sciences Research Institute, St George's
University of London, London, UK

Ruben Schleberger
Department of Cardiology, Albertinen Heart and Vascular
Center, Albertinen Hospital, Hamburg

Felix Schoenrath
Department of Cardiothoracic and Vascular Surgery,
Deutsches Herzzentrum der Charité, Berlin;
Charité – Universitätsmedizin Berlin,
corporate member of Freie Universität Berlin,
Humboldt-Universität zu Berlin, and Berlin Institute of
Health; DZHK (German Centre for Cardiovascular Research),
Partner Site Berlin, Germany

Jelena P Seferović
Endocrinology, Diabetes and Metabolic Disorder Clinic,
Clinical Center of Serbia, Belgrade, Serbia

Petar M Seferović
Faculty of Medicine, Belgrade University and Serbian Academy
of Science and Arts, Belgrade, Serbia

Michele Senni
University of Milano-Bicocca; Cardiovascular Department
and Cardiology Unit, ASST Papa Giovanni XXIII Hospital,
Bergamo, Italy

Noor Sharrack
Multidisciplinary Cardiovascular Research Centre and
Biomedical Imaging Science Department, Leeds Institute of
Cardiovascular and Metabolic Medicine, University of Leeds,
Leeds, UK

Evgeny Shlyakhtho
Almazov National Medical Research Centre, Saint-Petersburg,
Russian Federation

Arvind Singhal
Department of Cardiology, St Bartholomew's Hospital,
London, UK

Karen Sliwa
Cape Heart Institute, Department of Medicine and Cardiology,
Faculty of Health Sciences, University of Cape Town, Cape
Town, South Africa

Randall C Starling
Kaufman Center for Heart Failure Treatment and Recovery,
Cleveland Clinic, Cleveland Clinic Lerner College of Medicine,
Cleveland, Ohio, USA

Anna Strömberg
Department of Health, Medicine and Caring Sciences and
Department of Cardiology, Linkoping University, Sweden

Christian Templin
Department of Cardiology, University Heart Center Zurich,
University Hospital Zurich, Switzerland

Jelena-Rima Templin-Ghadri
Department of Cardiology, University Heart Center Zurich,
University Hospital Zurich, Switzerland

Thomas Thum
Institute of Molecular and Translational Therapeutic Strategies,
Hannover Medical School, Hannover; Fraunhofer Institute
for Toxicology and Experimental Medicine, Hannover; and
REBIRTH Center for Translational Regenerative Medicine,
Hannover Medical School, Hannover, Germany

Daniela Tomasoni
Institute of Cardiology, ASST Spedali Civili di Brescia and
Department of Medical and Surgical Specialties, Radiological
Sciences and Public Health, University of Brescia, Brescia, Italy

Alessandro Tomelleri
Unit of Immunology, Rheumatology, Allergy and Rare Diseases,
IRCCS San Raffaele Hospital, Milan and School of Medicine,
Vita-Salute San Raffaele University, Milan, Italy

Alessandro Trancuccio
University of Pavia, Pavia; Istituti Clinici Scientifici Maugeri,
IRCCS, Maugeri, Italy; and Centro Nacional de Investigaciones
Cardiovasculares (CNIC), Madrid, Spain

Miguel Sousa Uva
Cardiac Surgery Department, Hospital Santa Cruz, Carnaxide,
and Avenue Prof Reynaldo dos Santos, 2790-134 Carnaxide,
Portugal.Cardiovascular Research Centre, Department of
Surgery and Physiology, Faculty of Medicine-University of Porto,
Porto, Portugal

Cristiana Vitale
Department of Medical Sciences, St George's Hospital Medical
School, London, UK

Maurizio Volterrani
Cardiopulmonary Department, IRCCS San Raffaele, Rome;
Exercise Science and Medicine, San Raffaele Open University,
Rome, Italy

Adriaan Voors
Department of Cardiology, University of Groningen, University Medical Center Groningen, Groningen, the Netherlands

Michael Würdinger
Department of Cardiology, University Heart Center Zurich, University Hospital Zurich, Switzerland

Junjie Xiao
Institute of Cardiovascular Sciences, Shanghai Engineering Research Center of Organ Repair, School of Life Sciences, Shanghai University, Shanghai, China

Mehmet Birhan Yilmaz
Faculty of Medicine, Department of Cardiology, Dokuz Eylul University, Izmir, Turkey

José Luis Zamorano
Cardiology Department, University Hospital Ramon y Cajal, Madrid, Spain

Faiez Zannad
Université de Lorraine, Nancy, France

Jian Zhang
Fuwai Hospital Chinese Academy of Medical Science, Beijing, China

Shelley Zieroth
University of Manitoba, Cardiac Sciences Program, St. Boniface Hospital, Winnipeg, Canada

Symbols and abbreviations

➲	cross-reference	AIRE	Acute Infarction Ramipril Efficacy
~	approximately	AIT	amiodarone-induced thyrotoxicosis
≥	equal to or greater than	AJR	abdominal-jugular reflux
≤	equal to or less than	AKI	acute kidney injury
>	greater than	AL	amyloid light chain
<	less than	ALDOB	fructose-bisphosphate aldolase B
AAV	antineutrophil cytoplasmic antibody-associated vasculitides	ALLHAT	Antihypertensive and Lipid Lowering Treatment to Prevent Heart Attack Trial
AC	adenylyl cyclase	ALT	alanine aminotransferase
ACC	American College of Cardiology	ALVC	arrhythmogenic left ventricular cardiomyopathy
ACCF	American College of Cardiology Foundation		
ACCOMPLISH	Avoiding Cardiovascular Events through Combination Therapy in Patients Living with Systolic Hypertension (trial)	AMI	acute myocardial infarction
		AMP	adenosine monophosphate
		AMPK	adenosine monophosphate-activated protein kinase
ACE	angiotensin-converting enzyme		
ACEI	angiotensin-converting enzyme inhibitor	AMR	antibody-mediated rejection
ACEP	American College of Emergency Physicians	ANCA	antineutrophil cytoplasmic antibody
ACHD	adult congenital heart disease	ANDROMEDA	Antiarrhythmic trial with DROnedarone in Moderate to severe congestive heart failure Evaluating morbidity DecreAse (study)
ACLI	acute cardiogenic liver injury		
ACM	alcoholic cardiomyopathy; arrhythmogenic cardiomyopathy		
		ANP	atrial natriuretic peptide
ACPO	acute cardiogenic pulmonary oedema	APB	atrial premature beat
ACS	acute coronary syndrome	APD	action potential duration
ADHERE	Acute Decompensated Heart Failure National Registry	APO	acute pulmonary oedema
		APS	antiphospholipid syndrome
ADHF	acute decompensated heart failure	A1R	adenosine A1 receptor
ADP	adenosine diphosphate	AR	adrenergic receptor; aortic regurgitation
ADPR	ADP-ribose	ARB	angiotensin receptor blocker
AF	atrial fibrillation	ARDS	acute respiratory distress syndrome
AF-CHF	Atrial Fibrillation in Congestive Heart Failure (trial)	ARF	acute rheumatic fever
		ARIC	Atherosclerosis Risk in Communities
AHA	American Heart Association	ARNI	angiotensin receptor–neprilysin inhibitor
A-HeFT	African-American Heart Failure Trial	ARVC	arrhythmogenic right ventricular cardiomyopathy
AHF	acute heart failure		
AHI	apnoea–hypopnoea index	AS	aortic stenosis; antisynthetase syndrome
AI	artificial intelligence; angiotensin I	ASA	acetylsalicylic acid
AICD	automatic implantable cardioverter–defibrillator	ASCEND-HF	Acute Study of Clinical Effectiveness of Nesiritide in Decompensated Heart Failure
AII	angiotensin II		

ASD	atrial septal defect
AST	aspartate aminotransferase
ASV	adaptive servo-ventilation
AT	angiotensin
AT_1	angiotensin II type 1 (receptor)
AT_2	angiotensin II type 2 (receptor)
ATHENA-HF	Aldosterone Targeted Neurohormonal Combined with Natriuresis Therapy in Heart Failure
ATP	adenosine triphosphate; anti-tachycardia pacing
ATTR	amyloid transthyretin
ATTRv	variant ATTR
ATTRwt	wild-type ATTR
AUC	area under the curve
AV	atrioventricular
AVA	aortic valve area
AVAi	indexed aortic valve area
AVC	arrhythmogenic ventricular cardiomyopathy
AVP	arginine–vasopressin
β-OHB	β-hydroxybutyrate
BAT	baroreflex activation therapy
BB	beta blocker
BCAA	branched-chain amino acid
BCATm	branched-chain amino-transaminase
BCKDH	branched-chain α-keto acid dehydrogenase
BCKDK	branched-chain ketoacid dehydrogenase kinase
BDH1	β-hydroxybutyrate dehydrogenase 1
BEST	Beta-Blocker Evaluation in Survival Trial
beta3AR	beta-3 adrenergic receptor
BIMA	bilateral internal mammary artery
BiPAP	bilevel positive airway pressure
B2M	beta-2-microglobulin
BMI	body mass index
BNP	B-type/brain natriuretic peptide
BP	blood pressure
BPG	benzathine benzylpenicillin
BR	breathing reserve
B19V	parvovirus B19
Ca^{2+}	calcium
$[Ca^{2+}]_I$	intracellular calcium concentration
CA	central apnoea; cardiac amyloidosis
CABG	coronary artery bypass graft
CAD	coronary artery disease
CAMIAT	Canadian Amiodarone Myocardial Infarction Trial
CaMKII	Ca^{2+}/calmodulin-dependent protein kinase II
cAMP	cyclic adenosine monophosphate
CANVAS	CANagliflozin ardiovascular Assessment Study
CaO_2	arterial oxygen content
CAV	cardiac allograft vasculopathy
CCB	calcium channel blocker
CCL	CC-chemokine ligand
CCM	cardiac contractility modulation
CCS	Canadian Cardiovascular Society
CCT	cardiac computed tomography
ccTGA	congenitally corrected transposition of the great arteries
CCU	coronary care unit
CD38	cyclic ADP ribose hydrolase
CDS	clinical decision supports
CEC	Clinical Events Committee
CE-CMR	contrast-enhanced cardiac magnetic resonance
CFR	coronary flow reserve
CFVR	coronary flow velocity reserve
cGMP	cyclic guanosine monophosphate
CH	congestive hepatopathy
CHAMPION	CardioMEMS Heart Sensor Allows Monitoring of Pressure to Improve Outcomes in Class III Heart Failure
CHAMPIT	acute Coronary syndrome, Hypertension emergency, Arrhythmia, acute Mechanical cause, Pulmonary embolism, Infections and Tamponade
CHD	congenital heart disease
CHF	congestive heart failure
CHS	Cardiovascular Health Study
CI	cardiac index; confidence interval
CIBIS II	Cardiac Insufficiency Bisoprolol Study II
CIED	cardiac implantable electronic device
CK	creatine kinase
CKD	chronic kidney disease
CKD-EPI	Chronic Kidney Disease Epidemiology Collaboration
Cl^-	chloride
CLD	chronic lung disease
CMD	coronary microvascular dysfunction
CMR	cardiac magnetic resonance
CMR-FT	CMR feature tracking
CMRI	cardiac magnetic resonance imaging
CMV	cytomegalovirus
CNOS	constitutive nitric oxide synthase
CNP	C-type natriuretic peptide
CO	cardiac output; carbon monoxide
CO_2	carbon dioxide
CoA	coenzyme A
COAPT	Cardiovascular Outcomes Assessment of the MitraClip Percutaneous Therapy for Heart Failure Patients with Functional Mitral Regurgitation
COMET	Carvedilol Or Metoprolol European Trial
COMPASS	Cardiovascular Outcomes for People Using Anticoagulation Strategies (trial)

CONSENSUS	Cooperative North Scandinavian Enalapril Survival	DCM	dilated cardiomyopathy
COPD	chronic obstructive pulmonary disease	DD	diastolic dysfunction
COPERNICUS	Carvedilol Prospective Randomized Cumulative Survival (trial)	DECISION	Digoxin Evaluation in Chronic heart failure: Investigational Study In Outpatients in the Netherlands
CoQ10	coenzyme Q10	DI	dyssynchrony index
COVID-19	coronavirus disease 2019	DIAMOND	Danish Investigations of Arrhythmia and Mortality on Dofetilide (trial)
CP	constrictive pericarditis		
CPAP	continuous positive airway pressure	DIGIT-HF	DIGitoxin to Improve ouTcomes in patients with advanced chronic Heart Failure (trial)
CPB	cardiopulmonary bypass		
CpC-PH	combined precapillary and post-capillary pulmonary hypertension	DNP	D-type natriuretic peptide
		DOAC	direct-acting oral anticoagulant
CPET	cardiopulmonary exercise testing	DOSE	Diuretic Strategies in Patients with Acute Decompensated Heart Failure (trial)
CPFE	combined pulmonary fibrosis and emphysema		
CPT1	carnitine palmitoyltransferase 1	DPD	3,3-diphosphono-1,2-propanodicarboxylic acid
Cr	creatine	DPI	dual-pathway inhibition
CR	controlled release	DPP4	dipeptidyl peptidase 4
CrCl	creatinine clearance	DSA	donor-specific antibodies
CREDENCE	Canagliflozin and Renal Events in Diabetes with Established Nephropathy Clinical Evaluation (trial)	d-TGA	dextro-transposition of the great arteries
		Ea	arterial elastance
		EACTS	European Association for Cardio-Thoracic Surgery
CRF	cardiorespiratory fitness		
CRISPR	clustered regularly interspaced short palindromic repeats	EACVI	European Association of Cardiovascular Imaging
		EAPC	European Association of Preventive Cardiology
CRP	C-reactive protein		
CRT	cardiac resynchronization therapy	EC	excitation–contraction
CRT-D	CRT-defibrillator	ECG	electrocardiography
CRT-P	CRT-pacemaker	ECHO	echocardiography
CS	cardiogenic shock	ECMO	extracorporeal membrane oxygenation
CSA	central sleep apnoea	ecNOS	endothelial constitutive NO synthase
CSR	Cheyne–Stokes respiration	ECV	extracellular volume
CT	computed tomography	ED	Emergency Department
CTA	computed tomographic angiography	EDPVR	end-diastolic pressure–volume relationship
CTCA	CT coronary angiography	EDV	end-diastolic volume
CTEPH	chronic thromboembolic pulmonary hypertension	Ees	end-systolic elastance
		EF	ejection fraction
CTLA-4	cytotoxic lymphocyte-associated protein 4	eGFR	estimated glomerular filtration rate
cTn	cardiac troponin	EGFR	epidermal growth factor receptor
CTPA	computed tomography pulmonary angiography	EHRA	European Heart Rhythm Association
		EI	endotracheal intubation
CV	cardiovascular	ELISA	enzyme-linked immunosorbent assay
CVAE	cardiovascular adverse event	ELITE	Evaluation of Losartan in the Elderly (trial)
CVD	cardiovascular disease	EMA	European Medicines Agency
CvO_2	mixed venous oxygen content	Emax	elastance
CVOT	cardiovascular outcomes trial	EMB	endomyocardial biopsy
CVP	central venous pressure	EMCDDA	European Monitoring Centre for Drugs and Drug Addiction
CXCL12	CXC motif ligand-12		
2D	two-dimensional	EMF	endomyocardial fibrosis
3D	three-dimensional	eNAC	epithelial Na^+ channel
4D	four-dimensional	eNOS	endothelial nitric oxide synthase
DAMP	damage-associated molecular pattern	EORP	EURObservational Research Programme
DAPT	dual antiplatelet therapy	EOV	exertional oscillatory ventilation
DBP	diastolic blood pressure	Epac	exchange protein directly activated by cAMP
DCA	dichloroacetate	EROA	effective regurgitant orifice area

ERS	European Respiratory Society	G_s	stimulatory G protein
ESC	European Society of Cardiology	GSH	glutathione
ESH	European Society of Hypertension	GWAS	genome-wide association study
ESPVR	end-systolic pressure–volume relationship	GWTG-HF	Get With The Guidelines–Heart Failure (registry)
ESV	end-systolic volume		
ET	endothelin	HAPE	high-altitude pulmonary oedema
ETC	electron transport chain	Hb	haemoglobin
EURIDIS	EURopean trial In atrial fibrillation or flutter patients receiving Dronedarone for the maintenance of Sinus rhythm	HbA1c	glycosylated haemoglobin
		HBP	hexosamine biosynthetic pathway
		HCM	hypertrophic cardiomyopathy
EUROPA	EURopean trial On reduction of cardiac events with Perindopril in stable coronary Artery disease	HCN	hyperpolarization-activated cyclic nucleotide-gated (channel)
		HDAC	histone deacetylase
EuroSCORE II	European System for Cardiac Operative Risk Evaluation II	HDL-C	high-density lipoprotein cholesterol
		HED	hydroxyephedrine
EVALUATE-HF	Effects of Sacubitril/Valsartan vs. Enalapril on Aortic Stiffness in Patients With Mild to Moderate HF With Reduced Ejection Fraction	HER2	human epidermal growth factor receptor 2
		HES	hypereosinophilic syndrome
		HF	heart failure
		HFA	Heart Failure Association of European Society of Cardiology
EVEREST	Efficacy of Vasopressin Antagonism in Heart Failure Outcome Study With Tolvaptan	HfimpEF	heart failure with improved ejection fraction
EVM	endocardial voltage mapping		
EWGSOP	European Working Group on Sarcopenia in Older People	HfmrEF	heart failure with mildly reduced (mid-range) ejection fraction
FA	fatty acid	HfpEF	heart failure with preserved ejection fraction
FAC	fractional area change	HfrecEF	heart failure with recovered ejection fraction
FDA	Food and Drug Administration	HfrEF	heart failure with reduced ejection fraction
FDG	fluorodeoxyglucose	HFSA	Heart Failure Society of America
Fe^{2+}	ferrous ion	HH	hereditary haemochromatosis
FEV1	forced expiratory volume in 1 second	HHF	hospitalization for heart failure
FFA	free fatty acid	HHV	human herpesvirus
FFR	fractional flow reserve	HIF	hypoxia inducible factor
FGE	fast gradient echo	HIIT	high-intensity interval training
FGF	fibroblast growth factor	HIV	human immunodeficiency virus
FHS	Framingham Heart Study	HMDP	hydroxymethylene diphosphonate
FoCUS	focused cardiac ultrasound	HMG-CoA	hydroxymethylglutaryl coenzyme A
FSV	forward stroke volume	HMOD	hypertension-mediated organ damage
FVC	forced vital capacity	HNDC	hypokinetic non-dilated cardiomyopathy
GAG	glycosaminoglycan	HNO	nitroxyl
Gb_3	globotriaosylceramide	HNOCM	hypertrophic non-obstructive cardiomyopathy
GDMT	guideline-directed medical therapy		
GDT	guideline-directed therapies	H_2O	water
GESICA	Grupo de Estudio de la Sobrevida en la Insuficiencia Cardiaca en Argentina (trial)	H_2O_2	hydrogen peroxide
		HOCM	hypertrophic obstructive cardiomyopathy
		HOPE	Heart Outcomes Prevention Evaluation (trial)
GFR	glomerular filtration rate		
GH	growth hormone	HR	heart rate; hazard ratio
GISSI-3	3 Gruppo Italiano per lo Studio della Soprovvivenza nell'Infarto Miocardico	Hrmax	maximal heart rate
		HRR	heart rate recovery
		HRS	Heart Rhythm Society
GLP1	glucagon-like peptide 1	HRV	heart rate variability
GLS	global longitudinal strain	hs	high-sensitivity
GLUT	glucose transporter	hsCRP	high-sensitivity C-reactive protein
GPX	glutathione peroxidase	hs-cTn	high-sensitivity cardiac troponin
GRE	gradient echo		

HT	heart transplantation
HTN	hypertension
IABP	intra-aortic balloon pump
I_{Ca}	influx of calcium
ICA	invasive coronary angiography
ICD	International Classification of Disease; implantable cardioverter–defibrillator
ICI	immune checkpoint inhibitor
ICM	ischaemic cardiomyopathy
ICU	intensive care unit
ID	iron deficiency
IDH2	isocitrate dehydrogenase type 2
iFR	instantaneous wave-free ratio
IGF-1	insulin-like growth factor 1
IGFBP7	insulin-like growth factor binding protein 7
IgG	immunoglobulin G
IHD	ischaemic heart disease
IL-6	interleukin-6
IL-6R	interleukin-6 receptor
ILD	interstitial lung disease
IMA	internal mammary artery
IMAC	inner membrane anion channel
IMM	inner mitochondrial membrane
IMR	index of microvascular resistance
iNO	inhaled nitric oxide
INR	international normalized ratio
IOC	iron overload cardiomyopathy
IPAC	Investigations of Pregnancy-Associated Cardiomyopathy (study)
IpC-PH	isolated post-capillary pulmonary hypertension
IPD	individual patient data
IPF	idiopathic pulmonary fibrosis
IQR	interquartile range
IRD	incidence rate difference
IRR	incidence rate ratio
ISIS-4	4th International Study of Infarct Survival
ITF	International Task Force
ITT	intention-to-treat
IVIg	intravenous immunoglobulin
JHFS	Japanese Heart Failure Society
JVP	jugular venous pressure
K^+	potassium
KorAHF	Korean Acute Heart Failure
LA	left atrial/atrium
LAD	left anterior descending artery
LAP	left atrial pressure
LBBB	left bundle branch block
LDH	lactate dehydrogenase
LDL-C	low-density lipoprotein cholesterol
L-FABP	liver fatty acid-binding protein
LGE	late gadolinium enhancement
LIMA	left internal mammary artery
LMS	left main stem
LMWH	low-molecular weight heparin
LNA	locked nucleic acid
LPS	lipopolysaccharide
LTCC	L-type calcium channel
LV	left ventricular/left ventricle
LVAD	left ventricular assist device
LVD	left ventricular dysfunction
LVEDP	left ventricular end-diastolic pressure
LVEDVI	left ventricular end-diastolic volume index
LVEF	left ventricular ejection fraction
LVESD	left ventricular end-systolic diameter
LVESV	left ventricular end-systolic volume
LVESVI	left ventricular end-systolic volume index
LVFP	left ventricular diastolic filling pressure
LVH	left ventricular hypertrophy
LVOT	left ventricular outflow tract
LVOTO	left ventricular outflow tract obstruction
LVP	left ventricular pressure
LVSD	left ventricular systolic dysfunction
LVSWI	left ventricular stroke work index
LVWT	left ventricular wall thickness
m6A	N^6-methyladenosine
MACE	major adverse cardiovascular/cardiac events
MADIT-CRT	Multicenter Automatic Defibrillator Implantation with Cardiac Resynchronization Therapy
MAP	mitogen-activated protein
MAPK	mitogen-activated protein kinase
MasR	Mas receptor
MBF	myocardial blood flow
MCD	malonyl-CoA decarboxylase
MCE	moderate continuous exercise
MCP-1	monocyte chemoattractant protein 1
MCS	mechanical circulatory support
MCU	mitochondrial Ca^{2+} uniporter
MDCT	multidetector computed tomography
MDRD	Modification of Diet in Renal Disease
MECKI	Metabolic Exercise test data combined with Cardiac and Kidney Indexes score
MELD	Model for End Stage Liver Disease
MELD-XI	Model for End Stage Liver Disease excluding INR
MEF 2	myocyte enhancer factor 2
MERIT-HF	Metoprolol CR/XL Randomised Intervention Trial in Congestive Heart Failure
MESA	Multi-Ethnic Study of Atherosclerosis
MET	metabolic equivalent
Mg^{2+}	magnesium
MHD	mean heart dose
6MHW	6-minute hall walk
MI	myocardial infarction
MIBG	meta-iodobenzylguanidine
miRNA	microRNA
MLHFQ	Minnesota Living with Heart Failure Questionnaire

MMP	matrix metalloproteinase
MNA	Mini Nutritional Assessment
Mn-SOD	manganese-dependent superoxide dismutase
MODS	multiple organ dysfunction syndrome
MOLLI	modified look-locker inversion recovery
mPAP	mean pulmonary artery pressure
MPC	mitochondrial pyruvate carrier
mPCWP	mean pulmonary capillary wedge pressure
MPS	myocardial perfusion scintigraphy
mPTP	mitochondrial permeability transition pore
MR	mitral regurgitation; mineralocorticoid hormone receptor
MRA	mineralocorticoid receptor antagonist
mRAP	mean right atrial pressure
MRI	magnetic resonance imaging
mRNA	messenger RNA
Mrp4	multidrug resistance protein 4
MR-proANP	mid-regional pro-atrial natriuretic peptide
MT	metabolic threshold
mTOR	mechanistic/mammalian target of rapamycin
MVO	microvascular obstruction
MVO$_2$	oxygen consumption
MVR	mitral valve repair
MVV	maximal voluntary ventilation
6MWT	6-minute walking test
Na$^+$	sodium
NAD	nicotinamide adenine dinucleotide
NADPH	nicotinamide adenine dinucleotide phosphate
NAM	nicotinamide
NAMPT	nicotinamide phosphoribosyl transferase
nc	non-coding
NCC	Na$^+$/Cl$^-$ cotransporter
NCDR	National Cardiovascular Data Registry
NCLX	Na$^+$/Ca^{2+} exchanger
NCX	sodium–calcium exchanger
NDCC	non-dihydropyridine calcium channel blocker
NEPi	neprilysin inhibitor
NFAT	nuclear factor of activated T cells
NF-κB	nuclear factor kappa B
NHANES	National Health and Nutrition Examination Survey
NHE	Na$^+$/H$^+$ exchanger
NICE	National Institute for Health and Care Excellence
NIH	National Institutes of Health
NIPPV	non-invasive positive pressure ventilation
NIV	non-invasive ventilation
NKA	Na$^+$/K$^+$-ATPase
NKCC2	Na$^+$–K$^+$–2Cl$^-$ cotransporter 2
NMN	nicotinamide mononucleotide
NNT	nicotinamide nucleotide transhydrogenase
NO	nitric oxide

NOAC	non-vitamin K oral anticoagulant
NOS	nitric oxide synthase
NP	natriuretic peptide
N-3-PUFA	N-3 polyunsaturated fatty acids
NPY	neuropeptide Y
NR	nicotinamide riboside
NSAID	non-steroidal anti-inflammatory drug
NSAT	non-sustained atrial tachycardia
NSF	nephrogenic systemic fibrosis
NSVT	non-sustained ventricular tachycardia
NT-proBNP	N-terminal pro-B-type natriuretic peptide
NYHA	New York Heart Association
O$_2$	oxygen
O$_2^-$	superoxide
OAC	oral anticoagulant
OAT	organic anion transporter
OCTAVE	Omapatrilat Cardiovascular Treatment Versus Enalapril (trial)
OGlcNAcylation	Olinked glycosylation
OM	omecamtiv mecarbil
OMT	optimal medical therapy
ONPHEC	Ontario Population Health and Environment Cohort
OPTIC	Optimal Pharmacological Therapy in Cardioverter Defibrillator Patients (trial)
OPTIMIZE-HF	Organized Program to Initiate Lifesaving Treatment in Hospitalized Patients with Heart Failure
OR	odds ratio
OSA	obstructive sleep apnoea
OUES	oxygen uptake efficiency slope
OVERTURE	Omapatrilat Versus Enalapril Randomized Trial of Utility in Reducing events
PA	pulmonary artery
PAC	pulmonary artery catheterization
PAH	pulmonary arterial hypertension
PAI-1	plasminogen activator inhibitor 1
PALLAS	Permanent Atrial fibriLLAtion outcome Study using dronedarone on top of standard therapy
PaO$_2$	partial oxygen pressure
PAP	pulmonary artery pressure
PAR	population attributable risk
PARADIGM-HF	Prospective comparison of ARNI with ACEI to Determine Impact on Global Mortality and morbidity in Heart Failure (trial)
PARAGON-HF	Prospective Comparison of ARNI with ARB Global Outcomes in HF With Preserved Ejection Fraction (trial)
PARAMOUNT	Prospective comparison of ARNI with ARB on the Management Of heart failUre with preserved ejection fraction (trial)
PARP	poly (ADP-ribose) polymerase
PASP	pulmonary artery systolic pressure

PB	periodic breathing
PCI	percutaneous coronary intervention
PCr	phosphocreatine
PCWP	pulmonary capillary wedge pressure
PD-1	programmed cell death protein 1
PDE3	phosphodiesterase 3
PDE4	phosphodiesterase 4
PDGFR	platelet-derived growth factor receptor
PDH	pyruvate dehydrogenase
PD-L1	programmed cell death ligand 1
PE	pulmonary embolism
PEA	pulseless electrical activity
PEEP	positive end-expiratory pressure
PEF	peak expiratory flow
PESI	Pulmonary Embolism Severity Index
PET	positron emission tomography
PETCO$_2$	end-tidal partial pressure of carbon dioxide
PFK-1	phosphofructokinase 1
PGmean	mean pressure gradient
PH	pulmonary hypertension
PH-LHD	pulmonary hypertension with left heart disease
PHM	predicted heart mass
PI	proteasome inhibitor
PICP	procollagen type I carboxy-terminal propeptide
PI3K	phosphoinositide 3-kinase
PISA	proximal isovelocity surface area
PKA	protein kinase A
PKG	protein kinase G
PLB	phospholamban
PLE	protein-losing enteropathy
PLN	phospholamban
pMCS	percutaneous mechanical circulatory support
POCUS	point-of-care ultrasound
Pplat	plateau pressure
PPAR	peroxisome proliferator-activated receptor
ppb	part per billion
pPCI	primary percutaneous coronary intervention
PPCM	peripartum cardiomyopathy
PPG	photoplethysmography
ppm	part per million
PQC	protein quality control
PRA	panel reactive antibody
PREVEND	Prevention of Renal and Vascular End-stage Disease (study)
PRIME	Pharmacological Reduction of Functional, Ischemic Mitral Regurgitation (study)
PROVE-HF	Prospective Study of Biomarkers, Symptom Improvement, and Ventricular Remodeling During Sacubitril/Valsartan Therapy for HF
PRX	peroxiredoxin
PSRF	psychosocial risk factor
pSS	primary Sjogren syndrome
PTP	pretest probability
PV	pressure–volume (loop)

PVC	premature ventricular complex
PVR	pulmonary vascular resistance
PVRi	pulmonary vascular resistance index
PYP	pyrophosphate
QoL	quality of life
Qp/Qs	pulmonary-to-systemic flow ratio
QUIET	Quinapril Ischemic Event Trial
RA	radial artery; right atrium
RAID	Ranolazine Implantable Cardioverter–Defibrillator (study)
RAS	renin–angiotensin system
RAAS	renin–angiotensin–aldosterone system
RAP	right atrial pressure
RATE-AF	Rate Control Therapy Evaluation in Permanent Atrial Fibrillation (trial)
RBBB	right bundle branch block
RBM20	RNA-binding motif protein 20
RCM	restrictive cardiomyopathy
RCP	respiratory compensation point
RCT	randomized controlled trial
RDN	renal denervation
REALITY-AHF	Registry Focused on Very Early Presentation and Treatment in Emergency Department of Acute Heart Failure
RER	respiratory exchange ratio
REVERSE	REsynchronization reVErses Remodeling in Systolic left vEntricular dysfunction (trial)
RHC	right heart catheterization
RHD	rheumatic heart disease
RHR	resting heart rate
RIMP	RV index of myocardial performance
RNA	ribonucleic acid
ROS	reactive oxygen species
RPE	Rating of Perceived Exertion
RR	respiratory rate
RRT	renal replacement therapy
RV	right ventricle/right ventricular
RVD	right ventricular dysfunction
RVEDP	right ventricular end-diastolic pressure
RVEF	right ventricular ejection fraction
RVMI	right ventricular myocardial infarction
RVOT	right ventricular outflow tract
RVP	right ventricular pressure
RVSW	right ventricular stroke work
RVSWI	right ventricular stroke work index
RyR	ryanodine receptor
SAM	systolic anterior motion
SARF	severe acute respiratory failure
SARS-CoV-2	severe acute respiratory syndrome coronavirus 2
SAT	subcutaneous adipose tissue
SAVE	Survival and Ventricular Enlargement (trial)

SAVR	surgical aortic valve replacement	STS-PROM	Society of Thoracic Surgeons Predicted Risk of Mortality
SBP	systolic blood pressure	SV	stroke volume
SCAI	Society for Cardiovascular Angiography and Interventions	SVC	superior vena cava
SCD	sudden cardiac death	SVR	systemic vascular resistance; surgical ventricular reconstruction
SCOT	succinyl-CoA:3 oxoacid-CoA transferase	SVRi	systemic vascular resistance index
SCS	spinal cord stimulation	TAG	triacylglycerol
SD	systolic dysfunction; sudden death	TAPSE	tricuspid annular plane systolic excursion
SDF	stromal cell-derived factor	TAVI	transcatheter aortic valve implantation
SEE-HF	Screening for Advanced Heart Failure Treatment	TAVR	transcatheter aortic valve replacement
SENIORS	Study of the Effects of Nebivolol Intervention on Outcomes and Rehospitalisation in Seniors with Heart Failure	TCPC	total cavo-pulmonary connection
		TDI	tissue Doppler imaging
		T2DM	type 2 diabetes mellitus
SERCA	sarcoplasmic reticulum calcium-ATPase	T-DM1	trastuzumab-DM1
SET	systolic ejection time	TEER	transcatheter edge-to-edge repair
sGC	soluble guanylate cyclase	TGA	transposition of the great arteries
SGLT	sodium–glucose cotransporter	TGF-β	transforming growth factor beta
SGLT2i	sodium–glucose cotransporter 2 inhibitor	Th1	T helper 1
SHFM	Seattle Heart Failure Model	TIMI	Thrombolysis in Myocardial Infarction
SHIFT	Systolic Heart Failure Treatment with the I_f Inhibitor Ivabradine Trial	TIPS	trans-jugular intrahepatic portosystemic shunt
S-ICD	subcutaneous implantable cardioverter–defibrillator	TKI	tyrosine kinase inhibitor
		TLR	Toll-like receptor
SIRT	sirtuin	TMAO	trimethylamine N-oxide
SLE	systemic lupus erythematosus	TMZ	trimetazidine
sMDRD	simplified Modification of Diet in Renal Disease	TNF	tumour necrosis factor
		TPG	transpulmonary gradient
SMR	secondary mitral regurgitation	TR	tricuspid regurgitation
SNS	sympathetic nervous system	TRACE	Trandolapril Cardiac Evaluation (trial)
SNV	single-nucleotide variant	TRANSFORM-HF	ToRsemide compArisoN With furoSemide FORManagement of Heart Failure (trial)
SOLVD	Studies of Left Ventricular Dysfunction (trial)		
SPAP	systolic pulmonary artery pressure	Tregs	T regulatory cells
SPECT	single-photon emission computed tomography	TRUE-AHF	Trial of Ularitide Efficacy and Safety in Acute Heart Failure
SPRM	Seattle Proportional Risk Model	TRX	thioredoxin
SR	sarcoplasmic reticulum	TSE	turbo spin echo
SRV	systemic right ventricle	TSH	thyroid-stimulating hormone
SSc	systemic sclerosis	T2 STIR	T2-weighted short tau inversion recovery
SS-31	Szeto–Schiller peptide 31	TTE	transthoracic echocardiography
SSFP	steady-state free precession	TTNtv	*TTN*-truncating variants
SSRI	selective serotonin reuptake inhibitor	TTR	transthyretin
sST2	soluble ST2	TTS	Takotsubo syndrome
STAND-UP AHF	Study Assessing Nitroxyl Donor Upon Presentation with Acute Heart Failure	UDHF	universal definition of heart failure
		UDP-GlcNAc	uridine diphosphateβNacetylglucosamine
		UFH	unfractionated heparin
STE	speckle tracking echocardiography	VAC	ventricular–arterial coupling
STEMI	ST-segment elevation myocardial infarction	VAD	ventricular assist device
		VA ECMO	veno-arterial ECMO
STICH	Surgical Treatment for Ischaemic Heart Failure (trial)	Val-HeFT	Valsartan Heart Failure Trial
STICHES	STICH Extension Study (trial)	VANISH	Ventricular Tachycardia Ablation or Escalated aNtiarrhythmic Drugs in Ischemic Heart Disease (trial)
STS	Society of Thoracic Surgeons		

VAT	visceral adipose tissue; ventilatory anaerobic threshold
V_D	dead-space ventilation
VE	minute ventilation
VEGF	vascular endothelial growth factor
VF	ventricular fibrillation
VHD	valvular heart disease
V-HeFT	Veterans Administration Cooperative Study on Vasodilator Therapy of Heart Failure
VKA	vitamin K antagonist
VMAC	Vasodilatation in the Management of Acute Congestive Heart Failure
VO_2	oxygen uptake/consumption
VPC	ventricular premature complex
VRA	vasopressin receptor antagonists
VSD	ventricular septal defect
VT	ventricular tachycardia; tidal volume
VTE	venous thromboembolism
WARCEF	Warfarin versus Aspirin in Reduced Cardiac Ejection Fraction (trial)
WAT	white adipose tissue
WES	whole-exome sequencing
WGS	whole-genome sequencing
WHO	World Health Organization
WR	work rate
WRF	worsening renal function
WSPH	World Symposium on Pulmonary Hypertension
XL	extended release
XO	xanthine oxidase

SECTION 1

Universal definition of heart failure

CHAPTER 1.1

Universal definition of heart failure

Andrew JS Coats, Biykem Bozkurt, and
Petar M Seferović

Contents

Introduction

Defining a disease is essential for standardization of the criteria of the disease, so that accurate comparisons can be made across geographies, health systems, and timelines. Reliable criteria will also aid in research and for reviews of clinical practice that are essential for quality and safety improvement activities. There have been many definitions of heart failure (HF) over the decades, with significant changes being made as we understand more of the pathophysiology of the condition. Some of the early definitions tried to take a pathophysiological approach and incorporated terms and concepts that were impossible to apply in clinical practice, such as 'the inability of the heart to provide the circulatory needs of metabolizing tissues'. Alternative definitions were more pragmatic, as they were designed to be used in large-scale surveys or registries, and therefore it was necessary that they were easily understood by the non-expert and equally applicable, even when detailed clinical examination findings and investigations were not available. None of these previous definitions were necessarily incorrect, even when they took very different approaches to diagnosing HF, but rather they reflected the variety of needs that pertain to a diagnosis of heart failure. In 2020/1, a group of international HF associations, societies, and working groups partnered to develop an internationally collaborative venture that would, for the first time, standardize a definition of HF that could be applied worldwide and that could be used in a number of different settings and for multiple purposes (⊃ Figure 1.1.1). The reader is referred to the report of this meeting and the consensus paper that provided further information.[1]

How to define a disease

One primary consideration that is often missed is that we need to define the purpose, or purposes, we want our definition of HF to satisfy. Some disorders have a single identifiable aetiology, and hence the definition can be based on a precise pathway that identifies the causative agent that leads to a change in either physiology or pathology and which results in the clinical consequences recognized as the disease state. These disorders can be considered 'categorical' disorders in that they are either present or absent, and are defined by the above-mentioned sequence and diagnosed by the presence of the accepted aetiological agent. These include many infections and cancers. Other conditions may not have a single aetiology and are in reality disorders of physiological function, defined by a certain numerical abnormality in an aspect of bodily function. Many chronic disorders follow this pathway, particularly disorders of the ageing modern society, such as obesity, chronic kidney disease (CKD), and chronic lung disease, and disorders of physiological control such as blood sugar levels in type 2 diabetes, bone mineral density in osteoporosis, or skeletal muscle mass and function in sarcopenia. In this regard, HF has more in

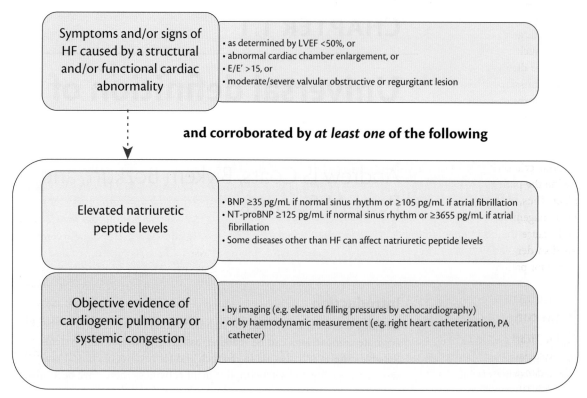

Figure 1.1.1 A simplified description of the universal definition of heart failure.

Bozkurt B, Coats AJS, Tsutsui H, *et al.* Universal definition and classification of heart failure: a report of the Heart Failure Society of America, Heart Failure Association of the European Society of Cardiology, Japanese Heart Failure Society and Writing Committee of the Universal Definition of Heart Failure: Endorsed by the Canadian Heart Failure Society, Heart Failure Association of India, Cardiac Society of Australia and New Zealand, and Chinese Heart Failure Association. *Eur J Heart Fail.* 2021 Mar;23(3):352–380. doi: 10.1002/ejhf.2115. Reprinted by permission of John Wiley and Sons on behalf of the European Society of Cardiology.

common with such a quantitative disorder, and less with categorical diseases, and the historical definitions of HF have tended to follow this path. There is, however, no single measure of organ function that can be used to define a 'failing' heart. Neither cardiac output or left ventricular ejection fraction (LVEF) can fulfil the role that the glomerular filtration rate (GFR) does for the diagnosis of CKD. For HF, we are left with using the third type of disease state—that of a recognized clinical syndrome involving a commonly accepted composite of signs, symptoms, and investigative findings that are recognized as forming the disease entity of HF.

Historical definitions

Early definitions of HF tended to focus on a physiological explanation for HF, such as a condition associated with a disorder of the circulation such that it cannot provide tissues with sufficient blood supply to satisfy their metabolic needs at rest or on exercise, which, although being conceptually attractive, had limitations in terms of its applicability in routine practice because of the difficulty of ascertaining the adequacy of the circulatory supply to exercising muscular tissue. More recent definitions of HF, such as those published by major international cardiology societies in their regular guidelines, have regarded HF as a complex clinical syndrome, encompassing multiple aspects and usually including the triad of: (1) some description of a structural and/or functional abnormality of the heart; (2) some classical symptoms; and (3)

some investigative parameters. Most, at some point, have also included a description of the process of fluid congestion as being either an absolute increase in blood volume or a redistribution of fluid that causes particular pathophysiology and, in many cases, symptoms of shortness of breath due to lung congestion. One criticism of these definitions is the lack of standardization, combined with poor applicability in routine clinical practice. Many require a definition of a physiological state that can rarely be verified in clinical practice and may be restricted to certain specialist fields or certain specialist hospitals. Other definitions of HF have been used for the purposes of disease coding in hospital systems, registries, and interventional clinical trials. For example, the Framingham Heart Study, an early and very influential epidemiological survey, utilized major and minor clinical criteria largely representing simple symptoms or clinical signs to define failure, based on a score made up of several less or more sensitive or specific parameters.[2] While this served the purposes of the epidemiological survey quite well, it was not considered accurate or reliable enough to be used either in routine clinical practice or for the purposes of recruiting patients to interventional trials. The emergence of randomized controlled trials to establish the efficacy of pharmacological and device-based treatments for HF has led to some standardization of the criteria for recruiting patients into such trials. These criteria, however, have been largely used to recruit patients at high risk of the type of subsequent clinical events against which the treatment is tested such as death or an unplanned HF-related hospitalization event. Certain 'enrichment' criteria were largely introduced to increase the risk of a patient experiencing such an event, without the intent of improving the specificity of the diagnosis. These include recruiting patients during an acute admission for HF, with very low LVEF and very elevated levels of natriuretic peptides or other markers of severe disease. The proponents of these criteria never initially suggested they should be used to define the disease, but the fact that a treatment has proven itself to be successful based on recruiting patients against these criteria has led some to consider they should be used to define the patient population that will likely respond to the treatment. Thus, we have recommended several treatments for use in the management of HF with reduced ejection fraction (HFrEF), not because the scientific community considered this was a separate disorder, but instead largely because trial evidence was accumulated for patients selected against such criteria.

A universal definition of heart failure: the 2021 international consensus

In early 2021, the Heart Failure Society of America (HFSA), the Heart Failure Association of European Society of Cardiology (HFA), and the Japanese Heart Failure Society (JHFS), as part of their ongoing trilateral agreement, agreed to review the proposed new universal definition of heart failure (UDHF) and decided to propose a consensus paper entitled '*Universal definition and classification of heart failure*'.[1] A working group was established that had representatives of these three associations/societies, as well as some from other HF associations and working groups representing groups from around the world. Four other associations endorsed the output of the working group; these were the Canadian Heart Failure Society, the Cardiac Society of Australia and New Zealand (CSANZ), the Heart Failure Association of India (HFAI), and the Chinese Heart Failure Association.

Staging

Any scheme for the diagnosis of HF can be improved by the ability to subdivide the diagnosis into other clinically meaningful subgroupings to aid in conversations among clinicians and also to assist in assessing clinical services or interventions. One such subgrouping is based on the severity of the disease, either cross-sectionally as how severely limited the patient is at a particular point in time, or longitudinally by defining the progression of the disorder, assuming that disease progression is, to some extent, predictable or in a certain direction. Many attempts have been made to stage HF, the two most common being the symptomatic stages of the New York Heart Association (NYHA) functional classes,[3] that has been in widespread clinical use for many years, and the more recent clinical staging of the American College of Cardiology Foundation/American Heart Association (ACCF/AHA) (➲ Figure 1.1.2).[4]

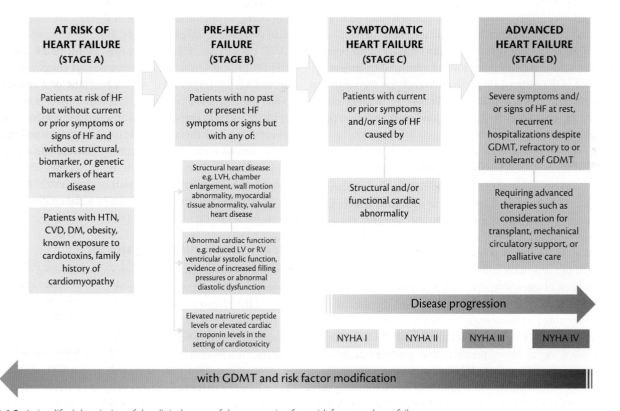

Figure 1.1.2 A simplified description of the clinical stages of the progression from risk factors to heart failure.

Bozkurt B, Coats AJS, Tsutsui H, *et al*. Universal definition and classification of heart failure: a report of the Heart Failure Society of America, Heart Failure Association of the European Society of Cardiology, Japanese Heart Failure Society and Writing Committee of the Universal Definition of Heart Failure: Endorsed by the Canadian Heart Failure Society, Heart Failure Association of India, Cardiac Society of Australia and New Zealand, and Chinese Heart Failure Association. *Eur J Heart Fail*. 2021 Mar;23(3):352–380. doi: 10.1002/ejhf.2115. Reprinted by permission of John Wiley and Sons on behalf of the European Society of Cardiology.

This four-stage classification into stages A to D has some advantages in that it recognizes the progression from risk factors for HF through early asymptomatic disease through to mildly and severely symptomatic disease. The staging system, however, has not been taken up extensively in routine practice and some people have felt it is suggesting that HF is a disease that can occur before symptoms, and this may be argued against the concept of HF as a symptomatic clinical syndrome. The consensus universal definition of HF paper proposes that stages A to D be incorporated into the new universal definition as a way of recognizing stages of disease that precede HF, translating stage A into 'at risk of HF' indicating patients with risk factors for the future development of HF, and stage B being called 'pre-HF' indicating established LV dysfunction that, in future, may lead to HF, but which is at the pre-symptomatic stage of the disorder. Stages C and D indicate the symptomatic stages of HF, with a rough translation being that stage C is similar to NYHA classes I, II, and IIIA, whereas stage D is more aligned to NYHA classes IIIB and IV or what is commonly called 'advanced HF'. Other staging systems that are popular include staging by degree of reduction in LVEF, which will be discussed in the next section, the MOGES system that defines HF further by its morpho-functional phenotype (M), organ involvement (O), genetic inheritance pattern (G), aetiological annotation (E), and functional status (S).[5] Another staging system in widespread use in the assessment of advanced HF, especially for patients being considered for transplantation or a mechanical circulatory support device, is the INTERMACS system, to which the reader is referred.[6] This system is a finer-grained subclassification of advanced HF that allows simplified descriptions of the clinical status of a patient, so that assessments can be made of the urgency of interventions and priority for limited advanced treatment options. None of the systems are perfect, but each has demonstrated value in aspects of clinical practice and research. The importance of the new proposed UDHF is that it could work in concert with these staging systems.

Left ventricular ejection fraction

The fractional emptying of the left ventricle with forward projection of the stroke volume into the aorta with each systole has a long history as a measure of cardiac systolic function. Folse and Braunwald (in *Circulation*, 1962) stated: 'The determination of the fraction of left ventricular end-diastolic volume ejected per beat and of the ventricle's end-diastolic and residual systolic volumes has been of interest to investigators for many years'.[7] It was calculated as forward stroke volume (FSV)/end-diastolic volume (EDV). They noted it was strongly inversely related to EDV. Bruce and Chapman[8] noted values of this fraction of 76.5% in normal males studied in the sitting position, thus realizing there was a normal range, even though, to this date, no universally accepted range of normal ejection fraction (EF) exists for all routinely used clinical imaging modalities. It was obvious that myocardial infarction, one of the most common causes of HF, often causes an enlarged, dilated, and remodelled left ventricle, with resulting low LVEF. The feature of low LVEF being a strong independent predictor of increased mortality risk was repeatedly identified and utilized in the design of clinical trials to recruit patients with a higher death rate. It was also recognized quite early on that the syndrome of HF could, in fact, present with low LVEF or could also present with higher, or even normal, LVEF. These latter patients were identified as having a different range of clinical characteristics, compared to the low LVEF HF patients. The higher LVEF HF patients tended to be older, more frequently female, and more likely to have an underlying aetiology of hypertensive heart disease than ischaemic heart disease, which was more common in the low LVEF type of HF patients. As stated earlier, very many of the intervention trials recruited HF patients preferentially with low LVEF, as this established a higher event rate population. Initially there was no consistency in the cut-off thresholds used for LVEF in such trials. Low LVEF trials used EF cut-offs of 25%, 35%, 40%, 45%, or occasionally 50%, and the much smaller number of trials that recruited HF patients with higher LVEF often used LVEF thresholds of above 40%, 45%, or 50%. Thus, although there was a spectrum of LVEF in patients diagnosed with HF, in common usage, two forms of HF were identified early on: one with reduced EF (HFrEF), and the other with preserved EF (HFpEF), although initially they were termed systolic and diastolic HF. More recently, the European HF guidelines initially recommended a third group called HF with mid-range EF (HFmrEF),[7,9] but which has now been revised to HF with mildly reduced EF (still termed HFmrEF),[9,10] in recognition of the fact that these patients pathophysiologically, and by their clinical characteristics and response to therapy, are more like HFrEF than they are like HFpEF patients. The now more widely accepted LVEF cut-offs are: HFrEF, EF ≤40%; HFmrEF, EF 41–49%; and HFpEF, EF ≥50%. A fourth category was specified as HF with improved EF (HFimpEF): HF with a baseline LVEF ≤40%, a ≥10-point increase from baseline LVEF, and a second measurement of LVEF >40% to emphasize the necessity to continue guideline-directed medical therapy (GDMT) among these patients. LVEF has shown its usefulness in recruiting patients into clinical trials, and as a result, many treatments are indicated only for selected subsets of HF patients on the basis of their LVEF. ➲ Table 1.1.1 demonstrates the prominent role LVEF has played in selecting patients for inclusion into clinical trials.

Heart failure disease trajectories

An important addition to the recently published UDHF is the concept of disease trajectories of HF. It is recognized with the extensive list of medications and devices that can modify outcomes in patients with HF that HF is not static in its severity. What previous definitions have failed to capture adequately is that patients can improve from more severe HF through the use of GDMT but remain at increased risk, compared to patients who never had HFrEF in the first place. Stages A to D of HF, classification systems based on LVEF, and the NYHA functional class classification schemes all failed to identify patients with improved or improving HF as a separate group. The UDHF paper included the concept of HFimpEF as a group defined as patients with an initial diagnosis

Table 1.1.1 The prominent role played by using LVEF to define a subset of HF patients recruited into clinical trials which subsequently have proved the value of the intervention (note that many more trials have selected patients with low LVEF (or using LVEF-like parameters), compared to trials that did not select on the basis of LVEF or which recruited only patients with higher LVEF)

Studies using LVEF-related measures to select	V-HeFT I (enlarged heart), CONSENSUS (enlarged heart size)
Studies using low LVEF as inclusion criterion	V-HeFT II (large heart or LVEF <45%), DIG (≤45%, and separate HFpEF trial), SOLVD (≤35%), USCP (≤35%), MERIT-HF (≤40%), CIBIS-II (≤35%), RALES (≤35%), ATLAS (≤30%), COPERNICUS (≤25%), VAL HeFT (≤40%), COMET (≤35%), CHARM-Alt (≤40%), HEALL (≤40%), EMPHASIS-HF (≤35%), SHIFT (≤35%), PARADIGM-HF (≤35%), DAPA-HF (≤40%), EMPEROR-REDUCED (≤40%), VICTORIA (<45%), GALACTIC-HF (≤35%),
Studies using high LVEF as inclusion criterion	CHARM-Pres (>40%), PEP-CHF (approximately >40%), I-PRESERVE (≥45%), PARAGON-HF (≥45%), TOPCAT (≥45%), EMPEROR-REDUCED (>40%)
Studies not restricted by LVEF as inclusion criterion	SENIORS, SOLOIST-WHF

Black = positive trials, orange = neutral trials.

of HFrEF, but in response to GDMT for HF have had an improvement, such that LVEF is increased by at least 10 percentage points and may now be in the range that would normally indicate HFpEF. These patients should not appropriately be classified as HFpEF but need a separate identity, which is why HFimpEF was introduced. Other terms that are used to describe the trajectory status of HF include a classification and whether HF is a new diagnosis or the patient previously had an established HF diagnosis (➲ Figure 1.1.3). The first is considered 'de novo' HF (also known as new-onset HF) and it carries a temporarily increased risk of adverse clinical outcomes, particularly as patients are unlikely to be treated with optimal GDMT at the beginning of the illness. When a patient has had a history of HF and is under treatment, this is commonly called 'chronic' HF and during this course of the disease, the patient has relatively minor symptoms and can be managed as an outpatient. Many people have called this 'stable' HF in the past, but the UDHF group felt this was a misleading term as it might be construed as indicating the patient no longer has significant disease or does not require optimization of GDMT or regular monitoring or observation. Therefore, instead of 'stable' HF, 'persistent' HF is recommended. Similarly, patients who have

had resolution of symptoms and signs and had normalization of LV function have been commonly called 'recovered' HF patients. The high risk of recurrence of symptoms and LV dysfunction upon withdrawal of pharmacological therapy[10] indicates that such patients should be continued on GDMT and should remain under regular review, and hence the term recovered HF is discouraged, with a preference for terms such as 'HF in remission' to suggest that the patient is at risk of deterioration at any time. The terms 'worsening HF' or acute decompensated HF (ADHF) are used for patients who have chronic HF but who subsequently develop an episode of acute or subacute decompensation, such as due to fluid retention or fluid maldistribution, leading to acute or subacute symptoms which may or may not require urgent hospital admission for increased treatment, particularly with use of intravenous diuretics and, in some cases, intravenous vasodilator or inotropic support. Because each episode of urgent admission for HF carries with it both short- and long-term increased risk, and each hospital admission is expensive and carries the opportunity for revising HF management, this has been a popular subclassification scheme for HF. By contrast, other markers of increasing risk, such as increasing levels of natriuretic peptides, have not translated

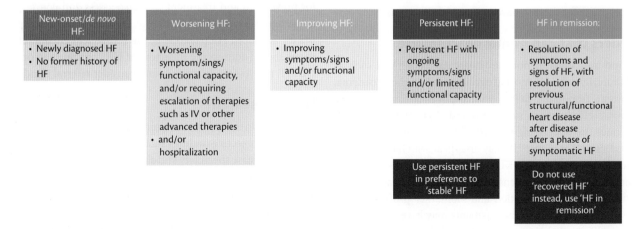

Figure 1.1.3 A nomenclature and classification for heart failure disease trajectories.

Bozkurt B, Coats AJS, Tsutsui H, et al. Universal definition and classification of heart failure: a report of the Heart Failure Society of America, Heart Failure Association of the European Society of Cardiology, Japanese Heart Failure Society and Writing Committee of the Universal Definition of Heart Failure: Endorsed by the Canadian Heart Failure Society, Heart Failure Association of India, Cardiac Society of Australia and New Zealand, and Chinese Heart Failure Association. Eur J Heart Fail. 2021 Mar;23(3):352–380. doi: 10.1002/ejhf.2115. Reprinted by permission of John Wiley and Sons on behalf of the European Society of Cardiology.

into clinically useful subclassifications. Subclassification of HF severity by the degree of elevation of natriuretic peptide levels may be something that develops in the future, but it has not been accepted widely to date.

Other subtypes of heart failure

There are other syndromes that fulfil the definition of HF but may require specific treatment and management strategies targeting the underlying or proximate cause, beyond treatment of HF itself. For example, right HF, acute myocardial infarction (AMI) or acute coronary syndrome, cardiogenic shock, hypertensive emergency, hypertensive heart disease, congenital heart disease, valvular heart disease, and high-output failure may fulfil the diagnostic criteria of HF but require specific treatment strategies beyond standard therapies of HF. The presence of right HF in the setting of left HF can be categorized as HF and may require modified treatment approaches. On the other hand, isolated right HF due to primary pulmonary hypertension aetiologies, although it may have symptoms or signs that mimic HF and may have elevated natriuretic peptide levels, would not be categorized under HF as the symptoms are not caused primarily by a structural and/or functional cardiac abnormality. On the other hand, right HF due to primary right ventricular conditions, such as arrhythmogenic right ventricular cardiomyopathy, would be categorized under HF. AMI would be the overarching definition of the clinical episode for any HF event in proximity to the infarction for those patients with HF during an AMI. It is also possible that these patients may progress to chronic HF. Though cardiogenic shock is an extreme form of HF, it requires urgent advanced therapies and needs to be specified. HF can be the preceding cause of shock in advanced HF patients, and identified as advanced HF complicated with cardiogenic shock. In hypertensive emergency and hypertensive heart disease complicated with HF, treatment of hypertension is critical. Similarly, valvular heart disease, congenital heart disease, and high-output cardiac failure can result in HF and require specific treatment strategies targeting the underlying anomaly and specific haemodynamic conditions. Given the unique nature of these diagnoses, it is appropriate for these to have unique identifications.

Disorders that can mimic heart failure

Symptoms and signs in non-cardiovascular conditions such as renal failure, liver failure, morbid obesity with peripheral oedema, and chronic respiratory failure with hypoventilation syndrome may mimic HF. In most, symptoms and signs of HF may disappear once the underlying primary cause is treated (e.g. symptoms and signs that mimic HF may disappear with haemodialysis in a patient with end-stage CKD). In some of these disease states, volume overload and compensatory mechanisms may result in haemodynamic characterization and biomarker profiles similar to HF, and in fact, some of these patients may have concomitant HF, since obesity, diabetes, and CKD are also risk factors for development of HF. In these conditions, objective markers such as natriuretic peptide levels and haemodynamic characterization of increased filling pressures can be helpful.

Disorders that can incorporate an element of heart failure

Certain disorders can be complicated with HF. The primary disease may require specific treatment strategies, but the development of HF as a complication usually confers a higher risk and worse prognosis, thus requiring treatment to also address the HF element. These can include cardiovascular causes such as AMI or acute coronary syndrome, hypertensive emergency as mentioned above, and also other cardiovascular diagnoses such as atrial fibrillation with a rapid ventricular response, prolonged ventricular arrhythmias, pulmonary embolus, pericardial diseases, and acute valvular dysfunction.

Use in practice

Despite guidelines and expansion of evidence for guideline-directed therapies, registries with real-world patients over the last 20 years have shown disappointing trends with little, if any, improvement in the use of GDMT, suggesting a lack of ability to standardize care in practice. Standardization of the definition of the HF syndrome is an important first step to enhance appropriate diagnosis and optimization of GDMT and achieve uniformity of care for HF universally. New revised terminologies of classification of HF as at risk of HF, pre-HF, HF, and advanced HF likely will be easier to understand for patients and clinicians alike, and will help clarify treatment indications for pre-HF, as well as for HF, along with incorporating asymptomatic phases under the UDHF umbrella without characterizing them as 'HF'. EF classifications provide clarity and standardization for targeting GDMT. Emphasis for trajectory terminologies for 'persistent' HF rather than 'stable' HF, and HF 'in remission' rather than 'recovered' HF, will prevent inertia and increase the likelihood of optimization and continuation of GDMT for indicated patients.

At the first encounter with the patient, clinicians should use the UDHF to diagnose, confirm, and document HF. They should then classify it according to LVEF to initiate and optimize GDMT. They should specify the stages of HF to initiate appropriate GDMT for prevention and treatment, and also assess and communicate the prognosis with the patient and consider referral to specialists for advanced HF patients. In the subsequent encounter, clinicians should address the trajectory of HF, continue and optimize GDMT, reassess the prognosis, and consider referral if indicated.

Use in research

Historically in the last 10 years, most clinical trials have already incorporated objective findings such as elevated natriuretic peptide levels to increase specificity and also to enrich patient populations for increased risk. The UDHF provides a simple, but conceptually comprehensive, definition with acceptable sensitivity and specificity. We believe the UDHF will help achieve uniformity for standard diagnostic criteria for research studies, as well as for registries and databases. The refined definitions of stages provide clarity for targeting treatment strategies for at-risk and pre-HF stages, which await development of new treatment strategies to prevent HF. This is a rapidly evolving field with advances in precision medicine. Genetic causes and biomarker characterization will help identify risk and targeted prevention and treatment strategies. The UDHF also provides a practical framework for modernization and harmonization of administrative codes for HF diagnosis and stages, and EF classification, which can impact the ability to capture quality measures and performance indicators in a reliable manner. The UDHF is envisioned to be very useful not only for clinicians, but also for researchers, administrators, regulatory agencies, and developers of performance measures, guidelines, and registries.

Summary

A UDHF is proposed that simplifies and democratizes the definition of HF, unifies different staging schemes, and forms a framework that can encompass disease staging and trajectories and aid clinical practice, research, and patient education.

Disclosures

Professor Coats declares no conflicts related to this work. Outside of this work, in the last 3 years, Professor Coats declares having received honoraria and/or lecture fees from: Astra Zeneca, Boehringer Ingelheim, Menarini, Novartis, Servier, Vifor, Abbott, Actimed, Arena, Cardiac Dimensions, Corvia, CVRx, Enopace, ESN Cleer, Faraday, Impulse Dynamics, Respicardia, and Viatris.

Professor Bozkurt declares no conflicts related to this work. Outside of this work, in the last 3 years, Professor Bozkurt declares having received consulting fees from Bristol Myers Squibb Pharmaceuticals, Baxter Healthcare Corporation, Sanofi-Aventis, Relypsa, and Amgen. She currently serves on the Clinical Event Committee for the GUIDE HF Trial sponsored by Abbott Vascular, and on the Data Safety Monitoring Committee of the ANTHEM (Autonomic REGULATION Therapy to Enhance Myocardial Function and Reduce progression of Heart Failure with reduced ejection fraction) trial sponsored by Liva Nova.

References

1. Bozkurt B, Coats AJS, Tsutsui H, *et al.* Universal definition and classification of heart failure: a report of the Heart Failure Society of America, Heart Failure Association of the European Society of Cardiology, Japanese Heart Failure Society and Writing Committee of the Universal Definition of Heart Failure: endorsed by the Canadian Heart Failure Society, Heart Failure Association of India, Cardiac Society of Australia and New Zealand, and Chinese Heart Failure Association. *Eur J Heart Fail.* 2021;23:352–80.
2. McKee PA, Castelli WP, McNamara PM, Kannel WB. The natural history of congestive heart failure: the Framingham study. *N Engl J Med.* 1971;285:1441–6.
3. White PD, Myers MM. The classification of cardiac diagnosis. *JAMA.* 1921;77:1414–15.
4. Yancy CW, Jessup M, Bozkurt B, *et al.* 2013 ACCF/AHA guideline for the management of heart failure. *Circulation.* 2013;128:e240–327.
5. Arbustini E, Narula N, Tavazzi L, *et al.* The MOGE(S) classification of cardiomyopathy for clinicians. *J Am Coll Cardiol.* 2014;64:304–18.
6. Stevenson LW, Pagani FD, Young JB, *et al.* INTERMACS profiles of advanced heart failure: the current picture. *J Heart Lung Transplant.* 2009;28:535–41.
7. Folse R, Braunwald E. Determination of fraction of left ventricular volume ejected per beat and of ventricular end-diastolic and residual volumes. Experimental and clinical observations with a precordial dilution technic. *Circulation.* 1962;25:674–85.
8. Bruce TA, Chapman CB. Left ventricular residual volume in the intact and denervated dog heart. *Circulation Res.* 1965;17:379–85.
9. Ponikowski P, Voors AA, Anker SD, *et al.* 2016 ESC Guidelines for the diagnosis and treatment of acute and chronic heart failure: the Task Force for the diagnosis and treatment of acute and chronic heart failure of the European Society of Cardiology (ESC). Developed with the special contribution of the Heart Failure Association (HFA) of the ESC. *Eur Heart J.* 2016;37:2129–200.
10. McDonagh TA, Metra M, Adamo M, *et al.*; ESC Scientific Document Group. 2021 ESC Guidelines for the diagnosis and treatment of acute and chronic heart failure: Developed by the Task Force for the diagnosis and treatment of acute and chronic heart failure of the European Society of Cardiology (ESC) With the special contribution of the Heart Failure Association (HFA) of the ESC. *Eur Heart J.* 2021;42:3599–726.

SECTION 2

Epidemiology of heart failure

CHAPTER 2.1

Epidemiology of heart failure

Amy Groenewegen, Ivan Milinković, Arno W Hoes, Arend Mosterd, and Frans H Rutten

Contents

Introduction

Heart failure has been described as an epidemic. It currently affects an estimated 64 million people worldwide, and the number of patients living with heart failure continues to increase due to a growing and ageing population. To quantify the exact burden of heart failure is challenging because it is a complex syndrome, and heart failure definitions have changed over time. This chapter provides an overview of heart failure occurrence and prognosis, and is a guide to the interpretation of differences across epidemiological reports.

Heart failure definitions and case ascertainment

Heart failure is not a single disease, but a heterogenous syndrome, and a generally accepted 'gold standard' for its diagnosis is lacking. Case ascertainment and categorization of patients, as well as comparison of epidemiological research studies in the literature, thus remain challenging. Echocardiography is the cornerstone of heart failure diagnosis, and left ventricular ejection fraction (LVEF) is generally viewed as a clinically useful phenotypic marker indicative of underlying pathophysiological mechanisms, prognosis, and sensitivity to therapy.[1] Heart failure patients are therefore most often categorized according to LVEF: heart failure with reduced (HFrEF, LVEF <40%), mildly reduced (HFmrEF, LVEF 40–49%), and preserved ejection fraction (HFpEF, LVEF ≥50%).[2]

HFrEF is the most well studied, and the only category for which clear prognostic benefits of therapy have been demonstrated in clinical trials. The decision to categorize by LVEF was originally based on the idea, among others, that systolic dysfunction was the primary cause of regressing pump function, and on the need to define heart failure populations with particularly high event rates (i.e. patients with low LVEF or 'systolic dysfunction') for enrolment in clinical trials. Clinical trials have used a range of LVEF cut-off values for inclusion criteria, with some as low as 25%, as an enrichment strategy to increase cardiovascular events, making comparison of earlier trial results even more difficult.[3] The current use of LVEF <40% as a criterion for HFrEF for clinical and epidemiological purposes is supported by evidence from several trials that showed dichotomizing patients based on LVEF <40% fairly reliably identified HFrEF patients who evidently would benefit from available pharmacological treatment.

Epidemiological studies appreciating HFpEF as an entity within the heart failure family are mainly from the last decade. Until 2013, when the American Heart Association (AHA) and American College of Cardiology Foundation (ACCF) published joint guidelines, there was no clearly defined cut-off for the ejection fraction for HFpEF. Thresholds for LVEF in the older literature varied between 40% and 55%, leading to large variations across epidemiological reports.[4] There is nowadays consensus on the key echocardiographic abnormalities that indicate left ventricular (LV) diastolic dysfunction in those with LVEF ≥50% (i.e. structural and functional abnormalities related to elevated LV filling pressures, impaired LV relaxation, concentric remodelling, and increased pulmonary artery pressures), but there is still ongoing debate on which combination is best and which cut-off points are to be used. In practice, concordance of the different echocardiographic parameters of diastolic dysfunction has been shown to be poor.[5] Variances in diagnostic criteria notwithstanding, it is estimated that over half of all heart failure patients in the general population have a preserved LVEF and this proportion is increasing.[6]

The term HFmrEF, for the previously ignored 'grey area' corresponding to an LVEF of 40–49%, was only recently introduced. This group comprises around 20% of all heart failure patients,[3] and was originally thought of as HFpEF patients whose LVEF declined secondarily. It has now become clear that patients with a 'mid-range' LVEF are intermediate regarding some characteristics, resembling HFrEF in age and with a male preponderance and prevalence of underlying ischaemic heart disease.[7] Moreover, recent post-hoc analyses of landmark trials showed that HFmrEF patients, unlike 'true' HFpEF patients, also significantly benefit from pharmacological therapy used in HFrEF.[8]

Classification based on LVEF comes with certain inherent limitations. Intra- and interobserver variability of echocardiographic LVEF assessment is reported to be 8–21% and 6–13%, respectively. The tendency to report LVEF in numbers ending with a 0 or a 5, known as the digit-rounding bias, is of particular importance in the HFmrEF group (most often defined as having an LVEF of 40–49%). Regression to the mean and measurement error (e.g. due to poor image quality) add to the echocardiographic measurement variability.[3] In the TOPCAT trial, for example, about 20% of participants would have been reclassified if LVEF measurements were repeated in a standard core laboratory.[9] In addition to difficulties of echocardiographic accuracy, LVEF is also notoriously dynamic and may change with treatment and over time: in nearly 40% of patients with HFrEF, LVEF will increase to >50% over 5 years with adequate treatment, while in nearly 40% of patients with HFpEF, LVEF will drop to <50% over the same period.[10] Therefore, prior knowledge about the LVEF trajectory is required in order to appreciate the LVEF and understand its impact on patient prognosis.

To measure an epidemic

Due to a lack of uniformity in the definition and diagnostic criteria of heart failure, especially of HFpEF and HFmrEF, estimations of prevalence and incidence vary widely and comparison across studies and over time is difficult.[11] Ideally, prevalence and incidence are measured in a random sample of the general population, using validated criteria to evaluate signs and symptoms and objective methods (such as natriuretic peptides and echocardiography or other forms of cardiac imaging) to assess cardiac dysfunction. In the absence of a generally accepted 'gold standard', the use of an expert panel to determine the presence of heart failure

based on multiple algorithms seems an appropriate method of case ascertainment. The number of studies applying this approach are limited and include the Olmsted County cohort, Prevention of Renal and Vascular End-stage Disease (PREVEND) study, the Framingham Heart Study (FHS), and the Atherosclerosis Risk in Communities (ARIC) study, among others.

Studies more often use registry data and billing codes, of which the accuracy and completeness may be unclear.[12] Misspecification of diagnoses and 'upcoding' for reimbursement incentives can lead to misrepresentation of trends in the prevalence and incidence over time. International Classification of Disease (ICD) codes are used worldwide in both primary and hospital care to facilitate comparability in epidemiological studies. ICD-10 codes are good at predicting the presence of heart failure (positive and negative predictive value of 90.2% and 97.2%, respectively), in comparison to chart reviewing,[13] but relevant ICD-9 codes were missing in approximately one-third of patients hospitalized with acute heart failure.[14] Self-report data, such as used by the large National Health and Nutrition Examination Survey (NHANES) registry, are potentially more inclusive, provided that patients have knowledge of their diagnosis.[11]

Hospital data on heart failure occurrence are nearly always incomplete, because chronic heart failure patients increasingly receive care in the primary care setting. In addition, heart failure patients are often admitted for non-cardiovascular causes and accurate identification of hospitalization for acute decompensated heart failure (as opposed to hospitalization for comorbidities) is challenging. Available heart failure classifications for the identification of acute decompensated heart failure (including Framingham criteria, modified Boston criteria, Gothenburg criteria, ICD-9 coding, and NHANES criteria) performed variably.[15] Lastly, hospital coding and claims data do not usually distinguish between first and subsequent admissions, counting multiple hospitalizations for the same individual as separate events. They therefore cannot reliably be used to estimate heart failure incidence.

Heart failure occurrence

Prevalence

In 2017, an estimated 64 million people were living with heart failure worldwide (⊙ Figure 2.1.1).[16] The prevalence of registered cases of heart failure is generally estimated at 1–2% of the general adult population in high-income countries (⊙ Table 2.1.1).[11] Population-based screening studies consequently have found a higher prevalence of around 4%.[17] Reliable estimates for developing regions are lacking, but current literature suggests that the number of patients living with heart failure might be even higher in low- and middle-income countries.[18]

Depending on the source data used, prevalence reports vary significantly within and across countries. Recently, the Heart Failure Association (HFA) of the European Society of Cardiology (ESC) conducted The Atlas Survey on heart failure burden across a wide range of European countries. The quality and completeness of source data varied across countries. Median heart failure

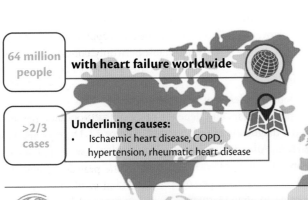

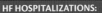

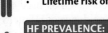

64 million people **with heart failure worldwide**

>2/3 cases

Underlining causes:
- Ischaemic heart disease, COPD, hypertension, rheumatic heart disease

HF INCIDENCE:
- **Global:** 1-9 cases per 1000 person-years
- **Europe:** ~3/1000 person-years (all age groups), ~5/1000 person-years (adults)
- **Age- and sex-standardized:** 0.7 for HFmrEF, 2.7 for HFpEF, 3.5 for HFrEF (per 1.000 person-years)
- **Lifetime risk of HF:** 33% for men vs 29% for women

HF PREVALENCE:
- **Population-based screening studies:** ~4%.
- **Age-stratified:** 0.7–1.3% for <55y, 4.7–13.3% for ≥65y
- **Age- and sex-adjusted:** 2.2%

HF HOSPITALIZATIONS:
- **1–2%** of all hospital admissions
- **Median number:** 2671 /million people per year
- **Admission rate:** ~once a year, regardless of LVEF (2/3 non-cardiovascular causes)
- **Age differences:** more than half >75 years
- **Sex differences:**
  - 144 women vs 186 men (per 100,000 persons)
  - 55% women of all HFpEF patients, 29% of all HFrEF patients, women:men with incident HFpEF -2:1.
- **LVEF distribution:** 60% HFrEF, 24% HFpEF, 16 HFmrEF
- **Median length of hospital stay:** 8.50 days
- **30-day readmission:** up to 30% (slightly higher in HFpEF vs HFrEF)
- **1-year readmission:** ~50%
- **5-year readmission:** 80%

MORTALITY:
- **In-hospital:** 2–17%
- **30-day:** 6.5% (5–20%)
- **All types of HF:** 20% for 1-year, 53% for 5-year, 75% for 10-year (death rate: 7.3% per year).
- **LVEF distribution (3 years):** 30.0% for HFrEF, 15.8% for HFmrEF, 16.6% for HFpEF

Predictors of mortality:
- age, renal function, blood pressure, sodium level, ejection fraction, male sex, natriuretic peptide levels, NYHA class, diabetes, BMI, and exercise capacity

Figure 2.1.1 Epidemiology of heart failure. BMI, body mass index; COPD, chronic obstructive pulmonary disease; HF, heart failure; HFmrEF, heart failure with mildly reduced ejection fraction; HFpEF, heart failure with preserved ejection fraction; HFrEF, heart failure with reduced ejection fraction; LVEF, left ventricular ejection fraction; NYHA, New York Heart Association.

Table 2.1.1 Overview of key community-based studies published from 2008 onwards reporting on the prevalence of heart failure, according to criteria used

First author	Years	Study population	Diagnostic criteria	Prevalence (%)
Studies using non-standardized criteria				
Curtis[20]	1994	USA, Medicare beneficiaries, age ≥65 years, age-adjusted	Inpatient and outpatient billing codes	9
	2003			12
Zarrinkoub[21]	2006–2010	Sweden, all ages, age- and sex-adjusted	Hospital, outpatient, and primary care registry	2.2
Conrad[22]	2002	UK, all ages, age- and sex-standardized	Hospital and primary care health records	1.5
	2014			1.6
Störk[23]	2009–2013	Germany, all ages, age- and sex-standardized	Health-care claims data	4.0
Benjamin[24]	2011–2014	USA, NHANES, age ≥20 years, age-adjusted	Self-report	Men: 2.4 Women: 2.6
Smeets[25]	2000	Belgium, aged ≥45 years, age-standardized	Primary care health registry	Men: 1.5 Women: 1.4
	2015			Men: 1.2 Women: 1.3
Meta-analysis of studies using rigorous echocardiographic case validation				
Van Riet[17]	1989–2010	28 articles, age ≥60 years	Echocardiographic validation	≥60 years: 11.8 (median) All ages: 4.2 (calculated)

NHANES, National Health and Nutrition Examination Survey.

This table includes key community-based studies published after January 2008. Studies that were included in the meta-analysis by Van Riet and colleagues are not represented separately.

prevalence was 1.7%, ranging from ≤1.2% in Greece and Spain to >3.0% in Lithuania and Germany.[19] Reasons for the heterogeneity include methodological issues with data collection and standardization. Differences in age structure of the included countries likely played a minor role, as the heart failure incidence was not above the median in countries with an older population. More likely, differences in socio-economic status, which has been related to risk factor management and age at onset of heart failure, played a role. Limited availability of diagnostic tools and a higher (financial) threshold to specialized heart failure care would have led to underreporting, particularly of HFpEF and HFmrEF.

A meta-analysis of population-based screening studies applying echocardiography to include unrecognized cases and exclude misclassified ones showed that the prevalence of all-type heart failure in high-income countries is around 11.8% in those aged 65 years and over. This accounts for a calculated prevalence in the general population of 4.2%—approximately twice as high as the prevalence estimated by studies using registry data only.[17] While this difference may be, in part, caused by poor accuracy of coding practices, it also illustrates that heart failure often remains undetected. Early recognition of non-acute onset is difficult because the symptoms are easily misclassified as chronic obstructive pulmonary disease (COPD), deconditioning, obesity, or simply ageing. In addition, echocardiography is often not readily available in primary care. Particularly HFpEF is easily missed; up to 76% of unrecognized cases of heart failure are patients with a preserved ejection fraction.[26]

Trends in heart failure prevalence

As a result of enhancement of echocardiographic imaging, as well as the more routine availability of natriuretic peptides, diagnosis of heart failure (notably HFpEF and HFmrEF) has increased over the last decade. This artificial increase in prevalence of heart failure influences the comparability of newer studies with earlier cohorts. Nonetheless, the number of patients living with heart failure has increased, even though incidence rates have stabilized or even may be declining, particularly in women. The increased prevalence reflects improved treatment options, a shift in age towards the right, and, ironically, improved survival after myocardial infarction.[11,27] HFpEF is likely the main driver behind the current overall prevalence, since studies over the past two decades have reported an increasing proportion of HFpEF among patients with new-onset heart failure.[6] Important risk factors for HFpEF include older age, hypertension, obesity, and obesity-related comorbidities such as type 2 diabetes mellitus. With ageing of the population and the relentless increase in obesity worldwide, the proportion of heart failure patients with HFpEF can only be expected to grow.

A community-based echocardiographic study in Spain in >250,000 low–middle-class people and defining heart failure according to the Framingham criteria, showed that heart failure prevalence steadily increased from 9 to 21 cases per 10,000 population between 2000 and 2007. Rates were higher in men than in women. The prevalence of HFpEF was higher than that of HFrEF, with the rates of HFpEF higher in women and HFrEF higher in men.[28] In a Swedish registry of primary and secondary care records of over 2 million inhabitants, the age- and sex-adjusted prevalence of 2.2% remained stable between 2006 and 2010.[21]

Incidence

The global incidence of heart failure ranges from 1 to 9 cases per 1000 person-years and depends again on the population studied and the diagnostic criteria used (➲ Figure 2.1.1).[11] According to the HFA's Atlas Survey, the median incidence of heart failure in European countries was 3.20 (interquartile range (IQR) 2.66–4.17) cases per 1000 person-years, ranging from ≤2 in Italy and Denmark to >6 in Germany.[19]

Recently, data from four community-based cohorts with prospective case validation and echocardiographic data (FHS, Cardiovascular Health Study (CHS), Multi-Ethnic Study of Atherosclerosis (MESA), PREVEND study) were pooled for evaluation of the respective contributions of HFpEF, HFmrEF, and HFrEF to the population burden of heart failure (➲ Table 2.1.2). Age- and sex-standardized incidence of HFmrEF was only 0.7 cases per 1000 person-years, compared to an incidence of 2.7 and 3.5 cases per 1000 person-years for HFpEF and HFrEF, respectively. Interestingly, predictors of incident heart failure did not differ across LVEF categories.[29]

Trends in heart failure incidence

High-income countries have seen a stabilization of incidence rates between 1970 and 1990, and some now even are experiencing a decrease.[11]

Between 2000 and 2010, there was a substantial decline in age- and sex-adjusted incidence of all-type heart failure in the Olmsted County Cohort study in the United States, from 3.2 to 2.2 cases per 1000 person-years.[6] Because diagnostic criteria, which include echocardiographic measures, have remained uniform over time in this cohort, its data can be used to reliably chart trends in incidence of heart failure stratified by LVEF. The decline was greater in HFrEF (45% decline) than in HFpEF (28% decline). The proportion of incident heart failure cases with HFpEF increased from 38% in 1986 to 52% in 2010, concurrently with an increase in heart failure patients with prevalent hypertension, atrial fibrillation, and diabetes. A decline of 7% of all-type heart failure was seen between 2002 and 2014 in the United Kingdom, based on primary care data from 4 million individuals, from 3.6 to 3.3 per 1000 person-years (adjusted incidence rate ratio (IRR) 0.93, 95% confidence interval (CI) 0.91–0.94).[22] The largest decline was observed in patients aged 60–84 years, whereas a worrying increase in incidence rate was reported in younger patients (<55 years). National data of heart failure occurrence in hospitalized patients in Denmark from 1994 to 2012 showed a similar trend.[33]

Heart failure in the young

The burden of heart failure lies predominantly among the elderly. Prevalence estimates of (all-type) heart failure range from 0.7% to 1.3% for those aged <55 years, and 4.7–13.3% for those aged ≥65 years, generally increasing with age.[17] Of patients hospitalized with heart failure, more than half are >75 years old.[38]

Table 2.1.2 Overview of key community-based studies published from 2008 onwards reporting on the incidence of heart failure, according to criteria used

First author	Years	Study population	Diagnostic criteria	Incidence
Studies using non-standardized criteria				
Loehr[30]	1987–2002	USA, ARIC study, age-adjusted	First heart failure hospitalization or death certificate	White men: 6.0/1000 p*y White women: 3.4/1000 p*y Black men: 9.1/1000 p*y Black women: 8.1/1000 p*y
Jhund[31]	1986	Scotland, age-adjusted	First heart failure hospitalization	Men: 1.2/1000 persons Women: 1.3/1000 persons
	2003			Men: 1.1/1000 persons Women: 1.0/1000 persons
Curtis[20]	1994	USA, Medicare beneficiaries, age ≥65 years, age-adjusted	Inpatient and outpatient billing codes	32/1000 p*y
	2003			29/1000 p*y
Yeung[32]	1997	Canada, age ≥20 years, age- and sex-standardized	Inpatient and outpatient billing codes	4.5/1000 persons
	2008			3.1/1000 persons
Zarrinkoub[21]	2006–2010	Sweden, all ages, age- and sex-adjusted	Hospital, outpatient, and primary care registry	3.8/1000 p*y
Christiansen[33]	1995	Denmark, age >18 years, age- and sex-adjusted	First-time in-hospital diagnosis of heart failure	>74 years: 16.4/1000 p*y 65–74 years: 6.3/1000 p*y 55–64 years: 2.0/1000 p*y 45–54 years: 0.50/1000 p*y 35–44 years: 0.13/1000 p*y 18–34 years: 0.04/1000 p*y
	2012			>74 years: 11.5/1000 p*y 65–74 years: 3.5/1000 p*y 55–64 years: 1.7/1000 p*y 45–54 years: 0.64/1000 p*y 35–44 years: 0.20/1000 p*y 18–34 years: 0.07/1000 p*y
Conrad[22]	2002	UK, all ages, age- and sex-standardized	Hospital and primary care health records	3.6/1000 p*y
	2014			3.3/1000 p*y
Störk[23]	2009–2013	Germany, all ages, age- and sex-standardized	Health-care claims data	6.6/1000 persons
Smeets[25]	2000	Belgium, aged ≥45 years, age-standardized	Primary care health registry	Men: 3.1/1000 persons Women: 2.2/1000 persons
	2015			Men: 2.8/1000 persons Women: 2.3/1000 persons
Studies using rigorous echocardiographic case validation				
Bahrami[34]	Enrolled 2000–2002, median follow-up 4 years	USA, MESA cohort, not adjusted	MESA criteria	African-American: 4.6/1000 p*y Hispanic: 3.5/1000 p*y White: 2.4/1000 p*y Chinese-American: 1.0/1000 p*y
Ho[35]	1981–2008	USA, FHS cohort	Framingham criteria	5/1000 p*y
Meyer[36]	1997–2010	Netherlands, PREVEND cohort	ESC criteria	Men: 3.7/1000 p*y Women: 2.4/1000 p*y
Tsao[37]	1990–1999	Combined FHS and CHS cohorts, age ≥60 years, age-standardized	Framingham and CHS criteria	19.7/1000 persons
	2000–2009			18.9/1000 persons
Gerber[6]	2000	USA, Olmsted County Cohort	Framingham criteria	3.2/1000 p*y
	2010			2.2/1000 p*y

ARIC, Atherosclerosis Risk in Communities; NHANES, National Health and Nutrition Examination Survey; MESA, Multi-Ethnic Study of Atherosclerosis; FHS, Framingham Heart Study; PREVEND, Prevention of Renal and Vascular End-stage Disease; CHS, Cardiovascular Health Study; p*y person-years.

However, recent studies suggest that the burden of heart failure in the younger population may be increasing. In a Danish nation-wide cohort study of hospitalized patients, the incidence rate of heart failure decreased substantially between 1995 and 2021 (IRR 0.90, 95% CI 0.88–0.93). The mean age simultaneously declined, however, and the proportion of patients with new-onset heart failure aged 50 years or younger doubled over the same time span (from 3% to 6%).[33] Similar trends were observed in Sweden—by linking nationwide hospital discharge and death registries between 1987 and 2006, investigators found a worrisome increase in heart failure incidence of 43% among people aged 35–44 years and even of 50% among people aged 18–34 years.[39] It remains unclear why heart failure incidence increases in the younger population, despite the overall observed decrease. The data may simply reflect better awareness and registration. Links have also been made with the higher prevalence of hypertension and obesity and obesity-related diseases, such as type 2 diabetes, which occur increasingly frequently in younger patients.

Lifetime risk

In the Cardiovascular Lifetime Risk Pooling project, using data from nearly 40,000 individuals included in American cohorts, the overall chance that a 45-year old develops heart failure before the age of 95 was 30–42% in white men, 20–29% in black men, 32–39% in white women, and 24–46% in black women.[40] The lower lifetime risk in black men, compared to white men, was attributed to competing risks, since black men have a higher risk of developing heart failure, according to community-based cohorts.[30] In contrast, from a British study of health records (from primary and hospital care and national registries) of 1.25 million inhabitants, the lifetime risk of developing heart failure at age 30 was only 5%. In hypertensive individuals (systolic blood pressure >140 mmHg), this risk increased to 7.8%.[41] The risks differ between these reports partly because of differences in the population under study—in the latter study, all individuals who had any type of pre-existing cardiovascular disease were excluded. Because heart failure is strongly associated with age and prior cardiovascular disease, the lower lifetime risks found in this study are not surprising.

The global burden of heart failure

Lower- and middle-income countries are estimated to carry over three-quarters of the cardiovascular disease burden, but very few studies provide reliable data on heart failure occurrence and outcomes in these regions.[11,42] Recently, a population-based study using insurance information in China estimated the prevalence to be 1.1% for both men and women, accounting for a total of 12.1 million Chinese inhabitants currently living with heart failure.[43] The incidence was 2 per 1000 person-years. In another report from China, the age-standardized rate increased by 5.4% between 2010 and 2015.[44] Based on scarce epidemiological data from other Asian regions, the prevalence ranges between 1% and 1.3%, similar to China. The only South American population-based study found a heart failure incidence of 2 per 1000 person-years,

based on self-reporting in Brazil. The prevalence was estimated to be 1% in Cuba. The prevalence in Australia is similar to that in Europe (1–2%), although much higher rates are found in echocardiographic screening studies among Indigenous communities (5.3%) despite a lower mean age. There are no population-based studies providing data on heart failure occurrence in African countries.

Over the last 15 years, clinical trials have enrolled an increasing number of patients from regions other than Europe and Northern America, promoting our understanding of regional differences in heart failure phenotypes. Based on data from the PARADIGM-HF trial, HFrEF patients from Latin America and the Asia-Pacific region are 10 years younger than their European and Northern American counterparts.[45] In South East Asia, the prevalence of overweight is much lower than in the United States, but the prevalence of diabetes is remarkably high and gives rise to a unique 'lean diabetic' HFpEF phenotype. This HFpEF phenotype is responsible for an estimated 20% of all heart failure cases in South East Asia and has a relatively high rate of all-cause mortality.[46] According to the Global Burden of Disease study, four underlying causes (ischaemic heart disease, COPD, hypertensive heart disease, and rheumatic heart disease) are responsible for over two-thirds of heart failure cases worldwide.[47] Undeveloped countries are disproportionally affected by rheumatic heart disease and hypertension. Infectious diseases, including human immunodeficiency virus (HIV), remain important causes of heart failure in lower-income countries worldwide. In Latin America, approximately half of heart failure cases are caused by Chagas' cardiomyopathy, a preventable parasitic disease.[48,49] Because infections occur at all ages, heart failure populations in developing regions tend to be relatively young. In sub-Saharan Africa, half of patients hospitalized for heart failure were aged 55 years or younger.[50] Simultaneously, diseases typically associated with a more Western-type lifestyle, such as diabetes and obesity, are increasingly common in low- and middle-income regions. This double disease burden is evidenced by data from the Global Burden of Disease Study that showed increased age-standardized rates of ischaemic heart disease in lower-income regions.[47]

Sex differences in heart failure epidemiology

Even though the incidence of all-type heart failure is fairly similar for men and women, the proportion of subtypes is decidedly different; notably HFpEF is more common in women.[6,22] In the Swedish Heart Failure registry, women accounted for 55% of all HFpEF patients and only 29% of all HFrEF patients.[51] In the Olmsted County Cohort study, women were over-represented among individuals with incident HFpEF by 2:1. Between 2000 and 2010, the proportion of patients with incident heart failure who had HFpEF increased from 48% to 52%. The overall heart failure incidence decreased for both men and women, but women exhibited a markedly larger decline in the incidence of HFrEF than HFpEF (−61% vs −27%), compared with men (−29% vs −27%).[6]

The relationship between hypertension and the development of LV hypertrophy, diastolic dysfunction, and HFpEF seems to be stronger in women than in men. Similarly, the excess risk associated with diabetes, which is a stronger risk factor for HFpEF than for HFrEF, is more pronounced in women,[52] also independent of age.[53] These findings led to the general idea that women are more susceptible to HFpEF than men. However, in pooled data from the CHS and MESA studies, female sex was not associated with a higher lifetime risk of HFpEF, but with a lower lifetime risk of HFrEF, compared to male sex (5.8% vs 10.6%).[54]

Prognosis of heart failure

Mortality of heart failure

Despite trials yielding effective treatments for HFrEF, and to a lesser extent HFmrEF, patients, heart failure prognosis remains poor. Estimates of the mortality associated with heart failure strongly depend on the baseline risk of the population under study, heart failure criteria and LVEF cut-off values used, as well as the introduction of bias through exclusion of patients with missing LVEF values.[11] Mortality rates are generally higher in observational studies than in clinical trial populations, which often include younger patients with fewer comorbidities.[55] Prognosis of the 'average' heart failure patient is therefore best evaluated in community-based cohorts, following up new cases of echocardiographically confirmed heart failure. Such studies include the Olmsted County Cohort, FHS, and CHS.

Combined data from the FHS and CHS cohorts, both of which use expert panels to determine the presence or absence of heart failure (HFpEF defined as LVEF ≥50%, and HFrEF as LVEF <50%), including elderly patients (aged 60 years and older) who were followed up between 1990 and 2009, showed that 67% of patients with heart failure died within 5 years of diagnosis, irrespective of LVEF.[37] The more dynamic Olmsted County Cohort study did not apply age restrictions. Incident cases of heart failure between 2000 and 2010 were followed up, and mortality rates for all-type heart failure were slightly lower: 20% at 1 year after diagnosis, and 53% at 5 years after diagnosis. Age-related hazard ratios tended to be lower in HFpEF (LVEF >50%, borderline significance), an effect that disappeared in multivariate analysis.[6] (See Table 2.1.3.)

Hospitalization is overall a strong prognostic predictor. In the Get With The Guidelines-Heart Failure cohort including 40,000 patients hospitalized with heart failure, aged ≥65 years,

stratified into HFrEF (46%), HFmrEF (8%), and HFpEF (46%), an alarming 5-year mortality rate of 75% was found, regardless of LVEF.[58] In a study of 2.1 million individuals in the United Kingdom, patients with heart failure newly recorded in primary care, and who had no prior hospital admission, had a 5-year mortality rate of 56%, compared to 78% in patients who were hospitalized for heart failure but did not have a primary care record.[59] In general, the steepest drop in the survival curve is during the initial weeks after admission. The value of in-hospital mortality estimates is dubious, as the length of hospital stay may, in part, depend on whether or not the patient is thought to have reached the palliative stage. Estimates of 30-day mortality rate are less susceptible to bias and range from 5% to 20% (Figure 2.1.1).[11,30,31]

How outcomes differ across the LVEF spectrum remains unclear. Some population-based studies report the risk of death to be as high, or nearly as high, in patients with HFpEF and HFmrEF, compared to HFrEF.[6,37] Randomized controlled trials, which tend to include only severe cases of heart failure as a strategy to increase cardiovascular outcomes, often find larger differences in survival between HFrEF patients and those with HFpEF and HFmrEF. In the CHARM trial, which included heart failure patients regardless of LVEF, the risk of all-cause death over 3 years of follow-up was 30.0%, 15.8%, and 16.6% in HFrEF, HFmrEF, and HFpEF patients, respectively. When LVEF was applied as a continuous variable, the risk decreased steeply with increasing ejection fraction until an ejection fraction of around 50%, and the risk was flat thereafter.[8]

Trends in mortality of heart failure

A recent meta-analysis pooling 60 observational studies, including 1.5 million ambulatory patients with chronic all-type heart failure, showed that survival rates have improved by approximately 20% since 1970. However, the decline in mortality has been only modest in the last decades, and 1- and 5-year mortality rates in heart failure remain high at 10.7% and 40.3%, respectively.[60] The reasons for this deflection remain uncertain, but it may include the shift from HFrEF to HFpEF (for which no evidence-based treatment is available) and the increased burden of comorbidities. The studies included in this meta-analysis were heterogeneous and often relied on primary care databases and health data registries. In lacking echocardiographic case validation, these

Table 2.1.3 Age-adjusted mortality (%) after onset of heart failure in women and men in population-based cohort studies during the period 1970–2010

Period	Olmsted County Cohort[6,56]				Framingham Heart Study[57]			
	1-year mortality		5-year mortality		1-year mortality		5-year mortality	
	Women	Men	Women	Men	Women	Men	Women	Men
1970–1979					28	41	59	75
1980–1989	20	30	51	65	27	33	51	65
1990–1999	17	21	46	50	24	28	45	59
2000–2010	20*		53*					

* No percentages were reported for men and women separately.

estimates are more susceptible to changes in coding practices and heart failure definitions over time.

In an echocardiographic study using a subsample of the FHS cohort and looking back across three decades (1985–2014), all-cause mortality did not change significantly over time or between the subgroups of HFrEF, HFmrEF, and HFpEF. However, cardiovascular mortality associated with HFrEF declined across the decades by 40% (hazard ratio 0.61, 95% CI 0.39–0.97), remaining unchanged in patients with HFmrEF and HFpEF. The absolute mortality rate in individuals with HFrEF was higher than in the other two groups in the initial decade (1985–1994) but converged thereafter, underscoring again the effectiveness of evidence-based strategies for HFrEF and the want of those for HFpEF.[61]

Hospitalizations

Heart failure hospitalizations represent 1–2% of all hospital admissions (⮕ Figure 2.1.1),[62] making it the most common diagnosis in hospitalized patients aged 65 years and older.[63] In the European Heart Failure Atlas Survey, the median number of heart failure discharges per million people was 2671 (IQR 1771–4317), ranging from <1000 in North Macedonia and the United Kingdom to >6000 in Romania, Norway, and Germany. The length of hospital stay also varied across countries, ranging from ≤6 days to ≥11 days, with a median of 8.5 days. The authors hypothesized that the heterogeneity reflects differences in hospital admission policies and criteria, access to, and quality of, hospital care and dedicated centres, and adherence to therapy.

In the community-based Olmsted County Cohort study, heart failure patients were admitted approximately once a year, regardless of LVEF.[6] By contrast, in the CHARM trial, the hospitalization rate declined with increasing LVEF until an LVEF of 40%, levelling off thereafter.[8] About two-thirds of heart failure hospitalization is for non-cardiovascular causes;[6] in some studies, this percentage is even higher in patients with HFpEF, reflecting older age and higher comorbidity burden.[64]

After a peak in the number of hospitalizations for heart failure during the 1990s in Europe and the United States, most community-based studies now show a marked decline. In a nationwide sample in Denmark, hospitalization rates decreased by 25% for women (from 192 to 144 per 100,000 persons) and by 14% for men (from 217 to 186) between 1983 and 2012.[33]

Heart failure is associated with the highest 30-day readmission rate of any diagnosis (approximately 20%, slightly higher in HFpEF compared to HFrEF).[64] Over half of patients will be rehospitalized during the first year after discharge, and over 80% within 5 years.[58,64] In the IMPACT-HF study, over half of all patients were discharged with unresolved symptoms. After 2 months of follow-up, half had worsening symptoms, a quarter were readmitted, and a little over 10% had died.[65]

Determinants of prognosis and prognostic models

Many determinants of prognosis have been identified. Because prognostic determinants are not necessarily causally related to the prognosis, correction does not always improve outcome. Age, New York Heart Association (NYHA) or AHA classification, and comorbidity burden are important indicators of severity and prognosis. The cause of heart failure also clearly relates to the prognosis—heart failure resulting from viral myocarditis or Takotsubo cardiomyopathy may be completely reversible, whereas patients with heart failure after a first myocardial infarction face a 5-year (age- and sex-adjusted) mortality rate of 39%.[66] Comorbidity is strongly associated with increased mortality. In a Danish nationwide cohort study, using low comorbidity as a reference, the 5-year mortality rate ratio was increased by 43% for moderate, 66% for severe, and 220% for very severe comorbidity.[67]

Several multivariable prognostic risk scores have been developed for different populations of heart failure patients. These may help predict mortality but are less useful for the prediction of hospitalization. The C-statistic, a measure of how well a model discriminates that varies from 0.5 (not better than a coin flip) to 1.0 (perfect prediction), seldom reaches 0.8 or higher in heart failure models. In a meta-analysis of 117 models (249 different variables), the prediction of death was only modestly accurate (average C-statistic 0.71). Models predicting the combined end point of death and heart failure hospitalization were even less discriminative (average C-statistic of 0.63).[68] In another systematic review of 64 models, a few variables emerged as consistent predictors of mortality: age, renal function, blood pressure, sodium level, ejection fraction, male sex, natriuretic peptide levels, NYHA class, diabetes, body mass index, and exercise capacity. Interestingly, only two of the included studies had used repeated measurements.[69]

As pointed out previously, one of the reasons why it is more difficult to predict mortality in heart failure populations than it is in the general population is that age and sex have a much lower C-statistic in heart failure patients. For example, in the Framingham cohort, a very simple model for predicting all-cause death in the general population containing only age and sex had a C-statistic of 0.75, which is already better than the average risk model for mortality in heart failure patients (average C-statistic of 0.71, often containing >10 factors).[70] In other words, once a patient develops severe heart failure, the risk of death is high, irrespective of age and sex.

Prevention of heart failure

The population attributable risk is the proportion of cases for an outcome that can be attributed to a certain risk factor among the entire population. Secular trends in population attributable risk are therefore particularly important from a prevention and public health point of view.

In the Olmsted County Cohort study, patients with coronary heart disease and diabetes had the highest risk of developing (all-type) heart failure. However, due to their very high prevalence, hypertension and coronary heart disease have a much greater population attributable risk than diabetes, each accounting for 20% of cases (against 12% for diabetes).[71] In the ARIC study, suboptimal control of five modifiable risk factors (smoking, diabetes, hypertension, hyperlipidaemia, and obesity) accounted for an estimated 88.8% of incident cases of heart failure.[72] Because of

Table 2.1.4 Comparison of non-standardized effects of reductions in systolic blood pressure on heart failure occurrence stratified by class of blood pressure-lowering drug

	Studies	Intervention		Control		RR (95% CI)
		Events	Participants	Events	Participants	
ACE inhibitor	13	1494	32,304	2706	50,277	0.98 (0.96–1.04)
ARB	8	1141	26,418	1187	26,311	0.81 (0.92–1.05)
Beta blocker	8	652	33,953	634	34,185	1.04 (0.93–1.16)
CCB	22	2104	72,323	2955	90,403	1.17 (1.11–1.24)
Diuretics	8	1108	32,580	1570	35,435	0.81 (0.75–0.88)

ACE, angiotensin-converting enzyme; ARB, angiotensin receptor blocker; CCB, calcium channel blocker; RR, relative risk; CI, confidence interval.
Reproduced from Ettehad D, Emdin CA, Kiran A, Anderson SG, Callender T, Emberson J, Chalmers J, Rodgers A, Rahimi K. Blood pressure lowering for prevention of cardiovascular disease and death: a systematic review and meta-analysis. *Lancet*. 2016 Mar 5;387(10022):957–967. doi: 10.1016/S0140-6736(15)01225-8 with permission from Elsevier.

the high prevalence of these risk factors, even a modest reduction may translate into a large improvement at population level. For example, a hypothetical reduction of 5% in diabetes prevalence among citizens in the United States was estimated to prevent 30,000 incident cases of hospitalization for heart failure per year. A 30% reduction in obesity and overweight could prevent 8.5% of incident heart failure cases.[73]

Every 10-mmHg systolic blood pressure reduction significantly reduces the risk of heart failure (RR 0.72, 95% CI 0.67–0.78).[74] However, not all antihypertensive drugs are equal in their propensity to prevent heart failure; diuretics seem the best (➲ Table 2.1.4).

Despite many strategies that might reduce the loss of disability-adjusted life-years due to heart failure, age remains the most important risk factor and will eventually take its toll. Simulation studies showed that, in a population of individuals with ideal risk factor profiles, heart failure incidence will only be about 25% less than in the current population.[75] Postponing heart failure, however, could still save hundreds of millions of years lived without disability and thereby reduce the burden of disease considerably.

Conclusions and future directions

The heart failure epidemic is changing. Incidence rates seem to have stabilized, but the number of patients living with heart failure is still increasing. Over the last decades, much better information is gathered about the heart failure epidemic, notably by large longitudinal population-based studies, although mainly in high-income countries. Special attention should be paid to the epidemiology of heart failure in low- and middle-income countries, which are disproportionally affected by preventable causes of heart failure. The case mix of heart failure is changing, with a larger proportion of patients with HFpEF. There is still much to learn in phenotyping beyond LVEF, and more information is needed on heart failure occurrence in specific populations, including women and the young. Before we can apply precision medicine, drug trials are needed to evaluate dosage of drugs in females and a more personalized treatment effect of a drug or a combination of drugs using individual patient data.

Key messages

- Heart failure affects an estimated 64 million people worldwide.
- Four underlying causes (ischaemic heart disease, COPD, hypertensive heart disease, and rheumatic heart disease) are responsible for over two-thirds of heart failure cases worldwide.
- Suboptimal control of five modifiable risk factors (smoking, diabetes, hypertension, hyperlipidaemia, and obesity) account for an estimated 88.8% of incident cases of heart failure.
- Estimations of prevalence and incidence vary widely due to a lack of uniformity in the definition and diagnostic criteria of heart failure.
- Global heart failure incidence ranges from 1 to 9 cases per 1000 person-years, depending on the population studied and the diagnostic criteria used. Age- and sex-standardized incidence of HFmrEF is only 0.7 cases per 1000 person-years, compared to an incidence of 2.7 and 3.5 cases per 1000 person-years for HFpEF and HFrEF, respectively. However, recent studies suggest that the heart failure burden in the younger population may be increasing.
- Heart failure prevalence is estimated at 1–2% of the general adult population, with an age- and sex-adjusted prevalence of 2.2%. All-type heart failure prevalence estimates range from 0.7% to 1.3% for those aged <55 years, and 4.7–13.3% for those aged ≥65 years.
- Women account for 55% of all HFpEF patients, and only 29% of all HFrEF patients. However, female sex does not seem to be associated with a higher lifetime risk of HFpEF, but with a lower HFrEF risk, compared to men (5.8% vs 10.6%).
- Heart failure hospitalizations represent 1–2% of all hospital admissions (median number of heart failure discharges of 2671 per million people (IQR 1771–4317). More than half are >75 years old. The median length of hospital stay is around 8.5 days. About two-thirds of heart failure hospitalizations is for non-cardiovascular causes, and in some studies higher in patients with HFpEF, reflecting older age and a higher comorbidity burden. Heart failure is associated with 30-day readmission rates of around 20%, with over half of patients rehospitalized during the first year, and over 80% within 5 years after discharge.
- One- and 5-year mortality rates are 10.7% and 40.3%, respectively.

◆ Determinants of prognosis: age, renal function, blood pressure, sodium level, ejection fraction, male sex, natriuretic peptide levels, NYHA class, diabetes, body mass index, and exercise capacity.

References

1. Borlaug BA, Redfield MM. Diastolic and Systolic Heart Failure Are Distinct Phenotypes Within the Heart Failure Spectrum. *Circulation* 2011;**123**:2006–14.

2. McDonagh TA, Metra M, Adamo M, et al. 2021 ESC Guidelines for the diagnosis and treatment of acute and chronic heart failure. *Eur Heart J* 2021;**42**:3599–726.

3. Savarese G, Stolfo D, Sinagra G, Lund LH. Heart failure with mid-range or mildly reduced ejection fraction. *Nat Rev Cardiol* 2022;**19**(2):100–16.

4. Selmeryd J, Henriksen E, Leppert J, Hedberg P. Interstudy heterogeneity of definitions of diastolic dysfunction severely affects reported prevalence. *Eur Heart J* 2016;**17**:892–9.

5. Petrie MC, Hogg K, Caruana L, McMurray JJ V. Poor concordance of commonly used echocardiographic measures of left ventricular diastolic function in patients with suspected heart failure but preserved systolic function: is there a reliable echocardiographic measure of diastolic dysfunction? *Heart* 2004;**90**:511–17.

6. Gerber Y, Weston SA, Redfield MM, et al. A contemporary appraisal of the heart failure epidemic in Olmsted County, Minnesota, 2000 to 2010. *JAMA* 2015;**175**:996–1004.

7. Lauritsen J, Gustafsson F, Abdulla J. Characteristics and long-term prognosis of patients with heart failure and mid-range ejection fraction compared with reduced and preserved ejection fraction: a systematic review and meta-analysis. *ESC Heart Fail* 2018;**5**:685–94.

8. Lund LH, Claggett B, Liu J, et al. Heart failure with mid-range ejection fraction in CHARM: characteristics, outcomes and effect of candesartan across the entire ejection fraction spectrum. *Eur J Heart Fail* 2018;**20**:1230–9.

9. Lam CSP, Solomon SD. Fussing Over the Middle Child: Heart Failure With Mid-Range Ejection Fraction. *Circulation* 2017;**135**:1279–80.

10. Dunlay SM, Roger VL, Weston SA, Jiang R, Redfield MM. Longitudinal Changes in Ejection Fraction in Heart Failure Patients With Preserved and Reduced Ejection Fraction. *Circ Heart Fail* 2012;**5**:720–6.

11. Groenewegen A, Rutten FH, Mosterd A, Hoes AW. Epidemiology of heart failure. *Eur J Heart Fail* 2020;**22**:1342–56.

12. Quach S, Blais C, Quan H. Administrative data have high variation in validity for recording heart failure. *Can J Cardiol* 2010;**26**:306–12.

13. Quan H, Li B, Saunders LD, et al.; IMECCHI Investigators. Assessing validity of ICD-9-CM and ICD-10 administrative data in recording clinical conditions in a unique dually coded database. *Health Serv Res* 2008;**43**:1424–41.

14. Goff DC, Pandey DK, Chan FA, Ortiz C, Nichaman MZ. Congestive Heart Failure in the United States. *Arch Intern Med* 2000;**160**:197.

15. Rosamond WD, Chang PP, Baggett C, et al. Classification of heart failure in the atherosclerosis risk in communities (ARIC) study a comparison of diagnostic criteria. *Circ Heart Fail* 2012;**5**:152–9.

16. James SL, Abate D, Abate KH, et al. Global, regional, and national incidence, prevalence, and years lived with disability for 354 Diseases and Injuries for 195 countries and territories, 1990-2017: A systematic analysis for the Global Burden of Disease Study 2017. *Lancet* 2018;**392**:1789–858.

17. Riet EES Van, Hoes AW, Wagenaar KP, et al. Epidemiology of heart failure: The prevalence of heart failure and ventricular dysfunction in older adults over time. A systematic review. *Eur J Heart Fail* 2016;**18**:242–52.

18. Banerjee A, Mendis S. Heart failure: the need for global health perspective. *Curr Cardiol Rev* 2013;**9**:97–8.

19. Seferović PM, Vardas P, Jankowska EA, et al. The Heart Failure Association Atlas: Heart Failure Epidemiology and Management Statistics 2019. *Eur J Heart Fail* 2021;**23**:906–14.

20. Curtis LH, Whellan DJ, Hammill BG, et al. Incidence and Prevalence of Heart Failure in Elderly Persons, 1994–2003. *Arch Intern Med* 2008;**168**:418.

21. Zarrinkoub R, Wettermark B, Wändell P, et al. The epidemiology of heart failure, based on data for 2.1 million inhabitants in Sweden. *Eur J Heart Fail* 2013;**15**:995–1002.

22. Conrad N, Judge A, Tran J, et al. Temporal trends and patterns in heart failure incidence: a population-based study of 4 million individuals. *Lancet* 2018;**391**:572–80.

23. Störk S, Handrock R, Jacob J, et al. Epidemiology of heart failure in Germany: a retrospective database study. *Clin Res Cardiol* 2017;**106**:913–22.

24. Benjamin EJ, Salim Virani CS, et al. Heart Disease and Stroke Statistics: 2018 Update A Report From the American Heart Association. *Circulation* 2018;**137**:67–492.

25. Smeets M, Vaes B, Mamouris P, et al. Burden of heart failure in Flemish general practices: a registry-based study in the Intego database. *BMJ Open* 2019;**9**:e022972.

26. Caruana L, Petrie MC, Davie AP, McMurray JJ. Do patients with suspected heart failure and preserved left ventricular systolic function suffer from 'diastolic heart failure'; or from misdiagnosis? A prospective descriptive study. *BMJ* 2000;**321**:215–18.

27. Dunlay SM, Roger VL. Understanding the Epidemic of Heart Failure: Past, Present, and Future. *Curr Heart Fail Rep* 2014;**11**:404–15.

28. Gomez-Soto FM, Andrey JL, Garcia-Egido AA, et al. Incidence and mortality of heart failure: A community-based study. *Int J Cardiol* 2011;**151**:40–5.

29. Bhambhani V, Kizer JR, Lima JAC, et al. Predictors and outcomes of heart failure with mid-range ejection fraction. *Eur J Heart Fail* 2018;**20**:651–9.

30. Loehr LR, Rosamond WD, Chang PP, Folsom AR, Chambless LE. Heart Failure Incidence and Survival (from the Atherosclerosis Risk in Communities Study). *Am J Cardiol* 2008;**101**:1016–22.

31. Jhund PS, Macintyre K, Simpson CR, et al. Long-Term Trends in First Hospitalization for Heart Failure and Subsequent Survival Between 1986 and 2003. *Circulation* 2009;**119**:515–23.

32. Yeung DF, Boom NK, Guo H, Lee DS, Schultz SE, Tu JV. Trends in the incidence and outcomes of heart failure in Ontario, Canada: 1997 to 2007. *CMAJ* 2012;**184**:E765–73.

33. Christiansen MN, Køber L, Weeke P, et al. Age-Specific Trends in Incidence, Mortality, and Comorbidities of Heart Failure in Denmark, 1995 to 2012. *Circulation* 2017;**135**:1214–23.

34. Bahrami H, Kronmal R, Bluemke DA, et al. Differences in the Incidence of Congestive Heart Failure by Ethnicity. *Arch Intern Med* 2008;**168**:2138.

35. Ho JE, Lyass A, Lee DS, et al. Predictors of new-onset heart failure: differences in preserved versus reduced ejection fraction. *Circ Heart Fail* 2013;**6**:279–86.

36. Meyer S, Brouwers FP, Voors AA, et al. Sex differences in new-onset heart failure. *Clin Res Cardiol* 2015;**104**:342–50.

37. Tsao CW, Lyass A, Enserro D, et al. Temporal Trends in the Incidence of and Mortality Associated With Heart Failure With Preserved and Reduced Ejection Fraction. *JACC Heart Fail* 2018;**6**:678–85.

38. Chen J, Normand S-LT, Wang Y, Krumholz HM. National and Regional Trends in Heart Failure Hospitalization and Mortality Rates for Medicare Beneficiaries, 1998–2008. *JAMA* 2011;**306**:1669.

39. Barasa A, Schaufelberger M, Lappas G, Swedberg K, Dellborg M, Rosengren A. Heart failure in young adults: 20-year trends in hospitalization, aetiology, and case fatality in Sweden. *Eur Heart J* 2014;**35**:25–32.

40. Huffman MD, Berry JD, Ning H, *et al.* Lifetime risk for heart failure among white and black Americans: cardiovascular lifetime risk pooling project. *J Am Coll Cardiol* 2013;**61**:1510–17.

41. Rapsomaniki E, Timmis A, George J, *et al.* Blood pressure and incidence of twelve cardiovascular diseases: lifetime risks, healthy life-years lost, and age-specific associations in 1.25 million people. *Lancet* 2014;**383**:1899–911.

42. Yusuf S, Rangarajan S, Teo K, *et al.* Cardiovascular risk and events in 17 low-, middle-, and high-income countries. *N Engl J Med* 2014;**371**:818–27.

43. Wang H, Chai K, Du M, *et al.* Prevalence and Incidence of Heart Failure Among Urban Patients in China: A National Population-Based Analysis. *Circ Heart Fail* 2021;**14**:e008406.

44. James SL, Abate D, Abate KH, *et al.* Global, regional, and national incidence, prevalence, and years lived with disability for 354 Diseases and Injuries for 195 countries and territories, 1990–2017: A systematic analysis for the Global Burden of Disease Study 2017. *Lancet* 2018;1789–858.

45. McMurray JJV, Packer M, Desai AS, *et al.* Angiotensin–Neprilysin Inhibition versus Enalapril in Heart Failure. *N Engl J Med* 2014;**371**:993–1004.

46. Tromp J, Tay WT, Ouwerkerk W, *et al.* Multimorbidity in patients with heart failure from 11 Asian regions: A prospective cohort study using the ASIAN-HF registry. *PLoS Med* 2018;**15**:1–22.

47. Vos T, Flaxman AD, Naghavi M, *et al.* Years lived with disability (YLDs) for 1160 sequelae of 289 diseases and injuries 1990–2010: a systematic analysis for the Global Burden of Disease Study 2010. *Lancet* 2012;**380**:2163–96.

48. Bocchi EA, Marcondes-Braga FG, Bacal F, *et al.* [Updating of the Brazilian guideline for chronic heart failure – 2012]. *Arq Bras Cardiol* 2012;**98**:1–33.

49. Ponikowski P, Anker SD, AlHabib KF, *et al.* Heart failure: preventing disease and death worldwide. *ESC Hear Fail* 2014;**1**:4–25.

50. Damasceno A, Mayosi BM, Sani M, *et al.* The Causes, Treatment, and Outcome of Acute Heart Failure in 1006 Africans From 9 Countries. *Arch Intern Med* 2012;**172**:1386.

51. Stolfo D, Uijl A, Vedin O, *et al.* Sex-Based Differences in Heart Failure Across the Ejection Fraction Spectrum: Phenotyping, and Prognostic and Therapeutic Implications. *JACC Heart Fail* 2019;**7**:505–15.

52. Vogel B, Acevedo M, Appelman Y, *et al.* The Lancet women and cardiovascular disease Commission: reducing the global burden by 2030. *Lancet* 2021;**397**:2385–438.

53. Boonman-De Winter LJM, Rutten FH, Cramer MJM, *et al.* High prevalence of previously unknown heart failure and left ventricular dysfunction in patients with type 2 diabetes. *Diabetologia* 2012;**55**:2154–62.

54. Pandey A, Omar W, Ayers C, *et al.* Sex and race differences in lifetime risk of heart failure with preserved ejection fraction and heart failure with reduced ejection fraction. *Circulation* 2018;**137**:1814–23.

55. Heiat A, Gross CP, Krumholz HM. Representation of the Elderly, Women, and Minorities in Heart Failure Clinical Trials. *Arch Intern Med* 2002;**162**:1682–8.

56. Roger VL, Weston SA, Redfield MM, *et al.* Trends in Heart Failure Incidence and Survival in a Community-Based Population. *JAMA* 2004;**292**:344.

57. Levy D, Kenchaiah S, Larson MG, *et al.* Long-Term Trends in the Incidence of and Survival with Heart Failure. *N Engl J Med* 2002;**347**:1397–402.

58. Shah KS, Xu H, Matsouaka RA, *et al.* Heart Failure With Preserved, Borderline, and Reduced Ejection Fraction: 5-Year Outcomes. *J Am Coll Cardiol* 2017;**70**:2476–86.

59. Koudstaal S, Pujades-Rodriguez M, Denaxas S, *et al.* Prognostic burden of heart failure recorded in primary care, acute hospital admissions, or both: a population-based linked electronic health record cohort study in 2.1 million people. *Eur J Heart Fail* 2017;**19**:1119–27.

60. Jones NRN, Roalfe AK, Adoki I, Hobbs FDR, Taylor CCJ. Survival of patients with chronic heart failure in the community: a systematic review and meta-analysis. *Eur J Heart Fail* 2019;**21**:1306–25.

61. Vasan RS, Xanthakis V, Lyass A, *et al.* Epidemiology of Left Ventricular Systolic Dysfunction and Heart Failure in the Framingham Study: An Echocardiographic Study Over 3 Decades. *JACC Cardiovasc Imaging* 2018;**11**:1–11.

62. Alla F, Zannad F, Filippatos G. Epidemiology of acute heart failure syndromes. *Heart Fail Rev* 2007;**12**:91–5.

63. Braunwald E. The war against heart failure: the Lancet lecture. *Lancet* 2015;**385**:812–24.

64. Cheng RK, Cox M, Neely ML, *et al.* Outcomes in patients with heart failure with preserved, borderline, and reduced ejection fraction in the Medicare population. *Am Heart J* 2014;**168**:721–30.e3.

65. Gheorghiade M, Filippatos G, De Luca L, Burnett J. Congestion in Acute Heart Failure Syndromes: An Essential Target of Evaluation and Treatment. *Am J Med* 2006;**119**:S3–10.

66. Gerber Y, Weston SA, Enriquez-Sarano M, *et al.* Mortality Associated With Heart Failure After Myocardial Infarction. *Circ Heart Fail* 2016;**9**:e002460.

67. Schmidt M, Ulrichsen SP, Pedersen L, Bøtker HE, Sørensen HT. Thirty-year trends in heart failure hospitalization and mortality rates and the prognostic impact of co-morbidity: a Danish nationwide cohort study. *Eur J Heart Fail* 2016;**18**:490–9.

68. Ouwerkerk W, Voors AA, Zwinderman AH. Factors Influencing the Predictive Power of Models for Predicting Mortality and/or Heart Failure Hospitalization in Patients With Heart Failure. *JACC Heart Fail* 2014;**2**:429–36.

69. Rahimi K, Bennett D, Conrad N, *et al.* Risk Prediction in Patients With Heart Failure: A Systematic Review and Analysis. *JACC Heart Fail* 2014;**2**:440–6.

70. Levy WC, Anand IS. Heart Failure Risk Prediction Models. *JACC Heart Fail* 2017;**2**:437–9.

71. Dunlay SM, Weston SA, Jacobsen SJ, Roger VL. Risk factors for heart failure: a population-based case-control study. *Am J Med* 2009;**122**:1023–8.

72. Folsom AR, Yamagishi K, Hozawa A, Chambless LE. Atherosclerosis Risk in Communities Study Investigators. Absolute and Attributable Risks of Heart Failure Incidence in Relation to Optimal Risk Factors. *Circ Heart Fail* 2009;**2**:11–17.

73. Avery CL, Loehr LR, Baggett C, *et al.* The Population Burden of Heart Failure Attributable to Modifiable Risk Factors. *J Am Coll Cardiol* 2012;**60**:1640–6.

74. Ettehad D, Emdin CA, Kiran A, *et al.* Blood pressure lowering for prevention of cardiovascular disease and death: A systematic review and meta-analysis. *Lancet* 2016;**387**:957–67.

75. Engelfriet PM, Hoogenveen RT, Poos MJJC, Blokstra A, van Baal PHM, Verschuren WMM. Heart failure: epidemiology, risk factors and future. [In Dutch]. Report by the Dutch National Institute for Public Health and the Environment (RIVM). 2012. Available from: https://www.rivm.nl/bibliotheek/rapporten/260401006.html.

SECTION 3

Aetiology of heart failure

CHAPTER 3.1

The role of ischaemic heart disease in heart failure

Rocco A Montone, Maurizio Volterrani, Jian Zhang, and Filippo Crea

Introduction

In last decades, ischaemic heart disease (IHD) emerged as the most important risk factor for the occurrence of heart failure (HF) because of improved survival following acute myocardial infarction (MI) and the declining prevalence of valvular heart disease.[1,2] According to contemporary reports, nearly two-thirds of HF cases are caused by IHD due to obstructive coronary artery disease (CAD). [1,2] However, these data may underestimate the prevalence of ischaemic mechanisms underlying HF. Indeed, it is worth noting that the presence of non-obstructive CAD at coronary angiography does not exclude the existence of alternative ischaemic mechanisms that may explain HF, in particular the presence of coronary microvascular dysfunction (CMD).[3] Thus, myocardial ischaemia may represent an important pathophysiological substrate along the entire spectrum of HF presentation, including both HF with reduced ejection fraction (EF) (HFrEF) and HF with preserved EF (HFpEF). Moreover, the presence of IHD has important prognostic implications, as it has been shown to be independently associated with a worsened long-term outcome both in HFpEF and HFrEF patients.[1,4]

In this chapter, we review the pathophysiological mechanisms underlying ischaemic HF, along with the diagnostic and therapeutic approaches.

Pathophysiological role of coronary artery disease in heart failure

Myocardial ischaemia is involved in the pathogenesis of HF across the entire spectrum of left ventricular (LV) function, including both HFrEF and HFpEF (➲ Figure 3.1.1).

Ischaemic mechanisms underlying HFrEF are mainly related to the consequences of acute MI, with LV remodelling occurring in the chronic phase after MI due to extensive scar formation. In particular, in patients with acute MI, prolonged ischaemia induces necrosis of different cellular lineages, including cardiomyocytes and endothelial cells.[5,6] This process triggers a pro-inflammatory response with recruitment of inflammatory cells not only into the infarcted zone, but also into the border zone, thereby extending the ischaemic area and promoting adverse myocardial remodelling.[2,6] Moreover, in the acute phase of MI, there is sudden modification in loading conditions of the left ventricle (LV) that triggers a cascade of neurohormonal activation that may contribute to the acute and chronic pathological changes underlying the occurrence of HF.[2] Primary percutaneous coronary intervention (PCI) emerged in

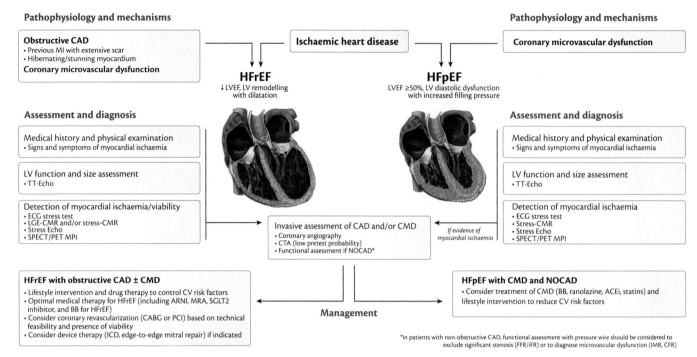

Figure 3.1.1 Pathophysiology, diagnosis, and management of coronary artery disease in patients with heart failure. CAD, coronary artery disease; MI, myocardial infarction; HFrEF, heart failure with reduced ejection fraction; HFpEF, heart failure with preserved ejection fraction; LVEF, left ventricular ejection fraction; LV, left ventricle; TT-Echo, transthoracic echocardiography; ECG, electrocardiogram; LGE-CMR, late gadolinium enhancement cardiac magnetic resonance; stress Echo, stress echocardiography; SPECT, single-photon emission computed tomography; PET, position emission tomography; MPI, myocardial perfusion imaging; CV, cardiovascular; ARNI, angiotensin receptor–neprilysin inhibitor; MRA, mineralocorticoid receptor; SGLT2I, sodium–glucose cotransporter 2 inhibitor; BB, beta-blocker; CABG, coronary artery bypass graft; PCI, percutaneous coronary intervention; ICD, implantable cardioverter–defibrillator; CTA, computed coronary angiography; NOCAD, non-obstructive coronary artery disease; ACEi, angiotensin-converting enzyme inhibitor; FFR, fractional flow reserve; IFR, instantaneous wave-free ratio; IMR, index of microvascular resistance; CFR, coronary flow reserve.

the last decades as the preferred strategy for revascularization in ST-segment elevation MI. However, even in the context of successful restoration of epicardial blood flow by primary PCI, a considerable proportion of patients, nearly 50%, still do not achieve optimal myocardial reperfusion,[5,6] due to the occurrence of coronary microvascular obstruction (MVO). Several interacting mechanisms have been suggested to be involved in the pathogenesis of MVO such as distal atherothrombotic embolization, ischaemia–reperfusion injury, and individual susceptibility to microvascular dysfunction.[6]

If prolonged ischaemia induces 'irreversible' damage resulting in cellular necrosis, brief episodes of acute myocardial ischaemia may cause a 'reversible' injury, the so-called myocardial stunning.[7] This is a condition characterized by prolonged and reversible contractile dysfunction in the presence of near-normal resting blood flow, but with a reduced coronary flow reserve (CFR), and usually results from transient severe ischaemia that persists after normal epicardial blood flow is restored. Stunned myocardium is mainly characterized by transient metabolic derangement at the cellular level.[8] Hibernating myocardium is another important phenomenon involving myocardial injury and dysfunction. Hibernating myocardium refers to a chronic condition characterized by a dysfunctional, but viable, myocardium with reduced coronary blood flow at rest.[7] Compared with myocardial stunning, in the

hibernating myocardium, there is extensive myocyte damage secondary to a longer duration of myocardial ischaemia and more severe reduction in myocardial perfusion. It is conceivable that stunning and hibernation represent a continuum of the same process, with repetitive episodes of stunning resulting in a progressive reduction in resting CFR and increased level of ultrastructural damage of cardiomyocytes.[7] The final common pathway of these ischaemic injuries at the myocardial level is the occurrence of LV adverse remodelling,[2,9] often associated with valvular abnormalities, such as functional mitral regurgitation (MR), that can further accelerate the deleterious structural changes in the LV through volume overload.[2]

The absence of obstructive coronary arteries does not rule out an ischaemic substrate underlying HF. Indeed, several studies suggest that CMD may play a key role in HFpEF and it should be considered as a possible contributor to myocardial dysfunction also in HFrEF.[3,10] Indeed, endothelial dysfunction reduces nitric oxide (NO) bioavailability, cyclic guanosine monophosphate content, and protein kinase G in adjacent cardiomyocytes. These changes are known to favour hypertrophy and fibrosis contributing to diastolic dysfunction.[10] In addition, microvascular inflammation contributes to the induction of cardiac fibrosis and vascular rarefaction. Transforming growth factor beta (TGF-β) is likely to play a major role in this setting, as suggested by the observation that disruption in TGF signalling attenuates cardiac pressure overload-induced interstitial fibrosis.[11] Accordingly, functional studies performed with use of pressure wires demonstrated a linear correlation between the index of microvascular resistance (IMR) and LV end-diastolic pressure (LVEDP) and a reduced endothelium-dependent vasodilator response to acetylcholine in HFpEF patients.[12] Moreover, Taqueti et al. documented that in patients with suspected angina, reduction in the CFR, together with diastolic dysfunction, predicted the risk of major adverse cardiovascular events (MACE) and hospitalizations due to HF during follow-up.[13]

Diagnostic approach in patients with coronary artery disease and heart failure

A detailed medical history and an accurate physical examination should always be carried out in all patients presenting with HF (➲ Figure 3.1.1). In particular, signs and symptoms of ischaemia should be carefully evaluated, along with assessment of a baseline ECG, a chest X-ray, and plasma biomarker levels (including high-sensitivity troponins and natriuretic peptides). Moreover, the use of non-invasive electrocardiography (ECG) or imaging stress tests, such as cardiac magnetic resonance (CMR), stress echocardiography, single-photon emission computed tomography (SPECT), or positron emission tomography, is recommended for the assessment of myocardial ischaemia and viability in patients with HF.[14]

Echocardiography represents a first-line investigation allowing quantification of LV systolic and diastolic function, along with segmental kinetic alterations, as well as assessing for the presence of concomitant valvular diseases. In HFrEF patients, severe LV dilatation is a marker of non-viable myocardium and LV wall thickness has been shown to be an important predictor of viability.[15] Stress echocardiography is important to evaluate the presence of ischaemic myocardium, by assessing the pathological response during exercise or during intravenous administration of dobutamine or dipyridamole. Moreover, dobutamine stress echocardiography is particularly indicated to assess for the presence of viable myocardium in patients with HFrEF, and is performed as a two-step assessment, first with low-dose (5–10 μg/kg/min) and then with high-dose (10–40 μg/kg/min) dobutamine. Biphasic response with increased myocardial contractility at low doses, and paradoxical deterioration of myocardial contractility at higher doses, is considered highly suggestive of viable myocardium.[16] Dipyridamole stress echocardiography allows also evaluating the coronary flow velocity reserve (CFVR) in the left anterior descending coronary artery and may be particularly useful in assessing for the presence of CMD.

SPECT is an imaging technique based on the assessment of myocardial uptake of radiotracer compounds (i.e. thallium-201 and technetium-99m). It is a widely available technique and provides an estimation of resting perfusion, stress-induced ischaemia, scar tissue, and cardiac systolic function. SPECT demonstrated high sensitivity (83–87%) and low specificity (53–68%)

for the prediction of recovery of contractile function following successful revascularization.[2,17] However, SPECT may underestimate tissue viability and its diagnostic accuracy is limited by lower-energy tracers, lower spatial resolution, and increased frequency of attenuation artefacts.[17]

CMR imaging is currently emerging as the most important examination in the assessment of myocardial ischaemia and viability. Indeed, along with information regarding cardiac structure and function, including shape, size, and wall thickness, CMR with gadolinium-chelated contrast enhancement (late gadolinium enhancement (LGE)) is important to evaluate the extent of non-viable myocardial scar tissue in HFrEF. In general, the absence of scar tissue is associated with a likelihood of myocardial contractile recovery of approximately 78%; however, when scar transmurality is >50%, the likelihood of functional recovery drops to approximately 8%.[18,19] In patients with scar transmurality of 1–50%, LGE CMR has a lower accuracy for predicting contractile recovery and additional evaluation with low-dose dobutamine stress CMR may be able to assess for the presence of contractile reserve and should be considered in order to improve the diagnostic accuracy of detecting myocardial viability.[20] Finally, stress CMR with adenosine administration may be useful in assessing for the presence of ischaemia due to CMD.

Coronary angiography is recommended in patients with HF who suffer from angina pectoris despite optimal medical therapy, provided the patient is otherwise suitable for coronary revascularization.[14] Coronary angiography should be considered in patients with HFrEF or HFpEF and those with intermediate-to-high pretest probability of CAD and the presence of ischaemia from non-invasive stress tests in order to establish the ischaemic aetiology and CAD severity.[14] In patients with angiographically non-obstructive CAD, functional assessment with pressure wire (i.e. fractional flow reserve (FFR) or instantaneous wave-free ratio (iFR)) should be considered to exclude significant stenosis or to diagnose the presence of CMD by evaluating the IMR and CFR, especially in patients with HFpEF. Coronary computed tomographic angiography (CTA) has been shown to have a very high negative predictive value and high sensitivity in evaluating severe stenosis. Thus, CTA may be considered in patients with a low-to-intermediate pretest probability of CAD or those with equivocal non-invasive stress tests.[14] CTA is not recommended in cases of extended coronary calcifications, irregular heart rate, significant obesity, or other conditions that prevent the acquisition of good-quality images.[14]

Management of patients with coronary artery disease and heart failure

Medical management remains the cornerstone for treatment of patients with HF across the wide spectrum of EF, and both in patients with HFrEF and in those with HFpEF, lifestyle intervention and drug therapy are of utmost importance to control existing cardiovascular risk factors. However, available therapeutic strategies are quite different for HFrEF compared with HFpEF.

In HFrEF patients, data from randomized trials have shown that three drug classes (mineralocorticoid receptor antagonists (MRAs), angiotensin receptor–neprilysin inhibitors (ARNIs), and sodium–glucose cotransporter 2 (SGLT2) inhibitors) reduce mortality beyond conventional therapy with either an angiotensin-converting enzyme (ACE) inhibitor or an angiotensin receptor blocker (ARB) plus a beta blocker (BB).[14,21,22,23] Of interest, the selective cardiac myosin activator omecamtiv mecarbil has also been shown to be effective in the recent GALACTIC-HF trial by stimulating the cardiac sarcomere, reducing the risk of HF events or cardiovascular death by 8% at 21.8 months.[24] However, in patients with HFrEF due to ischaemic heart disease, therapy requires a comprehensive approach that also includes secondary prevention measures (including lipid and antiplatelet therapy) and, if indicated, device therapies and coronary revascularization.[14] In particular, there is still ongoing debate regarding the prognostic benefit of revascularization therapy. Surgical revascularization (in addition to optimal medical therapy) has a class I, level of evidence A indication, according to the 2018 European Society of Cardiology (ESC) revascularization guidelines for patients with ischaemic cardiomyopathy with LVEF ≤35% and CAD (in particular those with two- or three-vessel CAD) amenable to surgical revascularization to improve prognosis.[25] The Surgical Treatment for Ischemic Heart Failure (STICH) trial, to date, is the largest randomized trial specifically addressing the role of revascularization in patients with LVEF ≤35% and CAD. The STICH trial randomly assigned 1212 patients to medical therapy plus coronary artery bypass graft (CABG) surgery or medical therapy alone. At a median follow-up of 56 months, all-cause mortality was not significantly different between the two arms (41% optimal medical therapy vs 36% CABG).[26] Regarding secondary outcomes, there was a trend towards reduced cardiovascular mortality in the CABG group that did not meet statistical significance. However, the STICH Extension Study (STICHES), which extended the follow-up to a median of 9.8 years in the same population, showed that the primary outcome of all-cause mortality was significantly lower in the CABG group, compared to the optimal medical therapy group, as well as the prespecified secondary outcomes of cardiovascular mortality and the combination of all-cause mortality with cardiovascular hospitalization.[27] Of note, in a viability substudy of the STICH trial, no significant interaction was observed between the presence or absence of myocardial viability and the beneficial effect of CABG plus medical therapy over medical therapy alone. An increase in LVEF was observed only among patients with myocardial viability, irrespective of treatment assignment. There was no association between changes in LVEF and subsequent death.[28] Of note, to date, there are no randomized controlled trials (RCTs) exploring the efficacy of PCI, compared to that of CABG, and the relative efficacy of PCI versus CABG for revascularization is unknown, although data from non-randomized registry suggest no difference in mortality between CABG and PCI.[29] Device therapy, such as implantable cardioverter–defibrillators (ICDs),

cardiac resynchronization therapy (CRT), and edge-to-edge repair of severe functional MR have also been shown to improve prognosis in patients with HFrEF and may be considered, if indicated, also in patients with HFrEF of ischaemic origin.[14]

Cardiogenic shock occurs in 7–10% of patients with acute MI and is associated with 40% mortality at 30 days.[30] In these patients, immediate coronary angiography is recommended (within 2 hours of hospital admission), with an intent to perform coronary revascularization, as early revascularization has been shown to reduce mortality.[14] Most patients with cardiogenic shock present with multivessel CAD, which is associated with higher mortality than single-vessel disease. The benefit of multivessel PCI in these patients has been a matter of debate for a long time. However, the recent CULPRIT-SHOCK trial demonstrated that the risk of death or renal replacement therapy at 30 days was lower with culprit lesion-only PCI than with immediate multivessel PCI, and mortality did not differ significantly between the two groups at 1-year follow-up.[31] In selected patients with acute MI and cardiogenic shock, short-term mechanical circulatory support may be considered. However, recently, the IABP-SHOCK II trial showed that use of an intra-aortic balloon pump (IABP) did not improve outcomes in this subset of patients,[30] and evidence for a clinical benefit of other devices (i.e. Impella® or extracorporeal membrane oxygenation (ECMO)) is still lacking.[32,33]

If several therapeutic strategies have been developed in the last decades for HFrEF, this has not been the case for HFpEF. Indeed, no medical treatment has been shown to improve all-cause mortality in the HFpEF population, as all failed to reduce their prespecified primary end points in their respective cardiovascular outcomes trials, although some have shown potential improvements in their secondary outcomes.[34] The presence of obstructive CAD is associated with increased mortality and greater deterioration in ventricular function, and complete revascularization may be associated with improved survival and less deterioration in LV function over time, even if these data need be confirmed in dedicated prospective trials.[35] CMD emerged in recent years as an important therapeutic target in HFpEF, and drugs that demonstrated a clinical benefit in patients with microvascular angina (i.e. BBs, ACE inhibitors, ranolazine, and statins) may be also considered for HFpEF patients. However, currently, there are no trials specifically evaluating the role of therapeutic strategies addressing CMD in this subset of patients.

Future directions

In last decades, much progress in the management of patients with ischaemic HF has been made. However, there are still many knowledge gaps that need to be addressed in future studies. Indeed, in HFrEF, the importance of myocardial viability as a guide for coronary revascularization needs to be clarified. Moreover, the benefit of PCI versus CABG in patients with multivessel disease and HFrEF should be evaluated in dedicated clinical trials.

Finally, further studies aiming at assessing the pathogenic role of CMD in the occurrence of HF are needed, as well as studies evaluating therapies targeting CMD. This latter point represents an important clinical need, especially in patients with HFpEF.

Summary

IHD represents the most important cause underlying the occurrence of HF. Multiple pathophysiological mechanisms may explain the association between myocardial ischaemia and HF, and understanding the exact mechanism of disease is crucial to obtaining a proper diagnosis and starting appropriate therapy. Medical management remains the cornerstone for treatment of patients with HF. Revascularization of obstructive CAD represents a possible solution when indicated. However, in HFrEF, the importance of myocardial viability as a guide for coronary revascularization needs to be clarified. Moreover, the benefit of PCI versus CABG in patients with multivessel disease and HFrEF is still a matter of debate. Finally, further studies aiming at assessing the pathogenic role of CMD in the occurrence of HF are needed, as well as studies evaluating therapies targeting CMD, especially in patients with HFpEF.

References

1. Gheorghiade M, Sopko G, De Luca L, et al. Navigating the crossroads of coronary artery disease and heart failure. Circulation. 2006;114:1202–13.
2. Cabac-Pogorevici I, Muk B, Rustamova Y, Kalogeropoulos A, Tzeis S, Vardas P. Ischaemic cardiomyopathy. Pathophysiological insights, diagnostic management and the roles of revascularisation and device treatment. Gaps and dilemmas in the era of advanced technology. Eur J Heart Fail. 2020;22:789–99.
3. Crea F, Bairey Merz CN, et al.; Coronary Vasomotion Disorders International Study Group (COVADIS). The parallel tales of microvascular angina and heart failure with preserved ejection fraction: a paradigm shift. Eur Heart J. 2017;38:473–7.
4. Hwang SJ, Melenovsky V, Borlaug BA. Implications of coronary artery disease in heart failure with preserved ejection fraction. J Am Coll Cardiol. 2014;63:2817–27.
5. Niccoli G, Montone RA, Ibanez B, et al. Optimized treatment of ST-elevation myocardial infarction. Circ Res. 2019;125:245–58.
6. Niccoli G, Scalone G, Lerman A, Crea F. Coronary microvascular obstruction in acute myocardial infarction. Eur Heart J. 2016;37:1024–33.
7. Kloner RA. Stunned and hibernating myocardium: where are we nearly 4 decades later? J Am Heart Assoc. 2020;9:e015502.
8. Poole-Wilson PA, Holmberg SR, Williams AJ. A possible molecular mechanism for 'stunning' of the myocardium. Eur Heart J. 1991;12:25–9.
9. Briceno N, Schuster A, Lumley M, Perera D. Ischaemic cardiomyopathy: pathophysiology, assessment and the role of revascularisation. Heart. 2016;102:397–406.
10. Mohammed SF, Hussain S, Mirzoyev SA, Edwards WD, Maleszewski JJ, Redfield MM. Coronary microvascular rarefaction and myocardial fibrosis in heart failure with preserved ejection fraction. Circulation. 2015;131:550–9.
11. Kuwahara F, Kai H, Tokuda K, et al. Transforming growth factor-beta function blocking prevents myocardial fibrosis and diastolic dysfunction in pressure-overloaded rats. Circulation. 2002;106:130–5.
12. D'Amario D, Migliaro S, Borovac JA, et al. Microvascular dysfunction in heart failure with preserved ejection fraction. Front Physiol. 2019;10:1347.
13. Taqueti VR, Solomon SD, Shah AM, et al. Coronary microvascular dysfunction and future risk of heart failure with preserved ejection fraction. Eur Heart J. 2018;39:840–9.
14. Ponikowski P, Voors AA, Anker SD, et al.; ESC Scientific Document Group. 2016 ESC Guidelines for the diagnosis and treatment of acute and chronic heart failure: The Task Force for the diagnosis and treatment of acute and chronic heart failure of the European Society of Cardiology (ESC) Developed with the special contribution of the Heart Failure Association (HFA) of the ESC. Eur Heart J. 2016;37:2129–200.
15. Cwajg JM, Cwajg E, Nagueh SF, et al. End-diastolic wall thickness as a predictor of recovery of function in myocardial hibernation: relation to rest-redistribution T1-201 tomography and dobutamine stress echocardiography. J Am Coll Cardiol. 2000;35:1152–61.
16. Cornel JH, Bax JJ, Elhendy A, et al. Biphasic response to dobutamine predicts improvement of global left ventricular function after surgical revascularization in patients with stable coronary artery disease: implications of time course of recovery on diagnostic accuracy. J Am Coll Cardiol. 1998;31:1002–10.
17. Schinkel AF, Bax JJ, Poldermans D, Elhendy A, Ferrari R, Rahimtoola SH. Hibernating myocardium: diagnosis and patient outcomes. Curr Probl Cardiol. 2007;32:375–410.
18. Romero J, Xue X, Gonzalez W, Garcia MJ. CMR imaging assessing viability in patients with chronic ventricular dysfunction due to coronary artery disease: a meta-analysis of prospective trials. JACC Cardiovasc Imaging. 2012;5:494–508.
19. Kim RJ, Wu E, Rafael A, et al. The use of contrast-enhanced magnetic resonance imaging to identify reversible myocardial dysfunction. N Engl J Med. 2000;343:1445–53.
20. Wellnhofer E, Olariu A, Klein C, et al. Magnetic resonance low-dose dobutamine test is superior to SCAR quantification for the prediction of functional recovery. Circulation. 2004;109:2172–4.
21. Packer M, Anker SD, Butler J, et al.; EMPEROR-Reduced Trial Investigators. Cardiovascular and renal outcomes with empagliflozin in heart failure. N Engl J Med. 2020;383:1413–24.
22. McMurray JJ, Packer M, Desai AS, et al.; PARADIGM-HF Investigators and Committees. Angiotensin–neprilysin inhibition versus enalapril in heart failure. N Engl J Med. 2014;371:993–1004.
23. Vaduganathan M, Claggett BL, Jhund PS, et al. Estimating lifetime benefits of comprehensive disease-modifying pharmacological therapies in patients with heart failure with reduced ejection fraction: a comparative analysis of three randomised controlled trials. Lancet. 2020;396:121–8.
24. Teerlink JR, Diaz R, Felker GM, et al.; GALACTIC-HF Investigators. Cardiac myosin activation with omecamtiv mecarbil in systolic heart failure. N Engl J Med. 2022;384:105–16.
25. Neumann FJ, Sousa-Uva M, Ahlsson A, et al.; ESC Scientific Document Group. 2018 ESC/EACTS Guidelines on myocardial revascularization. Eur Heart J. 2019;40:87–165.
26. Velazquez EJ, Lee KL, Deja MA, et al.; STICH Investigators. Coronary-artery bypass surgery in patients with left ventricular dysfunction. N Engl J Med. 2011;364:1607–16.
27. Petrie MC, Jhund PS, She L, et al.; STICH Trial Investigators. Ten-year outcomes after coronary artery bypass grafting according to age in patients with heart failure and left ventricular systolic dysfunction: an analysis of the extended follow-up of the STICH

Trial (Surgical Treatment for Ischemic Heart Failure). Circulation. 2016;134:1314–24.

28. Panza JA, Ellis AM, Al-Khalidi HR, *et al.* Myocardial viability and long-term outcomes in ischemic cardiomyopathy. N Engl J Med. 2019;381:739–48.

29. Bangalore S, Guo Y, Samadashvili Z, Blecker S, Hannan EL. Revascularization in patients with multivessel coronary artery disease and severe left ventricular systolic dysfunction: everolimus-eluting stents versus coronary artery bypass graft surgery. Circulation. 2016;133:2132–40.

30. Thiele H, Zeymer U, Neumann FJ, *et al.*; IABP-SHOCK II Trial Investigators. Intraaortic balloon support for myocardial infarction with cardiogenic shock. N Engl J Med. 2012;367:1287–96.

31. Thiele H, Akin I, Sandri M, *et al.*; CULPRIT-SHOCK Investigators. One-year outcomes after PCI strategies in cardiogenic shock. N Engl J Med. 2018;379:1699–710.

32. Schrage B, Ibrahim K, Loehn T, *et al.* Impella support for acute myocardial infarction complicated by cardiogenic shock. Circulation. 2019;139:1249–58.

33. Dhruva SS, Ross JS, Mortazavi BJ, *et al.* Association of use of an intravascular microaxial left ventricular assist device vs intra-aortic balloon pump with in-hospital mortality and major bleeding among patients with acute myocardial infarction complicated by cardiogenic shock. JAMA. 2020;323:734–45.

34. Del Buono MG, Iannaccone G, Scacciavillani R, *et al.* Heart failure with preserved ejection fraction diagnosis and treatment: an updated review of the evidence. Prog Cardiovasc Dis. 2020;63:570–84.

35. Hwang SJ, Melenovsky V, Borlaug BA. Implications of coronary artery disease in heart failure with preserved ejection fraction. J Am Coll Cardiol. 2014;63(25 Pt A):2817–27.

From hypertension to heart failure

Athanasios J Manolis and Yuri Lopatin

Contents

Introduction

According to recently published European Society of Cardiology (ESC)/European Society of Hypertension (ESH) hypertension (HTN) guidelines, HTN is defined as a systolic blood pressure (SBP) of 140 mmHg or more, or a diastolic blood pressure (DBP) of 90 mmHg or more, or where there is a requirement for antihypertensive medication.[1] In some cases, such as in the elderly or frail patients, these cut-offs are more flexible. According to ESC heart failure (HF) guidelines, HF is a clinical syndrome characterized by typical symptoms (e.g. breathlessness, ankle swelling, fatigue) that may be accompanied by signs (e.g. elevated jugular venous pressure, pulmonary crackles, peripheral oedema) caused by a structural and/or functional cardiac abnormality, resulting in a reduced cardiac output and/or elevated intracardiac pressures at rest or during stress.[2] HTN affects close to 1 billion adults worldwide, and this number is forecast to increase to over 1.5 billion by 2025.[3] More than 7.5 million deaths per year are attributable to HTN. HTN is the most important risk factor for cardiovascular (CV) morbidity and mortality. Untreated high blood pressure (BP) may progress, leading to many organ-specific changes, which are referred to in the new ESC/ESH hypertension guidelines as 'hypertension-mediated organ damage (HMOD)' (➲ Figure 3.2.1). HTN leads to endothelial dysfunction, subclinical or clinical organ damage such as left ventricular hypertrophy (LVH), microalbuminuria, increased intimal medial thickness, hypertensive retinopathy, coronary heart disease, chronic kidney disease, arrhythmias, stroke, HF with preserved (HFpEF) or reduced (HFrEF) ejection fraction, and neurovascular changes including stroke and dementia (➲ Figure 3.2.2). Individuals with high BP are more susceptible to ischaemic heart disease, and may have a 6-fold greater risk of myocardial infarction.[4] Due to its high prevalence, HTN carries the greatest risk of developing HF. HTN is also associated with the prevalence of atrial fibrillation and ventricular arrhythmias.[5] Increased left atrial pressure and left atrial enlargement are the most important risk factors for atrial fibrillation.

Various trials have shown an association between long-standing HTN and HF. There is a continuous relationship between BP and CV and renal events. Epidemiological data have shown a linear correlation between BP and CV risk from very low levels of BP (i.e. SBP >115 mmHg).[6] A meta-analysis of 23 trials including 193,424 patients with HTN or at 'high' CV risk, of whom the majority were hypertensive patients, showed that 28.9% developed HF, accounting for 9.1 events per 1000 patients. HF development was more prevalent among older subjects aged >65 years ($P<0.0001$), black versus non-black individuals ($P<0.0001$), diabetic versus non-diabetic patients ($P<0.0001$), and patients with 'very high' risk versus those with a 'high' risk profile ($P<0.0001$). This analysis

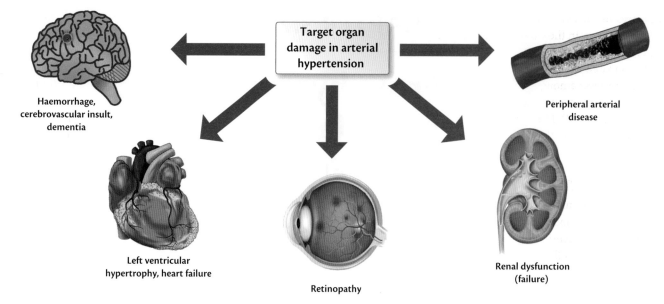

Figure 3.2.1 Possible complications of hypertension.

showed that HF development remains a major problem in pa-tients with HTN.[7] Indeed, among those who participated in the Framingham Heart Study with no history of HTN and CV dis-ease (*n* = 6859), the risk of developing CV disease in individuals with BP ≥130/85 mmHg was almost triple that in participants with BP <120/80 mmHg.[6] From the same study, 91% of partici-pants with HF who had a history of HTN had 2- (males) and 3-fold (females) increased risk of developing HF, compared to normotensives.[4] High BP directly correlates with a higher risk of developing HF. The risk of HF is doubled among patients with BP >160/100 mmHg, compared with those with BP <140/90 mmHg.[8] In addition, diabetes and dyslipidaemia often coexist with HTN,[9] which further increases the risk of CV disease. In the Avoiding Cardiovascular Events through Combination Therapy in Patients Living with Systolic Hypertension (ACCOMPLISH) trial, around 2% of high-risk hypertensive patients developed HF within 3 years.[10] In the Antihypertensive and Lipid-Lowering

Treatment to Prevent Heart Attack Trial (ALLHAT), in an average follow-up of 9 years, 1716 of 32,804 patients developed HF.[11] HTN causes remodelling of the structure and function of blood vessels and the left ventricle (LV), an adaptive mechanism in response to long-term HTN.[12] Previous studies have shown that around 36–41% of all hypertensives have LVH. In addition to high BP, other factors such as activation of the sympathetic ner-vous system (SNS) and renin–angiotensin–aldosterone system (RAAS), insulin resistance, and endothelin, among others,[6,9] are important causes for the development of hypertensive heart dis-ease (HHD). LVH, eccentric or concentric, is the initial step in the progression to HF.[13] Patients with concentric LVH usually develop HFpEF, whereas those with eccentric LVH will develop HFrEF. The classic course of left ventricular (LV) progression is the so-called 'burnt-out' LV, in which HTN leads to HFpEF or HFrEF.[14] However, ischaemic heart disease, and in particular myocardial infarction, leads directly to systolic HF.[15] There are

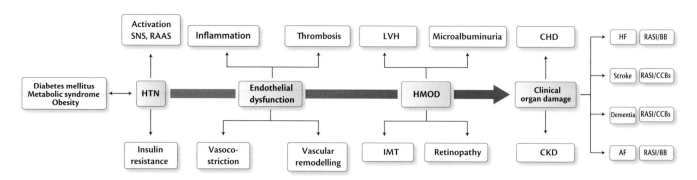

Figure 3.2.2 Pathophysiological mechanisms underlying arterial hypertension, subsequent progression to heart failure, and implications for treatment. BB, beta-blocker; CCB, calcium channel blocker; CHD, coronary heart disease; CKD, chronic kidney disease; IMT, intima media thickness; HTN, hypertension; LVH, left ventricular hypertrophy; HMOD, hypertension-mediated organ damage; RAAS, renin–angiotensin–aldosterone system; RASI, renin–angiotensin system inhibitor; SNS, sympathetic nervous system.

differences in the association between HTN and HF based on race, sex, and age. In the United States, there is a high prevalence of HTN among black patients, which is therefore more causative of HF, compared to ischaemic heart disease. Moreover, BP control rates are lower among black and Hispanic individuals, which is another reason accounting for the high risk of developing HF in these subgroups.[16] The 5-year mortality risk of HF is 50%, which is increased by the concomitant presence of both HTN and HF.[17]

Pathophysiology

The term of hypertensive heart disease (HHD) is commonly used to describe clinical manifestations of cardiac disease caused by the impact of hypertension on the heart. From a clinical point of view, Messerli and colleagues have divided HHD into four categories, which include isolated LV diastolic dysfunction, LV diastolic dysfunction with LVH, HFpEF, and HFrEF.[18] LV diastolic dysfunction is the first manifestation of HHD characterized by abnormalities in diastolic filling, distensibility, or relaxation of the LV.[19] In HTN, pressure and volume overload lead to structural and functional changes in the heart and blood vessels. These alterations are known as remodelling, which is considered as an adaptive mechanism, but also as a contributor to further progression of circulatory disorders.[20] Cardiac remodelling as a response to pressure overload results in concentric LVH, in which myocytes mainly increase in short-axis diameter.[21] By contrast, cardiac remodelling associated with chronic volume overload is characterized by increasing myocyte length, which ultimately causes dilatation of the LV with thin walls; this is defined as eccentric LVH.[22] The remodelling processes are not limited by the LV—enlargement of the left atrium and changes in the left atrial wall may create a substrate for the initiation of atrial fibrillation. Once LVH has manifested, the risk of HFpEF and HFrEF development increases significantly.[23] HFpEF is a more common consequence in long-standing hypertension than HFrEF. However, ischaemic events often instigate progression from HFpEF to HFrEF.[24]

In HTN, many pathophysiological mechanisms, including sympathetic overdrive, paracrine and autocrine signalling of RAAS activation, insulin resistance, endothelial dysfunction, and others, are responsible for the causation of, and subsequent progression to, HF (➲ Figure 3.2.2). [25-29] Involvement of these mechanisms in excessive BP elevation, development of LVH, myocardial fibrosis, vascular inflammation, and LV dysfunction has a complex character, which makes it difficult to determine the causal links among them. In this context, the long-standing paradigm of increased afterload as a major mechanism underlying the pathophysiology of the above-mentioned conditions has changed to a more multifaceted model describing the complexity of progression from HTN to HF.

According to this emerging model, comorbidity-associated systemic inflammation is the main driving factor impairing myocardial performance by inducing microvascular dysfunction.[13,30] This model presumes the following sequence of events leading to HF: (1) HTN as the most prevalent comorbidity induces a systemic pro-inflammatory state; (2) due to the pro-inflammatory state, coronary microvascular endothelial cells produce reactive oxygen species (ROS), limiting nitric oxide (NO) bioavailability for adjacent cardiomyocytes; (3) limited NO bioavailability, in turn, decreases protein kinase G (PKG) activity in cardiomyocytes; (4) low PKG activity leads to cardiomyocyte hypertrophy, thereby inducing concentric LV remodelling, and stiffens cardiomyocytes because of hypophosphorylation of the giant cytoskeletal protein titin; and (5) both stiffened cardiomyocytes and increased collagen deposition by myofibroblasts cause diastolic LV dysfunction.[30] All of the above-mentioned events are more strongly associated with the development of HFpEF—the most common consequence of HTN—than with HFrEF, in which LV remodelling is driven by progressive loss of cardiomyocytes.[31] Nevertheless, HFrEF, once developed, can also promote systemic and coronary endothelial dysfunction via neurohormonal activation and lead to altered shear stress, increased oxidative stress, and a decrease in the production of NO.[32] Attenuated endothelium-dependent vasodilatation was demonstrated in both patients with HFpEF and those with HFrEF. Endothelial dysfunction is also accompanied by other adverse effects at the vascular level, including alteration of anticoagulant properties, increased expression of adhesion molecules, and increased release of chemokines and cytokines.[33] It was found that different cytokines originating from intra- or extracardiac tissues may play an important role in the development and progression of HF, through their ability to modulate inflammation, myocyte stress and apoptosis, fibroblast activation, and extracellular matrix remodelling.[34]

The link between HTN and HF is also based on neurohumoral activation and insulin resistance. Activation of RAAS is one of the most important mechanisms contributing to vasoconstriction, ROS generation, vascular inflammation, and cardiac remodelling.[35] In addition, activation of the SNS plays an idiopathic role in the development of LVH, overt vasoconstriction, and retention of electrolytes such as sodium.[27] Moreover, the sympathetic overdrive is causally linked to endothelial dysfunction, the development of atherosclerosis, arrhythmias, and, in the case of extremely high SNS activation, even microscopic myocardial infarction.[36] In HTN, neurohumoral activation, inflammatory cytokines, oxidative stress, and haemodynamic disorders can lead to insulin resistance. In turn, increased insulin signalling may also drive HF progression via multiple mechanisms, including impaired metabolic efficacy, tissue fibrosis, apoptosis, and lipotoxicity.[28]

Prevention

Treating HTN intensively prevents and reverses myocardial and vessel changes in patients at risk of HF. Strict BP control with all classes of antihypertensive drugs prevents structural changes, LVH, and finally the development of HF (➲ Figure 3.2.2). Data have shown that all classes of antihypertensive drugs result in significant reduction in new onset of HF. However, in head-to-head comparisons, calcium channel blockers seem to be less effective in prevention of HF, compared to other classes.[1] It is well known that BP control reduces the incidence of HF by >50%.[1] Data have shown that for every 10 mmHg reduction in SBP, there is a 12% reduction in the risk of HF.[2]

Blood pressure targets in heart failure patients

Although signs and symptoms of HF are similar in both patients with HFpEF and those with HFrEF, those two entities require completely different therapeutic approaches, not only regarding pharmaceutical treatment, but also in terms of BP cutoffs. Usually not only do patients with HFpEF present with a past medical history of HTN, but also they have uncontrolled HTN requiring further antihypertensive treatment. On the other hand, although a significant proportion of HFrEF patients present with a past medical history of HTN, usually their BP levels are low because of substantial myocardial loss leading to reduced ejection fraction (EF). Unfortunately, the majority of studies assessing BP target levels in HF patients present data from both patients with HFrEF and those with HFpEF.

Data from the Organized Program to Initiate Lifesaving Treatment in Hospitalized Patients with Heart Failure (OPTIMIZE-HF) trial have shown that the higher the BP levels, the lower in-hospital mortality rates are.[37] A meta-analysis with a large number of patients with HF showed similar results.[38] A recent study showed a reverse J-curve association of high and low BPs with increased mortality in patients with HF with a BP threshold of 132.4/74.2 mmHg.[39] Low SBP was an independent predictor of morbidity and mortality in patients with reduced and preserved EF.[40] The Beta-Blocker Evaluation in Survival Trial (BEST) showed an increased risk of hospitalization due to HF, but not of all-cause mortality in patients with BP levels lower than 120 mmHg.[41] It has to be mentioned, however, that these controversial results of BP levels may be affected by the impaired clinical status of these patients (frailty, comorbidities, advanced age, disease severity, and cardiorenal syndrome) and there is not really a J-curve phenomenon. The benefits of treatment always must be weighed against the adverse events induced by low BP. Based on all the above, the ESC/ESH hypertension guidelines have proposed the following: (1) in patients with HFrEF, antihypertensive drug treatment should be commenced (if not already) when BP is >140/90 mmHg; (2) it is unclear how far BP should be lowered in patients with HF; and (3) outcomes for patients with HF have repeatedly been shown to be poor if BP levels are low, which suggests that it may be wise to avoid actively lowering BP to <120/70 mmHg.[38,40] It seems that the same J-curve exists in acute HF (AHF). Results from the Korean Acute Heart Failure (KorAHF) registry showed a reverse J-curve relationship between BP and the outcomes of patients who were hospitalized for HF, and the risk of mortality was similar for low and high BPs, both in HFrEF and HFpEF patients.[42] But also here, low BP levels may reflect the poor clinical condition of these patients. All the above recommendations seem to be applicable to patients with HFpEF. However, patients with HFrEF rarely have BP levels >140 mmHg. Usually their BP levels are low and if above 95–100 mmHg, physicians may start drug treatment with RAAS and/or beta-blockers (in low dose) in order to start

building HF treatment that would lead to an improvement in CV morbidity and mortality.

Treatment of arterial hypertension in patients with heart failure

The following drugs can be used in patients with HF and HTN: diuretics, beta-blockers, angiotensin-converting enzyme inhibitors (ACEIs), angiotensin receptor blockers (ARBs), mineralocorticoid receptor antagonists (MRAs), angiotensin receptor–neprilysin inhibitors (ARNIs; not yet approved for management of HTN). Also in some cases, hydralazine/nitrates, and recently sodium–glucose cotransporter 2 (SGLT2) inhibitors, can be used.

HFrEF develops when the cardiac output falls. This lead to a compensatory homeostatic response with the activation of the SNS and RAAS.[2] This activation induces a number of changes in the heart, kidneys, and vasculature in order to maintain CV homeostasis. However, with chronic activation, these responses result in increased haemodynamic stress and exert deleterious effects on the heart and the rest of the CV system. Numerous studies have shown that neurohormonal activation is now known to be one of the most important mechanisms underlying the progression of HF, and therapeutic antagonism of neurohormonal systems has become the cornerstone of contemporary pharmacotherapy for HF. Hence the gold standard treatment in almost all patients includes ACEIs or ARBs, beta-blockers, ARNIs, and MRAs. In patients with overload, the addition of torasemide or furosemide is important; if they remain hypertensive, addition of dihydropyridines should be considered.[1,2] Recently SGLT2 inhibitors have been shown to have beneficial effects in HF patients.

ACEIs and ARBs

ACEIs when given to patients with mild to advanced HF have been shown to reduce mortality and morbidity, increase cardiac output, decrease congestive symptoms, and delay HF progression in patients with HFrEF.[2] ACEIs are recommended, unless contraindicated or not tolerated, for all symptomatic patients—both normotensives and hypertensives. For patients in whom ACEIs are contraindicated or not tolerated, ARBs should be considered. ACEIs and ARBs should be uptitrated to the maximum tolerated dose in order to achieve adequate inhibition of RAAS. ACEIs are also recommended for patients with asymptomatic LV systolic dysfunction to reduce the risk of HF development, HF hospitalization, and death. ACEIs and ARBs does not need to be discontinued unless there is a significant increase in plasma creatinine concentration.[1,2]

Beta-blockers

Several randomized clinical trials that assessed the role of beta-blockers in HF showed an improvement in systolic function and a reversal of cardiac remodelling. The trials showed that adding a beta-blocker, on top of standard treatment, resulted in approximately 25–35% relative risk reduction in mortality, reduced the risk of hospitalization, and improved the quality of life.[43] According to ESC guidelines for HF, beta-blockers reduce mortality and morbidity in symptomatic patients with HFrEF despite treatment with an ACEI and, in most cases, a diuretic, although use of beta-blockers has not been tested in congested or decompensated patients. There is a consensus that beta-blockers and ACEIs are complementary and can be started together as soon as a diagnosis of HFrEF is made.[2] There is no evidence that favours initiation of treatment with a beta-blocker before commencing an ACEI. Beta-blockers should be initiated at a low dose in clinically stable patients and gradually uptitrated to the maximum tolerated dose. In patients hospitalized due to AHF, beta-blockers should be cautiously initiated in hospital once the patient is stabilized.[2]

ARNIs

Sacubitril/valsartan is the first agent to be approved in a new class of drugs called ARNIs. The medication is approved for treatment of HFrEF patients with New York Heart Association (NYHA) classes II, III, and IV. ARNIs can be used in place of ACEIs or ARBs, and in conjunction with other standard HF treatments. According to the 2016 ESC Heart Failure Guidelines,[2] ARNIs are now recommended in patients with chronic symptomatic HFrEF to reduce morbidity and mortality (class I recommendation). In addition to their beneficial effects in HF, ARNIs are very effective as antihypertensive drugs.

MRAs

The MRAs spironolactone and eplerenone are recommended for patients with symptomatic HF with EF of 35% or less. Although the role of MRAs in patients with EF >35% is unclear, they may benefit patients with comorbid HTN, diabetes mellitus, or renal insufficiency. MRAs can be used for BP management, regardless of HF status, as third- or fourth-line treatment. The risk of hyperkalaemia often limits the use of MRA therapy in patients with HF. Several factors increase the risk of hyperkalaemia, including renal insufficiency and diabetes mellitus. The presence of renal insufficiency or diabetes mellitus increases the risk of adverse events with MRA therapy in HF.[2]

Diuretics

Use of diuretics in patients with HTN is very common as monotherapy or in combination with other drug classes. Their use in patients with HF relieves congestive symptoms. Although they are widely used, there are limited data from randomized clinical trials regarding HF-related morbidity and mortality reduction. Diuretic efficacy may be limited by adverse neurohormonal activation and by 'congestion-like' symptoms. Diuretics are extremely useful and comprise various classes of agents for management of the hypervolaemic state (pulmonary and/or peripheral oedema). Loop diuretics produce a more intensive diuresis, and this drug class is preferred in HF patients with congestion. Current guidelines recommend the use of three loop diuretics in HF patients (furosemide, torasemide, and bumetanide) in order to reduce hospitalization due to HF, but also to improve symptoms and exercise capacity in patients with signs and/or symptoms of congestion. Thiazides and thiazide-like agents are less effective antihypertensive agents in patients with a reduced glomerular filtration rate (GFR) (estimated GFR (eGFR) <45 mL/min) and become ineffective when the eGFR is <30 mL/min. In such circumstances, loop diuretics such as furosemide and torasemide should replace thiazides and thiazide-like diuretics to achieve an antihypertensive effect.[2]

SGLT2 inhibitors

SGLT2 inhibitors are a novel generation of oral antihyperglycaemic drugs with a unique insulin-independent mechanism of action, and have been approved over the last decade for the management of type 2 diabetes. SGLT2 inhibitors have been shown to have not only antihyperglycaemic effects, but also beneficial antihypertensive effects in patients with HF. In a recent meta-analysis of two major outcome trials (DAPA-HF and EMPEROR-Reduced), empagliflozin or dapagliflozin, on top of standard treatment for HF, reduced all-cause mortality and CV death, hospitalizations for HF, and serious adverse renal outcomes, compared to placebo.[44,45] Many studies and meta-analyses have shown that administration of SGLT2 inhibitors in type 2 diabetes patients with or without HTN has a positive effect on BP, independent of the duration of treatment. Hypertensive patients at baseline achieve greater BP reductions, compared to normotensive subjects.[46,47] The precise pathophysiological mechanisms underlying the BP-lowering effects of SGLT2 inhibitors have not been fully elucidated. Various effects, such as diuretic and natriuretic action, weight loss, reduced arterial stiffness, and inhibition of sympathetic nervous activity, are likely to be involved.

Summary

Arterial HTN represents the main cause for the development of HF. A significant proportion of patients with HFpEF or HFrEF have a past medical history of HTN. Treating arterial HTN in these patients is often challenging.

References

1. Williams B, Mancia G, Spiering W, et al.; ESC Scientific Document Group. 2018 ESC/ESH Guidelines for the management of arterial hypertension. Eur Heart J. 2018;39(33):3021–104.
2. Ponikowski P, Voors AA, Anker SD, et al.; 2016 ESC Guidelines for the diagnosis and treatment of acute and chronic heart failure: The Task Force for the diagnosis and treatment of acute and chronic heart failure of the European Society of Cardiology (ESC) Developed with the special contribution of the Heart Failure Association (HFA) of the ESC. Eur Heart J. 2016;37(27):2129–200.
3. Keamey PM, Whelton M, Reynolds K, Muntner P, Whelton PK, He J. Global burden of hypertension: analysis of worldwide data. Lancet. 2005;365:217–23.
4. Levy D, Larson MG, Vasan RS, Kannel WB, Ho KK. The progression from hypertension to congestive heart failure. JAMA. 1996;275:1557–62.
5. Kallistratos MS, Poulimenos LE, Manolis AJ. Atrial fibrillation and arterial hypertension. Pharmacol Res. 2018;128:322–6.
6. Vasan RS, Larson MG, Leip EP, Evans JC, O'Donnell CJ, Kannel WB. Impact of high normal blood pressure on the risk of cardiovascular disease. N Engl J Med. 2001;345:1291–2.

7. Tocci G, Sciarreta S, Volpe M. Development of heart failure in recent hypertension trials. J Hypertens. 2008;26:1477–86.

8. Lloyd-Jones DM, Larson MG, Leip EP. Lifetime risk for developing congestive heart failure: the Framingham Heart Study. Circulation. 2002;106:3068–72.

9. de Boer IH, Bangalore S, Benetos A, Davis AM, Michos ED, Muntner P. Diabetes and hypertension: a position statement of American Diabetes Association. Diabetes Care. 2017;40:1273–84.

10. Jamerson K, Weber MA, Bakris GL, et al. Benazepril plus amlodipine or hydrochlorothiazide for hypertension in high risk patients. N Engl J Med. 2008;359:2417.

11. Piller LB, Baraniuk S, Simpson LM, et al. Long term follow-up of participants with heart failure in the antihypertensive and lipid lowering treatment to prevent heart attack trial (ALLHAT). Circulation. 2011;124:1811.

12. Cuspidi C, Sala C, Nrgri F, Mancia G, Morganti A. Prevalence of left ventricular hypertrophy in hypertension: an update review of echocardiographic studies. J Hum Hypertens. 2012;26:343–9.

13. Teo LY, Chan LL, Lam CS. Heart failure with preserved ejection fraction in hypertension. Curr Opin Cardiol. 2016;31:410–16.

14. Meerson FZ. Compensatory hyperfunction of the heart and cardiac insufficiency. Circ Res. 1962;10:250–8.

15. Drazner MH. The progression of hypertensive heart disease. Circulation. 2011;123:327–34.

16. Vivo RP, Krim SR, Cevik C, Witteles RM. Heart failure in Hispanics. J Am Coll Cardiol. 2009;53:1167–75.

17. Benjamin EJ, Muntner P, Bittencourt MS. Heart disease and stroke statistics2019 update: a report from the American Heart Association. Circulation. 2019;139:e56–528.

18. Messerli FH, Rimoldi SF, Bangalore S. The transition from hypertension to heart failure: contemporary update. JACC Heart Fail. 2017;5(8):543–51.

19. Sorrentino MJ. The evolution from hypertension to heart failure. Heart Fail Clin. 2019;15(4):447–53.

20. Gibbons GH, Dzau VJ. The emerging concept of vascular remodeling. N Engl J Med. 1994;330:1431–8.

21. Nakamura M, Sadoshima J. Mechanisms of physiological and pathological cardiac hypertrophy. Nat Rev Cardiol. 2018;15:387–407.

22. Gaasch WH, Zile MR. Left ventricular structural remodeling in health and disease: with special emphasis on volume, mass, and geometry. J Am Coll Cardiol. 2011;58:1733–40.

23. de Simone G, Gottdiener JS, Chinali M, Maurer MS. Left ventricular mass predicts heart failure not related to previous myocardial infarction: the Cardiovascular Health Study. Eur Heart J. 2008;29(6):741–7.

24. Borlaug BA, Redfield MM. Diastolic and systolic heart failure are distinct phenotypes within the heart failure spectrum. Circulation. 2011;123(18):2006–14.

25. Schlaich MP, Kaye DM, Lambert E, Sommerville M, Socratous F, Esler MD. Relation between cardiac sympathetic activity and hypertensive left ventricular hypertrophy. Circulation. 2003;108:560–5.

26. Wright JW, Mizutani S, Harding JW. Pathways involved in the transition from hypertension to hypertrophy to heart failure. Treatment strategies. Heart Fail Rev. 2008;13(3):367–75.

27. Sciarretta S, Paneni F, Palano F, et al. Role of the renin–angiotensin–aldosterone system and inflammatory processes in the development and progression of diastolic dysfunction. Clin Sci. 2009;116:467–77.

28. Doehner W, Frenneaux M, Anker SD. Metabolic impairment in heart failure: the myocardial and systemic perspective. J Am Coll Cardiol. 2014;64(13):1388–400.

29. Premer C, Kanelidis AJ, Hare JM, Schulman IH. Rethinking endothelial dysfunction as a crucial target in fighting heart failure. Mayo Clin Proc Innov Qual Outcomes. 2019;3(1):1–13.

30. Paulus WJ, Tschope C. A novel paradigm for heart failure with preserved ejection fraction: comorbidities drive myocardial dysfunction and remodeling through coronary microvascular endothelial inflammation. J Am Coll Cardiol. 2013;62:263–71.

31. González A, Ravassa S, Beaumont J, López B, Díez J. New targets to treat the structural remodeling of the myocardium. J Am Coll Cardiol. 2011;58:1833–43.

32. Marti CN, Gheorghiade M, Kalogeropoulos AP, Georgiopoulou VV, Quyyumi AA, Butler J. Endothelial dysfunction, arterial stiffness, and heart failure. J Am Coll Cardiol. 2012;60(16):1455–69.

33. Zuchi C, Tritto I, Carluccio E, Mattei C, Cattadori G, Ambrosio G. Role of endothelial dysfunction in heart failure. Heart Fail Rev. 2020;25(1):21–30.

34. Stanciu AE. Cytokines in heart failure. Adv Clin Chem. 2019;93:63–113.

35. Magyar R, Gal R, Riba A, Habo T, Halmosi R, Toth K. From hypertension to heart failure. World J Hypertens. 2015;5(2): 85–92.

36. Grassi G, Quarti-Trevano F, Esler MD. Sympathetic activation in congestive heart failure: an updated overview. Heart Fail Rev. 2021;26:173–82.

37. Tsimploulis A, Lam PH, Arundel C, et al. Systolic blood pressure and outcomes in patients with heart failure with preserved ejection fraction. JAMA Cardiol. 2018;3(4):288–97.

38. Zhang Y, Wang C, Zhang J, et al. Low systolic blood pressure for predicting all-cause mortality in patients hospitalised with heart failure: a systematic review and meta-analysis. Eur J Prev Cardiol. 2019;26(4):439–43.

39. Lee SE, Lee HY, Cho HJ, et al. Reverse J-curve relationship between on-treatment blood pressure and mortality in patients with heart failure. JACC Heart Fail. 2017;5(11):810–19.

40. Vidán MT, Bueno H, Wang Y, et al. The relationship between systolic blood pressure on admission and mortality in older patients with heart failure. Eur J Heart Fail. 2010;12(2):148–55.

41. White M, Desai RV, Guichard JL, et al. Bucindolol, systolic blood pressure, and outcomes in systolic heart failure: a prespecified post hoc analysis of BEST. Can J Cardiol. 2012;28(3):354–9.

42. Lee SE, Lee HY, Cho HJ, et al. Reverse J-curve relationship between on-treatment blood pressure and mortality in patients with heart failure. JACC Heart Fail. 2017;5(11):810–19.

43. Flather MD, Shibata MC, Coats AJ, et al.; SENIORS Investigators. Randomized trial to determine the effect of nebivolol on mortality and cardiovascular hospital admission in elderly patients with heart failure (SENIORS). Eur Heart J. 2005;26(3):215–25.

44. McMurray JJV, Solomon SD, Inzucchi SE, et al.; DAPA-HF Trial Committees and Investigators. Dapagliflozin in patients with heart failure and reduced ejection fraction. N Engl J Med. 2019;381(21):1995–2008.

45. Packer M, Anker SD, Butler J, et al.; EMPEROR-Reduced Trial Investigators. Cardiovascular and renal outcomes with empagliflozin in heart failure. N Engl J Med. 2020;383(15):1413–24.

46. Majewski C, Bakris GL. Blood pressure reduction: an added benefit of sodium–glucose cotransporter 2 inhibitors in patients with type 2 diabetes. Diabetes Care. 2015;38(3):429–30.

47. Kario K, Ferdinand KC, O'Keefe JH. Control of 24-hour blood pressure with SGLT2 inhibitors to prevent cardiovascular disease. Prog Cardiovasc Dis. 2020;63(3):249–62.

CHAPTER 3.3

Heart failure in valvular heart disease

Ana Pardo Sanz, Ivan Milinković, and José Luis Zamorano

Contents

Epidemiology of heart failure in valvular heart disease

Valvular heart disease (VHD) is an important cause of heart failure (HF).[1] Aortic stenosis and mitral regurgitation (MR) are the most common aetiologies of severe native VHD, frequently associated with congestive HF.[2] According to the EORP survey, congestive HF was present in 15.5% of patients with aortic stenosis, 11.5% of those with aortic regurgitation, 19.7% of those with mitral stenosis, 24.5% of those with primary MR, 50.0% of those with secondary MR, 29.0% of those with multiple left-sided valvular disease, and 44.8% of those with isolated right-sided valvular disease.[2]

Heart failure in aortic stenosis

Pathophysiology

HF in aortic stenosis can develop through several stages.[3] In the early stage, left ventricular (LV) mass is increased, which elevates LV filling pressures and causes systolic dysfunction, usually with a drop in left ventricular ejection fraction (LVEF) to below 50%. In later stages, dilatation of the left atrium and mitral valve dysfunction occur, followed by pulmonary vasculature changes and tricuspid valve dysfunction. In the final stages, the right ventricle is affected and biventricular dilatation develops. In addition, secondary ischaemia may contribute to evolution of the disease in all stages.[4]

Clinical presentation

Early symptoms of severe aortic stenosis are often mild, such as fatigue, dizziness, or breathlessness during exertion, particularly among elderly patients. When aortic stenosis becomes severe, angina, syncope, and HF symptoms appear.[5]

Diagnosis

Echocardiography, dobutamine stress echo, and computed tomography (CT) are used for the diagnosis and classification of aortic stenosis (⊃ Table 3.3.1).[1,6] Patients with primary contractile dysfunction (intrinsic contractility of the myocardium) and mild aortic stenosis can be falsely classified as having severe aortic stenosis. Aortic valve replacement or transcatheter aortic valve implantation (TAVI) may have no effect on the ejection fraction if decreased contractility coexists with 'pseudo'-stenosis. On the other hand, there are patients with a low stroke volume index ($<35\,\text{mL/m}^2$, low flow) and a low gradient with reduced (classical) or preserved (paradoxical) ejection fraction.[1,6]

Dobutamine stress echo is a valuable tool for differentiating pseudo-stenosis from actual stenosis. Intravenous administration of dobutamine in patients with aortic stenosis produces an increase in stroke volume and an increase in systolic pressure gradient across the aortic valve, with no influence on the calculated aortic valve area (AVA). Absence of

Table 3.3.1 Classification of aortic stenosis

	Mild	Moderate	Severe
Peak velocity (m/s)	2–2.9	3–4	>4
Mean gradient (mmHg)	<20	20–40	>40
Valve area (cm²)	>1.5	1–1.5	<1
Indexed valve area (cm²/m²)	>0.85	0.60–0.85	<0.60
Velocity ratio	>0.50	0.25–0.50	<0.25

a change in the valve area under different haemodynamic conditions indicates the presence of true severe aortic stenosis. A low gradient is the consequence of a low stroke volume, which results from increased systolic wall stress (afterload excess). This group of patients with low-flow aortic stenosis have a good response to percutaneous or surgical intervention (➡ Figure 3.3.1).[1,6,7]

Recent data suggest that more stringent LVEF cut-off of ≤60% in aortic stenosis may be used to precede the onset of symptoms and predict progression of the disease.[7] Therefore, regular LV function assessment in asymptomatic patients with aortic stenosis and early detection of dysfunction, especially in those with a history of decompensated HF episodes, can influence further treatment decisions.[1]

Treatment

Medical treatment of aortic stenosis does not improve outcomes. Guideline-directed therapy (GDT) for HF is indicated in all patients with symptomatic severe aortic stenosis and HF with reduced ejection fraction (HFrEF). Vasodilators should be used with caution in order to avoid hypotension, and improvement of symptoms after initiation of medical treatment should not delay any indicated intervention.[6]

If symptoms and severe high-gradient aortic stenosis are present (valve area ≤1 cm², mean gradient ≥40 mmHg), other potential sources of high-flow status must first be excluded and corrected (i.e. anaemia, hyperthyroidism, and arteriovenous shunts).[8] An aortic valve intervention is recommended in patients with HF symptoms and severe high-gradient aortic stenosis, regardless of LVEF. The management protocol of patients with low-flow low-gradient aortic stenosis is presented in ➡ Figure 3.3.1.[8] It is recommended to proceed with valvular intervention only in patients with a life expectancy of >1 year. TAVI is non-inferior to surgical aortic valve replacement (SAVR) in reducing mortality and disabling stroke in patients at high and intermediate risk of surgery.[9,10,11,12,13,14,15,16] SAVR is recommended in patients aged <75 years and at low surgical risk (STS-PROM score or EuroSCORE II <4%). TAVI is recommended in individuals aged >75 years or at

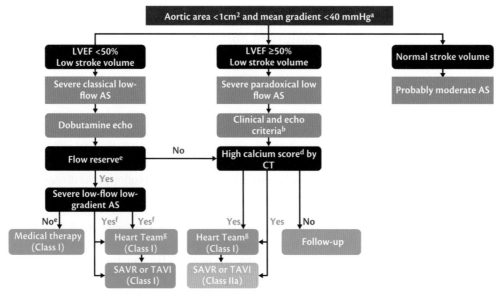

Figure 3.3.1 Management of low-gradient aortic stenosis.
AS, aortic stenosis; CT, computed tomography; EuroSCORE II, European System for Cardiac Operative Risk Evaluation II; LVEF, left ventricular ejection fraction; OMT, optimal medical therapy; SAVR, surgical aortic valve replacement; STS-PROM, Society of Thoracic Surgeons Predicted Risk of Mortality; TAVI, transcatheter aortic valve implantation. [a] Valve area ≤1 cm², peak velocity <4.0 m/s, mean gradient <40; stroke volume index ≤35 mL/m². [b] Age >70 years, typical symptoms without other explanations, left ventricular hypertrophy or reduced left ventricular longitudinal function, mean gradient 3040 mmHg, valve area ≤0.8 cm², stroke volume index ≤35 mL/m² assessed by techniques other than standard Doppler. [c] Flow reserve is defined as stroke volume index increase of >20%. [d] AS is very likely if the calcium score is ≥3000 in men and ≥1600 in women. AS is likely if the calcium score is ≥2000 in men and ≥1200 in women. AS is unlikely if the calcium score is <1600 in men and <800 in women. [e] Increase in valve area to >1.0 cm² in response to flow increase (flow reserve) during dobutamine stress echo. [f] Increase in mean gradient to at least 40 mmHg without significant change in valve area in response to flow increase (flow reserve) during dobutamine stress echo. [g] SAVR is recommended in patients aged <75 years and at low surgical risk (STS-PROM score or EuroSCORE II <4%), whereas TAVI in those aged >75 years or at high/prohibitive surgical risk (STS-PROM score or EuroSCORE II >8%). In all other cases, the choice between TAVI and SAVR is recommended to be decided by the heart team, weighing the pros and cons of each procedure, according to age, life expectancy, individual patient preference, and features including clinical and anatomical aspects. Colour code for classes of recommendation: green for class of recommendation I; yellow for class of recommendation IIa.
Modified from: 6. McDonagh TA et al. Eur Heart J. 2021 Sep 21;42(36):3599–3726. Saybolt MD, et al. Circ Cardiovasc Interv. 2017 Aug;10(8):e004838. doi:10.1161/CIRCINTERVENTIONS.117.004838.

high/prohibitive surgical risk (STS-PROM score or EuroSCORE II >8%). In other clinical scenarios, the choice between TAVI and SAVR should be made by the heart team, according to the patient's age, life expectancy, individual patient preference, and other clinical and anatomical aspects. Balloon aortic valvuloplasty may be considered in highly symptomatic patients with acute HF (i.e. cardiogenic shock) as a bridge to TAVI or SAVR, or in advanced HF as a bridge to transplantation or destination therapy.[9,10,11,12,13,14,15,16]

The ongoing Aortic Valve replAcemenT versus conservative treatment in Asymptomatic seveRe aortic stenosis (AVATAR) trial (NCT02436655)[17] will resolve a question of whether conservative treatment and watchful waiting till symptom onset is better than elective aortic valve surgery in severe aortic stenosis without symptoms (peak aortic valve flow velocity >4 m/s or mean pressure gradient ≥40 mmHg and AVA ≤1 cm^2 or indexed AVA (AVAi) ≤0.6 cm^2/m^2 at rest).

Prognosis

Aortic stenosis is a progressive disease that can remain asymptomatic for a long period of time. However, once it becomes symptomatic, and if left untreated, it is associated with poor prognosis. If there is no evident damage to the heart, 1-year mortality is as low as 4%. Patients in early stages with elevated filling pressures and a drop in LVEF to below 50% show increased mortality (9% vs 4%), hospitalization rate (17% vs 7%), and stroke rate (6% vs 2%), when compared to patients without cardiac damage. In patients with right ventricular damage, 1-year mortality can be up to 25%.[18]

The Long-term follow-up of the Placement of Aortic Transcatheter Valves (PARTNER 1B) trial showed that two-thirds of inoperable patients treated medically did not survive >2 years, whereas mortality was halved in those with transcatheter aortic valve replacement (TAVR).[19] The TAVR technique has progressed significantly over time, with indications for the procedure including patients with lower surgical risk.[20,21,22,23,24] This resulted in a decrease in overall rates of all-cause death at 1 year from 31% in the inoperable cohort of the PARTNER IB trial treated with TAVR to 7% in the Surgical Replacement and Transcatheter Aortic Valve Implantation (SURTAVI) trial targeting patients with an intermediate risk, and to 5% in the all-comers Nordic Aortic Valve Intervention (NOTION) trial.[13,23]

Heart failure in aortic regurgitation
Pathophysiology

Aortic regurgitation causes diastolic reflux of blood from the aorta into the LV due to malcoaptation of the aortic cusps. This can occur due to abnormalities of the aortic leaflets and/or their supporting structures (aortic root and annulus). Chronic severe aortic regurgitation causes volume and pressure overload on the LV. Volume overload is a consequence of the regurgitant volume and is directly related to the severity of the leak. Mild regurgitation causes minimal volume overload, and severe regurgitant volume produces massive overload and progressive chamber dilatation.

Pressure overload develops as a result of systolic hypertension caused by increased total aortic stroke volume, which is a result of simultaneous ejection of the regurgitant volume and forward stroke volume during systole.[25] Systolic hypertension may also contribute to progression of aortic root dilatation and worsening of regurgitation. In early stages of aortic regurgitation, the LV adapts to the volume overload by eccentric hypertrophy, which preserves LV diastolic compliance, keeping LV filling pressures normal or mildly increased. Eccentric hypertrophy also causes an increase in LV mass preserving normal LV volume/mass ratio and LVEF by increased preload.[26] In further stages, progressive LV dilatation and systolic hypertension increase wall stress and the volume/mass ratio, causing LV systolic dysfunction, a decline in LVEF, and severely reduced elastance (Emax). At this stage, it is highly unlikely that LVEF will increase after successful valve replacement. In later stages, end-systolic wall stress can be as high as in aortic stenosis and severe LV hypertrophy with fibrosis (cor bovinum) develops with increased LV volume and mass and spherical remodelling.[27]

Clinical presentation

Clinical presentation of aortic regurgitation in HF depends on a number of factors such as acuteness of onset, aortic and LV compliance, haemodynamic conditions, and severity of the lesion. Chronic aortic regurgitation is generally well tolerated and can be asymptomatic or with exertional dyspnoea as the most common manifestation. Angina can also occur because of a reduction in coronary flow reserve with predominantly systolic coronary flow. Conversely, acute aortic regurgitation leads to rapid cardiac decompensation and death if untreated.[1,6]

Diagnosis

Echocardiography allows assessment of the anatomy of the aortic leaflets and root, quantification of the severity of regurgitation, and characterization of LV size and function (➲ Table 3.3.2).[1,6,28] Magnetic resonance imaging (MRI) can also be used to detect and quantify regurgitation.[29] Exercise testing may be useful in some asymptomatic patients or those with mild symptoms to determine functional capacity and exercise-induced decrease in LVEF.[30]

Treatment

Vasodilators may be used in aortic regurgitation in order to decrease systolic hypertension, reduce wall stress, and delay the onset of LV dysfunction in asymptomatic patients, or to improve

Table 3.3.2 Classification of aortic regurgitation

	Jet size ratio	Pressure half-time	Regurgitant fraction (%)
Mild	<24	>500	<20
Moderate	25–45	500–349	20–35
Moderate to severe	46–64	349–200	56–50
Severe	>65	<200	>50

symptoms and LV function in those with dysfunction.[31] Renin–angiotensin–aldosterone (RAAS) inhibitors are preferred in HF patients with severe aortic regurgitation.[32] Medical therapy does not reduce significantly the regurgitant volume, because the regurgitant orifice area is relatively fixed and the diastolic blood pressure is already low.[31] Significant reduction in diastolic blood pressure should be avoided, since it might have adverse effects on coronary perfusion and worsen LV dysfunction.[31] Beta-blockers should be avoided in acute aortic regurgitation because they prolong diastole and may worsen the clinical course, and need to be used cautiously in chronic aortic regurgitation with HF. Aortic balloon counterpulsation is contraindicated because it worsens regurgitation. In non-severe aortic regurgitation, surgery needs to be performed if the LV end-diastolic diameter increases to 55 mm or 25 mm/m[2] or before LVEF falls to 55%.[33] Aortic valve surgery is recommended in patients with severe aortic regurgitation and HF symptoms, regardless of LVEF.[34] In cases of high or prohibitive surgical risk, TAVI also has been used to treat aortic regurgitation.[35] In acute aortic regurgitation, immediate surgical intervention is necessary because the acute volume overload results in severe hypotension and pulmonary oedema.[1]

Prognosis

In patients with chronic aortic regurgitation, operative mortality for isolated aortic valve replacement is 4% and rises if aortic root replacement or coronary bypass surgery is needed, or in elderly and comorbid patients.[36,37] The death rate for asymptomatic patients with normal LV size and function is 0.2% per year and rises to 10% per year in symptomatic patients with chronic severe aortic regurgitation. Surgery for symptomatic patients with severe aortic regurgitation has been shown to reduce symptoms, LV volume, LV mass, and wall stress, and to increase LVEF.[38]

Operative mortality is assessed to be 14%, 6.7%, and 3.7% for LVEF of 35%, 36–49%, and 50%, respectively.[39] Patients with severe LV dysfunction and a systolic blood pressure of 120 mmHg may be at high risk of adverse outcomes.[40]

Heart failure in mitral stenosis

Pathophysiology

The normal mitral orifice area is 4–6 cm[2]. If the area decreases to <2 cm[2], blood flow from the left atrium into the LV is impaired. This creates a pressure gradient across the mitral valve, and with the increase in gradient, the LV requires the atrial kick to fill with blood. When the mitral valve area is <1 cm[2], an increase in left atrial pressure occurs. A rise in pressure gradient of 20 mmHg across the mitral valve will cause a left atrial pressure of about 25 mmHg, which is transmitted to the pulmonary circulation, resulting in pulmonary hypertension, and, with further progression, will cause right ventricular failure. If the left atrial pressure remains elevated, the left atrium increases in size, resulting in a greater propensity to atrial fibrillation. If atrial fibrillation develops, the atrial kick is lost and LV filling is diminished, since patients with mitral stenosis rely on atrial contraction for about 20% of their cardiac output. This results in a decrease in cardiac output and the development of congestive HF (➲ Figure 3.3.2).[41,42]

Clinical presentation

The most common symptoms in mitral stenosis are dyspnoea, orthopnoea, and paroxysmal nocturnal dyspnoea. Patients may also have palpitations, chest pain, haemoptysis, light-headedness, syncope, and thromboembolism when the left atrial volume is increased. There is also an increase in symptoms of fatigue and weakness with exercise, pregnancy, emotional stress, anaemia, sepsis, and thyrotoxicosis. The enlarged left atrium compresses

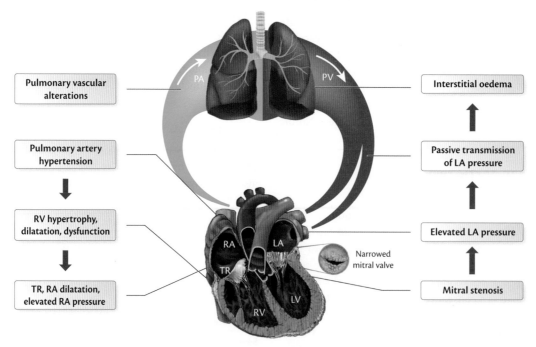

Figure 3.3.2 Pathophysiology of heart failure in mitral stenosis.

the left recurrent laryngeal nerve, leading to a hoarse voice. Advanced mitral stenosis often presents with right-sided heart failure (jugular venous distension, parasternal heave, hepatomegaly, ascites, oedema) and/or pulmonary hypertension.[6]

Diagnosis

Patients with mitral stenosis should undergo evaluation with an electrocardiogram (ECG), chest X-ray, echocardiography, stress exercise echocardiography, and cardiac catheterization.[43,44] The echocardiogram is useful for assessment of the aetiology, morphology, and severity of mitral stenosis, and for planning treatment (◆ Table 3.3.3). Analysis of the morphology of the mitral valve apparatus includes leaflet mobility and flexibility, leaflet thickness and calcification, subvalvular fusion, and appearance of commissures. The Wilkins score grades each of the components of the mitral apparatus from 1 to 4: leaflet mobility, thickness, and calcification, and impairment of the subvalvular apparatus. The Padial score grades leaflet thickening (each separately), commissural calcification, and subvalvular disease from 1 to 4. A Wilkins score of <8, a Padial score of <10, and less than moderate regurgitation have better outcomes.[43,44] An exercise echocardiogram measures the transmitral gradient and pulmonary artery systolic pressure at rest and on exercise. Cardiac catheterization should be performed when non-invasive tests are inconclusive or when there is a discrepancy between non-invasive tests and clinical findings regarding the severity of mitral stenosis (class I, level of evidence C).[1,6]

Treatment

Treatment of mitral stenosis involves medical therapy, percutaneous mitral valvuloplasty, and surgical therapy. Medical therapy cannot relieve a fixed obstruction of the mitral valve and is focused on improving symptoms, decreasing the thromboembolic risk, and preventing endocarditis and relapse of rheumatic fever in selected cases.[1,6] In patients in sinus rhythm and heart failure, diuretics help relieve congestion and beta-blockers help reduce symptoms associated with an elevated heart rate. In patients with atrial fibrillation, rate control agents such as beta-blockers and digitalis may also be used. Cardioversion is indicated in symptomatic and haemodynamically unstable patients. In stable patients, restoration of normal sinus rhythm is preferred over rate control to improve functional capacity and quality of life.

Anticoagulation is indicated in patients with paroxysmal, persistent, or permanent atrial fibrillation. Vitamin K antagonists are preferred, with a target international normalized ratio (INR) of 2.0–3.0.[1,6] Percutaneous mitral balloon valvuloplasty improves symptoms by increasing the mitral valve area and reducing the mitral valve gradient. It is indicated in symptomatic patients (New York Heart Association (NYHA) classes II–IV) with clinically significant mitral stenosis (valve area <1.5 cm²) or in asymptomatic patients with pulmonary hypertension with moderate or severe stenosis, and favourable valve morphology in the absence of left atrial thrombus, or moderate to severe MR. It may be considered also in symptomatic patients with a valve area larger than 1.5 cm² if symptoms cannot be explained by another cause and if the anatomy is favourable.[1,6] Mitral valve replacement surgery is indicated in patients with symptomatic moderate or severe mitral stenosis unsuitable for percutaneous mitral balloon valvuloplasty (class I, level of evidence B).[1,6] In such cases, tricuspid disease should be treated according to the recommendations.[1,6]

Prognosis

Prior to open heart surgery, the prognosis of mitral stenosis was poor. It has been reported that patients without complications have 10-year survival of 80%. However, patients who develop pulmonary hypertension have survival of <3 years. Other complications that may result in high morbidity include stroke and persistent atrial fibrillation.[45]

Heart failure in mitral regurgitation

Pathophysiology

Secondary MR may develop in patients with ischaemic or non-ischaemic LV remodelling and dilatation.[46] It occurs as a result of an imbalance between valve closure and leaflet tethering forces, and the dynamic impact of factors affecting LV preload and afterload. Secondary MR may also develop as a result of left atrial enlargement and mitral annular dilatation/flattening in patients with long-standing atrial fibrillation. In these patients, LVEF is often normal or mildly reduced. This so-called 'atrial' MR may also contribute to secondary MR in patients with HF and atrial fibrillation.[47]

In the initial phase, LV wall stress due to volume overload is countered by increased LV fractional shortening and low-resistance run-off into the low-pressure left atrium. In the compensated stage, LV dilatation maintains normal wall stress and diastolic pressures and patients remain asymptomatic during this phase for years. Persistent MR leads to progressive LV enlargement, and altered ventricular geometry and annular dilatation cause increasing degrees of MR, creating a vicious circle between MR and LV dilatation. Further on, systolic LV wall stress increases, which leads to an increase in end-diastolic pressure and eventually decreased contractility. As a consequence, irreversible LV dysfunction occurs, which leads to the decompensated stage of MR, HF, and poor prognosis (◆ Figure 3.3.3).[48]

Table 3.3.3 Classification of mitral stenosis

	Pressure gradient (mmHg)	Mitral valve area (cm²)	Pulmonary artery systolic pressure (mmHg)
Normal	0	>4.0	<14
Mild	1–5	2.5–4.0	<30
Moderate	6–10	1.0–2.5	30–50
Severe	>10	<1.0	>50

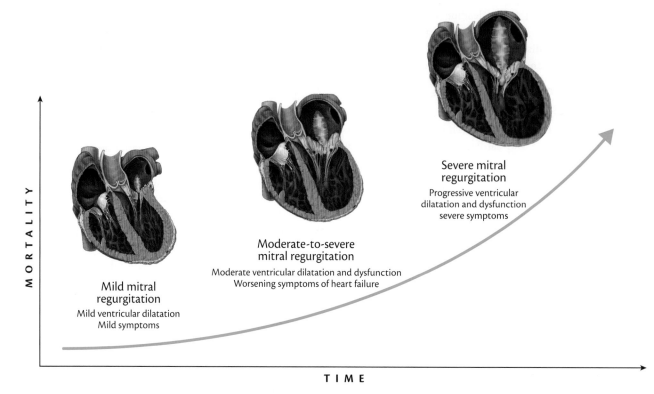

Figure 3.3.3 Pathophysiology of heart failure in mitral regurgitation.

LV and left atrial dilatation, remodelling, and dysfunction increase with increasing severity of MR.

Clinical presentation

Clinical presentation depends on the chronicity of MR. Acute severe MR can cause acute pulmonary oedema. On the other hand, chronic severe MR usually remains asymptomatic for years.[49] Typical symptoms include decreased exercise capacity and dyspnoea. In advanced stages, LV function could be affected, even in the absence of symptoms, but the majority of patients at this stage have symptoms of congestive HF. Due to left atrial dilatation, there is a predisposition to developing atrial fibrillation.[50]

Diagnosis

Differentiating primary MR and reduced LV function from true secondary MR is essential to define the optimal treatment strategy. Two-dimensional transthoracic echocardiography is an initial tool for the assessment of LV function and the aetiology and severity of MR. It allows structural and functional assessment of the mitral valve, LV, and left atrium (together with associated valve disease, right ventricular function, and estimated pulmonary pressure).[1,51] Three-dimensional transthoracic and transoesophageal echocardiography can provide more accurate anatomical information. However, use of sedation for transoesophageal examination may affect blood pressure, alter LV loading conditions, and result in underestimation of MR severity. Stress echocardiography may allow assessment of MR during exercise, as well as haemodynamic assessment of the interaction between MR severity and LV function.[52] In addition,

multidetector CT provides a more accurate anatomical insight,[53] and cardiac magnetic resonance allows more precise LV volume and ejection fraction measurements, identification of fibrosis or scar, and accurate quantification of MR severity.[54] The European Society of Cardiology (ESC) guidelines define secondary mitral regurgitation (SMR) as an effective regurgitant orifice area (EROA) of $\geq 20\,mm^2$ or a regurgitant volume of $\geq 30\,mL$, based on observational studies.[55] However, since quantitative assessment is highly operator-dependent, multiple parameters should also be assessed such as vena contracta, pulmonary vein systolic flow reversal, proximal isovelocity surface area (PISA) radius, and the subsequently derived EROA and regurgitant volume,[1,56] including three-dimensional imaging (three-dimensional vena contracta area) if diagnostic uncertainty exists (➲ Table 3.3.4).[57]

Treatment

In patients with severe primary MR and HF symptoms, surgery (preferably repair) is recommended as the first-line therapy. If surgery is contraindicated or considered high risk, percutaneous repair may be considered.[1,6,68]

Table 3.3.4 Classification of secondary mitral regurgitation

	Mild	Moderate	Severe
Vena contracta (mm)	<3	3–7	>7
Regurgitant volume (mL/beat)	<30	30–59	≥30
Regurgitant fraction (%)	<30	30–49	>50
Regurgitant orifice area (cm²)	<0.2	0.2–0.39	≥0/2

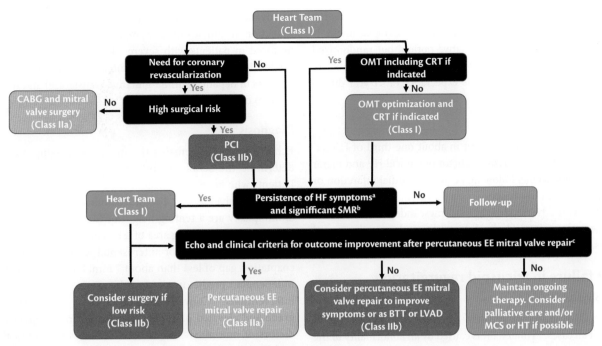

Figure 3.3.4 Management of secondary mitral regurgitation in patients with heart failure with reduced ejection fraction.
BTT, bridge to transplantation; CABG, coronary artery bypass graft; CRT, cardiac resynchronization therapy; EE, edge-to-edge; EROA, effective regurgitant orifice area; HF, heart failure; LVAD, left ventricular assist device; LVEF, left ventricular ejection fraction; LVESD, left ventricular end-systolic diameter; MCS, mechanical circulatory support; MT, medical therapy; NYHA, New York Heart Association; OMT, optimal medical therapy; PCI, percutaneous coronary intervention; SMR, secondary mitral regurgitation; TR, tricuspid regurgitation. [a] NYHA classes III and V. [b] Moderate-to-severe or severe (EROA ≥30 mm²). [c] All of the following criteria must be fulfilled: LVEF 20–50%, LVESD <70 mm, systolic pulmonary pressure <70 mmHg, absence of moderate or severe right ventricular dysfunction or severe TR, and absence of haemodynamic instability. Colour code for classes of recommendation: green for class of recommendation I; yellow for class of recommendation IIa; orange for class of recommendation IIb.
Modified from: 6. McDonagh TA *et al. Eur Heart J.* 2021 Sep 21;42(36):3599–3726.

In patients with secondary MR and HF, multidisciplinary management of HF is strongly recommended by the ESC guidelines (class I).[1,6] Optimization of guideline-directed medical therapy (GDMT) and cardiac resynchronization therapy (CRT) implantation (if indicated) are essential steps in the management of symptomatic moderate or severe secondary MR (➲ Figure 3.3.4).[1,6] All neurohormonal antagonists are mandatory in patients with HFrEF, unless contraindicated or intolerable, since they have a beneficial influence on LV dysfunction and remodelling.[58,59] In addition, angiotensin-converting enzyme inhibitors (ACEIs) and beta-blockers may reduce secondary MR through improvement of LV geometry and function.[60,61] Furthermore, sacubitril/valsartan can induce a significant reduction of EROA and regurgitant volume, on top of standard medical therapy.[62] Ivabradine has indications in sinus rhythm above ≥70 bpm despite beta-blockade or if beta-blockers are not tolerated.[6] Diuretics, nitrates, and hydralazine also reduce LV preload and afterload, and are associated with symptomatic improvement.[63] Oral anticoagulation is indicated in patients with atrial fibrillation and secondary MR. CRT improves global LV function, attenuates LV remodelling, and reduces papillary muscle dyssynchrony in patients with QRS prolongation.[64] Large randomized trials have confirmed a reduction of MR by 20–35% following CRT implantation as a result of LV reverse remodelling.[65,66]

Following myocardial revascularization with isolated coronary artery bypass graft (CABG) surgery, MR is improved in about 50% of cases.[67] Data concerning the effects of percutaneous coronary intervention in SMR are limited. In patients with severe secondary MR and HFrEF requiring revascularization, mitral valve surgery and CABG should be considered. Isolated mitral valve surgery may be considered in symptomatic patients with severe secondary MR despite optimal therapy and low surgical risk.[1,6,68] Percutaneous edge-to-edge mitral valve repair should be considered for outcome improvement only in carefully selected patients who remain symptomatic (NYHA classes III and IV) despite optimal medical therapy, with moderate-to-severe or severe secondary MR (EROA ≥30 mm²), favourable anatomical features, and fulfilling the inclusion criteria of the COAPT study (LVEF 20–50%, LV end-systolic diameter <70 mm, systolic pulmonary pressure <70 mmHg, absence of moderate or severe right ventricular dysfunction, absence of severe tricuspid regurgitation (TR), absence of haemodynamic instability).[69,70] Percutaneous edge-to-to edge mitral valve repair may also be considered to improve symptoms in patients with advanced HF, severe secondary MR, and severe symptoms despite medical therapy. In these patients, cardiac transplantation or left ventricular assist device (LVAD) implantation must also be considered.[71,72]

Other percutaneous mitral valve repair systems, such as indirect annuloplasty, can be an alternative for treatment, as they may reduce mitral regurgitant volume and produce reverse LV and left atrial remodelling,[73] as well as improve the 6-minute walking test (6MWT) distance and symptoms and reduce HF hospitalizations.[74,75] Transcatheter mitral valve replacement is also emerging as a possible alternative option, but randomized trials are still lacking.[76] Mitral valve interventions are not recommended in patients with a life expectancy of <1 year due to extracardiac conditions.[1,6]

Prognosis

Moderate or severe MR is present in about one-third of HF patients.[1] MR is an independent predictor of clinical HF and major cardiac outcome events following acute myocardial infarction or in patients with LV dysfunction.[77] In addition, secondary MR is associated with adverse clinical outcomes, independent of clinical, haemodynamic, echocardiographic, and neurohormonal findings.[78]

Heart failure in tricuspid regurgitation

Pathophysiology

Primary TR is less common than secondary TR, and occurs in 8–10% of all cases. Primary TR is caused by an abnormality of the tricuspid valve and/or its subvalvular apparatus, due to congenital or acquired causes.[79] Secondary (functional) TR accounts for 85–90% of all severe TR[80] and occurs predominantly as a result of left-sided heart disease. In patients with HF, chronic volume overload leads to ventricular distension and eccentric hypertrophy. With remodelling, the LV dilates more along its short axis and becomes more spherical, causing MR and increased left-sided ventricular or atrial hydrostatic pressure. The elevated pressure is transmitted passively to the pulmonary vasculature, resulting in increased right ventricular pressure work. Limited ability to increase right ventricular wall thickness in response to increased afterload leads to chronic increases in right ventricular chamber dimensions.[81] Concordantly, annular dilatation leads to inadequate coaptation of the tricuspid valve, resulting in TR. A positive feedback loop with increased volume work leads to further ventricular dilatation, annular dilatation, and regurgitation. Right ventricular dilatation and diastolic pressure increase, causing LV compression and restricted filling, with associated increase in LV diastolic and pulmonary artery systolic pressures.[82]

Clinical presentation

Symptoms may not appear until late stages of the disease. They could be related to right atrial hypertension and venous congestion (liver congestion, dyspepsia, anorexia, ascites, and oedema).

In advances stages, dyspnoea and fatigue could appear due to a reduction in cardiac output. Symptoms of right HF are more pronounced in patients with severe TR, with severe systemic congestion leading to multi-organ damage, as reflected by elevated markers of hepatic (gamma-glutamyl transferase) and renal (creatinine) dysfunction.[83]

Diagnosis

Echocardiography remains the mainstay imaging modality to determine the aetiology and characterize the severity of TR. Patients who have severe leaflet tethering may not benefit from tricuspid valve repair. Factors associated with unsuccessful annuloplasty are a tenting height of ≥0.8 cm, a tenting volume of ≥2 cm^3, and a tenting area of ≥1.8 cm^2. A coaptation depth of <10 mm and a central or anteroseptal jet location, as well as a coaptation gap of less than about 7 mm, have been identified as independent predictors of procedural success for transcatheter interventions.[84] Conversely, a reduction of TR of less than one grade and elevated pulmonary pressures are independent predictors of mortality.[85] It has been noticed that late in the natural history of the disease, patients fail to respond to diuretics and present with signs of severe right HF and low flow. Hahn and Zamorano[86] have proposed increasing the grades of TR severity to include very severe (or massive) TR, as well as torrential TR, to better characterize the severity of TR treated with transcatheter devices (➔ Table 3.3.5). The new grading scheme incorporates current knowledge about the baseline severity of disease and the clinically relevant reduction in TR severity with transcatheter intervention. Patients with massive and torrential TR and those with comorbidities, especially pulmonary disease, have been identified as populations at higher risk of death and readmission for HF.[87]

Treatment

Medical management of functional TR focuses on optimization of the underlying pathology, as well as on diuresis to reduce central venous congestion. In the case of HFrEF, this includes neurohumoral inhibitors and diuretics for symptom management.[88] Hydralazine or nitrates may be used to reduce afterload in black patients, ivabradine if patients are unable to achieve adequate heart rate reduction, and aldosterone receptor antagonists if renal function is not impaired significantly. Additionally, primary prevention of sudden cardiac death with implantation of a cardiac defibrillator is recommended when the LVEF remains

Table 3.3.5 Proposed expansion of the 'severe' grade

	Mild	Moderate	Severe	Massive	Torrential
Vena contracta (biplane)	<3 mm	3–6.9 mm	7–13 mm	14–20 mm	≥21 mm
EROA (PISA)	<20 mm^2	20–39 mm^2	40–59 mm^2	60–79 mm^2	≥80 mm^2
3D VCA or quantitative EROA			75–94 mm^2	95–114 mm^2	≥115 mm^2

3D VCA and quantitative Doppler EROA cut-offs may be greater than PISA EROA.
EROA, effective regurgitant orifice area; PISA, proximal isovelocity surface area; 3D VCA, three-dimensional vena contracta area.

below 35%, or CRT if QRS is >150 ms and a left bundle branch pattern is present.[89]

Transcatheter therapy and surgery may be considered in selected cases,[1,6] which need to be assessed by a multidisciplinary heart team. Tricuspid valve surgery is recommended in patients with severe TR requiring left-sided cardiac surgery. It should be considered also in patients with moderate TR and tricuspid annulus dilatation requiring left-sided cardiac surgery and in symptomatic patients with isolated severe TR. [1,6] However, surgery in isolated TR is burdened by high in-hospital mortality.[90] Transcatheter techniques have recently emerged as potential treatment options for TR. Preliminary results show improvement in TR severity and symptoms, with low complication rates (➲ Figure 3.3.5).[91] Further prospective studies are needed to show the prognostic impact of these treatments in HF patients.[92]

Prognosis

In patients with moderate or severe TR and HF, numerous observational studies showed an association with increased mortality in patients regardless of LVEF.[93,94,95,96] Increasing TR severity was also associated with an increased incidence of comorbidities, including pulmonary hypertension, diastolic dysfunction, NYHA class III symptoms, and reductions in LVEF. It has been reported that patients with trivial TR have a 5-year survival of close to 68%, as compared to 58%, 45%, and 34% for patients with mild, moderate, and severe TR, respectively.[93] Echocardiographic markers that correlate with the severity of TR and right ventricular failure, such as a baseline right atrial area of >27 cm^2, progressive increase in TR volume measured by a proximal isovelocity surface area of >15 mL, progressive right ventricular end-diastolic diameter mid increase of >10 mm, and reduction in systolic pulmonary artery pressure of >10 mmHg, have all been shown to be associated with increased 1-year mortality.[95]

Key messages

◆ In aortic stenosis, dobutamine stress echo is valuable for differentiating 'pseudo'-stenosis from actual stenosis. GDMT

is indicated in all patients with symptomatic severe aortic stenosis and HFrEF, although it does not improve outcomes. SAVR is recommended in patients aged <75 years and with STS-PROM scores or EuroSCORE II of <4%. TAVI is recommended in individuals aged >75 years or with STS-PROM scores or EuroSCORE II of >8%.

◆ In aortic regurgitation, RAAS inhibitors are preferred and beta-blockers should be avoided in the acute phase because they may worsen outcomes. Surgery is recommended in symptomatic severe aortic regurgitation, regardless of LVEF, and TAVI may be used in cases of high or prohibitive surgical risk. In non-severe aortic regurgitation, surgery needs to be performed if LV end-diastolic diameter increases to 55 mm or 25 mm/m^2 or before the LVEF falls to 55%.

◆ In mitral stenosis, medical therapy cannot relieve a fixed obstruction and it focuses on improving symptoms, decreasing the thromboembolic risk, and preventing endocarditis and relapse of rheumatic fever. Percutaneous mitral balloon valvuloplasty is indicated in symptomatic patients with a valve area of <1.5 cm^2 or in asymptomatic patients with pulmonary hypertension with moderate or severe stenosis and favourable valve morphology. Mitral valve replacement surgery is indicated in those unsuitable for percutaneous mitral balloon valvuloplasty.

◆ Differentiating primary MR with reduced LV function from true secondary MR is essential to define the optimal treatment strategy. In patients with severe primary MR and HF symptoms, surgery is recommended as the first-line therapy and percutaneous repair may be considered in high-risk patients. In secondary MR and HF, the first step is optimization of GDMT and CRT implantation. Percutaneous edge-to-edge mitral valve repair should be considered in those who are symptomatic despite OMT and with severe secondary MR (EROA ≥30 mm^2), LVEF 20–50%, LV end-systolic diameter <70 mm, systolic pulmonary pressure <70 mmHg, absence of moderate or severe right ventricular dysfunction, absence of severe TR, and absence of haemodynamic instability.

◆ Medical management of functional TR focuses on optimization of the underlying pathology, as well as on diuresis to reduce

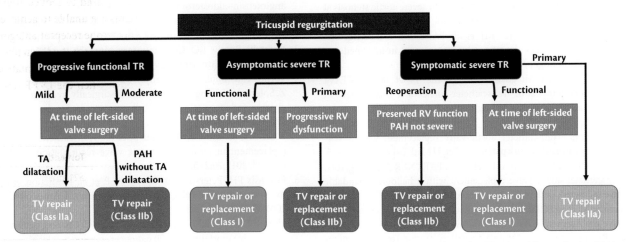

Figure 3.3.5 Management strategies for tricuspid regurgitation in heart failure. RV, right ventricle; TA, tricuspid annulus; TR, tricuspid regurgitation; PAH, pulmonary hypertension; TV, tricuspid valve.

central venous congestion. Implantation of a cardiac defibrillator is recommended when the LVEF remains below 35%, or CRT if QRS is >150 ms and a left bundle branch pattern is present. Transcatheter therapy and surgery may be considered by a multidisciplinary heart team.

References

1. Vahanian A, Beyersdorf F, Praz F, *et al.*; ESC/EACTS Scientific Document Group; ESC National Cardiac Societies. 2021 ESC/EACTS Guidelines for the management of valvular heart disease. Eur Heart J. 2022;43(7):561–632.

2. Iung B, Delgado V, Rosenhek R, *et al.*; EORP VHD II Investigators. Contemporary presentation and management of valvular heart disease: the EURObservational Research Programme Valvular Heart Disease II Survey. Circulation. 2019;140:1156–69.

3. Pardo Sanz A, Santoro C, Hinojar R, *et al.* Right ventricle assessment in patients with severe aortic stenosis undergoing transcatheter aortic valve implantation. Echocardiography. 2020;37:586–91.

4. Généreux P, Pibarot P, Redfors B, *et al.* Staging classification of aortic stenosis based on the extent of cardiac damage. Eur Heart J. 2017;38(45):3351–8.

5. Manning WJ. Asymptomatic aortic stenosis in the elderly: a clinical review. JAMA. 2013;310(14):1490–7.

6. McDonagh TA, Metra M, Adamo M, *et al.*; ESC Scientific Document Group. 2021 ESC Guidelines for the diagnosis and treatment of acute and chronic heart failure. Eur Heart J. 2021;42(36):3599–726.

7. Saybolt MD, Fiorilli PN, Gertz ZM, Herrmann HC. Low-flow severe aortic stenosis: evolving role of transcatheter aortic valve replacement. Circ Cardiovasc Interv. 2017;10(8):e004838.

8. Vahanian A, Beyersdorf F, Praz F, *et al.*; ESC/EACTS Scientific Document Group. 2021 ESC/EACTS Guidelines for the management of valvular heart disease. Eur Heart J. 2022;43(7):561–632.

9. Leon MB, Smith CR, Mack M, *et al.*; PARTNER Trial Investigators. Transcatheter aortic-valve implantation for aortic stenosis in patients who cannot undergo surgery. N Engl J Med. 2010;363:1597–607.

10. Smith CR, Leon MB, Mack MJ, *et al.*; PARTNER Trial Investigators. Transcatheter versus surgical aortic-valve replacement in high-risk patients. N Engl J Med. 2011;364:2187–98.

11. Adams DH, Popma JJ, Reardon MJ, *et al.*; US CoreValve Clinical Investigators. Transcatheter aortic-valve replacement with a self-expanding prosthesis. N Engl J Med. 2014;370:1790–8.

12. Popma JJ, Adams DH, Reardon MJ, *et al.*; CoreValve United States Clinical Investigators. Transcatheter aortic valve replacement using a self-expanding bioprosthesis in patients with severe aortic stenosis at extreme risk for surgery. J Am Coll Cardiol. 2014;63:1972–81.

13. Leon MB, Smith CR, Mack MJ, *et al.*; PARTNER 2 Investigators. Transcatheter or surgical aortic-valve replacement in intermediate-risk patients. N Engl J Med. 2016;374:1609–20.

14. Reardon MJ, Van Mieghem NM, Popma JJ, *et al.*; SURTAVI Investigators. Surgical or transcatheter aortic-valve replacement in intermediate-risk patients. N Engl J Med. 2017;376:1321–31.

15. Popma JJ, Deeb GM, Yakubov SJ, *et al.*; Evolut Low Risk Trial Investigators. Transcatheter aortic-valve replacement with a self-expanding valve in low-risk patients. N Engl J Med. 2019;380:1706–15.

16. Mack MJ, Leon MB, Thourani VH, *et al.*; PARTNER 3 Investigators. Transcatheter aortic-valve replacement with a balloon-expandable valve in lowrisk patients. N Engl J Med. 2019;380:1695–705.

17. Banovic M, Iung B, Bartunek J, *et al.* Rationale and design of the Aortic Valve replAcemenT versus conservative treatment in Asymptomatic seveRe aortic stenosis (AVATAR trial): a randomized multicenter controlled event-driven trial. Am Heart J. 2016;174:147–53.

18. Frank S, Johnson A, Ross J Jr. Natural history of valvular aortic stenosis. Br Heart J. 1973;35:41–6.

19. Kapadia SR, Leon MB, Makkar RR, *et al.* 5-year outcomes of transcatheter aortic valve replacement compared with standard treatment for patients with inoperable aortic stenosis (PARTNER 1): a randomised controlled trial. Lancet. 2015;385:2485–91.

20. Adams DH, Popma JJ, Reardon MJ, *et al.* Transcatheter aortic-valve replacement with a self-expanding prosthesis. N Engl J Med. 2014;370:1790–8.

21. Leon MB, Smith CR, Mack M, *et al.* Transcatheter aortic-valve implantation for aortic stenosis in patients who cannot undergo surgery. N Engl J Med. 2010;363:1597–607.

22. Leon MB, Smith CR, Mack MJ, *et al.* Transcatheter or surgical aortic-valve replacement in intermediate-risk patients. N Engl J Med. 2016;374:1609–20.

23. Reardon MJ, van Mieghem NM, Popma JJ, *et al.* Surgical or transcatheter aortic-valve replacement in intermediaterisk patients. N Engl J Med. 2017;376:1321–31.

24. Thyregod HG, Steinbruchel DA, Ihlemann N, *et al.* Transcatheter versus surgical aortic valve replacement in patients with severe aortic valve stenosis: 1-year results from the all-comers NOTION randomized clinical trial. J Am Coll Cardiol. 2015;65:2184–94.

25. Carabello BA. Aortic regurgitation: a lesion with similarities to both aortic stenosis and mitral regurgitation. Circulation. 1990;82:1051–3.

26. Starling MR, Kirsh MM, Montgomery DG, Gross MD. Mechanism for left ventricular systolic dysfunction in aortic regurgitation: importance for predicting the functional response to aortic valve replacement. J Am Coll Cardiol. 1991;17:887–97.

27. Magid NM, Young MS, Wallerson DC, *et al.* Hypertrophic and functional response to experimental chronic aortic regurgitation. J Mol Cell Cardiol. 1988;20:239–46.

28. Zoghbi WA, Enriquez-Sarano M, Foster E, *et al.* Recommendations for evaluation of the severity of native valvular regurgitation with two-dimensional and Doppler echocardiography. J Am Soc Echocardiogr. 2003;16:777–802.

29. Krombach GA, Kuhl H, Bucker A, *et al.* Cine MR imaging of heart valve dysfunction with segmented true fast imaging with steady state free precession. J Magn Reson Imaging. 2004;19:59–67.

30. Greenberg B, Massie B, Thomas D, *et al.* Association between the exercise ejection fraction response and systolic wall stress in patients with chronic aortic insufficiency. Circulation. 1985;71:458–65.

31. Grayburn PA. Vasodilator therapy for chronic aortic and mitral regurgitation. Am J Med Sci. 2000;320:202–8.

32. Elder DH, Wei L, Szwejkowski BR, *et al.* The impact of renin-angiotensin–aldosterone system blockade on heart failure outcomes and mortality in patients identified to have aortic regurgitation: a large population cohort study. J Am Coll Cardiol. 2011;58:2084–91.

33. Borer JS, Bonow RO. Contemporary approach to aortic and mitral regurgitation. Circulation. 2003;108:2432–8.

34. Tornos P, Sambola A, Permanyer-Miralda G, Evangelista A, Gomez Z, SolerSoler J. Long-term outcome of surgically treated aortic regurgitation: influence of guideline adherence toward early surgery. J Am Coll Cardiol. 2006;47:1012–17.

35. Yoon SH, Schmidt T, Bleiziffer S, *et al.* Transcatheter aortic valve replacement in pure native aortic valve regurgitation. J Am Coll Cardiol. 2017;70:2752–63.

36. Edwards FH, Peterson ED, Coombs LP, *et al.* Prediction of operative mortality after valve replacement surgery. J Am Coll Cardiol. 2001;37:885–92.

37. Florath I, Rosendahl UP, Mortasawi A, *et al.* Current determinants of operative mortality in 1400 patients requiring aortic valve replacement. Ann Thorac Surg. 2003;76:75–83.

38. Ishii K, Hirota Y, Suwa M, Kita Y, Onaka H, Kawamura K. Natural history and left ventricular response in chronic aortic regurgitation. Am J Cardiol. 1996;78:357–61.

39. Roman MJ, Klein L, Devereux RB, et al. Reversal of left ventricular dilatation, hypertrophy, and dysfunction by valve replacement in aortic regurgitation. Am Heart J. 1989;118:553–63.

40. Carabello BA. Is it ever too late to operate on the patient with valvular heart disease? J Am Coll Cardiol. 2004;44:376–83.

41. Imran TF, Awtry EH. Severe mitral stenosis. N Engl J Med. 2018;379(3):e6.

42. Banovic M, DaCosta M. Degenerative mitral stenosis: from pathophysiology to challenging interventional treatment. Curr Probl Cardiol. 2019;44(1):10–35.

43. Wunderlich NC, Beigel R, Ho SY, et al. Imaging for mitral interventions: methods and efficacy. JACC Cardiovasc Imaging. 2018;11(6):872–901.

44. Oktay AA, Gilliland YE, Lavie CJ, et al. Echocardiographic assessment of degenerative mitral stenosis: a diagnostic challenge of an emerging cardiac disease. Curr Probl Cardiol. 2017;42(3):71–100.

45. Russell EA, Walsh WF, Reid CM, et al. Outcomes after mitral valve surgery for rheumatic heart disease. Heart Asia. 2017;9(2):e010916.

46. Asgar AW, Mack MJ, Stone GW. Secondary mitral regurgitation in heart failure: pathophysiology, prognosis, and therapeutic considerations. J Am Coll Cardiol. 2015;65:1231–48.

47. Deferm S, Bertrand PB, Verbrugge FH, et al. Atrial functional mitral regurgitation: JACC review topic of the week. J Am Coll Cardiol. 2019;73:2465–76.

48. El Sabbagh A, Reddy YNV, Nishimura RA. Mitral valve regurgitation in the contemporary era. JACC Cardiovasc Imaging. 2018;11(4):628–43.

49. Rosenhek R, Rader F, Klaar U, et al. Outcome of watchful waiting in asymptomatic severe mitral regurgitation. Circulation. 2006;113(18):2238–44.

50. Piérard LA, Lancellotti P. The role of ischemic mitral regurgitation in the pathogenesis of acute pulmonary edema. N Engl J Med. 2004;351(16):1627–34.

51. Lancellotti P, Tribouilloy C, Hagendorff A, et al.; Scientific Document Committee of the European Association of Cardiovascular Imaging. Recommendations for the echocardiographic assessment of native valvular regurgitation: an executive summary from the European Association of Cardiovascular Imaging. Eur Heart J Cardiovasc Imaging. 2013;14:611–44.

52. Piérard LA, Lancellotti P. The role of ischemic mitral regurgitation in the pathogenesis of acute pulmonary edema. N Engl J Med. 2004;351:1627–34.

53. Theriault-Lauzier P, Dorfmeister M, Mylotte D, et al. Quantitative multi-slice computed tomography assessment of the mitral valvular complex for transcatheter mitral valve interventions part 2: geometrical measurements in patients with functional mitral regurgitation. EuroIntervention. 2016;12:e1021–30.

54. Thavendiranathan P, Phelan D, Thomas JD, Flamm SD, Marwick TH. Quantitative assessment of mitral regurgitation: validation of new methods. J Am Coll Cardiol. 2012;60:1470–83.

55. Rossi A, Dini FL, Faggiano P, et al. Independent prognostic value of functional mitral regurgitation in patients with heart failure. A quantitative analysis of 1256 patients with ischaemic and non-ischaemic dilated cardiomyopathy. Heart. 2011;97:1675–80.

56. Zoghbi WA, Adams D, Bonow RO, et al. Recommendations for non-invasive evaluation of native valvular regurgitation: a report from the American Society of Echocardiography developed in collaboration with the Society for Cardiovascular Magnetic Resonance. J Am Soc Echocardiogr. 2017;30:303–71.

57. Zeng X, Levine RA, Hua L, et al. Diagnostic value of vena contracta area in the quantification of mitral regurgitation severity by color Doppler 3D echocardiography. Circ Cardiovasc Imaging. 2011;4:506–13.

58. Doughty RN, Whalley GA, Walsh HA, Gamble GD, Lopez-Sendon J, Sharpe N; CAPRICORN Echo Substudy Investigators. Effects of carvedilol on left ventricular remodelling after acute myocardial infarction: the CAPRICORN Echo Substudy. Circulation. 2004;109:201–6.

59. Solomon SD, Skali H, Anavekar NS, et al. Changes in ventricular size and function in patients treated with valsartan, captopril, or both after myocardial infarction. Circulation. 2005;111:3411–19.

60. Lowes BD, Gill EA, Abraham WT, et al. Effects of carvedilol on left ventricular mass, chamber geometry, and mitral regurgitation in chronic heart failure. Am J Cardiol. 1999;83:1201–5.

61. Waagstein F, Stromblad O, Andersson B, et al. Increased exercise ejection fraction and reversed remodelling after long-term treatment with metoprolol in congestive heart failure: a randomized, stratified, double-blind, placebo controlled trial in mild to moderate heart failure due to ischemic or idiopathic dilated cardiomyopathy. Eur J Heart Fail. 2003;5:679–91.

62. Kang DH, Park SJ, Shin SH, et al. Angiotensin receptor neprilysin inhibitor for functional mitral regurgitation. Circulation. 2019;139:1354–65.

63. Palardy M, Stevenson LW, Tasissa G, et al.; ESCAPE Investigators. Reduction in mitral regurgitation during therapy guided by measured filling pressures in the ESCAPE trial. Circ Heart Fail. 2009;2:181–8.

64. Gertz ZM, Raina A, Saghy L, et al. Evidence of atrial functional mitral regurgitation due to atrial fibrillation: reversal with arrhythmia control. J Am Coll Cardiol. 2011;58:1474–81.

65. Cleland JG, Daubert JC, Erdmann E, et al.; Cardiac Resynchronization-Heart Failure (CARE-HF) Study Investigators. The effect of cardiac resynchronization on morbidity and mortality in heart failure. N Engl J Med. 2005;352:1539–49.

66. Ypenburg C, Lancellotti P, Tops LF, et al. Acute effects of initiation and withdrawal of cardiac resynchronization therapy on papillary muscle dyssynchrony and mitral regurgitation. J Am Coll Cardiol. 2007;50:2071–7.

67. Campwala SZ, Bansal RC, Wang N, Razzouk A, Pai RG. Factors affecting regression of mitral regurgitation following isolated coronary artery bypass surgery. Eur J Cardiothorac Surg. 2005;28:783–7.

68. Feldman T, Foster E, Glower DD, et al.; EVEREST II Investigators. Percutaneous repair or surgery for mitral regurgitation. N Engl J Med. 2011;364:1395–406.

69. Coats AJS, Anker SD, Baumbach A, et al. The management of secondary mitral regurgitation in patients with heart failure: a joint position statement from the Heart Failure Association (HFA), European Association of Cardiovascular Imaging (EACVI), European Heart Rhythm Association (EHRA), and European Association of Percutaneous Cardiovascular Interventions (EAPCI) of the ESC. Eur Heart J. 2021;42:1254–69.

70. Adamo M, Fiorelli F, Melica B, et al. COAPT-like profile predicts long-term outcomes in patients with secondary mitral regurgitation undergoing MitraClip implantation. JACC Cardiovasc Interv. 2021;14:15–25.

71. Crespo-Leiro MG, Metra M, Lund LH, et al. Advanced heart failure: a position statement of the Heart Failure Association of the European Society of Cardiology. Eur J Heart Fail. 2018;20:1505–35.

72. Godino C, Munafo A, Scotti A, et al. MitraClip in secondary mitral regurgitation as a bridge to heart transplantation: 1-year outcomes from the International MitraBridge Registry. J Heart Lung Transplant. 2020;39:1353–62.

73. Witte KK, Lipiecki J, Siminiak T, *et al.* The REDUCE FMR trial: a randomized sham-controlled study of percutaneous mitral annuloplasty in functional mitral regurgitation. JACC Heart Fail. 2019;7:945.

74. Geyer M, Keller K, Sotiriou E, *et al.* Association of transcatheter direct mitral annuloplasty with acute anatomic, haemodynamic, and clinical outcomes in severe mitral valve regurgitation. ESC Heart Fail. 2020;7:3336–44.

75. Ruf TF, Kreidel F, Tamm AR, *et al.* Transcatheter indirect mitral annuloplasty induces annular and left atrial remodelling in secondary mitral regurgitation. ESC Heart Fail. 2020;7:1400–8.

76. Sorajja P, Moat N, Badhwar V, *et al.* Initial feasibility study of a new transcatheter mitral prosthesis: the first 100 patients. J Am Coll Cardiol. 2019;73:1250–60.

77. Agricola E, Ielasi A, Oppizzi M, *et al.* Long-term prognosis of medically treated patients with functional mitral regurgitation and left ventricular dysfunction. Eur J Heart Fail. 2009;11:581–7.

78. Goliasch G, Bartko PE, Pavo N, *et al.* Refining the prognostic impact of functional mitral regurgitation in chronic heart failure. Eur Heart J. 2018;39:39–46.

79. Adler DS. Non-functional tricuspid valve disease. Ann Cardiothorac Surg. 2017;6(3):204–13.

80. Badano LP, Muraru D, Enriquez-Sarano M. Assessment of functional tricuspid regurgitation. Eur Heart J. 2013;34(25):1875–85.

81. Dahou A, Levin D, Reisman M, *et al.* Anatomy and physiology of the tricuspid valve. JACC Cardiovasc Imaging. 2019;12:458–68.

82. Antonio M, Claudio M, Matteo P, *et al.* Mechanism and implications of the tricuspid regurgitation. Circ Cardiovasc Interv. 2017;10(7):e005043.

83. Agricola E, Marini C, Stella S, *et al.* Effects of functional tricuspid regurgitation on renal function and long-term prognosis in patients with heart failure. J Cardiovasc Med (Hagerstown). 2017;18:60–8.

84. Min S-Y, Song J-M, Kim J-H, *et al.* Geometric changes after tricuspid annuloplasty and predictors of residual tricuspid regurgitation: a real-time three-dimensional echocardiography study. Eur Heart J. 2010;31(23):2871–80.

85. Taramasso M, Alessandrini H, Latib A, *et al.* Outcomes after current transcatheter tricuspid valve intervention: mid-term results from the International TriValve Registry. JACC Cardiovasc Interv. 2019;12(2):155–65.

86. Hahn RT, Zamorano JL. The need for a new tricuspid regurgitation grading scheme. Eur Heart J Cardiovasc Imaging. 2017;18(12):1342–43.

87. Santoro C, Marco Del Castillo A, González-Gómez A, *et al.* Mid-term outcome of severe tricuspid regurgitation: are there any differences according to mechanism and severity? Eur Heart J Cardiovasc Imaging. 2019;20(9):1035–42.

88. Yancy CW, Jessup M, Bozkurt B, *et al.* 2017 ACC/AHA/HFSA focused update of the 2013 ACCF/AHA Guideline for the management of heart failure: a report of the American College of Cardiology/American Heart Association Task Force on Clinical Practice Guidelines and the Heart Failure Society of America. J Card Fail. 2017;23:628–51.

89. American College of Cardiology Foundation/American Heart Association Task Force on Practice, American Association for Thoracic Surgery, American Society of Echocardiography. 2011 ACCF/AHA guideline for the diagnosis and treatment of hypertrophic cardiomyopathy: a report of the American College of Cardiology Foundation/American Heart Association Task Force on Practice Guidelines. J Thorac Cardiovasc Surg. 2011;142:e153–203.

90. Zack CJ, Fender EA, Chandrashekar P, *et al.* National trends and outcomes in isolated tricuspid valve surgery. J Am Coll Cardiol. 2017;70:2953–60.

91. Taramasso M, Benfari G, van der Bijl P, *et al.* Transcatheter versus medical treatment of patients with symptomatic severe tricuspid regurgitation. J Am Coll Cardiol. 2019;74:2998–3008.

92. Ramsdell GC, Nelson JA, Pislaru SV, Ramakrishna H. Tricuspid regurgitation in congestive heart failure: management strategies and analysis of outcomes. J Cardiothorac Vasc Anesth. 2021;35(4):1205–14.

93. Benfari G, Antoine C, Miller WL, *et al.* Excess mortality associated with functional tricuspid regurgitation complicating heart failure with reduced ejection fraction. Circulation. 2019;140:196–206.

94. Nath J, Foster E, Heidenreich PA. Impact of tricuspid regurgitation on long-term survival. J Am Coll Cardiol. 2004;43:405–9.

95. Hu K, Liu D, Stork S, *et al.* Echocardiographic determinants of one-year all-cause mortality in patients with chronic heart failure complicated by significant functional tricuspid regurgitation. J Card Fail. 2017;23:434–43.

96. Bartko PE, Arfsten H, Frey MK, *et al.* Natural history of functional tricuspid regurgitation: implications of quantitative Doppler assessment. JACC Cardiovasc Imaging. 2019;12:389–97.

CHAPTER 3.4

Cardiomyopathies

Contents

3.4.1 Genetic basis of cardiomyopathies

Thomas Thum, Stephane Heymans, and Johannes Backs

Introduction and genetic diversity of cardiomyopathies

Cardiomyopathies are a heterogeneous group of diseases affecting the cardiac muscle and are important drivers of heart failure (HF). A comprehensive understanding of the underlying mechanisms and natural courses has led to recent therapeutic advances with an important impact on management and prognosis.[1]

A major step forward in understanding the underlying genetic diversity was the initiation of the Human Genome Project in the nineties.[2,3] Here, more than 2 million single-nucleotide variants (SNVs) were discovered that showed a first glimpse of the huge genetic diversity. Interestingly, despite detection of many more variants within the last two decades,[4,5] only a fraction of genetic variants in human genomes have been detected so far. Among HF causes, genetic cardiomyopathies represent only a small, but very important, proportion of patients, and individualized treatment approaches are currently being developed. Among the cardiomyopathies, hypertrophic (HCM) and dilated cardiomyopathy (DCM) are the most prevalent. Recently, the epidemiology of genetic cardiomyopathies has extensively been reviewed and summarized.[6,7] In this chapter, we focus on genetic HCM and DCM, certain storage diseases, and peripartum cardiomyopathy (PPCM), and specifically highlight genetic mutations in which strong scientific interest exist, with recent progress, resulting in potential targeted therapeutic modalities, either in development or entering the clinical arena. We clearly acknowledge that many more (rare) forms of cardiomyopathies exist and are subject to intensive studies, with new treatments on the horizon.

Molecular and functional phenotyping of cardiomyopathies

Direct causes of cardiomyopathies include pathogenic gene variants (mutations), toxins (alcohol, chemotherapy, recreational drugs), autoimmunity, storage diseases (Fabry disease, amyloid), infections, and tachyarrhythmias.[8,9,10] Pregnancy and most cardiovascular comorbidities (diabetes, hypertension, kidney failure, anaemia) may accelerate HF. The combined presence of genetic and acquired causes is a key consideration during diagnostic workup, as both interact to worsen cardiac function.[11]

Clinical history, laboratory tests, and imaging are the first-line investigations. Echocardiography is central to diagnosis and monitoring of HCM, DCM, and arrhythmogenic cardiomyopathy. Cardiac magnetic resonance imaging provides more detailed morphological and prognostic information and should be performed at baseline. The prevalence of gene mutations may

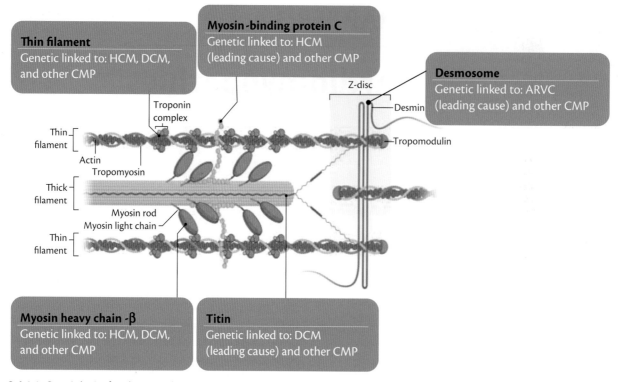

Figure 3.4.1.1 Genetic basis of cardiomyopathies. ARVC, arrhythmogenic right ventricular cardiomyopathy; CMP, cardiomyopathy; DCM, dilated cardiomyopathy; HCM, hypertrophic cardiomyopathy.

vary according to the morphological phenotype or underlying acquired cause: up to 40% in DCM, up to 60% in HCM, and up to 15% in chemotherapy-induced[12,13] and alcohol-induced cardiomyopathy[14] and PPCM.[15,16] In non-familial DCM, the prevalence of genetic mutations is over 10%.[11,12] Finding a pathogenic gene variant in a cardiomyopathy case will allow to better predict disease outcome and progression, refine the indication for device implantation, and also advise first-degree relatives on genetic counselling.[1] The most frequent genetic mutations responsible for some of the cardiomyopathies are presented in ➲ Figure 3.4.1.1.

Endomyocardial biopsy (EMB), with immunohistochemical quantification of inflammatory cells, remains the gold standard investigation for cardiac inflammation.[17,18] It is crucial to confirm the diagnosis of autoimmune disease in DCM patients with suspected giant cell myocarditis, eosinophilic myocarditis, vasculitis, sarcoidosis, or storage diseases, including amyloid or Fabry disease. In HCM, EMB might be considered if genetic or acquired causes cannot be identified. Risks and benefits of EBM should be evaluated and this procedure is reserved for specific situations where treatment may differ according to diagnosis.

Dilated cardiomyopathies

Definition and prevalence

DCM consists of left ventricular (LV) systolic dysfunction and LV dilatation in the absence of coronary artery disease or abnormal loading conditions (e.g. HF only caused by hypertension or cardiac valvular abnormalities). DCM often overlaps with hypokinetic non-dilated cardiomyopathy (HNDC), that is LV or biventricular global systolic dysfunction (left ventricular ejection fraction (LVEF) <45%) without dilatation.[9,10,11]

DCM has an estimated prevalence of between 1 in 250 to 1 in 500.[9] DCMs are heterogeneous diseases where genetic mutations (up to 40%) and acquired causes (toxic, storage disease, infectious, or metabolic) lead to cardiac dilatation, dysfunction, arrhythmias, and progressive HF. Symptoms reflective of HF or arrhythmias may prevail, but also muscle complaints may be present, as in Duchenne dystrophy, caused by a mutation in the dystrophin gene of the X chromosome. The association between common underlying genetic mutations and the pathophysiology and clinical presentation is presented in ➲ Figure 3.4.1.2.

Titin truncation cardiomyopathy

The most common mutations in DCM are within the titin gene. Titin (*TTN*) is one of the largest proteins encoded by the human genome and is essential for cardiomyocyte structure and function.[19] In up to 25% of patients with DCM, heterozygous *TTN*-truncating variants (TTNtv) underlie the disease that tend to accumulate and induce cardiotoxic reactions.[15,20,21] Interestingly, TTNtv are also present at a rate of 0.5–3% in the healthy population, and here they are a risk factor for future adverse cardiac remodelling.[12] Moreover, acquired/environmental factors can add to a genetic background, eventually leading to disease onset and development.[11] In addition, TTNtv are present in up to 15% of patients with 'acquired DCM', including pregnancy-,[15] alcohol-,[14] and chemotherapy-induced[22] cardiomyopathy.

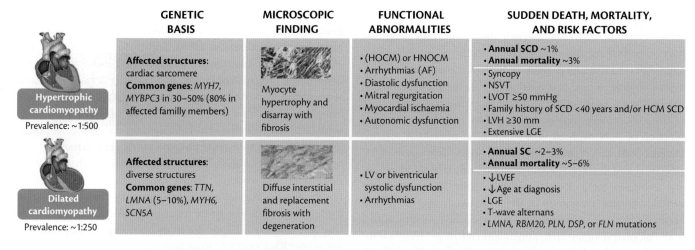

	GENETIC BASIS	MICROSCOPIC FINDING	FUNCTIONAL ABNORMALITIES	SUDDEN DEATH, MORTALITY, AND RISK FACTORS
Hypertrophic cardiomyopathy Prevalence: ~1:500	**Affected structures:** cardiac sarcomere **Common genes:** MYH7, MYBPC3 in 30–50% (80% in affected family members)	Myocyte hypertrophy and disarray with fibrosis	• (HOCM) or HNOCM • Arrhythmias (AF) • Diastolic dysfunction • Mitral regurgitation • Myocardial ischaemia • Autonomic dysfunction	• **Annual SCD** ~1% • **Annual mortality** ~3% • Syncope • NSVT • LVOT ≥50 mmHg • Family history of SCD <40 years and/or HCM SCD • LVH ≥30 mm • Extensive LGE
Dilated cardiomyopathy Prevalence: ~1:250	**Affected structures:** diverse structures **Common genes:** TTN, LMNA (5–10%), MYH6, SCN5A	Diffuse interstitial and replacement fibrosis with degeneration	• LV or biventricular systolic dysfunction • Arrhythmias	• **Annual SC** ~2–3% • **Annual mortality** ~5–6% • ↓LVEF • ↓Age at diagnosis • LGE • T-wave alternans • LMNA, RBM20, PLN, DSP, or FLN mutations

Cardiomyopathies in storage diseases: Lysosomal storage disorders most prevalent (Pompeand Danondisease); mucopolysaccharidoses and glycosphingolipids (Anderson–Fabry disease). Fabry disease most common (undetectable α-galactosidase A enzyme -GLA gene). **Peripartum cardiomyopathy:** Typical observed mutation in the sarcomere gene titin (TTN), ~0–15% of PPCM.

Figure 3.4.1.2 Link between genetic basis, pathophysiology, and outcomes in cardiomyopathies. AF atrial fibrillation; DSP, desmoplakin; FLN, filamin; HCM, hypertrophic cardiomyopathy; HNOCM, hypertrophic non-obstructive cardiomyopathy; HOCM, hypertrophic obstructive cardiomyopathy; LGE, late gadolinium enhancement; LMNA, lamin; LVH, left ventricular hypertrophy; LVOT, left ventricular outflow tract; MYBPC3, myosin-binding protein C; MYH6, α-myosin heavy chain; MYH7, β-myosin heavy chain; NSVT, non-sustained ventricular tachycardia; PLN, phospholamban; RBM20, RNA-binding motif protein 20; SCD, sudden cardiac death; SCN5A, sodium channel; TTN, titin.

TTNtv additionally predispose to a number of other cardiac rhythmological diseases such as early or familial atrial fibrillation (AF)[23] and ventricular tachyarrhythmias.[24,25] TTNtv thus should be seen as a common genetic risk factor for the development of HF and/or arrhythmias when combined with additional acquired (or genetic) disease factors.

Importantly, cardiac function improves in up to 80% of TTNtv cardiomyopathy patients upon optimal HF treatment, but the remaining 20% still follow a more malignant clinical course, with persistent cardiac dysfunction and life-threatening arrhythmias.[10] RNA sequencing (RNA-seq) identified at least two distinct subgroups among TTNtv patients: a 'benign' form of TTNtv-DCM, and a 'malignant' TTNtv group (lower LVEF, increased cardiac fibrosis, more arrhythmias, higher concentration of blood inflammatory markers, and increased concentration of N-terminal pro-B-type natriuretic peptide) that had close gene expression similarities to those of LMNA patients, with similarities in their clinical phenotype.[26]

Key pathomechanisms of TTNtv-DCM suggest that titin haploinsufficiency is present in TTNtv hearts and causes loss of sarcomeres.[27,28] Contractile deficiency was also shown to be present in human induced pluripotent stem cardiomyocytes, with a heterozygous TTNtv engineered into three-dimensional heart muscle.[27,28] Of translational importance, repair of the TTNtv by CRISPR (Clustered Regularly Interspaced Short Palindromic Repeats)/Cas9 gene editing in engineered heart muscle fully rescued contractility.[27]

DCM laminopathies (LMNA)

LMNA is a nuclear protein and mutations cause structural abnormalities in the nuclear envelope, triggering different molecular events underlying LMNA-related DCM.[29] Mutations in the lamin A/C (LMNA) gene cause laminopathies, a group of disorders characterized by phenotypically heterogeneous manifestations. Laminopathies can affect distinct tissues (striated muscles, peripheral nerves, adipose tissue) or can present as a systemic disease (progeria, or accelerated ageing) involving several organs in parallel. Cardiac involvement often presents as a rapidly progressing DCM associated with conduction system disease, AF, and malignant ventricular tachyarrhythmias.[30] In DCM patients with pathogenic LMNA variants, between 15% and 40% will develop life-threatening ventricular arrhythmias (approximately 15% will die) or HF progression within 5 years. Non-sustained ventricular tachycardia, decreased LVEF, male sex, and non-missense mutations are the main risk factors.[31] Mechanistically involved in LMNA-DCM is activation of mitogen-activated protein (MAP) kinases (Ras, ERK1/2, p38 MAPK) and AKT/mTOR and chromatin disorganization, as well as increased platelet-derived growth factor receptor (PDGFR) expression, leading to progression to myocyte death and fibrosis.[32] Thus, clinical trials have focused on inhibition of p38 MAPK, Ras, mTOR, and PDGFR, with an ongoing phase 3 trial involving a selective oral inhibitor of the p38 MAPK pathway in symptomatic LMNA-DCM (ARRY-371797, also PF-07265803; available from: https://clinicaltrials.gov/ct2/show/NCT0 3439514). Recently, a Ras inhibitor (lonafarnib)—with Ras/MAPK being crucial to signal transduction for cell growth and differentiation—has been approved to reduce mortality in LMNA-related progeria (Hutchinson–Gilford progeria syndrome and progeroid laminopathies).[33] Its benefit in LMNA-DCM, however, remains to be tested.

Phospholamban cardiomyopathy

Phospholamban (PLN) is a protein in the sarcoplasmic reticulum membrane that regulates the sarco-/endoplasmic reticulum calcium ATPase (SERCA) protein. PLN plays a crucial role in calcium handling in health and disease.[34,35] A specific mutation in the *PLN* gene, in which the arginine in amino acid position 14 of the PLN protein is deleted (p.Arg14del), results in a gain of function of PLN, with chronic suppression of SERCA activity. Patients with a *PLN* mutation have a higher frequency of LV structural and functional abnormalities, compared to other genetic arrhythmogenic cardiomyopathy patients.[36] The consequent cardiomyopathy is common in the Netherlands and the United States, and gives rise to a severe form of cardiomyopathy with a high risk of developing arrhythmias and end-stage HF.[37,38] Of individuals with the PLN p.Arg14del variant, between 20% and 40% will develop life-threatening ventricular arrhythmia or HF (of whom approximately 15% will die) within 5 years. The exact rate will depend on the extent of family screening, with identification of phenotype-negative mutation carriers. Decreased LVEF, the number of premature ventricular contractions, and the presence of negative T-waves on the electrocardiogram (ECG) are the main predictors of malignant ventricular arrhythmias and death.[31] Thus, the reported rate of cardiac mortality will depend on the functional/electrical penetrance of the mutation into the extent of family screening (asymptomatic vs symptomatic; phenotype-negative vs positive).

PLN cardiomyopathy is characterized by common features of severe HF such as cellular loss, fibrosis, and impaired calcium handling. In addition, the heart muscle shows PLN aggregates that localize with the endoplasmic reticulum and nucleus.[39] A mouse model with the murine variant of the p.Arg14del mutation almost completely mimics human cardiomyopathy.[40] These mouse studies showed that PLN aggregates may occur already in the disease process before the development of an overt cardiac phenotype.[41,42] This 'cardiodegenerative' phenotype prompts the need for further studies and may provide novel targets for disease monitoring and therapy. Currently, a large number of preclinical studies are being conducted on compounds that aim to repair the genetic defect (e.g. antisense and gene therapy), but also that target protein aggregation and integrity, as these appear highly crucial to PLN cardiomyopathy.[43,44]

Other mutations underlying dilated cardiomyopathy

Sarcomeric (motor) genes encoding proteins that form thick and thin sarcomeric filaments are involved not only in HCM, but also in DCM. These proteins include myosin heavy chain α and β (*MYH6* and *MYH7*, respectively), MYBPC3, troponins (*TNNT2*, *TNNI3*, and *TNNC1*), tropomyosin 1 (*TPM1*), cardiac actin 1 (*ACTC1*), myopalladin (*MYPN*), and possibly many more.[45] Up to 10% of familial DCM cases result from genetic variants that encode contractile proteins, with substantial phenotypic variability.[46] Other genetic variants have been described in *FLNC* encoding filamin C, in the context of DCM.[47] It is well known that in both long QT syndrome and Brugada syndrome, heterozygous autosomal dominant pathological variants are found in the sodium channel gene *SCN5A*. Missense variants in *SCN5A* have been described in familial DCM, and these carry a higher risk of arrhythmias.[48] Additionally, mutations in genes coding for the desmosome proteins are known in DCM; the desmosome has a symmetrical myocyte structure, in which each part resides in the cytoplasm of one of a pair of adjacent cells, anchoring the intermediate filaments in the cytoskeleton to the cell surface. A prevalence of 5% of desmosomal protein-coding gene variants in 100 unrelated patients with DCM have been discovered that, however, need functional workup.[49] Recent evidence suggests a contribution from splice regulatory networks in many diseases, including cardiomyopathies. The splice regulator RNA-binding motif protein 20 (RBM20) is important in determining the physiological messenger RNA (mRNA) landscape formation; interestingly, rare variants in the *RBM20* gene explain up to 6% of genetic DCM cases.[50]

Phenomapping and diagnosis of dilated cardiomyopathy

The minimal set of genes to be analysed in DCM or hypokinetic non-DCM[8,11,51] should include titin, lamin A/C, myosin heavy chain, troponin T, troponin-C myosin-binding protein C, RBM20, PLN, sodium channel α unit, BaCl2-associated athanogene 3, actin α cardiac muscle, nexilin, tropomyosin 1, and vinculin.[52,53] EMB quantifies the amount of inflammation and reveals storage diseases in cases of suspected phenotypes requiring specific treatments (i.e. giant cell myocarditis, eosinophilic myocarditis, sarcoidosis, vasculitis, lupus erythematosus, storage diseases, or any other systemic, autoimmune, or inflammatory conditions).[1,18,54] Biopsies also help in detecting and classifying DCM subtypes. Additionally, infectious triggers can be determined such as common cardiotrophic viruses (parvovirus B19, human herpesvirus (HHV) 4, HHV6, and enteroviruses (adenovirus and Coxsackie virus) by reverse transcriptase polymerase chain reaction; viral mRNA for active viral replication, if possible; and, on indication, cytomegalovirus (CMV), human immunodeficiency virus (HIV), *Borrelia burgdorferi* (Lyme disease), *Coxiella burnetii* (Q fever), *Trypanosoma cruzi* (Chagas disease, (migrant of) South American origin), and severe acute respiratory syndrome coronavirus 2 (SARS-CoV-2).[55] The use of additional gene sequencing and familial segregation may be considered in cases of a clear family history or structural phenotype. If neuromuscular complaints or disorders are present, cardiac forms of Duchenne muscular dystrophy should be considered, and mutations in the dystrophin gene on the X chromosome should be assessed for. The described heterogeneity in DCM phenotypes, however, makes it difficult to classify DCM with great precision and impairs clinical decision-making, including the decision on adequate (if available) therapy. Deep phenomapping of DCM was recently performed in 795 consecutive DCM patients comprising extensive clinical data on aetiology and comorbidities, imaging, genetics, and EMB.[56] In this cohort, four clinically distinct phenogroups (PGs) were identified, based upon unsupervised hierarchical clustering of the principal components, that is, patients with: (1) mild systolic dysfunction; (2) autoimmune; (3) genetic and arrhythmias; and (4) severe systolic dysfunction. RNA-seq of cardiac samples revealed a distinct underlying molecular profile per group: pro-inflammatory (2, autoimmune); pro-fibrotic (3, genetic and arrhythmias); and metabolic (4, low ejection fraction) gene expression patterns. Identification of DCM phenogroups associated with significant differences in clinical presentation, underlying molecular profiles, and outcome will help to pave the way for individual treatment. In particular, genetic modifiers may be discovered by large genome-wide association studies (GWAS), which have already generated several genetic loci associated with early-onset DCM.[57,58] Therefore, more studies to determine additional genetics (epigenetic and transcriptional) in different cells (single cell/nuclear sequencing), together with epidemiological data (acquired risk factors and family screening), are required to enable individualized therapy for DCM patients.

Treatment of dilated cardiomyopathy

In the case of DCM, standard HF treatment should be started according to existing guidelines. Even after recovery of the ejection fraction, HF drugs should be continued, as relapse may occur in up to 40% of patients with treatment cessation.[59] Patients with LMNA, RBM20, PLN, or FLN mutations carry a higher risk of sudden cardiac death (SCD), and therefore, an early indication for primary prevention by use of an implantable cardioverter–defibrillator (ICD) should be considered (guided by risk factors, as detailed).[60] Titin (TTN) mutations have a higher rate of LV reverse remodelling (in up to 70–80% of cases), but a paradoxically increased risk of atrial and ventricular tachyarrhythmias; thus, close arrhythmia monitoring and treatment are required.[12,23,25,61,62] Lyme disease (B. burgdorferi) should be treated with antibiotics (doxycycline), and Chagas disease (T. cruzi) according to current recommendations.[63] Autoimmune/inflammatory conditions, including giant cell and eosinophilic myocarditis, sarcoidosis, and vasculitis, require immunosuppressive therapy.

The indication for ICD implantation in patients with a low ejection fraction (≤35%) is still valid in DCM patients with a high relative likelihood of SCD, according to the DANISH trial.[64,65] Specific treatments for DCM are currently not available, but under development.

Hypertrophic cardiomyopathies
Definition and prevalence

HCM has a prevalence of approximately 1 in 500 and thus is the most common inherited cardiac disease.[66] The hallmark of HCM includes massive myocardial hypertrophy that develops usually in the absence of any pressure overload or other hypertrophy-related conditions (no detection of hypertension or aortic stenosis, no form of infiltration such as amyloidosis or storage diseases). HCM is divided into cases with LV outflow tract obstruction (hypertrophic obstructive cardiomyopathy (HOCM)) or without (HNOCM), and other forms appear as apical, segmental, or concentric forms of hypertrophy. Histologically, typical findings include various degrees of interstitial fibrosis, myocyte enlargement, and cardiomyocyte disarray.[67,68] Common underlying genetic mutations, pathophysiology, and clinical presentation are depicted in ➲ Figure 3.4.1.2.

Underlying causal mutations in hypertrophic cardiomyopathy

Up to 60% of gene mutations in HCM occur in cardiac contractile proteins, and phenotypically this results in various degrees of LV hypertrophy, increased interstitial fibrosis, and diastolic dysfunction.[69] MYBPC3 and MYH7, encoding cardiac myosin-binding protein C (cMyBP-C) and β-myosin heavy chain, are the most prevalently affected genes, containing approximately 30–40% of all pathogenic or likely pathogenic HCM variants, respectively.[70] TNNT2 encoding cardiac troponin T is the main affected thin filament gene. Most MYBPC3 mutations are truncating (75%),[71,72,73] leading to the absence of mutant protein and cMyBP-C haploinsufficiency.[74,75,76] HCM-involved non-sarcomeric genes include those encoding proteins found in the Z-disk, sarcoplasmic reticulum, and plasma membrane. These variants are rare and include myozenin 2 (MYOZ2), ubiquitin E3 ligase tripartite motif protein 63 (TRIM63), and four-and-a-half LIM domains 1 (FHL1), which have been described as causes of HCM.[77,78] Other genes recently described to be involved in HCM include long non-coding RNAs. Indeed, the long non-coding RNA H19 have been found repressed in cardiac hypertrophy and HF tissues.[79] Interestingly, in sarcomere no-mutation patients, there was an enrichment with patients showing an H19 mutation, suggesting a significant association between H19 variants and the risk of developing HCM.[80] Dozens of additional genes have been implicated in HCM in recent years, although these reports varied considerably in their study design and strength of evidence (the findings of candidate gene studies, in particular, often failed to be replicated). Comprehensive reappraisal of these associations has been performed in recent years by rare variant association studies[51,81] and curation of published evidence through the National Institutes of Health (NIH)-funded ClinGen initiative.[82,83] Validated gene–disease associations arising from these efforts reveal different genetic architectures that better reflect the distinctive phenotypes of the major cardiomyopathies, and enable more focused and accurate genetic testing for cardiomyopathy patients.

Mechanistically, the ubiquitin–proteasome system and autophagy–lysosomal pathway are impaired in HCM, and activation of autophagy partially restores the pathological phenotype in mouse models.[84,85] Mutations also lead to altered calcium sensitivity, perturbed length-dependent activation, increased cross-bridge kinetics, and increased tension cost of myofilament contraction,[86] leading to increased adenosine triphosphate (ATP) utilization by sarcomeres. Indeed, mutation-induced sarcomere changes have a negative impact on cellular energetics and may be targeted by interventions aimed to correct the sarcomere deficit, or by optimizing processes involved in metabolism and mitochondrial function.[87]

Phenomapping and diagnosis

HCM is a typical single-gene disorder with an autosomal dominant pattern of inheritance.[88] Usually a single mutation is sufficient to cause HCM, albeit with variable penetrance and expression. The clinical diagnosis of HCM is based on the presence of LV hypertrophy, defined by an end-diastolic ventricular septal thickness of ≥13 mm in adults, occurring in the absence of abnormal loading conditions or other secondary causes such as hypertension or aortic stenosis. The first suspicion usually stems from imaging analyses such as echocardiography or magnetic resonance imaging (MRI), followed by genetic testing. Genetic testing is part of the standard of care in the diagnosis and management of HCM, especially in the presence of a positive family history. Genetic testing for HCM is routinely available and typically includes sequencing a panel of HCM-associated genes, although the number of investigated genes varies a lot across countries and providers. In the last years, whole-exome and whole-genome sequencing has been increasingly available.[89] To date, these more comprehensive testing approaches are still expensive and more commonly used in research settings.

Current and future therapy of hypertrophic cardiomyopathy

HCM management has three important aims including symptom reduction, prevention of SCD and thus prolongation of lifespan. Symptomatic management primarily involves pharmacologic therapy with calcium antagonists and/or beta-blockers, septal reduction, or in individuals with severe refractory symptoms, ultimately cardiac transplantation or LVAD implantation. Recently, also novel therapies that directly target one of the underlying molecular mechanisms of the disease have been developed. Mavacamten (previously known as MYK-461) is a first-in-class allosteric inhibitor of cardiac-specific myosin ATP with the aim to reduce pathological hypercontractility in HCM. In EXPLORER-HCM, mavacamten markedly improved the health status of patients with symptomatic obstructive hypertrophic cardiomyopathy compared with placebo, with a low number needed to treat for marked improvement.[90,91] Mechanistically, mavacamten reduces excessive cross-bridging between myosin and actin and restore the capacity of myosin interacting-heads motif to sequester myosin from its disordered relaxed state to the super relaxed state.[92] Genotype–phenotype relationships are present also in HCM but still not completely understood. For instance, *MYH7* variants seem to have an earlier onset of disease higher, an incidence of atrial fibrillation, and greater risk of cardiac events.[93,94] Preclinical data of *MYBPC3* gene therapy in HCM mouse models, mouse and human engineered heart tissues (EHTs) and human induced pluripotent stem cell-derived cardiomyocytes (hiPSC-CMs) illustrate that *MYBPC3* gene replacement therapy via adeno-associated virus (AAV) vector transfer is appropriate to replace the deficient protein in cardiomyocytes for severe forms of HCM.[95,96,97,98,99,100] The positive association of patients with H19 mutations and higher occurrence of HCM suggest the long non-coding RNA H19 as a potential additional target. Indeed in mouse models and human cardiomyocytes and engineered heart tissue, H19 overexpression results in marked reductions in cardiac hypertrophy and fibrosis.[79] Future research may allow clinicians with improved decision making regarding management and therapies in selected HCM individuals.

Cardiomyopathies in storage diseases
Definition and prevalence

There are many forms of cardiac storage diseases and here we will focus only on the most common form of lysosomal storage disorders that comprise a group of diseases caused by a deficiency of lysosomal enzymes, membrane transporters, or other proteins involved in lysosomal biology. Cardiac phenotypes of those diseases can be observed in lysosomal glycogen storage diseases (Pompe and Danon disease) and mucopolysaccharidoses, as well as in glycosphingolipidoses (Anderson–Fabry disease).[101] Indeed, Fabry disease is the most common form of storage disease with a cardiac phenotype. It is an X-linked lysosomal storage disorder caused by pathogenic variants in the α-galactosidase A (*GLA*) gene, leading to reduced or undetectable α-galactosidase A enzyme activity and progressive accumulation of globotriaosylceramide (Gb_3) and its deacylated form globotriaosylsphingosine (lyso-Gb_3) in cells throughout the body, including the kidneys and heart tissue.[102] More than 1000 variants within the *GLA* gene have been identified, and the prevalence of Fabry disease varies according to the screening method employed. Neonatal screening programmes have reported a relative high incidence of disease-causing variants, ranging from 1:1250 to 1:7800.[103,104] The usual diagnosis is absence or severely reduced (<1% of normal) α-galactosidase A enzyme activity.[105] Typical clinical manifestations include skin signs such as angiokeratoma or hypohidrosis, peripheral neuropathy, premature stroke, kidney involvement with microalbuminuria and proteinuria or kidney insufficiency, and finally cardiomyopathy. In addition to imaging analyses, genetic testing is important both in the index patients, but also in family relatives. Especially in female Fabry patients, gene sequencing is the first-choice method for screening, as well as for confirmation of the diagnosis in males with low α-galactosidase A activity. Also, in many patients, the level of Gb_3 is elevated in the plasma or urine but may be normal in patients with isolated cardiac involvement.[106] Importantly, pathogenic Fabry genetic variants leading to classical disease are associated with higher lyso-Gb_3 levels, compared to later-onset variants, which may be associated even with normal lyso-Gb_3 levels.[107] For treatment of Fabry disease, several options are available. Since 2001, enzyme replacement therapy has been available and is indicated in all symptomatic patients with classical disease, including children, at the earliest signs of organ involvement.[103] With respect to cardiac involvement, data suggest that early initiation of enzyme replacement therapy is crucial. Indeed, data indicate that the heart responds less well to therapy when disease is advanced,[108] and there is limited evidence for a beneficial effect of enzyme replacement therapy in late-onset cardiac variants.[109] Likewise, patients with extensive myocardial fibrosis seem to respond less to therapy in terms of functional improvement.[108] Comprehensive phenotyping is crucial for grading the severity of pathogenic *GLA* variants, to clarify the phenotypic correlations of hypomorphic alleles and to define benign polymorphisms, as well as to establish the pathogenicity of variants of uncertain significance.[110]

Peripartum cardiomyopathy

PPCM occurs globally in all ethnic groups and should be suspected in any peripartum woman presenting with symptoms and signs of HF. This phenotype occurs mostly towards the end of pregnancy or in the months following delivery, and is confirmed by new LV dysfunction. PPCM has substantial maternal and neonatal morbidity and mortality, with maternal mortality ranging widely from 0% to 30%, depending on the ethnic background and geographical region.[111] Importantly, patients with abnormal cardiac findings should be urgently referred to a cardiology team for expert management. A detailed genetic workup should be considered if there is a family history of cardiomyopathy or sudden death. Typical mutations can be found in the sarcomeric gene titin (*TTN*), a well-established disease gene for DCM. Here, several rare truncating mutations in *TTN* were reported in PPCM patients from European and American populations.[15,16] These mutations comprise approximately 10–15% of a PPCM cohort, suggesting many other gene mutations might be present in PPCM cohorts. Details about current strategies for diagnosis and disease management have been published recently.[111]

Future treatment options for cardiomyopathies

There are several exciting developments in the field of cardiomyopathy treatment, many of which are disease-specific rather than symptomatic in nature. They include genome editing that holds the potential to correct a pathogenic variant early before it manifests clinically.[112] Many current approaches to gene editing use the CRISPR technique to induce sequence-dependent strand breaks that may then be repaired by either endogenous repair mechanisms or homology-directed repair, thereby correcting the pathogenic variant.[112] Other techniques, especially in the field of HCM, include gene therapy and gene replacement. However, although such approaches are promising, most have produced either small or transient effects, and further significant work is needed before their clinical application is considered a real possibility.[112] In Fabry disease, a first gene therapy pilot project was completed, in which efficient LV-mediated gene transfer into enriched CD34+ cells in patients with Fabry disease was performed. In this study, increased circulating and intracellular α-galactosidase A activity, without serious safety concerns, was reported.[113] All patients produced α-galactosidase A to near-normal level within 1 week. Plasma and leucocytes showed α-galactosidase A activity within or above the reference range, and reductions in plasma and urine levels of Gb$_3$ and lyso-Gb$_3$ were demonstrated. However, before gene therapy can be adopted as a therapeutic intervention for Fabry disease, it remains to be shown whether the current gene therapy approaches will achieve sufficient α-galactosidase A activity in different tissues.[114] Another investigational approach includes administration of α-galactosidase A mRNA to stimulate the production of α-galactosidase A. In this mouse and non-human primate study, mRNA for human α-galactosidase A encapsulated in lipid nanoparticles also increased α-galactosidase A levels expressed in cardiac, kidney, and liver tissues, resulting in enhanced Gb$_3$ clearance.[115] In conclusion, there are many disease-directed novel therapeutic approaches currently being developed in the field of cardiomyopathies, and clinicians are eagerly awaiting these next-generation therapeutics.

References

1. Seferović PM, Polovina M, Bauersachs J, et al. Heart failure in cardiomyopathies: a position paper from the Heart Failure Association of the European Society of Cardiology. *Eur J Heart Fail.* 2019;21:553–76.
2. Craig Venter J, Adams MD, Myers EW, et al. The sequence of the human genome. *Science.* 2001;291:1304–51.
3. Lander ES, Linton LM, Birren B, et al. Initial sequencing and analysis of the human genome. *Nature.* 2001;409:860–921.
4. Auton A, Abecasis GR, Altshuler DM, et al. A global reference for human genetic variation. *Nature.* 2015;526:68–74.
5. Wheeler DA, Srinivasan M, Egholm M, et al. The complete genome of an individual by massively parallel DNA sequencing. *Nature.* 2008;452:872–6.
6. Pasqualucci D, Iacovoni A, Palmieri V, et al. Epidemiology of cardiomyopathies: essential context knowledge for a tailored clinical workup. *Eur J Prev Cardiol.* 2022;29:1190–9
7. Elliott P, Andersson B, Arbustini E, et al. Classification of the cardiomyopathies: a position statement from the European Society Of Cardiology Working Group on Myocardial and Pericardial Diseases. *Eur Heart J.* 2008;29:270–6.
8. Arbustini E, Narula N, Dec GW, et al. The MOGE(S) classification for a phenotype–genotype nomenclature of cardiomyopathy: endorsed by the World Heart Federation. *J Am Coll Cardiol.* 2013;62:2046–72.
9. Pinto YM, Elliott PM, Arbustini E, et al. Proposal for a revised definition of dilated cardiomyopathy, hypokinetic non-dilated cardiomyopathy, and its implications for clinical practice: a position statement of the ESC working group on myocardial and pericardial diseases. *Eur Heart J.* 2016;37:1850–8.
10. Verdonschot JAJ, Hazebroek MR, Wang P, et al. Clinical phenotype and genotype associations with improvement in left ventricular function in dilated cardiomyopathy. *Circ Heart Fail.* 2018;11:e005220.
11. Hazebroek MR, Moors S, Dennert R, et al. Prognostic relevance of gene–environment interactions in patients with dilated cardiomyopathy: applying the MOGE(S) Classification. *J Am Coll Cardiol.* 2015;66:1313–23.
12. Schafer S, De Marvao A, Adami E, et al. Titin-truncating variants affect heart function in disease cohorts and the general population. *Nat Genet.* 2017;49:46–53.
13. Linschoten M, Teske AJ, Baas AF, et al. Truncating titin (TTN) variants in chemotherapy-induced cardiomyopathy. *J Card Fail.* 2017;23:476–9.
14. Ware JS, Amor-Salamanca A, Tayal U, et al. Genetic etiology for alcohol-induced cardiac toxicity. *J Am Coll Cardiol.* 2018;71:2293–302.
15. Ware JS, Li J, Mazaika E, et al. Shared genetic predisposition in peripartum and dilated cardiomyopathies. *N Engl J Med.* 2016;374:233–41.
16. Van Spaendonck-Zwarts KY, Posafalvi A, van Den Berg MP, et al. Titin gene mutations are common in families with both peripartum cardiomyopathy and dilated cardiomyopathy. *Eur Heart J.* 2014;35:2165–73.

17. Leone O, Veinot JP, Angelini A, *et al.* 2011 consensus statement on endomyocardial biopsy from the Association for European Cardiovascular Pathology and the Society for Cardiovascular Pathology. *Cardiovasc Pathol.* 2012;21:245–74.

18. Seferović PM, Tsutsui H, Mcnamara DM, *et al.* Heart Failure Association, Heart Failure Society of America, and Japanese Heart Failure Society position statement on endomyocardial biopsy. *J Card Fail.* 2021;27:727–43.

19. Linke WA. Titin gene and protein functions in passive and active muscle. *Annu Rev Physiol.* 2018;80:389–411.

20. Herman DS, Lam L, Taylor MRG, *et al.* Truncations of titin causing dilated cardiomyopathy. *N Engl J Med.* 2012;366:619–28.

21. Roberts AM, Ware JS, Herman DS, *et al.* Integrated allelic, transcriptional, and phenomic dissection of the cardiac effects of titin truncations in health and disease. *Sci Transl Med.* 2015;7:270ra6.

22. Garcia-Pavia P, Kim Y, Restrepo-Cordoba MA, *et al.* Genetic variants associated with cancer therapy-induced cardiomyopathy. *Circulation.* 2019;140:31–41.

23. Ahlberg G, Refsgaard L, Lundegaard PR, *et al.* Rare truncating variants in the sarcomeric protein titin associate with familial and early-onset atrial fibrillation. *Nat Commun.* 2018;9:4316.

24. Tayal U, Newsome S, Buchan R, *et al.* Truncating variants in titin independently predict early arrhythmias in patients with dilated cardiomyopathy. *J Am Coll Cardiol.* 2017;69:2466–8.

25. Verdonschot JAJ, Hazebroek MR, Derks KWJ, *et al.* Titin cardiomyopathy leads to altered mitochondrial energetics, increased fibrosis and long-term life-threatening arrhythmias. *Eur Heart J.* 2018;39:864–73.

26. Verdonschot JAJ, Derks KWJ, Hazebroek MR, *et al.* Distinct cardiac transcriptomic clustering in titin and lamin A/C-associated dilated cardiomyopathy patients. *Circulation.* 2020;142:1230–2.

27. Fomin A, Gärtner A, Cyganek L, *et al.* Truncated titin proteins and titin haploinsufficiency are targets for functional recovery in human cardiomyopathy due to *TTN* mutations. 2021;13:eabd3079.

28. Hinson JT, Chopra A, Nafissi N, *et al.* Titin mutations in iPS cells define sarcomere insufficiency as a cause of dilated cardiomyopathy. *Science.* 2015;349:982–6.

29. Nikolova V, Leimena C, McMahon AC, *et al.* Defects in nuclear structure and function promote dilated cardiomyopathy in lamin A/C-deficient mice. 2004;113:357–69.

30. Arbustini E, Pilotto A, Repetto A, *et al.* Autosomal dominant dilated cardiomyopathy with atrioventricular block: a lamin A/C defect-related disease. *J Am Coll Cardiol.* 2002;39:981–90.

31. Verstraelen TE, van Lint FHM, Bosman LP, *et al.* Prediction of ventricular arrhythmia in phospholamban p.Arg14del mutation carriers: reaching the frontiers of individual risk prediction. *Eur Heart J.* 2021;42:2842–50.

32. Crasto S, My I, Di Pasquale E. The broad spectrum of LMNA cardiac diseases: from molecular mechanisms to clinical phenotype. *Front Physiol.* 2020;11:761.

33. Kahn J. FDA approves first treatment for Hutchinson–Gilford progeria syndrome and some progeroid laminopathies. US Food and Drug Administration: 2020.

34. MacLennan DH, Kranias EG. Phospholamban: a crucial regulator of cardiac contractility. *Nat Rev Mol Cell Biol.* 2003;4:566–77.

35. Schmitt JP, Kamisago M, Asahi M, *et al.* Dilated cardiomyopathy and heart failure caused by a mutation in phospholamban. *Science.* 2003;299:1410–13.

36. Bhonsale A, Groeneweg JA, James CA, *et al.* Impact of genotype on clinical course in arrhythmogenic right ventricular dysplasia/cardiomyopathy-associated mutation carriers. *Eur Heart J.* 2015;36:847–55.

37. Van Der Zwaag PA, van Rijsingen IAW, Asimaki A *et al.* Phospholamban R14del mutation in patients diagnosed with dilated cardiomyopathy or arrhythmogenic right ventricular cardiomyopathy: evidence supporting the concept of arrhythmogenic cardiomyopathy. *Eur J Heart Fail.* 2012;14:1199–207.

38. Van Rijsingen IAW, van Der Zwaag PA, Groeneweg JA, *et al.* Outcome in phospholamban R14del carriers: results of a large multicentre cohort study. *Circ Cardiovasc Genet.* 2014;7:455–65.

39. Te Rijdt WP, van Tintelen JP, Vink A, *et al.* Phospholamban p.Arg14del cardiomyopathy is characterized by phospholamban aggregates, aggresomes, and autophagic degradation. *Histopathology.* 2016;69:542–50.

40. Eijgenraam TR, Boukens BJ, Boogerd CJ, *et al.* The phospholamban p.(Arg14del) pathogenic variant leads to cardiomyopathy with heart failure and is unresponsive to standard heart failure therapy. *Sci Rep.* 2020;10:16710.

41. Eijgenraam TR, Boogerd CJ, Stege NM, *et al.* Protein aggregation is an early manifestation of phospholamban p.(Arg14del)-related cardiomyopathy: development of PLN-R14del-cardiomyopathy. *Circ Heart Fail.* 2021;14:e008532.

42. Karakikes I, Stillitano F, Nonnenmacher M, *et al.* Correction of human phospholamban R14del mutation associated with cardiomyopathy using targeted nucleases and combination therapy. *Nat Commun.* 2015;6:6955.

43. Doevendans PA, Glijnis PC, Kranias EG. Leducq Transatlantic Network of Excellence to Cure phospholamban-Induced Cardiomyopathy (CURE-PLaN). *Circ Res.* 2019;125:720–4.

44. Grote Beverborg N, Später D, Knöll R, *et al.* Phospholamban antisense oligonucleotides improve cardiac function in murine cardiomyopathy. *Nat Commun.* 2021;12:5180.

45. Kim KH, Pereira NL. Genetics of cardiomyopathy: clinical and mechanistic implications for heart failure. *Korean Circ J.* 2021;51:797–836.

46. Kamisago M, Sharma SD, DePalma SR, *et al.* Mutations in sarcomere protein genes as a cause of dilated cardiomyopathy. *N Engl J Med.* 2000;343:1688–96.

47. Ortiz-Genga MF, Cuenca S, Dal Ferro M, *et al.* Truncating *FLNC* mutations are associated with high-risk dilated and arrhythmogenic cardiomyopathies. *J Am Coll Cardiol.* 2016;68:2440–51.

48. McNair WP, Sinagra G, Taylor MRG, *et al. SCN5A* mutations associate with arrhythmic dilated cardiomyopathy and commonly localize to the voltage-sensing mechanism. *J Am Coll Cardiol.* 2011;57:2160–8.

49. Elliott P, O'Mahony C, Syrris P, *et al.* Prevalence of desmosomal protein gene mutations in patients with dilated cardiomyopathy. *Circ Cardiovasc Genet.* 2010;3:314–22.

50. Koelemen J, Gotthardt M, Steinmetz LM, Meder B. RBM20-related cardiomyopathy: current understanding and future options. *J Clin Med.* 2021;10:4101.

51. Mazzarotto F, Tayal U, Buchan RJ, *et al.* Reevaluating the genetic contribution of monogenic dilated cardiomyopathy. *Circulation.* 2020;141:387–98.

52. Haas J, Frese KS, Peil B, *et al.* Atlas of the clinical genetics of human dilated cardiomyopathy. *Eur Heart J.* 2015;36:1123–35.

53. Verdonschot JAJ, Hazebroek MR, Ware JS, Prasad SK, Heymans SRB. Role of targeted therapy in dilated cardiomyopathy: the challenging road toward a personalized approach. *J Am Heart Assoc.* 2019;8:e012514.

54. Caforio ALP, Pankuweit S, Arbustini E, *et al.* Current state of knowledge on aetiology, diagnosis, management, and therapy of myocarditis: a position statement of the European Society of Cardiology Working Group on Myocardial and Pericardial Diseases. *Eur Heart J.* 2013;34:2636–48.

55. Thum T. SARS-CoV-2 receptor ACE2 expression in the human heart: cause of a post-pandemic wave of heart failure? *Eur Heart J.* 2020;41:1807–9.

56. Verdonschot JAJ, Merlo M, Dominguez F, *et al.* Phenotypic clustering of dilated cardiomyopathy patients highlights important pathophysiological differences. *Eur Heart J.* 2021;42:162–74.

57. Garnier S, Harakalova M, Weiss S, *et al.* Genome-wide association analysis in dilated cardiomyopathy reveals two new players in systolic heart failure on chromosomes 3p25.1 and 22q11.23. *Eur Heart J.* 2021;42:2000–11.

58. Villard E, Perret C, Gary F, *et al.* A genome-wide association study identifies two loci associated with heart failure due to dilated cardiomyopathy. *Eur Heart J.* 2011;32:1065–76.

59. Halliday BP, Wassall R, Lota AS, *et al.* Withdrawal of pharmacological treatment for heart failure in patients with recovered dilated cardiomyopathy (TRED-HF): an open-label, pilot, randomised trial. *Lancet.* 2019;393:61–73.

60. Van Rijsingen IAW, Arbustini E, Elliott PM, *et al.* Risk factors for malignant ventricular arrhythmias in lamin A/C mutation carriers a European cohort study. *J Am Coll Cardiol.* 2012;59: 493–500.

61. Corden B, Jarman J, Whiffin N, *et al.* Association of titin-truncating genetic variants with life-threatening cardiac arrhythmias in patients with dilated cardiomyopathy and implanted defibrillators. *JAMA Netw Open.* 2019;2:e196520.

62. Ware JS, Cook SA. Role of titin in cardiomyopathy: from DNA variants to patient stratification. *Nat Rev Cardiol.* 2018;15:241–52.

63. Echeverría LE, Marcus R, Novick G, *et al.* WHF IASC roadmap on Chagas disease. *Glob Heart.* 2020;15:26.

64. Kristensen SL, Levy WC, Shadman R, *et al.* Risk models for prediction of implantable cardioverter–defibrillator benefit: insights from the DANISH trial. *JACC Heart Fail.* 2019;7:717–24.

65. Køber L, Thune JJ, Nielsen JC, *et al.* Defibrillator implantation in patients with nonischemic systolic heart failure. *N Engl J Med.* 2016;375:1221–30.

66. Maron BJ, Gardin JM, Flack JM, Gidding SS, Kurosaki TT, Bild DE. Prevalence of hypertrophic cardiomyopathy in a general population of young adults. Echocardiographic analysis of 4111 subjects in the CARDIA Study. Coronary Artery Risk Development in (Young) Adults. *Circulation.* 1995;92:785–9.

67. Marian AJ, Braunwald E. Hypertrophic cardiomyopathy: genetics, pathogenesis, clinical manifestations, diagnosis, and therapy. *Circ Res.* 2017;121:749–70.

68. Cahill TJ, Ashrafian H, Watkins H. Genetic cardiomyopathies causing heart failure. *Circ Res.* 2013;113:660–75.

69. McKenna WJ, Judge DP. Epidemiology of the inherited cardiomyopathies. *Nat Rev Cardiol.* 2021;18:22–36.

70. Ingles J, Semsarian C. Making the case for cascade screening among families with inherited heart disease. *Hear Rhythm.* 2020;17: 113–14.

71. Behrens-Gawlik V, Mearini G, Gedicke-Hornung C, Richard P, Carrier L. *MYBPC3* in hypertrophic cardiomyopathy: from mutation identification to RNA-based correction. *Pflugers Arch.* 2014;466:215–23.

72. Carrier L, Mearini G, Stathopoulou K, Cuello F. Cardiac myosin-binding protein C (*MYBPC3*) in cardiac pathophysiology. *Gene.* 2015;573:188–97.

73. Carrier L. Targeting the population for gene therapy with *MYBPC3.* *J Mol Cell Cardiol.* 2021;150:101–8.

74. Marston S, Copeland O, Gehmlich K, Schlossarek S, Carrier L. How do *MYBPC3* mutations cause hypertrophic cardiomyopathy? 2012;33:75–80.

75. Marston S, Copeland O, Jacques A, *et al.* Evidence from human myectomy samples that *MYBPC3* mutations cause hypertrophic cardiomyopathy through haploinsufficiency. *Circ Res.* 2009;105:219–22.

76. Van Dijk SJ, Dooijes D, Dos Remedios C, *et al.* Cardiac myosin-binding protein C mutations and hypertrophic cardiomyopathy: haploinsufficiency, deranged phosphorylation, and cardiomyocyte dysfunction. *Circulation.* 2009;119:1473–83.

77. Friedrich FW, Wilding BR, Reischmann S, *et al.* Evidence for *FHL1* as a novel disease gene for isolated hypertrophic cardiomyopathy. *Hum Mol Genet.* 2012;21:3237–54.

78. Osio A, Tan L, Chen SN, *et al.* Myozenin 2 is a novel gene for human hypertrophic cardiomyopathy. *Circ Res.* 2007;100:766–8.

79. Viereck J, Bührke A, Foinquinos A, *et al.* Targeting muscle-enriched long non-coding RNA H19 reverses pathological cardiac hypertrophy. *Eur Heart J.* 2020;41:3462–74.

80. Gómez J, Lorca R, Reguero JR, *et al.* Genetic variation at the long noncoding RNA H19 gene is associated with the risk of hypertrophic cardiomyopathy. *Epigenomics.* 2018;10:865–73.

81. Walsh R, Thomson KL, Ware JS, *et al.* Reassessment of Mendelian gene pathogenicity using 7,855 cardiomyopathy cases and 60,706 reference samples. 2017;19:192–203.

82. Ingles J, Goldstein J, Thaxton C, *et al.* Evaluating the clinical validity of hypertrophic cardiomyopathy genes. *Circ Genomic Precis Med.* 2019;12:57–64.

83. Jordan E, Peterson L, Ai T, *et al.* An evidence-based assessment of genes in dilated cardiomyopathy. *Circulation.* 2021;144:7–19.

84. Schlossarek S, Englmann DR, Sultan KR, Sauer M, Eschenhagen T, Carrier L. Defective proteolytic systems in *Mybpc3*-targeted mice with cardiac hypertrophy. *Basic Res Cardiol.* 2012;107:235.

85. Singh SR, Zech ATL, Geertz B, *et al.* Activation of autophagy ameliorates cardiomyopathy in *Mybpc3*-targeted knockin mice. *Circ Heart Fail.* 2017;10:e004140.

86. Nollet EE, Daan Westenbrink B, de Boer RA, Kuster DWD, van der Velden J. Unraveling the genotype–phenotype relationship in hypertrophic cardiomyopathy: obesity-related cardiac defects as a major disease modifier. *J Am Heart Assoc.* 2020;9:e01864.

87. Van Der Velden J, Tocchetti CG, Varricchi G, *et al.* Metabolic changes in hypertrophic cardiomyopathies: scientific update from the working group of myocardial function of the European Society of Cardiology. *Cardiovasc Res.* 2018;114:1273–80.

88. Greaves SC, Roche AHG, Neutze JM, Whitlock RML, Veale AMO. Inheritance of hypertrophic cardiomyopathy: a cross sectional and M mode echocardiographic study of 50 families. *Br Heart J.* 1987;58:259–66.

89. Bagnall RD, Ingles J, Dinger ME, *et al.* Whole genome sequencing improves outcomes of genetic testing in patients with hypertrophic cardiomyopathy. *J Am Coll Cardiol.* 2018;72:419–29.

90. Spertus JA, Fine JT, Elliott P, *et al.* Mavacamten for treatment of symptomatic obstructive hypertrophic cardiomyopathy (EXPLORER-HCM): health status analysis of a randomised, double-blind, placebo-controlled, phase 3 trial. *Lancet.* 2021;397: 2467–75.

91. Olivotto I, Oreziak A, Barriales-Villa R, *et al.* Mavacamten for treatment of symptomatic obstructive hypertrophic cardiomyopathy (EXPLORER-HCM): a randomised, double-blind, placebo-controlled, phase 3 trial. *Lancet.* 2020;396:759–69.

92. Rohde JA, Roopnarine O, Thomas DD, Muretta JM. Mavacamten stabilizes an autoinhibited state of two-headed cardiac myosin. *Proc Natl Acad Sci U S A.* 2018;115:E7486–94.

93. Mathew J, Zahavich L, Lafreniere-Roula M, *et al.* Utility of genetics for risk stratification in pediatric hypertrophic cardiomyopathy. *Clin Genet.* 2018;93:310–19.

94. Ho CY, Day SM, Ashley EA, *et al.* Genotype and lifetime burden of disease in hypertrophic cardiomyopathy: insights from the sarcomeric human cardiomyopathy registry (SHaRe). *Circulation.* 2018;138:1387–98.

95. Mearini G, Stimpel D, Geertz B, *et al. Mybpc3* gene therapy for neonatal cardiomyopathy enables long-term disease prevention in mice. *Nat Commun.* 2014;5:5515.

96. Mearini G, Stimpel D, Krämer E, *et al.* Repair of Mybpc3 mRNA by 5′-trans-splicing in a mouse model of hypertrophic cardiomyopathy. *Mol Ther Nucleic Acids.* 2013;2:e102.

97. Dutsch A, Wijnker PJM, Schlossarek S, *et al.* Phosphomimetic cardiac myosin-binding protein C partially rescues a cardiomyopathy phenotype in murine engineered heart tissue. *Sci Rep.* 2019;9:18152.

98. Wijnker PJM, Friedrich FW, Dutsch A, *et al.* Comparison of the effects of a truncating and a missense *MYBPC3* mutation on contractile parameters of engineered heart tissue. *J Mol Cell Cardiol.* 2016;97:82–92.

99. Prondzynski M, Krämer E, Laufer SD, *et al.* Evaluation of *MYBPC3* trans-splicing and gene replacement as therapeutic options in human iPSC-derived cardiomyocytes. *Mol Ther Nucleic Acids.* 2017;7:475–86.

100. Li J, Mamidi R, Doh CY, *et al.* AAV9 gene transfer of cMyBPC N-terminal domains ameliorates cardiomyopathy in cMyBPC-deficient mice. *JCI Insight.* 2020;5:e130182.

101. Nair V, Belanger EC, Veinot JP. Lysosomal storage disorders affecting the heart: a review. *Cardiovasc Pathol.* 2019;39:12–24.

102. Aerts JM, Groener JE, Kuiper S, *et al.* Elevated globotriaosylsphingosine is a hallmark of Fabry disease. *Proc Natl Acad Sci U S A.* 2008;105:2812–17.

103. Linhart A, Germain DP, Olivotto I, *et al.* An expert consensus document on the management of cardiovascular manifestations of Fabry disease. *Eur J Heart Fail.* 2020;22:1076–96.

104. Lin HY, Chong KW, Hsu JH, *et al.* High incidence of the cardiac variant of Fabry disease revealed by newborn screening in the Taiwan Chinese population. *Circ Cardiovasc Genet.* 2009;2:450–6.

105. Doheny D, Srinivasan R, Pagant S, Chen B, Yasuda M, Desnick RJ. Fabry disease: prevalence of affected males and heterozygotes with pathogenic *GLA* mutations identified by screening renal, cardiac and stroke clinics, 1995–2017. *J Med Genet.* 2018;55:261–8.

106. Ferreira S, Auray-Blais C, Boutin M, *et al.* Variations in the *GLA* gene correlate with globotriaosylceramide and globotriaosylsphingosine analog levels in urine and plasma. *Clin Chim Acta.* 2015;447:96–104.

107. Maruyama H, Miyata K, Mikame M, *et al.* Effectiveness of plasma lyso-Gb3 as a biomarker for selecting high-risk patients with Fabry disease from multispecialty clinics for genetic analysis. *Genet Med.* 2019;21:44–52.

108. Weidemann F, Niemann M, Breunig F, *et al.* Long-term effects of enzyme replacement therapy on Fabry cardiomyopathy: evidence for a better outcome with early treatment. *Circulation.* 2009;119:524–9.

109. Liu HC, Lin HY, Yang CF, *et al.* Globotriaosylsphingosine (lyso-Gb3) might not be a reliable marker for monitoring the long-term therapeutic outcomes of enzyme replacement therapy for late-onset Fabry patients with the Chinese hotspot mutation (IVS4+919G>A). *Orphanet J Rare Dis.* 2014;9:111.

110. Oliveira JP, Ferreira S. Multiple phenotypic domains of Fabry disease and their relevance for establishing genotype–phenotype correlations. *Appl Clin Genet.* 2019;12:35–50.

111. Sliwa K, Bauersachs J, Arany Z, Spracklen TF, Hilfiker-Kleiner D. Peripartum cardiomyopathy: from genetics to management. *Eur Heart J.* 2021;42:3094–102.

112. Repetti GG, Toepfer CN, Seidman JG, Seidman CE. Novel therapies for prevention and early treatment of cardiomyopathies. *Circ Res.* 2019;124:1536–50.

113. Khan A, Barber DL, Huang J, *et al.* Lentivirus-mediated gene therapy for Fabry disease. *Nat Commun.* 2021;12:1178.

114. Vardarli I, Weber M, Rischpler C, Führer D, Herrmann K, Weidemann F. Fabry cardiomyopathy: current treatment and future options. *J Clin Med.* 2021;10:3026.

115. DeRosa F, Smith L, Shen Y, *et al.* Improved efficacy in a Fabry disease model using a systemic mRNA liver depot system as compared to enzyme replacement therapy. *Mol Ther.* 2019;27:878–89.

3.4.2 Dilated and hypokinetic non-dilated cardiomyopathy

Petar M Seferović, Biykem Bozkurt, and Marija Polovina

Definition

Dilated cardiomyopathy (DCM) refers to a variety of heterogeneous myocardial disorders that result in left ventricular (LV) or biventricular dilatation associated with systolic dysfunction, in the absence of abnormal loading conditions (hypertension, valvular or congenital heart disease) and significant ischaemic heart disease.[1,2] Hypokinetic non-DCM is defined as LV or biventricular global systolic dysfunction (i.e. left ventricular ejection fraction (LVEF) <45%) without chamber dilatation.[1] The clinical presentation, natural course, and treatment possibilities are significantly influenced by the diverse aetiologies of DCM (e.g. genetic, inflammatory, infectious, cardiotoxicity, endocrine, or neuromuscular abnormalities, cardiotoxicity) and variable underlying mechanisms responsible for the disease. In addition, other cardiomyopathies (e.g. hypertrophic or infiltrative cardiomyopathies) can evolve into a dilated form over time.[3] In order to improve diagnostic and prognostic precision in DCM, the MOGE(S) classification of cardiomyopathies has been proposed, which includes assessment of the morphofunctional phenotype (M), organ involvement (O), genetic inheritance (G), aetiology (E), and functional status (S) of the disease.[4]

Epidemiology

The reported incidence of DCM varies across the continents, which may be due to underreporting, changes in definition and diagnostic capabilities, and geographical, environmental, and genetic variation.[3] In Western populations, the annual incidence of DCM is about 5–8 cases per 100,000 people and the prevalence is 36 patients per 100,000 of the population.[2] Compared with Western countries, the reported prevalence of DCM may be lower in Eastern Asia (14 cases per 100,000 people in Japan) and higher in some parts of Africa and Latin America.[2] With increasing rates of predisposing risk factors (e.g. obesity, diabetes, cardiotoxicity, rise in infectious aetiologies) and an improvement in diagnostic capabilities, the prevalence of DCM will likely increase.

DCM is one of the leading causes of heart failure with reduced ejection fraction (HFrEF). In most multicentre randomized trials on HFrEF, approximately 12–35% of enrolled patients had DCM.[2] These estimates are approximate because of a lack of full diagnostic assessment for DCM in most trials. Likewise, the prevalence of DCM in observational studies of patients with heart failure (HF) varies broadly (8–47%), which reflects considerable heterogeneity in diagnostic precision in different clinical settings.[2] According to the Acute Decompensated Heart Failure National Registry (ADHERE) from the United States, 47% of patients admitted to hospital with HF have DCM.[5] Similarly, in a large HF registry encompassing the European Society of Cardiology (ESC) member countries, non-ischaemic aetiologies account for 46% of patients with acute HF, and for 57% of those with chronic HF, but the true prevalence of DCM remains unclear.[6] According to the ESC Cardiomyopathy Registry, DCM is the second most frequent cardiomyopathy (preceded by hypertrophic cardiomyopathy) identified in 39% of enrolled patients.[7] Data from observational studies suggest that the incidence of DCM is higher in men, compared to women.[8]

Aetiology and pathophysiology

A wide spectrum of aetiologies have been identified in DCM, including pathogenic gene variants, infections, autoimmunity, toxins, medications, and endocrine and metabolic abnormalities (➔ Figure 3.4.2.1). In some instances, DCM becomes clinically manifest following an interaction of multiple factors, including a predisposing pathogenic gene variant and subsequent exposure to acquired causes (e.g. toxins, tachyarrhythmias, alcohol abuse, pregnancy, etc.) and/or disease modifiers (i.e. conditions that can aggravate DCM such as systemic infection, common comorbidities, etc.). Regardless of the inciting event(s), the development of DCM is perpetuated by maladaptive mechanisms, including alterations in signal transduction, contractile performance, neurohormonal processes, and cardiac metabolism, biomechanical defects, and cardiac fibrosis.

Most cases of DCM are non-familial (sporadic), whereas a familial form (defined as the presence of DCM in two or more first- or second-degree relatives, or the presence of autopsy-proven DCM in a first-degree relative with sudden cardiac death (SCD) at <50 years of age) accounts for 30–50% of cases.[1,9] Genetic causes can be determined in approximately 40% of patients, including approximately 10% of those with sporadic DCM.[10] Pathogenic variants encompass mutations in genes encoding sarcomere proteins, the cytoskeleton, nuclear envelope, and sarcolemma, ion channels, and/or intercellular junction molecules. Over 100 genes have been implicated in the development of DCM, either as an isolated condition or as part of a clinical syndrome (e.g. Duchenne/Becker muscular dystrophy, Emery–Dreifuss muscular dystrophy, spinocerebellar ataxia, Barth syndrome, etc.).[11] Most mutations follow an autosomal dominant pattern of inheritance, but autosomal recessive, X-linked, and matrilineal patterns of inheritance (i.e. affecting mitochondrial DNA) have been described. Truncating mutations in the titin gene are the most common, accounting for approximately 25% and 18% of familial and sporadic cases of DCM, respectively.[12] Titin-truncating variants can be associated with ventricular arrhythmias and enhanced cardiac fibrosis. Mutations in genes encoding nuclear envelope proteins (*LMNA* and *EMD*), filamin (*FLN*), ribonucleic acid binding motif 20 (*RBM20*), and phospholamban (*PLN*) have been associated with conduction abnormalities and a high risk of supraventricular and ventricular arrhythmias.[13] Of note, malignant ventricular

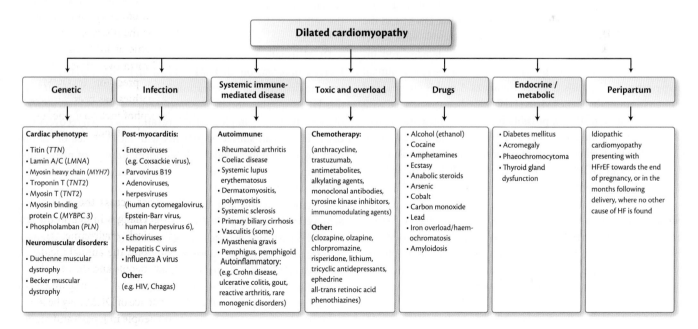

Figure 3.4.2.1 Aetiologies of dilated cardiomyopathy.

Seferović PM, Polovina M, Bauersachs J, *et al.* Heart failure in cardiomyopathies: a position paper from the Heart Failure Association of the European Society of Cardiology. *Eur J Heart Fail.* 2019 May;21(5):553–576. doi: 10.1002/ejhf.1461. Reprinted by permission of John Wiley and Sons on behalf of the European Society of Cardiology.

arrhythmias can occur regardless of the severity of LV dysfunction in carriers of those gene mutations, which underlies the significance of genetic testing for risk stratification of SCD in affected patients. An overlap in genetic causes of different cardiomyopathies is possible, depending on the type and position of the mutations. Pathological genetic variants in sarcomeric proteins (troponin, β-myosin heavy chain, or α-myosin heavy chain) can cause DCM or hypertrophic (or less frequently restrictive) cardiomyopathy,[14,15] whereas mutations in desmosomal proteins, usually associated with arrhythmogenic right ventricular cardiomyopathy, have been identified as a cause of DCM with a high risk of malignant arrhythmias.[16,17] As a further illustration of the genetic complexity in DCM, a multinational study including 639 patients with sporadic and familial DCM demonstrated that approximately 38% of patients had compound (multiple disease) mutations or combined heterozygous mutations, and approximately 13% had ≥3 mutations.[18]

Viral infection with activation of immune-mediated myocardial damage is also an important cause of DCM. Enteroviruses (e.g. Coxsackie B virus) and adenoviruses can cause myocarditis that can progress to DCM, involving three phases.[19] Firstly, viral infection causes acute myocyte damage, leading to activation of the innate and acquired immune systems. In the second phase, immune system activation can lead to viral clearance and recovery (healed myocarditis), or it can perpetuate myocardial damage by direct cytotoxicity (due to viral persistence) or immune-mediated mechanisms such as molecular mimicry (i.e. immune-mediated attack on myocardial proteins that bear similarities to viral proteins) and autoantibodies directed against cellular molecules. These processes can cause substantial myocardial loss and replacement fibrosis, leading to the development of DCM in the final phase. The role of parvovirus B19 infection in myocarditis and the development of DCM has not been confirmed, but it is suggested that high copy numbers of viral DNA (>500 viral DNA copies per microgram of cardiac DNA) and the presence of actively replicating virus (with detectible viral RNA) could be implicated in severe endothelial cell damage and inflammatory myocardial response.[20,21] Herpesviruses (e.g. human herpesvirus 6), hepatitis C virus, influenza A and B viruses, and human immunodeficiency virus (HIV) have been associated with the development of DCM, possibly by immune-mediated mechanisms. Severe acute respiratory syndrome coronavirus 2 (SARS-CoV-2) has been shown to cause myocarditis,[22] but its role in the development of DCM has not yet been established. In addition to being caused by viruses, DCM can rarely result from bacterial infection with *Borrelia burgdorferi* in Lyme disease and from parasitic infestation with *Trypanosoma cruzi* in Chagas disease. Immune-mediated mechanisms are responsible for the development of DCM in autoimmune diseases (e.g. rheumatoid arthritis, systemic lupus erythematosus, dermatomyositis, polymyositis) and autoinflammatory disorders (e.g. inflammatory bowel disease, vasculitis).[23]

DCM can occur following exposure to toxic agents (e.g. alcohol abuse, illicit drugs, iron overload/haemochromatosis) and medications (Figure 3.4.2.1). In particular, cardiotoxicity of cancer therapies has become an important cause of serious adverse effects responsible for premature treatment discontinuation and increased mortality. Multiple cancer therapies have been implicated in the development of myocardial dysfunction and HF. The most investigated is anthracycline cardiotoxicity (doxorubicin, idarubicin, daunorubicin, and epirubicin), which results from impairment in mitochondrial function and cellular membrane damage caused by increased production of reactive oxygen species.[24] Myocardial damage becomes irreversible following administration of a cumulative lifetime dose of an anthracycline, with considerable variability in individual susceptibility, likely reflecting differences in genetic predisposition and acquired risk factors (such as pre-existing cardiovascular disease and radiotherapy).[25] Other cancer therapies that can cause myocardial dysfunction and HF include alkylating agents (cyclophosphamide), cisplatin, taxanes (paclitaxel and docetaxel), growth-promoting human epidermal growth factor receptor 2 (HER2)-targeted therapies (trastuzumab, pertuzumab), tyrosine kinase inhibitors (sunitinib, pazopanib, sorafenib), and immune checkpoint inhibitors.[25,26]

In some instances, DCM can be caused by endocrine and metabolic abnormalities, nutritional deficiencies, and persistent or repetitive supraventricular/ventricular tachycardia (tachycardia-induced cardiomyopathy) (Figure 3.4.2.1). DCM occurring towards the end of pregnancy or in the months following delivery is defined as peripartum cardiomyopathy. Other causes of cardiomyopathy should be ruled out in these patients.

The characteristic pathological changes in cardiac anatomy associated with DCM are presented in Figure 3.4.2.2.

Natural history

The natural course of DCM, including development and progression of HF, and the risk of SCD vary significantly, depending on the aetiology, age of onset (paediatric DCM tends to have a worse prognosis), sex, and impact of treatment.[27,28]

DCM usually presents with symptomatic HF. A study of patients with recent-onset DCM (<6 months) demonstrated that HF was the first clinical presentation in 32%, while 66% had at least one HF hospitalization before enrolment.[29] Following an episode of new-onset HF, complete structural and functional recovery can occur in a small subset of patients without evidence of significant myocardial loss, which allows normalization of myocardial function upon cessation of the inciting event (e.g. intoxication, inflammation, arrhythmias). More frequently, stabilization of contractile function and remission of HF symptoms could be achieved with use of guideline-directed therapies (GDT) for HF. Over the past four decades, the prognosis of DCM has become more favourable, reflecting earlier diagnosis and wider implementation of GDT.[12] Accordingly, a single-centre study demonstrated a substantial improvement in survival free of HF death/heart transplantation in DCM (i.e. 55%, 71%, and 87% survival rates, respectively, at 8-yearly intervals between 1978 and 2007) with use of GDT, while the risk of SCD declined substantially in recent

Dilated cardiomyopathy

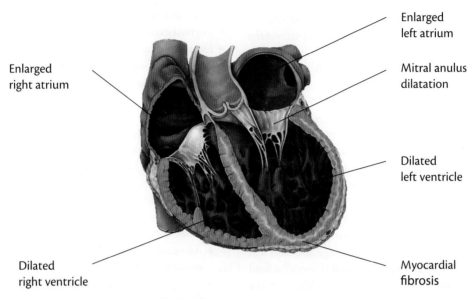

Enlarged left atrium

Mitral anulus dilatation

Dilated left ventricle

Myocardial fibrosis

Dilated right ventricle

Enlarged right atrium

Enlarged left atrium

Figure 3.4.2.2 Characteristic pathoanatomical changes in dilated cardiomyopathy.
Seferović PM, Polovina M, Bauersachs J, *et al*. Heart failure in cardiomyopathies: a position paper from the Heart Failure Association of the European Society of Cardiology. *Eur J Heart Fail*. 2019 May;21(5):553–576. doi: 10.1002/ejhf.1461. Reprinted by permission of John Wiley and Sons on behalf of the European Society of Cardiology.

years, with more widespread use of implantable cardioverter–defibrillators (ICDs).[30] Timely GDT implementation provides an opportunity for improvement in LV contractile function. Indeed, a significant proportion of patients (approximately 30–70%, depending on the criteria) with newly diagnosed DCM experience LV reverse remodelling, which is associated with a lower risk of mortality, including SCD.[29,31,32] LV reverse remodelling occurs more frequently in women and patients with higher baseline LVEF, lesser degree of LV enlargement,[32] and lower extent of late gadolinium enhancement (LGE) on cardiac magnetic resonance (CMR) imaging.[29] Importantly, in those individuals who experience recovery of LV function, continuation of GDT is crucial, as a randomized study (TRED HF) indicated that withdrawal of GDT resulted in a relapse of LV dysfunction in 40% of patients at 6 months.[33]

Despite advances in HF treatment, a significant proportion of patients with DCM will progress to advanced HF. DCM accounts for >40% of patients receiving long-term mechanical circulatory support and represents the most frequent indication for heart transplantation and the third most frequent indication for heart and lung transplantation in adults.[34,35] As shown in ❯ Box 3.4.2.1, there are a number of parameters, in addition to GDT, that predict the progression of HF in patients with DCM.

The risk of arrhythmia is also high in DCM. According to the ESC Cardiomyopathy Registry, the rate of major arrhythmic events (i.e. SCD or resuscitated ventricular fibrillation/cardiac arrest or sustained ventricular tachycardia) in a contemporary

Box 3.4.2.1 Factors associated with poor prognosis in patients with dilated cardiomyopathy

- Older age (>60 years)
- Significant left ventricular enlargement
- Significant right ventricular enlargement
- Reduced left and/or right ventricular ejection fraction
- Right-sided heart failure
- Advanced New York Heart Association class (NYHA class III or IV)
- Peak oxygen consumption <10–12 mL/kg/min
- Recurrent heart failure hospitalizations
- Persistent S_3 gallop
- Pulmonary hypertension
- Hypotension
- Moderate-to-severe mitral regurgitation
- ECG findings of LBBB, persistent tachycardia, and wide QRS
- Recurrent ventricular tachycardia
- Elevated levels of natriuretic peptides (NT-proBNP or BNP)
- Elevated cardiac troponin
- Reduced eGFR
- Elevated transaminase and bilirubin levels
- Hyponatraemia
- Pronounced mid-wall myocardial LGE on CMR imaging

ECG, electrocardiogram; LBBB, left bundle branch block; NT-proBNP, N-terminal pro-B-type natriuretic peptide; BNP, B-type natriuretic peptide; eGFR, estimated glomerular filtration rate; LGE, late gadolinium contrast; CMR, cardiac magnetic resonance.

cohort of 1105 adults with DCM was 6.1% per year, slightly exceeding the annual rate (5.1%) of major HF events (i.e. HF death or heart transplant or ventricular assist device implantation).[36] Almost 30% of patients had a history of atrial fibrillation (AF) at baseline, and new-onset AF was documented in 5.5% at 1-year follow-up.[36] Ventricular arrhythmias occurred at 1-year follow-up in 8.2% and 15.1% of ICD carriers for primary and secondary prevention, respectively.

The rate of total cardiovascular mortality (3.3% per year) is higher in patients with DCM, compared to that in patients with other cardiomyopathies (hypertrophic and arrhythmogenic),[36] and pump failure in advanced HF remains the most prevalent cause of death responsible for approximately 70% of cardiovascular deaths, while SCD accounts for the remaining approximately 30%.[37] There is also a high risk of non-cardiovascular mortality (deaths due to cancer, infections, pulmonary disease, or haemorrhage), which increases with older age and greater severity of HF and accounts for approximately a third of total deaths in patients with DCM.[38,39] Registry data also indicated that patients with familial DCM tend to be diagnosed at a younger age and with less severe phenotype, unlike patients with a sporadic form who tend to be older and with more cardiovascular comorbidities at the time of diagnosis. Nevertheless, 1-year outcomes were similar for both the familial and sporadic forms.[40]

Diagnostic strategies

Patients with DCM should undergo thorough diagnostic evaluation, including a common diagnostic approach appropriate for all patients with HF, and further targeted assessment to establish a specific aetiology (or aetiologies) of DCM.[1] Diagnostic assessment of patients with DCM is summarized in ➲ Box 3.4.2.2.

Baseline evaluation should include a detailed history, including detailed family history for hereditary causes, complete physical examination, assessment of comorbidities, diagnostic tests, including an electrocardiogram (ECG), chest X-ray, and baseline laboratory analysis, as well as standard transthoracic echocardiographic examination.

ECG has a low specificity for DCM, but a completely normal ECG is infrequent (10%) and therefore has a high negative predictive value to rule out DCM. The most frequent ECG abnormalities include non-specific QRS prolongation and fragmentation, bundle branch blocks, T-wave inversion, unexplained LV hypertrophy, atrioventricular conduction abnormalities, ventricular premature complexes (VPCs), and AF.[41]

Transthoracic echocardiographic examination is the first-line imaging tool for diagnosis, follow-up, and planning of treatment (e.g. valve interventions, mechanical circulatory support) in patients with DCM and for screening of their family members. Echocardiographic diagnostic criteria for DCM are presented in ➲ Box 3.4.2.3.

The echocardiographic hallmark of DCM is LV systolic disfunction, defined as reduced LVEF of <45% and LV (or biventricular) dilatation. Hypokinetic non-DCM is characterized by LV or biventricular global systolic dysfunction (defined as

Box 3.4.2.2 Diagnostic assessment in patients with suspected dilated cardiomyopathy

- Patient history and family history (know cardiomyopathy, neuromuscular disease, sudden cardiac death in relatives <50 years old), review of comorbidities
- Physical examination
- Electrocardiography
- Transthoracic echocardiography
- Ambulatory electrocardiogram (Holter) monitoring (24- or 48-hour)
- Chest X-ray
- Laboratory analysis: troponin, creatine kinase, natriuretic peptides, liver and renal function, full blood count, glycosylated haemoglobin (HbA1c), thyroid function, iron status (ferritin and transferrin saturation), markers of autoimmune diseases
- Invasive coronary angiography or computed tomography coronary angiography
- Cardiac magnetic resonance imaging:
  - Assessment of left and right ventricular volumes, mass, and ejection fraction
  - Tissue characterization: storage infiltration inflammation, fibrosis, and scarring
- Endomyocardial biopsy:
  - Histopathology: standard plus specific staining techniques
  - Immunohistochemistry: standard plus additional immunohistochemical staining for lamin A/C, dystrophin, etc.
  - Quantitative RT-PCR: viruses and *Borrelia*
  - Genetic testing: *TTN*, *LMNA*, *MHC*, *TNNT*, troponin-C, *MYBPC1*, *RBM20*, *PLN*, sodium channel α unit, BAG3, actin α cardiac muscle, nexilin, tropomyosin-1, vinculin

TTN, gene encoding titin; *LMNA*, gene encoding lamin A/C; *TNNT*; gene encoding troponin T; *MYBPC1*, gene encoding myosin-binding protein C1; *RBM20*, gene encoding RNA-binding motif protein 20; *PLN*, gene encoding phospholamban; *BAG3*, gene encoding co-chaperone 3.

Source data from McDonagh TA, Metra M, Adamo M, Gardner RS, Baumbach A, Böhm M, et al. 2021 ESC Guidelines for the diagnosis and treatment of acute and chronic heart failure: Developed by the Task Force for the diagnosis and treatment of acute and chronic heart failure of the European Society of Cardiology (ESC) With the special contribution of the Heart Failure Association (HFA) of the ESC. *European Heart Journal*. 2021.

LVEF <45%) without dilatation. With progression of the disease, the geometry of the left ventricle assumes a more spherical shape (an increase in the sphericity index—a ratio between the short and long axis of the left ventricle). LV wall thickness is normal or only slightly increased and there is global LV hypocontractility and sometimes regional wall motion abnormalities (hypokinesis/akinesis) that do not follow the coronary artery distribution. In some cases, evidence of LV mechanical dyssynchrony is also present. LV enlargement leads to mitral annulus dilatation, papillary apparatus displacement, leaflet tethering and malcoaptation that result in secondary (functional) mitral regurgitation (MR) and left atrial enlargement. Evidence of LV diastolic dysfunction is also present. In some cases, loss of LV contractile function leads to spontaneous echo contrast and LV thrombi formation. The

Box 3.4.2.3 Echocardiographic diagnostic criteria for (1) dilated cardiomyopathy and (2) non-dilated hypokinetic cardiomyopathy

1. LV or biventricular systolic dysfunction (defined as LVEF <45%) and dilatation* that are not explained by abnormal loading conditions or coronary heart disease
2. LV or biventricular global systolic dysfunction (defined as LVEF <45%) without dilatation, that is not explained by abnormal loading conditions or coronary heart disease

*LV dilatation is defined as: LV end-diastolic volume or diameter >2 standard deviations from normal, according to nomograms corrected for body surface area and age or for body surface area and gender.

LV, left ventricular; LVEF, left ventricular ejection fraction.

Source data from Donal E, Delgado V, Bucciarelli-Ducci C, Galli E, Haugaa KH, Charron P, et al. Multimodality imaging in the diagnosis, risk stratification, and management of patients with dilated cardiomyopathies: an expert consensus document from the European Association of Cardiovascular Imaging. *Eur Heart J Cardiovasc Imaging.* 2019;20(10):1075–93.

right ventricle may be normal, or right ventricular enlargement and dysfunction can occur because of biventricular involvement or pulmonary hypertension. RV dilatation/dysfunction is frequently accompanied by functional tricuspid regurgitation.

ECG Holter monitoring (24-hour or 48-hour) is useful for the assessment of cardiac rhythm disorders, in particular, in patients suspected of having tachycardia-induced cardiomyopathy and arrhythmogenic cardiomyopathy.

In all patients, visualization of coronary arteries is mandatory to rule out ischaemic heart disease. The diagnostic test of choice (e.g. non-invasive testing with stress echocardiography, nuclear stress testing, computed tomography (CT) angiography, invasive coronary angiography) may vary according to the pretest probability of coronary heart disease and risk factors. In patients with a low to intermediate pretest probability or those with an equivocal non-invasive stress test, CT coronary angiography may be utilized, whereas in those with a high pretest probability or a positive non-invasive stress test, invasive coronary angiography should be performed.[1]

CMR imaging with T1 and T2 sequencing and LGE is the most precise imaging tool in the assessment of LV and right ventricular volumes, mass, and ejection fraction, but also for tissue characterization. CMR can provide evidence of myocardial inflammation (in myocarditis and inflammatory cardiomyopathy), based on specific diagnostic criteria with T1-weighted and T2-weighted mapping techniques and use of LGE. Apparently, myocardial inflammation is present if at least one T2-weighted criterion (i.e. global or regional increase of myocardial T2 relaxation time or increased signal intensity in T2-weighted images) and at least one T1-based criterion (increased myocardial T1, extracellular volume, or LGE) are present.[42] Even if only one criterion is present, there is a strong possibility of inflammation. CMR imaging can be useful in the diagnosis of infiltrative cardiomyopathies (sarcoidosis, amyloidosis, haemochromatosis with T2* imaging, storage diseases such as Fabry disease), structural anomalies such as non-compaction cardiomyopathy, and

arrhythmogenic cardiomyopathy. It is the preferred imaging method to assess myocardial fibrosis using LGE along with T1 mapping. Moreover, CMR imaging can provide important prognostic information, given that approximately one-third of DCM patients demonstrate mid-wall interventricular LGE (i.e. a sign of replacement fibrosis), which has an incremental predictive value to LVEF for a higher risk of all-cause and cardiovascular mortality, including SCD.[43]

Endomyocardial biopsy (EMB) can be useful in selected patients presenting with recent-onset HF refractory to standard treatment, after exclusion of other specific aetiologies. In this setting, EMB can be useful to confirm a specific diagnosis that would influence therapy, such as giant cell myocarditis, myocardial infiltrative processes (e.g. cardiac sarcoidosis, cardiac amyloidosis), and inflammatory cardiomyopathy, when a diagnosis cannot be achieved by other non-invasive means.[44]

Identification of pathological gene variants can aid in diagnostic and prognostic assessment, including disease progression and the risk of SCD. All patients with DCM or hypokinetic non-DCM and all first-degree adult relatives of patients with diagnosed cardiomyopathy should undergo genetic testing and counselling.[1]

When suspected, additional laboratory testing for aetiologies such as infections (e.g. HIV, Lyme disease, Chagas disease), illicit drugs (e.g. cocaine, metamphetamine), autoimmune diseases (serology), haemochromatosis (e.g. ferritin level, genetic testing), and cardiac amyloidosis (serum and urine monoclonal light chains, serum and urine immunofixation electrophoresis, serum free light chains) can be useful.

Management strategies

Two important aspects need to be considered in the treatment of patients with DCM. Firstly, contemporary guidelines recommend the use of HF-related treatment, which includes pharmacological and device therapies with a proven benefit in HFrEF, in all patients with DCM. Additionally, when a specific management strategy is available for a specific aetiology, aetiology-related therapy should be considered.

Heart-failure related therapy

Available evidence indicates that pharmacological therapies, including angiotensin-converting enzyme inhibitors (ACEIs) or angiotensin receptor–neprilysin inhibitors (or angiotensin receptor blockers), beta-blockers, mineralocorticoid receptor antagonists, and sodium–glucose cotransporter 2 inhibitors, are beneficial in both ischaemic and non-ischaemic HFrEF, including patients with DCM. Major clinical trials of those medications included a substantial proportion (approximately 20–50%) of patients with non-ischaemic HFrEF or idiopathic DCM, and there was no evidence of heterogeneity (or difference) according to HF aetiology (ischaemic vs non-ischaemic). As noted above, the TRED-HF trial demonstrated a risk of relapse following withdrawal of GDT in patients with recovered LV function,[33] suggesting that improvement in function represents remission, rather than permanent recovery, for many patients with DCM and that therapy for HF should be continued unless the aetiology is fully reversible.

Furthermore, device therapy (ICDs and cardiac resynchronization therapy (CRT)) should be considered in indicated patients with DCM. The DANISH trial raised concerns that primary ICD implantation in patients with non-ischaemic HF (including DCM) does not reduce all-cause mortality.[39] However, a sub-analysis of that trial suggested there was a significant benefit for all-cause mortality in individuals ≤70 years old.[45] Survival benefit was also confirmed in a meta-analysis (including six primary and two secondary prevention trials enrolling patients with non-ischaemic HF) that assessed effects on survival with primary ICD implantation in non-ischaemic HF.[46] Nevertheless, favourable effects were reduced by inclusion of the DANISH trial where background use of contemporary pharmacological therapy and CRT was high, and both treatment modalities have proven benefit for decreasing mortality.[46] Therefore, the ESC guidelines recommend ICD implantation for risk reduction of SCD and all-cause mortality in symptomatic patients with DCM with an LVEF of ≤35% (despite receiving GDT for ≥3 months), provided that their life expectancy is longer than 1 year.[1]

Furthermore, in patients with DCM and confirmed *LMNA* gene mutations, early implantation of an ICD may be considered in primary prevention of SCD, guided by risk factor assessment.[1] Accordingly, a risk prediction model to estimate the absolute 5-year risk of malignant ventricular arrhythmias has been validated and is available online (available from: https://lmna-risk-vta.fr). The score is derived from readily assessable risk predictors, including male sex, non-missense *LMNA* mutations, first-degree or higher atrioventricular block, non-sustained ventricular tachycardia, and LVEF <45%.[47]

CRT is also a viable treatment option in patients with DCM. It is indicated if LVEF is ≤35% (despite receiving GDT for ≥3 months) and QRS duration is ≥150 ms with a left bundle branch block (LBBB) QRS morphology. Besides, CRT should be considered in patients with a QRS duration of ≥150 ms with a non-LBBB morphology, as well as in those with a QRS duration of 130–149 ms and LBBB.[1]

Severe functional (secondary) MR is frequent in DCM and is associated with impaired prognosis. Percutaneous edge-to-edge mitral valve repair (MVR) may be considered as a treatment option in selected patients with DCM and moderate-to-severe functional MR. Two randomized trials have compared the effectiveness of percutaneous MVR with the MitraClip device (in addition to GDT), compared to medical treatment alone, with diverging results. The MITRA-FR study demonstrated neutral results in terms of risk reduction in mortality or HF hospitalization with MitraClip, compared to GDT alone, at 1 and 2 years.[48,49] Conversely, the COAPT trial demonstrated a significant reduction in hospitalization for HF and all-cause mortality at 2 years with MitraClip, compared to GDT.[50] The difference in outcomes may be explained by differences in study populations, as patients in the COAPT trial had more severe MR and less advanced LV remodelling (i.e. dilatation and dysfunction), compared to MITRA-FR patients. This suggests that too advanced LV dilatation or dysfunction may not derive benefit from the MitraClip procedure.[51]

In patients with DCM and advanced HFrEF with persistent severe symptoms and recurrent HF hospitalizations, implantation of a left ventricular assist device (LVAD) should be considered. Presently, continuous-flow LVADs are the most commonly used devices that are indicated as a bridge-to-transplantation, a bridge-to-candidacy, or destination therapy. In rare cases, an LVAD may be implanted as a bridge-to-recovery. Apparently, patients with DCM may have greater potential to improve contractile function upon LVAD implantation, compared to those with ischaemic HF, which may allow successful weaning from LVAD in selected patients. The results of a multicentre study involving 40 highly selected younger patients (average age of 35 years) with DCM and a short duration of HF symptoms showed that optimized LVAD speed, combined with GDT, resulted in sustained improvement in LVEF.[52] This allowed LVAD explantation in half of those patients after 18 months, with subsequent 1-year survival free from LVAD/transplantation in 90%, and in 77% of patients at 2 and 3 years.[52]

Heart transplantation remains the gold standard therapy for advanced HF in patients with DCM. DCM is the most frequent indication for heart transplantation in younger and middle-aged adults, and the second most frequent indication (following ischaemic heart disease) in older adults (aged ≥60 years).[53] Compared with ischaemic HF, patients with DCM are often younger and with fewer comorbidities at the time of transplantation, and after transplantation, they generally have a good prognosis, with a median survival of approximately 12 years.[53]

Aetiology-related therapy

Identification of a specific aetiology in a patient with DCM provides an opportunity for aetiology-related management, in addition to GDT. However, aetiology-related therapy in many instances is still an evolving concept that requires further confirmation. In patients with inflammatory DCM without viral persistence, two clinical trials demonstrated that 3–6 months of immunosuppressive treatment (with prednisone and azathioprine) resulted in a sustained improvement in LVEF, albeit without an effect on survival.[54,55] Moreover, immunosuppression has shown beneficial effects in patients with giant cell and eosinophilic myocarditis and cardiac sarcoidosis.[56,57,58] Removal of circulating anti-myocardial autoantibodies (e.g. anti-β1-adrenoreceptor antibodies) by immunoadsorption, followed by substitution of immunoglobulins, represents another approach to immunomodulation in DCM. A meta-analysis of five studies with a total of 395 patients with DCM, that assessed the effectiveness of immunoadsorption, demonstrated that this strategy is safe and associated with an improvement in LV size and LVEF, as well as relief of symptoms.[59]

In patients with proven Lyme disease-related DCM, antibiotic treatment can result in improvement in LV performance and symptoms.[60] Likewise, HIV-positive patients and those with

Chagas disease should be treated according to specific recommendations. In patients with tachycardia-induced cardiomyopathy, due to fast-rate atrial tachyarrhythmias (i.e. AF) or increased burden of VPCs (exceeding 20% of all cardiac contractions), treatment of cardiac rhythm disorders can provide significant LV reverse remodelling and even complete normalization of contractile function. Clinical trial data support catheter ablation of AF as the preferred method of treating patients with HF, given the greater success rate of sinus rhythm maintenance compared with antiarrhythmic drugs.[61,62] Catheter ablation is also highly effective in VPC suppression.[63] However, GDT should be continued in patients with recovered arrhythmia-induced cardiomyopathy, as there may be a risk of HF relapse with arrhythmia recurrence, with a similar or worse clinical presentation and a high risk of SCD.[64]

Chelation therapy, including newer forms of oral chelators (deferoxamine), and phlebotomy can be helpful in patients with iron overload/haemochromatosis and an early diagnosis of DCM. In addition, abstinence from alcohol and/or illicit drugs and management of the underlying nutritional deficits and endocrine or metabolic disorders offer possibilities for aetiology-related therapy in selected patients with DCM.

Future directions

Extensive phenotyping can provide an aetiology of DCM and characterization of downstream molecular processes involved in the pathogenesis of the disease, with possible implications for treatment.[65] Several pharmacological interventions in this field have been explored such as increasing cardiac contractility, decreasing fibrosis, and replacing cardiac myocytes by stem cells.[65]

Increasing cardiac contractile performance

Increasing cardiac contractility with danicamtiv (a selective cardiac myosin activator) has shown favourable results in improving LV systolic function in patients with HFrEF (approximately 50% with a non-ischaemic aetiology) in a phase 2 trial.[66] There is an ongoing randomized controlled study with danicamtiv in patients with DCM due to genetic variants of myosin heavy chain-7 or titin truncating variants (NCT04572893). Furthermore, treatment with omecamtiv mecarbil, another cardiac myosin activator, has resulted in a modest reduction in the composite end point of HF events and cardiovascular death in the GALACTIC HF Trial.[67] This trial included approximately 46% of patients with non-ischaemic HFrEF, and no evidence of heterogeneity for subgroups of patients with an ischaemic versus a non-ischaemic aetiology was revealed.[67] These medications await further data on safety and efficacy in specific phenotypes of DCM patients, especially those with genetic cardiomyopathies and severe systolic dysfunction.

Targeting myocardial fibrosis

There have been attempts to influence the main pathways involved in the development of myocardial fibrosis (e.g. mineralocorticoid receptors, transforming growth factor beta (TGF-β), matrix proteins, and expression of pro-fibrotic microRNAs). These strategies are currently in experimental or early trial phase with several tested agents (e.g. mineralocorticoid receptor antagonists, citrus pectin, anti-fibrotic microRNA, pirfenidone). Pirfenidone is an orally bioavailable anti-fibrotic agent that inhibits the synthesis and secretion of TGF-β1. It is successfully used in the treatment of idiopathic pulmonary fibrosis and has shown promising results in reducing myocardial fibrosis in patients with heart failure with preserved ejection fraction (HFpEF), but its safety and efficacy in DCM await further trials.[68]

Stem cell therapy

Though stem cell therapy was initially reported to have favourable effects on LV function, it failed as a definitive treatment strategy due to challenges in homing and retention of stem cells and a lack of large-scale trials showing long-term safety and efficacy.[69]

Treatment related to pathogenic gene mutations

Promising strategies are evolving for downstream molecular targeting of specific gene mutations. Experimental studies demonstrated that pathological *LMNA* mutations result in increased cardiac activity of mitogen-activated protein (MAP) kinases. In experimental models, treatment with a MAP kinase inhibitor prevented LV dilatation and contractile deterioration. The first international phase 3 clinical trial involving genotype-specific therapy is under way, investigating the benefits of MAP kinase inhibition on functional capacity in patients with DCM caused by an *LMNA* mutation (NCT03439514).

Clustering of specific phenotypes

Better understanding of the clustering of similar phenotypes in DCM (i.e. pheno-groups), by integrating aetiologies, comorbidities, cardiac function, and genetic expression, may offer possibilities for targeted therapy. In a study of 800 patients who underwent in-depth phenotyping, four distinct pheno-groups were identified: (1) mild systolic dysfunction; (2) autoimmune; (3) arrhythmia; and (4) severe systolic dysfunction. Specific molecular changes have been associated with these pheno-groups that may present future treatment targets.[70]

Key messages

- DCM includes a variety of heterogeneous myocardial disorders that result in LV (or biventricular) dilatation and systolic dysfunction in the absence of abnormal loading conditions. Hypokinetic non-DCM is defined as LV or biventricular global systolic dysfunction (i.e. LVEF <45%) without chamber dilatation.

- DCM can have a variety of aetiologies, including gene mutations, infections, autoimmunity, toxins, medications, and endocrine and metabolic abnormalities.

- DCM is an important cause of HFrEF. Despite progress in treatment, many patients develop advanced HF, and DCM is one of the leading indications for long-term mechanical circulatory support or heart transplantation. Advanced HF remains the most frequent cause of death (approximately 70% of cardiovascular mortality) in DCM, whereas SCD accounts for the remaining approximately 30%.

♦ Patients with DCM should undergo thorough diagnostic evaluation, including a common diagnostic approach indicated for all patients with HF and a targeted assessment to establish a specific aetiology (or aetiologies) of DCM. Exclusion of coronary artery disease is mandatory.

♦ Management includes standard pharmacological and device treatment for HFrEF (HF-related therapy). All patients should receive ACEIs or angiotensin receptor–neprilysin inhibitor (or angiotensin receptor blockers), beta-blockers, mineralocorticoid receptor antagonists, and sodium–glucose cotransporter 2 inhibitors. If indicated, ICD and CRT should be considered. In patients with advanced HF, LVAD and heart transplantation are important treatment options.

♦ When a specific treatment strategy is available for a specific aetiology, it should be considered (aetiology-related therapies), in addition to standard therapy for HFrEF. These treatment modalities include (but are not limited to) immunosuppression, immunoadsorption, treatment of infectious causes (e.g. Lyme disease, Chagas disease, and HIV infection), alcohol and drug abstinence, chelation therapy, and correction of nutritional, metabolic, and endocrine disorders in selected cases.

References

1. McDonagh TA, Metra M, Adamo M, et al. 2021 ESC Guidelines for the diagnosis and treatment of acute and chronic heart failure: developed by the Task Force for the diagnosis and treatment of acute and chronic heart failure of the European Society of Cardiology (ESC) with the special contribution of the Heart Failure Association (HFA) of the ESC. Eur Heart J. 2021;42(36):3599–726.

2. Seferović PM, Polovina M, Bauersachs J, et al. Heart failure in cardiomyopathies: a position paper from the Heart Failure Association of the European Society of Cardiology. Eur J Heart Fail. 2019;21(5):553–76.

3. Bozkurt B, Colvin M, Cook J, et al. Current diagnostic and treatment strategies for specific dilated cardiomyopathies: a scientific statement from the American Heart Association. Circulation. 2016;134(23):e579–646.

4. Arbustini E, Narula N, Tavazzi L, et al. The MOGE(S) classification of cardiomyopathy for clinicians. J Am Coll Cardiol. 2014;64(3):304–18.

5. Adams KF Jr, Fonarow GC, Emerman CL, et al. Characteristics and outcomes of patients hospitalized for heart failure in the United States: rationale, design, and preliminary observations from the first 100,000 cases in the Acute Decompensated Heart Failure National Registry (ADHERE). Am Heart J. 2005;149(2):209–16.

6. Crespo-Leiro MG, Anker SD, Maggioni AP, et al. European Society of Cardiology Heart Failure Long-Term Registry (ESC-HF-LT): 1-year follow-up outcomes and differences across regions. Eur J Heart Fail. 2016;18(6):613–25.

7. Charron P, Elliott PM, Gimeno JR, et al. The Cardiomyopathy Registry of the EURObservational Research Programme of the European Society of Cardiology: baseline data and contemporary management of adult patients with cardiomyopathies. Eur Heart J. 2018;39(20):1784–93.

8. Nieminen MS, Harjola V-P, Hochadel M, et al. Gender related differences in patients presenting with acute heart failure. Results from EuroHeart Failure Survey II. Eur J Heart Fail. 2008;10(2):140–8.

9. Pinto YM, Elliott PM, Arbustini E, et al. Proposal for a revised definition of dilated cardiomyopathy, hypokinetic non-dilated cardiomyopathy, and its implications for clinical practice: a position statement of the ESC working group on myocardial and pericardial diseases. Eur Heart J. 2016;37(23):1850–8.

10. Bondue A, Arbustini E, Bianco A, et al. Complex roads from genotype to phenotype in dilated cardiomyopathy: scientific update from the Working Group of Myocardial Function of the European Society of Cardiology. Cardiovasc Res. 2018;114(10):1287–303.

11. Favalli V, Serio A, Grasso M, Arbustini E. Genetic causes of dilated cardiomyopathy. Heart. 2016;102(24):2004–14.

12. Herman DS, Lam L, Taylor MR, et al. Truncations of titin causing dilated cardiomyopathy. N Engl J Med. 2012;366(7):619–28.

13. van Rijsingen IAW, Arbustini E, Elliott PM, et al. Risk factors for malignant ventricular arrhythmias in lamin A/C mutation carriers:a European cohort study. J Am Coll Cardiol. 2012;59(5):493–500.

14. Carniel E, Taylor MR, Sinagra G, et al. Alpha-myosin heavy chain: a sarcomeric gene associated with dilated and hypertrophic phenotypes of cardiomyopathy. Circulation. 2005;112(1):54–9.

15. Møller DV, Andersen PS, Hedley P, et al. The role of sarcomere gene mutations in patients with idiopathic dilated cardiomyopathy. Eur J Hum Genet. 2009;17(10):1241–9.

16. Elliott P, O'Mahony C, Syrris P, et al. Prevalence of desmosomal protein gene mutations in patients with dilated cardiomyopathy. Circ Cardiovasc Genet. 2010;3(4):314–22.

17. Spezzacatene A, Sinagra G, Merlo M, et al. Arrhythmogenic phenotype in dilated cardiomyopathy: natural history and predictors of life-threatening arrhythmias. J Am Heart Assoc. 2015;4(10):e002149.

18. Haas J, Frese KS, Peil B, et al. Atlas of the clinical genetics of human dilated cardiomyopathy. Eur Heart J. 2015;36(18):1123–35a.

19. Tschöpe C, Ammirati E, Bozkurt B, et al. Myocarditis and inflammatory cardiomyopathy: current evidence and future directions. Nat Rev Cardiol. 2021;18(3):169–93.

20. Bock CT, Klingel K, Kandolf R. Human parvovirus B19-associated myocarditis. N Engl J Med. 2010;362(13):1248–9.

21. Bock CT, Düchting A, Utta F, et al. Molecular phenotypes of human parvovirus B19 in patients with myocarditis. World J Cardiol. 2014;6(4):183–95.

22. Bojkova D, Wagner JUG, Shumliakivska M, et al. SARS-CoV-2 infects and induces cytotoxic effects in human cardiomyocytes. Cardiovasc Res. 2020;116(14):2207–15.

23. Caforio ALP, Adler Y, Agostini C, et al. Diagnosis and management of myocardial involvement in systemic immune-mediated diseases: a position statement of the European Society of Cardiology Working Group on Myocardial and Pericardial Disease. Eur Heart J. 2017;38(35):2649–62.

24. Hahn VS, Lenihan DJ, Ky B. Cancer therapy-induced cardiotoxicity: basic mechanisms and potential cardioprotective therapies. J Am Heart Assoc. 2014;3(2):e000665.

25. Zamorano JL, Lancellotti P, Rodriguez Muñoz D, et al. 2016 ESC Position Paper on cancer treatments and cardiovascular toxicity developed under the auspices of the ESC Committee for Practice Guidelines: the Task Force for cancer treatments and cardiovascular toxicity of the European Society of Cardiology (ESC). Eur Heart J. 2016;37(36):2768–801.

26. Lyon AR, Dent S, Stanway S, et al. Baseline cardiovascular risk assessment in cancer patients scheduled to receive cardiotoxic cancer therapies: a position statement and new risk assessment tools from the Cardio-Oncology Study Group of the Heart Failure Association of the European Society of Cardiology in collaboration with the International Cardio-Oncology Society. Eur J Heart Fail. 2020;22(11):1945–60.

27. Rusconi P, Wilkinson JD, Sleeper LA, *et al.* Differences in presentation and outcomes between children with familial dilated cardiomyopathy and children with idiopathic dilated cardiomyopathy: a report from the Pediatric Cardiomyopathy Registry Study Group. Circ Heart Fail. 2017;10(2):e002637.

28. Felker GM, Thompson RE, Hare JM, *et al.* Underlying causes and long-term survival in patients with initially unexplained cardiomyopathy. N Engl J Med. 2000;342(15):1077–84.

29. Kubanek M, Sramko M, Maluskova J, *et al.* Novel predictors of left ventricular reverse remodeling in individuals with recent-onset dilated cardiomyopathy. J Am Coll Cardiol. 2013;61(1):54–63.

30. Merlo M, Pivetta A, Pinamonti B, *et al.* Long-term prognostic impact of therapeutic strategies in patients with idiopathic dilated cardiomyopathy: changing mortality over the last 30 years. Eur J Heart Fail. 2014;16(3):317–24.

31. Merlo M, Pyxaras SA, Pinamonti B, Barbati G, Di Lenarda A, Sinagra G. Prevalence and prognostic significance of left ventricular reverse remodeling in dilated cardiomyopathy receiving tailored medical treatment. J Am Coll Cardiol. 2011;57(13):1468–76.

32. McNamara DM, Starling RC, Cooper LT, *et al.* Clinical and demographic predictors of outcomes in recent onset dilated cardiomyopathy: results of the IMAC (Intervention in Myocarditis and Acute Cardiomyopathy)-2 study. J Am Coll Cardiol. 2011;58(11):1112–18.

33. Halliday BP, Wassall R, Lota AS, *et al.* Withdrawal of pharmacological treatment for heart failure in patients with recovered dilated cardiomyopathy (TRED-HF): an open-label, pilot, randomised trial. Lancet. 2019;393(10166):61–73.

34. Rose EA, Gelijns AC, Moskowitz AJ, *et al.* Long-term use of a left ventricular assist device for end-stage heart failure. N Engl J Med. 2001;345(20):1435–43.

35. Yoshioka D, Li B, Takayama H, *et al.* Outcome of heart transplantation after bridge-to-transplant strategy using various mechanical circulatory support devices. Interact Cardiovasc Thorac Surg. 2017;25(6):918–24.

36. Gimeno JR, Elliott PM, Tavazzi L, *et al.* Prospective follow-up in various subtypes of cardiomyopathies: insights from the ESC EORP Cardiomyopathy Registry. Eur Heart J Qual Care Clin Outcomes. 2021;7(2):134–42.

37. Schultheiss HP, Fairweather D, Caforio ALP, *et al.* Dilated cardiomyopathy. Nat Rev Dis Primers. 2019;5(1):32.

38. Halliday BP, Gulati A, Ali A, *et al.* Sex- and age-based differences in the natural history and outcome of dilated cardiomyopathy. Eur J Heart Fail. 2018;20(10):1392–400.

39. Køber L, Thune JJ, Nielsen JC, *et al.* Defibrillator implantation in patients with nonischemic systolic heart failure. N Engl J Med. 2016;375(13):1221–30.

40. Asselbergs FW, Sammani A, Elliott P, *et al.* Differences between familial and sporadic dilated cardiomyopathy: ESC EORP Cardiomyopathy & Myocarditis registry. ESC Heart Fail. 2021;8(1):95–105.

41. Finocchiaro G, Merlo M, Sheikh N, *et al.* The electrocardiogram in the diagnosis and management of patients with dilated cardiomyopathy. Eur J Heart Fail. 2020;22(7):1097–107.

42. Ferreira VM, Schulz-Menger J, Holmvang G, *et al.* Cardiovascular magnetic resonance in nonischemic myocardial inflammation: expert recommendations. J Am Coll Cardiol. 2018;72(24):3158–76.

43. Donal E, Delgado V, Bucciarelli-Ducci C, *et al.* Multimodality imaging in the diagnosis, risk stratification, and management of patients with dilated cardiomyopathies: an expert consensus document from the European Association of Cardiovascular Imaging. Eur Heart J Cardiovasc Imaging. 2019;20(10):1075–93.

44. Seferović PM, Tsutsui H, McNamara DM, *et al.* Heart Failure Association of the ESC, Heart Failure Society of America and Japanese Heart Failure Society Position statement on endomyocardial biopsy. Eur J Heart Fail. 2021;23(6):854–71.

45. Elming MB, Nielsen JC, Haarbo J, *et al.* Age and outcomes of primary prevention implantable cardioverter–defibrillators in patients with nonischemic systolic heart failure. Circulation. 2017;136(19):1772–80.

46. Beggs SAS, Jhund PS, Jackson CE, McMurray JJV, Gardner RS. Non-ischaemic cardiomyopathy, sudden death and implantable defibrillators: a review and meta-analysis. Heart. 2018;104(2):144–50.

47. Wahbi K, Ben Yaou R, Gandjbakhch E, *et al.* Development and validation of a new risk prediction score for life-threatening ventricular tachyarrhythmias in laminopathies. Circulation. 2019;140(4):293–302.

48. Obadia JF, Messika-Zeitoun D, Leurent G, *et al.* Percutaneous repair or medical treatment for secondary mitral regurgitation. N Engl J Med. 2018;379(24):2297–306.

49. Iung B, Armoiry X, Vahanian A, *et al.* Percutaneous repair or medical treatment for secondary mitral regurgitation: outcomes at 2 years. Eur J Heart Fail. 2019;21(12):1619–27.

50. Stone GW, Lindenfeld J, Abraham WT, *et al.* Transcatheter mitral-valve repair in patients with heart failure. N Engl J Med. 2018;379(24):2307–18.

51. Pibarot P, Delgado V, Bax JJ. MITRA-FR vs. COAPT: lessons from two trials with diametrically opposed results. Eur Heart J Cardiovasc Imaging. 2019;20(6):620–4.

52. Birks EJ, Drakos SG, Patel SR, *et al.* Prospective multicenter study of myocardial recovery using left ventricular assist devices (RESTAGE-HF [Remission from Stage D Heart Failure]): medium-term and primary end point results. Circulation. 2020;142(21):2016–28.

53. Lund LH, Edwards LB, Dipchand AI, *et al.* The Registry of the International Society for Heart and Lung Transplantation: Thirty-third Adult Heart Transplantation Report-2016; Focus Theme: primary diagnostic indications for transplant. J Heart Lung Transplant. 2016;35(10):1158–69.

54. Frustaci A, Russo MA, Chimenti C. Randomized study on the efficacy of immunosuppressive therapy in patients with virus-negative inflammatory cardiomyopathy: the TIMIC study. Eur Heart J. 2009;30(16):1995–2002.

55. Wojnicz R, Nowalany-Kozielska E, Wojciechowska C, *et al.* Randomized, placebo-controlled study for immunosuppressive treatment of inflammatory dilated cardiomyopathy: two-year follow-up results. Circulation. 2001;104(1):39–45.

56. Cooper LT, Jr., Hare JM, Tazelaar HD, *et al.* Usefulness of immunosuppression for giant cell myocarditis. Am J Cardiol. 2008;102(11):1535–9.

57. Bleeker JS, Syed FF, Cooper LT, Weiler CR, Tefferi A, Pardanani A. Treatment-refractory idiopathic hypereosinophilic syndrome: pitfalls and progress with use of novel drugs. Am J Hematol. 2012;87(7):703–6.

58. Rosenthal DG, Parwani P, Murray TO, *et al.* Long-term corticosteroid-sparing immunosuppression for cardiac sarcoidosis. J Am Heart Assoc. 2019;8(18):e010952.

59. Bian R-t, Wang Z-t, Li W-y. Immunoadsorption treatment for dilated cardiomyopathy: a PRISMA-compliant systematic review and meta-analysis. Medicine. 2021;100(26):e26475.

60. Kuchynka P, Palecek T, Havranek S, *et al.* Recent-onset dilated cardiomyopathy associated with *Borrelia burgdorferi* infection. Herz. 2015;40(6):892–7.

61. Marrouche NF, Brachmann J, Andresen D, *et al.* Catheter ablation for atrial fibrillation with heart failure. N Engl J Med. 2018;378(5):417–27.

62. Di Biase L, Mohanty P, Mohanty S, *et al*. Ablation versus amiodarone for treatment of persistent atrial fibrillation in patients with congestive heart failure and an implanted device: results from the AATAC multicenter randomized trial. Circulation. 2016;133(17):1637–44.

63. Takemoto M, Yoshimura H, Ohba Y, *et al*. Radiofrequency catheter ablation of premature ventricular complexes from right ventricular outflow tract improves left ventricular dilation and clinical status in patients without structural heart disease. J Am Coll Cardiol. 2005;45(8):1259–65.

64. Nerheim P, Birger-Botkin S, Piracha L, Olshansky B. Heart failure and sudden death in patients with tachycardia-induced cardiomyopathy and recurrent tachycardia. Circulation. 2004;110(3):247–52.

65. Verdonschot JAJ, Hazebroek MR, Ware JS, Prasad SK, Heymans SRB. Role of targeted therapy in dilated cardiomyopathy: the challenging road toward a personalized approach. J Am Heart Assoc. 2019;8(11):e012514.

66. Voors AA, Tamby JF, Cleland JG, *et al*. Effects of danicamtiv, a novel cardiac myosin activator, in heart failure with reduced ejection fraction: experimental data and clinical results from a phase 2a trial. Eur J Heart Fail. 2020;22(9):1649–58.

67. Teerlink JR, Diaz R, Felker GM, *et al*. Cardiac myosin activation with omecamtiv mecarbil in systolic heart failure. N Engl J Med. 2021;384(2):105–16.

68. Lewis GA, Schelbert EB, Naish JH, *et al*. Pirfenidone in heart failure with preserved ejection fraction: rationale and design of the PIROUETTE Trial. Cardiovasc Drugs Ther. 2019;33(4):461–70.

69. Hamshere S, Arnous S, Choudhury T, *et al*. Randomized trial of combination cytokine and adult autologous bone marrow progenitor cell administration in patients with non-ischaemic dilated cardiomyopathy: the REGENERATE-DCM clinical trial. Eur Heart J. 2015;36(44):3061–9.

70. Verdonschot JAJ, Merlo M, Dominguez F, *et al*. Phenotypic clustering of dilated cardiomyopathy patients highlights important pathophysiological differences. Eur Heart J. 2021;42(2):162–74.

3.4.3 Hypertrophic cardiomyopathy

Perry Elliott, Michel Noutsias, and
Aris Anastasakis

Introduction

The term cardiomyopathies comprises a group of disorders characterized by structural and functional abnormalities of the myocardium that are unexplained by abnormal loading conditions or coronary artery disease.[1,2,3] In the past, cardiomyopathies were further subclassified into primary forms in which the heart is the only involved organ, and secondary forms in which cardiomyopathy is a manifestation of a systemic disorder.[1] Current European Society of Cardiology (ESC) recommendations are to group cardiomyopathies into familial/genetic and non-familial/non-genetic subtypes, irrespective of the presence of extracardiac manifestations.[2] Hypertrophic cardiomyopathy (HCM) is defined by increased thickness of the left ventricular (LV) wall that cannot be explained solely by abnormal loading conditions.[2]

HCM is most often inherited as an autosomal dominant trait, but the disorder encompasses a wide group of conditions that lead to left ventricular hypertrophy (LVH) through different pathophysiological mechanisms. HCM is most commonly caused by mutations in sarcomeric protein genes, but phenocopies caused by rarer genetic variants, as well as acquired disease mimics such as amyloidosis, are not infrequent.[1,2,3]

Epidemiology

The estimated population prevalence of HCM in adults ranges from 1:300 to 1:600.[2,3,4,5,6,7,8,9,10,11] There is no specific distribution of HCM according to race or geography, but most studies report a male predominance. The prevalence of HCM in children is unknown, but two studies have reported an annual incidence of 0.3–0.5 per 100,000.[12,13]

Inheritance

HCM is usually inherited as an autosomal dominant trait, whereby a single mutation is usually sufficient to cause the disease, albeit with variable penetrance and clinical expression. The variability of the phenotype is, at least in part, due to the causal mutation acting in concert with a number of other genetic and of non-genetic influences. Autosomal recessive, X-linked, and matrilinear modes of inheritance are described but are rare. X-linked inheritance raises the possibility of specific genocopies such as Fabry disease.[14]

Pathophysiology

A diverse array of mechanisms, mirroring the diversity of the causal genes and mutations, are implicated in the pathogenesis of HCM. Initial or proximal phenotypes result from the direct effects of mutations on the structure and function of the encoded proteins; intermediary (or secondary) phenotypes include molecular changes that occur in response to the changes in protein structure and function. Examples of the latter include altered gene expression and activation of signalling pathways such as the mitogen-activated protein kinase (MAPK) and transforming growth factor beta 1 (TGF-β1) pathways. Finally, tertiary effects include histological and pathological phenotypes which are a consequence of the perturbation of a myriad of secondary molecular events in the myocardium such as activation of hypertrophic signalling pathways. It is important to note that there is a distinction between cases of HCM caused by sarcomere protein mutations and those caused by other phenocopies, since ventricular hypertrophy in the latter may, in some cases, result from storage of material such as glycogen.

About 35–60% of patients with HCM are heterozygous for missense or truncating mutations in genes encoding one of eight cardiac sarcomeric proteins, mostly MYH7 (β-myosin heavy chain), MYBPC3 (cardiac myosin-binding protein C), and TNNT2 (troponin T2).[14,15,16,17] Mutations in sarcomere genes cause alterations in the myocardium that result in myocyte disarray, hypertrophy, and fibrosis, which, in turn, lead to impaired systolic and diastolic function.[18,19,20,21,22,23,24]

Septal hypertrophy leads to narrowing of the LV outflow tract (LVOT), which, together with abnormal blood flow vectors that dynamically displace the mitral valve leaflets anteriorly, and anatomical changes in the mitral valve and apparatus such as leaflet elongation and anterior displacement of the papillary muscles, result in systolic anterior motion (SAM) of the mitral valve leaflets, such that they make contact with the interventricular septum and cause left ventricular outflow tract obstruction (LVOTO).[25,26,27,28,29,30] SAM is usually associated with mitral regurgitation (MR) due to loss of leaflet coaptation. The severity of LVOTO varies with preload, afterload, and LV contractility. LVOTO causes an increase in LV systolic pressure, myocardial ischaemia, and prolonged ventricular relaxation (➲ Figure 3.4.3.1). By convention, a peak LVOT gradient of ≥30 mmHg defines LVOTO, with resting or provoked gradients of ≥50 mmHg usually considered the threshold for interventional treatment.

Diastolic dysfunction is the result of altered ventricular load, high intracavitary pressures, non-uniformity in ventricular contraction and relaxation, and delayed inactivation from abnormal intracellular calcium reuptake.[31,32,33] Myocardial hypertrophy, ischaemia, and fibrosis lead to increased chamber stiffness. Left atrial dilatation caused by increased filling pressures and MR predisposes to atrial fibrillation (AF). Exercise intolerance or symptoms of heart failure (HF) in the absence of LVOTO occur because of diastolic dysfunction and decreased ventricular cavity size and stroke volume.

MR may result from SAM of the mitral valve or from primary leaflet abnormalities. SAM of the mitral valve causes loss of leaflet coaptation, and mitral regurgitation that is predominantly mid-to-late systolic and posterior or lateral in orientation. Significant MR may not be evident without provocation for LVOTO. Primary abnormalities of the mitral valve apparatus, such as excessive leaflet length, anomalous papillary muscle insertion, and anteriorly displaced papillary muscles, are common.[34,35,36,37]

Myocardial ischaemia is frequent and caused by a mismatch between myocardial oxygen supply and demand.[38,39,40,41,42,43,44,45] Mechanisms include myocardial hypertrophy and microvascular dysfunction with impaired coronary flow reserve caused by medial hypertrophy of the intramural arterioles, reduced capillary density, and high intracavitary pressures. Myocardial bridges can cause systolic compression of epicardial coronary vessels that may persist into diastole, impairing blood flow.[44] Apical myocardial ischaemia may contribute to the development of LV aneurysms.[46]

Diagnosis

The general approach to diagnosis of HCM is shown in ➲ Figure 3.4.3.2. HCM is characterized by LVH, a non-dilated

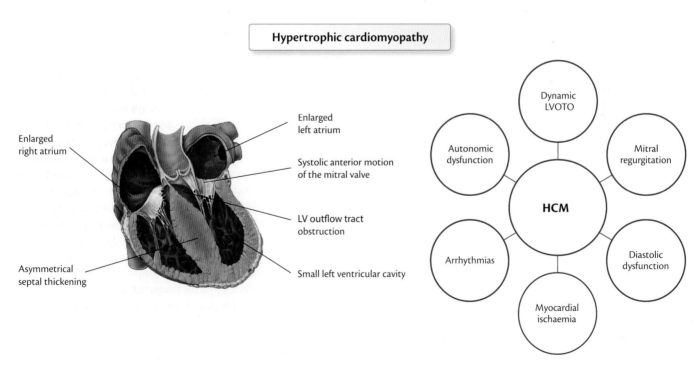

Figure 3.4.3.1 Clinical pathology and pathophysiology of hypertrophic cardiomyopathy. HCM, hypertrophic cardiomyopathy; LVOTO, left ventricular outflow tract obstruction.

Source data from Seferović PM, Polovina M, Bauersachs J, *et al*. Heart failure in cardiomyopathies: a position paper from the Heart Failure Association of the European Society of Cardiology. *Eur J Heart Fail*. 2019 May;21(5):553–576. doi: 10.1002/ejhf.1461.

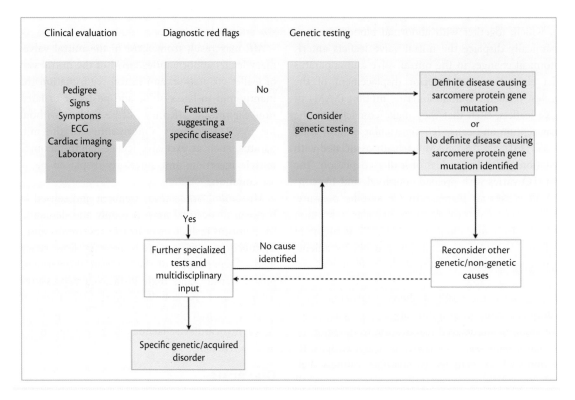

Figure 3.4.3.2 Hypertrophic cardiomyopathy diagnostic pathway (ESC, 2014).

Elliott PM, Anastasakis A, Borger MA, *et al.* 2014 ESC Guidelines on diagnosis and management of hypertrophic cardiomyopathy: the Task Force for the Diagnosis and Management of Hypertrophic Cardiomyopathy of the European Society of Cardiology (ESC). *Eur Heart J.* 2014 Oct 14;35(39):2733–79. doi: 10.1093/eurheartj/ehu284. © The European Society of Cardiology. Reprinted by permission of Oxford University Press.

left ventricle, and a normal or increased LVEF. LVH is usually asymmetric, with involvement most commonly of the basal interventricular septum. It is occasionally restricted to other myocardial regions such as the apex and the mid portion, as well as the posterior wall, of the left ventricle.

The clinical diagnosis of HCM in an adult requires demonstration of an end-diastolic LV wall thickness of ≥15 mm by any imaging technique.[2,4] In first-degree relatives, the threshold is lower, with an LV wall thickness of ≥13 mm sufficient for diagnosis.[2,3] In children, a diagnosis of HCM has been defined as an LV wall thickness of >2 standard deviations than the predicted mean (z-score >2).[2,3]

In families with genetic forms of HCM, relatives may have non-diagnostic electrocardiogram (ECG) and imaging findings. While the specificity of such abnormalities is low, in the context of familial disease, they can represent early or mild expression of the disease, and the presence of multiple features increases the accuracy for predicting the disease in genotyped populations. In general, the presence of any abnormality (e.g. abnormal myocardial Doppler imaging and strain, incomplete SAM or elongation of the mitral valve leaflet(s), and abnormal papillary muscles), particularly in the presence of an abnormal ECG, increases the probability of the disease in relatives. Inverted T-waves in leads II, III, aVF and V5–V6 or I, aVL, and V5–V6,

and pathological Q-waves are consistent with subclinical HCM (➲ Figure 3.4.3.3).

Clinical evaluation

Age and pattern of inheritance

One of the most important factors to take into consideration during the workup of HCM and its possible phenocopies is the age of the patient.[47] For example, some inherited metabolic disorders are much more likely to appear in neonates or infants, whereas diseases such as wild-type transthyretin (TTR)-related amyloidosis is mostly seen in men over 65 years old. Construction of a three- or four-generation family pedigree is vital, as it will depict the likely pattern of inheritance. The pedigree is also valuable in identifying relatives at risk of disease inheritance (➲ Table 3.4.3.1).

History and physical examination

Most people affected by HCM are asymptomatic or complain of few symptoms. In such cases, the diagnosis is usually incidental or results from family screening. Some patients complain of angina, dyspnoea, palpitations, or syncope, and non-cardiac symptoms can point to other systemic diagnoses (➲ Table 3.4.3.2). General physical examination is often normal in patients without systemic or syndromic disease, although some disease manifestations

Subclinical phase and evolution of the disease

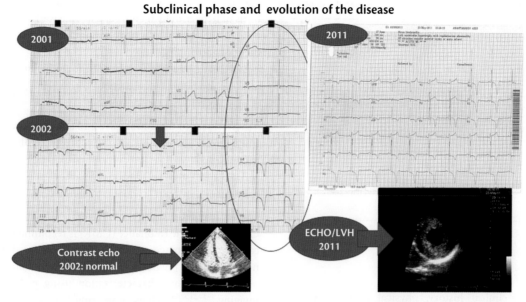

Figure 3.4.3.3 A typical subclinical phenotype, with ECG evolution during serial evaluation, borderline left ventricular wall thickness, incomplete systolic motion of the mitral valve, and abnormal tissue Doppler of the mitral annulus. 2001: minor repolarization abnormalities in leads II,II,AVF, V5,V6/normal ECHO; 2002: giant negative T waves/normal ECHO; 2011: typical clinical expression of hypertrophic cardiomyopathy: abnormal ECG/ECHO/LVH.

such as deafness and peripheral neuropathy require specific questioning.

Most of the classical cardiac signs of HCM relate to the presence of LVOTO. There is a rapid up-and-down stroke to the arterial pulse and an ejection systolic murmur heard best at the left sternal edge, with radiation to the right upper sternal edge and apex. Manoeuvres reducing the ventricular preload or afterload, such as standing up from a squatting position or the Valsalva manoeuvre, increase the intensity of the murmur. Most patients with LVOTO have signs of MR.

Specific clinical features that constitute red flags for HCM phenocopies and systemic disease such as skeletal muscle weakness, diabetes, and renal failure should be noted. For a more comprehensive list of red flags for HCM phenocopies, see ➲ Table 3.4.3.2.

Table 3.4.3.1 Differential diagnosis based on pattern of inheritance

AD	◆ Sarcomere HCM ◆ Familial transthyretin-related amyloidosis ◆ Noonan/LEOPARD syndrome ◆ Mitochondrial cardiomyopathy (nuclear DNA mutations)
AR	◆ Friedreich's ataxia ◆ Mitochondrial cardiomyopathy (nuclear DNA mutations, TRIM63, GSD)
X-linked	◆ Anderson–Fabry disease ◆ Danon disease ◆ Mitochondrial cardiomyopathy (nuclear DNA mutations)
Matrilinear	◆ Mitochondrial cardiomyopathy (mitochondrial DNA mutations)

AD, autosomal dominant; AR, autosomal recessive; HCM hypertrophic cardiomyopathy; GSD, glycogen storage disorder.
Source data from Rapezzi C, Arbustini E, Caforio AL. Diagnostic work-up in cardiomyopathies: bridging the gap between clinical phenotypes and final diagnosis. A position statement from the ESC Working Group on Myocardial and Pericardial Diseases. *Eur Heart J.* 2013 May;34(19):1448–58. doi: 10.1093/eurheartj/ehs397.

Table 3.4.3.2 Examples of clinical diagnostic red flags

Learning difficulties	Mitochondrial diseases Noonan syndrome Danon disease
Sensorineural deafness	Mitochondrial diseases Anderson–Fabry disease LEOPARD syndrome
Visual impairment	Mitochondrial diseases (retinal disease, optic nerve atrophy) TTR-related amyloidosis (vitreous opacities) Danon disease (retinitis pigmentosa) Anderson–Fabry disease (cataracts, corneal opacities)
Gait disturbance	Friedreich's ataxia
Paraesthesiae/sensory abnormalities/neuropathic pain	Amyloidosis, Anderson–Fabry disease
Carpal tunnel syndrome (bilateral)	TTR-related amyloidosis
Muscle weakness	Mitochondrial diseases, glycogen storage disorders, *FHL1* mutation, Danon disease
Palpebral ptosis	Mitochondrial diseases, myotonic dystrophy
Cutaneous	Anderson–Fabry disease (angiokeratomata), cardiocutaneous facial syndromes (lentigines)

TTR, transthyretin.
Source data from Rapezzi C, Arbustini E, Caforio AL. Diagnostic work-up in cardiomyopathies: bridging the gap between clinical phenotypes and final diagnosis. A position statement from the ESC Working Group on Myocardial and Pericardial Diseases. *Eur Heart J.* 2013 May;34(19):1448–58. doi: 10.1093/eurheartj/ehs397.

Table 3.4.3.3 Examples of ECG features suggesting specific diagnoses

Short P-R/pre-excitation	Glycogenosis Danon disease PRKAG2 Anderson–Fabry disease
AV block	Amyloidosis Late-stage Anderson–Fabry disease Danon disease Acute myocarditis
Extreme LVH (Sokolow >100)	Danon disease Pompe
Low QRS voltage (or normal voltages despite increased LV wall thickness)	Amyloidosis

AV, atrioventricular; LVH, left ventricular hypertrophy; LV, left ventricular.

Electrocardiogram

Along with the clinical history, physical examination, and imaging, the ECG helps to direct the diagnosis towards HCM and aids in the detection of HCM phenocopies.[47] The ECG is a sensitive diagnostic test for HCM, as a normal ECG is present in only 5–10% of patients. Possible findings are LVH by voltage criteria with widespread repolarization abnormalities, lateral and inferior Q-waves, and deep negative T-waves in the precordial leads. There may be also left axis deviation and evidence of left and/or right atrial enlargement. ➲ Table 3.4.3.3 shows specific ECG findings and their associations with specific HCM phenocopies.

Cardiac imaging

Echocardiography

Classically, HCM is characterized by asymmetrical septal hypertrophy (➲ Figure 3.4.3.4), with SAM of the mitral valve leaflet (➲ Figure 3.4.3.5), LVOTO in 70% of cases, and MR. Other patterns of hypertrophy include apical, free wall, or concentric LVH. LVOTO is defined as a peak instantaneous Doppler LVOT gradient of >30 mmHg.[48]

Systematic imaging assessment should include:[48]

- LVH distribution and severity
- Left atrial enlargement
- Assessment of the mitral valve and any associated anatomical or functional abnormalities such as SAM, papillary muscle thickening or abnormal insertions, and MR
- Assessment of LVOTO with and without provocation
- Evaluation of systolic and diastolic function.

Cardiac magnetic resonance imaging

Cardiac magnetic resonance (CMR) is recommended when echocardiographic images are suboptimal and for differential diagnosis of HCM phenocopies. The most valuable additive value of CMR is tissue characterization using gadolinium contrast imaging.[49,50,51,52,53] Extensive scarring (≥15% of LV mass) may be associated with an increased risk of sudden cardiac death (SCD) (➲ Figure 3.4.3.6) Ventricular apical aneurysms are more easily seen with CMR than with echocardiography.

Laboratory tests

Routine laboratory tests help in detecting systemic disease or comorbidities (➲ Table 3.4.3.4). Increased levels of natriuretic peptides[54,55] and high-sensitivity cardiac troponin T (hs-cTnT) are markers of poor prognosis (➲ Table 3.4.3.3).

Exercise stress testing

In patients with symptomatic HF despite optimal medical therapy, a cardiopulmonary exercise stress test should be performed to evaluate functional status. An exercise stress test may

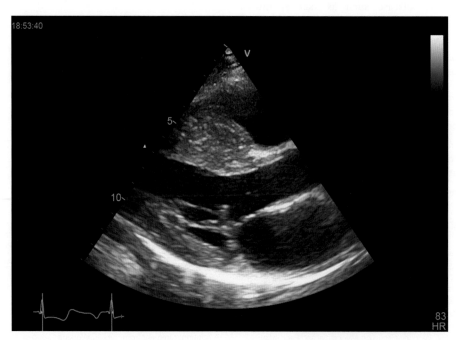

Figure 3.4.3.4 Hypertrophic cardiomyopathy. Two-dimensional echocardiogram showing asymmetric septal hypertrophy.

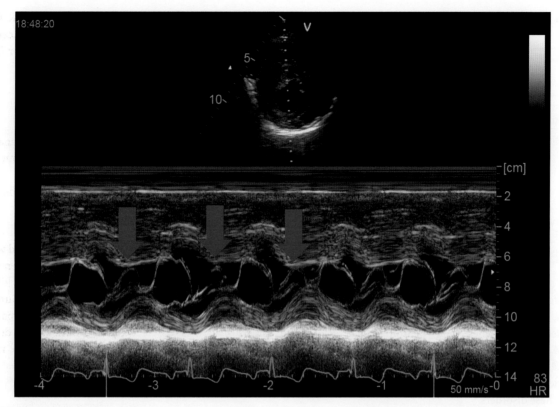

Figure 3.4.3.5 M-mode echocardiogram showing systolic anterior motion of the mitral valve in hypertrophic obstructive cardiomyopathy.

be considered for risk stratification prior to sports participation, and symptomatic patients without a resting or provocable LVOT gradient of >50 mmHg on transthoracic echocardiography (TTE) should undergo an exercise TTE to detect and quantify latent LVOTO.[2,4] An abnormal blood pressure response to exercise, which is present in about one-third of patients, is a marker of poor prognosis.[56,57,58]

Differential diagnosis

Conditions that produce secondary LVH can overlap phenotypically with HCM, such as remodelling secondary to intense exercise, as well as morphological changes related to long-standing systemic hypertension. HCM subtypes not caused by cardiac sarcomere mutations are often referred to as HCM phenocopies and include a variety of disorders such as glycogen storage disorders,

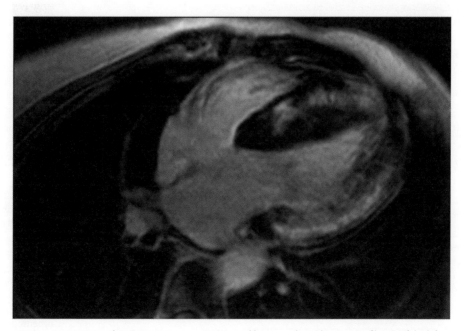

Figure 3.4.3.6 Cardiac magnetic resonance scan showing severe asymmetric septal hypertrophy with extensive fibrosis of the left ventricle.

Table 3.4.3.4 Differential diagnosis based on routine laboratory findings

Elevated transaminase levels	Mitochondrial diseases Glycogenosis Danon disease
Proteinuria with/without decreased glomerular filtration rate	Anderson–Fabry disease Amyloidosis
Elevated creatine kinase levels	Mitochondrial diseases Glycogenosis Danon disease ALPK3 mutations
Lactic acidosis	Mitochondrial diseases
Leucocytopenia	Mitochondrial diseases (TAZ gene/Barth syndrome)
Myoglobinuria	Mitochondrial diseases

lysosomal storage disorders, mitochondrial cytopathies, cardiac amyloidosis, disorders of fatty acid metabolism, neuro-cardio-facial-cutaneous syndromes, and neuromuscular disorders (➲ Table 3.4.3.5). Patterns of inheritance, multi-organ (especially neurological, musculoskeletal, and renal) involvement, and ECG characteristics, such as pre-excitation, are useful to differentiate HCM from these disorders.[47]

Table 3.4.3.5 Differential diagnosis of hypertrophic cardiomyopathy

Disease	Clinical features
Glycogen storage diseases	
Type II (Pompe)	Hypotonia, failure to thrive
Type III (Cori or Forbes disease)	Hypoglycaemia, failure to thrive, hepatomegaly
Type IX (cardiac phosphorylase kinase deficiency)	Hepatomegaly, growth retardation
Congenital disorder of glycosylation type 1a	Neurodevelopmental delay
Disorders of amino acid metabolism	
Type 1 tyrosinaemia	Failure to thrive
Dihydrolipoamide dehydrogenase deficiency	Maple syrup urine disease
Disorders of fatty acid metabolism	
Very long-chain acyl CoA dehydrogenase deficiency (VLCAD)	Fatigue, muscle weakness, hepatomegaly, metabolic crisis
Malonyl-CoA decarboxylase deficiency	Hypotonia, developmental delay, hypoglycaemia
Systemic primary carnitine deficiency	Variable—metabolic or cardiac presentation
Lysosomal storage diseases	
Mucolipidosis type II α/β	Short stature, skeletal abnormalities
Mucopolysaccharidosis type VII (Sly syndrome)	Macrocephaly, hepatosplenomegaly
Gangliosidosis type 1	HCM or DCM

Disease	Clinical features
Mitochondrial disorders	
Complex I, II, III, IV, and V deficiency	Variable presentations
ACAD9 deficiency (complex I)	
ATP synthase deficiency (complex V)	Hypotonia, hypertrophic cardiomyopathy, lactic acidosis, hyperammonaemia, and 3-methylglutaconic aciduria
Cytochrome C oxidase deficiency (complex IV)	
Mitochondrial disorders	
Combined oxidative phosphorylation deficiency (types 3, 5, 8, 9, and 10)	Fatal infantile HCM
Kearns–Sayre syndrome	Chronic progressive external ophthalmoplegia, bilateral pigmentary retinopathy, and cardiac conduction abnormalities
Leber's hereditary optic neuropathy	Acute loss of central vision
Leigh syndrome (pyruvate dehydrogenase complex deficiency)	Movement disorders
Friedreich's ataxia	Most common inherited ataxia, often non-ambulatory by mid-twenties; major cause of death is heart failure. Estimated carrier frequency 1/100. Due to mutation or trinucleotide repeat expansion (GAA)
Sengers syndrome	Congenital cataracts, skeletal myopathy, lactic acidosis
Pyruvate dehydrogenase lipoic acid synthetase deficiency	Neonatal encephalomyopathy, lactic acidosis
Primary coenzyme Q10 deficiency	Encephalopathy, myopathy
Cardiocutaneous syndromes or RASopathies	
LEOPARD syndrome	Lentigines, ECG abnormalities, ocular hypertelorism, pulmonary valve stenosis, abnormalities of genitalia in males, growth retardation, deafness
Noonan syndrome	Pulmonary stenosis, atrial septal defect, short stature, learning difficulties, pectus excavatum, impaired blood clotting, webbed neck, flat nose bridge
Costello syndrome	Fetal overgrowth, postnatal growth retardation, coarse face, loose skin, developmental delay
Cardiofaciocutaneous syndrome	Overlap with Costello and Noonan syndrome
Neurofibromatosis type I	Neurofibromas, café-au-lait patches, high blood pressure
Lipodystrophic syndromes	
Congenital generalized lipodystrophy	
Type 1 (Berardinelli–Seip syndrome)	Lipoatrophy, hepatomegaly, acromegaloid features, insulin resistance, skeletal muscle hypertrophy

Disease	Clinical features
Type 2 (Seip syndrome)	
Neuromuscular disorders	
Myofibrillar myopathy type 2	Early cataracts
Myofibrillar myopathy type 1	HCM, DCM, or RCM. Initially distal, then proximal muscle weakness. Onset in second or third decade
Myopathy, X-linked, with postural muscle atrophy or Emery–Dreifuss muscular dystrophy type 6	Progressive muscular dystrophy with onset in adulthood. Patients may show muscle hypertrophy in early stages of the disorder
Congenital myopathy 2a, typical autosomal dominant (nemaline myopathy type 3 (NEM3))	Skeletal myopathy with variable age of onset and severity. Also DCM

HCM, hypertrophic cardiomyopathy; DCM, dilated cardiomyopathy; ATP, adenosine triphosphate; RCM, restrictive cardiomyopathy.

Hypertension

Systemic hypertension is the most common cause of acquired LVH but frequently coexists with HCM. Hypertension alone typically produces concentric remodelling of the left ventricle, as opposed to asymmetric septal hypertrophy with a small cavity size in HCM.[59,60,61,62] Moderate to severe hypertrophy (≥15 mm) is rare in Caucasians with hypertension but occurs more frequently in black patients. A normal 12-lead ECG or increased QRS voltage without repolarization abnormality favours hypertensive disease. SAM of the mitral valve or dynamic LVOTO may be seen in some patients with LVH secondary to hypertension but tends to occur later in systole, compared to HCM. Tissue Doppler imaging may show greater impairment of diastolic function in HCM, with lower early diastolic velocities and greater reductions in radial and longitudinal strain. CMR imaging can be helpful in identifying patterns of fibrosis that are more typical of HCM, and levels of serum markers, such as brain natriuretic peptide, tend to be higher in HCM than in hypertensive LVH patients. Good blood pressure control with antihypertensive agents can lead to reverse ventricular remodelling, with regression of hypertrophy over 6–12 months, in patients with hypertensive heart disease.

Athletic adaptation

Some highly trained athletes, especially weightlifters, rowers, and cyclists, have physiological hypertrophy. However, this will regress if training is discontinued and a septal thickness of >16 mm is likely to be pathological.[63,64,65,66,67,68] Several features such as a family history of HCM or SCD, symptoms, ECG findings (abnormal Q-waves, inverted T-waves), echocardiographic findings (asymmetrical septal LVH, SAM of the mitral valve), a lack of response to detraining for 3 months, and positive genetic testing favour a diagnosis of HCM. Additionally, LVH in female athletes does not usually reach the severity found in HCM. Black athletes may demonstrate a greater LV wall thickness of up to 16 mm. Doppler evidence of abnormal filling patterns with impaired diastolic function is not usually seen in the athlete's heart.

Cardiac amyloidosis

Light chain amyloidosis (AL) and TTR amyloidosis (mutant and wild-type) are commonly associated with HCM and restrictive cardiomyopathy.[69] TTR amyloid cardiomyopathy (➔ Figure 3.4.3.7), caused by deposition of TTR amyloid fibrils in the myocardium, is a common cause of HF with preserved ejection fraction in the elderly. Clues to the diagnosis include a history of bilateral carpal tunnel syndrome, biceps tendon rupture, and lumbar spinal stenosis. Echocardiographic features suggestive of the disease include pericardial effusion with bi-atrial dilatation, restrictive LV physiology, apical sparing on global longitudinal strain, and a granular sparkling appearance of the myocardium. On CMR imaging, increased T1 signal and marked extracellular volume expansion are highly suggestive of cardiac amyloidosis. This may occur with subendocardial enhancement on gadolinium-enhanced imaging. TTR cardiac amyloidosis is particularly avid for ^{99m}Tc-phosphate derivatives used for bone imaging, and increased cardiac uptake in the absence of evidence for plasma cell dyscrasia is pathognomonic for the disease (➔ Figure 3.4.3.8).[69]

Treatment of TTR amyloid cardiomyopathy with tafamidis, a novel drug that binds to the thyroxine-binding site on the TTR tetramer and inhibits its dissociation into monomers, is associated with reductions in all-cause mortality and cardiovascular-related hospitalizations and reduces the decline in functional capacity and quality of life, as compared to placebo.[70]

Genetic testing

Clinical genetic testing supports a diagnosis of HCM and guides individualized treatment decisions for specific disease subtypes. It also underpins screening and management strategies for families. Depending on the gene panel and genetic screening method used, a disease-causing genetic variant is found in between 34% and 60% of cases.[71,72,73] Variants responsible for HCM can be found in various genes, but the majority occur in those encoding sarcomeric proteins.

Clinical scenarios influenced by genetic test results include:

♦ Presymptomatic diagnosis: early clinical manifestations in asymptomatic carriers of pathogenic variants may be subtle and may only become apparent with serial monitoring

♦ Clinical monitoring: monitoring of affected and healthy variant carriers is tailored to age, baseline tests, symptoms, and other non-cardiac traits in cases of syndromic cardiomyopathies

♦ Therapy: examples of diagnoses that have specific drug therapies include some storage disorders (e.g. Fabry disease) and RASopathies (e.g. MEK inhibitors such as selumetinib)

♦ Prenatal diagnosis and preimplantation diagnoses: identification of a pathogenic variant provides the opportunity for preimplantation genetic testing.

In the past, genetic analysis was performed using Sanger sequencing whereby the order of nucleotides is analysed in series, one after the other, in each gene of interest. While this method is accurate and reproducible, it is also time-consuming and expensive, and so most clinical diagnostic testing is performed using a highly parallelized sequencing process (next-generation sequencing), which permits rapid and simultaneous investigation of large numbers of genes using targeted gene panels (a set of known disease-causing genes). Whole-exome sequencing (WES), which covers almost all protein-coding sequences, or whole-genome sequencing (WGS),

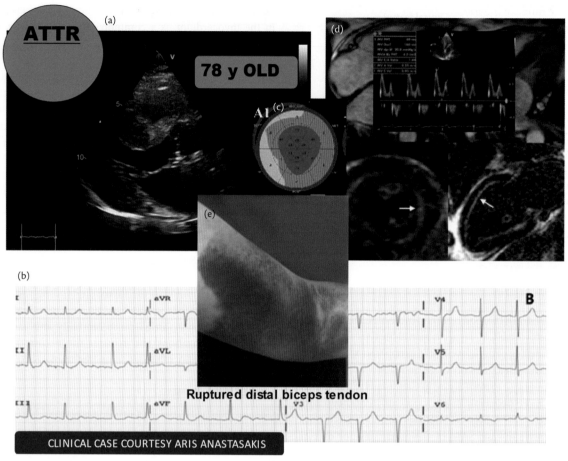

Figure 3.4.3.7 A 78-year-old male patient (ATTR amyloidosis, wild-type). (a) Left ventricular hypertrophy. (b) ECG: QS in leads V1 to V3. (c) Restrictive diastolic function. (d) Cardiac magnetic resonance: subendocardial fibrosis. (e) Ruptured distal biceps tendon.

which also includes nearly all non-coding sequences, are rapidly transitioning into routine diagnosis.

Genetic counselling is an essential component of the diagnostic process and management of HCM. This should include creation of a three-generation family pedigree to provide information on the heritability of the disease and inform recommendations for screening of relatives.[2,4] Whenever genetic testing is offered, individuals should be informed about the purpose of the test, the

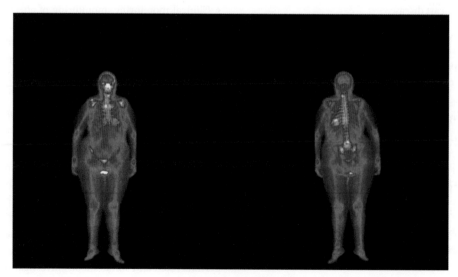

Figure 3.4.3.8 DPD cardiac uptake grade III.
Courtesy of Dr Koutelou (Onassis Cardiac Surgery Centre).

most probable mode of inheritance, the reliability of the test, and the potential hazards, including the psychological and social impact of a test result.

Treatment and management

Management of symptoms

Symptomatic patients with LVOTO should be treated with non-vasodilating beta-blockers.[2,3,74,75,76,77,78,79,80] If beta-blockers are not tolerated or are ineffective, then disopyramide, verapamil, or diltiazem can be used. Low-dose loop or thiazide diuretics can be considered with caution to improve breathlessness, but while avoiding hypovolaemia. Patients who remain symptomatic, with LVOTO of >50 mmHg, New York Heart Association (NYHA) class III–IV symptoms, and/or recurrent exertional syncope despite maximum tolerated medical therapy, should be considered for invasive treatment.[2,3] The main invasive methods for relieving LVOTO are surgical myectomy and septal alcohol ablation. Surgical septal myectomy involves resection of a rectangular trough from the basal septum below the aortic valve to beyond the point of the mitral leaflet–septal contact. Septal alcohol ablation is the process by which a localized septal scar is created following selective injection of alcohol into a septal perforator artery. This relieves the LVOTO, but potential issues with the papillary muscles or the mitral valve cannot be addressed. The mortality rate is similar to that with surgical myomectomy (1–3%), with the main complications being atrioventricular (AV) block (7–20%).[81,82,83,84,85,86,87]

In non-obstructive HCM, the main therapies to improve symptoms include beta-blockers, verapamil, and diltiazem. Symptoms of HF should be treated according to standard guidelines. ACE inhibitors (ACEIs) and mineralocorticoid receptor antagonists are indicated if the LVEF is <50%.[2,3]

Emerging pharmacological therapies

Mavacamten is a novel, first-in-class allosteric inhibitor of cardiac myosin ATPase, which selectively reduces myocardial contractility by decreasing actin–myosin affinity and restoring the ratio of myosin heads in the super-relaxed state.[88] CK274 is also a drug with a similar action, but with a different pharmacokinetic profile, currently undergoing phase 2 clinical experimentation (ClinicalTrials.gov identifier: NCT04219826). EXPLORER-HCM, a multicentre phase 3 study, evaluated the efficacy and safety of mavacamten in adults with symptomatic obstructive HCM and showed improvement in peak oxygen consumption during exercise, NYHA functional class, and post-exercise LVOTO gradient, compared to placebo. The drug was generally well tolerated and a decrease in LVEF to <50% on mavacamten was observed in 6% of patients, which resolved in all patients with temporary treatment discontinuation.

Sudden cardiac death prevention

Systematic identification and management of patients at high risk of SCD is central to management of HCM.[2,3] The risk of SCD ranges from 0.5% to 2% per year in adults with HCM.[89,90,91,92,93,94,95,96,97] There appears to be no sex- or race-based differences in absolute SCD risk, but women may have a higher rate than general

population controls, compared to men.[97,98,99] Several clinical risk factors are used to identify high-risk patients who may be candidates for SCD prevention with implantable cardioverter–defibrillators (ICDs).[2,3] Current ESC guidelines recommend the use of a disease-specific prediction tool (HCM Risk-SCD Score) that is used to calculate a 5-year risk estimate for SCD, based on age, family history of SCD, unexplained syncope, LVOT gradient, maximum LV wall thickness, left atrial diameter, and the presence of non-sustained ventricular tachycardia (NSVT). Treatment thresholds for ICD implantation are guided by the 5-year risk estimate (➲ Figure 3.4.3.9).[2] The score is validated only in adults, but similar risk tools have been developed for children and adolescents.[96] In addition, it does not apply to rarer phenocopies. Other potential risk markers considered in American guidelines include potential prognostic markers such as extensive late gadolinium enhancement, LV apical aneurysms, or impaired ejection fraction, and these may be helpful in borderline or uncertain cases.[3]

Atrial fibrillation

The most common arrhythmia in HCM patients is AF, which is associated with reduced quality of life, HF, and stroke.[100,101,102] Restoration of sinus rhythm may reduce AF-related symptoms and functional decline. Both European and American guidelines initially recommend a pharmacological approach to maintain sinus rhythm, with amiodarone considered to be the most effective. Other options include sotalol and disopyramide.[2,3] Anticoagulation using direct-acting oral anticoagulants (DOACs) as a first-line option and vitamin K antagonists as a second-line option, independent of the CHA2DS2-VASc score, is indicated in all patients with AF.[2,3] Rate control can be achieved with beta-blockers, verapamil, or diltiazem.[2,3] Non-pharmacological treatment of AF by catheter-based or surgical ablation may be considered in symptomatic patients with relapses despite adequate medical therapy. Nonetheless, repeat procedures are frequently needed, as mid-term recurrence despite continuing antiarrhythmic drugs is common.[103,104]

Exercise recommendations

Until recently, guidelines prohibited competitive sports in all individuals with HCM. However, recent data showed that individuals who continued participating in sports after ICD implantation had no increase in appropriate device therapies and demonstrated that patients with HCM who participated in rehabilitation programmes had significantly improved functional capacity without any adverse events,[105,106,107,108] thus leading to relaxation of this advice. The latest ESC guidelines on sports participation recommend a more liberal approach, suggesting a more tailored approach after careful evaluation[109] and discussion with the patient and family.

Conclusions

Since its modern characterization more than half a century ago, progress in the diagnosis and management of patients with HCM has paralleled technological advances in genetic testing, cardiac imaging, prevention of serious arrhythmias, cardiac surgery, and interventional cardiology. Enhanced annotation of the human

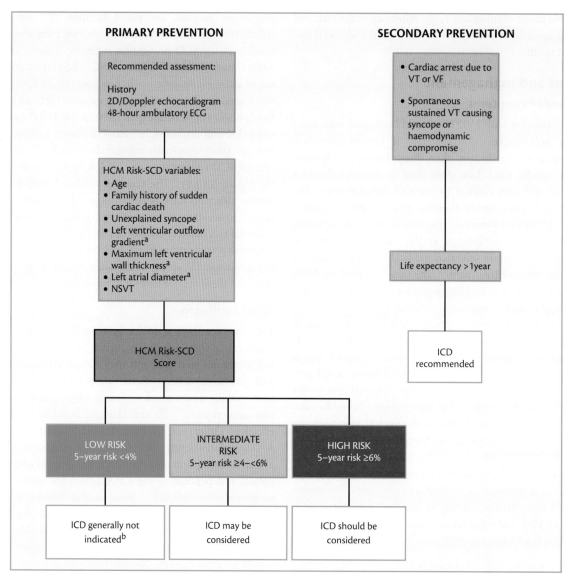

Figure 3.4.3.9 Risk stratification for sudden cardiac death.

Elliott PM, Anastasakis A, Borger MA, *et al.* 2014 ESC Guidelines on diagnosis and management of hypertrophic cardiomyopathy: the Task Force for the Diagnosis and Management of Hypertrophic Cardiomyopathy of the European Society of Cardiology (ESC). *Eur Heart J.* 2014 Oct 14;35(39):2733–79. doi: 10.1093/eurheartj/ehu284. © The European Society of Cardiology. Reprinted by permission of Oxford University Press.

genetic variants and their variable relation to clinical expression is likely to facilitate identification of individuals who carry pathogenic variants, allowing precise identification of patients prone to complications and enabling the development of new modifying therapies.

References

1. Elliott P, *et al.* Classification of the cardiomyopathies: a position statement from the European Society of Cardiology Working Group on Myocardial and Pericardial Diseases. *Eur Heart J.* 2008;29(2):270–6.

2. Elliott P, *et al.* 2014 ESC Guidelines on diagnosis and management of hypertrophic cardiomyopathy: the Task Force for the Diagnosis and Management of Hypertrophic Cardiomyopathy of the European Society of Cardiology (ESC). *Eur Heart J.* 2014;35(39):2733–79.

3. Ommen SR, *et al.* 2020 AHA/ACC Guideline for the diagnosis and treatment of patients with hypertrophic cardiomyopathy: executive summary: a Report of the American College of Cardiology/American Heart Association Joint Committee on Clinical Practice Guidelines. *J Am Coll Cardiol.* 2020;76(25):3022–55.

4. Semsarian C, *et al.* New perspectives on the prevalence of hypertrophic cardiomyopathy. *J Am Coll Cardiol.* 2015;65(12):1249–54.

5. Maron BJ, *et al.* Prevalence of hypertrophic cardiomyopathy in a general population of young adults. Echocardiographic analysis of 4111 subjects in the CARDIA Study. Coronary Artery Risk Development in (Young) Adults. *Circulation.* 1995;92(4):785–9.

6. Maron BJ, *et al.* Clinical profile of hypertrophic cardiomyopathy identified *de novo* in rural communities. *J Am Coll Cardiol.* 1999;33(6):1590–5.

7. Zou Y, *et al.* Prevalence of idiopathic hypertrophic cardiomyopathy in China: a population-based echocardiographic analysis of 8080 adults. *Am J Med.* 2004;116(1):14–18.

8. Maron BJ, *et al.* Prevalence of hypertrophic cardiomyopathy in a population-based sample of American Indians aged 51 to 77 years (the Strong Heart Study). *Am J Cardiol.* 2004;93(12):1510–14.

9. Corrado D, *et al.* Screening for hypertrophic cardiomyopathy in young athletes. *N Engl J Med.* 1998;339(6):364–9.

10. Nistri S, *et al.* Screening for hypertrophic cardiomyopathy in a young male military population. *Am J Cardiol.* 2003;91(8):1021–3, A8.

11. Maron BJ, *et al.* Genetics of hypertrophic cardiomyopathy after 20 years: clinical perspectives. *J Am Coll Cardiol.* 2012;60:705–15.

12. Nugent AW, *et al.* The epidemiology of childhood cardiomyopathy in Australia. *N Engl J Med.* 2003;348:1639–46.

13. Lipshultz SE, *et al.* The incidence of pediatric cardiomyopathy in two regions of the United States. *N Engl J Med.* 2003;348:1647–55.

14. Ho CY, *et al.* Genetic advances in sarcomeric cardiomyopathies: state of the art. *Cardiovasc Res.* 2015;105:397–408.

15. Thierfelder L, *et al.* α-tropomyosin and cardiac troponin T mutations cause familial hypertrophic cardiomyopathy: a disease of the sarcomere. *Cell.* 1994;77:701–12.

16. Van Driest SL, *et al.* Prevalence and spectrum of thin filament mutations in an outpatient referral population with hypertrophic cardiomyopathy. *Circulation.* 2003;108:445–51.

17. Coppini R, *et al.* Clinical phenotype and outcome of hypertrophic cardiomyopathy associated with thin-filament gene mutations. *J Am Coll Cardiol.* 2014;64:2589–600.

18. Belus A, *et al.* The familial hypertrophic cardiomyopathy-associated myosin mutation R403Q accelerates tension generation and relaxation of human cardiac myofibrils. *J Physiol.* 2008;586:3639–44.

19. Ferrantini C, *et al.* Mechanical and energetic consequences of HCM-causing mutations. *J Cardiovasc Transl Res.* 2009;2:441–51.

20. Spudich JA. Three perspectives on the molecular basis of hypercontractility caused by hypertrophic cardiomyopathy mutations. *Arch Eur J Physiol.* 2019;471:701–17.

21. Tardiff JC, *et al.* Targets for therapy in sarcomeric cardiomyopathies. *Cardiovasc Res.* 2015;105(4):457–70.

22. Ashrafian H, *et al.* Hypertrophic cardiomyopathy: a paradigm for myocardial energy depletion. *Trends Genet.* 2003;19:263–8.

23. Hoskins AC, *et al.* Normal passive viscoelasticity but abnormal myofibrillar force generation in human hypertrophic cardiomyopathy. *J Mol Cell Cardiol.* 2010;49(5):737–45.

24. Schotten U, *et al.* Altered force-frequency relation in hypertrophic obstructive cardiomyopathy. *Basic Res Cardiol.* 1999;94(2):120–7.

25. Kim D-H, *et al.* *In vivo* measurement of mitral leaflet surface area and subvalvular geometry in patients with asymmetrical septal hypertrophy: insights into the mechanism of outflow tract obstruction. *Circulation.* 2010;122:1298–307.

26. Sherrid MV, *et al.* Systolic anterior motion begins at low left ventricular outflow tract velocity in obstructive hypertrophic cardiomyopathy. *J Am Coll Cardiol.* 2000;36:1344–54.

27. Maron MS, *et al.* Hypertrophic cardiomyopathy is predominantly a disease of left ventricular outflow tract obstruction. *Circulation.* 2006;114(21):2232–9.

28. Shah JS, *et al.* Prevalence of exercise-induced left ventricular outflow tract obstruction in symptomatic patients with non-obstructive hypertrophic cardiomyopathy. *Heart.* 2008;94(10):1288–94.

29. Patel P, *et al.* Left ventricular outflow tract obstruction in hypertrophic cardiomyopathy patients without severe septal hypertrophy: implications of mitral valve and papillary muscle abnormalities assessed using cardiac magnetic resonance and echocardiography. *Circ Cardiovasc Imaging.* 2015;8:e003132.

30. Numata S, *et al.* Excess anterior mitral leaflet in a patient with hypertrophic obstructive cardiomyopathy and systolic anterior motion. *Circulation.* 2015;131:1605–7.

31. Bonow RO, *et al.* Regional left ventricular asynchrony and impaired global left ventricular filling in hypertrophic cardiomyopathy: effect of verapamil. *J Am Coll Cardiol.* 1987;9(5):1108–16.

32. Nihoyannopoulos P, *et al.* Diastolic function in hypertrophic cardiomyopathy: relation to exercise capacity. *J Am Coll Cardiol.* 1992;19(3):536–40.

33. Villemain O, *et al.* Myocardial stiffness evaluation using noninvasive shear wave imaging in healthy and hypertrophic cardiomyopathic adults. *J Am Coll Cardiol Imaging.* 2019;12:1135–45.

34. Hang D, *et al.* Accuracy of jet direction on Doppler echocardiography in identifying the etiology of mitral regurgitation in obstructive hypertrophic cardiomyopathy. *J Am Soc Echocardiogr.* 2019;32:333–40.

35. Maron MS, *et al.* Mitral valve abnormalities identified by cardiovascular magnetic resonance represent a primary phenotypic expression of hypertrophic cardiomyopathy. *Circulation.* 2011;124:40–7.

36. Groarke JD, *et al.* Intrinsic mitral valve alterations in hypertrophic cardiomyopathy sarcomere mutation carriers. *Eur Heart J Cardiovasc Imaging.* 2018;19:1109–16.

37. Sherrid MV, *et al.* The mitral valve in obstructive hypertrophic cardiomyopathy: a test in context. *J Am Coll Cardiol.* 2016;67:1846–58.

38. Cannon RO 3rd, *et al.* Myocardial ischemia in patients with hypertrophic cardiomyopathy: contribution of inadequate vasodilator reserve and elevated left ventricular filling pressures. *Circulation.* 1985;71(2):234–43.

39. Maron BJ, *et al.* Intramural ('small vessel') coronary artery disease in hypertrophic cardiomyopathy. *J Am Coll Cardiol.* 1986;8:545–57.

40. Karamitsos TD, *et al.* Blunted myocardial oxygenation response during vasodilator stress in patients with hypertrophic cardiomyopathy. *J Am Coll Cardiol.* 2013;61:1169–76.

41. Raphael CE, *et al.* Mechanisms of myocardial ischemia in hypertrophic cardiomyopathy: insights from wave intensity analysis and magnetic resonance. *J Am Coll Cardiol.* 2016;68:1651–60.

42. Bravo PE, *et al.* Relationship of delayed enhancement by magnetic resonance to myocardial perfusion by positron emission tomography in hypertrophic cardiomyopathy. *Circ Cardiovasc Imaging.* 2013;6:210–17.

43. Binder J, *et al.* Apical hypertrophic cardiomyopathy: prevalence and correlates of apical outpouching. *J Am Soc Echocardiogr.* 2011;24:775–81.

44. Hostiuc S, *et al.* Cardiovascular consequences of myocardial bridging: a meta-analysis and meta-regression. *Sci Rep.* 2017;7:14644.

45. Sharzehee M, *et al.* Hemodynamic effects of myocardial bridging in patients with hypertrophic cardiomyopathy. *Am J Physiol Heart Circ Physiol.* 2019;317:H1282–91.

46. Rowin EJ, *et al.* Hypertrophic cardiomyopathy with left ventricular apical aneurysm: implications for risk stratification and management. *J Am Coll Cardiol.* 2017;69:761–73.

47. Rapezzi C, *et al.* Diagnostic work-up in cardiomyopathies: bridging the gap between clinical phenotypes and final diagnosis. A position statement from the ESC Working Group on Myocardial and Pericardial Diseases. *Eur Heart J.* 2013;34(19):1448–58.

48. Williams LK, *et al.* Echocardiography in hypertrophic cardiomyopathy diagnosis, prognosis, and role in management. *Eur J Echocardiogr* 2009;10:iii9–14.

49. Neubauer S, *et al.* Distinct subgroups in hypertrophic cardiomyopathy in the NHLBI HCM Registry. *J Am Coll Cardiol.* 2019;74(19):2333–45.

50. Briasoulis A, *et al.* Myocardial fibrosis on cardiac magnetic resonance and cardiac outcomes in hypertrophic cardiomyopathy: a meta-analysis. *Heart.* 2015;101(17):1406–11.

51. Maron MS. Clinical utility of cardiovascular magnetic resonance in hypertrophic cardiomyopathy. *J Cardiovasc Magn Reson.* 2012;14(1):13.

52. Chan RH, *et al.* Prognostic value of quantitative contrast-enhanced cardiovascular magnetic resonance for the evaluation of sudden death risk in patients with hypertrophic cardiomyopathy. *Circulation.* 2014;130(6):484–95.

53. Radenkovic D, et al. T1 mapping in cardiac MRI. Heart Fail Rev. 2017;22(4):415–30.

54. Geske JB, et al. B-type natriuretic peptide and survival in hypertrophic cardiomyopathy. J Am Coll Cardiol. 2013;61(24):2456–60.

55. Coats CJ, et al. Relation between serum N-terminal pro-brain natriuretic peptide and prognosis in patients with hypertrophic cardiomyopathy. Eur Heart J. 2013;34(32):2529–37.

56. Coats CJ, et al. Cardiopulmonary exercise testing and prognosis in hypertrophic cardiomyopathy. Circ Heart Fail. 2015;8(6):1022–31.

57. Magrì D, et al. Heart failure progression in hypertrophic cardiomyopathy: possible insights from cardiopulmonary exercise testing. Circ J. 2016;80(10):2204–11.

58. Sadoul N, et al. Prospective prognostic assessment of blood pressure response during exercise in patients with hypertrophic cardiomyopathy. Circulation. 1997;96(9):2987–91.

59. Kato TS, et al. Discrimination of nonobstructive hypertrophic cardiomyopathy from hypertensive left ventricular hypertrophy on the basis of strain rate imaging by tissue Doppler ultrasonography. Circulation. 2004;110:3808–14.

60. Doi YL, et al. 'Pseudo' systolic anterior motion in patients with hypertensive heart disease. Eur Heart J. 1983;4:838–45.

61. Nagakura T, et al. Hypertrophic cardiomyopathy is associated with more severe left ventricular dyssynchrony than is hypertensive left ventricular hypertrophy. Echocardiography. 2007;24:677–84.

62. Ogino K, et al. Neurohumoral profiles in patients with hypertrophic cardiomyopathy: differences to hypertensive left ventricular hypertrophy. Circ J. 2004;68:444–50.

63. Pelliccia A, et al. European Association of Preventive Cardiology (EAPC) and European Association of Cardiovascular Imaging (EACVI) joint position statement: recommendations for the indication and interpretation of cardiovascular imaging in the evaluation of the athlete's heart. Eur Heart J. 2018;39(21):1949–69.

64. Basavarajaiah S, et al. Ethnic differences in left ventricular remodeling in highly-trained athletes. J Am Coll Cardiol. 2008;51(23): 2256–62.

65. Sharma S, et al. International recommendations for electrocardiographic interpretation in athletes. Eur Heart J. 2018;39(16): 1466–80.

66. Pelliccia A, et al. Remodeling of left ventricular hypertrophy in elite athletes after long-term deconditioning. Circulation. 2002; 105(8):944–9.

67. Weiner RB, et al. Regression of 'gray zone' exercise-induced concentric left ventricular hypertrophy during prescribed detraining. J Am Coll Cardiol. 2012;59(22):1992–4.

68. Maron BJ. Distinguishing hypertrophic cardiomyopathy from athlete's heart: a clinical problem of increasing magnitude and significance. Heart. 2005;91:1380–2.

69. Maurer MS, et al. Addressing common questions encountered in the diagnosis and management of cardiac amyloidosis. Circulation. 2017;135(14):1357–77.

70. Maurer MS, et al.; ATTR-ACT Study Investigators. Tafamidis treatment for patients with transthyretin amyloid cardiomyopathy. N Engl J Med. 2018;379(11):1007–16.

71. Alfares AA, et al. Results of clinical genetic testing of 2,912 probands with hypertrophic cardiomyopathy: expanded panels offer limited additional sensitivity. Genet Med. 2015;17(11):880–8.

72. Ingles J, et al. Evaluating the clinical validity of hypertrophic cardiomyopathy genes. Circ Genomic Precis Med. 2019;12(2):e002460.

73. Ingles J, et al. A cost-effectiveness model of genetic testing for the evaluation of families with hypertrophic cardiomyopathy. Heart. 2012;98(8):625–30.

74. Ammirati E, et al. Pharmacological treatment of hypertrophic cardiomyopathy: current practice and novel perspectives. Eur J Heart Fail. 2016;18:1106–18.

75. Nistri S, et al. β blockers for prevention of exercise-induced left ventricular outflow tract obstruction in patients with hypertrophic cardiomyopathy. Am J Cardiol. 2012;110:715–19.

76. Moran AM, Colan SD. Verapamil therapy in infants with hypertrophic cardiomyopathy. Cardiol Young. 1998;8:310–19.

77. Bonow RO, et al. Effects of verapamil on left ventricular systolic function and diastolic filling in patients with hypertrophic cardiomyopathy. Circulation. 1981;64:787–96.

78. Coppini R, et al. Electrophysiological and contractile effects of disopyramide in patients with obstructive hypertrophic cardiomyopathy: a translational study. JACC Basic to Transl Sci. 2019;4:795–813.

79. Sherrid MV, et al. Multicenter study of the efficacy and safety of disopyramide in obstructive hypertrophic cardiomyopathy. J Am Coll Cardiol. 2005;45:1251–8.

80. Zampieri M, et al. Pathophysiology and treatment of hypertrophic cardiomyopathy: new perspectives. Curr Heart Fail Rep. 2021;18:169–79.

81. Rastegar H, et al. Results of surgical septal myectomy for obstructive hypertrophic cardiomyopathy: the Tufts experience. Ann Cardiothorac Surg. 2017;6:353–63.

82. Maron BJ, et al. Low operative mortality achieved with surgical septal myectomy: role of dedicated hypertrophic cardiomyopathy centers in the management of dynamic subaortic obstruction. J Am Coll Cardiol. 2015;66(11):1307–8.

83. Kwon DH, et al. Characteristics and surgical outcomes of symptomatic patients with hypertrophic cardiomyopathy with abnormal papillary muscle morphology undergoing papillary muscle reorientation. J Thorac Cardiovasc Surg. 2010;140(2):317–24.

84. Hong JH, et al. Mitral regurgitation in patients with hypertrophic obstructive cardiomyopathy: implications for concomitant valve procedures. J Am Coll Cardiol. 2016;68:1497–504.

85. Veselka J, et al. Long-term survival after alcohol septal ablation for hypertrophic obstructive cardiomyopathy: a comparison with general population. Eur Heart J. 2014;35(30):2040–5.

86. Liebregts M, et al. A systematic review and meta-analysis of long-term outcomes after septal reduction therapy in patients with hypertrophic cardiomyopathy. JACC Heart Fail. 2015;3(11): 896–905.

87. Agarwal S, et al. Updated meta-analysis of septal alcohol ablation versus myectomy for hypertrophic cardiomyopathy. J Am Coll Cardiol. 2010;55(8):823–34.

88. Olivotto I, et al. Mavacamten for treatment of symptomatic obstructive hypertrophic cardiomyopathy (EXPLORER-HCM): a randomised, double-blind, placebo-controlled, phase 3 trial. Lancet. 2020;396:759–69.

89. O'Mahony C, Elliott PM. Prevention of sudden cardiac death in hypertrophic cardiomyopathy. Heart. 2014;100(3):254–60.

90. Maron BJ. Contemporary insights and strategies for risk stratification and prevention of sudden death in hypertrophic cardiomyopathy. Circulation. 2010;121(3):445–56. Erratum in: Circulation. 2010;122(1):e7.

91. Elliott PM, et al. Sudden death in hypertrophic cardiomyopathy: identification of high risk patients. J Am Coll Cardiol. 2000;36:2212–18.

92. Maron BJ. Risk stratification and role of implantable defibrillators for prevention of sudden death in patients with hypertrophic cardiomyopathy. Circulation. 2010;74:2271–82.

93. Ho CY, et al. Genotype and lifetime burden of disease in hypertrophic cardiomyopathy: insights from the sarcomeric human cardiomyopathy Registry (SHaRe). Circulation. 2018;138(14):1387–98.

94. O'Mahony C, et al.; Hypertrophic Cardiomyopathy Outcomes Investigators. A novel clinical risk prediction model for sudden cardiac death in hypertrophic cardiomyopathy (HCM risk-SCD). Eur Heart J. 2014;35(30):2010–20.

95. O'Mahony C, et al. International External Validation Study of the 2014 European Society of Cardiology Guidelines on Sudden Cardiac Death Prevention in Hypertrophic Cardiomyopathy (EVIDENCE-HCM). Circulation. 2018;137(10):1015–23.

96. Norrish G, *et al.* Development of a novel risk prediction model for sudden cardiac death in childhood hypertrophic cardiomyopathy (HCM Risk-Kids). *JAMA Cardiol.* 2019;4(9):918.

97. Lorenzini M, *et al.* Mortality among referral patients with hypertrophic cardiomyopathy vs the general European population. *JAMA Cardiol.* 2020;5(1):73.

98. Wells S, *et al.* Association between race and clinical profile of patients referred for hypertrophic cardiomyopathy. *Circulation.* 2018;137:1973–5.

99. Olivotto I, *et al.* Gender-related differences in the clinical presentation and outcome of hypertrophic cardiomyopathy. *J Am Coll Cardiol.* 2005;46:480–7.

100. Maron BJ, *et al.* Clinical profile of stroke in 900 patients with hypertrophic cardiomyopathy. *J Am Coll Cardiol.* 2002;39(2):301–7.

101. Guttmann OP, *et al.* Atrial fibrillation and thromboembolism in patients with hypertrophic cardiomyopathy: systematic review. *Heart.* 2014;100(6):465–72.

102. Guttmann OP, *et al.* Predictors of atrial fibrillation in hypertrophic cardiomyopathy. *Heart.* 2017;103(9):672–8.

103. Zhao D-S, *et al.* Outcomes of catheter ablation of atrial fibrillation in patients with hypertrophic cardiomyopathy: a systematic review and meta-analysis. *Europace.* 2016;18:508–20.

104. Creta A, *et al.* Catheter ablation of atrial fibrillation in patients with hypertrophic cardiomyopathy: a European observational multicentre study. *Europace.* 2021;23(9):1409–17.

105. Dejgaard LA, *et al.* Vigorous exercise in patients with hypertrophic cardiomyopathy. *Int J Cardiol.* 2018;250:157–63.

106. Lampert R, *et al.* Safety of sports for athletes with implantable cardioverter-defibrillators: long-term results of a prospective multinational registry. *Circulation.* 2017;135(23):2310–12.

107. Klempfner R, *et al.* Efficacy of exercise training in symptomatic patients with hypertrophic cardiomyopathy: results of a structured exercise training program in a cardiac rehabilitation center. *Eur J Prev Cardiol.* 2015;22(1):13–19.

108. Saberi S, *et al.* Effect of moderate-intensity exercise training on peak oxygen consumption in patients with hypertrophic cardiomyopathy: a randomized clinical trial. *JAMA.* 2017;317(13):1349.

109. Pelliccia A, *et al.* 2020 ESC Guidelines on sports cardiology and exercise in patients with cardiovascular disease. *Eur Heart J.* 2021;42(1):17–96.

3.4.4 **Restrictive cardiomyopathy**

Claudio Rapezzi[†], Alberto Aimo, Ales Linhart, and Andre Keren

Definition and classification of restrictive cardiomyopathies: open issues

Restrictive cardiomyopathy (RCM) is probably the least common form of heart muscle disease, but also the most difficult to define and classify. Whereas the defining features of hypertrophic cardiomyopathy (HCM), dilated cardiomyopathy (DCM), and

[†]Author deceased.

some cases of arrhythmogenic cardiomyopathy can be easily detected by transthoracic echocardiography, the same is not true for RCM.

A 2008 position statement by the European Society of Cardiology (ESC) identified 'restrictive left ventricular (LV) physiology' as a hallmark of RCM (➲ Figure 3.4.4.1).

This physiology is characterized by increased myocardial stiffness causing a rapid rise in ventricular pressure, with only small increases in filling volumes.[1] According to the ESC definition, RCM is also characterized by 'normal or reduced systolic and diastolic volumes (of one or both ventricles)' and 'normal ventricular wall thickness'.[1] While this definition is accurate from a theoretical perspective, it does not capture some characteristics of several forms of RCM listed in the same position statement. For example, patients with cardiac amyloidosis (CA) nearly always show an increased LV wall thickness and their systolic function may be depressed; patients with cardiac sarcoidosis or advanced haemochromatosis almost always show dilated and hypokinetic ventricles. If we rely on restrictive physiology as a defining feature of RCM and we want to consider the disorders reported in ➲ Table 3.4.4.1 as forms of RCM, we must acknowledge that LV wall thickness can be increased, although such increase may not be due to cardiomyocyte hypertrophy, but rather due to interstitial infiltration (in CA) or intracellular storage (in glycogenosis, haemochromatosis, and sphingolipidoses). Indeed, in some disorders, the two phenotypes (hypertrophic and restrictive) may coexist in the same patient, making the classification challenging. Another important point is that many conditions traditionally classified as RCM do not show a restrictive physiology throughout their natural history (i.e. from early-stage to advanced disease), but only in the initial phase (with evolution towards a hypokinetic and dilated stage) or in the terminal phase (often starting from a HCM phenotype). This is, for example, the case of iron overload cardiomyopathy (IOC) and cardiac sarcoidosis, in which the overt cardiac phenotype is dilated and hypokinetic, but which can display a restrictive physiology in the initial phase when the LV is not dilated and LV ejection fraction (LVEF) is still preserved.

Another limitation of the current classification is that it does not refer to the type of myocardial substrate that is instead quite heterogeneous (➲ Figure 3.4.4.2). In some forms, there are abnormalities at the myocardial level, and in others at the endomyocardial level. Among the former conditions, we have disorders where the abnormality lies in cardiomyocyte functioning (without gross morphological abnormalities), and others with variable degrees of intramyocardial fibrosis, or with extracellular infiltration, or with intracellular accumulation.

A classification taking into account all these variables can be helpful to clinicians who must diagnose the patient and make appropriate treatment decisions. ➲ Figure 3.4.4.3 proposes a classification of RCM according to the substrate and the transitory or structural nature of the restrictive pathophysiology. The most frequent diseases will be examined in the second part of the chapter.

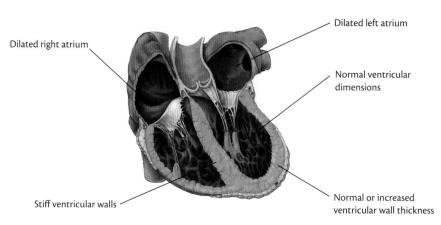

Restrictive cardiomyopathy

Dilated left atrium

Dilated right atrium

Normal ventricular dimensions

Stiff ventricular walls

Normal or increased ventricular wall thickness

Figure 3.4.4.1 Illustration of typical morphological features of restrictive cardiomyopathy.

The restrictive phenotype: haemodynamic, clinical, and imaging features

Patients with RCM have a rigid, non-compliant LV, with impaired diastolic filling and high filling pressures (central figure). Chronically elevated LV diastolic pressures commonly induce pulmonary hypertension, which tends to exacerbate right heart failure (HF), especially when the right ventricle (RV) is affected

Table 3.4.4.1 Possible causes of restrictive cardiomyopathy

Familial	Non-familial
Familial, unknown gene	Amyloid (AL/prealbumin)
Sarcomeric protein mutations	Scleroderma
Troponin I (RCM ± HCM)	Endomyocardial fibrosis
Essential light chain of myosin	Hypereosinophilic syndrome
Familial amyloidosis	Idiopathic
Transthyretin (RCM + neuropathy)	Chromosomal cause
Apolipoprotein (RCM + nephropathy)	Drugs (serotonin,
Desminopathy	methysergide, ergotamine,
Pseudoxanthoma elasticum	mercurial agents, busulfan)
Haemochromatosis	Carcinoid heart disease
Anderson–Fabry disease	Metastatic cancers
Glycogen storage disease	Radiation
Primary hyperoxaluria	Drugs (anthracyclines,
Gaucher disease	chloroquine/
Mucopolysaccharidosis types I and II	hydroxychloroquine)
Niemann–Pick disease	*Diabetic cardiomyopathy*
Myofibrillar myopathies	*Sarcoidosis*
Werner's syndrome	
Endocardial fibroelastosis	

Conditions not listed in the European Society of Cardiology position statement are shown in italics.

AL, amyloid light chain; HCM, hypertrophic cardiomyopathy; RCM, restrictive cardiomyopathy.

Reproduced from Elliott P, Andersson B, Arbustini E, *et al*. Classification of the cardiomyopathies: a position statement from the European Society of Cardiology Working Group on Myocardial and Pericardial Diseases. *Eur Heart J*. 2008 Jan;29(2):270–6. doi: 10.1093/eurheartj/ehm342 with permission from Oxford University Press.

by the disease process (as in CA). In the early stages of RCM, LV systolic function is typically preserved, at least when assessed in terms of LVEF, but tends to deteriorate over time. Despite preserved systolic function, the LV cannot fill adequately and therefore, the stroke volume cannot increase during exercise. The only adaptive response to exercise is an increase in heart rate, which can be blunted in patients with autonomic dysfunction such as some patients with CA. Low cardiac output and possibly also autonomic dysfunction make patients susceptible to hypotension. Furthermore, atrial dilatation often leads to atrial fibrillation (AF), which causes the loss of atrial contribution to LV filling.[2]

On *invasive haemodynamic assessment*, RCM is characterized by elevated diastolic filling pressures and rapid equalization of filling pressures of the four cardiac chambers during diastole, with a 'dip and plateau' or a 'square root' pattern on pressure tracings (➜ Figure 3.4.4).[3] This pattern may be amplified by manoeuvres that augment ventricular filling such as volume infusion or leg raising. As these findings are common in constrictive pericarditis (CP), several haemodynamic patterns allowing a differential diagnosis have been identified (➜ Table 3.4.4.2).[4] Atrial *x* and *y* descents tend to be relatively blunted compared with CP, and the *a* wave may be depressed when the atria are primarily affected (as in CA). Disproportionate left heart stiffness may also result in moderate pulmonary hypertension, which is not found in CP. Dynamic respiratory variations allow differentiation of RCM from CP. Indeed, the RCM process renders the chambers minimally distensible; therefore, there is little respiratory variation in flow or pressure, as opposite to CP. Additionally, in RCM, there is minimal ventricular interdependence, and thus inspiratory effects on ventricular systolic pressures are concordant, that is, there is little change in peak ventricular systolic pressures with respiration and they move in the same direction.[2,5]

With respect to *clinical features*, patients with RCM often complain of exercise intolerance due to inability of the ventricles to fill adequately at higher heart rates. Fatigue and lower extremity

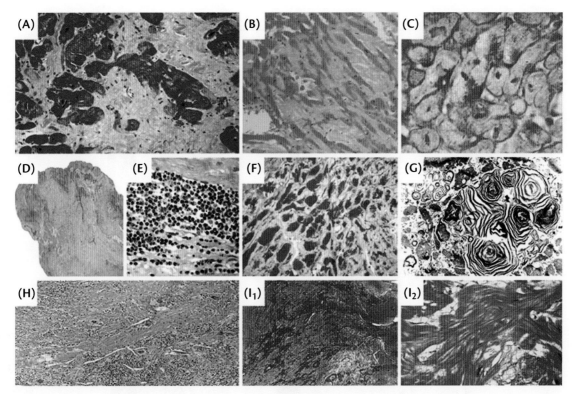

Figure 3.4.4.2 Myocardial tissue in nine different forms of restrictive cardiomyopathy (RCM). (A) Idiopathic RCM. (B) Cardiac amyloidosis. (C) Danon disease. (D) Endomyocardial fibrosis. (E) Hypereosinophilic syndrome. (F) Glycogenosis. (G) Anderson–Fabry disease. (H) Sarcoidosis. (I) End-stage hypertrophic cardiomyopathy.
Courtesy of Dr Ornella Leone, Bologna, Italy.

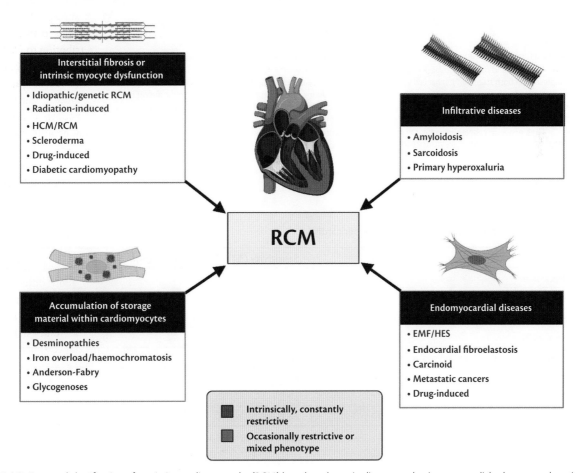

Figure 3.4.4.3 Proposed classification of restrictive cardiomyopathy (RCM) based on the main disease mechanism, myocardial substrate, and persistency of restriction over time. See text for details. EMF, endomyocardial fibrosis; HES, hypereosinophilic syndrome.

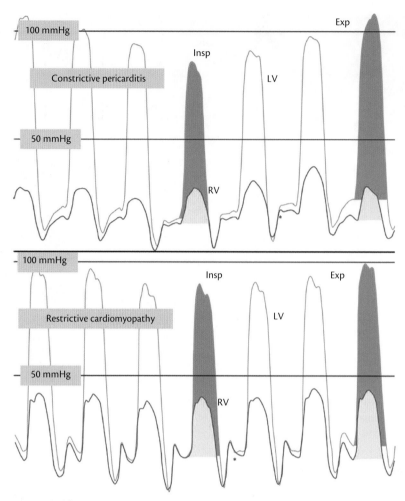

Figure 3.4.4.4 Simultaneous right and left ventricular haemodynamic assessment in constrictive pericarditis and restrictive cardiomyopathy.
(*Top*) Left ventricular (LV) (*blue*) and right ventricular (RV) (*orange*) haemodynamic pressure tracings in constrictive pericarditis. End-diastolic filling pressures are elevated, and a 'square root' sign is present on both tracings (*). Enhanced ventricular interdependence is present, demonstrated by visualization of the systolic area index, RV (*light grey*) and LV (*dark grey*) areas under the curve for both inspiration (*Insp*) and expiration (*Exp*). During inspiration, there is an increase in the area of the RV pressure curve and a decrease in the area of the LV pressure curve. (*Bottom*) LV and RV pressure tracings in restrictive cardiomyopathy. End-diastolic pressures are elevated and a square root sign (*) is seen; there is no evidence of enhanced ventricular interdependence, with parallel changes in LV and RV pressure curve areas.
Reproduced from Geske JB, Anavekar NS, Nishimura RA, Oh JK, Gersh BJ. Differentiation of Constriction and Restriction: Complex Cardiovascular Hemodynamics. *J Am Coll Cardiol.* 2016 Nov 29;68(21):2329–2347. doi: 10.1016/j.jacc.2016.08.050 with permission from Elsevier.

Table 3.4.4.2 Echocardiographic features of constrictive pericarditis

	Sensitivity (%)	Specificity (%)	PPV (%)	NPV (%)
1 Ventricular septal shift	93	69	92	74
2 Changes in mitral E velocity >14.6%	84	73	92	55
3 Medial e′ velocity >9 cm/s	83	81	94	57
4 Medial e′/lateral ≥0.91	75	85	95	50
5 Hepatic vein diastolic reversal velocity/forward velocity in expiration ≥0.79	76	88	96	49
1 and 3	80	92	97	56
1 with 3 or 5	87	91	97	65
1 with 3 and 5	64	97	99	42

E, early diastolic mitral inflow Doppler velocity; e′, early diastolic mitral annular tissue Doppler velocity; NPV, negative predictive value; PPV, positive predictive value.
Reproduced from Welch TD, Ling LH, Espinosa RE, Anavekar NS, Wiste HJ, Lahr BD, Schaff HV, Oh JK. Echocardiographic diagnosis of constrictive pericarditis: Mayo Clinic criteria. *Circ Cardiovasc Imaging.* 2014 May;7(3):526–34. doi: 10.1161/CIRCIMAGING.113.001613 with permission from Wolters Kluwer.

oedema are other prominent features. Chest pain is infrequent. Physical examination may reveal jugular venous distension, a third heart sound (produced by accelerated early diastolic LV filling—equivalent of a prominent E wave on transmitral Doppler recording), and less frequently a fourth heart sound (related to vigorous atrial contraction, rather encountered in early stages of the disease). Hepatomegaly, ascites, and marked oedema of the lower extremities may occur in more advanced cases. Mitral, as well as tricuspid, regurgitation is often present. The electrocardiogram shows sinus rhythm, with large P-waves indicative of bi-atrial enlargement, accompanied by non-specific repolarization abnormalities; AF is not uncommon. Low voltages, a pseudo-infarction pattern, bundle branch block, and atrioventricular block may point to specific aetiologies, as explained below. The chest X-ray usually shows a normal-sized ventricular silhouette, with enlarged atria, lack of calcification, and varying degrees of pulmonary congestion.[6,7,8]

Transthoracic echocardiography is the first-line imaging technique in the diagnostic workup of RCM, and enables both morphological characterization of the specific underlying cardiomyopathy and quite detailed characterization of cardiac haemodynamics, which has greatly reduced the need for invasive catheterization. Echocardiography in RCM typically demonstrates normal or borderline LVEF and RV ejection fraction (RVEF) values, normal chamber volumes, and bi-atrial enlargement. LV wall thickness is often increased, with different severity and patterns of hypertrophy according to the specific condition. The restrictive filling pattern is characterized by increased early diastolic filling velocity (E waves) because of elevated left atrial (LA) pressure, decreased atrial filling velocity (A waves) due to high ventricular diastolic pressure, E/A ratios of >1.5, decreased mitral deceleration time (<160 ms), and shortened isovolumetric relaxation time. The systolic-to-diastolic pulmonary venous flow ratio is markedly decreased as a result of high LA pressures. Tissue Doppler typically demonstrates reduced early diastolic myocardial velocity (e'), with an elevated E/e' ratio (➲ Figure 3.4.4.5).[5,6,8] Specific findings such as endomyocardial infiltration in endomyocardial fibrosis (EMF), scarring in sarcoidosis, or apical sparing phenomenon on strain analysis in CA may be helpful in elucidating the underlying aetiology.

Cardiac magnetic resonance (CMR) imaging is the gold standard technique for non-invasive characterization of cardiac tissues (the myocardium, as well as the endocardium and pericardium), based upon the intrinsic magnetic properties of different tissues and the distribution patterns of gadolinium-based contrast agents. Increased signal on T2-weighted sequences or quantitative T2 mapping may indicate myocardial oedema and inflammation. Late gadolinium enhancement denotes fibrotic tissue, and native or contrast-enhanced T1 mapping is useful in quantifying diffuse myocardial fibrosis.[9] Native T1 mapping is markedly increased in CA, whereas it is decreased in Anderson–Fabry disease and haemochromatosis.[10] Other patterns of tissue signal may point to specific aetiologies, as discussed below.

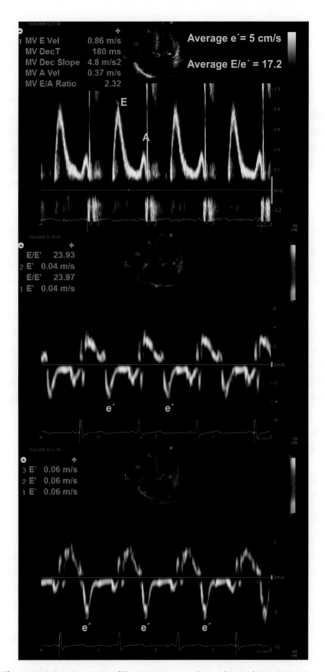

Figure 3.4.4.5 Restrictive filling pattern on echocardiographic examination. Typical restrictive left ventricular filling demonstrated by echocardiography with a high E-to-A ratio (>2) and increased E/e' ratios both on septal and lateral mitral annulus corners (typically >15).

Treatment of heart failure in restrictive cardiomyopathies: general principles

Given the peculiar pathophysiology of RCM, HF treatment relies on principles which are different from those for HF with reduced or preserved ejection fraction (EF). Two characteristics of RCM are particularly relevant and influence the therapeutic strategy:

◆ The restrictive physiology implies that the duration of diastole has a relatively limited impact on the amount of ventricular filling and cardiac output becomes crucially dependent on the heart rate.

◆ Reverse remodelling of the LV (i.e. reduction of ventricular volumes and LVEF recovery) is not a therapeutic goal. On the contrary, clinical improvement may be accompanied by a small increase in LV end-diastolic volume.[11]

Therapy for RCM should aim first at relieving congestion. Loop diuretics are essential in reducing pulmonary and peripheral oedema, as well as ascites. Care should be taken to avoid overdiuresis because even mild hypovolaemia may cause a fall in stroke volume and a low output state. In cases with a clear restrictive physiology, the strict dependence of cardiac output on the heart rate implies that beta-blockers may worsen the haemodynamic function and induce hypotension. Similarly, drugs acting on the renin–angiotensin–aldosterone system may be poorly tolerated because of hypotension.

Patients with an overt restrictive physiology are poorly tolerant to bradycardia, and bradyarrhythmias may require the implantation of an atrioventricular sequential pacemaker. AF is common and often poorly tolerated because of the loss of atrial contribution to ventricular filling. Rhythm control should be preferred over rate control, but achieving and maintaining sinus rhythm may be difficult. The thromboembolic risk is very high in patients with AF, and anticoagulation should be started in all patients with AF regardless of their CHA_2DS_2-VASc score. There are not enough data to recommend direct oral anticoagulants over vitamin K antagonists, or vice versa, and both options are valid. Finally, therapy should be targeted to the specific aetiology when identified.[6]

Diagnosis and management of the most frequent restrictive cardiomyopathies

Idiopathic or genetic RCM (primary RCM)

The definition of primary RCM encompasses idiopathic and definitely genetic RCMs. In cases of idiopathic RCM, familial aggregation or absence of any identifiable cause may suggest a possible genetic disorder, but the search for gene mutations is negative. Familial cases generally display a pattern of autosomal dominant inheritance with variable penetrance. RCM-associated mutations have been currently described in several genes encoding sarcomeric and non-sarcomeric proteins (➲ Figure 3.4.4.6).[12] A search on the Leiden Open Variation Database (available from: https://www.lovd.nl/) on 13 December 2021 identified mutations in *MYPN* (myopalladin), *FLNC* (filamin-C), *TNNI3* (troponin I3), and *TNNT2* (troponin T2) as causes of genetic RCM. Other genes associated with RCM are *ACTC1* (cardiac actin),[13] *ACTN2* (cardiac actinin 2),[14] *TTN* (titin),[15] and *CRYAB* (αB-crystallin).[16] In both idiopathic and genetic RCMs, disease mechanisms likely include abnormal functioning of sarcomere proteins and activation of fibrotic pathways following tissue damage.[5,17,18]

Most patients are diagnosed in the paediatric age due to a clinical picture of severe chronic HF. Skeletal myopathy, particularly affecting distal muscles of the extremities, and atrioventricular block are present in some familial cases. The electrocardiogram shows signs of atrial enlargement (either left or bi-atrial). The echocardiogram shows functional alterations common to other forms of RCM (➲ Figure 3.4.4.7). No disease-modifying therapy is currently available. HF treatment follows the general principles discussed above.

Considerable genotypic and phenotypic overlap exists between RCM and HCM. At the gene level, the two different phenotypes can be expressed by the same mutations; in a number of cases, the phenotype is mixed from the beginning (overtly restrictive haemodynamics with generally modest LV hypertrophy); in others, there is a restrictive evolution starting from a classic HCM phenotype (➲ Figure 3.4.4.8). Myocardial disarray is not pathognomonic for HCM, as it can also occur in RCM.[19,20,21]

The reference to RCM as 'non-dilated cardiomyopathy' has also limited diagnostic value, as a lack of ventricular dilatation is a hallmark of HCM, can occur in arrhythmogenic cardiomyopathy, and is a central feature of 'hypokinetic non-dilated cardiomyopathy'.[22] This entity was initially described in heart transplant recipients with end-stage HF and included in the 2008 ESC classification of cardiomyopathies as 'mildly dilated cardiomyopathy', a subtype of DCM.[1,22] Ventricular size was normal or mildly dilated, with severe LV systolic dysfunction, but without restrictive haemodynamics on catheterization (➲ Figure 3.4.4.9). Except for heart size, the morphological, haemodynamic, and histopathological features were undistinguishable from those of typical DCM.[23] The clinical course and prognosis are also very similar to DCM, particularly in the advanced phase of the disease.[24,25] Familial occurrence of this entity was associated with mutations in lamin A/C.[26]

Desminopathies

Desminopathies are genetic RCM that should be considered separately because they are characterized by the accumulation of material within the cardiomyocytes. Desmin is a 53-kDa intermediate filament of myocardial, skeletal, and smooth muscle that connects myofibrils and anchors them to the sarcolemma, thus stabilizing the sarcomeres. Pathogenic *DES* mutations may induce the formation of cellular aggregates that disrupt the cardiomyocyte architecture or alter the nanomechanical properties of intermediate filaments. The hereditary pattern may be either autosomal dominant or autosomal recessive. The spectrum of cardiac phenotypes includes dilated, arrhythmogenic, noncompaction, hypertrophic, and also restrictive cardiomyopathies; the latter may be associated with atrioventricular block and variables degrees of skeletal myopathy.[6,27] In a subject with apparently idiopathic RCM, the coexistence of advanced atrioventricular block acts as a red flag raising suspicion for desminopathy.[28]

Radiation-induced restrictive cardiomyopathy

Radiation therapy is still widely used in the treatment of numerous cancers. Recent modifications in radiation dose and delivery have reduced the incidence of cardiac complications, but the risk of contemporary regimens remains unknown, also because of a lack of standardized echocardiographic screening and the often long latent period.[29] At sufficient doses, radiation of the mediastinum can damage virtually any component of the heart. Radiation-related RCM is due to early inflammation, microvascular injury, and reduced capillary density, which lead to ischaemia and myocyte replacement with diffuse bands of collagen replacement fibrosis.[30]

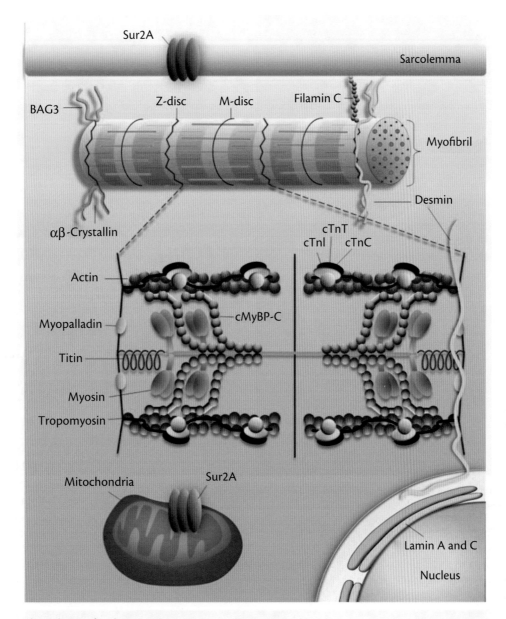

Figure 3.4.4.6 Contractile machinery of cardiomyocytes.
Cardiomyocytes are thickly packed with contractile elements, the myofibrils, which are connected to each other and via the cytoskeleton to the extracellular matrix and to the nucleus. Myofibrils are composed of sarcomeres, the smallest contractile units of the cardiac muscle cell. Proteins whose genes are targets for mutations leading to restrictive cardiomyopathy are indicated. cMyBP-C, myosin binding protein C; cTnI, cTnT, cTnC, cardiac troponin subunits I, T and C; Sur2A, sulfonylurea receptor isoform 2A; BAG3, Bcl2-associated athanogene 3.
Reproduced from Cimiotti D, Budde H, Hassoun R, Jaquet K. Genetic Restrictive Cardiomyopathy: Causes and Consequences-An Integrative Approach. *Int J Mol Sci*. 2021 Jan 8;22(2):558. doi: 10.3390/ijms22020558 with permission from MDPI https://creativecommons.org/licenses/by/4.0/ Attribution 4.0 International (CC BY 4.0).

Radiation predominantly causes RCM with diastolic dysfunction, usually with a latent period of 10–15 years.[31] Differentiation between RCM and CP may be difficult, even with advanced imaging and heart catheterization, also because these conditions may coexist. An endomyocardial biopsy (EMB) may be required in selected cases, especially if surgical pericardiectomy is considered. No specific therapies exist for this form of RCM. Clinical management of established disease is symptomatic and consists largely of diuretics to control volume overload.[7] Heart transplantation has been performed successfully in a limited number of patients with advanced disease. However, the reported 5-year post-transplant survival was 58%, which was lower than in transplant for other types of RCM, likely because of a detrimental effect of mediastinal fibrosis and radiation lung disease on outcome.[32]

Endomyocardial diseases

Both EMF and hypereosinophilic syndrome (HES) are currently considered secondary to proteotoxic damage produced on the endocardium by eosinophils.

EMF is commonly seen in equatorial countries and accounts for approximately 20% of HF cases and 15% of cardiac deaths in equatorial Africa. EMF typically affects impoverished young

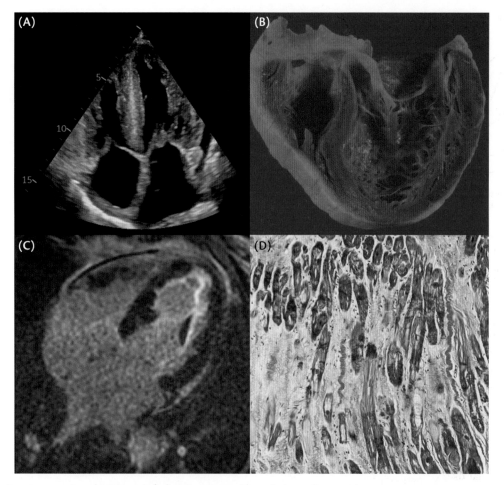

Figure 3.4.4.7 Imaging, macroscopic and microscopic findings in patients with restrictive cardiomyopathy.
(A) Four-chamber echocardiographic view of a 52-year-old man with light chain cardiac amyloidosis. (B) Late gadolinium enhancement acquisition of a 62-year-old woman with endomyocardial fibrosis. (C) Explanted heart of a 55-year-old man with primary restrictive cardiomyopathy. (D) Myocardial histology of a 45-year-old man with primary restrictive cardiomyopathy; a large amount of interstitial fibrosis (in blue on Mallory staining) is evident within the left ventricular myocardium.

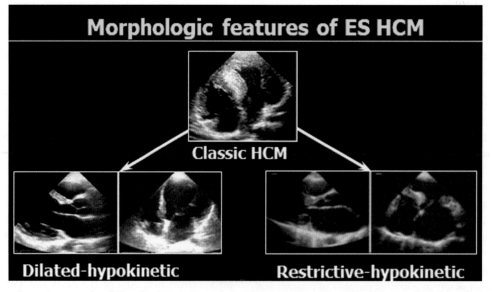

Figure 3.4.4.8 Echocardiographic examples of dilated and restrictive evolutions from a classic hypertrophic phenotype (HCM).
ES, end-stage.

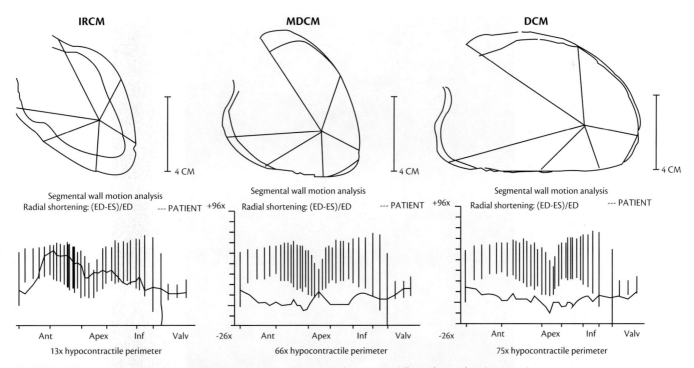

Figure 3.4.4.9 Ventricular size and contractility patterns prior to heart transplantation in different forms of cardiomyopathy. Systolic and diastolic angiographic contours in the upper panels, and segmental contractility projected against the normal range (hatched areas) in the lower panels, in idiopathic restrictive CM (IRCM), mildly dilated CM (MDCM), currently known as 'hypokinetic non-dilated CM' (see text), and typical dilated CM (DCM). In IRCM, the ventricular cavity was small and contractility was normal, with minimal segmental asynergy. Note the similar poor contractility pattern in patients with MDCM and DCM, but different ventricular size. Reproduced from Keren A, Billingham ME, Popp RL. Features of mildly dilated congestive cardiomyopathy compared with idiopathic restrictive cardiomyopathy and typical dilated cardiomyopathy. J Am Soc Echocardiogr. 1988 Jan–Feb;1(1):78–87. doi: 10.1016/s0894-7317(88)80066-x with permission from Elsevier.

adults, with a bimodal distribution peaking at 10 and 30 years of age. A combination of dietary, environmental, and infectious factors may elicit an inflammatory process, leading to progressive endomyocardial damage and scarring. The natural history of EMF includes an active phase with inflammation and eosinophilia that progresses to restrictive heart disease. In the chronic phase, biventricular involvement is found in more than half of cases, followed by isolated right-sided or left-sided heart involvement (➲ Figure 3.4.4.10). AF occurs in >30% of patients and embolic complications are common.[7]

HES affecting the heart, formerly known as Loeffler's endocarditis, is a very rare condition caused by the release of highly active biological substances that damage the endothelium and myocardium. Most patients are diagnosed between 20 and 50 years of age. Mechanisms of eosinophilia include helminthic and parasitic infections, malignancies, eosinophilic leukaemia, allergic drug reactions, hypersensitivity, and eosinophilic granulomatosis with polyangiitis. The natural history of HES includes the same three phases as described for EMF. The fibrotic stage results in RCM due to extensive endomyocardial fibrosis, and resembles EMF.[7] Interestingly, peripheral eosinophilia was absent on admission in up to 25% of cases during the acute inflammatory phase of eosinophilic myocarditis, and EMB was required to reach the correct diagnosis.[33]

The acute phase of endomyocardial damage is rarely detected in time for a dedicated intervention. In HES, corticosteroids alone or in combination with cytolytic therapies have been associated with LVEF recovery and improved symptoms. Some molecules that block different pathways of eosinophilic inflammation

are under investigation. Imatinib is a monoclonal antibody that blocks FIP1L1–PDGFR tyrosine kinase, an essential enzyme in the pathophysiology of idiopathic HES, which could be useful in treatment of early stages of EMF.[34]

Medical management of the fibrotic stage may include diuretics, and aspirin or anticoagulation to prevent intracardiac thrombi. Anticoagulation can promote the reabsorption of thrombosis, even in non-acute phases of the disease.[35] The fibrotic stage may occasionally require surgical therapy, which may include resection of endocardial scar, as well as subchordal repair and/or valve repair or replacement.[7] Surgical resection of subendocardial fibrosis is rarely curative, even in centres of expertise, and cardiac transplantation is an option in advanced cases.

Iron overload cardiomyopathy

Iron overload disorders are characterized by the appearance of non-transferrin-bound iron, an expansion of the labile intracellular iron pool, and formation of reactive oxygen species causing oxidative damage to lipid membranes and cellular proteins.[36] Furthermore, ferrous (Fe^{2+}) ions induce an increase in calcium influx in cardiomyocytes, which may contribute to diastolic dysfunction.[37] Pathological iron deposition begins in the epicardium, then extends to the myocardium and finally to the endocardium. IOC manifests in early stages as RCM; systolic function is preserved until late disease stages.[38]

Excessive iron accumulation may occur due to increased gastrointestinal iron absorption or, much more frequently, following repeated blood transfusions.[39] Hereditary haemochromatosis (HH) is

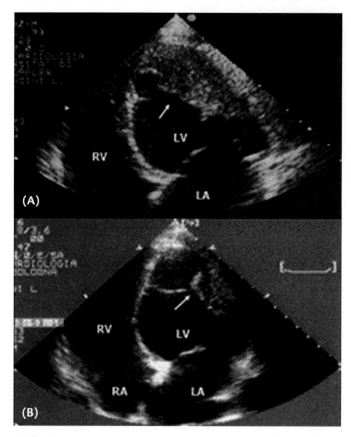

Figure 3.4.4.10 A case of endomyocardial fibrosis.
Echocardiographic findings in a 58-year-old male with endomyocardial fibrosis involving the left ventricular apex and lateral apical wall (A). The volume of the fibro-thrombotic mass was greatly reduced after 4 months of anticoagulation therapy with warfarin (B).

an autosomal disorder due to mutations in genes involved in iron metabolism causing increased iron absorption.[40] Type 1 HH is an autosomal recessive disorder due to mutations in the *HFE* gene that encodes a protein controlling gastrointestinal iron absorption. Type 2 HH is associated with mutations in the genes encoding hepcidin, a regulator of circulating iron, or hemojuvelin (a protein that interacts with hepcidin). Type 3 HH results from mutations in the gene encoding transferrin receptor 2. Type 4 HH is caused by mutations in the gene that encodes ferroportin, a protein controlling iron efflux.[41] Type 1 and 4 HH usually manifest during the fourth or fifth decades of life, whereas type 2 HH typically presents by the second decade. Type 3 HH usually manifests before 30 years. Secondary iron overload occurs primarily in patients with hereditary anaemias, particularly alpha-thalassaemia, beta-thalassaemia, and sickle cell anaemia, who receive unopposed transfusion therapy.[39,40]

Plasma B-type natriuretic peptide should be measured in all suspected cases and holds prognostic significance.[42,43] Echocardiography is the main imaging modality to screen patients with suspected IOC and for follow-up. LV wall thickness is not increased. Diastolic dysfunction with a restrictive filling pattern, with or without LA enlargement, is an early finding.[44,45] IOC may progress towards a dilated phenotype with biventricular dilatation and LVEF reduction, or a restrictive phenotype with RV dilatation, increased pulmonary artery pressures, and preserved LVEF.[41] EMB is no longer routinely utilized, and CMR imaging has become the non-invasive procedure of choice for estimating

overall myocardial iron content. T2* relaxation time is an excellent measure of myocardial iron deposition and is useful for serial assessment of response to iron chelation therapy. T2* values in the interventricular septum are typically <20 ms. A T2* value of <10 ms is indicative of severe iron overload and predicts HF development with a sensitivity of 98% and a specificity of 83%.[46]

The mainstay of treatment in patients with haemochromatosis is phlebotomy.[39,40,41] Aggressive iron removal initiated early in the disease process may achieve an improvement in cardiac function.[47,48] Chelation therapy is an effective alternative option when phlebotomy is not feasible. In transfusion-dependent patients with acquired haematological conditions, iron chelation therapy is generally initiated after 10–20 transfusions to prevent myocardial iron accumulation.[48] Three chelators are available: parenteral deferoxamine, and oral deferiprone and deferasirox. Chelation therapy improves systolic and diastolic LV function, and reduces mortality.[49,50] A small minority of patients now progress to the dilated phenotype and overt symptomatic HF.[7]

Cardiac amyloidosis

Amyloidosis is a condition where one of >30 different precursor proteins with an unstable tertiary structure misfolds and aggregates into amyloid fibrils that accumulate in the extracellular space of organs and tissues.[51] All amyloid deposits stained with Congo red dye display a typical apple-green birefringence under polarized light microscopy, and show a β-pleated sheet configuration under electron microscopy. Over 95% of cases of CA are represented by light chain (AL) amyloidosis or transthyretin (TTR) amyloidosis (ATTR).[52,53] AL amyloidosis results from deposition of immuno-globulin light chains from plasma cell dyscrasia. It is a rare condition, with an incidence of approximately 1 per 100,000.[54] TTR is a protein synthetized in the liver that circulates as a tetramer and transports thyroxin and retinol. TTR may dissociate into monomers and deposits as amyloid fibrils, either because of mutations that reduce the stability of TTR tetramers (variant ATTR (ATTRv)) or as an age-related overproduction phenomenon (wild-type ATTR (ATTRwt)). ATTRv is generally rare, but some genetic variants are endemic in specific geographical regions or ethnic groups. ATTRwt is an underdiagnosed cause of HF, with a prevalence of 13% among patients with HF with preserved EF.[55]

The clinical presentation of amyloidosis is highly variable, according to the pattern of organ involvement.[54] Systemic AL amyloidosis is a multisystem disorder commonly affecting the liver, kidneys, autonomic and peripheral nervous systems, and heart. Cardiac involvement is present in 50–70% of patients with AL amyloidosis and is the main determinant of prognosis.[56,57] Patients with AL-CA typically are aged over 40 years. CA is the dominant feature of ATTRwt and some variants (e.g. Val122Ile).[58,59] Patients with ATTR-CA most commonly are aged over 70 years. Various *TTR* mutations are associated with differing ages of onset (from 30 to 70 years) and different risks of cardiomyopathy.[53]

CA often presents with dyspnoea and signs of systemic venous congestion. Patients may also present with syncope because of bradyarrhythmias or advanced atrioventricular block,[60] but also excessive diuresis or autonomic neuropathy. Patients with CA have a high risk of systemic thromboembolism. The haemodynamic consequences of diastolic dysfunction and amyloid infiltration of atrial walls contribute to atrial dysfunction, with a risk of atrial thrombus formation, even in sinus rhythm.[61,62] Cardiac ATTR has been identified in a substantial minority of patients with severe aortic stenosis undergoing surgical (6–12%)[63,64] or percutaneous valve replacement (16%).[65] ATTR with associated RCM may contribute to low-flow, low-gradient aortic stenosis.[66]

Clinical manifestations of AL amyloidosis include non-specific symptoms (fatigue, poor appetite, early satiety, and weight loss), as well as symptoms and signs of kidney disease, peripheral neuropathy, carpal tunnel syndrome, gastrointestinal involvement, macroglossia, purpura, and bleeding diathesis. Bilateral carpal tunnel syndrome, spinal stenosis, and biceps tendon rupture are relatively common in patients with ATTRwt.[67]

Natriuretic peptide and troponin levels are commonly elevated in patients with CA, particularly those with AL-CA.[67] A hallmark of CA is discordance between increased LV wall thickness and QRS voltage, which is often reduced; low QRS voltage is more frequent in patients with AL-CA (60%) than those with ATTR-CA (20%).[68] Among patients with ATTRwt, 30% have voltage criteria for LV hypertrophy or left bundle branch block, and 70% have pseudo-infarction patterns. AF is more common in ATTRwt (40%) than in ATTRv (11%) or AL (9%).[52,53,67]

Echocardiography is the first-line imaging technique. Reduction in global longitudinal strain is one of the earliest markers of CA and presents with a characteristic pattern of relative apical sparing, which has 93% sensitivity and 82% specificity for CA.[69,70] Infiltration of ventricular walls produces an appearance of hypertrophy with non-dilated or small ventricles. LV hypertrophy is typically symmetrical in AL-CA, and asymmetrical with predominantly septal hypertrophy in ATTR-CA. Stroke volume index is invariably reduced, even in the very early stages of infiltration.[71] Diastolic dysfunction is almost invariably present with early impaired relaxation, which then invariably progresses to typical restrictive physiology.[71] Non-specific findings include thickening of the valves and interatrial septum and a speckled appearance of the myocardium. The atria are almost invariably dilated. Small pericardial and pleural effusions are common findings, especially in AL amyloidosis. The main echocardiographic findings in CA are summarized in ➔ Figure 3.4.4.11.

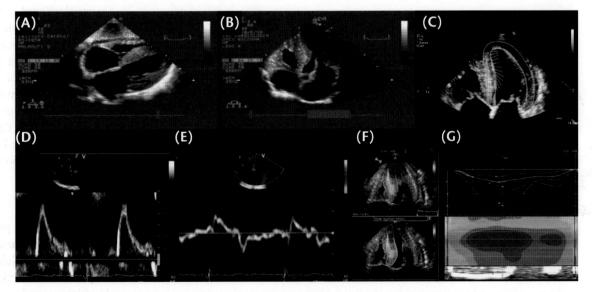

Figure 3.4.4.11 Echocardiographic features in patients with cardiac amyloidosis. Biventricular wall thickening (A, B), bi-atrial enlargement (A, B), small pericardial effusion (A), abnormal contraction (C, E, F), and relaxation (D) patterns, and apical sparing on speckle tracking analysis (G).

CMR typically shows diffuse subendocardial or transmural late gadolinium enhancement, associated with abnormal gadolinium kinetics that may manifest as simultaneous myocardial and blood nulling or suboptimal myocardial nulling. Native myocardial T1 elevation is an early disease marker. Extracellular volume fraction measurement using a contrast agent may quantify the cardiac amyloid burden and response to therapy.[72,73]

Cardiac scintigraphy using [99m]technetium-labelled tracers is a pivotal test for identifying ATTR-CA. The Perugini staging system relies on simple visual scoring of the planar image: grade 0 corresponds to no cardiac uptake, and grades 1–3 to progressively greater cardiac uptake, compared to bone uptake.[74] ATTR-CA is particularly avid for bone tracers, whereas uptake in AL-CA is absent or low.[75] A grade 2 or 3 positive bone tracer cardiac scintigraphy in a patient without monoclonal protein is highly specific for ATTR-CA, and thus sufficient for diagnosis of this condition without tissue biopsy.[75] The main limitation of bone tracer scintigraphy is lack of quantification of the amyloid burden, a parameter that might prove useful for assessing response to therapy.

Identification of monoclonal protein (by serum protein immunofixation, urine protein immunofixation, or serum free light chain ratio analysis), along with echocardiographic or CMR imaging findings consistent with CA, is suggestive of AL but may also be caused by ATTR with an unrelated monoclonal gammopathy of undetermined significance.[76] When a monoclonal protein is found, evaluation typically includes tissue biopsy (e.g. periumbilical fat, renal, or endomyocardial). Mass spectrometry is the golden standard for identifying the precursor protein and amyloidosis type.[77]

According to the diagnostic algorithm recently introduced by an ESC consensus document,[78] in the presence of cardiac and other findings suggestive of amyloidosis, the next step is to search for a monoclonal protein (through serum kappa/lambda free light chain ratio analysis, serum protein immunofixation, and urine protein immunofixation) and to perform bone scintigraphy with [99m]technetium-labelled tracers. If no monoclonal protein is found and there is an intense cardiac uptake of the bone tracer, ATTR-CA can be diagnosed, with no need for histological confirmation; in cases with a less intense tracer uptake (i.e. lower than bone), EMB is needed for diagnosis. When a monoclonal protein is identified and bone scintigraphy is positive, a tissue biopsy (usually cardiac) is required. When there is a monoclonal protein, but scintigraphy is negative, CMR imaging may be considered to exclude CA (when negative) or to refer the patient for tissue biopsy (when positive). Finally, when no monoclonal protein is found and bone scintigraphy is negative, CA is unlikely (➲ Figure 3.4.4.12).[78,79]

Patients with ATTRwt-CA have a median survival of 3.5 years.[80] The clinical phenotype of ATTRv varies among TTR variants and includes primary polyneuropathy (Val30Met), cardiomyopathy (Val122Ile, Leu111Met, Ile68Leu), and mixed phenotype (T60A). Peripheral neuropathy and autonomic dysfunction have a significant impact on quality of life, but cardiac involvement is the main determinant of prognosis, with a median survival of 4–5 years when cardiac amyloidosis is present.[51] Natural history studies found that patients with cardiac AL amyloidosis and HF without disease-specific treatment had an overall median survival of only 6 months.[57] With contemporary management, the median survival for AL amyloidosis with cardiac involvement has significantly improved (e.g. 5.5 years after diagnosis).[81]

A staging system validated in both ATTRwt and ATTRv is based on serum levels of N-terminal pro-B-type natriuretic peptide (NT-proBNP) and estimated glomerular filtration rate (eGFR).[82] Stage I is defined as NT-proBNP ≤3000 ng/L and eGFR ≥45 mL/min/

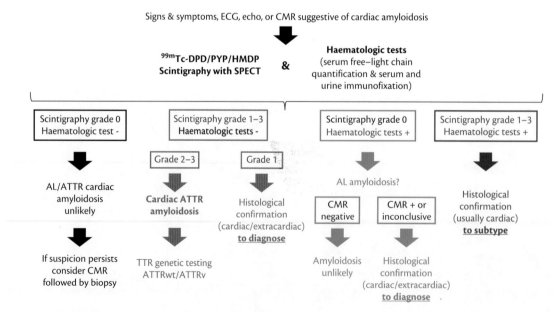

Figure 3.4.4.12 Diagnostic algorithm for cardiac amyloidosis according to the European Society of Cardiology.

AL, amyloid light chain; ATTR, amyloid transthyretin (v, variant; wt, wild-type); CMR, cardiac magnetic resonance; DPD, diphosphonate; ECG, electrocardiogram; HMDP, hydroxymethylene diphosphonate; PYP, pyrophosphate; SPECT, single-photon emission computed tomography.

Reproduced from Garcia-Pavia P, Rapezzi C, Adler Y, et al. Diagnosis and treatment of cardiac amyloidosis. A position statement of the European Society of Cardiology Working Group on Myocardial and Pericardial Diseases. Eur J Heart Fail. 2021 Apr;23(4):512–526. doi: 10.1002/ejhf.2140 with permission from John Wiley and Sons.

1.73 m²; stage III is defined as NT-proBNP >3000 ng/L and eGFR <45 mL/min/1.73 m², and the other patients were in stage II. Median survival among stage I patients was 69 months, stage II patients 47 months, and stage III patients 24 months.[82] The Revised Mayo Stage system for AL amyloidosis assigns 1 point for NT-proBNP ≥1800 ng/L, troponin T ≥25 ng/L, and difference of ≥18 mg/dL between the kappa and lambda free light chains, which means stages I–IV carry scores of 0 to 3 points, respectively. Median survival from diagnosis was 94.1, 40.3, 14, and 5.8 months, respectively.[83] In AL amyloidosis, changes in NT-proBNP have also been used to predict response to treatment and disease progression, with a decrease in NT-proBNP of >30% and >300 ng/L from a baseline value of ≥650 ng/L associated with better prognosis.[84]

Treatment of CA should relieve HF symptoms and target the underlying disease. Loop diuretics are the mainstay of HF management. Mineralocorticoid receptor antagonists are generally well tolerated. Beta-blockers have no proven benefit and may be poorly tolerated when cardiac output is dependent on the heart rate because of a low, fixed stroke volume. Angiotensin-converting enzyme inhibitors or angiotensin receptor blockers may induce hypotension, especially in patients with autonomic neuropathy. Digoxin may be carefully used in patients with AF and a rapid ventricular response. Amiodarone is well tolerated. Verapamil and diltiazem are contraindicated. Experience with catheter ablation

for atrial arrhythmias is limited. Anticoagulation is indicated in patients with AF; the role of anticoagulation in patients in sinus rhythm is uncertain. Either warfarin or one of the newer oral anticoagulants have been used. General indications for cardiac pacing should be applied. The efficacy of implantable cardioverter–defibrillator therapy is uncertain. Heart transplantation in AL-CA should be followed by high-dose chemotherapy and autologous haematopoietic stem cell transplantation within 12 months.

Disease-modifying therapies for AL-CA involves administration of chemotherapy and/or autologous stem cell transplantation in an attempt to treat the underlying plasma cell clone, and requires close collaboration between cardiologists and haematologists. The most common initial chemotherapy regimens used are now bortezomib-based. In eligible patients, autologous stem cell transplantation involves administration of high-dose melphalan followed by stem cell rescue.[52]

Disease-modifying treatments acting on several steps of the amyloidogenic cascade of ATTR-CA are now available (→ Figure 3.4.4.13). Tafamidis stabilizes the TTR tetramer and may thus reduce the formation of TTR amyloid. It prolongs survival in patients with ATTR-CA,[11,85] and is the only approved treatment (61 mg once daily) for patients in New York Heart Association (NYHA) classes I–III with ATTRwt-CA or ATTRv-CA without polyneuropathy.[79,86,87,88,89] ESC HF guidelines include a class I, level

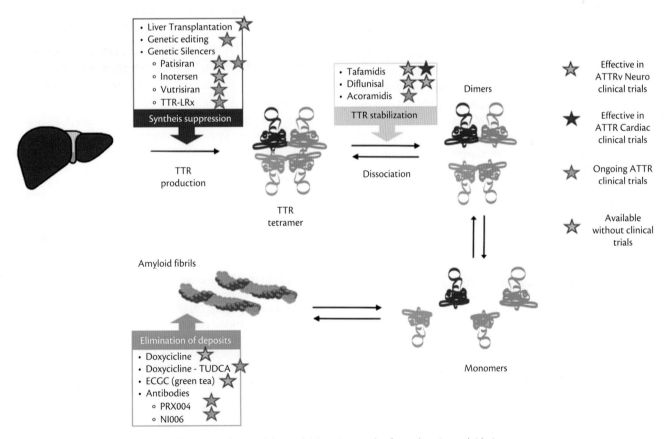

Figure 3.4.4.13 Proposed therapies acting on several steps of the amyloidogenic cascade of transthyretin amyloidosis.
ATTR(v), (variant) amyloid transthyretin amyloidosis; EGCG, epigallocatechin gallate; TTR, transthyretin; TUDCA, tauroursodeoxycholic acid.
Reproduced from Garcia-Pavia P, Rapezzi C, Adler Y, *et al*. Diagnosis and treatment of cardiac amyloidosis. A position statement of the European Society of Cardiology Working Group on Myocardial and Pericardial Diseases. *Eur J Heart Fail*. 2021 Apr;23(4):512–526. doi: 10.1002/ejhf.2140 with permission from John Wiley and Sons.

of evidence B recommendation for tafamidis in patients with NYHA class I or II, without explicitly addressing the issue of patients in NYHA class III who showed less convincing results in the ATTR ACT trial in terms of hospitalizations.[11,85] In cases with a mixed neurological and cardiological phenotype, patisiran and inotersen can also be considered,[79] but phase 3 trials specifically dedicated to CA are still ongoing. Several novel therapies (e.g. acoramidis/AG10/ or antibody-based therapy PRX004) are under development.

Liver transplantation removes the mutant amyloidogenic TTR in ATTRv, but in ATTRwt, the precursor protein is native TTR and thus liver transplantation is not indicated. Patients with ATTRv-CA may be candidates for heart transplantation if amyloid neuropathy is absent or mild. Most mutations may need a combined liver and heart transplantation to prevent recurrence in the transplanted heart.[90] Unfortunately, cardiac disease may progress after liver transplantation in some patients with ATTRv.[53] Heart transplantation can be considered in selected cases, although patients with isolated ATTRwt-CA are often too old.

Future directions

There are several grey zones and unmet needs in the current definition and classification of RCM (➲ Box 3.4.4.1). We can first envisage a redefinition of RCM, focusing on the main disease mechanisms and conditions where restrictive physiology is a central and constant feature. Such classification would identify four subgroups of disorders sharing at least some pathophysiological elements (impairment of the sarcomere and/or interstitial fibrosis, infiltration of extracellular spaces, accumulation of storage material within cardiomyocytes, or EMF) and narrow the spectrum of RCM. An effort is warranted to better elucidate genotype–phenotype correlations in RCM and the degree of overlap with mutations causing HCM or other cardiomyopathies. Loop diuretics will likely remain the mainstay of treatment for pulmonary and systemic congestion; sodium–glucose cotransporter 1 inhibitors might play some role, given their diuretic and cardioprotective effects and their ability to improve diastolic function[91] and to improve the clinical outcome of patients with HF with preserved EF.[92] Many disease-modifying treatments for CA are now available or are being investigated, whereas research on other forms of RCM is languishing and should receive a new impulse.

Box 3.4.4.1 Issues with the current definition and classification of RCM

- Both 'inclusion and exclusion' criteria are not specific.
- The definition is based on haemodynamic criteria that are not completely verifiable with non-invasive techniques.
- Restrictive physiology may be present only in a temporal phase in disease evolution.
- 'Restrictive physiology' is shared by other cardiomyopathies with different phenotypes.
- The highly heterogeneous spectrum of myocardial substrates and morphological phenotypes is not adequately considered.

Key messages

- RCM encompasses a group of extremely heterogeneous disorders.
- The unifying feature is a restrictive physiology, with a rapid rise in ventricular pressure, with only small increases in filling volumes, as a result of increased myocardial stiffness.
- We may identify four subsets of conditions according to the main disease mechanism: (1) interstitial fibrosis or intrinsic myocardial dysfunction; (2) infiltration of the extracellular spaces; (3) accumulation of storage material within cardiomyocytes; and (4) EMF.
- Many conditions traditionally considered as forms of RCM do not show a restrictive physiology throughout their history, but only in the initial phase (with subsequent evolution towards a hypokinetic and dilated phenotype) or the terminal phase (often starting from a hypertrophic phenotype).
- In paediatric and young individuals, the most common forms of RCM are those caused by mutations in sarcomeric or non-sarcomeric genes. Atrioventricular conduction disturbances are particularly common in desminopathies.
- CA, and particularly ATTR-CA, is the most common form of RCM in adults and the elderly.
- Some cardiological or non-cardiological features are red flags raising suspicion for CA; the definite diagnosis of ATTR-CA can be reached through a non-invasive algorithm.
- Tafamidis, a TTR tetramer stabilizer, is currently the only approved disease-modifying treatment for ATTR-CA.

References

1. Elliott P, Andersson B, Arbustini E, *et al.* Classification of the cardiomyopathies: a position statement from the European Society Of Cardiology Working Group on Myocardial and Pericardial Diseases. *European Heart Journal.* 2008;29:270–6.
2. Goldstein JA and Kern MJ. Hemodynamics of constrictive pericarditis and restrictive cardiomyopathy. *Catheterization and Cardiovascular Interventions.* 2020;95:1240–8.
3. Geske JB, Anavekar NS, Nishimura RA, Oh JK, and Gersh BJ. Differentiation of constriction and restriction: complex cardiovascular hemodynamics. *Journal of the American College of Cardiology.* 2016;68:2329–47.
4. Welch TD, Ling LH, Espinosa RE, *et al.* Echocardiographic diagnosis of constrictive pericarditis: Mayo Clinic criteria. *Circulation Cardiovascular Imaging.* 2014;7:526–34.
5. Garcia MJ. Constrictive pericarditis versus restrictive cardiomyopathy? *Journal of the American College of Cardiology.* 2016;67:2061–76.
6. Pereira NL, Grogan M, and Dec GW. Spectrum of restrictive and infiltrative cardiomyopathies: part 1 of a 2-part series. *Journal of the American College of Cardiology.* 2018;71:1130–48.
7. Pereira NL, Grogan M, and Dec GW. Spectrum of restrictive and infiltrative cardiomyopathies: part 2 of a 2-part series. *Journal of the American College of Cardiology.* 2018;71:1149–66.
8. Zwas DR, Gotsman I, Admon D, and Keren A. Advances in the differentiation of constrictive pericarditis and restrictive cardiomyopathy. *Herz.* 2012;37:664–73.

9. Iles L, Pfluger H, Phrommintikul A, *et al.* Evaluation of diffuse myocardial fibrosis in heart failure with cardiac magnetic resonance contrast-enhanced T1 mapping. *Journal of the American College of Cardiology.* 2008;52:1574–80.

10. Galea N, Polizzi G, Gatti M, Cundari G, Figuera M, and Faletti R. Cardiovascular magnetic resonance (CMR) in restrictive cardiomyopathies. *La Radiologia Medica.* 2020;125:1072–86.

11. Maurer MS, Schwartz JH, Gundapaneni B, *et al.* Tafamidis treatment for patients with transthyretin amyloid cardiomyopathy. *The New England Journal of Medicine.* 2018;379:1007–16.

12. Cimiotti D, Budde H, Hassoun R, and Jaquet K. Genetic restrictive cardiomyopathy: causes and consequences: an integrative approach. *International Journal of Molecular Sciences.* 2021;22:558.

13. Kaski JP, Syrris P, Burch M, *et al.* Idiopathic restrictive cardiomyopathy in children is caused by mutations in cardiac sarcomere protein genes. *Heart.* 2008;94:1478–84.

14. Kostareva A, Kiselev A, Gudkova A, *et al.* Genetic spectrum of idiopathic restrictive cardiomyopathy uncovered by next-generation sequencing. *PLoS One.* 2016;11:e0163362.

15. Peled Y, Gramlich M, Yoskovitz G, *et al.* Titin mutation in familial restrictive cardiomyopathy. *International Journal of Cardiology.* 2014;171:24–30.

16. Brodehl A, Gaertner-Rommel A, Klauke B, *et al.* The novel αB-crystallin (CRYAB) mutation p.D109G causes restrictive cardiomyopathy. *Human Mutation.* 2017;38:947–52.

17. Yumoto F, Lu QW, Morimoto S, *et al.* Drastic Ca^{2+} sensitization of myofilament associated with a small structural change in troponin I in inherited restrictive cardiomyopathy. *Biochemical and Biophysical Research Communications.* 2005;338:1519–26.

18. Hayashi T, Shimomura H, Terasaki F, *et al.* Collagen subtypes and matrix metalloproteinase in idiopathic restrictive cardiomyopathy. *International Journal of Cardiology.* 1998;64:109–16.

19. Mogensen J, Kubo T, Duque M, *et al.* Idiopathic restrictive cardiomyopathy is part of the clinical expression of cardiac troponin I mutations. *Journal of Clinical Investigation.* 2003;111:209–16.

20. Gambarin FI, Tagliani M, and Arbustini E. Pure restrictive cardiomyopathy associated with cardiac troponin I gene mutation: mismatch between the lack of hypertrophy and the presence of disarray. *Heart.* 2008;94:1257.

21. Angelini A, Calzolari V, Thiene G, *et al.* Morphologic spectrum of primary restrictive cardiomyopathy. *American Journal of Cardiology.* 1997;80:1046–50.

22. Pinto YM, Elliott PM, Arbustini E, *et al.* Proposal for a revised definition of dilated cardiomyopathy, hypokinetic non-dilated cardiomyopathy, and its implications for clinical practice: a position statement of the ESC working group on myocardial and pericardial diseases. *European Heart Journal.* 2016;37:1850–8.

23. Keren A, Billingham ME, and Popp RL. Features of mildly dilated congestive cardiomyopathy compared with idiopathic restrictive cardiomyopathy and typical dilated cardiomyopathy. *Journal of the American Society of Echocardiography.* 1988;1:78–87.

24. Keren A, Gottlieb S, Tzivoni D, *et al.* Mildly dilated congestive cardiomyopathy. Use of prospective diagnostic criteria and description of the clinical course without heart transplantation. *Circulation.* 1990;81:506–17.

25. Gigli M, Stolfo D, Merlo M, *et al.* Insights into mildly dilated cardiomyopathy: temporal evolution and long-term prognosis. *European Journal of Heart Failure.* 2017;19:531–9.

26. Taylor MR, Fain PR, Sinagra G, *et al.* Natural history of dilated cardiomyopathy due to lamin A/C gene mutations. *Journal of the American College of Cardiology.* 2003;41:771–80.

27. Brodehl A, Hakimi SAP, Stanasiuk C, *et al.* Restrictive cardiomyopathy is caused by a novel homozygous desmin (*DES*) mutation

28. Arbustini E, Morbini P, Grasso M, *et al.* Restrictive cardiomyopathy, atrioventricular block and mild to subclinical myopathy in patients with desmin-immunoreactive material deposits. *Journal of the American College of Cardiology.* 1998;31:645–53.

29. Belzile-Dugas E and Eisenberg MJ. Radiation-induced cardiovascular disease: review of an underrecognized pathology. *Journal of the American Heart Association.* 2021;10:e021686.

30. Chello M, Mastroroberto P, Romano R, Zofrea S, Bevacqua I, and Marchese AR. Changes in the proportion of types I and III collagen in the left ventricular wall of patients with post-irradiative pericarditis. *Cardiovascular Surgery.* 1996;4:222–6.

31. Heidenreich PA, Hancock SL, Lee BK, Mariscal CS, and Schnittger I. Asymptomatic cardiac disease following mediastinal irradiation. *Journal of the American College of Cardiology.* 2003;42:743–9.

32. Al-Kindi SG and Oliveira GH. Heart transplantation outcomes in radiation-induced restrictive cardiomyopathy. *Journal of Cardiac Failure.* 2016;22:475–8.

33. Brambatti M, Matassini MV, Adler ED, Klingel K, Camici PG, and Ammirati E. Eosinophilic myocarditis: characteristics, treatment, and outcomes. *Journal of the American College of Cardiology.* 2017;70:2363–75.

34. Rotoli B, Catalano L, Galderisi M, *et al.* Rapid reversion of Loeffler's endocarditis by imatinib in early stage clonal hypereosinophilic syndrome. *Leukemia and Lymphoma.* 2004;45:2503–7.

35. Lofiego C, Ferlito M, Rocchi G, *et al.* Ventricular remodeling in Loeffler endocarditis: implications for therapeutic decision making. *European Journal of Heart Failure.* 2005;7:1023–6.

36. Andrews NC. Disorders of iron metabolism. *The New England Journal of Medicine.* 1999;341:1986–95.

37. Oudit GY, Sun H, Trivieri MG, *et al.* L-type Ca^{2+} channels provide a major pathway for iron entry into cardiomyocytes in iron-overload cardiomyopathy. *Nature Medicine.* 2003;9:1187–94.

38. Liu P and Olivieri N. Iron overload cardiomyopathies: new insights into an old disease. *Cardiovascular Drugs and Therapy.* 1994;8:101–10.

39. Murphy CJ and Oudit GY. Iron-overload cardiomyopathy: pathophysiology, diagnosis, and treatment. *Journal of Cardiac Failure.* 2010;16:888–900.

40. Gujja P, Rosing DR, Tripodi DJ, and Shizukuda Y. Iron overload cardiomyopathy: better understanding of an increasing disorder. *Journal of the American College of Cardiology.* 2010;56:1001–12.

41. Kremastinos DT and Farmakis D. Iron overload cardiomyopathy in clinical practice. *Circulation.* 2011;124:2253–63.

42. Machado RF, Anthi A, Steinberg MH, *et al.* N-terminal pro-brain natriuretic peptide levels and risk of death in sickle cell disease. *JAMA.* 2006;296:310–18.

43. Isma'eel H, Chafic AH, El Rassi F, *et al.* Relation between iron-overload indices, cardiac echo-Doppler, and biochemical markers in thalassemia intermedia. *American Journal of Cardiology.* 2008;102:363–7.

44. Kremastinos DT, Tsiapras DP, Tsetsos GA, *et al.* Left ventricular diastolic Doppler characteristics in beta-thalassemia major. *Circulation.* 1993;88:1127–35.

45. Spirito P, Lupi G, Melevendi C, and Vecchio C. Restrictive diastolic abnormalities identified by Doppler echocardiography in patients with thalassemia major. *Circulation.* 1990;82:88–94.

46. Kirk P, Roughton M, Porter JB, *et al.* Cardiac T2* magnetic resonance for prediction of cardiac complications in thalassemia major. *Circulation.* 2009;120:1961–8.

p.Y122H leading to a severe filament assembly defect. *Genes (Basel).* 2019;10:918.

47. Candell-Riera J, Lu L, Serés L, *et al.* Cardiac hemochromatosis: beneficial effects of iron removal therapy. An echocardiographic study. *American Journal of Cardiology.* 1983;52:824–9.

48. Rivers J, Garrahy P, Robinson W, and Murphy A. Reversible cardiac dysfunction in hemochromatosis. *American Heart Journal.* 1987;113:216–17.

49. Tanner MA, Galanello R, Dessi C, *et al.* A randomized, placebo-controlled, double-blind trial of the effect of combined therapy with deferoxamine and deferiprone on myocardial iron in thalassemia major using cardiovascular magnetic resonance. *Circulation.* 2007;115:1876–84.

50. Pennell DJ, Berdoukas V, Karagiorga M, *et al.* Randomized controlled trial of deferiprone or deferoxamine in beta-thalassemia major patients with asymptomatic myocardial siderosis. *Blood.* 2006;107:3738–44.

51. Fontana M, Ćorović A, Scully P, and Moon JC. Myocardial amyloidosis: the exemplar interstitial disease. *JACC Cardiovascular Imaging.* 2019;12:2345–56.

52. Falk RH, Alexander KM, Liao R, and Dorbala S. AL (light-chain) cardiac amyloidosis: a review of diagnosis and therapy. *Journal of the American College of Cardiology.* 2016;68:1323–41.

53. Ruberg FL, Grogan M, Hanna M, Kelly JW, and Maurer MS. Transthyretin amyloid cardiomyopathy: JACC state-of-the-art review. *Journal of the American College of Cardiology.* 2019;73:2872–91.

54. Wechalekar AD, Gillmore JD, and Hawkins PN. Systemic amyloidosis. *The Lancet.* 2016;387:2641–54.

55. González-López E, Gallego-Delgado M, Guzzo-Merello G, *et al.* Wild-type transthyretin amyloidosis as a cause of heart failure with preserved ejection fraction. *European Heart Journal.* 2015;36:2585–94.

56. Merlini G and Bellotti V. Molecular mechanisms of amyloidosis. *The New England Journal of Medicine.* 2003;349:583–96.

57. Kyle RA, Linos A, Beard CM, *et al.* Incidence and natural history of primary systemic amyloidosis in Olmsted County, Minnesota, 1950 through 1989. *Blood.* 1992;79:1817–22.

58. Rapezzi C, Quarta CC, Obici L, *et al.* Disease profile and differential diagnosis of hereditary transthyretin-related amyloidosis with exclusively cardiac phenotype: an Italian perspective. *European Heart Journal.* 2013;34:520–8.

59. Gagliardi C, Perfetto F, Lorenzini M, *et al.* Phenotypic profile of Ile68Leu transthyretin amyloidosis: an underdiagnosed cause of heart failure. *European Journal of Heart Failure.* 2018;20:1417–1425.

60. Chamarthi B, Dubrey SW, Cha K, Skinner M, and Falk RH. Features and prognosis of exertional syncope in light-chain associated AL cardiac amyloidosis. *American Journal of Cardiology.* 1997;80:1242–5.

61. Martinez-Naharro A, Gonzalez-Lopez E, Corovic A, *et al.* High prevalence of intracardiac thrombi in cardiac amyloidosis. *Journal of the American College of Cardiology.* 2019;73:1733–4.

62. El-Am EA, Dispenzieri A, Melduni RM, *et al.* Direct current cardioversion of atrial arrhythmias in adults with cardiac amyloidosis. *Journal of the American College of Cardiology.* 2019;73: 589–97.

63. Longhi S, Lorenzini M, Gagliardi C, *et al.* Coexistence of degenerative aortic stenosis and wild-type transthyretin-related cardiac amyloidosis. *JACC Cardiovascular Imaging.* 2016;9:325–7.

64. Treibel TA, Fontana M, Gilbertson JA, *et al.* Occult transthyretin cardiac amyloid in severe calcific aortic stenosis: prevalence and prognosis in patients undergoing surgical aortic valve replacement. *Circulation Cardiovascular Imaging.* 2016;9:e005066.

65. Cavalcante JL, Rijal S, Abdelkarim I, *et al.* Cardiac amyloidosis is prevalent in older patients with aortic stenosis and carries worse prognosis. *Journal of Cardiovascular Magnetic Resonance.* 2017;19:98.

66. Castaño A, Narotsky DL, Hamid N, *et al.* Unveiling transthyretin cardiac amyloidosis and its predictors among elderly patients with severe aortic stenosis undergoing transcatheter aortic valve replacement. *European Heart Journal.* 2017;38:2879–87.

67. Vergaro G, Aimo A, Barison A, *et al.* Keys to early diagnosis of cardiac amyloidosis: red flags from clinical, laboratory and imaging findings. *European Journal of Preventive Cardiology.* 2020;27:1806–15.

68. Mussinelli R, Salinaro F, Alogna A, *et al.* Diagnostic and prognostic value of low QRS voltages in cardiac AL amyloidosis. *Annals of Noninvasive Electrocardiology.* 2013;18:271–80.

69. Phelan D, Collier P, Thavendiranathan P, *et al.* Relative apical sparing of longitudinal strain using two-dimensional speckle-tracking echocardiography is both sensitive and specific for the diagnosis of cardiac amyloidosis. *Heart.* 2012;98:1442–8.

70. Phelan D, Thavendiranathan P, Popovic Z, *et al.* Application of a parametric display of two-dimensional speckle-tracking longitudinal strain to improve the etiologic diagnosis of mild to moderate left ventricular hypertrophy. *Journal of the American Society of Echocardiography.* 2014;27:888–95.

71. Knight DS, Zumbo G, Barcella W, *et al.* Cardiac structural and functional consequences of amyloid deposition by cardiac magnetic resonance and echocardiography and their prognostic roles. *JACC Cardiovascular Imaging.* 2019;12:823–33.

72. Martinez-Naharro A, Baksi AJ, Hawkins PN, and Fontana M. Diagnostic imaging of cardiac amyloidosis. *Nature Reviews Cardiology.* 2020;17:413–26.

73. Martinez-Naharro A, Treibel TA, Abdel-Gadir A, *et al.* Magnetic resonance in transthyretin cardiac amyloidosis. *Journal of the American College of Cardiology.* 2017;70:466–77.

74. Perugini E, Guidalotti PL, Salvi F, *et al.* Noninvasive etiologic diagnosis of cardiac amyloidosis using 99mTc-3,3-diphosphono-1,2-propanodicarboxylic acid scintigraphy. *Journal of the American College of Cardiology.* 2005;46:1076–84.

75. Gillmore JD, Maurer MS, Falk RH, *et al.* Nonbiopsy diagnosis of cardiac transthyretin amyloidosis. *Circulation.* 2016;133:2404–12.

76. Lachmann HJ, Booth DR, Booth SE, *et al.* Misdiagnosis of hereditary amyloidosis as AL (primary) amyloidosis. *The New England Journal of Medicine.* 2002;346:1786–91.

77. Nativi-Nicolau J and Maurer MS. Amyloidosis cardiomyopathy: update in the diagnosis and treatment of the most common types. *Current Opinion in Cardiology.* 2018;33:571–9.

78. Garcia-Pavia P, Rapezzi C, Adler Y, *et al.* Diagnosis and treatment of cardiac amyloidosis. A position statement of the European Society of Cardiology Working Group on Myocardial and Pericardial Diseases. *European Journal of Heart Failure.* 2021;23:512–26.

79. Garcia-Pavia P, Rapezzi C, Adler Y, *et al.* Diagnosis and treatment of cardiac amyloidosis. A position statement of the Eurojpean Society of Cardiology Working Group on Myocardial and Pericardial Diseases. *European Heart Journal.* 2021;42:1554–68.

80. Grogan M, Scott CG, Kyle RA, *et al.* Natural history of wild-type transthyretin cardiac amyloidosis and risk stratification using a novel staging system. *Journal of the American College of Cardiology.* 2016;68:1014–20.

81. Madan S, Kumar SK, Dispenzieri A, *et al.* High-dose melphalan and peripheral blood stem cell transplantation for light-chain amyloidosis with cardiac involvement. *Blood.* 2012;119:1117–22.

82. Gillmore JD, Damy T, Fontana M, *et al.* A new staging system for cardiac transthyretin amyloidosis. *European Heart Journal.* 2018;39:2799–806.

83. Kumar S, Dispenzieri A, Lacy MQ, *et al.* Revised prognostic staging system for light chain amyloidosis incorporating cardiac biomarkers and serum free light chain measurements. *Journal of Clinical Oncology.* 2012;30:989–95.

84. Palladini G, Dispenzieri A, Gertz MA, *et al*. New criteria for response to treatment in immunoglobulin light chain amyloidosis based on free light chain measurement and cardiac biomarkers: impact on survival outcomes. *Journal of Clinical Oncology*. 2012;30:4541–9.

85. Elliott P, Drachman BM, Gottlieb SS, *et al*. Long-term survival with tafamidis in patients with transthyretin amyloid cardiomyopathy. *Circulation Heart Failure*. 2022;15:e008193.

86. Yilmaz A, Bauersachs J, Bengel F, *et al*. Diagnosis and treatment of cardiac amyloidosis: position statement of the German Cardiac Society (DGK). *Clinical Research in Cardiology*. 2021;110:479–506.

87. Kittleson MM, Maurer MS, Ambardekar AV, *et al*. Cardiac amyloidosis: evolving diagnosis and management: a scientific statement from the American Heart Association. *Circulation*. 2020;142:e7–22.

88. Kitaoka H, Izumi C, Izumiya Y, *et al*. CS 2020 guideline on diagnosis and treatment of cardiac amyloidosis. *Circulation Journal*. 2020;84:1610–71.

89. Fine NM, Davis MK, Anderson K, *et al*. Canadian Cardiovascular Society/Canadian Heart Failure Society Joint position statement on the evaluation and management of patients with cardiac amyloidosis. *Canadian Journal of Cardiology*. 2020;36:322–34.

90. Aimo A, Rapezzi C, Vergaro G, *et al*. Management of complications of cardiac amyloidosis: 10 questions and answers. *European Journal of Preventive Cardiology*. 2021;28:1000–5.

91. Santos-Gallego CG, Requena-Ibanez JA, San Antonio R, *et al*. Empagliflozin ameliorates diastolic dysfunction and left ventricular fibrosis/stiffness in nondiabetic heart failure: a multimodality study. *JACC Cardiovascular Imaging*. 2021;14:393–407.

92. Anker SD, Butler J, Filippatos G, *et al*. Empagliflozin in heart failure with a preserved ejection fraction. *The New England Journal of Medicine*. 2021;385:1451–61.

3.4.5 Arrhythmogenic right ventricular cardiomyopathy

Cristina Basso, Hugh Calkins, and Domenico Corrado

Introduction

Arrhythmogenic right ventricular cardiomyopathy (ARVC) is a rare heart muscle disease characterized by progressive myocardial atrophy with fibrofatty replacement.[1,2,3,4] The estimated prevalence in the general population ranges from 1:2000 to 1:5000.[3,5] Considered in the past to be an endemic disease in North East Italy, ARVC is now well recognized worldwide.

It is a genetically determined heredo-familial cardiomyopathy caused by mutations in genes encoding mostly desmosomal proteins (about 50% of probands). ARVC affects more frequently males,[3,5] despite a similar prevalence of mutations in both sexes. The disease usually becomes clinically overt in the second to fourth decade of life, with palpitations, syncope, or sudden death (SD), particularly during effort in the young and athletes.[1,5,6,7] An age-related penetrance has been demonstrated, with high clinical and genetic variability. More rarely, clinical presentation occurs before puberty or in the elderly.

Since there is no single gold standard, diagnostic criteria have been put forward, including various sources of information, such as morpho-functional abnormalities of the right ventricle (RV), tissue characterization of the myocardium through endomyocardial biopsy (EMB), depolarization and repolarization abnormalities, left bundle branch block (LBBB) morphology, ventricular arrhythmias, and family history.[8,9]

The identification of biventricular and left ventricular variants through genotype–phenotype correlation studies, including contrast-enhanced cardiac magnetic resonance (CE-CMR), supports the use of the broader term arrhythmogenic cardiomyopathy.[4] A proposal for modification of the international guidelines for the diagnosis of the entire spectrum of the disease has been recently put forward.[10]

Pathology

ARVC is a cardiomyopathy characterized by atrophy of the ventricular myocardium, with fibrofatty replacement in its overt form.[1,2,11] The disease has nothing in common with Uhl's disease, a congenital heart defect with total absence of the right ventricular (RV) myocardium since birth.[12] In fact, cardiomyocyte death occurs progressively with time, leading to myocardial atrophy starting from the epicardium towards the endocardium, to become eventually transmural. In the classical RV variant, wall thinning can lead to the pathognomonic features of the disease, that is, RV aneurysms in the inflow, apex, and outflow tract (the so-called 'triangle of dysplasia').[2,13]

However, concealed variants do exist, characterized by a grossly normal heart in the absence of wall thinning and/or aneurysm, where only a careful histopathology study can reveal fibrofatty replacement of the myocardium that is not necessarily transmural. Moreover, subepicardial and/or mid-myocardial myocyte necrosis with inflammation has been reported in the early stages of the disease in the context of a positive family history and/or genetic test.[14] Finally, variants with isolated or predominant LV involvement, where the process is usually limited to the subepicardium or mid-mural layers, have been increasingly recognized, particularly in the posterolateral region.[2,15] The ventricular septum is mostly spared. Chamber dilatation is observed in diffuse forms, typically with biventricular involvement (➲ Figure 3.4.5.1).

Histologically, besides fibrofatty replacement and cardiomyocyte abnormalities, inflammation has been described both in the human heart and in experimental models.[2,16,17] Disease progression may occur through periodic 'bursts' of a stable disease, with a 'myocarditis-like' clinical picture, consisting of chest pain, electrocardiogram (ECG) changes, and enzyme release, in the setting of normal coronary arteries.[18]

Genetic background

Although the familial background has been recognized since the eighties,[19] the first disease-causing gene was discovered in 2000.[20] ARVC is now reported as a heredo-familial disease, mostly due to pathogenic mutations of genes encoding proteins of the intercellular junctions, more frequently desmosomal proteins such as plakophilin (*PKP2*), desmoplakin (*DSP*), desmoglein (*DSG2*), and

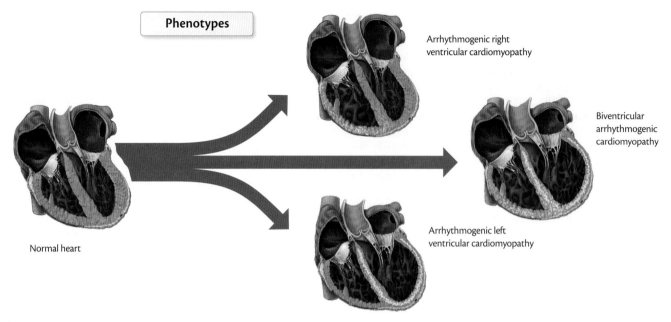

Phenotypes

Normal heart

Arrhythmogenic right ventricular cardiomyopathy

Biventricular arrhythmogenic cardiomyopathy

Arrhythmogenic left ventricular cardiomyopathy

Figure 3.4.5.1 Diagram illustrating the development of distinct phenotypes of arrhythmogenic cardiomyopathy.
Source: Corrado D, Perazzolo Marra M, Zorzi A, et al. Diagnosis of arrhythmogenic cardiomyopathy: The Padua criteria. *Int J Cardiol.* 2020 Nov 15;319:106–114.

desmocollin (*DSC2*) (➲ Table 3.4.5.1).[19,20,21,22,23,24,25] Exceptionally, genes encoding proteins of the 'area composita', such as αT-catenin (*CTNNA3*) and N-cadherin (*CDH2*), are involved.[26,27] Non-desmosomal gene mutations also have been described in ARVC probands, such as phospholamban (*PLN*), filamin C (*FLNC*), desmin (*DES*), titin (*TTN*), lamin A/C (*LMNA*), transmembrane protein 43 (*TMEM43*), and transforming growth factor beta-3 (*TGF-3*) genes,[28,29,30,31,32,33,34,35] some of which are also associated with other cardiomyopathies with overlapping phenotypes.

Comprehensive analysis of known desmosomal ARVC-causing genes currently identifies approximately 50% of probands.[36,37] Genetic testing and its interpretation should be performed by genetic counsellors in dedicated cardiogenetic centres with counselling facilities. Due to the limited diagnostic yield from screening of known causal genes, a negative genetic test does not exclude a genetic background. On the other hand, a positive genetic test opens the door to early identification of asymptomatic carriers by cascade genetic screening. Increasing awareness that

Table 3.4.5.1 Genetic background of arrhythmogenic cardiomyopathy

Gene	Reference	Year	Protein	Chromosomal location	Prevalence (%)
ARVC genes encoding desmosomal proteins					
PKP2	23	2005	Plakophilin-2	12p11.21	30–40
DSP	22	2002	Desmoplakin	6p24.3	10-15
DSG2	24	2006	Desmoglein-2	18q12.1	3–8
DSC2	25	2006	Desmocollin-2	18q12.1	1–5
JUP	20	2000	Plakoglobin	17q21.2	<1
Other non-desmosomal ARVC genes					
CTNNA3	26	2013	αT-catenin	10q21.3	<1
CDH2	27	2017	N-cadherin	18q12.1	<1
TMEM43	28	2008	Transmembrane protein 43	3p25.1	<1
TTN	30	2011	Titin	2q31.2	<1
FLNC	34	2016	Filamin C	7q32.1	<1
LMNA	32	2012	Lamin A/C	1q22	<1
TGF-β3	33	2005	Transforming growth factor β3	14q24.3	<1
PLN	31	2012	Phospholamban	6q22.31	<1
DES	29	2009	Desmin	2q35	<1
SCN5A	35	2017	Voltage-gated sodium channel subunit α Nav 1.5	3p22.2	<1

many variants are of uncertain significance and the low sensitivity of molecular genetics have recently raised concerns about its role in the diagnosis of ARVC.[38,39] Unlike other cardiomyopathies, the demonstration of a pathogenic variant in ARVC-related genes is listed as a major criterion in the 2010 Task Force Criteria.[9] Accordingly, genetic testing should be reserved to probands with a 'phenotypic' diagnosis of ARVC and to their family members for cascade screening. Carriers of multiple mutations show wide variability in clinical expression and the extent of the disease is greater, compared to that in single-mutation carriers.[40,41]

Pathogenesis

The detection of inflammatory cells and viral genomes in the myocardium of ARVC patients led to the early theory of an infective aetiopathogenesis, in the era preceding the discovery of the disease-causing genes.[2,17] Viruses are now considered as innocent bystanders or superimposed to a disease-prone myocardium.[42] Recently, the role of autoimmunity in disease pathogenesis has been addressed, although the exact trigger and mechanisms for autoimmunity in arrhythmogenic cardiomyopathy are still unknown.[43]

With ARVC being a cardiomyopathy linked to mutations mostly in desmosomal genes, loss of adhesion between cardiomyocytes, predisposing to cell detachment and death, has been advocated as the most obvious pathogenetic theory.[4,44] This theory could also explain the role of exercise as a disease modifier by exacerbating the cell adhesion defect, as demonstrated in multiple experimental murine models (→ Figure 3.4.5.2).[45] However, besides mechanical cell attachment, desmosomes are also mediators of signal transduction pathways. In ARVC experimental models, redistribution of plakoglobin (also known as γ-catenin) from the cell membrane to the nucleus, where it competes with β-catenin, has been proven.[46,47] This accounts for dysregulation of canonical Wnt, Hippo, and TGF-β signalling pathways as responsible for the development of the ARVC phenotype, mainly fibroadiposis.[48]

To discover the cell origin of fatty tissue in ARVC, several theories have been postulated, from transdifferentiation of adult cardiomyocytes[49] to abnormal differentiation of cardiac stem cells.[50,51,52] However, the cell source of fibrosis and adiposis is still debated. Recently, it has been demonstrated that cardiac-resident mesenchymal cells express desmosome proteins and can be a source of adipocytes in ARVC.[53] The effects of signal transduction pathways in different cell types have not been studied in detail. Since it has been shown that desmosomal proteins are not expressed exclusively in cardiomyocytes, but also in other cell types, these may also respond to the presence of gene mutations. Ongoing experimental studies are now addressing this hypothesis.

There is also evidence that both desmosomal and non-desmosomal gene mutations cause electromechanical dysfunction in ARVC, even independently from structural abnormalities.[54,55,56,57,58] Whereas scar-related re-entrant ventricular tachycardia (VT) usually occurs in patients with overt disease, ventricular fibrillation (VF) can occur in early stages or during evolutive poussées due to acute myocyte death and reactive inflammation.[59] More recently, gap junction remodelling and sodium channel interference have been advanced in experimental models as alternative substrates for life-threatening arrhythmias, even in the pre-phenotypic disease stage, but this occurrence has to be confirmed in both the clinical and pathological setting. Moreover, mutations in non-desmosomal genes, such as PLN and RYR2, could directly impair calcium handling.

Clinical picture

Clinical presentation varies with age and stage of disease. ARVC usually manifests with heart palpitations, syncope, or cardiac arrest. However, four phases have been classically recognized in the natural history of ARVC, including: the 'concealed' phase with subtle RV structural changes, with or without ventricular arrhythmias; an 'overt electrical disorder' with life-threatening ventricular arrhythmias and RV morpho-functional abnormalities; and RV, or even biventricular,

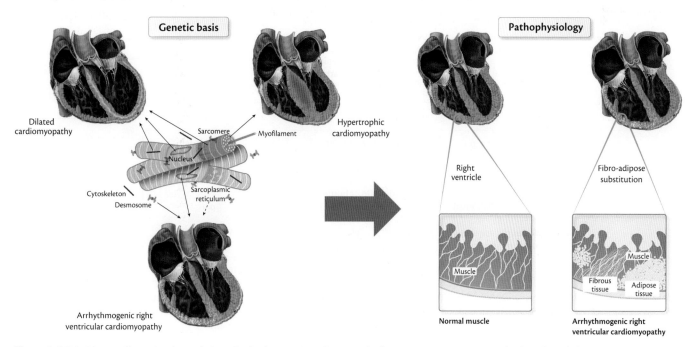

Figure 3.4.5.2 Diagram illustrating the evolution of arrhythmogenic cardiomyopathy from genetic mutations to pathophysiological alterations.

'failure' mimicking dilated cardiomyopathy.[3,4] Electrical instability is a risk factor for SD which can occur at any time in the disease course.[59] The incidence of SD ranges from 0.08% to 3.6% per year in adults with ARVC. Age-related prevalence is well recognized.[5,60]

Findings from a 12-lead ECG, such as depolarization abnormalities, QRS widening, epsilon waves, and repolarization changes with inverted T-waves on precordial leads, as well as ventricular arrhythmias with an LBBB morphology, are the most typical changes that warrant a cardiology referral. Less common presentations are RV or biventricular dilatation, with or without heart failure (HF) symptoms, mimicking dilated cardiomyopathy.[61]

In the paediatric age group, the disease rarely appears before the age of 10 years due to the well-known age-related penetrance.[62,63,64] Chest pain, dynamic ECG changes, myocardial enzyme release, and normal coronary arteries are often observed that mimic myocarditis or myocardial infarction.[3,17,62,63] Follow-up with non-invasive clinical investigation of children with a positive family history or those suspicious for ARVC is recommended on a regular basis, to monitor the impending disease onset in the pubertal period.

It is well known that competitive sports activity leads to a 5-fold increase in SD risk in young people affected by ARVC.[6] Sports activity and strenuous physical exercise increase both disease penetrance and the risk of occurrence of ventricular arrhythmias and HF in desmosomal gene mutation carriers.[65,66]

Although the usual clinical picture of ARVC consists of life-threatening arrhythmias and SD, less frequently, patients present with congestive HF that can even mimic dilated cardiomyopathy. The incidence of HF and that of heart transplantation in ARVC are largely variable in the literature, depending mostly on the selection criteria of patients, whether referred for ventricular arrhythmias or HF. Although the most common indication for heart transplantation is HF, patients can be referred also due to refractory electrical storms. In a large cohort of ARVC patients, the HF incidence was 13%, with 4% eventually having heart transplantation.[67] Patients with multiple mutations are thought to develop a more severe phenotype, with those with *DSP* mutations more prone to developing HF.[68,69,70] More recently, Vischer *et al.*[71] reported that 5.9% of ARVC patients reached the composite endpoint of heart transplantation and death due to HF. According to their data, patients with HF predominantly carried *PKP2* mutations and often had multiple variants. Moreover, RV dysfunction appears to be a determinant of heart transplantation and death during follow-up. Similar results with predominantly *PKP2* mutations were found in an American and a Nordic Registry series,[72,73] whereas in the largest cohort of patients with heart transplantation due to ARVC, there was no information on genetic data.[74]

Diagnosis

The absence of a single gold standard for ARVC diagnosis led to the introduction of the original scoring system of the International Task Force (ITF) Criteria in 1994.[8] These diagnostic criteria combined different sources of information, such as RV morpho-functional abnormalities, myocardial tissue abnormalities, ECG changes, and arrhythmic and familial findings. The original diagnostic criteria were revised in 2010 to improve diagnostic sensitivity, by maintaining diagnostic specificity,[9] while also introducing quantitative parameters based on comparison with normal subject data.

However, the 1994 and 2010 ITF criteria exclusively targeted the classical RV phenotype, without providing criteria for diagnosis of left-sided variants.[10] Moreover, tissue characterization was still based only upon EMB findings,[75] without taking into account the role of CE-CMR for detection of myocardial fibrosis, which is a determinant for an accurate diagnosis of the LV phenotype.[65,74,75] For these reasons, in 2020, an international expert consensus document proposed an upgrade of the diagnostic criteria (the so-called 'Padua criteria'), introducing specific criteria for the diagnosis of the LV phenotype (➲ Figure 3.4.5.3).[10] The same multiparametric approach recommended in 2010 for classic ARVC has been utilized, with six categories of diagnostic information (➲ Table 3.4.5.2). The diagnostic criteria for LV involvement are classified

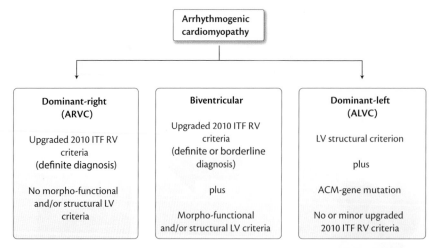

Figure 3.4.5.3 Diagnosis of phenotypic variants of arrhythmogenic cardiomyopathy. Demonstration of morpho-functional and/or structural abnormalities of the right and/or left ventricle is required. ITF, International Task Force Criteria; LV, left ventricle; RV, right ventricle; ALVC, arrhythmiogenic left ventricular cardiomyopathy; ARVC, arrhythmogenic right ventricular cardiomyopathy; ACM, arrhythmogenic cardiomyopathy.
Reproduced from Corrado D, Perazzolo Marra M, Zorzi A, *et al.* Diagnosis of arrhythmogenic cardiomyopathy: The Padua criteria. *Int J Cardiol.* 2020 Nov 15;319:106–114. doi: 10.1016/j.ijcard.2020.06.005 with permission from Elsevier.

Table 3.4.5.2 Diagnosis of arrhythmogenic cardiomyopathy: the proposed 'Padua criteria'

Category	Right ventricle (upgraded 2010 ITF diagnostic criteria)	Left ventricle (new diagnostic criteria)
I. Morpho-functional ventricular abnormalities	By two-dimensional echocardiography, CMR, or angiography: Major: ♦ Regional RV akinesia, dyskinesia, or bulging PLUS one of the following: ♦ Global RV dilatation (increase of RV EDV according to imaging test-specific monograms for age and gender) ♦ Global RV systolic dysfunction (reduction of RVEF according to imaging test-specific monograms for age, sex, and BSA) Minor: ♦ Regional RV akinesia, dyskinesia, or aneurysm of RV free wall	By two-dimensional echocardiography, CMR, or angiography: Major: ♦ Global LV systolic dysfunction (reduction in LVEF according to imaging test-specific monograms for age, sex, and BSA), with or without LV dilatation (increase in LV EDV according to imaging test-specific monograms for age, sex, and BSA) Minor: ♦ Regional LV hypokinesia or akinesia of LV free wall, septum, or both
II. Structural myocardial abnormalities	By CE-CMR: Major: ♦ Transmural LGE (stria pattern) of ≥1 RV region(s) (inlet, outlet, and apex in two orthogonal views) By EMB (limited indications): Major: ♦ Fibrous replacement of myocardium in ≥1 sample, with or without fatty tissue	By CE-CMR: Major: ♦ LV LGE (stria pattern) of ≥1 bullseye segment(s) (in two orthogonal views) of the free wall (subepicardial or mid-myocardial) or septum, or both (excluding septal junctional LGE)
III. Repolarization abnormalities	Major: ♦ Inverted T-waves in right precordial leads (V1, V2, and V3) or beyond in individuals with completed pubertal development (in the absence of complete RBBB) Minor: ♦ Inverted T-waves in leads V1 and V2 in individuals with completed pubertal development (in the absence of complete RBBB) ♦ Inverted T-waves in leads V1, V2, V3, and V4 in individuals with completed pubertal development in the presence of complete RBBB	Minor: ♦ Inverted T-waves in left precordial leads (V4 to V6) (in the absence of complete LBBB)
IV. Depolarization abnormalities	Minor ♦ Epsilon wave (reproducible low-amplitude signals between end of QRS complex to onset of T-wave) in the right precordial leads (leads V1 to V3) ♦ Terminal activation duration of QRS ≥55 ms measured from nadir of S wave to end of QRS, including R', in leads V1, V2, or V3 (in the absence of complete RBBB)	Minor: ♦ Low QRS voltages (<0.5 mV peak to peak) in limb leads (in the absence of obesity, emphysema, or pericardial effusion)
V. Ventricular arrhythmias	Major: ♦ Frequent ventricular extrasystoles (>500 per 24 hours), non-sustained or sustained ventricular tachycardia of LBBB morphology Minor: ♦ Frequent ventricular extrasystoles (>500 per 24 hours), non-sustained or sustained ventricular tachycardia of LBBB morphology with inferior axis ('RVOT pattern')	Minor: ♦ Frequent ventricular extrasystoles (>500 per 24 hours), non-sustained or sustained ventricular tachycardia with RBBB morphology (excluding the 'fascicular pattern')
VI. Family history/genetics		Major: ♦ Disease confirmed in a first-degree relative who meets diagnostic criteria ♦ Disease confirmed pathologically at autopsy or surgery in a first-degree relative ♦ Identification of a pathogenic or likely pathogenetic AC mutation in the patient under evaluation Minor: ♦ History of AC in a first-degree relative in whom it is not possible or practical to determine whether the family member meets diagnostic criteria ♦ Premature sudden death (<35 years of age) due to suspected AC in a first-degree relative ♦ AC confirmed pathologically or by diagnostic criteria in a second-degree relative

AC, arrhythmogenic cardiomyopathy; BSA, body surface area; EDV, end-diastolic volume; EF, ejection fraction; ITF, International Task Force; LBBB, left bundle branch block; LGE, late gadolinium enhancement; LV, left ventricle; RBBB, right bundle branch block; RV, right ventricle; RVOT, right ventricular outflow tract.

Reproduced from Corrado D, Perazzolo Marra M, Zorzi A, *et al*. Diagnosis of arrhythmogenic cardiomyopathy: The Padua criteria. *Int J Cardiol*. 2020 Nov 15;319:106–114. doi: 10.1016/j.ijcard.2020.06.005 with permission from Elsevier.

as 'major' when they are *essential*, and 'minor' when they are *not necessary but contribute* to characterize the LV phenotype. While in the *biventricular* ARVC variant, the left-sided abnormalities are easily considered specific due to the concomitant fulfilment of criteria for the RV phenotype, the diagnosis of arrhythmogenic left ventricular cardiomyopathy (ALVC) in patients without clinically detectable RV abnormalities cannot be achieved on the basis of isolated LV 'phenotypic' criteria, because of a possible overlap with other myocardial diseases such as dilated and inflammatory cardiomyopathies. Thus, a definite diagnosis of 'left dominant' disease requires positive genetic testing for ARVC-causing gene mutation or evidence of familial disease, besides structural and/or morpho-functional LV abnormalities.

According to these criteria, the diagnosis of ARVC (dominant right) variant is reached when fulfilling the criteria for: *definite* ARVC, that is, two major, one major and two minor, or four minor criteria from different categories; *borderline* ARVC, that is, one major and one minor, or three minor criteria from different categories; and *possible* ARVC, that is, one major, or two minor criteria (≥1 morpho-functional and/or structural criterion, either major or minor needed for each diagnosis), in the absence of LV involvement. The diagnosis of 'biventricular' variant is reached when fulfilling the criteria for definite, borderline, or possible ARVC (≥1 criterion, either major or minor, from categories I or II needed), along with LV morpho-functional and/or structural abnormalities. The diagnosis of ALVC variant is reached in the setting of structural (and/or morpho-functional) LV abnormalities *plus* demonstration of a disease-causing gene mutation or evidence of familial disease, in the absence of RV involvement.

Differential diagnosis/disease phenocopies

Differential diagnosis in patients with suspected ARVC includes myocarditis, sarcoidosis, RV infarction, dilated cardiomyopathy, Chagas disease, pulmonary hypertension, and congenital heart disease with volume overload (such as Ebstein anomaly, atrial septal defect, partial anomalous venous return, and left-to-right shunt).[3] In some instances, especially when dealing with probands with a sporadic form, EMB can be crucial to rule out myocarditis and sarcoidosis.[10,75] Tissue characterization can be achieved also by CE-CMR[67,76,77] or indirectly by electroanatomical voltage mapping where abnormal low-voltage areas correspond to loss of electrically active myocardium caused by fibrofatty replacement.[78,79,80,81]

Disease phenocopies include also non-structural diseases. In fact, one of the main diagnostic dilemma is to distinguish ARVC from idiopathic RV outflow tract VT, since the latter is usually benign.[79] The idiopathic nature of VT is supported by the absence of family history, a normal basal 12-lead ECG, a normal ventricular structure on cardiac imaging and electroanatomic mapping, a single VT morphology and non-inducibility at programmed ventricular stimulation. Finally, in highly trained competitive athletes, a differential diagnosis with physiological adaptation to training can be required. RV enlargement, ECG abnormalities, and arrhythmias reflect the increased haemodynamic load during exercise.[81,82,83] While global RV systolic dysfunction and/or regional wall motion abnormalities, such as bulging or aneurysms, are more in keeping with ARVC, the absence of overt structural changes of the RV, frequent premature ventricular complexes, or inverted T-waves in precordial leads all support a benign nature (so-called 'athlete heart'). The proposed flow chart for clinical diagnosis of arrhythmogenic cardiomyopathy is shown in ⮕ Figure 3.4.5.4.

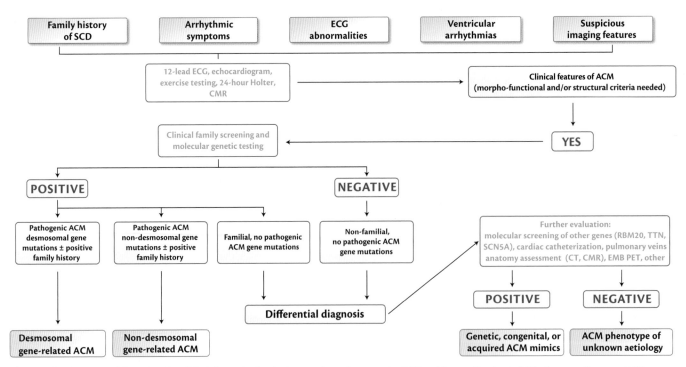

Figure 3.4.5.4 Proposed flow chart for clinical diagnosis of arrhythmogenic cardiomyopathy. SCD, sudden cardiac death; ECG, electrocardiogram; ACM, arrhythmogenic cardiomyopathy; RBM20, RNA-binding motif protein 20; TTN, titin; SCN5A, sodium voltage-gated channel α subunit 5; CT, computed tomography; CMR, cardiac magnetic resonance; EMB, endomyocardial biopsy; PET, positron emission tomography.

Therapy

The arrhythmogenic cardiomyopathy management options regard lifestyle modifications, pharmacological treatment, catheter ablation, implantable cardioverter–defibrillator (ICD), and exceptionally heart transplantation.

Lifestyle modification is the first and easy tool to prevent SD. The significant reduction in death rates from ARVC recorded after the introduction of pre-participation screening in young athletes supports the concept that sports restriction is lifesaving.[7] Moreover, endurance sports and frequent exercise increase disease penetrance, as well as the occurrence of VT and HF in desmosomal gene carriers.[81,82,83]. Although pregnancy is well tolerated, evaluation for risk stratification and strict surveillance are recommended.[84]

Beta-blocker therapy is recommended as an anti-adrenergic treatment in all ARVC patients, regardless of symptoms and arrhythmic manifestations.[85,86,87,88] However, prophylactic use in healthy gene mutation carriers is not justified. Even left cardiac sympathetic denervation has been proposed in ARVC patients with refractory adrenergic-dependent ventricular arrhythmias. Antiarrhythmic drug therapy does not protect adequately against SD and is used to reduce the arrhythmia burden in patients with frequent premature ventricular beats and non-sustained VT. It is also useful as an adjunct treatment to catheter ablation and ICD therapy to reduce VT recurrences and device discharges. Sotalol and amiodarone are the most effective drugs with a relatively low proarrhythmic risk.

Catheter ablation of the macro-re-entry circuit is a non-pharmacological therapeutic option for ARVC patients with VT and should not be considered as an alternative strategy to ICD therapy.[89,90] Catheter ablation is recommended in the presence of incessant or frequent VT triggering ICD interventions refractory to maximal antiarrhythmic drug therapy.[88] Despite the high acute success rate, a high rate of recurrence has been reported using conventional electrophysiological mapping and an endocardial approach. A combined endo-epicardial approach is now used by referral centres to reduce the rate of recurrences.

ICD therapy is the first-line approach for high-risk patients.[91,92,93] Despite its well-known benefit on survival, lead- and device-related complications, as well as inappropriate intervention, usually caused by sinus tachycardia or atrial tachyarrhythmia, should be taken into account and justify risk stratification in ARVC patients.

Several risk factors for SD have been identified from follow-up studies. While a history of cardiac arrest due to VF or sustained VT confers the highest risk, the prognostic role of syncope and non-sustained VT remains controversial. Moreover, conflicting results about the prognostic role of VT/VF inducibility by programmed ventricular stimulation come from different studies.

On the basis of annual rates of malignant arrhythmic events, three risk categories have been identified. ARVC patients with a history of cardiac arrest or sustained VT, or with severe dysfunction of the RV, LV, or both, represent the high-risk category (event rate of >10% per year), with a class I recommendation for ICD therapy.

The intermediate-risk category (event rate of 1–10% per year) includes patients with ≥1 risk factors and no previous malignant arrhythmias—the indication for ICD therapy remains uncertain. ICD therapy can be recommended (class IIa) in the presence of major risk factors such as syncope, non-sustained VT, or moderate ventricular dysfunction; ICD treatment may also be considered (class IIb) in selected patients with ≥1 minor risk factors, in whom the arrhythmic risk is not sufficiently high or defined. The decision is on an individual basis, taking into account all the following: statistical risk, socio-economic factors, psychological impact, patient preferences, and high rate of device-related adverse effects over time. Finally, in asymptomatic patients with no risk factors and in healthy gene carriers (low-risk category; event rate of <10% per year), prophylactic ICD therapy is not recommended (class III). The performance of the 'three categories' risk stratification has been validated by outcome studies among ARVC patients who received ICD implantation.[94]

Subcutaneous ICD implantation has been proven to substantially reduce lead-related complications, but while maintaining efficacy.[95,96] ICDs are particularly implanted for primary prevention in young ARVC patients who do not need ventricular pacing for bradycardia or cardiac resynchronization therapy. Recently, a calculator has been proposed for 'primary' risk stratification of patients with ARVC.[97,98] However, its use is associated with potential overestimation of the risk of VT or VF, which may translate into overtreatment with ICD of asymptomatic patients (ARVC Risk Calculator disclaimer available from: https://arvcrisk.com/disclaimer/).

Heart failure and antithrombotic drug therapy

In ARVC patients with right- and/or left-sided HF, standard drug therapy with angiotensin-converting enzyme inhibitors, angiotensin II receptor blockers, beta-blockers, and diuretics is recommended.[88] In the setting of asymptomatic RV and/or LV dysfunction, angiotensin-converting enzyme inhibitors or angiotensin II receptor blockers also may be considered. Oral anticoagulation is generally indicated for secondary prevention in patients with intracardiac thrombosis or venous/systemic thromboembolism.

Despite some experimental evidence, preload-reducing drug therapy is not part of the routine clinical approach and requires validation in other ARVC models and patients.[99]

Future directions

Despite decades of research, there is yet no curative treatment for arrhythmogenic cardiomyopathy and all available therapeutic tools are still focused on prevention or attenuation of disease symptoms and signs. Ongoing investigations on the cellular and molecular pathways of disease pathogenesis, following the identification of genetic mutations, aim to discover new therapies targeting specific pathways involved in arrhythmogenic cardiomyopathy. Modification of environmental factors could also play a role.

On the diagnostic front, efforts should be made to understand the precise role of genetic screening not only in early identification, but also in risk stratification. Moreover, CMR should be considered the main imaging tool in patients with a suspicion for arrhythmogenic cardiomyopathy.

Summary

Arrhythmogenic cardiomyopathy is a genetically determined cardiomyopathy, with an estimated prevalence of 1:2000 to 1:5000, and pathogenic mutations are found in at least 50% of probands, mostly in genes encoding desmosomal proteins. It is characterized by progressive myocardial atrophy, with fibrofatty replacement of the ventricular myocardium leading to wall thinning and aneurysms when transmural in advanced forms.

In this chapter, we address the wide spectrum of clinical presentation, which is more often associated with ECG abnormalities and ventricular arrhythmias, although HF is not uncommon. Moreover, we focus on lifestyle modifications and therapy to prevent SD (including antiarrhythmic drugs, catheter ablation, and ICD).

The evolution of the concept from the originally described RV variant towards a wider phenotype including biventricular and LV variants has led to the recent proposal of updated diagnostic criteria. Inclusion of tissue characterization through CMR imaging is mandatory in the clinical workup to assess for LV involvement.

Key messages

◆ Arrhythmogenic cardiomyopathy is a genetically determined cardiomyopathy, and genetic screening of family members is needed for early diagnosis.

◆ The spectrum of the disease is wider than previously thought, and includes RV, LV, and biventricular variants.

◆ Diagnostic criteria have been updated to include identification of LV variants.

◆ CMR is an essential imaging tool to assess for the presence of LV involvement.

◆ Differential diagnosis with disease phenocopies is needed, particularly in sporadic forms.

◆ Prevention of SD and disease evolution can be achieved also through lifestyle modifications, including sports activity restriction.

◆ Ongoing research on the cellular and molecular pathways of disease pathogenesis point to discovering target therapies to prevent disease onset and progression in gene mutation carriers.

Acknowledgements

This work has been supported by Registry for Cardio-cerebrovascular Pathology, Veneto Region, Venice, Italy; PRIN Ministry of Education, University and Research, Rome, Italy; and CARIPARO Foundation, Padova, Italy.

References

1. Thiene G, Nava A, Corrado D, Rossi L, Pennelli N. Right ventricular cardiomyopathy and sudden death in young people. N Engl J Med. 1988; 318:129–33.
2. Basso C, Thiene G, Corrado D, Angelini A, Nava A, Valente M. Arrhythmogenic right ventricular cardiomyopathy. Dysplasia, dystrophy, or myocarditis? Circulation. 1996; 94:983–91.
3. Basso C, Corrado D, Marcus FI, Nava A, Thiene G. Arrhythmogenic right ventricular cardiomyopathy. Lancet. 2009; 373:1289–300.
4. Basso C, Bauce B, Corrado D, Thiene G. Pathophysiology of arrhythmogenic cardiomyopathy. Nat Rev Cardiol. 2011; 9:223–33.
5. Nava A, Bauce B, Basso C, et al. Clinical profile and long-term follow-up of 37 families with arrhythmogenic right ventricular cardiomyopathy. J Am Coll Cardiol. 2000; 36:2226–33.
6. Corrado D, Basso C, Rizzoli G, Schiavon M, Thiene G. Does sports activity enhance the risk of sudden death in adolescents and young adults? J Am Coll Cardiol. 2003; 42:1959–63.
7. Corrado D, Basso C, Pavei A, Michieli P, Schiavon M, Thiene G. Trends in sudden cardiovascular death in young competitive athletes after implementation of a preparticipation screening program. JAMA. 2006; 296:1593–601.
8. McKenna WJ, Thiene G, Nava A, et al. Diagnosis of arrhythmogenic right ventricular dysplasia/cardiomyopathy. Task Force of the Working Group Myocardial and Pericardial Disease of the European Society of Cardiology and of the Scientific Council on Cardiomyopathies of the International Society and Federation of Cardiology. Br Heart J. 1994; 71:215–18.
9. Marcus FI, McKenna WJ, Sherrill D, et al. Diagnosis of arrhythmogenic right ventricular cardiomyopathy/dysplasia: proposed modification of the Task Force Criteria. Eur Heart J. 2010; 31:806–14.
10. Corrado D, Perazzolo Marra M, Zorzi A, et al. Diagnosis of arrhythmogenic cardiomyopathy: the Padua criteria. Int J Cardiol. 2020; 319:106–14.
11. Richardson P, McKenna W, Bristow M, et al. Report of the 1995 World Health Organization/International Society and Federation of Cardiology Task Force on the Definition and Classification of cardiomyopathies. Circulation. 1996; 93:841–2.
12. Uhl HSM. A previously undescribed congenital malformation of the heart: almost total absence of the myocardium of the right ventricle. Bull Johns Hopkins Hosp. 1952; 91:197–209.
13. Marcus FI, Fontaine GH, Guiraudon G, et al. Right ventricular dysplasia: a report of 24 adult cases. Circulation. 1982; 65:384–98.
14. Bauce B, Basso C, Rampazzo A, et al. Clinical profile of four families with arrhythmogenic right ventricular cardiomyopathy caused by dominant desmoplakin mutations. Eur Heart J. 2005; 26:1666–75.
15. Corrado D, Basso C, Thiene G, et al. Spectrum of clinicopathologic manifestations of arrhythmogenic right ventricular cardiomyopathy/dysplasia: a multicenter study. J Am Coll Cardiol. 1997; 30:1512–20.
16. Pilichou K, Remme CA, Basso C, et al. Myocyte necrosis underlies progressive myocardial dystrophy in mouse dsg2-related arrhythmogenic right ventricular cardiomyopathy. J Exp Med. 2009; 206:1787–802.
17. Thiene G, Corrado D, Nava A, et al. Right ventricular cardiomyopathy: is there evidence of an inflammatory aetiology? Eur Heart J. 1991; 12 Suppl D:22–5.
18. Bariani R, Cipriani A, Rizzo S, et al. 'Hot phase' clinical presentation in arrhythmogenic cardiomyopathy. EP Europace. 2021; 23:907–17.
19. Nava A, Thiene G, Canciani B, et al. Familial occurrence of right ventricular dysplasia: a study involving nine families. J Am Coll Cardiol. 1988; 12:1222–8.

20. McKoy G, Protonotarios N, Crosby A, *et al.* Identification of a deletion in plakoglobin in arrhythmogenic right ventricular cardiomyopathy with palmoplantar keratoderma and woolly hair (Naxos disease). Lancet. 2000; 355:2119–24.

21. Norgett EE, Hatsell SJ, Carvajal-Huerta L, *et al.* Recessive mutation in desmoplakin disrupts desmoplakin-intermediate filament interactions and causes dilated cardiomyopathy, woolly hair and keratoderma. Hum Mol Genet. 2000; 9:2761–6.

22. Rampazzo A, Nava A, Malacrida S, *et al.* Mutation in human desmoplakin domain binding to plakoglobin causes a dominant form of arrhythmogenic right ventricular cardiomyopathy. Am J Hum Genet. 2002; 71:1200–6.

23. Gerull B, Heuser A, Wichter T, *et al.* Mutations in the desmosomal protein plakophilin-2 are common in arrhythmogenic right ventricular cardiomyopathy. Nat Genet. 2005; 37:106.

24. Pilichou K, Nava A, Basso C, *et al.* Mutations in desmoglein-2 gene are associated with arrhythmogenic right ventricular cardiomyopathy. Circulation. 2006; 113:1171–9.

25. Syrris P, Ward D, Evans A, *et al.* Arrhythmogenic right ventricular dysplasia/cardiomyopathy associated with mutations in the desmosomal gene desmocollin-2. Am J Hum Genet. 2006; 79:978–84.

26. Van Hengel J, Calore M, Bauce B, *et al.* Mutations in the area composita protein αT-catenin are associated with arrhythmogenic right ventricular cardiomyopathy. Eur Heart J. 2013; 34:201–10.

27. Mayosi BM, Fish M, Shaboodien G, *et al.* Identification of cadherin 2 (*CDH2*) mutations in arrhythmogenic right ventricular cardiomyopathy. Circ Cardiovasc Genet 2017; 10:e001605.

28. Merner ND, Hodgkinson KA, Haywood AF, *et al.* Arrhythmogenic right ventricular cardiomyopathy type 5 is a fully penetrant, lethal arrhythmic disorder caused by a missense mutation in the *TMEM43* gene. Am J Hum Genet. 2008; 82:809–21.

29. van Tintelen JP, Van Gelder IC, Asimaki A *et al.* Severe cardiac phenotype with right ventricular predominance in a large cohort of patients with a single missense mutation in the *DES* gene. Heart Rhythm. 2009; 6:1574–83.

30. Taylor M, Graw S, Sinagra G, *et al.* Genetic variation in titin in arrhythmogenic right ventricular cardiomyopathy-overlap syndromes. Circulation. 2011; 124:876–85.

31. van der Zwaag PA, van Rijsingen IA, Asimaki A, *et al.* Phospholamban R14del mutation in patients diagnosed with dilated cardiomyopathy or arrhythmogenic right ventricular cardiomyopathy: evidence supporting the concept of arrhythmogenic cardiomyopathy. Eur J Heart Fail. 2012; 14:1199–207.

32. Quarta G, Syrris P, Ashworth M, *et al.* Mutations in the lamin A/C gene mimic arrhythmogenic right ventricular cardiomyopathy. Eur Heart J. 2012; 33:1128–36.

33. Beffagna G, Occhi G, Nava A, *et al.* Regulatory mutations in transforming growth factor-beta 3 gene cause arrhythmogenic right ventricular cardiomyopathy type 1. Cardiovasc Res. 2005; 65:366–73.

34. Ortiz-Genga MF, Cuenca S, Dal Ferro M, *et al.* Truncating *FLNC* mutations are associated with high-risk dilated and arrhythmogenic cardiomyopathies. J AmColl Cardiol 2016; 68:2440–51.

35. Te Riele AS, Agullo-Pascual E, James CA, *et al.* Multilevel analyses of SCN5A mutations in arrhythmogenic right ventricular dysplasia/cardiomyopathy suggest noncanonical mechanisms for disease pathogenesis. Cardiovasc Res. 2017; 113:102–11.

36. Pilichou K, Thiene G, Bauce B, *et al.* Arrhythmogenic cardiomyopathy. Orphanet J Rare Dis. 2016; 11:33.

37. James CA, Syrris P, van Tintelen JP, Calkins H. The role of genetics in cardiovascular disease: arrhythmogenic cardiomyopathy. Eur Heart J. 2020; 41:1393–400.

38. Kapplinger JD, Landstrom AP, Salisbury BA, *et al.* Distinguishing arrhythmogenic right ventricular cardiomyopathy/dysplasia-associated mutations from background genetic noise. J Am Coll Cardiol. 2011; 57:2317–27.

39. Andreasen C, Nielsen JB, Refsgaard L, *et al.* New population-based exome data are questioning the pathogenicity of previously cardiomyopathy-associated genetic variants. Eur J Hum Genet. 2013; 21:918–28.

40. Bauce B, Nava A, Beffagna G, *et al.* Multiple mutations in desmosomal proteins encoding genes in arrhythmogenic right ventricular cardiomyopathy/dysplasia. Heart Rhythm. 2010; 7:22–9.

41. Rigato I, Bauce B, Rampazzo A, *et al.* Compound and digenic heterozygosity predicts lifetime arrhythmic outcome and sudden cardiac death in desmosomal gene-related arrhythmogenic right ventricular cardiomyopathy. Circ Cardiovasc Genet. 2013; 6:533–42.

42. Calabrese F, Basso C, Carturan E, Valente M, Thiene G. Arrhythmogenic right ventricular cardiomyopathy/dysplasia: is there a role for viruses? Cardiovasc Pathol. 2006; 15:11–17.

43. Caforio ALP, Re F, Avella A, *et al.* Evidence from family studies for autoimmunity in arrhythmogenic right ventricular cardiomyopathy: associations of circulating anti-heart and anti-intercalated disk autoantibodies with disease severity and family history. Circulation. 2020; 141:1238–48.

44. Basso C, Czarnowska E, Della Barbera M, *et al.* Ultrastructural evidence of intercalated disc remodelling in arrhythmogenic right ventricular cardiomyopathy: an electron microscopy investigation on endomyocardial biopsies. Eur Heart J. 2006; 27:1847–54.

45. Kirchhof P, Fabritz L, Zwiener M, *et al.* Age- and training-dependent development of arrhythmogenic right ventricular cardiomyopathy in heterozygous plakoglobin-deficient mice. Circulation. 2006; 114:1799–806.

46. Garcia-Gras E, Lombardi R, Giocondo MJ, *et al.* Suppression of canonical Wnt/beta-catenin signaling by nuclear plakoglobin recapitulates phenotype of arrhythmogenic right ventricular cardiomyopathy. J Clin Invest. 2006; 116:2012–21.

47. Lombardi R, da Graca Cabreira-Hansen M, Bell A, Fromm RR, Willerson JT, Marian AJ. Nuclear plakoglobin is essential for differentiation of cardiac progenitor cells to adipocytes in arrhythmogenic right ventricular cardiomyopathy. Circ Res. 2011; 109:1342–53.

48. Chen SN, Gurha P, Lombardi R, Ruggiero A, Willerson JT, Marian AJ. The hippo pathway is activated and is a causal mechanism for adipogenesis in arrhythmogenic cardiomyopathy. Circ Res. 2014; 114:454–68.

49. d'Amati G, di Gioia CR, Giordano C, Gallo P. Myocyte transdifferentiation: a possible pathogenetic mechanism for arrhythmogenic right ventricular cardiomyopathy. Arch Pathol Lab Med. 2000; 124:287–90.

50. Kim C, Wong J, Wen J, *et al.* Studying arrhythmogenic right ventricular dysplasia with patient-specific iPSCs. Nature. 2013; 494:105–10.

51. Wen JY, Wei CY, Shah K, Wong J, Wang C, Chen HS. Maturation-based model of arrhythmogenic right ventricular dysplasia using patient-specific induced pluripotent stem cells. Circ J. 2015; 79:1402–8.

52. Lombardi R, Dong J, Rodriguez G, *et al.* Genetic fate mapping identifies second heart field progenitor cells as a source of adipocytes in arrhythmogenic right ventricular cardiomyopathy. Circ Res. 2009; 104:1076–84.

53. Sommariva E, Brambilla S, Carbucicchio C, *et al.* Cardiac mesenchymal stromal cells are a source of adipocytes in arrhythmogenic cardiomyopathy. Eur Heart J. 2016; 37:1835–46.

54. Sato PY, Coombs W, Lin X, *et al*. Interactions between ankyrin-G, plakophilin-2, and connexin43 at the cardiac intercalated disc. Circ Res. 2011; 109:193–201.

55. Zhang Q, Deng C, Rao F, *et al*. Silencing of desmoplakin decreases connexin43/Nav1.5 expression and sodium current in HL-1 cardiomyocytes. Mol Med Rep. 2013; 8:780–6.

56. Noorman M, Hakim S, Kessler E, *et al*. Remodeling of the cardiac sodium channel, connexin43, and plakoglobin at the intercalated disk in patients with arrhythmogenic cardiomyopathy. Heart Rhythm. 2013; 10:412–19.

57. Rizzo S, Lodder EM, Verkerk AO, *et al*. Intercalated disc abnormalities, reduced Na(+) current density, and conduction slowing in desmoglein-2 mutant mice prior to cardiomyopathic changes. Cardiovasc Res. 2012; 95:409–18.

58. Cerrone M, Noorman M, Lin X, *et al*. Sodium current deficit and arrhythmogenesis in a murine model of plakophilin-2 haploinsufficiency. Cardiovasc Res. 2012; 95:460–8.

59. Basso C, Corrado D, Bauce B, Thiene G. Arrhythmogenic right ventricular cardiomyopathy. Circ Arrhythm Electrophysiol. 2012; 5:1233–46.

60. Mast TP, James CA, Calkins H, *et al*. Evaluation of structural progression in arrhythmogenic right ventricular dysplasia/cardiomyopathy. JAMA Cardiol. 2017; 2:293–302.

61. Gilotra NA, Bhonsale A, James CA, *et al*. Heart failure is common and under-recognized in patients with arrhythmogenic right ventricular cardiomyopathy/dysplasia. Circ Heart Fail. 2017; 10:e003819.

62. Daliento L, Turrini P, Nava A, *et al*. Arrhythmogenic right ventricular cardiomyopathy in young versus adult patients: similarities and differences. J Am Coll Cardiol. 1995; 25:655–64.

63. Bauce B, Rampazzo A, Basso C, *et al*. Clinical phenotype and diagnosis of arrhythmogenic right ventricular cardiomyopathy in pediatric patients carrying desmosomal gene mutations. Heart Rhythm. 2011; 8:1686–95.

64. Te Riele ASJM, James CA, Sawant AC, *et al*. Arrhythmogenic right ventricular dysplasia/cardiomyopathy in the pediatric population: clinical characterization and comparison with adult-onset disease. JACC Clin Electrophysiol. 2015; 1:551–60.

65. Wang W, Tichnell C, Murray BA, *et al*. Exercise restriction is protective for genotype-positive family members of arrhythmogenic right ventricular cardiomyopathy patients. Europace. 2020; 22:1270–8.

66. James CA, Bhonsale A, Tichnell C, *et al*. Exercise increases age-related penetrance and arrhythmic risk in arrhythmogenic right ventricular dysplasia/cardiomyopathy-associated desmosomal mutation carriers. J Am Coll Cardiol. 2013; 62:1290–7.

67. Groeneweg JA, Bhonsale A, James, CA, *et al*. Clinical presentation, long-term follow-up, and outcomes of 1001 arrhythmogenic right ventricular dysplasia/cardiomyopathy patients and family members. Circ Cardiovasc Genet. 2015; 8:437–46.

68. Bhonsale A, Groeneweg JA, James CA, *et al*. Impact of genotype on clinical course in arrhythmogenic right ventricular dysplasia/cardiomyopathy-associated mutation carriers. Eur Heart J. 2015; 36:847–55.

69. Sen-Chowdhry S, Syrris P, Ward D, Asimaki A, Sevdalis E, McKenna WJ. Clinical and genetic characterization of families with arrhythmogenic right ventricular dysplasia/cardiomyopathy provides novel insights into patterns of disease expression. Circulation. 2007; 115:1710–20.

70. Bauce B, Nava A, Beffagna G, *et al*. Multiple mutations in desmosomal proteins encoding genes in arrhythmogenic right ventricular cardiomyopathy/dysplasia. Heart Rhythm. 2010; 7:22–9.

71. Vischer AS, Castelletti S, Syrris P, McKenna WJ, Pantazis A. Heart failure in patients with arrhythmogenic right ventricular cardiomyopathy: genetic characteristics. Int J Cardiol. 2019; 286:99–103.

72. Tedford RJ, James C, Judge DP, *et al*. Cardiac transplantation in arrhythmogenic right ventricular dysplasia/cardiomyopathy. J Am Coll Cardiol. 2012; 59:289–90.

73. Gilljam T, Haugaa KH, Jensen HK, *et al*. Heart transplantation in arrhythmogenic right ventricular cardiomyopathy: experience from the Nordic ARVC Registry. Int J Cardiol. 2018; 250:201–6.

74. DePasquale EC, Cheng RK, Deng MC, *et al*. Survival after heart transplantation in patients with arrhythmogenic right ventricular cardiomyopathy. J Card Fail. 2017; 23:107–12.

75. Basso C, Ronco F, Marcus F, *et al*. Quantitative assessment of endomyocardial biopsy in arrhythmogenic right ventricular cardiomyopathy/dysplasia: an *in vitro* validation of diagnostic criteria. Eur Heart J. 2008; 29:2760–71.

76. Sen-Chowdhry S, Syrris P, Prasad SK, *et al*. Left-dominant arrhythmogenic cardiomyopathy: an under-recognized clinical entity. J Am Coll Cardiol. 2008; 52:2175–87.

77. Perazzolo Marra M, Leoni L, Bauce B, *et al*. Imaging study of ventricular scar in arrhythmogenic right ventricular cardiomyopathy: comparison of 3D standard electroanatomical voltage mapping and contrast-enhanced cardiac magnetic resonance. Circ Arrhythm Electrophysiol. 2012; 5:91–100.

78. Corrado D, Basso C, Leoni L, *et al*. Three-dimensional electroanatomic voltage mapping increases accuracy of diagnosing arrhythmogenic right ventricular cardiomyopathy/dysplasia. Circulation. 2005; 111:3042–50.

79. Corrado D, Basso C, Leoni L, *et al*. Three-dimensional electroanatomical voltage mapping and histologic evaluation of myocardial substrate in right ventricular outflow tract tachycardia. J Am Coll Cardiol. 2008; 51:731–9.

80. Migliore F, Zorzi A, Silvano M, *et al*. Prognostic value of endocardial voltage mapping in patients with arrhythmogenic right ventricular cardiomyopathy/dysplasia. Circ Arrhythm Electrophysiol. 2013; 6:167–76.

81. La Gerche A, Burns AT, Mooney DJ, *et al*. Exercise-induced right ventricular dysfunction and structural remodelling in endurance athletes. Eur Heart J. 2012; 33:998–1006.

82. Zaidi A, Sheikh N, Jongman JK, *et al*. Clinical differentiation between physiological remodeling and arrhythmogenic right ventricular cardiomyopathy in athletes with marked electrocardiographic repolarization anomalies. J Am Coll Cardiol. 2015; 65:2702–11.

83. Ruwald AC, Marcus F, Estes NA 3rd, *et al*. Association of competitive and recreational sport participation with cardiac events in patients with arrhythmogenic right ventricular cardiomyopathy: results from the North American multidisciplinary study of arrhythmogenic right ventricular cardiomyopathy. Eur Heart J. 2015; 36:1735–43.

84. Bauce B, Daliento L, Frigo G, Russo G, Nava A. Pregnancy in women with arrhythmogenic right ventricular cardiomyopathy/dysplasia. Eur J Obstet Gynecol Reprod Biol. 2006; 127:186–9.

85. Wichter T, Paul TM, Eckardt L, *et al*. Arrhythmogenic right ventricular cardiomyopathy. Antiarrhythmic drugs, catheter ablation, or ICD? Herz. 2005; 30:91–101.

86. Marcus GM, Glidden DV, Polonsky B, *et al*.; Multidisciplinary Study of Right Ventricular Dysplasia Investigators. Efficacy of antiarrhythmic drugs in arrhythmogenic right ventricular cardiomyopathy: a report from the North American ARVC Registry. J Am Coll Cardiol. 2009; 54:609–15.

87. Rigato I, Corrado D, Basso C, *et al*. Pharmacotherapy and other therapeutic modalities for managing arrhythmogenic right ventricular cardiomyopathy. Cardiovasc Drugs Ther. 2015; 29:171–7.

88. Corrado D, Wichter T, Link MS, *et al*. Treatment of arrhythmogenic right ventricular cardiomyopathy/dysplasia: an International Task Force consensus statement. Circulation. 2015; 132:441–53.

89. Dalal D, Jain R, Tandri H, *et al.* Longterm efficacy of catheter ablation of ventricular tachycardia in patients with arrhythmogenic right ventricular dysplasia/cardiomyopathy. J Am Coll Cardiol. 2007; 50:432–40.

90. Garcia FC, Bazan V, Zado ES, Ren JF, Marchlinski FE. Epicardial substrate and outcome with epicardial ablation of ventricular tachycardia in arrhythmogenic right ventricular cardiomyopathy/dysplasia. Circulation. 2009; 120:366–75.

91. Corrado D, Leoni L, Link MS, *et al.* Implantable cardioverter–defibrillator therapy for prevention of sudden death in patients with arrhythmogenic right ventricular cardiomyopathy/dysplasia. Circulation. 2003; 108:3084–91.

92. Corrado D, Calkins H, Link MS, *et al.* Prophylactic implantable defibrillator in patients with arrhythmogenic right ventricular cardiomyopathy/dysplasia and no prior ventricular fibrillation or sustained ventricular tachycardia. Circulation. 2010; 122:1144–52.

93. Bhonsale A, James CA, Tichnell C, *et al.* Incidence and predictors of implantable cardioverter–defibrillator therapy in patients with arrhythmogenic right ventricular dysplasia/cardiomyopathy undergoing implantable cardioverter–defibrillator implantation for primary prevention. J Am Coll Cardiol. 2011; 58:1485–96.

94. Orgeron GM, Te Riele A, Tichnell C, *et al.* Performance of the 2015 International Task Force consensus statement risk stratification algorithm for implantable cardioverter–defibrillator placement in arrhythmogenic right ventricular dysplasia/cardiomyopathy. Circ Arrhythm Electrophysiol. 2018;11:e005593.

95. Migliore F, Viani S, Bongiorni MG, *et al.* Subcutaneous implantable cardioverter defibrillator in patients with arrhythmogenic right ventricular cardiomyopathy: results from an Italian multicenter registry. Int J Cardiol. 2019;280:74–9.

96. Orgeron GM, Bhonsale A, Migliore F, *et al.* Subcutaneous implantable cardioverter–defibrillator in patients with arrhythmogenic right ventricular cardiomyopathy/dysplasia: a transatlantic experience. J Am Heart Assoc. 2018;7:e008782.

97. Cadrin-Tourigny J, Bosman LP, Nozza A, *et al.* A new prediction model for ventricular arrhythmias in arrhythmogenic right ventricular cardiomyopathy. Eur Heart J. 2019; 40:1850–8.

98. Cadrin-Tourigny J, Bosman LP, Wang W, *et al.* Sudden cardiac death prediction in arrhythmogenic right ventricular cardiomyopathy: a multinational collaboration. Circ Arrhythm Electrophysiol. 2021; 14:e008509.

99. Fabritz L, Hoogendijk MG, Scicluna BP, *et al.* Load-reducing therapy prevents development of arrhythmogenic right ventricular cardiomyopathy in plakoglobin-deficient mice. J Am Coll Cardiol. 2011; 57:740–50.

3.4.6 Peripartum cardiomyopathy

Karen Sliwa and Johann Bauersachs

What is PPCM and how does it present?

Peripartum cardiomyopathy (PPCM) is a life-threatening cardiomyopathy characterized by acute or slowly progressing left ventricular (LV) dysfunction—late in pregnancy, during delivery, or in the first post-partum months—in women with no previously known heart disease.[1,2] Recent publications have shown that PPCM occurs globally in all ethnic groups.[3] Women often present with non-specific symptoms of heart failure during or after pregnancy to medical professionals from various disciplines.

Distinguishing signs and symptoms of PPCM from the spectrum of normal pregnancy can be challenging, but a low threshold of suspicion of heart failure is crucial in women with suggestive clinical features. Shortness of breath, fatigue, and mild ankle swelling are less specific symptoms of heart failure during pregnancy, whereas orthopnoea and paroxysmal nocturnal dyspnoea are more specific. The majority of women with PPCM present with severe symptoms (New York Heart Association class III or IV).[4] PPCM is a diagnosis of exclusion and, as such, a detailed medical history, in addition to exploration of symptoms, is essential to identify other factors that could cause dilated cardiomyopathy. These include, but are not limited to, viruses, alcohol, and medication (particularly cardiotoxic chemotherapy).

How should one investigate?

Any woman with signs or symptoms suggestive of PPCM should undergo urgent cardiac investigation, with prompt referral to a specialist when indicated by an abnormal test result. Once a diagnosis of PPCM is reached, additional tests can be considered to allow more sophisticated phenotyping and prognostication.

Electrocardiography (ECG) is a widely available, cheap, and powerful diagnostic tool in heart failure. It should form the basis of clinical workup in all women with a potential cardiac-related complaint and, in particular, those with suspected PPCM. To a varying degree, the ECG is abnormal in the vast majority of women with PPCM at the time of diagnosis. In a prospective study of women with PPCM in South Africa, 96% had at least one ECG abnormality and 49% had a significant ECG abnormality (e.g. Q-wave abnormality, ST-segment depression, T-wave inversion, bundle branch block, second- or third-degree atrioventricular block, frequent ectopy, brady- or tachyarrhythmia.[5]

Chest X-rays are helpful in identifying alternative causes for breathlessness or hypoxia, such as infection, effusion, or pneumothorax, but can be normal in PPCM. When positive findings do exist, they include cardiomegaly and/or features of pulmonary congestion.

After ECG, echocardiography is the main diagnostic modality used to confirm the presence of cardiac dysfunction in PPCM and quantify its severity. Importantly, it also excludes alternative causes of heart failure such as primary valvular disease, a number of inherited or acquired cardiomyopathies, and congenital heart disease. In patients with PPCM, LV end-diastolic and end-systolic volumes are commonly pathologically enlarged. The mean left ventricular ejection fraction (LVEF) at the time of diagnosis in a global study on PPCM was around 30% in all ethnic groups.[3] Coexisting functional mitral regurgitation and right ventricular dysfunction are common. A comprehensive assessment of the right heart is important if advanced heart failure therapies are likely to be required. Furthermore, reduced baseline right ventricular function has also been shown to be an independent predictor of a worse outcome.[6,7]

In addition to assessing cardiac structure and function, echocardiography is an important tool in the identification of heart failure sequelae such as intracardiac thrombi. Access to cardiac magnetic resonance imaging (MRI) is often prohibited by cost and geographical location, and thus it is not widely used in the diagnosis of PPCM. Cardiac MRI can be useful to exclude other aetiologies, such as ischaemic cardiomyopathy or infiltrative diseases, and to supplement information provided by echocardiography.

As with heart failure due to other causes, routine haematological and biochemical testing can provide information on potentially reversible contributory factors, such as clinically significant anaemia, and help to establish the presence of end-organ damage. Natriuretic peptide levels (where available) should be measured in women with suspected PPCM.

There appears to be a genetic overlap between inherited dilated cardiomyopathy and PPCM. Approximately 1 in 7 women with PPCM will have a truncating gene variant, the majority of which will be in the titin (*TTN*) gene. It is unknown whether this represents the same disease, or rather a genetic predisposition to PPCM. The presence of a *TTN* variant is not associated with more severe cardiac dysfunction at the time of diagnosis but is associated with a lower chance of LV improvement and lower LVEF at 1 year. In health-care systems which offer it, genetic testing should be considered in all cases of PPCM to facilitate family screening.

How to risk-stratify a woman with newly diagnosed peripartum cardiomyopathy

As soon as PPCM is suspected, risk stratification should be performed immediately to assess the risk of major complications and identify the appropriate level of care. Risk stratification should gather and integrate several different parameters, as outlined in ➲ Table 3.4.6.1.

The strongest parameters in identifying patients at risk of complications are non-Caucasian race, ECG QT-interval prolongation, LVEF <30% and LV end-diastolic parameter of >60 mm at the time of disease diagnosis, the degree of alteration of LVEF after treatment, biventricular dysfunction, and delay of diagnosis. Other parameters, including older age, antepartum diagnosis, haemodynamic parameters at presentation, and cardiac biomarkers, may help refine the risk stratification.[8] Patients with a history of a previous diagnosis of PPCM have a particularly high risk of poor outcome and careful history taking must always be part of the first assessment.[9] In all women with PPCM and a subsequent pregnancy, the key parameter is pre-pregnancy LVEF since the risk of deterioration, and even death, is significant in cases of persistent LV dysfunction before subsequent pregnancies. However, even patients with recovered LV function are still at risk of relapse.

PPCM is associated with significant morbidity and mortality. Most of the life-threatening complications, including severe heart failure, cardiogenic shock, arrhythmias, thromboembolic complications, and death, can be prevented with early aggressive treatment.[2]

How to manage a woman presenting with acute peripartum cardiomyopathy

Managing women presenting with severe forms of acute PPCM leading to cardiopulmonary instability is challenging. Practical

Table 3.4.6.1 Prognostic risk stratification in women presenting with peripartum cardiomyopathy

	Parameter	Reference
Medical history	Subsequent pregnancy	Elkayam et al.[44] Hilfiker-Kleiner et al.[45]
Patient characteristics	Non-Caucasian Age >35 years	McNamara et al.[35] Blauwet et al.[33]
Presentation	Delayed diagnosis >1 week after symptoms	Goland et al.[46]
Physical examination	SBP <110 mmHg HR >100 bpm NYHA classes III–IV	Libhaber et al.[39]
ECG	Sinus tachycardia Left atrial abnormality QRS >120 ms QTc >460 ms	Honigberg[47] Hoevelmann et al.[5]
Echocardiography	LVEF <30% LVEDD >60 mm Decreased RVEF	Goland et al.[48] Haghikia et al.[7] Blauwet et al.[6] Karaye[49]
MRI	LVEF <30% LV thrombus	Mouquet et al.[50]
Cardiac markers	NT-proBNP	Forster et al.[51]

ECG, echocardiogram; MRI, magnetic resonance imaging; SBP, systolic blood pressure; HR, heart rate; NYHA, New York Heart Association; LVEF, left ventricular ejection fraction; LVEDD, left ventricular end-diastolic diameter; RVEF, right ventricular ejection fraction; LV, left ventricular; NT-proBNP, N-terminal pro-B-type natriuretic peptide.

recommendations for acute treatment of PPCM causing acute heart failure (AHF) are based on recent data and clinical experience.[10,11,12]

Interdisciplinary approaches from cardiologists, intensivists, obstetricians, neonatologists, and anaesthetists are necessary to interact jointly in cases of acute PPCM. Most women admitted with acute PPCM present with symptoms and signs of AHF, related primarily to systemic congestion.

The initial evaluation of patients with suspected acute PPCM needs to include two components, which should be performed simultaneously, to allow timely diagnosis and treatment delivery: evaluation of the cardiopulmonary distress and confirmation of the diagnosis. Since PPCM is a diagnosis of exclusion, several additional tests should be performed. The differential diagnosis of acute PPCM includes myocarditis, pulmonary embolism, aggravation of pre-existing cardiomyopathy, valve disease, congenital heart disease, and amniotic liquid embolism, among others. The diagnostic process should not delay the start of treatment, which should commence as soon as AHF is suspected.

The presence of cardiopulmonary distress criteria should lead to intensive cardiac care unit admission: haemodynamic instability (systolic blood pressure <90 mmHg, heart rate >130 bpm or <45 bpm), respiratory distress (respiratory rate >25 breaths/min; peripheral oxygen saturation <90%) or signs of tissue hypoperfusion with abnormal cellular oxygen metabolism (increased blood lactate >2.0 mmol/L; altered mental state and oliguria <0.5 mL/kg/h).[13,14]

⟳ Figure 3.4.6.1A and B summarizes the recommended treatment algorithm for patients with acute PPCM. Women presenting with acute PPCM should benefit, as for other forms of AHF, from adequate non-invasive monitoring, oxygen supplementation in cases of hypoxia, or non-invasive ventilation (NIV) in cases of respiratory distress. The initial decongestive treatment depends on the time point of onset. For women presenting during pregnancy, joint cardiac and obstetric care and observance of the European Society of Cardiology (ESC) guidelines for the management of cardiovascular diseases in pregnancy are recommended.[15] Conversely, women presenting after delivery should be treated according to the ESC guidelines for heart failure.[16] Decongestive treatment should be tailored according to the haemodynamic profile and includes vasodilators (in the presence of systolic blood pressure >110 mmHg, more cautiously between 90 and 110 mmHg) and/or diuretics to reduce fluid overload. However, diuretics need to be administered with caution during pregnancy, as they may impair perfusion of the placenta and should be tapered, when possible, after stabilization. Use of inotropes should be restricted to patients in cardiogenic shock.

Patients with severe distress should be transferred early to an experienced centre whenever possible. For patients with persistent haemodynamic instability despite medical treatment, mechanical circulatory support should be considered, such as implantation of a temporary mechanical circulatory support system, either as 'bridge-to-recovery' if ventricular function improves during subsequent days and weaning can be achieved or

as 'bridge-to-bridge' if haemodynamic impairment persists and circulatory support has to be ensured by switching to a more durable device. Because of the higher proportion of patients with at least partial recovery of ventricular function, compared to other cardiomyopathies, an initial 'bridge-to-transplantation' strategy is seldom necessary. Cardiac transplantation is reserved for the minority of patients in whom ventricular recovery after 6–12 months is not sufficient, but it has to be considered that post-transplant outcomes in women with PPCM appear to be worse than in other recipients (i.e. higher mortality, higher incidence of rejection with shorter graft survival, and higher rates of retransplantation).[17]

The Impella® rotary pump is a percutaneous device for temporary support. It is inserted percutaneously from the femoral artery or operatively via the axillary/subclavian artery and placed in the left ventricle through the aortic valve. Depending on the model, it provides a substantially higher degree of haemodynamic support, compared to an intra-aortic balloon pump (IABP) (up to 5.5 L/min), but requires a stricter anticoagulation regime than an IABP and is associated with haemolysis.[18,19]

During pregnancy, angiotensin-converting enzyme (ACE) inhibitors and angiotensin receptor blockers (ARBs) are contraindicated because of fetal toxicity, and hydralazine and nitrates should be used instead. After delivery, ACE inhibitors should be started. Despite an increased risk of fetal growth restriction, beta-blockers are indicated in all stable patients with marked systolic dysfunction while pregnant and in all patients postpartum.[11] Mineralocorticoid receptor antagonists (MRAs) should be avoided during pregnancy and lactation, but should be started afterward in symptomatic women—especially in women with LVEF <35%. No data exist for the use of sacubitril/valsartan in women during pregnancy or breastfeeding.

Bromocriptine, a substance used for many years to stop lactation in post-partum women by suppressing prolactin production, was evaluated as adjunctive treatment of PPCM in a proof-of-concept, open-label clinical study[1] and a recent randomized study by comparing two different dose regimes of bromocriptine (2.5 mg daily for 1 week vs 5 mg daily for 2 weeks, followed by 2.5 mg daily for 6 weeks) in severe PPCM patients. The women included in this study displayed a high LV recovery rate at 6 months, indicating a beneficial association between use of bromocriptine in acute PPCM and clinical outcome. The improvement in LVEF was similar in the short-term (1 week) and long-term (8 weeks) bromocriptine groups, albeit a not statistically significant trend for more patients reaching full recovery at 6 months found in the long-term group. Based on these data, bromocriptine has been added as a therapy that may be considered in women with newly diagnosed PPCM.[15] Furthermore, bromocriptine-induced ablactation may have another beneficial effect of allowing the introduction of oral heart failure therapies without harming the newborn. Indeed, several drug classes (e.g. MRAs and sacubitril/valsartan) are contraindicated during lactation because of safety concerns. Bromocriptine treatment should always be accompanied by anticoagulation, with heparin at least at prophylactic dose, to reduce the thromboembolic risk.

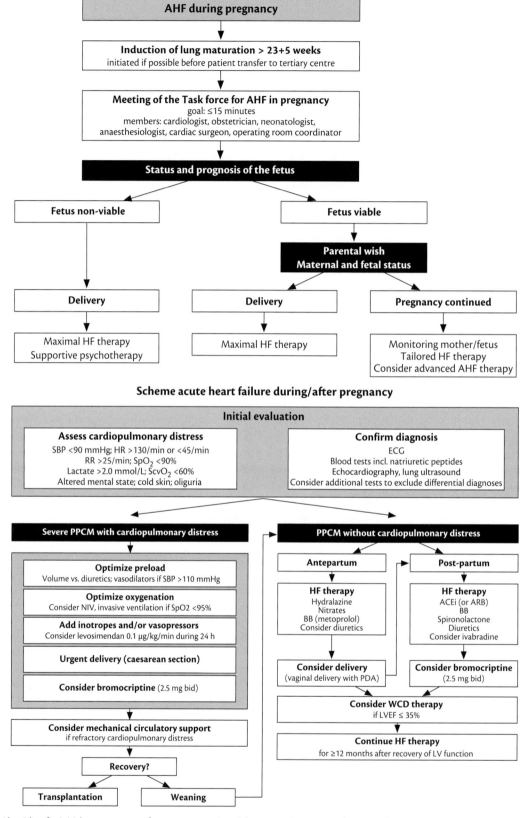

Figure 3.4.6.1 Algorithm for initial management of women presenting with acute peripartum cardiomyopathy. ACEi, angiotensin-converting enzyme inhibitor; ARB, angiotensin receptor blocker; BB, beta-blocker; ECG, electrocardiogram; HF, heart failure; HR, heart rate; LVEF, left ventricular ejection fraction; NIV, non-invasive ventilation; PDA, peridural anaesthesia; RR, respiratory rate; SBP, systolic blood pressure; SpO$_2$, peripheral oxygen saturation; WCD, wearable cardioverter–defibrillator.

Reproduced from Bauersachs J, Arrigo M, Hilfiker-Kleiner D, et al. Current management of patients with severe acute peripartum cardiomyopathy: practical guidance from the Heart Failure Association of the European Society of Cardiology Study Group on peripartum cardiomyopathy. *Eur J Heart Fail*. 2016 Sep;18(9):1096–105. doi: 10.1002/ejhf.586 with permission from John Wiley and Sons.

In summary, recently, a therapeutic algorithm has been proposed to regroup all essential and concomitant therapies under the BOARD acronym: *B*romocriptine, *O*ral heart failure therapies, *A*nticoagulants, vaso*R*elaxing agents, and *D*iuretics (➲ Figure 3.4.6.2).[21]

ACE inhibitors, beta-blockers, and MRAs should probably be given in guideline-based dosages and not discontinued during the first year after complete recovery of LV function. Earlier, stepwise discontinuation of heart failure therapy might be considered if both complete recovery of ventricular function and normal exercise response are achieved. Since relapses have been observed after recovery, tapering of disease-modifying heart failure drugs should be performed under close observation of LV function.[22] Joint cardiologic and obstetric management, including counselling on the potential risk of PPCM recurrence in future pregnancies, is recommended.

What is known of the short- and longer-term prognosis?

Although the prognosis of PPCM patients is more favourable, compared to that of patients with other cardiomyopathies (e.g. familial dilated cardiomyopathy), outcomes (particularly recovery of LV function and mortality) significantly differ globally (➲ Figure 3.4.6.3).[2,9] Patients with African and African-American backgrounds are at higher risk of developing PPCM. Until recently, it was thought that women of African ethnicity always experience worse outcomes.[23,24,25] However, recently published data from the global European Society of Cardiology EuroObservational research programme demonstrated a worse outcome in women from the Middle East (compared to African patients) who were entered into this study that included >700 women with newly diagnosed PPCM.[3] Currently, it is unknown whether different genetic backgrounds play a key role in defining prognosis or whether the main determinants are also influenced by access to health-care systems and heart failure therapy.

Many studies have focused on the assessment of LV function at 6 months' follow-up. Full recovery (mostly defined as LVEF >50–55%) ranges widely, depending on racial background and geographical region. Data from China, Japan, Turkey, the United States, and Germany demonstrate recovery rates of between 44% and 63% after 6 months.[9,26,27,28,29,30] Women in Pakistan, the Philippines, Nigeria, and South Africa display a lower chance of full recovery rates, ranging from 21% to 36%.[9,31,32,33,34]

Prospective studies and registries that included patients with a follow-up of ≥12 months demonstrated relatively high rates of LV recovery in PPCM patients. The multicentre Investigations of Pregnancy-Associated Cardiomyopathy (IPAC) study analysed 100 American women with PPCM.[35] LV recovery was observed in 72% of women after 12 months. In a Turkish study, LV recovery was present in 44% of women.[28] It is of note that >50% of patients who recovered did so beyond 12 months after initial diagnosis.

Only very few prospective data have reported on the long-term follow-up of PPCM patients beyond 5 years after initial diagnosis. A German study prospectively investigated outcome of 67 patients, with a mean follow-up of 63 ± 11 months.[36] The LV function improved from 26% at initial diagnosis to 50% after 12

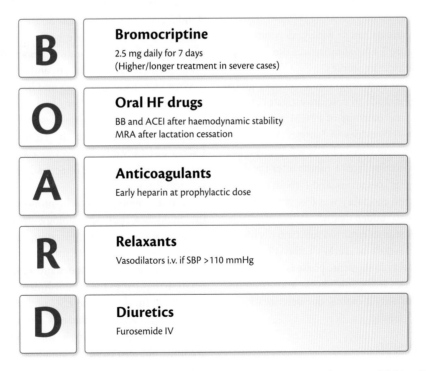

Figure 3.4.6.2 BOARD algorithm for treatment of peripartum cardiomyopathy. ACEI, angiotensin-converting enzyme inhibitor; BB, beta-blocker; IV, intravenous; MRA, mineralocorticoid receptor antagonist; SBP, systolic blood pressure.

Reproduced from Karen Sliwa, Johann Bauersachs, Zolt Arany, *et al.* Peripartum cardiomyopathy: from genetics to management, *European Heart Journal*, Volume 42, Issue 32, 21 August 2021, Pages 3094–3102, https://doi.org/10.1093/eurheartj/ehab458 with permission from Oxford University Press.

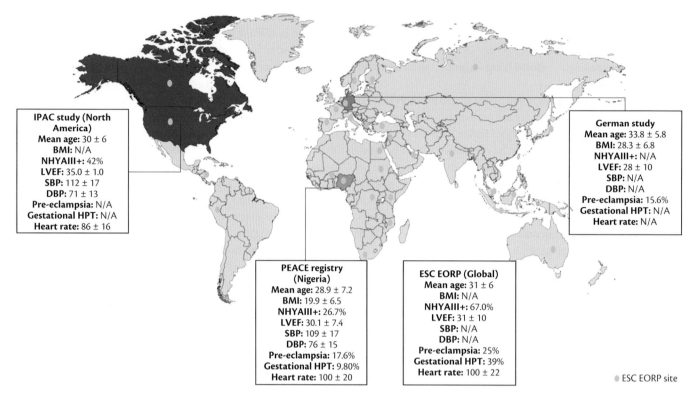

IPAC study (North America)
Mean age: 30 ± 6
BMI: N/A
NHYAIII+: 42%
LVEF: 35.0 ± 1.0
SBP: 112 ± 17
DBP: 71 ± 13
Pre-eclampsia: N/A
Gestational HPT: N/A
Heart rate: 86 ± 16

German study
Mean age: 33.8 ± 5.8
BMI: 28.3 ± 6.8
NHYAIII+: N/A
LVEF: 28 ± 10
SBP: N/A
DBP: N/A
Pre-eclampsia: 15.6%
Gestational HPT: N/A
Heart rate: N/A

PEACE registry (Nigeria)
Mean age: 28.9 ± 7.2
BMI: 19.9 ± 6.5
NHYAIII+: 26.7%
LVEF: 30.1 ± 7.4
SBP: 109 ± 17
DBP: 76 ± 15
Pre-eclampsia: 17.6%
Gestational HPT: 9.80%
Heart rate: 100 ± 20

ESC EORP (Global)
Mean age: 31 ± 6
BMI: N/A
NHYAIII+: 67.0%
LVEF: 31 ± 10
SBP: N/A
DBP: N/A
Pre-eclampsia: 25%
Gestational HPT: 39%
Heart rate: 100 ± 22

● ESC EORP site

Figure 3.4.6.3 Comparison of clinical presentation and outcome of multicentre PPCM studies.

months, and 54% after 5 years. The number of patients experiencing full recovery was 48% after 6 months, further rising to 60% and 72% after 1 and 5 years, respectively.

Mortality

Mortality rates of PPCM patients range widely, depending on geographical regions. ⮞ Figure 3.4.6.2 summarizes the mortality rates from several recent multicentre studies.

The EURObservational Research Programme (EORP) global registry on PPCM, the largest study to date, investigates clinical presentation, management, and outcome of PPCM patients.[14] A total of 743 patients from >40 countries in Europe, Africa, Asia Pacific, and the Middle East were enrolled over a 6-year period. Initial results showed low mortality rates 1 month after the diagnosis (2.4% overall, 3.4% in ESC countries, and 1.4% in non-ESC countries).[4] However, 6-month mortality was 6%, with 42% due to heart failure and 30% due to sudden death.[3]

Mortality rates from other studies reported substantially higher mortality ranges, such as 15–30% in Turkey[37] and 12–28% in South Africa.[38,39] Early mortality in the acute phase is often due to AHF, malignant arrhythmias, cardiogenic shock, and thromboembolic events.[11,40] Later mortality is mainly due deterioration of LV function leading to heart failure.

Summary and conclusion

PPCM is a global disease that is often not diagnosed timely, leading to significant morbidity and mortality. It is an important contributor to early (<42 days) and late (up to 1 year) post-partum maternal death. The reported 1-year mortality ranges from 5% to 25%.

In the last two decades, remarkable advances in the understanding of the pathogenesis and improvement in patient management and therapy have been achieved, largely due to team efforts and close collaboration among basic scientists, cardiologists, intensive care specialists, and obstetricians.

With increasing awareness and better diagnostic tools, the disease has moved from a 'rare' to a 'relatively frequent' pregnancy complication, thereby raising research interest in this field.

Under the umbrella of the Heart Failure Association of the ESC, a PPCM Study Group was established in 2009, which has led to several research projects advancing the knowledge about this condition.[41]

Despite ongoing research, numerous uncertainties regarding the incidence, pathophysiology, treatment, and prognosis of PPCM patients persist, indicating the need for further investigation. The need to create more awareness about this condition globally, as well as to understand differences in mode and presentation, has led to the establishment of an international registry on PPCM, funded by the ESC under the umbrella of the *EORP*, which recruited >700 patients from >40 countries. Follow-up concluded in 2021. Many lessons will be learnt from this programme, but also from the multicentre Nigerian PEACE PPCM registry[42] and the large clinical service dedicated to women with PPCM in Iraq.[43]

Key messages

- PPCM is a global disease with substantial morbidity and mortality.
- Women with PPCM have a risk of dying due to heart failure and sudden cardiac death.
- Family screening for familial cardiomyopathy and genetic testing could be considered, as 1 in 7 patients with PPCM have a significant variant.

References

1. Sliwa K, Blauwet L, Tibazarwa K, *et al.* Evaluation of bromocriptine in the treatment of acute severe peripartum cardiomyopathy: a proof-of-concept pilot study. Circulation 2010;121:1465–73.

2. Bauersachs J, Konig T, van der Meer P, *et al.* Pathophysiology, diagnosis and management of peripartum cardiomyopathy: a position statement from the Heart Failure Association of the European Society of Cardiology Study Group on peripartum cardiomyopathy. Eur J Heart Fail. 2019;21:827–43.

3. Sliwa K, Petrie MC, van der Meer P, *et al.* Clinical presentation, management, and 6-month outcomes in women with peripartum cardiomyopathy: an ESC EORP registry. Eur Heart J 2020;41:3787–97.

4. Sliwa K, Mebazaa A, Hilfiker-Kleiner D, *et al.* Clinical characteristics of patients from the worldwide registry on peripartum cardiomyopathy (PPCM): EURObservational Research Programme in conjunction with the Heart Failure Association of the European Society of Cardiology Study Group on PPCM. Eur J Heart Fail. 2017;19:1131–41.

5. Hoevelmann J, Viljoen CA, Manning K, *et al.* The prognostic significance of the 12-lead ECG in peripartum cardiomyopathy. Int J Cardiol. 2019;276:177–84.

6. Blauwet LA, Delgado-Montero A, Ryo K, *et al.*; IPAC Investigators. Right ventricular function in peripartum cardiomyopathy at presentation is associated with subsequent left ventricular recovery and clinical outcomes. Circ Heart Fail. 2016;9:e002756.

7. Haghikia A, Rontgen P, Vogel-Claussen J, *et al.* Prognostic implication of right ventricular involvement in peripartum cardiomyopathy: a cardiovascular magnetic resonance study. ESC Heart Fail. 2015;2:139–49.

8. Goland S, Mouquet F. Risk stratification in patients with newly diagnosed PPCM. In: Sliwa K, ed. *Peripartum Cardiomyopathy: From Pathophysiology to Management.* New York, NY: Elsevier; 2021, in press.

9. Sliwa K, Petrie MC, Hilfiker-Kleiner D, *et al.* Long-term prognosis, subsequent pregnancy, contraception and overall management of peripartum cardiomyopathy: practical guidance paper from the Heart Failure Association of the European Society of Cardiology Study Group on Peripartum Cardiomyopathy. Eur J Heart Fail. 2018;20:951–62.

10. Arrigo M, Mebazaa A. How to manage a woman presenting with acute PPCM? In: Sliwa K, ed. *Peripartum Cardiomyopathy: From Pathophysiology to Management.* New York, NY: Elsevier; 2021, in press.

11. Bauersachs J, Arrigo M, Hilfiker-Kleiner D, *et al.* Current management of patients with severe acute peripartum cardiomyopathy: practical guidance from the Heart Failure Association of the European Society of Cardiology Study Group on peripartum cardiomyopathy. Eur J Heart Fail. 2016;18:1096–105.

12. Mebazaa A, Yilmaz MB, Levy P, *et al.* Recommendations on prehospital and early hospital management of acute heart failure: a consensus paper from the Heart Failure Association of the European Society of Cardiology, the European Society of Emergency Medicine and the Society of Academic Emergency Medicine. Eur J Heart Fail. 2015;17:544–58.

13. Mebazaa A, Tolppanen H, Mueller C, *et al.* Acute heart failure and cardiogenic shock: a multidisciplinary practical guidance. Intensive Care Med. 2016;42:147–63.

14. Sliwa K, Hilfiker-Kleiner D, Mebazaa A, *et al.* EURObservational Research Programme: a worldwide registry on peripartum cardiomyopathy (PPCM) in conjunction with the Heart Failure Association of the European Society of Cardiology Working Group on PPCM. Eur J Heart Fail. 2014;16:583–91.

15. Regitz-Zagrosek V, Roos-Hesselink JW, Bauersachs J, *et al.*; ESC Scientific Document Group. 2018 ESC Guidelines for the management of cardiovascular diseases during pregnancy. Eur Heart J. 2018;39:3165–241.

16. McDonagh TA, Metra M, Adamo M, *et al.*; ESC Scientific Document Group. 2021 ESC Guidelines for the diagnosis and treatment of acute and chronic heart failure. Eur Heart J. 2021;42:3599–726.

17. Rasmusson K, Brunisholz K, Budge D, *et al.* Peripartum cardiomyopathy: post-transplant outcomes from the United Network for Organ Sharing Database. J Heart Lung Transplant. 2012;31:180–6.

18. Schroeter MR, Unsold B, Holke K, Schillinger W. Pro-thrombotic condition in a woman with peripartum cardiomyopathy treated with bromocriptine and an Impella LP 2.5 heart pump. Clin Res Cardiol. 2013;102:155–7.

19. Sieweke JT, Pfeffer TJ, Berliner D, *et al.* Cardiogenic shock complicating peripartum cardiomyopathy: importance of early left ventricular unloading and bromocriptine therapy. Eur Heart J Acute Cardiovasc Care 2020;9:173–82.

20. Hilfiker-Kleiner D, Haghikia A, Berliner D, *et al.* Bromocriptine for the treatment of peripartum cardiomyopathy: a multicentre randomized study. Eur Heart J. 2017;38:2671–9.

21. Arrigo M, Blet A, Mebazaa A. Bromocriptine for the treatment of peripartum cardiomyopathy: welcome on BOARD. Eur Heart J. 2017;38:2680–2.

22. Hilfiker-Kleiner D, Haghikia A, Nonhoff J, Bauersachs J. Peripartum cardiomyopathy: current management and future perspectives. Eur Heart J. 2015;36:1090–7.

23. Kao DP, Hsich E, Lindenfeld J. Characteristics, adverse events, and racial differences among delivering mothers with peripartum cardiomyopathy. JACC Heart Fail. 2013;1:409–16.

24. Irizarry OC, Levine LD, Lewey J, *et al.* Comparison of clinical characteristics and outcomes of peripartum cardiomyopathy between African American and Non-African American women. JAMA Cardiol. 2017;2:1256–60.

25. Bauersachs J. Poor outcomes in poor patients?: peripartum cardiomyopathy—not just black and white. JAMA Cardiol. 2017;2:1261–2.

26. Hu CL, Li YB, Zou YG, *et al.* Troponin T measurement can predict persistent left ventricular dysfunction in peripartum cardiomyopathy. Heart 2007;93:488–90.

27. Kamiya CA, Kitakaze M, Ishibashi-Ueda H, *et al.* Different characteristics of peripartum cardiomyopathy between patients complicated with and without hypertensive disorders. Results from the Japanese Nationwide survey of peripartum cardiomyopathy. Circ J. 2011;75:1975–81.

28. Biteker M, Ilhan E, Biteker G, Duman D, Bozkurt B. Delayed recovery in peripartum cardiomyopathy: an indication for long-term follow-up and sustained therapy. Eur J Heart Fail. 2012;14:895–901.

29. Cooper LT, Mather PJ, Alexis JD, *et al.* Myocardial recovery in peripartum cardiomyopathy: prospective comparison with recent

onset cardiomyopathy in men and nonperipartum women. J Card Fail. 2012;18:28–33.

30. Duncker D, Haghikia A, Konig T, et al. Risk for ventricular fibrillation in peripartum cardiomyopathy with severely reduced left ventricular function-value of the wearable cardioverter/defibrillator. Eur J Heart Fail. 2014;16:1331–6.

31. Sharieff S, Zaman K. Prognostic factors at initial presentation in patients with peripartum cardiomyopathy. J Pak Med Assoc. 2003;53:297–300.

32. Sliwa K, Forster O, Libhaber E, et al. Peripartum cardiomyopathy: inflammatory markers as predictors of outcome in 100 prospectively studied patients. Eur Heart J. 2006;27:441–6.

33. Blauwet LA, Libhaber E, Forster O, et al. Predictors of outcome in 176 South African patients with peripartum cardiomyopathy. Heart. 2013;99:308–13.

34. Cuenza LR, Manapat N, Jalique JR. Clinical profile and predictors of outcomes of patients with peripartum cardiomyopathy: The Philippine Heart Center Experience. ASEAN Heart J. 2016;24:9.

35. McNamara DM, Elkayam U, Alharethi R, et al.; IPAC Investigators. Clinical outcomes for peripartum cardiomyopathy in North America: results of the IPAC Study (Investigations of Pregnancy-Associated Cardiomyopathy). J Am Coll Cardiol. 2015;66:905–14.

36. Moulig V, Pfeffer TJ, Ricke-Hoch M, et al. Long-term follow-up in peripartum cardiomyopathy patients with contemporary treatment: low mortality, high cardiac recovery, but significant cardiovascular co-morbidities. Eur J Heart Fail. 2019;21:1534–42.

37. Duran N, Gunes H, Duran I, Biteker M, Ozkan M. Predictors of prognosis in patients with peripartum cardiomyopathy. Int J Gynaecol Obstet. 2008;101:137–40.

38. Sliwa K, Forster O, Tibazarwa K, et al. Long-term outcome of peripartum cardiomyopathy in a population with high seropositivity for human immunodeficiency virus. Int J Cardiol. 2011;147:202–8.

39. Libhaber E, Sliwa K, Bachelier K, Lamont K, Bohm M. Low systolic blood pressure and high resting heart rate as predictors of outcome in patients with peripartum cardiomyopathy. Int J Cardiol. 2015;190:376–82.

40. Duncker D, Westenfeld R, Konrad T, et al. Risk for life-threatening arrhythmia in newly diagnosed peripartum cardiomyopathy with low ejection fraction: a German multi-centre analysis. Clin Res Cardiol. 2017;106:582–9.

41. Sliwa K, Bauersachs J, Coats AJS. The European Society of Cardiology Heart Failure Association Study Group on Peripartum Cardiomyopathy: what has been achieved in 10 years. Eur J Heart Fail. 2020;22:1060–4.

42. Karaye KM, Sa'idu H, Balarabe SA, et al.; Peace Registry Investigators. Clinical features and outcomes of peripartum cardiomyopathy in Nigeria. J Am Coll Cardiol. 2020;76:2352–64.

43. Al Farhan A, Yaseen I. Setting up a clinical service for PPCM in Iraq. In: Sliwa K, ed. Peripartum Cardiomyopathy: From Pathophysiology to Management. New York, NY: Elsevier; 2021, pp. 91–124.

44. Elkayam U, Tummala PP, Rao K, et al. Maternal and fetal outcomes of subsequent pregnancies in women with peripartum cardiomyopathy. N Engl J Med. 2001;344:1567–71.

45. Hilfiker-Kleiner D, Haghikia A, Masuko D, et al. Outcome of subsequent pregnancies in patients with peripartum cardiomyopathy in relation to medical therapy. Eur J Heart Fail. 2017;19:1723–28.

46. Goland S, Modi K, Bitar F, et al. Clinical profile and predictors of complications in peripartum cardiomyopathy. J Card Fail. 2009;15:645–50.

47. Honigberg MC, Elkayam U, Rajagopalan N, et al.; IPAC Investigators. Electrocardiographic findings in peripartum cardiomyopathy. Clin Cardiol. 2019;42:524–9.

48. Goland S, Bitar F, Modi K, et al. Evaluation of the clinical relevance of baseline left ventricular ejection fraction as a predictor of recovery or persistence of severe dysfunction in women in the United States with peripartum cardiomyopathy. J Card Fail. 2011;17:426–30.

49. Karaye KM. Right ventricular systolic function in peripartum and dilated cardiomyopathies. Eur J Echocardiogr. 2011;12:372–4.

50. Mouquet F, Lions C, de Groote P, et al. Characterisation of peripartum cardiomyopathy by cardiac magnetic resonance imaging. Eur Radiol 2008;18:2765–9.

51. Forster O, Hilfiker-Kleiner D, Ansari AA, et al. Reversal of IFN-gamma, oxLDL and prolactin serum levels correlate with clinical improvement in patients with peripartum cardiomyopathy. Eur J Heart Fail. 2008;10:861–8.

3.4.7 Takotsubo syndrome

Jelena Templin-Ghadri, Michael Würdinger, Johann Bauersachs, and Christian Templin

Introduction

Takotsubo syndrome (TTS) was first described by Sato and colleagues in Japan in 1990. They reported a case series of women who presented with unusual left ventricular wall motion abnormalities after severe emotional stress. The morphological resemblance to a traditional octopus trap led them to the term 'takotsubo' syndrome.[1] Although TTS is increasingly recognized, the true prevalence of TTS might still be underestimated. Increasing research effort over the last years has contributed to a better understanding of TTS. It is no longer a disease of postmenopausal women with an emotional stressor, an apical ballooning pattern, and a benign prognosis.[2] TTS has a diverse clinical picture, with significant mortality and morbidity, comparable to that of acute myocardial infarction (AMI).[3,4] Therapeutic management of TTS is still challenging, and evidence-based treatment is entirely lacking.[5] Further research is needed to assess different treatment options in order to improve the outcome of TTS patients.

Nomenclature, definition, and classification of takotsubo syndrome

Nomenclature

TTS was often referred to as an apical ballooning syndrome or stress cardiomyopathy. Other less frequently used terms were broken heart syndrome and neurogenic stunned myocardium. Moreover, it was estimated that no less than 75 individual descriptive names have been used in the literature for this rather newly recognized disease.[6] The term 'takotsubo' was initially used in a Japanese case series in 1990 and was referring to a traditional Japanese fishing pot that resembles the characteristic wall motion abnormalities during systole.[1] TTS was incorporated into the American Heart Association's classification of cardiomyopathies as an acquired primary cardiomyopathy in 2006.[7] However, current pathophysiological understanding challenges this categorization. Therefore, and due to variable patterns of TTS, there recently has been a consensus to call this disease 'takotsubo syndrome' instead of the previous mentioned terms.[8]

Definition

TTS is defined as an acute, transient left ventricular dysfunction with distinct wall motion abnormalities that extend beyond the territory of a single coronary artery. These wall motion abnormalities appear in a typical circumferential pattern. Accountable stenoses of the coronary arteries and myocarditis must be ruled out for the diagnosis.[8] However, coincident coronary artery disease (CAD) can be found in a majority of the patients and does not rule out the diagnosis of TTS.[9]

Different diagnostic criteria have been established for TTS such as the InterTAK diagnostic criteria, established by an international expert consensus committee, that implement current concepts of TTS (➡ Table 3.4.7.1).[8]

Classification

TTS is classified into four types, depending on the region of wall motion abnormalities. The typical form of TTS is the apical type, which accounts for 82% of all cases. It presents with apical akinesis and basal hypercontractility. Atypical TTS forms include the mid-ventricular, basal, and focal types that are present in 15%, 2%, and 2% of cases, respectively.[3] In all TTS types, except the focal type, wall motion abnormalities extend beyond a single coronary artery vessel. Cardiac magnetic resonance imaging (CMRI) might be useful to distinguish the focal type from AMI.[10] ➡ Figure 3.4.7.1 shows the four different TTS types.[3]

Patients with atypical TTS types often present with different clinical characteristics: patients are younger; they more often have neurological comorbidities; left ventricular ejection fraction (LVEF) is less reduced; brain natriuretic peptide (BNP) levels are lower; and the electrocardiogram (ECG) shows more often ST-segment depression.[11]

In about one-third of cases, the right ventricle is also involved, which is a predictor of worse outcome.[12,13] Isolated right ventricular dysfunction has been reported as an extremely rare variant.[14]

Epidemiology

TTS is estimated to account for 1–3% of all patients who are admitted with suspected ST-segment elevation myocardial infarction (STEMI).[15,16] The proportion among female patients might be as high as 5–6%.[17] However, an underdiagnosis of TTS is likely. The incidence has increased by almost 20-fold between 2006 and 2012, presumably due to increased awareness of the condition.[18]

TTS has been reported worldwide and occurs in various ethnic groups.[3] Women are predominantly affected and account for approximately 90% of cases, with the majority of cases reported in postmenopausal women. However, any age group can be affected and TTS has been described even in children.[19,20]

Risk factors

It is obvious that individuals have different vulnerability to developing TTS in certain situations. A predilection of postmenopausal female patients[3] and familial cases[8] indicate an impact of female sex hormones and genetic factors.

In addition, patients frequently present with comorbidities that might act as risk factors for the development of TTS. Among the wide range of comorbidities reported, psychiatric and

Table 3.4.7.1 InterTAK Diagnostic Criteria

1	Patients show transient[a] left ventricular dysfunction (hypokinesia, akinesia, or dyskinesia) presenting as apical ballooning or mid-ventricular, basal, or focal wall motion abnormalities. Right ventricular involvement can be present. Besides these regional wall motion patterns, transitions between all types can exist. The regional wall motion abnormality usually extends beyond a single epicardial vascular distribution; however, rare cases can exist where the regional wall motion abnormality is present in the subtended myocardial territory of a single coronary artery (focal takotsubo syndrome)[b]
2	An emotional, physical, or combined trigger can precede the takotsubo syndrome event, but this is not obligatory
3	Neurological disorders (e.g. subarachnoid haemorrhage, stroke/transient ischaemic attack, or seizures), as well as phaeochromocytoma, may serve as triggers for takotsubo syndrome
4	New ECG abnormalities are present (ST-segment elevation, ST-segment depression, T-wave inversion, and QTc prolongation); however, rare cases exist without any ECG changes
5	Levels of cardiac biomarkers (troponin and creatine kinase) are moderately elevated in most cases; significant elevation in brain natriuretic peptide levels is common
6	Significant coronary artery disease is not a contradiction in takotsubo syndrome
7	Patients have no evidence of infectious myocarditis[b]
8	Postmenopausal women are predominantly affected

[a] Wall motion abnormalities may remain for a prolonged period of time, or documentation of recovery may not be possible, for example, death before evidence of recovery could be captured.
[b] Cardiac magnetic resonance imaging is recommended to exclude infectious myocarditis and confirm a diagnosis of takotsubo syndrome.

Reproduced from Ghadri JR, Wittstein IS, Prasad A, *et al*. International Expert Consensus Document on Takotsubo Syndrome (Part II): Diagnostic Workup, Outcome, and Management. *Eur Heart J*. 2018 Jun 7;39(22):2047–2062. doi: 10.1093/eurheartj/ehy077 with permission from Oxford University Press.

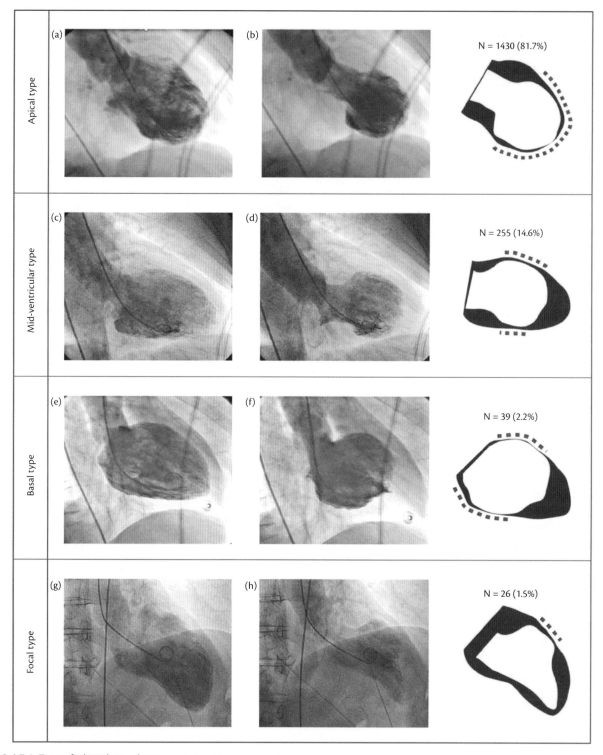

Figure 3.4.7.1 Types of takotsubo syndrome.
Reproduced from Templin C, Ghadri JR, Diekmann J, *et al*. Clinical Features and Outcomes of Takotsubo (Stress) Cardiomyopathy. *N Engl J Med*. 2015 Sep 3;373(10):929–38. doi: 10.1056/NEJMoa1406761 with permission from Massachusetts Medical Society.

neurological disorders are the most common. More than half of the patients in the InterTAK Registry have an acute, chronic, or previous neurological or psychiatric disorder.

There was a prevalence of 30% for chronic psychiatric disorders, particularly affective, anxiety, and adjustment disorders. The prevalence was significantly higher than in

age- and gender-matched patients with acute coronary syndrome (ACS).[3]

TTS has been reported in central neurological disorders such as stroke, subarachnoid haemorrhage, and seizures.[21] The insula and posterior fossa are mainly affected in patients with ischaemic stroke and epileptic events who develop TTS.[22] Furthermore, a heart–brain interaction in TTS is assumed, since substantial structural differences in the limbic network between TTS and healthy controls have been shown.[23]

Other frequently observed predisposing factors are chronic obstructive lung diseases and malignancy. Chronic pulmonary diseases have been found in 13–15% of patients, including chronic obstructive pulmonary disease, asthma, and pulmonary circulatory disorders.[20,24] The prevalence of malignancies in TTS was reported to be 17–30%.[25,26,27]

The exact pathophysiological implication of these predisposing comorbidities is not established. However, an increase in catecholamine levels and changes in the autonomic nervous system might be mechanisms leading to a higher susceptibility to TTS.

Traditional cardiovascular risk factors do not appear to play a role in the pathophysiology but are common in patients with TTS.[20] Interestingly, the reported prevalence of diabetes mellitus is lower than expected for an age-matched population. This fact has led to the hypothesis that diabetic autonomic neuropathy might have a protective effect against TTS.[28] However, supportive data are sparse and further studies are necessary to prove this hypothesis.

Trigger factors

A typical feature of TTS is the association with an emotional or a physical triggering event, which can be found in two-thirds of patients[3] and led to the terms 'broken heart syndrome' and 'stress cardiomyopathy'.[6,29]

Early reports highlighted, in particular, emotional triggers. However, an increasing number of physical triggers have also been described over the last years.[6] Data from the InterTAK Registry demonstrated a higher prevalence of physical triggers. Physical triggers were identified in 36%, and emotional triggers in 27.7%, of cases.[3] Physical triggers can be associated with every organ system and medical condition. Common physical triggers include central neurological disorders (e.g. stroke, seizure, subarachnoid hemorrhage), respiratory diseases (e.g. pneumonia, chronic obstructive lung disease exacerbation, pneumothorax), anaesthesia, and surgical procedures.[30] Physical triggers are an independent predictor of worse in-hospital outcome.[3]

Any kind of emotion can trigger TTS. Unlike previous assumptions, positive emotional triggers can also be found in TTS ('happy heart-syndrome').[29]

Emotional triggers appear to be more prevalent among women, whereas physical triggers are more frequent in men. Interestingly, in a third of TTS patients, no triggering factor was present.[31]

Pathophysiology

The pathophysiology of TTS is not yet completely understood. The sympathetic nervous system seems to play a central role in the pathophysiology, and TTS might be the result of a catecholamine surge in predisposed and susceptible individuals. Besides other preclinical and clinical hints for this pathomechanism, levels of plasma catecholamine are substantially elevated in TTS. Emotional and physical triggers are a frequent phenomenon and include medical conditions with elevated plasma catecholamine

levels such as phaeochromocytoma and subarachnoid haemorrhage. Furthermore, TTS has been reported as a complication of administered catecholamines or beta-receptor agonists. Typical histopathological findings are contraction band necroses, which previously were associated with conditions of catecholamine excess.[32] In addition, structural abnormalities of the autonomic nervous system have been found in TTS.[23]

Several pathomechanisms that might eventually lead to TTS have been proposed. However, none can explain the development of TTS on its own. Among these, most evidence has been found for microvascular dysfunction and a direct effect on cardiomyocytes.[32] Many findings indicate that microvascular dysfunction may play a major role in the pathophysiology of TTS. Reversible microvascular dysfunction has been found in several invasive and non-invasive imaging studies. Thrombolysis in Myocardial Infarction (TIMI) flow and TIMI myocardial perfusion grades were found to be impaired in TTS in the acute phase, with normalization during follow-up. Coronary flow reserve was found to be reduced both in invasive and non-invasive measurements. Myocardial contrast echocardiography showed impaired myocardial perfusion in areas with wall motion abnormalities, which improved during follow-up.[32] Besides these microvascular effects, catecholamine excess could cause cardiomyocyte toxicity through direct myocardial cell injury, either by cyclic adenosine monophosphate (cAMP)-mediated calcium overload of cells that produces a concentration-dependent decrease in cardiomyocyte viability, or by a switch from β2-adrenergic receptor Gs protein with a positive inotropic response to a β2-adrenergic receptor Gi protein with a negative inotropic response.[33] Other mechanisms that might be involved in TTS are reduced metabolism, myocardial oedema, and inflammation in areas of wall motion abnormalities.[32]

The lacking oestrogen-mediated downregulation of beta-receptors on cardiomyocytes may be a pathomechanism in postmenopausal patients. However, this cannot be an explanation for TTS in men and premenopausal women.[32]

Clinical presentation

Patients with TTS typically present with symptoms and signs of ACS. The most common symptoms are chest pain, shortness of breath, and syncope.[3]

Patients who develop TTS after a physical trigger (e.g. sepsis, respiratory failure, neurological injury) might lack typical symptoms, as manifestation of the underlying disease is predominant. In these situations, TTS is often detected by the presence of acute heart failure, elevated cardiac biomarker levels, abnormal ECG findings, or newly discovered cardiac dysfunction.[8]

A proportion of patients present with symptoms of complications of TTS such as acute heart failure with congestion, pulmonary oedema, or cardiogenic shock, cardiac arrest, or stroke.[3] About 10% of patients will present with haemodynamic instability requiring either mechanical or pharmacological circulatory support.[3,34] Cardiac arrest at presentation was reported in 4% of patients with TTS. Of these, 57% had ventricular fibrillation or tachycardia, and 43% had asystole or pulseless electrical activity (PEA).[35]

Diagnostic testing

Since the clinical presentation of TTS is comparable to that of ACS, the most important diagnostic step is to rule out myocardial infarction. Therefore, coronary angiography with ventriculography remains the diagnostic tool of choice at the early stage of diagnosis. In patients with ST-segment elevation or haemodynamic instability, emergency coronary angiography should be performed to rule out myocardial infarction and mechanical complications of TTS by invasive haemodynamic measurements. In the same step, typical wall motion abnormalities can be visualized by ventriculography. In stable patients without ST-segment elevation, the diagnostic approach depends on the pretest probability of TTS.[5] The pretest probability can be estimated by the InterTAK Diagnostic Score (available from: http://www.takotsubo-registry.com/takotsubo-score.html). A score ≤70 points hints to a low or intermediate likelihood, whereas a score >70 points hints to a high pretest probability (the cut-off of 70 points means a probability of 90% of TTS).[36] If the pretest probability is high, ruling out of coronary stenoses by coronary computed tomography, instead of using invasive diagnostics, might be justified, and typical wall motion abnormalities can be visualized by transthoracic echocardiography (TTE) in this situation. Since TTS is a diagnosis of exclusion, CMRI is recommended to rule out myocarditis, especially if there are red flags such as signs of viral infection, increased inflammation parameters, or pericardial effusion. ➔ Figure 3.4.7.2 provides an algorithm for the diagnosis of TTS.[5]

Electrocardiography

In most patients, ECG abnormalities are detectable at presentation. ST-segment elevation can be found in 44% of cases, T-wave inversions in 41%, and QT prolongation in 50%. Less typical are ST-segment depression (5%) and left bundle branch block (5%), and even normal ECGs without repolarization abnormalities can be found.[3] ST-segment elevation is more common in the lateral leads, and reciprocal ST-segment depression is less typical in TTS compared to STEMI.[37]

Dynamic repolarization changes over time are an important element of TTS. ST-segment elevation at presentation typically develops into deep, symmetrical T-wave inversion and QT interval prolongation within 24–48 hours. These ECG changes commonly persist for weeks to months and normalize along with wall motion abnormalities.[37]

Recently, ECG criteria have been proposed to differentiate TTS from ACS in patients with and those without ST-segment elevation. In the ST-segment elevation setting, ST-segment elevation in lead –aVR, combined with ST-segment elevation in the anteroseptal leads, was 100% specific for TTS, with a positive predictive value of 100%. In the non-ST-segment elevation setting, ST-segment elevation in lead –aVR, combined with T-wave inversion in any lead, was 100% specific for TTS, with a positive predictive value of 100%. However, sensitivity was very low in both cases.[38]

Cardiac biomarkers

Cardiac biomarker levels are elevated in about 90% of patients. However, peak troponin levels are lower than in AMI, and creatine kinase levels are often not, or only slightly, elevated compared to troponin levels. On the other hand, natriuretic peptides (BNP, NT-proBNP) are typically distinctly elevated due to left ventricular dysfunction. A high BNP/troponin ratio has been reported to have a high accuracy in the differential diagnosis between TTS and AMI, and can help in the diagnostic workup.[39,40]

As future perspective for the diagnosis of TTS, a pattern of four distinct circulating microRNAs (miRNAs) (miR-1, miR-16, miR-26a, and miR-133a) has been identified as a robust marker for distinction of TTS from acute STEMI.[41]

Coronary angiography and ventriculography

The basic component of TTS diagnosis is absence of a culprit lesion in the epicardial coronary arteries on coronary angiography. This is essential even if clinical, laboratory, and non-invasive imaging findings are suggestive of TTS, since myocardial infarction can mimic the wall motion abnormalities of TTS.[3] A common angiographic finding in TTS is absence of critical stenoses of coronary arteries. However, the coexistence of CAD does not exclude TTS and even obstructive concomitant CAD has been found in 23.0% of TTS patients.[9] Despite non-obstructive epicardial arteries, abnormal coronary flow, likely due to acute microcirculatory dysfunction, can be found in many patients at the time of presentation.[16,42]

Ventriculography allows assessment of left ventricular global function and the typical wall motion abnormalities, and thus the diagnosis of TTS. Furthermore, invasive haemodynamic measurements during ventriculography facilitate the detection of complications such as left ventricular outflow tract obstruction (LVOTO) and acute mitral regurgitation.[43]

Non-invasive imaging studies

Transthoracic echocardiography

TTE is the non-invasive imaging method of choice in TTS due to its widespread availability and feasibility. It allows evaluation of global left ventricular systolic function and detection of the typical patterns of wall motion abnormalities in TTS in the acute phase. Right ventricular involvement can be evaluated by visualization of right ventricular dilatation and hypo- or akinesia of the free wall. Impaired coronary microcirculation in the acute phase could be demonstrated by assessment of the coronary blood flow reserve with Doppler TTE and myocardial contrast echocardiography. Besides evaluation of ventricular function, TTE facilitates the detection of complications of TTS such as LVOTO, mitral regurgitation, and ventricular thrombi in the acute phase. Furthermore, it is recommended for follow-up observation of recovery of wall motion abnormalities, which resolve typically after several weeks.[44]

Cardiac computed tomography

Cardiac computed tomography (CCT) allows non-invasive assessment of coronary arteries. However, there is no opportunity for intervention in CCT. Thus, this modality is an alternative to

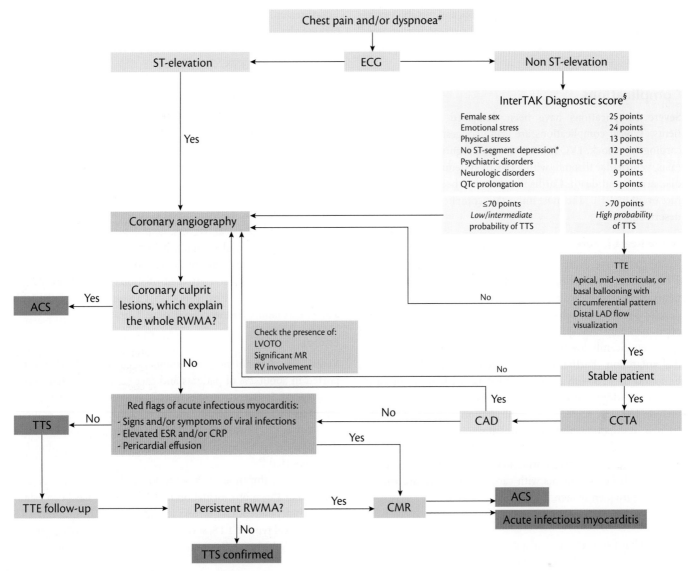

Figure 3.4.7.2 Algorithm for the diagnosis of takotsubo syndrome. #Applied to patients who are seeking medical emergency departments with, for example, chest pain and/or dyspnoea. §The InterTAK Diagnostic Score did not include patients with phaeochromocytoma-induced takotsubo syndrome in which atypical patterns are more frequently noted. *Except in lead aVR. ACS, acute coronary syndrome; CAD, coronary artery disease; CCTA, coronary computed tomography angiography; CMR, cardiac magnetic resonance; CRP, C-reactive protein; ECG, electrocardiogram; ESR, erythrocyte sedimentation rate; InterTAK, International Takotsubo Registry; LAD, left anterior descending coronary artery; LVOTO, left ventricular outflow tract obstruction; MR, mitral regurgitation; QTc, QT-time corrected for heart rate; RV, right ventricle; RWMA, regional wall motion abnormality; TTE, transthoracic echocardiography; TTS, takotsubo syndrome. Reproduced from Ghadri JR, Wittstein IS, Prasad A, et al. International Expert Consensus Document on Takotsubo Syndrome (Part II): Diagnostic Workup, Outcome, and Management. Eur Heart J. 2018 Jun 7;39(22):2047–2062. doi: 10.1093/eurheartj/ehy077 with permission from Oxford University Press.

coronary angiography to rule out coronary stenoses in patients with low pretest probability for CAD or in critically ill patients in whom wall motion abnormalities typical for TTS have been found in echocardiography.[44]

Cardiac magnetic resonance imaging

CMRI is useful for further diagnosis in the subacute phase of TTS. It allows reproducible evaluation of biventricular cardiac function, as well as identification of the typical wall motion abnormalities and right ventricular involvement. CMRI might serve as a second-line imaging tool and an alternative to echocardiography in patients with poor acoustic windows. CMRI enables the detection of myocardial oedema and necrosis, and by the latter, the differentiation from myocardial infarction and myocarditis. Myocardial oedema presents as a high-intensity area in

T2-weighted sequences and typically matches the wall motion abnormality regions in the acute phase. It disappears within a few weeks in TTS. Late gadolinium enhancement, which would suggest myocardial fibrosis or necrosis, is typically absent in TTS. This finding is important for differentiation from myocardial infarction or myocarditis, in which areas of late gadolinium enhancement are detected.

Furthermore, CMRI is a reliable method to detect complications such as valvular dysfunction or intracardiac thrombi. It has been shown that left ventricular thrombi are detectable with higher sensitivity and specificity with CMRI than with TTE.[44]

Nuclear imaging

The application of single-photon emission computed tomography (SPECT) and positron emission tomography in TTS for assessment of cardiac innervation, perfusion, and metabolism has been analysed in several studies, mainly for research purposes.[43] However, they have not been implemented in clinical practice to date.

Complications

Severe complications have been described in 20% of patients. Typical complications are acute congestive heart failure, cardiogenic shock, LVOTO, acute mitral regurgitation, arrhythmias, ventricular thrombi with a risk of systemic embolism, cardiac arrest, and death. Cardiac rupture has been described as a rare event in TTS.[3] The most important complications of TTS are described below.

Acute heart failure

Acute congestive heart failure has been reported in 12–45% of TTS patients, and cardiogenic shock in 6–20%.[5] Most of these patients present with cardiogenic shock at admission, whereas 30% develop shock in the subacute phase.[34] Left ventricular function is often markedly reduced, and the reported mean LVEF was found to be significantly lower than in matched patients with myocardial infarction. Furthermore, impaired diastolic function can be found in TTS with an elevated left ventricular end-diastolic pressure.[3] Additional factors contributing to acute heart failure include LVOTO, acute mitral regurgitation, regional right ventricular dysfunction, and atrial fibrillation. Independent risk factors for development of cardiogenic shock are the apical type of TTS, LVEF of <45%, atrial fibrillation on admission, physical triggers, and diabetes. Patients with cardiogenic shock are younger and more frequently men.[34]

Left ventricular outflow tract obstruction

LVOTO has been reported in approximately 20% of patients and is more common in the apical type of TTS. Patients with LVOTO are older, often with modest proximal septal hypertrophy (septal bulge), providing an anatomical substrate for dynamic LVOTO.[45] Systolic gradients >100 mmHg have been observed.[6,45] LVOTO may be exacerbated by catecholaminergic drugs and could be one mechanism for increased in-hospital mortality with catecholamine administration in TTS.[31] Furthermore, LVOTO is associated with mitral regurgitation in TTS. Systolic anterior motion (SAM) of the anterior leaflet of the mitral valve might be one mechanism underlying this correlation.[45]

Acute mitral regurgitation

Significant transient acute mitral valve regurgitation occurs in 14–25% of TTS patients and is associated with the apical type of TTS, lower LVEF, acute pulmonary oedema, cardiogenic shock, and an overall worse outcome.[5,46]

Mechanisms include mitral valve SAM associated with LVOTO, and leaflet tethering.[45,47] Mitral regurgitation typically improves or resolves with normalization of wall motion abnormalities.[46]

Arrhythmias

Cardiac arrhythmias are an important aspect of complications of TTS, as well as determinants of the short-term disease outcome.

Life-threatening ventricular arrhythmias, such as ventricular tachycardia, torsades de pointes, and ventricular fibrillation, have been reported in 3–9% of patients and occur most often in the subacute phase of TTS.[5]

Torsades de pointes tachycardia is associated with QT interval prolongation of >500 ms.[48,49] Male sex, bradycardia, and atrial fibrillation have been reported to increase the risk of TTS-associated torsades de pointes.[49]

Cardiac arrest was reported in 6% of patients with TTS. Most cardiac arrests occurred at presentation, but 19% were documented in the subacute phase of TTS. Ventricular fibrillation or tachycardia and asystole or PEA account for about half of cardiac arrests, respectively. Cardiac arrest is more frequent in men and in patients with physical triggers, neurological comorbidities, an apical type of TTS, and atrial fibrillation.[35]

Other arrhythmias that are associated with TTS are atrioventricular (AV) blocks and atrial fibrillation.[5,50] Atrial fibrillation can be found in 7% of patients with TTS and is associated with acute heart failure and worse outcome.[50]

Embolic events

Ventricular thrombi next to akinetic segments in TTS are reported in about 2% of patients and carry a risk of systemic embolic events. Ischaemic strokes in association with TTS have been reported in 1% of patients, and rarely other systemic embolic events occur.[51] Thrombi usually form within the first few days, although delayed formation with subsequent embolization has been reported.[39]

Recently, a thrombus risk score for evaluation of the risk of ventricular thrombus formation in TTS patients has been established. Independent risk factors for intracardiac thrombi in TTS are the apical type of TTS, severe left ventricular systolic dysfunction, elevated white cell counts, and previous vascular disease.[51]

Management

Since the pathophysiological perceptions of TTS are still vague, contemporary management of TTS is non-specific. It is based on a combination of heart failure treatment, prevention of recurrence, and therapy for pre-existing medical conditions.

Acute treatment

Acute treatment of TTS particularly consists of treatment of acute complications of the disease and the underlying medical condition. Outcome in patients with secondary TTS might depend on the course of the underlying condition.

Considering the pathophysiology of TTS, it is recommended to avoid catecholamine therapy whenever possible, and its use has been associated with a mortality of 20%. This principle becomes mostly important in patients with LVOTO, as the pressure gradient in the outflow tract increases with administration of catecholamines.[31] On the other hand, beta-blockers have not been associated with a benefit on mortality or recurrence rates,[33] but are frequently implemented in the therapy of TTS. Angiotensin-converting enzyme inhibitors (ACEIs) and angiotensin receptor blockers (ARBs) are widely administered to patients with TTS and have been shown to have a beneficial effect on the outcome of TTS in a retrospective analysis.[3]

Treatment of acute congestive heart failure consists of diuretics and nitroglycerin preparations. Cardiogenic shock requires intensive care and pharmacological or mechanical circulatory support. In systolic heart failure, catecholamines should be avoided, as mentioned previously. Instead levosimendan, a calcium sensitizer, is recommended as the positive inotropic medication of choice.[52] In LVOTO, inotropic agents, diuretics, and nitroglycerin should be discontinued to prevent an increase in the pressure gradient and deterioration of cardiogenic shock. Medical treatment options for reduction in the pressure gradient in LVOTO are short-acting beta-blockers or, as an alternative, verapamil and diltiazem, and intravenous fluids if necessary.[53] Microaxial pumps (Impella®) might be a valuable treatment option in severe cases with LVOTO and cardiogenic shock.[54] Other mechanical support devices are intra-aortic balloon pumps (IABPs) and extracorporeal venoarterial membrane oxygenators.[34]

QT-prolonging drugs should be avoided in patients with TTS, as QT prolongation can persist in these patients and increase the risk of torsades de pointes tachycardia. Hypokalaemia, hypomagnesaemia, and use of bradycardic and antiarrhythmic drugs may aggravate QTc interval prolongation and should be avoided.

Monitoring of the heart rhythm is recommended until normalization of the QT interval is demonstrated.[48] Tachycardic rhythm disorders should be treated with beta-blockers. The value of using implantable cardioverter–defibrillators is unclear.[55] Therefore, and due to the reversible nature of TTS, they should be avoided and wearable defibrillators can be considered as an alternative in individual cases.

Anticoagulation should be considered in patients with TTS at high risk of thromboembolic complications until recovery of wall motion abnormalities. In patients with ventricular thrombi, therapeutic anticoagulation with heparin and oral vitamin K antagonists is recommended. Temporary therapeutic anticoagulation may also be considered in patients with a high thrombus risk score (→ Complications, p. 122).

Long-term management

TTS is an acute, transient impairment of left ventricular function, with complete recovery typically within several weeks.[8] Therefore, long-term management focuses on treatment of heart failure and comorbidities, and the prevention of recurrence.

Beta-blockers and ACEIs/ARBs are most frequently administered at discharge.[33] ACEIs/ARBs are associated with improved 1-year survival, whereas beta-blockers have not been shown to have any benefit.[3] To date, there is no evidence for a beneficial effect of any drug on recurrence of TTS.[33] Nevertheless, all data originate from observational analyses, as no prospective studies on treatment have been conducted. Therefore, treatment with beta-blockers and ACEIs/ARBs is recommended until short-term follow-up after approximately 8 weeks. Long-term continuation of these drugs cannot be

recommended for TTS on the basis of available data, and is advised if other indications, such as hypertension or persisting heart failure, are present.

Since psychiatric comorbidities are a frequent trigger of TTS, all patients should be screened for those diseases and be offered psychiatric care. However, the effect of psychiatric treatment on recurrence rates is still unclear. Substitution of oestrogen in postmenopausal women is in discussion, although data on this topic are lacking.[5]

Outcome and prognosis

Unlike initially assumed, TTS cannot be considered a benign disease. Its morbidity and mortality are comparable to that of AMI. Newer findings have highlighted a number of severe cardiovascular complications and occurrence of adverse outcomes, including death.[3,39,56]

Short-term outcome

Short-term outcome of TTS is determined by the presence of acute complications and the underlying disease in patients with physical triggers. In-hospital mortality has been reported at around 4% and comparable to that of AMI.[3] Over 80% of TTS related in-hospital deaths occur in the setting of an underlying critical illness, which often includes subarachnoid haemorrhage, acute respiratory failure, and sepsis.[56] Hospital death is usually attributable to congestive heart failure, cardiogenic shock, or cardiac arrest.[17,56]

Predictors of unfavourable outcome are male sex, physical trigger factors, acute neurological or psychiatric diseases, troponin levels of more than 10 times the normal level, high BNP/NT-proBNP levels, initial LVEF <45%, moderate to severe mitral regurgitation, and right ventricular involvement.[3,5]

Long-term outcome and recurrence

Patients who survive an acute event typically show complete recovery of LVEF and regional wall motion within several weeks.[8] However, long-term mortality of TTS is comparable to that in patients with ACS,[3,57] and higher than in an age- and sex-matched general population.[6,56] The annual mortality rate is 5.6%. The rate of major adverse cardiovascular events is 9.9% per year.[3] Mortality is highest during the first year after the TTS event and is more commonly associated with the underlying disease. However, approximately 40% of TTS-related deaths are attributable to a cardiovascular cause, less than in patients with ACS treated with percutaneous coronary intervention, but greater than in the general population.[17] Predictors of increased 5-year mortality are male sex, age >70 years, physical or no identified triggers, neurological disorders, cancer, and LVEF <45%. These have led to TTS classification (InterTAK classification) according to its outcome prognosis.[57] Recently, the InterTAK Prognosis Score has been developed, which allows identification of high-risk patients.[58] → Figure 3.4.7.3 shows long-term mortality of TTS, compared to ACS.

Approximately 5% of patients develop recurrent TTS within 30 days to several years after their index admission. The recurrence

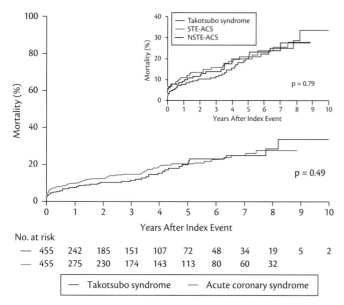

Figure 3.4.7.3 Long-term mortality in takotsubo syndrome compared to acute coronary syndrome. Kaplan–Meier curve for long-term mortality in patients with Takotsubo syndrome compared to an age- and sex-matched cohort of patients with acute coronary syndrome (ACS), including ST-segment elevation (STE) ACS (*n* = 233) and non-ST-segment elevation (NSTE) ACS (*n* = 222). Patients with takotsubo syndrome had long-term mortality risk comparable to those with ACS (*P* = 0.49) or with STE- and NSTE-ACS (*P* = 0.79).
Reproduced from Ghadri JR, Kato K, Cammann VL, *et al.* Long-Term Prognosis of Patients With Takotsubo Syndrome. *J Am Coll Cardiol.* 2018 Aug 21;72(8):874–882. doi: 10.1016/j.jacc.2018.06.016 with permission from Elsevier.

rate is reported at 1.8% per year. Recurrence can occur in all age groups and sex categories, and multiple TTS events have been described. The trigger factor may be different in index and recurrent events, and the TTS type changes in approximately 30%. Neurological and psychiatric disorders have been found to be independent risk factors for recurrence.[59]

Future directions

Increasing research efforts over the last years have led to a change in many assumptions about TTS. It is much more frequent than previously thought and affects all age groups, sexes, and ethnic groups. Unlike previous notions, TTS is not a benign disease and has noteworthy morbidity and mortality, which is comparable to AMI. However, many aspects in TTS remain unclear. The exact pathophysiological mechanisms of TTS are not yet understood. It is not completely known why some people are more susceptible to TTS. A potential influence of oestrogen deficiency might not explain the cases in younger females and males. To date, treatment options for prevention of recurrence and long-term mortality are lacking and additional research needs to be conducted. Finally, patients with incomplete recovery have received more attention recently. Further research needs to elucidate the causes and significance of persistent symptoms, higher long-term morbidity and mortality, and diagnostic results hinting to structural myocardial changes, such as late gadolinium enhancement, in certain patients.

References

1. Sato, H., Tako-tsubo-like left ventricular dysfunction due to multivessel coronary spasm. In: Kodama K, Haze K, Hori M, eds. *Clinical Aspect of Myocardial Injury: From Ischemia to Heart Failure.* [Chapter in Japanese] Tokyo: Kagakuhyoronsha Publishing Co, 1990: pp. 56–64.
2. Cammann, V.L., *et al.*, Takotsubo syndrome: uncovering myths and misconceptions. Curr Atheroscler Rep, 2021. **23**(9): p. 53.
3. Templin, C., *et al.*, Clinical features and outcomes of takotsubo (stress) cardiomyopathy. N Engl J Med, 2015. **373**(10): p. 929–38.
4. Napp, L.C. and J. Bauersachs, Takotsubo syndrome: between evidence, myths, and misunderstandings. Herz, 2020. **45**(3): p. 252–66.
5. Ghadri, J.R., *et al.*, International expert consensus document on takotsubo syndrome (part II): diagnostic workup, outcome, and management. Eur Heart J, 2018. **39**(22): p. 2047–62.
6. Sharkey, S.W., *et al.*, Natural history and expansive clinical profile of stress (takotsubo) cardiomyopathy. J Am Coll Cardiol, 2010. **55**(4): p. 333–41.
7. Maron, B.J., *et al.*, Contemporary definitions and classification of the cardiomyopathies: an American Heart Association Scientific Statement from the Council on Clinical Cardiology, Heart Failure and Transplantation Committee; Quality of Care and Outcomes Research and Functional Genomics and Translational Biology Interdisciplinary Working Groups; and Council on Epidemiology and Prevention. Circulation, 2006. **113**(14): p. 1807–16.
8. Ghadri, J.R., *et al.*, International expert consensus document on takotsubo syndrome (part I): clinical characteristics, diagnostic criteria, and pathophysiology. Eur Heart J, 2018. **39**(22): p. 2032–46.
9. Napp, L.C., *et al.*, Coexistence and outcome of coronary artery disease in takotsubo syndrome. Eur Heart J, 2020. **41**(34): p. 3255–68.
10. Kato, K., *et al.*, Prevalence and clinical features of focal takotsubo cardiomyopathy. Circ J, 2016. **80**(8): p. 1824–9.
11. Ghadri, J.R., *et al.*, Differences in the clinical profile and outcomes of typical and atypical takotsubo syndrome: data from the International Takotsubo Registry. JAMA Cardiol, 2016. **1**(3): p. 335–40.
12. Elesber, A.A., *et al.*, Transient cardiac apical ballooning syndrome: prevalence and clinical implications of right ventricular involvement. J Am Coll Cardiol, 2006. **47**(5): p. 1082–3.
13. Citro, R., *et al.*, Clinical profile and in-hospital outcome of Caucasian patients with takotsubo syndrome and right ventricular involvement. Int J Cardiol, 2016. **219**: p. 455–61.
14. Stahli, B.E., F. Ruschitzka, and F. Enseleit, Isolated right ventricular ballooning syndrome: a new variant of transient cardiomyopathy. Eur Heart J, 2011. **32**(14): p. 1821.
15. Prasad, A., *et al.*, Incidence and angiographic characteristics of patients with apical ballooning syndrome (takotsubo/stress cardiomyopathy) in the HORIZONS-AMI trial: an analysis from a multicenter, international study of ST-elevation myocardial infarction. Catheter Cardiovasc Interv, 2014. **83**(3): p. 343–8.
16. Bybee, K.A., *et al.*, Clinical characteristics and thrombolysis in myocardial infarction frame counts in women with transient left ventricular apical ballooning syndrome. Am J Cardiol, 2004. **94**(3): p. 343–6.
17. Redfors, B., *et al.*, Mortality in takotsubo syndrome is similar to mortality in myocardial infarction: a report from the SWEDEHEART registry. Int J Cardiol, 2015. **185**: p. 282–9.
18. Minhas, A.S., A.B. Hughey, and T.J. Kolias, Nationwide trends in reported incidence of takotsubo cardiomyopathy from 2006 to 2012. Am J Cardiol, 2015. **116**(7): p. 1128–31.
19. Pilgrim, T.M. and T.R. Wyss, Takotsubo cardiomyopathy or transient left ventricular apical ballooning syndrome: a systematic review. Int J Cardiol, 2008. **124**(3): p. 283–92.

20. Pelliccia, F., *et al.*, Comorbidities frequency in takotsubo syndrome: an international collaborative systematic review including 1109 patients. Am J Med, 2015. **128**(6): p. 654.e11–19.

21. Porto, I., *et al.*, Stress cardiomyopathy (tako-tsubo) triggered by nervous system diseases: a systematic review of the reported cases. Int J Cardiol, 2013. **167**(6): p. 2441–8.

22. Blanc, C., *et al.*, Takotsubo cardiomyopathy following acute cerebral events. Eur Neurol, 2015. **74**(3–4): p. 163–8.

23. Hiestand, T., *et al.*, Takotsubo syndrome associated with structural brain alterations of the limbic system. J Am Coll Cardiol, 2018. **71**(7): p. 809–11.

24. Kato, K., *et al.*, Prognostic impact of acute pulmonary triggers in patients with takotsubo syndrome: new insights from the International Takotsubo Registry. ESC Heart Fail, 2021. **8**(3): p. 1924–32.

25. Sattler, K., *et al.*, Prevalence of cancer in takotsubo cardiomyopathy: short and long-term outcome. Int J Cardiol, 2017. <u>**238**</u>: p. 159–65.

26. Girardey, M., *et al.*, Impact of malignancies in the early and late time course of takotsubo cardiomyopathy. Circ J, 2016. **80**(10): p. 2192–8.

27. Cammann, V.L., *et al.*, Clinical features and outcomes of patients with malignancy and takotsubo syndrome: observations from the International Takotsubo Registry. J Am Heart Assoc, 2019. **8**(15): p. e010881.

28. Pop-Busui, R., Cardiac autonomic neuropathy in diabetes: a clinical perspective. Diabetes Care, 2010. **33**(2): p. 434–41.

29. Ghadri, J.R., *et al.*, Happy heart syndrome: role of positive emotional stress in takotsubo syndrome. Eur Heart J, 2016. **37**(37): p. 2823–9.

30. Schlossbauer, S.A., J.R. Ghadri, and C. Templin, [Takotsubo-Syndrom: ein haufig verkanntes Krankheitsbild]. Praxis (Bern 1994), 2016. **105**(20): p. 1185–92.

31. Templin, C., J.R. Ghadri, and L.C. Napp, Takotsubo (stress) cardiomyopathy. N Engl J Med, 2015. **373**(27): p. 2689–91.

32. Lyon, A.R., *et al.*, Pathophysiology of takotsubo syndrome: JACC state-of-the-art review. J Am Coll Cardiol, 2021. **77**(7): p. 902–21.

33. Kato, K., *et al.*, Takotsubo syndrome: aetiology, presentation and treatment. Heart, 2017. **103**(18): p. 1461–9.

34. Di Vece, D., *et al.*, Outcomes associated with cardiogenic shock in takotsubo syndrome. Circulation, 2019. **139**(3): p. 413–15.

35. Gili, S., *et al.*, Cardiac arrest in takotsubo syndrome: results from the InterTAK Registry. Eur Heart J, 2019. **40**(26): p. 2142–51.

36. Ghadri, J.R., *et al.*, A novel clinical score (InterTAK Diagnostic Score) to differentiate takotsubo syndrome from acute coronary syndrome: results from the International Takotsubo Registry. Eur J Heart Fail, 2017. **19**(8): p. 1036–42.

37. Duran-Cambra, A., *et al.*, Systematic review of the electrocardiographic changes in the takotsubo syndrome. Ann Noninvasive Electrocardiol, 2015. **20**(1): p. 1–6.

38. Frangieh, A.H., *et al.*, ECG criteria to differentiate between takotsubo (stress) cardiomyopathy and myocardial infarction. J Am Heart Assoc, 2016. **5**(6): p. e003418.

39. Lyon, A.R., *et al.*, Current state of knowledge on takotsubo syndrome: a position statement from the Taskforce on Takotsubo Syndrome of the Heart Failure Association of the European Society of Cardiology. Eur J Heart Fail, 2016. **18**(1): p. 8–27.

40. Frohlich, G.M., *et al.*, Takotsubo cardiomyopathy has a unique cardiac biomarker profile: NT-proBNP/myoglobin and NT-proBNP/troponin T ratios for the differential diagnosis of acute coronary syndromes and stress induced cardiomyopathy. Int J Cardiol, 2012. **154**(3): p. 328–32.

41. Jaguszewski, M., *et al.*, A signature of circulating microRNAs differentiates takotsubo cardiomyopathy from acute myocardial infarction. Eur Heart J, 2014. **35**(15): p. 999–1006.

42. Rigo, F., *et al.*, Diffuse, marked, reversible impairment in coronary microcirculation in stress cardiomyopathy: a Doppler transthoracic echo study. Ann Med, 2009. **41**(6): p. 462–70.

43. Bossone, E., *et al.*, Takotsubo cardiomyopathy: an integrated multi-imaging approach. Eur Heart J Cardiovasc Imaging, 2014. **15**(4): p. 366–77.

44. Citro, R., *et al.*, Multimodality imaging in takotsubo syndrome: a joint consensus document of the European Association of Cardiovascular Imaging (EACVI) and the Japanese Society of Echocardiography (JSE). Eur Heart J Cardiovasc Imaging, 2020. **21**(11): p. 1184–207.

45. De Backer, O., *et al.*, Prevalence, associated factors and management implications of left ventricular outflow tract obstruction in takotsubo cardiomyopathy: a two-year, two-center experience. BMC Cardiovasc Disord, 2014. **14**: p. 147.

46. Citro, R., *et al.*, Echocardiographic correlates of acute heart failure, cardiogenic shock, and in-hospital mortality in tako-tsubo cardiomyopathy. JACC Cardiovasc Imaging, 2014. **7**(2): p. 119–29.

47. Izumo, M., *et al.*, Mechanisms of acute mitral regurgitation in patients with takotsubo cardiomyopathy: an echocardiographic study. Circ Cardiovasc Imaging, 2011. **4**(4): p. 392–8.

48. Madias, C., *et al.*, Acquired long QT syndrome from stress cardiomyopathy is associated with ventricular arrhythmias and torsades de pointes. Heart Rhythm, 2011. **8**(4): p. 555–61.

49. Samuelov-Kinori, L., *et al.*, Takotsubo cardiomyopathy and QT interval prolongation: who are the patients at risk for torsades de pointes? J Electrocardiol, 2009. **42**(4): p. 353–7.e1.

50. El-Battrawy, I., *et al.*, Impact of atrial fibrillation on outcome in takotsubo syndrome: data from the International Takotsubo Registry. J Am Heart Assoc, 2021. **10**(15): p. e014059.

51. Ding, K.J., *et al.*, Intraventricular thrombus formation and embolism in takotsubo syndrome: insights from the International Takotsubo Registry. Arterioscler Thromb Vasc Biol, 2020. **40**(1): p. 279–87.

52. Santoro, F., *et al.*, Safety and feasibility of levosimendan administration in takotsubo cardiomyopathy: a case series. Cardiovasc Ther, 2013. **31**(6): p. e133–7.

53. Palecek, T., P. Kuchynka, and A. Linhart, Treatment of takotsubo cardiomyopathy. Curr Pharm Des, 2010. **16**(26): p. 2905–9.

54. Napp, L.C., *et al.*, Impella mechanical circulatory support for takotsubo syndrome with shock: a retrospective multicenter analysis. Cardiovasc Revasc Med, 2022. **40**: p. 113–19.

55. Stiermaier, T., *et al.*, Prevalence and clinical significance of life-threatening arrhythmias in takotsubo cardiomyopathy. J Am Coll Cardiol, 2015. **65**(19): p. 2148–50.

56. Sharkey, S.W., *et al.*, Clinical profile of patients with high-risk takotsubo cardiomyopathy. Am J Cardiol, 2015. **116**(5): p. 765–72.

57. Ghadri, J.R., *et al.*, Long-term prognosis of patients with takotsubo syndrome. J Am Coll Cardiol, 2018. **72**(8): p. 874–82.

58. Wischnewsky, M.B., *et al.*, Prediction of short- and long-term mortality in takotsubo syndrome: the InterTAK Prognostic Score. Eur J Heart Fail, 2019. **21**(11): p. 1469–72.

59. Kato, K., *et al.*, Takotsubo recurrence: morphological types and triggers and identification of risk factors. J Am Coll Cardiol, 2019. **73**(8): p. 982–4.

CHAPTER 3.5

Myocarditis and pericarditis

Stephane Heymans, Arsen D Ristić,
Yehuda Adler, and Massimo Imazio

Contents

Introduction: myocarditis and myopericarditis as a cause of heart failure

Myocarditis can cause transient or chronic and progressive heart failure, depending on the causative agent, the extent and duration of inflammation of the heart, and the response of the immune system. Infectious triggers are most commonly viruses, and less frequently bacteria, fungi, and parasites (➲ Table 3.5.1).[1] Systemic diseases and toxic agents are important non-infectious causes of myocarditis. The incidence of acute myocarditis is estimated to be 1.5 million cases per year in the world population.[2] Endomyocardial biopsy (EMB)-proven chronic inflammation can be found in 9–30% of adult patients with dilated cardiomyopathy (DCM).[3,4] In 20–30% of cases, myocarditis and pericarditis may co-occur. As the viral triggers in peri- and myocarditis are common cough viruses, with only a minority of infected persons developing peri- or myocarditis, a certain immune–genetic susceptibility—including coding and non-coding genes—of the affected person is key.[5,6] The proposed pathophysiology of myocarditis and the trajectory of the disease are presented in ➲ Figure 3.5.1. The most frequent causes of myocarditis are shown in ➲ Table 3.5.1.[1,7]

Clinical presentation and diagnosis of myocarditis

Myocarditis has an extensively variable clinical presentation, with the following main patterns: (1) chest pain (pseudoacute myocardial infarction); (2) heart failure; and (3) arrhythmias or even sudden death.[3,7,8] A flu-like febrile syndrome (respiratory infection or gastroenteritis) usually precedes pericarditis/myocarditis for 1–2 weeks. Alternatively, symptoms of an underlying disease with pericardial/myocardial involvement (e.g. systemic inflammatory disease, cancer) should be enquired about. In clinically evident cases of (sub)acute myocarditis, C-reactive protein (CRP) and troponin levels are usually elevated.

On the electrocardiogram (ECG), the classical feature of acute (myo-)pericarditis is '*widespread concave ST-segment elevation*' (➲ Figure 3.5.2). However, the earliest ECG sign of an atrial current of injury is *PR depression* (➲ Figure 3.5.2). Both signs demonstrate subepicardial involvement and are absent in isolated 'pure pericarditis', as the pericardium is electrically silent.[6] The ECG evolves according to the classical four Spodick stages. Early presentation is associated with ST-segment elevation, whereas late presentation or chronic forms may result in a normal ECG or negative T-waves (reflecting an ECG in evolution). The risk of cardiac arrhythmias is very low in the absence of myocarditis or structural heart disease.[9]

An echocardiogram is mandatory in patients with suspected acute myocarditis or pericarditis to assess myocardial function and the presence, size, and haemodynamic

Table 3.5.1 Most frequent causes of myocarditis and myopericarditis

Infectious	
Viral	Parvovirus B19, human herpesvirus 6, Epstein–Barr virus, enteroviruses (Coxsackie virus A and B), adenovirus, cytomegalovirus, HIV, SARS-CoV-2
Other (myocarditis)	*Borrelia burgdorferi*, *Coxiella burnetii* (Q fever)
Autoimmune	
Systemic autoimmune disease	Sarcoidosis, giant cell myocarditis, systemic lupus erythematosus, ANCA-positive vasculitis, rheumatoid arthritis, any other autoimmune disease
Toxic	
Medications	Immune checkpoint inhibitors, anthracyclines, clozapine, adrenergic drugs, 5-fluorouracil
Other toxic agents	Alcohol, amphetamines, cocaine, crack

HIV, human immunodeficiency virus; SARS-CoV-2, severe acute respiratory syndrome coronavirus 2; ANCA, antineutrophil cytoplasmic antibody.

importance of possible pericardial effusion. In the majority of patients, echocardiography findings are normal or almost normal. Global or regional impairment of contractility without overt dilatation of cardiac chambers is revealed in patients with more extensive inflammation at initial presentation, followed by complete, or almost complete, recovery in the next few weeks in >50% of patients with enterovirus or adenovirus infection.[1,7,10]

Rarely the disease may progress to inflammatory cardiomyopathy, presenting as acute or chronic heart failure, across a wide spectrum ranging from heart failure with preserved ejection fraction (HFpEF) to advanced heart failure with reduced ejection fraction (HFrEF) requiring intensive care, mechanical circulatory support, or heart transplantation. Cardiac magnetic resonance (CMR) may allow non-invasive assessment of myocardial inflammation according to recently revised criteria (➲ Table 3.5.2).[11]

CMR provides strong evidence for myocardial inflammation, with high specificity, if the scan demonstrates a combination of myocardial oedema and the presence of other CMR markers of inflammatory myocardial injury. This is based on at least one T2-based criterion (global or regional increase of myocardial T2 relaxation time or increased signal intensity on T2-weighted CMR images), with at least one T1-based criterion (increased myocardial T1, extracellular volume, or late gadolinium enhancement; see ➲ Table 3.5.2).

The diagnosis of 'clinically suspected myocarditis' can be established in the presence of at least two diagnostic criteria from

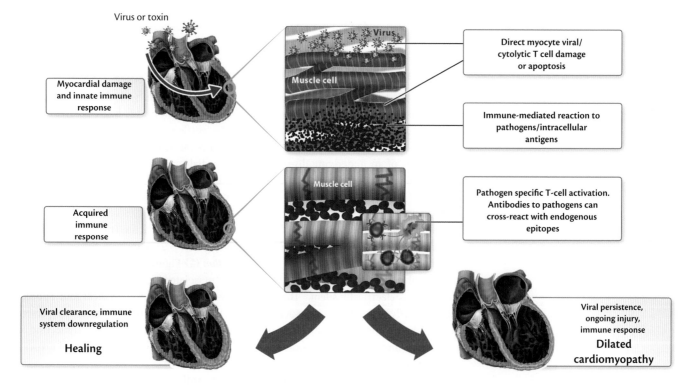

Figure 3.5.1 Proposed pathophysiology of myocarditis and the evolution of inflammation.

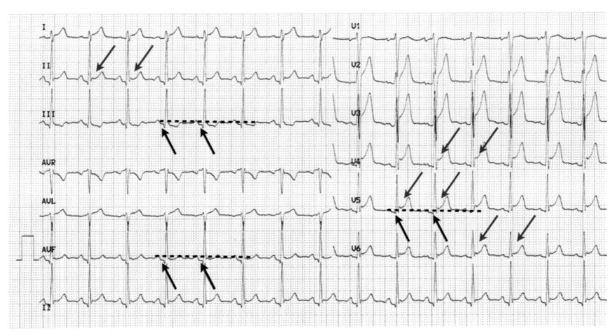

Figure 3.5.2 Classical ECG with 'widespread ST-segment elevation' (red arrows) and PR depression (black arrows) in a young patient with acute myopericarditis (mixed form with myocarditis and pericarditis and preserved biventricular function).

different categories (typical clinical presentation with one or more positive mandatory diagnostic tests, preferably CMR) in the absence of significant coronary artery, valvular, or congenital heart disease, or hereditary cardiomyopathies (→ Table 3.5.3).[1,4,7,10,12,13,14,15] Non-invasive testing may be sufficient to support a diagnosis of 'clinically suspected myocarditis', after exclusion of coronary artery disease by coronary angiography or computed tomography (CT). However, EMB remains the gold standard for the final diagnosis, but will only be performed in those cases with persistent cardiac dysfunction within days after initial presentation or when myocarditis is recurrent.

According to the 2021 Heart Failure Association (HFA)/Heart Failure Society of America (HFSA)/Japanese Heart Failure Society (JHFS) position statement on EMB[16] and the 2013 position statement of the European Society of Cardiology (ESC) Working Group on myocardial and pericardial diseases,[7] EMB is mandatory to confirm a clinically suspected diagnosis of myocarditis, especially in those cases with persistent left ventricular dysfunction or recurrent myocarditis. Up to 80% of acute myocarditis patients will functionally recover within several days after the initial symptoms, and therefore may not require EMB in the acute situation. By contrast, EMBs are recommended in patients with fulminant myocarditis and cardiogenic shock, as well as in patients with severe and progressive acute heart failure or left ventricular dysfunction, and/or cardiac rhythm disorders (frequent ventricular premature complexes, ventricular tachycardia, conduction abnormalities) (→ Table 3.5.4).[1,4,10,16,17,18,19,20,21] Typical pathohistological findings in myocarditis include lymphocytic myocarditis (the

Table 3.5.2 Cardiac magnetic resonance in myocarditis patients

Cardiac magnetic resonance in line with updated 2018 Lake Louis Criteria[11]	
When?	At baseline in all patients with clinical history + ECG, troponin, or echocardiographic abnormalities, and significant coronary artery disease excluded or unlikely At follow-up in those patients with persistent myocardial dysfunction at echocardiography, arrhythmias, or ECG abnormalities
What?	At baseline: T1, T2, and late enhancement within 2 weeks after onset in order to evaluate cardiac oedema and injury, according to the Lake Louise criteria At follow-up: late enhancement to evaluate the degree of scarring; T1 or T2 only if persistent inflammation is suspected
Evidence of myocarditis?	Acute phase: at least one T2-based criterion (global or regional increase of myocardial T2 relaxation time or increased signal intensity in T2-weighted CMR images), with at least one T1-based criterion (increased myocardial T1, extracellular volume, or late gadolinium enhancement) Acute phase: only one (i.e. T2- or T1-based) marker may still support a diagnosis of acute myocardial inflammation in an appropriate clinical scenario, albeit with lower specificity Chronic phase: a negative T1/T2 scan does not exclude a still ongoing inflammatory process
Follow-up CMR	Follow-up with CMR is advised after treatment in those patients with persistent dysfunction on echocardiography, arrhythmias, or ECG abnormalities

CMR, cardiac magnetic resonance.

Table 3.5.3 Diagnostic criteria for acute myocarditis

Definition of clinically suspect acute myocarditis: clinical presentation + ≥ 1 mandatory diagnostic test being positive (by preference CMR) in the absence of significant coronary artery, valvular or congenital heart disease, or other causes

		Sensitivity	Specificity
Signs and symptoms			
Clinical presentation	Acute/ new onset chest pain, dyspnoea, signs of left and/or right HF, and unexplained arrhythmias or aborted sudden death	Low	Low
Mandatory diagnostic tests			
ECG	New and dynamic ECG ST-T abnormalities, atrial or ventricular arrhythmias, or QRS abnormalities	High	Low
Laboratory	Elevated troponins, dynamic over time. BNP and nt pro BNP may be elevated reflecting the degree of concomitant heart failure. In the presence of haemodynamically significant pericardial effusion BNP and nt pro BNP are lower that it would be expected according to the level of myocardial dysfunction (12)	Intermediate[a]	Low
Cardiac function	New structural or function abnormalities (regional wall motion abnormalities or global ventricular dysfunction with or without ventricular dilatation, increased wall thickness, pericardial effusion, of intracardiac thrombi), not explained by other conditions (e.g. valvular heart disease)	High	Low
Oedema/ fibrosis-CMR	T1 or T2 (oedema) increased. Gadolinium late enhancement in line with T1 or T2 increase	High	Intermediate
Additional diagnostic tests			
Coronary angiography	To exclude significant coronary artery disease or acute coronary syndrome		
Endomyocardial biopsies (➲ Table 3.5.4)	*Immunostaining of T-lymphocytes, monocytes, macrophages *Presence of infection (PCR for common cardiotropic viruses)	Low	High
Laboratory test	*Muscular enzymes, liver and renal function, haemoglobin and white blood cell counts, natriuretic peptides, thyroid stimulating hormones, iron status and indicators of systemic autoimmune disease *Borrelia burdorferi, HIV, CMV or SARS-CoV-2 if clinical suspicion *Viral serology should not be performed in view of the high prevalence of circulating immunoglobulin G antibodies to cardiotropic viruses in the absence of viral myocarditis MicroRNA (hsa-miR-Chr8:96) could be a novel technique to distinguish patients with myocarditis from those with myocardial infarction (4,13)		
Genetic testing and counselling	In those cases with a familial history of an (inherited) non-ischemic cardiomyopathy (2 or more relatives) (14,15)		

DNA= deoxyribonucleic acid; ECG = electrocardiogram; EMB = endomyocardial biopsy; h = hours; HF = heart failure; MCS = mechanical circulatory support; MR = magnetic resonance. [a] Negative troponins do not exclude acute myocarditis, but indicate the absence of direct cardiomyocyte injury due to inflammation.

Table 3.5.4 Indications for endomyocardial biopsy in patients with clinically suspected myocarditis

Endomyocardial biopsy, left or right ventricle, or both	
When?	Suspected fulminant myocarditis or acute myocarditis with severe acute heart failure, persistent left ventricular dysfunction, and/or cardiac rhythm disorders Suspected myocarditis in haemodynamically stable patients
How many?	At least five samples from different sites to reduce the risk of sampling error. Sample processing and analysis include staining for histopathology, quantitative real-time PCR for viruses and *Borrelia*, and immunohistochemical analysis
Infectious	Common cardiotropic viruses (parvovirus B19, HHV4, HHV6, enteroviruses (adenovirus and Coxsackie virus) by real-time PCR Viral mRNA for active viral replication, but low sensitivity On indication: CMV, HIV, *Borrelia burgdorferi* (Lyme disease), *Coxiella burnetii* (Q fever), and SARS-CoV-2
Staining/pathology	CD3, CD4, CD8, or CD45 staining for lymphocytes and CD68 staining for macrophages; anti-HLA-DR; fibrosis (Masson's trichrome and picrosirius red), amyloid fibrils (Congo red)
Therapeutic consequences?	Immunosuppressive therapy in giant cell or eosinophilic myocarditis, sarcoidosis, or vasculitis, and in patients with persistent cardiac inflammation in the absence of active viral infection Antibiotics: *B. burgdorferi* (Lyme disease) Antiviral therapy: HIV, CMV, HHV6 pending load and viral replication (mRNA)

CD, cluster of differentiation; CMV, cytomegalovirus; HIV, human immunodeficiency virus; HHV4, human herpesvirus 4; HHV6, human herpesvirus 6; HLA, human leucocyte antigen; mRNA, messenger ribonucleic acid; PCR, polymerase chain reaction; SARS-CoV-2, severe acute respiratory syndrome coronavirus 2.

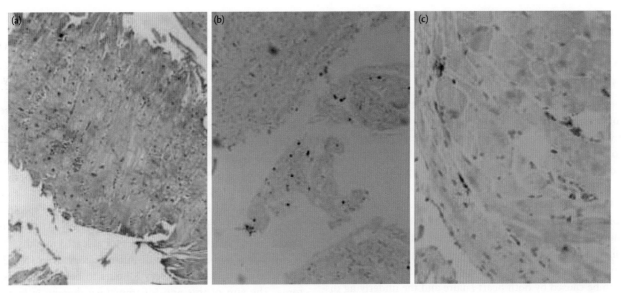

Figure 3.5.3 Endomyocardial biopsy in a patient with lymphocytic myocarditis. (a) Interstitial lymphocytic infiltrate in the myocardium (haematoxylin and eosin stain, magnification ×160). (b) Immunohistochemistry revealing CD3+ T-lymphocytic inflammatory infiltrate (magnification ×250). (c) CD68+ macrophages in the inflammatory infiltrate (magnification ×400).
Courtesy of Dr. Vesna Božić, cardiopathologist, University Clinical Center of Serbia, Belgrade.

most common form) (➲ Figure 3.5.3), eosinophilic myocarditis (often accompanied by peripheral blood eosinophilia), giant cell myocarditis (frequently with a fulminant course), and granulomatous myocarditis (e.g. in cardiac sarcoidosis).[16]

In some instances, autoimmune myocarditis may cause progressive heart failure that is unresponsive to treatment and/or cardiac rhythm disorders in patients with autoimmune diseases (polymyositis, dermatomyositis, systemic lupus erythematosus, rheumatoid arthritis, etc.).[1,18]

Management of patients with myocarditis and perimyocarditis

Patients with clinically suspected myocarditis should be hospitalized and monitored for at least 48 hours, especially when troponin levels are elevated or when cardiac dysfunction and/or arrhythmias are present.[1,10,21] Despite the lack of evidence in this specific setting, heart failure therapy should be given in the presence of HFrEF or heart failure with mildly reduced ejection fraction (HFmrEF) and continued for at least 3 months after normalization of cardiac function.[10,17,18] Patients can be discharged from hospital once cardiac enzyme levels have decreased, arrhythmias have disappeared, and cardiac systolic dysfunction has stabilized. Immunosuppression for at least 12 months is required in acute myocarditis with EMB evidence of autoimmune disease, including giant cell myocarditis, vasculitis, sarcoidosis, and myocarditis associated with known extracardiac autoimmune disease.[7,10,16,20] Steroid therapy is indicated in cardiac sarcoidosis regardless of the degree of ventricular dysfunction and in infection-negative eosinophilic or toxic myocarditis with heart failure and arrhythmia. Immunosuppression may be considered for 6 months in patients with infection-negative lymphocytic myocarditis.[7,22] Immunosuppression should be started only after

ruling out active infection on EMB by polymerase chain reaction (PCR). Intense sports activities should be avoided as long as symptoms are present, cardiac enzyme levels are elevated, or ECG/imaging abnormalities are not completely recovered, and for 6 months after their recovery/normalization.[23] A yearly follow-up for at least 4 years, including an ECG and echocardiography after the initial acute myocarditis, should be performed, as myocarditis may lead to DCM in up to 20% of cases.[7,18,24]

Different retrospective studies observed a beneficial effect of immunosuppression not only on functional recovery,[24,25] but also on mortality[18] in patients with inflammatory cardiomyopathy or chronic myocarditis (with a calcineurin inhibitor, azathioprine or mycophenolate mofetil, and corticosteroids for at least 12 months). Prospective blinded, randomized, and placebo-controlled trials with old or new immunosuppressive/immunomodulatory drugs are lacking and required.

A recent randomized, double-blind, placebo-controlled single-centre trial investigated the benefits of intravenous immunoglobulin (IVIg) beyond conventional therapy in patients with parvovirus B19 (B19V) persistence and idiopathic chronic DCM.[26] IVIg therapy did not significantly improve cardiac systolic function or functional capacity beyond standard medical therapy in patients with idiopathic chronic DCM and cardiac B19V persistence.[26] As corticosteroids facilitate the replication of herpesviruses, they should be avoided in patients with clinically suspected myocarditis in whom EMB has not been performed to exclude the presence of herpesviruses (HHV4 or HHV6).[1,7,10,16]

Non-pharmacological recommendations include restriction of physical activity beyond ordinary sedentary life until resolution of symptoms and normalization of CRP levels for patients not involved in competitive sports, and for an arbitrary term of 6 months for athletes. For athletes, return to competitive sports is allowed only after symptoms have resolved and diagnostic tests (i.e. CRP, ECG, and echocardiogram) have normalized.[23]

Role of the pericardium and pericardial effusion in heart failure

The pericardium exerts a compressive contact force on the surface of the myocardium that becomes more substantial when heart volume increases, as in patients with heart failure.[27] Small or moderate pericardial transudates frequently accompany advanced heart failure, especially in patients with pulmonary hypertension, and is a marker of poor prognosis. On the other hand, patients with myopericarditis can also progress to inflammatory cardiomyopathy and HFrEF, as patients with isolated myocarditis occasionally do. Furthermore, in patients with acute myocardial infarction or acute pericarditis–myocarditis, and those with systemic or metabolic disease or active cancer, pericardial effusion can be caused by both heart failure and the underlying disease. Hypothyroidism, a condition that frequently accompanies chronic heart failure, should always be considered in the differential diagnosis, as well as coronavirus disease 2019 (Covid-19).[28,29]

Pericarditis is an inflammatory pericardial syndrome, with or without pericardial effusion.[6,28] The annual incidence of acute pericarditis is approximately 27.7 per 100,000 individuals.[28] The usual presentation is acute, with retrosternal 'chest pain' and pleuritic features (>85% of cases), worsening with inspiration and in the supine position. A pericardial friction rub on physical examination that sounds like walking in fresh snow is present in a minority of patients. Pericarditis may also result in a non-specific increase in pericardial echogenicity, probably related to oedema and fibrinous exudation in the pericardial layers. However, this finding is non-specific, as it is frequently present in healthy young, non-obese people. Importantly, the absence of a pericardial effusion does not exclude pericarditis. Chemistry may show elevation of inflammatory markers (CRP and white cell count) in most cases within 6 hours from onset of symptoms, but not in all cases because of a possible early presentation or effects of empirical anti-inflammatory therapies. Normal markers of inflammation do not exclude pericarditis.[28,30] In developing countries, tuberculosis is the most common cause of pericarditis and pericardial diseases, and is often associated with human immunodeficiency virus (HIV) infection, especially in specific geographical areas such as sub-Saharan Africa.[31] Clinical diagnosis of pericarditis can be made *with at least two of the criteria* shown in ⊃ Table 3.5.5.[28]

In cases of atypical or doubtful presentation, elevation of inflammatory markers or imaging evidence of pericardial inflammation may be helpful. CMR is the preferred technique, with evidence of oedema on T2-weighted dark blood images and the presence of late gadolinium enhancement.[32]

In pericarditis, the main aim of this diagnostic workup is to exclude the most common important aetiologies:

1 Bacterial (especially tuberculosis and purulent pericarditis)

2 Cancer (usually secondary pericardial involvement from lung and breast cancer or lymphomas, leukaemia, contiguous cancer, for example, oesophageal or gastric cancer, pleural

mesothelioma, and melanoma; rare as primary—mainly pericardial mesothelioma)

3 Systemic inflammatory diseases.

For bacterial and neoplastic pericarditis, a *definite diagnosis* consists of identification of the aetiological agent in the pericardial fluid or tissue, whereas a *probable diagnosis* is based on assessment of markers (e.g. adenosine deaminase, unstimulated interferon gamma, tumour markers) in the pericardial fluid or on evidence of the disease elsewhere in patients with concomitant pericarditis and usually moderate to large pericardial effusions.[28]

For patients with pericarditis, in the absence of a specific aetiology other than viral (idiopathic), the *mainstay of therapy* is colchicine using weight-adjusted doses for at least 3 months.[6,28,33,34,35] Aspirin or a non-steroidal anti-inflammatory drug (NSAID) is provided as attack doses every 8 hours to better control symptoms. The aim of this anti-inflammatory therapy is to control chest pain, improve remission rates over short-term follow-up (1 week), and prevent recurrence of pericarditis with colchicine. In patients with a second episode after 3 months' therapy, colchicine and an NSAID should be given for 1 year, or lifelong after a third episode.[36,37,38] Corticosteroids should NOT be considered as a first-line therapy, except in patients with a history of allergy or hypersensitivity to aspirin/NSAIDs or those already on corticosteroids for a specific indication (e.g. systemic inflammatory disease on steroids, pregnancy).[28,39]

In pericarditis not responding sufficiently to colchicine, corticosteroids are given on top of colchicine. Low to moderate doses (e.g. prednisone 0.2–0.5 mg/kg/day or equivalent) should be provided for 2–4 weeks, followed by slow and gradual tapering.[28,39] If a specific aetiology is identified, targeted therapy is warranted. Recently, anti-interleukin-1 receptor antagonists (anakinra, rilonacept) emerged as a promising novel therapeutic approach in colchicine-resistant recurrent pericarditis.[39,40,41] Larger studies are needed to replicate findings, as well as to assess safety and longer-term efficacy.

The choice of drug should be based on the history of the patient (contraindications, previous efficacy, or side effects), the presence of concomitant diseases (favouring aspirin over other NSAIDs

Table 3.5.5 Definitions and diagnostic criteria for acute pericarditis

Pericarditis	Definition and diagnostic criteria
Acute	At least two of the four following criteria should be present: 1. Pericarditic chest pain 2. Pericardial rubs 3. New widespread ST-segment elevation or PR depression on ECG 4. Pericardial effusion (new or worsening) Additional supporting findings: ◆ Elevation of markers of inflammation (i.e. C-reactive protein, erythrocyte sedimentation rate, and white cell count) ◆ Evidence of pericardial inflammation by an imaging technique (computed tomography, cardiac magnetic resonance)

when aspirin is already needed as antiplatelet treatment), and physician expertise.

Percutaneous pericardiotomy is an evolving and potentially promising mode of treatment in HFpEF, with a successful experimental proof-of-concept which is yet to be proven in the clinical setting. This minimally invasive procedure mitigates elevation in left ventricular filling pressures with volume loading in diastolic dysfunction and could be especially beneficial in right heart failure (with or without pulmonary hypertension) and in obese HFpEF patients.[42,43,44]

Heart failure in constrictive pericarditis

Constrictive pericarditis is a potentially curable form of heart failure caused by fibrotic changes (with or without calcification) and/or thickening of the pericardium. Transient constriction is frequently unrecognized in acute pericarditis or iatrogenic pericardial injury or trauma. Constrictive pericarditis may resolve spontaneously within 6–12 weeks, but its resolution can be facilitated by anti-inflammatory medications (colchicine, NSAIDs, and more recently anakinra).[28,45,46,47] The probability of recovery is higher in patients with markedly elevated CRP levels and signs of pericardial inflammation on CMR.[48,49] Chronic constrictive pericarditis is caused by previous infectious or tuberculous pericarditis, acute cardiac surgery, connective tissue diseases, or radiation therapy. Clinical manifestations include progressive fatigue, breathlessness, and poor effort tolerance, along with signs of right heart failure, including jugular venous distension, peripheral oedema, liver enlargement, ascites, and cardiac cachexia. Main changes in cardiac haemodynamics comprise rapid rise in diastolic pressures and their equalization at end-diastole in both ventricles.[50] More specific invasive haemodynamic criteria for constrictive pericarditis are based on discordant left and right ventricular systolic pressure changes with respiration.[51,52] Respiratory variation in ventricular filling and interventricular dependence are part of the specific diagnostic criteria for constrictive pericarditis.[53] Respiratory variations of 30% or more in mitral inflow and hepatic vein velocity patterns and early diastolic velocity of the mitral annulus are also contributing to the diagnosis.[53,54] The differential diagnosis should include restrictive cardiomyopathy, amyloidosis, chronic obstructive lung disease, and pulmonary arterial hypertension. However, the pulmonary artery systolic pressure is usually lower than 50 mmHg in constrictive pericarditis. Combined post-capillary and precapillary pulmonary hypertension develops in a subset of patients with constrictive pericarditis and is associated with long-term mortality after pericardiectomy.[55]

For chronic constrictive pericarditis, complete pericardiectomy is the treatment of choice, resulting in complete recovery if the procedure is timely and successfully performed. Before surgery, anti-inflammatory treatment should be applied for at least 3–6 months to facilitate recovery in transient constriction (>20% of patients).[28,45] Patients with advanced disease with extensive myocardial fibrosis have very high perioperative mortality and a poor prognosis.[55,56,57,58,59] Residual constriction can persist after incomplete pericardiectomy, and recurrent constrictive pericarditis can occur if the aetiology of the disease has not been treated (e.g. tuberculosis).[56] After a successful and timely pericardiectomy, a large majority of patients can fully recover, but not to the level to be involved in competitive sports.[23,60]

Key messages

- Myocarditis is a heterogeneous disease with great variability in clinical presentation and evolution.
- Myocarditis may be caused by many aetiological agents, with distinct immunophenotypes, being mostly the result of patient-dependent immune susceptibility.
- Patients with a pseudo-myocardial infarction presentation, preserved biventricular function, and concomitant pericarditis (myopericarditis) usually have an uncomplicated course, with a good prognosis.
- Patients with persistent heart failure, left ventricular dysfunction, and arrhythmias require a targeted approach with specific diagnostics (EMB), therapies, and prolonged follow-up.
- Although EBM provides definite confirmation of myocarditis, non-invasive imaging with CMR may be sufficient for a clinical diagnosis and follow-up in uncomplicated cases.
- EMB is strongly indicated in patients with recurrent myocarditis, persistent systolic dysfunction, or suspected giant cell myocarditis, or sarcoidosis of the heart.
- Small or moderate pericardial transudate frequently accompanies advanced heart failure, especially in patients with pulmonary hypertension, and is a marker of poor prognosis.
- Viral and idiopathic pericarditis are the most common forms of acute pericarditis encountered in clinical practice in developed countries with a low prevalence of tuberculosis.
- Specific features at presentation may suggest an increased risk of complications during follow-up: non-viral aetiologies (e.g. high fever >38°C (100.4 °F)), a subacute course with symptoms over several days without a clear-cut acute onset, evidence of large pericardial effusion with diastolic echo-free space of >20 mm, cardiac tamponade, failure to respond within 7 days to aspirin/NSAID, associated myocarditis (myopericarditis), immunodepression, trauma, and oral anticoagulant therapy.
- The presence of one or more of these features identifies a potentially high-risk case of acute pericarditis for admission. In these cases, searching for the aetiology is mandatory.
- Patients with acute pericarditis and no risk features can be considered at low risk and managed as outpatients. In these cases, follow-up is mandatory after 1 week to assess the response to empirical anti-inflammatory therapy.
- Mainstay of therapy in pericarditis is anti-inflammatory therapy with colchicine plus aspirin or an NSAID.
- The course of acute pericarditis is relatively benign and self-limiting, and is rarely complicated with recurrences or pericardial constriction.
- For chronic constrictive pericarditis, complete pericardiectomy is the treatment of choice, resulting in complete recovery if the procedure is timely and successfully performed.

Before surgery, anti-inflammatory treatment should be given for at least 3–6 months to facilitate recovery in transient forms of constriction.

References

1. Heymans S, Eriksson U, Lehtonen J, Cooper LT Jr. The quest for new approaches in myocarditis and inflammatory cardiomyopathy. J Am Coll Cardiol. 2016;68(21):2348–64.

2. Global Burden of Disease Study 2013 Collaborators. Global, regional, and national incidence, prevalence, and years lived with disability for 301 acute and chronic diseases and injuries in 188 countries, 1990–2013: a systematic analysis for the Global Burden of Disease Study 2013. Lancet. 2015;386(9995):743–800.

3. Hazebroek MR, Moors S, Dennert R, et al. Prognostic relevance of gene–environment interactions in patients with dilated cardiomyopathy: applying the MOGE(S) Classification. J Am Coll Cardiol. 2015;66(12):1313–23.

4. Corsten MF, Papageorgiou A, Verhesen W, et al. MicroRNA profiling identifies microRNA-155 as an adverse mediator of cardiac injury and dysfunction during acute viral myocarditis. Circ Res. 2012;111(4):415–25.

5. Hazebroek M, Dennert R, Heymans S. Virus infection of the heart: unmet therapeutic needs. Antivir Chem Chemother. 2012;22(6):249–53.

6. Imazio M, Gaita F, LeWinter M. Evaluation and treatment of pericarditis: a systematic review. JAMA. 2015;314(14):1498–506.

7. Caforio AL, Pankuweit S, Arbustini E, et al.; European Society of Cardiology Working Group on Myocardial and Pericardial Diseases. Current state of knowledge on aetiology, diagnosis, management, and therapy of myocarditis: a position statement of the European Society of Cardiology Working Group on Myocardial and Pericardial Diseases. Eur Heart J. 2013;34(33):2636–48, 2648a–d.

8. Ammirati E, Cipriani M, Moro C, et al.; Registro Lombardo delle Miocarditi. Clinical presentation and outcome in a contemporary cohort of patients with acute myocarditis: Multicenter Lombardy Registry. Circulation. 2018;138(11):1088–99.

9. Imazio M, Lazaros G, Picardi E, et al. Incidence and prognostic significance of new onset atrial fibrillation/flutter in acute pericarditis. Heart. 2015;101(18):1463–7.

10. Tschöpe C, Ammirati E, Bozkurt B, et al. Myocarditis and inflammatory cardiomyopathy: current evidence and future directions. Nat Rev Cardiol. 2021;18(3):169–93.

11. Ferreira VM, Schulz-Menger J, Holmvang G, et al. Cardiovascular magnetic resonance in nonischemic myocardial inflammation: expert recommendations. J Am Coll Cardiol. 2018;72(24):3158–76.

12. Lauri G, Rossi C, Rubino M, et al. B-type natriuretic peptide levels in patients with pericardial effusion undergoing pericardiocentesis. Int J Cardiol. 2016;212:318–23.

13. Blanco-Domínguez R, Sánchez-Díaz R, de la Fuente H, et al. A novel circulating microRNA for the detection of acute myocarditis. N Engl J Med. 2021;384(21):2014–27.

14. Ader F, Surget E, Charron P, et al. Inherited cardiomyopathies revealed by clinically suspected myocarditis: highlights from genetic testing. Circ Genom Precis Med. 2020;13(4):e002744.

15. Wilde AAM, Semsarian C, Márquez MF, et al. ESC Scientific Document Group. European Heart Rhythm Association (EHRA)/Heart Rhythm Society (HRS)/Asia Pacific Heart Rhythm Society (APHRS)/Latin American Heart Rhythm Society (LAHRS) Expert Consensus Statement on the state of genetic testing for cardiac diseases. Europace. 2022:euac030.

16. Seferović PM, Tsutsui H, McNamara DM, et al. Heart Failure Association of the ESC, Heart Failure Society of America and Japanese Heart Failure Society position statement on endomyocardial biopsy. Eur J Heart Fail. 2021;23(6):854–71.

17. McDonagh TA, Metra M, Adamo M, et al.; ESC Scientific Document Group. 2021 ESC Guidelines for the diagnosis and treatment of acute and chronic heart failure. Eur Heart J. 2021;42(36):3599–726.

18. Merken J, Hazebroek M, Van Paassen P, et al. Immunosuppressive therapy improves both short- and long-term prognosis in patients with virus-negative nonfulminant inflammatory cardiomyopathy. Circ Heart Fail. 2018;11(2):e004228.

19. Cheng CY, Baritussio A, Giordani AS, Iliceto S, Marcolongo R, Caforio ALP. Myocarditis in systemic immune-mediated diseases: prevalence, characteristics and prognosis. A systematic review. Autoimmun Rev. 2022;21(4):103037.

20. Cheng CY, Cheng GY, Shan ZG, et al. Efficacy of immunosuppressive therapy in myocarditis: a 30-year systematic review and meta analysis. Autoimmun Rev. 2021;20(1):102710.

21. Sinagra G, Anzini M, Pereira NL, et al. Myocarditis in clinical practice. Mayo Clin Proc. 2016;91(9):1256–66.

22. Frustaci A, Russo MA, Chimenti C. Randomized study on the efficacy of immunosuppressive therapy in patients with virus-negative inflammatory cardiomyopathy: the TIMIC study. Eur Heart J. 2009;30(16):1995–2002.

23. Pelliccia A, Solberg EE, Papadakis M, et al. Recommendations for participation in competitive and leisure time sport in athletes with cardiomyopathies, myocarditis, and pericarditis: position statement of the Sport Cardiology Section of the European Association of Preventive Cardiology (EAPC). Eur Heart J. 2019;40(1):19–33.

24. Sotiriou E, Heiner S, Jansen T, et al. Therapeutic implications of a combined diagnostic workup including endomyocardial biopsy in an all-comer population of patients with heart failure: a retrospective analysis. ESC Heart Fail. 2018;5(4):630–41.

25. Maisch B, Hufnagel G, Kölsch S, et al. Treatment of inflammatory dilated cardiomyopathy and (peri)myocarditis with immunosuppression and i.v. immunoglobulins. Herz. 2004;29(6):624–36.

26. Hazebroek MR, Henkens M, Raafs AG, et al. Intravenous immunoglobulin therapy in adult patients with idiopathic chronic cardiomyopathy and cardiac parvovirus B19 persistence: a prospective, double-blind, randomized, placebo-controlled clinical trial. Eur J Heart Fail. 2021;23:302–9.

27. Borlaug BA, Reddy YNV. The role of the pericardium in heart failure: implications for pathophysiology and treatment. JACC Heart Fail. 2019;7(7):574–85.

28. Adler Y, Charron P, Imazio M, et al.; ESC Scientific Document Group. 2015 ESC Guidelines for the diagnosis and management of pericardial diseases: The Task Force for the Diagnosis and Management of Pericardial Diseases of the European Society of Cardiology (ESC) Endorsed by: The European Association for Cardio-Thoracic Surgery (EACTS). Eur Heart J. 2015;36(42):2921–64.

29. Miró Ò, Sabaté M, Jiménez S, et al.; Spanish Investigators on Emergency Situations TeAm (SIESTA) network; SIESTA network. A case-control, multicentre study of consecutive patients with COVID-19 and acute (myo)pericarditis: incidence, risk factors, clinical characteristics and outcomes. Emerg Med J. 2022;39(5):402–10.

30. Imazio M, Brucato A, Maestroni S, et al. Prevalence of C-reactive protein elevation and time course of normalization in acute pericarditis: implications for the diagnosis, therapy, and prognosis of pericarditis. Circulation. 2011;123(10):1092–7.

31. Mayosi BM. Contemporary trends in the epidemiology and management of cardiomyopathy and pericarditis in sub-Saharan Africa. Heart. 2007;93(10):1176–83.

32. Cosyns B, Plein S, Nihoyanopoulos P, *et al.*; European Association of Cardiovascular Imaging (EACVI); European Society of Cardiology Working Group (ESC WG) on Myocardial and Pericardial diseases. European Association of Cardiovascular Imaging (EACVI) position paper: multimodality imaging in pericardial disease. Eur Heart J Cardiovasc Imaging. 2015;16(1):12–31.

33. Imazio M, Brucato A, Cemin R, *et al.*; ICAP Investigators. A randomized trial of colchicine for acute pericarditis. N Engl J Med. 2013;369(16):1522–8.

34. Imazio M, Bobbio M, Cecchi E, *et al.* Colchicine in addition to conventional therapy for acute pericarditis: results of the COlchicine for acute PEricarditis (COPE) trial. Circulation. 2005;112(13):2012–16.

35. Chiabrando JG, Bonaventura A, Vecchié A, *et al.* Management of acute and recurrent pericarditis: JACC state-of-the-art review. J Am Coll Cardiol. 2020;75(1):76–92.

36. Imazio M, Brucato A, Ferrazzi P, *et al.*; COPPS-2 Investigators. Colchicine for prevention of postpericardiotomy syndrome and postoperative atrial fibrillation: the COPPS-2 randomized clinical trial. JAMA. 2014;312(10):1016–23.

37. Imazio M, Brucato A, Cemin R, *et al.*; CORP (COlchicine for Recurrent Pericarditis) Investigators. Colchicine for recurrent pericarditis (CORP): a randomized trial. Ann Intern Med. 2011;155(7):409–14.

38. Imazio M, Bobbio M, Cecchi E, *et al.* Colchicine as first-choice therapy for recurrent pericarditis: results of the CORE (COlchicine for REcurrent pericarditis) trial. Arch Intern Med. 2005;165(17):1987–91.

39. Imazio M. Pharmacologic therapies for pericarditis: the past, the present, and the future. Trends Cardiovasc Med. 2022;S1050-1738(22)00044-5.

40. Brucato A, Imazio M, Gattorno M, *et al.* Effect of anakinra on recurrent pericarditis among patients with colchicine resistance and corticosteroid dependence: the AIRTRIP randomized clinical trial. JAMA. 2016;316(18):1906–12.

41. Klein AL, Imazio M, Cremer P, *et al.*; RHAPSODY Investigators. Phase 3 trial of interleukin-1 trap rilonacept in recurrent pericarditis. N Engl J Med. 2021;384(1):31–41.

42. Borlaug BA, Carter RE, Melenovsky V, *et al.* Percutaneous pericardial resection: a novel potential treatment for heart failure with preserved ejection fraction. Circ Heart Fail. 2017;10(4):e003612.

43. Borlaug BA, Schaff HV, Pochettino A, *et al.* Pericardiotomy enhances left ventricular diastolic reserve with volume loading in humans. Circulation. 2018;138(20):2295–7.

44. Jain CC, Pedrotty D, Araoz PA, *et al.* Sustained improvement in diastolic reserve following percutaneous pericardiotomy in a porcine model of heart failure with preserved ejection fraction. Circ Heart Fail. 2021;14(2):e007530.

45. Haley JH, Tajik AJ, Danielson GK, Schaff HV, Mulvagh SL, Oh JK. Transient constrictive pericarditis: causes and natural history. J Am Coll Cardiol. 2004;43(2):271–5.

46. Gentry J, Klein AL, Jellis CL. Transient constrictive pericarditis: current diagnostic and therapeutic strategies. Curr Cardiol Rep. 2016;18(5):41.

47. Andreis A, Imazio M, Giustetto C, Brucato A, Adler Y, De Ferrari GM. Anakinra for constrictive pericarditis associated with incessant or recurrent pericarditis. Heart. 2020;106(20):1561–5.

48. Cremer PC, Tariq MU, Karwa A, *et al.* Quantitative assessment of pericardial delayed hyperenhancement predicts clinical improvement in patients with constrictive pericarditis treated with anti-inflammatory therapy. Circ Cardiovasc Imaging. 2015;8(5): e003125.

49. Feng D, Glockner J, Kim K, *et al.* Cardiac magnetic resonance imaging pericardial late gadolinium enhancement and elevated inflammatory markers can predict the reversibility of constrictive pericarditis after antiinflammatory medical therapy: a pilot study. Circulation. 2011;124:1830–7.

50. Tzani A, Doulamis IP, Tzoumas A, *et al.* Meta-analysis of population characteristics and outcomes of patients undergoing pericardiectomy for constrictive pericarditis. Am J Cardiol. 2021; 146:120–7.

51. Talreja DR, Nishimura RA, Oh JK, Holmes DR. Constrictive pericarditis in the modern era: novel criteria for diagnosis in the cardiac catheterization laboratory. J Am Coll Cardiol. 2008;51(3):315–19.

52. Yang JH, Miranda WR, Borlaug BA, *et al.* Right atrial/pulmonary arterial wedge pressure ratio in primary and mixed constrictive pericarditis. J Am Coll Cardiol. 2019;73(25):3312–21.

53. Welch TD, Ling LH, Espinosa RE, *et al.* Echocardiographic diagnosis of constrictive pericarditis: Mayo Clinic criteria. Circ Cardiovasc Imaging. 2014;7(3):526–34.

54. Chetrit M, Xu B, Verma BR, Klein AL. Multimodality imaging for the assessment of pericardial diseases. Curr Cardiol Rep. 2019; 21(5):41.

55. Lim K, Yang JH, Miranda WR, *et al.* Clinical significance of pulmonary hypertension in patients with constrictive pericarditis. Heart. 2021;107(20):1651–6.

56. Murashita T, Schaff HV, Daly RC, *et al.* Experience with pericardiectomy for constrictive pericarditis over eight decades. Ann Thorac Surg. 2017;104(3):742–50.

57. Liu VC, Fritz AV, Burtoft MA, Martin AK, Greason KL, Ramakrishna H. Pericardiectomy for constrictive pericarditis: analysis of outcomes. J Cardiothorac Vasc Anesth. 2021;35(12):3797–805.

58. Yadav S, Shah S, Iqbal Z, *et al.* Pericardiectomy for constrictive tuberculous pericarditis: a systematic review and meta-analysis on the etiology, patients' characteristics, and the outcomes. Cureus. 2021;13(9):e18252.

59. Huang JB, Wen ZK, Yang JR, *et al.* Analysis of risk factors of early mortality after pericardiectomy for constrictive pericarditis. Heart Surg Forum. 2022;25(1):E056–64.

60. Seidenberg PH, Haynes J. Pericarditis: diagnosis, management, and return to play. Curr Sports Med Rep. 2006;5(2):74–9.

CHAPTER 3.6

Congenital heart disease

Werner Budts and Jolien Roos-Hesselink

Contents

Introduction

The number of patients with congenital heart disease (CHD) who reach adulthood is continuously increasing. It can be stated that 90% of children with CHD survive into adulthood.[1] Moreover, in the last few years, the number of adults with CHD has exceeded the number of children with a congenital heart defect. As a consequence, today, increasing care is needed for adult congenital heart disease (ACHD). Although the majority of ACHD patients have a stable health, many will develop complications later in life (◗ Figure 3.6.1), of which arrhythmia and heart failure (HF) are the two most common. The literature reports an overall prevalence of complications in one-quarter of patients after a median follow-up of 35 years.[2,3] However, the prevalence might even rise to 60% according to the underlying ACHD diagnosis.[4] These complications are associated with premature death and increased hospitalization, and negatively impact the quality of life. There is a tendency to extrapolate the treatment strategy used in patients with acquired heart disease to ACHD patients with HF. In some cases, this is acceptable and could have beneficial effects on clinical outcome, but in other cases, this standard approach to treat HF might have adverse effects, with progressive deterioration of the clinical status of the patient. The reason for this phenomenon is that ACHD patients are a highly heterogenous population, with failure of not only a systemic left ventricle (LV), but also of a systemic subpulmonary right ventricle (RV) or a single ventricle, with or without persistent left-to-right or right-to-left shunting. It is obvious that standard drug therapy could cause adverse effects. Today all therapeutic suggestions are based on expert opinion (level of evidence C).[5] Even use of resynchronization therapy, the criteria for, and timing of, ventricular assist device (VAD) implantation, and timing of (combined) transplantation are unexplored in larger ACHD series. The relatively low number of ACHD patients per expert centre and the high heterogeneity of the ACHD HF population make it almost impossible to set up randomized controlled trials (RCTs) with a view to ameliorate the level of evidence from C to A. This chapter provides an overview of the complexity of ACHD HF patients and proposes some treatment recommendations. These recommendations must be appreciated on top of existing guidelines. In addition, emphasis is put on the clear need for further studies, preferably RCTs.

Heterogeneity and pathophysiology

In general cardiology, HF is in the majority of cases related to a failing systemic LV. Failing might occur in systole and/or in diastole, known as HF with reduced ejection fraction (EF) and HF with preserved EF, respectively. There are many ACHD patients who might fit in these HF categories, in relation to impaired systemic LV function, such as those with aortic coarctation or aortic stenosis. A failing subpulmonary RV is also

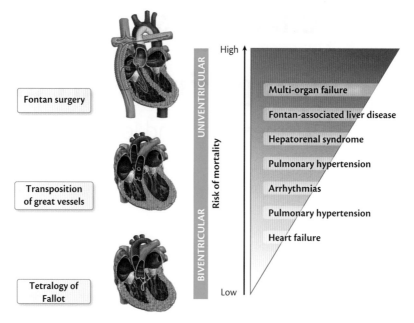

Figure 3.6.1 Congenital heart disease and mortality/complication risks.

not that uncommon in general cardiology and is mostly related to pressure load on the RV secondary to moderate to severe pulmonary hypertension or volume load caused by severe tricuspid valve regurgitation. The subpulmonary RV in ACHD patients might also be volume-loaded due to a significant supratricuspid left-to-right shunt or moderate to severe long-standing pulmonary valve regurgitation (e.g. tetralogy of Fallot). These causes are rather rare in acquired heart disease. Moreover, not all subpulmonary ventricles in ACHD are morphological RVs, but LVs (after atrial switch repair for transposition of the great arteries (dextro (d)-TGA) and in congenitally corrected transposition of the great arteries (ccTGA)). The haemodynamic effects of pressure and/or volume overload in these cases differ from those on a subpulmonary RV and might need an altered therapeutic approach. As a consequence, many ACHD patients have a systemic RV instead of an LV (TGA with atrial switch or ccTGA). Which structural and functional parameters are considered to be normal for a systemic RV are unknown, and this knowledge gap makes it difficult to define a failing systemic RV and determine when to diagnose HF.[6] Therefore, it still remains unclear when to start HF therapy and, if commenced, what kind of therapy should be given. General cardiology is dealing with a typical biventricular circulation: two pumps—one for the systemic circulation and one for the pulmonary circulation. In more complex ACHD, a univentricular circulation or a one and a half circulation might be present (e.g. tricuspid atresia). These ventricles might also become dysfunctional and lead to clinical signs of HF. However, these signs could be misleading, and be related to circulatory failure (which differs from HF), and not to ventricular dysfunction, but rather be caused by circulatory obstructions in the circuit. A typical example is an obstruction to the systemic venous return in a Fontan circuit. Clinical signs of HF might be present but should be considered as due to circulatory failure.[7] Obviously,

HF in ACHD might also occur due to tachyarrhythmias or even ischaemic heart disease.[8] The incidence of acquired heart disease is rising because of the ageing ACHD population. Moreover, it is hypothesized that ACHD patients might have a genetic predisposition for an abnormal haemodynamic reaction, which might explain the faster progression to HF in some specific patients.

Finally, similar to HF in acquired heart disease, HF in ACHD has to be considered as a multi-organ disease. HF in ACHD might be related to impaired renal function, and cardiac liver cirrhosis is not uncommon in a failing Fontan circuit or in ACHD pathology with elevated systemic atrial pressures. Protein-losing enteropathy might occur in a failing Fontan circuit. Chronic elevated systemic venous filling pressures are considered to trigger the development of protein-losing enteropathy (PLE) and plastic bronchitis. The literature reports that, in some cases, approximately 30–50% of ACHD patients show significantly impaired renal function.[9] Haematological disorders occur often in cyanotic patients with elevated haematocrit levels, triggering symptoms and complications related to hyperviscosity.

Diagnosis

The diagnostic process of symptomatic and clinical HF in ACHD basically is similar to diagnosing HF in acquired heart disease. Progressive impairment of functional capacity and typical signs of systemic and/or subpulmonary HF make the diagnosis quite clear. However, exercise capacity can also be lower in ACHD patients without obvious HF,[10] which sometimes makes the diagnosis of HF very difficult. Moreover, clinical signs in ACHD might be misleading. Patients who underwent a bidirectional Glenn procedure have—even in the absence of HF—an increased jugular venous pressure because of the connection of the superior vena cava (SVC) to the pulmonary circulation. Also, in Fontan patients in whom both the SVC and the inferior vena cava are connected to the pulmonary circulation, more congestion occurs—in many cases, without signs of circulatory failure. Electrocardiography, echocardiography, and, if requested, cardiac magnetic resonance imaging or computed tomography might help to confirm a clinical diagnosis of HF and to identify the triggering aetiology. Measuring biomarker levels (B-type natriuretic peptide and N-terminal pro-B-type natriuretic peptide) in these patients is of utmost importance by confirming the diagnosis of HF and has added value in determining the prognosis and outcome. However, biomarker levels might be moderately increased in more complex ACHD without signs or symptoms of HF. The latter can also complicate the diagnosis of HF.

The diagnosis of HF in asymptomatic patients is less evident, especially when clinical signs of HF are absent. Technical examinations might help in assessing for signs of HF, but in many cases, only ventricular performance is impaired. In acquired heart disease, when the systemic LV function is reduced to an EF <50%, it can be considered as preclinical HF, in which case, treatment is generally initiated. However, whereas in acquired heart disease, myocardial dysfunction is progressing, this is not usually the case in typical ACHD patients with a systemic LV; for example, a patient who underwent a ventricular septal defect closure with a large patch might have an EF <50% and remain stable for many years or even lifelong, without the need for drug treatment. Thus, EF as an only parameter is not sufficiently reliable to confirm a diagnosis of HF. Here, changes in biomarker levels and/or changes in exercise capacity (measured on cardiopulmonary exercise testing) might help to identify the transition from still normal ventricular function to pathological ventricular dysfunction with output failure. A position paper from the Working Group of Grown-Up Congenital Heart Disease and the Heart Failure Association of the European Society of Cardiology (ESC) has proposed an algorithm that could be applied in daily practice.[8] A more recent review by Leusveld et al. and the new ESC guidelines on ACHD[5] recommend to shift the use of biomarkers earlier in the diagnostic algorithm for HF in ACHD.[11]

The same problem occurs and is even more prominent in patients with a systemic RV. The systemic RV in ACHD patients has rarely an EF ≥50% and this is often the reason why patients with a systemic RV are too quickly and unjustifiably considered to be in HF. Also, the EF measurements obtained from patients with a single ventricle or with a one and a half circulation may not really help in identifying a deterioration of myocardial function. In both cases, changes in biomarker levels and/or changes in exercise capacity might help to identify the first stage in the evolution to symptomatic and clinical HF.[8] An example of a diagnostic algorithm that could be applied is presented in ⊃ Figure 3.6.2.

Medical treatment

Before medical treatment is started, structural optimization always needs to be considered and performed when possible. As in acquired heart disease, pressure and/or volume unloading of a ventricle by carrying out a surgical or interventional procedure might lead to positive remodelling of the systemic or subpulmonary ventricle and prevent the development of clinically evident HF. In addition, arrhythmias need to be treated when and where possible. Although the ESC HF guidelines[12] recommended for patients with acquired heart disease are frequently also applied to ACHD patients, the level of evidence for doing so is still lacking. Therefore, extrapolation of recommendations may not be appropriate and an individualized approach is warranted for ACHD patients.

Failure of the systemic left ventricle in adult congenital heart disease

In ACHD with output failure from a systemic LV, neurohormonal and cardiac autonomic activity is increased. With the diagnostic criteria in mind, initiation of standard HF therapy can

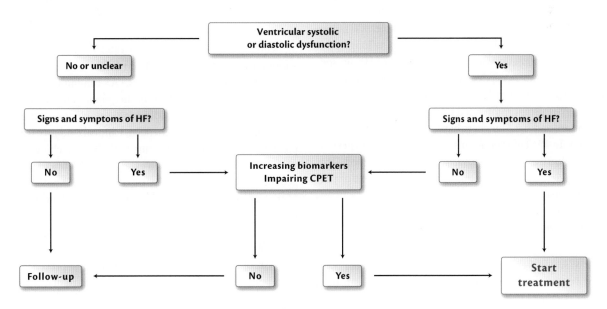

Figure 3.6.2 Example of a diagnostic algorithm to diagnose and treat heart failure. This algorithm begins with imaging as the first step. Different variants of this algorithm exist and are mainly centre- or opinion-based.

be considered, more specifically renin–angiotensin–aldosterone system (RAAS) inhibitors, beta-blockers, mineralocorticoid receptor antagonists, and diuretics. Although use of digoxin remains controversial, it may be beneficial in patients with diminished ventricular function and atrial fibrillation with increased ventricular response. The decision to start treatment is straightforward when symptoms and clinical signs are present. However, the benefit of medical treatment in ACHD patients with impaired systemic LV function with no increase in biomarker levels or decrease in exercise capacity has never been documented.

Failure of the systemic right ventricle in adult congenital heart disease

Although not supported by any scientific evidence, standard HF therapy is initiated as part of routine management of most patients with a failing systemic RV. Beneficial effects are expected in theory, based on increased neurohormonal and autonomic activity. However, it remains unclear whether patients with a systemic RV and reduced EF, with or without an increase in biomarker levels and/or impaired exercise capacity, would benefit from standard HF therapy. Many centres do not initiate treatment if there is no change in functional status and no increase in biomarker levels. It remains doubtful of whether to initiate standard HF treatment even when patients remain completely asymptomatic, with increasing biomarker levels. RAAS inhibitors have not been proven to show clear clinical benefits, except in some symptomatic patients,[13,14,15] whereas beta-blockers might have a positive effect on functional capacity, atrioventricular valve regurgitation, and RV remodelling.[16,17,18] Use of diuretics achieves the most rapid subjective positive response, and when there is evidence of fluid retention, diuretics should be prescribed.

Failure of the subpulmonary right ventricle in adult congenital heart disease

The subpulmonary RV in ACHD is more frequently exposed to volume and/or pressure overload than in acquired heart disease. When timely structural optimization is not possible, RV failure can occur, leading to systemic venous congestion. As long as patients remain asymptomatic, with no clinical signs of HF, no specific medical treatment is needed. When symptoms and clinical signs of HF are present, loop diuretics are the preferred choice. In cases of therapy-resistant right-sided HF, thiazides may be added. RAAS inhibitors and beta-blockers have never been investigated in this setting. In RV failure due to severe pulmonary hypertension, use of selective pulmonary vasodilators is preferred. This is discussed in detail in the ESC guidelines on treatment of pulmonary hypertension.[19]

Failure of the single ventricle in adult congenital heart disease

Failure of a single ventricle usually occurs in patients who underwent Fontan palliation. The dominant ventricle can be a morphological RV or LV. When the single ventricle becomes dysfunctional, pressures in the Fontan circuit increase, the circulation fails, and the patient becomes symptomatic. Loop diuretics are mostly used to lower the filling pressures and achieve symptomatic relief. However, overuse of diuretics can reduce the preload and cause a cardiorenal imbalance. Mineralocorticoid receptor antagonists can have a positive impact on PLE. There are no data to suggest a beneficial effect of RAAS inhibitors in Fontan patients. Only carvedilol has proven effects on symptoms and signs of HF. If the Fontan circuit fails due to progressive increase in pulmonary vascular resistance, selective pulmonary vasodilators, such as endothelin receptor antagonists or phosphodiesterase-5 inhibitors, can be considered.

Heart failure in ACHD patients with persistent right-to-left shunt

In more complex congenital heart defects, pulmonary blood flow might be decreased due to high pulmonary vascular resistance or mechanical outflow tract obstruction. Co-occurrence of an intra- or extracardiac shunt mediates right-to-left shunting, resulting in central cyanosis. Moreover, the systemic, subpulmonary, or single ventricle can also fail in these patients. In contrast to patients without shunting, reduced systemic afterload can further exacerbate right-to-left shunting and progressive systemic desaturation. In these patients, medical HF therapy always needs to be initiated with great caution.

The above paragraphs have mainly focused on therapeutic regimens for systolic dysfunction. However, HF with preserved EF can also occur in ACHD patients. LV outflow tract obstruction, including (sub)valvular aortic stenosis and coarctation, and genetic predisposition, chronic cyanosis, and chronic deprived ventricular filling, are potential causes of diastolic dysfunction of the ventricle. To date, no studies on medical treatment for diastolic HF have reported a beneficial effect on outcome. Again, data from general cardiology are extrapolated for application in the treatment of patients with ACHD, but without proven benefit. Diuretics might improve signs and symptoms, and use of beta-blockers is expected to prolong the ventricular filling time.[8]

Besides standard HF therapy, other pharmacological agents are also used in patients with ACHD. When beta-blockers prove inadequate in lowering the heart rate, ivabradine can be given, although the latter has only been tested in acquired heart disease.[20] When HF is resistant to RAAS inhibitors, a combination of valsartan and sacubitril could help maintain therapy-resistant patients compensated.[21] Adding sodium–glucose cotransporter 2 inhibitors might also be beneficial. Clinical evidence for iron supplementation in ACHD patients with HF is lacking, although it sounds scientifically logical to extend this treatment approach for general cardiology patients with HF to ACHD patients with HF. Moreover, iron deficiency is not that uncommon in ACHD patients[22] and needs to be treated to improve functional capacity.[23] Antiplatelet therapy or oral anticoagulation is only indicated in cases of coronary or peripheral atherosclerosis, or where there is a risk of local thrombus formation, in the presence of mechanical valves, or thrombogenic supraventricular arrhythmias, respectively.

A summary of medical treatment in ACHD patients with HF is provided in ➲ Table 3.6.1.

Table 3.6.1 Summary of medical treatment options in patients with heart failure and adult congenital heart disease

Systemic left ventricle	Extrapolation of standard heart failure therapy	RAAS inhibitors
		Beta-blockers
		MRAs
		Diuretics
		Digoxin in cases of atrial fibrillation with rapid ventricular response
	Start treatment	Signs and symptoms of HF
		Decreased exercise performance
		Increased biomarker levels
Systemic right ventricle	Extrapolation of standard heart failure therapy	RAAS inhibitors: no clear clinical benefit
		MRAs: effect unknown
		Beta-blockers: improve surrogate endpoints
		Diuretics to control signs/symptoms and if fluid retention
	Start treatment	Signs and symptoms of HF
		Decreased exercise performance
		Increased biomarkers
		Asymptomatic patient with increased biomarker levels: unknown
Subpulmonary right ventricle		RAAS inhibitors: never investigated
		Beta-blockers: never investigated
		Loop diuretics ± thiazides preferred if fluid retention
		Pulmonary vasodilators in cases of PAH
	Start treatment	Signs and symptoms of HF
Single ventricle	Applicable for Fontan circulation	RAAS inhibitors: no clear clinical benefit
		MRAs in cases of PLE
		Carvedilol with effect on signs and symptoms
		Balanced use of loop diruretics
		Selective pulmonary vasodilators in cases of increased PVR
	Start treatment	Signs and symptoms of circulatory failure
Persistent right left shunt	Central cyanosis	Avoid excessive systemic afterload reduction
	Start treatment	Signs and symptoms of HF

RAAS, renin–angiotensin–aldosterone system; MRA, mineralocorticoid receptor antagonist; HF, heart failure; PAH, pulmonary arterial hypertension; PLE, protein-losing enteropathy; PVR, pulmonary vascular resistance.

Device therapy

Cardiac resynchronization therapy

In patients who are unresponsive to medical treatment or in whom significant electromechanical dyssynchrony is present, cardiac resynchronization therapy (CRT) could play a beneficial role. CRT has been proven effective in the failing systemic LV where it can lead to functional improvement and a reduction in HF-associated morbidity and mortality. CRT is frequently associated with the implantation of an automatic defibrillator when the patient is at high risk of malignant arrhythmia and sudden cardiac death. In general, the proportion of non-responders are higher among ACHD patients, compared to patients with ischaemic heart disease and idiopathic dilated cardiomyopathy. Moreover, the long-term effects of CRT in ACHD patients are currently still unknown. However, there are some positive features that have been observed in ACHD patients treated with CRT. A systemic LV resynchronizes better than a systemic RV.[24] Also, when only the RV is continuously paced, the risk of dyssynchrony increases, in which case applying CRT could improve the resynchronization parameters.[25] CRT is also recommended for patients with double discordance and complete atrioventricular block, although anatomical issues may hamper device implantation. The pacing site for optimal results is of utmost importance, particularly in patients with single ventricle physiology.[25] In functional class IV patients, CRT can serve as a bridge to mechanical assist devices and/or heart transplantation. Remote monitoring, such as with use of implantable loop recorders, might help in early detection of malignant arrhythmia. More details on CRT and ACHD can be found in the respective guideline.[26]

Ventricular assist devices

Use of VADs is also applicable in ACHD patients with a failing systemic LV. They can be used as destination therapy or as a bridge to transplantation.[27] Use of VAD therapy has been described in some patients with a failing systolic RV, but success rates can be compromised by anatomical complexity, trabecularization of the RV, and associated comorbidity,[28,29] and even more so in patients with a failing Fontan circulation. The function of a single ventricle, both morphological LV and RV, can be supported by VAD therapy. However, liver cirrhosis, associated haematological and coagulations disorders, and anatomical/technical issues can undermine feasibility and beneficial clinical outcome.[30,31] Finally, VAD therapy can also be applied in cases of a failing subpulmonary ventricle, but again here no hard clinical outcome data are available to support a definite level of evidence.[27]

Assist devices and transplantation

The number of ACHD patients with end-stage HF is continuously increasing. In general, when the systemic LV or RV starts to fail in biventricular circulation, pulmonary vascular resistance is meticulously monitored to avoid a combined heart–lung transplantation. It has been suggested that the short-term outcome of transplantation in ACHD patients is worse, compared to that in patients with non-ACHD pathology (20–30% 30-day mortality in ACHD patients). However, long-term outcome seems to be similar to, or even better than, that in patients with acquired heart disease. Following the first year post-transplantation, ACHD patients showed improved survival: 5-year survival ranged from 69% to 80%, compared to approximately 72% in non-ACHD patients, whereas 10-year survival was even further improved, ranging from 52.8% to 57.4%, compared with 50.9% to 53.6% in non-ACHD transplant recipients.[32] The transplant risk is higher in ACHD patients with single-ventricle lesions, compared to those with a biventricular circulation.[33] Moreover, human leucocyte antigen sensitization is detrimental to transplant outcome and is a specific concern in patients with ACHD who already underwent several surgical procedures or blood transfusion, and/or had pregnancies in the past.[34] Assist devices might be used as a bridge to transplantation or as destination therapy. The results of heart transplantation for both failing LV and RV are good. In some patients, only a heart–lung transplantation is an option, especially in patients with Eisenmenger syndrome or those in whom the pulmonary vascular circulation remains immature. The high number of bronchial collateral arteries, and consequently associated high intraoperative bleeding risk, could reduce the success rate of a heart–lung transplantation down to only 50%. Moreover, there is the constant ethical balance between the number of donors and the number of patients on the waiting list. A heart–lung transplantation uses three organs that could be implanted in three other patients. Many centres have abandoned combined heart–lung transplantation because of the high operative risk and the shortage of donors. Some specific cases are chosen for double lung transplantation and repair of (simple) underlying congenital heart defects. Most of these results are similar to, or even worse than, standard heart–lung transplantation. Long bypass time, as well as longer ischaemic time, compromises, in most of these cases, this type of approach. An emerging issue is progressive failure of the Fontan circulation. A single heart transplantation should be the most effective approach, but a failing Fontan circuit is frequently associated with liver cirrhosis. Many transplant centres opt for combined heart–liver transplantation, but this intervention has to be seen as high risk and relevant experience is very limited. A failing Fontan circulation is characterized by multi-organ dysfunction, which, in turn, influences the clinical outcome. Finally, the anatomical complexity and the number of previous interventions have to be taken into account for risk estimation. Timely counselling offered by expert transplant centres is needed in this complex decision-making process.

Cardiopulmonary rehabilitation

The beneficial effect of cardiopulmonary rehabilitation has been proven in HF patients with acquired heart disease. A minimum of physical activity or recreational sports is also recommended in stable HF patients. Although there are no specific studies that investigated the impact of exercise in ACHD patients with HF, the position paper of the ESC Working Group on Adult Congenital Heart Disease and the Section of Sports Cardiology promote at least minimal physical activity for all ACHD patients, including those with stable HF.[35] If the type and intensity of exercise are aligned with the haemodynamic and electrophysiological status of the patient, it is assumed that exercising can be done in a safe manner. A group from Rotterdam followed up a cohort of ACHD patients for 10 years and concluded that a required minimum of exercise is not related to impaired outcome.[36] Moreover, the risk of sudden death during exercise is low for the overall ACHD population. Sudden cardiac events are very rare, occurring in only 10% of patients, during exercise.[37] Obviously, when new symptoms occur, patients need to be re-evaluated, and the individualized exercise prescription adapted accordingly.[35]

Management of acute heart failure

Approximately 7% of all hospital admissions of patients with ACHD are related to HF.[38] With an ageing population, it is expected that this number will increase further over time.

Van De Bruaene *et al.* have proposed treatment algorithms for acute subaortic and acute subpulmonary ventricular failure.[34] Both algorithms distinguish between the presence and absence of shunt lesions. Further differentiation in shunt lesions is made between patients with high pulmonary vascular resistance (with a predominant right-to-left shunt) and those with low pulmonary vascular resistance (with a predominant left-to-right shunt).

Oxygen has to be given to all hypoxic HF patients, including those with ACHD. In patients with a right-to-left shunt, it might be that the systemic saturation does not increase much because of the extra-pulmonary shunt; this patient group is not influenced by oxygen therapy. Similar to acute HF in acquired heart disease, oxygen is not indicated in patients with a failing systemic ventricle. However, regardless of the systemic saturation, oxygen therapy has to be instituted in ACHD patients with a failing subpulmonary ventricle, as oxygen lowers the pulmonary vascular resistance and reduces afterload.

Use of diuretics—both loop diuretics and, in some cases, in combination with thiazides—is very important in ACHD patients with failing systemic and/or subpulmonary ventricles. However, this population also has to deal with the typical heart–kidney balance: the lower the circulating volume, the higher the risk of insufficient renal perfusion and renal function impairment. If requested, dialysis should be commenced. Focus on this heart–kidney balance is even more important in patients with a Fontan circulation in whom a minimum volume load is required as the driving force for circulation. Too high doses of diuretics might significantly decrease the single-ventricle cardiac output.[39]

Similar to treatment of patients with acquired HF, vasodilators play a major role in treatment of a failing systemic ventricle. The benefit of using vasodilators in a failing subpulmonary ventricle or a single ventricle is not proven. As in chronic heart failure, vasodilators might aggravate a right-to-left shunt, resulting in further systemic desaturation.

Vasopressors, such as noradrenaline, are also indicated in some specific ACHD patients who present with acute HF. Severe hypotension can lead to impaired perfusion of the coronary arteries; vasopressors help to redistribute blood from the extremities to the vital organs. In patients with right-to-left shunting, vasopressors are used to increase the systemic vascular resistance, in general more so than the pulmonary vascular resistance. As a consequence, the right-to-left shunt improves, as well as the systemic saturation. Low to moderate doses of noradrenaline are most effective in controlling the balance between the systemic and pulmonary vascular resistance.

Inotropes are also beneficial. Besides the general use of milrinone in the post-operative intensive care setting, it increases the contractility of the volume-loaded subpulmonary RV and reduces the systemic and pulmonary vascular resistance in ACHD patients. Low-dose dobutamine decreases the systemic and pulmonary vascular resistance, in addition to improving myocardial dysfunction. High-dose dobutamine increases the pulmonary vascular resistance and can have an adverse effect on afterload of the subpulmonary ventricle. Finally, levosimendan, a calcium sensitizer, has both a positive inotropic effect and a vasodilatory effect. In patients with severe low-output HF, levosimendan seems to be more efficient than dobutamine.[40] ACHD patients with end-stage HF can be treated with levosimendan as outpatients on a regular basis.[41]

Selective pulmonary vasodilators are specifically used in patients with high pulmonary vascular resistance. Inhaled nitric oxide and inhaled iloprost, a prostacyclin analogue, are the most commonly used. When inhaled, they have no effect on the systemic vascular resistance, but only on the pulmonary vascular resistance. Intravenous pulmonary vasodilators, such as prostacyclin, can cause systemic hypotension and, if possible, should be avoided. Moreover, as a precaution, with respect to all intravenous therapy in ACHD patients with shunt lesions, paradoxical air and/or thrombus embolism should be avoided.

Psychological support and end-of-life management

Depending on the severity of their symptoms, ACHD patients with HF face limitations in their daily life. These limitations not only involve reduced physical capacity, but also impact the patients' mental health and social life. Such limitations and the need for hospitalizations can negatively affect the quality of life. In addition to systematic medical follow-up, psychological support is often required. Symptomatic relief and mitigating the need for regular hospitalizations could help stabilize patients' mental health. Psychologists and nurse practitioners play an important role in achieving these goals. CHD patients are considered to have a chronic disease condition, particularly those with HF. It is advocated that these patients are offered advanced care management, initiated during the transition period from paediatric CHD to ACHD. Where at the beginning this advanced care management still may focus on reparative interventions, it is possible that, after a while, a palliative approach is needed and a dialogue about end-of-life care is initiated.[42,43] This is a rather difficult process that can be organized by a palliative care support team with sufficient expertise in this matter. Some of these approaches have been described for HF patients with acquired heart disease and could be applied to the ACHD population.[42,43] However, there are no clinical data that justify implementing this approach without the requested critical background.

Future directions

Looking for the right definition of heart failure

The heterogeneity of the ACHD population means that only one definition of HF for all types of ACHD will not suffice. One does not fit all. The scientific community has to continue to search for definitions adapted to specific pathologies, so these disease-oriented definitions can be used for diagnosis, therapy, and evaluation of treatment effect.

Prevention of heart failure

In many cases, the original cause of HF is known. Early structural optimization, modified surgical approaches, and more appropriate interventional procedures may contribute to a lower risk of developing HF later in life. Continuing feedback from the adult programme to congenital surgeons, paediatric cardiologists, and all health-care professionals involved helps in the process for treatment optimalization.

Preclinical detection by deep phenotyping

As in many disease processes, there would be added value in being able to predict adverse cardiovascular events before obvious structural, functional, or biochemical abnormalities become apparent. A combination of minimal changes in variables could provide the opportunity to predict adverse cardiovascular events and consequently anticipate them in a timely manner.[44] Early therapeutic strategies based on data obtained by deep phenotyping is one of future possibilities, but the development is still in its infancy.

Randomized controlled trials

RCTs represent the only way to improve the level of evidence of ACHD therapy. While RCTs usually include relatively homogeneous patient groups, this is not always the case in daily clinical practice. Patient characteristics often differ from those of the original study patients. This is especially true for the ACHD patient group where there is pronounced heterogeneity. Despite the fact that RCTs represent the only way to achieve a higher level of evidence, it would be very difficult in practice to set up RCTs in the ACHD population. To recruit enough patients and achieve the necessary statistical power, multicentre collaboration is needed. The will is certainly not lacking among the ACHD community, but the road to its achievement is difficult (logistically and financially).

Big data and artificial intelligence

One option to address the problems associated with RCTs is to analyse large data sets with use of artificial intelligence. Hospitals, governments, and scientific organizations have large databases, longitudinal in time. A combination of these databases can simulate a patient's digital life course via deep learning.[45] Using the principle of evidence-based medicine, a prediction model can then be created for the real patient, with particular attention to the therapeutic approach and outcome. This too is still in its infancy, but it will be an important step towards personalized medicine. Especially in a heterogeneous group of patients, this approach will have a clear added value.

Summary

HF is a common problem in ACHD patients, and with ageing of the population and the rise in the number of complex cases, the incidence will increase further. In addition to clinical signs and symptoms, significant impairment in exercise performance and a clear increase in circulating biomarker levels make a diagnosis of HF more likely, although the diagnosis remains challenging in this specific group. The heterogeneity of the ACHD patient population hinders the 'blind' application of HF in acquired heart disease guidelines in CHD patients. Moreover, even drug trials in more homogeneous groups of ACHD failed to show any positive effect on clinical outcome. Only surrogate endpoints were achieved. The more complex the CHD, the more the treating physician has to be aware of adverse effects of the interventions used. In-depth knowledge of the underlying disease is of utmost importance, and if lacking, a referral to, or at least advice from, an expert centre is required. In addition to drugs, device therapy and transplantation can both still offer alternative, albeit temporary, treatment solutions. Unfortunately, for some patients who end up on a palliative trajectory, end-of-life care management should be offered. Many aspects discussed in this chapter are based on small studies and expert opinion. Large multicentre trials are warranted to answer the remaining questions.

Key messages

- The number of ACHD patients is increasing.
- HF is one of the most common complications and has a direct impact on life expectancy and quality of life.
- Medical treatment of HF in ACHD patients is not supported by clinical evidence.
- Early recognition of HF and a personalized approach are crucial.
- Heart transplantation and assist device treatment should be considered in a timely manner.
- Increased focus on advanced care planning is warranted.

References

1. Moons P, Bovijn L, Budts W, Belmans A, Gewillig M. Temporal trends in survival to adulthood among patients born with congenital heart disease from 1970 to 1992 in Belgium. Circulation 2010;**122**(22):2264–72.
2. Piran S, Veldtman G, Siu S, Webb GD, Liu PP. Heart failure and ventricular dysfunction in patients with single or systemic right ventricles. Circulation 2002;**105**(10):1189–94.
3. Cuypers JA, Eindhoven JA, Slager MA, et al. The natural and unnatural history of the Mustard procedure: long-term outcome up to 40 years. Eur Heart J 2014;**35**(25):1666–74.
4. Norozi K, Wessel A, Alpers V, et al. Incidence and risk distribution of heart failure in adolescents and adults with congenital heart disease after cardiac surgery. Am J Cardiol 2006;**97**(8):1238–43.
5. Baumgartner H, De Backer J, Babu-Narayan SV, et al.; ESC Scientific Document Group. 2020 ESC Guidelines for the management of adult congenital heart disease. Eur Heart J 2021;**25**(4):543–645.
6. Bolger AP, Gatzoulis MA. Towards defining heart failure in adults with congenital heart disease. Int J Cardiol 2004;**97**(Suppl 1):15–23.
7. Broda CR, Downing TE, John AS. Diagnosis and management of the adult patient with a failing Fontan circulation. Heart Fail Rev 2020;**25**(4):633–46.
8. Budts W, Roos-Hesselink J, Rädle-Hurst T, et al. Treatment of heart failure in adult congenital heart disease: a position paper of the Working Group of Grown-Up Congenital Heart Disease and the Heart Failure Association of the European Society of Cardiology. Eur Heart J 2016;**37**(18):1419–27.
9. Saiki H, Kuwata S, Kurishima C, et al. Prevalence, implication, and determinants of worsening renal function after surgery for congenital heart disease. Heart Vessels 2016;**31**(8):1313–18.
10. Diller GP, Dimopoulos K, Okonko D, et al. Exercise intolerance in adult congenital heart disease: comparative severity, correlates, and prognostic implication. Circulation 2005;**112**(6):828–35.
11. Leusveld EM, Kauling RM, Geenen LW, Roos-Hesselink JW. Heart failure in congenital heart disease: management options and clinical challenges. Expert Rev Cardiovasc Ther 2020;**18**(8):503–16.
12. Ponikowski P, Voors AA, Anker SD, et al. 2016 ESC Guidelines for the diagnosis and treatment of acute and chronic heart failure. Rev Esp Cardiol (Engl Ed) 2016;**69**(12):1167.
13. Dore A, Houde C, Chan KL, et al. Angiotensin receptor blockade and exercise capacity in adults with systemic right ventricles: a multicenter, randomized, placebo-controlled clinical trial. Circulation 2005;**112**(16):2411–16.
14. van der Bom T, Winter MM, Bouma BJ, et al. Effect of valsartan on systemic right ventricular function: a double-blind, randomized, placebo-controlled pilot trial. Circulation 2013;**127**(3):322–30.

15. van Dissel AC, Winter MM, van der Bom T, *et al.* Long-term clinical outcomes of valsartan in patients with a systemic right ventricle: follow-up of a multicenter randomized controlled trial. Int J Cardiol 2019;**278**:84–7.

16. Doughan AR, McConnell ME, Book WM. Effect of beta blockers (carvedilol or metoprolol XL) in patients with transposition of great arteries and dysfunction of the systemic right ventricle. Am J Cardiol 2007;**99**(5):704–6.

17. Giardini A, Lovato L, Donti A, *et al.* A pilot study on the effects of carvedilol on right ventricular remodelling and exercise tolerance in patients with systemic right ventricle. Int J Cardiol 2007;**114**(2):241–6.

18. Bouallal R, Godart F, Francart C, Richard A, Foucher-Hossein C, Lions C. Interest of β-blockers in patients with right ventricular systemic dysfunction. Cardiol Young 2010;**20**(6):615–19.

19. Galiè N, Humbert M, Vachiery JL, *et al.*; Members: ATF, Members ATF. 2015 ESC/ERS Guidelines for the diagnosis and treatment of pulmonary hypertension: The Joint Task Force for the Diagnosis and Treatment of Pulmonary Hypertension of the European Society of Cardiology (ESC) and the European Respiratory Society (ERS)Endorsed by: Association for European Paediatric and Congenital Cardiology (AEPC), International Society for Heart and Lung Transplantation (ISHLT). Eur Heart J 2016;**37**(1):67–119.

20. Bouabdallaoui N, O'Meara E, Bernier V, *et al.* Beneficial effects of ivabradine in patients with heart failure, low ejection fraction, and heart rate above 77 b.p.m. ESC Heart Fail 2019;**6**(6):1199–207.

21. Maurer SJ, Pujol Salvador C, Schiele S, Hager A, Ewert P, Tutarel O. Sacubitril/valsartan for heart failure in adults with complex congenital heart disease. Int J Cardiol 2020;**300**:137–40.

22. Van De Bruaene A, Delcroix M, Pasquet A, *et al.* Iron deficiency is associated with adverse outcome in Eisenmenger patients. Eur Heart J 2011;**32**(22):2790–9.

23. Tay EL, Peset A, Papaphylactou M, *et al.* Replacement therapy for iron deficiency improves exercise capacity and quality of life in patients with cyanotic congenital heart disease and/or the Eisenmenger syndrome. Int J Cardiol 2011;**151**(3):307–12.

24. Janousek J, Gebauer RA, Abdul-Khaliq H, *et al.* Cardiac resynchronisation therapy in paediatric and congenital heart disease: differential effects in various anatomical and functional substrates. Heart 2009;**95**(14):1165–71.

25. Khairy P, Fournier A, Thibault B, Dubuc M, Therien J, Vobecky SJ. Cardiac resynchronization therapy in congenital heart disease. Int J Cardiol 2006;**109**(2):160–8.

26. European Society of Cardiology (ESC); European Heart Rhythm Association EHRA); Brignole M, Auricchio A, Baron-Esquivias G, *et al.*. 2013 ESC guidelines on cardiac pacing and cardiac resynchronization therapy: the task force on cardiac pacing and resynchronization therapy of the European Society of Cardiology (ESC). Developed in collaboration with the European Heart Rhythm Association (EHRA). Europace 2013;**15**(8):1070–118.

27. Mulukutla V, Franklin WJ, Villa CR, Morales DL. Surgical device therapy for heart failure in the adult with congenital heart disease. Heart Fail Clin 2014;**10**(1):197–206.

28. Joyce DL, Crow SS, John R, *et al.* Mechanical circulatory support in patients with heart failure secondary to transposition of the great arteries. J Heart Lung Transplant 2010;**29**(11):1302–5.

29. Shah NR, Lam WW, Rodriguez FH, *et al.* Clinical outcomes after ventricular assist device implantation in adults with complex congenital heart disease. J Heart Lung Transplant 2013;**32**(6):615–20.

30. Rodefeld MD, Boyd JH, Myers CD, *et al.* Cavopulmonary assist: circulatory support for the univentricular Fontan circulation. Ann Thorac Surg 2003;**76**(6):1911–16; discussion 1916.

31. Russo P, Wheeler A, Russo J, Tobias JD. Use of a ventricular assist device as a bridge to transplantation in a patient with single ventricle physiology and total cavopulmonary anastomosis. Paediatr Anaesth 2008;**18**(4):320–4.

32. Goldberg SW, Fisher SA, Wehman B, Mehra MR. Adults with congenital heart disease and heart transplantation: optimizing outcomes. J Heart Lung Transplant 2014;**33**(9):873–7.

33. Kirk R, Dipchand AI, Edwards LB, *et al.*; International Society for Heart and Lung Transplantation. The Registry of the International Society for Heart and Lung Transplantation: fifteenth pediatric heart transplantation report--2012. J Heart Lung Transplant 2012;**31**(10):1065–72.

34. Van De Bruaene A, Meier L, Droogne W, *et al.* Management of acute heart failure in adult patients with congenital heart disease. Heart Fail Rev 2018;**23**(1):1–14.

35. Budts W, Börjesson M, Chessa M, *et al.* Physical activity in adolescents and adults with congenital heart defects: individualized exercise prescription. Eur Heart J 2013;**34**(47):3669–74.

36. Opić P, Utens EM, Cuypers JA, *et al.* Sports participation in adults with congenital heart disease. Int J Cardiol 2015;**187**:175–82.

37. Koyak Z, Harris L, de Groot JR, *et al.* Sudden cardiac death in adult congenital heart disease. Circulation 2012;**126**(16):1944–54.

38. Verheugt CL, Uiterwaal CS, van der Velde ET, *et al.* The emerging burden of hospital admissions of adults with congenital heart disease. Heart 2010;**96**(11):872–8.

39. Dimopoulos K, Diller GP, Koltsida E, *et al.* Prevalence, predictors, and prognostic value of renal dysfunction in adults with congenital heart disease. Circulation 2008;**117**(18):2320–8.

40. Ricci Z, Garisto C, Favia I, Vitale V, Di Chiara L, Cogo PE. Levosimendan infusion in newborns after corrective surgery for congenital heart disease: randomized controlled trial. Intensive Care Med 2012;**38**(7):1198–204.

41. Cranley J, Hardiman A, Freeman LJ. Pulsed levosimendan in advanced heart failure due to congenital heart disease: a case series. Eur Heart J Case Rep 2020;**4**(3):1–6.

42. Troost E, Roggen L, Goossens E, *et al.* Advanced care planning in adult congenital heart disease: transitioning from repair to palliation and end-of-life care. Int J Cardiol 2019;**279**:57–61.

43. Schwerzmann M, Goossens E, Gallego P, *et al.* Recommendations for advance care planning in adults with congenital heart disease: a position paper from the ESC Working Group of Adult Congenital Heart Disease, the Association of Cardiovascular Nursing and Allied Professions (ACNAP), the European Association for Palliative Care (EAPC), and the International Society for Adult Congenital Heart Disease (ISACHD). Eur Heart J 2020;**41**:4200–10.

44. Santens B, Helsen F, Van De Bruaene A, *et al.* Adverse functional remodelling of the subpulmonary left ventricle in patients with a systemic right ventricle is associated with clinical outcome. Eur Heart J Cardiovasc Imaging 2021;**23**(5):680–8.

45. Corral-Acero J, Margara F, Marciniak M, *et al.* The 'Digital Twin' to enable the vision of precision cardiology. Eur Heart J 2020;**41**(48):4556–64.

CHAPTER 3.7

Endocrine and metabolic abnormalities

Martin Huelsmann, Jelena P Seferović, and Francesco Cosentino

Contents

Introduction

Endocrine and metabolic diseases can affect the structure and/or function of the heart. The most common endocrine diseases causing heart failure (HF) are thyroid disorders, phaeochromocytoma, and primary hyperaldosteronism. Other endocrine diseases related to HF are rare and include parathyroid, pituitary, as well as adrenal gland, abnormalities. Endocrine diseases may worsen pre-existing HF. Treatment of underlying disorders usually improves HF. Diabetes is the most common endocrine disease among patients with HF and will be discussed in ⊃ Chapter 12.8. A brief summary of these diseases, along with common signs/symptoms, is given in ⊃ Table 3.7.1.

Thyroid gland

Introduction

Thyroid hormones may play an essential role in the function of the heart and in the cardiovascular (CV) system, in both physiological and pathological conditions. Via various signalling pathways, thyroid hormones significantly affect cardiac morphology and function, as well as cell metabolism. Thyroid hormones, via direct and indirect mechanisms, control the heart rate, myocardial systolic and diastolic function, and systemic vascular resistance (⊃ Figure 3.7.1).[1]

The clinical presentation of thyroid dysfunction may depend on the underlying heart disease and the severity of HF, as patients in higher New York Heart Association (NYHA) classes may tolerate poorly even minor changes in thyroid hormone levels. Thyroid dysfunction is considered to be an important risk factor for cardiovascular disease (CVD) and HF. In a meta-analysis of 25,390 participants, subclinical hyper- and hypothyroidism have been associated with an increased risk of HF.[2] In another large cohort of HF patients, thyroid dysfunction (both hyper- and hypothyroidism) was prevalent in about 14% of subjects and was significantly associated with more severe HF symptoms, as well as an increased risk of left ventricular assist device (LVAD) implantation and cardiac transplantation. Furthermore, thyroid dysfunction in patients with HF was associated with 60% higher risk of mortality, compared to euthyroid patients.[3]

When a diagnosis of HF is made, thyroid function tests are recommended.[4] Treatment of underlying thyroid disturbances can reverse associated cardiac abnormalities.

Hyperthyroidism

Hyperthyroidism is a rare (about 1%) cause,[3] but nevertheless can have dramatic effects on the heart. Toxic effects (positive chronotropic, inotropic, and dromotropic) of excessive thyroid hormones include tachycardia, increased cardiac contractility, and elevated cardiac output. Increased cardiac output (2–3 times higher compared to normal) is the

Table 3.7.1 Summary of endocrine diseases leading to heart failure

Endocrine disease	Key signs and symptoms
Thyroid gland	
Hyperthyroidism	Tachycardia, increased cardiac contractility, elevated cardiac output
Hypothyroidism	Hoarse voice, slow mentation and movement, pedal oedema, coarse, dry, and pale skin, delayed knee jerk Cold intolerance, fatigue, bradycardia, diastolic hypertension, distant heart sounds
Phaeochromocytoma	Episodic sweating, palpitation, headache, sustained or episodic severe hypertension Tachycardia, hypertension, panic or anxiety
Adrenal gland	
Primary hyperaldosteronism	Hypertension, hypokalaemia, suppressed renin levels
Primary hypoaldosteronism	Severe sustained hypertension, hypokalaemia Intravascular volume depletion, hyponatraemia, hyperkalaemia
Hypercortisolaemia	Hypertension, hyperglycaemia, dyslipidaemia, obesity, prothrombotic state—all contribute to accelerated atherosclerosis and myocardial structural and functional abnormalities such as hypertrophy, concentric remodelling, and fibrosis
Parathyroid disease	
Hyperparathyroidism	Hyperparathyroidism or other hypercalcaemic aetiology, polyuria and dehydration, acute kidney injury, short QTc interval Increased cardiac contractility, shortening of PR and QT intervals, ST-segment and T-wave changes. Concomitant increase in blood pressure, as well as calcification of cardiac valves, may contribute to the onset of arrhythmias and heart failure
Hypoparathyroidism	Tetany, positive Trousseau and Chvostek signs, known hypoparathyroidism, long QTc interval Tetany, stridor, and carpopedal spasm by reducing cardiac contractility may favour the onset of dilated cardiomyopathy ECG changes include prolonged QTc interval and non-specific T-wave abnormalities
Vitamin D metabolism	Hypertension, ST-segment depression, shortened QT interval, bradycardia
Pituitary gland	
Acromegaly	Left axis deviation, septal Q-waves, ST-segment and T-wave depression, as well as atrial and ventricular arrhythmias, concentric biventricular hypertrophy, diastolic and systolic dysfunction, arrhythmias, and congestive heart failure

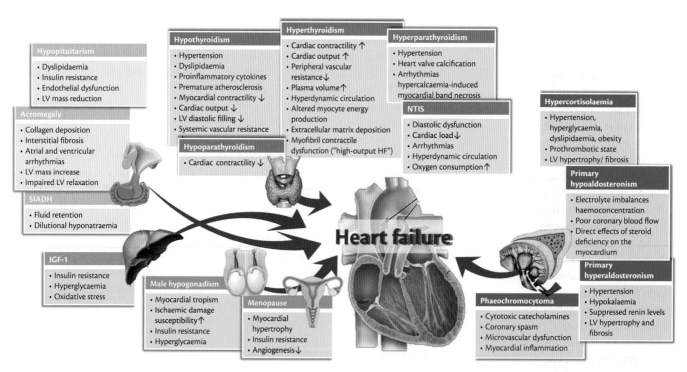

Figure 3.7.1 Pathophysiology of heart failure in endocrine diseases. IGF-1, insulin-like growth factor 1; NTIS, non-thyroidal illness syndrome; SIADH, syndrome of inappropriate antidiuretic hormone secretion; GH, growth hormone.
Modified from: Endocrine system dysfunction and chronic heart failure: a clinical perspective, *Endocrine* Volume 75, pages 360–376 (2022).

result of elevated heart rate and reduced peripheral vascular resistance. The decrease in peripheral vascular resistance and mean arterial pressure develops to allow relaxation of arteriolar vascular smooth muscle. These haemodynamic changes lead to decreased renal perfusion pressure, increased sodium reabsorption, activation of the renin–angiotensin–aldosterone system, expansion of plasma volume, and increased preload.

An untreated high-output state and sustained haemodynamic load in hyperthyroidism result in hyperdynamic circulation which, in turn, may lead to altered myocyte energy production. It may further cause myocyte damage, extracellular matrix deposition, and myofibril contractile dysfunction ('high-output HF'). If the increase in cardiac output is significant, particularly in older patients, it can precipitate systolic hypertension in up to 30% of cases.[5,6] As the disease progresses, tachycardia and increased cardiac contractility deplete myocardial energy potential, resulting in left ventricular (LV) hypertrophy, myocardial remodelling, pulmonary congestion, and atrial fibrillation.[7] In later stages, decreased cardiac contractility, abnormal diastolic compliance, and LV dilatation occur. In about 20% of patients with hyperthyroidism, pulmonary hypertension may develop due to increased pulmonary flow and pressure, resulting in jugular venous hypertension, hepatic congestion, and peripheral oedema (➔ Figure 3.7.1).

The main symptoms in the majority of these patients include palpitations, irregular heartbeat, and shortness of breath. Dyspnoea on exertion, orthopnoea, and paroxysmal nocturnal dyspnoea may also develop. In later stages, peripheral oedema, elevated jugular venous pressure, or S3 may occur. Exercise intolerance and exertional dyspnoea are predominantly caused by skeletal and respiratory muscle weakness and pulmonary hypertension.

A differential diagnosis between HF and hyperthyroidism may be challenging. In about 6% of patients, HF occurs as an initial presentation of hyperthyroidism and half of these patients have LV dysfunction.[8] An increased incidence of LV hypertrophy and HF with preserved ejection fraction are also frequently reported in association with hyperthyroidism.[9] The elderly population with previous ischaemic hypertensive and/or valvular heart disease are particularly vulnerable, with a high risk of developing HF. Therefore, early diagnosis of hyperthyroidism is needed to prevent clinical worsening.

The most common rhythm disturbance in hyperthyroidism is sinus tachycardia, although the most clinically significant is atrial fibrillation, which occurs in 2–20% of patients. Atrial fibrillation is also common in HF, with a high occurrence in the presence of hyperthyroidism. The type of atrial fibrillation present is usually persistent rather than paroxysmal. The causes of atrial fibrillation in these patients include tachycardia, increased sympathetic drive, and atrial ectopic activity, as well as a rise in left atrial pressure. Risk factors for the development of atrial fibrillation in patients with hyperthyroidism and HF are advanced age, male gender, ischaemic heart disease, chronic kidney disease, and valvular heart disease. In HF patients, fast and sustained atrial fibrillation results in LV systolic and diastolic dysfunction, as well

as pulmonary congestion, which worsens the clinical course.[10] In these patients, timely rate and/or rhythm control, as well as proper anticoagulation treatment, are necessary.

Amiodarone is a very effective antiarrhythmic agent in the treatment of ventricular and atrial tachyarrhythmias in HF. However, treatment with amiodarone may cause hyperthyroidism in 8% of patients, amplifying the underlying endocrine disorder. Amiodarone-induced thyrotoxicosis (AIT) is associated with a 3-fold increase in major adverse CV events and may also present with worsening of HF symptoms. Although medical management with anti-thyroidal agents and steroids are treatment cornerstones, thyroidectomy may be considered in severe cases,[11] especially where amiodarone therapy cannot be stopped.

Management of HF in hyperthyroidism includes restoration of the euthyroid state, beta-adrenergic blockade for reduction of heart rate, and diuretics to improve congestive symptoms. Prompt initiation of treatment after a HF diagnosis is essential because of a significant incidence of CV adverse events.[3] LV function recovery depends on patient characteristics, including age, comorbidities, diabetes, and coronary artery disease. Heart rate reduction and control of the ventricular response in atrial fibrillation lead to fast recovery of LV function. Treatment with beta-blockers results in prompt improvement, whereas anti-thyroid treatment requires more time. Digitalis and anticoagulation may also be indicated. Definitive treatment of hyperthyroidism with radioactive iodine ablation or thyroidectomy may lead to prompt recovery of cardiac function. HF in hyperthyroidism has historically been considered a reversible cause of LV dysfunction. In these patients, several studies have validated a reversal of echocardiographic abnormalities as well as improved CV outcomes.[12,13]

Hypothyroidism

Hypothyroidism is associated with a significant number of CV risk factors, including hypertension, dyslipidaemia, and alterations in pro-inflammatory cytokines, all of which play a role in triggering premature atherosclerosis and coronary artery disease. This may indirectly cause and accelerate LV systolic and diastolic dysfunction and neurohumoral activation, and hence the development of HF.[14] Mild CV signs and symptoms, such as cold intolerance, fatigue, bradycardia, diastolic hypertension, and distant heart sounds, are clinical manifestations of hypothyroidism. The most frequent ECG changes include sinus bradycardia, low QRS voltage, atrioventricular block, and prolongation of the QT interval. QT interval prolongation may predispose to ventricular arrhythmias (torsades de pointes).[15]

Haemodynamic changes in hypothyroidism are characterized by bradycardia, decreased myocardial contractility, reduction in cardiac output, impaired LV diastolic filling, and increased systemic vascular resistance. The latter (by as much as 30%) results in diastolic hypertension in about 25% of patients. Increased arterial stiffness may also contribute to high blood pressure and vascular dysregulation (➔ Figure 3.7.1).

Pooled analysis from six prospective cohorts demonstrated an increased risk of HF events, as well as all-cause mortality, in hypothyroidism.[3,16] In addition, hypothyroidism was found to be an independent predictor of HF hospitalization and CV death. HF hospitalization in hypothyroidism was more frequent in subjects older than 65 years and in those with previously established HF.

Interestingly, long-term hypothyroidism could result in the development of constrictive pericarditis and ultimately cause HF.[17] Echocardiography may not always be sensitive enough for diagnosing this disorder, and invasive haemodynamic evaluation may be required. Thyroid hormone replacement improves CV risk factors as well as LV function.

Subclinical thyroid disease

Subclinical thyroid disease is characterized by thyroid dysfunction in the absence of typical symptoms of hyper- or hypothyroid disease. Subclinical hypo- and hyperthyroidism are associated with an increased risk of developing HF and adverse prognosis. Subclinical thyroid dysfunction may be potentially a useful and promising predictor for long-term prognosis in HF patients.

Patients with subclinical hyperthyroidism, especially those older than 65 years, have a higher incidence of HF hospitalization, all-cause mortality, and CV events.[18] In addition, a significant association between subclinical hyperthyroidism and atrial fibrillation has been shown, with an inverse correlation between thyroid-stimulating hormone (TSH) level and the risk of atrial fibrillation.[19] Subclinical hypothyroidism predominantly occurs in younger women, and correlates with an increased risk of both HF hospitalization and/or all-cause mortality.[20]

Taking into account these associations, early diagnosis and timely initiation of adequate treatment for subclinical thyroid dysfunction are indicated.

Phaeochromocytoma

Phaeochromocytoma is a rare neuroendocrine catecholamine-secreting tumour that arises from chromaffin cells in the sympathetic nervous system. It accounts for 0.5% of secondary hypertension in general practice. Ten to 20% of patients with phaeochromocytoma present with HF. Clinical manifestations of phaeochromocytoma include tachycardia, hypertension, panic, and anxiety, while nausea, fever, and flushing are less common. CV manifestations of this endocrine disorder include myocardial infarction, cardiac arrhythmias, and HF.[21]

Although the majority of patients with phaeochromocytoma have normal or increased LV systolic function, the pattern of LV dysfunction may be variable (⮞ Figure 3.7.1). Phenotypically, HF may present as dilated cardiomyopathy, Takotsubo cardiomyopathy, and hypertrophic obstructive cardiomyopathy.[22] When transient LV dysfunction is present (Takotsubo cardiomyopathy),[23,24] patients usually recover within several days. The pathophysiology of Takotsubo cardiomyopathy includes direct cytotoxic catecholamine injury, coronary spasm, microvascular dysfunction, and myocardial inflammation.[23,24]

Treatment of phaeochromocytoma consists of initial alpha-blockade, followed by beta-blockade. Beta-blockade should always be given together with alpha-blockade, as otherwise this could worsen hypertensive episodes. Medical management of

these tumours prior to surgery may be challenging in the context of HF.[25,26] Surgical removal of phaeochromocytoma is a recommended treatment.

Adrenal gland
Primary hyperaldosteronism

Primary hyperaldosteronism (Conn's disease) is characterized by increased secretion of aldosterone, usually caused by adrenal adenoma or bilateral adrenal hyperplasia. As HF is a syndrome accompanied by secondary hyperaldosteronism, an overlap of typical signs can occur and clinical cases may be overseen. The disease usually presents with hypertension (about 10% of patients), hypokalaemia, and suppressed renin levels.[27]

Increased aldosterone levels have detrimental effects on the myocardium and vascular smooth muscle, causing LV hypertrophy and fibrosis. They also induce endothelial dysfunction, increased arterial stiffness, and peripheral vascular resistance (⮞ Figure 3.7.1).

Furthermore, these patients frequently have renal dysfunction, as well as coronary and cerebrovascular disease.[28,29] Patients with primary hyperaldosteronism may present rarely (4.1%) with HF, but have a 4-fold higher risk of HF development. Treatment of primary hyperaldosteronism is surgical (unilateral or bilateral adrenalectomy). Medical treatment for HF includes mineralocorticoid receptor antagonists, angiotensin-converting enzyme (ACE) inhibitors/angiotensin II receptor blockers, potassium-sparing diuretics, and calcium channel blockers.[27]

Primary hypoaldosteronism

Primary hypoaldosteronism (Addison's disease) is a rare disorder characterized by insufficient cortisol and aldosterone production by the adrenal glands, most frequently due to autoimmune disease. It often presents with intravascular volume depletion, hyponatraemia, and hyperkalaemia.[30] Primary adrenal insufficiency can cause CV abnormalities, mostly due to reduced plasma volume and electrolyte disturbances. Although considered a rare cause of HF, adrenal insufficiency may present as new-onset systolic HF. The pathophysiology of this type of HF involves electrolyte imbalances, haemoconcentration causing poor coronary blood flow, and also direct effects of steroid deficiency on the myocardium (⮞ Figure 3.7.1).[31]

Treatment for primary adrenal insufficiency includes optimal doses of glucocorticoids, loop diuretics, and ACE inhibitors. Aldosterone receptor antagonists are not recommended in this setting. Adrenal replacement therapy in this condition may lead to rapid improvement of cardiac function. Replacement of mineralocorticoids is still under debate. As cases are rare, there is no clear evidence, but dosages should be as low as possible in case HF is not reversible. This is also true for glucocorticoids, as discussed below.

Hypercortisolaemia

Excessive cortisol secretion is caused by pituitary adenoma (Cushing's disease) or adrenal gland adenoma (Cushing's syndrome). Hypercortisolaemia is associated with hypertension, hyperglycaemia, dyslipidaemia, obesity, and a prothrombotic state, all of which contribute to accelerated atherosclerosis. On the other hand, excessive cortisol secretion can also cause myocardial structural and functional abnormalities such as hypertrophy, concentric remodelling, and fibrosis.[32,33] In 40% of patients with hypercortisolaemia, global LV dysfunction may be present. In rare cases, dilated cardiomyopathy can develop.[34] Concomitant ECG changes affect the duration of PR and QT intervals (➲ Figure 3.7.1).

Treatment includes surgical removal of the pituitary or adrenal gland adenoma, followed by careful cortisol and mineralocorticoid supplementation. Treatment of hypercortisolaemia has been shown to improve myocardial function.

Parathyroid disease

Parathyroid glands secrete parathyroid hormone, which is responsible for control of calcium homeostasis. Diseases of the parathyroid glands impact cardiac function through direct effects on the myocardium, vascular smooth muscle, and endothelial cells, but also through impairment of serum calcium levels. The association between parathyroid hormone levels and HF risk with adverse outcomes has been thoroughly investigated.[35,36,37,38]

Hyperparathyroidism

Primary hyperparathyroidism is usually caused by parathyroid gland adenoma leading to increased levels of parathyroid hormone and serum calcium levels. Hypercalcaemia may increase cardiac contractility and induce shortening of PR and QT intervals, as well as ST-segment and T-wave changes.[39] Concomitant increase in blood pressure, as well as calcification of cardiac valves, may contribute to the onset of arrhythmias and HF. Hypercalcaemia-induced myocardial band necrosis has been described as a putative cause of acute decompensation in pre-existing HF (➲ Figure 3.7.1). Primary hyperparathyroidism is an independent predictor of HF.[40,41,42] A prospective study showed LV hypertrophy in 82% of patients with hyperparathyroidism. Although LV systolic function is maintained in these patients, long-standing or severe hyperparathyroidism may cause LV diastolic dysfunction. Interestingly, LV dysfunction may not be reversed by parathyroidectomy.[39,42] Diagnosis of primary and secondary hyperparathyroidism in the presence of manifest HF is often difficult.[43]

Hypoparathyroidism

Hypocalcaemia (hypoparathyroidism) is a rare condition that is usually diagnosed by low calcium levels, after surgical removal of the parathyroid glands. Also, chronic kidney failure causes low serum calcium and parathyroid hormone levels. Hypocalcaemia typically associated with tetany, stridor, and carpopedal spasm by reducing cardiac contractility may favour the onset of dilated cardiomyopathy (➲ Figure 3.7.1). ECG changes include prolonged QTc interval and non-specific T-wave abnormalities.

Clinical improvement is obtained with calcium and vitamin D supplementation.[44,45]

Vitamin D metabolism

Vitamin D deficiency is associated with increased CV morbidity.[46] In the VINDICATE trial, vitamin D supplementation was associated with improvement of chamber geometry and ejection fraction, but no change in functional status of HF patients or outcome.[47] Available studies are small, and larger studies are urgently warranted in this setting.

Increased levels of vitamin D may be associated with hypertension, while ECG changes include ST-segment depression, shortened QT interval, and bradycardia (➲ Figure 3.7.1). In addition, vitamin D toxicity induces hypercalcaemia, causing acute kidney injury and eventually HF exacerbation.[48]

Pituitary gland

Both excess and deficiency of the growth hormone (GH)/insulin-like growth factor 1 (IGF-1) axis are associated with an increased risk of CV morbidity. Indeed, these conditions correlate with CV risk factors such as hypertension, dyslipidaemia, insulin resistance, atherosclerosis, and HF.

Acromegaly

Acromegaly is a rare condition predominantly caused by a GH-secreting pituitary adenoma. It is associated with hypertension, type 2 diabetes, and dyslipidaemia, which have detrimental effects on the myocardium (cardiomyocyte increase, collagen deposition, and interstitial fibrosis).[49]

The prevalence of congestive HF in patients with acromegaly ranges from 1% to 10%. The clinical course of CV abnormalities and HF in acromegaly depend on age, as well as on the severity and duration of the disease. Severe and advanced HF is associated with poor prognosis. HF symptoms and signs are found only in 10% of patients. ECG findings include left axis deviation, septal Q-waves, and ST- and T-wave depression as well as atrial and ventricular arrhythmias in up to 50% of patients. Echocardiography usually reveals LV hypertrophy, LV mass increase, and impaired LV relaxation (➲ Figure 3.7.1).[50]

In rare cases, a specific acromegalic cardiomyopathy has been described presenting with concentric biventricular hypertrophy, diastolic and systolic dysfunction, arrhythmias, and congestive HF.[51,52] Successful treatment of acromegaly results in improvement of both CV risk factors and cardiac function.

Growth hormone deficiency

GH deficiency is a clinical condition characterized by decreased production of GH and IGF-1. GH deficiency is associated with an increased CV risk profile, including increased body fat, dyslipidaemia, insulin resistance, and endothelial dysfunction (➲ Figure 3.7.1). Myocardial abnormalities include a reduction of LV cardiac mass and decreased LV wall and interventricular septal thickness.[53,54,55] Treatment with recombinant GH in patients with GH deficiency improves the CV risk pattern and cardiac mass and performance.

Summary

Although HF in endocrine disease is rare, it may have an adverse prognostic impact. Therefore, careful screening with natriuretic peptides and/or echocardiographic assessment is mandatory. In the setting of HF, endocrine causes are often reversible. Therefore, the differential diagnosis of causes of congestive heart failure should always include an endocrinological pattern of laboratory tests.

References

1. Biondi B. Mechanisms in endocrinology: heart failure and thyroid dysfunction. Eur J Endocrinol. 2012;167:609–18.

2. Gencer B, Collet TH, Virgini V, et al. Subclinical thyroid dysfunction and the risk of heart failure events: an individual participant data analysis from 6 prospective cohorts. Circulation. 2012;126:1040–9.

3. Mitchell JE, Hellkamp AS, Mark DB, et al. Thyroid function in heart failure and impact on mortality. JACC Heart Fail. 2013;1:48–55.

4. Hunt SA, Abraham WT, Chin MH, et al. 2009 focused update incorporated into the ACC/AHA 2005 guidelines for the diagnosis and management of heart failure in adults: a report of the American College of Cardiology Foundation/American Heart Association Task Force on Practice Guidelines developed in collaboration with the International Society for Heart and Lung Transplantation. Circulation. 2009; 119:e391–479.

5. Danzi S, Klein I. Thyroid hormone and the cardiovascular system. Med Clin North Am. 2012; 96:257–68.

6. Biondi B, Palmieri EA, Lombardi G, Fazio S. Effects of thyroid hormone on cardiac function: the relative importance of heart rate, loading conditions, and myocardial contractility in the regulation of cardiac performance in human hyperthyroidism. J Clin Endocrinol Metab. 2002;87:968–74.

7. Weltman NY, Wang D, Redetzke RA, Gerdes AM. Long-standing hyperthyroidism is associated with normal or enhanced intrinsic cardiomyocyte function despite decline in global cardiac function. PLoS One. 2012;7:e46655

8. Siu CW, Yeung CY, Lau CP, Kung AW, Tse HF. Incidence, clinical characteristics and outcome of congestive heart failure as the initial presentation in patients with primary hyperthyroidism. Heart. 2007;93:483–7.

9. Pearce EN, Yang Q, Benjamin EJ, Aragam J, Vasan RS. Thyroid function and left ventricular structure and function in the Framingham Heart Study. Thyroid. 2010;20:369–73.

10. Shimizu T, Koide S, Noh JY, Sugino K, Ito K, Nakazawa H. Hyperthyroidism and the management of atrial fibrillation. Thyroid. 2002;12:489–93.

11. Bahn RS, Burch HB, Cooper DS, et al.; American Thyroid Association, American Association of Clinical Endocrinologists. Hyperthyroidism and other causes of thyrotoxicosis: management guidelines of the American Thyroid Association and American Association of Clinical Endocrinologists. Endocr Pract. 2011;17:456–520.

12. Osuna PM, Udovcic M, Sharma MD. Hyperthyroidism and the heart. Methodist Debakey Cardiovasc J. 2017;13:60–3.

13. Choudhury RP, MacDermot J. Heart failure in thyrotoxicosis, an approach to management. Br J Clin Pharmacol. 1998;46:421–4.

14. Pasqualetti G, Niccolai F, Calsolaro V, et al. Relationship between thyroid dysfunction and heart failure in older people. J Clin Gerontol Geriatr. 2017; 65:184–91.

15. Klein I, Danzi S. Thyroid disease and the heart. Circulation 2007;116:1725–35.

16. Chen S, Shauer A, Zwas DR, et al. The effect of thyroid function on clinical outcome in patients with heart failure. Eur J Heart Fail. 2014;16:217–26.

17. Tyagi G, Doctorian T, Rabkin D, Hilliard A. Constrictive pericarditis in a patient with long standing hypothyroidism. J Am Coll Cardiol. 2015; 65:A758.

18. Nanchen D, Gussekloo J, Westendorp RG, et al. Subclinical thyroid dysfunction and the risk of heart failure in older per- sons at high cardiovascular risk. J Clin Endocrinol Metab. 2012;97:852–61.

19. Selmer C, Olesen JB, Hansen ML, et al. The spectrum of thyroid disease and risk of new onset atrial fibrillation: a large population cohort study BMJ. 2012;345:e7895.

20. Iacoviello M, Guida P, Guastamacchia E, et al. Prognostic role of subclinical hypothyroidism in chronic heart failure outpatients. Curr Pharm Des. 2008;14: 2686–92.

21. Reyes HA, Paquin JJ, Harris DM. Pheochromocytoma, 'the great masquerader,' presenting as severe acute decompensated heart failure in a young patient. Case Rep Cardiol. 2018;2018:8767801.

22. Agrawal S, Shirani J, Garg L, et al. Pheochromocytoma and stress cardiomyopathy: insight into pathogenesis. World J Cardiol. 2017;9(3):255–60.

23. Batisse-Lignier M, Pereira B, Motreff P, et al. Acute and chronic pheochromocytoma-induced cardiomyopathies: different prognoses?: a systematic analytical review. Medicine (Baltimore). 2015;94:e2198.

24. Park JH, Kim KS, Sul JY, et al. Prevalence and patterns of left ventricular dysfunction in patients with pheochromocytoma. J Cardiovasc Ultrasound. 2011;19:76–82.

25. Sanna GD, Talanas G, Fiore G, Canu A, Terrosu P. Pheochromocytoma presenting as an acute coronary syn- drome complicated by acute heart failure: the challenge of a great mimic. J Saudi Heart Assoc. 2016;28:278–82.

26. Mamoojee Y, Arham M, Elsaify W, Nag S. Lesson of the month 2: catecholamine-induced cardiomyopathy: pitfalls in diagnosis and medical management. Clin Med. 2016;16:201–3.

27. Funder JW, Carey RM, Mantero F, et al. The management of primary aldosteronism: case detection, diagnosis, and treatment: an endocrine society clinical practice guideline. J Clin Endocrinol Metab. 2016;101:1889–916.

28. Rossi GP, Bernini G, Caliumi C, et al.; PAPY Study Investigators. A prospective study of the prevalence of primary aldosteronism in 1,125 hypertensive patients. J Am Coll Cardiol. 2006;48: 2293–300.

29. White PC. Aldosterone: direct effects on and production by the heart. J Clin Endocrinol Metab. 2003;88:2376–83.

30. Pitt B, Zannad F, Remme WJ, et al. The effect of spironolactone on morbidity and mortality in patients with severe heart failure. Randomized Aldactone Evaluation Study Investigators. N Engl J Med. 1999;341:709–17.

31. Ross, IL, Bergthorsdottir R, Levitt N, et al. Cardiovascular risk factors in patients with Addison's disease: a comparative study of South African and Swedish patients. PLoS One. 2014;9:e90768.

32. Yiu KH, Marsan NA, Delgado V, et al. Increased myocardial fibrosis and left ventricular dysfunction in Cushing's syndrome. Eur J Endocrinol. 2012;166:27–34.

33. Kamenicky P, Redheuil A, Roux C, et al. Cardiac structure and function in Cushing's syndrome: a cardiac magnetic resonance imaging study. J Clin Endocrinol Metab. 2014;99:E2144–53.

34. Muiesan ML, Lupia M, Salvetti M, et al. Left ventricular structural and functional characteristics in Cushing's syndrome. J Am Coll Cardiol. 2003;41:2275–9.

35. Hagstrom E, Ingelsson E, Sundstrom J, *et al.* Plasma parathyroid hormone and risk of congestive heart failure in the community. Eur J Heart Fail. 2010;12:1186–92.

36. Kestenbaum B, Katz R, de Boer I, *et al.* Vitamin D, parathyroid hormone, and cardiovascular events among older adults. J Am Coll Cardiol. 2011;58:1433–41.

37. di Giuseppe R, Buijsse B, Hirche F, *et al.* Plasma fibroblast growth factor 23, parathyroid hormone, 25-hydroxyvitamin D3, and risk of heart failure: a prospective, case-cohort study. J Clin Endocrinol Metab. 2014;99:947–55.

38. Schierbeck LL, Jensen TS, Bang U, Jensen G, Køber L, Jensen JEB. Parathyroid hormone and vitamin D: markers for cardiovascular and all-cause mortality in heart failure. Eur J Heart Fail 2011;13:626–32.

39. Birgander M, Bondeson AG, Bondeson L, Willenheimer R, Rydberg E. Cardiac structure and function before and after parathyroidectomy in patients with asymptomatic primary hyperparathyroidism. Endocrinologist. 2009;19:154.

40. Knoll K, Kurowski V, Schunkert H, Sager HB. Management of hypercalcaemia-induced heart failure using mechanical circulatory support. Eur J Cardio Thorac Surg. 2018;54:784–5.

41. Bansal N, Zelnick L, Robinson-Cohen C, *et al.* Serum parathyroid hormone and 25-hydroxyvitamin D concentrations and risk of incident heart failure: the multi-ethnic study of atherosclerosis. J Am Heart Assoc. 2014;3:e001278.

42. Bollerslev J, Rosen T, Mollerup CL, *et al.*; SIPH Study Group. Effect of surgery on cardiovascular risk factors in mild primary hyperparathyroidism. J Clin Endocrinol Metab. 2009;94:2255–61.

43. Oliveira Martins Duarte J, Pestana Pereira PML, Sobral ASG, *et al.* A rare and reversible case of heart failure hypocalcemia due to hypoparathyroidism. Clin Case Rep. 2019;7:1932–4.

44. Anderson JL, Vanwoerkom RC, Horne BD, *et al.* Parathyroid hormone, vitamin D, renal dysfunction and cardiovascular disease: dependent or independent risk factors? Am Heart J. 2011;162:331–9.

45. Parepa I. Hypocalcemic cardiomyopathy: a rare heart failure etiology in adult. Acta Endocrinol. 2019;15:107–12.

46. Holick MF. Vitamin D deficiency. N Engl J Med. 2007;357:266–81.

47. Witte KK, Byrom R, Gierula J, *et al.* Effects of vitamin D on cardiac function in patients with chronic HF. J Am Coll Cardiol. 2016;67:2593–603.

48. Marcinowska-Suchowierska E, Kupisz-Urbanska M, Łukaszkiewicz J, Płudowski P, Jones G. Vitamin D toxicity. A clinical perspective. Front Endocrinol. 2018;9:550.

49. Sharma AN, Tan M, Amsterdam EA, Singh GD. Acromegalic cardiomyopathy: epidemiology, diagnosis, and management. Clin Cardiol. 2018;41:419–25.

50. Lugo G, Pena L, Cordido F. Clinical manifestations and diagnosis of acromegaly. Int J Endocrinol. 2012;2012:540398.

51. Clayton RN. Cardiovascular function in acromegaly. Endocr Rev. 2003;24:272–7.

52. Bruch C, Herrmann B, Schmermund A, Bartel T, Mann K, Erbel R. Impact of disease activity on left ventricular performance in patients with acromegaly. Am Heart J. 2002;144:538–43.

53. Verhelst J, Abs R. Cardiovascular risk factors in hypopituitary GH-deficient adults. Eur J Endocrinol. 2009;161:S41–9.

54. Colao A. The GH-IGF-I axis and the cardiovascular system: clinical implications. Clin Endocrinol (Oxf). 2008;69:347–58.

55. Colao A, Di Somma C, Savanelli MC, De Leo M, Lombardi G. Beginning to end: cardiovascular implications of growth hormone (GH) deficiency and GH therapy. Growth Horm IGF Res. 2006;16:S41–8.

CHAPTER 3.8

Obesity

Lina Badimon, Stefan D Anker, and Stephan von Haehling

Contents

Introduction

Obesity is a growing cardiovascular health problem of epidemic proportions, with the World Health Organization (WHO) estimating more than 1 billion adults to be overweight, of whom 300 million are actually obese. Obesity has been known to be a direct cause of, but also a risk factor for, heart failure (HF). However, the situation appears to change once HF is clinically manifest, a situation known as the 'obesity paradox'. Usually, obesity is defined using the body mass index (BMI; kg/m^2), which was originally suggested in 1832 by the Belgian mathematician Adolphe Quételet (1796–1874).[1] The index formerly known as the Quételet index passed on to be called the BMI.[1] A BMI of ≥30 kg/ m^2 usually identifies obesity, and several grades have been defined (⮕ Table 3.8.1).

Epidemiology of obesity and heart failure

The prevalence of obesity in HF is higher in HF with preserved ejection fraction (HFpEF) than in HF with reduced ejection fraction (HFrEF). It has been reported to reach an average of 45% in HFpEF and 36% in HFrEF in hospital cohorts, 36% in HFpEF and 26% in HFrEF in randomized controlled trials, and 51% in HFpEF and 37% in HFrEF in community care.[2] The epidemic of obesity is an important public health problem. According to WHO data from 2016, 39% of adults worldwide are overweight (BMI ≥25 kg/m^2) and 13% of adults are obese (BMI ≥30 kg/m^2).[3] Determinants of the prevalence of obesity are geography, sex, and income level. The highest prevalence is found in the Americas (63% overweight, 29% obese), followed by Europe (62% overweight, 25% obese) and the low-end South East Asia (22% overweight, 5% obese). In America, Europe, and the Western Pacific, men are more likely to be overweight, whereas in the Eastern Mediterranean region, Asia, and Africa, the prevalence is higher in women. In contrast, the prevalence of obesity is higher in women in all regions. Thus, in Europe and the Eastern Mediterranean regions and America, over 50% of women are overweight, of whom about half are obese (obese women: 25% in the European region, 24% in the Eastern Mediterranean region, 30% in America). The most striking difference in obesity according to gender is seen in Africa, South East Asia, and the Eastern Mediterranean region where obesity prevalence in women is roughly double that in men.[3] If countries are stratified by income, overweight prevalence increases from low- (21%), lower middle- (28%), and upper middle- (43%) to high-income countries (57%). Similarly, the prevalence of obesity is four times higher in high-income (24%) than in low-income (5%) countries.[3] The dramatic development of overweight and obesity from 1980 to 2013 was recently described in a systematic analysis in the Global Burden of Disease Study 2013.[2] In both developed and developing countries, successive cohorts (birth years from 1935 to 2005) appeared to be gaining weight at all ages (including childhood and adolescence), with the most rapid weight gain at the age of 20–40 years. Furthermore, the prevalence of obesity in developed countries is moving towards younger ages.[3]

Table 3.8.1 Classification of body weight according to BMI

Classification term	BMI (kg/m²)
Underweight	<18.5
Normal weight	18.5–24.9
Overweight	25.0–29.9
Obesity grade 1	30.0–34.9
Obesity grade 2	35.0–39.9
Obesity grade 3 (morbid obesity)	≥40.0

Source data from Poirier P, Eckel RH. Cardiovascular consequences of obesity. *Drug Discovery Today: Therapeutic Strategies* 2008; 5:45–51.

Obesity is an independent risk factor for HF. Myocardial remodelling and diastolic dysfunction due to increased haemodynamic load, endothelial dysfunction, neurohormonal activation, and increased oxidative stress may result in congestive HF. However, no effect of obesity has been found on long-term survival. In many studies, a better outcome has been shown even in patients with increased BMI. This phenomenon, called the 'obesity paradox', is described in this chapter, but the underlying mechanisms remain elusive. Most of these studies have focused on the BMI, and a few on the percentage of body fat, but there is little information regarding other parameters such as the role of different adipose tissue depots (subcutaneous vs visceral vs ectopic) and their biochemical characteristics.

Obesity as a risk factor for heart disease and heart failure

Obesity and overweight are risk factors for heart disease. The adipose tissue has been traditionally considered an energy storage organ, but at present the existing evidence highlights the adipose tissue as an active endocrine organ that secretes numerous hormones and bioactive molecules called adipokines.[4] Adipokines regulate in an endocrine, autocrine, and paracrine manner not only adipose tissue metabolism, but also other main organs in the body, because they are key regulators of glucose, lipid metabolism, blood pressure, inflammation, and oxidative stress. Data also suggest that adipokine dysregulation may be the link between obesity and the development of cardiovascular diseases. Various adipokines, including adiponectin, leptin, omentin, and resistin, have been shown to affect the function of endothelial cells, smooth muscle cells, and innate immunity cells.[5]

Interestingly, certain adipose tissue depots are more strongly correlated with obesity-associated comorbidities than total adipose tissue mass, reinforcing the concept of depot-specific metabolic functions.[6] The principal depots of white adipose tissue (WAT) include visceral adipose tissue (VAT) which surrounds the visceral organs, subcutaneous adipose tissue (SAT) located below the skin, and ectopic adipose tissue which consists of non-storage depots. Although overall fat mass is important for the development of obesity-associated comorbidities, VAT accumulation is an independent risk factor for obesity-related metabolic and cardiovascular disorders. This differential impact on cardiovascular risk seems to be related to adipokines secreted from different fat depots. Specifically, leptin, mainly secreted by SAT, is positively correlated with body fat, whereas adiponectin which is more influenced by VAT is reduced in obesity. A recent finding from the Multi-Ethnic Study of Atherosclerosis (MESA) describes that only visceral fat was associated with incident HF, whereas subcutaneous fat was not.[7] More information on the effects of fat depots, including epicardial fat, on the development of HF is needed.

Pathophysiology: obesity and comorbidities in heart failure

In healthy conditions, adipose tissue is composed of a variety of cells, in addition to mature adipocytes. These include adipocyte progenitors, endothelial cells, fibroblasts, and immune cells (M2-like macrophages, T regulatory cells (Tregs), and eosinophils) (⮑ Figure 3.8.1). When adipose tissue expands, adipocytes

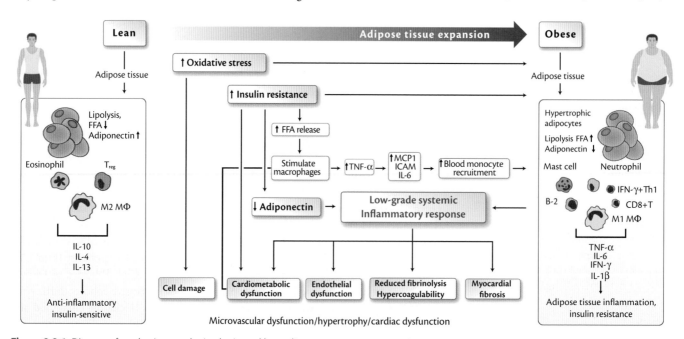

Figure 3.8.1 Diagram of mechanisms at play in obesity and heart disease.

enlarge, storing fat, and monocytes are recruited from blood into the obese adipose tissue where they differentiate into M1 macrophages with pro-inflammatory activity. Adipocytes release free fatty acids (FFAs) and stimulate macrophages via Toll-like receptor (TLR) 4, resulting in NF-κB activation (master transcription factor for inflammatory responses) and tumour necrosis factor alpha (TNF-α) production. In turn, macrophage-derived TNF-α activates adipocytes to secrete monocyte chemoattractant protein 1 (MCP-1) and interleukin-6 (IL-6), promoting further monocyte infiltration.[8] In addition, expansion of adipose tissue is accompanied by a reduction in eosinophils and Tregs and an increase in neutrophils, B cells, mast cells, and interferon gamma-producing T helper 1 (Th1) and CD8+ T cells that together create an overall pro-inflammatory milieu. This inflammatory response is further enhanced by a decrease in adiponectin, a key adipose tissue-secreted anti-inflammatory protein that inhibits TLR-activated NF-κB activity.[9] Neuroendocrine alterations and enhanced oxidative stress seem to induce the decline in adiponectin release. Perpetuation of this cycle triggers a local pro-inflammatory response that propagates into low-grade systemic inflammation.[5]

The different fat depots (visceral vs subcutaneous) are heterogeneous not only in terms of metabolic capacities, but also in macrophage abundance and secretome patterns. As such, M2 macrophage infiltration and secretion of pro-inflammatory mediators are more pronounced in VAT than in SAT.[10] The role of the different adipose tissue depots in organ function and the potential role for microRNAs (miRNAs) in the pathogenesis of obesity and their effects on the myocardium are matters of active investigation.

Hypertension, diabetes mellitus, hyperlipidaemia, and metabolic syndrome are common comorbidities in obesity that also have a high impact on the development of HF and affect clinical outcomes. Control of these different cardiovascular risk factors by coordinated prevention strategies will help to reduce the burden of HF.

Cardiometabolic dysfunction and heart failure

Obesity has a high influence on the regulation of cardiac metabolism. The normal heart uses both FFAs and glucose as substrates to maintain its energy balance. In obesity, plasma levels of FFAs and triacylglycerol increase, modifying not only uptake of FFAs, but also that of glucose.[11] Intracellular accumulation of lipids, and thus alterations in cardiac metabolism, occurs due to excessive fatty acid utilization as substrate (➲ Figure 3.8.1).

Increased FFA oxidation still cannot keep up with the accumulation of FFAs, resulting in the formation and accumulation of lipotoxins such as ceramides. A more detailed picture emerged from studies showing that increased levels of FFA inhibit glucose uptake driven by insulin.[12] In addition, mitochondrial oxidative capacity is reduced, whereas mitochondrial uncoupling is increased, which—together with decreased glucose utilization—impairs myocardial energetics and consequently mechanical performance.[11] Finally, increased levels of FFAs inhibit oxidation of pyruvate and pyruvate dehydrogenase activity. These mechanisms may contribute to systolic dysfunction, increased end-diastolic volume, and cardiac hypertrophy that can be observed in obesity.[13,14] Furthermore, adipokines also exert effects on cardiac metabolism; although the exact role of adiponectin remains incompletely understood, it appears to increase FFA oxidation in the heart and skeletal muscle. Leptin also increases FFA oxidation and associated oxygen consumption, which decreases cardiac efficiency, in part attributable to mitochondrial uncoupling.[13,14] Moreover, leptin may increase blood pressure by increasing sympathetic vasomotor tone, which could promote cardiac hypertrophy.

Vascular effects and microvascular dysfunction

Obesity is associated with altered endothelial function that shifts the balance towards constriction by impairing the release and activity of relaxing factors and concomitantly enhancing the production of vasoconstrictors. The resulting enhanced vascular tone compromises regional blood flow to different tissues and organs (including the coronary circulation) and consequently impairs organ function. The vasoconstrictor influence is enhanced, in part, by an enhanced sympathetic tone in obese subjects, but also because the endothelium releases potent vasoconstrictors.[15] Impaired endothelial function is aggravated as obesity progresses towards insulin resistance.

Classical adipokines also exert detrimental effects on endothelial cells. Leptin was initially described as a peptide stimulating endothelial dilator mechanisms (at high concentrations), but such effects are lost in obese individuals. Conversely, adiponectin has been found to exert beneficial effects on endothelial dilator functions.[16] The discrepant effects of these two adipokines on vascular function may add up to worsen the vascular dilator capacity in obesity, because leptin levels are enhanced (suggested to be a consequence of leptin resistance) whereas adiponectin levels are decreased in obese individuals. There is ample evidence from both clinical and experimental studies that obesity is an independent risk factor for coronary microvascular dysfunction.[17,18,19] In addition, obesity is associated with perturbations in adjustments to coronary blood flow with increased metabolic demands.[17] Obesity-associated abnormalities in coronary blood flow regulation can result from either functional changes, that is, regulation of vascular tone, or structural changes within the coronary microcirculation, for example, rarefaction and/or inward remodelling.[20,21,22] Alterations in the control of coronary microvascular tone are characterized by loss of endothelial vasodilator influence, as well as by increased neurohumoral and endothelium-derived (ROS, endothelin, prostanoids) vasoconstrictor influences, resulting in a shift in the vasomotor balance towards increased vasoconstriction. In addition to the functional changes in the control of vascular tone, obesity can also result in structural remodelling of coronary microcirculation. Further research is needed to understand the underlying mechanisms, from inflammation to substrate provision to microvascular cell in-depth regulation, that trigger coronary microvascular abnormalities in obesity and how this impacts the development of HF.

Obesity and changes in cardiac haemodynamics

Obesity causes a vast array of haemodynamic alterations that can lead to changes in cardiac morphology and ventricular function. First and foremost, excessive adipose tissue accumulation yields an increase in total and central blood volume. However, because adipose tissue is not normally highly perfused, the relationship between the BMI and blood volume is non-linear. Still, the altered blood volume triggers an increased preload and stroke volume, ultimately leading to an increase in cardiac output. As there is only minimal change in the heart rate, changes in stroke volume are the main drivers of this haemodynamic adaptation.[23] Using data from 700 patients without coronary artery disease who underwent coronary angiography, Stelfox et al.[23] reported an increase of 0.08 L/min in cardiac output, with each increase per BMI-unit. The corresponding increase in stroke volume was 1.35 mL per BMI-unit. In this study, cardiac index and stroke volume index were less reliable than the absolute values (→ Figure 3.8.2). Adipose tissue has little metabolic demand, but obesity also comes with increased lean tissue, which is associated with increased oxygen requirements and carbon dioxide production.

Early reports noted excessive cardiac fat accumulation leading to an increase in heart weight.[24] Post-mortem studies revealed that increased heart weight is associated with increased left ventricular wall thickness and left ventricular hypertrophy in almost all cases. Increased right ventricular wall thickness affects only 15% of cases, but excessive epicardial fat has been reported in 64% of cases.[25] Left ventricular mass is consistently correlated with body weight and BMI, which has mostly been attributed to increased pre- and afterload-associated ventricular remodelling. Another important predictor of increased left ventricular mass is the duration of obesity, particularly when present for more than 15 years.[25] Haemodynamic changes include increased resting left ventricular and diastolic pressure as a result of poor left ventricular compliance, increased pulmonary artery and right atrial pressures, and increased pulmonary capillary wedge pressure, even though the latter finding was inconsistent. One study found that exercise in morbidly obese subjects yielded an increase in central blood volume of about 20%, an increase in left ventricular dp/dt of 57%, and an increase in left ventricular end-diastolic pressure of about 48%. Resulting changes in blood flow include, for example, changes in cerebral blood flow, which seems to be low-normal or low. Splanchnic blood flow, on the other hand, is increased, whereas renal blood flow is reduced. Interestingly, left ventricular systolic function parameters show mixed results when obese and non-obese patients are compared. Some studies showed lower mean left ventricular ejection fraction values in obese subjects, whereas others failed to find significant differences. Conduction abnormalities typically lead to increases in QRS and QT duration; other changes are rather inconsistent.[26]

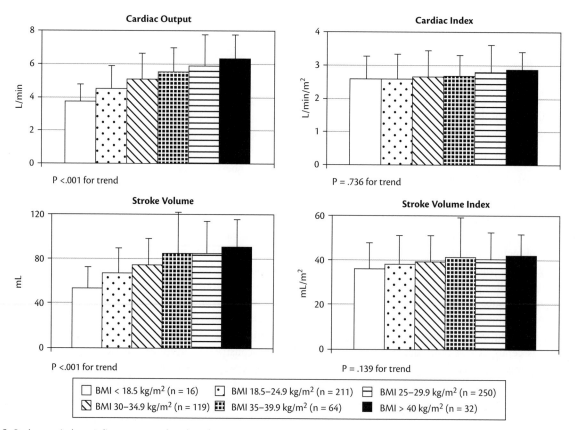

Figure 3.8.2 Body mass index, cardiac output, and stroke volume.

Reproduced from Stelfox HT, Ahmed SB, Ribeiro RA, Gettings EM, Pomerantsev E, Schmidt U. Hemodynamic monitoring in obese patients: the impact of body mass index on cardiac output and stroke volume. *Crit Care Med.* 2006 Apr;34(4):1243–6. doi: 10.1097/01.CCM.0000208358.27005.F4 with permission from Wolters Kluwer.

The obesity paradox revisited

The term obesity paradox has received tremendous interest in recent years. It describes a phenomenon that is reproducible across a wide range of large-scale trial databases in HF, as well as other cardiovascular disorders. Conditions that have been associated with the obesity paradox include coronary artery disease, acute myocardial infarction, acute cerebral stroke or transient ischaemic attack, atrial fibrillation, percutaneous coronary intervention, and transcatheter aortic valve implantation, as well as several types of cardiovascular surgery.[27] Here the term obesity paradox describes a state in which mild obesity is associated with better survival than normal weight or underweight. The prerequisite for the occurrence of this phenomenon is always the presence of chronic disease, usually associated with at least subclinical inflammatory processes. Therefore, it is not surprising that the obesity paradox is reproducible not only in chronic cardiovascular disease, but also in cancer and pulmonary and kidney diseases, as well as in patients on intensive care units.[28]

The obesity paradox was first described in patients on haemodialysis in the late 1990s,[29] only to be validated in cardiac patients by Gruberg and colleagues in 2002 when they studied 633 consecutive patients undergoing percutaneous coronary intervention and divided them into three groups according to BMI: 18.5–24.9, 25–30, and >30 kg/m². [30] Interestingly, they found that among these patients, underweight subjects and those with a BMI in the normal range had the highest risk of in-hospital complications and cardiac death, as well as increased 1-year mortality. Based on this observation, researchers started to undertake validation studies from available databases, for example, using the ADHERE database that includes data from 108,927 patients hospitalized for acute HF in 263 hospitals.[31] They found that patients in the highest quartile of BMI above 30.4 kg/m² had the lowest mortality rate, independent of whether the left ventricular ejection fraction was <40% or ≥40% (◉ Figure 3.8.3). Overall, the authors noted that for every 5-unit increase in BMI, the odds of risk-adjusted mortality were 10% lower (95% confidence interval 0.88–0.93; P <0.0001). A meta-analysis of nine observational studies to investigate the relationship between increased BMI and mortality in 28,209 patients with HF, with a mean follow-up duration of 2.7 years, found that both overweight and obesity were associated with lower all-cause mortality, as well as with lower cardiovascular mortality.[32] Data from 6632 patients enrolled into the EPHESUS trial of eplerenone post-acute myocardial infarction found similar results. Of the patients enrolled, 1573 were obese with a BMI of ≥30 kg/m². Interestingly, the authors used a propensity score matching analysis pattern and found that the paradoxical pre-match associates between obesity and reduced mortality disappeared when the analysis was adjusted only for age, but not for gender. The authors concluded that paradoxical unadjusted survival associated with obesity may be largely explained by the younger age of obese patients. Indeed, a number of mechanisms have been suggested to explain the protective

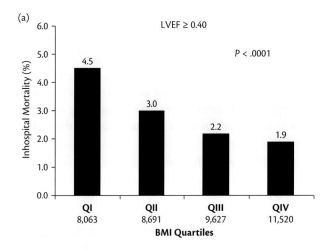

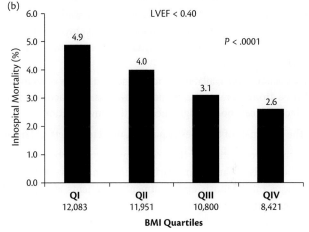

Figure 3.8.3 Obesity paradox. Body mass index and mortality risk.
Reproduced from Fonarow GC, Srikanthan P, Costanzo MR, Cintron GB, Lopatin M; ADHERE Scientific Advisory Committee and Investigators. An obesity paradox in acute heart failure: analysis of body mass index and inhospital mortality for 108,927 patients in the Acute Decompensated Heart Failure National Registry. *Am Heart J.* 2007 Jan;153(1):74–81. doi: 10.1016/j.ahj.2006.09.007 with permission from Elsevier.

effect of higher BMI, including factors such as storage of fat or muscle mass, potentially more aggressive treatment in obese subjects, or even selection bias.[33] Others have suggested the existence of a 'lean paradox', with normal weight or underweight having a poorer prognosis.[34] The ongoing debate, however, is continuously fuelled by additional data published on the presence of an obesity paradox also for patients with HFpEF. Data from the I-PRESERVE trial showed a U-shaped relationship between BMI category and adverse outcomes.[35] In this analysis, patients with BMI of 26.5–30.9 kg/m² had the lowest rate of the primary composite outcome of death or cardiovascular hospitalization. This relationship remained robust, even after adjusting for 21 risk variables, including age, gender, and N-terminal pro-B-type natriuretic peptide.

With the obesity paradox being highly reproducible across databases, the European Society of Cardiology's guidelines for HF state that in HF patients with moderate degrees of obesity (BMI <35 kg/m²), weight loss cannot be recommended. In those with more advanced obesity (35–45 kg/m²), weight loss may be considered to manage symptoms and exercise capacity.[36]

Summary and key messages

Obesity is a risk factor for the development of HF, with a higher impact in HFpEF than in HFrEF. However, this effect is diluted in patients with HF, with the best prognosis observed in overweight and obese patients and the worst prognosis observed in underweight or cachectic patients. We are missing information to be able to have an in-depth understanding of these clinical observations:

◆ While BMI is a clinically easy and non-invasive parameter to determine obesity, it is imprecise and possibly outdated. Other scores are needed.

◆ Currently, we know that the different fat depots are metabolically distinct. The different adipose tissue depots may have differential effects in HF and on its development and severity.

◆ Future studies should aim at enhancing our understanding of the specific role of epicardial adipose tissue on myocardial function and on functional and structural alterations of myocardial perfusion.

◆ Excess fatty acid availability and the indirect effects of factors released from extracardiac tissues, as well as the haemodynamic effect of excess body weight, need further investigation.

◆ The dynamics of the obesity paradox need to be better clarified.

Active investigation of the cross-regulation of obesity-driven metabolic disturbances in heart function may have future implications on diagnosis and treatment of patients at risk of HF development.

References

1. Eknoyan G. Adolpfe Quetelet (1796–1874): the average man and indices of obesity. Nephrol Dial Transplant. 2008;23(1):47–51.

2. Triposkiadis F, Giamouzis G, Parissis J, et al. Reframing the association and significance of co-morbidities in heart failure. Eur J Heart Fail. 2016;18(7):744–58.

3. World Health Organization. The Global Health Observatory [online database]. Available from: http://apps.who.int/gho/data/view.main

4. Scherer PE. Adipose tissue: from lipid storage compartment to endocrine organ. Diabetes. 2006;55:1537–45.

5. Badimon L, Bugiardini R, Cenko E, et al. Obesity and heart disease. Eur Heart J. 2017;38(25):1951–8.

6. Ferrer-Lorente R, Bejar MT, Tous M, Vilahur G, Badimon L. Systems biology approach to identify alterations in the stem cell reservoir of subcutaneous adipose tissue in a rat model of diabetes: effects on differentiation potential and function. Diabetologia. 2014;57:246–56.

7. Rao VN, Zhao D, Allison MA, et al. Adiposity and incident heart failure and its subtypes: MESA (Multi-Ethnic Study of Atherosclerosis). JACC Heart Fail. 2018;6:999–1007.

8. Han MS, Jung DY, Morel C, et al. JNK expression by macrophages promotes obesity-induced insulin resistance and inflammation. Science. 2013;339:218–22.

9. Wensveen FM, Valentic S, Sestan M, Turk Wensveen T, Polic B. The 'Big Bang' in obese fat: events initiating obesity-induced adipose tissue inflammation. Eur J Immunol. 2015;45:2446–56.

10. Zhu Y, Tchkonia T, Stout MB, et al. Inflammation and the depot-specific secretome of human preadipocytes. Obesity (Silver Spring). 2015;23:989–99.

11. Lopaschuk GD, Ussher JR, Folmes CD, Jaswal JS, Stanley WC. Myocardial fatty acid metabolism in health and disease. Physiol Rev. 2010;90:207–25.

12. Peterson LR, Soto PF, Herrero P, et al. Impact of gender on the myocardial metabolic response to obesity. JACC Cardiovasc Imaging. 2008;1:424–33.

13. Boudina S, Sena S, O'Neill BT, Tathireddy P, Young ME, Abel ED. Reduced mitochondrial oxidative capacity and increased mitochondrial uncoupling impair myocardial energetics in obesity. Circulation. 2005;112:2686–95.

14. Guarini G, Kiyooka T, Ohanyan V, et al. Impaired coronary metabolic dilation in the metabolic syndrome is linked to mitochondrial dysfunction and mitochondrial DNA damage. Basic Res Cardiol. 2016;111:29.

15. Bagi Z, Feher A, Cassuto J. Microvascular responsiveness in obesity: implications for therapeutic intervention. Br J Pharmacol. 2012;165:544–60.

16. Margaritis M, Antonopoulos AS, Digby J, et al. Interactions between vascular wall and perivascular adipose tissue reveal novel roles for adiponectin in the regulation of endothelial nitric oxide synthase function in human vessels. Circulation. 2013;127:2209–21.

17. Romero-Corral A, Sert-Kuniyoshi FH, Sierra-Johnson J, et al. Modest visceral fat gain causes endothelial dysfunction in healthy humans. J Am Coll Cardiol. 2010;56:662–6.

18. Koller A, Balasko M, Bagi Z. Endothelial regulation of coronary microcirculation in health and cardiometabolic diseases. Intern Emerg Med. 2013;8 Suppl 1:S51–4.

19. Berwick ZC, Dick GM, Tune JD. Heart of the matter: coronary dysfunction in metabolic syndrome. J Mol Cell Cardiol. 2012;52:848–56.

20. Belin de Chantemele EJ, Stepp DW. Influence of obesity and metabolic dysfunction on the endothelial control in the coronary circulation. J Mol Cell Cardiol. 2012;52:840–7.

21. Duncker DJ, Koller A, Merkus D, Canty JM, Jr. Regulation of coronary blood flow in health and ischemic heart disease. Prog Cardiovasc Dis. 2015;57:409–22.

22. Pries AR, Badimon L, Bugiardini R, et al. Coronary vascular regulation, remodelling, and collateralization: mechanisms and clinical implications on behalf of the working group on coronary pathophysiology and microcirculation. Eur Heart J. 2015;36:3134–46.

23. Stelfox HT, Ahmed SB, Ribeiro RA, Gettings EM, Pomerantsev E, Schmidt U. Hemodynamic monitoring in obese patients: the impact of body mass index on cardiac output and stroke volume. Crit Care Med. 2006;34(4):1243–6.

24. Bedford E. The story of fatty heart. A disease of Victorian times. Br Heart J. 1972;34(1):23–8.

25. Nakajima T, Fujioka S, Tokunaga K, Hirobe K, Matsuzawa Y, Tarui S. Noninvasive study of left ventricular performance in obese patients: influence of duration of obesity. Circulation. 1985;71(3):481–6.

26. Poirier P, Eckel RH. Cardiovascular consequences of obesity. Drug Discovery Today: Therapeutic Strategies. 2008; 5:45–51.

27. Doehner W. Critical appraisal of the obesity paradox in cardiovascular disease: how to manage patients with overweight in heart failure? Heart Fail Rev. 2014;19(5):637–44.

28. Lainscak M, von Haehling S, Doehner W, Anker SD. The obesity paradox in chronic disease: facts and numbers. J Cachexia Sarcopenia Muscle. 2012;3(1):1–4.

29. Fleischmann E, Teal N, Dudley J, May W, Bower JD, Salahudeen AK. Influence of excess weight on mortality and hospital stay in 1346 hemodialysis patients. Kidney Int. 1999;55(4):1560–7.

30. Gruberg L, Weissman NJ, Waksman R, *et al.* The impact of obesity on the short-term and long-term outcomes after percutaneous coronary intervention: the obesity paradox? J Am Coll Cardiol. 2002;39(4):578–84.

31. Fonarow GC, Srikanthan P, Costanzo MR, Cintron GB, Lopatin M; ADHERE Scientific Advisory Committee and Investigators. An obesity paradox in acute heart failure: analysis of body mass index and inhospital mortality for 108,927 patients in the Acute Decompensated Heart Failure National Registry. Am Heart J. 2007;153(1):74–81.

32. Oreopoulos A, Padwal R, Kalantar-Zadeh K, Fonarow GC, Norris C, McAlister FA. Body mass index and mortality in heart failure: a meta-analysis. Am Heart J. 2008;156(1):13–22.

33. Da Fonseca GWP, von Haehling S. An overview of anamorelin as a treatment option for cancer-associated anorexia and cachexia. Expert Opin Pharmacother. 2021;22(7):889–95.

34. Elagizi A, Kachur S, Lavie CJ, *et al.* An overview and update on obesity and the obesity paradox in cardiovascular diseases. Prog Cardiovasc Dis. 2018;61(2):142–50.

35. Haass M, Kithman DW, Anand IS, *et al.* Body mass index and adverse cardiovascular outcomes in heart failure patients with preserved ejection fraction: results from the Irbesartan in Heart Failure with Preserved Ejection Fraction (I-PRESERVE) trial. Circ Heart Fail. 2011;4(3):324–31.

36. Ponikowski P, Voors AA, Anker SD, *et al.*; ESC Scientific Document Group. 2016 ESC Guidelines for the diagnosis and treatment of acute and chronic heart failure: The Task Force for the diagnosis and treatment of acute and chronic heart failure of the European Society of Cardiology (ESC) Developed with the special contribution of the Heart Failure Association (HFA) of the ESC. Eur Heart J. 2016;37(27):2129–200. Erratum in: Eur Heart J. 2016; PMID: 27206819.

CHAPTER 3.9

Cancer and cancer therapy

Dimitrios Farmakis*, Alexander Lyon*,
Teresa Lopez Fernandez, and
Daniela Cardinale

Contents

Introduction

Cancer and cancer therapies increase the vulnerability of the cardiovascular (CV) system, and are well-established risk factors for heart failure (HF) and left ventricular (LV) dysfunction during and after treatment.[1] In a recent observational study including >3 million cancer survivors, 11% died from CV diseases (two-thirds with HF). CV mortality risk was highest within the first year following cancer diagnosis, although it remained elevated throughout follow-up.[2] There are a range of effective cancer treatments recognized to cause LV dysfunction and HF (➲ Table 3.9.1). HF may manifest during cancer treatment, whereas close monitoring with echocardiography, including myocardial strain imaging, and cardiac biomarkers allows early detection of preclinical myocardial dysfunction. This is important as early detection allows implementation of cardioprotective strategies to mitigate the risk of developing clinical HF. HF can also present in cancer survivors following completion of cancer treatment. The delay in presentation can range from within 12 months of the last cancer treatment to 20+ years later, particularly in young patients.

Historically, anthracycline chemotherapy has been identified as a cause of HF in cancer patients and survivors since its introduction in the 1960s. The first reports of cardiotoxicity appeared in the 1960s, and more detailed studies, with recognition of increased risk with increasing dose, began in the 1970s. High-dose radiation therapy to a field involving the heart has now been identified to cause HF via a range of pathophysiological mechanisms in cancer survivors, often presenting late, up to more than 10 years, after their radiation therapy.

The monoclonal antibody trastuzumab is an effective treatment for human epidermal growth factor receptor 2 (HER2)-positive breast cancer, and the observation of trastuzumab-induced LV dysfunction and HF began in the late 1990s and the 2000–10 era from large randomized trials when cardiac surveillance became mandatory. In the last 20 years, there has been an explosion of new cancer therapies which are now recognized to cause LV dysfunction and HF, including tyrosine kinase inhibitors (TKIs) blocking specific cellular growth and signalling pathways, RAF–MEK inhibitors, proteasome inhibitors (PIs), and drugs activating the immune system (immune checkpoint inhibitors (ICIs)).

---

* DF and AL have contributed equally and share the lead author role.

Table 3.9.1 Main systemic anticancer agents causing left ventricular dysfunction and heart failure

Drug class	Drug names	Main indications
Anthracyclines	Doxorubicin, epirubicin, daunorubicin, idarubicin	Breast cancer, lymphoma, acute leukaemia, sarcoma
Alkylating agents	Cyclophosphamide, ifosfamide, melphalan	Breast cancer, lung cancer, ovarian cancer, sarcomas, leukaemia, lymphomas, multiple myeloma
HER2-targeted therapies	Trastuzumab, pertuzumab, emtansine (T-DM1), lapatinib, neratinib, tucatinib	HER2+ breast cancer HER2+ gastric cancer
VEGF inhibitors	TKIs: sunitinib, pazopanib, sorafenib, axitinib, tivozanib, cabozantinib, regorafenib, lenvatinib, vandetinib Antibodies: bevacizumab, ramucirumab	VEGF TKIs: renal cancer, hepatocellular cancer, thyroid cancer, colon cancer, sarcoma, GIST Antibodies: breast cancer, ovarian cancer, gastric cancer, gastro-oesophageal cancer, colon cancer
Multi-targeted kinase inhibitors	First generation: imatinib Second generation: nilotinib, dasatinib, bosutinib Third generation: ponatinib	Chronic myeloid leukaemia
Proteasome inhibitors	Carfilzomib, bortezomib, ixazomib	Multiple myeloma
Immunomodulatory drugs	Lenalidomide, pomalidomide	Multiple myeloma
Combination RAF and MEK inhibitors	Dabrafenib + trametinib, vemurafenib + cobimetinib, encorafenib + binimetinib	RAF-mutant melanoma
Immune checkpoint inhibitors	Anti-programmed cell death 1 inhibitors: nivolumab, pembrolizumab Anti-cytotoxic T lymphocyte-associated protein 4 inhibitor: ipilimumab Anti-programmed death ligand 1 inhibitor: avelumab, atezolizumab, durvalumab	Melanoma (metastatic and adjuvant) Metastatic renal cancer, non-small cell lung cancer, small cell lung cancer, refractory Hodgkin's lymphoma, metastatic triple negative breast cancer, metastatic urothelial cancer, liver cancer, MMR-deficient cancer
Anti-androgrens	Abiraterone	Prostate cancer
GnRH agonists	Goserelin	ER+ breast cancer
EGFR inhibitors	Osimertinib	EGFR-mutant non-small cell lung cancer

HER2, human epidermal growth factor receptor 2; T-DM1, trastuzumab-DM1; VEGF, vascular endothelial growth factor; TKI, tyrosine kinase inhibitor; GIST, gastrointestinal stromal tumour; GnRH, gonadotropin-releasing hormone; ER, (o)estrogen receptor; MMR, mismatch repair; EGFR, epidermal growth factor receptor.
Source data from Baseline cardiovascular risk assessment in cancer patients scheduled to receive cardiotoxic cancer therapies: a position statement and new risk assessment tools from the Cardio-Oncology Study Group of the Heart Failure Association of the European Society of Cardiology in collaboration with the International Cardio-Oncology Society. *Eur J Heart Fail.* 2020 Nov;22(11):1945–1960. doi: 10.1002/ejhf.1920.

Heart failure and left ventricular dysfunction during cancer treatment

Definition of cancer therapy-related cardiac dysfunction

According to the International Cardio-Oncology Society 2021 consensus statement, cancer therapy-related cardiac dysfunction is defined as, and classified according to, the presence or absence of HF symptoms, the degree of LV ejection fraction (LVEF) decline, and the presence or absence of LV global longitudinal strain (GLS) decrease or cardiac biomarker (troponins, natriuretic peptides) elevation.[3] This definition is presented in ◗ Table 3.9.2.

Table 3.9.2 Definition and classification of cancer therapy-related cardiac dysfunction according to the International Society of Cardio-Oncology 2021 consensus statement

	Mild	Moderate	Severe	Very severe
Asymptomatic CTRCD	LVEF ≥50% AND new relative decline in GLS by >15% from baseline AND/OR new rise in cardiac biomarker levels	New LVEF reduction by ≥10% to LVEF of 40–49% OR new LVEF reduction by 15% from baseline AND/OR new rise in cardiac biomarker levels	New LVEF reduction to <40%	
Symptomatic CTRCD	Mild HF symptoms, no intensification of therapy required	Need for outpatient intensification of diuretic and HF therapy	HF hospitalization	Requiring inotropic support, mechanical circulatory support, or consideration for transplantation

CTRD, cancer therapy-related cardiac dysfunction; LVEF, left ventricular ejection fraction; GLS, global longitudinal strain; HF, heart failure.
Source data from Herrmann J, Lenihan D, Armenian S, *et al.* Defining cardiovascular toxicities of cancer therapies: an International Cardio-Oncology Society (IC-OS) consensus statement. *Eur Heart J.* 2022 Jan 31;43(4):280–299. doi: 10.1093/eurheartj/ehab674.

Anthracyclines

Anthracycline chemotherapies, including doxorubicin, epirubicin, idarubicin, and daunorubicin, are part of evidence-based treatments for a range of malignancies, including breast cancer, lymphomas, leukaemias, and sarcomas. These are used for patients with potentially curable cancers, as well as those with metastatic disease. Anthracycline chemotherapy is cardiotoxic via inhibition of topoisomerase IIβ in cardiomyocytes, leading to increased oxidative stress, decreased mitochondrial function, and apoptosis or necrosis.[4]

In modern series, a 9% incidence of LV dysfunction was observed in adult patients during the first year after completion of therapy, with >75% of whom being asymptomatic at diagnosis.[5,6] Although HF can occur at any anthracycline dose, patients receiving >250 mg/m^2 of doxorubicin or equivalent or combination therapy (chemotherapy, HER2-therapies, or mediastinal irradiation) are at higher risk.[7] The presence of pre-existing CV conditions[8] and premature occurrence of conventional CV risk factors[9] increase patient susceptibility to develop long-term HF.[10] Adult survivors of childhood and adolescent cancer treated with anthracyclines and radiotherapy have a high dose-dependent HF risk (incidence of grade ≥3 CV diseases at 40 years of 7.4%).[11,12]

Risk stratification before starting treatment followed by close surveillance in medium- and high-risk patients is recommended, according to the European Society of Cardiology (ESC) 2021 heart failure guidelines and the 2022 ESC guidelines on cardio-oncology (⊃ Figure 3.9.1).[13a,13b]

During treatment, a rise in cardiac troponin level or a fall in GLS is an early sign of cardiotoxicity, predicting a later LVEF decline and further CV events.[14] Using high-sensitivity (hs)-troponin, up to 50% of patients receiving six cycles of R-CHOP chemotherapy have a detectable rise in their cardiac troponin level during treatment.[15] Specific guidance on risk stratification and patient monitoring is provided in a series of ESC Heart Failure Association (HFA) position statements.[16,17,18]

Trastuzumab and HER2-targeted therapies

Trastuzumab was the first monoclonal antibody developed to target the HER2 receptor expressed on HER2+ breast cancer cells. There are now a range of other agents used in combination with trastuzumab (pertuzumab) or in place of trastuzumab (trastuzumab emtansine and trastuzumab deruxtecan), and also small-molecule HER2 TKIs (lapatinib, neratinib, tucatinib). These treatments are proven to improve survival in women with early invasive or metastatic HER2+ breast cancer, but cause LV systolic dysfunction in up to 15% of cases. After the initially high rates of fatal HF (5%) in the first trials of metastatic HER2+ breast cancer where trastuzumab and anthracycline chemotherapy were given concordantly, trastuzumab administration was delayed until after completion of anthracycline chemotherapy in subsequent trials and real-world practice.

The overall incidence of trastuzumab-induced cardiotoxicity varies according to the definition used in different studies: the rate of LV dysfunction ranges from 2% to 7% when trastuzumab is used as monotherapy; from 2% to 13% when trastuzumab is used

in combination with paclitaxel; and up to 28% when trastuzumab is used concurrently with anthracyclines plus cyclophosphamide.[19,20,21,22,23,24,25,26,27] The rate and severity of trastuzumab-related LV dysfunction and HF are higher at approximately 10–16% in real-world cohorts, compared to breast cancer trials.[28]

Trastuzumab causes a different form of cardiotoxicity from that of anthracyclines: it typically manifests during treatment and is not dose-dependent, and anthracycline-like changes are not seen on biopsy. Differently from anthracyclines, which are directly cytotoxic, trastuzumab decreases cardiomyocyte resilience to other stressors by hindering cellular survival mechanisms downstream of the HER2 receptor, blocking neuregulin function, released by endothelial cells, that is pivotal for normal cardiac growth and survival (⊃ Figure 3.9.2).[29,30,31]

The clinical outcome of patients with trastuzumab-induced cardiotoxicity seems more favourable than that associated with anthracycline: LV dysfunction usually recovers after drug withdrawal and HF therapy initiation.[32]

Recognized factors associated with an increased risk of developing trastuzumab cardiotoxicity include older age, pre-existing CV comorbid conditions (e.g. hypertension, coronary artery disease), low-normal baseline LVEF, obesity, black race, previous treatment with anthracycline chemotherapy, and short time interval between anthracycline treatment and trastuzumab administration.[29] In 251 women with breast cancer, high baseline level of troponin I showed to be a predictor of trastuzumab-induced cardiac dysfunction.[33] These findings were confirmed in a subsequent study including 533 breast cancer patients receiving trastuzumab: an increased baseline level of troponin I (or T) was associated with a 4-fold risk of developing LV dysfunction.[34]

Trastuzumab-DM1 (T-DM1) is an immunoconjugate consisting of trastuzumab and emtansine, a chemotherapeutic agent with potent cytotoxic activity on microtubules.[35]

Pertuzumab is a fully humanized monoclonal antibody that, after binding to the HER2 receptor, causes activation of antibody-mediated cellular cytotoxicity, similarly to trastuzumab. Pertuzumab and trastuzumab, by targeting different HER2 epitopes, seem to express complementary and synergistic activity.[36,37]

The incidence of T-DM1 and pertuzumab cardiotoxic effects, in comparison with trastuzumab, was evaluated in large clinical trials.[38,39,40,41,42,43] In summary, T-DM1 showed a lower rate of LV dysfunction than trastuzumab, and might be the choice for patients needing long-term treatment with trastuzumab and who are at high risk of cardiotoxicity. Pertuzumab seems to add only little additional risk of cardiotoxicity to trastuzumab, with which it is nearly always administered.

Lapatinib is an oral small-molecule inhibitor of the HER1/ErbB1 and HER2/ErbB2 receptor tyrosine kinases, approved for metastatic breast cancer.[44,45] The overall cardiotoxicity rate related to lapatinib is 2.7%.[46] Lapatinib was found in a phase 3 randomized clinical trial to increase the rate of cardiac events (decreased LVEF and HF) from 5% to 9% when given with paclitaxel in metastatic breast cancer.[47] Similar to trastuzumab, the cardiotoxic effects of lapatinib are exacerbated by concomitant anthracycline

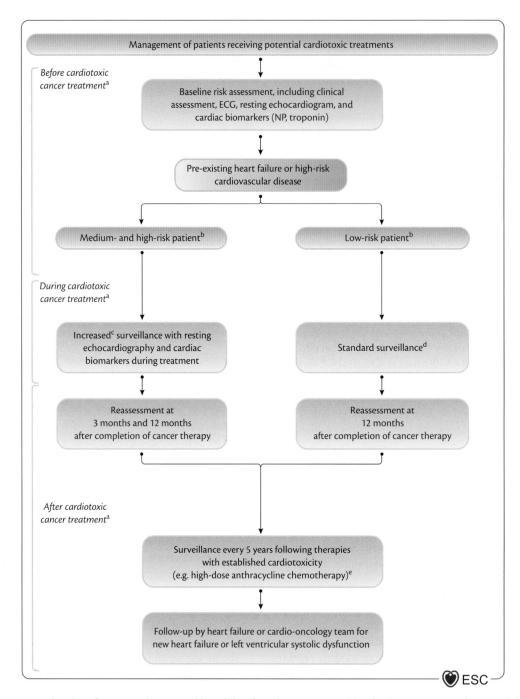

Figure 3.9.1 Management algorithm of patients with cancer and heart failure, from the 2021 ESC Guideline for the management of acute and chronic heart failure.
[a]Anthracycline chemotherapy, trastuzumab and HER2-targeted therapies, VEGF inhibitors, proteasome inhibitors, combination RAF/MEK inhibitors. [b] Low, medium and high risk may be calculated using the HFA-ICOS baseline cardiovascular risk proformas. [c] Increased surveillance is intended between 1 and 4 weeks. [d] Standard surveillance is intended every 3 months. [e] 5-yearly surveillance at follow-up = clinical review every 5 years with history, examination, NP and troponin levels, and echocardiogram.
Reproduced from McDonagh TA, Metra M, Adamo M, *et al*; ESC Scientific Document Group. 2021 ESC Guidelines for the diagnosis and treatment of acute and chronic heart failure. *Eur Heart J.* 2021 Sep 21;42(36):3599–3726. doi: 10.1093/eurheartj/ehab368 with permission from Oxford University Press.

use.[48] The risk of LV dysfunction and HF induced by lapatinib seems to be significantly lower than that induced by trastuzumab and is generally reversible after HF treatment initiation.[29]

Vascular endothelial growth factor inhibitors

Agents targeting the vascular endothelial growth factor (VEGF) receptor are licensed treatments for a range of solid tumours, including metastatic renal cancer, metastatic thyroid cancer,

metastatic colon cancer, metastatic hepatocellular carcinoma, gastrointestinal stromal tumour, and metastatic sarcoma. These drugs include monoclonal antibodies (bevacizumab) and TKIs (sorafenib, sunitinib, axitinib, pazopanib, regorafenib, lenvatinib, and vandetinib). Anti-VEGF drugs, by blocking the action of VEGF and its receptor, hamper the formation of new blood vessels that are essential for development of the microenvironment indispensable for tumour growth and spread.[49,50] These drugs

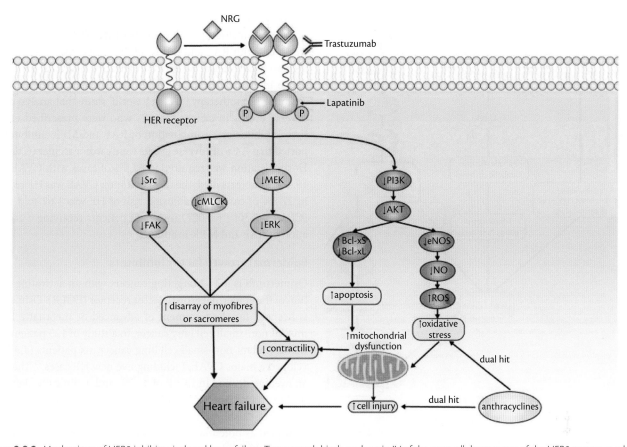

Figure 3.9.2 Mechanisms of HER2 inhibitor-induced heart failure. Trastuzumab binds to domain IV of the extracellular segment of the HER2 receptors, which inhibits the downstream HER2 pathway. Inhibition of PI3K/Akt signalling results in accumulation of ROS and activation of apoptosis, which subsequently leads to mitochondrial impairment. The decreased activity of MEK/Erk and Src/FAK pathway results in disarray of myofibres and sarcomeres. Furthermore, mitochondrial dysfunction and myocardial structure disorder lead to heart failure. Anthracycline could augment the cardiotoxicity of trastuzumab by aggravating mitochondrial dysfunction and cell injury. HER2, human epidermal growth factor receptor 2; ROS, reactive oxygen species.
Reproduced from Wu Q, Bai B, Tian C, Li D, Yu H, Song B, Li B, Chu X. The Molecular Mechanisms of Cardiotoxicity Induced by HER2, VEGF, and Tyrosine Kinase Inhibitors: an Updated Review. *Cardiovasc Drugs Ther*. 2021 Apr 13. doi: 10.1007/s10557-021-07181-3 with permission from Springer.

reduce nitric oxide bioavailability, which can cause vasoconstriction, capillary rarefaction, and abnormal glomerular function, leading to hypertension and proteinuria.[51] They also have a direct cardiotoxic effect leading to impaired cardiomyocyte mitochondrial function in preclinical models.[51] Most of these drugs block multiple kinases, and may cause cardiotoxicity and HF by both on- and off-target kinase inhibition.

VEGF inhibitor-induced hypertension has elicited the most attention, as it appears in up to 80–90% of cases.[52] Data from large clinical trials indicated, however, that some VEGF, in particular bevacizumab, sunitinib, sorafenib, pazopanib, axitinib, and vandetanib, are also associated with the development of LV dysfunction (2–19%) and HF (1–10%).[53,54,55,56,57,58,59] Cardiotoxicity may be exerted directly on cardiomyocytes or indirectly via the toxic effect on coronary microvascular vasculature.[49] Moreover, inhibition of VEGF induces hypertension and increases cardiac afterload, potentially affecting cardiac function (→ Figure 3.9.3).[31,60] The risk of cardiotoxicity may be worsened by previous or concurrent cardiac injury elicited by other anticancer therapies such as anthracyclines and ICIs. The presence of baseline CV comorbidities is a recognized additional risk factor.

Cardiac dysfunction associated with VEGF inhibitors seems, at least in part, reversible if promptly identified and treated.[61]

Multi-targeted kinase inhibitors targeting BCR–ABL

Inhibitors of the chimeric protein BCR–ABL, which is implicated in the pathogenesis of chronic myeloid leukaemia, include the TKIs imatinib (first generation), nilotinib, dasatinib, bosutinib (second generation), and ponatinib (third generation). Among other forms of cardiotoxicities, including arterial hypertension, arterial and venous thromboembolism, peripheral arterial disease, atrial fibrillation, pericardial effusion, and pulmonary hypertension (dasatinib), these agents may also cause LV dysfunction and HF.[62] More specifically, dasanitib and ponatinib, as well as, to a lesser extent, imatinib, have been associated with HF.

Proteasome inhibitors

PIs, including bortezomib, carfilzomib, and ixazomib, block the action of the proteasome that is responsible for the degradation of dysfunctional or unnecessary proteins, and are licensed for the treatment of multiple myeloma. PIs have been associated with a spectrum of CV toxicities, including LV dysfunction and

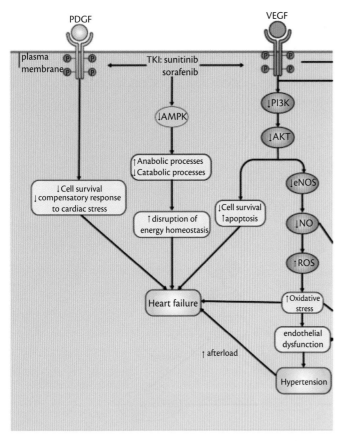

Figure 3.9.3 Mechanisms of VEGFi-induced heart failure. Sorafenib or sunitinib are TKIs targeting VEGFR and PDGFR. Inhibition of VEGF induces hypertension and increases cardiac afterload, bringing burden to the heart. PDGFR, platelet-derived growth factor receptor; TKI, tyrosine kinase inhibitor; VEGF, vascular endothelial growth factor; VEGFi, VEGF inhibitor; VEGFR, VEGF receptor.
Reproduced from Wu Q, Bai B, Tian C, Li D, Yu H, Song B, Li B, Chu X. The Molecular Mechanisms of Cardiotoxicity Induced by HER2, VEGF, and Tyrosine Kinase Inhibitors: an Updated Review. *Cardiovasc Drugs Ther.* 2021 Apr 13. doi: 10.1007/s10557-021-07181-3 with permission from Springer.

HF.[63,64,65] Of these, carfilzomib is associated with the highest risk of cardiotoxicity.[64,65,66] The reported incidence of LV dysfunction or HF is up to 23% of patients.[67] Carfilzomib-related HF develops rather early after treatment initiation; a median time of approximately 2 weeks has been reported.[68] Hypertension has also been associated with PIs and may contribute to the development of HF, particularly HF with preserved ejection fraction (HFpEF).

RAF and MEK inhibitors

RAF and MEK inhibitors are licensed for the treatment of BRAF-mutant melanomas and other rarer RAF-mutant malignancies (RAF-mutant colorectal, non-small cell lung, and thyroid cancers). Some patients receive a single RAF inhibitor (vemurafenib, dabrafenib, encorafenib), but now combinations of RAF and MEK inhibitors (vemurafenib/cobimetinib; dabrafenib/trametinib; encorafenib/binimetinib) are superior.

There is now recognition that these cancer drugs can cause LV dysfunction and HF, particularly when given as a combination of RAF and MEK inhibitors. In randomized controlled trials, the rate of new LV dysfunction or HF was 5–11%.[69,70] A meta-analysis of five trials including 2317 patients with melanoma reported that treatment with RAF and lMEK inhibitors was associated with an increased risk of LVEF reduction (relative risk 3.72, 95% confidence interval (CI) 1.74–7.94; $P <0.001$), compared with RAF inhibitor monotherapy.[71] A 'real-world' study that analysed 7712 adverse events in cancer patients who were prescribed either a RAF inhibitor or a combination of RAF and MEK inhibitors reported that 7.4% of adverse events were cardiovascular (CVAEs).[72] Hospitalization was required in 64.8% of cases with CVAEs, and 18.4% of subjects died; the most common CVAE was HF reported in 27.2% of cases. The adjusted risk of HF was 1.62-fold higher (CI 1.14–2.30; $P = 0.007$) in cancer patients receiving a combination of RAF and MEK inhibitors.

Epidermal growth factor inhibitors

Osimertinib is a TKI targeting cancers with an activating mutation of the epidermal growth factor receptor (EGFR). Osimertinib is licensed for the treatment of advanced or metastatic EGFR-mutant non-small cell lung cancer. In a study of 123 patients with EGFR-mutant non-small cell lung cancer, six patients (4.9%) developed a major CVAE, including five new HF cases.[73] There was an average decline in LVEF of 4–5%, and a clinically significant decline in LVEF of >10% and up to <53% was observed in 11% of cases. Pre-existing CV diseases, including valvular disease, were identified as potential risk factors. The LV impairment seems to be reversible with drug cessation.

Immune checkpoint inhibitors

ICIs are a rapidly expanding class of cancer drugs which activate the immune system to target cancer cells. ICIs are antibodies targeted against immune checkpoints, which include cytotoxic lymphocyte-associated protein 4 (CTLA-4; e.g. ipilimumab), programmed cell death protein 1 (PD-1; e.g. nivolumab, pembrolizumab) expressed by T lymphocytes, and programmed cell death ligand 1 (PD-L1; e.g. atezolizumab, avelumab) expressed on tumour cells.

ICIs can cause LV dysfunction and HF via a range of mechanisms.[74] The most widely recognized mechanism is myocarditis, which can present as fulminant myocarditis with cardiogenic shock and ventricular tachyarrhythmias and may be fatal in up to 25–50% of cases.[75,76] ICI-mediated myocarditis typically occurs during the first four cycles of treatment, with most cases after the first or second cycle, but 25% of cases occur later during treatment or rarely after completion of treatment. ICI-mediated myocarditis usually presents with clinical symptoms and raised cardiac troponin levels, and 50% of cases have reduced LVEF. QRS prolongation on the electrocardiogram (ECG) is the most common ECG abnormality and is associated with major adverse cardiac events (MACE).[77] Diagnosis is usually confirmed by cardiac magnetic resonance imaging (MRI), and a recent study identified elevated myocardial T1 and T2 levels as more sensitive than T2-weighted short tau inversion recovery (T2 STIR) for the diagnosis of acute ICI-mediated myocarditis.[78]

Other causes of HF in patients receiving ICIs include a non-inflammatory HF syndrome seen in patients on longer courses of treatment, presenting typically after 6 months; troponin levels may be normal and cardiac magnetic resonance (CMR) evidence of inflammation is absent.[76] HF may also result acutely due to cardiac tamponade secondary to ICI-mediated pericarditis or ICI-induced complete heart block.[79] Takotsubo syndrome may also be triggered by ICI treatment and present with acute HF.[80] ICIs may cause acute atherosclerotic plaque rupture and acute coronary syndrome that may be complicated by HF, while the potential long-term effects of ICIs on atherosclerosis acceleration and CV ageing are currently being discussed.[81]

Radiotherapy to a volume including the heart

Radiotherapy-induced HF typically develops several years or decades after exposure due to direct myocardial damage or as a consequence of radiation-induced myocardial ischaemia, valvular heart disease, pericardial constriction, and direct myocardial injury causing restrictive cardiomyopathy.[82] HFpEF appears to be more common than LV dysfunction, and the relative risk increases in proportion to the received mean heart dose (MHD) and the presence of HF risk factors such as AC.[83] High risk patients were those treated with ≥35 Gy to a volume including the heart (or ≥10 Gy MHD) or combination therapies. In childhood cancer survivors the CV risk was multiplied by 60 in patients who had received ≥30 Gy, and 61 in those who had received both anthracycline chemotherapy and radiotherapy.[9] Although there is no safe MHD, there is little evidence that a MHD of <5 Gy alone can significantly increase the long-term risk of HF.[12]

Cancer-induced cardiac dysfunction and heart failure

Cancer itself may affect the CV system, independent of cardiotoxicity of anticancer therapies. A series of metabolic, inflammatory, autonomic, and other mechanisms are believed to possibly cause CV abnormalities such as arrhythmias, that may, in turn, contribute to the development or exacerbation of HF.[84] Takotsubo syndrome, that may be manifested as acute HF, has also been associated with cancer.[85] It should also be taken under consideration that cancer and HF share many common risk factors and pathogenetic mechanisms, with a central role of inflammation, that may concurrently lead to both conditions.[86] In addition, the presence of cancer may further lead to HF deterioration by depriving patients of specific HF therapies such as device implantation.[87] Finally, advanced cancer is often followed by progressive muscle wasting and cachexia that may also affect the heart, causing myocardial atrophy and energy depletion that may, in turn, lead to cardiac dysfunction and HF.[88,89]

Summary and key messages

A range of cancer therapies can cause new LV dysfunction and HF, either during cancer treatment or, in the case of anthracycline chemotherapy and radiation therapy, many years or even decades later. It is important to have a high index of suspicion for new HF in a cancer patient presenting with new symptoms while receiving a cancer treatment recognized to cause HF. The risk depends upon the interaction with baseline risk factors, including previous cardiotoxic cancer treatments, age, pre-existing CV diseases, and baseline LVEF and natriuretic peptide levels. Genetic risk also appears to be important, particularly in patients presenting with new HF who have an otherwise low-risk profile.

The mechanism of HF differs according to cancer drug and dose/duration of exposure, including myocyte necrosis and injury (anthracycline chemotherapy), functional impairment which is reversible with drug cessation (trastuzumab and TKIs), ischaemia (VEGF TKIs), and myocarditis (ICIs). However, the degree of recovery versus permanent injury varies and can be observed in each of these classes of cardiotoxic cancer therapy.

Future directions

Large registries and real-world studies collecting epidemiology data on the incidence and risk factors for HF secondary to cancer therapies, particularly recently licensed ones, are required. As the range and number of new cancer therapies with potential cardiotoxicity, including HF, are growing rapidly, collecting data on CV events and outcomes with appropriate adjudication during cancer trials is crucial. Novel biomarkers and cardiac imaging techniques will help in understanding the nature of cancer therapy-related HF, and define optimal surveillance strategies for early identification of cardiac dysfunction during and after treatment. Structured monitoring and treatment strategies need to be developed and evaluated in clinical trials. The role of cardioprotective interventions started before cancer therapy in targeted patient subgroups also needs to be tested in clinical studies.

References

1. Zamorano JL, Lancellotti P, Rodriguez Muñoz D, et al.; ESC Scientific Document Group. 2016 ESC Position Paper on cancer treatments and cardiovascular toxicity developed under the auspices of the ESC Committee for Practice Guidelines: The Task Force for cancer treatments and cardiovascular toxicity of the European Society of Cardiology (ESC). *Eur Heart J* 2016;**37**:2768–801.
2. Sturgeon KM, Deng L, Bluethmann SM, et al. A population-based study of cardiovascular disease mortality risk in US cancer patients. *Eur Heart J* 2019;**40**:3889–97.
3. Herrmann J, Lenihan D, Armenian S, et al. Defining cardiovascular toxicities of cancer therapies: an International Cardio-Oncology Society (IC-OS) consensus statement. *Eur Heart J* 2022;**43**:280–99.
4. Zhang S, Liu X, Bawa-Khalfe T, et al. Identification of the molecular basis of doxorubicin-induced cardiotoxicity. *Nat Med* 2012;**18**:1639–42.
5. Cardinale D, Colombo A, Bacchiani G, et al. Early detection of anthracycline cardiotoxicity and improvement with heart failure therapy. *Circulation* 2015;**131**:1981–8.
6. Demissei BG, Finkelman BS, Hubbard RA, et al. Cardiovascular function phenotypes in response to cardiotoxic breast cancer therapy. *J Am Coll Cardiol* 2019;**73**:248–9.
7. Smith LA, Cornelius VR, Plummer CJ, et al. Cardiotoxicity of anthracycline agents for the treatment of cancer: systematic review and meta-analysis of randomised controlled trials. *BMC Cancer* 2010;**10**:337.

8. Abdel-Qadir H, Thavendiranathan P, Austin PC, et al. Development and validation of a multivariable prediction model for major adverse cardiovascular events after early stage breast cancer: a population-based cohort study. *Eur Heart J* 2019;**40**:3913–20.

9. Faber J, Wingerter A, Neu MA, et al. Burden of cardiovascular risk factors and cardiovascular disease in childhood cancer survivors: data from the German CVSS-study. *Eur Heart J* 2018;**39**:1555–62.

10. Farmakis D, Mantzourani M, Filippatos G. Anthracycline-induced cardiomyopathy: secrets and lies. *Eur J Heart Fail* 2018;**20**:907–9.

11. Haddy N, Diallo S, El-Fayech C, et al. Cardiac diseases following childhood cancer treatment: cohort study. *Circulation* 2016;**133**:31–8.

12. Wang L, Wang F, Chen L, Geng Y, Yu S, Chen Z. Long-term cardiovascular disease mortality among 160 834 5-year survivors of adolescent and young adult cancer: an American population-based cohort study. *Eur Heart J* 2021;**42**:101–9.

13a. McDonagh TA, Metra M, Adamo M, et al. 2021 ESC Guidelines for the diagnosis and treatment of acute and chronic heart failure. *Eur Heart J* 2021;**42**:3599–726.

13b. Lyon AR, Lopez-Fernandez T, Couch LS, et al.; ESC Scientific Document Group. 2022 ESC Guidelines on cardio-oncology developed in collaboration with the European Hematology Association (EHA), the European Society for Therapeutic Radiology and Oncology (ESTRO) and the International Cardio-Oncology Society (IC-OS). *Eur Heart J* 2022;**43**:4229–361.

14. Cardinale D, Sandri MT, Colombo A, et al. Prognostic value of troponin I in cardiac risk stratification of cancer patients undergoing high-dose chemotherapy. *Circulation* 2004;**109**:2749–54.

15. Jones M, O'Gorman P, Kelly C, Mahon N, Fitzgibbon MC. High-sensitive cardiac troponin-I facilitates timely detection of subclinical anthracycline-mediated cardiac injury. *Ann Clin Biochem* 2017;**54**:149–57.

16. Lyon AR, Dent S, Stanway S, et al. Baseline cardiovascular risk assessment in cancer patients scheduled to receive cardiotoxic cancer therapies: a position statement and new risk assessment tools from the Cardio-Oncology Study Group of the Heart Failure Association of the European Society of Cardiology in collaboration with the International Cardio-Oncology Society. *Eur J Heart Fail* 2020;**22**:1945–60.

17. Pudil R, Mueller C, Čelutkienė J, et al. Role of serum biomarkers in cancer patients receiving cardiotoxic cancer therapies: a position statement from the Cardio-Oncology Study Group of the Heart Failure Association and the Cardio-Oncology Council of the European Society of Cardiology. *Eur J Heart Fail* 2020;**22**:1966–83.

18. Čelutkienė J, Pudil R, López-Fernández T, et al. Role of cardiovascular imaging in cancer patients receiving cardiotoxic therapies: a position statement on behalf of the Heart Failure Association (HFA), the European Association of Cardiovascular Imaging (EACVI) and the Cardio-Oncology Council of the European Society of Cardiology (ESC). *Eur J Heart Fail* 2020;**22**:1504–24.

19. Seidman A, Hudis C, Pierri MK, et al. Cardiac dysfunction in the trastuzumab clinical trials experience. *J Clin Oncol* 2002;**20**:1215–21.

20. Slamon DJ, Leyland-Jones B, Shak S, et al. Use of chemotherapy plus a monoclonal antibody against HER2 for metastatic breast cancer that overexpresses HER2. *N Engl J Med* 2001;**344**:783–92.

21. Ewer MS, O'Shaughnessy JA. Cardiac toxicity of trastuzumab-related regimens in HER2-overexpressing breast cancer. *Clin Breast Cancer* 2007;**7**:22–9.

22. Romond EH, Perez EA, Bryant J, et al. Trastuzumab plus adjuvant chemotherapy for operable HER2-positive breast cancer. *N Engl J Med* 2005;**353**:1673–84.

23. Suter TM, Procter M, van Veldhuisen DJ, et al. Trastuzumab-associated cardiac adverse effects in the herceptin adjuvant trial. *J Clin Oncol* 2007;**25**:3859–65.

24. Vogel CL, Cobleigh MA, Tripathy D, et al. Efficacy and safety of trastuzumab as a single agent in first-line treatment of HER2-overexpressing metastatic breast cancer. *J Clin Oncol* 2002;**20**:719–26.

25. Perez EA, Suman VJ, Davidson NE, et al. Cardiac safety analysis of doxorubicin and cyclophosphamide followed by paclitaxel with or without trastuzumab in the North Central Cancer Treatment Group N9831 adjuvant breast cancer trial. *J Clin Oncol* 2008;**26**:1231–8.

26. Tripathy D, Slamon DJ, Cobleigh M, et al. Safety of treatment of metastatic breast cancer with trastuzumab beyond disease progression. *J Clin Oncol* 2004;**22**:1063–70.

27. Yeh ETH, Bickford CL. Cardiovascular complications of cancer therapy: incidence, pathogenesis, diagnosis, and management. *J Am Coll Cardiol* 2009;**53**:2231–47.

28. Battisti NML, Andres MS, Lee KA, et al. Incidence of cardiotoxicity and validation of the Heart Failure Association-International Cardio-Oncology Society risk stratification tool in patients treated with trastuzumab for HER2-positive early breast cancer. *Breast Cancer Res Treat* 2021;**188**:149–63.

29. Dempsey N, Rosenthal A, Dabas N, Kropotova Y, Lippman M, Bishopric NH. Trastuzumab-induced cardiotoxicity: a review of clinical risk factors, pharmacologic prevention, and cardiotoxicity of other HER2-directed therapies. *Breast Cancer Res Treat* 2021;**188**:21–36.

30. Gonciar D, Mocan L, Zlibut A, Mocan T, Agoston-Coldea L. Cardiotoxicity in HER2-positive breast cancer patients. *Heart Fail Rev* 2021;**26**:919–35.

31. Wu Q, Bai B, Tian C, et al. The Molecular Mechanisms of Cardiotoxicity Induced by HER2, VEGF, and Tyrosine Kinase Inhibitors: an Updated Review. *Cardiovasc Drugs Ther* 2022;**36**:511–24.

32. Ewer SM, Ewer MS. Cardiotoxicity profile of trastuzumab. *Drug Saf* 2008;**31**:459–67.

33. Cardinale D, Colombo A, Torrisi R, et al. Trastuzumab-induced cardiotoxicity: clinical and prognostic implications of troponin I evaluation. *J Clin Oncol* 2010;**28**:3910–16.

34. Zardavas D, Suter TM, van Veldhuisen DJ, et al. Role of troponins I and T and N-terminal prohormone of brain natriuretic peptide in monitoring cardiac safety of patients with early-stage human epidermal growth factor receptor 2-positive breast cancer receiving trastuzumab: a herceptin adjuvant study cardiac marker substudy. *J Clin Oncol* 2017;**35**:878–84.

35. Barok M, Joensuu H, Isola J. Trastuzumab emtansine: mechanisms of action and drug resistance. *Breast Cancer Res* 2014;**16**:209.

36. Scheuer W, Friess T, Burtscher H, Bossenmaier B, Endl J, Hasmann M. Strongly enhanced antitumor activity of trastuzumab and pertuzumab combination treatment on HER2-positive human xenograft tumor models. *Cancer Res* 2009;**69**:9330–6.

37. Baselga J, Swain SM. Novel anticancer targets: revisiting ERBB2 and discovering ERBB3. *Nat Rev Cancer* 2009;**9**:463–75.

38. Baselga J, Cortés J, Kim S-B, et al. Pertuzumab plus trastuzumab plus docetaxel for metastatic breast cancer. *N Engl J Med* 2012;**366**:109–19.

39. Perez EA, Barrios C, Eiermann W, et al. Trastuzumab emtansine with or without pertuzumab versus trastuzumab plus taxane for human epidermal growth factor receptor 2-positive, advanced breast cancer: primary results from the phase III MARIANNE study. *J Clin Oncol* 2017;**35**:141–8.

40. Gianni L, Pienkowski T, Im YH, et al. 5-year analysis of neoadjuvant pertuzumab and trastuzumab in patients with locally advanced, inflammatory, or early-stage HER2-positive breast cancer (NeoSphere): a multicentre, open-label, phase 2 randomised trial. *Lancet Oncol* 2016;**17**:791–800.

41. Von Minckwitz G, Procter M, de Azambuja E, et al. Adjuvant pertuzumab and trastuzumab in early HER2-positive breast cancer. *N Engl J Med* 2017;**377**:122–31.

42. Hurvitz SA, Martin M, Symmans WF, et al. Neoadjuvant trastuzumab, pertuzumab, and chemotherapy versus trastuzumab emtansine plus pertuzumab in patients with HER2-positive breast cancer (KRISTINE): a randomised, open-label, multicentre, phase 3 trial. *Lancet Oncol* 2018;**19**:115–26.

43. Von Minckwitz G, Huang C-S, Mano MS, et al. Trastuzumab emtansine for residual invasive HER2-positive breast cancer. *N Engl J Med* 2019;**380**:617–28.

44. Konecny GE, Pegram MD, Venkatesan N, et al. Activity of the dual kinase inhibitor lapatinib (GW572016) against HER-2-overexpressing and trastuzumab-treated breast cancer cells. *Cancer Res* 2006;**66**:1630–9.

45. Geyer CE, Forster J, Lindquist D, et al. Lapatinib plus capecitabine for HER2-positive advanced breast cancer. *N Engl J Med* 2006;**355**:2733–43.

46. Choi HD, Chang MJ. Cardiac toxicities of lapatinib in patients with breast cancer and other HER2-positive cancers: a meta-analysis. *Breast Cancer Res Treat* 2017;**166**:927–36.

47. Guan Z, Xu B, Desilvio ML, et al. Randomized trial of lapatinib versus placebo added to paclitaxel in the treatment of human epidermal growth factor receptor 2-overexpressing metastatic breast cancer. *J Clin Oncol* 2013;**31**:1947–53.

48. Hsu WT, Huang CY, Yen CYT, Cheng AL, Hsieh PCH. The HER2 inhibitor lapatinib potentiates doxorubicin-induced cardiotoxicity through iNOS signaling. *Theranostics* 2018;**8**:3176–88.

49. Dobbin SJH, Petrie MC, Myles RC, Touyz RM, Lang NN. Cardiotoxic effects of angiogenesis inhibitors. *Clin Sci (Lond)* 2021;**135**:71–100.

50. Hurtado-de-Mendoza D, Loaiza-Bonilla A, Bonilla-Reyes PA, Alcorta R. Cardio-oncology: cancer therapy-related cardiovascular complications in a molecular targeted era: new concepts and perspectives. *Cureus* 2017;**9**:e1258.

51. Herrmann J, Yang EH, Iliescu CA, et al. Vascular toxicities of cancer therapies: the old and the new: an evolving avenue. *Circulation* 2016;**133**:1272–89.

52. Small HY, Montezano AC, Rios FJ, Savoia C, Touyz RM. Hypertension due to antiangiogenic cancer therapy with vascular endothelial growth factor inhibitors: understanding and managing a new syndrome. *Can J Cardiol* 2014;**30**:534–43.

53. Steingart RM, Bakris GL, Chen HX, et al. Management of cardiac toxicity in patients receiving vascular endothelial growth factor signaling pathway inhibitors. *Am Heart J* 2012;**163**:156–63.

54. Cameron D, Brown J, Dent R, et al. Adjuvant bevacizumab-containing therapy in triple-negative breast cancer (BEATRICE): primary results of a randomised, phase 3 trial. *Lancet Oncol* 2013;**14**:933–42.

55. Motzer RJ, Hutson TE, Cella D, et al. Pazopanib versus sunitinib in metastatic renal-cell carcinoma. *N Engl J Med* 2013;**369**:722–31.

56. Motzer RJ, Escudier B, Tomczak P, et al. Axitinib versus sorafenib as second-line treatment for advanced renal cell carcinoma: overall survival analysis and updated results from a randomised phase 3 trial. *Lancet Oncol* 2013;**14**:552–62.

57. Qi WX, Shen Z, Tang LN, Yao Y. Congestive heart failure risk in cancer patients treated with vascular endothelial growth factor tyrosine kinase inhibitors: a systematic review and meta-analysis of 36 clinical trials. *Br J Clin Pharmacol* 2014;**78**:748–62.

58. Hahn VS, Zhang KW, Sun L, Narayan V, Lenihan DJ, Ky B. Heart failure with targeted cancer therapies: mechanisms and cardioprotection. *Circ Res* 2021;**128**:1576–93.

59. Goldman A, Bomze D, Dankner R, et al. Cardiovascular toxicities of antiangiogenic tyrosine kinase inhibitors: a retrospective, pharmacovigilance study. *Target Oncol* 2021;**16**:471–83.

60. Ewer MS, Suter TM, Lenihan DJ, et al. Cardiovascular events among 1090 cancer patients treated with sunitinib, interferon, or placebo: a comprehensive adjudicated database analysis demonstrating clinically meaningful reversibility of cardiac events. *Eur J Cancer* 2014;**50**:2162–70.

61. Shelburne N, Adhikari B, Brell J, et al. Cancer treatment-related cardiotoxicity: current state of knowledge and future research priorities. *J Natl Cancer Inst* 2014;**106**:dju232.

62. Moslehi JJ, Deininger M. Tyrosine kinase inhibitor-associated cardiovascular toxicity in chronic myeloid leukemia. *J Clin Oncol* 2015;**33**:4210–18.

63. Siegel D, Martin T, Nooka A, et al. Integrated safety profile of single-agent carfilzomib: experience from 526 patients enrolled in 4 phase II clinical studies. *Haematologica* 2013;**98**:1753–61.

64. Dimopoulos MA, Moreau P, Palumbo A, et al.; ENDEAVOR Investigators. Carfilzomib and dexamethasone versus bortezomib and dexamethasone for patients with relapsed or refractory multiple myeloma (ENDEAVOR): a randomised, phase 3, open-label, multicentre study. *Lancet Oncol* 2016;**17**:27–38.

65. Stewart AK, Rajkumar SV, Dimopoulos MA, et al.; ASPIRE Investigators. Carfilzomib, lenalidomide, and dexamethasone for relapsed multiple myeloma. *N Engl J Med* 2015;**372**:142–52.

66. Das A, Dasgupta S, Gong Y, et al. Cardiotoxicity as an adverse effect of immunomodulatory drugs and proteasome inhibitors in multiple myeloma: a network meta-analysis of randomized clinical trials. *Hematol Oncol* 2022;**40**:233–42.

67. Danhof S, Schreder M, Rasche L, Strifler S, Einsele H, Knop S. 'Real-life' experience of preapproval carfilzomib-based therapy in myeloma: analysis of cardiac toxicity and predisposing factors. *Eur J Haematol* 2016;**97**:25–32.

68. Nakao S, Uchida M, Satoki A, Okamoto K, Uesawa Y, Shimizu T. Evaluation of cardiac adverse events associated with carfilzomib using a Japanese real-world database. *Oncology* 2022;**100**:60–4.

69. Ascierto PA, McArthur GA, Dréno B, et al. Cobimetinib combined with vemurafenib in advanced BRAFV600-mutant melanoma (coBRIM): updated efficacy results from a randomised, double-blind, phase 3 trial. *Lancet Oncol* 2016;**17**:1248–60.

70. Long V, Flaherty KT, Stroyakovskiy D, et al. Erratum: Dabrafenib plus trametinib versus dabrafenib monotherapy in patients with metastatic BRAF V600E/K-mutant melanoma: long-term survival and safety analysis of a phase 3 study. *Ann Oncol* 2019;**30**:1848.

71. Mincu RI, Mahabadi AA, Michel L, et al. Cardiovascular adverse events associated with BRAF and MEK inhibitors: a systematic review and meta-analysis. *JAMA Netw Open* 2019;**2**:e198890.

72. Guha A, Jain P, Fradley MG, et al. Cardiovascular adverse events associated with BRAF versus BRAF/MEK inhibitor: cross-sectional and longitudinal analysis using two large national registries. *Cancer Med* 2021;**10**:3862–72.

73. Kunimasa K, Kamada R, Oka T, et al. Cardiac adverse events in EGFR-mutated non-small cell lung cancer treated with osimertinib. *JACC CardioOncology* 2020;**2**:1–10.

74. Lyon AR, Yousaf N, Battisti NML, Moslehi J, Larkin J. Immune checkpoint inhibitors and cardiovascular toxicity. *Lancet Oncol* 2018;**19**:e447–58.

75. Mahmood SS, Fradley MG, Cohen JV, et al. Myocarditis in patients treated with immune checkpoint inhibitors. *J Am Coll Cardiol* 2018;**71**:1755–64.

76. Hu J-R, Florido R, Lipson EJ, et al. Cardiovascular toxicities associated with immune checkpoint inhibitors. *Cardiovasc Res* 2019;**115**:854–68.

77. Zlotoff DA, Hassan MZO, Zafar A, et al. Electrocardiographic features of immune checkpoint inhibitor associated myocarditis. *J Immunother Cancer* 2021;**9**:e002007.

78. Thavendiranathan P, Zhang L, Zafar A, *et al.* Myocardial T1 and T2 mapping by magnetic resonance in patients with immune checkpoint inhibitor-associated myocarditis. *J Am Coll Cardiol* 2021;**77**: 1503–16.

79. Ball S, Ghosh RK, Wongsaengsak S, *et al.* Cardiovascular toxicities of immune checkpoint inhibitors: JACC Review Topic of the Week. *J Am Coll Cardiol* 2019;**74**:1714–27.

80. Serzan M, Rapisuwon S, Krishnan J, Chang IC, Barac A. Takotsubo cardiomyopathy associated with checkpoint inhibitor therapy: endomyocardial biopsy provides pathological insights to dual diseases. *JACC CardioOncology* 2021;**3**:330–4.

81. Zhang L, Reynolds KL, Lyon AR, Palaskas N, Neilan TG. The evolving immunotherapy landscape and the epidemiology, diagnosis, and management of cardiotoxicity: JACC: CardioOncology Primer. *JACC CardioOncology* 2021;**3**:35–47.

82. Lancellotti P, Nkomo VT, Badano LP, *et al.* Expert Consensus for multi-modality imaging evaluation of cardiovascular complications of radiotherapy in adults: a report from the European Association of Cardiovascular Imaging and the American Society of Echocardiography. *J Am Soc Echocardiogr* 2013;**26**:1013–32.

83. Desai MY, Windecker S, Lancellotti P, *et al.* Prevention, diagnosis, and management of radiation-associated cardiac disease: JACC Scientific Expert Panel. *J Am Coll Cardiol* 2019;**74**:905–27.

84. Farmakis D, Parissis J, Filippatos G. Insights into onco-cardiology: atrial fibrillation in cancer. *J Am Coll Cardiol* 2014;**63**:945–53.

85. Desai A, Noor A, Joshi S, Kim AS. Takotsubo cardiomyopathy in cancer patients. *Cardiooncology* 2019;**5**:7.

86. Farmakis D, Stafylas P, Giamouzis G, Maniadakis N, Parissis J. The medical and socioeconomic burden of heart failure: a comparative delineation with cancer. *Int J Cardiol* 2016;**203**:279–81.

87. Ameri P, Canepa M, Anker MS, *et al.*; Heart Failure Association Cardio-Oncology Study Group of the European Society of Cardiology. Cancer diagnosis in patients with heart failure: epidemiology, clinical implications and gaps in knowledge. *Eur J Heart Fail* 2018;**20**:879–87.

88. Belloum Y, Rannou-Bekono F, Favier FB. Cancer-induced cardiac cachexia: pathogenesis and impact of physical activity (review). *Oncol Rep* 2017;**37**:2543–52.

89. Anker MS, Sanz AP, Zamorano JL, *et al.* Advanced cancer is also a heart failure syndrome: a hypothesis. *J Cachexia Sarcopenia Muscle* 2021;**12**:533–7.

CHAPTER 3.10

Toxins and infections

Antonello Gavazzi, Maria Carmo Nunes, and Fausto Pinto

Contents

Introduction

There are several uncommon causes of impaired cardiac structure and function leading to heart failure (HF), such as toxins, systemic infections, and cardiac infections, as reported in ⮞ Box 3.10.1.

The mechanisms of cardiotoxicity due to these causes are multiple and complex, involving direct and indirect interactions with the cardiovascular system, resulting in structural alterations and functional manifestations (⮞ Figure 3.10.1).

Because of limited space, each of these causes cannot be extensively examined, but the most clinically relevant and prevalent ones are analysed.

Toxins

Several exogenous and endogenous toxins have been described as responsible for cardiac dysfunction (⮞ Box 3.10.1). The true prevalence of toxin-related left ventricular (LV) dysfunction and HF in the general population is not known. Substances of abuse, drugs, and environmental agents are the most frequently involved.

Alcohol

The underlying mechanism responsible for alcohol-related cardiotoxicity, due to ethanol as the active ingredient, is multifactorial and still poorly understood. It includes increased oxidative stress, alterations of the excitation–contraction coupling in cardiac myocytes, changes in calcium sensitivity of myofilaments, alterations in structure and function of the mitochondria and sarcoplasmic reticulum, deregulation of protein synthesis with decrease of contractile proteins, interference in carbohydrate metabolism, disruption of transduction signals, and induction of apoptosis. Activation of the sympathetic nervous system, the renin–angiotensin system, and cytokines may contribute to the overall myocardial injury. The negative effects on myocardial function of chronic alcohol abuse seem to be neither beverage- nor amount-specific, but to depend on environmental factors such as cobalt and arsenic, age, and gender.[1,2,3] Moreover, individual susceptibility is relevant, probably related to genetic factors. There have been reports of 5-year average alcohol consumption of >90 g/day inducing preclinical and symptomatic HF. Alcohol is a major cause of dilated cardiomyopathy (DCM), with a reported incidence of around 30%. Alcohol abstinence has been associated with amelioration of LV function and improvement of symptoms and signs of HF. However, the degree of reversibility is variable. In chronic alcoholism, nutritional deficiencies (vitamins such as thiamine, and minerals, such as selenium and zinc) may be present, facilitating the development of HF, and may require appropriate supplement.

Box 3.10.1 Toxins and infections that may cause myocardial dysfunction and heart failure

- ◆ Toxins
  - Alcohol
  - Recreational sympathomimetic drugs (cocaine, amphetamines, ecstasy)
  - Catecholamines (adrenaline, noradrenaline, dopamine)
  - Uraemic toxins (parathyroid hormone, phosphate, FGF23, Klotho, sclerostin)
  - Thyroid hormone
  - Anticancer drugs (anthracyclines, trastuzumab, imatinib, sunitinib, bortezomib)
  - Antiretroviral drugs (azidothymidine)
  - Antidiabetic drugs (rosiglitazone)
  - Antidepressant and antipsychotic drugs (clozapine, fluvoxamine, imipramine, olanzapine, venlafaxine)
  - Androgenic anabolic steroids
  - Environmental agents (air particulates, carbon monoxide, metal)
  - Scorpion venom
- ◆ Systemic infections
- ◆ Cardiac infections
  - Virus (adenovirus, enteroviruses, parvovirus B19, cytomegalovirus, Epstein–Barr virus, hepatitis C virus, influenza viruses, coronaviruses, HIV)
  - Bacteria (*Staphylococcus*, *Streptococcus*, *Mycobacterium*, *Legionella*, *Corynebacterium diphtheriae*)
  - Fungus (*Aspergillus*, *Nocardia*)
  - Ricketsia (Rocky Mountain spotted fever, Q fever, typhus)
  - Spirochaetes (*Borrelia*–Lyme disease, *Leptospira*, syphilis)
  - Helminths (*Echinococcus*, *Trichinella*, *Schistosoma*)
  - Protozoa (*Trypanosoma*, *Toxoplasma*, *Leishmania*, *Entamoeba*)

Recreational sympathomimetic drugs

Recreational sympathomimetic drugs include cocaine, amphetamines, and ecstasy. Illegal use of sympathomimetic agents is highly prevalent in developed countries and after cannabis, this class of drugs are the most often seized by law enforcement authorities.

Cocaine

Cocaine is a strong stimulant of the central nervous system and induces potentially lethal cardiovascular effects, with multiple mechanisms involved in cocaine-related cardiotoxicity.[4] The drug mainly acts by inhibiting the presynaptic reuptake of catecholamines and dopamine, leading to post-synaptic overactivation of sympathetic and dopaminergic receptors.

Cocaine at high doses can block fast sodium and potassium channels, and inhibit calcium entry into myocytes, impairing myocyte electrical activity and contractility. Furthermore, cocaine promotes formation of intracoronary thrombus, inducing platelet hyperaggregability, increased production of thromboxane, and coronary vasospasm. As a consequence, a high incidence of transient myocardial ischaemia and recurrent myocardial infarction has been reported in cocaine users, causing ventricular dysfunction and symptomatic HF. The amount and duration of cocaine use necessary to develop these negative cardiac effects have not been clearly determined.

Cocaine and concomitant alcohol consumption may potentiate the cardiotoxic effects of cocaine and ethanol by forming cocaethylene, a more potent cardiotoxic metabolite.[5] Cannabis also potentiates the cardiotoxic effect of cocaine via increasing plasma concentrations of the drug.

Cocaine abstinence has been shown to reverse cardiac dysfunction.[6]

Amphetamines and metamphetamines

Amphetamines and metamphetamines, which are synthetic derivatives of phenethylamines, are potent stimulators of the central nervous system. Ecstasy is a derivative of amphetamines and exerts a similar sympathomimetic effect. The cardiotoxicity has been attributed to both direct and indirect effects of these drugs. Oxidative stress and catecholaminergic stimulation are operative, with cellular death, fibrosis, and contraction band necrosis, but at high doses, disruption of microtubules and actin occurs. Genetic susceptibility has been hypothesized. Amphetamines induce hypertension, myocardial ischaemia, inflammatory infiltrates, and areas of necrosis, resulting in diastolic and systolic ventricular dysfunction. Cardiomyopathy has been reported in 18% of subjects consuming metamphetamines. The negative impact of amphetamines is potentiated by concomitant use of alcohol or cannabis. Amphetamine abstinence has been associated with some reversibility of cardiac lesions.[6]

Catecholamines

After persistent exposure to increased levels of catecholamines, patterns of myocarditis, myocardial fibrosis, or myocyte hypertrophy have been described. Adrenaline, noradrenaline, and dopamine in excess can induce ventricular dysfunction and symptomatic HF.[7] Phaeochromocytomas produce, store, and secrete catecholamines, usually noradrenaline and adrenaline, whereas production of dopamine is uncommon. Hypertension is the initial most common manifestation, and angina and acute myocardial infarction may occur even in the absence of coronary artery disease. Clinical phenotypes of dilated and hypertrophic cardiomyopathies may develop.

Uraemic toxins

Uraemic toxins with presumed cardiotoxicity start to accumulate in the body since early stages of renal disease. Vitamin D deficiency, secondary hyperparathyroidism, hyperphosphataemia, and newly described toxins, such as fibroblast growth factor 23 (FGF23), Klotho, and sclerostin, are reported as the most relevant contributing factors, with distinct pathophysiological mechanisms, to cardiac remodelling, including LV hypertrophy, declining of LV ejection fraction (EF), and symptomatic HF.

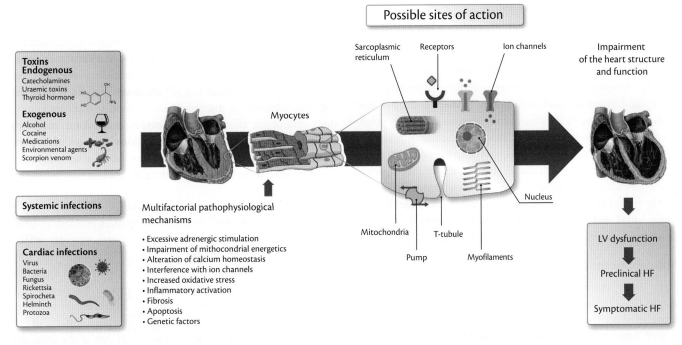

Figure 3.10.1 Overview of the effects of toxins and systemic and cardiac infections on cardiac structure and function. The pathophysiological mechanisms are multifactorial, and the sites of action at myocyte-level include the nucleus, myofilaments, mitochondria, T-tubules, sarcoplasmic reticulum, ion channels, pumps, and receptors. The negative effects of toxins and infections on left ventricular (LV) function lead to various degrees of heart failure (HF).

Thyroid hormone

Thyroid hormone exerts direct and complex effects on the cardiovascular system, and in dysthyroidism has been implicated in causing various degrees of ventricular dysfunction till overt HF. In hyperthyroidism, there is a hyperdynamic status due to a primary cardiac effect of the thyroid hormone with catecholamine contribution. The histological pattern is non-specific, with focal lymphocytic or eosinophilic infiltration, myocardial fibrosis, fatty storage, and myofibril hypertrophy. High cardiac output, persistent sinus tachycardia, and atrial fibrillation are the usual clinical findings, but poor cardiac contractility and low cardiac output have been described in long-standing forms. In hypothyroidism, abnormalities of diastolic and systolic indices, bradycardia, mild hypertension, and reduced cardiac output have been reported, but symptomatic HF is rare.

Medications

Anticancer drugs

Anticancer drugs may have a variety of cardiovascular secondary effects, in particular LV dysfunction and HF. In a European prospective registry, among patients scheduled for anticancer therapy, cardiotoxicity was identified in 37.5% during follow-up, with 31.6% with mild, 2.8% with moderate, and 3.1% with severe myocardial damage/dysfunction.[8] Two distinct types of anticancer drug-induced cardiac dysfunction have been described.[9]

Type I is induced by classic chemotherapeutic agents, typically anthracyclines, and to a lesser extent by high-dose cyclophosphamide or taxanes. The main mechanism is cleavage of DNA by inhibition of topoisomerase IIb and disruption of neuregulin–Erb

receptor signalling involved in cardiomyocyte growth and survival. Additional determinants are oxidative stress, cardiomyocyte apoptosis, impaired synthesis of DNA, RNA, and transcription factors, and changes in mitochondrial bioenergetics and calcium homeostasis.

Cardiac damage is characterized by loss of myofibrils and cytoplasmic vacuolization of the cardiomyocytes, and is largely irreversible. The entity of cardiotoxicity depends on the drug cumulative dose administered. Several risk factors have been established, such as concomitant cardiac irradiation or association with another cardiotoxic drug, age over 65 years, female gender, and cardiovascular comorbidity. Genetic factors may contribute.

Type II cardiotoxicity is mainly associated with the more recent biologically targeted antiblastic drugs such as the monoclonal antibody trastuzumab, small-molecule tyrosine kinase inhibitors (e.g. imatinib, lapatinib, sunitinib), and proteasome inhibitors (e.g. bortezomib). Trastuzumab, which targets the human epidermal growth factor receptor 2 (HER2), inhibits the activation of a tyrosine protein kinase receptor, triggers cellular oxidative stress, and alters the expression of myocardial genes essential for DNA repair and cardiac and mitochondrial function. Decreased LVEF during therapy occurs in up to 28% of patients and is usually reversible.[10] Cardiotoxicity mechanisms of other new anticancer drugs are still largely hypothetical.

Antiretroviral drugs

Exposure to antiretroviral therapy has been associated with an increased cardiovascular risk.[10] Among these drugs, a clear cardiotoxic effect has been described for azidothymidine, as a result of mitochondrial toxicity and an increased production of mitochondrial reactive oxygen species (ROS).

Antidiabetic drugs

Thiazolidinediones, which are insulin sensitizers widely used to lower blood glucose levels in type 2 diabetes mellitus, can cause fluid retention and induce HF. Suspected drug-related cardiotoxicity arose in the case of rosiglitazone. The exact mechanism is not known; no direct effect on cardiac function or structure has been demonstrated, and interference with mitochondrial respiration or oxidative stress is under investigation. In the RECORD trial, rosiglitazone was associated with a 2-fold higher risk of HF hospitalizations or death.[11] Therefore, it is recommended that rosiglitazone should be discontinued in patients developing symptomatic HF while using the medication.

Antidepressant and antipsychotic drugs

Some antidepressants and antipsychotic drugs (clozapine, fluvoxamine, imipramine, olanzapine, venlafaxine) can cause decreased myocardial contractility and HF.[10] Catecholamine-induced myocardial damage, in conjunction with inhibition of noradrenaline and dopamine reuptake, has been hypothesized, but a possible role for CYP2D6 polymorphism has also been proposed. Tricyclic antidepressants can exert a cardiotoxic effect, with multiple sites of action, including direct action on membrane-bound receptors, ion channels, and intracellular organelles.

Androgenic anabolic steroids

Cardiovascular toxicities of androgenic anabolic steroids, which are illegally misused at high doses in professional sport to enhance physical performance, have not been systematically explored. Alterations of cardiac structure occur with maladaptive cardiac hypertrophy—which is initially concentric and then eccentric—increased fibrosis, diastolic dysfunction, and finally overt HF occurrence.[7] With anabolic steroid discontinuation, the negative cardiovascular effects are reversible, but it is not clear whether restoration of full cardiac function and structure can be achieved.

Environmental agents

Air pollution with excessive exposure to particulate matter is responsible for increased cardiovascular morbidity and mortality. Inhalation of air particulate induces systemic inflammation, oxidative stress, vascular injury, and autonomic dysfunction. HF hospitalizations increase when levels of particulate air pollution are elevated.

Carbon monoxide

Carbon monoxide exposure leads to hypoxic injury, impairment of the mitochondrial respiratory chain at the cytochrome c oxidase level, and decrease in glutathione concentrations and ATP production. After carbon monoxide poisoning, myocarditis and LV systolic dysfunction have been reported.[12]

Metals

Cobalt-related DCM is caused probably by interference with energy production and contractile mechanisms, along with additional factors (nutrition, hypothyroidism, polycythaemia, elevated liver enzymes).[13] Cobalt is commonly used in nutritional supplements, recreational or medicine products, or alloys for prostheses. Antimony, present in many commercial and domestic products, may cause lethal oxidative stress and cell death mediated by elevation in intracellular calcium levels. Association between antimony exposure and HF occurrence has been reported. Lithium, which is the drug of choice for bipolar disorder, can induce cardiotoxic effects through several mechanisms, including depletion of intracellular potassium and displacement of intracellular calcium.[14] Both therapeutic and toxic levels of serum lithium were reported to be associated with cardiomyopathy.

Scorpion venom

Scorpion envenomation is a common medical problem in tropical and subtropical areas worldwide. Cardiovascular effects include hypertension, pulmonary oedema, and depressed ventricular function.[15] Myocardial damage is represented by diffuse mononuclear infiltrates, subendocardial haemorrhages, and focal necrosis. The probable pathophysiological mechanism is related to an abrupt and massive catecholamine release. Effects of envenomation are variable and depend on the age of the scorpion, the amount of venom injected, and the victim's body size.

Systemic infections

Any severe systemic infection may induce HF through different pathophysiological mechanisms such as increased haemodynamic burden on the heart, persistently augmented heart rate, and raised levels of pro-inflammatory cytokines (e.g. tumour necrosis factor alpha, interleukins). Infection is frequently the precipitating cause of HF in a patient with underlying cardiac disease. Description of causative agents that, during systemic infections, may produce cardiac damage is beyond the scope of this chapter.

Cardiac infections

Cardiac infections may be due to several different agents, including viruses, bacteria, fungi, helminths, and protozoa, with distinct pathophysiological mechanisms causing significant damage to cardiac structure and function.

Viral myocarditis

Among viral cardiac infections, the most clinically relevant are myocarditis caused usually by enteroviruses, specifically Coxsackie group B serotypes and, less commonly, adenoviruses, parvovirus B19, hepatitis C virus, cytomegalovirus, and human immunodeficiency virus (HIV).[16,17] More recently, severe acute respiratory syndrome coronavirus 2 (SARS-CoV-2) has been added as a new causative agent. Viral myocarditis accounts for about 20% of cases of DCM. The pathogenesis is thought to begin with direct viral invasion of the myocardium and subsequent immunological activation. Normal cellular and antibody-mediated immune responses lead to viral clearing and myocardial healing. However, a few patients go on to develop DCM and HF due to an abnormal immune response, furthering myocardial damage. The exact mechanisms are unknown but involve cytokines, autoantibodies, and possibly other processes associated with persistent low-level viral replication in myocytes, causing myocyte atrophy, apoptosis, and adverse ventricular remodelling.

Giant cell myocarditis is a rare disorder of uncertain origin, usually associated with ventricular arrhythmias and progressive HF, and can be rapidly fatal.[18] Multinucleated giant cells seen on endomyocardial biopsy (EMB) are pathognomonic.

Clinical manifestations range from asymptomatic ECG abnormalities to cardiogenic shock. Myocarditis can also masquerade and present as acute coronary syndrome.

Serum cardiac enzymes (e.g. troponin, creatine kinase) are measured when myocarditis is suspected. Rising viral titres are inconclusive. Sinus tachycardia and non-specific ST-segment and T-wave abnormalities are common ECG findings. When the pericardium is involved, diffuse ST-segment elevations typical for acute pericarditis are also seen. Ventricular ectopy is common, and atrioventricular (AV) conduction defects can also be observed.

Echocardiography is recommended in the initial diagnostic evaluation to assess cardiac function. Cardiac magnetic resonance imaging (MRI) is considered by many as the gold standard for myocarditis, in order to detect myocardial inflammation and injury.[19]

EMB should be performed when there is rapid clinical deterioration. Histopathological abnormalities, such as infiltrating white cells (i.e. macrophages, lymphocytes, and eosinophils), myocardial damage, and interstitial fibrosis, are used for diagnosis. Polymerase chain reaction can detect specific viral genomes in the myocardium.

Supportive care is the mainstay of treatment. Tailored immunosuppression may be considered, depending on the phase of the disease and the type of underlying autoimmune or immune-mediated form.

About one-third of patients fully recover; one-third have some sequelae in the form of LV systolic dysfunction but are stable on medical therapy, and one-third progress to advanced HF.

SARS-CoV-2

Coronavirus disease 2019 (Covid-19) is caused by SARS-CoV-2. It began in December 2019 in Wuhan, China and rapidly expanded to become a global pandemic, resulting in significant morbidity and mortality. Pre-existing cardiovascular conditions are predictors of adverse outcomes and are more frequent in patients with severe forms of Covid-19.[20,21] The risk of Covid-19 infection may be higher in chronic HF patients who are elderly and often have comorbidities. Biopsy-proven myocardial localization of viral particles with morphology and size typical of coronavirus was first described in a Covid-19 patient presenting with cardiogenic shock.[22]

Cardiovascular complications associated with Covid-19 include acute cardiac injury, myocarditis, stress cardiomyopathy, ischaemic myocardial injury, cytokine release syndrome, cardiac arrhythmias, thrombotic disease, acute HF, and cardiogenic shock. Covid-19 pneumonia, inducing hypoxaemia, dehydration, and hypoperfusion, may lead to worsening haemodynamic status.

In initial reports, HF was observed in 23% of Covid-19 patients (52% in non-survivors vs 12% in survivors).[23] In another study, among patients with a previously normal LVEF admitted to the intensive care unit, one-third evolved with acute HF and cardiogenic shock.[24] Covid-19-induced massive pulmonary embolism complicated by acute right-sided HF has been also reported.

The long-term consequences in patients previously infected are still unknown. In a cohort of patients recently recovered from Covid-19 infection, cardiac magnetic resonance (CMR) revealed cardiac involvement in 78% of cases and ongoing myocardial inflammation in 60%, independent of pre-existing conditions, severity, and overall course of the acute illness, and time from the original diagnosis. Thus, further investigation on this area is needed.[25]

Human immunodeficiency virus

The HIV syndrome affects nearly 70 million people, with over 30 million deaths and 36.7 million currently living with the condition.[26] Individuals with HIV are at increased risk of developing cardiovascular disease (CVD). HIV is recognized as a potential cause of myocarditis and DCM, especially in developing countries where a high mortality rate for HF is reported. A clinical diagnosis of myocarditis or HF may be difficult in an HIV-infected patient because of confounding symptoms due to concomitant bronchopulmonary complications and/or wasting syndromes, especially in advanced stages of the disease.[27] HIV-1 virions appear to infect myocytes in a patchy distribution, without a direct association between the virus presence and cardiac dysfunction. The effects of chronic HIV infection include increased inflammation, immune activation, and immunosenescence.[28] Myocardial dendritic cells play a major role by activating multifunctional cytokines and the inducible form of nitric oxide synthase, promoting progressive myocardial damage. Co-infection with other viruses (generally Coxsackie virus B3 and cytomegalovirus) may also contribute to the process.[27] Furthermore, HIV has been linked to the presence of large-vessel vasculopathy, with ectasia and aneurysm formation, with both phenomena associated with the development of ischaemic stroke and intracranial haemorrhage.[29]

Ricketsia

Myocarditis is a rare disease manifestation of acute Q fever caused by *Coxiella burnetii*, an infectious Gram-negative proteobacteria. *C. burnetii* has a large animal reservoir and is often transmitted to humans during animal birth.

Its presentation is non-specific, often delaying diagnosis and resulting in morbidity and mortality. Diagnosis is routinely achieved after ruling out more common causes of cardiomyopathy, followed by confirmatory serological testing for *C. burnetii*. However, diagnosis can be difficult, as *C. burnetii* does not routinely grow in blood cultures. Thus, serology is often used for diagnostic purposes. Ideally, two serum samples should be obtained—the first at symptom onset and the second at 2–4 weeks after antibiotic initiation. *C. burnetii* exhibits a two-phase antigenic variation caused by changes in lipopolysaccharide C antigens: phase I (often seen in chronic Q fever) and phase II (often seen in acute Q fever). Indirect immunofluorescence assay is used for serological detection of Q fever.[30] Cardiac MRI can be a helpful diagnostic tool, recording subepicardial abnormalities with myocardial oedema and inflammation. The pericardium often demonstrates a normal appearance.[31] EMB is a useful diagnostic modality when a clinical scenario includes idiopathic HF of under 2 weeks' duration unresponsive to conventional therapy.

Borrelia

Lyme disease is caused by spirochaete bacteria (usually *Borrelia burgdorferi*), most commonly transmitted by the *Ixodes scapularis* tick (the blacklegged tick). It is endemic to some regions of Canada, the United States, Central Europe, and Asia. Annual incidence is estimated at 300,000 cases in the United States and 200,000 cases in Western Europe.[32,33] As migratory birds carrying *I. scapularis* are affected by climate change, the geographical spread of the disease is expected to increase.[34] Studies in non-human primates demonstrate a relationship between conduction disturbances, the intensity of myocardial inflammation, and the number of spirochaetes in the cardiac tissue. The chronic sequelae of Lyme disease and potential long-term effects on the heart are less well understood. Acute infection is often asymptomatic or mistaken for a viral infection. Early disseminated Lyme disease can present dramatically with high-degree AV block or neurological symptoms (nerve palsy), whereas the late-disseminated form occurs months after the initial infection, most often presenting as Lyme arthritis.[34]

Fulminant myocarditis and acute HF have been reported.[35] A provocative link between Lyme disease and DCM was first suggested in the 1990s, after *B. burgdorferi* was cultured and spirochaetes identified from EMBs of patients with idiopathic DCM and positive Lyme serology. However, the correlation between *Borrelia* infection and the development of DCM has not been subsequently confirmed.

Parasitic infections

Parasitic infections account for a great burden of morbidity and mortality, especially in developing countries.[36] The heart may be affected by a variety of helminthic or protozoal infections, as shown in ⊃ Table 3.10.1, triggering an inflammatory response,

Table 3.10.1 Helminthic and protozoal infections that may present with heart involvement

Main helminthic infections	Parasite	Cardiovascular features
Schistosomiasis	*Schistosoma mansoni* *S. japonicum* *S. intercalatum* *S. mekongi*	PH with right-sided HF
Tropical endomyocardial fibrosis	Helminths, especially filarial infections	Biventricular involvement as the most common presentation, bi-atrial dilatation and atrial fibrillation
Cysticercosis	*Cysticercus cellulosae* (larval cyst of *Taenia solium*)	Multiple and randomly distributed cysts in the sub-pericardium, sub-endocardium, and myocardium
Echinococcosis	*Echinococcus granulosus* (cystic echinococcosis)	Cysts discovered incidentally, manifest as arrhythmias, myocardial infarction, cardiac tamponade, PH, purulent pericarditis, and sudden death
Trichinellosis	*Trichinella spiralis* and other species	Cardiomegaly, eosinophilic myocarditis, arrhythmias, AV block, non-specific ECG changes and pericardial effusions
Main protozoal infections	**Parasite**	**Cardiovascular features**
Chagas disease	*Trypanosoma cruzi*	Myocarditis, DCM with HF, arrhythmias, thromboembolism, sudden death
Human African trypanosomiasis	*T. brucei gambiense* *T. brucei rhodesiense*	Stage I: myocarditis and occasionally pancarditis, involvement of the conduction system, ECG changes Stage II: pancarditis (rare)
Leishmaniasis	*Leishmania major* (cutaneous) *L. braziliensis* (mucosal) *L. donovani, L. infantum, L. chagasi* (visceral)	Cardiotoxicity due to pentavalent antimony treatment, including ECG changes and arrhythmias
Toxoplasmosis	*Toxoplasma gondii*	Cardiac involvement frequently asymptomatic; myocarditis and pericarditis more frequent in immunodeficient individuals (arrhythmias and HF)
Amoebiasis	*Entamoeba histolytica*	Amebic pericarditis is a serious and rare complication, which may present as purulent pericarditis
Malaria	*Plasmodium* spp.	Non-cardiogenic pulmonary oedema; septic shock-like syndrome, severe metabolic disturbances, and severe anaemia that may precipitate HF

AV, atrioventricular; DCM, dilated cardiomyopathy; HF, heart failure; PH, pulmonary hypertension.
Source data from Nunes MCP, Guimarães Júnior MH, Diamantino AC, *et al.* Cardiac manifestations of parasitic diseases. *Heart* 2017;103:651–658.

with subsequent myocardial injury.[17] Although unusual causes of cardiac disease outside endemic areas, heart involvement due to parasites should be considered in the differential diagnosis, especially of myocardial and/or pericardial diseases of unknown aetiology.

Helminthic infections

Schistosomiasis is a tropical helminthic infection caused by the digenetic trematode of the genus *Schistosoma*, and is the second most prevalent endemic parasitic disease in the world, with Africa being the geographical area most affected.[37] Schistosome infections are classified as acute and chronic phases and as different clinical forms.[38] The acute phase is usually unapparent in people living in endemic areas. The chronic form may cause pulmonary hypertension (PH), and schistosomiasis is one of the most common aetiologies of PH worldwide.[39] Potential major pathophysiological mechanisms, although largely unknown, are mechanical obstruction of the pulmonary arteries by parasite egg embolization and pulmonary vascular changes, including inflammation, medial thickening, and intimal remodelling.

Patients who develop schistosomiasis-associated PH have signs and symptoms primarily resulting from progressive right-sided HF.

Other helminthic infections that may cause myocardial injury are shown in ⊃ Table 3.10.1.

Protozoal infections

Chagas disease, caused by the protozoan *Trypanosoma cruzi*, is the main cause of infectious myocarditis[40] and remains one of the most prevalent parasitic diseases in Latin America.[41] The pathophysiology of myocardial damage is complex and multifactorial, including inflammation, necrosis, and fibrosis, and parasite persistence is central by driving the immune response.[42] Discrepancy between the severity of tissue damage and parasite load has led to the suggestion that immune-mediated myocardial injury plays a pivotal pathogenetic role.[42] The balance between immune-mediated parasite containment and damaging inflammation of host tissues likely determines the course of disease. Additionally, autonomic nervous system derangements and microvascular disturbances may contribute to the pathogenesis. Chronic myocarditis involves all cardiac chambers and the conduction system. The clinical expression of Chagas disease and its prognosis result from multiple factors linked to the parasite, the host, the interaction between the two, and environmental factors. Clinical presentation varies widely, ranging from asymptomatic to severe forms, with HF, cardiac arrhythmias, thromboembolism, or sudden death.[40,43] DCM is the most severe manifestation, which develops in 20–40% of infected individuals over the years.[40,44] Specific patterns of segmental myocardial contractility abnormalities mainly localized in the LV apex and inferolateral walls are common, and LV apical aneurysm is a typical finding ⊃ Figure 3.10.2).

The diagnosis is based on demonstration of antibodies directed against *T. cruzi* antigens by at least two different serological tests. The most commonly used serological tests are an enzyme-linked

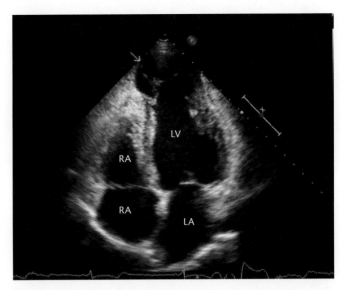

Figure 3.10.2 Two-dimensional echocardiogram with the apical four-chamber view showing left ventricular apical aneurysm (arrow) in a patient with Chagas disease. LA, left atrium; LV, left ventricle; RA, right atrium; RV, right ventricle.

immunosorbent assay, indirect immunofluorescence, and haemagglutination.[45]

African trypanosomiasis, also known as sleeping sickness, is a neglected tropical disease present in sub-Saharan Africa and caused by the *Trypanosoma* genus,[46] protozoan parasites classically transmitted through the bite of blood-sucking tsetse flies. There are two forms: the slow-progressing form, caused by *T. brucei gambiense*, endemic in western and central Africa, and the faster progressing form, caused by *T. brucei rhodesiense*, found in eastern and southern Africa. Despite reduced tsetse populations and interrupted *T. brucei* transmission over the last years, the disease is a considerable burden on rural communities. In a globalized world, cases are also diagnosed outside endemic countries among travellers, tourists, expatriates, and migrants.

Clinical presentation depends on the *T brucei* subspecies, host response, and disease stage, but the disease progresses to death if untreated. Clinical evolution occurs in two stages: the first, or early, haemolymphatic stage, followed by the second, or late, meningoencephalitic stage, in which trypanosomes cross the blood–brain barrier and invade the central nervous system, with typical neurological disturbances, including sleep disorder. In *T. rhodesiense* infection, a more acute course, without a clear distinction between stages, occurs.[47]

Although neurological symptoms are prevalent, cardiac involvement has been reported, especially during the haemolymphatic stage. Myocarditis and occasionally pancarditis leading to arrhythmias and HF have been described. Chronic pancarditis and, as the infection progresses, myocytolysis and fibrosis may develop.[48] HF has also been occasionally reported in association with late *T. rhodesiense* infection.

Cardiac involvement, as demonstrated by ECG alterations, appears early and precedes central nervous system involvement.[49] Diagnosis requires direct visualization of trypanosomes in the blood or lymphonode aspirates, blood, or cerebrospinal fluid.[47] This is possible in *T. brucei rhodesiense* infection because of high levels of parasitaemia, but not in the case of *T. brucei gambiense* where parasitaemia is cyclical.[46] Reliable serodiagnostic tests exist for *T. brucei gambiense* infection, based on detection of specific antibodies, and recently rapid diagnostic tests have been developed.

Future directions

In the field of toxins and infections as possible causes of HF, the pathogenetic mechanisms are not fully understood. The emerging innovative technologies applied to a specific approach in these particular forms of HF will help in the future to address these knowledge gaps.

Summary

The heart may be affected by a variety of viral, bacterial, fungal, protozoal, and helminthic infections, with predominant cardiac involvement, leading to progressive ventricular dysfunction and HF.

Several exogenous and endogenous toxins have been reported as possible causes.

Cardiac infection with various viruses may induce myocarditis, subsequent myocardial dysfunction, and overt HF.

Parasitic infections, in particular Chagas disease, which cause myocarditis leading to cardiomyopathy, and helminthic infections including schistosomiasis, causing PH and right ventricular HF, are the most prevalent.

Different and complex pathophysiological mechanisms, involving inflammation, immunity, and genetic susceptibility, are operative.

Key messages

- Exogenous and endogenous toxins, systemic infections, and cardiac infections represent relatively uncommon causes of impaired cardiac function and HF.
- Different and complex pathophysiological mechanisms leading to myocardial dysfunction are operative.
- Reversibility of cardiac dysfunction after removal of the causative agent depends on several factors.
- In cases of myocardial and/or pericardial diseases of unknown aetiology, heart involvement due to parasitic infection, although unusual outside endemic areas, should be considered in the differential diagnosis.

References

1. George A, Figueredo VM. Alcoholic cardiomyopathy: a review. J Card Fail. 2011;17: 844–9.
2. Iacovoni A, De Maria R, Gavazzi A. Alcoholic cardiomyopathy. J Cardiovasc Med. 2010;11:884–92
3. Gavazzi A, De Maria R, Parolini M, Porcu M. Italian multicentre cardiomyopathy study group: alcohol abuse and dilated cardiomyopathy in men. Am J Cardiol. 2000;85:1114–18.
4. Maraj S, Figueredo VM, Lynn MD. Cocaine and the heart. Clin Cardiol. 2010;33:264–9.
5. Henning RJ, Wilson LD, Glauser JM. Cocaine plus ethanol is more cardiotoxic than cocaine or ethanol alone. Crit Care Med. 1994;22:1896–906.
6. Morris P, Robinson T, Channer K. Reversible heart failure: toxins, tachycardiomyopathy and mitochondrial abnormalities. Postgrad Med J. 2012;88:706–12.
7. Albakri A. Toxin-induced cardiomyopathy: a review and pooled analysis of pathophysiology, diagnosis and clinical management. Res Rev Insights. 2019;3:1–21.
8. Lopez-Sendon J, Alvarez-Ortega C, Aunon PZ, et al. Classification, prevalence, and outcomes of anticancer therapy-induced cardiotoxicity: the CARDIOTOX registry. Eur Heart J. 2020; 41:1720–9.
9. Ewer MS, Ewer SM. Cardiotoxicity of anticancer treatments. Nat Rev Cardiol. 2015;12:547–58.
10. Hantson P. Mechanisms of toxic cardiomyopathy. Clin Toxicol. 2019;57:1–9.
11. Komajda M, McMurray JJV, Beck-Nielsen HB, et al. Heart failure events with rosiglitazone in type 2 diabetes: data from the RECORD clinical trial. Eur Heart J. 2010;31:824–31.
12. Lippi G, Rastelli G, Meschi T, et al. Pathophysiology, clinics, diagnosis and treatment of heart involvement in carbon monoxide poisoning. Clin Biochem. 2012;45:1278–85.
13. Packer M. Cobalt cardiomyopathy: a critical reappraisal in light of a recent resurgence. Circ Heart Fail. 2016;9:e003604. pii: e00360.
14. Rosero Enriquez AS, Ballesteros Prados A, Petcu AS. Cardiomyopathy secondary to long-term treatment with lithium: a case report and literature review. J Clin Psychopharmacol. 2018;38:157–9.
15. Abroug F, Souheil E, Ouanes I, et al. Scorpion-related cardiomyopathy: clinical characteristics, pathophysiology, and treatment. Clin Toxicol. 2015;53:511–18.
16. Caforio ALP, Pankuweit S, Arbustini E, et al. Current state of knowledge on aetiology, diagnosis, management, and therapy of myocarditis: a position statement of the European Society of Cardiology Working Group on Myocardial and Pericardial Diseases. Eur Heart J. 2013; 34:2636–48.
17. Tschöpe C, Ammirati E, Bozkurt B, et al. Myocarditis and inflammatory cardiomyopathy: current evidence and future directions. Nat Rev Cardiol. 2021;18:169–93.
18. Cooper LT. Giant cell myocarditis: diagnosis and treatment. Herz. 2000;25:291–8.
19. Bucciarelli-Ducci C. Diagnosing myocarditis with magnetic resonance. J Cardiovasc Med. 2017;18 Suppl 1:e75–6.
20a. Task Force for the management of COVID-19 of the European Society of Cardiology. European Society of Cardiology guidance for the diagnosis and management of cardiovascular disease during the COVID-19 pandemic: part 1—epidemiology, pathophysiology, and diagnosis. Eur Heart J. 2022;43:1033–58.
20b. Task Force for the management of COVID-19 of the European Society of Cardiology. ESC guidance for the diagnosis and management of cardiovascular disease during the COVID-19 pandemic: part 2—care pathways, treatment, and follow-up. Eur Heart J. 2022;43:1059–103.
21. Yang J, Zheng Y, Gou X, et al. Prevalence of comorbidities and its effects in patients infected with SARS-CoV-2: a systematic review and meta-analysis. Int J Infect Dis. 2020;94:91–5.
22. Tavazzi G, Pellegrini C, Maurelli M, et al. Myocardial localization of coronavirus in COVID-19 cardiogenic shock. Eur J Heart Fail. 2020;2:911–15.

23. Zhou F, Yu T, Du R, *et al*. Clinical course and risk factors for mortality of adult inpatients with COVID-19 in Wuhan, China: a retrospective cohort study. Lancet. 2020;395:1054–62.

24. Arentz M, Yim E, Klaff L, *et al*. Characteristics and outcomes of 21 critically ill patients with COVID-19 in Washington state. JAMA. 2020;323:1613–14.

25. Puntmann VO, Carerj ML, Wieters I, *et al*. Outcomes of cardiovascular magnetic resonance imaging in patients recently recovered from coronavirus disease 2019 (COVID-19). JAMA Cardiol. 2020;5(11):1265–73.

26. Fajardo-Ortiz D, Lopez-Cervantes M, Duran L, *et al*. The emergence and evolution of the research fronts in HIV/AIDS research. PLoS One. 2017;12(5):e0178293

27. Barbaro G. HIV-associated cardiomyopathy. Etiopathogenesis and clinical aspects. Herz. 2005;30:486–92.

28. Eckard AR, Meissner EG, Singh I, McComsey GA. Cardiovascular disease, statins, and HIV. J Infect Dis. 2017;215:496.

29. Avan A, Digaleh H, Di Napoli M, *et al*. Socioeconomic status and stroke incidence, prevalence, mortality, and worldwide burden: an ecological analysis from the Global Burden of Disease Study 2017. BMC Med. 2019;17(1):191.

30. Scott JW, Baddour LM, Tleyjeh IM, Moustafa S, Sun YG, Mookadam F. Q fever endocarditis: the Mayo clinic experience. Am J Med Sci. 2008;336:53–7.

31. Canga-Villegas A. Acute Q fever myocarditis: thinking about a life-threatening but potentially curable condition. Int J Cardiol. 2012;158:e17–19.

32. Hinckley AF, Connally NP, Meek JI, *et al*. Lyme disease testing by large commercial laboratories in the United States. Clin Infect Dis. 2014;59(5):676–81.

33. Sykes RA, Makiello P. An estimate of Lyme borreliosis incidence in Western Europe. J Public Health (Oxf). 2017;39 (1):74–81.

34. Yeung C, Baranchuk A. Diagnosis and treatment of Lyme carditis: JACC review topic of the week. J Am Coll Cardiol. 2019;73(6):717–26.

35. Zupan Z, Mijatovic D, Medved I, *et al*. Successful treatment of fulminant Lyme myocarditis with mechanical circulatory support in a young male adult: a case report. Croat Med J. 2017;58(2):185–93.

36. Nunes MCP, Júnior MHG, Diamantino AC, Gelape CL, Ferrari TCA. Cardiac manifestations of parasitic diseases. Heart. 2017;103:651–8.

37. Chitsulo L, Engels D, Montresor A, Savioli L. The global status of schistosomiasis and its control. Acta Tropica. 2000;77:41–5.

38. Ferrari TCA, Moreira PRR. Neuroschistosomiasis: clinical symptoms and pathogenesis. Lancet Neurology. 2011;10:853–64.

39. Papamatheakis DG, Mocumbi AOH, Kim NH, Mandel J. Schistosomiasis-associated pulmonary hypertension. Pulmonary Circulation. 2014;4:596–611.

40. Nunes MCP, Dones W, Morillo CA, Encina JJ, Ribeiro AL; Council on Chagas Disease of the Interamerican Society of Cardiology. Chagas disease: An overview of clinical and epidemiological aspects. J Am Coll Cardiol. 2013;62:767–76.

41. World Health Organization. Chagas disease in Latin America: an epidemiological update based on 2010 estimates. Geneva: World Health Organization; 2015.

42. Marin-Neto JA, Cunha-Neto E, Maciel BC, Simoes MV. Pathogenesis of chronic Chagas heart disease. Circulation. 2007;115:1109–23.

43. Nunes MCP, Beaton A, Acquatella H, *et al*. Chagas cardiomyopathy: an update of current clinical knowledge and management: a scientific statement from the American Heart Association. Circulation. 2018;138:e169–209.

44. Ribeiro AL, Nunes MP, Teixeira MM, Rocha MO. Diagnosis and management of Chagas disease and cardiomyopathy. Nat Rev Cardiol. 2012;9:576–89.

45. Otani MM, Vinelli E, Kirchhoff LV, *et al*. Who comparative evaluation of serologic assays for Chagas disease. Transfusion. 2009;49:1076–82.

46. Büscher P, Cecchi G, Jamonneau V, Priotto G. Human African trypanosomiasis. Lancet. 2017;390:2397–409.

47. Bennett J, Dolin R, Mondell G, Mandell D. *Bennett's Principles and Practice of Infectious Diseases*, 8th edition. Philadelphia, PA: Elsevier; 2014.

48. Poltera A, Cox J, Owor R. Pancarditis affecting the conducting system and all valves in human African trypanosomiasis. Brit Heart J. 1976;38:827–37.

49. Blum JA, Schmid C, Burri C, *et al*. Cardiac alterations in human african trypanosomiasis (*T.b gambiense*) with respect to the disease stage and antiparasitic treatment. PLoS Negl Trop Dis. 2009;3:e383.

SECTION 4

Prevention of heart failure

CHAPTER 4.1

Prevention of heart failure

Massimo Francesco Piepoli, Maria Benedetta Matrone, Paul Dendale, and Shelley Zieroth

Contents

Introduction

Heart failure (HF) is a chronic condition, with increasing consequences in terms of the number of patients affected, its associated clinical consequences, and its implications in health-care expenditure.[1] Despite the development of disease-modifying therapies for HF, clinical outcomes have remained poor. Because of rapid ageing of the population, the incidence of HF will be increasing in the coming years. Therefore, a key issue in modern medicine is prevention of the development of HF in order to reduce hospital admission rates, clinical sequelae, and economic consequences. So far, preventive measures have acquired a fundamental role and made it necessary to draft a guide document drawn from evidence-based information.

This chapter focuses on primary prevention of the development of HF, and thus *not* on preventing its complications in those with established HF. Because of the pervasive aspects of economic transition, twenty-first-century lifestyles, and rapid urbanization, some new behavioural risk indicators are gaining importance such as excessive alcohol consumption and unhealthy diet habits. These are added to the well-established risk factors known to the entire scientific community such as hypertension, type 2 diabetes mellitus (T2DM), smoking, dyslipidaemia, and a sedentary lifestyle. In general, analyses from European, as well North American, populations have provided evidence that implementation of healthy behaviours lowers the risk of HF development in both men and women.[2,3]

In this chapter, we present potential interventions that have been shown to prevent the development of HF, as recommended by the European Guidelines of Cardiovascular Prevention in Clinical Practice,[4] and the more recent European Society of Cardiology (ESC) guidelines for the management of dyslipidaemias[5] (➲ Tables 4.1.1 and 4.1.2).

Classical modifiable risk factors

Arterial hypertension

Arterial hypertension is the most common modifiable risk factor for HF and is one which has been increasing in relevance over time among patients with HF. In a population-based case-control study in Olmsted County, a history of hypertension was present in 66% of patients with HF from 1985 to 1990, and increased to 74% from 1997 to 2002.[6] The population attributable risk (PAR) for HF conferred by hypertension has been estimated at 20%.

In the general population, the prevalence of hypertension is approximately 30–45% and the lifetime probability of developing hypertension is >75%.[7] Strategies to control hypertension are a vital part of any public health effort to prevent HF.

Table 4.1.1 Risk factor goals and target levels for important cardiovascular risk factors

Smoking	No exposure to tobacco in any form
Diet	Healthy diet low in saturated fat, with a focus on wholegrain products, vegetables, fruit, and fish
Physical activity	3.5–7 hours of moderately vigorous physical activity per week or 30–60 minutes on most days
Body weight	BMI 20–25 kg/m^2 and waist circumference <94 cm (men) and <80 cm (women)
Blood pressure	<140/90 mmHg[a]
LDL-C	**Very high risk in primary or secondary prevention:** a therapeutic regimen that achieves ≥50% LDL-C reduction from baseline[b] and an LDL-C goal of <1.4 mmol/L (<55 mg/dL) No current statin use: this is likely to require high-intensity LDL-loweing therapy Current LDL-lowering treatment: increased treatment intensity is required **High risk:** a therapeutic regimen that achieves ≥50% LDL-C reduction from baseline[b] and an LDL-C goal of <1.8 mmol/L (<70 mg/dL) **Moderate risk:** a goal of <2.6 mmol/L (<100 mg/dL) **Low risk:** a goal of <3.0 mmol/L (<116 mg/dL)
Non-HDL-C	Non-HDL-C secondary goals are <2.2, 2.6, and 3.4 mmol/L (<85, 100, and 130 mg/dL) for very high-, high-, and moderate-risk individuals, respectively
ApoB	ApoB secondary goals are <65, 80, and 100 mg/dL for very high- and moderate-risk individuals, respectively
Triglycerides	No goal, but <1.7 mmol/L (<150 mg/dL) indicates lower risk and higher levels indicate a need to assess for other risk factors
Diabetes	HbA1c <7% (<53 mmol/mol)

[a] Lower treatment targets are recommended for most treated hypertensive patients, provided the treatment is well tolerated.
[b] The term 'baseline' refers to the LDL-C level in a person not taking any lipid-lowering medication, or to the extrapolated baseline value for those who are on current treatment.
Apo, apolipoprotein; BMI, body mass index; HbA1c, glycated haemoglobin; HDL-C, high-density lipoprotein cholesterol; LDL-C, low-density lipoprotein cholesterol.
Source data from Piepoli MF, Hoes AW, Agewall S, *et al.* 2016 European Guidelines on cardiovascular disease prevention in clinical practice. *European Heart Journal*, 2016; 37(29), 2315–2381 and Mach F, Baigent C, Catapano AL, *et al.* 2019 ESC/EAS Guidelines for the management of dyslipidaemias: lipid modification to reduce cardiovascular risk. *European Heart Journal*, 2020; 41(1), 111–188.

Hypertensive subjects have a substantially greater risk of developing HF than normotensive men and women.[8] Elevated diastolic, and especially systolic, blood pressures are major risk factors for incident HF.[9]

Arterial hypertension has a bidirectional effect in the context of HF with reduced ejection fraction (HFrEF) and HF with preserved ejection fraction (HFpEF). The mechanism

Table 4.1.2 Healthy diet characteristics

Saturated fatty acids to account for <10% of total energy intake through replacement by polyunsaturated fatty acids
Trans-unsaturated fatty acids: as little as possible, preferably no intake from processed food, and <1% of total energy intake from natural sources
<5 g of salt per day
30–45 g of fibre per day, preferably from wholegrain products
≥200 g of fruit per day (2–3 servings)
≥200 g of vegetables per day (2–3 servings)
Fish 1–2 times per week, one of which to be oily fish
30 g of unsalted nuts per day
Consumption of alcoholic beverages should be limited to two glasses per day (20 g/day of alcohol) for men and one glass per day (10 g/day of alcohol) for women
Consumption of sugar-sweetened soft drinks and alcoholic beverages must be discouraged

Reproduced from Piepoli MF, Hoes AW, Agewall S, *et al.* 2016 European Guidelines on cardiovascular disease prevention in clinical practice. *European Heart Journal*, 2016; 37(29), 2315–2381 with permission from Oxford University Press.

by which arterial hypertension triggers HFrEF is through incident coronary artery disease (CAD), with hypertension representing the initial trigger, whereas CAD is the clinical event driving the development of decompensated HF. Hypertension can also lead to HFpEF in patients without CAD through hypertension-mediated organ damage, in particular left ventricular hypertrophy.

The effect of hypertension treatment on the development of HF has been evaluated in several clinical trials. Long-term treatment of hypertension reduces the risk of HF by approximately 50% and is associated with lower HF mortality. From 14,709 ARIC (Atherosclerosis Risk in Communities) study participants, the incidence rate differences (IRDs) for the association between five modifiable risk factors and HF were estimated. A 5% proportional reduction in the prevalence of hypertension would lead to the prevention of 28 cases of incident HF/100,000 persons per year in African-American cohorts and 19/100,000 persons per year in Caucasians (➲ Table 4.1.3).[10] A comparative meta-analysis on antihypertensive drugs showed that diuretics (with an odds ratio (OR) of 0.59), angiotensin-converting enzyme inhibitors (ACEIs; OR 0.70), and angiotensin II receptor blockers (ARBs; OR 0.79) were more effective in reducing the incidence of HF, compared to placebo and also to calcium channel blockers, beta-blockers, and alpha-blockers.[11] Another meta-analysis evaluating the effect of beta-blockers found that the degree of blood pressure reduction was the main determinant of success in reducing subsequent HF: beta-blockers did not seem to have a significant effect on reducing HF beyond blood pressure reduction.[12]

Table 4.1.3 Race-specific estimates of the preventable number of heart failure cases, years of life lost lived with disability that would result from a 5% proportional reduction in the prevalence of five common cardiovascular risk factors in the United States from the ARIC cohort study, 1987–2008

Exposure	African-Americans				Caucasians			
	Disability-adjusted life years				Disability-adjusted life years			
	Period prevalence, 1987–1998*	Preventable number of heart failure cases†	Number of years of life lost‡	Number of years of life with disability†	Period prevalence, 1987–1998*	Preventable number of heart failure cases†	Number of years of life lost‡	Number of years of life with disability‡
Current smoking	32.4	15	28	6	26.8	10	63	19
Diabetes	31.0	53	65	13	17.1	33	81	24
Elevated LDL-C	65.4	23	60	12	60.5	11	120	36
Hypertension	71.1	28	68	14	45.3	19	102	31
Obesity	50.2	16	39	8	33.9	15	69	21

* Assessed at baseline and on three triennial visits.
‡ Per year for all participants with heart failure.
† Per 100,000 person-years.
ARIC, Atherosclerosis Risk in Communities study; LDL-C, low-density lipoprotein cholesterol.
Reproduced from Avery CL, Loehr LR, Baggett C, *et al.* The population burden of heart failure attributable to modifiable risk factors: the ARIC (Atherosclerosis Risk in Communities) study. *J Am Coll Cardiol.* 2012;60(17):1640–1646 with permission from Elsevier.

Diabetes mellitus

Diabetes mellitus and HF are closely interconnected. HF is one of the most frequent cardiovascular (CV) complications of T2DM, regardless of the baseline CV risk.[13,14] Studies demonstrated that treatment of T2DM is a viable strategy for preventing HF.

In a recent community-based study of 1.9 million people without CV disease (CVD), with a median follow-up of 5.5 years, people with T2DM frequently developed HF as the first CV presentation, with a hazard ratio (HR) for incident HF of 1.56 (95% confidence interval (CI) 1.45–1.69), compared to those without T2DM.[13] In a meta-analysis of 16 CV outcome trials in T2DM versus placebo, both patients with and those without prior CVD had more frequent hospitalization for HF than for stroke and only marginally less frequent hospitalization for HF than for myocardial infarction (MI).[14] Several risk factors and comorbidities contribute to the development of HF in T2DM, such as myocardial ischaemia, hypertension, obesity, and chronic kidney disease, in association with possible direct myocardial impairment caused by T2DM.[15,16,17]

Despite the use of insulin and insulin secretagogues for tight glycaemic control (i.e. targeting normal levels of glycosylated haemoglobin (HbA1c)), there is no proven efficacy in reducing the risk of developing HF;[18] indeed intensive glycaemic control has been shown to increase mortality.[19] Other therapies (e.g. rosiglitazone) may increase the risk of HF.[20]

Nevertheless, a major breakthrough in HF prevention has come from recent CV outcome trials with a novel class of glucose-lowering medications: sodium–glucose cotransporter 2 (SGLT2) inhibitors. In multiple clinical trials of patients with T2DM and either established CVD or with multiple risk factors, SGLT2 inhibitors (empagliflozin, canagliflozin, dapagliflozin, and ertugliflozin) have shown a consistent risk reduction in HF hospitalization, whereas their effects on mortality and other outcomes of interest have varied across the trials (⊙ Table 4.1.4).[21,22,23,24] High-risk individuals with T2DM and nephropathy also benefited from a reduction in HF complications.[25] This was later confirmed in a broader population of patients with chronic kidney disease with and without T2DM.[26] Dapagliflozin, canagliflozin, and empagliflozin were evaluated in a recent meta-analysis and shown to have a significant risk reduction for the combined endpoint of CV death or hospitalization for HF (HR 0.77, 95% CI 0.71–0.84; $P<0.0001$), as well as for hospitalization for HF (HR 0.69, 95% CI 0.61–0.79; $P<0.0001$), in both patients with and those without CVD.[27] The beneficial effect on HF hospitalizations has been further confirmed in a subsequent study.[24] Based on these findings, recent practice guidelines[28] and expert consensus documents[29,30,31] have strengthened the role of SGLT2 inhibitors in the prevention of HF in T2DM. The proposed mechanisms are multiple; first of all, a mediation analysis of clinical trial data on empagliflozin has suggested a reduction in intravascular volume (clinically demonstrated by an increase in haematocrit and haemoglobin levels).[32] Metabolism activation (with reduction in uric acid levels, fasting glycaemia, and HbA1c levels), modulation of inflammation, adipose tissue and adipokines, fluid excretion, tubuloglomerular feedback, and nephroprotection are other mechanisms probably involved.[32]

Other hypoglycaemic drugs, for example, dipeptidyl peptidase 4 (DPP4) inhibitors and glucagon-like peptide 1 (GLP1) receptor agonists, have not proven effective in the prevention of HF in T2DM. In their respective CV outcome trials, DPP4 inhibitors were associated either with no effect on,[33,34,35] or with a higher risk of (saxagliptin, vildagliptin, and a non-statistically significant trend with alogliptin), HF hospitalization,[36,37] whereas use of GLP1 receptor agonists had a neutral effect on HF risk.[38,39,40,41,42]

T2DM is usually part of the metabolic syndrome, so patients with T2DM may benefit from overall management of risk factors and comorbidities. Indeed, in the Cardiovascular outcomes

Table 4.1.4 Cardiovascular and renal outcome trials on SGTL2 inhibitors in patients with type 2 diabetes mellitus

Medication	Trial	Patients, n	Patient characteristics	Follow-up (mean or median), years	Primary outcome (HR, 95% CI; P-value)	HF hospitalization (HR, 95% CI; P-value)
Empagliflozin	EMPA-REG OUTCOME[21]	7020	Established CVD	3.1	3-point MACE* (0.86, 0.74–0.99; P <0.001 for non-inferiority; P = 0.04 for superiority)	0.65, 0.50–0.85; P = 0.002
Canagliflozin	CANVAS Program[22]	10,142	Established CVD (66%); CV risk factors (34%)	3.2	3-point MACE* (0.86, 0.75–0.97; P <0.001 for non-inferiority; P = 0.02 for superiority)	0.67, 0.52–0.87
Dapagliflozin	DECLARE TIMI-58[23]	17,160	Established CVD (41%); CV risk factors (59%)	4.2	Co-primary outcome: 3-point MACE* (0.93, 0.84–1.03; P = 0.17) Co-primary outcome: CV death or HF hospitalization (0.83, 0.73–0.95; P = 0.005)	0.73, 0.61–0.88
Ertugliflozin	VERTIS-CV[24]	8246	Established CVD	3.5	3-point MACE* (0.97, 0.85–1.11; P <0.001 for non-inferiority)	0.70, 95% CI 0.54–0.90; P = 0.006
Canagliflozin	CREDENCE[25]	4401	Chronic kidney disease (eGFR 30 to <90 mL/ min per 1.73 m² of body surface area and ratio of albumin-to-creatinine >300–5000 mg/g)	2.6	Composite of end-stage kidney disease (dialysis, transplantation, or sustained eGFR of <15 mL/min per 1.73 m²), doubling of serum creatinine level, or death from renal or cardiovascular causes (0.70, 0.59–0.82; P <0.001)	0.61, 0.47–0.80; P <0.001
Dapagliflozin	DAPA-CKD[26]	4304 (2906 with T2DM)	Chronic kidney disease (eGFR ≥25 and ≥75 mL/ min per 1.73 m2; urinary albumin-to-creatinine ratio between ≥200 mg/g and ≤5000 mg/g)	2.4	Worsening kidney function (defined as >50% sustained decline in eGFR or onset of end-stage kidney disease) or death due to kidney disease or cardiovascular disease (0.61, 0.51–0.72; P <0.001)	0.71, 0.55–0.92; P <0.001

* Three-point MACE (major adverse cardiovascular events): cardiovascular death, non-fatal myocardial infarction, and stroke.
CI, confidence interval; CV, cardiovascular; CVD, cardiovascular disease; eGFR, estimated glomerular filtration rate; HF, heart failure; HR, hazard ratio; T2DM, type 2 diabetes mellitus.

in the Irbesartan Diabetic Nephropathy Trial of patients with T2DM and overt nephropathy, treatment with irbesartan reduced the incidence of HF, compared with placebo (HR 0.72, 95% CI 0.52–1.00; P = 0.048) and amlodipine (HR 0.65, 95% CI 0.48–0.87; P = 0.004).[43] Data from real-world practice are conflicting. A recent cohort study of >270,000 individuals with T2DM demonstrated that this approach may be insufficient in those who have five risk factors (elevated HbA1c, elevated low-density lipoprotein cholesterol level, albuminuria, smoking, and elevated blood pressure) within guideline-directed target ranges.[44] In this population, the risk of HF remained elevated (HR 1.45, 95% CI 1.34–1.57) despite a reduction in other CV outcomes (MI, stroke, and mortality).[44] Other real-world data, on the other hand, corroborate findings from CV outcome trials on SGLT2 inhibitors regarding their effectiveness in risk reduction of HF, compared with other glucose-lowering agents.[45,46]

Sedentary habits

Exercise tolerance is another risk factor for HF; physically active individuals have a significantly lower risk of HF, when compared to those with low exercise tolerance, and the risk reduction may be dose-sensitive.[47,48] A simple metric such as (self-reported)

ability to walk at pace (>5 km or 3 miles per hour) was related to reduced HF risk. In the Women's Health Initiative, after adjustment for other risk factors, the HF risk for active adults was 0.66 (95% CI 0.58–0.75), and 0.77 (95% CI 0.67–0.87) for somewhat active adults, compared with inactive adults.[49] The incidence of HF in the same study ranged from 1.55 per 1000 person-years for physically active individuals (defined as >150 minutes/week of moderate physical activity, or >75 minutes/week of vigorous physical activity) to 2.15 per 1000 person-years for those who were somewhat active (less than the activity thresholds for 'active', but >0), and to 3.29 per 1000 person-years for those who were inactive.[49]

Endocrine and metabolic factors

Lipid concentrations

In a follow-up (mean of 26 years) of 6860 Framingham Heart Study participants (mean age of 44 years; 54% of women) free of baseline coronary heart disease, 680 participants (10% of total; 49% of women) developed HF.[50] Participants with high baseline levels of non-high-density lipoprotein cholesterol (non-HDL-C; >190 mg/dL) and those with low levels of HDL-C (<40 mg/dL in men, <50 mg/dL in women) experienced a 29% and 40% higher HF risk, respectively, compared to those in the desirable lipid categories; the PARs for high non-HDL-C levels and low HDL-C levels were 7.5% and 15%, respectively. After additional adjustment for interim MI, hazards associated with high non-HDL-C and low HDL-C levels remained statistically significant. In the recent Multiethnic Study of Atherosclerosis, only lipid measures from T2DM patients were associated with incident HF.[51]

Hydroxymethylglutaryl coenzyme A (HMG-CoA) reductase inhibitors (statins) reduce CV events in patients with and those without previously diagnosed CVD, and consequently may prevent HF development. The absolute risk reduction is proportional to the baseline CV risk and lipid blood levels. Initiating drug therapy in elderly individuals, however, requires caution.[5]

Finally, a meta-analysis of unpublished data from major randomized trials has shown that statins modestly reduce the occurrence of a first non-fatal HF hospitalization not preceded by MI (risk ratio 0.91, 95% CI 0.84–0.98).[52]

Obesity

Overweight and obesity adversely affect many CVDs, including HF. Body weight and body mass index (BMI) are specifically associated with the risk of HF development,[53,54] which has been estimated to increase by 5–7% with each increment of $1 kg/m^2$ in BMI.[53] The contribution of obesity (BMI >30 kg/m^2) to the development of HFpEF is greater than to that of HFrEF; nevertheless, body weight is a risk factor in both scenarios.[55] In a population study from Rochester, Minnesota, obesity was present in 20.5% of patients newly diagnosed with HF from 1985 to 1990, compared to 29.5% from 1997 to 2002 ($P = 0.003$ for trend). HF was found to develop about 16 years from onset of obesity.[53] The PAR of obesity for incident HF was estimated at 12%. According to a study from the Women's Health Initiative, the incidence of HF increased from 1.32 per 1000 person-years for patients with a BMI of between 18.5 and 25 kg/m^2 to 1.72 per 1000 person-years for those with a BMI of between 25 and 30 kg/m^2, and to 3.37 per 1000 person-years for those with a BMI of >30 kg/m^2.[53] After adjusting

for classical and acquired risk factors, the risk of developing HF for patients with a BMI of between 18.5 and 25 kg/m^2 was 0.43 (95% CI 0.38–0.48), and 0.50 (95% CI 0.45–0.56) for those with a BMI of between 25 and 30 kg/m^2, compared to those with a BMI of >30 kg/m^2.

The exact mechanisms underlying obesity-related HF are still unknown. Excessive adipose tissue accumulation results in an increase in circulating blood volume. A successive, persistent increase in cardiac output, cardiac work, and systemic blood pressure,[56] lipotoxicity-induced cardiac myocyte injury and myocardial lipid accumulation,[57] as well as oxidative stress, have been implicated as multiple potential mechanisms leading to overt HF.[58] There is a close pathophysiological link between excess fat tissue and metabolic syndrome and HF at the molecular, neurohormonal, and central haemodynamic levels.[57,59] Weight loss is undoubtedly related to favourable haemodynamic effects. Further research and large-scale studies are needed on safety or efficacy of weight loss through diet and exercise or bariatric surgery in obese patients with HF. However, a healthy weight is important for overall health, and weight control has been confirmed to reduce the risk of HF in large cohort analyses.[60]

Thyroid disease and other endocrine disorders

Multiple endocrine dysfunctions have an adverse impact on the CV system and occasionally can be associated with HF (➔ Table 4.1.5).[61,62] Endocrine disease can be a truly reversible factor in cardiac dysfunction, thus offering the possibility of aetiological treatment of HF or even prevention. Many studies have recently confirmed that persistent subclinical thyroid dysfunction is associated with the development of HF. Hypothyroidism is common, as it affects 4–10% of the general population, but the prevalence of subclinical hypothyroidism is about 5–15%.[62] It can affect the heart and circulatory system in a number of ways, as it may trigger rhythm disturbances including sinus bradycardia, QT prolongation, and atrioventricular block, diastolic hypertension, low cardiac output with narrow pulse pressure, and hypercholesterolaemia with accelerated atherosclerosis. HF in this case

Table 4.1.5 Main endocrine disorders that may lead or contribute to the development of heart failure

Hormone	Endocrinopathy	Main mechanisms of heart failure
Aldosterone	Hyperaldosteronism	Hypertension, myocardial fibrosis, diastolic LV dysfunction, volume overload
Catecholamines	Phaeochromocytoma	Hypertension, catecholamine-induced cardiomyopathy
Cortisol	Cushing's syndrome (endogenous or iatrogenic)	Hypertension, LV hypertrophy, diastolic LV dysfunction, metabolic alterations
Growth hormone	Acromegaly	Acromegalic cardiomyopathy
	Growth hormone deficiency	Reduced LV mass with impaired myocardial contractility and cardiac output
Parathyroid hormone	Hypoparathyroidism	Hypocalcaemia-induced myocardial dysfunction (possibly due to disrupted excitation–contraction coupling)
Prolactin	[18-kDa prolactin fragment]	Peripartum cardiomyopathy
Thyroid hormone	Hypothyroidism	Diastolic LV dysfunction, decreased cardiac output
	Hyperthyroidism	Tachyarrhythmia, hypertension, LV hypertrophy, diastolic LV dysfunction, increased cardiac output

LV, left ventricle/ventricular.

may be related to diastolic left ventricular (LV) dysfunction and low cardiac output.[63] Data from the Healthy Aging and Body Composition Study, an interdisciplinary population-based study of 2730 men and women aged 70–79 years, revealed that subclinical hypothyroidism (thyroid-stimulating hormone (TSH) levels of 7.0–9.9 mIU/L) was associated with a 2.6-fold increased risk of developing HF, compared to normal TSH levels; this relative risk increased to 3.3-fold in patients with TSH levels of ≥10 mIU/L.[62] Several subsequent studies, such as the Cardiovascular Health Study, confirmed these results.[63]

Hyperthyroidism has important CV consequences, as it results in an increased heart rate due to sinus tachycardia or atrial fibrillation, and a decrease in systemic vascular resistance with subsequent renin–angiotensin–aldosterone system activation and increased preload. These changes, in turn, lead to increased cardiac output (increased preload and decreased afterload) and systolic hypertension (increased heart rate and cardiac output), with subsequent LV hypertrophy and diastolic LV dysfunction.[63] These abnormalities may lead to HF, but they are reversible if detected early and the underlying endocrinopathy is corrected.[64]

Toxic factors

Alcohol abuse

Among the consequences of excessive alcohol consumption, dilated cardiomyopathy (defined as alcoholic cardiomyopathy (ACM)) is definitely one of the most relevant. It has been estimated that up to 40% of cases of dilated cardiomyopathy can be attributed to excessive alcohol consumption.[65]

Even though mild alcohol consumption was reported to be protective against HF development,[66] recent studies have challenged this concept with the observation that low-volume drinkers may appear healthy only because the 'abstainers' to whom they are compared are biased towards ill health.[67]

In contrast, long-term heavy alcohol use (>40 g of alcohol daily, approximately 2.5–3 standard drinks per day) for >5 years has been associated with a higher risk.[67] This was confirmed by a large combined analysis of individual participant data from more than half a million current drinkers; this study showed that the risk of mortality increased over the entire range of alcohol intake of above 45 g daily.[68] In addition, individual genetic susceptibility is believed to play a major role in the pathogenesis of ACM in patients who consume alcohol above recommended levels.[69]

A clinical diagnosis of ACM is suspected when biventricular dysfunction and dilatation are persistently observed in a hard drinker in the absence of other known causes for myocardial disease. ACM is more prevalent in men aged 30–55 years who have been heavy consumers of alcohol for >10 years. Women represent approximately 14% of ACM cases but are likely to be more vulnerable with less lifetime alcohol consumption.[70]

Recovery of LV function has been described after alcohol withdrawal,[71] and in this case, ACM has a better prognosis than dilated cardiomyopathy in alcohol abstainers.[65] Although more evidence is needed on the risk thresholds for alcohol consumption in order to prevent HF, the available data support the adoption of lower limits of alcohol consumption than those recommended in most current guidelines and strongly suggest that ACM patients should be advised to stop drinking.[72]

Smoking

Among the risk factors for CVD, smoking is certainly modifiable. Several studies have associated smoking with a higher risk of developing HFrEF, independently of other lifestyle risk factors.[49,73,74,75,76] In the Women's Health Initiative study, the adjusted risk of incident HFrEF for never-smokers was 0.43 (95% CI 0.33–0.55) and 0.47 (95% CI 0.37–0.60) for former smokers, compared to current smokers.[49] In this study, smoking was also associated with HFpEF, with similar HRs.

Whereas smoking increases the risk of ischaemic heart disease, indirectly causing HF, there are also direct effects of smoking that result in cardiac dysfunction and HF. In healthy individuals, greater LV mass, poorer systolic function of the left and right ventricles, and also worse diastolic function as reflected by a higher E/e′ were observed in smokers, compared to non-smokers.[77,78,79,80,81] A recent meta-analysis has found fairly strong evidence that continued smoking after HF had been diagnosed was associated with 38% increased mortality risk and 45% increased risk of hospital readmission.[82]

E-cigarettes and vaping have been proposed as a way to ease the transition to quitting smoking and could thus be helpful to prevent CVD, including HF. However, they can pose a health risk to the user for several reasons, including a higher risk of CVDs in dual users of e-cigarettes plus combustible cigarettes, compared with smoking alone.[83,84]

The increasing use of waterpipe (Hookah/Shisha/Hubble bubble) is worrying, because this form of smoking exposes smokers to significantly higher levels of constituents of cigarette smoke, along with several toxic and hazardous materials, many of which are known to be harmful to CV health.[85,86]

Cocaine

Cocaine remains the second most commonly used illicit drug in Europe overall, after cannabis, according to the latest European Monitoring Centre for Drugs and Drug Addiction (EMCDDA) report.

It is estimated to be used by around 13 million Europeans at least once in their lifetime (3.9% of adults aged 15–64 years).[87] Cocaine enhances monoamine neurotransmitter activity in the central and peripheral nervous systems, blocking the reuptake of dopamine, noradrenaline, and serotonin, and modulates endogenous opioid receptors, giving rise to a sensation of increased energy, alertness, euphoria, and reduced tiredness.[88] Studies have consistently reported the wide-reaching effects of cocaine on the heart and blood vessels. The use of cocaine causes sympathetic-mediated CV complications, including coronary and peripheral vasoconstriction, tachyarrhythmias, increased myocardial oxygen consumption, and hypertension. Cocaine also induces a pro-inflammatory and prothrombotic state by activating mast cells, platelets, and the coagulation cascade. Moreover, it causes direct damage to endothelial cells (by blocking nitric oxide synthase and promoting endothelin-1 release), vascular smooth muscle cells (by impairing acetylcholine-induced vasorelaxation and intracellular calcium handling), and cardiomyocytes (by directly blocking sodium, potassium, and calcium channels, with direct negative inotropic and proarrhythmic effects). As such, cocaine promotes even early-onset atherosclerosis, as well as cystic medial necrosis, and a hypersensitivity reaction (enhanced by contaminants such as amphetamine, sugars, and talc) that may further aggravate CV damage. All these multifactorial mechanisms cause acute coronary syndromes and early-onset atherosclerosis, but also non-ischaemic complications such as takotsubo cardiomyopathy, myocarditis, cardiac hypertrophy, dilated cardiomyopathy, arrhythmias, endocarditis, hypertensive crises, aortic dissection or rupture, ischaemic and haemorrhagic stroke, pulmonary hypertension, and vasculitis.[88] Twenty-five per cent of cases of MI occurring in adults aged 18–45 years are caused by cocaine abuse.[89] LV dysfunction has been reported in 4–18% of cocaine abusers with no evidence of HF symptoms and independently of CAD. Furthermore, several CV magnetic resonance studies have confirmed the presence of myocardial oedema in up to 47%, and fibrosis in up to 73%, of asymptomatic cocaine users.[90] ⟴ Figure 4.1.1 summarizes the pathophysiology and clinical manifestations of CV damages related to acute and chronic cocaine abuse.

Cardiotoxic and nutritional factors

Extensive evidence indicates that many toxic factors are associated with HF development, such as chloroquine, cobalt, clozapine, and catecholamines, but any list will likely be incomplete. It is worth mentioning here that several medicaments can also be associated with a true toxic cardiomyopathy, most notably anticancer drugs (see also below), antiretroviral agents, and thiazolidinedione antidiabetic drugs.[91] Furthermore, some substances prescribed for athletic performance enhancement (e.g. anabolic steroids) and weight loss (e.g. ephedra, amphetamine) are associated with LV dysfunction and sudden cardiac death.

Severe nutritional deficiencies, such as those occurring in eating disorders like anorexia nervosa, can also account for the development of cardiomyopathy.[92]

Chemotherapy

Trends in long-term survival of patients with cancer have considerably increased, thanks to aggressive anticancer treatment which, conversely, is associated with an increased risk of both short- and long-term adverse CV effects. Cardiotoxicity is a major adverse effect of some of these drugs and has an important impact on patients' survival and quality of life, independent of the oncologic process. Cardiotoxicity related to chemotherapy leads mainly to LV dysfunction. LV dysfunction and HF are known consequences associated with exposure to several chemotherapy agents. The classic description of cardiomyopathy related to chemotherapy stems from anthracyclines. With this class of drugs, the typically dose-related onset of cardiomyopathy can occur acutely (even during or shortly after treatment), subacutely (days or weeks after treatment), or chronically (months to years after treatment).

Newer agents, such as trastuzumab, appear to have a different pattern of cardiac dysfunction that is not necessarily dose-related and is supposedly due to alterations in myocardial signalling without apoptosis, which is often reversible. A newer class of chemotherapy drugs that target and inhibit vascular endothelial growth factor (VEGF) very frequently can result in severe hypertension. Commonly, this occurs before the development of cardiomyopathy and diastolic HF may be an early clinical manifestation. Also small molecules with anti-vascular endothelial

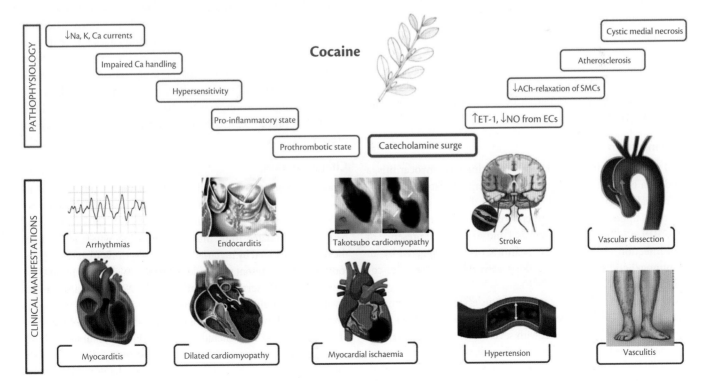

Figure 4.1.1 A summary of the pathophysiology and clinical manifestations of cardiovascular involvement in acute and chronic cocaine abuse.

growth factor activity (tyrosine kinase inhibitors) can induce LV dysfunction.[93] Moreover, immune checkpoint inhibitors, a newer class of anticancer agents, have been associated with cardiotoxicity mainly in the form of myocarditis and HF.

Regular exercise training has been associated with protective effects in the prevention of LV dysfunction in breast cancer patients, but the use of CV drugs for cardioprotection in oncological patients has not been recommended so far.[94] Baseline risk stratification and regular clinical, imaging, and laboratory follow-up are highly required to facilitate prevention and early detection of HF, with the aim of CV optimization, proper design of anticancer regimens, and monitoring of side effects. A baseline risk stratification tool has been proposed by the Heart Failure Association (HFA) of the ESC.[95]

Radiotherapy

Hodgkin's lymphoma and cancers of the lung, oesophagus, and breast often require radiation therapy to the breast area. A high dose of radiation on a large volume of heart muscle carries a great risk of cardiotoxicity. Marked interstitial myocardial fibrosis is quite common in radiotherapy-induced cardiotoxicity, with lesions of variable volumes and distribution. Studies found a relative risk of fatal CV events of between 2.2 and 12.7 in survivors of Hodgkin's lymphoma, and between 1.0 and 2.2 in patients with breast cancer. The risk of HF among survivors was increased 4.9-fold.[96,97] Systolic dysfunction is generally observed when patients are treated with radiotherapy combined with anthracyclines. A restrictive haemodynamic pattern can occur in the absence of prior treatment with an anthracycline; on a microscopic level, collagen synthesis not only increases as a whole, but the proportion of type I collagen increases proportionally to type III. This significant alteration in collagen synthesis may contribute to impaired diastolic distensibility of the ventricles seen in this group of patients.[98] Patients with myocardial involvement often have interstitial fibrosis. Loss of myocardium results in renin–angiotensin–aldosterone system- and adrenergic system-driven myocardial remodelling, which is progressive and results in end-stage symptoms.[99]

Alteration in the radiotherapy field or targeted radiation, with avoidance and/or shielding of the heart, remains a fundamental issue in prevention of radiation-induced cardiac damage and eventually HF.[100]

Viral infection

Viral infection may lead to HF by provoking viral myocarditis, a condition brought about by an excessive inflammatory response upon viral infection of the heart. Among the most common are common upper respiratory tract viruses, enteroviruses, parvovirus B19, and human herpesvirus 4 and 6. With the presence of viral infection in the heart, myocarditis may be triggered by an immunogenetic susceptibility, along with other factors, e.g. co-infection with other viruses.[101]

Other systemic conditions, such as lupus erythematosus, muscle disease, and HIV, can involve viral myocarditis. Its clinical presentation may vary from acute, with severe haemodynamic failure, such as in acute fulminant cases, to subacute, with a better tolerated status. Prognosis therefore can vary from spontaneous complete resolution to, in up to 20% of cases, the development of severe HF.

Yearly follow-up of cardiac function and symptoms for 4 years at least after viral myocarditis is essential in order to prevent HF recurrences.[102] Also endomyocardial biopsies are recommended in the event of recurrent myocarditis, persistent or progressive systolic dysfunction, or suspicion of possible underlying (auto) immune problems.[101,103] In those cases with persistent immune activation and in cases of autoimmune disease, identified by an increase in cytotoxic T-cells quantified from endomyocardial biopsies, HF may be prevented through immunosuppressive therapy.[104] In cases of high cardiac copy numbers and active viral replication, antiviral therapy may help to decrease the viral presence and, as such, might prevent HF development.[104] Given the high prevalence of circulating immunoglobulin G (IgG) antibodies to cardiotrophic viruses in the absence of viral myocarditis, viral serology is not useful.

Direct data on the incidence of *de novo* HF and influenza vaccination in the general population are unavailable as yet. In contrast, influenza vaccination has been proven to reduce the risk of CV events (including HF hospitalizations) in some populations, but there is no direct evidence of influenza-triggered myocarditis.[105,106]

Management is based on both preventive strategies and curative modalities for clinically evident viral disease (➲ Figure 4.1.2).

In recent times, coronavirus disease 2019 (Covid-19) has been shown to be a possible cause of HF.[107] Myocardial injury has been observed in a relevant number of patients, 10–60% or more, depending on age and comorbidities. It may be consequent to non-specific mechanisms, such as fever and adrenergic activation, as well as mechanisms typically related to Covid-19, such as angiotensin II release and an uncontrolled inflammatory response also causing pneumonia and acute respiratory distress syndrome in many patients.[108] In most cases, typical histopathological signs of myocarditis have not been demonstrated as yet. Covid-19 infection of the myocardium has been shown to be most likely localized in interstitial cells or macrophages rather than in myocytes.[109] Although some abnormalities have been shown by cardiac imaging,[110] nevertheless the long-term consequences of Covid-19 on cardiac function have not been made fully clear. Hence it is of utmost importance that proper measures should be adopted to prevent Covid-19 from spreading, and hence also to prevent HF.[108]

Chagas disease

Chagas disease is a potentially life-threatening illness caused by the protozoan parasite *Trypanosoma cruzi*, transmitted by contact with infected faeces of haematophagous insects. Over five million people are estimated to be infected worldwide, which is 7.5 times the number affected by malaria.[111] Acute infections are often asymptomatic but can present with mild or atypical flu-like symptoms. The most serious long-term complication of the disease is Chagas cardiomyopathy, occurring in up to 30% of infected patients up to 20 years after the initial infection. Signs and symptoms of the chronic phase of Chagas disease may include: HFrEF, conduction abnormalities, arrhythmias, thromboembolic phenomena, precordial chest pain, and sudden death. The main underlying mechanisms are cardiac dysautonomia, microvascular disturbances, parasite-dependent

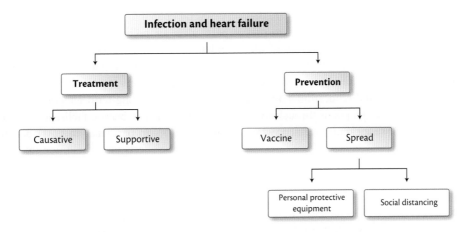

Figure 4.1.2 Viral infections: preventive strategies and treatment.

myocardial damage, and immune-mediated myocardial injury. Myocarditis is key and parallels HF development.[112]

The best approach to preventing Chagas disease-related HF is prevention of the disease itself. Although Chagas disease has usually been confined to endemic rural areas in Latin America, migration movements have caused urbanization of the disease, followed by its spread to other continents. Currently, Chagas disease is not only a major cause of death in endemic countries, but also an important cause of morbidity and mortality among immigrant populations in non-endemic countries such as the United States, Spain, and other European countries.

Control strategies, including early detection—by either serological or PCR testing—of *T. cruzi* infection and treatment of new cases, are essential. Currently, Chagas disease caused by *T. cruzi* is treated with only two drugs—nifurtimox and benznidazole, but their efficacy in preventing specifically HF has not been proven. In patients older than 50 years, or those with cardiomyopathy already present, treatment will not cure the cardiomyopathy or reduce mortality. The role played by concomitant comorbidities or genetics in the clinical progression from asymptomatic status to overt HF is unknown. Infected patients with no initial cardiac manifestations should undergo yearly follow-up to assess for cardiac symptoms and electrocardiogram (ECG) abnormalities; abnormal findings should prompt cardiac workup, including echocardiography and ECG monitoring. Since the ECG is normal in about 10% of patients with LV abnormalities, echocardiography to detect LV abnormalities is a better choice.[113]

Rheumatic heart disease

Acute rheumatic fever (ARF), commonly called rheumatic fever, is a reaction of the body's immune system to an untreated infection with group A streptococcal bacteria (Strep A) that commonly cause throat infection and some skin infections.[114] Severe or recurrent episodes of ARF can lead to rheumatic heart disease (RHD), which can involve permanent heart valve damage, with complications including HF, stroke, arrhythmias, and premature death.[115] To date, RHD affects approximately 40 million people, almost all in low- and middle-income countries, causing more than 300,000 deaths each year.[116]

Nevertheless, there are many opportunities to intervene and reduce incident disease, as the causal pathway of RHD is quite protracted. There are some specific prevention strategies for RHD. First, strategies must act on the indirect causes of the disease, with primary, secondary, and tertiary prevention addressing the direct biomedical causes.

Transmission of Strep A typically occurs through large airborne droplets and skin-to-skin contact.[117] It follows that some settings may influence the risk of Strep A infection—in particular, households which provide an extended duration of exposure to individuals with Strep A is associated with an increased risk of transmission and infection. Action must be taken to address the environmental and socio-economic causes of Strep A infections leading to ARF and RHD, in particular reducing household crowding and improving hygiene infrastructure.

Primary prevention of ARF, and subsequent RHD, involves identification of Strep A infections and delivery of appropriate antibiotic treatment. Prompt treatment with oral penicillin is reported to reduce the attack rate of ARF following Strep A pharyngitis by approximately 70%, increasing to 80% if a single intramuscular injection of benzathine benzylpenicillin (BPG) is given.[118]

Secondary prevention is the strategy with the best-proven efficacy and cost-effectiveness. This comprises regular antibiotic prophylaxis to prevent further streptococcal infections, and hence ARF recurrences, among individuals who have had ARF or live with RHD. Administration of intramuscular injections of BPG at appropriate 3- or 4-week intervals remains the mainstay of disease-altering therapy for RHD since the drug's development in the 1950s. Receiving more than 80% of scheduled injections appears to prevent Strep A infections and be protective against recurrent episodes of ARF,[116] which, in turn, leads to better clinical outcomes, including reduced overall mortality.[119,120,121,122,123] Hence, early and accurate diagnosis of ARF is a critical opportunity to prevent RHD because it allows for disease-altering secondary prophylaxis to be initiated as soon as possible. Similarly, early diagnosis of RHD is important as secondary prophylaxis can be started as soon as possible to help prevent the progression of valve disease and heart damage, allowing regression or even complete resolution of RHD.

People living with RHD require access to appropriate care that is safe and effective, and affordable essential medicines to prevent complications and ensure the best possible quality of life. Tertiary care aims to prevent premature death and reduce the level of disability inflicted by RHD. This is done by monitoring of valve function through clinical review and echocardiography, as well as by managing and treating RHD symptoms through therapies such as advanced medical and surgical management when appropriate.[124,125]

Sleep apnoea

Patients with overt HF show a high prevalence of periodic breathing (PB) and Cheyne–Stokes respiration (CSR) with alternating central apnoea (CA) and hyperpnoea, not only during sleep (central sleep apnoea (CSA)), but also in daytime in awake patients.[130,131] Severe CA is associated with increased mortality.[129,130,131] HF affects control of breathing and thereby predisposes to CSA. Thus, CA can be considered more a consequence of HF than a cause. CA is triggered by increased isolated or combined peripheral and central chemosensitivity (increased controller gain), increased lung-to-chemoreceptor circulatory delay, and reduced damping of blood gas levels (increased plant gain).[132] On the other hand, obstructive sleep apnoea (OSA) and hypopnoea result from complete or partial repetitive collapse of the upper airways during sleep and are associated with increased breathing effort, reduced oxygen saturation, increased arterial carbon dioxide, LV afterload and wall tension, and myocardial oxygen needs, alterations in autonomic nervous tone, and arousal from sleep.[133]

In patients with asymptomatic LV dysfunction, there is a high prevalence of CSA where the severity of CSA may not be related to the severity of haemodynamic impairment.[134] Severe CSA is associated with impaired cardiac autonomic control and increased cardiac arrhythmias.[134] The risk of progression to overt HF or sudden death for patients with asymptomatic dysfunction is quite high, particularly in the setting of ischaemic cardiomyopathy.

On the other hand, a Danish nationwide database, covering the entire Danish population (including 4.9 million individuals, average age of 53.4 years), established that OSA is associated with an increased risk of incident HF in patients of all ages. Moreover, another large study, including a total of 1927 men and 2495 women, with an average age of 40 years and free of CAD and HF at the time of baseline polysomnography over a median follow-up period of 9 years, showed an increased risk of incident HF in community-dwelling middle-aged and older men with OSA.[135] Continuous positive airway pressure (CPAP) therapy was associated with a lower risk of incident HF in elderly patients, especially those aged over 60 years.[136]

Environmental and air pollution

Experimental and epidemiological studies in the recent decade have investigated the health effects of exposure to environmental risk factors, particularly ambient air pollution.[137] More than 20% of all CV deaths are caused by air pollution, according to the World Health Organization (WHO),[137] while the Global Burden of Disease Study ranked ambient air pollution ninth among modifiable risk factors.[138]

Several epidemiological studies suggest that exposure to fine particulate air pollution can lead to oxidative stress, systemic inflammation, and vasoconstriction, which may increase blood pressure and result in atherosclerosis, ultimately increasing the risk of adverse effects of CVD.[139,140]

The impact of long-term air pollution on CV mortality and hospitalization has been established in epidemiological cohort studies,[141,142,143] in particular in CAD patients.[144] Although evidence for the effects of air pollution on the development of HF is less clear, a systematic review and meta-analysis[145] on the association between acute exposure to air pollution and HF showed that increased concentrations of gaseous components and particulate matter were associated with HF hospitalization or death. The percentage risk increase for carbon monoxide was 3.52 (95% CI 2.52–4.54) per 1 part per million (ppm); for sulfur dioxide 2.36 (95% CI 1.35–3.38) per 10 parts per billion (ppb); for nitrogen dioxide 1.70 (95% CI 125–2.16) per 10 ppb; for ozone 0.46 (95% CI 0.10–1.02) per 10 ppb; for $PM_{2.5}$ 2.12 (95% CI 1.42–2.82) per 10 $\mu g/m^3$; and for PM_{10} 1.63 (95% CI 1.20–2.07) per 10 $\mu g/m^3$.

There is growing evidence for a dose–response relationship between long-term exposure to ambient air pollution and HF. One epidemiological cohort study in the United Kingdom found that the HRs of HF for a 10 $\mu g/m^3$ increase in $PM_{2.5}$, PM_{10}, $PM_{2.5-10}$, nitrogen dioxide, and nitrogen oxides were 1.85 (95% CI 1.34–2.55), 1.61 (95% CI 1.30–2.00), 1.13 (95% CI 0.80–1.59), 1.10 (95% CI 1.04–1.15), and 1.04 (95% CI 1.02–1.06), respectively.[146] The Ontario Population Health and Environment Cohort (ONPHEC) study on the roles of different pollutants in the development and progression of chronic diseases reported that the HRs of incident HF responding with every interquartile range increase in exposure were 1.05 (95% CI 1.04–1.05) for $PM_{2.5}$, 1.02 (95% CI 1.01–1.04) for nitrogen dioxide, 1.03 (95% CI 1.02–1.03) for ozone (O_3), and 1.02 (95% CI 1.02–1.03) for oxides, respectively.[147] A separate study within ONPHEC reported that the HR for each interquartile-range increase in ultrafine particle matter exposure was 1.03 (95% CI 1.02–1.05) and exposure to nitrogen dioxide was also independently associated with a higher risk of HF incidence (HR for each increase in interquartile range 1.04, 95% CI 1.03–1.06).[148]

Sex-based predispositions

The overall lifetime risk of HF is comparable between the sexes. However, there are notable sex differences in the landscape of this condition (➡ Figure 4.1.3).[149] Men are predisposed to HFrEF, whereas HFpEF is more prevalent among women (for individuals aged ≥80 years, HFpEF prevalence is 4–6% among men and 8–10% among women).

Sex differences are also influenced by how 'traditional' risk factors confer risk between the sexes; for example, T2DM, obesity, hypertension, and tobacco smoking are stronger risk factors in women.

Other sex-specific clinical conditions predispose to HF in women. Peripartum cardiomyopathy is a potentially life-threatening condition which occurs in the last month of pregnancy or in the months following delivery in women without other known causes of HF, and affects 1:1000 pregnancies. Several factors may contribute, including environmental factors (e.g. infections), pregnancy-associated conditions such as pre-eclampsia,

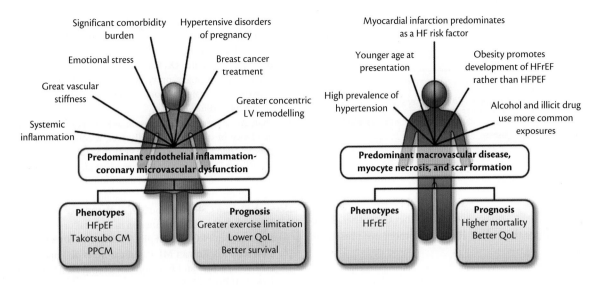

Figure 4.1.3 Sex differences in heart failure.
Reproduced Lam CSP, Arnott C, Beale AL, *et al.* Sex differences in heart failure. *Eur Heart J.* 2019 Dec 14;40(47):3859–3868c. doi: 10.1093/eurheartj/ehz835 with permission from Oxford University Press.

mode of delivery, and genetic predisposition. Furthermore, breast cancer is the most common cancer in women and shares common risk factors with CVD, including age, obesity, and tobacco use. A stable to increasing incidence, coupled with a decrease in mortality, has resulted in a growing population of survivors at risk of cardiotoxicity from systemic anticancer therapies (anthracyclines, radiation, trastuzumab, and endocrine therapy). In epidemiological studies of breast cancer survivors, late CV mortality exceeds oncological mortality.

Future directions

HF is a major and growing public health problem worldwide and its prevention is a key issue in modern medicine. There is undeniable evidence for the efficacy of therapies and the role of a healthy lifestyle. Nevertheless, the gap between recommendations and their clinical implementation is rising. Along with uncontrolled risk factors (including diabetes and obesity), there are other increasingly important behavioural risk indicators related to the pervasive aspects of economic development, rapid urbanization, and twenty-first-century lifestyles (in particular, concerning unhealthy diet habits, malnutrition, alcohol consumption, smoking, drug abuse, stress, and pollution). This unmet need is particularly evident in the less fortunate sections of the population. The central role of scientific communities, among which are the ESC and its associations (HFA and the European Association of Preventive Cardiology (EAPC)) is to spread the message of the importance of the culture of prevention.

Summary and key messages

Overall, modifiable risk factors play an important role and reducing these risk factors is crucial to the prevention of HF. Comorbidities are also important contributors to the HF epidemic. A summary list of the risk factors and comorbidities promoting the development of HF, as well as potential interventions, is provided in ⊃ Table 4.1.6. It should be emphasized, however, that the preventive potential of optimal management of comorbidities, in terms of lowering the incidence of HF, is less

Table 4.1.6 Risk factors and comorbidities promoting the development of heart failure, and potential interventions

Risk factor	Potential interventions
Arterial hypertension	Healthy lifestyle*, antihypertensive medications (mainly diuretics and ACEIs/ARBs)
Diabetes mellitus	Healthy lifestyle*, SGLT2 inhibitors
Sedentary habits	Regular physical activity*
Dyslipidaemia	Healthy diet, statins or other lipid-lowering drugs
Obesity	Healthy diet*, bariatric surgery
Endocrine disorders	Early diagnosis, specific therapy for treatment
Alcohol intake/abuse	General population: no or light alcohol intake. Patients with toxic cardiomyopathy: complete abstention
Smoking	No exposure in any form, nicotine replacement therapy
Cocaine	Supervised detoxification and medical treatment
Cardiotoxic drugs (e.g. anabolic steroids, anorectics)	Supervised cessation
Chemotherapy	Dose optimization, monitoring of side effects
Chest radiation	Dose and localization optimization
Viral infections	Influenza vaccination, early diagnosis
Microbial infection (e.g. Chagas disease, rheumatic heart disease)	Early diagnosis, specific antimicrobial therapy for either prevention or/and treatment
Sleep apnoea	CPAP therapy for individuals aged >60 years with an obstructive form
Environmental and air pollution	Measures to reduce or prevent pollution
Hypertensive disorders in pregnancy	Early diagnosis, specific therapy for treatment

* Refer to Tables 4.3.1 and 4.3.2.

ACEI, angiotensin-converting enzyme inhibitor; ARB, angiotensin receptor blocker, SGLT2, sodium–glucose cotransporter 2; CPAP, continuous positive airway pressure.
Modified from references 61 and 62.

Table 4.1.7 Drugs reducing the risk of heart failure development or hospitalization

Drugs/interventions	Comments
Diuretics	In patients with hypertension
ACEI/ARB	In patients with hypertension
Statins	In patients at high risk of cardiovascular disease
SGLT2 inhibitors	In patients with DM at high risk of cardiovascular disease

straightforward. Finally, pharmacological therapies that have been shown to reduce the risk of HF development are presented (◑ Table 4.1.7).

Note

This chapter is reproduced from Piepoli MF, Adamo M, Barison A, et al. Preventing heart failure: a position paper of the Heart Failure Association in collaboration with the European Association of Preventive Cardiology. *Eur J Prev Cardiol.* 2022 Feb 19;29(1):275–300. doi: 10.1093/eurjpc/zwab147 (C) European Society of Cardiology by permission of Oxford University Press.

References

1. Groenewegen A, Rutten FH, Mosterd A, Hoes AW. Epidemiology of heart failure. Eur J Heart Fail. 2020;22(8):1342–56.
2. Uijl A, Koudstaal S, Direk K, et al. Risk factors for incident heart failure in age- and sex-specific strata: a population-based cohort using linked electronic health records. *Eur J Heart Fail.* 2019;21(10):1197–206.
3. Del Gobbo LC, Kalantarian S, Imamura F, et al. Contribution of major lifestyle risk factors for incident heart failure in older adults: the Cardiovascular Health Study. *JACC Heart Fail.* 2015;3(7):520–8.
4. Piepoli MF, Hoes AW, Agewall S, et al. 2016 European Guidelines on cardiovascular disease prevention in clinical practice. *Eur Heart J.* 2016;37(29):2315–81.
5. Mach F, Baigent C, Catapano AL, et al. 2019 ESC/EAS Guidelines for the management of dyslipidaemias: lipid modification to reduce cardiovascular risk. *Eur Heart J.* 2020;41(1):111–88.
6. Dunlay SM, Weston SA, Jacobsen SJ, Roger VL. Risk factors for heart failure: a population-based case-control study. *Am J Med.* 2009;122(11):1023–8.
7. Vasan RS, Beiser A, Seshadri S, et al. Residual lifetime risk for developing hypertension in middle-aged women and men: the Framingham Heart Study. *JAMA.* 2002;287(8):1003–10.
8. Levy D, Larson MG, Vasan RS, Kannel WB, Ho KK. The progression from hypertension to congestive heart failure. *JAMA.* 1996;275(20):1557–62.
9. Wilhelmsen L, Rosengren A, Eriksson H, Lappas G. Heart failure in the general population of men: morbidity, risk factors and prognosis. *J Intern Med.* 2001;249(3):253–61.
10. Avery CL, Loehr LR, Baggett C, et al. The population burden of heart failure attributable to modifiable risk factors: the ARIC (Atherosclerosis Risk in Communities) study. *J Am Coll Cardiol.* 2012;60(17):1640–6.
11. Sciarretta S, Palano F, Tocci G, Baldini R, Volpe M. Antihypertensive treatment and development of heart failure in hypertension:
a Bayesian network meta-analysis of studies in patients with hypertension and high cardiovascular risk. *Arch Intern Med.* 2011;171(5):384–94.
12. Bangalore S, Wild D, Parkar S, Kukin M, Messerli FH. Beta-blockers for primary prevention of heart failure in patients with hypertension insights from a meta-analysis. *J Am Coll Cardiol.* 2008;52(13):1062–72.
13. Shah A, Langenberg C, Rapsomaniki E, et al. Type 2 diabetes and incidence of cardiovascular diseases: a cohort study in 1.9 million people. *Diab Endocrinol.* 2015;3:(2):105–13.
14. McAllister DA, Read SH, Kerssens J, et al. Incidence of hospitalization for heart failure and case-fatality among 3.25 million people with and without diabetes mellitus. *Circulation.* 2018;138(24):2774–86.
15. Shah SJ, Lam CSP, Svedlund S, et al. Prevalence and correlates of coronary microvascular dysfunction in heart failure with preserved ejection fraction: PROMIS-HFpEF. *Eur Heart J.* 2018;39(37): 3439–50.
16. Devereux RB, Roman MJ, Paranicas M, et al. Impact of diabetes on cardiac structure and function: the Strong Heart Study. *Circulation.* 2000;101(19):2271–6.
17. Van Melle JP, Bot M, de Jonge P, de Boer RA, van Veldhuisen DJ, Whooley MA. Diabetes, glycemic control, and new-onset heart failure in patients with stable coronary artery disease: data from the heart and soul study. *Diabetes Care.* 2010;33(9):2084–9.
18. Rosano GM, Vitale C, Seferovic P. Heart failure in patients with diabetes mellitus. *Card Fail Rev.* 2017;3(1):52–5.
19. Gerstein HC, Miller ME, Byington RP, et al. Effects of intensive glucose lowering in type 2 diabetes. *N Engl J Med.* 2008;358(24):2545–59.
20. Komajda M, McMurray JJ, Beck-Nielsen H, et al. Heart failure events with rosiglitazone in type 2 diabetes: data from the RECORD clinical trial. *Eur Heart J.* 2010;31(7):824–31.
21. Zinman B, Wanner C, Lachin JM, et al.; EMPA-REG OUTCOME Investigators. Empagliflozin, cardiovascular outcomes, and mortality in type 2 diabetes. *N Engl J Med.* 2015;373(22):2117–28.
22. Neal B, Perkovic V, Mahaffey KW, et al.; CANVAS Program Collaborative Group. Canagliflozin and cardiovascular and renal events in type 2 diabetes. *N Engl J Med.* 2017;377(7):644–57.
23. Wiviott SD, Raz I, Bonaca MP, et al.; DECLARE–TIMI 58 Investigators. Dapagliflozin and cardiovascular outcomes in type 2 diabetes. *N Engl J Med.* 2019;380(4):347–57.
24. Cannon CP, Pratley R, Dagogo-Jack S, et al.; VERTIS CV Investigators. Cardiovascular outcomes with ertugliflozin in type 2 diabetes. *N Engl J Med.* 2020;383(15):1425–35.
25. Perkovic V, Jardine MJ, Neal B, et al.; CREDENCE Trial Investigators. Canagliflozin and renal outcomes in type 2 diabetes and nephropathy. *N Engl J Med.* 2019;380(24):2295–306.
26. Heerspink HJL, Stefánsson BV, Correa-Rotter R, et al.; DAPA-CKD Trial Committees and Investigators. Dapagliflozin in patients with chronic kidney disease. *N Engl J Med.* 2020;383(15):1436–46.
27. Zelniker TA, Wiviott SD, Raz I, et al.; TIMI Study Group. SGLT2 inhibitors for primary and secondary prevention of cardiovascular and renal outcomes in type 2 diabetes: a systematic review and meta-analysis of cardiovascular outcome trials. *Lancet.* 2019;393(10166):31–9.
28. Rydén L, Grant PJ, Anker SD, ESC Committee for Practice Guidelines (CPG), et al. ESC Guidelines on diabetes, pre-diabetes, and cardiovascular diseases developed in collaboration with the EASD: the Task Force on diabetes, pre-diabetes, and cardiovascular diseases of the European Society of Cardiology (ESC) and developed in collaboration with the European Association for the Study of Diabetes (EASD). *Eur Heart J.* 2020;41(2):255–323.
29. Seferović PM, Coats AJS, Ponikowski P, et al. European Society of Cardiology/Heart Failure Association position paper on the role and

safety of new glucose-lowering drugs in patients with heart failure. *Eur J Heart Fail.* 2020;22(2):196–213.

30. Seferović PM, Fragasso G, Petrie M, *et al.* Sodium-glucose co-transporter 2 inhibitors in heart failure: beyond glycaemic control. A position paper of the Heart Failure Association of the European Society of Cardiology. *Eur J Heart Fail.* 2020;22(9):1495–503.

31. Seferovic PM, Ponikowski P, Anker SD, *et al.* Clinical practice update on heart failure 2019: pharmacotherapy, procedures, devices and patient management. An expert consensus meeting report of the Heart Failure Association of the European Society of Cardiology. *Eur J Heart Fail.* 2019;21(10):1169–86.

32. Inzucchi SE, Zinman B, Fitchett D, *et al.* How does empagliflozin reduce cardiovascular mortality? Insights from a mediation analysis of the EMPA-REG OUTCOME Trial. *Diabetes Care.* 2018;41(2):356–63.

33. Green JB, Bethel MA, Armstrong PW, *et al.*; TECOS Study Group. Effect of sitagliptin on cardiovascular outcomes in type 2 diabetes. *N Engl J Med.* 2015;373(3):232–42.

34. McGuire DK, Alexander JH, Johansen OE, *et al.*; CARMELINA Investigators. Linagliptin effects on heart failure and related outcomes in individuals with type 2 diabetes mellitus at high cardiovascular and renal risk in CARMELINA. *Circulation.* 2019;139(3):351–61.

35. Zannad F, Cannon CP, Cushman WC, *et al.*; EXAMINE Investigators. Heart failure and mortality outcomes in patients with type 2 diabetes taking alogliptin versus placebo in EXAMINE: a multicentre, randomised, double-blind trial. *Lancet.* 2015;385(9982):2067–76.

36. Scirica BM, Braunwald E, Raz I, *et al.*; SAVOR-TIMI 53 Steering Committee and Investigators. Heart failure, saxagliptin, and diabetes mellitus: observations from the SAVOR-TIMI 53 randomized trial. *Circulation.* 2014;130(18):1579–88.

37. McMurray JJV, Ponikowski P, Bolli GB, *et al.*; VIVIDD Trial Committees and Investigators. Effects of vildagliptin on ventricular function in patients with type 2 diabetes mellitus and heart failure: a randomized placebo-controlled trial. *JACC Heart Fail.* 2018;6(1):8–17.

38. Pfeffer MA, Claggett B, Diaz R, *et al.*; ELIXA Investigators. Lixisenatide in patients with type 2 diabetes and acute coronary syndrome. *N Engl J Med.* 2015;373(23):2247–57.

39. Holman RR, Bethel MA, Mentz RJ, *et al.*; EXSCEL Study Group. Effects of once-weekly exenatide on cardiovascular outcomes in type 2 diabetes. *N Engl J Med.* 2017;377(13):1228–39.

40. Husain M, Birkenfeld AL, Donsmark M, *et al.*; for the PIONEER 6 Investigators. Oral semaglutide and cardiovascular outcomes in patients with type 2 diabetes. *N Engl J Med.* 2019;381(9):841–51.

41. Marso SP, Daniels GH, Brown-Frandsen K, *et al.*; LEADER Steering Committee; LEADER Trial Investigators. Liraglutide and cardiovascular outcomes in type 2 diabetes. *N Engl J Med.* 2016;375(4):311–22.

42. Hernandez AF, Green JB, Janmohamed S, *et al.*; Harmony Outcomes Committees and Investigators. Albiglutide and cardiovascular outcomes in patients with type 2 diabetes and cardiovascular disease (Harmony Outcomes): a double-blind, randomised placebo-controlled trial. *Lancet.* 2018;392(10157):1519–29.

43. Berl T, Hunsicker LG, Lewis JB, *et al.*; Irbesartan Diabetic Nephropathy Trial. Collaborative Study Group. Cardiovascular outcomes in the Irbesartan Diabetic Nephropathy Trial of patients with type 2 diabetes and overt nephropathy. *Ann Intern Med.* 2003;138(7):542–9.

44. Rawshani A, Rawshani A, Franzén S, *et al.* Risk factors, mortality, and cardiovascular outcomes in patients with type 2 diabetes. *N Engl J Med.* 2018;379(7):633–44.

45. Kosiborod M, Lam CSP, Kohsaka S, *et al.*; CVD-REAL Investigators and Study Group. Cardiovascular events associated with SGLT-2 inhibitors versus other glucose-lowering drugs: the CVD-REAL 2 study. *J Am Coll Cardiol.* 2018;71(23):2628–39.

46. Patorno E, Pawar A, Franklin JM, *et al.* Empagliflozin and the risk of heart failure hospitalization in routine clinical care. *Circulation.* 2019;139(25):2822–30.

47. Pandey A, Garg S, Khunger M, *et al.* Dose–response relationship between physical activity and risk of heart failure: a meta-analysis. *Circulation.* 2015;132(19):1786–94.

48. He J, Ogden LG, Bazzano LA, Vupputuri S, Loria C, Whelton PK. Risk factors for congestive heart failure in US men and women: NHANES I epidemiologic follow-up study. *Arch Intern Med.* 2001;161(7):996–1002.

49. Agha G, Loucks EB, Tinker LF, *et al.* Healthy lifestyle and decreasing risk of heart failure in women: the Women's Health Initiative observational study. *J Am Coll Cardiol.* 2014;64(17):1777–85.

50. Velagaleti RS, Massaro J, Vasan RS, Robins SJ, Kannel WB, Levy D. Relations of lipid concentrations to heart failure incidence: the Framingham Heart Study. *Circulation.* 2009;120(23):2345–51.

51. Ebong IA, Goff DC Jr, Rodriguez CJ, Chen H, Sibley CT, Bertoni AG. Association of lipids with incident heart failure among adults with and without diabetes mellitus: Multiethnic Study of Atherosclerosis. *Circ Heart Fail.* 2013;6(3):371–8.

52. Preiss D, Campbell RT, Murray HM, *et al.* The effect of statin therapy on heart failure events: a collaborative meta-analysis of unpublished data from major randomized trials. *Eur Heart J.* 2015;36(24):1536–46.

53. Kenchaiah S, Evans JC, Levy D, *et al.* Obesity and the risk of heart failure. *N Engl J Med.* 2002;347(5):305–13.

54. Chen X, Thunström E, Hansson P-O, *et al.* High prevalence of cardiac dysfunction or overt heart failure in 71-year-old men: a 21-year follow-up of 'The Study of men born in 1943'. *Eur J Prev Cardiol.* 2020;27(7):717–25.

55. Eaton CB, Pettinger M, Rossouw J, *et al.* Risk factors for incident hospitalized heart failure with preserved versus reduced ejection fraction in a multiracial cohort of postmenopausal women. *Circ Heart Fail.* 2016;9(10):e002883.

56. Alpert MA. Obesity cardiomyopathy: pathophysiology and evolution of the clinical syndrome. *Am J Med Sci.* 2001;321(4):225–36.

57. Marfella R, Di Filippo C, Portoghese M, *et al.* Myocardial lipid accumulation in patients with pressure-overloaded heart and metabolic syndrome. *J Lipid Res.* 2009;50(11):2314–23.

58. Aimo A, Castiglione V, Borrelli C, *et al.* Oxidative stress and inflammation in the evolution of heart failure: from pathophysiology to therapeutic strategies. *Eur J Prev Cardiol.* 2020;27(5):494–510.

59. Reddy YNV, Anantha-Narayanan M, Obokata M, *et al.* Hemodynamic effects of weight loss in obesity: a systematic review and meta-analysis. *JACC Heart Fail.* 2019;7(8):678–87.

60. Wang Y, Tuomilehto J, Jousilahti P, *et al.* Lifestyle factors in relation to heart failure among Finnish men and women. *Circ Heart Fail.* 2011;4(5):607–12.

61. Favuzzi AMR, Venuti A, Bruno C, *et al.* Hormonal deficiencies in heart failure with preserved ejection fraction: prevalence and impact on diastolic dysfunction: a pilot study. *Eur Rev Med Pharmacol Sci.* 2020;24(1):352–6.

62. Bielecka-Dabrowa A, Godoy B, Suzuki T, Banach M, von Haehling S. Subclinical hypothyroidism and the development of heart failure: an overview of risk and effects on cardiac function. *Clin Res Cardiol.* 2019;108(3):225–33.

63. Rhee SS, Pearce EN. Update: systemic diseases and the cardiovascular system (II). The endocrine system and the heart: a review. *Rev Esp Cardiol.* 2011;64(3):220–31.

64. Rodondi N, Newman AB, Vittinghoff E, *et al.* Subclinical hypothyroidism and the risk of heart failure, other cardiovascular events, and death. *Arch Intern Med.* 2005;165(21):2460–6.

65. Piano MR. Alcoholic cardiomyopathy: incidence, clinical characteristics, and pathophysiology. *Chest*. 2002;121(5):1638–50.

66. Guzzo-Merello G, Segovia J, Dominguez F, et al. Natural history and prognostic factors in alcoholic cardiomyopathy. *JACC Heart Fail*. 2015;3(1):78–86.

67. Larsson SC, Orsini N, Wolk A. Alcohol consumption and risk of heart failure: a dose–response meta-analysis of prospective studies. *Eur J Heart Fail*. 2015;17(4):367–73.

68. Stockwell T, Zhao J, Panwar S, Roemer A, Naimi T, Chikritzhs T. Do 'moderate' drinkers have reduced mortality risk? A systematic review and meta-analysis of alcohol consumption and all-cause mortality. *J Stud Alcohol Drugs*. 2016;77(2):185–98.

69. Wood AM, Kaptoge S, Butterworth AS, et al.; Emerging Risk Factors Collaboration/EPIC-CVD/UK Biobank Alcohol Study Group. Risk thresholds for alcohol consumption: combined analysis of individual-participant data for 599 912 current drinkers in 83 prospective studies. *Lancet*. 2018;391(10129):1513–23.

70. Ware JS, Amor-Salamanca A, Tayal U, et al. Genetic etiology for alcohol-induced cardiac toxicity. *J Am Coll Cardiol*. 2018;71(20):2293–302.

71. Pavan D, Nicolosi GL, Lestuzzi C, Burelli C, Zardo F, Zanuttini D. Normalization of variables of left ventricular function in patients with alcoholic cardiomyopathy after cessation of excessive alcohol intake: an echocardiographic study. *Eur Heart J*. 1987;8(5):535–40.

72. Golder C, Gaziano JM. Should people with heart failure avoid alcohol? An evidence review. *Nursing Times*. 2018;114;3:43–5.

73. Garwal SK, Chambless LE, Ballantyne CM, et al. Prediction of incident heart failure in general practice: the Atherosclerosis Risk in Communities (ARIC) Study. *Circ Heart Fail*. 2012;5(4):422–9.

74. Gopal DM, Kalogeropoulos AP, Georgiopoulou VV, et al. Cigarette smoking exposure and heart failure risk in older adults: the Health, Aging, and Body Composition Study. *Am Heart J*. 2012;164(2):236–42.

75. Kamimura D, Cain LR, Mentz RJ, et al. Cigarette smoking and incident heart failure: insights from the Jackson Heart Study. *Circulation*. 2018;137(24):2572–82.

76. Aune D, Schlesinger S, Norat T, Riboli E. Tobacco smoking and the risk of heart failure: a systematic review and meta-analysis of prospective studies. *Eur J Prev Cardiol*. 2019;26(3):279–88.

77. Ambrose JA, Barua SR. The pathophysiology of cigarette smoking and cardiovascular disease: an update. *J Am Coll Cardiol*. 2004;43(10):1731–7.

78. Nadruz W Jr, Claggett B, Gonçalves A, et al. Smoking and cardiac structure and function in the elderly: The ARIC Study (Atherosclerosis Risk in Communities). *Circ Cardiovasc Imaging*. 2016;9(9):e004950.

79. Moreira HT, Armstrong AC, Nwabuo CC, et al. Association of smoking and right ventricular function in middle age: CARDIA study. *Open Heart*. 2020;7(1):e001270.

80. Hendriks T, van Dijk R, Alsabaan NA, van der Harst P. Active tobacco smoking impairs cardiac systolic function. *Sci Rep*. 2020;10(1):6608.

81. Rosen BD, Saad MF, Shea S, et al. Hypertension and smoking are associated with reduced regional left ventricular function in asymptomatic: individuals the Multi-Ethnic Study of Atherosclerosis. *J Am Coll Cardiol*. 2006;47(6):1150–8.

82. Son YJ, Lee HJ. Association between persistent smoking after a diagnosis of heart failure and adverse health outcomes: a systematic review and meta-analysis. *Tob Induc Dis*. 2020;18:1–11.

83. Kim C-Y, Paek Y-J, Seo HG, et al. Dual use of electronic and conventional cigarettes is associated with higher cardiovascular risk factors in Korean men. *Sci Rep*. 2020;10(1):1–10.

84. Kavousi M, Pisinger C, Barthelemy JC, et al. Electronic cigarettes and health with special focus on cardiovascular effects: position paper of the European Association of Preventive Cardiology (EAPC). *Eur J Prev Cardiol*. 2021;28(14):1552–66.

85. Osei AD, Mirbolouk M, Orimoloye OA. The association between e-cigarette use and asthma among never combustible cigarette smokers: behavioral risk factor surveillance system (BRFSS) 2016 & 2017. *BMC Pulm Med*. 2019;19:180.

86. Rezk-Hanna M, Benowitz NL. Cardiovascular effects of hookah smoking: potential implications for cardiovascular risk. *Nicotine Tob Res*. 2019;21(9):1151–61.

87. European Monitoring Centre for Drugs and Drug Addiction. The state of the drugs problem in Europe. Luxembourg: Publications Office of the European Union; 2009.

88. Havakuk O, Rezkalla SH, Kloner RA. The cardiovascular effects of cocaine. *J Am Coll Cardiol*. 2017;70(1):101–13.

89. Qureshi AI, Suri MF, Guterman LR, Hopkins LN. Cocaine use and the likelihood of nonfatal myocardial infarction and stroke: data from the Third National Health and Nutrition Examination Survey. *Circulation*. 2001;103(4):502–6.

90. Aquaro GD, Gabutti A, Meini M, et al. Silent myocardial damage in cocaine addicts. *Heart*. 2011;97(24):2056–62.

91. Hantson P. Mechanisms of toxic cardiomyopathy. *Clin Toxicol (Phila)*. 2019;57(1):1–9.

92. Becker AE, Grinspoon SK, Klibanski A, Herzog DB. Eating disorders. *N Engl J Med*. 1999;340(14):1092–8.

93. Totzek M, Muncu RI, Mrotzek S, Schadendorf D, Rassaf T. Cardiovascular diseases in patients receiving small molecules with anti-vascular endothelial growth factor activity: a meta-analysis of approximately 29,000 cancer patients. *Eur J Prev Cardiol*. 2018;25(5):482–94.

94. Howden EJ, Bigaran A, Beaudry R, et al. Exercise as a diagnostic and therapeutic tool for the prevention of cardiovascular dysfunction in breast cancer patients. *Eur J Prev Cardiol*. 2019;26(3):305–15.

95. Lyon AR, Dent S, Stanway S, et al. Baseline cardiovascular risk assessment in cancer patients scheduled to receive cardiotoxic cancer therapies: a position statement and new risk assessment tools from the Cardio-Oncology Study Group of the Heart Failure Association of the European Society of Cardiology in collaboration with the International Cardio-Oncology Society. *Eur J Heart Fail*. 2020;22(11):1945–60.

96. Aleman BM, van den Belt-Dusebout AW, De Bruin ML, et al. Late cardiotoxicity after treatment for Hodgkin lymphoma. *Blood*. 2007;109(5):1878–86.

97. Hooning MJ, Botma A, Aleman BM, et al. Long-term risk of cardiovascular disease in 10-year survivors of breast cancer. *J Natl Cancer Inst*. 2007;99(5):365–75.

98. Chello M, Mastroroberto P, Romano R, Zofrea S, Bevacqua I, Marchese AR. Changes in the proportion of types I and III collagen in the left ventricular wall of patients with post-irradiative pericarditis. *Cardiovasc Surg*. 1996;4(2):222–6.

99. Veinot J. Pathology of radiation-induced heart disease: a surgical and autopsy study of 27 cases. *Hum Pathol*. 1996;27(8):766–73.

100. Menezes KM, Wang H, Hada M, Saganti PB. Radiation matters of the heart: a mini review. *Front Cardiovasc Med*. 2018;5:83.

101. Heymans S, Eriksson U, Lehtonen J, Cooper LT Jr. The quest for new approaches in myocarditis and inflammatory cardiomyopathy. *J Am Coll Cardiol*. 2016;68(21):2348–64.

102. Ammirati E, Frigerio M, Adler ED, et al. Management of acute myocarditis and chronic inflammatory cardiomyopathy: an expert consensus document. *Circ Heart Fail*. 2020;13(11):e007405.

103. Tschöpe C, Cooper LT, Torre-Amione G, Van Linthout S. Management of myocarditis-related cardiomyopathy in adults. *Circ Res*. 2019;124(11):1568–83.

104. Caforio AL, Pankuweit S, Arbustini E, *et al*.; European Society of Cardiology Working Group on Myocardial and Pericardial Diseases. Current state of knowledge on aetiology, diagnosis, management, and therapy of myocarditis: a position statement of the European Society of Cardiology Working Group on Myocardial and Pericardial Diseases. *Eur Heart J*. 2013;34(33):2636–48, 2648a–d.

105. Wu H-H, Chang Y-Y, Kuo S-C, Chen Y-T. Influenza vaccination and secondary prevention of cardiovascular disease among Taiwanese elders—a propensity score-matched follow-up study. *PLoS One*. 2019;14(7):e0219172.

106. Kadoglou NPE, Bracke F, Simmers T, Tsiodras S, Parissis J. Influenza infection and heart failure-vaccination may change heart failure prognosis? *Heart Fail Rev*. 2017;22(3):329–36.

107. Barison A, Aimo A, Castiglione V, *et al*. Cardiovascular disease and COVID-19: les liaisons dangereuses. *Eur J Prev Cardiol*. 2020;27(10):1017–25.

108. Zhang Y, Coats AJS, Zheng Z, *et al*. Management of heart failure patients with COVID-19: a joint position paper of the Chinese Heart Failure Association & National Heart Failure Committee and the Heart Failure Association of the European Society of Cardiology. *Eur J Heart Fail*. 2020;22(6):941–56.

109. Lindner D, Fitzek A, Bräuninger H, *et al*. Association of cardiac infection with SARS-CoV-2 in confirmed COVID-19 autopsy cases. *JAMA Cardiol*. 2020;5(11):1281–5.

110. Puntmann VO, Carerj ML, Wieters I, *et al*. Outcomes of cardiovascular magnetic resonance imaging in patients recently recovered from coronavirus disease 2019 (COVID-19). *JAMA Cardiol*. 2020;5(11):1265–73.

111. Bern C. Chagas' disease. *N Engl J Med*. 2015;373(5):456–66.

112. Marin-Neto JA, Cunha-Neto E, Maciel BC, Simões MV. Pathogenesis of chronic Chagas heart disease. *Circulation*. 2007;115(9): 1109–23.

113. Echeverría LE, Rojas LZ, Villamizar MC, *et al*. Echocardiographic parameters, speckle tracking, and brain natriuretic peptide levels as indicators of progression of indeterminate stage to Chagas cardiomyopathy. *Echocardiography*. 2020;37(3):429–38.

114. Carapetis JR, McDonald M, Wilson NJ. Acute rheumatic fever. *Lancet*. 2005;366(9480):155–68.

115. Carapetis JR, Steer AC, Mulholland EK, Weber M. The global burden of group A streptococcal diseases. *Lancet Infect Dis*. 2005;5(11):685–94.

116. GBD 2017 Disease and Injury Incidence and Prevalence Collaborators. Global, regional, and national incidence, prevalence, and years lived with disability for 354 diseases and injuries for 195 countries and territories, 1990–2017: a systematic analysis for the Global Burden of Disease Study 2017. *Lancet*. 2018;392(10159):1789–858.

117. Barth DD, Daw J, Xu R, *et al*. Modes of transmission and attack rates of group A Streptococcal infection: a protocol for a systematic review and meta-analysis. *Syst Rev*. 2021;10(1):90.

118. Robertson KA, Volmink JA, Mayosi BM. Antibiotics for the primary prevention of acute rheumatic fever: a meta-analysis. *BMC Cardiovasc Disord*. 2005;5(1):1–9.

119. Mota CC, Meira ZM, Graciano RN, Graciano FF, Araújo FD. Rheumatic fever prevention program: long-term evolution and outcomes. *Front Pediatr*. 2015;2:141.

120. Mirabel M, Tafflet M, Noël B, *et al*. Newly diagnosed rheumatic heart disease among indigenous populations in the Pacific. *Heart*. 2015;101(23):1901–6.

121. de Dassel JL, de Klerk N, Carapetis JR, Ralph AP. How many doses make a difference? An analysis of secondary prevention of rheumatic fever and rheumatic heart disease. *J Am Heart Assoc Cardiovasc Cerebrovasc Dis*. 2018;7(24):e010223.

122. Okello E, Longenecker CT, Beaton A, Kamya MR, Lwabi P. Rheumatic heart disease in Uganda: predictors of morbidity and mortality one year after presentation. *BMC Cardiovasc Disord*. 2017;17:20.

123. WHO Study Group on Rheumatic Fever and Rheumatic Heart Disease, World Health Organization. Rheumatic fever and rheumatic heart disease: report of a WHO Expert Consultation, Geneva, 20 October–1 November 2001. Technical report series; no. 923. Geneva: World Health Organization; 2001.

124. Carapetis JR, Beaton A, Cunningham MW, *et al*. Acute rheumatic fever and rheumatic heart disease. *Nat Rev Dis Primers*. 2016;2:15084.

125. Bowen A, Currie B, Katzenellenbogen J, *et al*. The 2020 Australian guideline for prevention, diagnosis and management of acute rheumatic fever and rheumatic heart disease. Darwin: Menzies School of Health Research; 2020.

130. Ponikowski P, Anker SD, Chua TP, *et al*. Oscillatory breathing patterns during wakefulness in patients with chronic heart failure: clinical implications and role of augmented peripheral chemosensitivity. *Circulation*. 1999;100(24):2418–24.

131. Emdin M, Mirizzi G, Giannoni A, *et al*. Prognostic significance of central apneas throughout a 24-hour period in patients with heart failure. *J Am Coll Cardiol*. 2017;70(11):1351–64.

132. Giannoni A, Morelli MS, Francis D. *Pathophysiology of central apneas in heart failure*. In: Emdin M, Giannoni A, Morelli MS, Francis D, eds. *The Breathless Heart: Apneas in Heart Failure*. Cham: Springer; 2016, pp. 91–124.

133. Bradley TD, Floras JS. Sleep apnea and heart failure: part I: obstructive sleep apnea. *Circulation*. 2003;107(12):1671–8.

134. Lanfranchi PA, Somers VK, Braghiroli A, Corra U, Eleuteri E, Giannuzzi P. Central sleep apnea in left ventricular dysfunction: prevalence and implications for arrhythmic risk. *Circulation*. 2003;107(5):727–32.

135. Gottlieb DJ, Yenokyan G, Newman AB, *et al*. Prospective study of obstructive sleep apnea and incident coronary heart disease and heart failure: the Sleep Heart Health Study. *Circulation*. 2010;122(4):352–60.

136. Holt A, Bjerre J, Zareini B, *et al*. Sleep apnea, the risk of developing heart failure, and potential benefits of continuous positive airway pressure (CPAP) therapy. *J Am Heart Assoc Cardiovasc Cerebrovasc Dis*. 2018;7(13):e008684.

137. World Health Organization. Ambient air pollution: a global assessment of exposure and burden of disease. Geneva, World Health Organization; 2016.

138. Cohen AJ, Brauer M, Burnett R, *et al*. Estimates and 25-year trends of the global burden of disease attributable to ambient air pollution: an analysis of data from the Global Burden of Diseases Study 2015. *Lancet*. 2017;389(10082):1907–18.

139. Yixing Du, Xiaohan Xu, Chu M, Guo Y, Wang J. Air particulate matter and cardiovascular disease: the epidemiological, biomedical and clinical evidence. *J Thorac Dis*. 2016;8(1):E8–19.

140. Pope CA 3rd, Dockery DW. Health effects of fine particulate air pollution: lines that connect. *J Air Waste Manag Assoc*. 2006;56(6):709–42.

141. Brook RD, Rajagopalan S, Pope CA 3rd, *et al*.; American Heart Association Council on Epidemiology and Prevention, Council on the Kidney in Cardiovascular Disease, and Council on

Nutrition, Physical Activity and Metabolism. Particulate matter air pollution and cardiovascular disease: an update to the scientific statement from the American Heart Association. *Circulation*. 2010;121(21):2331–78.

142. Hoek G, Brunekreef B, Goldbohm S, Fischer P, van den Brandt PA. Association between mortality and indicators of traffic-related air pollution in the Netherlands: a cohort study. *Lancet* 2002;360:1203–9.

143. Pope CA 3rd, Burnett RT, Thurston GD, *et al*. Cardiovascular mortality and long-term exposure to particulate air pollution: epidemiological evidence of general pathophysiological pathways of disease. *Circulation*. 2004;109(1):71–7.

144. Cohen G, Steinberg DM, Keinan-Boker L, *et al*. Preexisting coronary heart disease and susceptibility to long-term effects of traffic-related air pollution: a matched cohort analysis. *Eur J Prev Cardiol*. 2021;28(13):1475–86.

145. Shah AS, Langrish JP, Nair H, *et al*. Global association of air pollution and heart failure: a systematic review and meta-analysis. *Lancet*. 2013;382(9897):1039–48.

146. Wang M, Zhou T, Song Y, *et al*. Joint exposure to various ambient air pollutants and incident heart failure: a prospective analysis in UK Biobank. *Eur Heart J*. 2021;42(16):1582–91.

147. Bai L, Shin S, Burnett RT, *et al*. Exposure to ambient air pollution and the incidence of congestive heart failure and acute myocardial infarction: a population-based study of 5.1 million Canadian adults living in Ontario. *Environ Int*. 2019;132:105004.

148. Bai L, Weichenthal S, Kwong JC, *et al*. Associations of long-term exposure to ultrafine particles and nitrogen dioxide with increased incidence of congestive heart failure and acute myocardial infarction. *Am J Epidemiol*. 2019;188(1):151–9.

149. Lam CSP, Arnott C, Beale AL, *et al*. Sex differences in heart failure. *Eur Heart J*. 2019;40:3859–68c.

SECTION 5

Pathophysiology of heart failure

CHAPTER 5.1

Molecular and cellular mechanisms

Junjie Xiao, Thomas Thum, Gianluigi Condorelli, and Johannes Backs

Contents

Introduction

The last three decades have been characterized by three major developments. In the 1990s, we started to realize—partly through coincidental findings—that changes in gene expression are associated with heart failure.[1] In the 2000s, several molecular pathways and processes were identified and proven to be critical for heart function, but remained partly fragmented and disconnected from other pathways.[2] The last decade was characterized by a revolution in multi-omics technologies that has allowed us today to detect and integrate nearly any change in gene expression and to identify signatures of heart disease at several levels, such as the genome, epigenome, transcriptome, spliceosome, translatome, proteome, and metabolome.[3] Importantly, the genomic era has led to improved understanding of the genetic causes of heart failure, pointing out important players of processes that are critical for cardiac homeostasis and function.[4] For example, mutations in genes encoding sarcomeric or calcium (Ca^{2+}) handling proteins (e.g. *MYBPC, MYH7, TTN, RYR2*) lead to various forms of cardiomyopathies, thereby intuitively pointing to the relative importance of the functional role of the related processes. But mutations in genes encoding transcriptional and splicing regulators or proteins controlling chromatin architecture (e.g. *GATA4, RBM20, LMNA*) cause cardiomyopathies too. Importantly, we have started to identify shared pathways that are also affected by acquired causes of heart failure such as haemodynamic, neurohormonal, and metabolic stress. In this chapter, we will briefly summarize only some milestone discoveries that highlight the importance of selected biological processes and mediators, as it is impossible to review all the important work that today is at the basis of our understanding of cardiac biology and disease.

Excitation–contraction coupling

Excitation–contraction (EC) coupling is an essential process that links electrical excitation of the surface membrane to contraction of cardiac myocytes. Intracellular Ca^{2+} movements and concentration ($[Ca^{2+}]_I$) play a crucial role in contraction and relaxation of cardiac myocytes. In normal heart, the action potential of the surface membrane opens the voltage-gated L-type Ca^{2+} channels, leading to an influx of small amounts of Ca^{2+} (I_{Ca}) that then activates ryanodine receptors (RyRs) on the sarcoplasmic reticulum (SR) to release large amounts of Ca^{2+} into the cytosol, directly visualized as Ca^{2+} sparks. This Ca^{2+}-induced Ca^{2+} release is closely related to the dyadic structure space where the T-tubules and SR are located in close proximity. After contraction, Ca^{2+} must be removed from the cytosol to ensure effective relaxation of cardiac myocytes. This is predominantly regulated by SR Ca^{2+}-ATPase (SERCA), which recycles Ca^{2+} back to the SR, and to a lesser extent by the sodium–calcium exchanger (NCX) which pumps Ca^{2+} into the extracellular space.

In heart failure, changes in either structural or functional coupling contribute to altered cardiac contractility. The loss of T-tubules and L-type Ca^{2+} channels and/or altered coupling with RyRs is critically responsible for dyssynchrony of the systolic Ca^{2+} transient during heart failure.[5] During the early hypertrophy stage, when I_{Ca} is normal, the reduced ability of this current to trigger SR Ca^{2+} release contributes to progression of heart failure.[6] Upon cardiac stress, reduced expression of junctophilin-2 on the SR is involved in disrupting junctional membrane complexes between the sarcolemmal membrane and the SR.[7] In addition, downregulation and/or dysfunction of SERCA can occur during heart failure, causing blunted cardiac relaxation. Indeed, transgenic and gene knockout animal models showed that increasing the expressional level or function of SERCA increases Ca^{2+} transport and improves cardiac contractility during cardiac hypertrophy and heart failure, whereas downregulating the SERCA pump has detrimental effects.[8] Reduced SERCA expression or activity is related to altered expression or phosphorylation of phospholamban (PLB) and sarcolipin during heart failure;[9] these control systolic and diastolic $[Ca^{2+}]_i$, and both are important for maintaining EC coupling and cardiac contractility, a fact that can be exploited for the treatment of heart failure.

Sarcomere function

The sarcomere is the basic unit of contraction of striated muscle. Delimited by the Z-lines, it is mainly formed from actin and myosin filaments: the thinner actin filaments are bound directly to the Z-line, whereas the thicker myosin filaments are connected to the Z-line by the elastic, elongated protein titin. In the heart, tropomyosin and three major types of cardiac troponin (TnC, TnT, and TnI) are bound to actin.

During diastole, the binding sites between the actin filaments and the myosin heads are covered by tropomyosin. When $[Ca^{2+}]_i$ increases and activates TnC, TnI moves closer to TnC, reducing the interaction between TnI and actin, while the interaction between TnC and TnT is strengthened. These conformational changes of the cardiac troponin complex lead to repositioning of tropomyosin, exposing the binding sites between actin and the myosin heads. In turn, the myosin heads attach to the actin filaments to form cross-bridges, initiating sliding of actin and myosin relative to each other, and hence shortening the sarcomere.

Protein quality control (PQC) is important for the sarcomere. The process is effected by molecular chaperones, the calpain and ubiquitin–proteasomes systems, and the autophagy–lysosome pathway. Indeed, disturbance of PQC leads to structural and functional alterations of the sarcomere.[10] Hypertrophic cardiomyopathy (HCM) and dilated cardiomyopathy (DCM) are the most prevalent types of cardiomyopathy, and are closely related to mutations and the ensuing dysfunction of sarcomeric proteins. Among the sarcomeric genes, *MYBPC3*—which encodes cardiac myosin binding protein C—is the most frequently mutated gene in HCM. Usually, truncating mutations are responsible for the absence of the protein. Patients with homozygous mutations in *MYBPC3* usually have more severe clinical manifestations and are at high risk of sudden death, and preclinical studies have demonstrated that gene therapy targeting *MYBPC3* can prevent cardiac dysfunction and left ventricular hypertrophy in mice with HCM.[11] But apart from genetics-based therapy, contractile activators, such as the myosin activators omecamtiv mecarbil and danicamtiv (MYK-491), as well as the Ca^{2+} sensitizer and troponin activator AMG594, have been developed for the treatment of DCM and heart failure with reduced ejection fraction (HFrEF); moreover, the myosin inhibitors mavacamten, CK-274, and MYK-581 have been developed to treat HCM when hypercontractility is present. These small molecules, which act directly on the contractile apparatus, are emerging as promising tools to control cardiac contractility during heart failure.

Autophagy

Autophagy is an evolutionarily conserved catabolic process directed at the preservation of cellular homeostasis in response to stress. Indeed, post-mitotic cardiomyocytes require autophagic flux quality control mechanisms to prevent cell death and replacement with fibrotic material.[12] Autophagic protein turnover depends on lysosomes and can be divided into macro-autophagy, micro-autophagy, and chaperone-mediated autophagy. In macro-autophagy, big pieces of cytosolic material, including organelles, are packed into autophagosomes, which then fuse with lysosomes. After degradation, the material is released from the lysosomes for intracellular recycling. This process is essential for cardiomyocytes to adapt to stress. In micro-autophagy, small cytoplasmic pieces are directly invaginated into the lysosomal or late endosomal membrane. In chaperone-mediated autophagy, substrate proteins containing a specific pentapeptide sequence are recognized by cytosolic co-chaperones before they translocate into the lysosomal lumen. All three forms of autophagy result in the release of amino acids that can be used for protein synthesis or energy production.

Autophagy plays a fundamental role in regulating cardiomyocyte survival and cardiac function in normal and diseased conditions.[13] For example, cardiac-specific loss of autophagy induced by cardiac-specific deletion of *Atg5* in adult mice led to cardiac hypertrophy, left ventricular dilatation, and contractile dysfunction, highlighting the essential role of autophagy in cardiac homeostasis.[14] Similarly, exaggerated autophagy also leads to cardiac dysfunction. Of importance, histone deacetylases have been found to be required for the autophagic response in cardiomyocytes, pointing to a link between epigenetic processes and autophagy. Indeed, by suppressing autophagy, pan-histone deacetylase (HDAC) inhibition reduces the increase in ventricular mass in response to pressure overload.[15] FYCO1, which binds to LC3, another key player in autophagy, has also been found to be essential for adaptation to cardiac stress.[16] FYCO1 gain-of-function is sufficient to improve cardiac function in response to biomechanical stress, thereby establishing components of the autophagic machinery as potential therapeutic targets.

Cell–cell communication

Cellular heterogeneity is increasingly recognized and has become detectable by the emergence of single-cell sequencing technology.[17] In the heart, communication between myocytes and non-myocytes is essential for cardiac homeostasis, and several studies using new technologies have identified key mechanisms for short- and long-distance communication in heart disease. For instance, secretome analysis has led to the identification of PCSK6 as a cardiomyocyte-secreted factor that induces fibroblast activation and subsequent cardiac fibrosis.[18] Similarly, cardiomyocyte-derived chemokines released in a CaM kinase II-dependent manner attract inflammatory cells post-myocardial infarction to trigger myocardial scar formation and dysfunction.[19,20]

As well as secreting polypeptides and chemokines, cardiac cells can actively release extracellular vesicles and exosomes, which are small membrane-bound vesicles of endocytic origin. Exosomes can contain different types of components as cargo, such as non-coding (nc)RNAs, and can therefore transfer signalling information from one cell type to another or from one cell type to the same cell type. This phenomenon is being exploited for biomarker development and novel therapeutic applications in cardiovascular diseases.[21] For instance, exosomes enriched in cardiac fibroblast-derived microRNA passenger strands were shown to mediate cardiomyocyte hypertrophy; in particular, fibroblast exosomal-derived microRNA-21-3p was identified as a potent paracrine-acting RNA molecule that induces cardiomyocyte hypertrophy.[22] Thus, exosomes hold translational potential for targeted delivery of therapeutic agents to the heart.[23]

Signal transduction

Transduction of signals within cardiomyocytes and between different cardiac cells is essential for cardiac homeostasis; when perturbed, it can lead to heart dysfunction. Several adaptive and maladaptive signalling pathways have been described over the last three decades.[24] Many of them are induced by neurohormonal activation, but it is increasingly recognized that metabolic and inflammatory factors talk to cardiomyocytes too and can induce changes in cell morphology and function.[25,26] For instance, catecholamines, angiotensin II, and prostaglandins signal through G protein-coupled receptors to modulate, for example, EC coupling, sarcomere function, and gene expression (for more details, see below).[27, 28]

Signalling molecules are diverse and include: enzymes such as protein kinases/phosphatases, acetyltransferases/deacetylases, de-/ubiquitinases, and many others that are still emerging; metabolites that serve as second messengers or as substrates for post-translational modifications; and scaffold proteins that orchestrate microdomains and bring together important signalling mediators.[29,30,31,32] It is beyond the scope of this chapter to comprehensively summarize all the essential signalling mediators of cardiomyocyte homeostasis and dysfunction. Moreover, the hope that any of these mediators might reveal to be targetable for reversal of heart failure has unfortunately not been fulfilled yet. However, it is worthwhile speculating on the underlying reasons for this and to critically question the conclusions that have been made.

Although there is an overwhelming body of work that has led to proof-of-principle experiments showing that, for example,

protein kinase C, calcineurin, or CaM kinase II are required for heart failure sub-phenotypes,[33,34,35] inhibitors of these enzymes have yet not reached the clinical heart failure arena. Moreover, mouse models with gene deletions certainly do not mimic enzymatic inhibition accurately, so there may be many reasons for the full translational potential having not been reached yet: species differences between model systems and patients, compensation in chronic disease versus the more acute nature of model systems, neglected complexity and comorbidities in model systems, biased approaches, and reproducibility issues may all have contributed to this situation. Successful drug development programmes are also underrepresented because of a lack of assays and missed opportunities in precisely defining druggable signalling events. With regard to the latter, it is important to understand that many signalling transduction enzymes are multifunctional and have many targets, and that some may be adaptive, while others are maladaptive, depending on the situation. Besides careful consideration of the preclinical model, which can be more tailored or more complex, future signalling transduction research should more closely focus on signalling events instead of on entire functions of an enzyme. Of note, protein–protein interaction inhibitors have not been fully explored in cardiovascular medicine, so they might yet be found to more precisely target the causes of heart disease, as has been the case in oncology, for example.[36]

Transcription and translation

The morphological and functional phenotypes of the heart are governed by genes that are transcribed and translated into proteins. Thus, the mechanisms that control transcription and translation are key in homeostasis and disease. In fact, changes in gene expression are functionally more relevant to the control of cardiac function than previously assumed. Within days or weeks, gene misexpression can contribute to cardiac dysfunction by promoting cardiac remodelling, including cardiomyocyte hypertrophy and fibrosis; within hours or even minutes, misexpression can lead to dysregulation of Ca^{2+} handling and contractility.[37] Thus, transcription and translation factors, as well as the regulatory upstream mechanism, are potential targets for novel therapeutic strategies.

Twenty-five years ago, calcineurin signalling and dephosphorylation of nuclear factor of activated T cells (NFAT), resulting in nuclear accumulation of NFAT, were shown to drive cardiac hypertrophy.[38] Another landmark discovery was that the transcription factor myocyte enhancer factor 2 (MEF2) drives cardiac hypertrophy and dysfunction when unleashed from its repression by class IIa histone deacetylases.[39,40] The concept of 'reactivation of a fetal gene programme' dominated conceptual thinking two to three decades ago,[1,2] but today the emergence of unbiased multi-omics sequencing technologies has meant that the underlying target genes and related pathways can be described in more detail, down to the single-cell level.[3,17]

Several transcription factors and co-factors have been identified to regulate various aspects of cardiac function.[41] For example, nuclear receptors, including peroxisome proliferator-activated receptors (PPARs), control the selection of myocardial substrates for energy production, a phenomenon that is decisive for cardiac dysfunction.[42] Members of the nuclear receptor subfamily 4 group A, in particular Nr4A1, have emerged as critical regulators of cardiac function by promoting the production of glucose metabolites, in particular O-GlcNAc, which is used for post-translational modifications and thereby controls contractility of the heart.[37]

Changes in messenger RNA (mRNA) levels do not necessarily reflect changes in protein levels because translational efficacy depends on the activity of the translational machinery, which also underlies regulatory mechanisms and provides specificity. Recent advances in ribosomal profiling have also led to the identification of translational programmes at this layer of gene expression control.[43] A prominent regulator of translation is mTOR (mechanistic target of rapamycin) signalling, which, however, regulates both physiological and pathological growth at the level of translation in the heart.[44] A better understanding of the specific mechanisms involved in disease states might lead to new therapeutic approaches at this level of gene expression regulation.[45]

Taken together, transcriptional and translational factors, as well as upstream signals, are promising targets to regulate gene expression programmes that today can be detected by multi-omics technology. However, the mode of the druggable action needs to be narrowed down by mechanistic and biochemical studies.

Epigenetics and epitranscriptomics

The cells of all organs share the same DNA sequence but present with fundamentally different phenotypes. During cell differentiation, modifications of chromatin (epigenetics) and RNA (epitranscriptomics) lead to activation or inactivation of specific gene programmes, thereby defining the identities and functions of cell types. Chromatin is the combination of DNA and histones, the proteins around which the DNA is wound, and its opening and closing regulates transcription. Covalent modifications occur at the level of DNA and histones—for the former through methylation or demethylation, and for the latter through acetylation, methylation, and other post-translational modifications.[46]

The modifications are mediated by different classes of enzymes that have been studied over the last two decades, among which HDACs and methyltransferases have gained the most attention because of their signal responsiveness and their critical roles for cardiac growth.[39,46] Class IIa HDACs inhibit the transcription factor MEF2 via their non-enzymatic domains. Class I, IIb, and IV HDACs have higher deacetylase activity than class IIa. This activity, unlike the non-enzymatic function of class IIa HDACs, seems to damage the heart. Indeed, pan-HDAC inhibitors have been shown to be cardioprotective.[47] However, the cardio-detrimental substrates of pan-HDAC inhibitors have remained elusive. Nevertheless, over the last decade, a multitude of isoform-selective inhibitors have been developed and are now ready to be studied in different forms of heart failure, such as HFpEF in which pan-HDAC inhibitors have recently been reported to be effective in rodent and large animal models.[48,49] Identification of

the underlying isoforms therefore holds potential for future therapies for HFpEF.

Other research has demonstrated that the acetyl-lysine reader proteins, named BET family bromodomain proteins, drive cardiac fibrosis and hypertrophy.[50] Importantly, JQ1, a small-molecule inhibitor of BET family bromodomain proteins, has been shown to counteract cardiac hypertrophy and therefore represents a new modality to combat heart failure.

These examples highlight that we are only at the beginning of developing small-molecule inhibitors of epigenetic enzymes and readers for therapy of heart failure. Medicinal chemistry will be key to developing further isoform-selective inhibitors with optimized modes of action.

Reports are published on how epitranscriptomic modifications and the underlying enzymes affect gene expression.[51] N^6-methyladenosine (m6A) methylation is the most prevalent internal post-transcriptional modification on mammalian mRNA and is driven by the m6A RNA methylase methyltransferase-like 3 (METTL3). Remarkably, deletion of *Mettl3* abrogated the ability of cardiomyocytes to undergo hypertrophy when stimulated to grow, pointing to yet another layer of gene expression that is interesting as a target for treating heart failure.

Non-coding RNAs

Vast parts of the mammalian genome are actively transcribed, predominantly giving rise to ncRNA transcripts, such as microRNAs, long ncRNAs, and circular RNAs (circRNAs), among others,[52] all of which are today recognized as critical regulators of cardiac homeostasis and disease. MicroRNAs are short sequences of about only 20 nucleotides, and they mainly interact with the 3′-untranslated region of the mRNA they target, thereby inhibiting protein translation. They are involved in a multitude of cardiovascular processes in normal and disease conditions.[53] Long ncRNAs comprise a large group of extremely diverse molecules of >200 nucleotides in length; they regulate gene expression at the nuclear and cytoplasmic levels.[54] CircRNAs are covalently closed RNA rings formed through alternative back-splicing of protein-coding exons, and either regulate host gene expression or serve as scaffolds and molecular sponges.[55]

The history of ncRNAs in cardiac research is relatively young, but preclinical and clinical translation has already begun. Differential expression of microRNAs was reported for the first time only 15 years ago, and since then their essential role in cardiac homeostasis has been widely described.[56,57,58] To date, many ncRNAs have been identified to play adaptive and maladaptive roles in the heart and are suggested as promising targets to combat heart failure.[52] One prototypical example is inhibition of microRNA-132 via a synthetic locked nucleic acid antisense oligonucleotide inhibitor (anti-miR-132; CDR132L), which was effective in blunting post-myocardial infarction heart failure in pigs.[59] In a first-in-human phase 1b study, CDR132L was found to be safe and well tolerated.[60] Thus, additional clinical studies are awaited to confirm the beneficial pharmacodynamic effects of CDR132L in treatment of heart failure in patients.

It is exciting that within 15 years from the discovery of the functional relevance of ncRNAs for heart disease, translational developments are already under way in the form of clinical trials. Hopefully, these approaches will soon reach the clinical arena for routine treatment of heart failure.

Future directions

As outlined, we live in exciting times during which basic research has progressed to new translational concepts and clinical trials in a relatively short period of time. This is best exemplified by microRNA-132. Several other microRNA-based approaches will likely follow because the design of the actual therapeutic is based on the nucleotide sequence of microRNA itself. Other new therapeutic approaches require precise definition of the mode of action and development of the therapeutic modality. One example in this regard is mavacamten for the treatment of HCM. HDAC inhibitors also hold promise, for example in the treatment of HFpEF, as does targeting protein–protein interactions, which might be superior to inhibiting enzymatic functions of multifunctional enzymes. But despite the many conceptual breakthroughs, which we have been able to only partly summarize above, we are still only at the beginning of combining certain research directions. Today's challenge is to bring diverse research strategies together to identify the mechanisms of disease-causing 'ome' programmes and to precisely define the mode of action for drug development. Hopefully, the latter will take place in the next decade, moving us beyond the current pharmacological approaches.

In this chapter, we have highlighted the interconnection of many processes and mediators, a phenomenon that will be increasingly recognized by further integration of the multi-omics technology and artificial intelligence. One promising conceptual approach is to identify shared pathways that originate from inherited and acquired causes of heart failure, thereby potentially unmasking unifying themes in the regulation of cardiac function. In contrast, but requiring similar research strategies, are tailored approaches, which should be comprehensively tested in the future.

Today, we can define cardiomyopathies based on the mutated causative gene, rather than on the morphological or functional phenotype. For instance, RBM20- and lamin A-related cardiomyopathies both present with a DCM phenotype but may respond differently to the manipulation of, for example, a disease-causing splice event of RBM20. A better understanding of the pathogenesis of cardiomyopathies caused by gene mutations will move our field towards precision medicine and tailored therapies.

Summary and key messages

This chapter summarizes key molecular and cellular mechanisms leading to heart failure and provides an overview of selected translational programmes. Two key messages are: (1) different molecular and cellular mechanisms should not be viewed as disconnected processes, but should be integrated to discover unifying themes (➲ Figure 5.1.1); and (2) today's detailed understanding of the causes of heart failure should now be used to move to genotype-informed mechanistic research in order to enable

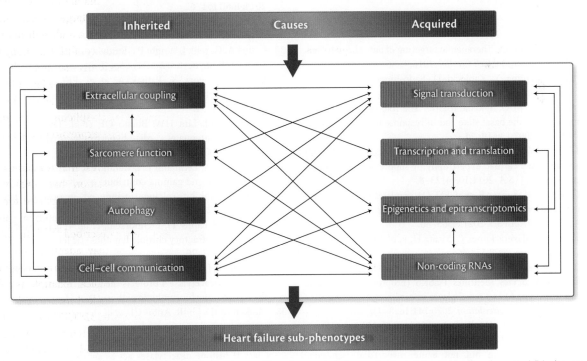

Figure 5.1.1 Cartoon highlighting the topics discussed in this chapter. The colour code indicates that both inherited (red) and acquired (blue) causes of heart failure result in shared processes (shown on the left) and use shared mediators (shown on the right) that eventually lead to heart failure sub-phenotypes such as cardiac remodelling, cardiac dysfunction, and arrhythmias. Several examples are highlighted, showing the interconnection of the processes and mediators and suggesting the existence of common mechanisms.

tailored therapies to be tested in smaller, but more focused, clinical trials in the future.

References

1. Kurabayashi M, Shibasaki Y, Komuro I, Tsuchimochi H, Yazaki Y. The myosin gene switching in human cardiac hypertrophy. *Jpn Circ J.* 1990;54:1192–205.

2. Frey N, Olson EN. Cardiac hypertrophy: the good, the bad, and the ugly. *Annu Rev Physiol.* 2003;65:45–79.

3. Rajewsky N, Almouzni G, Gorski SA, et al.; LifeTime Community Working Group. LifeTime and improving European healthcare through cell-based interceptive medicine. *Nature.* 2020;587:377–86.

4. Seferovic PM, Polovina M, Bauersachs J, et al. Heart failure in cardiomyopathies: a position paper from the Heart Failure Association of the European Society of Cardiology. *Eur J Heart Fail.* 2019;21:553–76.

5. Setterberg IE, Le C, Frisk M, Li J, Louch WE. The physiology and pathophysiology of T-tubules in the heart. *Front Physiol.* 2021;12:718404.

6. Gomez AM, Valdivia HH, Cheng H, et al. Defective excitation–contraction coupling in experimental cardiac hypertrophy and heart failure. *Science.* 1997;276:800–6.

7. van Oort RJ, Garbino A, Wang W, et al. Disrupted junctional membrane complexes and hyperactive ryanodine receptors after acute junctophilin knockdown in mice. *Circulation.* 2011;123:979–88.

8. Miyamoto MI, del Monte F, Schmidt U, et al. Adenoviral gene transfer of SERCA2a improves left-ventricular function in aortic-banded rats in transition to heart failure. *Proc Natl Acad Sci U S A.* 2000;97:793–8.

9. Periasamy M, Bhupathy P, Babu GJ. Regulation of sarcoplasmic reticulum Ca^{2+} ATPase pump expression and its relevance to cardiac muscle physiology and pathology. *Cardiovasc Res.* 2008;77:265–73.

10. Martin TG, Kirk JA. Under construction: the dynamic assembly, maintenance, and degradation of the cardiac sarcomere. *J Mol Cell Cardiol.* 2020;148:89–102.

11. Carrier L. Targeting the population for gene therapy with MYBPC3. *J Mol Cell Cardiol.* 2021;150:101–8.

12. Schiattarella GG, Hill JA. Therapeutic targeting of autophagy in cardiovascular disease. *J Mol Cell Cardiol.* 2016;95:86–93.

13. Sciarretta S, Maejima Y, Zablocki D, Sadoshima J. The role of autophagy in the heart. *Annu Rev Physiol.* 2018;80:1–26.

14. Nakai A, Yamaguchi O, Takeda T, et al. The role of autophagy in cardiomyocytes in the basal state and in response to hemodynamic stress. *Nat Med.* 2007;13:619–24.

15. Cao DJ, Wang ZV, Battiprolu PK, et al. Histone deacetylase (HDAC) inhibitors attenuate cardiac hypertrophy by suppressing autophagy. *Proc Natl Acad Sci U S A.* 2011;108:4123–8.

16. Kuhn C, Menke M, Senger F, et al. FYCO1 regulates cardiomyocyte autophagy and prevents heart failure due to pressure overload *in vivo. JACC Basic Transl Sci.* 2021;6:365–80.

17. Litvinukova M, Talavera-Lopez C, Maatz H, et al. Cells of the adult human heart. *Nature.* 2020;588:466–72.

18. Kuhn TC, Knobel J, Burkert-Rettenmaier S, et al. Secretome analysis of cardiomyocytes identifies PCSK6 (proprotein convertase subtilisin/kexin type 6) as a novel player in cardiac remodeling after myocardial infarction. *Circulation.* 2020;141:1628–44.

19. Weinreuter M, Kreusser MM, Beckendorf J, et al. CaM kinase II mediates maladaptive post-infarct remodeling and pro-inflammatory chemoattractant signaling but not acute myocardial ischemia/reperfusion injury. *EMBO Mol Med.* 2014;6:1231–45.

20. Suetomi T, Willeford A, Brand CS, et al. Inflammation and NLRP3 inflammasome activation initiated in response to pressure overload by Ca$^{(2+)}$/calmodulin-dependent protein kinase II delta signaling in cardiomyocytes are essential for adverse cardiac remodeling. *Circulation.* 2018;138:2530–44.

21. Sahoo S, Adamiak M, Mathiyalagan P, Kenneweg F, Kafert-Kasting S, Thum T. Therapeutic and diagnostic translation of extracellular vesicles in cardiovascular diseases: roadmap to the clinic. *Circulation.* 2021;143:1426–49.

22. Bang C, Batkai S, Dangwal S, et al. Cardiac fibroblast-derived microRNA passenger strand-enriched exosomes mediate cardiomyocyte hypertrophy. *J Clin Invest.* 2014;124:2136–46.

23. Sahoo S, Kariya T, Ishikawa K. Targeted delivery of therapeutic agents to the heart. *Nat Rev Cardiol.* 2021;18:389–99.

24. Maillet M, van Berlo JH, Molkentin JD. Molecular basis of physiological heart growth: fundamental concepts and new players. *Nat Rev Mol Cell Biol.* 2013;14:38–48.

25. Karlstaedt A, Zhang X, Vitrac H, et al. Oncometabolite d-2-hydroxyglutarate impairs alpha-ketoglutarate dehydrogenase and contractile function in rodent heart. *Proc Natl Acad Sci U S A.* 2016;113:10436–41.

26. Meijers WC, Maglione M, Bakker SJL, et al. Heart failure stimulates tumor growth by circulating factors. *Circulation.* 2018;138:678–91.

27. Pfleger J, Gresham K, Koch WJ. G protein-coupled receptor kinases as therapeutic targets in the heart. *Nat Rev Cardiol.* 2019;16:612–22.

28. Toth AD, Schell R, Levay M, et al. Inflammation leads through PGE/EP3 signaling to HDAC5/MEF2-dependent transcription in cardiac myocytes. *EMBO Mol Med.* 2018;10:e8536.

29. Dodge-Kafka K, Gildart M, Tokarski K, Kapiloff MS. mAKAPbeta signalosomes: a nodal regulator of gene transcription associated with pathological cardiac remodeling. *Cell Signal.* 2019;63:109357.

30. Lorenz K, Stathopoulou K, Schmid E, Eder P, Cuello F. Heart failure-specific changes in protein kinase signalling. *Pflugers Arch.* 2014;466:1151–62.

31. Li P, Ge J, Li H. Lysine acetyltransferases and lysine deacetylases as targets for cardiovascular disease. *Nat Rev Cardiol.* 2020;17:96–115.

32. Judina A, Gorelik J, Wright PT. Studying signal compartmentation in adult cardiomyocytes. *Biochem Soc Trans.* 2020;48:61–70.

33. Braz JC, Gregory K, Pathak A, et al. PKC-alpha regulates cardiac contractility and propensity toward heart failure. *Nat Med.* 2004;10:248–54.

34. De Windt LJ, Lim HW, Bueno OF, et al. Targeted inhibition of calcineurin attenuates cardiac hypertrophy *in vivo. Proc Natl Acad Sci U S A.* 2001;98:3322–7.

35. Kreusser MM, Lehmann LH, Keranov S, et al. Cardiac CaM kinase II genes delta and gamma contribute to adverse remodeling but redundantly inhibit calcineurin-induced myocardial hypertrophy. *Circulation.* 2014;130:1262–73.

36. Seymour JF, Kipps TJ, Eichhorst B, et al. Venetoclax–rituximab in relapsed or refractory chronic lymphocytic leukemia. *N Engl J Med.* 2018;378:1107–20.

37. Lehmann LH, Jebessa ZH, Kreusser MM, et al. A proteolytic fragment of histone deacetylase 4 protects the heart from failure by regulating the hexosamine biosynthetic pathway. *Nat Med.* 2018;24:62–72.

38. Molkentin JD, Lu JR, Antos CL, et al. A calcineurin-dependent transcriptional pathway for cardiac hypertrophy. *Cell.* 1998;93:215–28.

39. Zhang CL, McKinsey TA, Chang S, Antos CL, Hill JA, Olson EN. Class II histone deacetylases act as signal-responsive repressors of cardiac hypertrophy. *Cell.* 2002;110:479–88.

40. Kim Y, Phan D, van Rooij E, *et al*. The MEF2D transcription factor mediates stress-dependent cardiac remodeling in mice. *J Clin Invest*. 2008;118:124–32.

41. McKinsey TA, Olson EN. Toward transcriptional therapies for the failing heart: chemical screens to modulate genes. *J Clin Invest*. 2005;115:538–46.

42. Vega RB, Kelly DP. Cardiac nuclear receptors: architects of mitochondrial structure and function. *J Clin Invest*. 2017;127:1155–64.

43. Doroudgar S, Hofmann C, Boileau E, *et al*. Monitoring cell-type-specific gene expression using ribosome profiling in vivo during cardiac hemodynamic stress. *Circ Res*. 2019;125:431–48.

44. Sciarretta S, Forte M, Frati G, Sadoshima J. New insights into the role of mTOR signaling in the cardiovascular system. *Circ Res*. 2018;122:489–505.

45. Volkers M, Konstandin MH, Doroudgar S, *et al*. Mechanistic target of rapamycin complex 2 protects the heart from ischemic damage. *Circulation*. 2013;128:2132–44.

46. Papait R, Serio S, Condorelli G. Role of the epigenome in heart failure. *Physiol Rev*. 2020;100:1753–77.

47. Kong Y, Tannous P, Lu G, *et al*. Suppression of class I and II histone deacetylases blunts pressure-overload cardiac hypertrophy. *Circulation*. 2006;113:2579–88.

48. Jeong MY, Lin YH, Wennersten SA, *et al*. Histone deacetylase activity governs diastolic dysfunction through a nongenomic mechanism. *Sci Transl Med*. 2018;10:eaao0144.

49. Wallner M, Eaton DM, Berretta RM, *et al*. HDAC inhibition improves cardiopulmonary function in a feline model of diastolic dysfunction. *Sci Transl Med*. 2020;12:eaay7205.

50. Haldar SM, McKinsey TA. BET-ting on chromatin-based therapeutics for heart failure. *J Mol Cell Cardiol*. 2014;74:98–102.

51. Dorn LE, Lasman L, Chen J, *et al*. The N(6)-methyladenosine mRNA methylase METTL3 controls cardiac homeostasis and hypertrophy. *Circulation*. 2019;139:533–45.

52. Bar C, Chatterjee S, Falcao Pires I, *et al*. Non-coding RNAs: update on mechanisms and therapeutic targets from the ESC Working Groups of Myocardial Function and Cellular Biology of the Heart. *Cardiovasc Res*. 2020;116:1805–19.

53. Condorelli G, Latronico MV, Cavarretta E. microRNAs in cardiovascular diseases: current knowledge and the road ahead. *J Am Coll Cardiol*. 2014;63:2177–87.

54. Yao RW, Wang Y, Chen LL. Cellular functions of long noncoding RNAs. *Nat Cell Biol*. 2019;21:542–51.

55. Kristensen LS, Andersen MS, Stagsted LVW, Ebbesen KK, Hansen TB, Kjems J. The biogenesis, biology and characterization of circular RNAs. *Nat Rev Genet*. 2019;20:675–91.

56. van Rooij E, Sutherland LB, Qi X, Richardson JA, Hill J, Olson EN. Control of stress-dependent cardiac growth and gene expression by a microRNA. *Science*. 2007;316:575–9.

57. Care A, Catalucci D, Felicetti F, *et al*. MicroRNA-133 controls cardiac hypertrophy. *Nat Med*. 2007;13:613–18.

58. Thum T, Gross C, Fiedler J, *et al*. MicroRNA-21 contributes to myocardial disease by stimulating MAP kinase signalling in fibroblasts. *Nature*. 2008;456:980–4.

59. Foinquinos A, Batkai S, Genschel C, *et al*. Preclinical development of a miR-132 inhibitor for heart failure treatment. *Nat Commun*. 2020; 11:633.

60. Taubel J, Hauke W, Rump S, *et al*. Novel antisense therapy targeting microRNA-132 in patients with heart failure: results of a first-in-human phase 1b randomized, double-blind, placebo-controlled study. *Eur Heart J*. 2021;42:178–88.

CHAPTER 5.2

Alterations in myocardial metabolism

Edoardo Bertero and Christoph Maack

Contents

Introduction

Cardiac contraction and relaxation are energy-consuming processes that are sustained by continuous regeneration of adenosine triphosphate (ATP) from adenosine diphosphate (ADP). Most (approximately 95%) of ATP produced in the heart is derived from mitochondrial oxidative phosphorylation, whereas the remaining 5% is produced by glucose oxidation to pyruvate via glycolysis. If these processes were to stop, the average ATP content of cardiac myocytes (approximately 10 mM) would be sufficient to support only a few heartbeats. Thus, evolution has devised a complex machinery that continuously extracts chemical energy from circulating substrates such as glucose and fatty acids (FAs) to maintain the reaction of ATP hydrolysis to ADP far from its thermodynamic equilibrium, thus keeping ATP breakdown highly exergonic. Cardiac energy metabolism can be schematically divided into three components (⊃ Figure 5.2.1):

1 Cellular internalization of circulating substrates and their 'priming' for oxidation inside mitochondria

2 The process of oxidative phosphorylation, whereby chemical energy extracted from circulating substrates is stored in a chemical and electrical potential across the inner mitochondrial membrane, and subsequently harnessed to catalyse ADP phosphorylation to form ATP

3 Transfer of the phosphoryl group of ATP from the site of its synthesis to that of its utilization via the creatine shuttle.

In this chapter, we give an overview of cardiac substrate metabolism in the healthy heart, its interconnection with the processes that govern cardiac contraction and relaxation, and how these processes are altered in, and contribute to the progression of, heart failure (HF).

Cardiac energy metabolism in the normal heart

Substrate uptake and utilization

The first step in cardiac energy metabolism involves uptake of carbon substrates from the bloodstream and their priming for oxidation in mitochondria. One remarkable property of the healthy heart is its capability to shift between different substrates for ATP production, depending on their availability and the hormonal milieu, without consequences on mechanical performance—a property coined *metabolic flexibility*.[1] In fact, fluxes through ATP-producing pathways continuously change even in the normal heart, while ATP concentration is maintained constant on a beat-to-beat basis. Although

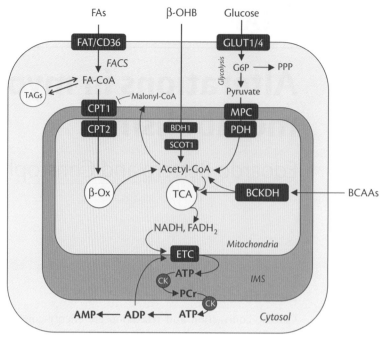

Figure 5.2.1 Cardiac substrate uptake and utilization. The heart uses primarily fatty acids (FAs) and glucose for ATP production. FAs are taken up via the FA translocase (FA/CD36), conjugated with coenzyme A (CoA), and then imported in the mitochondrial matrix via the carnitine shuttle. The rate-limiting reaction of the shuttle and of FA oxidation, catalysed by carnitine palmitoyltransferase 1 (CPT1), is inhibited by malonyl-CoA, the product of acetyl-CoA carboxylation. Glucose is taken up via the glucose transporters GLUT1 and GLUT4, and subsequently phosphorylated to form glucose-6-phosphate (G6P). Glucose and glycolytic intermediates can be channelled into non-oxidative pathways (E Figure 5.2.3) such as the pentose phosphate pathway (PPP). When used for ATP production, glucose is imported in the mitochondrial matrix via the mitochondrial pyruvate carrier (MPC), converted to acetyl-CoA by pyruvate dehydrogenase (PDH), and then channelled into the Krebs cycle. In heart failure, the contribution of ketone oxidation to ATP production is increased. The ketone β-hydroxybutyrate (β-OHB) is converted to acetoacetate by the β-hydroxybutyrate dehydrogenase 1 (BDH1). Subsequently, acetoacetate is bound to CoA by the succinyl-CoA:3 oxoacid-CoA transferase (SCOT1), and then channelled into the Krebs cycle in the form of acetyl-CoA. Branched-chain amino acids (BCAAs) are also channelled into the Krebs cycle upon oxidation by branched chain α-keto acid dehydrogenase (BCKDH). The reducing equivalents derived from terminal oxidation of acetyl-CoA via the Krebs cycle are transferred to the electron transport chain (ETC) via the reduced forms of NAD (NADH) and FAD (FADH₂). The ATP produced by oxidative phosphorylation is transferred to the cytosol via the creatine kinase (CK) shuttle, which entails transfer of the phosphoryl group of ATP to creatine (Cr), producing phosphocreatine (PCr) and ADP. PCr is smaller than ATP and diffuses into the cytosol where its phosphoryl group is transferred back to ADP. Other abbreviations: AMP, adenosine monophosphate.

glucose was initially identified as 'the origin of muscular force', the concept that cardiac oxidative metabolism is fuelled by more than one carbon source had already been proposed in 1914 by Charles Lovatt Evans, who conducted pioneering experiments with the heart–lung preparation established by Starling.[2] Major advances in the field were brought about in the 1950s by the development of coronary sinus catheterization, which allowed the measurement of transcardiac (i.e. arteriovenous) gradients of metabolites *in situ*.[3] Combined with the infusion of isotope-labelled substrates, cardiac catheterization also enabled assessment of myocardial production of $^{14}CO_2$ derived from terminal mitochondrial oxidation of ^{14}C-labelled glucose or FAs, thus providing a quantitative measure of cardiac combustion of substrates extracted from the circulation.[4,5,6] While cardiac uptake of metabolites was previously equated to their complete oxidation, these studies revealed that approximately 20% and 80% of extracted glucose and FAs, respectively, are oxidized in the human myocardium. Altogether, these studies established the widely accepted view that in the healthy heart, 60–90% of ATP production is sustained by FA oxidation and the remaining 10–40% derives from pyruvate oxidation, whereas the contribution

of ketones and amino acids is minor.[7,8,9] However, substantial variations in substrate preference can occur in physiological or pathological conditions such as diabetes, prolonged fasting, or HF.[7,8,9]

Fatty acids

FAs enter cardiac myocytes predominantly via the FA translocase (FAT/CD36). Although the translocation of FAT/CD36 from cytosolic vesicles to the sarcolemmal membrane is controlled by insulin, FA uptake into the heart is mainly determined by the plasmatic concentrations of FAs. In the cytosol, FAs are converted to long-chain acyl-CoA esters, the majority of which (approximately 75%) is immediately transferred into mitochondria via a series of three enzymatic reactions denoted as the carnitine shuttle. The second step of the shuttle, which entails conversion of acyl-CoA esters into long-chain acylcarnitines by carnitine palmitoyltransferase 1 (CPT1), is the rate-limiting step of FA oxidation in mitochondria (➲ Figure 5.2.1). In the mitochondrial matrix, FAs are oxidized to acetyl-CoA to fuel the Krebs cycle. In fed states, excess acetyl-CoA is carboxylated to form malonyl-CoA, which, in turn, limits FA entry into the mitochondrial matrix via allosteric inhibition of CPT1. The remaining 25% of long-chain acyl-CoA esters is stored in the intramyocardial triacylglycerol (TAG) pool, which is continuously turned over and represents an important source of FAs for oxidation.[9,10] FAs have the highest ATP yield per two-carbon unit, and on a molar basis, the amount of ATP produced from FA oxidation is several-fold higher than for glucose oxidation; however, FAs are the least efficient substrates in terms of ATP produced per oxygen (O_2) consumed (P/O ratio).

Glucose

Cardiac myocytes import glucose from the bloodstream via the sarcolemmal glucose transporter GLUT4, whose expression and membrane translocation are enhanced by insulin and, to a lesser extent, via the constitutively active transporter GLUT1. Furthermore, cardiac myocytes can also derive glucose from a modest intracellular glycogen pool. After phosphorylation in the cytosol, glucose enters glycolysis. Pyruvate, the terminal product of glycolysis, has two possible fates: conversion to lactate or uptake and oxidation in mitochondria. Under normoxic conditions, mitochondrial pyruvate carriers (MPCs) transfer pyruvate into mitochondria[11,12] where it undergoes oxidative decarboxylation to acetyl-CoA, a reaction catalysed by the pyruvate dehydrogenase (PDH) enzyme complex (➲ Figure 5.2.1). This step is finely tuned by a kinase, which inhibits PDH upon phosphorylation, and a phosphatase, which, in contrast, promotes pyruvate entry into the Krebs cycle by dephosphorylating PDH.[13] In addition to glycolysis and glycogen synthesis, glucose can also be channelled into the pentose phosphate pathway, whose first reaction is the main cytosolic source of nicotinamide adenine dinucleotide phosphate (NADPH).

Ketones

Ketones are produced from acetyl-CoA in the liver during states of caloric restriction, and are used for ATP production by other tissues (primarily skeletal muscle, but also the brain) where they are converted to acetyl-CoA and oxidized via the Krebs cycle. Ketones represent a negligible source of ATP in the healthy heart but can be used for this purpose under fasting conditions. The ketone β-hydroxybutyrate (β-OHB) is converted to acetoacetate by the β-hydroxybutyrate dehydrogenase 1 (BDH1). Subsequently, acetoacetate is bound to coenzyme A (CoA) by succinyl-CoA:3 oxoacid-CoA transferase (SCOT1), which uses the Krebs cycle intermediate succinyl-CoA as a CoA donor and produces succinate and acetoacetate-CoA; the latter undergoes thiolytic reduction to produce acetyl-CoA (➲ Figure 5.2.1).

Amino acids

Oxidation of substrates other than FAs, glucose, and lactate accounts only for a minority of ATP production in the normal heart. Indeed, studies in humans indicate that the heart secretes most amino acids, reflecting active proteolysis.[14] Amino acid excretion from the heart might serve different purposes such as removal of nitrogen derived from protein turnover. Because most human studies are based on transcardiac gradients of metabolite concentrations assessed in blood samples collected after overnight fasting, under fed conditions, the opposite trend, that is, an imbalance towards protein synthesis, would be expected.

Impaired catabolism of branched-chain amino acids (BCAAs) has been implicated in maladaptive cardiac remodelling, and thus this pathway has been extensively studied in the heart. The first step in BCAA catabolism involves the transfer of one amino group to α-ketoglutarate, a reaction catalysed by the mitochondrial branched-chain amino-transaminase (BCATm). The product of this reaction is one α-keto acid, which undergoes oxidative decarboxylation by the mitochondrial branched-chain α-keto acid dehydrogenase (BCKDH). BCKDH shares structural and functional similarities with PDH, including its post-translational regulation by phosphorylation. BCKDH produces either acetyl-CoA or succinyl-CoA, which can be channelled into the Krebs cycle (➲ Figure 5.2.1).

Regulation of substrate preference

Cardiac substrate preference is determined by multiple factors: (1) substrate availability; (2) expression of membrane transporters for substrate internalization; and (3) expression and activity of oxidative enzymes. In turn, the latter is controlled by numerous mechanisms operating on different timescales: in the short term, the catalytic activity of rate-limiting enzymes is inhibited by the abundance of their products or a shift in the NADH redox state towards reduction; alternatively, post-translational modifications (e.g. phosphorylation or acetylation) or interaction with regulatory proteins can switch on or off specific enzymes. On a longer timescale, the number of enzyme molecules is determined by transcription factors that regulate the expression of wide sets of genes in a coordinated fashion. For instance, FA utilization is regulated by malonyl-CoA-dependent inhibition of CPT1, which limits import of acyl-CoA inside the mitochondrial matrix when acetyl-CoA is abundant; additionally, rate-limiting enzymes of FA oxidation are inhibited by high acetyl-CoA/CoA and NADH/NAD$^+$ ratios. A longer-term control of FA oxidation is mediated by the peroxisome proliferator-activated receptor α (PPARα), which induces the expression of FA oxidative enzymes.

A concept for the mutual control of glucose and FA oxidation in cardiac muscle has been coined by Philip Randle in 1963[15] who described the 'glucose–fatty acid cycle', which was thereafter often referred to as the 'Randle cycle'. In essence, it describes a mechanism by which glucose, when taken up into adipose tissue under the control of insulin, prevents lipolysis and thereby reduces circulating levels of FAs. Conversely, when circulating FA levels are high, the uptake of FAs into cardiac muscle inhibits glucose oxidation through acetyl-CoA-mediated inhibition of PDH, 6-phosphofructo-1-kinase, and glucose uptake,[15,16] shifting substrate utilization even more strongly towards FA oxidation. While these processes govern metabolic flexibility in the short term, longer-term priming towards FA oxidation, with less metabolic flexibility, occurs in the diabetic heart mostly through chronic activation of PPARα.[17]

Mitochondrial oxidative metabolism

Oxidative phosphorylation

In cardiac myocytes, as much as 95% of ATP is produced in mitochondria, which occupy up to 35% of cell volume. Mitochondria are surrounded by two membranes, the innermost of which is impermeable to ions and displays profound invaginations denoted as *cristae*. This inner mitochondrial membrane (IMM) contains four types of protein complexes that comprise electron acceptors, together assembling the electron transport chain (ETC). The reducing equivalents derived from terminal oxidation of acetyl-CoA via the Krebs cycle are transferred to the ETC via the reduced forms of NAD (NADH) and FAD (FADH$_2$), and subsequently channelled through the electron acceptors contained in the ETC. Because each acceptor has a slightly higher affinity for electrons than the previous one, each electron transfer releases a small amount of energy, which is used to translocate hydride ions (H$^+$) into the space between the two mitochondrial membranes (intermembrane space). Molecular oxygen (O$_2$) is the terminal electron acceptor at complex IV (cytochrome oxidase) and is reduced to water (H$_2$O) upon acceptance of two electrons. The chemical (ΔpH) and electrical ($\Delta\Psi_m$) potential generated by the activity of the ETC complexes, together denoted as the proton motive force ($\Delta\mu_H$), is used by another membrane-embedded enzyme, the F$_1$-F$_o$ ATP synthase or complex V, to catalyse the phosphorylation of ADP to ATP. Subsequently, ATP is translocated by the adenine nucleotide translocator to the intermembrane space in exchange for ADP.

The creatine shuttle

The ATP produced in mitochondria is shuttled to the site of its utilization by means of phosphoryl transferase reactions catalysed by creatine kinase (CK), which transfer the phosphoryl group of ATP to creatine (Cr), producing phosphocreatine (PCr) and ADP. PCr is smaller than ATP and rapidly diffuses to the cytosol, where its phosphoryl group is transferred back to ADP (➲ Figure 5.2.1). The CK reaction is approximately ten times faster than ATP synthesis by oxidative phosphorylation and functions as an efficient 'energy buffer', preventing fluctuations in ADP levels when ATP consumption exceeds ATP supply. Adenylate kinase is another phosphoryl transferase that contributes to maintain high ATP levels by transferring phosphoryl groups among adenine nucleotides.

Cardiac mechano-energetic coupling

Parallel activation of mitochondrial oxidative metabolism by ADP and Ca^{2+}

During physical exercise, cardiac output can rapidly increase 4- to 6-fold, paralleled by an increase in myocardial work and oxygen consumption (MVO$_2$). The changes in excitation–contraction (EC) coupling occurring during physical exercise are accompanied by a surge in ATP turnover, primarily by myosin and ion channels, which needs to be matched by an increase in ATP production via oxidative phosphorylation and glycolysis. Oxidative phosphorylation is fine-tuned to swiftly adapt to the continuous variations of ATP consumption of the cardiac myocyte. When ATP turnover increases, the accelerated ADP flux into mitochondria via the creatine shuttle stimulates the F$_1$-F$_o$ ATP synthase to regenerate ATP. In parallel, the activity of the Krebs cycle dehydrogenases is stimulated by the accumulation of calcium (Ca^{2+}) in the mitochondrial matrix, which provides the ETC with the supply of reducing equivalents needed to maintain the proton motive force (➲ Figure 5.2.2). Therefore, ADP and Ca^{2+} are central modulators of the metabolic adaptation to elevations in cardiac workload, where ADP accelerates the electron flux along the ETC and Ca^{2+} provides *parallel activation* of mitochondrial oxidative metabolism.[18]

Mitochondrial Ca^{2+} handling

The primary pathway of rapid mitochondrial Ca^{2+} uptake is via the mitochondrial Ca^{2+} uniporter (MCU) complex, a macromolecular complex residing in the IMM. The MCU comprises five subunit types, two spanning the IMM (MCUa and EMRE) and three located in the intermembrane space (MICU1, 2, and 3) that modulate MCU complex activity in response to changes in cytosolic [Ca^{2+}]. To prevent mitochondrial Ca^{2+} overload and consequent dissipation of the proton motive force, the MCU complex has a low apparent affinity for Ca^{2+} (k_D 20–30 μM), which implies that the [Ca^{2+}] required for Ca^{2+} influx into the mitochondrial matrix is higher than the physiological cytosolic [Ca^{2+}] range.[19] The close apposition of mitochondria and the sarcoplasmic reticulum (SR) creates a spatially localized 'microdomain' where [Ca^{2+}] is substantially higher than in the bulk cytosol. Therefore, the spatial proximity between sites of Ca^{2+} release from the SR and mitochondria is essential for the Ca^{2+}-dependent adaptation of oxidative metabolism.[20]

Ca^{2+} efflux from mitochondria is mediated by another IMM-resident protein, the Na$^+$/Ca^{2+} exchanger (NCLX), the activity of which is primarily determined by the [Na$^+$] gradient across the IMM.[21] Kinetics of Ca^{2+} efflux via the NCLX are much slower than of MCU-mediated Ca^{2+} uptake, accounting for the accumulation of free matrix Ca^{2+} during elevations in cardiac workload. While there is general agreement that mitochondria can take up Ca^{2+} rapidly, also on a beat-to-beat basis, the absolute amounts taken up, and whether these contribute to cytosolic Ca^{2+} buffering, are more controversial, although most evidence suggests that mitochondrial Ca^{2+} handling is rather inconsequential for EC coupling.[18,22] Irrespective of these controversies, the key physiological trigger for activation of the Krebs cycle dehydrogenases is likely the cumulative increase in diastolic matrix [Ca^{2+}].

Mitochondrial Ca^{2+} in rodents and humans

The role of Ca^{2+} in the rapid adaptation of oxidative metabolism has been mostly studied in small rodents (mice and rats), but it is likely more relevant in humans than in mice because of the larger chronotropic and inotropic reserve of the human heart. The heart rate in mice can increase from 500–600 bpm at rest to 700–800 bpm during exercise, whereas humans can increase the heart rate 3- to 4-fold during exercise. Similarly, isometric force development (measured *ex vivo*) increases marginally when the stimulation frequency increases from 8 to 12 Hz in murine cardiac trabeculae, whereas human cardiac trabeculae develop 81–168% more force when the stimulation frequency is increased from 0.5 to 2.5 Hz.[23] Furthermore, cytosolic [Na$^+$] is markedly higher in mice (9–14 mmol/L) than in humans (4–8 mmol/L), where it falls within the steep part of the Na$^+$-dependent regulation of NCLX activity.[24] Therefore, the rate of Ca^{2+} extrusion should be more sensitive to changes in cytosolic [Na$^+$] in humans, compared to

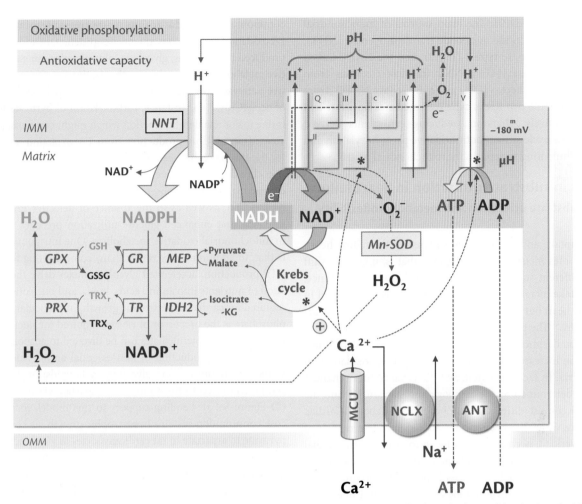

Figure 5.2.2 Cardiac mechano-energetic coupling. Metabolic adaptation to elevations in cardiac workload is driven by the parallel activation of oxidative phosphorylation and the Krebs cycle dehydrogenases by adenosine diphosphate (ADP) and Ca^{2+}, respectively. Ca^{2+} is taken up in the mitochondrial matrix via the mitochondrial Ca^{2+} uniporter (MCU), a multiprotein complex residing in the inner mitochondrial membrane (IMM), and is extruded in exchange for Na^+ via the mitochondrial Na^+/Ca^{2+} exchanger (NCLX). In the matrix, Ca^{2+} stimulates Krebs cycle dehydrogenases to regenerate the reduced forms of nicotinamide adenine dinucleotide (NADH) and nicotinamide adenine dinucleotide phosphate (NADPH), thereby providing reducing equivalents to the electron transport chain (ETC) for adenosine triphosphate (ATP) production and to the mitochondrial H_2O_2-eliminating systems, including glutathione peroxidase (GPX) and the peroxiredoxin (PRX)/thioredoxin (TRX) system. In addition to the isocitrate dehydrogenase type 2 (IDH2) and malate dehydrogenase (MEP), a major source of NADPH in the heart is the nicotinamide nucleotide transhydrogenase (NNT) reaction, which harnesses the proton motive force to transfer hydride ion equivalents from NADH to $NADP^+$. Other abbreviations: ANT, adenine nucleotide translocator; GR, glutathione reductase; GSSG, oxidized form of glutathione; TR, thioredoxin reductase.
Reproduced from Bertero E, Maack C. Calcium Signaling and Reactive Oxygen Species in Mitochondria. *Circ Res*. 2018 May 11;122(10):1460–1478. doi: 10.1161/CIRCRESAHA.118.310082 from Wolters Kluwer.

rodents. Overall, these differences imply that the variations in ATP consumption during workload transitions are larger, and consequently the Ca^{2+}-dependent modulation of oxidative metabolism more relevant, in humans than in mice.

Mitochondrial reactive oxygen species

The high electron affinity of O_2 accounts for the large amount of energy released upon reduction of one molecule of O_2 to two molecules of H_2O, resulting in a substantially larger ATP yield of aerobic, compared with anaerobic, metabolism. The incomplete reduction of O_2, however, can lead to the generation of reactive oxygen species (ROS) that can wreak havoc in the cell by subtracting electrons to lipids, amino acids, or nucleotides. Mitochondria, and the ETC in particular, represent a major source of ROS in cardiac myocytes. To protect cellular components from oxidative damage, mitochondria are equipped with an efficient antioxidative machinery. Superoxide (O_2^-), the product of incomplete O_2 reduction, is converted to hydrogen peroxide (H_2O_2) by the manganese-dependent superoxide dismutase (Mn-SOD), the enzyme with the highest catalytic efficiency described thus far ($k \simeq 2 \times 10^9 M^{-1} \times s^{-1}$). In turn, H_2O_2 is eliminated via reduction to H_2O catalysed by matrix peroxidases, including peroxiredoxin (PRX) and glutathione peroxidases (GPX). The conversion of H_2O_2 to H_2O catalysed by PRX and GPX is coupled to the oxidation of thioredoxin (TRX) and glutathione (GSH), respectively, that, in turn, are maintained in their reduced (i.e. active) form by a cascade of redox reactions that derive reducing equivalents from NADPH. The main sources of mitochondrial NADPH are nicotinamide nucleotide transhydrogenase (NNT), isocitrate dehydrogenase type 2 (IDH2), and the NADP-linked malate dehydrogenase (MEP). NNT transfers electrons from NADH to $NADP^+$, whereas IDH2 and MEP reduce $NADP^+$ from the oxidation of the two Krebs cycle intermediates isocitrate and malate, respectively. Therefore, reducing equivalents derived from the Krebs cycle sustain both oxidative phosphorylation and the H_2O_2-eliminating systems in the mitochondrial matrix.

Changes in substrate utilization in heart failure

Altered substrate utilization and metabolic inflexibility

Fatty acids

Substrate uptake and utilization are altered in the failing heart, which becomes metabolically 'inflexible', that is, unable to shift between different substrates for ATP production. For instance, glucose uptake increases 2-fold during elevations of workload in the healthy heart but does not change in patients with dilated cardiomyopathy.[25] The prevailing view in the field is that the rate of FA oxidation declines with progression of HF, and this is accompanied by an increase in glycolysis, but not glucose oxidation, in mitochondria. In fact, the extent and direction of these changes are largely determined by the aetiology and stage of HF and the presence of comorbidities such as obesity and diabetes. Cardiac hypertrophy, which has been mostly studied in rodent models of pressure overload, is characterized by an increase in myocardial glucose uptake, whereas FA uptake and oxidation are unchanged or only mildly reduced.[26,27,28,29,30] As hypertrophy progresses towards left ventricular (LV) systolic dysfunction and dilatation, the rate of FA oxidation progressively declines and yet remains the major source of ATP in the heart.[14] The decreased reliance on FAs for ATP production was reported also in animal models of ischaemic and pacing-induced HF,[31] as well as in humans with dilated cardiomyopathy.[32,33] Accumulation of incompletely oxidized FAs and toxic lipid species, such as ceramides, might directly damage cellular components and contribute to cardiac myocyte dysfunction, a phenomenon termed *lipotoxicity*. Decreased FA utilization in the failing heart can be traced to suppression of transcriptional regulators such as PPARα and ERRα/ERRγ[34,35] and concomitant activation of the PPARγ hypoxia inducible factor (HIF)-1α signalling axis,[36] resulting in downregulation of rate-limiting FA oxidation enzymes. However, other studies reported an opposite pattern, that is, unchanged or even increased uptake of FAs in patients with HF.[37] In patients with obesity and diabetes, which are important risk factors for the development of HF, insulin resistance and PPARα activation hamper metabolic flexibility and shift substrate utilization towards FA oxidation.[17] Therefore, the underlying aetiology and stage of HF play an important role for the mode of metabolic dysregulation.

Glucose

Glucose uptake and rates of glycolysis are often increased in animal models and patients with HF, which has been attributed to increased GLUT1 expression and to enhanced activity of the rate-limiting glycolysis enzyme phosphofructokinase 1 (PFK-1).[25,38,39] This is commonly interpreted as a compensatory response to impairment in FA oxidation and the consequent energy deficit. In addition to ATP produced by glycolysis, glycolytic intermediates can sustain oxidative metabolism via anaplerosis, that is, the recruitment of alternative pathways to generate Krebs cycle intermediates independent of acetylCoA.[40] For instance, carboxylation of pyruvate to malate is one major anaplerotic reaction which might compensate the decreased acetyl-CoA production from FA oxidation and account for the mismatch between glycolytic flux and glucose oxidation in mitochondria.[40,41] However, as noted above, increased glycolysis in cardiac hypertrophy is observed prior to the progression to systolic dysfunction, as well as in the absence of defective FA oxidation, implying that enhanced glucose utilization precedes the decline in mitochondrial oxidative metabolism. One intriguing possibility is that, in addition to (or rather than) compensating for deficient ATP production, accelerated glycolytic fluxes drive the incorporation of nutrients into amino acids, lipids, and nucleotides that are required for cardiac hypertrophic growth. In particular, glucose-6-phosphate is the precursor of ribose, required for nucleotide synthesis; glycolytic intermediates can be diverted to anabolic pathways leading to the production of non-essential amino acids (such as serine), hexosamines, and glycerophospholipids; finally, pyruvate can be converted to the amino acid aspartate via transamination (➔ Figure 5.2.3). Lending support to this model, increased glucose consumption sustains hypertrophic growth via conversion of pyruvate to aspartate in rat cardiomyocytes *in vitro* and in mice *in vivo*.[42] One key regulatory step that determines the anabolic or catabolic fate of glucose is pyruvate import into mitochondria: MPC downregulation, which has been associated with pressure overload in rodents and humans, decreases pyruvate oxidation and promotes cardiomyocyte growth. Intriguingly, cardiomyocyte-specific knockout of MPC subunits is sufficient to induce cardiac hypertrophy and ultimately leads to LV dysfunction in mice, whereas MPC overexpression protects from hypertrophic remodelling during pressure overload.[43]

Ketones

Cardiac hypertrophy and failure are accompanied by an increased abundance of intermediates and upregulation of enzymes involved in uptake and oxidation of ketones.[32,44] Furthermore, HF patients exhibit higher levels of circulating ketones during fasting[45] and an increased myocardial uptake of the ketone β-OHB, compared to healthy individuals.[37] Altogether, these findings indicate that ketone oxidation might become a relevant source of ATP in the failing heart. This metabolic shift is energetically advantageous, since ketone oxidation produces more energy per two-carbon unit, compared to glucose, and the ATP production/oxygen consumption (P/O) ratio of β-OHB (2.50) is comparable to that of glucose (2.53) and substantially higher than that of palmitate (2.33). On these grounds, it was proposed that β-OHB represents a 'super-fuel',[46] and that promoting ketones over FA oxidation increases cardiac metabolic efficiency. Corroborating this concept, a 3-hour infusion of β-OHB acutely increased cardiac output in patients with HF with reduced ejection fraction (HFrEF) and healthy controls, compared to placebo.[47] However, this effect was

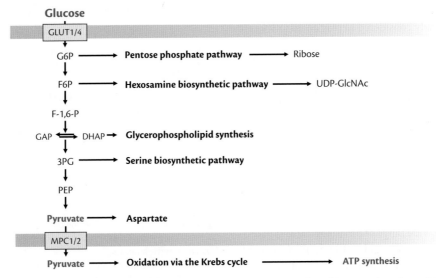

Figure 5.2.3 Pathways of non-oxidative glucose metabolism. The mitochondrial pyruvate carrier (MPC) is a central regulator of the fate of glucose in cardiac myocytes. During pressure overload, increased glucose consumption sustains hypertrophic growth via conversion of pyruvate to aspartate. In heart failure, the mismatch between glycolysis and pyruvate oxidation in mitochondria results in the accumulation of glycolytic intermediates that fuel accessory anabolic pathways such as the pentose phosphate pathway and the hexosamine biosynthetic pathway (HBP).

accompanied by an increase in heart rate, which argues against a mere inotropic effect through improvement of energetics, which would have rather *reduced* heart rate by reflex withdrawal of the sympathetic tone. In contrast, the haemodynamic effect of β-OHB is more likely the result of vasodilatation, as peripheral vascular resistance decreased after β-OHB infusion, which may have triggered sympathetic activation, explaining the increase in heart rate and stroke volume.[47]

Amino acids

During fasting, patients with HFrEF have a 2-fold higher rate of amino acid-derived nitrogen release from the heart, compared to healthy individuals, indicating accelerated proteolysis.[14] However, specific amino acid oxidative pathways, such as BCAA catabolism, are impaired in HF.[48,49] Accumulation of BCAAs has detrimental consequences on cardiac function, sensitizing the heart to ischaemic injury[49] and promoting cardiac hypertrophy via activation of mechanistic target of rapamycin (mTOR) signalling.[48] This might explain why elevated levels of circulating BCAAs portend an increased risk of developing cardiovascular disease, including HF.[50,51] Pharmacological interventions promoting BCAA degradation via branched-chain ketoacid dehydrogenase kinase (BCKDK) inhibition improve cardiac function and insulin sensitivity, thereby increasing glucose oxidation.[52]

Intermediary metabolism dictates signalling responses and gene expression

Changes in the metabolic status of a cell have important consequences on cellular signalling and gene expression. The link between the cellular metabolic and transcriptional machinery is provided by enzymes that modify the packaging of DNA using metabolic intermediates such as acetyl-CoA, α-ketoglutarate, or nicotinamide adenine dinucleotide (NAD) as substrates or cofactors. The abundance of these metabolites varies according to

changes in substrate preference, consequently affecting the organization of chromatin, that is, the complex of DNA and histones that regulates the accessibility of the genome to transcriptional enzymes. In addition, metabolic intermediates can be used for post-translational modification of proteins other than histones, including enzymes involved in oxidative metabolism. Therefore, the activity of metabolic pathways and the levels of metabolic intermediates dictate signalling responses and gene expression by inducing post-translational modification of proteins.

O-linked glycosylation

The hexosamine biosynthetic pathway (HBP) is a metabolic pathway that converts glucose to uridine diphosphate-β-N-acetylglucosamine (UDP-GlcNAc), which serves as a substrate for O-linked glycosylation (O-GlcNAcylation) of proteins. Flux through the HBP is critical to cardiac homeostatic responses and maladaptive remodelling by regulating UDP-GlcNAc availability, and thereby the level of O-GlcNAcylation of the cardiac myocyte proteome. Sustained high plasma glucose levels, as seen in diabetes mellitus, activate the HBP, inducing protein O-GlcNAcylation. Counterintuitively, increased O-GlcNAcylation is seen also in response to glucose deprivation, indicating that this is a response to nutrient stress rather than a direct consequence of hyperglycaemia. Although the HBP takes place in the cytosol, cardiac mitochondria can import UDP-GlcNAc and contain the enzymatic machinery required to regulate O-GlcNAcylation. In diabetes, O-GlcNAcylation of Ca^{2+}/calmodulin-dependent protein kinase II (CaMKII) activates spontaneous SR Ca^{2+} release events that predispose to cardiac mechanical dysfunction and arrhythmia.[53] At the same time, O-GlcNAcylation of histone deacetylase 4 (HDAC4) at Ser-642 is required for production of the cardioprotective N-terminal proteolytic fragment of HDAC4.[54] Overall, O-GlcNAcylation modulates the activity of proteins involved in essential cardiac myocyte functions. Depending on the target protein, O-GlcNAcylation can have both adaptive and mal-adaptive effects; it is generally considered to play an adaptive role in response to acute stressors such as ischaemia/reperfusion, but in the long run, it becomes detrimental to cardiac function.

Protein acetylation and sirtuins

Lysine acetylation is a post-translational modification that was pinpointed as a regulator of cardiac energy metabolism.[55] Acetylation targets include virtually all proteins, regardless of the cellular compartment in which they are located. The level of protein acetylation is determined by the balance between the activity of acetyl-transferases, which use acetyl-CoA as a donor of acetyl groups, and of deacetylases such as sirtuins (SIRTs). SIRTs are a family of enzymes catalysing NAD-dependent deacylation of proteins and are involved in a wide range of physiological and pathological processes. SIRT activity is regulated by multiple factors, including the availability of the co-substrate NAD and the redox state of the NAD pool.[56] Mitochondrial protein acetylation is increased in the failing myocardium, possibly as a consequence of acetyl-CoA accumulation or reduced expression and activity of SIRT3, the sirtuin isoform found in the mitochondrial matrix.[57,58] SIRT3 activity protects mitochondria from oxidative stress and increases ATP production via deacetylation of Mn-SOD and of specific subunits of ETC complexes I and II. However, it remains unclear whether protein acetylation, as observed in HF, has an impact on mitochondrial function. Increased acetylation of mitochondrial proteins is accompanied by disruption of cardiac mitochondrial and contractile function in *Sirt3*-knockout mice,[59] whereas an even more robust increase in acetylation of the mitochondrial proteome obtained by concomitant genetic deletion of SIRT3 and carnitine acetyltransferase had no effect on mitochondrial oxidative metabolism in another study.[60] Therefore, conflicting evidence exists regarding the role of protein acetylation in mitochondrial oxidative metabolism.

NAD synthesis and consumption

The pyridine nucleotide NAD is the coenzyme of dehydrogenase reactions of both glycolysis and the Krebs cycle, and thus plays a central role in oxidative metabolism. NAD exists in two forms, oxidized (NAD^+) and reduced (NADH), and the $NADH/NAD^+$ ratio modulates the activity of numerous enzymes; for example, when the mitochondrial $NADH/NAD^+$ ratio is high (more reduced), the rate-limiting reactions of FA oxidation are inhibited, and vice versa. Furthermore, NAD is the co-substrate of three classes of enzymes involved in essential cellular functions: SIRTs, poly (ADP-ribose) polymerase (PARP), and cyclic ADP ribose hydrolase (also known as CD38); these enzymes degrade NAD to nicotinamide (NAM) and ADP-ribose (ADPR). NAD is produced by three independent pathways: the Preiss–Handler pathway, which uses nicotinic acid (one form of vitamin B_3); the *de novo* biosynthetic pathway, which synthesizes NAD from the essential amino acid tryptophan; and the salvage pathway, which recycles NAM and represents the major source of cellular NAD (➲ Figure 5.2.4). While NAD degradation is matched by NAD recycling or *de novo* synthesis under normal conditions, this equilibrium is altered with ageing and in chronic diseases such as HF.

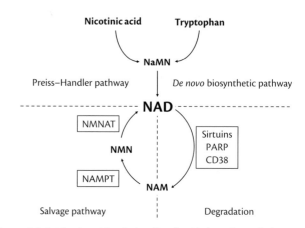

Figure 5.2.4 Nicotinamide adenine dinucleotide (NAD) metabolism. NAD can be synthetized from nicotinic acid via the Preiss–Handler pathway or *de novo* from the amino acid tryptophan. NAD is the substrate of multiple enzymes, including sirtuins, poly (ADP-ribose) polymerases (PARP), and cyclic ADP-ribose hydrolase (also known as CD38); these enzymes degrade NAD to nicotinamide (NAM) and ADP-ribose. NAM can be recycled via the salvage pathway, which consists of two reactions catalysed by nicotinamide phosphoribosyl transferase (NAMPT) and nicotinamide mononucleotide adenyltransferase (NMNAT). Other abbreviations: NaMN, nicotinic acid mononucleotide; NMN, nicotinamide mononucleotide.

Mechano-energetic uncoupling in heart failure

Alterations in excitation–contraction coupling in heart failure

In the failing heart, alterations in cellular Na^+ and Ca^{2+} handling contribute to the development and progression of HF by uncoupling the ATP-consuming processes in the cytosol from mitochondrial oxidative metabolism.[18] In HFrEF, the amplitude of cytosolic Ca^{2+} transients is decreased, which can be traced primarily to decreased activity of the SR Ca^{2+}-ATPase (SERCA) and Ca^{2+} leak from type 2 ryanodine receptors (RyR2), leading to a reduced SR Ca^{2+} load.[61] Furthermore, the heightened diastolic $[Ca^{2+}]$ and slowed cytosolic Ca^{2+} removal increases ventricular wall tension during diastole, thus imposing additional ATP consumption.[62] One central defect in cellular ion handling in animals and humans with systolic HF is the elevation in cytosolic $[Na^+]$ in cardiac myocytes. Multiple factors likely contribute to increased cytosolic $[Na^+]$ in HFrEF, including: (1) reduced Na^+/K^+ ATPase activity; (2) increased Na^+/H^+ exchanger (NHE) activity;[63,64] and (3) prolongation of the late Na^+ current (I_{Na}).[65] Elevated $[Na^+]$ and diminished $[Ca^{2+}]$ shift the reversal potential of the sarcolemmal Na^+/Ca^{2+} exchanger (NCX) towards a more hyperpolarized state; as a result, the NCX operates in *reverse* mode (i.e. importing Ca^{2+} from the extracellular space) during the initial phases of the action potential. On the one hand, Ca^{2+} influx via the NCX partly compensates for decreased SR Ca^{2+} release, but on the other hand, it further hinders diastolic Ca^{2+} removal and thus increases diastolic tension.[66]

Altered excitation–contraction coupling affecting mitochondrial redox regulation

Derangements in EC coupling have important consequences on mitochondrial function. First, decreased Ca^{2+} release from the SR,

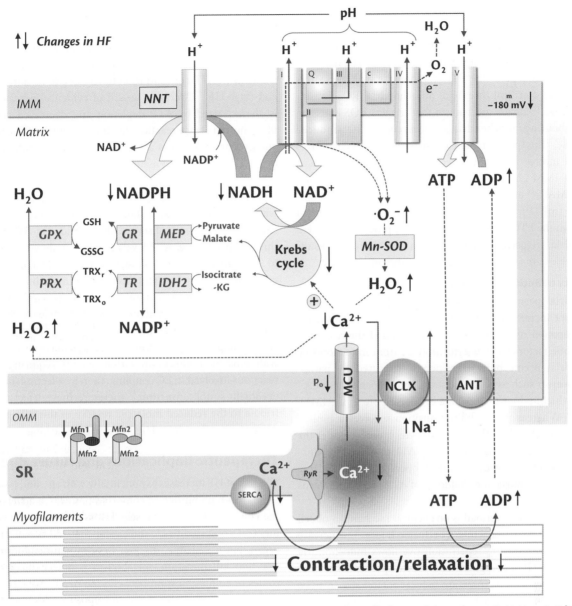

Figure 5.2.5 Cardiac mechano-energetic uncoupling in heart failure. In heart failure, reduced SR Ca^{2+} release and elevated cytosolic Na^+ impair Ca^{2+} accumulation in the mitochondrial matrix, thereby hindering the Ca^{2+}-dependent stimulation of the Krebs cycle. The shortage of reducing equivalents to the electron transport chain and to mitochondrial H_2O_2-eliminating systems causes bioenergetic mismatch and oxidative stress. Red arrows ($\uparrow$ and $\downarrow$) indicate changes in heart failure. Other abbreviations: ANT, adenine nucleotide translocator; GR, glutathione reductase; GSSG, oxidized form of glutathione; Mfn1/2, mitofusin 1/2; TR, thioredoxin reductase.

Reproduced from Bertero E, Maack C. Calcium Signaling and Reactive Oxygen Species in Mitochondria. *Circ Res.* 2018 May 11;122(10):1460–1478. doi: 10.1161/ CIRCRESAHA.118.310082 from Wolters Kluwer.

together with structural alterations of the SR–mitochondria contact sites,[67] hinders mitochondrial Ca^{2+} uptake.[68] Furthermore, increased cytosolic $[Na^+]$ accelerates Ca^{2+} efflux from the mitochondrial matrix by increasing the driving force for Ca^{2+} extrusion via the NCLX.[69] As a consequence, mitochondrial Ca^{2+} accumulation is impaired in HF, resulting in insufficient regeneration of reducing equivalents required to fuel ATP production via oxidative phosphorylation and to support the NADPH-dependent elimination of H_2O_2.[70] In addition, during pathological afterload elevations, reversal of the NNT reaction becomes thermodynamically favourable, and thus contributes to depleting mitochondrial

antioxidative capacity by regenerating reduced NADH from NADPH.[71] Altogether, alterations in EC coupling in HF compromise the finely tuned regulation of mitochondrial oxidative metabolism, provoking oxidation of the mitochondrial pyridine nucleotide pool that leads to bioenergetic mismatch and mitochondrial emission of ROS (➲ Figure 5.2.5).

Mitochondria as regulators of cell death

Mitochondrial ROS-induced ROS release

Mitochondrial dysfunction in HF cannot be exclusively attributed to alterations in EC and mechano-energetic coupling, as numerous other mitochondrial processes are disrupted. First, ROS production at the ETC, and not only emission from the mitochondrial matrix, is increased in failing cardiac myocytes. Superoxide formation at complex I is increased in HF, likely reflecting direct damage to the ETC.[72] When the oxidative stress burden reaches a critical threshold, mitochondrial ROS can induce a positive feedback mechanism that triggers ROS emission from neighbouring mitochondria, a process coined 'ROS-induced ROS release'. This phenomenon consists of the dissipation of the proton motive force ($\Delta\mu_H$) secondary to the ROS-induced opening of IMM channels such as the inner membrane anion channel (IMAC)[73] and/or the mitochondrial permeability transition pore (mPTP).[74] Collapse of $\Delta\mu_H$ is accompanied by a burst of ROS from the ETC that can elicit the same process in adjacent mitochondria, triggering a chain reaction that ultimately results in irreversible damage to cellular components and cell death.[74]

Permeability transition and cell death

Mitochondrial permeability transition is a process consisting of an abrupt increase in permeability of the IMM that results in the dissipation of the proton motive force and the release of pro-apoptotic factors such as cytochrome c from mitochondria. Mitochondrial permeability transition is triggered by pathological processes such as oxidative stress and mitochondrial Ca^{2+} overload, which induce the opening of a large pore in the IMM, the mPTP. Whereas permeability transition involves a limited number of mitochondria, the release of cytochrome c ignites the apoptotic cascade, which is sustained by ATP produced by functional mitochondria. However, if mPTP opening involves a large number of mitochondria, the shutdown of ATP production leads to necrotic cell death.

Mitochondrial Ca^{2+} overload is one central mechanism of cell death in the context of ischaemia/reperfusion injury. The increase in cytosolic $[Ca^{2+}]$ during reperfusion overflows mitochondria and leads to mPTP opening. Cardiomyocyte-specific ablation of the MCU or NCLX overexpression reduces infarct size in mice by preventing mitochondrial Ca^{2+} overload or accelerating Ca^{2+} clearance, respectively, thus preventing mitochondrial permeability transition.[75,76] Therefore, while in chronic HF, reduced mitochondrial Ca^{2+} contributes to altering oxidative metabolism and ROS elimination, *excess* mitochondrial Ca^{2+} plays a pathological role by inducing mPTP opening and cell death in the setting of ischaemia/reperfusion.

The energetic basis of heart failure

The concept that the failing heart is 'an engine out of fuel' has been a central dogma in the field of cardiac energy metabolism since decades.[77] The first report documenting decreased Cr levels in the failing myocardium dates back to 1939; since then, a wealth of studies—mostly based on phosphorus-31 magnetic resonance (^{31}P-MR) spectroscopy—have demonstrated that HF is characterized by a progressive decline in the myocardial PCr/ATP ratio, which correlates with indicators of LV dysfunction and portends poor outcomes. Indeed, because the CK reaction favours ATP over PCr synthesis by a factor of approximately 100, the decline

in PCr levels precedes ATP depletion, accounting for the decrease in the PCr/ATP ratio. This is exacerbated by the concomitant depletion of total Cr levels, which accompanies HF progression. In addition, the ATP backbone is progressively degraded, leading to a decline in ATP concentration to 60–70% of its normal value in end-stage HF.[78] Overall, a wealth of evidence indicates that HF is characterized by ATP depletion and decreased capacity for phosphotransferase reaction, lending support to the concept that energy starvation plays a causative role in the pathophysiology of HF. The underlying assumption is that ATP supply becomes a limiting factor for cardiac contraction and relaxation in the failing heart; however, not all lines of evidence are fully consistent with this concept. First, a significant drop in ATP concentration (by 30–40%) has been observed only in end-stage HF, and even at this advanced stage, ATP levels remain far above those required to sustain cardiac function at rest. Cr and PCr levels decrease earlier and to a larger extent; however, animal studies have shown that severe Cr depletion in mice does not alter cardiac function at baseline.[79] A more relevant problem is that while [ATP] is in much excess of [ADP], a micromolar increase in [ADP] lowers the free Gibbs energy (ΔG_{ATP}) without tangible reductions in [ATP], but with substantial effects on various energy-requiring enzymatic reactions involved in EC coupling, thereby affecting diastolic, and eventually systolic, function.[80] Therefore, these defects might contribute to the reduced inotropic reserve of the failing heart, but evidence that they drive HF progression is lacking.

Therapeutic implications and future directions

The risk of HF increases exponentially with age, and patients with HF have a high burden of comorbidities, which adversely affects the course of HF.[81] Conversely, HF predisposes to the development of comorbidities,[17] indicating that HF is not an isolated organ, but a systemic, disease. Besides neuroendocrine activation and inflammation, metabolism is one of the three major routes of communication between the heart and other organs,[82] and obesity and diabetes are independent risk factors for HF development.[17,83,84,85,86]

Medical treatment of patients with HFrEF has long been limited to drugs interfering with neuroendocrine activation.[87] Various approaches to targeting metabolism at the level of mitochondria, substrate utilization, dietary supplementations, and systemic metabolism have been developed, but with variable results in patients with HF.[88] In the following section, a selection of these approaches is presented.

Improving electron transport chain function
Szeto–Schiller peptide 31

The Szeto–Schiller peptide 31 (SS-31, also known as elamipretide) accumulates approximately 1000-fold in mitochondria, protects the mitochondrial phospholipid cardiolipin from damage by oxidative stress,[89,90] and thereby maintains proper function of the respiratory chain, avoiding aberrant slippage of electrons to O_2 to produce superoxide anion radicals (O_2^-). Furthermore, SS-31 prevents cardiolipin from converting cytochrome c into a peroxidase, while protecting its electron-carrying function.[91,92] In various preclinical animal models of HF, SS-31 ameliorated maladaptive cardiac remodelling, improved cardiac function, and prolonged survival.[93,94] Whereas also in a dog model of HFrEF, short- (48 hours) or long-term treatment with SS-31 (for 3 months) increased LV ejection fraction and reduced LV volumes, these effects were not observed in humans with HFrEF treated with SS-31 after 28 days of treatment,[95] despite initial promising effects of short-term infusion of elamipretide on LV volumes.[96]

Coenzyme Q$_{10}$

Other approaches target nutrient deficiencies in HF. Coenzyme Q$_{10}$ is a component of the ETC in mitochondria,[97] but also other cellular membranes where it maintains endothelial nitric oxide synthase (eNOS) function to prevent its uncoupling and ROS generation.[98] In patients with HF, decreased coenzyme Q$_{10}$ levels correlate with the severity of disease.[99,100] In 420 patients with HFrEF, coenzyme Q$_{10}$ improved symptoms and reduced major adverse cardiovascular events, including total mortality,[101] effects that were supported by additional (and recent) meta-analyses.[102,103] However, larger clinical outcome trials are required to confirm these promising results.

Targeting substrate preference

The idea of the failing heart as an energy-starved engine provides the conceptual framework for therapeutic approaches targeting substrate preference to improve cardiac efficiency. Because FA oxidation requires more oxygen than glucose oxidation for any given quantity of ATP produced (i.e. FAs have a lower P/O ratio than glucose), pharmacological agents inhibiting FA utilization and/or promoting glucose oxidation were tested in animal models and patients with HF.

Inhibiting fatty acid oxidation

Trimetazidine (TMZ) reduces FA utilization via competitive inhibition of the long-chain 3-ketoacyl-CoA thiolase, the enzyme catalysing the last step of FA oxidation.[104,105] TMZ is recommended by the current European Society of Cardiology (ESC) guidelines as a second-line treatment to reduce angina frequency in patients whose symptoms are not controlled with other antianginal medications. Studies in patients with ischaemic HF reported that TMZ improves the PCr/ATP ratio, consequently improving symptoms and exercise capacity.[106] Similar effects were also observed in patients with idiopathic dilated cardiomyopathy.[107] However, these studies were limited by the small population and the observational design, and no large clinical trials have been conducted to test the effects of TMZ in HFrEF.

Pharmacological agents inhibiting malonyl-CoA degradation were developed as an alternative approach to inhibiting FA oxidation. Malonyl-CoA is a potent endogenous inhibitor of CPT1, the rate-limiting step of FA import in mitochondria, and is degraded by malonyl-CoA decarboxylase (MCD). MCD inhibitors were shown to improve cardiac function by ameliorating myocardial efficiency in a rat model of myocardial infarction.[108] MCD inhibitors have not yet been tested in humans.

Stimulating glucose utilization

Dichloroacetate (DCA) promotes glucose utilization by inhibiting PDH kinase, thereby restoring the coupling of glycolysis with pyruvate oxidation in mitochondria in HF. In rodents, DCA improves cardiac efficiency and prevents maladaptive remodelling induced by ischaemia/reperfusion injury[109] and chronic pressure overload.[110] Short-term treatment with DCA was tested in small clinical trials, which could recapitulate some of the promising observations of preclinical studies. In patients with stable angina and coronary artery disease, DCA stimulated myocardial lactate utilization, increased stroke volume, and enhanced myocardial efficiency.[111] Similarly, DCA increased myocardial lactate consumption and improved LV mechanical efficiency in patients with HFrEF.[112] However, other studies yielded conflicting results,[113] and research on this agent and therapeutic approach has been abandoned.

Iron supplementation

Iron is essential to mitochondrial function, where it is complexed in iron–sulfur clusters that govern electron-transferring redox reactions at the ETC, but also in Krebs cycle dehydrogenases. About one-third of all patients with HF have serum iron deficiency, which is associated with decreased exercise capacity and adverse outcome.[114,115] Intravenous application of ferric carboxymaltose improves exercise capacity, symptoms, and quality of life, and reduces hospitalizations in patients with HF,[116,117,118,119] whereas total or cardiovascular mortality remained unaffected.[117,119] It is still unresolved whether the beneficial effects of iron are mediated by improvement of cardiac or skeletal muscle function, or both.[88,120] Although in the human failing heart, *total* iron content is reduced, this decrease may not occur in mitochondria[121] and appears unrelated to serum iron status,[122] severity of the disease,[123] or the activity of ETC complexes.[124] On the other hand, reduced myocardial iron content was associated with decreased Krebs cycle and antioxidative enzyme activities.[124] Interestingly, ferric carboxymaltose improves LV ejection fraction in patients with HFrEF and cardiac resynchronization therapy, suggesting benefits also on the heart itself.[125] Current ESC guidelines for the diagnosis and treatment of acute and chronic HF recommend to regularly screen for anaemia and iron deficiency in patients with HF, and to use ferric carboxymaltose in patients with HF (LV ejection fraction <45%) and iron deficiency to improve symptoms, exercise capacity, and quality of life.[87] Ongoing phase 3 clinical trials currently are evaluating the impact of iron carboxymaltose on cardiovascular mortality and hospitalization for HF (NCT03037931 and FAIR-HF2-DZHK5).

Nicotinamide adenine dinucleotide supplementation

Supplementations with NAD precursors, such as nicotinamide riboside (NR) and nicotinamide mononucleotide (NMN), prevented maladaptive remodelling in various preclinical models of HF with preserved ejection fraction (HFpEF) or HFrEF.[58,126,127,128,129] Supplementation of mouse models of genetic dilated cardiomyopathy or of pathological cardiac hypertrophy maintains the cardiac pool of NAD, which is otherwise 30% lower in untreated sick animals, compared to controls.[126,130] Most interestingly, this treatment preserved cardiac function, while limiting eccentric remodelling of the left ventricle, raising the interest in translating this approach to clinics. Reduced NAD availability in HF is associated with reduced expression of the gene encoding nicotinamide phosphoribosyl transferase (NAMPT), the rate-limiting enzyme of the NAD salvage pathway,[131] indicating that impaired NAM recycling contributes to depleting NAD in failing cardiac myocytes. However, the effect of NAMPT overexpression was cardioprotective in response to certain stressors, such as ischaemic injury,[131] but detrimental in the context of chronic pressure overload.[132] Increased degradation might also contribute to NAD depletion, but the role of the NAD-consuming enzymes in HF has been less investigated thus far. Furthermore, the mechanisms of how decreased NAD availability contributes to HF are not completely understood. It has been proposed that decreased NAD levels and a shift towards a more reduced $NADH/NAD^+$ redox state hinder SIRT3 activity, resulting in mitochondrial protein hyperacetylation. However, effects of NR/NMN supplementation on acetylation of the mitochondrial proteome differed, depending on the mouse model,[58,127] and it remains unclear whether mitochondrial protein acetylation has relevant consequences on mitochondrial function.[60] Overall, supplementation of NAD precursors is emerging as a potential therapeutic strategy for HFrEF and HFpEF, and there are numerous ongoing clinical trials testing this approach in humans; however, the mechanism of how rescuing NAD levels is beneficial in HF is not fully resolved.

SGLT2 inhibitors

Only recently, clinical studies with inhibitors of sodium–glucose cotransporter 2 (SGLT2) revealed that metabolic interventions provide substantial benefit for patients with HFrEF, even in the absence of diabetes.[133] Moreover, for patients with HFpEF, SGLT2 inhibitors (SGLT2i) became the first approach to improving outcome in this growing patient population.[134] SGLT2i induce urinary excretion of glucose and Na^+ by inhibiting their reabsorption via SGLT2 in the proximal tubule. Glucosuria improves glycaemic control and induces weight loss, and the accompanying natriuresis lowers blood pressure and reduces volume overload. It is poorly understood how these effects translate into a large and rapid improvement in cardiovascular outcomes regardless of diabetes, but the underlying mechanisms likely involve improvements in systemic and cardiac metabolism.

The increase in glucose excretion induced by SGLT2i produces a fasting-like state that stimulates lipolysis and ketogenesis. It has been proposed that the ensuing increase in plasma ketone levels provides the energy-starved failing heart with a 'thrifty substrate'.[135] In a porcine model of myocardial infarction, treatment with empagliflozin enhanced cardiac efficiency by inducing a substrate shift towards ketone, FA, and BCAA utilization for ATP production.[136] Furthermore, ketones might ameliorate maladaptive cardiac remodelling by virtue of their anti-inflammatory properties.[137] Studies in humans, however, indicate that the ketogenic effect of SGLT2i is primarily seen in diabetic subjects,

whereas the increase in plasma ketones induced in non-diabetic HF patients is low or null.[138,139]

Another intriguing possibility is that the fasting-like state induced by SGLT2i switches on cellular sensors that mediate responses to nutrient deprivation such as SIRT1 and adenosine monophosphate-activated protein kinase (AMPK).[140] Activation of SIRT1 and AMPK has manifold consequences that could contribute to the cardioprotective effect of SGLT2i. For instance, SIRT1 activates the transcription factor PGC-1α by deacetylation. PGC-1α is a master regulator of mitochondrial biogenesis and stimulates autophagy, an essential homeostatic process that entails degradation of dysfunctional cellular components. In the heart, autophagic removal of dysfunctional mitochondria is protective against various types of cardiac stressors.[141,142,143]

In addition, SGLT2i might have beneficial effects on cardiac myocyte ion homeostasis. SGLT2i were initially shown to inhibit NHE,[144] and although this observation was subsequently refuted by others,[145] SGLT2i were recently reported to inhibit the late sodium current (I_{Na}).[146] Both NHE and I_{Na} contribute to the increase in cytosolic $[Na^+]$ in HFrEF, which causes diastolic dysfunction and prevents the Ca^{2+}-dependent stimulation of the Krebs cycle. Therefore, SGLT2i might improve ATP production and reduce oxidative stress in HFrEF by lowering cytosolic $[Na^+]$ via NHE and/or I_{Na} inhibition.[130]

Conclusions

The heart as a flexible omnivore has optimized its fuel utilization and adaptation of ATP production in mitochondria during great variations of cardiac workload. In HF and its metabolic comorbidities, cardiac metabolism loses metabolic flexibility and suffers disturbance in intermediate metabolism, redox state, and energetic efficiency. The clinical success of SGLT2i is a proof-of-concept that therapeutic interference with cardiac metabolism can further improve outcome in patients with HF beyond neuroendocrine blockade. Further research is needed to better understand the actual underlying mechanisms of these benefits, with a view to developing additional treatment approaches for patients with HF.

References

1. Taegtmeyer H. Carbohydrate interconversions and energy production. Circulation 1985;72:IV1–8.
2. Taegtmeyer H, Lam T, Davogustto G. Cardiac metabolism in perspective. Compr Physiol 2016;6:1675–99.
3. Bing RJ. Myocardial metabolism. Circulation 1955;12:635–47.
4. Wisneski JA, Gertz EW, Neese RA, Gruenke LD, Morris DL, Craig JC. Metabolic fate of extracted glucose in normal human myocardium. J Clin Invest 1985;76:1819–27.
5. Wisneski JA, Gertz EW, Neese RA, Mayr M. Myocardial metabolism of free fatty acids. Studies with 14C-labeled substrates in humans. J Clin Invest 1987;79:359–66.
6. Wisneski JA, Gertz EW, Neese RA, Gruenke LD, Craig JC. Dual carbon-labeled isotope experiments using D-[6–14C] glucose and L-[1,2,3–13C3] lactate: a new approach for investigating human myocardial metabolism during ischemia. J Am Coll Cardiol 1985;5:1138–46.

7. Bertero E, Maack C. Metabolic remodelling in heart failure. Nat Rev Cardiol 2018;15:457–470.

8. Gertz EW, Wisneski JA, Stanley WC, Neese RA. Myocardial substrate utilization during exercise in humans. Dual carbon-labeled carbohydrate isotope experiments. J Clin Invest 1988;82:2017–25.

9. Lopaschuk GD, Ussher JR, Folmes CD, Jaswal JS, Stanley WC. Myocardial fatty acid metabolism in health and disease. Physiol Rev 2010;90:207–58.

10. Banke NH, Wende AR, Leone TC, et al. Preferential oxidation of triacylglyceride-derived fatty acids in heart is augmented by the nuclear receptor PPARalpha. Circ Res 2010;107:233–41.

11. Bricker DK, Taylor EB, Schell JC, et al. A mitochondrial pyruvate carrier required for pyruvate uptake in yeast, Drosophila, and humans. Science 2012;337:96–100.

12. Herzig S, Raemy E, Montessuit S, et al. Identification and functional expression of the mitochondrial pyruvate carrier. Science 2012;337:93–6.

13. Stanley WC, Recchia FA, Lopaschuk GD. Myocardial substrate metabolism in the normal and failing heart. Physiol Rev 2005;85:1093–129.

14. Murashige D, Jang C, Neinast M, et al. Comprehensive quantification of fuel use by the failing and nonfailing human heart. Science 2020;370:364–8.

15. Randle PJ, Garland PB, Hales CN, Newsholme EA. The glucose fatty-acid cycle. Its role in insulin sensitivity and the metabolic disturbances of diabetes mellitus. Lancet 1963;1:785–9.

16. Hue L, Taegtmeyer H. The Randle cycle revisited: a new head for an old hat. Am J Physiol Endocrinol Metab 2009;297:E578–91.

17. Maack C, Lehrke M, Backs J, et al. Heart failure and diabetes: metabolic alterations and therapeutic interventions: a state-of-the-art review from the Translational Research Committee of the Heart Failure Association–European Society of Cardiology. Eur Heart J 2018;39:4243–54.

18. Bertero E, Maack C. Calcium signaling and reactive oxygen species in mitochondria. Circ Res 2018;122:1460–78.

19. Kirichok Y, Krapivinsky G, Clapham DE. The mitochondrial calcium uniporter is a highly selective ion channel. Nature 2004;427:360–4.

20. Rizzuto R, Pinton P, Carrington W, et al. Close contacts with the endoplasmic reticulum as determinants of mitochondrial Ca^{2+} responses. Science 1998;280:1763–6.

21. Paucek P, Jaburek M. Kinetics and ion specificity of $Na^{(+)}/Ca^{(2+)}$ exchange mediated by the reconstituted beef heart mitochondrial $Na^{(+)}/Ca^{(2+)}$ antiporter. Biochim Biophys Acta 2004;1659:83–91.

22. Boyman L, Williams GS, Lederer WJ. The growing importance of mitochondrial calcium in health and disease. Proc Natl Acad Sci U S A 2015;112:11150–1.

23. Milani-Nejad N, Janssen PM. Small and large animal models in cardiac contraction research: advantages and disadvantages. Pharmacol Ther 2014;141:235–49.

24. Bers DM. Excitation–Contraction Coupling and Cardiac Contractile Force, 2nd edition. Dordrecht: Kluwer Academic Publisher; 2001.

25. Neglia D, De Caterina A, Marraccini P, et al. Impaired myocardial metabolic reserve and substrate selection flexibility during stress in patients with idiopathic dilated cardiomyopathy. Am J Physiol Heart Circ Physiol 2007;293:H3270–8.

26. Grover-McKay M, Schwaiger M, Krivokapich J, Perloff JK, Phelps ME, Schelbert HR. Regional myocardial blood flow and metabolism at rest in mildly symptomatic patients with hypertrophic cardiomyopathy. J Am Coll Cardiol 1989;13:317–24.

27. Rosenblatt-Velin N, Montessuit C, Papageorgiou I, Terrand J, Lerch R. Postinfarction heart failure in rats is associated with upregulation of GLUT-1 and downregulation of genes of fatty acid metabolism. Cardiovasc Res 2001;52:407–16.

28. Kato T, Niizuma S, Inuzuka Y, et al. Analysis of metabolic remodeling in compensated left ventricular hypertrophy and heart failure. Circ Heart Fail 2010;3:420–30.

29. Degens H, de Brouwer KF, Gilde AJ, et al. Cardiac fatty acid metabolism is preserved in the compensated hypertrophic rat heart. Basic Res Cardiol 2006;101:17–26.

30. Chandler MP, Kerner J, Huang H, et al. Moderate severity heart failure does not involve a downregulation of myocardial fatty acid oxidation. Am J Physiol Heart Circ Physiol 2004;287:H1538–43.

31. Osorio JC, Stanley WC, Linke A, et al. Impaired myocardial fatty acid oxidation and reduced protein expression of retinoid X receptor-alpha in pacing-induced heart failure. Circulation 2002;106:606–12.

32. Bedi KC Jr, Snyder NW, Brandimarto J, et al. Evidence for intramyocardial disruption of lipid metabolism and increased myocardial ketone utilization in advanced human heart failure. Circulation 2016;133:706–16.

33. Davila-Roman VG, Vedala G, Herrero P, et al. Altered myocardial fatty acid and glucose metabolism in idiopathic dilated cardiomyopathy. J Am Coll Cardiol 2002;40:271–7.

34. Barger PM, Brandt JM, Leone TC, Weinheimer CJ, Kelly DP. Deactivation of peroxisome proliferator-activated receptor-alpha during cardiac hypertrophic growth. J Clin Invest 2000;105:1723–30.

35. Lahey R, Wang X, Carley AN, Lewandowski ED. Dietary fat supply to failing hearts determines dynamic lipid signaling for nuclear receptor activation and oxidation of stored triglyceride. Circulation 2014;130:1790–9.

36. Krishnan J, Suter M, Windak R, et al. Activation of a HIF1alpha-PPARgamma axis underlies the integration of glycolytic and lipid anabolic pathways in pathologic cardiac hypertrophy. Cell Metab 2009;9:512–24.

37. Voros G, Ector J, Garweg C, et al. Increased cardiac uptake of ketone bodies and free fatty acids in human heart failure and hypertrophic left ventricular remodeling. Circ Heart Fail 2018;11:e004953.

38. Diakos NA, Navankasattusas S, Abel ED, et al. Evidence of glycolysis up-regulation and pyruvate mitochondrial oxidation mismatch during mechanical unloading of the failing human heart: implications for cardiac reloading and conditioning. JACC Basic Transl Sci 2016;1:432–44.

39. Lei B, Lionetti V, Young ME, et al. Paradoxical downregulation of the glucose oxidation pathway despite enhanced flux in severe heart failure. J Mol Cell Cardiol 2004;36:567–76.

40. Sorokina N, O'Donnell JM, McKinney RD, et al. Recruitment of compensatory pathways to sustain oxidative flux with reduced carnitine palmitoyltransferase I activity characterizes inefficiency in energy metabolism in hypertrophied hearts. Circulation 2007;115:2033–41.

41. Pound KM, Sorokina N, Ballal K, et al. Substrate-enzyme competition attenuates upregulated anaplerotic flux through malic enzyme in hypertrophied rat heart and restores triacylglyceride content: attenuating upregulated anaplerosis in hypertrophy. Circ Res 2009;104:805–12.

42. Ritterhoff J, Young S, Villet O, et al. Metabolic remodeling promotes cardiac hypertrophy by directing glucose to aspartate biosynthesis. Circ Res 2020;126:182–96.

43. Fernandez-Caggiano M, Kamynina A, Francois AA, et al. Mitochondrial pyruvate carrier abundance mediates pathological cardiac hypertrophy. Nat Metab 2020;2:1223–31.

44. Aubert G, Martin OJ, Horton JL, et al. The failing heart relies on ketone bodies as a fuel. Circulation 2016;133:698–705.

45. Lommi J, Koskinen P, Naveri H, Harkonen M, Kupari M. Heart failure ketosis. J Intern Med 1997;242:231–8.

46. Cahill GF, Jr. Fuel metabolism in starvation. Annu Rev Nutr 2006;26:1–22.

47. Nielsen R, Moller N, Gormsen LC, *et al.* Cardiovascular effects of treatment with the ketone body 3-hydroxybutyrate in chronic heart failure patients. Circulation 2019;139:2129–41.

48. Sun H, Olson KC, Gao C, *et al.* Catabolic defect of branched-chain amino acids promotes heart failure. Circulation 2016;133:2038–49.

49. Li T, Zhang Z, Kolwicz SC, Jr. et al. Defective branched-chain amino acid catabolism disrupts glucose metabolism and sensitizes the heart to ischemia-reperfusion injury. Cell Metab 2017;25:374–85.

50. Magnusson M, Lewis GD, Ericson U, *et al.* A diabetes-predictive amino acid score and future cardiovascular disease. Eur Heart J 2013;34:1982–9.

51. Ruiz-Canela M, Toledo E, Clish CB, *et al.* Plasma branched-chain amino acids and incident cardiovascular disease in the PREDIMED Trial. Clin Chem 2016;62:582–92.

52. Chen M, Gao C, Yu J, *et al.* Therapeutic effect of targeting branched-chain amino acid catabolic flux in pressure-overload induced heart failure. J Am Heart Assoc 2019;8:e011625.

53. Erickson JR, Pereira L, Wang L, *et al.* Diabetic hyperglycaemia activates CaMKII and arrhythmias by O-linked glycosylation. Nature 2013;502:372–6.

54. Kronlage M, Dewenter M, Grosso J, *et al.* O-GlcNAcylation of histone deacetylase 4 protects the diabetic heart from failure. Circulation 2019;140:580–94.

55. Matsuhashi T, Hishiki T, Zhou H, *et al.* Activation of pyruvate dehydrogenase by dichloroacetate has the potential to induce epigenetic remodeling in the heart. J Mol Cell Cardiol 2015;82:116–24.

56. Karamanlidis G, Lee CF, Garcia-Menendez L, *et al.* Mitochondrial complex I deficiency increases protein acetylation and accelerates heart failure. Cell Metab 2013;18:239–50.

57. Horton JL, Martin OJ, Lai L, *et al.* Mitochondrial protein hyperacetylation in the failing heart. JCI Insight 2016;2:e84897.

58. Tong D, Schiattarella GG, Jiang N, *et al.* NAD(+) repletion reverses heart failure with preserved ejection fraction. Circ Res 2021;128:1629–41.

59. Koentges C, Pfeil K, Schnick T, *et al.* SIRT3 deficiency impairs mitochondrial and contractile function in the heart. Basic Res Cardiol 2015;110:36.

60. Davidson MT, Grimsrud PA, Lai L, *et al.* Extreme acetylation of the cardiac mitochondrial proteome does not promote heart failure. Circ Res 2020;127:1094–108.

61. Hobai IA, O'Rourke B. Decreased sarcoplasmic reticulum calcium content is responsible for defective excitation-contraction coupling in canine heart failure. Circulation 2001;103:1577–84.

62. Bers DM. Altered cardiac myocyte Ca regulation in heart failure. Physiology (Bethesda) 2006;21:380–7.

63. Schwinger RH, Wang J, Frank K, *et al.* Reduced sodium pump alpha1, alpha3, and beta1-isoform protein levels and Na$^+$, K$^+$-ATPase activity but unchanged Na$^+$-Ca^{2+} exchanger protein levels in human heart failure. Circulation 1999;99:2105–12.

64. Baartscheer A, Schumacher CA, van Borren MM, Belterman CN, Coronel R, Fiolet JW. Increased Na$^+$/H$^+$-exchange activity is the cause of increased [Na$^+$]i and underlies disturbed calcium handling in the rabbit pressure and volume overload heart failure model. Cardiovasc Res 2003;57:1015–24.

65. Valdivia CR, Chu WW, Pu J, *et al.* Increased late sodium current in myocytes from a canine heart failure model and from failing human heart. J Mol Cell Cardiol 2005;38:475–83.

66. Pieske B, Maier LS, Piacentino V 3rd, Weisser J, Hasenfuss G, Houser S. Rate dependence of [Na$^+$]i and contractility in nonfailing and failing human myocardium. Circulation 2002;106:447–53.

67. Pinali C, Bennett H, Davenport JB, Trafford AW, Kitmitto A. Three-dimensional reconstruction of cardiac sarcoplasmic reticulum reveals a continuous network linking transverse-tubules: this organization is perturbed in heart failure. Circ Res 2013;113:1219–30.

68. Kohlhaas M, Maack C. Adverse bioenergetic consequences of Na$^+$-Ca^{2+} exchanger-mediated Ca^{2+} influx in cardiac myocytes. Circulation 2010;122:2273–80.

69. Maack C, Cortassa S, Aon MA, Ganesan AN, Liu T, O'Rourke B. Elevated cytosolic Na$^+$ decreases mitochondrial Ca^{2+} uptake during excitation-contraction coupling and impairs energetic adaptation in cardiac myocytes. Circ Res 2006;99:172–82.

70. Kohlhaas M, Liu T, Knopp A, *et al.* Elevated cytosolic Na$^+$ increases mitochondrial formation of reactive oxygen species in failing cardiac myocytes. Circulation 2010;121:1606–13.

71. Nickel AG, von Hardenberg A, Hohl M, *et al.* Reversal of mitochondrial transhydrogenase causes oxidative stress in heart failure. Cell Metab 2015;22:472–84.

72. Ide T, Tsutsui H, Kinugawa S, *et al.* Mitochondrial electron transport complex I is a potential source of oxygen free radicals in the failing myocardium. Circ Res 1999;85:357–63.

73. Aon MA, Cortassa S, Marban E, O'Rourke B. Synchronized whole cell oscillations in mitochondrial metabolism triggered by a local release of reactive oxygen species in cardiac myocytes. J Biol Chem 2003;278:44735–44.

74. Zorov DB, Filburn CR, Klotz L-O, Zweier JL, Sollott SJ. Reactive oxygen species (ROS-induced) ROS release. A new phenomenon accompanying induction of the mitochondrial permeability transition in cardiac myocytes. J Exp Med 2000;192:1001–14.

75. Kwong JQ, Lu X, Correll RN, *et al.* The mitochondrial calcium uniporter selectively matches metabolic output to acute contractile stress in the heart. Cell Rep 2015;12:15–22.

76. Luongo TS, Lambert JP, Gross P, *et al.* The mitochondrial Na(+)/Ca(2+) exchanger is essential for Ca(2+) homeostasis and viability. Nature 2017;545:93–7.

77. Neubauer S. The failing heart: an engine out of fuel. N Engl J Med 2007;356:1140–51.

78. Nascimben L, Ingwall JS, Pauletto P, *et al.* Creatine kinase system in failing and nonfailing human myocardium. Circulation 1996;94:1894–901.

79. Lygate CA, Aksentijevic D, Dawson D, *et al.* Living without creatine: unchanged exercise capacity and response to chronic myocardial infarction in creatine-deficient mice. Circ Res 2013;112:945–55.

80. Sequeira V, Bertero E, Maack C. Energetic drain driving hypertrophic cardiomyopathy. FEBS Lett 2019;593:1616–26.

81. Störk S, Hense HW, Zentgraf C, *et al.* Pharmacotherapy according to treatment guidelines is associated with lower mortality in a community-based sample of patients with chronic heart failure: a prospective cohort study. Eur J Heart Fail 2008;10:1236–45.

82. Bertero E, Dudek J, Cochain C, *et al.* Immuno-metabolic interfaces in cardiac disease and failure. Cardiovasc Res 2022;118:37–52.

83. Ng M, Fleming T, Robinson M, *et al.* Global, regional, and national prevalence of overweight and obesity in children and adults during 1980–2013: a systematic analysis for the Global Burden of Disease Study 2013. Lancet 2014;384:766–81.

84. Braunwald E. Diabetes, heart failure, and renal dysfunction: the vicious circles. Progr Cardiovasc Dis 2019;62:298–302.

85. Robertson J, Lindgren M, Schaufelberger M, *et al.* Body mass index in young women and risk of cardiomyopathy: a long-term follow-up study in Sweden. Circulation 2020;141:520–9.

86. Robertson J, Schaufelberger M, Lindgren M, *et al.* Higher body mass index in adolescence predicts cardiomyopathy risk in midlife. Circulation 2019;140:117–25.

87. McDonagh TA, Metra M, Adamo M, *et al.* 2021 ESC Guidelines for the diagnosis and treatment of acute and chronic heart failure. Eur Heart J 2021;42:3599–726.

88. von Hardenberg A, Maack C. Mitochondrial therapies in heart failure. Handb Exp Pharmacol 2017;243:491–514.

89. Zhao K, Zhao G-M, Wu D, *et al.* Cell-permeable peptide antioxidants targeted to inner mitochondrial membrane inhibit mitochondrial swelling, oxidative cell death, and reperfusion injury. J Biol Chem 2004;279:34682–90.

90. Szeto HH. First-in-class cardiolipin-protective compound as a therapeutic agent to restore mitochondrial bioenergetics. Br J Pharmacol 2014;171:2029–50.

91. Szeto HH, Schiller PW. Novel therapies targeting inner mitochondrial membrane—from discovery to clinical development. Pharm Res 2011;28:2669–79.

92. Szeto HH. First-in-class cardiolipin-protective compound as a therapeutic agent to restore mitochondrial bioenergetics. Br J Pharmacol 2014;171:2029–50.

93. Dai D-F, Chen T, Szeto H, *et al.* Mitochondrial targeted antioxidant peptide ameliorates hypertensive cardiomyopathy. J Am Coll Cardiol 2011;58:73–82.

94. Nickel AG, von Hardenberg A, Hohl M, *et al.* Reversal of mitochondrial transhydrogenase causes oxidative stress in heart failure. Cell Metab 2015;22:472–84.

95. Butler J, Khan MS, Anker SD, *et al.* Effects of elamipretide on left ventricular function in patients with heart failure with reduced ejection fraction: the PROGRESS-HF phase 2 yrial. J Card Fail 2020;26:429–37.

96. Daubert MA, Yow E, Dunn G, *et al.* Novel mitochondria-targeting peptide in heart failure treatment: a randomized, placebo-controlled trial of elamipretide. Circ Heart Fail 2017;10:e004389.

97. Schwarz K, Siddiqi N, Singh S, Neil CJ, Dawson DK, Frenneaux MP. The breathing heart: mitochondrial respiratory chain dysfunction in cardiac disease. Int J Cardiol 2014;171:134–43.

98. Mugoni V, Postel R, Catanzaro V, *et al.* Ubiad1 is an antioxidant enzyme that regulates eNOS activity by CoQ10 synthesis. Cell 2013;152:504–18.

99. Mortensen SA. Coenzyme Q10: will this natural substance become a guideline-directed adjunctive therapy in heart failure? JACC Heart Failure 2015;3:270–1.

100. Mortensen SA, Vadhanavikit S, Muratsu K, Folkers K. Coenzyme Q10: clinical benefits with biochemical correlates suggesting a scientific breakthrough in the management of chronic heart failure. Int J Tissue React 1990;12:155–62.

101. Mortensen SA, Rosenfeldt F, Kumar A, *et al.* The effect of coenzyme Q10 on morbidity and mortality in chronic heart failure: results from Q-SYMBIO: a randomized double-blind trial. JACC: Heart Failure 2014;2:641–9.

102. Khan MS, Khan F, Fonarow GC, *et al.* Dietary interventions and nutritional supplements for heart failure: a systematic appraisal and evidence map. Eur J Heart Fail 2021;23:1468–76.

103. Fotino AD, Thompson-Paul AM, Bazzano LA. Effect of coenzyme Q(1)(0) supplementation on heart failure: a meta-analysis. Am J Clin Nutr 2013;97:268–75.

104. Kantor PF, Lucien A, Kozak R, Lopaschuk GD. The antianginal drug trimetazidine shifts cardiac energy metabolism from fatty acid oxidation to glucose oxidation by inhibiting mitochondrial long-chain 3-ketoacyl coenzyme A thiolase. Circ Res 2000; 86:580–8.

105. Lopaschuk GD, Barr R, Thomas PD, Dyck JR. Beneficial effects of trimetazidine in *ex vivo* working ischemic hearts are due to a stimulation of glucose oxidation secondary to inhibition of long-chain 3-ketoacyl coenzyme a thiolase. Circ Res 2003;93:e33–7.

106. Fragasso G, Perseghin G, De Cobelli F, *et al.* Effects of metabolic modulation by trimetazidine on left ventricular function and phosphocreatine/adenosine triphosphate ratio in patients with heart failure. Eur Heart J 2006;27:942–8.

107. Tuunanen H, Engblom E, Naum A, *et al.* Trimetazidine, a metabolic modulator, has cardiac and extracardiac benefits in idiopathic dilated cardiomyopathy. Circulation 2008;118:1250–8.

108. Wang W, Zhang L, Battiprolu PK, *et al.* Malonyl CoA decarboxylase inhibition improves cardiac function post-myocardial infarction. JACC Basic Transl Sci 2019;4:385–400.

109. Liu B, Clanachan AS, Schulz R, Lopaschuk GD. Cardiac efficiency is improved after ischemia by altering both the source and fate of protons. Circ Res 1996;79:940–8.

110. Lydell CP, Chan A, Wambolt RB, *et al.* Pyruvate dehydrogenase and the regulation of glucose oxidation in hypertrophied rat hearts. Cardiovasc Res 2002;53:841–51.

111. Wargovich TJ, MacDonald RG, Hill JA, Feldman RL, Stacpoole PW, Pepine CJ. Myocardial metabolic and hemodynamic effects of dichloroacetate in coronary artery disease. Am J Cardiol 1988;61:65–70.

112. Bersin RM, Wolfe C, Kwasman M, *et al.* Improved hemodynamic function and mechanical efficiency in congestive heart failure with sodium dichloroacetate. J Am Coll Cardiol 1994;23:1617–24.

113. Lewis JF, DaCosta M, Wargowich T, Stacpoole P. Effects of dichloroacetate in patients with congestive heart failure. Clin Cardiol 1998;21:888–92.

114. Von Haehling S, Jankowska EA, van Veldhuisen DJ, Ponikowski P, Anker SD. Iron deficiency and cardiovascular disease. Nat Rev Cardiol 2015;12:659–69.

115. Jankowska EA, Rozentryt P, Witkowska A, *et al.* Iron deficiency: an ominous sign in patients with systolic chronic heart failure. Eur Heart J 2010;31:1872–80.

116. Anker SD, Comin Colet J, Filippatos G, *et al.* Ferric carboxymaltose in patients with heart failure and iron deficiency. N Engl J Med 2009;361:2436–48.

117. Jankowska EA, Tkaczyszyn M, Suchocki, *et al.* Effects of intravenous iron therapy in iron-deficient patients with systolic heart failure: a meta-analysis of randomized controlled trials. Eur J Heart Fail 2016;18:786–95.

118. Ponikowski P, van Veldhuisen DJ, Comin Colet J, *et al.* Beneficial effects of long-term intravenous iron therapy with ferric carboxymaltose in patients with symptomatic heart failure and iron deficiency. Eur Heart J 2015;36:657–68.

119. Ponikowski P, Kirwan BA, Anker SD, *et al.* Ferric carboxymaltose for iron deficiency at discharge after acute heart failure: a multicentre, double-blind, randomised, controlled trial. Lancet 2020;396:1895–904.

120. Stugiewicz M, Tkaczyszyn M, Kasztura M, Banasiak W, Ponikowski P, Jankowska EA. The influence of iron deficiency on the functioning of skeletal muscles: experimental evidence and clinical implications. Eur J Heart Fail 2016;18:762–73.

121. Khechaduri A, Bayeva M, Chang H-C, Ardehali H. Heme levels are increased in human failing hearts. J Am Coll Cardiol 2013;61:1884–93.

122. Leszek P, Sochanowicz B, Szperl M, *et al.* Myocardial iron homeostasis in advanced chronic heart failure patients. Int J Cardiol 2012;159:47–52.

123. Leszek P, Sochanowicz B, Brzóska K, *et al.* Does myocardial iron load determine the severity of heart insufficiency? Int J Cardiol 2015;182:191–3.

124. Melenovsky V, Petrak J, Mracek T, *et al.* Myocardial iron content and mitochondrial function in human heart failure: a direct tissue analysis. Eur J Heart Fail 2017;19:522–30.

125. Martens P, Dupont M, Dauw J, *et al.* The effect of intravenous ferric carboxymaltose on cardiac reverse remodelling following cardiac resynchronization therapy-the IRON-CRT trial. Eur Heart J 2021;42:4905–14.

126. Diguet N, Trammell SAJ, Tannous C, *et al.* Nicotinamide riboside preserves cardiac function in a mouse model of dilated cardiomyopathy. Circulation 2018;137:2256–73.

127. Lee CF, Chavez JD, Garcia-Menendez L, *et al.* Normalization of NAD^+ redox balance as a therapy for heart failure. Circulation 2016;134:883–94.

128. Abdellatif M, Trummer-Herbst V, Koser F, *et al.* Nicotinamide for the treatment of heart failure with preserved ejection fraction. Sci Transl Med 2021;13:eabd7064.

129. O'Brien KD, Tian R. Boosting mitochondrial metabolism with dietary supplements in heart failure. Nat Rev Cardiol 2021; 18:685–6.

130. Vignier N, Chatzifrangkeskou M, Morales Rodriguez B, *et al.* Rescue of biosynthesis of nicotinamide adenine dinucleotide protects the heart in cardiomyopathy caused by lamin A/C gene mutation. Hum Mol Genet 2018;27:3870–80.

131. Hsu CP, Oka S, Shao D, Hariharan N, Sadoshima J. Nicotinamide phosphoribosyltransferase regulates cell survival through NAD^+ synthesis in cardiac myocytes. Circ Res 2009;105:481–91.

132. Byun J, Oka SI, Imai N, *et al.* Both gain and loss of NAMPT function promote pressure overload-induced heart failure. Am J Physiol Heart Circ Physiol 2019;317:H711–25.

133. Zannad F, Ferreira JP, Pocock SJ, *et al.* SGLT2 inhibitors in patients with heart failure with reduced ejection fraction: a meta-analysis of the EMPEROR-Reduced and DAPA-HF trials. Lancet 2020;396:819–29.

134. Anker SD, Butler J, Filippatos G, *et al.* Empagliflozin in heart failure with a preserved ejection fraction. N Engl J Med 2021;385:1451–61.

135. Beadle RM, Williams LK, Kuehl M, *et al.* Improvement in cardiac energetics by perhexiline in heart failure due to dilated cardiomyopathy. JACC Heart Fail 2015;3:202–11

136. Santos-Gallego CG, Requena-Ibanez JA, San Antonio R, *et al.* Empagliflozin ameliorates adverse left ventricular remodeling in nondiabetic heart failure by enhancing myocardial energetics. J Am Coll Cardiol 2019;73:1931–44.

137. Deng Y, Xie M, Li Q, *et al.* Targeting mitochondria-inflammation circuit by β-hydroxybutyrate mitigates HFpEF. Circ Res 2021;128:232–45.

138. Al Jobori H, Daniele G, Adams J, *et al.* Determinants of the increase in ketone concentration during SGLT2 inhibition in NGT, IFG and T2DM patients. Diabetes Obes Metab 2017;19:809–13.

139. Ferrannini E, Baldi S, Frascerra S, *et al.* Shift to fatty substrate utilization in response to sodium–glucose cotransporter 2 inhibition in subjects without diabetes and patients with type 2 diabetes. Diabetes 2016;65:1190–5.

140. Packer M. Role of deranged energy deprivation signaling in the pathogenesis of cardiac and renal disease in states of perceived nNutrient overabundance. Circulation 2020;141:2095–105.

141. Shirakabe A, Zhai P, Ikeda Y, *et al.* Drp1-dependent mitochondrial autophagy plays a protective role against pressure overload-induced mitochondrial dysfunction and heart failure. Circulation 2016;133:1249–63.

142. Wang B, Nie J, Wu L, *et al.* AMPKalpha2 protects against the development of heart failure by enhancing mitophagy via PINK1 phosphorylation. Circ Res 2018;122:712–29.

143. Eisenberg T, Abdellatif M, Schroeder S, *et al.* Cardioprotection and lifespan extension by the natural polyamine spermidine. Nat Med 2016;22:1428–38.

144. Baartscheer A, Schumacher CA, Wüst RC, *et al.* Empagliflozin decreases myocardial cytoplasmic Na(+) through inhibition of the cardiac Na(+)/H(+) exchanger in rats and rabbits. Diabetologia 2017;60:568–73.

145. Chung YJ, Park KC, Tokar S, *et al.* Off-target effects of SGLT2 blockers: empagliflozin does not inhibit Na^+/H^+ exchanger-1 or lower $[Na^+]i$ in the heart. Cardiovasc Res 2021;117:2794–806.

146. Philippaert K, Kalyaanamoorthy S, Fatehi M, *et al.* Cardiac late sodium channel current is a molecular target for the sodium/glucose cotransporter 2 inhibitor empagliflozin. Circulation 2021;143:2188–204.

CHAPTER 5.3

Ventricular remodelling

Javier Díez and Hans-Peter
Brunner-La Rocca

Contents

Introduction

Although often used in the context of eccentric hypertrophy, ventricular remodelling is defined as any phenotypic changes to ventricular chamber geometry and function that occur in response to sustained physiological or pathological stress.[1] Ventricular remodelling related to pathological stress is associated with progressive development of heart failure (HF) and poor clinical outcomes (➲ Figure 5.3.1). The progressive impairment of function in the remodelled ventricle is likely due to a number of alterations in the histological structure, oxygen and nutrition supply, energy efficiency, and electrical activity of the myocardium (➲ Figure 5.3.1).[2] Of note, remodelling is a dynamic process. For example, a patient can have progressive adverse remodelling over time after the onset of HF, and then experience reverse remodelling with guideline-directed therapy. Adverse remodelling can recur when guideline-directed medical therapy is withdrawn or there is further progression of HF due to a new trigger.[3]

This chapter is divided into three parts. In the first part, the causes and mechanisms triggering and influencing adverse ventricular remodelling, as well as the variable resulting geometric and functional phenotypes, are discussed. In the second part, the diverse myocardial cellular and molecular alterations underlying the deleterious consequences of the remodelling process for the heart are reviewed. In the third part, an outlook on therapeutic interventions related to ventricular remodelling is given.

Remodelling responses of the ventricle to pathological stress

Ventricular remodelling can be roughly divided into two groups—concentric and eccentric—although there is some overlap. Concentric remodelling is defined as ventricular hypertrophy with increased wall thickness, but without dilatation and usually with normal systolic function. If symptoms of HF are present, these patients have HF with preserved ejection fraction (HFpEF), previously called diastolic HF. Still, systolic function may be reduced in HFpEF if measures other than left ventricular ejection fraction (LVEF) are considered. Thus, systolic longitudinal strain may be reduced in a significant number of HFpEF patients and seems to be related to the severity of HF.[4] Moreover, LVEF may be slightly reduced in HF patients with concentric remodelling, that is, having HF with mid-range LVEF (HFmrEF).[5] Eccentric remodelling is defined as ventricular hypertrophy with significant dilatation. Systolic function can be either normal or reduced, although eccentric remodelling is typically seen in patients with reduced LVEF (HF with reduced ejection fraction (HFrEF)), previously called systolic HF. Wall thickness is often normal, but muscle mass is increased due to ventricular dilatation.

The resulting adaptation of the ventricle(s) largely depends on the underlying cause, but genetic predisposition also plays a role, most likely not only in genetically related

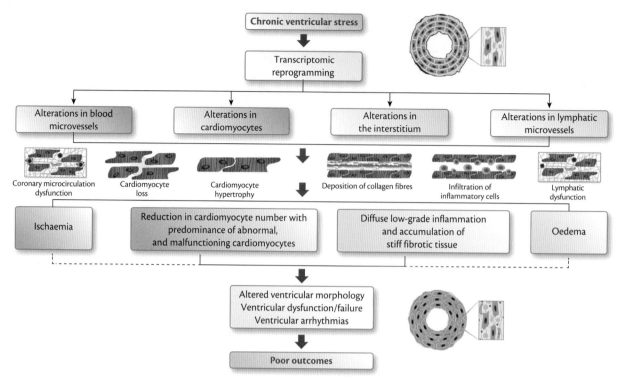

Figure 5.3.1 Sequence of alterations that develop in the microstructural components of the myocardium in the chronically stressed ventricle and that, in turn, contribute to the development of alterations in ventricular morphology and function associated with poor outcomes of ventricular remodelling.

cardiomyopathies. Pressure overload primarily results in concentric hypertrophy, whereas volume overload and myocardial injury typically result in eccentric hypertrophy.[6] Therefore, the most important underlying causes of concentric left ventricular (LV) remodelling are arterial hypertension and aortic stenosis. The most important genetic cause is hypertrophic cardiomyopathy (HCM), with a link between significant concentric remodelling in HCM gene carriers and hypertension.[7] However, a relatively common and previously underestimated cause of HFpEF can also be amyloid deposition.[8]

The most common causes of eccentric remodelling are volume overload (e.g. due to mitral or aortic regurgitation) and loss of myocardium (e.g. due to myocardial infarction or myocarditis).[9] Importantly, the remodelling process requires time. Accordingly, early phases of myocardial injury may result in reduction of cardiac function without changes in size or structure, whereas eccentric remodelling occurs within weeks, months, or even years. Neurohumoral activation plays an important role in this adaptation process. Its inhibition not only may improve outcome, but also may even prevent or reverse, at least in part, eccentric remodelling.[10]

Traditionally, eccentric hypertrophy was seen as the final common pathway of all cardiac injury, that is, also in underlying diseases primarily resulting in concentric hypertrophy, and the LVEF seen as a continuum related to the severity of HF. This might be true in some patients with, for example, aortic stenosis. However, even in aortic stenosis, the development of reduced LVEF may begin early and before aortic stenosis becomes severe in some patients.[11] Thus, such patients may develop an eccentric phenotype even with pressure overload, possibly determined by

the underlying (genetic) predisposition. The recent findings in HFpEF question the common pathophysiology of concentric and eccentric remodelling, as the neurohumoral concept is obviously wrong in HFpEF. All therapies being beneficial in HFrEF failed in HFpEF,[12] indicating that the two must be seen as distinct disease entities. The pathophysiology and adaptive mechanism in HFrEF and eccentric remodelling seem to be relatively homogeneous and related to the neurohumoral concept, independently of the underlying disease in HFrEF.[5] However, many of the neurohumoral pathways are also altered in HFpEF, but their treatment obviously has no or very little effects clinically. Alternative pathways such as inflammation have been suggested as a central mechanism in HFpEF.[13] However, results regarding their role in HFpEF are not uniform.[14] Importantly, inhibition of neurohumoral stimulation reduces inflammation but has no effect in HFpEF.[15] Similarly, fibrosis is considered a central factor in HFpEF, but inhibition by mineralocorticoid receptor antagonism has little, if any, effect in HFpEF.[16] Taken together, whereas important factors with resulting microstructural and electrophysiological alterations in eccentric remodelling are well understood, the pathophysiological key factors in understanding pathological concentric remodelling are less clear.

Myocardial alterations during the remodelling process

The process of adverse ventricular remodelling entails substantial transcriptional reprogramming mainly due to altered epigenetic regulation of gene expression.[17] The transcriptomic reprogramming, combined with age-, sex-, and environment-related influences, triggers the activation of a complex series of signalling pathways, leading to a number of interrelated microstructural, metabolic, and electrophysiological alterations (➲ Figure 5.3.1).[18]

Microstructural alterations

The main alterations of the myocardium in the remodelled ventricle include cardiomyocyte hypertrophy and death, interstitial inflammation and alterations in the collagen matrix, and changes in blood and lymphatic microvessels.

In the adult stressed ventricle, individual cardiomyocytes increase in size as a result of *de novo* protein synthesis and spatial reorganization of sarcomeres, and the ventricular wall develops hypertrophy to reduce ventricular wall stress.[19] The hypertrophic geometry varies according to the type of stress and resulting hypertrophy, as discussed above. Whereas in eccentric hypertrophy cardiomyocytes grow in length, in concentric hypertrophy they grow in width. Recent investigation has identified phosphoinositide 3-kinase (PI3K), Akt, and mammalian target of rapamycin (mTOR) as a major downstream effector pathway involved in cardiomyocyte hypertrophy.[20] Dysregulation of mechanisms involved in cardiomyocyte contractility, such as excitation–contraction coupling, a process that tightly regulates calcium (Ca^{2+}) influx and uptake, is a common feature of pathological cardiomyocyte hypertrophy.[21]

Cardiomyocyte death due to necrosis, apoptosis, or autophagy is a typical feature of ventricular remodelling.[22] Whereas necrosis is critical in HF associated with ischaemia in myocardial infarction or myocarditis, apoptosis plays a role in ventricular remodelling associated with haemodynamic overload.[23] Cardiomyocyte loss due to high rates of cell death may facilitate adverse remodelling through both a reduction in the number of contractile cells and side-to-side slippage of cells resulting in mural thinning and chamber dilatation.[24] Mitochondrial alterations (i.e. loss of transmembrane proton gradient and accumulation of misfolded proteins) are key players in cell death.[25]

Immune cells are recruited to the myocardial interstitium to remove dead cardiomyocytes, which is essential for healing.[26] Insufficient clearance of dying cardiomyocytes has been shown to promote unfavourable remodelling through unresolved immune reaction. Additionally, cardiomyocyte mitochondrial DNA that escapes from autophagy causes inflammation during the remodelling process.[27] Recent evidence supports a pivotal role for CCR2+ macrophages that interact with other immune cell populations, including infiltrating monocytes, through the Toll-like receptor and trigger interleukin-1-mediated cascades, inducing the synthesis of cytokines and chemokines involved in apoptosis and fibrosis.[28]

Alterations of the collagen matrix are important in the remodelled ventricle in a double sense. On the one hand, focal post-infarct scar and diffuse interstitial fibrosis result from excessive *de novo* synthesis of highly cross-linked and stiff collagen type I and III fibres by activated fibroblasts and fibroblasts differentiated to myofibroblasts under the influence of transforming growth factor beta (TGF-β), among many other pro-fibrotic factors.[29] Diffuse fibrosis is associated with increased passive stiffness and filling pressures that contribute to diastolic dysfunction. On the other hand, excessive degradation of the physiological endomysial and perimysial collagen scaffold surrounding groups of cardiomyocytes and individual cardiomyocytes, respectively, with subsequent cell slippage and loss of synchrony and synergy during contraction, might facilitate LV dilatation and impair systolic function.[29]

Structural changes of the coronary microcirculation in ventricular remodelling include reduced maximal cross-sectional area of pre-arterioles and arterioles due to hyperplasia, hypertrophy, and altered alignment of vascular smooth muscle cells, with encroachment of the tunica media into the lumen, and reduced capillary density.[30] Whereas persistent changes in tone and circumferential wall tension drive arteriolar changes, rarefaction or inadequate vascular growth is involved in the diminution of capillaries.[30] Structural alterations in coronary microcirculation facilitate myocardial ischaemia/hypoxia, namely when endothelial dysfunction is also present.

In the remodelled ventricle, there is a reduction in the number of lymphatic microvessels that leads to interstitial accumulation of fluids, proteins, lipids, and immune cells, resulting in myocardial oedema and inflammation.[31] Both stimulate the differentiation of fibroblasts into myofibroblasts, triggering a pro-fibrotic response and diffuse interstitial fibrosis that may further limit lymphatic uptake.[32] All the microstructural alterations reviewed here can coexist in the remodelled myocardium, regardless of the type of stress leading to the remodelling process, and ➲ Table 5.3.1 shows how they are distributed according to the clinical phenotype of ventricular remodelling.

Metabolic alterations

Adverse ventricular remodelling is accompanied by alterations of substrate uptake and utilization, oxidative phosphorylation, and energy shuttling via phosphotransfer systems.[33] In spite of the switching of the main energy substrates from fatty acids to glycolysis, the relative contribution of glucose utilization to adenosine triphosphate (ATP) production is not increased, as this change is not matched by an increase in pyruvate oxidation in the mitochondria. In addition, the concomitant decrease in fatty acid oxidation is not matched by a decrease in fatty acid uptake, resulting in the accumulation of toxic lipid intermediates. Furthermore, shuttling of high-energy phosphates via the creatine shuttle is impaired. Altogether, these alterations manifest as a 30% decrease in ATP concentration.

Besides impaired ATP production, mitochondrial dysfunction also results in the generation of mitochondrial reactive oxygen species, which contribute to various cellular dysfunctions in the remodelled ventricle, including stimulation of cardiomyocyte hypertrophy and death,[34] as well as activation of fibroblasts and their differentiation into myofibroblasts.[35]

Table 5.3.1 Alterations of myocardial microstructure according to the clinical phenotype of ventricular remodelling

		Clinical phenotype	
		Eccentric hypertrophy with reduced LVEF	**Concentric hypertrophy with preserved LVEF**
Microstructural alterations	Alterations of cardiomyocyte	Longitudinal hypertrophy Severe necrosis Presence of apoptosis Presence of autophagy? Severe reduction in cell number	Transversal hypertrophy Non-severe necrosis Presence of apoptosis Presence of autophagy? Non-severe reduction in cell number
	Alterations of interstitium	Oedema Severe inflammation Focal post-infarct scarring Non-severe diffuse interstitial fibrosis Collagen scaffold disruption	Oedema Non-severe inflammation Severe diffuse interstitial fibrosis
	Alterations of microvasculature	Non-severe pre-arteriolar and arteriolar wall changes Non-severe blood capillary rarefaction Decreased lymphangiogenesis	Severe arteriolar and arteriolar wall changes Severe blood capillary rarefaction Decreased lymphangiogenesis

Electrophysiological alterations

The electrical activity of the remodelled ventricle is altered via two main mechanisms: distortion of the electrophysiological harmony of the myocardium caused by fibrosis,[36] and alteration of the electrical activity of the cardiomyocyte due to changes in density and spatial distribution of multiple electrogenic transport processes (e.g. outward potassium (K^+) currents, inward Ca^{2+} currents, the late component of the inward sodium (Na^+) current).[37] Whereas the former induces a myocardial arrhythmogenic substrate by slowing action potential propagation and facilitating re-entry, the latter promotes repolarization abnormalities, specifically prolongation of action potential duration. These electrophysiological alterations are not restricted to the ventricular myocardium but are frequently present in the atrial myocardium, thus increasing susceptibility to atrial fibrillation in patients with ventricular remodelling and HF.[38]

Impact of therapy on ventricular remodelling and future directions

Ventricular remodelling is associated with poor prognosis, whereas reverse remodelling indicates improved outcome, particularly in HFrEF.[5] In HFpEF, the association between reverse remodelling and better outcome is less clear.

Novel therapies may act via different pathways than neurohumoral blockade. Thus, sodium–glucose cotransporter 2 (SGLT2) inhibitors were found to improve outcome significantly in patients with HFrEF.[39] In addition to increased natriuresis, they have multiple potentially beneficial effects, such as improved cardiac metabolism, improved autophagy and lysosomal degradation, and reduced oxidative stress and inflammation, resulting in improved remodelling.[40] Whether SGLT2 inhibitors are also effective in facilitating reverse modelling in patients with HFpEF is not yet known.

In HFrEF patients not eligible for cardiac resynchronization therapy (i.e. those with narrow QRS complex), cardiac contractility modulation (CCM) might be an option, which consists of biphasic high-voltage bipolar signals delivered to the right ventricular septum during the absolute refractory period.[41] Although large endpoint trials are not yet available, results from smaller studies are promising. In particular, CCM may result not only in improved symptoms, quality of life, and potentially HF hospitalizations, but also in reverse remodelling.[41] Recent progress in understanding the molecular and cellular basis of ventricular remodelling is paving the way for development of novel gene-, small molecule-, and extracellular vesicle- and cell-based treatment strategies capable of repairing the myocardial microstructure and restoring normal metabolism and electrical activity.[31,33,42] Thus, there are a large number of additional experimental therapies that have the potential to improve remodelling, in both reduced and preserved LVEF.

Summary and key messages

The failing heart is characterized by complex ventricular remodelling, involving alterations in gross morphology, tissue microstructure, metabolism, and electrical activity of the ventricles. Current therapy for HF still has a limited capacity to reverse ventricular remodelling and restore cardiac function fully, and the development of adequate therapeutic strategies is still an important unmet medical need, particularly for patients with HFpEF. Because of the diversity of intricate and interlacing cellular and molecular pathways involved in the pathogenesis of adverse ventricular remodelling, the currently accepted practice of aggregating all phenotypes of remodelling together, regardless of the underlying mechanisms, no longer holds to treat this complex pathophysiological condition. Thus, it is conceivable that some of the therapies that have failed in clinical trials target relevant mechanisms that are not common to all subsets of remodelling. In this conceptual framework, the necessity exists to personalize the treatment of patients with specific subsets of ventricular remodelling, which, in turn, implies identifying these patients through the use of panels of biomarkers reflecting the diversity of alterations present in the remodelled myocardium.

References

1. Cohn JN, Ferrari R, Sharpe N. Cardiac remodeling: concepts and clinical implications: a consensus paper from an international forum on cardiac remodeling. Behalf of an International Forum on Cardiac Remodeling. J Am Coll Cardiol. 2000;35(3):569–82.

2. Burchfield JS, Xie M, Hill JA. Pathological ventricular remodeling: mechanisms: part 1 of 2. Circulation. 2013;128(4):388–400.

3. Halliday BP, Wassall R, Lota AS, et al. Withdrawal of pharmacological treatment for heart failure in patients with recovered dilated cardiomyopathy (TRED-HF): an open-label, pilot, randomised trial. Lancet. 2019;393(10166):61–73.

4. Shah AM, Claggett B, Sweitzer NK, et al. Prognostic importance of impaired systolic function in heart failure with preserved ejection fraction and the impact of spironolactone. Circulation. 2015;132(5):402–14.

5. Ponikowski P, Voors AA, Anker SD, et al. 2016 ESC Guidelines for the diagnosis and treatment of acute and chronic heart failure: The Task Force for the diagnosis and treatment of acute and chronic heart failure of the European Society of Cardiology (ESC) Developed with the special contribution of the Heart Failure Association (HFA) of the ESC. Eur Heart J. 2016;37(27):2129–200.

6. Jessup M, Brozena S. Heart failure. N Engl J Med. 2003; 348(20):2007–18.

7. Claes GR, van Tienen FH, Lindsey P, et al. Hypertrophic remodelling in cardiac regulatory myosin light chain (MYL2) founder mutation carriers. Eur Heart J. 2016;37(23):1815–22.

8. Manolis AS, Manolis AA, Manolis TA, Melita H. Cardiac amyloidosis: an underdiagnosed/underappreciated disease. Eur J Intern Med. 2019;67:1–13.

9. Bhatt AS, Ambrosy AP, Velazquez EJ. Adverse remodeling and reverse remodeling after myocardial infarction. Curr Cardiol Rep. 2017;19(8):71.

10. Landmesser U, Wollert KC, Drexler H. Potential novel pharmacological therapies for myocardial remodelling. Cardiovasc Res. 2009;81(3):519–27.

11. Ito S, Miranda WR, Nkomo VT, et al. Reduced left ventricular ejection fraction in patients with aortic stenosis. J Am Coll Cardiol. 2018;71(12):1313–21.

12. Seferovic PM, Ponikowski P, Anker SD, et al. Clinical practice update on heart failure 2019: pharmacotherapy, procedures, devices and patient management. An expert consensus meeting report of the Heart Failure Association of the European Society of Cardiology. Eur J Heart Fail. 2019;21(10):1169–86.

13. Paulus WJ, Tschope C. A novel paradigm for heart failure with preserved ejection fraction: comorbidities drive myocardial dysfunction and remodeling through coronary microvascular endothelial inflammation. J Am Coll Cardiol. 2013;62(4):263–71.

14. Van Empel V, Brunner-La Rocca HP. Inflammation in HFpEF: key or circumstantial? Int J Cardiol. 2015;189:259–63.

15. Solomon SD, Vaduganathan M, Claggett BL, et al. Sacubitril/valsartan across the spectrum of ejection fraction in heart failure. Circulation. 2020;141(5):352–61.

16. Solomon SD, Claggett B, Lewis EF, et al. Influence of ejection fraction on outcomes and efficacy of spironolactone in patients with heart failure with preserved ejection fraction. Eur Heart J. 2016;37(5):455–62.

17. Kim SY, Morales CR, Gillette TG, Hill JA. Epigenetic regulation in heart failure. Curr Opin Cardiol. 2016;31(3):255–65.

18. Schirone L, Forte M, Palmerio S, et al. A review of the molecular mechanisms underlying the development and progression of cardiac remodeling. Oxid Med Cell Longev. 2017;2017:3920195.

19. Nakamura M, Sadoshima J. Mechanisms of physiological and pathological cardiac hypertrophy. Nat Rev Cardiol. 2018;15(7):387–407.

20. Aoyagi T, Matsui T. Phosphoinositide-3 kinase signaling in cardiac hypertrophy and heart failure. Curr Pharm Des. 2011;17(18):1818–24.

21. Lehnart SE, Maier LS, Hasenfuss G. Abnormalities of calcium metabolism and myocardial contractility depression in the failing heart. Heart Fail Rev. 2009;14(4):213–24.

22. Whelan RS, Kaplinskiy V, Kitsis RN. Cell death in the pathogenesis of heart disease: mechanisms and significance. Annu Rev Physiol. 2010;72:19–44.

23. Del Re DP, Amgalan D, Linkermann A, Liu Q, Kitsis RN. Fundamental mechanisms of regulated cell death and implications for heart disease. Physiol Rev. 2019;99(4):1765–817.

24. Dorn GW, 2nd. Apoptotic and non-apoptotic programmed cardiomyocyte death in ventricular remodelling. Cardiovasc Res. 2009;81(3):465–73.

25. Di Lisa F, Carpi A, Giorgio V, Bernardi P. The mitochondrial permeability transition pore and cyclophilin D in cardioprotection. Biochim Biophys Acta. 2011;1813(7):1316–22.

26. Frangogiannis NG. The inflammatory response in myocardial injury, repair, and remodelling. Nat Rev Cardiol. 2014 11(5):255–65.

27. Nishida K, Otsu K. Autophagy during cardiac remodeling. J Mol Cell Cardiol. 2016;95:11–18.

28. Rhee AJ, Lavine KJ. New Approaches to target inflammation in heart failure: harnessing insights from studies of immune cell diversity. Annu Rev Physiol. 2020;82:1–20.

29. López B, Ravassa S, Moreno MU, et al. Diffuse myocardial fibrosis: mechanisms, diagnosis and therapeutic approaches. Nat Rev Cardiol. 2021;18:479–98.

30. Pries AR, Badimon L, Bugiardini R, et al. Coronary vascular regulation, remodelling, and collateralization: mechanisms and clinical implications on behalf of the working group on coronary pathophysiology and microcirculation. Eur Heart J. 2015;36(45):3134–46.

31. Brakenhielm E, Alitalo K. Cardiac lymphatics in health and disease. Nat Rev Cardiol. 2019;16(1):56–68.

32. Brakenhielm E, González A, Díez J. Role of cardiac lymphatics in myocardial edema and fibrosis: JACC Review Topic of the Week. J Am Coll Cardiol. 2020;76(6):735–44.

33. Bertero E, Maack C. Metabolic remodelling in heart failure. Nat Rev Cardiol. 2018;15(8):457–70.

34. Kolwicz SC, Jr., Purohit S, Tian R. Cardiac metabolism and its interactions with contraction, growth, and survival of cardiomyocytes. Circ Res. 2013;113(5):603–16.

35. Gibb AA, Lazaropoulos MP, Elrod JW. Myofibroblasts and fibrosis: mitochondrial and metabolic control of cellular differentiation. Circ Res. 2020;127(3):427–47.

36. Nguyen MN, Kiriazis H, Gao XM, Du XJ. Cardiac fibrosis and arrhythmogenesis. Compr Physiol. 2017;7(3):1009–49.

37. Cutler MJ, Jeyaraj D, Rosenbaum DS. Cardiac electrical remodelling in health and sisease. Trends Pharmacol Sci. 2011;32(3):174–80.

38. Hohendanner F, Heinzel FR, Blaschke F, et al. Pathophysiological and therapeutic implications in patients with atrial fibrillation and heart failure. Heart Fail Rev. 2018;23(1):27–36.

39. Packer M, Anker SD, Butler J, et al. Cardiovascular and renal outcomes with empagliflozin in heart failure. N Engl J Med. 2020;383(15):1413–24.

40. Lopaschuk GD, Verma S. Mechanisms of cardiovascular benefits of sodium glucose co-transporter 2 (SGLT2) inhibitors: a state-of-the-art review. JACC Basic Transl Sci. 2020;5(6):632–44.

41. Tschöpe C, Kherad B, Klein O, *et al.* Cardiac contractility modulation: mechanisms of action in heart failure with reduced ejection fraction and beyond. Eur J Heart Fail. 2019;21(1):14–22.

42. Steffens S, Van Linthout S, Sluijter JPG, Tocchetti CG, Thum T, Madonna R. Stimulating pro-reparative immune responses to prevent adverse cardiac remodelling: consensus document from the joint 2019 meeting of the ESC Working Groups of cellular biology of the heart and myocardial function. Cardiovasc Res. 2020;116(11):1850–62.

CHAPTER 5.4

Neurohormonal activation in heart failure

Antoni Bayes-Genis and Faiez Zannad

Contents

Introduction

Heart failure (HF) with reduced ejection fraction (HFrEF) has many aetiologies, including derangement of the myocardium and/or great vessels and structural/metabolic abnormalities. Although the aetiology of HFrEF can vary widely, molecular and biochemical pathways and mechanical factors involved in cardiac remodelling are thought to be similar. Over the past few decades, there has been a profound evolution in the knowledge of HF pathobiology. From the traditional vision of HF as a problem exclusively of cardiac origin, it has evolved to an integrated model in which the progressive nature of the HF syndrome is seen as complex structural and functional changes in response to multiple regulatory and counter-regulatory neurohormonal systems acting in an autocrine, paracrine, and endocrine manner.[1]

The neurohormonal response aids the body in responding to challenges that impair the circulation, notably underfilling of the systemic arterial system or a decrease in blood pressure. In short-term emergencies, this response is adaptive, in that it helps the body meet the challenges posed such as by exercise and blood loss. However, in the context of HF, which also causes underfilling of the systemic arterial system, the haemodynamic reaction becomes maladaptive and significantly contributes to the long-term problems of HF. The neurohormonal systems involved in HF exert opposing counter-regulatory effects. On one hand, the sympathetic nervous system (SNS), renin–angiotensin–aldosterone system (RAAS), and arginine–vasopressin (AVP) system maintain cardiac output through increased retention of salt and water, peripheral arterial vasoconstriction, and increased contractility. Other neurohormonal systems have essentially vasodilator and natriuretic functions, namely the natriuretic peptide (NP) system. Remarkably, HFrEF is also characterized by important changes in several systems that normally antagonize SNS and RAAS activation such as loss of parasympathetic tone and increased resistance to NPs.[2]

This chapter will focus on neurohormonal activation in HFrEF. The pathobiology of HF with preserved ejection fraction (HFpEF) seems to be less dependent on neurohormonal activation and more intermingled with other systemic pathways, including systemic inflammation, renal dysfunction, and pulmonary hypertension, among others.[3] The neurohormonal hypothesis of HFrEF has been validated in multiple landmark clinical trials. The combined antagonism of the RAAS and SNS by angiotensin-converting enzyme inhibitors (ACEIs)[4,5] or angiotensin receptor blockers (ARBs),[6] beta-blockers,[7,8,9] and mineralocorticoid receptor antagonists (MRAs)[10,11] forms the basis for evidence-based treatment of patients with HFrEF. More recently, results using angiotensin receptor–neprilysin inhibitors (ARNIs) have enhanced our understanding of the counter-regulatory pathways provided by the NP system.[12] In sharp contrast, none of the clinical trials that aimed to modulate the neurohormonal activation system in HFpEF have yielded a significant reduction in events or a substantial modulation of disease progression.[13,14,15]

The sympathetic nervous system

The SNS was one of the first mechanisms to be studied in the context of HF. In 1897, Starling associated tachycardia and vasoconstriction typical of HF with a reflex mechanism.[16] Nearly 70 years later, Chidsey *et al.* showed that HF is intrinsically associated with SNS activation and increased levels of circulating noradrenaline.[16] Reduced clearance of noradrenaline due to low cardiac output may contribute to its high levels, but most of the increase in plasma noradrenaline levels is due to excessive secretion by cardiac sympathetic nerve endings. The stimulus for this sympathetic surge is sustained attenuation of 'high-pressure' carotid sinus and aortic arch baroreceptors and 'low-pressure' cardiopulmonary mechanoreceptors, resulting in withdrawal of the parasympathetic tone and a reflex increase in the sympathetic tone. Additional neurogenic inputs in HF include increased chemosensitivity to hypoxia and hypercapnia, and enhanced ergoreceptor reflexes (i.e. enhanced sensitivity to the metabolic effects of muscle work).[2]

The SNS is initially activated as it increases the heart rate to compensate for arterial underfilling. This increases cardiac output and redistributes blood flow from the splanchnic area to the heart and skeletal muscle. Renal vasoconstriction leads to salt and water retention, which improves the perfusion of vital organs.

However, as HF progresses, increased levels of local and circulating catecholamines are directly associated with accelerated progression of HF through induction of fetal gene programmes, downregulation of calcium-regulating genes, myocyte hypertrophy, apoptosis, and necrosis, and also indirectly by activating the RAAS. Myocyte loss due to continuous sympathetic toxicity may stimulate further hypertrophy of the remaining myocardium,

leading to progressive remodelling of the ventricle. Furthermore, sustained sympathetic stimulation leads to progressive salt and water retention, vasoconstriction, oedema, and increased pre- and afterload. These, in turn, increase ventricular wall stress, resulting in higher myocardial oxygen demand and myocardial ischaemia. Excess sympathetic activity may also predispose to ventricular arrhythmias.[17]

Paradoxically, the failing heart exhibits greatly decreased responsiveness to endogenous catecholamines. Chronic SNS activation is associated with decreased β-adrenergic receptor density and sensitivity, accompanied by a proportional decrease in the activity of adenylyl cyclase and agonist-stimulated muscle contractility.[18] Expression of the β1-receptor is decreased to approximately 50% in HF, whereas the β1-adrenergic receptor is the predominant subtype (approximately 70–80%) in the healthy human heart. Moreover, adrenergic receptors undergo functional desensitization, leading to uncoupling from downstream G protein activation. As this phenomenon is non-uniformly distributed across the myocardium, it contributes to the mechanical and electrophysiological derangements that are typical of HF (➲ Figure 5.4.1). We refer the reader to Lymeropoulos *et al.* for a comprehensive review of the adrenergic nervous system in HF.[19]

Overall, from a clinical perspective, elevated plasma noradrenaline levels are associated with decreased survival in HF patients.[20] To counteract the deleterious effects of SNS activation, treatment with beta-blockers attenuates cardiac remodelling, thereby preserving cardiac function and improving survival.[7,8,9]

The renin–angiotensin–aldosterone system

The RAAS is a central feature in the pathophysiology of HF and has been studied extensively. With the inclusion of novel components, it has become evident that the RAAS is much more complex than originally anticipated. There are two main axes of the RAAS which counteract each other in terms of vascular control:

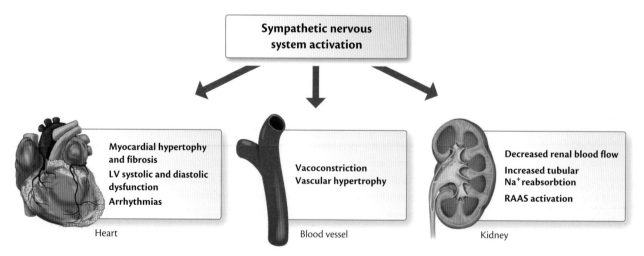

Figure 5.4.1 Effects of sympathetic nervous system activation. Increased sympathetic nervous system activity contributes to the pathophysiology of heart failure via multiple mechanisms involving cardiac, renal, and vascular function. RAAS, renin–angiotensin–aldosterone system.

Source data from Hartupee J, Mann DL. Neurohormonal activation in heart failure with reduced ejection fraction. *Nat Rev Cardiol.* 2017 Jan;14(1):30–38. doi: 10.1038/nrcardio.2016.163.

the classical vasoconstrictive axis and the opposing vasorelaxant axis. The relevance of the vasorelaxant axis in HF homeostasis control is still unclear. Furthermore, evolving knowledge has expanded the RAAS from a systemic or typically endocrine system to organ or tissue paracrine and autocrine systems that strongly interact.

⮕ Figure 5.4.2 illustrates the principal effects of RAAS activation and the sites of its blockade. Briefly, the classical RAAS consists of a cascade of enzymatic reactions involving three components: angiotensinogen, renin, and angiotensin-converting enzyme (ACE), which generate angiotensin (AT)-II as the biologically active product. AT-II binds to two types of specific receptors: angiotensin receptor type 1 (AT_1R) and angiotensin receptor type 2 (AT_2R). Both receptors belong to the family of heterotrimeric G protein-coupled receptors. Most of the deleterious actions of AT-II have been attributed to interaction with AT_1R, which is the predominant receptor in adult tissues, whereas AT_2R generally produces beneficial effects. The other RAAS axis, according to current knowledge, counteracts the classical axis in terms of vascular control. This opposing vasorelaxant axis involves ACE-2, and AT-I to VII interacting with the Mas receptor (MasR). The MasR signalling pathways are being uncovered, but they currently have unclear clinical potential. Finally, the contribution of other short-chain peptides derived from AT-II, including AT-III and AT-IV, as effectors in the RAAS is evolving, but they seem to play relevant and complementary roles to AT-II.[2]

Interest was raised in the RAAS over a century ago, in 1898, when Tigerstedt and Bergman identified a substance produced by the renal cortex in rabbits that triggers a vasoconstrictor response, a substance they called renin. However, it was not until the 1940s that the substance responsible for vasoconstriction, known today as AT-II, was identified.[21] Based on these and other basic studies, the traditional endocrine pathway of the RAAS was born. This systemic RAAS is activated in response to the presence of renal hypoperfusion, and the baroreceptors present in the renal afferent arteriole stimulate secretory granules to produce renin. Renin is responsible for catalysing the transformation of angiotensinogen (of liver origin) into AT-I (decapeptide), which, in turn, is catalysed into AT-II (octapeptide) by ACE (membrane-bound on endothelial cells). Systemic AT-II is mainly involved in acute responses to maintain plasma volume and electrolyte homeostasis, including vasoconstriction, a direct effect on tubular sodium reabsorption, and aldosterone secretion through AT-II-mediated stimulation of AT_1Rs in the zona glomerulosa of the adrenal glands.[22]

The notion of a systemic RAAS evolved in the early 1980s, when a series of experiments suggested the existence of paracrine and autocrine RAAS. Local RAAS have tissue-specific roles and are regulated independently of the circulating system. Evidence suggests that AT-II production occurs in different organs at the tissue level, including the brain, heart, and vasculature, and that local AT-II levels could even exceed plasma AT-II levels. Tissue AT-II is associated with target organ damage such as renal failure and cardiac remodelling. Local system functions of the RAAS include cell growth and remodelling in the heart, regulation of blood pressure, central effects on food and water

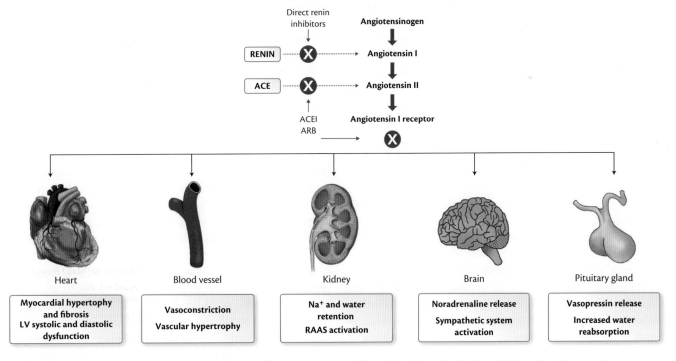

Figure 5.4.2 Effects of activation of the renin–angiotensin–aldosterone system and the principal sites of its blockade. ACE, angiotensin-converting enzyme; ACEI, angiotensin-converting enzyme inhibitor; ARB, angiotensin receptor blocker; LV, left ventricular; Na⁺, sodium; RAAS, renin–angiotensin–aldosterone system.

Source data from Mangiafico S, Costello-Boerrigter LC, Andersen IA, Cataliotti A, Burnett JC Jr. Neutral endopeptidase inhibition and the natriuretic peptide system: an evolving strategy in cardiovascular therapeutics. *Eur Heart J.* 2013 Mar;34(12):886–893c. doi: 10.1093/eurheartj/ehs262.

intake, and hormone secretion in the pancreas. The pathophysiological significance of the intracellular cardiac RAAS is more recent and incomplete, but diabetes seems to be a major stimulus for the activation of the intracellular RAAS. We refer the reader to the review by Hartupee and Mann[2] for further elaboration of the RAAS in HFrEF.

At the renal level, activation of the RAAS leads to increased salt and water retention through multiple mechanisms. AT-II directly causes sodium retention at the proximal tubule, whereas aldosterone causes increased sodium resorption in the distal tubule. AT-II also stimulates the release of arginine–vasopressin (AVP), which contributes to the development of hyponatraemia in patients with HF.[2]

At the vascular level, the effects of AT-II are varied and include increased peripheral vascular resistance, vasoconstriction of the glomerular efferent arteriole, contraction of vascular smooth muscle, and pro-inflammatory effects by activation of the nuclear factor kappa B (NF-κB) inflammatory pathway, as well as elevation of the pro-inflammatory mediators interleukin (IL)-6, tumour necrosis factor alpha (TNF-α), and monocyte chemoattractant protein 1 (MCP-1).[23] AT-II alters endothelial function by attenuating both nitric oxide (NO) production and endothelium-dependent vasodilatation, as well as by generating reactive oxygen species (ROS) in blood vessels, which inactivates endothelial NO synthase (eNOS), decreasing NO production.[24] Furthermore, the effects of AT-II on the vessel wall stimulate collagen synthesis and smooth muscle cell proliferation, leading to vascular remodelling.[25]

At the cardiac level, AT-II has been both directly and indirectly implicated in cardiac remodelling. AT-II increases myocardial oxidative stress, which further augments the hypertrophic signalling programme with fibrosis[26] and left ventricular dysfunction.[27] AT-II acts directly through AT_1R to drive fibroblast division and collagen production. AT-II activation also leads to necrotic and apoptotic myocyte cell death. Furthermore, AT-II induces haemodynamic changes as it promotes systemic vasoconstriction and fluid retention, which places haemodynamic stress on the heart, resulting in pathological cardiac remodelling.[28,29] In some cases, remodelling likely occurs indirectly as a consequence of increased afterload on the basis of hypertension and alterations in arterial stiffness.

Aldosterone isolation and adrenal origin and structure date back nearly 70 years.[30] At the distal nephron, aldosterone increases sodium and water reabsorption, leading to an increase in extracellular fluid volume. Mineralocorticoid hormone receptors (MRs) have been detected in human cardiomyocytes and cardiac fibroblasts,[31] and their exposure to elevated circulating levels of aldosterone leads to myocardial damage that is unrelated to changes in blood pressure.[32] Chronic aldosterone exposure causes fibrosis in the heart, vascular remodelling, and inflammation of the perivascular tissue.[33,34,35] Further evidence indicates that aldosterone contributes to both systolic and diastolic myocardial dysfunction via mechanisms related to induction of oxidative

stress. Most importantly, cardiac and vascular derangements caused by aldosterone are prevented or attenuated by administration of MRAs in animal models.

Renin inhibitors block the conversion of angiotensinogen to AT-I. Given their low potency and lack of specificity, as well as their low bioavailability and short half-life, these drugs are not currently indicated for HF treatment. ACEIs reduce the amount of AT-II available by inhibiting its synthesis from AT-I. ARBs act downstream of ACEIs, inhibiting AT-II signal transduction when stimulating AT_1R. ARBs are not superior to ACEIs in reducing mortality associated with HFrEF, and are recommended when patients are intolerant to ACEIs. Unlike ACEIs, ARBs do not practically inhibit degradation of bradykinin. MRAs inhibit transduction of the aldosterone signal (➲ Figure 5.4.2). They are associated with a reduction in cardiovascular mortality and, together with ACEIs and beta-blockers, received a IA indication in European Society of Cardiology (ESC) guidelines.[36]

The natriuretic peptide system

The discovery and relevance of the NP system in the context of HF are relatively more recent concepts. In 1956, Kisch described granules in the atria, but it was not until 1978 that De Bold suggested that these atrial granules are storage sites for a protein or polypeptide. De Bold also reported a massive and rapid increase in excretion of water and sodium when homogenized granules were injected into rats, naming the substance responsible for these effects atrial natriuretic peptide (ANP).[21] In 1986, Burnett et al. detected high plasma levels of ANP in patients with HF.[37] In 1988, Sudoh et al. identified a new peptide isolated from pig brain that had properties similar to ANP, which was termed brain NP (now called B-type natriuretic peptide, or BNP).[38] It is now recognized that BNP production mainly occurs in the ventricular tissue. More recently, the C-type NP (CNP)[39] and a D-type NP (DNP) have been reported.

The NPs play key roles in HF, counteracting the effects of overstimulation of the SNS, RAAS, and AVP system.[40] ANP and BNP are predominantly of cardiac origin, whereas CNP is largely sourced from endothelial cells throughout the systemic vasculature. Bioactive NPs act via G protein-coupled transmembrane receptors activating cyclic guanosine monophosphate (cGMP) as a second messenger.[41] ANP and BNP act via the NPR-A receptor to exert natriuretic, diuretic, haemo-concentrating, and vasodilating effects, in association with suppression of the RAAS and SNS, as well as trophic effects that oppose cardiac hypertrophy and fibrosis. CNP, operating via the NPR-B receptor, is not natriuretic but is central to vasomotion and opposes vascular cell hyperplasia (➲ Figure 5.4.3). All three of these NPs are cleared via the NPR-C receptor, in concert with proteolysis.[41,42] Neprilysin is responsible for the initial proteolytic cleavage of ANP and CNP and plays a role in processing BNP, but it does not cleave the amino-terminal prohormone fragments (NT-proANP and NT-proBNP).[43] Much of the impact of inhibiting neprilysin

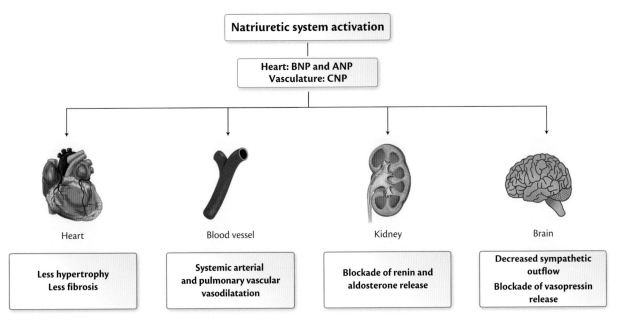

Figure 5.4.3 Effects of activation of the natriuretic peptide system. ANP, atrial natriuretic peptide; BNP, B-type natriuretic peptide; CNP, C-type natriuretic peptide.

in preclinical and clinical settings has been presumed to be due to enhanced bioactivity of NPs. The ranking of avidity of neprilysin is CNP > ANP > BNP. In healthy conditions, proteolytic cleavage and removal by the 'clearance' NP receptor NPR-C play equal roles in the metabolism of NPs, but in high-NP states, such as HF, it seems likely that neprilysin plays an increasingly important role.[43]

In the early stage of HF, NPs play a beneficial role in maintaining homeostasis. However, with progressive deterioration of cardiac function, NPs lose efficiency by one of the following mechanisms: a decrease in NP availability due to reduced production, increased removal, or enzymatic degradation through neprilysin; a reduced NP response due to reduced expression or sensitization of NPRs or inhibition of downstream signalling pathways; and/or an overlap of the effects of neurohormonal systems with functions contrary to NPs, namely the RAAS and SNS. Nevertheless, elevation in plasma levels of NPs is frequently observed in HF, so measurement of plasma levels of BNP (and NT-proBNP) constitutes a marker of disease severity and predictor of prognosis.

The recent incorporation of ARNIs into the HF armamentarium follows the already long-lasting trend in the modulation of neurohormonal pathways to achieve therapeutic goals in HF. Their innovative character lies not in the identity of the molecules that compose them (sacubitril, a neprilysin inhibitor (NEPi), and valsartan, a previously tested ARB marketed individually), but rather in their combination in a single drug (➲ Table 5.4.1). Thus, this therapy for HF aims not only to attenuate potentially harmful neurohormonal mechanisms, but also to amplify the protective NP mechanisms at the cardiovascular level (see ➲ Chapter 8.3 for more details on the sacubitril/valsartan mechanism of action and clinical evidence).

Other neurohormonal systems activated in heart failure

Arginine–vasopressin system

The first studies on the impact of AVP on HF date back to the early 1980s. Szatalowicz *et al.* in 1981 published the first observation that vasopressin levels were generally elevated in patients with HF.[44]

AVP is a nonapeptide synthesized in the hypothalamus and stored in the posterior pituitary for release in response to both osmotic and non-osmotic factors. The dominant stimulus for AVP secretion is serum osmolality. Non-osmotic factors, including cardiac filling pressure, arterial pressure, and other influences, such as the effects of adrenergic stimuli and AT-II on the central nervous system, can modulate the osmotic control of AVP to varying degrees.[45]

Plasma levels of AVP are elevated in the presence of left ventricular dysfunction, correlating with poor outcomes. Its major actions relevant to HF are signalling at the V1a and V2 receptors. The V1a receptor is a G protein-coupled receptor that, when activated, increases intracellular calcium through the inositol triphosphate pathway. The result is constriction of smooth muscle and a positive inotropic effect on cardiac muscle.[46] Prolonged V1a stimulation leads to synthesis of proteins involved in cellular hypertrophy in both vascular and myocardial tissue. Activation of the V2 receptor alters the expression of aquaporin channels, increasing the permeability of the renal collecting tubular cells to water, resulting in water retention. Excess AVP secretion could contribute to the pathophysiology of HF by several distinct load-dependent and load-independent mechanisms (➲ Figure 5.4.4).

Several inhibitors of vasopressin receptors (namely conivaptan, a V1a/V2 receptor inhibitor, and the V2e receptor

Table 5.4.1 Impact of neurohormonal blockade on peptide levels and physiological effects

	NEPi	ACEI	NEPi + ACEI (omapatrilat)	ARNI (sacubitril/valsartan)
Effects on hormones				
Angiotensin II	↑	↓	↓	↑
Renin	↓	↑	↔ ↑	↑
Aldosterone	↓	↔	↓	↓
NPs or cGMP	↑	↓/↔	↑	↑
Endothelin-1	↑	↔	↑	↓
Bradykinin	↑	↑	↑↑	↑
Physiological effects				
Blood pressure	↔	↓	↓	↓
Sodium excretion	↑	↑	↑	↑↑
Cardiac hypertrophy	↔ ↓	↓	↓↓	↓↓
Cardiac fibrosis	↓	↓	↓↓	↓↓

Angiotensin receptor–neprilysin inhibitors (ARNIs) overcome increased RAAS activation seen with neprilysin inhibition (NEPi) monotherapy, and are not associated with the excessive increase in bradykinin seen with angiotensin-converting enzyme inhibitors (ACEIs) + NEPi.

NP, natriuretic peptide; cGMP, cyclic guanosine monophosphate.

inhibitors lixivaptan and tolvaptan) have been developed and tested in several clinical trials. The results are promising, showing an improvement in dyspnoea and hyponatraemia, but there is no evidence of benefits in cardiovascular morbidity and mortality.[45]

Endothelin

Endothelin (ET) is a 21-amino acid peptide discovered in 1988 by Yanagisawa *et al.*[47] ET derives from the big-ET, a larger precursor, by action of the ET-converting enzyme family. Three isoforms of ET, named ET-1, ET-2, and ET-3, have been identified. ET-1 is generated mainly by vascular endothelial cells and exerts various important biological actions mediated by two receptor subtypes, ET-A and ET-B, belonging to the G protein-coupled receptor family. ET-1 is a potent vasoconstrictive agent that has inotropic and mitogenic actions, modulates salt and water homeostasis, and plays an important role in the maintenance of vascular tone and blood pressure.[48]

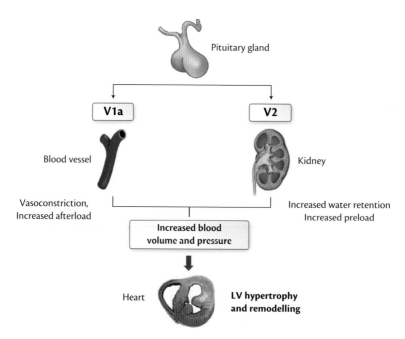

Figure 5.4.4 Effects of activation of the arginine–vasopressin system.

V1a, vasopressin 1a receptor; V2, vasopressin 2; LV, left ventricular.

Source data from Szatalowicz VL, Arnold PE, Chaimovitz C, Bichet D, Berl T, Schrier RW. Radioimmunoassay of plasma arginine vasopressin in hyponatremic patients with congestive heart failure. *N Engl J Med*. 1981 Jul 30;305(5):263–6. doi: 10.1056/NEJM198107303050506.

ET signalling has been proposed as a mediator of combined pre- and post-capillary pulmonary hypertension, and elevated levels of ET-1 are associated with worse morbidity and mortality in individuals with HF. Despite this, and in contrast to individuals with pulmonary arterial hypertension, ET receptor antagonism in patients with HF has not shown any benefit and may be harmful.[49]

Oxidative stress and nitrosative stress in heart failure

Over the past few decades, clinical and experimental studies have provided substantial evidence that oxidative stress, defined as an excess production of ROS relative to antioxidant defence, is enhanced in HF. The cause of increased ROS in this setting is still not completely understood, but it may include increased production of ROS due to increased metabolic activity, stimulated production by mechanical strain, neurohormonal activation, inflammatory cytokines, and decreased antioxidant activity.

ROS are derived from several intracellular sources, including mitochondria, NAD(P)H oxidase, xanthine oxidase, and uncoupled NO synthase (NOS). ROS can directly impair contractile function by modifying proteins central to excitation–contraction coupling. Moreover, ROS activate a broad variety of hypertrophy signalling kinases and transcription factors, and mediate apoptosis. They also stimulate cardiac fibroblast proliferation and activate matrix metalloproteinases, leading to extracellular matrix remodelling. These cellular events are involved in the development and progression of maladaptive myocardial remodelling and failure.[50]

NO is a free radical that can both directly and indirectly modify the myocardial response to oxidative stress. NO is synthesized in the conversion of L-arginine to L-citrulline by a family of NOS. Through chemical reactions with ROS, NO can either decrease or increase oxidative stress at the cellular or tissue level. Low levels of NO, as are formed by NOS 3, may reduce the level of oxidative stress by decreasing the production of O_2^- through inhibition of oxidative enzymes.[51] Higher levels of NO may increase oxidative stress by reacting with O_2^- to generate peroxynitrite ($ONOO^-$), a toxic free radical.[52]

Many questions about the role of oxidative stress in HF remain to be answered. In addition, the results of applying preclinical observations to the development of therapeutic strategies for patients with HF have been disappointing.

Future directions

Whether additional neurohormonal modulation to the current armamentarium will yield further benefit in the future is not certain. Nevertheless, novel mechanisms may arise, such as sodium–glucose cotransporter 2 (SGLT2) receptor inhibition, which are also proving to prolong survival and increase the quality of life of patients with HF.

Summary

HF is a clinical syndrome involving multiple pathogenic pathways, but with the central player of neurohormonal activation, particularly in HFrEF. Over the past few decades, a profound understanding of the interplay between the different neurohormonal axes has developed, paralleled by an immense increase in the complexity of each system, with endocrine, paracrine, and autocrine effectors. Such gain in pathobiology comprehension has culminated with the development of drugs with major clinical relevance.

Key messages

◆ The neurohormonal response aids the body in responding to challenges that impair the circulation. In the short term, this response helps the body to meet the challenges posed. In the context of HF, the haemodynamic reaction becomes maladaptive and significantly contributes to the long-term problems of HF.

◆ The neurohormonal systems involved in HF exert opposing counter-regulatory effects.

◆ The SNS, RAAS, and AVP system maintain cardiac output through increased retention of salt and water, peripheral arterial vasoconstriction, and increased contractility.

◆ The NP system has essentially vasodilator and natriuretic functions.

◆ The combined antagonism of the neurohormonal systems involved in HF forms the basis for evidence-based treatment of patients with HFrEF.

References

1. Packer M. The neurohormonal hypothesis: a theory to explain the mechanism of disease progression in heart failure. J Am Coll Cardiol. 1992;20(1):248–54.
2. Hartupee J, Mann DL. Neurohormonal activation in heart failure with reduced ejection fraction. Nat Rev Cardiol. 2017;14(1):30–8.
3. Bayes-Genis A, Bisbal F, Núñez J, et al. Transitioning from preclinical to clinical heart failure with preserved ejection fraction: a mechanistic approach. J Clin Med. 2020;9(4):1110.
4. Cohn JN, Johnson G, Ziesche S, et al. A comparison of enalapril with hydralazine–isosorbide dinitrate in the treatment of chronic congestive heart failure. N Engl J Med. 1991;325(5):303–10.
5. SOLVD Investigators; Yusuf S, Pitt B, Davis CE, Hood WB, Cohn JN. Effect of enalapril on survival in patients with reduced left ventricular ejection fractions and congestive heart failure. N Engl J Med. 1991;325(5):293–302.
6. Cohn JN, Tognoni G; Valsartan Heart Failure Trial Investigators. A randomized trial of the angiotensin-receptor blocker valsartan in chronic heart failure. N Engl J Med. 2001;345(23):1667–75.
7. Packer M, Bristow MR, Cohn JN, et al. The effect of carvedilol on morbidity and mortality in patients with chronic heart failure. U.S. Carvedilol Heart Failure Study Group. N Engl J Med. 1996;334(21):1349–55.
8. MERIT-HF Study Group. Effect of metoprolol CR/XL in chronic heart failure: Metoprolol CR/XL Randomised Intervention Trial in Congestive Heart Failure (MERIT-HF). Lancet. 1999;353(9169):2001–7.
9. Bristow MR, Gilbert EM, Abraham WT, et al. Carvedilol produces dose-related improvements in left ventricular function and survival in subjects with chronic heart failure. MOCHA Investigators. Circulation. 1996;94(11):2807–16.

10. Pitt B, Zannad F, Remme WJ, *et al*. The effect of spironolactone on morbidity and mortality in patients with severe heart failure. Randomized Aldactone Evaluation Study Investigators. N Engl J Med. 1999;341(10):709–17.

11. Zannad F, McMurray JJ, Krum H, *et al*.; EMPHASIS-HF Study Group. Eplerenone in patients with systolic heart failure and mild symptoms. N Engl J Med. 2011;364(1):11–21.

12. McMurray JJ, Packer M, Desai AS, *et al*.; PARADIGM-HF Investigators and Committees. Angiotensin–neprilysin inhibition versus enalapril in heart failure. N Engl J Med. 2014;371(11):993–1004.

13. Pitt B, Pfeffer MA, Assmann SF, *et al*.; TOPCAT Investigators. Spironolactone for heart failure with preserved ejection fraction. N Engl J Med. 2014;370(15):1383–92.

14. Massie BM, Carson PE, McMurray JJ, *et al*.; I-PRESERVE Investigators. Irbesartan in patients with heart failure and preserved ejection fraction. N Engl J Med. 2008;359(23):2456–67.

15. Solomon SD, McMurray JJV, Anand IS, *et al*.; PARAGON-HF Investigators and Committees. Angiotensin–neprilysin inhibition in heart failure with preserved ejection fraction. N Engl J Med. 2019;381(17):1609–20.

16. Chidsey CA, Braunwald E, Morrow AG. Catecholamine excretion and cardiac stores of norepinephrine in congestive heart failure. Am J Med. 1965;39:442–51.

17. Florea VG, Cohn JN. The autonomic nervous system and heart failure. Circ Res. 2014;114(11):1815–26.

18. Bristow MR, Ginsburg R, Minobe W, *et al*. Decreased catecholamine sensitivity and beta-adrenergic-receptor density in failing human hearts. N Engl J Med. 1982;307(4):205–11.

19. Lymperopoulos A, Rengo G, Koch WJ. Adrenergic nervous system in heart failure: pathophysiology and therapy. Circ Res. 2013;113(6):739–53.

20. Cohn JN, Levine TB, Olivari MT, *et al*. Plasma norepinephrine as a guide to prognosis in patients with chronic congestive heart failure. N Engl J Med. 1984;311(13):819–23.

21. Braunwald E. The path to an angiotensin receptor antagonist–neprilysin inhibitor in the treatment of heart failure. J Am Coll Cardiol. 2015;65(10):1029–41.

22. Polónia J, Gonçalves FR. The historical evolution of knowledge of the involvement of neurohormonal systems in the pathophysiology and treatment of heart failure. Rev Port Cardiol. 2019;38(12):883–95.

23. Grosman-Rimon L, Billia F, Wright E, *et al*. Neurohormones, inflammatory mediators, and cardiovascular injury in the setting of heart failure. Heart Fail Rev. 2020;25(5):685–701.

24. Loot AE, Schreiber JG, Fisslthaler B, Fleming I. Angiotensin II impairs endothelial function via tyrosine phosphorylation of the endothelial nitric oxide synthase. J Exp Med. 2009;206(13):2889–96.

25. Daemen MJ, Lombardi DM, Bosman FT, Schwartz SM. Angiotensin II induces smooth muscle cell proliferation in the normal and injured rat arterial wall. Circ Res. 1991;68(2):450–6.

26. Kawano H, Do YS, Kawano Y, *et al*. Angiotensin II has multiple profibrotic effects in human cardiac fibroblasts. Circulation. 2000;101(10):1130–7.

27. Booz GW, Baker KM. Molecular signalling mechanisms controlling growth and function of cardiac fibroblasts. Cardiovasc Res. 1995;30(4):537–43.

28. Harada K, Komuro I, Shiojima I, *et al*. Pressure overload induces cardiac hypertrophy in angiotensin II type 1A receptor knockout mice. Circulation. 1998;97(19):1952–9.

29. Ruzicka M, Leenen FH. Relevance of blockade of cardiac and circulatory angiotensin-converting enzyme for the prevention of volume overload-induced cardiac hypertrophy. Circulation. 1995;91(1):16–19.

30. Weber KT. Aldosterone in congestive heart failure. N Engl J Med. 2001;345(23):1689–97.

31. Lombès M, Alfaidy N, Eugene E, Lessana A, Farman N, Bonvalet JP. Prerequisite for cardiac aldosterone action. Mineralocorticoid receptor and 11 beta-hydroxysteroid dehydrogenase in the human heart. Circulation. 1995;92(2):175–82.

32. Marney AM, Brown NJ. Aldosterone and end-organ damage. Clin Sci (Lond). 2007;113(6):267–78.

33. Rocha R, Rudolph AE, Frierdich GE, *et al*. Aldosterone induces a vascular inflammatory phenotype in the rat heart. Am J Physiol Heart Circ Physiol. 2002;283(5):H1802–10.

34. Jaffe IZ, Mendelsohn ME. Angiotensin II and aldosterone regulate gene transcription via functional mineralocortoicoid receptors in human coronary artery smooth muscle cells. Circ Res. 2005;96(6):643–50.

35. Neves MF, Amiri F, Virdis A, Diep QN, Schiffrin EL; CIHR Multidisciplinary Research Group on Hypertension. Role of aldosterone in angiotensin II-induced cardiac and aortic inflammation, fibrosis, and hypertrophy. Can J Physiol Pharmacol. 2005;83(11):999–1006.

36. McDonagh TA, Metra M, Adamo M, *et al*.; ESC Scientific Document Group. 2021 ESC Guidelines for the diagnosis and treatment of acute and chronic heart failure: Developed by The Task Force for the diagnosis and treatment of acute and chronic heart failure of the European Society of Cardiology (ESC). With the special contribution of the Heart Failure Association (HFA) of the ESC. Eur J Heart Fail. 2022;24(1):4–131.

37. Burnett JC Jr, Kao PC, Hu DC, *et al*. Atrial natriuretic peptide elevation in congestive heart failure in the human. Science. 1986;231(4742):1145–7.

38. Sudoh T, Kangawa K, Minamino N, Matsuo H. A new natriuretic peptide in porcine brain. Nature. 1988;332(6159):78–81.

39. Sudoh T, Minamino N, Kangawa K, Matsuo H. C-type natriuretic peptide (CNP): a new member of natriuretic peptide family identified in porcine brain. Biochem Biophys Res Commun. 1990;168(2):863–70.

40. Bayes-Genis A, Morant-Talamante N, Lupón J. Neprilysin and natriuretic peptide regulation in heart failure. Curr Heart Fail Rep. 2016;13(4):151–7.

41. Potter LR. Natriuretic peptide metabolism, clearance and degradation. FEBS J. 2011;278(11):1808–17.

42. Mangiafico S, Costello-Boerrigter LC, Andersen IA, Cataliotti A, Burnett JC Jr. Neutral endopeptidase inhibition and the natriuretic peptide system: an evolving strategy in cardiovascular therapeutics. Eur Heart J. 2013;34(12):886–93c.

43. Bayes-Genis A, Barallat J, Richards AM. A test in context: neprilysin: function, inhibition, and biomarker. J Am Coll Cardiol. 2016;68(6):639–53.

44. Szatalowicz VL, Arnold PE, Chaimovitz C, Bichet D, Berl T, Schrier RW. Radioimmunoassay of plasma arginine vasopressin in hyponatremic patients with congestive heart failure. N Engl J Med. 1981;305(5):263–6.

45. Goldsmith SR, Gheorghiade M. Vasopressin antagonism in heart failure. J Am Coll Cardiol. 2005;46(10):1785–91.

46. Xu YJ, Gopalakrishnan V. Vasopressin increases cytosolic free [Ca2+] in the neonatal rat cardiomyocyte. Evidence for V1 subtype receptors. Circ Res. 1991;69(1):239–45.

47. Yanagisawa M, Kurihara H, Kimura S, *et al*. A novel potent vasoconstrictor peptide produced by vascular endothelial cells. Nature. 1988;332(6163):411–15.

48. Giannessi D, Del Ry S, Vitale RL. The role of endothelins and their receptors in heart failure. Pharmacol Res. 2001;43(2):111–26.

49. Kelso EJ, Geraghty RF, McDermott BJ, Trimble ER, Nicholls DP, Silke B. Mechanical effects of ET-1 in cardiomyocytes isolated from normal and heart-failed rabbits. Mol Cell Biochem. 1996;157(1–2): 149–55.

50. Dhalla AK, Hill MF, Singal PK. Role of oxidative stress in transition of hypertrophy to heart failure. J Am Coll Cardiol. 1996;28(2):506–14.

51. Palacios-Callender M, Quintero M, Hollis VS, Springett RJ, Moncada S. Endogenous NO regulates superoxide production at low oxygen concentrations by modifying the redox state of cytochrome c oxidase. Proc Natl Acad Sci U S A. 2004;101(20):7630–5.

52. Pacher P, Beckman JS, Liaudet L. Nitric oxide and peroxynitrite in health and disease. Physiol Rev. 2007;87(1):315–424.

CHAPTER 5.5

Immune-mediated mechanisms

Ulrich Hofmann, Stefan Frantz, and
Nikolaos Frangogiannis

Contents

Introduction

For nearly the whole spectrum of heart failure, spanning from heart failure with preserved ejection fraction (HFpEF) to heart failure with reduced ejection fraction (HFrEF), and a variety of aetiologies, including ischaemic, inherited, and metabolic cardiomyopathies, there is solid mechanistic evidence linking the involvement of the immune system to disease pathology, as recently reviewed in the literature.[1,2] Animal models of heart disease have revealed a variety of mechanisms that explain how non-infectious triggers in the diseased myocardium elicit an immune response, including both innate and adaptive immune activation. However, there is still very limited evidence regarding the role of inflammation as a therapeutic target in human heart disease. Only a limited number of prospective clinical trials were specifically designed to study the impact of drugs interfering with inflammation in patients with heart failure, as reviewed recently.[1,3] Unfortunately, none of the approaches showed a convincing clinical benefit. However, it should be noted that most of the clinical studies testing targeted anti-cytokine approaches in human patients were performed more than 10 years ago and focused on very specific mediators. Large-scale interventions testing effects of other immune-modulatory therapeutics in heart failure populations are widely lacking. Since the first anti-cytokine trials, the field has tremendously developed. Progress in fundamental immunology has led to major advances in our understanding of the cellular immunobiology of the myocardium. Experimental studies have contributed new insights into the role of adaptive immune responses in myocardial disease. Finally, yet importantly, our therapeutic armamentarium has been expanded beyond neutralization of cytokines and chemokines to include a broad range of agents for targeted immuno-modulation. Significant challenges remain. In the upcoming era of 'precision medicine', the design of new interventional studies is hampered by limitations of tools for pathophysiological stratification of heart failure patients. In particular, we lack established biomarkers to identify subpopulations of heart failure patients who might benefit from specific therapeutic approaches.

In this chapter, we summarize the basic mechanisms of immune activation in heart failure, and highlight the clinical implications of inflammatory pathways in heart failure therapeutics.

Inflammation as a common feature across the heart failure syndrome in humans

A large amount of mostly correlative data show that elevated circulating markers of inflammation, such as, for example, tumour necrosis factor (TNF), high-sensitivity C-reactive protein (hsCRP), and interleukin-6 (IL-6), are associated with worsening myocardial function and predict outcomes in both patients with HFpEF and those with

HFrEF. Our current pathophysiological concept of the role of inflammation in heart failure follows to some extent the former quasi-binary classification of heart failure in HFpEF and HFrEF, whereas its role in HFmrEF is still elusive. HFpEF is often associated with, and is most likely causally promoted by, all components of the metabolic syndrome that finally lead to systemic inflammation and vascular disease. Moreover, there are other non-metabolic systemic and heart disease entities presenting with an HFpEF phenotype, for example, amyloidosis, for which the role of inflammation is not yet well established. The heterogeneity and phenotypic complexity of the clinical HFpEF syndrome pose challenges for preclinical research. In particular, there is no standard HFpEF animal model to study pathophysiological mechanisms and therapeutic approaches *in vivo*. Therefore, our pathophysiological understanding of how systemic inflammation and vascular disease lead to the HFpEF phenotype and how this could translate into anti-inflammatory approaches to mitigate HFpEF is still quite rudimentary.

In contrast to HFpEF, mostly pathophysiological processes *within* the myocardium that lead to loss of contractile tissue initiate the development of HFrEF. In HFrEF, systemic inflammation is more often a secondary phenomenon initiated by several factors, including local sterile inflammation initiated by acute and chronic myocardial damage and by systemic haemodynamic changes and neurohumoral responses.

The relative contribution of inflammatory signalling in heart failure progression likely depends on the underlying aetiology of the disease. For example, in patients with myocarditis, inflammatory injury is the primary cause of adverse remodelling, contractile dysfunction, and heart failure.[4] In contrast, in other heart failure aetiologies, the role of inflammatory responses in the pathogenesis of cardiac dysfunction is less convincingly documented. All forms of myocardial injury result in activation of a secondary immune response that may play a role in heart failure progression. It should be emphasized that inflammatory mediators in failing hearts may also transduce protective signals, promoting cardiomyocyte survival and activating an angiogenic programme. To what extent the detrimental actions of inflammatory mediators outweigh their protective effects may be dependent on the pathophysiological context and on cytokine-specific patterns of inflammatory activation.

Basic principles of immune activation in heart failure

Regardless of the aetiology of heart failure, activation of inflammatory mediators may be involved in the pathogenesis of heart failure progression through several different mechanisms, including negative inotropic, pro-apoptotic, and matrix-degrading actions of inflammatory cytokines[5,6] and downstream activation of a fibrogenic programme that leads to stimulation of interstitial fibroblasts and deposition of extracellular matrix in the cardiac interstitium (➲ Figure 5.5.1). Inflammation-mediated myocardial fibrosis increases ventricular stiffness and may play an important role in the pathogenesis of HFpEF.[7]

Several different myocardial cell types may contribute to activation of inflammatory pathways in the failing heart. Injured cardiomyocytes release damage-associated molecular patterns (DAMPs) that activate innate immune responses, leading to induction of inflammatory cytokines and chemokines. Mechanical stress, neurohumoral activation, and ischaemia may directly induce expression of pro-inflammatory cytokines in cardiomyocytes, promoting local activation of inflammatory signalling.[8] Vascular endothelial cells are also capable of secreting large amounts of chemokines and cytokines and may be highly responsive to ischaemic injury, playing an important role in activation of inflammatory responses in ischaemic cardiomyopathy. The heart also contains a sizeable population of macrophages[9] and mast cells[10] that may respond to cardiomyocyte-derived DAMPs, acquiring a pro-inflammatory phenotype. A growing body of evidence suggests that lymphocytes are recruited in the failing heart and orchestrate macrophage-mediated inflammation and fibrogenesis.[11,12] Although fibroblasts are capable of secreting inflammatory mediators following activation, their contribution in the inflammatory response in the failing heart remains unknown. Fibroblasts are more prominently involved as targets of inflammatory cytokines that deposit and remodel the extracellular matrix, contributing to the pathogenesis of fibrosis and diastolic dysfunction.[13]

Specific cytokines and chemokines involved in the pathogenesis of heart failure

Extensive experimental evidence suggests an important role for the inflammatory cytokines TNF, IL-1β, and IL-6 in the remodelling and failing heart (➲ Figure 5.5.1). The multifunctional cytokine TNF is the best-studied inflammatory cytokine in heart failure. Expression of TNF is markedly increased in the failing heart.[14] Numerous experimental studies have suggested a critical role for TNF in the pathogenesis of heart failure. Both genetic and antibody inhibition studies in heart failure models showed that TNF contributes to the pathogenesis of systolic dysfunction.[15,16,17] The adverse effects of TNF on cardiac remodelling may involve negative inotropic and pro-apoptotic actions in cardiomyocytes,[18,19] matrix-degrading effects through induction and activation of matrix metalloproteinases (MMPs),[20,21] stimulation of inflammatory cell recruitment through expression of endothelial adhesion molecules,[22] and accentuation of microvascular dysfunction.[23] Studies in human heart failure support the notion that TNF may contribute to cardiac dysfunction. Higher circulating levels of TNF were associated with increased mortality in both HFrEF and HFpEF patients.[24] However, it should be emphasized that the role of TNF in heart failure is not unidimensional. Several investigations have suggested that, in addition to its effects on progression of adverse remodelling and dysfunction, TNF may also exert protective effects on stressed or injured cardiomyocytes[25] by reducing intracellular calcium overload or by attenuating mitochondrial dysfunction. The basis for the conflicting findings suggesting both protective and injurious effects of TNF *in vivo* is unclear, but may reflect context- and

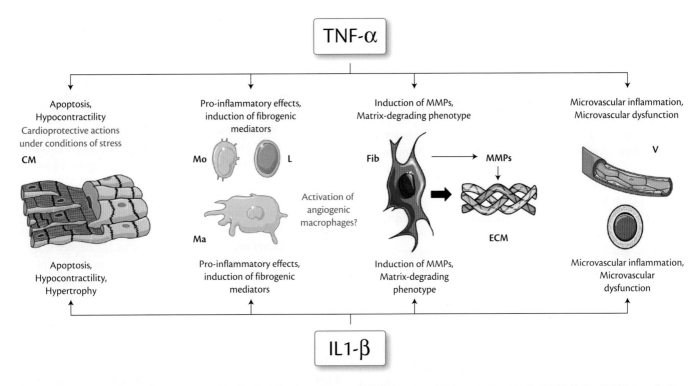

Figure 5.5.1 Actions of pro-inflammatory cytokines in the failing heart. The pro-inflammatory cytokines tumour necrosis factor alpha (TNF-α) and interleukin (IL)-1β play an important role in the pathogenesis of heart failure by: inducing cardiomyocyte (CM) apoptosis; exerting negative inotropic actions; stimulating monocyte (Mo), lymphocyte (L), and macrophage (Ma) activation; promoting a matrix-degrading fibroblast (Fib) phenotype; and stimulating microvascular inflammation and dysfunction. Pro-inflammatory cytokines may also trigger fibrosis by inducing the synthesis of fibrogenic mediators such as TGF-β. It should be emphasized that the effects of pro-inflammatory cytokines are not exclusively detrimental. TNF may also protect ischaemic or stressed cardiomyocytes by attenuating mitochondrial dysfunction. Cytokine-mediated inflammation may also play a role in angiogenesis. V, vessel; ECM, extracellular matrix; MMP, matrix metalloproteinase.

This image was designed using Servier Medical Art (https://smart.servier.com/).

dose-dependent actions of the cytokine through different TNF receptors.[26]

Several members of the IL-1 family, including IL-1α/IL-1β, and IL-18, and the IL-33/soluble IL-1 receptor-like 1 (ST2) axis have been implicated in the pathogenesis of heart failure. Myocardial IL-1β expression is consistently upregulated in experimental models of heart failure[27] and in patients with cardiomyopathic conditions.[28] Heart failure is also associated with activation of the inflammasome,[29] the molecular platform responsible for caspase-1-mediated processing of pro-IL-1β into its active form. Both genetic and pharmacological approaches have suggested an important role for IL-1β signalling cascades in mediating adverse remodelling and dysfunction in experimental models of heart failure.[30] The effects of IL-1β on the failing heart may involve negative inotropic actions, pro-apoptotic effects on cardiomyocytes, mobilization and activation of leucocytes,[31] induction of adhesion molecules in endothelial cells, stimulation of a matrix-degrading phenotype in fibroblasts,[31] and pro-fibrotic effects mediated through increased expression of growth factors such as transforming growth factor beta (TGF-β).[32] The fibrogenic, microvascular, and inflammatory effects of IL-1β may contribute to the pathogenesis of HFpEF.

Studies on the role of IL-6 in heart failure have produced conflicting results, depending on the pathophysiological context, the model, and the type of experiment used to study the role of the cytokine. Most of the evidence suggests that activation of IL-6 signalling in the failing heart promotes dysfunction through pro-inflammatory actions of downstream gp130/STAT3 signalling.[33] In contrast, other investigations found no significant effects of IL-6 in the pressure-overloaded failing heart.[34] The pleiotropic actions of IL-6 on many different cell types that involve both classic IL-6 receptor (IL-6R)-mediated cascades and trans-signalling may explain the conflicting findings. IL-6 exerts its actions not only through binding to the cell surface IL-6R and subsequent association of the IL-6/IL-6R complex with glycoprotein 130, but also through association with soluble protease-derived IL-6R and subsequent stimulation of glycoprotein 130 cascades in cells lacking the receptor.[35] This mechanism of action is called 'trans-signaling' and may significantly contribute to the *in vivo* effects of the cytokine. Unfortunately, very limited information is available on the relative *in vivo* role of classic and trans-IL-6 signalling in heart failure.

Members of the chemokine family of chemotactic cytokines are also involved in the pathogenesis of heart failure, acting through chemotactic recruitment of leucocytes. The CC-chemokine ligand (CCL)-2 (also known as monocyte chemoattractant protein (MCP-) 1) is the best studied member of the CC-chemokine subfamily in heart failure and contributes to the pathogenesis of cardiac remodelling and fibrosis in models of ischaemic and non-ischaemic heart failure.[36] The fibrogenic effects of CCL2 in the failing heart may predominantly involve recruitment of monocytes capable of secreting fibrogenic mediators, rather than direct effects on resident cardiac fibroblasts.[37] Stromal cell-derived factor (SDF)-1 (also known as CXC motif ligand-12 (CXCL12)) is a chemokine with a critical role in cardiovascular development and disease. CXCL12 is markedly induced in injured hearts and exerts a wide range of actions on vascular cells, cardiomyocytes, immune cells, and progenitor cells. Pharmacological and genetic studies have produced conflicting evidence on the *in vivo* effects of CXCL12 in heart failure. In addition to its angiogenic actions, CXCL12 has been suggested to exert dose-dependent protective and pro-apoptotic effects on cardiomyocytes,[38] and may also stimulate immune cell activation, thus promoting inflammatory injury. The conflicting findings may reflect distinct cell- and context-specific actions of CXCL12 through its two main receptors CXCR4 and CXCR7.

Translational gaps and roadblocks

In the 1990s, the extensive experimental and clinical evidence implicating TNF as a central mediator in the pathogenesis of heart failure led to the conduction of several large prospective clinical trials aiming at neutralization of TNF in HFrEF. A pooled analysis showed that the compound etanercept had no effect on death and heart failure hospitalizations in HFrEF patients.[39] Infliximab, another TNF antagonist, even seemed to dose-dependently increase mortality in HFrEF patients.[40] Conflicting findings between promising preclinical data and disappointing clinical trials dampened for many years the enthusiasm to invest in further preclinical research and especially in clinical studies testing anti-inflammatory interventions in heart failure patients.

Since then, most progress on the role of the immune system in the pathogenesis of HFrEF has been derived from preclinical myocardial infarction (MI) models. Considering that MI is a major cause for chronic heart failure and that therapeutic interventions of limited duration (i.e. during the healing phase) might suffice to improve an individual patient's prognosis, acute MI seems currently to be the most promising disease state for immune-therapeutic approaches. A large body of preclinical evidence indicates that therapeutic interventions blocking excessive inflammation reduce the risk of maladaptive healing and consequent progression to chronic adverse remodelling as a cause for heart failure. However, experimental studies also showed that a tightly controlled balance between pro- and anti-inflammatory mechanisms is essential for wound healing after MI. Therefore, inflammation cannot be regarded simply as a maladaptive process, especially in the early stages after MI. Key questions on timing, duration, and proper identification of MI patients who would benefit from an immuno-therapeutic intervention are still open. Some of these questions cannot be properly addressed in standard rodent models of MI. Therefore, we currently face huge translational roadblocks, which have slowed advancement in the field for a long time.

Future directions: diagnostic and therapeutic horizons

Recently, the CANTOS trial showed that pharmacological blockade of IL-1β reduces the risk of recurrent vascular events, HF hospitalization, and mortality in patients with prior MI,[41] lending renewed support to the hypothesis that inflammatory mediators (cytokines and chemokines) are promising therapeutic targets in selected patients. However, the CANTOS trial was primarily designed to test the hypothesis that anti-IL-1β treatment reduces the incidence of vascular events in patients with a recent MI[42] and the data on HF were derived from a secondary endpoint analysis. The patient cohort was not properly characterized with respect to the prevalence and aetiology of baseline myocardial function and incident HF. Therefore, a prospective trial would be needed to make definite conclusions on the efficacy of the approach on clinically relevant HF endpoints. Unfortunately, the company decided not to study the drug canakinumab further in the cardiovascular field. However, other IL-1-binding compounds are available for clinical use. There are some preliminary data from relatively small clinical HF trials available for the compound anakinra.[43]

Within the innate immune system, inflammasome activation is a key event for IL-1β release in acute and chronic disease states. Colchicine has pleiotropic anti-inflammatory effects, including inhibitory action on inflammasomes. The drug showed favourable effects on cardiovascular events in several large prospective, placebo-controlled trials in coronary heart disease patients, including patients with recent acute MI. The benefits were more marked when treatment was initiated within the first 3 days after MI, as compared to within days 4–30, supporting the strategy of early initiation of colchicine in order to improve cardiovascular outcomes post-MI.[44] It is tempting to speculate that early colchicine initiation would also beneficially affect HF endpoints. Therefore, drugs targeting the inflammasome–IL-1β axis seem to be highly promising candidates for clinical trials in post-MI patients.

The innate immune system offers a plethora of therapeutic targets beyond pro-inflammatory cytokines. Upstream activation pathways, like pattern recognition receptors and inflammasomes, and regulators of leucocyte migration, including chemokine receptor antagonists and cell adhesion molecules merit further translational studies. Besides these targeted approaches, broader anti-inflammatory interventions include drugs such as adenosine receptor agonists and methotrexate that modulate the activity of leucocytes and non-leucocytes. Of note, compounds approved for clinical application are available for many of these targets, as they have been developed for other indications. However, only a minority of these were tested in advanced preclinical or early clinical HF trials. Many of these drugs have been developed for autoimmune arthritis. Fitting into the concept that systemic inflammation and vascular disease can lead to the HFpEF phenotype, patients with rheumatoid arthritis show increased cardiovascular mortality and seem to also have a higher risk of HFpEF.[45] Retrospective analysis showed that some drugs approved for rheumatoid arthritis could also be protective against cardiovascular events and HFpEF.[46]

Besides the innate mechanism of inflammation, the adaptive immune response to cardiac injury came into focus only recently. Rodent models showed that the injured heart is a target for antigen-specific autoimmune responses. However, for several reasons, the standard mouse models have serious limitations, especially regarding adaptive immune responses. Therefore, more reassuring data describing adaptive immune responses in humans would be of high value. Despite limited understanding of the relevance of adaptive immune responses in humans, early clinical trials targeting B and T lymphocytes are ongoing.[47,48]

Novel diagnostic strategies are now required that allow for personalized decisions on which individual patients might benefit from specific approaches. In the field of myocarditis, an inflammatory cardiomyopathy, myocardial biopsy is still regarded as the diagnostic gold standard for decision on immuno-modulatory treatment, but this approach has inherent limitations. Blood biomarkers and imaging might offer information to guide therapeutic decisions on immuno-modulatory treatment. However, there is a general lack of clinical trials that study interventions guided by biomarkers. Just to bring one example—the chemokine receptor CXCR4 is expressed on a variety of cells, including leucocytes. It was recently shown in patients after MI that activated mediastinal lymph nodes, indicative of an adaptive immune response, can be detected with a specific CXCR4 positron emission tomography (PET) tracer by using a PET/computed tomography (CT) approach.[49] Another experimental study demonstrated that PET/CT imaging-guided CXCR4 inhibition accelerates inflammation resolution in the infarcted myocardium and improves outcome.[50] As a matter of course, this innovative approach needs to be validated in a prospective clinical trial.

Moreover, unbiased omics approaches hold great promise to identify markers that allow for the identification of HF patients with high inflammatory burden. However, clinical trials testing immuno-modulatory approaches in patients selected by established or novel inflammation imaging techniques or other biomarkers are still pending.

Summary and key messages

Preclinical studies have raised hopes for new immuno-modulatory approaches that target very different components of the immune system that are relevant mostly for ischaemic HF. However, our understanding of the therapeutic potential of immuno-modulation in non-ischaemic HF, and especially in inherited cardiomyopathies, is still rudimentary. Given the resources needed to conduct an early clinical trial, or even a HF outcome trial, it is currently still a major challenge to select promising approaches as advanced translational data, for example, from large animal experiments, are widely lacking. Biomarker-guided approaches could help to limit sample size by identifying those patients most likely to benefit from immuno-modulation.

References

1. Adamo L, Rocha-Resende C, Prabhu SD, Mann DL. Reappraising the role of inflammation in heart failure. Nat Rev Cardiol. 2020;17(5):269–85.
2. Castillo EC, Vazquez-Garza E, Yee-Trejo D, Garcia-Rivas G, Torre-Amione G. What is the role of the inflammation in the pathogenesis of heart failure? Curr Cardiol Rep. 2020;22(11):139.
3. Panahi M, Papanikolaou A, Torabi A, et al. Immunomodulatory interventions in myocardial infarction and heart failure: a systematic review of clinical trials and meta-analysis of IL-1 inhibition. Cardiovasc Res. 2018;114(11):1445–61.
4. Trachtenberg BH, Hare JM. Inflammatory cardiomyopathic syndromes. Circ Res. 2017;121(7):803–18.
5. Finkel MS, Oddis CV, Jacob TD, Watkins SC, Hattler BG, Simmons RL. Negative inotropic effects of cytokines on the heart mediated by nitric oxide. Science. 1992;257(5068):387–9.
6. Siwik DA, Chang DL, Colucci WS. Interleukin-1beta and tumor necrosis factor-alpha decrease collagen synthesis and increase matrix metalloproteinase activity in cardiac fibroblasts in vitro. Circ Res. 2000;86(12):1259–65.
7. Frangogiannis NG. The extracellular matrix in ischemic and nonischemic heart failure. Circ Res. 2019;125(1):117–46.
8. Kapadia SR, Oral H, Lee J, Nakano M, Taffet GE, Mann DL. Hemodynamic regulation of tumor necrosis factor-alpha gene and protein expression in adult feline myocardium. Circ Res. 1997;81(2):187–95.
9. Epelman S, Lavine KJ, Beaudin AE, et al. Embryonic and adult-derived resident cardiac macrophages are maintained through distinct mechanisms at steady state and during inflammation. Immunity. 2014;40(1):91–104.
10. Frangogiannis NG, Lindsey ML, Michael LH, et al. Resident cardiac mast cells degranulate and release preformed TNF-alpha, initiating the cytokine cascade in experimental canine myocardial ischemia/reperfusion. Circulation. 1998;98(7):699–710.
11. Hofmann U, Frantz S. Role of lymphocytes in myocardial injury, healing, and remodeling after myocardial infarction. Circ Res. 2015;116(2):354–67.
12. Blanton RM, Carrillo-Salinas FJ, Alcaide P. T-cell recruitment to the heart: friendly guests or unwelcome visitors? Am J Physiol Heart Circ Physiol. 2019;317(1):H124–40.
13. Humeres C, Frangogiannis NG. Fibroblasts in the infarcted, remodeling, and failing heart. JACC Basic Transl Sci. 2019;4(3):449–67.
14. Torre-Amione G, Kapadia S, Lee J, et al. Tumor necrosis factor-alpha and tumor necrosis factor receptors in the failing human heart. Circulation. 1996;93(4):704–11.
15. Sun M, Chen M, Dawood F, et al. Tumor necrosis factor-alpha mediates cardiac remodeling and ventricular dysfunction after pressure overload state. Circulation. 2007;115(11):1398–407.
16. Jobe LJ, Melendez GC, Levick SP, Du Y, Brower GL, Janicki JS. TNF-alpha inhibition attenuates adverse myocardial remodeling in a rat model of volume overload. Am J Physiol Heart Circ Physiol. 2009;297(4):H1462–8.
17. Berry MF, Woo YJ, Pirolli TJ, et al. Administration of a tumor necrosis factor inhibitor at the time of myocardial infarction attenuates subsequent ventricular remodeling. J Heart Lung Transplant. 2004;23(9):1061–8.
18. Yokoyama T, Vaca L, Rossen RD, Durante W, Hazarika P, Mann DL. Cellular basis for the negative inotropic effects of tumor necrosis factor-alpha in the adult mammalian heart. J Clin Invest. 1993;92(5):2303–12.
19. Haudek SB, Taffet GE, Schneider MD, Mann DL. TNF provokes cardiomyocyte apoptosis and cardiac remodeling through

activation of multiple cell death pathways. J Clin Invest. 2007;117(9): 2692–701.

20. Sivasubramanian N, Coker ML, Kurrelmeyer KM, et al. Left ventricular remodeling in transgenic mice with cardiac restricted overexpression of tumor necrosis factor. Circulation. 2001;104(7):826–31.

21. Li YY, Feng YQ, Kadokami T, et al. Myocardial extracellular matrix remodeling in transgenic mice overexpressing tumor necrosis factor alpha can be modulated by anti-tumor necrosis factor alpha therapy. Proc Natl Acad Sci U S A. 2000;97(23):12746–51.

22. Mattila P, Majuri ML, Mattila PS, Renkonen R. TNF alpha-induced expression of endothelial adhesion molecules, ICAM-1 and VCAM-1, is linked to protein kinase C activation. Scand J Immunol. 1992;36(2):159–65.

23. Mark KS, Trickler WJ, Miller DW. Tumor necrosis factor-alpha induces cyclooxygenase-2 expression and prostaglandin release in brain microvessel endothelial cells. J Pharmacol Exp Ther. 2001;297(3):1051–8.

24. Dunlay SM, Weston SA, Redfield MM, Killian JM, Roger VL. Tumor necrosis factor-alpha and mortality in heart failure: a community study. Circulation. 2008;118(6):625–31.

25. Kurrelmeyer KM, Michael LH, Baumgarten G, et al. Endogenous tumor necrosis factor protects the adult cardiac myocyte against ischemic-induced apoptosis in a murine model of acute myocardial infarction. Proc Natl Acad Sci U S A. 2000;97(10):5456–61.

26. Hamid T, Gu Y, Ortines RV, et al. Divergent tumor necrosis factor receptor-related remodeling responses in heart failure: role of nuclear factor-kappaB and inflammatory activation. Circulation. 2009;119(10):1386–97.

27. Dewald O, Ren G, Duerr GD, et al. Of mice and dogs: species-specific differences in the inflammatory response following myocardial infarction. Am J Pathol. 2004;164(2):665–77.

28. Francis SE, Holden H, Holt CM, Duff GW. Interleukin-1 in myocardium and coronary arteries of patients with dilated cardiomyopathy. J Mol Cell Cardiol. 1998;30(2):215–23.

29. Suetomi T, Willeford A, Brand CS, et al. Inflammation and NLRP3 inflammasome activation initiated in response to pressure overload by Ca(2+)/calmodulin-dependent protein kinase II delta signaling in cardiomyocytes are essential for adverse cardiac remodeling. Circulation. 2018;138(22):2530–44.

30. Bujak M, Dobaczewski M, Chatila K, et al. Interleukin-1 receptor type I signaling critically regulates infarct healing and cardiac remodeling. Am J Pathol. 2008;173(1):57–67.

31. Saxena A, Chen W, Su Y, et al. IL-1 induces proinflammatory leukocyte infiltration and regulates fibroblast phenotype in the infarcted myocardium. J Immunol. 2013;191(9):4838–48.

32. Bageghni SA, Hemmings KE, Yuldasheva NY, et al. Fibroblast-specific deletion of interleukin-1 receptor-1 reduces adverse cardiac remodeling following myocardial infarction. JCI Insight. 2019;5(17):e125074.

33. Hilfiker-Kleiner D, Shukla P, Klein G, et al. Continuous glycoprotein-130-mediated signal transducer and activator of transcription-3 activation promotes inflammation, left ventricular rupture, and adverse outcome in subacute myocardial infarction. Circulation. 2010;122(2):145–55.

34. Lai NC, Gao MH, Tang E, et al. Pressure overload-induced cardiac remodeling and dysfunction in the absence of interleukin 6 in mice. Lab Invest. 2012;92(11):1518–26.

35. Mackiewicz A, Schooltink H, Heinrich PC, Rose-John S. Complex of soluble human IL-6-receptor/IL-6 up-regulates expression of acute-phase proteins. J Immunol. 1992;149(6):2021–7.

36. Hanna A, Frangogiannis NG. Inflammatory cytokines and chemokines as therapeutic targets in heart failure. Cardiovasc Drugs Ther. 2020;34(6):849–63.

37. Frangogiannis NG, Dewald O, Xia Y, et al. Critical role of monocyte chemoattractant protein-1/CC chemokine ligand 2 in the pathogenesis of ischemic cardiomyopathy. Circulation. 2007;115(5): 584–92.

38. Hu X, Dai S, Wu WJ, et al. Stromal cell derived factor-1 alpha confers protection against myocardial ischemia/reperfusion injury: role of the cardiac stromal cell derived factor-1 alpha CXCR4 axis. Circulation. 2007;116(6):654–63.

39. Mann DL, McMurray JJ, Packer M, et al. Targeted anticytokine therapy in patients with chronic heart failure: results of the Randomized Etanercept Worldwide Evaluation (RENEWAL). Circulation. 2004;109(13):1594–602.

40. Chung ES, Packer M, Lo KH, Fasanmade AA, Willerson JT; Anti-TNF Therapy Against Congestive Heart Failure Investigators. Randomized, double-blind, placebo-controlled, pilot trial of infliximab, a chimeric monoclonal antibody to tumor necrosis factor-alpha, in patients with moderate-to-severe heart failure: results of the anti-TNF Therapy Against Congestive Heart Failure (ATTACH) trial. Circulation. 2003;107(25):3133–40.

41. Everett BM, Cornel JH, Lainscak M, et al. Anti-inflammatory therapy with canakinumab for the prevention of hospitalization for heart failure. Circulation. 2019;139(10):1289–99.

42. Ridker PM, Everett BM, Thuren T, et al. Antiinflammatory therapy with canakinumab for atherosclerotic disease. N Engl J Med. 2017;377(12):1119–31.

43. Buckley LF, Carbone S, Trankle CR, et al. Effect of interleukin-1 blockade on left ventricular systolic performance and work: a post hoc pooled analysis of 2 clinical trials. J Cardiovasc Pharmacol. 2018;72(1):68–70.

44. Bouabdallaoui N, Tardif JC, Waters DD, et al. Time-to-treatment initiation of colchicine and cardiovascular outcomes after myocardial infarction in the Colchicine Cardiovascular Outcomes Trial (COLCOT). Eur Heart J. 2020;41(42):4092–9.

45. Logstrup BB, Ellingsen T, Pedersen AB, Kjaersgaard A, Botker HE, Maeng M. Development of heart failure in patients with rheumatoid arthritis: a Danish population-based study. Eur J Clin Invest. 2018;48(5):e12915.

46. Roubille C, Richer V, Starnino T, et al. The effects of tumour necrosis factor inhibitors, methotrexate, non-steroidal anti-inflammatory drugs and corticosteroids on cardiovascular events in rheumatoid arthritis, psoriasis and psoriatic arthritis: a systematic review and meta-analysis. Ann Rheum Dis. 2015;74(3):480–9.

47. Sanchez-Trujillo L, Jerjes-Sanchez C, Rodriguez D, et al. Phase II clinical trial testing the safety of a humanised monoclonal anti body anti-CD20 in patients with heart failure with reduced ejection fraction, ICFEr-RITU2: study protocol. BMJ Open. 2019;9(3): e022826.

48. Zhao TX, Kostapanos M, Griffiths C, et al. Low-dose interleukin-2 in patients with stable ischaemic heart disease and acute coronary syndromes (LILACS): protocol and study rationale for a randomised, double-blind, placebo-controlled, phase I/II clinical trial. BMJ open. 2018;8(9):e022452.

49. Rieckmann M, Delgobo M, Gaal C, et al. Myocardial infarction triggers cardioprotective antigen-specific T helper cell responses. J Clin Invest. 2019;129(11):4922–36.

50. Hess A, Derlin T, Koenig T, et al. Molecular imaging-guided repair after acute myocardial infarction by targeting the chemokine receptor CXCR4. Eur Heart J. 2020;41(37):3564–75.

CHAPTER 5.6

Inflammation, oxidative stress, and endothelial dysfunction

Stephane Heymans

Contents

Introduction

Vascular endothelial cells constitute the majority of the non-cardiomyocyte population of the heart. Therefore, their structural and/or functional abnormalities will have a strong impact on overall cardiac function and structure.[1] The microvascular bed, consisting of capillaries and arterioles, connects circulating inflammatory cells—the chronic systemic low-grade inflammation, together with heart failure (HF)—with the function of cardiomyocytes and fibroblasts. This chronic systemic inflammation and endothelial dysfunction go hand in hand with increased oxidative stress in endothelial cells and cardiomyocytes. Chronic oxidative stress and inflammation impact the main cell populations of the heart, including cardiomyocytes, fibroblasts, and the vascular bed itself. Therefore, the microvascular paradigm proposes endothelial dysfunction as the central mediator between chronic systemic low-grade inflammation and cardiac hypertrophy and fibrosis in HF.[2]

Metabolic and immune-mediated comorbidities are central in causing endothelial dysfunction and oxidative stress in HF. The metabolic syndrome (MetS: diabetes, hypertension, hyperlipidaemia), chronic kidney disease, and autoimmune diseases all trigger chronic systemic low-grade inflammation, characterized by elevated levels of circulating immune cells and pro-inflammatory cytokines (➲ Figure 5.6.1). Microvascular dysfunction may also occur in the context of cardiomyopathies or in the presence of obstructive epicardial coronary artery disease, or may even have a genetic origin.[3]

In this section, we will describe the impact of endothelial dysfunction and oxidative stress on the different cardiac compartments, starting with the microvascular bed through to cardiomyocytes and fibroblasts, and ending with the beginning, that is, inflammation and all its functional and morphological consequences on the heart.

The microvascular bed: molecular dysfunction and its rarefaction in heart failure

MetS-related comorbidities, such as obesity, type 2 diabetes (T2DM), and hypertension, trigger chronic systemic low-grade inflammation, with the release of pro-inflammatory cytokines and upregulation of endothelial adhesion molecules (➲ Figure 5.6.2). As a result, leucocytes, especially monocytes, invade the myocardium. Systemic inflammation co-occurs with upregulation of endothelial adhesion molecules, such as intercellular adhesion molecule 1 (ICAM-1) and vascular cellular adhesion molecule 1 (VCAM-1), and corresponding ligands on circulating monocytes. These monocytes produce pro-fibrotic factors, including transforming growth factor beta (TGFβ) and SPARC (osteonectin), among others, thereby inducing cardiac fibrosis. Furthermore, the systemic pro-inflammatory state induces coronary microvascular endothelial cells to produce

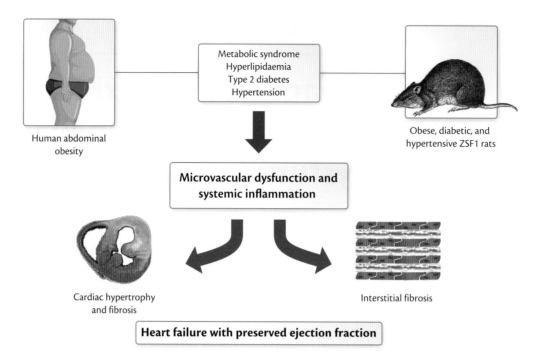

Figure 5.6.1 The metabolic syndrome (obesity, diabetes, hypertension, and hyperlipidaemia) is the main driver of endothelial dysfunction and related systemic inflammation. Locally, in the heart, it induces cardiac hypertrophy and fibrosis, leading to heart failure with preserved ejection fraction.

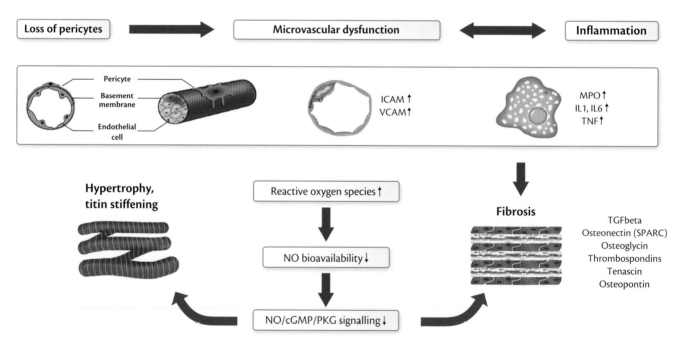

Figure 5.6.2 Metabolic syndrome (MetS)-related comorbidities trigger chronic systemic low-grade inflammation, characterised by elevated levels of circulating immune cells and pro-inflammatory cytokines and upregulation of endothelial adhesion molecules, such as intercellular and vascular cellular adhesion molecule-1 (ICAM-1 and VCAM-1), and corresponding ligands on circulating leucocytes. The resultant increased myocardial infiltration of leucocytes, especially monocytes, elevates cardiac transforming growth factor beta (TGFβ) levels and matricellular proteins, thereby inducing cardiac fibrosis. Furthermore, the systemic pro-inflammatory state causes coronary microvascular endothelial cells to produce excessive reactive oxygen species (ROS), contributing to cardiac oxidative stress resulting in oxidation of nitric oxide (NO). Consequently, the reduced NO bioavailability leads to impaired nitric oxide/cyclic guanosine monophosphate/protein kinase G (NO/cGMP/PKG) signalling, causing vascular endothelial dysfunction and cardiomyocyte hypertrophy and titin stiffening. Decreased NO bioavailability, increased leucocyte infiltration, oxidative stress, and/or neurohormonal activation trigger coronary microvascular endothelial dysfunction and reduced flow-mediated dilatation, which adversely impact cardiac perfusion, as observed in most HFpEF comorbidities.

excessive reactive oxygen species (ROS), contributing to cardiac oxidative stress and oxidation of nitric oxide (NO). The resulting impaired NO bioavailability reduces nitric oxide/cyclic guanosine monophosphate/protein kinase G (NO/cGMP/PKG) signalling, further aggravating the vascular endothelial dysfunction and leading to cardiomyocyte hypertrophy and overall stiffening.

NO is crucial to the normal function of the endothelium: it mediates vasodilatation, prevents platelet aggregation, and preserves the integrity of the endothelial layer via its anti-inflammatory, pro-angiogenic, anti-apoptotic, and anti-fibrotic properties.[4] An imbalance between endothelium-derived relaxing factors (primarily NO) and constrictors (e.g. endothelin-1)[5] also reduces flow-mediated dilatation of the microvascular bed, which adversely impacts cardiac perfusion.[6] Reduced NO bioavailability leads to: (1) a reduction in endothelial NO synthase (eNOS); (2) an increase in expression/activity of arginase, the natural competitor of eNOS; (3) deprivation of the substrate L-arginine via impaired recycling of L-citrulline; (4) a lack of the eNOS cofactor tetrahydrobiopterin; (5) a low eNOS/inducible NO synthase (iNOS) ratio; and (6) uncoupling of eNOS, a phenomenon via which eNOS produces superoxide ($O_2 \bullet$) rather than NO.[7,8]

In parallel with detrimental microvascular molecular alterations, a reduction in myocardial microvascular density, called microvascular rarefaction, occurs in HF patients.[9] Impaired coronary flow reserve relates to obesity, hypertension, increased subepicardial adipose tissue, T2DM, and advance ageing.[10,11] Capillary rarefaction contributes to insufficient cardiac perfusion by impairing myocardial oxygen delivery and increasing microvascular coronary resistance in HF patients. Reduced cardiac perfusion leads to a local blood supply–demand imbalance and energy metabolite deficiency, causing cardiac metabolic reprogramming and dysfunction.[12] More than 50% of patients with coronary microvascular dysfunction have an impaired capillary flow, which is independently associated with worsening diastolic function and HF hospitalization.[13] Microvascular rarefaction also correlates with reduced insulin delivery to muscles and adipose tissue.[14] Despite accumulating evidence for coronary microvascular rarefaction during HF development—in particular heart failure with preserved ejection fraction (HFpEF), its exact role in disease progression is still unknown.

The microvascular endothelial barrier

The microvascular endothelial barrier, which consists of the glycocalyx and intercellular tight junctions, is a barrier against free exchange between blood and tissues; a lack of NO due to endothelial dysfunction and oxidative stress will harm the integrity of the glycocalyx,[15] inducing pro-adhesion mediators of inflammatory cells.[16] In addition to its well-known role in heart failure with reduced ejection fraction (HFrEF), thinning of, and damage to, the glycocalyx occurs in most HFpEF-associated comorbidities. The glycocalyx acts as a mechanotransducer and controls vasoreactivity and peripheral resistance.[1] Its disruption induces detrimental alteration to coagulation and increases leucocyte adhesion to the endothelium. In particular, increased circulating levels of syndecan-1, a glycocalyx-shedding regulator and

biomarker,[17] are associated with endothelial dysfunction and an increased risk of all-cause mortality and HF rehospitalization.[18]

Impact of microvascular dysfunction on cardiomyocytes

Cardiomyocyte–endothelial cross-talk

Cardiomyocytes are in close spatial and anatomical contact with the coronary microvascular bed, allowing adequate oxygen and food supply, as well as bidirectional communication. Cardiomyocytes, in turn, also regulate the tone, growth, and development of the microvasculature via endothelin-1, fibroblast growth factor 2, and vascular endothelial growth factor A (VEGF-A), among others.[19] Endothelin-1 strongly contributes to cardiomyocyte hypertrophy as a result of inflammation or pressure load.[20] Insufficient cardiomyocyte–vascular cross-talk due to microvascular dysfunction may impair the compensatory growth of small vessels, together with myocyte hypertrophy, again resulting in relative hypoperfusion of the myocardium. This imbalance between vasculature and cardiomyocyte growth further induces progressive cardiac dysfunction by increasing cardiac hypertrophy and fibrosis, a maladaptive vicious circle.[1]

Titin alterations

The giant sarcomeric protein titin is not only a force-transducing protein, but also the main determinant of cardiomyocyte stiffness. Titin spans the sarcomere from the Z disk to the M line. It functions as a molecular spring supporting early diastolic recoil and late diastolic distensibility of cardiomyocytes.[21] Changes in cGMP/PKG signalling, increased oxidative stress, and impaired NO bioavailability make the titin protein less flexible, contributing to cardiac stiffness and diastolic dysfunction, often preceding cardiac fibrosis.[22] How do microvascular dysfunction and oxidative stress increase titin stiffness? First, oxidative stress induces the formation of disulfide bridges within the titin molecule, and causes isoform shifts and post-transcriptional modifications and aggregation of titin.[21] Alternative splicing of titin messenger ribonucleic acid (mRNA) creates isoforms with differing degrees of stiffness: the short, stiffer N2B isoform; and the longer, more compliant N2BA isoform. Increased PKG signalling, together with microvascular dysfunction, also induces increased phosphorylation of titin's PEVK element (domain rich in proline (P), glutamate (E), valine (V), and lysine (K)), augmenting cardiomyocyte stiffness. A decrease in protein kinase A, PKG, or calcium (Ca^{2+})/calmodulin-dependent protein kinase II activity under metabolic and inflammatory conditions results in hypophosphorylation of the N2B domain within titin, causing an increase in resting tension of titin.[21,23] Whereas post-translational modifications of titin increase cardiac stiffness in the short term, isotype switching does so in the long term.[21,23] In conclusion, microvascular dysfunction strongly impacts titin relaxation, resulting in cardiomyocyte stiffness, which leads to diastolic dysfunction, even in the absence of—or preceding and/or occurring in parallel with—cardiac fibrosis.

Impact of microvascular dysfunction on the fibroblast compartment

Oxidative stress and endothelial dysfunction induce cellular changes in fibroblasts, leading to increased interstitial fibrosis. Reduced NO bioavailability directly accelerates the conversion of fibroblasts into matrix-producing myofibroblasts. Fibrosis consists of the production of structural collagen fibres, as well as that of non-structural glycoproteins/proteoglycans. The latter have a pleiotropic function, as they act as a kind of interface among different cardiac cells, affecting inflammation, angiogenesis, cardiomyocyte function, and fibroblast proliferation.[24,25] Decreased cGMP induces phosphodiesterase 2-mediated degradation of cyclic adenosine monophosphate (cAMP) and also stimulates the differentiation of fibroblasts into myofibroblasts.[26] NO deprivation may also help the transdifferentiation of endothelial cells into myofibroblasts—so-called endothelial-to-mesenchymal transition (EndMT).[27] Finally, decreased NO bioavailability triggers the inflammation-related release of cytokines and chemokines, that in turn promote cardiac fibrosis.[28] Decreased NO bioavailability increases the expression of monocyte chemoattractant protein 1 (MCP-1) and VCAM-1, and subsequent adhesion of immune cells, which further triggers cardiac fibrosis and diastolic dysfunction via the release of TGFβ.[28] (Myo) fibroblasts further modulate the inflammatory process via the expression of matricellular proteins, chemokines, and matrix metalloproteinases (MMPs). MMPs produced by monocytes facilitate the degradation of the basement membrane and consequent transendothelial migration.[29,30,31] Myocardial fibrosis and dynamic changes in protein composition of the extracellular matrix are well-known pathological hallmarks of HF.[25]

Collagen

The quantity, type, and degree of cross-linking of collagen impact cardiac stiffness. Increased collagen deposition, switching from more flexible collagen type III to stiffer collagen type I, as well as collagen cross-linking, all induce cardiac stiffening and diastolic dysfunction. Lysyl oxidases (LOXs) are the main enzymes that cross-link collagen. Non-structural glycoproteins, such as SPARC (osteonectin) and osteoglycin (also called mimecan), also increase stiffening of collagen fibrils by stimulating their juxtaposition, making the fibrils thicker and less flexible.[32]

Non-structural matricellular proteins

HF and its comorbidities may induce a marked increase of several members of the matricellular family, including thrombospondins (TSPs), tenascin-C, osteopontin, SPARC, and periostin. These matricellular proteins regulate fibroblast proliferation and activation, and fibroblast conversion to myofibroblasts.[25,33,34] They all also induce the fibrogenic programme in cardiac fibroblasts, mostly by increasing the expression of TGFβ. Although the traditional definition of a matricellular protein implies the absence of a structural role, several members of the matricellular family (such as SPARC, TSP-1, and TSP-2) have been implicated in collagen fibril assembly and in regulation of extracellular matrix cross-linking.

TSP-2 and TSP-4 also improve survival of cardiomyocytes; absence of TSP-2 in mice results in reduced cardiomyocyte survival, as well as ageing,[35] whereas a lack of TSP-4 causes cardiomyocyte death due to loss of a TSP-4-dependent protective endoplasmic reticulum stress response.[36] Considering the diverse functions of matricellular proteins also on other cardiac cell types, their multiple functional domains, and their context-dependent effects, understanding the relative contribution of each matricellular protein in cardiac fibrosis and dysfunction in human HF remains challenging.

Inflammation

HF-related comorbidities are associated with chronic systemic low-grade inflammation, together with endothelial dysfunction and increased oxidative stress. The latter relates to augmented levels of systemic inflammatory markers, such as acute inflammatory C-reactive protein (CRP), interleukin (IL) 1, IL6, tumour necrosis factor (TNF), and myeloperoxidase (MPO), with its extent paralleling the number of comorbidities in HF patients. Circulating inflammatory factors, together with MetS and autoimmune disease, increase the systemic levels of neutrophils and monocytes, and facilitate the adhesion and transmigration of these cells into the cardiac tissue.[37] The role of activation and homing of splenic monocytes is central in this chronic inflammation, with a positive correlation between diastolic dysfunction and the release of splenic myeloid cells in HFpEF.[38] Activation of the renin–angiotensin–aldosterone system (RAAS) may also lead to endothelial cell activation, and upregulates inflammatory factors and their adhesion molecules. In T2DM, elevated advanced glycation end products (AGEs)/AGE receptor (RAGE) signalling stimulate the nuclear factor kappa-B (NFκB) signalling pathway, inducing pro-inflammatory genes and RAGE, forming a vicious cycle of self-renewing pro-inflammatory signals.[39]

Methods for measuring endothelial dysfunction

Numerous methods for measuring endothelial function exist,[40] most notably intracoronary arterial infusions combined with quantitative coronary angiography and Doppler imaging, flow-mediated vasodilation (FMD), peripheral arterial tonometry (PAT), endothelial progenitor cell colony-forming unit (EPC-CFU) assay, and circulating endothelial progenitor cells (EPCs). Whereas most of these methods are able to distinguish between patients with cardiovascular disease (CVD) and healthy controls, their diagnostic value in follow-up of endothelial dysfunction in individual patients is limited. Intracoronary acetylcholine (ACh) infusion was the first method discovered for measuring endothelial function; however, due to its invasive nature, FMD has largely replaced ACh infusion as the most widely used method. PAT is a newly emerging non-invasive method that is currently under investigation as an adjunct to FMD. Lastly, EPC measurements are generally considered a less direct method of measuring dysfunction, but studies have shown their important prognostic role in CVD. In conclusion, reliable methods to study and prospectively follow up endothelial dysfunction in individual patients are lacking, which limits the possibility of developing new therapies targeting microvascular dysfunction.

Heart failure treatment by targeting endothelial dysfunction and oxidative stress

Research into novel treatments for microvascular dysfunction is an unmet clinical need and is made more difficult due to the lack of reliable biomarkers/methods to measure endothelial dysfunction. Classical drugs, such as statins, angiotensin-converting enzyme (ACE) inhibitors, and beta-blockers, may all directly or mostly indirectly improve endothelial function, with associated upregulation of NO bioavailability and an inhibitory effect on vascular inflammation. Novel drugs targeting NO bioavailability, PKG expression, and cGMP signalling are the mostly focused research areas.[41]

Augmentation of cGMP signalling is recognized as a potential therapeutic strategy in HFpEF, based on several preclinical and clinical studies that have investigated various mechanisms and effects of cGMP enhancement.[42] However, the recent neutral result of the Effect of Phosphodiesterase-5 Inhibition on Exercise Capacity and Clinical Status in Heart Failure with Preserved Ejection Fraction (RELAX) trial with the phosphodiesterase type 5 (PDE-5) inhibitor sildenafil has challenged this strategy.[43] An alternative explanation focuses on the lack of significant increase in plasma cGMP with sildenafil, suggesting failure to adequately test the cGMP enhancement hypothesis. The discovery of soluble guanylate cyclase (sGC) stimulators and sGC activators is a milestone in the field of NO/sGC/cGMP pharmacology. The sGC stimulators and activators bind directly to reduced heme-containing and oxidized heme-free sGC, respectively, which results in an increase in cGMP production. The sGC stimulators and activators have a unique mode of action, with a broad treatment potential in CVD and beyond, but definite evidence is still needed from clinical trials.[44]

Given the plethora of cardiac detrimental effects triggered by chronic systemic low-grade inflammation alongside endothelial dysfunction-related systemic inflammation, the use of cytokine inhibitors has been extensively investigated in HF patients. IL-1β blockage (anakinra), for example, improved aerobic exercise capacity in HFpEF patients and is currently being investigated in a phase 2 clinical trial.[45] Furthermore, the multi-cytokine blocker pentoxifylline was found to reduce vascular events, systemic inflammation, and all-cause mortality, and to improve prognosis in HFrEF patients.[46] Despite all this, currently no effective anti-inflammatory drug has been approved for the treatment or prevention of HFpEF.

In conclusion, treatment of chronic inflammation and endothelial dysfunction depends on underlying comorbidities and disease triggers of HFpEF. In those patients with MetS, drugs targeting metabolism in different organs will most probably be effective. As HFpEF is part of a multi-organ disease, a systemic pill targeting the triad of inflammation, metabolism, and fibrosis in different organs will be most successful.

Summary and key messages

◆ The microvascular bed, consisting of capillaries and arterioles, connects circulating inflammatory cells—the chronic systemic low-grade inflammation, together with HF—with the function of cardiomyocytes and fibroblasts.

◆ Microvascular dysfunction mainly results from MetS—diabetes, hypertension, and hyperlipidaemia, together with obesity—and drives cardiac hypertrophy and diastolic dysfunction, leading to HFpEF.

◆ Members of the matricellular family, including TSPs, tenascin-C, osteopontin, SPARC, and periostin, regulate cardiac fibrosis, cardiomyocyte survival, and inflammation.

◆ Drugs that are beneficial in decreasing this metabolic load, such as sodium–glucose cotransporter 2 (SGLT2) inhibitors, have been proven to be beneficial in treating HFpEF.

Future directions

◆ Whether immune-regulating drugs, such as MPO inhibitors, or any other chemokine/cytokine-modulating drugs may be beneficial in treating endothelial dysfunction-related HFpEF remains unclear.

◆ Future clinical trials will address whether reducing the metabolic load via lowering of lipids or treating obesity may also be beneficial in treating endothelial dysfunction and related HFpEF progression.

◆ Reducing fibrosis may require controlled regulation of both inflammation and fibrosis. It is unclear whether reducing fibrosis only would be beneficial, due to the increased risk of cardiac dilatation.

References

1. Cuijpers I, Simmonds SJ, van Bilsen M, et al. Microvascular and lymphatic dysfunction in HFpEF and its associated comorbidities. *Basic Res Cardiol.* 2020;115:39.

2. Paulus WJ, Tschope C. A novel paradigm for heart failure with preserved ejection fraction: comorbidities drive myocardial dysfunction and remodeling through coronary microvascular endothelial inflammation. *J Am Coll Cardiol.* 2013;62:263–71.

3. Fedele F, Mancone M, Chilian WM, et al. Role of genetic polymorphisms of ion channels in the pathophysiology of coronary microvascular dysfunction and ischemic heart disease. *Basic Res Cardiol.* 2013;108:387.

4. Tschope C, Van Linthout S. New insights in (inter)cellular mechanisms by heart failure with preserved ejection fraction. *Curr Heart Fail Rep.* 2014;11:436–44.

5. Versari D, Daghini E, Virdis A, Ghiadoni L, Taddei S. Endothelium-dependent contractions and endothelial dysfunction in human hypertension. *Br J Pharmacol.* 2009;157:527–36.

6. Forrester SJ, Kikuchi DS, Hernandes MS, Xu Q, Griendling KK. Reactive oxygen species in metabolic and inflammatory signaling. *Circ Res.* 2018;122:877–902.

7. Braunwald E. Diabetes, heart failure, and renal dysfunction: the vicious circles. *Prog Cardiovasc Dis.* 2019;62:298–302.

8. Camici PG, Tschope C, Di Carli MF, Rimoldi O, Van Linthout S. Coronary microvascular dysfunction in hypertrophy and heart failure. *Cardiovasc Res.* 2020;116:806–16.

9. Mohammed SF, Hussain S, Mirzoyev SA, Edwards WD, Maleszewski JJ, Redfield MM. Coronary microvascular rarefaction and myocardial fibrosis in heart failure with preserved ejection fraction. *Circulation.* 2015;131:550–9.

10. Campbell DJ, Somaratne JB, Prior DL, *et al.* Obesity is associated with lower coronary microvascular density. *PLoS One.* 2013;8:e81798.

11. Nakanishi K, Fukuda S, Tanaka A, Otsuka K, Taguchi H, Shimada K. Relationships between periventricular epicardial adipose tissue accumulation, coronary microcirculation, and left ventricular diastolic dysfunction. *Can J Cardiol.* 2017;33:1489–97.

12. van de Wouw J, Sorop O, van Drie RWA, *et al.* Perturbations in myocardial perfusion and oxygen balance in swine with multiple risk factors: a novel model of ischemia and no obstructive coronary artery disease. *Basic Res Cardiol.* 2020;115:21.

13. Taqueti VR, Solomon SD, Shah AM, *et al.* Coronary microvascular dysfunction and future risk of heart failure with preserved ejection fraction. *Eur Heart J.* 2018;39:840–9.

14. Baron AD, Tarshoby M, Hook G, *et al.* Interaction between insulin sensitivity and muscle perfusion on glucose uptake in human skeletal muscle: evidence for capillary recruitment. *Diabetes.* 2000;49:768–74.

15. Bruegger D, Rehm M, Jacob M, *et al.* Exogenous nitric oxide requires an endothelial glycocalyx to prevent postischemic coronary vascular leak in guinea pig hearts. *Crit Care.* 2008;12:R73.

16. Jacob M, Paul O, Mehringer L, *et al.* Albumin augmentation improves condition of guinea pig hearts after 4 hr of cold ischemia. *Transplantation.* 2009;87:956–65.

17. Schellings MW, Vanhoutte D, van Almen GC, *et al.* Syndecan-1 amplifies angiotensin II-induced cardiac fibrosis. *Hypertension.* 2010;55:249–56.

18. Tromp J, van der Pol A, Klip IT, *et al.* Fibrosis marker syndecan-1 and outcome in patients with heart failure with reduced and preserved ejection fraction. *Circ Heart Fail.* 2014;7:457–62.

19. Tirziu D, Giordano FJ, Simons M. Cell communications in the heart. *Circulation.* 2010;122:928–37.

20. Heymans S, Hirsch E, Anker SD, *et al.* Inflammation as a therapeutic target in heart failure? A scientific statement from the Translational Research Committee of the Heart Failure Association of the European Society of Cardiology. *Eur J Heart Fail.* 2009;11:119–29.

21. Hamdani N, Paulus WJ. Myocardial titin and collagen in cardiac diastolic dysfunction: partners in crime. *Circulation.* 2013;128:5–8.

22. Chung CS, Hutchinson KR, Methawasin M, *et al.* Shortening of the elastic tandem immunoglobulin segment of titin leads to diastolic dysfunction. *Circulation.* 2013;128:19–28.

23. van Heerebeek L, Hamdani N, Falcao-Pires I, *et al.* Low myocardial protein kinase G activity in heart failure with preserved ejection fraction. *Circulation.* 2012;126:830–9.

24. Schellings MW, Pinto YM, Heymans S. Matricellular proteins in the heart: possible role during stress and remodeling. *Cardiovasc Res.* 2004;64:24–31.

25. Rienks M, Papageorgiou AP, Frangogiannis NG, Heymans S. Myocardial extracellular matrix: an ever-changing and diverse entity. *Circ Res.* 2014;114:872–88.

26. Vettel C, Lammle S, Ewens S, *et al.* PDE2-mediated cAMP hydrolysis accelerates cardiac fibroblast to myofibroblast conversion and is antagonized by exogenous activation of cGMP signaling pathways. *Am J Physiol Heart Circ Physiol.* 2014;306:H1246–52.

27. Murdoch CE, Chaubey S, Zeng L, *et al.* Endothelial NADPH oxidase-2 promotes interstitial cardiac fibrosis and diastolic dysfunction through proinflammatory effects and endothelial-mesenchymal transition. *J Am Coll Cardiol.* 2014;63:2734–41.

28. Khan BV, Harrison DG, Olbrych MT, Alexander RW, Medford RM. Nitric oxide regulates vascular cell adhesion molecule 1 gene expression and redox-sensitive transcriptional events in human vascular endothelial cells. *Proc Natl Acad Sci U S A.* 1996;93:9114–19.

29. Heymans S, Lupu F, Terclavers S, *et al.* Loss or inhibition of uPA or MMP-9 attenuates LV remodeling and dysfunction after acute pressure overload in ice. *Am J Pathol.* 2005;166:15–25.

30. Heymans S, Luttun A, Nuyens D, *et al.* Inhibition of plasminogen activators or matrix metalloproteinases prevents cardiac rupture but impairs therapeutic angiogenesis and causes cardiac failure. *Nat Med.* 1999;5:1135–42.

31. Creemers E, Cleutjens J, Smits J, *et al.* Disruption of the plasminogen gene in mice abolishes wound healing after myocardial infarction. *Am J Pathol.* 2000;156:1865–73.

32. Vanhoutte D, van Almen GC, Van Aelst LN, *et al.* Matricellular proteins and matrix metalloproteinases mark the inflammatory and fibrotic response in human cardiac allograft rejection. *Eur Heart J.* 2013;34:1930–41.

33. Papageorgiou AP, Heymans S. Interactions between the extracellular matrix and inflammation during viral myocarditis. *Immunobiology.* 2012;217:503–10.

34. Vanhoutte D, van Almen GC, Van Aelst LN, *et al.* Matricellular proteins and matrix metalloproteinases mark the inflammatory and fibrotic response in human cardiac allograft rejection. *Eur Heart J.* 2013;34:1930–41.

35. Swinnen M, Vanhoutte D, Van Almen GC, *et al.* Absence of thrombospondin-2 causes age-related dilated cardiomyopathy. *Circulation.* 2009;120:1585–97.

36. Lynch JM, Maillet M, Vanhoutte D, *et al.* A thrombospondin-dependent pathway for a protective ER stress response. *Cell.* 2012;149:1257–68.

37. Glezeva N, Voon V, Watson C, *et al.* Exaggerated inflammation and monocytosis associate with diastolic dysfunction in heart failure with preserved ejection fraction: evidence of M2 macrophage activation in disease pathogenesis. *J Card Fail.* 2015;21:167–77.

38. Hulsmans M, Sager HB, Roh JD, *et al.* Cardiac macrophages promote diastolic dysfunction. *J Exp Med.* 2018;215:423–40.

39. Bierhaus A, Humpert PM, Morcos M, *et al.* Understanding RAGE, the receptor for advanced glycation end products. *J Mol Med (Berl).* 2005;83:876–86.

40. Chia PY, Teo A, Yeo TW. Overview of the assessment of endothelial function in humans. *Front Med (Lausanne).* 2020;7:542567.

41. Maack C, Lehrke M, Backs J, *et al.* Heart failure and diabetes: metabolic alterations and therapeutic interventions: a state-of-the-art review from the Translational Research Committee of the Heart Failure Association-European Society of Cardiology. *Eur Heart J.* 2018;39:4243–54.

42. Greene SJ, Gheorghiade M, Borlaug BA, *et al.* The cGMP signaling pathway as a therapeutic target in heart failure with preserved ejection fraction. *J Am Heart Assoc.* 2013;2:e000536.

43. Redfield MM, Chen HH, Borlaug BA, *et al.* Effect of phosphodiesterase-5 inhibition on exercise capacity and clinical status in heart failure with preserved ejection fraction: a randomized clinical trial. *JAMA.* 2013;309:1268–77.

44. Sandner P, Zimmer DP, Milne GT, Follmann M, Hobbs A, Stasch JP. Soluble guanylate cyclase stimulators and activators. *Handb Exp Pharmacol.* 2021;264:355–94.

45. Van Tassell BW, Trankle CR, Canada JM, *et al.* IL-1 blockade in patients with heart failure with preserved ejection fraction. *Circ Heart Fail.* 2018;11:e005036.

46. Champion S, Lapidus N, Cherie G, Spagnoli V, Oliary J, Solal AC. Pentoxifylline in heart failure: a meta-analysis of clinical trials. *Cardiovasc Ther.* 2014;32:159–62.

CHAPTER 5.7

Alterations in renal haemodynamics and function in heart failure

Patrick Rossignol and Kevin Damman

Introduction

Interactions between chronic or acute heart failure (HF) and chronic kidney disease (CKD) or acute kidney injury are usually described as cardiorenal syndromes.[1,2] Although this term is not practical for clinical use, as it encompasses the entire spectrum of heart and kidney diseases, it is a fair representation of the close interaction between HF and accompanying renal dysfunction. CKD, mostly defined as an estimated glomerular filtration rate (eGFR) of <60 mL/min/1.73 m^2, is a highly prevalent condition among patients with acute and chronic HF. According to a meta-analysis of 57 studies comprising 1,076,104 patients,[3] 32% of HF patients presented with CKD. Both CKD and worsening renal function (WRF) were found to be associated with a 2-fold increase in mortality rate.[3] A number of factors were also found to be associated with WRF, including non-modifiable factors (e.g. age), cardiovascular risk factors (diabetes, hypertension), congestion or hypotension as hallmarks of HF severity, and drug use.[3] On the other hand, hypotension, kidney dysfunction, and hyperkalaemia are the main triggers for renin–angiotensin–aldosterone system (RAAS) inhibitor non-use, underdosing, and discontinuation.[4,5,6]

Kidney function estimation

In routine practice, while acknowledging the shortcomings of using serum creatinine level as a marker of glomerular filtration, kidney function is usually estimated by the creatinine-derived eGFR using the simplified Modification of Diet in Renal Disease (sMDRD) or the Chronic Kidney Disease Epidemiology Collaboration (CKD-EPI) formula. The latter has the best accuracy in the chronic HF setting.[7] Of importance, the presence of a steady state is a prerequisite for using such formulae, which precludes using the latter in the context of acute kidney injury where use of serum creatinine level and/or urinary output is considered instead.[7,8]

Pathophysiology of renal impairment in heart failure

Haemodynamic alterations that occur in HF, such as reduced cardiac output and increased filling pressures (especially central venous pressure), are the main determinants of renal dysfunction in HF (➲ Figure 5.7.1).[9,10,11,12] In the setting of chronic HF with reduced ejection fraction (HFrEF), reduced renal perfusion is mainly responsible for the reduction in the glomerular filtration rate (GFR), and renal autoregulation (counteracted by evidence-based therapies) preserves the GFR to some extent.[9,13] In the setting of volume overload, such as in acute HF, the relative contributions of low cardiac output and low renal blood flow are less important, and it is hypothesized that increased central and renal venous pressures are the main driving force of a low GFR and the development of WRF.[10,11,12] Increased

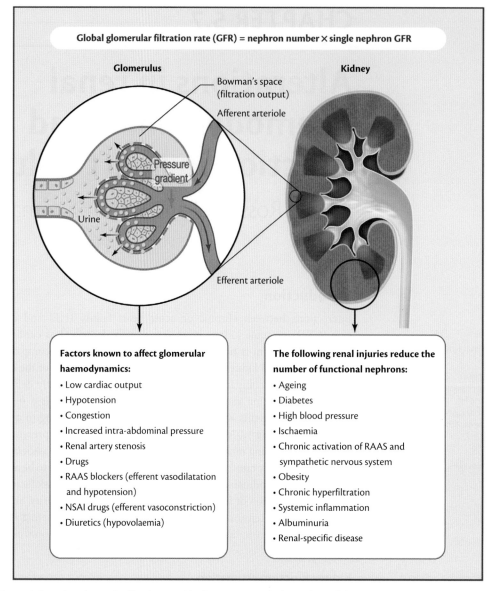

Figure 5.7.1 Main factors influencing glomerular filtration rate (GFR) in patients with chronic heart failure. RAAS, renin–angiotensin–aldosterone system; NSAI, non-steroidal anti-inflammatory.

Reproduced from Mewton N, Girerd N, Boffa JJ, *et al*. Practical management of worsening renal function in outpatients with heart failure and reduced ejection fraction: Statement from a panel of multidisciplinary experts and the Heart Failure Working Group of the French Society of Cardiology. *Arch Cardiovasc Dis*. 2020 Oct;**113**(10):660–670. doi: 10.1016/j.acvd.2020.03.018 with permission from Elsevier.

renal venous pressures not only influence renal perfusion pressure, but are also linked to intrarenal hypertension in the encapsulated kidney and renal interstitial fibrosis, and can also exert pressure on the renal tubular system and collecting ducts, which can collapse under increased intrarenal pressures.[14] During treatment of volume overload and congestion, the effects of increased renal venous pressures become less important and renal perfusion will be the main contributing factor to renal dysfunction.

It is important to realize that these haemodynamic concepts are the basis of cardiorenal interactions, but that there are many interindividual differences. For example, HF patients who have either long-standing diabetes mellitus or hypertension, and/or an atherosclerotic risk profile are at greater risk of glomerulosclerosis, loss of nephrons, and renal fibrosis. Different concomitant therapies also have their influence on renal perfusion and filtration (such as angiotensin-converting enzyme inhibitors (ACEIs), angiotensin receptor blockers (ARBs), angiotensin receptor–neprilysin inhibitors (ARNIs), mineralocorticoid receptor antagonists (MRAs), and sodium–glucose cotransporter 2 (SGLT2) inhibitors), which means that the haemodynamic equilibrium that eventually leads to renal filtration will be a more dynamic process and differ in each individual.[7] Unfortunately, to date, it is impossible to measure or calculate single-nephron GFR in humans.

Worsening renal function

In relatively stable chronic HF patients with reduced ejection fraction, the slope in eGFR decline can be as high as 2 mL/min/

$1.73\,m^2$ per year, as compared to 0.5–1.0 mL/min/$1.73\,m^2$ per year in healthy individuals.[7] In acute HF, changes in renal function are much more difficult to investigate, as there is no steady state to allow appropriate use of creatinine-based formulae of eGFR. However, changes in serum creatinine concentration during treatment of acute HF can be large and variable, suggesting a large variation in individual changes in the GFR in this high-risk population.[15]

When the serum creatinine level increases or the eGFR decreases more than expected, the literature on renal disease advocates the use of the term acute kidney injury (AKI).[8] Yet, the occurrence of true AKI in the setting of HF is rare, and the pathophysiology of AKI in renal disease is entirely different as compared to acute renal changes in HF. The former represents intrarenal changes, whereas the haemodynamics are responsible for most changes in renal function in (acute) HF. Therefore, the HF literature has adopted the term worsening renal function (WRF).[7,16] As mentioned, WRF per se is associated with worse clinical outcomes, but more recent research and consensus statements have clearly shown that it is even more important to consider the context in which WRF develops. As such, WRF can be a representation of a worsening condition (true WRF), whereas we also observe WRF in the setting of initiation of lifesaving therapies or during decongestive treatment (pseudo-WRF).[7] In the former situation, WRF is associated with worse outcomes, whereas this is not the case (or at least less so) in the latter setting.

In the chronic HF setting, total GFR is the product of both the number of functioning nephrons and the single-nephron GFR[7] (➲ Figure 5.7.1), according to a recent position paper.[17] Chronic HF and CKD share common risk factors (e.g. hypertension, obesity, diabetes) and interrelated comorbidities (e.g. coronary artery disease), with the latter contributing to the frequently observed impairment in kidney function in HF patients. In both conditions, there is often overactivation of the RAAS, which can be amplified by loop or thiazide diuretic use. Initiation of lifesaving therapies (with RAAS and SGLT-2 inhibitors) is usually associated with a rise in serum creatinine level, due to renal haemodynamic alterations, which ultimately does not impair the beneficial cardiovascular effects of these drugs.[18] A meta-analysis showed that WRF in patients with HFrEF randomized to RAAS inhibitor therapy was associated with a greater mortality risk, compared to patients without WRF (relative risk 1.19, 95% confidence interval (CI) 1.08–1.31; $P<0.001$), although this risk was lower than the mortality risk associated with WRF in patients randomized to placebo (relative risk 1.48, 95% CI 1.35–1.62; $P<0.001$; $P=0.005$ for interaction with patients randomized to RAAS inhibitors). In contrast, WRF in patients with HF with preserved ejection fraction (HFpEF) randomized to RAAS inhibitor therapy was associated with a greater mortality risk, whereas in patients with HFpEF randomized to placebo, it was not significantly associated with mortality.[2,19] There is no evidence, to date, that RAAS inhibitors may ultimately improve kidney function in

chronic HFrEF in the long term, although it is hypothesized that they may limit progression of eGFR decline.

In contrast, despite the initial reduction in eGFR, HFrEF patients with and those without diabetes under treatment with SGLT2 inhibitors ultimately showed a more preserved eGFR in the long term and a concomitant improvement in cardiovascular and renal outcomes.[20] The exact mechanisms by which SGLT2 inhibitors exert their renal and cardiovascular benefits are not fully established but are probably related to their effects on sodium balance, energy homeostasis, and mitigation of cellular stress.[20] The effects of SGLT2 inhibitors on renal haemodynamics in HF are under investigation, but given the decrease in GFR in the context of higher natriuresis and pronounced RAAS inhibition, they are likely the result of afferent arteriolar constriction due to tubuloglomerular feedback. Results of cardiovascular (and renal) outcome trials with SGLT-2 inhibitors in HFpEF are eagerly awaited.[21]

Insights into the pathophysiology of the WRF phenomenon in acute HF

The pathophysiology of WRF in acute HF is depicted in ➲ Figure 5.7.2.[7] Venous congestion—rather than low cardiac output alone—is the major contributor of the observed WRF in acute HF.[11] Decongestion strategies (e.g. with loop diuretics) may ultimately lead to improved kidney function but also may worsen it (pseudo-WRF, which—in the context of a favourable diuretic response—is not associated with clinical outcome), and in the event of dehydration and/or hypotension associated with hypovolaemia, it should be considered as true WRF which is associated with worse outcomes.

Practical management of (pseudo-)WRF/dyskalaemia: the Assess, Adapt, Monitor (A2M) algorithm

Should (pseudo-)WRF and/or hyperkalaemia (an inherent risk from using RAAS inhibitors) or hypokalaemia occur (while using non-potassium-sparing (loop) diuretics), the interplay between HF and kidney disease in patients with chronic cardiorenal syndrome can lead to highly complex and challenging clinical scenarios.[2] The 2016 European Society of Cardiology (ESC)/Heart Failure Association (HFA) guidelines published two insightful web appendix tables (Tables 7.4 and 7.6) on kidney function/potassium management in HFrEF patients treated with ACEIs/ARBs or MRAs, respectively.[22] These guidelines can be summarized as three general rules (➲ Figure 5.7.3, thus proposing a simple and pragmatic algorithm in various clinical settings for use by clinicians faced with WRF in chronic HFrEF outpatients):

- An increase in creatinine concentration following RAAS inhibitor initiation is common, and is acceptable up to 50% above the baseline value; in the same manner, an increase in potassium concentration of up to ≤5.5 mmol/L is acceptable;

- For increases in creatinine concentration of >50% and below 100% of the baseline value, the clinical situation should be assessed using a systematic approach (congestion, dehydration, blood pressure, concomitant interaction), and medications

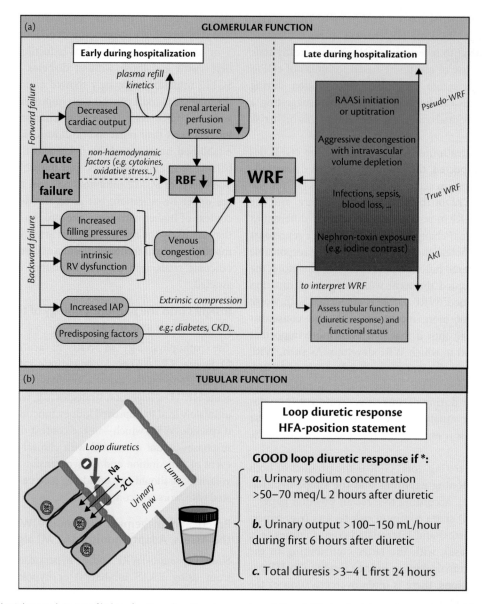

Figure 5.7.2 Pathophysiology and timing of kidney function alterations in acute heart failure. (a) Pathophysiology of worsening renal function (WRF) in relation to timing of hospitalization. Later in hospitalization, changes in serum creatinine concentration can occur (WRF); while some cases are not associated with worse outcome (pseudo-WRF = green), others are (true WRF/acute kidney injury). To understand pseudo-WRF, assessment of tubular function (diuretic response, b) is necessary. AKI, acute kidney injury; CKD, chronic kidney disease; HFA, Heart Failure Association; IAP, intra-abdominal pressure; RAASi, renin–angiotensin–aldosterone system inhibitor; RBF, renal blood flow; RV, right ventricular.

Reproduced from Mullens W, Damman K, Testani JM, et al. Evaluation of kidney function throughout the heart failure trajectory—a position statement from the Heart Failure Association of the European Society of Cardiology. Eur J Heart Fail. 2020 Apr;22(4):584–603. doi: 10.1002/ejhf.1697. wth permission from John Wiley and Sons.

should be adjusted accordingly (halving of usual doses can be considered), with careful and close follow-up after any change in treatment strategy; and

- If the potassium concentration rises to >5.5 mmol/L, or the creatinine concentration increases by >100% of the baseline value or is >310 µmol/L, or the eGFR is <20 mL/min/1.73 m², current ACEIs (or ARBs or ARNIs) and MRAs should be stopped and specialist advice from a nephrologist should be sought; in all cases of hyperkalaemia of >5.5 mmol/L, a second blood sample should be taken for confirmation, due to potential confounders such as haemolysis.

In any instance, non-cardiac aetiologies of WRF must be sought (e.g. acute intercurrent illness, drugs such as non-steroidal anti-inflammatory drugs and antibiotics, contrast agent exposure, etc.).

Future directions

Research priorities may include:[21]

- Defining the best monitoring strategies for decongestion or recurrent congestion[23]
- Identifying the most effective components of disease management programmes

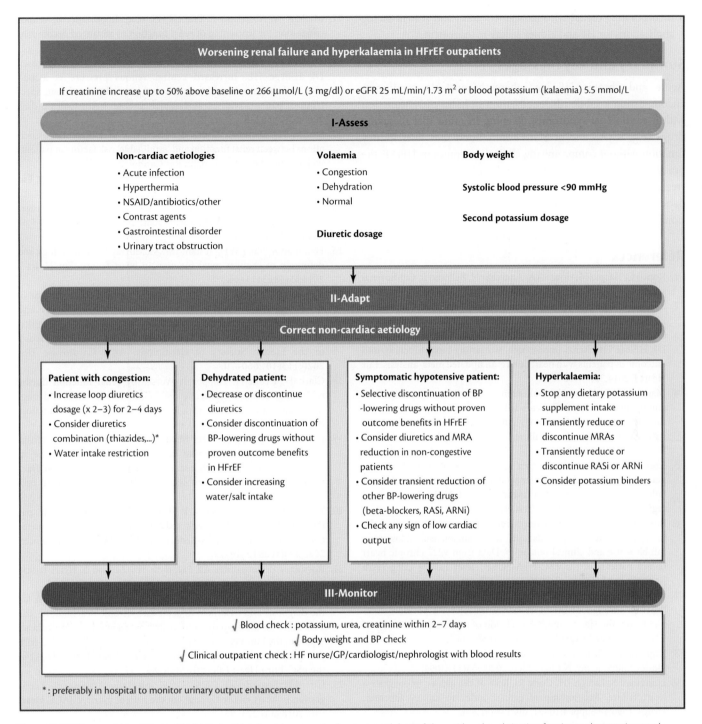

Figure 5.7.3 'Assess, Adapt, Monitor' (A2 M) algorithm for management of patients with heart failure with reduced ejection fraction and worsening renal function and/or hyperkalaemia. ARNi, angiotensin receptor–neprilysin inhibitor; BP, blood pressure; eGFR, estimated glomerular filtration rate; GP, general practitioner; HF, heart failure; HFrEF, heart failure with reduced ejection fraction; MRA, mineralocorticoid receptor antagonist; NSAID, non-steroidal anti-inflammatory drug; RASi, renin–angiotensin system inhibitor.

Reproduced from Mewton N, Girerd N, Boffa JJ, et al. Practical management of worsening renal function in outpatients with heart failure and reduced ejection fraction: Statement from a panel of multidisciplinary experts and the Heart Failure Working Group of the French Society of Cardiology. Arch Cardiovasc Dis. 2020 Oct;**113**(10):660–670. doi: 10.1016/j.acvd.2020.03.018 with permission from Elsevier.

◆ Incorporating digital self-management tools and patient-facing applications for HF and kidney failure management.[24]

Summary and key messages

Acute and chronic HF are inherently unstable conditions, encompassing a subtle (dis)equilibrium in kidney (dys)function within cardiorenal syndromes. Keeping in mind that lifesaving drugs (e.g. RAAS and/or SGLT2 inhibitors) may alter kidney function without compromising clinical outcomes in HFrEF, the practising physician must be ready to adapt ongoing HF drug treatment (especially with loop diuretics) at any time of their patient's clinical status, while properly interpreting kidney function variations.

References

1. Ronco C, Haapio M, House AA, Anavekar N, Bellomo R. Cardiorenal syndrome. J Am Coll Cardiol. 2008;52(19):1527–39.

2. Zannad F, Rossignol P. Cardiorenal syndrome revisited. Circulation. 2018;138(9):929–44.

3. Damman K, Valente MA, Voors AA, O'Connor CM, van Veldhuisen DJ, Hillege HL. Renal impairment, worsening renal function, and outcome in patients with heart failure: an updated meta-analysis. Eur Heart J. 2014;35(7):455–69.

4. Maggioni AP, Anker SD, Dahlstrom U, et al. Are hospitalized or ambulatory patients with heart failure treated in accordance with European Society of Cardiology guidelines? Evidence from 12,440 patients of the ESC Heart Failure Long-Term Registry. Eur J Heart Fail. 2013;15(10):1173–84.

5. Komajda M, Cowie MR, Tavazzi L, et al. Physicians' guideline adherence is associated with better prognosis in outpatients with heart failure with reduced ejection fraction: the QUALIFY international registry. Eur J Heart Fail. 2017;19(11):1414–23.

6. Rossignol P, Lainscak M, Crespo-Leiro MG, et al. Unravelling the interplay between hyperkalaemia, renin–angiotensin–aldosterone inhibitor use and clinical outcomes. Data from 9222 chronic heart failure patients of the ESC-HFA-EORP Heart Failure Long-Term Registry. Eur J Heart Fail. 2020;22(8):1378–89.

7. Mullens W, Damman K, Testani JM, et al. Evaluation of kidney function throughout the heart failure trajectory: a position statement from the Heart Failure Association of the European Society of Cardiology. Eur J Heart Fail. 2020;22(4):584–603.

8. Legrand M, Rossignol P. Cardiovascular consequences of acute kidney injury. Reply. N Engl J Med. 2020;383(11):1094.

9. Ljungman S, Laragh JH, Cody RJ. Role of the kidney in congestive heart failure. Relationship of cardiac index to kidney function. Drugs. 1990;39 Suppl 4:10–21; discussion 2–4.

10. Damman K, Navis G, Smilde TD, et al. Decreased cardiac output, venous congestion and the association with renal impairment in patients with cardiac dysfunction. Eur J Heart Fail. 2007;9(9):872–8.

11. Mullens W, Abrahams Z, Francis GS, et al. Importance of venous congestion for worsening of renal function in advanced decompensated heart failure. J Am Coll Cardiol. 2009;53(7):589–96.

12. Damman K, van Deursen VM, Navis G, Voors AA, van Veldhuisen DJ, Hillege HL. Increased central venous pressure is associated with impaired renal function and mortality in a broad spectrum of patients with cardiovascular disease. J Am Coll Cardiol. 2009;53(7):582–8.

13. Smilde TD, Damman K, van der Harst P, et al. Differential associations between renal function and 'modifiable' risk factors in patients with chronic heart failure. Clin Res Cardiol. 2009;98(2):121–9.

14. Damman K, Testani JM. The kidney in heart failure: an update. Eur Heart J. 2015;36(23):1437–44.

15. Beldhuis IE, Streng KW, van der Meer P, et al. Trajectories of changes in renal function in patients with acute heart failure. J Card Fail. 2019;25(11):866–74.

16. Damman K, Tang WH, Testani JM, McMurray JJ. Terminology and definition of changes renal function in heart failure. Eur Heart J. 2014;35(48):3413–16.

17. Mewton N, Girerd N, Boffa JJ, et al. Practical management of worsening renal function in outpatients with heart failure and reduced ejection fraction: statement from a panel of multidisciplinary experts and the Heart Failure Working Group of the French Society of Cardiology. Arch Cardiovasc Dis. 2020;113(10):660–70.

18. Clark H, Krum H, Hopper I. Worsening renal function during renin–angiotensin–aldosterone system inhibitor initiation and long-term outcomes in patients with left ventricular systolic dysfunction. Eur J Heart Fail. 2014;16(1):41–8.

19. Beldhuis IE, Streng KW, Ter Maaten JM, et al. Renin–angiotensin system inhibition, worsening renal function, and outcome in heart failure patients with reduced and preserved ejection fraction: a meta-analysis of published study data. Circ Heart Fail. 2017;10(2):e003588.

20. Zannad F, Ferreira JP, Pocock SJ, et al. SGLT2 inhibitors in patients with heart failure with reduced ejection fraction: a meta-analysis of the EMPEROR-Reduced and DAPA-HF trials. Lancet. 2020;396(10254):819–29.

21. Rossignol P, Hernandez AF, Solomon SD, Zannad F. Heart failure drug treatment. Lancet. 2019;393(10175):1034–44.

22. Ponikowski P, Voors AA, Anker SD, et al. 2016 ESC Guidelines for the diagnosis and treatment of acute and chronic heart failure: The Task Force for the diagnosis and treatment of acute and chronic heart failure of the European Society of Cardiology (ESC). Developed with the special contribution of the Heart Failure Association (HFA) of the ESC. Eur J Heart Fail. 2016;18(8):891–975.

23. Girerd N, Seronde MF, Coiro S, et al. Integrative assessment of congestion in heart failure throughout the patient journey. JACC Heart Fail. 2018;6(4):273–85.

24. Rossignol P, Coats AJ, Chioncel O, Spoletini I, Rosano G. Renal function, electrolytes, and congestion monitoring in heart failure. Eur Heart J Suppl. 2019;21(Suppl M):M25–31.

CHAPTER 5.8

Systemic adaptations in metabolism and nutritional status

Stephan von Haehling and Wolfram Doehner

Contents

Introduction

Chronic heart failure (HF) is a systemic and multifaceted syndrome involving maladaptation and impairment of metabolic regulation in multiple organs and systems. Metabolic imbalance affects both energy metabolism and structural metabolism that can be best described as anabolic blunting and catabolic dominance.[1] This imbalance intensifies body wasting processes leading to sarcopenia and cachexia. While some of these tissue wasting processes are related to the ageing process, others are more disease-related. Recent research data have buttressed the view that a variety of factors contribute to catabolic wasting, in particular neurohormonal, pro-inflammatory, and immune activation and an imbalance between anabolic and catabolic activity, as well as nutritional aspects and a sedentary lifestyle. Since the processes involved in wasting are closely intertwined, the presence of a wasting continuum has been proposed for HF.[2] Unfortunately, it is unclear what the determinants of manifest wasting in HF are, but skeletal muscle wasting—also known as sarcopenia—affects 20–50% of all HF patients, while overt weight loss affects approximately 10–15% of ambulatory patients. It has been well established that quality of life and mobility are significantly affected when skeletal muscle is lost as part of the wasting process.[3] The aim of this chapter is to provide an overview of metabolic pathways, including nutritional aspects, that interact in patients with advanced HF.

Muscle wasting

The term muscle wasting refers primarily to the loss of skeletal muscle. However, cardiac muscle can also be affected as part of catabolic processes during the course of the disease. It is important to acknowledge that the ageing process per se is usually associated with loss of 1–2% of skeletal muscle per year.[4] Therefore, skeletal muscle wasting beyond certain cut-off values—in geriatrics usually termed sarcopenia—affects 5–13% of 60- to 70-year-old subjects and up to 50% of all octogenerians.[1] The term sarcopenia was originally suggested in 1989.[5] It describes a clinical condition that is different from cachexia, because sarcopenia implies the loss of skeletal muscle's functional tissue that may be compensated for by adipose tissue or other non-functional tissue inside skeletal muscle. While the term cachexia refers to easily measurable loss of body weight as a consequence of global tissue wasting that includes adipose tissue, skeletal muscle, and bone tissue, sarcopenia is not usually associated with weight loss. The common definition of sarcopenia is too low lean (fat-free) appendicular mass where the lean mass corrected for height squared is lower than two standard deviations below the mean value of healthy individuals from the same ethnic group aged 20–30 years.[6] Cut points defined by this criterion and used in studies of HF were <7.26 kg for appendicular lean mass in men and <5.45 kg in women.[6] Thus, sarcopenia affects approximately 20% of patients with HF with reduced ejection fraction,[7] and about the same percentage of patients with HF with preserved ejection fraction.[8] One study in patients with dilated cardiomyopathy found higher values, reaching a prevalence of 47.3%.[9] However, it is unclear if patients with genetically determined cardiomyopathy may have myositis or other muscle disorders playing a role. Importantly, the presence of sarcopenia represents an independent predictor of survival (⊃ Figure 5.8.1),[10] but sarcopenia in HF is also associated with reduced exercise capacity and muscle strength,[7,8] endothelial dysfunction,[11] low quality of life, and altered resting energy expenditure (⊃ Figure 5.8.2).

Cardiac cachexia

The term cachexia was first used by the French physician Charles Mauriac, who mentioned it in his medical dissertation in 1860.[12] Cardiac cachexia describes involuntary weight loss as the cardinal symptom in the context of HF. Several cut-off values and time courses of weight loss have been proposed to define cachexia,[13,14] but the most appropriate cut-off is 6% loss in body weight over the preceding 12 months.[15] Notably, involuntary weight loss of this degree, even in obese subjects, can be a sign of an anabolic/catabolic imbalance and thus be referred to as cachexia, which is always a *signum mali ominis*, and in HF an independent predictor of death.[16] Cardiac cachexia affects all body compartments, including skeletal muscle, in which case its presence is associated with reduced muscle mass, muscle strength, and exercise capacity.[2] However, pro-inflammatory activation and other components of the wasting process described below contribute to the overall clinical picture with anorexia, anaemia, hypogonadism, and insulin resistance.[12,17]

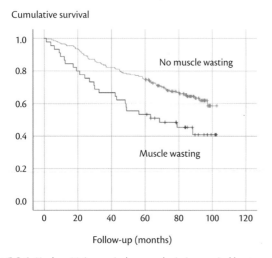

Cumulative survival

No muscle wasting

Muscle wasting

Follow-up (months)

Figure 5.8.1 Kaplan–Meier survival curves depicting survival by status of muscle wasting in a mixed cohort of patients with heart failure.
Reproduced from von Haehling S, Garfias Macedo T, Valentova M, Anker MS, Ebner N, Bekfani et al. Muscle wasting as an independent predictor of survival in patients with chronic heart failure. *J Cachexia Sarcopenia Muscle*. 2020;11(5):1242–1249. doi: 10.1002/jcsm.12603 with permission from John Wiley and Sons.

Anabolic/catabolic imbalance

As mentioned before, an imbalance between anabolic and catabolic mechanisms contributes to body wasting in HF. Energy expenditure and appetite are regulated in a complex manner in humans (⊃ Figure 5.8.3).[18] It is still not fully uncovered how the derangement of the mediators involved in this system is principally triggered. However, it appears that pro-inflammatory activation, with increases in circulating cytokines and reactive oxygen species (ROS), does play a role. The net result is a metabolic imbalance that depends, on one side, on blunted signals of anabolic factors such as insulin, testosterone, and growth hormone (GH). A typical pathology observed in this context is the development of hormonal resistance of tissues such as that described for insulin resistance[19] and GH resistance[20] in patients with HF. Cachectic HF patients were found to present with reduced plasma levels of insulin-like growth factor 1 (IGF-1), indicating acquired GH resistance[21] that has been reported for many catabolic disease states, including sepsis or chronic obstructive pulmonary disease (COPD).[21]

Other signalling factors may also be relevant to impaired metabolic balance, such as neuropeptide Y (NPY), leptin, and adiponectin, but their roles in HF are not fully understood. NPY is a potent stimulator of food intake in the hypothalamus. In patients with HF, elevated levels of NPY have been reported, in comparison to healthy control subjects, even though only small amounts of the peptide cross the blood–brain barrier.[22] Leptin, a protein hormone exclusively secreted from fat tissue, directly inhibits the effects of NPY and relates to the GH-binding protein, the cleaved extracellular domain of the GH receptor, which suggests an interaction with the GH signalling pathway. Leptin levels are elevated in HF when corrected for adipose tissue mass,[22] which is viewed as a negative feedback link between adipose tissue and food intake. In the periphery, leptin, together with adiponectin, another adipocyte-derived hormone, sensitizes tissue for the action of insulin.[23] Insulin is another important mediator centrally involved in abnormal metabolic balance in HF. Besides its role in the regulation of glucose balance, insulin has a strong anabolic capacity. Insulin resistance has been observed as an intrinsic pathophysiological feature of HF that is associated with symptomatic severity of HF, as well as with reduced muscle strength,[24] increased vascular resistance, and higher mortality.[25]

Nutritional aspects

A number of nutritional deficits have been reported in patients with HF. Another frequent finding in patients with HF is anorexia, that is, loss of appetite. Unsurprisingly, a higher risk of malnutrition has been reported in patients with HF, even without manifest wasting processes.[26] Nutritional deficits embrace magnesium, calcium, zinc, copper, manganese, energy, and vitamins B_1, B_2, and B_9 (folic acid).[27] Deficiencies in micronutrients are frequently the result of use of loop and thiazide diuretics, and a study of 404 patients who received furosemide over at least 3 months found that 12.3% had manifest magnesium deficiency. Women, patients with diabetes, and patients with coincident

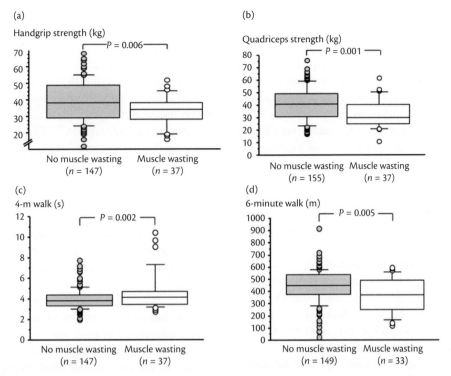

Figure 5.8.2 Measures of skeletal muscle function in patients with heart failure with or without sarcopenia (skeletal muscle wasting). (a) Handgrip strength, as assessed by a handgrip dynamometer, in patients with and without sarcopenia (muscle wasting). (b) Quadriceps strength, as assessed by an isokinetic dynamometer, in patients with and without sarcopenia (muscle wasting). (c) Exercise capacity, as assessed by time taken in the 4-metre walk test. (d) Exercise capacity, as assessed by distance walked in the 6-minute walk test.

Reproduced from Fülster S, Tacke M, Sandek A, *et al*. Muscle wasting in patients with chronic heart failure: results from the studies investigating co-morbidities aggravating heart failure (SICA-HF). *Eur Heart J*. 2013 Feb;34(7):512–19. doi: 10.1093/eurheartj/ehs381 with permission from Oxford University Press.

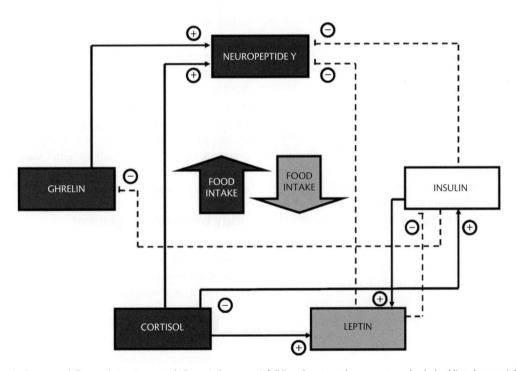

Figure 5.8.3 Interplay between different players in energy balance in humans. A full line denotes enhancement, and a dashed line denotes inhibition.

Reproduced from von Haehling S, Doehner W, Anker SD. Nutrition, metabolism, and the complex pathophysiology of cachexia in chronic heart failure. *Cardiovasc Res*. 2007 Jan 15;73(2):298–309. doi: 10.1016/j.cardiores.2006.08.018 with permission from Oxford University Press.

hyponatraemia and/or hypocalcaemia were the most frequently affected.[28] Unfortunately, it is difficult to predict who will likely develop such micronutrient deficiencies, because in this study, almost 5% of patients had hypermagnesaemia despite use of loop diuretics. A small randomized, double-blind controlled trial found that daily intake of high doses of the trace elements calcium, magnesium, zinc, and selenium, as well as vitamins A, B_6, B_{12}, C, D, and E, thiamine, riboflavin, and folic acid, over 9 month led to a reduction in left ventricular volume and an improvement in ejection fraction.[29] Altogether, evidence remains very limited, which has led to a recommendation in the guidelines from the American Heart Association stating that only manifest deficiencies in trace elements or vitamins should be treated. Guidelines from the European Society of Cardiology do not provide recommendations in this regard.[30]

Some studies have investigated the effect of nutraceuticals in the context of HF. The data have recently been reviewed by the International Lipid Expert Panel.[31] Even though studies for the use of coenzyme Q_{10} suggest a beneficial effect, the overall availability of data, particularly from randomized controlled trials, is not robust enough to give valid recommendations.

Iron deficiency (ID) is one of the most common nutritional deficiencies in the world, and it has been shown that this has a major impact on functional capacity and symptomatic status in patients with HF.[32,33] Consequently, substantial evidence has been accumulated from a series of controlled clinical trials to show that replenishment of iron stores in patients with HF and ID results in clinically relevant improvement of functional status and reduced hospitalization for HF. Notably, oral administration of iron has not yielded beneficial effects, as these preparations are not sufficiently absorbed[34] in the gastrointestinal tract in patients with HF who often have bowel wall oedema. Administration of intravenous ferric carboxymaltose in patients with ID is best supported by randomized clinical trials.[35,36,37] ID in patients with HF is usually defined as serum ferritin level of <100 ng/L, or serum ferritin level of 100–299 ng/L together with a transferrin saturation of <20%. Using these criteria, up to 50% of all ambulatory patients with HF might be affected and treatable with intravenous ferric carboxymaltose for symptomatic improvement.[38,39] Indeed, repletion of iron stores in affected patients leads to improved functional states, as assessed by using the 6-minute corridor walk test, and improved quality of life, as well as reduced hospitalization rates.[40] Beneficial effects are corroborated by effects on skeletal and cardiac muscle physiology.[41,42] Limited data are available for other novel intravenous iron preparations that also suggest a beneficial effect.[43,44] A robust evidence base is also available for use of N-3 polyunsaturated fatty acids (N-3-PUFA), which has been validated in a large-scale trial comparing 1 g of N-3 PUFA to placebo. Treatment led to a significant reduction in the risk of death or cardiovascular hospitalization.[45]

Malabsorption

Malabsorption is another important factor to be considered in patients with metabolic disorders and/or manifest wasting disorders. Bowel wall oedema play the most important part in this consideration. Blood shunting from arterioles to venules as a result of ischaemia at the tip of villi can be observed in patients with low cardiac output.[46,47] An increased bowel wall thickness, suggestive of bowel wall oedema, has been reported in patients with HF,[48] which can ultimately lead to fat malabsorption and protein loss, with the latter particularly contributing to the development of cardiac cachexia.[49,50] Finally, bowel wall oedema has been suggested to cause translocation of bacterial endotoxin, thus triggering pro-inflammatory cytokine activation.[51]

Macronutrients

The wasting process in HF is maintained through protein degradation by the proteasome, particularly in skeletal muscle. Amino acid supplementation may be beneficial, in particular by using branched-chain amino acids (leucine, isoleucine, and valine). Other essential amino acids may also confirm beneficial effects. A small investigator-blinded and randomized study of 38 patients with HF showed that a mix of all essential amino acids resulted in an improvement in peak oxygen consumption and distance walked in the 6-minute walk test over 2 months of oral treatment. Another randomized, double-blind, placebo-controlled study of oral amino acid supplementation in patients with chronic HF was able to show a small improvement in peak oxygen consumption after 30 days of treatment.[52,53] Other studies, however, had difficulties in validating these findings.[54] Other potential treatment approaches have used, for example, a high-calorie, protein-rich nutritional supplement in patients with cardiac cachexia. A 6-week intervention, followed by an additional 18 weeks of follow-up without intervention, showed an increase in the 6-minute walk test distance and fat tissue, as well as an improvement in quality of life. No change was reported in left ventricular ejection fraction or peak oxygen consumption.[55] Other potential anabolic approaches embrace testosterone administration, which has been used mostly in male patients, even though one study administered in women a small dose of testosterone via a transdermal patch. A general recommendation is available for protein intake. This recommendation is 0.8 g/kg of body weight per day, even though patients with HF may require higher doses. Experts recommend 1.0–1.2 g/kg of body weight.[56] Calorie intake of up to 35 kcal/kg of body weight seems to be safe, but other sources recommend a maximum of 28 kcal/kg per day.

Body weight management

There is no compelling evidence in support of weight reduction in patients with manifest HF to improve mortality outcome.[57] By contrast, observed weight loss in the course of HF was shown to predict increased mortality.[58] Details are discussed in Chapter 5.2. This finding is widely discussed as the obesity paradox, but given the bulk and variety of evidence, rather an obesity paradigm should be concluded.[59] In fact, there is compelling evidence for a benefit from some excessive body weight on mortality outcomes in HF because higher body weight has been included in several risk scores for HF as an anti-risk factor, that is, higher body weight

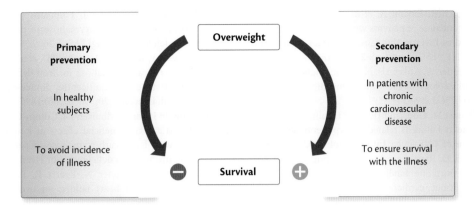

Figure 5.8.4 The obesity paradigm in cardiovascular disease. Weight management recommendation should clearly differentiate between primary prevention in healthy subjects and secondary outcome prevention in patients with established cardiovascular disease.
Reproduced from Doehner W, von Haehling S, Anker SD. Protective overweight in cardiovascular disease: moving from 'paradox' to 'paradigm'. *Eur Heart J.* 2015 Oct 21;36(40):2729–32. doi: 10.1093/eurheartj/ehv414 with permission from Oxford University Press.

predicts better survival.[60,61] Importantly, body weight management recommendations in patients with HF should adopt a clearly differentiating approach, with a distinction between primary prevention (i.e. in healthy subjects), where excessive body weight should be avoided, and secondary outcome prevention in patients with established HF where longest survival with the existing disease is the treatment goal (⊃ Figure 5.8.4).

Future directions

Cachexia and sarcopenia have been identified as important comorbidities of HF. Several pathophysiological aspects have been elucidated in order to better understand the metabolic pathways that lead to body wasting. Unfortunately, this understanding has not yielded positive treatment trials, even though several attempts have been made. Possibly, a multifactorial approach with using a yet unidentified drug together with nutritional support and an exercise intervention would be helpful. Clinical trials in this regard are eagerly awaited.

Conclusions

Sarcopenia affects 20–50% of patients, and cardiac cachexia 10–15%. No recommendations can be made based on robust clinical evidence, but overt deficiencies in trace elements should be replenished and malnutrition and weight loss may be treated with high-calorie nutritional supplements; small doses of N3-PUFA seem to be beneficial, and patients with muscle wasting may have some benefit from essential amino acid administration. It is also important to bear in mind the pivotal role of exercise training in the treatment of muscle wasting. This point is discussed in detail in ⊃ Chapter 9.6.

References

1. Doehner W, Frenneaux M, Anker SD. Metabolic impairment in heart failure. The myocardial and systemic perspective. J Am Coll Cardiol. 2014;64:1388–400.
2. Von Haehling S. The wasting continuum in heart failure: from sarcopenia to cachexia. Proc Nutr Soc. 2015;74(4):367–77.
3. Emami A, Saitoh M, Valentova M, *et al.* Comparison of sarcopenia and cachexia in men with chronic heart failure: results from the Studies Investigating Co-morbidities Aggravating Heart Failure (SICA-HF). Eur J Heart Fail. 2018;20(11):1580–7.
4. Doherty TJ. Invited review: aging and sarcopenia. J Appl Physiol. 2003;95:1717–27.
5. Rosenberg ICH. Sarcopenia: origins and clinical relevance. Clin Geriatr Med. 2011;27:337–9.
6. Von Haehling S, Ebner N, Dos Santos MR, Springer J, Anker SD. Muscle wasting and cachexia in heart failure: mechanisms and therapies. Nat Rev Cardiol. 2017;14(6):323–41.
7. Fülster S, Tacke M, Sandek A, *et al.* Muscle wasting in patients with chronic heart failure: results from the studies investigating co-morbidities aggravating heart failure (SICA-HF). Eur Heart J. 2013;34(7):512–19.
8. Bekfani T, Pellicori P, Morris DA, *et al.* Sarcopenia in patients with heart failure with preserved ejection fraction: impact on muscle strength, exercise capacity and quality of life. Int J Cardiol. 2016;222:41–6.
9. Hajahmadi M, Shemshadi S, Khalilipur E, *et al.* Muscle wasting in young patients with dilated cardiomyopathy. J Cachexia Sarcopenia Muscle. 2017;8(4):542–8.
10. Von Haehling S, Garfias Macedo T, Valentova M, *et al.* Muscle wasting as an independent predictor of survival in patients with chronic heart failure. J Cachexia Sarcopenia Muscle. 2020;11(5):1242–9.
11. Dos Santos MR, Saitoh M, Ebner N, *et al.* Sarcopenia and endothelial function in patients with chronic heart failure: results from the Studies Investigating Comorbidities Aggravating Heart Failure (SICA-HF). J Am Med Dir Assoc. 2017;18(3):240–5.
12. Doehner W, Anker SD. Cardiac cachexia in early literature: a review of research prior to Medline. Int J Cardiol. 2002;85:7–14.
13. Evans WJ, Morley JE, Argilés J, *et al.* Cachexia: a new definition. Clin Nutr. 2008;27(6):793–9.
14. Von Haehling S, Anker SD. Cachexia as a major underestimated and unmet medical need: facts and numbers. J Cachexia Sarcopenia Muscle. 2010;1(1):1–5.
15. Anker SD, Negassa A, Coats AJ, *et al.* Prognostic importance of weight loss in chronic heart failure and the effect of treatment with angiotensin-converting-enzyme inhibitors: an observational study. Lancet. 2003;361(9363):1077–83.
16. Anker SD, Ponikowski P, Varney S, *et al.* Wasting as independent risk factor for mortality in chronic heart failure. Lancet. 1997;349(9058):1050–3.

17. Saitoh M, Dos Santos MR, Emami A, et al. Anorexia, functional capacity, and clinical outcome in patients with chronic heart failure: results from the Studies Investigating Co-morbidities Aggravating Heart Failure (SICA-HF). ESC Heart Fail. 2017;4(4):448–57.

18. Von Haehling S, Doehner W, Anker SD. Nutrition, metabolism, and the complex pathophysiology of cachexia in chronic heart failure. Cardiovasc Res. 2007;73(2):298–309.

19. Doehner W, Rauchhaus M, Godsland IF, et al. Insulin resistance in moderate chronic heart failure is related to hyperleptinaemia, but not to norepinephrine or TNF-alpha. Int J Cardiol. 2002;83:73–81.

20. Doehner W, Pflaum CD, Rauchhaus M, et al. Leptin, insulin sensitivity and growth hormone binding protein in chronic heart failure with and without cardiac cachexia. Eur J Endocrinol. 2001;145:727–35.

21. Anker SD, Volterrani M, Pflaum CD, et al. Acquired growth hormone resistance in patients with chronic heart failure: implications for therapy with growth hormone. J Am Coll Cardiol. 2001;38:443–52.

22. Feng Q, Lambert ML, Callow ID, Arnold JM. Venous neuropeptide Y receptor responsiveness in patients with chronic heart failure. Clin Pharmacol Ther. 2000;67(3):292–8.

23. Ronti T, Lupattelli G, Mannarino E. The endocrine function of adipose tissue: an update. Clin Endocrinol (Oxf). 2006;64(4):355–65.

24. Doehner W, Turhan G, Leyva F, et al. Skeletal muscle weakness is related to insulin resistance in patients with chronic heart failure. ESC Heart Fail. 2015;2:85–9.

25. Doehner W, Rauchhaus M, Ponikowski P, et al. Impaired insulin sensitivity as an independent risk factor for mortality in patients with stable chronic heart failure. J Am Coll Cardiol. 2005;46(6):1019–26.

26. Saitoh M, Dos Santos MR, Ebner N, et al. Nutritional status and its effects on muscle wasting in patients with chronic heart failure: insights from Studies Investigating Co-morbidities Aggravating Heart Failure. Wien Klin Wochenschr. 2016;128(Suppl 7):497–504.

27. Gorelik O, Almoznino-Sarafian D, Feder I, et al. Dietary intake of various nutrients in older patients with congestive heart failure. Cardiology. 2003;99(4):177–81.

28. Cohen N, Almoznino-Sarafian D, Zaidenstein R, et al. Serum magnesium aberrations in furosemide (frusemide) treated patients with congestive heart failure: pathophysiological correlates and prognostic evaluation. Heart. 2003;89(4):411–16.

29. Witte KK, Nikitin NP, Parker AC, et al. The effect of micronutrient supplementation on quality-of-life and left ventricular function in elderly patients with chronic heart failure. Eur Heart J. 2005;26(21):2238–44.

30. McDonagh TA, Metra M, Adamo M, et al.; ESC Scientific Document Group. 2021 ESC Guidelines for the diagnosis and treatment of acute and chronic heart failure. Eur Heart J. 2021;42(36):3599–726.

31. Cicero AFG, Colletti A, von Haehling S, et al.; International Lipid Expert Panel. Nutraceutical support in heart failure: a position paper of the International Lipid Expert Panel (ILEP). Nutr Res Rev. 2020;33(1):155–79.

32. Jankowska EA, Rozentryt P, Witkowska A, et al. Iron deficiency predicts impaired exercise capacity in patients with systolic chronic heart failure. J Card Fail. 2011;17:899–906.

33. Ebner N, Jankowska EA, Ponikowski P, et al. The impact of iron deficiency and anaemia on exercise capacity and outcomes in patients with chronic heart failure. Results from the Studies Investigating Co-morbidities Aggravating Heart Failure. Int J Cardiol. 2016;205:6–12.

34. Lewis GD, Malhotra R, Hernandez AF, et al.; NHLBI Heart Failure Clinical Research Network. Effect of oral iron repletion on exercise capacity in patients with heart failure with reduced ejection fraction and iron deficiency: The IRONOUT HF Randomized Clinical Trial. JAMA. 2017;317(19):1958–966. Erratum in: JAMA. 2017;317(23):2453.

35. Anker SD, Comin Colet J, Filippatos G, et al.; FAIR-HF Trial Investigators. Ferric carboxymaltose in patients with heart failure and iron deficiency. N Engl J Med. 2009;361(25):2436–48.

36. Ponikowski P, Kirwan BA, Anker SD, et al.; AFFIRM-AHF investigators. Ferric carboxymaltose for iron deficiency at discharge after acute heart failure: a multicentre, double-blind, randomised, controlled trial. Lancet. 2020;396(10266):1895–904.

37. Ponikowski P, van Veldhuisen DJ, Comin-Colet J, et al.; CONFIRM-HF Investigators. Beneficial effects of long-term intravenous iron therapy with ferric carboxymaltose in patients with symptomatic heart failure and iron deficiency. Eur Heart J. 2015;36(11):657–68.

38. Von Haehling S, Ebner N, Evertz R, Ponikowski P, Anker SD. Iron deficiency in heart failure: an overview. JACC Heart Fail. 2019;7(1):36–46.

39. Von Haehling S, Arzt M, Doehner W, et al. Improving exercise capacity and quality of life using non-invasive heart failure treatments: evidence from clinical trials. Eur J Heart Fail. 2021;23(1):92–113.

40. Graham FJ, Pellicori P, Ford I, Petrie MC, Kalra PR, Cleland JGF. Intravenous iron for heart failure with evidence of iron deficiency: a meta-analysis of randomised trials. Clin Res Cardiol. 2021;110(8):1299–307.

41. Haddad S, Wang Y, Galy B, et al. Iron-regulatory proteins secure iron availability in cardiomyocytes to prevent heart failure. Eur Heart J. 2017;38(5):362–72.

42. Hirsch VG, Tongers J, Bode J, et al. Cardiac iron concentration in relation to systemic iron status and disease severity in non-ischaemic heart failure with reduced ejection fraction. Eur J Heart Fail. 2020;22(11):2038–46.

43. Charles-Edwards G, Amaral N, Sleigh A, et al. Effect of iron isomaltoside on skeletal muscle energetics in patients with chronic heart failure and iron deficiency. Circulation. 2019;139(21):2386–98.

44. Ambrosy AP, von Haehling S, Kalra PR, et al. Safety and efficacy of intravenous ferric derisomaltose compared to iron sucrose for iron deficiency anemia in patients with chronic kidney disease with and without heart failure. Am J Cardiol. 2021;152:138–45.

45. Tavazzi L, Maggioni AP, Marchioli R, et al.; Gissi-HF Investigators. Effect of n-3 polyunsaturated fatty acids in patients with chronic heart failure (the GISSI-HF trial): a randomised, double-blind, placebo-controlled trial. Lancet. 2008;372(9645):1223–30.

46. Takala J. Determinants of splanchnic blood flow. Br J Anaesth. 1996;77(1):50–8.

47. Krack A, Sharma R, Figulla HR, Anker SD. The importance of the gastrointestinal system in the pathogenesis of heart failure. Eur Heart J. 2005;26(22):2368–74.

48. Sandek A, Bauditz J, Swidsinski A, et al. Altered intestinal function in patients with chronic heart failure. J Am Coll Cardiol. 2007;50(16):1561–9.

49. King D, Smith ML, Chapman TJ, Stockdale HR, Lye M. Fat malabsorption in elderly patients with cardiac cachexia. Age Ageing. 1996;25(2):144–9.

50. King D, Smith ML, Lye M. Gastro-intestinal protein loss in elderly patients with cardiac cachexia. Age Ageing. 1996;25(3):221–3.

51. Rauchhaus M, Coats AJ, Anker SD. The endotoxin–lipoprotein hypothesis. Lancet. 2000;356(9233):930–3.

52. Aquilani R, Opasich C, Gualco A, et al. Adequate energy–protein intake is not enough to improve nutritional and metabolic status in muscle-depleted patients with chronic heart failure. Eur J Heart Fail. 2008;10(11):1127–35.

53. Aquilani R, Viglio S, Iadarola P, et al. Oral amino acid supplements improve exercise capacities in elderly patients with chronic heart failure. Am J Cardiol. 2008;101(11A):104E–10E.

54. Pineda-Juárez JA, Sánchez-Ortiz NA, Castillo-Martínez L, *et al.* Changes in body composition in heart failure patients after a resistance exercise program and branched chain amino acid supplementation. Clin Nutr. 2016;35(1):41–7.

55. Rozentryt P, von Haehling S, Lainscak M, *et al.* The effects of a high-caloric protein-rich oral nutritional supplement in patients with chronic heart failure and cachexia on quality of life, body composition, and inflammation markers: a randomized, double-blind pilot study. J Cachexia Sarcopenia Muscle. 2010;1(1):35–42.

56. Payne-Emerson H, Lennie TA. Nutritional considerations in heart failure. Nurs Clin North Am. 2008;43(1):117–32; vii.

57. Jordan J, Toplak H, Grassi G, *et al.* Joint statement of the European Association for the Study of Obesity and the European Society of Hypertension: obesity and heart failure. J Hypertens. 2016;34:1678–88.

58. Anker SD, Negassa A, Coats AJ, *et al.* Prognostic importance of weight loss in chronic heart failure and the effect of treatment with angiotensin-converting-enzyme inhibitors: an observational study. Lancet. 2003;361:1077–83.

59. Doehner W, von Haehling S, Anker SD. Protective overweight in cardiovascular disease: moving from 'paradox' to 'paradigm'. Eur Heart J. 2015;36:2729–32.

60. Levy WC, Mozaffarian D, Linker DT, *et al.* The Seattle Heart Failure Model: prediction of survival in heart failure. Circulation. 2006;113:1424–33.

61. Pocock SJ, Ariti CA, McMurray JJ, *et al.* Predicting survival in heart failure: a risk score based on 39 372 patients from 30 studies. Meta-Analysis Global Group in Chronic Heart Failure. Eur Heart J. 2013;34:1404–13.

SECTION 6

Clinical phenotypes of chronic heart failure

CHAPTER 6.1

Clinical phenotypes of heart failure with reduced ejection fraction

Brian P Halliday and Thomas F Lüscher

Contents

Introduction

When the English physician William Withering, inspired by old folk herbalist mother Hutton in Shropshire, started to use foxglove in patients who had 'dropsy', he was amazed by its favourable effects. As he reported in his seminal monograph published in 1786 '*An account of the Foxglove and some of its medical uses with practical remarks on dropsy, and other diseases*',[1] his patients with peripheral oedema, ascites, and pulmonary congestion started to diurese after ingesting his herbal extract. He was amazed that their oedema vanished and proposed that the condition was due to water retention. Over two centuries later, our understanding and treatment of heart failure have advanced considerably, but his basic observation remains important.

At that moment in history, it was not possible to assess cardiac function using cardiac imaging. With the advent of imaging techniques, initially chest X-rays discovered by Wilhelm Röntgen more than a century later, and then contrast ventriculography, nuclear techniques, echocardiography, and eventually cardiac magnetic resonance (CMR), it became clear that most patients with this condition had enlarged ventricles with reduced systolic function, leading to the use of the term heart failure, and more recently heart failure with reduced ejection fraction (HFrEF).

However, there was little progress in the understanding and management of the condition until the 1970s. Indeed, initially, besides digitalis and later mercury diuretics, bedrest was the predominant recommendation for many decades. As the pump function of the heart was reduced, stimulating the heart intuitively appeared to be the most promising approach; however, all such attempts, using inotropes and phosphodiesterase inhibitors, proved deleterious for clinical outcomes, although they at first improved exercise performance of patients. In a seminal paradigm shift, Jay Cohn showed in his landmark studies that unloading of the heart, rather than stimulating it, was effective. Indeed, the degree of sympathetic activation was predictive of mortality. For the first time, peripheral vasodilators such as hydralazine and nitrates that counteracted the peripheral vasoconstriction induced by sympathetic activation provided beneficial outcomes in patients with HFrEF.

Defining heart failure with reduced ejection fraction

With the widespread availability of echocardiography, diagnosing heart failure focused on characterizing left ventricular (LV) systolic function. This allowed for the recruitment of large numbers of patients into seminal trials. In most cases, trialists selected a left ventricular ejection fraction (LVEF) of <40% or <35% as an entry criterion, as this patient group were expected to have a high event rate and a therapeutic effect may therefore become obvious with relatively small numbers (➲ Figure 6.1.1).[2,3,4] Thus, heart failure was

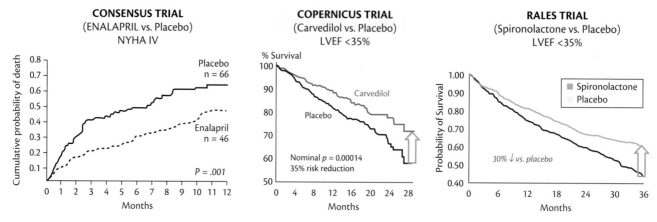

Figure 6.1.1 Seminal trials in heart failure with reduced ejection fraction (HFrEF).

Source data from CONSENSUS Trial Study Group. Effects of enalapril on mortality in severe congestive heart failure. Results of the Cooperative North Scandinavian Enalapril Survival Study (CONSENSUS). *N Engl J Med*. 1987 Jun 4;316(23):1429–35. doi: 10.1056/NEJM198706043162301. Pitt B, Zannad F, Remme WJ, et al. The effect of spironolactone on morbidity and mortality in patients with severe heart failure. Randomized Aldactone Evaluation Study Investigators. *N Engl J Med*. 1999 Sep 2;341(10):709–17. doi: 10.1056/NEJM199909023411001. Packer M, Fowler MB, Roecker EB, *et al*.; Carvedilol Prospective Randomized Cumulative Survival (COPERNICUS) Study Group. Effect of carvedilol on the morbidity of patients with severe chronic heart failure: results of the carvedilol prospective randomized cumulative survival (COPERNICUS) study. *Circulation*. 2002 Oct 22;106(17):2194–9. doi: 10.1161/01.cir.0000035653.72855.bf. PMID: 12390947.

phenotypically characterized by LVEF rather than based on its cause or pathophysiology. Based on the emphatic results of trials that followed, this approach appeared to be successful.

However, it was later recognized that signs and symptoms of heart failure (➲ Chapter 7.1) also occurred in patients with preserved LVEF, many of whom were obese, diabetic, and/or hypertensive, and more commonly among women. As a consequence, the current classification into HFrEF and heart failure with preserved ejection fraction (HFpEF) evolved. Later, it was also recognized that patients initially classified as HFpEF who had an LVEF of 40–50% may, in fact, have an intermediate phenotype closer to HFrEF. This led to the term heart failure with mid-range ejection fraction, which has since been superseded by the term heart failure with mildly reduced ejection fraction (HFmrEF) (➲ Table 6.1.1).[5,6] This group is made up of patients with *de novo* myocardial dysfunction, as well as those with previous severe reductions

in LVEF who have subsequently improved on medical therapy. The latter group was previously termed heart failure with recovered ejection fraction (HFrecEF). However, heart failure with improved ejection fraction is likely to be more accurate, given the ongoing risk of future relapse.[7]

The three forms of heart failure are defined based on: (1) symptoms (see ➲ Chapter 7.1) and (2) LVEF. For HFmrEF and HFpEF, elevated natriuretic peptide concentrations and the presence of structural heart disease and/or diastolic dysfunction are also required. However, the 2016 classification has been increasingly criticized for several reasons. First, the LVEF cut-off of <40% was arbitrarily chosen by trialists in the past, whereas most physicians would consider an LVEF of below 50% as abnormal.[8] Second, mortality continuously increases with declining LVEF below 60% with no apparent step-up.[9] Third, the results of the EMPEROR,[10] TOPCAT,[11] and PARAGON trial[12] strongly

Table 6.1.1 Classification of heart failure according to the 2021 ESC Guidelines

Criteria	HFrEF	HFmrEF	HFpEF
1	Symptoms ± signs*	Symptoms ± signs*	Symptoms ± signs*
2	LVEF ≤40%	LVEF 41–49%†	LVEF ≥50%
3	–	–	Objective evidence of cardiac structural and/or functional abnormalities consistent with the presence of LV diastolic dysfunction/ raised LV filling pressures, including raised natriuretic peptide levels‡

* Signs may not be present in the early stages of heart failure (especially in HFpEF) and in optimally treated patients.

† For a diagnosis of HFmrEF, the presence of other evidence of structural heart disease (e.g. increased left atrial size, LV hypertrophy, or echocardiographic measures of impaired LV filling) makes the diagnosis more likely.

‡ For a diagnosis of HFpEF, the greater the number of abnormalities present, the higher the likelihood of HFpEF.

HF, heart failure; HFmrEF, heart failure with mildly reduced ejection fraction; HFpEF, heart failure with preserved ejection fraction; HFrEF, heart failure with reduced ejection fraction; LV, left ventricle; LVEF, left ventricular ejection fraction.

McDonagh TA, Metra M, Adamo M, et al; ESC Scientific Document Group. 2021 ESC Guidelines for the diagnosis and treatment of acute and chronic heart failure. *Eur Heart J*. 2021 Sep 21;42(36):3599–3726. doi: 10.1093/eurheartj/ehab368. © The European Society of Cardiology. Reprinted by permission of Oxford University Press.

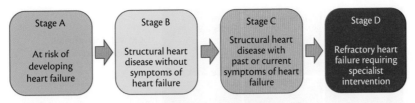

Figure 6.1.2 American College of Cardiology/American Heart Association stages of heart failure.

suggested that empagliflozin, spironolactone, and sacubitril/valsartan, respectively, reduce the event rate primarily in patients with HFmrEF, as well as those with HFrEF. Thus, it appears that HFmrEF is simply a milder form of HFrEF, and mortality and the benefit of heart failure drugs increase continuously and become more pronounced, respectively, as LVEF decreases.

Clinical presentation

Heart failure is a clinical syndrome rather than a disease. It presents with typical symptoms such as reduced exercise capacity, breathlessness on exertion, fatigue, and later at rest, when lying flat (orthopnoea) or when stooping or tying shoes (bendopnoea).

Symptoms can be assessed objectively using the *Minnesota Living with Heart Failure Questionnaire* or *Kansas City Cardiomyopathy Questionnaire*. Furthermore, exercise tests (i.e. treadmill or bicycle) and the *6-minute walking test* can be used.

Usually, the severity of symptoms is described using the New York Heart Association (NYHA) classification, with class I defining patients without symptoms, class II those with symptoms upon heavy exercise, class III those with symptoms on light exercise, and class IV those with symptoms at rest. The American Heart Association and American College of Cardiology have also proposed stages A to D where A describes patients without objective evidence of structural heart disease and without signs or symptoms of heart failure, but who are at increased risk of developing heart failure based on risk factors; stage B those with evidence of structural heart disease, but without signs or symptoms of heart failure; stage C those with evidence of structural heart disease with signs or symptoms of heart failure; and stage D those with refractory heart failure requiring specialized interventions (➲ Figure 6.1.2).[13]

Causes of heart failure with reduced ejection fraction

Ischaemic cardiomyopathy

Ischaemic heart disease is the most common cause of HFrEF.[14,15] Its incidence is likely to continue to rise, given the combination of improved survival of patients following acute myocardial infarction (MI) with the widespread use of primary percutaneous coronary intervention and the ageing population.

The diagnosis of ischaemic cardiomyopathy is based on evidence of previous MI and/or coronary artery disease (CAD) significant enough to result in LV systolic dysfunction. Determination of aetiology may not always be straightforward; many patients with non-ischaemic heart failure will have bystander CAD or regional wall motion abnormalities on echocardiography that may be interpreted as evidence of previous infarction. A standardized definition for ischaemic cardiomyopathy has been proposed for use in clinical research, which differentiates patients with HFrEF based on the clinical history and anatomical severity of CAD.[16] This defines it as LV systolic dysfunction (LVEF <40%) in a patient with prior MI or coronary revascularization, or ≥75% stenosis in the proximal left anterior descending artery (LAD) or left main stem (LMS), or ≥75% stenosis in two or more epicardial vessels. In a study of almost 2000 patients, individuals with less severe CAD who did not meet this definition were found to have comparable survival to patients with non-ischaemic heart failure, and better survival to those with more severe CAD who met the proposed definition.[16] This definition is therefore primarily based on prognosis for the purposes of selecting patients for research. Whether individual cases have a predominant ischaemic or non-ischaemic contribution is still frequently debated. Patients with both ischaemic heart disease and risk factors for non-ischaemic disease are common among an ageing population and in an era when genetic predisposition to developing heart failure is increasingly recognized. A 'one size fits all' definition to define the cause of HFrEF may therefore be unrealistic.

Another limitation of this definition, which is almost 20 years old, is the imperfect reproducibility of determining the anatomical severity of stenoses on angiography. The role of invasive functional testing, which has become more common over the last 10 years, is also unclear. Confirmation of prior unrecognized MI is now also established by CMR imaging, which may detect previous asymptomatic MI among patients with unobstructed coronary arteries where the infarct-related artery has recanalized (➲ Figure 6.1.3).[17]

Three concepts have been described that are central to the development of myocardial dysfunction among patients with CAD: myocardial stunning, hibernation, and scarring.[18,19] Rather than distinct processes, it is best to view these phenomena as a continuum, representing different stages of myocardial adaptation to ischaemia. Myocardial stunning typically occurs after a single episode of ischaemia and is characterized by reduced myocardial contractility with normal resting myocardial blood flow.[19,20] Coronary flow reserve may be reduced and myocardial energetics are typically impaired, possibly contributed to by excess generation of reactive oxygen species.[21] Ultrastructural changes are absent. Hibernation develops in cases of recurrent or persistent ischaemia with reduced regional myocardial blood flow at rest. It has been proposed that this hypocontractile state is an adaptive response to ischaemia, downregulating energy consumption in an act of 'self-preservation'.[18] Hibernation is characterized by structural changes with loss of sarcomeres, sarcoplasmic reticulum

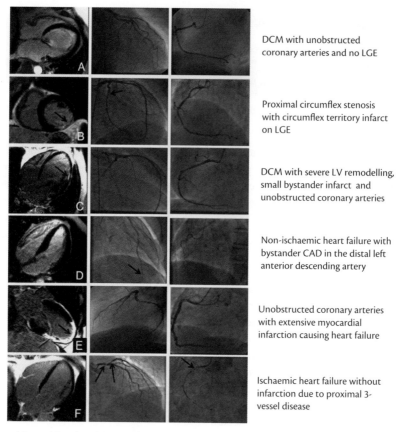

DCM with unobstructed
coronary arteries and no LGE

Proximal circumflex stenosis
with circumflex territory infarct
on LGE

DCM with severe LV remodelling,
small bystander infarct and
unobstructed coronary arteries

Non-ischaemic heart failure with
bystander CAD in the distal left
anterior descending artery

Unobstructed coronary arteries
with extensive myocardial
infarction causing heart failure

Ischaemic heart failure without
infarction due to proximal 3-
vessel disease

Figure 6.1.3 Phenotypes of heart failure with reduced ejection fraction characterized by late gadolinium enhanced (LGE) cardiovascular magnetic resonance and coronary angiography.

Reproduced from Assomull RG, Shakespeare C, Kalra PR, Lloyd G, Gulati A, Strange J, Bradlow WM, Lyne J, Keegan J, Poole-Wilson P, Cowie MR, Pennell DJ, Prasad SK. Role of cardiovascular magnetic resonance as a gatekeeper to invasive coronary angiography in patients presenting with heart failure of unknown etiology. *Circulation*. 2011 Sep 20;124(12):1351–60. doi: 10.1161/CIRCULATIONAHA.110.011346 with permission from Wolters Kluwer.

disarray, and abnormal mitochondria; metabolic shifts with an increase in glucose utilization, a reduction in beta-oxidation of fatty acid intermediates, and reduced mitochondrial oxidation; abnormal calcium handling; and, in more severe cases, interstitial fibrosis.[19] In cases of persistent ischaemia with progressive remodelling or in the case of untreated infarction, myocyte cell death occurs, with collagen replacement and scar formation.

These concepts have been considered key to decision-making regarding the treatment of ischaemic cardiomyopathy, specifically the selection of patients for revascularization. While myocyte replacement with scar is considered an irreversible phenomenon, restoration of myocardial contractility occurs following revascularization of hibernating or stunned myocardium.[22,23] Indeed, this forms the basis of the retrospective definition of hibernation following successful revascularization. Several imaging techniques, including stress echocardiography, CMR, and nuclear methods, identify areas of dysfunctional viable myocardium and this may be viewed as a surrogate for hibernation prior to revascularization.

Non-ischaemic cardiomyopathy

Non-ischaemic cardiomyopathy is a broad term that encompasses many different diseases. This group may be further subdivided, based on the morphological phenotype, into dilated, restrictive, and hypertrophic cardiomyopathies.[24] As the latter two groups of conditions are typically associated with preserved ejection fraction, the most common non-ischaemic cause of HFrEF is the family of conditions referred to as dilated cardiomyopathy.

Dilated cardiomyopathy (DCM) encompasses myocardial diseases with a reduction in LV systolic dysfunction and LV dilation that cannot be explained by abnormal loading or ischaemic injury.[25] HFrEF secondary to valvular heart disease and that to hypertension are typically considered separate entities. More recently, a spectrum of non-ischaemic diseases including patients with non-dilated left ventricle (LV) has been recognized, leading to the creation of another term 'hypokinetic non-dilated cardiomyopathy'.[25] This includes patients with unexplained LV systolic dysfunction without dilatation.

There are many possible causes of DCM and related phenotypes, including genetic, toxic, endocrinological, infective, and autoimmune triggers. While many triggers are recognized, in clinical practice, most patients are still diagnosed with idiopathic DCM, as the cause remains unexplained. While DCM has often been divided into separate diseases based on the perceived aetiology, recent work has highlighted considerable overlap between different groups. A similar background of oligogenic susceptibility

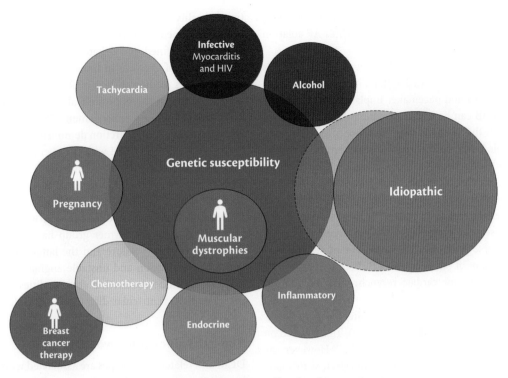

Figure 6.1.4 Overlap between environmental triggers and genetic susceptibility in dilated cardiomyopathy.

is found among patients labelled as having peripartum cardio-myopathy, alcohol-related DCM, or cardiomyopathy secondary to chemotherapy cardiotoxicity, compared to those patients with idiopathic disease.[26,27,28] DCM is therefore best considered a het-erogeneous family of diseases with multiple possible aetiological insults and a spectrum of genetic susceptibility ranging from an oligogenic to a monogenic basis. Overlap between environ-mental triggers and an inheritable component appears frequent (➲ Figure 6.1.4).[29]

Multiple disease mechanisms may contribute to the develop-ment of LV systolic dysfunction and many are shared between different forms of the disease. The most commonly recognized genetic forms of the disease arise from rare variants in sarcomeric genes, resulting in reduced actin–myosin cross-bridging, hypocontractility, and increased susceptibility to haemodynamic load. Extrinsic triggers, such as alcohol and cardiotoxic chemo-therapy, lead to increased oxidative stress, impaired mitochon-drial energetics, and metabolic shifts, which reduce adenosine triphosphate (ATP) delivery to the sarcomere and promote the formation of myocardial fibrosis.[26,27] Multiple different mechan-isms have been suggested to play a role in peripartum cardiomy-opathy, including oxidative stress, angiogenic imbalances, and increased susceptibility to haemodynamic loads.[30] Activation of the inflammasome and pro-fibrotic networks play a prominent role in myocarditis and autoimmune disease.

These mechanisms produce a common phenotype character-ized by the structural, functional, and pathological hallmarks of DCM. The pathological features include myocyte hypertrophy, cell death, and fibrosis.[31] Interstitial fibrosis is ubiquitous beyond early forms of the disease and describes accumulation of collagen in the extracellular and perivascular space in the absence of cell death.[32] Replacement fibrosis describes areas of collagen replace-ment following widespread myocyte death and is characteristic of severe disease with advanced LV remodelling.[32] It occurs in around 30–50% of cases and identifies a group of patients at high risk of adverse outcomes, specifically major arrhythmic events.[33,34] Extensive myocardial fibrosis may be present with specific genetic phenotypes.[35] Microvascular dysfunction and reduced myocar-dial perfusion reserve, likely secondary to increased wall stress and interstitial fibrosis, may also be present.[36]

In this chapter, we will move forward to discuss additional spe-cific features of the phenotypes of HFrEF, including characteristic appearances on electrocardiography (ECG) and cardiovascular imaging, as well as typical biomarker profiles and the findings of genetic testing.

Electrocardiographic phenotypes in HFrEF
Ischaemic cardiomyopathy

The 12-lead ECG is a mainstay investigation for the investigation of patients with HFrEF. ECG abnormalities are common among patients with CAD, including rhythm disturbances such as atrial fibrillation (AF), conduction abnormalities such as left bundle branch block (LBBB), and signs of previous MI such as Q-waves. On the other hand, a completely normal ECG makes the diag-nosis of HFrEF unlikely.

The prevalence of AF among heart failure patients is around 30%.[37,38] Whereas AF is an independent predictor of adverse outcome among patients with HFpEF, this is not consistently the case among patients with HFrEF.[37,38] A prompt diagnosis of AF in patients with ischaemic cardiomyopathy is nevertheless essential to enable appropriate thromboprophylaxis and selection of appropriate patients for specific therapies such as AF ablation (◆ Chapter 12.7).[39]

Among patients with stable CAD, the prevalence of LBBB is around 4–5%[40] and this is associated with an increased risk of future heart failure events and pacemaker implantation. While the development of LBBB can be a sign of acute infarction, registry studies confirm that this is an uncommon cause of LBBB among patients with stable CAD, with chronic disease progression and ventricular remodelling being a more common contributor.[40] Among patients with chronic stable heart failure, the prevalence of LBBB is higher at around 20–30%, with a crude incidence of 10% at 1 year after the initial diagnosis.[41,42] It is associated with more severe disease, and progression of QRS duration is associated with an adverse prognosis.[41,42] Measurement of QRS duration and identification of patients with LBBB are important for the selection of patients for cardiac resynchronization therapy (◆ Chapter 9.2).[5,6,43]

The identification of Q-waves on an ECG often prompts suspicion of previous transmural MI (◆ Figure 6.1.5). This is based on initial animal work published almost 70 years ago.[44] However, the sensitivity and specificity of this sign are imperfect, with many other recognized causes of Q-waves. The relationship between transmurality of infarction and the presence of Q-waves has been questioned, and what constitutes a pathological Q-wave is also poorly defined and debated.[45] The theoretical basis for the development of Q-waves in transmural MI is the loss of electromotive forces leading to loss of R-wave and the recognition of depolarization in the opposite wall of the LV. However, a study using late gadolinium enhancement CMR to measure the extent and transmurality of infarction demonstrated that the occurrence of Q-waves was associated with the overall size of infarction, rather than with transmurality.[45] Indeed, Q-waves were present in 28% of cases with subendocardial MI and absent in 29% of cases with transmural MI.[45] Nevertheless, large population studies have demonstrated prognostic differences between Q-wave and non-Q-wave MI, with the former group having a higher incidence of subsequent heart failure and the latter having a higher incidence of reinfarction and unstable angina.[46] Mimics of Q-wave infarction include conduction abnormalities such as ventricular pre-excitation, ventricular dilatation in DCM, and hypertrophic cardiomyopathy.

Non-ischaemic cardiomyopathy

DCM and related phenotypes are associated with ECG abnormalities in 80% of cases.[47] While these may be non-specific, they may

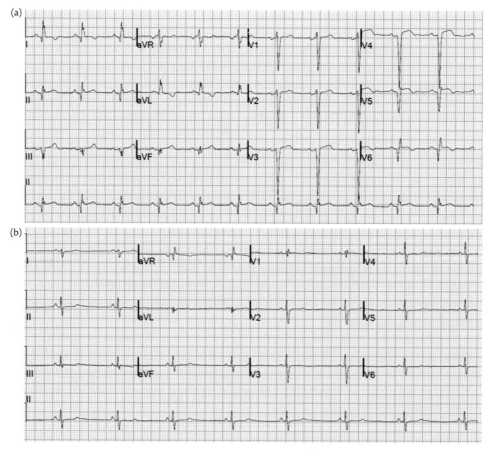

Figure 6.1.5 (a) A 12-lead ECG of a patient with a previous large apical myocardial infarction with ST-segment elevation in leads V3–V5 and Q-waves in leads V4, V5, II, III, and aVF. (b) A 12-lead ECG of a patient with non-ischaemic dilated cardiomyopathy with extensive myocardial fibrosis. Small QRS voltages with flattening of the T-waves are noted.

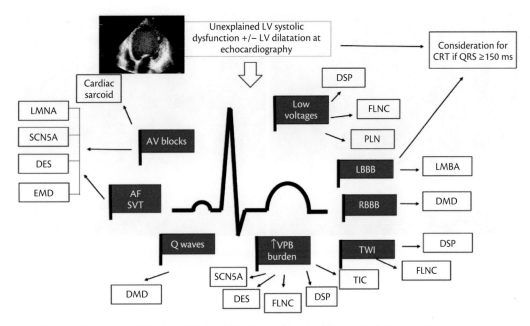

Figure 6.1.6 Electrocardiographic features which may provide diagnostic clues to the underlying cause of dilated cardiomyopathy.
Reproduced from Finocchiaro G, Merlo M, Sheikh N, *et al*. The electrocardiogram in the diagnosis and management of patients with dilated cardiomyopathy. *Eur J Heart Fail*. 2020 Jul;22(7):1097–1107. doi: 10.1002/ejhf.1815 with permission from John Wiley and Sons.

provide clues to the underlying aetiology when combined with other clinical information (➡ Figure 6.1.6).

As with other HFrEF phenotypes, LBBB is found in around a third of patients.[48] Although a feature seen commonly across many diseases, LBBB occurring early in the disease course, particularly if there is coexisting atrioventricular (AV) block, may increase suspicion of DCM secondary to variants in the lamin A/C gene (*LMNA*). This is particularly relevant in the presence of a family history of DCM and/or sudden cardiac death or a high burden of ventricular arrhythmia and AF, all common features of laminopathy.[49] Other common causes of AV block include cardiac sarcoidosis, whereas AF has also been recognized as an early feature of DCM secondary to truncating variants in the gene for titin (*TTN*), the most common genetic cause of DCM.[50] Right bundle branch block is seen less commonly, affecting around 2–6% of patients,[48] but is frequently found in patients with dystrophinopathies and neuromuscular disease.[51] Tall R-waves in the right precordial leads are another feature of dystrophinopathies, possibly reflecting the high burden of myocardial replacement fibrosis in the lateral wall.

An overlap between arrhythmogenic ventricular cardiomyopathy (AVC) (➡ Chapters 3.4.2 and 3.4.5) and DCM is increasingly recognized, with the vast majority of AVC cases demonstrating LV involvement and a proportion showing predominant changes in the LV.[52] Genetic variants in the genes for desmoplakin (*DSP)* and filamin C (*FLNC*) are perhaps the best recognized forms of left dominant disease, characterized by extensive myocardial fibrosis, often circumferential in its distribution (➡ Figure 6.1.7).[35] Repolarization abnormalities, particularly T-wave inversion, are frequently seen in the lateral and limb leads, combined with small QRS complexes, reflecting the regional differences in fibrotic burden.

Imaging phenotypes in HFrEF
Left ventricular assessment

Given the importance of the LV in the classification of heart failure, much attention is often paid to this chamber during an imaging examination. Accurate and precise measurement of LVEF is a key component, given the importance of this variable to treatment decisions and the close correlation between this measurement and the prognostic benefit of heart failure therapy.[53] Cardiac imaging has developed rapidly since the early heart failure trials where LVEF was a key inclusion criterion. Alongside this, the methods currently used to assess LVEF are much different. For example, in the Studies of Left Ventricular Dysfunction (SOLVD) trial, only a minority of patients (21%) had LVEF measured using echocardiography, with nuclear methods being more common.[54] Three-dimensional assessment methods including CMR or echocardiography are now the most commonly used and afford greater precision. However, interstudy and interobserver variability is still approximately 3–5% (and probably higher with echocardiography) and this should be borne in mind when using these measures to make therapy decisions in clinical practice.

Assessment of systolic function, however, extends well beyond the measurement of a single variable.[55] Assessment of myocardial deformation and regional myocardial function plays increasingly important roles. The value of myocardial deformation assessment is perhaps greatest in cases with preserved LVEF, to identify the subset of these patients with abnormal ventricular geometry and impaired systolic function. Nevertheless, global longitudinal strain, the assessment of longitudinal myocardial shortening, also adds incremental prognostic value in patients with HFrEF.[56] Visual assessment of morphology often provides clues towards helping to define the aetiology. Areas of regional thinning

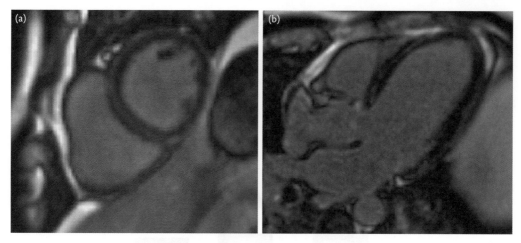

Figure 6.1.7 Late gadolinium enhancement cardiovascular magnetic resonance images of a patient with a pathogenic nonsense variant in *FLNC*, demonstrating extensive mid-wall/subepicardial myocardial fibrosis in the septum and basal lateral wall.

and/or dysfunction following a coronary distribution may identify areas of non-viable or hibernating myocardium due to previous infarction or ischaemia. This often leads to the diagnosis of ischaemic cardiomyopathy in a patient with new-onset heart failure. However, similar appearances may also be seen in patients with cardiac sarcoidosis. Lateral wall thinning, combined with regional dysfunction, is also frequently seen in genetic cardiomyopathies, particularly those associated with muscular dystrophies.[51]

Another aspect of the assessment of LV performance is the evaluation of LV diastolic function. While less important for securing a diagnosis in HFrEF, compared to HFpEF, assessment of LV relaxation provides incremental prognostic information in HFrEF and therefore adds to the overall phenotypic assessment within this group of patients.[57]

Characterization of myocardial viability and scar

Tissue characterization, particularly assessment of myocardial scar using CMR, is another important element of LV assessment. The detection of subendocardial or transmural infarction using CMR has at least as good sensitivity and specificity as invasive coronary angiography for the diagnosis of ischaemic cardiomyopathy, and it has been suggested that this may be used as a gatekeeper to invasive investigations.[17] Whereas magnetic resonance coronary angiography has also been shown to be effective in identifying rare cases of proximal three-vessel disease with widespread hibernation and without infarction, this is not commonly performed in clinical practice.[17] The transmural extent of myocardial scar in patients with ischaemic cardiomyopathy has been shown to determine the likelihood of improved contractility following revascularization.[58] This forms the basis of myocardial viability assessment using contrast-enhanced CMR, with dysfunctional segments without scar or only thin layers of partial-thickness scar having the greatest chance of showing improved contractility following successful revascularization. Other commonly used techniques to assess myocardial viability include dobutamine stress echocardiography and positron emission tomography (PET). An improvement in contraction during low-dose

dobutamine stress echocardiography, followed by a deterioration at higher doses as ischaemia develops, is a strong predictor of recovery in function following revascularization.[59] PET imaging enables the assessment of both perfusion (using tracers such as rubidium-82) and metabolism (using 18-fluorodeoxyglucose. Reduced perfusion with maintained metabolism is characteristic of viable myocardium.

Scar in mid-myocardial or subepicardial distributions may also be detected in non-ischaemic cardiomyopathies. As well as identifying patterns and distributions of scar typical of specific genetic or acquired cardiomyopathies (➲ Figure 6.1.7),[35] this also provides incremental prognostic information.[60] Patients with DCM and mid-wall fibrosis have been shown to have a 5- to 8-fold increase in the risk of sudden cardiac death events, compared to those without.[60,61] This may therefore have an important role in treatment stratification, specifically the selection of patients for implantable cardioverter–defibrillators. Detection of scar in the posterior wall may also predict a lower chance of gaining benefit from cardiac resynchronization therapy.[62,63]

Functional mitral regurgitation

Functional mitral regurgitation (MR) is commonly seen among patients with LV systolic dysfunction. This occurs in the context of a structurally normal mitral valve secondary to annular dilatation and leaflet tenting, tethering, and restriction due to regional myocardial dysfunction. Greater attention is being paid to the evaluation of functional MR following the emergence of percutaneous treatments that may reduce its severity. The recent COAPT trial confirmed that, at least for a subset of patients with HFrEF, functional MR leads to a poorer outcome.[64] In this trial, use of the MitraClip improved outcomes.[64] Comparison of the patient population with other trials of percutaneous intervention, which proved neutral, suggests that patients with the most severe MR who do not have advanced LV remodelling (i.e. a disproportionate degree of MR) may be the most likely to gain benefit from this treatment.[64,65] This emphasizes the importance of a comprehensive phenotypic assessment.

Left atrial assessment

The left atrium (LA) plays an important role in maintaining cardiac function, acting as an elastic reservoir and contributing to LV stroke volume during atrial contraction, as well as playing a role in regulating volume status through secretion of atrial natriuretic peptide. Dilatation, elevation of left atrial (LA) pressure, and reduction in LA function are commonly seen among patients with HFrEF and independently predict adverse prognosis.[66,67,68] Dilatation of the LA appears to be a more prominent feature of HFrEF, with increases in LA pressure and less prominent dilatation typical of HFpEF.[66] This may represent a difference in atrial fibrotic remodelling and varying responses adapting to elevated LV filling pressures and MR. The LA also serves as a buffer between the pulmonary circulation and the LV. It therefore follows that impairment of LA function is closely associated with pulmonary vascular resistance (PVR).[66]

Pulmonary vascular assessment

Estimation of pulmonary pressures is frequently made using echocardiography, based on Doppler assessments of the pulmonary and tricuspid valves. However, invasive catheter studies remain the gold standard for pulmonary vascular assessment, with better precision, compared to echocardiography. Pulmonary hypertension is a common feature of advanced HFrEF and is included within group 2 of the World Health Organization classification.[69] Elevated LA pressure is considered the primary mechanism. However, around 20% of patients have a mixed phenotype with elevated PVR.[70] This is associated with worse functional status, lower cardiac output, and worse survival.[70] It may be related to vasoconstriction due to reduced nitric oxide availability, and to pulmonary venous and arterial remodelling due to prolonged exposure to elevated pressures.[71,72] Given the importance of PVR in selecting patients for heart transplantation, defining the specific pulmonary vascular phenotype of patients using invasive catheter studies, including vasodilator testing, remains an important part of investigation of patients with HFrEF.[73]

Right ventricular assessment

Whereas the diagnosis of HFrEF relies on the assessment of LV systolic dysfunction, evaluation of the right ventricle (RV) remains an important part of the phenotypic assessment of HFrEF (➲ Chapter 6.4). This is frequently challenging due to its thin walls and triangular shape, which wraps around the LV. Three-dimensional volumetric assessment with CMR is perhaps the most precise technique.[74] Right ventricular (RV) dysfunction is common, affecting 30–60% of cases. This may be due to intrinsic myocardial disease, ischaemia, previous infarction, or increased afterload due to post-capillary pulmonary hypertension secondary to left heart disease.[75,76,77] Evaluating morphology, as well as function, is an important element of phenotypic assessment. The presence of regional wall motion abnormalities, wall thinning, aneurysms, or fibrofatty infiltration raises suspicion of biventricular forms of arrhythmogenic cardiomyopathies (➲ Chapter 3.4.5).[52] Discriminating these forms

of the disease from other causes of HFrEF is important due to the malignant disease course, characterized by a high incidence of sudden cardiac death, as well as the implications for family members.

Genetic phenotyping in HFrEF

Familial DCM, defined as DCM occurring in at least two closely related relatives, accounts for around 25–50% of cases.[78] It therefore represents a relatively small proportion of HFrEF cases. With the introduction of next-generation sequencing panel testing and reductions in costs, the use of genetic testing in DCM and HFrEF has increased. Commonly sequenced genes in panel testing for DCM are included in ➲ Box 6.1.1.[79] In the most recent guidelines, testing has been recommended in all cases of DCM and hypokinetic non-DCM.[6] In areas where resources may not enable this volume of testing, cases with clinical features suspicious of a genetic phenotype or those with a confirmed family history may be prioritized.[80,81] A likely pathogenic or pathogenic variant may be identified in 30–40% of familial cases and in 15–20% of all cases.[78,81,82]

Whereas genetic DCM has traditionally been considered a monogenic disease with Mendelian inheritance, recent research, predominantly on carriers of truncating variants in the

---

Box 6.1.1 Genes most robustly associated with dilated cardiomyopathy

Sarcomeric

- *TTN* (titin)
- *MYH7* (β-myosin heavy chain)
- *TNNT2* (troponin T)
- *TNNC1* (troponin C)
- *TPM1* (tropomyosin)
- *FLNC* (filamin C)
- *ACTC1* (α-actin)
- *NEXN* (nexilin)

Nuclear envelope

- *LMNA* (lamin A/C)

Desmosomal

- *DSP* (desmoplakin)

Cytoskeleton

- *DMD* (dystrophin)
- *VCL* (vinculin)

Sarcoplasmic reticulum

- *PLN* (phospholamban)

Spliceosomal

- *RBM20* (RNA-binding protein 20)

Molecular chaperone/autophagy

- *BAG3* (*BCL2*-associated athanogene 3)

titin gene (*TTN*), has confirmed an oligogenic basis for many patients with DCM, including those who were initially perceived to have a non-genetic basis to their disease such as peripartum or chemotherapy-associated cardiomyopathy.[26,27,28] Families with incomplete penetrance and variable expression are commonly encountered. This emphasizes the importance of appropriate genetic counselling prior to undertaking predictive testing in family members.

While the main purpose of genetic testing is to enable cascade predictive testing in unaffected family members to determine future risk and follow-up, the identification of variants in a smaller number of specific genes can inform prognosis and influence management. Variants in the lamin A/C gene (*LMNA*) have almost complete penetrance and are associated with premature AV block, ventricular arrhythmia, and a high incidence of sudden cardiac death and heart failure.[49,83] Use of implantable cardioverter–defibrillators before traditional thresholds is reached based on LVEF is advocated, particularly in patients requiring pacing for bradyarrhythmia indications. Similarly, variants in desmosomal genes or the filamin C gene (*FLNC*) are associated with fibrotic phenotypes of disease with a more malignant prognosis linked with a high incidence of major arrhythmia and sudden death.[84,85] A more aggressive approach towards primary prevention of sudden cardiac death appears sensible in such genotypes.[84,85]

A genetic contribution to ischaemic HFrEF is also increasingly recognized. This may be related to the cumulative effects of common genetic variation. Indeed, a genome-wide association study identified 12 variants associated with modifiable risk factors, as well as traits related to LV structure and function that were associated with the development of heart failure among 47,000 patients with heart failure.[86] While not imminently foreseeable, this raises the future possibility of incorporating a polygenic risk score to estimate the risk of developing heart failure in at-risk populations. Another study suggested a contribution from rare genetic variation in genes associated with DCM in a small proportion of patients with ischaemic HFrEF. It demonstrated that 2.8% of patients diagnosed with HFrEF secondary to ischaemic

heart disease in two randomized controlled trials carried a rare variant associated with cardiomyopathy that was classified as likely pathogenic or pathogenic.[87] The majority of rare variants were in *TTN* and these variants were enriched, compared to control populations where they are found in <1% of people. This supports the concept that relatively rare variation in genes associated with DCM may create an oligogenic susceptibility to developing contractile impairment that is unmasked by various 'second hits', including ischaemic heart disease. It also emphasizes the possibility of there being more than one factor contributing to the development of HFrEF and the need to comprehensively assess the phenotype before attaching a diagnostic label.

Natural history

The natural history of HRrEF may be characterized by progressive enlargement of cardiac chambers, declining contractility of the LV, and later also of the RV, with increasing regurgitation of the AV valves. Clinically this is associated with increasing symptoms, initially during exercise and later at rest. Typically, this decline is intertwined by episodes of decompensation due to water retention with increased LV filling pressures and pulmonary hypertension, and pulmonary and peripheral oedema leading to frequent hospitalizations (➔ Figure 6.1.8). With appropriate treatment, including diuretics and guideline-directed medical and device therapy (➔ Chapters 9.1 and 9.2), patients are discharged, only to be readmitted with further decompensations due to progressive pump failure. The risk of mortality from both non-sudden and sudden causes steadily increases and cardiac transplantation or mechanical circulatory support becomes the only additional treatment options available.

Fortunately, with the development of an array of effective heart failure drugs, the clinical outcomes of patients with HFrEF have markedly improved and progressive, refractory disease is less common. One-year mortality in patients with HFrEF declined from 16% to 12% with the introduction of angiotensin-converting enzyme (ACE) inhibitors, to 8% with the introduction of beta-blockers on top of ACE inhibitors, and to 6% with the addition

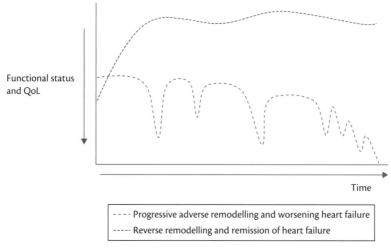

Functional status and QoL

Time

- - - - Progressive adverse remodelling and worsening heart failure
——— Reverse remodelling and remission of heart failure

Figure 6.1.8 Natural history of heart failure with reduced ejection fraction.

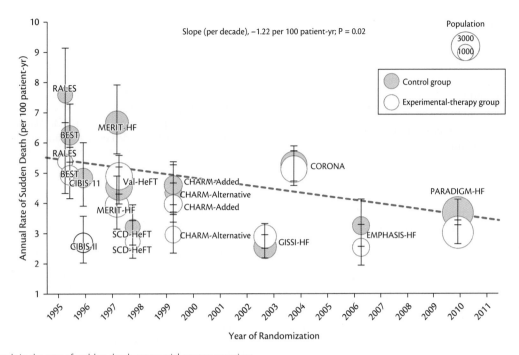

Figure 6.1.9 Trends in the rate of sudden death across trial groups over time.

Reproduced from Shen L, Jhund PS, Petrie MC, *et al*. Declining Risk of Sudden Death in Heart Failure. *N Engl J Med*. 2017 Jul 6;377(1):41–51. doi: 10.1056/NEJMoa1609758 with permission from Massachusetts Medical Society.

of mineralocorticoid receptor antagonists.[88] With the further addition of angiotensin receptor–neprilysin inhibitors (ARNIs) and sodium–glucose cotransporter 2 (SGLT2) inhibitors, on top of conventional triple therapy, the mean life expectancy of a 55-year old patient with HFrEF is increased by around 6 years, with a mean survival of almost 18 years.[89] Furthermore, a 44% decline in sudden cardiac death has been noted in patients enrolled in the early to the most recent trials (➲ Figure 6.1.9).[90] Medical therapy is frequently accompanied by LV reverse remodelling, characterized by a reduction in LV cavity size and improved systolic function.[91] This is most frequently seen among patients with DCM, compared to those with ischaemic cardiomyopathy, and may occur in as many as 40–50% of patients.[92,93] This is frequently associated with resolution of symptoms and good long-term outcomes.[92,93] A recent randomized trial has confirmed that despite improvement in cardiac function and resolution of symptoms, many patients continue to benefit from pharmacological therapy and have a high risk of relapse if therapy is withdrawn.[7] It is therefore best to view this phenomenon as heart failure remission, as opposed to recovery.

Future directions

Further improvement of clinical outcomes in patients with HFrEF is an unmet need, as many patients suffer from progressive disease in spite of current management. What is currently missing, at least for the vast majority of patients, is true recovery of LV and RV pump function as provided by heart transplantation. Heart transplantation, however, can only be considered for highly selected patients with end-stage heart failure, due to limited organ availability, as well as side effects and risks of immunosuppression

required for graft survival. The totally implantable artificial heart still remains an ambition, although progress has been made with LV assist devices in patients with advanced HFrEF.[94]

With cardiac myosin activators, a novel approach to improving outcomes by increasing myocardial pump function has been recently investigated. Although the selective cardiac myosin activator omecamtiv mecarbil improves cardiac performance in patients with HFrEF, the drug reduced the primary outcome, a composite of a heart failure event or cardiovascular death, by only 8% in the GALACTIC-HF trial [95] Nevertheless, this is the first agent acting on the heart itself that proved safe and somewhat effective on top of current guideline-recommended therapy.

Stem cells have been a great hope, particularly in patients with reduced LVEF after an ST-segment elevation MI, to prevent and/or reverse LV remodelling and heart failure. Unfortunately, the effects of intracoronary infusion of bone marrow-derived stem cells had only minor or no effects on LVEF.[96] Whether mesenchymal or genetically engineered stem cells might provide better results remains to be shown.[97]

Finally, targeted genetic therapies are a big hope for monogenetic non-ischaemic cardiomyopathies, particularly since the development of gene editing techniques such as CRISPR (clustered regularly interspaced short palindromic repeats)/Cas-9.[98] Indeed, in human embryos, this technique has already been successfully used to correct a mutation in the gene encoding myocardial contractile protein leading to hypertrophic cardiomyopathy.[99] Therapies targeting the molecular pathways that mediate the effects of specific genetic variants also provide hope for modifying the disease course of some of the most malignant genetic forms of the disease.[100]

Summary and key messages

Heart failure has traditionally been classified on the basis of the LVEF due to the remarkable ability to predict the likelihood of benefit from prognostic heart failure therapies. Following the PARAGON-HF trial and the EMPEROR programme of studies, ARNIs and SGLT2 inhibitors will be used increasingly in patients with the mildest reductions in ejection fraction.

Ischaemic cardiomyopathy is the most common cause of HFrEF caused by myocardial dysfunction driven by previous infarction and scar formation and persistent or recurrent ischaemia causing hibernation. Non-ischaemic cardiomyopathy is a heterogeneous group of different diseases driven by environmental insults, genetic susceptibility, or frequently a combination of the two. With the pursuit of precision medicine, characterization of the disease substrate and phenotype is likely to play an increasing role in the selection of patients for specific therapies such as implantable cardioverter–defibrillators or those targeting important specific disease mechanisms. Multimodality imaging, genetic testing, and biomarkers will be at the centre of advances in precision medicine.

References

1. Withering W. *An Account of the Foxglove and Some of Its Medical Uses: With Practical Remarks on Dropsy and Other Diseases*. London: G. G. J. and J. Robinson; 1785.

2. Packer M, Fowler MB, Roecker EB, *et al.* Effect of carvedilol on the morbidity of patients with severe chronic heart failure: results of the carvedilol prospective randomized cumulative survival (COPERNICUS) study. *Circulation*. 2002;106:2194–9.

3. Consensus Trial Study Group. Effects of enalapril on mortality in severe congestive heart failure. Results of the Cooperative North Scandinavian Enalapril Survival Study (CONSENSUS). *N Engl J Med*. 1987;316:1429–35.

4. Pitt B, Zannad F, Remme WJ, *et al.* The effect of spironolactone on morbidity and mortality in patients with severe heart failure. Randomized Aldactone Evaluation Study Investigators. *N Engl J Med*. 1999;341:709–17.

5. Ponikowski P, Voors AA, Anker SD, *et al.* 2016 ESC Guidelines for the diagnosis and treatment of acute and chronic heart failure. *Eur Heart J*. 2016;37:2129–200.

6. McDonagh TA, Metra M, Adamo M, *et al.* 2021 ESC Guidelines for the diagnosis and treatment of acute and chronic heart failure. *Eur Heart J*. 2021;42:3599–726.

7. Halliday BP, Wassall R, Lota AS, *et al.* Withdrawal of pharmacological treatment for heart failure in patients with recovered dilated cardiomyopathy (TRED-HF): an open-label, pilot, randomised trial. *Lancet*. 2019;393:61–73.

8. Luscher TF. Lumpers and splitters: the bumpy road to precision medicine. *Eur Heart J*. 2019;40:3292–6.

9. Wehner GJ, Jing L, Haggerty CM, *et al.* Routinely reported ejection fraction and mortality in clinical practice: where does the nadir of risk lie? *Eur Heart J*. 2020;41:1249–57.

10. Anker SD, Butler J, Filippatos G, *et al.* Empagliflozin in heart failure with a preserved ejection fraction. *N Engl J Med*. 2022;386:e57.

11. Solomon SD, Claggett B, Lewis EF, *et al.* Influence of ejection fraction on outcomes and efficacy of spironolactone in patients with heart failure with preserved ejection fraction. *Eur Heart J*. 2016;37:455–62.

12. Solomon SD, McMurray JJV, Anand IS, *et al.* Angiotensin-neprilysin inhibition in heart failure with preserved ejection fraction. *N Engl J Med*. 2019;381:1609–20.

13. Yancy CW, Jessup M, Bozkurt B, *et al.* 2013 ACCF/AHA guideline for the management of heart failure. *Circulation*. 2013;128:e240–327.

14. Mosterd A and Hoes AW. Clinical epidemiology of heart failure. *Heart*. 2007;93:1137–46.

15. Redfield MM, Jacobsen SJ, Burnett JC Jr, Mahoney DW, Bailey KR, and Rodeheffer RJ. Burden of systolic and diastolic ventricular dysfunction in the community: appreciating the scope of the heart failure epidemic. *JAMA*. 2003;289:194–202.

16. Felker GM, Shaw LK, and O'Connor CM. A standardized definition of ischemic cardiomyopathy for use in clinical research. *J Am Coll Cardiol*. 2002;39:210–18.

17. Assomull RG, Shakespeare C, Kalra PR, *et al.* Role of cardiovascular magnetic resonance as a gatekeeper to invasive coronary angiography in patients presenting with heart failure of unknown etiology. *Circulation*. 2011;124:1351–60.

18. Rahimtoola SH. The hibernating myocardium. *Am Heart J*. 1989;117:211–21.

19. Bayeva M, Sawicki KT, Butler J, Gheorghiade M, and Ardehali H. Molecular and cellular basis of viable dysfunctional myocardium. *Circ Heart Fail*. 2014;7:680–91.

20. Briceno N, Schuster A, Lumley M, and Perera D. Ischaemic cardiomyopathy: pathophysiology, assessment and the role of revascularisation. *Heart*. 2016;102:397–406.

21. Poole-Wilson PA, Holmberg SR, and Williams AJ. A possible molecular mechanism for 'stunning' of the myocardium. *Eur Heart J*. 1991;12 Suppl F:25–9.

22. Carluccio E, Biagioli P, Alunni G, *et al.* Patients with hibernating myocardium show altered left ventricular volumes and shape, which revert after revascularization: evidence that dyssynergy might directly induce cardiac remodeling. *J Am Coll Cardiol*. 2006;47:969–77.

23. Rahimtoola SH, La Canna G, and Ferrari R. Hibernating myocardium: another piece of the puzzle falls into place. *J Am Coll Cardiol*. 2006;47:978–80.

24. Arbustini E, Narula N, Tavazzi L, *et al.* The MOGE(S) classification of cardiomyopathy for clinicians. *J Am Coll Cardiol*. 2014;64:304–18.

25. Pinto YM, Elliott PM, Arbustini E, *et al.* Proposal for a revised definition of dilated cardiomyopathy, hypokinetic non-dilated cardiomyopathy, and its implications for clinical practice. *Eur Heart J*. 2016;37:1850–8.

26. Garcia-Pavia P, Kim Y, Alejandra Restrepo-Cordoba M, *et al.* Genetic variants associated with cancer therapy-induced cardiomyopathy. *Circulation*. 2019;140:31–41.

27. Ware JS, Amor-Salamanca A, Tayal U, *et al.* Genetic etiology for alcohol-induced cardiac toxicity. *J Am Coll Cardiol*. 2018;71:2293–302.

28. Ware JS, Li J, Mazaika E, *et al.* Shared genetic predisposition in peripartum and dilated cardiomyopathies. *N Engl J Med*. 2016;374:233–41.

29. Halliday BP, Jones RE, Hammersley DJ. Dilated cardiomyopathy. In: Malik M, ed. Sex Differences in Cardiac Electrophysiology. London: Elsevier; 2020, pp. 363–73.

30. Hilfiker-Kleiner D and Sliwa K. Pathophysiology and epidemiology of peripartum cardiomyopathy. *Nat Rev Cardiol*. 2014;11:364–70.

31. Beltrami CA, Finato N, Rocco M, *et al.* The cellular basis of dilated cardiomyopathy in humans. *J Mol Cell Cardiol*. 1995;27:291–305.

32. Halliday BP and Prasad SK. The interstitium in the hypertrophied heart. *JACC Cardiovasc Imaging*. 2019;12:2357–68.

33. Halliday B, Gulati A, Ali A, *et al.* Association between mid-wall late gadolinium enhancement and sudden cardiac death in patients with

dilated cardiomyopathy and mild and moderate left ventricular systolic dysfunction. *Circulation*. 2017;135:2106–15.

34. Halliday BP, Baksi AJ, Gulati A, *et al.* Outcome in dilated cardiomyopathy related to the extent, location, and pattern of late gadolinium enhancement. *JACC Cardiovasc Imaging*. 2019;12:1645–55.

35. Augusto JB, Eiros R, Nakou E, *et al.* Dilated cardiomyopathy and arrhythmogenic left ventricular cardiomyopathy: a comprehensive genotype-imaging phenotype study. *Eur Heart J Cardiovasc Imaging*. 2020;21:326–36.

36. Gulati A, Ismail TF, Ali A, *et al.* Microvascular dysfunction in dilated cardiomyopathy: a quantitative stress perfusion cardiovascular magnetic resonance study. *JACC Cardiovasc Imaging*. 2019;12:1699–708.

37. Linssen GC, Rienstra M, Jaarsma T, *et al.* Clinical and prognostic effects of atrial fibrillation in heart failure patients with reduced and preserved left ventricular ejection fraction. *Eur J Heart Fail*. 2011;13:1111–20.

38. Zafrir B, Lund LH, Laroche C, *et al.* Prognostic implications of atrial fibrillation in heart failure with reduced, mid-range, and preserved ejection fraction: a report from 14 964 patients in the European Society of Cardiology Heart Failure Long-Term Registry. *Eur Heart J*. 2018;39:4277–84.

39. Marrouche NF, Kheirkhahan M, and Brachmann J. Catheter ablation for atrial fibrillation with heart failure. *N Engl J Med*. 2018; 379:492.

40. Darmon A, Ducroqc G, Elbez Y, *et al.* Prevalence, incidence and prognostic implications of left bundle branch block in patients with stable coronary artery disease. An analysis from the CLARIFY registry. *Arch Cardiovasc Dis*. 2020;12:107–8.

41. Baldasseroni S, Opasich C, Gorini M, *et al.* Left bundle-branch block is associated with increased 1-year sudden and total mortality rate in 5517 outpatients with congestive heart failure: a report from the Italian network on congestive heart failure. *Am Heart J*. 2002;143:398–405.

42. Clark AL, Goode K, and Cleland JG. The prevalence and incidence of left bundle branch block in ambulant patients with chronic heart failure. *Eur J Heart Fail*. 2008;10:696–702.

43. Cleland JG, Daubert JC, Erdmann E, *et al.* The effect of cardiac resynchronization on morbidity and mortality in heart failure. *N Engl J Med*. 2005;352:1539–49.

44. Prinzmetal M, Shaw CM Jr, Maxwell MH, *et al.* Studies on the mechanism of ventricular activity. VI. The depolarization complex in pure subendocardial infarction; role of the subendocardial region in the normal electrocardiogram. *Am J Med*. 1954;16:469–89.

45. Moon JC, De Arenaza DP, Elkington AG, *et al.* The pathologic basis of Q-wave and non-Q-wave myocardial infarction: a cardiovascular magnetic resonance study. *J Am Coll Cardiol*. 2004;44:554–60.

46. Berger CJ, Murabito JM, Evans JC, Anderson KM, and Levy D. Prognosis after first myocardial infarction. Comparison of Q-wave and non-Q-wave myocardial infarction in the Framingham Heart Study. *JAMA*. 1992;268:1545–51.

47. Finocchiaro G, Merlo M, Sheikh N, *et al.* The electrocardiogram in the diagnosis and management of patients with dilated cardiomyopathy. *Eur J Heart Fail*. 2020;22:1097–107.

48. Weintraub RG, Semsarian C, and Macdonald P. Dilated cardiomyopathy. *Lancet*. 2017;390:400–14.

49. Pasotti M, Klersy C, Pilotto A, *et al.* Long-term outcome and risk stratification in dilated cardiolaminopathies. *J Am Coll Cardiol*. 2008;52:1250–60.

50. Tayal U, Newsome S, Buchan R, *et al.* Truncating variants in titin independently predict early arrhythmias in patients with dilated cardiomyopathy. *J Am Coll Cardiol*. 2017;69:2466–8.

51. Diegoli M, Grasso M, Favalli V, *et al.* Diagnostic work-up and risk stratification in X-linked dilated cardiomyopathies caused by dystrophin defects. *J Am Coll Cardiol*. 2011;58:925–34.

52. Miles C, Finocchiaro G, Papadakis M, *et al.* Sudden death and left ventricular involvement in arrhythmogenic cardiomyopathy. *Circulation*. 2019;139:1786–97.

53. Solomon SD, Vaduganathan M, Claggett BL, *et al.* Sacubitril/valsartan across the spectrum of ejection fraction in heart failure. *Circulation*. 2020;141:352–61.

54. The SOLVD Investigators. Effect of enalapril on survival in patients with reduced left ventricular ejection fractions and congestive heart failure. *N Engl J Med*. 1991;325:293–302.

55. Halliday BP, Senior R, and Pennell DJ. Assessing left ventricular systolic function: from ejection fraction to strain analysis. *Eur Heart J*. 2021;42:789–97.

56. Kalam K, Otahal P, and Marwick TH. Prognostic implications of global LV dysfunction: a systematic review and meta-analysis of global longitudinal strain and ejection fraction. *Heart*. 2014;100:1673–80.

57. Hansen S, Brainin P, Sengelov M, *et al.* Prognostic utility of diastolic dysfunction and speckle tracking echocardiography in heart failure with reduced ejection fraction. *ESC Heart Fail*. 2020;7:147–57.

58. Kim RJ, Wu E, Rafael A, *et al.* The use of contrast-enhanced magnetic resonance imaging to identify reversible myocardial dysfunction. *N Engl J Med*. 2000;343:1445–53.

59. La Canna G, Alfieri O, Giubbini R, Gargano M, Ferrari R, and Visioli O. Echocardiography during infusion of dobutamine for identification of reversibly dysfunction in patients with chronic coronary artery disease. *J Am Coll Cardiol*. 1994;23:617–26.

60. Halliday BP, Gulati A, Ali A, *et al.* Association between midwall late gadolinium enhancement and sudden cardiac death in patients with dilated cardiomyopathy and mild and moderate left ventricular systolic dysfunction. *Circulation*. 2017;135:2106–15.

61. Gulati A, Jabbour A, Ismail TF, *et al.* Association of fibrosis with mortality and sudden cardiac death in patients with nonischemic dilated cardiomyopathy. *JAMA*. 2013;309:896–908.

62. Chalil S, Foley PW, Muyhaldeen SA, *et al.* Late gadolinium enhancement-cardiovascular magnetic resonance as a predictor of response to cardiac resynchronization therapy in patients with ischaemic cardiomyopathy. *Europace*. 2007;9:1031–7.

63. Leyva F. The role of cardiovascular magnetic resonance in cardiac resynchronization therapy. *Heart Fail Clin*. 2017;13:63–77.

64. Stone GW, Lindenfeld J, Abraham WT, *et al.* Transcatheter mitral-valve repair in patients with heart failure. *N Engl J Med*. 2018;379:2307–18.

65. Obadia JF, Messika-Zeitoun D, Leurent G, *et al.* Percutaneous repair or medical treatment for secondary mitral regurgitation. *N Engl J Med*. 2018;379:2297–306.

66. Melenovsky V, Hwang SJ, Redfield MM, Zakeri R, Lin G, and Borlaug BA. Left atrial remodeling and function in advanced heart failure with preserved or reduced ejection fraction. *Circ Heart Fail*. 2015;8:295–303.

67. Modin D, Sengelov M, Jorgensen PG, *et al.* Prognostic value of left atrial functional measures in heart failure with reduced ejection fraction. *J Card Fail*. 2019;25:87–96.

68. Gulati A, Ismail TF, Jabbour A, *et al.* Clinical utility and prognostic value of left atrial volume assessment by cardiovascular magnetic resonance in non-ischaemic dilated cardiomyopathy. *Eur J Heart Fail*. 2013;15:660–70.

69. Simonneau G, Gatzoulis MA, Adatia I, *et al.* Updated clinical classification of pulmonary hypertension. *J Am Coll Cardiol*. 2013;62:D34–41.

70. Miller WL, Grill DE, and Borlaug BA. Clinical features, hemodynamics, and outcomes of pulmonary hypertension due to chronic heart failure with reduced ejection fraction: pulmonary hypertension and heart failure. *JACC Heart Fail*. 2013;1:290–9.

71. Fayyaz AU, Edwards WD, Maleszewski JJ, *et al*. Global pulmonary vascular remodeling in pulmonary hypertension associated with heart failure and preserved or reduced ejection fraction. *Circulation*. 2018;137:1796–810.

72. Verbrugge FH, Dupont M, Bertrand PB, *et al*. Pulmonary vascular response to exercise in symptomatic heart failure with reduced ejection fraction and pulmonary hypertension. *Eur J Heart Fail*. 2015;17:320–8.

73. Crawford TC, Leary PJ, Fraser CD 3rd, *et al*. Impact of the new pulmonary hypertension definition on heart transplant outcomes: expanding the hemodynamic risk profile. *Chest*. 2020;157:151–61.

74. Globits S, Pacher R, Frank H, *et al*. Comparative assessment of right ventricular volumes and ejection fraction by thermodilution and magnetic resonance imaging in dilated cardiomyopathy. *Cardiology*. 1995;86:67–72.

75. Gulati A, Ismail TF, Jabbour A, *et al*. The prevalence and prognostic significance of right ventricular systolic dysfunction in nonischemic dilated cardiomyopathy. *Circulation*. 2013;128:1623–33.

76. La Vecchia L, Paccanaro M, Bonanno C, Varotto L, Ometto R, and Vincenzi M. Left ventricular versus biventricular dysfunction in idiopathic dilated cardiomyopathy. *Am J Cardiol*. 1999;83:120–2, A9.

77. Pueschner A, Chattranukulchai P, Heitner JF, *et al*. The prevalence, correlates, and impact on cardiac mortality of right ventricular dysfunction in nonischemic cardiomyopathy. *JACC Cardiovasc Imaging*. 2017;10:1225–36.

78. Hershberger RE, Hedges DJ, and Morales A. Dilated cardiomyopathy: the complexity of a diverse genetic architecture. *Nat Rev Cardiol*. 2013;10:531–47.

79. Mazzarotto F, Tayal U, Buchan RJ, *et al*. Reevaluating the genetic contribution of monogenic dilated cardiomyopathy. *Circulation*. 2020;141:387–98.

80. Rosenbaum AN, Agre KE, and Pereira NL. Genetics of dilated cardiomyopathy: practical implications for heart failure management. *Nat Rev Cardiol*. 2020;17:286–97.

81. Hershberger RE, Lindenfeld J, Mestroni L, Seidman CE, Taylor MR, Towbin JA, and Heart Failure Society of America. Genetic evaluation of cardiomyopathy: a Heart Failure Society of America practice guideline. *J Card Fail*. 2009;15:83–97.

82. McNally EM, Golbus JR, and Puckelwartz MJ. Genetic mutations and mechanisms in dilated cardiomyopathy. *J Clin Invest*. 2013;123:19–26.

83. Meune C, van Berlo JH, Anselme F, Bonne G, Pinto YM, and Duboc D. Primary prevention of sudden death in patients with lamin A/C gene mutations. *N Engl J Med*. 2006;354:209–10.

84. Ortiz-Genga MF, Cuenca S, Dal Ferro M, *et al*. Truncating *FLNC* mutations are associated with high-risk dilated and arrhythmogenic cardiomyopathies. *J Am Coll Cardiol*. 2016;68:2440–51.

85. Gigli M, Merlo M, Graw SL, *et al*. Genetic risk of arrhythmic phenotypes in patients with dilated cardiomyopathy. *J Am Coll Cardiol*. 2019;74:1480–90.

86. Shah S, Henry A, Roselli C, *et al*. Genome-wide association and Mendelian randomisation analysis provide insights into the pathogenesis of heart failure. *Nat Commun*. 2020;11:163.

87. Povysil G, Chazara O, Carss KJ, *et al*. Assessing the role of rare genetic variation in patients with heart failure. *JAMA Cardiol*. 2021;6:379–86.

88. McMurray JJ. CONSENSUS to EMPHASIS: the overwhelming evidence which makes blockade of the renin-angiotensin-aldosterone system the cornerstone of therapy for systolic heart failure. *Eur J Heart Fail*. 2011;13:929–36.

89. Vaduganathan M, Claggett BL, Jhund PS, *et al*. Estimating lifetime benefits of comprehensive disease-modifying pharmacological therapies in patients with heart failure with reduced ejection fraction: a comparative analysis of three randomised controlled trials. *Lancet*. 2020;396:121–8.

90. Shen L, Jhund PS, Petrie MC, *et al*. Declining risk of sudden death in heart failure. *N Engl J Med*. 2017;377:41–51.

91. Aimo A, Gaggin HK, Barison A, Emdin M, and Januzzi JL Jr. Imaging, biomarker, and clinical predictors of cardiac remodeling in heart failure with reduced ejection fraction. *JACC Heart Fail*. 2019;7:782–94.

92. Merlo M, Pyxaras SA, Pinamonti B, Barbati G, Di Lenarda A, and Sinagra G. Prevalence and prognostic significance of left ventricular reverse remodeling in dilated cardiomyopathy receiving tailored medical treatment. *J Am Coll Cardiol*. 2011;57:1468–76.

93. Tayal U, Wage R, Newsome S, *et al*. Predictors of left ventricular remodelling in patients with dilated cardiomyopathy: a cardiovascular magnetic resonance study. *Eur J Heart Fail*. 2020;22:1160–70.

94. Mehra MR, Naka Y, Uriel N, *et al*. A fully magnetically levitated circulatory pump for advanced heart failure. *N Engl J Med*. 2017;376:440–50.

95. Teerlink JR, Diaz R, Felker GM, *et al*. Cardiac myosin activation with omecamtiv mecarbil in systolic heart failure. *N Engl J Med*. 2021;384:105–16.

96. Schachinger V, Erbs S, Elsasser A, *et al*. Intracoronary bone marrow-derived progenitor cells in acute myocardial infarction. *N Engl J Med*. 2006;355:1210–21.

97. Fan M, Huang Y, Chen Z, *et al*. Efficacy of mesenchymal stem cell therapy in systolic heart failure: a systematic review and meta-analysis. *Stem Cell Res Ther*. 2019;10:150.

98. Lander ES. The heroes of CRISPR. *Cell*. 2016;164:18–28.

99. Ma H, Marti-Gutierrez N, Park SW, *et al*. Correction of a pathogenic gene mutation in human embryos. *Nature*. 2017;548:413–19.

100. Wu W, Muchir A, Shan J, Bonne G, and Worman HJ. Mitogen-activated protein kinase inhibitors improve heart function and prevent fibrosis in cardiomyopathy caused by mutation in lamin A/C gene. *Circulation*. 2011;123:53–61.

CHAPTER 6.2

Heart failure with mildly reduced ejection fraction

Adriaan A Voors, Benda Moura, Lars Lund, and Carolyn SP Lam

Contents

Introduction

One of the first scientific documents on diastolic heart failure (HF) was a review paper published by Pravin Shah and Ramdas Pai in 1992.[1] Three remarkable quotes from that paper are:

1. 'Diastolic heart failure is a distinct clinical entity increasingly seen in older patients and requires special awareness to make the diagnosis.'

2. 'It appears that prognosis is significantly better for those with normal systolic function.'

3. 'Diastolic heart failure is difficult to treat.'

Twenty-eight years later, we have to acknowledge that only little progression has been made. One important change is related to the nomenclature and definitions of categories of HF according to the left ventricular ejection fraction (LVEF). Since diastolic dysfunction was found across the whole spectrum of LVEF, and since it appeared that systolic function was also impaired in patients with normal LVEF, the task force of the 2008 European Society of Cardiology (ESC) HF Guidelines decided to change the name of 'diastolic heart failure' into 'heart failure with preserved ejection fraction (HFpEF)'.[2] As quoted in the 2008 ESC HF Guidelines: 'Other phrases have been used to describe diastolic HF, such as HF with preserved ejection fraction (HFPEF), HF with normal ejection fraction (HFNEF), or HF with preserved systolic function (HFPSF). We have elected to use the abbreviation HFPEF in this document.' Although this name became widely accepted, inconsistency remained regarding the cut-off of LVEF. The definition of HFpEF ranges from LVEF >35%, 40%, 45%, and 50% to 55%. The 2012 ESC HF Guidelines quoted: 'Patients with an EF in the range 35–50% therefore represent a "grey area" and most probably have primarily mild systolic dysfunction.'[3] Similarly, the 2013 American College of Cardiology Foundation (ACCF)/American Heart Association (AHA) HF Guidelines acknowledged that 'HFpEF has been variably classified as EF >40%, >45%, >50%, and >55%' and '[p]atients with an EF in the range of 40% to 50% represent an intermediate group. These patients are often treated for underlying risk factors and comorbidities and with GDMT similar to that used in patients with HFrEF.'[4]

In 2014, Carolyn Lam and Scott Solomon published an editorial entitled 'The middle child in heart failure: heart failure with midrange ejection fraction'.[5] In their editorial, they concluded that patients with HF and an LVEF of between 40% and 50% constitute a sizeable proportion (10–20%) of the HF population, have a unique clinical, echocardiographic, haemodynamic, and biomarker profile, compared to patients with HFrEF and HFpEF, and carry a poor prognosis. Importantly, they noted large gaps in evidence regarding its treatment. Therefore, the task force of the 2016 ESC HF Guidelines[6] concluded that:

1. There was a grey area of between 40% and 50% where the definition of HFrEF and HFpEF remained unclear and inconsistent

2. Patients with an LVEF of 40–49% have a different phenotype, compared to those with an LVEF of >50%

3. There are potentially differential treatment effects for patients with an LVEF of 40–50%, compared to those with an LVEF of >50%.

Based on these conclusions, the task force of the 2016 ESC HF Guidelines decided to formally identify HFmrEF as a separate group. HFmrEF was defined as patients with typical symptoms (and signs) of HF, an N-terminal pro-B-type natriuretic peptide (NT-proBNP) level of >125 pg/mL, and evidence of structural or functional cardiac abnormalities. In the 2021 ESC HF Guidelines, an LVEF of <50% was sufficient evidence of a functional cardiac abnormality and no additional requirements needed to be met.[7]

Structural or functional cardiac abnormalities included either left ventricular hypertrophy (defined as a left ventricular mass index of >95 g/m^2 in women, and >115 g/m^2 in men), a left atrial volume index of >34 mL/m^2, a mean septal/lateral tissue velocity of <9 cm/s, or E/e′ of ≥13. The additional natriuretic peptide level and echocardiographic criteria were similar to HFpEP, but not required for HFrEF where typical symptoms (± signs) and an LVEF of <40% were sufficient to establish a diagnosis of HFrEF.

The task force of the 2016 ESC HF guidelines had carefully considered the advantages and disadvantages of introducing another HF category. One of the most important arguments in favour was that '[i]dentifying HFmrEF as a separate group will stimulate research into the underlying characteristics, pathophysiology[,] and treatment of this group of patients.'[6] Four years after its introduction, we have to conclude that our knowledge of this 'middle child' has substantially increased and will be summarized in this chapter. This chapter will discuss the epidemiology and clinical characteristics of HFmrEF, followed by the evidence for potential treatments. Finally, we will focus on the sex differences and propose a modest renaming from 'HF with mid-range ejection fraction' to 'HF with mildly reduced ejection fraction'.

Epidemiology of heart failure with mildly reduced ejection fraction

The definition of HF with mildly reduced ejection fraction (HFmrEF) in the ESC guidelines had as a main objective to shed light on a cohort of patients who had not been, until then, specifically studied in randomized clinical trials, resulting in a lack of knowledge of the clinical characteristics and prognosis of, and treatment for, HFmrEF.[6] The aim was not to assume the existence of a new entity with different phenotype characteristics or pathophysiology, but to have investigations focused on these particular patients, allowing better profiling of this cohort, and thus more accurate management leading to an improved outcome.

Several publications have since addressed HFmrEF patients, allowing a deeper understanding of this group. Present knowledge is derived from registries and clinical trials focusing on patients with HFrEF or HFpEF that included some patients with this intermediate ejection fraction (EF). For a better description of this cohort, we only included those of patients across the whole spectrum of EF and with a definition of HFmrEF as in the ESC Guidelines.

Prevalence

In large trials and real-world registries, the prevalence of HFmrEF ranges from 12% to 14% among patients hospitalized for HF,[8,9] and between 17% and 24% among outpatients.[10,11,12,13]

In the large Get With The Guidelines–Heart Failure (GWTG-HF) registry, within the short time frame from 2005 to 2010, the proportion of patients hospitalized for HFmrEF remained stable (around 15%), whereas that of patients hospitalized for HFpEF increased from 33% to 39%, and for HFrEF it decreased from 52% to 47%.[14]

Patient characteristics

The ESC Heart Failure Long Term Registry, conducted from 2011 to 2015, enrolled 9134 outpatients with HF.[11] Patients in the HFmrEF group (24% of the population) had several characteristics in common with HFrEF patients: they were, on average, 4 years younger than those with HFpEF and more frequently male, and presented more often with an ischaemic aetiology. On the other hand, these patients had a higher body mass index (BMI), closer to that of the HFpEF group, but with respect to systolic blood pressure, the prevalence of smoking habits, atrial fibrillation, and left ventricular hypertrophy was intermediate between that in the HFrEF and HFpEF groups.

The Swedish Heart Failure Registry included both outpatients and hospitalized patients. In this database comprising a total of 42,061 patients, 21% of patients had HFmrEF.[15] Most clinical characteristics, such as age, proportion of women, systolic blood pressure, atrial fibrillation, hypertension, and NT-proBNP levels, were present as a continuum across HFpEF, HFmrEF, and HFrEF. HFmrEF resembled HFrEF with a lower prevalence of diabetes and a higher prevalence of coronary artery disease (CAD).

The CHART-2 observational study included 3480 outpatients from Japan, of whom 17% had HFmrEF.[13] HFmrEF patients had largely intermediate characteristics between HFpEF and HFrEF: the proportion of women, age, BMI, hypertension, atrial fibrillation, and systolic and diastolic blood pressures increased significantly from HFrEF, through to HFmrEF, and to HFpEF, whereas a history of admission for HF, heart rate, haemoglobin level, and serum levels of blood urea nitrogen (BUN), creatinine, and brain natriuretic peptide (BNP) decreased. CAD was the most frequent aetiology across all LVEF values, but significantly higher in HFmrEF and HFrEF.

In the large GWTG-HF database[8] that included 99,825 patients admitted for acute HF from 2005 to 2013, 13% had HFmrEF. These patients were more similar to those with HFpEF than to those with HFrEF with respect to age and several comorbidities (such as anaemia, atrial fibrillation, diabetes, hypertension, and renal disease). However, the prevalence of diabetes, peripheral vascular disease, hyperlipidaemia, renal insufficiency, and dialysis was higher among HFmrEF patients, compared to the other groups. A history of acute myocardial infarction (AMI) or CAD and an ischaemic aetiology of HF were more frequent among HFmrEF patients, and identical to those with HFrEF. Precipitating factors of hospitalization were mainly similar to those of HFpEF, such as uncontrolled hypertension or non-compliance to diet, except again for ischaemia where it resembled more HFrEF.

In two trials including patients across all LVEF values,[10,12] HFmrEF was more similar to HFrEF with respect to several clinical characteristics such as age, gender, systolic blood pressure, atrial fibrillation, and a history of AMI. With respect to BMI, the distribution of New York Heart Association (NYHA) class, and a history of hypertension, the HFmrEF group had intermediate values between HFrEF and HFpEF. The prevalence of other comorbidities, such as diabetes and stroke, was the same across all groups. Interestingly, in one study, NT-proBNP levels were significantly higher in HFrEF and HFmrEF patients, compared to HFpEF patients, and NT-proBNP-guided therapy had a beneficial effect on reducing the risk of HF hospitalization among HFrEF and HFmrEF patients, but not among HFpEF patients.[12]

The large heterogeneity of patients with HFmrEF becomes evident from different publications. Despite this variability in clinical characteristics, it seems reasonably fair to acknowledge HFmrEF as a cohort of patients with a clinical phenotype that is most often intermediate between that of HFrEF and HFpEF.[16] There is a closer similarity between HFmrEF and HFrEF with respect to an ischaemic aetiology. The GWTG-HF registry is the only study in which HFmrEF more closely resembles HFpEF. This registry includes patients hospitalized for HF, whereas other registries and trials include exclusively outpatients (except the Swedish registry which includes both outpatients and hospitalized patients). This discrepancy might therefore be explained by the inclusion of different populations (◑ Table 6.2.1).

Prognosis

In the ESC Heart Failure Long Term Registry, 1-year all-cause mortality in patients with HFmrEF was 7.6%, compared to

Table 6.2.1 Prevalence of HFmrEF (large trials and real-world registries)

	Rickenbacher et al., 2017[12]	Toma et al., 2014[9]	Lund et al., 2018[10]	Chioncel et al., 2017[11]	Tsuji et al., 2017[13]	Koh et al., 2017[15]	Kapoor et al., 2016[8]
Age (years), mean ± SD	79	73	65 ± 11	64.2 ± 14.2	69.0 ± 11.6	74	77
Female gender, (%)	46.3	41.1	29.9	31.5	28.2	39	48.85
BMI (kg/m²), mean ± SD or median (IQR)	25.5	31.5 ± 7.2	27.8 (25.0–31.2)	28.6 ± 5.4	22.8 ± 5.3	27	
SBP (mmHg), mean ± SD or median (IQR)	127	130 (117–147)	130 (120–145)	126.5 ± 21.1	124.7 ± 19.3	131	
Heart rate (bpm), mean ± SD or median (IQR)	76	78 (68–90)		73.2 ± 15.9	73.4 ± 14.7	57	
NYHA class ≥ III (%)	71.3		42.3	18.4	11.8	31.2	
Oedema	49			26.0			
eGFR (mL/min/1.73 m²), mean ± SD or median (IQR)	49	53.8 (38.5–69.9)			58.6 ± 22.1	62	
NT-proBNP (pg/mL), median (IQR)	3941 (2247–6760)	3931 (1933–8269)				2160 (938–4763)	
BNP (pg/mL)		898			164.5 (83.4, 310.7)		
CAD	56.5	69	66.9	41.8	52.9		68.95
Hypertensive heart disease	27.8		12.7	9.6	14.3		
Atrial fibrillation	39.6	49.9	25.6	22.3	43.5	58	41.76
Diabetes mellitus	39.8	50.2	28.6	30.5	36.1	27	50.16
Hypertension	82.4	81.9	56.2		89.8	64	82.18
Myocardial infarction	45.4	36.5	57.6		41.1	53 (CAD)	25.46 / 59.89 (CAD)
Chronic kidney disease	63.9			16.5			31.15
Anaemia	38					35	27.2
COPD	21.3	20.3		11.6		30	36.43

SD, standard deviation; BMI, body mass index; IQR, interquartile range; SBP, systolic blood pressure; NYHA, New York Heart Association; eGFR, estimated glomerular filtration rate; NT-proBNP, N-terminal pro-B-type natriuretic peptide; BNP, brain natriuretic peptide; HF, heart failure; CAD, coronary artery disease; COPD, chronic obstructive pulmonary disease.

8.8% in patients with HFrEF and 6.4% in patients with HFpEF. In HFmrEF patients, all-cause hospitalization and hospitalization for HF (HHF) were closer to HFpEF and significantly lower than in HFrEF. In all three LVEF categories, age, NYHA classes III and IV, and chronic kidney disease (CKD) were predictors of mortality.

In the Swedish registry, after multivariate adjustments, mortality was numerically higher in HFmrEF, compared to HFpEF, but this difference was not statistically significant. The presence of CAD, however, had an impact on prognosis in patients with HFmrEF. Patients with HFmrEF and CAD had a higher mortality rate at 1 and 3 years than those with HFpEF. In the absence of CAD, HFmrEF patients had a similar mortality rate to HFpEF patients. CKD, defined as an estimated glomerular filtration rate (eGFR) of $\leq 60\,\text{mL/min/1.73\,m}^2$, was a stronger predictor of death in HFrEF and HFmrEF patients than in HFpEF patients,[17] suggesting that the interaction between HF and CKD may be similar in HFrEF and HFmrEF, and may be different in HFpEF.

In the GWTG-HF registry, the median length of stay in patients hospitalized for HF was similar in the HFrEF, HFmrEF, and HFpEF groups.[8] In-hospital mortality was 3.1% in the overall population during the study, with a slightly higher unadjusted death rate in the HFrEF group (3.2%), compared to the population with HFmrEF (2.6%). In patients with HFmrEF, pneumonia was associated with longer hospital stay, whereas dietary and medication non-compliance was associated with reduced length of stay.

Another analysis of GWTG-HF[7] examined the relationship between EF and outcomes at 30 days and 1 year. Mortality in the total cohort was 8.8% at 30 days, and 36% at 1 year. Mortality at 1 year, after risk adjustment, was not significantly different between HFrEF, HFmrEF, and HFpEF patients. Those with HFpEF and HFmrEF had an increased risk of all-cause readmission, compared to patients with HFrEF. Conversely, the risk of cardiovascular (CV) and HF readmissions was higher in HFrEF and HFmrEF, compared to HFpEF.

In patients with hospitalization for HF, mortality at 5 years was 75% and remained similar across all LVEF groups.[18] Readmission rate by 5 years was 80.4% for the total cohort. Patients with HFrEF and HFmrEF maintained higher CV and HF readmission rates than those with HFpEF.[18]

Patients with HFmrEF enrolled in the CHARM Programme had a prognosis closer to that of patients with HFpEF, with a lower risk of HF and CV events than in HFrEF patients. In fact, the composite endpoint of CV death/HF hospitalization declined with increasing EF, up to an EF of 50%, and remained stable for higher EF. With respect to first HF hospitalization, first all-cause hospitalization, and recurrent HF hospitalization, the risk decreased with increasing LVEF up to an EF of around 40%.[10]

An age- and sex-matched analysis of the ASCEND trial[9] showed that 180-day mortality was lower in patients with HFmrEF than in those with HFrEF. When analysing the LVEF as a continuous variable, a U-shape mortality pattern was identified. After age and sex adjustments, the mortality rate above an LVEF of 35% was attenuated, but for EF <35%, the mortality risk increased as the EF declined.

Clearly, the picture emerging from multiple studies comparing the epidemiology of patients with HFrEF, HFmrEF, and HFpEF is not homogeneous. ● Table 6.2.2 summarizes the prevalence and prognosis of patients with HFmrEF. Despite this variability of results, HFmrEF patients show event rates that range from similar to rates in both HFrEF and HFpEF patients, to better than in those with HFrEF, resembling HFpEF. In patients with HFmrEF of ischaemic aetiology, the prognosis is worse than in those with HFpEF.

Transition from LVEF category

HF is an evolving condition and during the course of the disease, patients may transition in or out of the HFmrEF phenotype. On the one hand, evaluation of EF not only has significant inter- and intraobserver variability, but also varies with different modalities. Further, some physiological variables can temporarily influence the LVEF such as preload, systolic blood pressure, and heart rate.[19] All these may lead HFrEF patients to progress to the higher end of EF, and HFpEF patients to the lower end of EF, to be included in the HFmrEF group. This could, at least partially, explain the heterogeneity of HFmrEF patients in different studies.

On the other hand, it is now clear that patients may experience changes in LVEF over time as a result of disease progression/regression or therapy. In many patients with HFrEF, the LVEF can improve significantly such as in younger patients, women, those with no CAD, and those achieving higher doses of guideline-directed medical therapy (GDMT). These patients may thus leave the HFrEF range and enter the HFmrEF range. Conversely, in HFpEF patients, a deterioration in the LVEF may occur, especially in the presence of CAD,[20,21] moving these patients into the HFmrEF range. In the CHART-2 study, at 3-year follow-up, only 34% of patients initially with HFmrEF were still classified as having HFmrEF. From the original group of HFmrEF patients, around 45% had an improvement in EF and were in the HFpEF group, although some exhibited deterioration, with 21% of patients moving into the HFrEF group. An ischaemic aetiology was found to be independently associated with a decrease in LVEF from HFpEF to HFmrEF.[13] This finding can help explain the results in the Swedish registry where HFmrEF mortality was closer to that of HFpEF, except in the presence of CAD. Instead of a single evaluation of the LVEF at baseline, a longitudinal assessment of the LVEF, and taking into consideration other factors such as aetiology, is of utmost importance for assessing prognosis in patients with HFmrEF.

Treatment of HFmrEF

Treatment of risk factors, symptoms, and precipitants

In ● Transition from LVEF category (above), we discussed that HFmrEF appears to share the pathophysiology and clinical characteristics with both HFrEF and HFpEF.[11,15,17,22] Some risk factors such as hypertension and diabetes are common, regardless of the EF, and should be aggressively treated in HFmrEF as well. Similarly,

Table 6.2.2 Summary of studies describing the prevalence and prognosis of patients with HFmrEF

Study characteristics	Inclusion criteria	Number of patients	Prevalence of HFmrEF (%)	Outcomes, HFrEF	Outcomes, HFmrEF	Outcomes, HFpEF
Lund et al., 2018[10] TRIAL Follow-up of 38 months	Patients enrolled in CHARM Programme Chronic HF, outpatients	7598	17	All-cause mortality: 10.7 per 100 patient-years CV death/HHF: 15.9 per 100 patient-years HHF: 10.5 per 100 patient-years CV death: 8.9 per 100 patient-years	All-cause mortality: 5.4 per 100 patient-years CV death/HHF: 8.5 per 100 patient-years HHF: 6.0 per 100 patient-years CV death: 4.3 per 100 patient-years (non-significantly different from HFpEF)	All-cause mortality: 5.7 per 100 patient-years CV death/HHF:8.9 per 100 patient-years HHF: 6.6 per 100 patient-years CV death: 3.8 per 100 patient-years
Rickenbacher et al., 2017[12] TRIAL Follow-up of 794 days	TIME-CHF patients Chronic HF, outpatients	622	17	Survival free of all-cause hospitalization: 25% Survival free of HHF: 51% Overall survival: 62%	Mortality: 40% (no significant differences) Survival free of all-cause hospitalization: 19% Survival free of HHF: 44% Overall survival: 58% No significant differences between HFrEF, HFmrEF, and HFpEF	Survival free of all-cause hospitalization: 21% Survival free of HHF: 48% Overall survival: 61%
Toma et al., 2014[9] TRIAL Follow-up of 180 days	Inclusion criteria of ASCEND-HF trial with LVEF recorded (ADHF)	5687	12	Mortality at 180 days, sex- and age-matched analysis of 674 patients: 18% (HFrEF vs HFmrEF; P = 0.01)	After adjustment for baseline characteristics using the ASCEND-HF model, 30- and 180-day mortality was similar across LVEF groups Mortality at 180 days, sex- and age-matched analysis of 674 patients: 13%	
Chioncel et al., 2017[11] REGISTRY Follow-up of 1 year	ESC HF long-term registry Outpatients	9134	24	Mortality at 1 year: 8.8% All-cause death or HHF: 21% HHF: 15% All-cause hospitalization: 32%	Mortality at 1 year: 7.6% (not statistically significantly different from HFrEF or HFpEF) All-cause death or HHF: 15% HHF: 8.7% All-cause hospitalization: 22%	Mortality at 1 year: 6.3% All-cause death or HHF: 15% HHF: 9.7% All-cause hospitalization: 24%
Tsuji et al., 2017[13] REGISTRY Follow-up of 3 years	CHART-2 registry Outpatients	3480	17	1-year transition HFmrEF → HFrEF: 22% 3-year transition HFmrEF → HFrEF: 21%	Intermediate incidences of all-cause death, CV death, and HF admission (all P-values for trend <0.001) 1-year transition HFmrEF → HFpEF: 44%; HFmrEF → HFrEF: 16% 3-year transition HFmrEF → HFpEF: 45% HFmrEF → HFrEF: 21%	1-year transition HFpEF → HFmrEF: 8% 3-year transition HFpEF → HFmrEF: 8%
Koh et al., 2017[15] Follow-up of 3 years	Chronic Outpatients + at discharge after HHF	42,061	21	All-cause mortality: 146.55 per 1000 person-years	All-cause mortality: 140.65 per 1000 person-years HFmrEF and HFpEF had similar 1-year mortality (HR 1.08 (1.00–1.18); P = 0.052); and 3-year mortality (HR 1.06 (1.00–1.12); P=0.066) With CAD, mortality was higher in HFmrEF than in HFpEF at 1 year (HR 1.14 (1.02–1.28); P = 0.026) and at 3 years (HR 1.11 (1.02–1.21); P = 0.011), but not in the absence of CAD	All-cause mortality: 175.79 per 1000 person-years
Kapoor et al., 2016[8] Hospitalization	Patients hospitalized for HF GWTG-HF	99,825	13	In-hospital death: 3.2%	In-hospital death: 2.6% Factors associated with in-hospital death: WRF (OR 1.53, 95% CI 1.02–2.28); pneumonia (OR 1.48, 95% CI 1.05–2.10); medication non-compliance (OR 0.52, 95% CI 0.27–0.98) Factors associated with hospital stay of >4 days: pneumonia (OR 1.31, 95% CI 1.18–1.45); dyspnoea (OR 1.31, 95% CI 1.18–1.45); dietary non-compliance: (OR 0.672, 95% CI 0.75–0.99)	In-hospital death: 3.0%

HFmrEF, heart failure with mid-range ejection fraction; HFrEF, heart failure with reduced ejection fraction; HFpEF, heart failure with preserved ejection fraction; CV, cardiovascular; HHF, hospitalization for heart failure; HF, heart failure; ADHF, acutely decompensated heart failure; LVEF, left ventricular ejection fraction; CAD, coronary artery disease; GWTG-HF, Get With The Guidelines-Heart Failure; WRF, worsening renal function; OR, odds ratio; CI, confidence interval.

the HF syndrome is not defined by the EF, but rather by compensatory neurohormonal activation to restore or maintain cardiac output, leading to volume retention and elevated left ventricular filling pressures. Thus, diuretics and, in the acute setting, intravenous vasodilators (if blood pressure allows) are indicated for symptom relief in all patients with HF, irrespective of the LVEF. Finally, precipitants such as ischaemia and rapid atrial fibrillation should also be prevented and treated.

Evidence from observational studies and randomized controlled trials in HF, also including HFmrEF

No randomized clinical trial has been performed specifically in patients with HFmrEF. Several HFpEF trials used cut-offs of ≥40% or ≥45% and therefore partly included patients with HFmrEF. These trials were overall neutral (most importantly, CHARM-Preserved,[23] I-PRESERVE,[24] PEP-CHF,[25] TOPCAT,[26] and PARAGON-HF[27]). Thus, until recently, there was no evidence-based disease-modifying therapy to improve long-term outcomes in patients with HFmrEF or HFpEF. In recent years, it has become evident that sodium–glucose cotransporter 2 (SGLT2) inhibitors are effective in HFrEF patients, with and without diabetes. The first randomized controlled trial (RCT) data to support SGLT2 inhibitors in HFmrEF and HFpEF come from SOLOIST-WHF.[28] The combined SGLT2 and sodium–glucose cotransporter 1 (SGLT1) inhibitor sotagliflozin was superior to placebo in patients with diabetes and HF (across the entire EF spectrum) after a worsening HF episode (hazard ratio (HR) for the primary endpoint a composite of CV death and total HHF and urgent visits for HF 0.67 (0.52–0.85); P 0.001). In a prespecified subgroup analysis of EF <50% versus EF ≥50%, there was no treatment–EF interaction and HRs were similar in both groups,

suggesting sotagliflozin is effective in HFrEF/HFmrEF, as well as in HFpEF (➲ Figure 6.2.1). The SGLT2 inhibitors dapagliflozin and empagliflozin are currently being tested in HF patients with EF >40%, with and without diabetes. If these trials are positive, SGLT2 inhibitors may be the first firmly established therapy in HFrEF, HFmrEF, and HFpEF.

Several proven therapies for HFrEF, such as angiotensin-converting enzyme (ACE) inhibitors, angiotensin receptor blockers (ARBs), beta-blockers, and mineralocorticoid receptor antagonists, did not clearly show beneficial outcomes in patients with HFpEF. However, modest potential benefits were observed in studies that included patients with an LVEF of >40%.[29,30] The first analyses of randomized data were post hoc analyses from RCTs that included patients with an LVEF of 40% and higher. In CHARM-Overall (candesartan vs placebo in HF across the EF spectrum), candesartan was overall effective and there was no interaction with EF.[31] In CHARM-Preserved (HF with EF >40%), a covariate-adjusted analysis suggested that candesartan was effective (HR for the primary composite outcome 0.86, 95% confidence interval (CI) 0.74–1.0; P = 0.051),[23] and when all cumulative, rather than only the first, HHFs were counted, the benefit was statistically significant (rate ratio for total HHFs 0.75 (0.62–0.91); P = 0.003).[32] In PEP-CHF (HF and an echocardiogram suggesting diastolic dysfunction and excluding substantial left ventricular systolic dysfunction or valve disease), perindopril appeared effective at 1 year, but there was extensive crossover and the trial was ultimately neutral.[25] In I-PRESERVE (HF with EF ≥45%; irbesartan vs placebo), covariate-adjusted analyses suggested potential efficacy.[24] Finally, in TOPCAT (HF with EF ≥45%; spironolactone vs placebo), spironolactone appeared effective when the North and South America strata were analysed separately (HR for the primary outcome

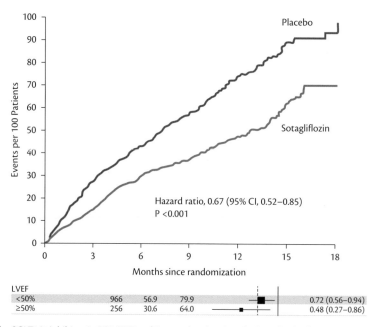

Figure 6.2.1 Main outcomes of the SGLT1/2 inhibitor in SOLOIST and Forest plot showing the beneficial effects in both patients with HFpEF and those with HFrEF.

Reproduced from Bhatt DL, Szarek M, Steg PG, *et al.*; SOLOIST-WHF Trial Investigators. Sotagliflozin in Patients with Diabetes and Recent Worsening Heart Failure. *N Engl J Med.* 2021 Jan 14;384(2):117–128. doi: 10.1056/NEJMoa2030183. with permission from Massachusettes Medical Society.

0.82 (0.69–0.98); $P=0.026$,[26] and when the stratum of patients included was based on natriuretic peptide levels (confirming the presence of HF) (HR 0.65 (0.49–0.87); $P<0.01$), rather than when the stratum of patients with a history of HF hospitalization (which is less reliable) was analysed separately.[33]

Post hoc efficacy data from subgroup analyses of randomized controlled trials

After the HFmrEF category was proposed in the 2016 ESC HF guidelines[6] and clinical characterization (discussed above) suggested that HFmrEF has much in common with HFrEF, several sub-analyses and meta-analyses specifically on patients with HFmrEF were performed. These suggested that some drugs that are effective in HFrEF may be effective also in HFmrEF (but generally not in HFpEF). Indeed, the EF cut-off of 30%, 35%, or 40% used in most of the HFrEF trials over the last generation was arbitrary and not selected for any pathophysiological reason, but to enrich for risk and events.

Treatment effect with ejection fraction as continuous splines

Assessing the effect of therapy in HFmrEF by EF analysed as a continuous spline variable recognizes the continuous nature of the EF and the arbitrariness of distinct cut-offs. ➲ Figure 6.2.2 shows the treatment effect on primary outcomes by EF splines in the CHARM Programme,[31] TOPCAT,[26] DIG,[34] and PARADIGM-HF/PARAGON-HF combined.[35] These show the treatment effect (HR or incidence rate ratio) with 95% CIs in relation to the EF on a continuous scale. The CHARM Programme suggested that candesartan significantly reduced the composite of CV death and first HF hospitalization and first and recurrent HF hospitalization to an EF of well above 50%.[36] TOPCAT suggested that spironolactone significantly reduced the primary composite outcome of CV death, HF hospitalization, or aborted cardiac arrest, as well as HF hospitalization alone again to an EF of well above 50%.[37] In the DIG trial of patients with HF in sinus rhythm, overall, digoxin did not affect mortality, but there was a trend towards a reduction in death from HF and a significant reduction in HHF.[38] In spline analyses, the effect was less clear-cut than in CHARM and TOPCAT, but digoxin appeared to significantly reduce the composite of CV death or HF hospitalization in the EF range of 40–50%.[34]

Finally, in the PARAGON-HF (Prospective Comparison of Angiotensin Receptor Neprilysin Inhibitor With Angiotensin Receptor Blocker Global Outcomes in Heart Failure and Preserved Left Ventricular Ejection Fraction) trial,[27] the prespecified subgroup analysis by EF showed that patients with

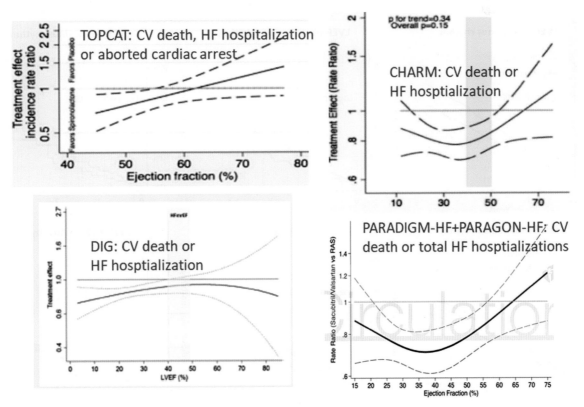

Figure 6.2.2 Treatment effect on the primary outcomes by EF splines in the CHARM Programme,[31] TOPCAT,[26] DIG,[34] and PARADIGM-HF/PARAGON-HF combined.

Reproduced from Pfeffer MA, Swedberg K, Granger CB, et al.; CHARM Investigators and Committees. Effects of candesartan on mortality and morbidity in patients with chronic heart failure: the CHARM-Overall programme. Lancet. 2003 Sep 6;362(9386):759–66. doi: 10.1016/s0140-6736(03)14282-1 with permission from Elsevier. Pitt B, Pfeffer MA, Assmann SF, et al.; TOPCAT Investigators. Spironolactone for heart failure with preserved ejection fraction. N Engl J Med. 2014 Apr 10;370(15):1383–92. doi: 10.1056/NEJMoa1313731. Reproduced from Abdul-Rahim AH, Shen L, Rush CJ, et al.; VICCTA-Heart Failure Collaborators. Effect of digoxin in patients with heart failure and mid-range (borderline) left ventricular ejection fraction. Eur J Heart Fail. 2018 Jul;20(7):1139–1145. doi: 10.1002/ejhf.1160 with permission from John Wiley and Sons.

an EF of below the median of 57% appeared to benefit from sacubitril/valsartan (vs valsartan) in terms of reduction in the primary composite outcome of CV death and total HHFs, whereas there was essentially no effect in those with an EF of >57%—a significant EF-by-treatment interaction. Taken in the context of the PARADIGM-HF (Prospective Comparison of ARNI With ACEI to Determine Impact on Global Mortality and Morbidity in Heart Failure) trial showing robust reductions in the primary composite endpoint of CV death or first HHF by 20% with sacubitril/valsartan (vs enalapril) in patients with an EF of ≤40%, patients with an EF in the mid range of 40–50% may also benefit from sacubitril/valsartan, compared to renin–angiotensin–aldosterone system inhibitors without neprilysin inhibition.[35]

Treatment effect with ejection fraction as a distinct HFmrEF category

Assessing the effect of therapy in HFmrEF by EF categories may be more clinically palatable and allows for establishing treatment criteria. ➲ Figure 6.2.3 shows a distinct effect of candesartan on the composite of CV death or HF hospitalization,[36] and of beta-blockers (in sinus rhythm) on all-cause mortality and CV mortality[39] (unfortunately, the beta-blocker analyses did not include HF hospitalization). In DIG, there was no distinct difference in effect in HFmrEF versus in HFpEF.[34] ➲ Table 6.2.3 provides comprehensive data on potential treatment effect specifically in HFmrEF (with effect in HFrEF and HFpEF provided for comparison) from primary, post hoc, and subgroup analyses from

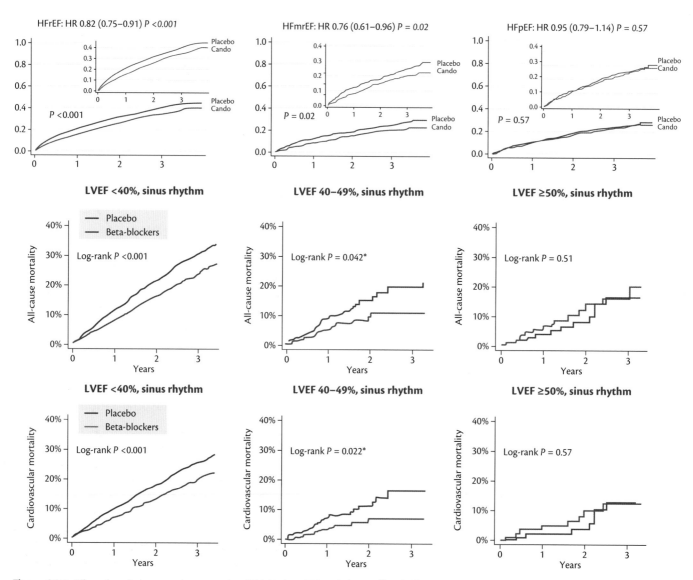

Figure 6.2.3 Effect of candesartan on the composite of CV death or HF hospitalization,[36] and of beta-blockers (in sinus rhythm) on all-cause mortality and CV mortality.[39]

Reproduced from Lund LH, Claggett B, Liu J, et al. Heart failure with mid-range ejection fraction in CHARM: characteristics, outcomes and effect of candesartan across the entire ejection fraction spectrum. *Eur J Heart Fail*. 2018 Aug;20(8):1230–1239. doi: 10.1002/ejhf.1149 with permission from John Wiley and Sons. Reproduced from Cleland JGF, Bunting KV, Flather MD, et al.; Beta-blockers in Heart Failure Collaborative Group. Beta-blockers for heart failure with reduced, mid-range, and preserved ejection fraction: an individual patient-level analysis of double-blind randomized trials. *Eur Heart J*. 2018 Jan 1;39(1):26–35. doi: 10.1093/eurheartj/ehx564 with permission from Oxford University Press.

Table 6.2.3 Post hoc or subgroup analyses*

EF group	Endpoint	HR or RR (95% CI)
CHARM Programme: HF across the EF spectrum (PMID: 29431256)		
<40%	CV death or HHF	0.82 (0.75–0.91)
40–49%		0.76 (0.61–0.96)
≥50%		0.95 (0.79–1.14)
<40%	Recurrent HHF	0.68 (0.58–0.80)
40–49%		0.48 (0.33–0.70)
≥50%		0.78 (0.59–1.03)
Beta-blockers in Heart Failure Collaborative Group: meta-analysis of beta-blocker RCTs (showing sinus rhythm) (PMID: 29040525)		
<40%	All-cause mortality	0.67–0.76 (0.50–0.65 to 0.83–0.90)
40–49%		0.59 (0.34–1.03)
≥50%		1.79 (0.78–4.10)
<40%	CV death	0.67–0.78 (0.52–0.65 to 0.80–0.99)
40–49%		0.48 (0.24–0.97)
≥50%		1.77 (0.61–5.14)
<40%	Composite CV death or CV hospitalization	0.68–0.80 (0.60–0.72 to 0.77–0.88)
40–49%		0.83 (0.60–1.13)
≥50%		0.66 (0.38–1.15)
DIG trial post hoc analysis across the EF spectrum (PMID: 29493058)		
<40%	CV death or HHF	0.83 (0.77–0.89)
40–49%		0.96 (0.79–1.17)
≥50%		0.92 (0.71–1.20)
<40%	HF death or HHF	0.74 (0.68–0.81)
40–49%		0.83 (0.66–1.05)
≥50%		0.88 (0.65–1.19)
PARADIGM-HF + PARAGON-HF analysis across the EF spectrum (PMID: 31736342)		
≤42.5%	CV death or first HHF	HR 0.77–0.81 (0.63–0.71 to 0.92–0.94)
>42.5–52.5		0.89 (0.73–1.10)
>52.5		0.89–1.03 (0.74–0.80 to 1.06–1.32)
≤42.5%	Total HHF	0.75–0.82 (0.60–0.63 to 0.90–1.11)
>42.5–52.5		0.77 (0.58–1.02)
>52.5		0.81–1.04 (0.63–0.76 to 1.05–1.44)

* This table shows EF groups, endpoints, and treatment effect for the respective endpoints in the respective EF groups. Only selected endpoints are shown. In the beta-blocker collaborative and combined PARADIGM-HF/PARAGON-HF, the HFrEF, HFmrEF, and/or HFpEF groups were further subdivided into smaller EF increments. For these, the treatment effect column shows the range for the HRs/RRs and the range for the 95% CIs for these EF groups.
HR, hazard ratio; CI, confidence interval; HF, heart failure; EF, ejection fraction; CV, cardiovascular; HHF, hospitalization for heart failure; RCT, randomized controlled trial.

HFpEF trials and HF programmes and meta-analyses across the EF spectrum.

Caution in interpretation of post hoc and subgroup analyses

Subgroups are intended to assess consistency across multiple patient phenotypes, rather than to identify potential unique responders. Furthermore, even if prespecified, findings in subgroups may occur by chance and they should be interpreted with caution and not used to guide therapy. Nevertheless, in certain situations, a subgroup finding, if properly interpreted and taken together with other evidence, may provide sufficient evidence for treatment recommendations of modest grade and level of evidence. The subgroup with EF below the median in PARAGON-HF was large (including half of the patients in the trial); the test for interaction was statistically significant; it was internally consistent with adjacent subgroups, that is, across PARADIGM-HF and PARAGON-HF together, the efficacy of sacubitril/valsartan was progressively greater as the EF declined.[35] Furthermore, as discussed above, the results were externally consistent with results from the post hoc analyses in HFmrEF from the trials discussed above. Finally, since HFmrEF in many ways clinically and pathophysiologically resembles HFrEF, but not HFpEF, an effect of sacubitril/valsartan in HFmrEF is also biologically plausible.

Summary of treatment recommendations in HFmrEF

The above data are not fully consistent and should be interpreted with caution. Nevertheless, taken together, these data suggest that ARBs, spironolactone, beta-blockers (in sinus rhythm), sacubitril/valsartan, and SGLT2 inhibitors, as well as potentially also digoxin, are effective in HFmrEF. Thus, prior HF trials may have used too low a cut-off of EF to define 'reduced' EF and a recent consensus statement of the Heart Failure Association of the ESC suggested that mineralocorticoid receptor antagonists, ARBs, and beta-blockers may be considered in patients with HFmrEF. A similar recommendation for these therapies was provided in the 2021 ESC HF Guidelines.[7] In addition, the recent results of EMPEROR-preserved provide compelling evidence for a beneficial effect of the SGLT2 inhibitor empagliflozin to reduce CV mortality or HF hospitalization in patients with HFmrEF.[40]

Sex differences and implications of renaming as 'heart failure with mildly reduced ejection fraction'

The observation that patients with HFmrEF may benefit from mineralocorticoid receptor antagonists,[37] ARBs,[36] beta-blockers,[39] and digoxin,[34] in sharp distinction from patients defined as HFpEF according to the 2016 ESC HF Guidelines (LVEF ≥50%) and more similar to patients with EF <40%, has led to questioning of the EF cut-off with which we define 'mid-range' or 'mildly reduced' EF. Since EF is a continuous variable with a normal distribution within the population, the cut-off value to define 'normal' versus 'reduced' EF is arbitrary. In guidelines from the American Society of Echocardiography and the European Society of Echocardiography, a normal EF is defined as >55%. Population-based data support this threshold to define 'normal' EF. In the Framingham Heart Study, participants with an EF of 50–55% were at greater risk of HF and death, compared to those with an EF of >55%. More recently, in a large US regional healthcare system, the relationship between clinically assessed EF and survival was found to be u-shaped, with a nadir of risk at an LVEF of 60–65%.[41] Similar relationships were observed in a large validation data set from New Zealand when restricted to patients reported to have HF, as well as after adjustments for conditions associated with an elevated EF such as mitral regurgitation.[41] This suggests that the 'sweet spot' to define normal versus reduced EF may be 60%—notably higher than in prior definitions used in

HF—and also highlights that it is not only reduced EF that is a problem, but too high an EF may also be harmful.[42]

Importantly, the 'normal' distribution of EF increases with age and is higher in women than in men in the general population.[43] This makes sense when considering that the EF is a fraction which increases as the heart remodels with age, with shrinkage of left ventricular end-diastolic volume (denominator) being greater than reduction in stroke volume (numerator). Thus, a common EF cut-off for 'normal' of 50%, regardless of age or sex, would end up including elderly women who actually have relatively reduced EF for their age and sex. Such sex differences may explain the observation in the PARAMOUNT (Prospective comparison of ARNi with ARB on Management Of heart failUre with preserved ejectioN fracTion) trial where subtle left ventricular systolic dysfunction was more apparent in women than in men with HFpEF.[44] Furthermore, in combined analyses of PARAGON-HF and PARADIGM-HF data, sex-specific treatment effect splines across the entire EF spectrum showed efficacy of sacubitril/valsartan in the EF range of 40–50% in both sexes, with the upper 95% CI boundary of the rate ratio for sacubitril/valsartan versus the comparator renin–angiotensin blockade remaining below 1.0 (indicating benefit with sacubitril/valsartan) up to higher EFs in women, compared to men.[45] When such sex–EF interaction analyses were extended in pooled patient-level data analyses from trials of ARBs and mineralocorticoid receptor antagonists across the entire EF spectrum of HF,[46] similar patterns were observed (➲ Figure 6.2.4). Treatment with neurohormonal blockade was found to be beneficial beyond the upper limit of EF eligibility used in contemporary HFrEF clinical trials (40%), with benefit extending to the EF range of 40–50%. Of note, the benefit of each treatment seemed to extend to higher EFs in women, compared to men (➲ Figure 6.2.4).

How may these data inform our EF classification or nomenclature in HF? More straightforward and easy to implement may be to lump HFmrEF under 'reduced' EF (using a cut-off of, say, <50%), thus simplifying the classification into two, instead of three, categories. However, combining patients with 'mid-range' or 'mildly reduced' and more severely reduced EF into one group would fail to acknowledge the limited strength of trial evidence in HFmrEF versus those with lower EFs. On the other hand, naming patients with EF below 50% (or 55%) under the common term 'reduced', while still making a distinction between 'mildly reduced' versus more severely reduced EF, would recognize the smaller relative and absolute benefits of neurohormonal antagonists, as well as the lower strength of supporting evidence, in HFmrEF compared to HF with EF <40%. Therefore, the task force of the 2021 ESC HF Guidelines have decided to rename 'heart failure with mid-range ejection fraction' to 'heart failure with mildly reduced ejection fraction'.[7]

There are several important clinical implications of the new nomenclature 'heart failure with mildly reduced ejection fraction'. The inclusion of the term 'reduced' in 'mildly reduced' would signal clinicians to consider treating these patients with neurohormonal agents known to be beneficial in patients with

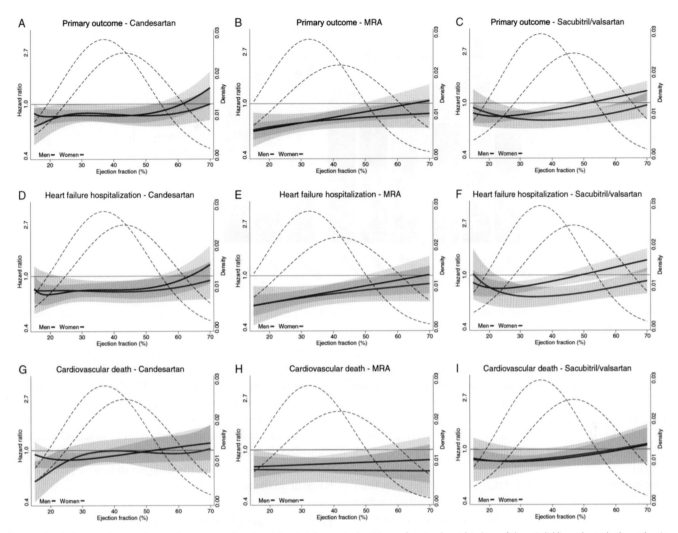

Figure 6.2.4 Sex-specific association of treatment effect (*y*-axis) with left ventricular ejection fraction (*x*-axis) in heart failure. Solid lines show the hazard ratio for the primary composite outcome (A–C) and its components (D–I), according to treatment group in the CHARM Programme for candesartan versus placebo (A, D, G); RALES, EMPHASIS-HF, and TOPCAT (Americas) for mineralocorticoid receptor antagonist (MRA) versus placebo (B, E, H); and PARADIGM-HF and PARAGON-HF for sacubitril/valsartan versus renin–angiotensin–aldosterone system inhibitor (C, F, I); in men (blue) and women (red). Dotted curves show the normalized distribution of the ejection fraction in men (blue) and women (red). Shaded areas represent the 95% confidence intervals.
Reproduced from Dewan P, Jackson A, Lam CSP, *et al.* Interactions between left ventricular ejection fraction, sex and effect of neurohumoral modulators in heart failure. *Eur J Heart Fail.* 2020 May;22(5):898–901. doi: 10.1002/ejhf.1776 with permission from John Wiley and Sons.

HF and more severely reduced EF. This approach gives the patient the benefit of the doubt, reducing the risk of patients with mildly reduced EF, especially women, being possibly deprived of potentially beneficial therapies. While enlarging the treatment population, the reclassification accordingly reduces the population of HF with higher EFs, for which we still have no evidence of treatment outcome benefits—those with EF ≥50% or 55% in men and ≥55 or 60% in women who may be aptly renamed 'heart failure with normal EF'. In recognizing the known imprecision and variability of EF measurements by current clinical methods,[47,48,49] the new nomenclature also reminds clinicians to pay attention to measurements in the borderline EF zone of 40–50%. Attempts should be made to obtain as precise a measurement of EF as possible, to avoid misclassification. Finally, these considerations are expected to impact future HF clinical trial designs, whereby trials targeting 'reduced' EF may enrol patients with up to a higher EF cut-off than in prior trials.

Summary and future perspectives

The introduction of HFmrEF in the 2016 ESC HF Guidelines resulted in a tremendous increase in our knowledge on this 'middle child'. A large number of studies have been published on the characteristics, clinical outcome, and potential treatment of these patients. What are the main lessons that we have learnt? First, approximately one out of five patients has HFmrEF. Second, the clinical characteristics are often in between those of HFrEF and HFpEF. However, an ischaemic aetiology is present more often in HFmrEF than in HFpEF, and is very similar to HFrEF (⊃ Figure 6.2.5).

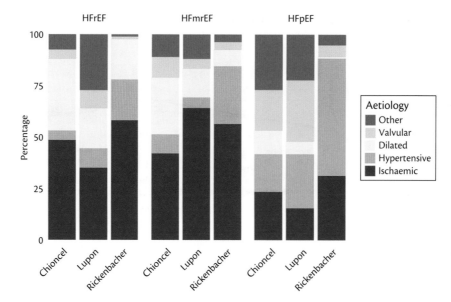

Figure 6.2.5 Hypertensive and ischaemic aetiologies for heart failure with reduced (HFrEF), mildly reduced (HFmrEF), and preserved (HFpEF) ejection fraction in four recent studies.

Patients with HFrEF and HFmrEF more often have ischaemic heart disease and idiopathic dilated cardiomyopathy, whereas hypertensive heart disease and valvular heart disease are more common aetiologies in HFpEF. Clinical outcome of patients with HFmrEF is slightly better than those with HFrEF, especially when corrected for the higher mean age in patients with HFmrEF.

Importantly, it should be noted that LVEF changes over time. In patients with new-onset HFrEF, and especially those with a non-ischaemic aetiology, LVEF often improves after treatment and patients shift from HFrEF to HFmrEF or even HFpEF. Conversely, some patients deteriorate from HFpEF to HFmrEF or HFrEF. Several studies have shown that improvement in LVEF is related to a better prognosis and deterioration of LVEF is related to a worse prognosis. Also, measurement of LVEF is often not very precise and sometimes a range of 5–10 is used. Taken together, these observations question whether HFmrEF should be considered as a separate entity at all. While there are valid arguments for not considering HFmrEF as a separate category, there is one important finding supported by several studies that is in favour of considering HFmrEF as a separate entity. Treatments that have been shown to improve clinical outcome in patients with HFrEF, such as ARBs, beta-blockers, and mineralocorticoid receptor antagonists, also seem to benefit patients with HFmrEF, but not those with HFpEF. This suggests that the pathophysiology behind HFmrEF is more similar to HFrEF than to HFpEF, which was confirmed in observational studies where an ischaemic aetiology of HF was more often present in patients with HFmrEF than in those with HFpEF. So, instead of adding HFmrEF as a separate category of patients, one might also question whether an LVEF of 40% is the right cut-off to identify patients with HFrEF. Maybe a better cut-off for HFrEF should be <50%. The downside to this is that the identification of the cut-off of 35–40% for HFrEF is driven by the trial enrolment criteria. But probably any EF below 50% (and maybe below 55% for women) might be considered as HFrEF also. That is why we have proposed to rename 'heart failure with mid-range ejection fraction' to 'heart failure with mildly reduced ejection fraction' to emphasize this similarity with HFrEF. Practical considerations and clinical consequences of categorizing or grouping patients will ultimately drive the decision of how to proceed with HFmrEF in the future.

Summary and key messages

- The introduction of HFmrEF in the 2016 ESC HF Guidelines resulted in a tremendous increase in our knowledge on patients with HF and an LVEF of between 40% and 50%.

- Patients with HFmrEF more often have an ischaemic aetiology, compared to patients with HFpEF.

- Post hoc data suggest that ARBs, spironolactone, beta-blockers (in sinus rhythm), sacubitril/valsartan, and SGLT2 inhibitors are effective not only in HFrEF patients, but also in those with HFmrEF.

- Since an ischaemic aetiology and response to therapy in patients with HFmrEF more closely resemble HFrEF, the 2021 ESC HF Guidelines task force decided to rename 'heart failure with mid-range ejection fraction' to 'heart failure with mildly reduced ejection fraction'.

- ACE inhibitors, ARBs, sacubitril/valsartan, mineralocorticoid receptor antagonists, and beta-blockers have now received a class IIb (level of evidence C) recommendation for the treatment of patients with HFmrEF.

References

1. Shah PM, Pai RG. Diastolic heart failure. Curr Probl Cardiol. 1992;17:781–868.

2. Dickstein K, Cohen-Solal A, Filippatos G, et al.; ESC Committee for Practice Guidelines (CPG). ESC Guidelines for the diagnosis and treatment of acute and chronic heart failure 2008: the Task Force for the Diagnosis and Treatment of Acute and Chronic Heart Failure 2008 of the European Society of Cardiology. Developed in collaboration with the Heart Failure Association of the ESC (HFA) and endorsed by the European Society of Intensive Care Medicine (ESICM). Eur Heart J. 2008;29:2388–442.

3. McMurray JJ, Adamopoulos S, Anker SD, et al.; ESC Committee for Practice Guidelines. ESC Guidelines for the diagnosis and treatment of acute and chronic heart failure 2012: The Task Force for the Diagnosis and Treatment of Acute and Chronic Heart Failure 2012 of the European Society of Cardiology. Developed in collaboration with the Heart Failure Association (HFA) of the ESC. Eur Heart J. 2012;33:1787–847.

4. Yancy CW, Jessup M, Bozkurt B, et al.; American College of Cardiology Foundation; American Heart Association Task Force on Practice Guidelines. 2013 ACCF/AHA guideline for the management of heart failure: a report of the American College of Cardiology Foundation/American Heart Association Task Force on Practice Guidelines. J Am Coll Cardiol. 2013;15:e147–239.

5. Lam CS, Solomon SD. The middle child in heart failure: heart failure with mid-range ejection fraction (40–50%). Eur J Heart Fail. 2014;16:1049–55.

6. Ponikowski P, Voors AA, Anker SD, et al.; ESC Scientific Document Group. 2016 ESC Guidelines for the diagnosis and treatment of acute and chronic heart failure: the Task Force for the diagnosis and treatment of acute and chronic heart failure of the European Society of Cardiology (ESC) Developed with the special contribution of the Heart Failure Association (HFA) of the ESC. Eur Heart J. 2016;37:2129–200.

7. McDonagh TA, Metra M, Adamo M, et al.; ESC Scientific Document Group. 2021 ESC Guidelines for the diagnosis and treatment of acute and chronic heart failure. Eur Heart J. 2021;42:3599–726.

8. Kapoor JR, Kapoor R, Ju C, et al. Precipitating clinical factors, heart failure characterization, and outcomes in patients hospitalized with heart failure with reduced, borderline, and preserved ejection fraction. JACC Heart Fail. 2016;4:464–72.

9. Toma M, Ezekowitz JA, Bakal JA, et al. The relationship between left ventricular ejection fraction and mortality in patients with acute heart failure: insights from the ASCEND-HF Trial. Eur J Heart Fail. 2014;16:334–41.

10. Lund LH, Claggett B, Liu J, et al. Heart failure with mid-range ejection fraction in CHARM: characteristics, outcomes and effect of candesartan across the entire ejection fraction spectrum. Eur J Heart Fail. 2018;20:1230–9.

11. Chioncel O, Lainscak M, Seferovic PM, et al. Epidemiology and one-year outcomes in patients with chronic heart failure and preserved, mid-range and reduced ejection fraction: an analysis of the ESC Heart Failure Long-Term Registry. Eur J Heart Fail. 2017;19:1574–85.

12. Rickenbacher P, Kaufmann BA, Maeder MT, et al.; TIME-CHF Investigators. Heart failure with mid-range ejection fraction: a distinct clinical entity? Insights from the Trial of Intensified versus standard Medical therapy in Elderly patients with Congestive Heart Failure (TIME-CHF). Eur J Heart Fail. 2017;19:1586–96.

13. Tsuji K, Sakata Y, Nochioka K, et al.; CHART-2 Investigators. Characterization of heart failure patients with mid-range left ventricular ejection fraction: a report from the CHART-2 Study. Eur J Heart Fail. 2017;19:1258–69.

14. Steinberg BA, Zhao X, Heidenreich PA, et al.; Get With the Guidelines Scientific Advisory Committee and Investigators. Trends in patients hospitalized with heart failure and preserved left ventricular ejection fraction: prevalence, therapies, and outcomes. Circulation. 2012;126:65–75.

15. Koh AS, Tay WT, Teng THK, et al. A comprehensive population-based characterization of heart failure with mid-range ejection fraction. Eur J Heart Fail. 2017;19:1624–34.

16. Lauritsen J, Gustafsson F, Abdulla J. Characteristics and long-term prognosis of patients with heart failure and mid-range ejection fraction compared with reduced and preserved ejection fraction: a systematic review and meta-analysis. ESC Heart Fail. 2018;5:685–94.

17. Löfman I, Szummer K, Dahlström U, Jernberg T, Lund LH. Associations with and prognostic impact of chronic kidney disease in heart failure with preserved, mid-range, and reduced ejection fraction. Eur J Heart Fail. 2017;19:1606–14.

18. Shah KS, Xu H, Matsouaka RA, et al. Heart failure with preserved, borderline, and reduced ejection fraction: 5-year outcomes. J Am Coll Cardiol. 2017;70:2476–86.

19. Marwick TH. Ejection fraction pros and cons: JACC state-of-the-art review. J Am Coll Cardiol. 2018;72:2360–79.

20. Dunlay SM, Roger VL, Weston SA, Jiang R, Redfield MM. Longitudinal changes in ejection fraction in heart failure patients with preserved and reduced ejection fraction. Circ Heart Fail. 2012;5:720–6.

21. Savarese G, Vedin O, D'Amario D, et al. Prevalence and prognostic implications of longitudinal ejection fraction change in heart failure. JACC Heart Fail. 2019;7:306–17.

22. Vedin O, Lam CSP, Koh AS, et al. Significance of ischemic heart disease in patients with heart failure and preserved, midrange, and reduced ejection fraction: a nationwide cohort study. Circ Heart Fail. 2017;10:e003875.

23. Yusuf S, Pfeffer MA, Swedberg K, et al.; CHARM Investigators and Committees. Effects of candesartan in patients with chronic heart failure and preserved left-ventricular ejection fraction: the CHARM-Preserved Trial. Lancet. 2003;362:777–81.

24. Massie BM, Carson PE, McMurray JJ, et al.; I-PRESERVE Investigators. Irbesartan in patients with heart failure and preserved ejection fraction. N Engl J Med. 2008;359:2456–67.

25. Cleland JG, Tendera M, Adamus J, Freemantle N, Polonski L, Taylor J; PEP-CHF Investigators. The perindopril in elderly people with chronic heart failure (PEP-CHF) study. Eur Heart J. 2006;27:2338–45.

26. Pitt B, Pfeffer MA, Assmann SF, et al.; TOPCAT Investigators. Spironolactone for heart failure with preserved ejection fraction. N Engl J Med. 2014;370:1383–92.

27. Solomon SD, McMurray JJV, Anand IS, et al.; PARAGON-HF Investigators and Committees. Angiotensin–neprilysin inhibition in heart failure with preserved ejection fraction. N Engl J Med. 2019;381:1609–20.

28. Bhatt DL, Szarek M, Steg PG, et al.; SOLOIST-WHF Trial Investigators. Sotagliflozin in patients with diabetes and recent worsening heart failure. N Engl J Med. 2021;384:117–28.

29. Lund LH, Benson L, Dahlström U, Edner M, Friberg L. Association between use of β-blockers and outcomes in patients with heart failure and preserved ejection fraction. JAMA. 2014;312:2008–18.

30. Lund LH, Benson L, Dahlström U, Edner M. Association between use of renin–angiotensin system antagonists and mortality in patients with heart failure and preserved ejection fraction. JAMA. 2012;308:2108–17.

31. Pfeffer MA, Swedberg K, Granger CB, et al.; CHARM Investigators and Committees. Effects of candesartan on mortality and morbidity in patients with chronic heart failure: the CHARM-Overall programme. Lancet. 2003;362:759–66.

32. Rogers JK, Pocock SJ, McMurray JJ, *et al*. Analysing recurrent hospitalizations in heart failure: a review of statistical methodology, with application to CHARM-Preserved. Eur J Heart Fail. 2014;16:33–40.

33. Girerd N, Ferreira JP, Rossignol P, Zannad F. A tentative interpretation of the TOPCAT trial based on randomized evidence from the brain natriuretic peptide stratum analysis. Eur J Heart Fail. 2016;18:1411–14.

34. Abdul-Rahim AH, Shen L, Rush CJ, *et al*.; VICCTA-Heart Failure Collaborators. Effect of digoxin in patients with heart failure and mid-range (borderline) left ventricular ejection fraction. Eur J Heart Fail. 2018;20:1139–45.

35. Solomon SD, Vaduganathan M, Claggett BL, *et al*. Sacubitril/valsartan across the spectrum of ejection fraction in heart failure. Circulation. 2020;141:352–61.

36. Lund LH, Claggett B, Liu J, *et al*. Heart failure with mid-range ejection fraction in CHARM: characteristics, outcomes and effect of candesartan across the entire ejection fraction spectrum. Eur J Heart Fail. 2018;20:1230–9.

37. Solomon SD, Claggett B, Lewis EF, *et al*.; TOPCAT Investigators. Influence of ejection fraction on outcomes and efficacy of spironolactone in patients with heart failure with preserved ejection fraction. Eur Heart J. 2016;37:455–62.

38. Digitalis Investigation Group. The effect of digoxin on mortality and morbidity in patients with heart failure. N Engl J Med. 1997;336:525–33.

39. Cleland JGF, Bunting KV, Flather MD, *et al*.; Beta-blockers in Heart Failure Collaborative Group. Beta-blockers for heart failure with reduced, mid-range, and preserved ejection fraction: an individual patient-level analysis of double-blind randomized trials. Eur Heart J. 2018;39:26–35.

40. Anker SD, Butler J, Filippatos G, *et al*.; EMPEROR-Preserved Trial Investigators. Empagliflozin in heart failure with a preserved ejection fraction. N Engl J Med. 2021;385:1451–61.

41. Wehner GJ, Jing L, Haggerty CM, *et al*. Routinely reported ejection fraction and mortality in clinical practice: where does the nadir of risk lie? Eur Heart J. 2020;41:1249–57.

42. Luscher TF. Lumpers and splitters: the bumpy road to precision medicine. Eur Heart J. 2019;40:3292–6.

43. Echocardiographic Normal Ranges Meta-Analysis of the Left Heart Collaboration. Ethnic-specific normative reference values for echocardiographic LA and LV size, LV mass, and systolic function: the EchoNoRMAL Study. JACC Cardiovasc Imaging. 2015;8:656–65.

44. Gori M, Lam CS, Gupta DK, *et al*. Sex-specific cardiovascular structure and function in heart failure with preserved ejection fraction. Eur J Heart Fail. 2014;16:535–42.

45. McMurray JJV, Jackson AM, Lam CSP, *et al*. Effects of sacubitril-valsartan versus valsartan in women compared with men with heart failure and preserved ejection fraction: insights from PARAGON-HF. Circulation. 2020;141:338–51.

46. Dewan P, Jackson A, Lam CSP, *et al*. Interactions between left ventricular ejection fraction, sex and effect of neurohumoral modulators in heart failure. Eur J Heart Fail. 2020;22:898–901.

47. Campbell RT, Petrie MC, McMurray JJV. Redefining heart failure phenotypes based on ejection fraction. Eur J Heart Fail. 2018;20:1634–5.

48. McGowan JH, Cleland JG. Reliability of reporting left ventricular systolic function by echocardiography: a systematic review of 3 methods. Am Heart J. 2003;146:388–97.

49. Lam CS, Solomon SD. Fussing over the middle child: heart failure with mid-range ejection fraction. Circulation. 2017;135:1279–80.

CHAPTER 6.3

Heart failure with preserved ejection fraction

Rudolf A de Boer, Burkert Pieske, and
Barry A Borlaug

Contents

Introduction

Heart failure (HF) is a clinical syndrome characterized by signs such as dyspnoea, exertional dyspnoea, and orthopnoea, and by symptoms such as oedema and fluid retention. HF is not a diagnosis, but rather a consequence of one or more aetiological factors such as myocardial infarction, valvular heart disease, and hypertension. As a consequence, changes in the myocardial tissue occur, with functional consequences. Left ventricular ejection fraction (LVEF) is a measure of myocardial performance and since has long been used to define HF. Although heavily disputed, almost all diagnostic and therapeutic algorithms for HF lean heavily on LVEF, and the current European Society of Cardiology (ESC) (and American College of Cardiology (ACC)/American Heart Association (AHA)) guidelines define HF with reduced, mildly reduced, and preserved ejection fraction (generally referred to as HFrEF, HFmrEF, and HFpEF, as HF with LVEF ≤40%, 41–49%, and ≥50%, respectively).[1]

Strikingly, about 50% of all patients with HF present with HFpEF. HFpEF has long been considered an ageing-associated phenomenon, but patients with HFpEF have a high burden of disease and clinical outcomes are poor (although better than in patients with HFrEF). Whereas diagnosis, workup, treatment, and long-term surveillance have been studied in detail in HFrEF, there is far less knowledge and consensus on how to approach HFpEF. Perhaps as a consequence, most trials with cardiovascular (CV) drugs showed neutral results. So evidently, there are numerous gaps in evidence for HFpEF, and in the coming decades, we will hopefully see that our understanding deepens and that we will be able to develop treatments to provide hope for the millions of patients with this subform of HF.

Epidemiology of heart failure with preserved ejection fraction

Prevalence

It has been difficult to exactly map the incidence and prevalence of HFpEF. Because of the various diagnostic algorithms that are in use, reported incidence and prevalence rates vary substantially. Furthermore, HF often is a secondary diagnosis during hospitalization and HFpEF may more often be overlooked than HFrEF, which has a more clear and straightforward presentation and diagnosis. However, in the last decades, large-scale programmes, such as the ESC's Euro Heart Failure Survey and the AHA's Get With The Guidelines program, in concert with better registration in national health registries, have provided far better insight into the incidence and prevalence. Since long, the prevalence of HF in the population has been estimated to be 1–2%. Further, it has been reported that of all HF cases, approximately 30% are due to HFrEF, 14–25% due to HFmrEF, and 50–60% due to HFpEF.[2] This is also supported by the American OPTIMIZE-HF Registry,

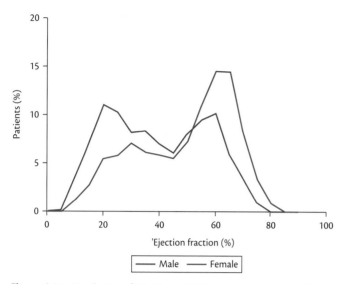

Figure 6.3.1 Distribution of HFpEF and HFrEF among patients hospitalized for HF (presented for men and women).
Reproduced from Borlaug BA, Redfield MM. Diastolic and systolic heart failure are distinct phenotypes within the heart failure spectrum. *Circulation*. 2011 May 10;123(18):2006–13; discussion 2014. doi: 10.1161/CIRCULATIONAHA.110.954388 with permission from Wolters Kluwer.

with more women affected by HFpEF than men (➲ Figure 6.3.1). Importantly, over the course of the last decades, we see a clear shift in the proportion of HFpEF cases of the total HF diagnoses,

with fewer HFrEF diagnoses and more HFpEF diagnoses (➲ Figure 6.3.2).[2]

Incidence rates are even more difficult to estimate, as HFpEF very often does not present as an acute event, but rather as a slowly progressive disorder without a clear onset. As such, a diagnostic code may not be added and the diagnosis of HFpEF may be obscured by, for example, hypertension, chronic obstructive pulmonary disease (COPD), atrial fibrillation (AF), and frailty in the elderly. A recent review by Groenewegen summarized the most recent data on incident HF, and incident HFpEF in particular.[3] It was reported that incident HF in Europe and the United States varies widely from 1 to 9 cases per 1000 person-years. It depends on the populations that were studied, particularly community-dwelling cohorts and at-risk populations such as the elderly and hypertensive patients, and the diagnostic criteria used.[3,4,5] Roughly 30–50% of incident HF cases are due to HFpEF.

Prognosis and survival

Mortality associated with HFpEF is substantial, ranging from 10% to 30% annually, and is higher in epidemiological studies than in clinical trials. A recent comparison between randomized controlled trials (RCTs) with patients enrolled for uncomplicated hypertension or for elevated CV risk and patients enrolled for HFpEF showed almost 100% higher mortality in HFpEF, compared to hypertension or increased CV risk (➲ Figure 6.3.3). However, the mode of death is more diverse than in HFrEF

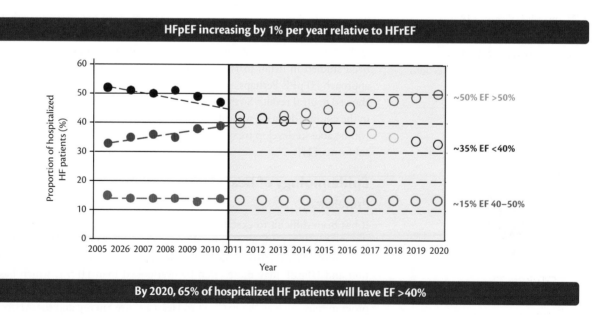

EF, ejection fraction; HF, heart failure; HFpEF, heart failure with preserved ejection fraction; HFrEF, heart failure with reduced ejection fraction

Figure 6.3.2 Trends in prevalence of HF, divided into HFrEF, HFmrEF, and HFpEF. In 2013, the year of publication of this article, it was predicted that at round 2020, HFpEF would become the dominant form of HF, and this has become true.
Reproduced from Oktay AA, Rich JD, Shah SJ. The emerging epidemic of heart failure with preserved ejection fraction. *Curr Heart Fail Rep*. 2013 Dec;10(4):401–10. doi: 10.1007/s11897-013-0155-7 with permission from Springer.

Mortality in HFpEF trials was higher than that observed in other CV trials

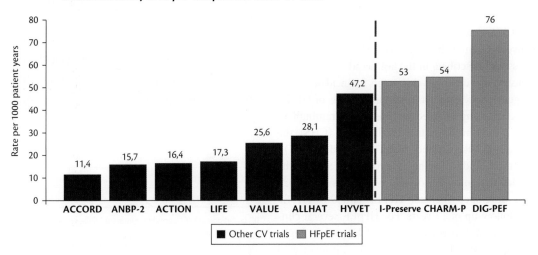

Overall mortality in HFpEF compared to other CV trials

ACCORD, Action to Control Cardiovascular Risk in Diabetes; ANBP-2, second Australian National Blood Pressure trial; ACTION, A Coronary disease Trial Investigating Outcome with Nifedipine; CV, cardiovascular; LIFE, Losartan Intervention for Endpoint reduction in hypertension; VALUE, Valsartan Antihypertensive Long-term Use Evaluation; ALLHAT, Antihypertensive and Lipid-Lowering Treatment to Prevent Heart Attack Trial; HFpEF, heart failure with preserved ejection fraction; HYVET, Hypertension in the Very Elderly Trial; DIG-PEF, digitalis investigation group; CHARM-Preserved, Candesartan in Heart failure: Assessment of Reduction in Mortality and morbidity; I-PRESERVE, Irbesartanin Heart Failure with Preserved Systolic Function

Figure 6.3.3 Mortality in randomized clinical trials (RCTs) enrolling patients with hypertension or increased cardiovascular (CV) risk (red bars), and in RCTs enrolling patients with HFpEF (blue bars). Clearly, mortality is much higher in HFpEF.
Reproduced from Campbell RT, Jhund PS, Castagno D, et al. What have we learned about patients with heart failure and preserved ejection fraction from DIG-PEF, CHARM-preserved, and I-PRESERVE? *J Am Coll Cardiol.* 2012 Dec 11;60(23):2349–56. doi: 10.1016/j.jacc.2012.04.064 with permission from Elsevier.

(➲ Figure 6.3.4). CV causes, including coronary artery disease (CAD), stroke, progressive pump failure, arrhythmias, or sudden cardiac death, are still the primary mode of death in HFpEF.[6] However, non-CV deaths were also observed in observational studies (32–49%)[4,7] and clinical trials (28–30%).[8] Common comorbidities, such as stroke, cancer, respiratory disease, sepsis, and renal disease, and other causes are crucial determinants of outcome.

Hospitalization for HF or other CV causes is a frequent problem for patients with HF. Again, the rate of hospitalization varies widely, depending on the patient category studied. In some high-risk populations, it may be as high as 50% within 6 months, and admission rate by 5 years has been reported to be up to 85%.[8] Approximately 10–30% of all admissions have HF as the primary diagnosis, but non-CV reasons for hospitalizations are common.

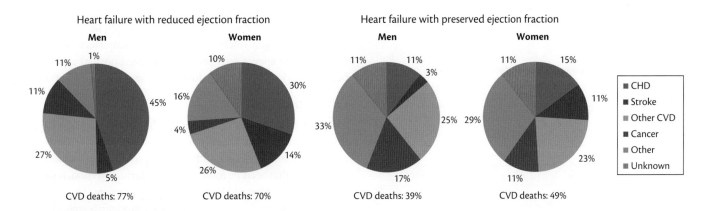

Underlying causes of death by gender and left ventricular ejection fraction in 463 patients in the Framingham Heart Study. CVD, cardiovascular disease; CHD, coronary heart disease.

Figure 6.3.4 Modes of death in HFrEF and HFpEF. In HFrEF, only 25% or less of all mortality is from non-cardiovascular (CV) causes. However, in HFpEF, with a much more heterogeneous pathophysiology, non-CV mortality is about 30–45%.
Reproduced from Lee DS, Gona P, Albano I, et al. A systematic assessment of causes of death after heart failure onset in the community: impact of age at death, time period, and left ventricular systolic dysfunction. *Circ Heart Fail.* 2011 Jan;4(1):36–43. doi: 10.1161/CIRCHEARTFAILURE.110.957480 with permission from Wolters Kluwer.

Risk factors for incident heart failure with preserved ejection fraction

As discussed, HF is not a single diagnosis, but a consequence of various diseases—CV and non-CV. HFpEF shares several risk factors with HFrEF but overall is a more heterogeneous disease, and as such, risk factors are less well described. In the last decade, several large studies were published that described risk factors for incident HF.[9]

Ho and colleagues[10] were the first to publish models of HFrEF and HFpEF prediction using a pooled analysis of the Framingham Heart Study (FHS), the Cardiovascular Health Study (CHS), the Prevention of Renal and Vascular End-stage Disease (PREVEND), and the Multi-Ethnic Study of Atherosclerosis (MESA) in the International Collaboration on Heart Failure Subtypes. Of 28,820 participants, 982 developed incident HFpEF and 909 HFrEF during a median follow-up of 12 years. For HFpEF, several clinical predictors significantly predicted incident HFpEF, as highlighted in ➲ Table 6.3.1. More factors were significantly associated with incident HFrEF (➲ Table 6.3.2). Strikingly, male sex, current smoking status, previous myocardial infarction (MI), and electrocardiographic (ECG) left ventricular (LV) hypertrophy, and left bundle branch block were more strongly associated with incident HFrEF, whereas advanced age, female sex, and increased body mass index (BMI) were more strongly associated with incident HFpEF. Risk predictors for HFmrEF have been separately described, and as this phenotype seems to lean more towards HFrEF than towards HFpEF, risk predictors are also more in line with HFrEF.[11] Furthermore, CV biomarkers, such natriuretic peptides, may be used to improve diagnostic performance in HFpEF, as they were shown to be predictive on top of a clinical model for incident HFpEF (➲ Figure 6.3.5).[12] In addition to natriuretic peptides, urinary albumin excretion was predictive for HFpEF and suggestive associations for high-sensitivity troponins, plasminogen activator inhibitor 1 (PAI-1), and fibrinogen were observed. Again, the predictive values of several CV biomarkers for incident HFrEF were stronger than for HFpEF, underscoring the complex and heterogeneous nature of HFpEF. Ever since, several other risk models of incident HF have been published, mostly reporting on the same

Table 6.3.1 Clinical predictors for incident HFpEF

HFpEF	HR (95% CI)	*P*-value
Age, per 10 years	1.90 (1.74–2.07)	<0.0001
Male sex	0.93 (0.78–1.11)	0.43
Systolic BP, per 20 mmHg	1.14 (1.05–1.37)	0.003
Body mass index, per 4 kg/m²	1.28 (1.21–1.37)	<0.0001
Antihypertensive treatment	1.42 (1.18–1.71)	0.0002
Previous myocardial infarction	1.48 (1.12–1.96)	0.006

BP, blood pressure; CI, confidence interval; HFpEF, heart failure with preserved ejection fraction; HR, hazard ratio.

Reproduction from Ho JE, Enserro D, Brouwers FP, *et al*. Predicting Heart Failure With Preserved and Reduced Ejection Fraction: The International Collaboration on Heart Failure Subtypes. *Circ Heart Fail*. 2016 Jun;9(6):10.1161/CIRCHEARTFAILURE.115.003116 e003116. doi: 10.1161/CIRCHEARTFAILURE.115.003116 with permissions from Wolters Kluwer.

Table 6.3.2 Clinical predictors for incident HFrEF

HFrEF	HR (95% CI)	*P*-value
Age, per 10 years	1.66 (1.52–1.80)	<0.0001
Male sex	1.84 (1.55–2.19)	<0.0001
Systolic BP, per 20 mmHg	1.14 (1.10–1.30)	<0.0001
Body mass index, per 4 kg/m²	1.19 (1.11–1.28)	<0.0001
Antihypertensive treatment	1.35 (1.13–1.63)	0.0001
Diabetes	1.83 (1.48–2.26)	<0.0001
Current smoker	1.41 (1.14–1.75)	0.0015
Previous myocardial infarction	2.60 (2.08–3.25)	<0.0001
ECG LV hypertrophy	2.12 (1.55–2.90)	<0.0001
Left bundle branch block	3.17 (2.11–4.78)	<0.0001

BP, blood pressure; CI, confidence interval; HFrEF, heart failure with reduced ejection fraction; HR, hazard ratio.

Reproduction from Ho JE, Enserro D, Brouwers FP, *et al*. Predicting Heart Failure With Preserved and Reduced Ejection Fraction: The International Collaboration on Heart Failure Subtypes. *Circ Heart Fail*. 2016 Jun;9(6):10.1161/CIRCHEARTFAILURE.115.003116 e003116. doi: 10.1161/CIRCHEARTFAILURE.115.003116 with permissions from Wolters Kluwer.

risk factors, although their associations may differ according to age strata, male and female sex, and race.[13,14]

Pathophysiology

HFpEF is often conceptualized as an isolated disorder of LV diastolic dysfunction. However, studies over the past two decades have shown that the pathophysiology is much more complex, extending to include LV systolic dysfunction, as well as structural and functional abnormalities involving the left atrium (LA) and right ventricle (RV).[15] There are also important abnormalities outside the heart, particularly involving the lungs, vasculature (endothelium, arteries, and veins), skeletal muscle, kidneys, and adipose tissue. These cardiac and non-cardiac abnormalities are believed to be caused by chronic systemic inflammation related to ageing and comorbidities such as obesity and diabetes.[16] An overarching theme that is crucial to the pathophysiology is an abnormality in organ reserve. For example, many facets of cardiac function may appear well preserved or even normal at rest, but become markedly abnormal during stresses such as with exercise.

Left ventricle

The most consistent and conspicuous abnormality in HFpEF is LV diastolic dysfunction. On average, patients with HFpEF display increased diastolic chamber stiffness and prolonged relaxation, abnormalities that become more profound during exertion, resulting in marked elevation in LV diastolic filling pressure (LVFP).[15] The increase in LVFP causes an elevation in pulmonary capillary pressures, unfavourably altering the Starling forces to promote dynamic lung congestion.[17] Diastolic dysfunction in HFpEF is associated with abnormalities in the cardiac myocyte related to altered energy metabolism, abnormal calcium handling, and alterations in the giant macromolecule titin, which importantly regulates myocyte stiffness.[16] Increases in chamber stiffness also develop secondary

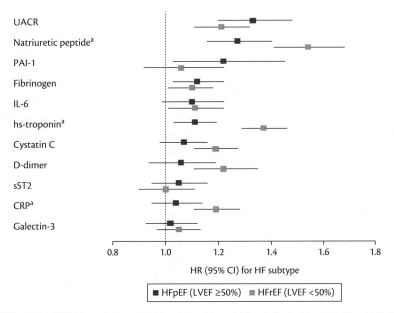

Figure 6.3.5 Associations of cardiovascular (CV) biomarkers and incident heart failure (HF), split for incident HFpEF and HFrEF. Natriuretic peptides and urinary albumin-to-creatinine ratio (UACR) are independently associated with incident HFpEF, with suggestive signals for high-sensitivity troponin and for plasminogen activator inhibitor 1 (PAI-1) and fibrinogen. CI, confidence interval; CRP, C-reactive protein; HR, hazard ratio; hs-IL-6, interleukin-6; LVEF, left ventricular ejection fraction.

Reproduced from de Boer RA, Nayor M, deFilippi CR, *et al.* Association of Cardiovascular Biomarkers With Incident Heart Failure With Preserved and Reduced Ejection Fraction. *JAMA Cardiol.* 2018 Mar 1;3(3):215–224. doi: 10.1001/jamacardio.2017.4987 with permission from JAMA Network.

to changes in the extracellular matrix, including quantitative and qualitative changes in fibrillar collagen.

In addition to diastolic dysfunction, patients with HFpEF display subtle abnormalities in LV systolic function. While the global ejection fraction (EF) is (by definition) normal, systolic mechanics assessed using tissue Doppler and strain echocardiography or by cardiac magnetic resonance imaging (MRI) are frequently abnormal. These abnormalities that are mild at rest often become marked during exercise.[18,19] This is important because inability to contract to low end-systolic volume limits recoil forces that favourably affect filling in subsequent diastole, further increasing the LVFP. Limited contractile reserve also limits the stroke volume response to exercise in patients with HFpEF, contributing to cardiac output limitation that limits peak aerobic capacity.[19]

Left atrium

In addition to LV dysfunction, patients with HFpEF characteristically display abnormalities in left atrial (LA) structure and function, including excessive LA dilatation and impairment in LA reservoir, conduit, and booster strain.[20] LA stiffness is often increased in patients with HFpEF, leading to a prominent V wave on the pulmonary capillary wedge tracing. LA remodelling stretches the mitral annulus, leading to development of atrial functional mitral regurgitation (MR) in patients with HFpEF, which is usually mild to moderate in severity.[21] LA dysfunction also drives the genesis of AF, which develops in two-thirds of patients with HFpEF. The presence of LA remodelling, dysfunction, and AF (collectively termed LA myopathy) is strongly associated with the development of more severe pulmonary vascular disease, pulmonary hypertension (PH), and the development of right ventricular dysfunction.[20]

Pulmonary hypertension

The majority of patients with HFpEF have at least mild PH, defined by a mean pulmonary artery (PA) pressure of >20 mmHg.[1] This is most commonly caused by passive transmission of elevated LA pressure (isolated post-capillary PH (IpC-PH)), but in a sizeable minority of patients (approximately 20%), there may be secondary changes in the pulmonary vasculature that lead to combined precapillary and post-capillary PH (CpC-PH). The precapillary component is caused, in part, by vasoconstriction and also by structural remodelling in both the small arteries and veins. Patients with HFpEF and CpC-PH typically have a history of AF and display greater neurohormonal activation (higher endothelin-1 levels) and poorer outcomes, in tandem with distinct pathophysiological features, including more severe right HF and enhanced ventricular interdependence (discussed below).[22,23]

Right heart failure

RV dysfunction develops in approximately one-third of patients with HFpEF due to chronic increases in LA and PA pressures.[24,25] Development of RV dysfunction is strongly associated with the presence of obesity, as well as with the development of incident AF. Patients with RV failure frequently develop significant functional tricuspid regurgitation related to annular dilatation, worsening right heart volume load and promoting right atrial dilatation.[25] Patients with HFpEF and right HF develop more lung congestion, likely due to impaired pulmonary lymphatic drainage, as well as kidney dysfunction, congestive hepatopathy, altered gut absorption, and eventually cardiac cachexia.[17,26] As such, RV failure is typically an expression of advanced HFpEF,[25] but clinically relevant abnormalities in RV function may be observed during exercise, even among patients with early-stage HFpEF.[19]

Pericardial restraint and ventricular interdependence

Elevation in LVFP is typically considered only in light of abnormal LV diastolic properties, but 40% of intracavitary LVFP is related to pressure applied externally to the LV from the right heart and pericardium.[27] When amplified, this pericardial restraining effect leads to increased competition or coupling between the right and left sides of the heart, termed enhanced ventricular interdependence. Ventricular interdependence is heightened in patients with PH and right HF (due to dilatation of the RV and right atrium), those with LA myopathy (due to the latter plus LA dilatation), and in patients with obesity who display increased total heart volume in tandem with increases in epicardial adipose tissue volume.[27,28] Patients with increased ventricular interdependence require a higher LVFP to achieve a given LV transmural distending pressure, which determines the preload volume.[28]

Vascular dysfunction

Systemic arterial stiffening is frequently increased in patients with HFpEF, particularly during the stress of exercise, where it is associated with more dramatic elevations in LVFP.[29,30] Endothelial dysfunction is common in HFpEF, both in the systemic arteries and also in the coronary microvasculature.[31] While little studied, it is also likely that abnormalities in the veins play an important role in HFpEF, whereby reductions in venous compliance or capacitance lead to overly exuberant increases in venous return to the heart, amplifying increases in LVFP caused by diastolic dysfunction and pericardial restraint.

Non-cardiovascular organ involvement

In addition to pulmonary vascular changes, chronic exposure to high LVFP causes structural remodelling in the alveolar capillary interface, compromising pulmonary gas diffusion.[26] Systemic inflammation, metabolic stress, and elevated systemic venous pressures promote kidney dysfunction, favouring volume retention that further exacerbates congestion, particularly among obese patients.[25,32] A number of patients display sarcopenia and abnormalities in the ability to utilize and extract oxygen in skeletal muscle, which may be related, in part, to mitochondrial dysfunction, as well as to microvascular rarefaction and alterations in myofibre isotype expression.[15,16]

Diagnosis

Diagnosis of HFpEF is straightforward when clinical evidence of congestion is present, but becomes challenging in euvolaemic patients with exertional dyspnoea.[33,34,35] One major factor that confounds diagnosis is the observation that many patients with HFpEF display normal haemodynamics at rest, with elevations in LVFP that develop exclusively during the stress of exercise.[36] As such, exercise stress testing has become essential in the diagnostic evaluation.[33,34,35,36]

HFpEF is defined haemodynamically as an inability of the heart to pump blood to the body at a rate commensurate with its needs at rest or during exercise at normal LVFP. This haemodynamic definition ties in closely with the current diagnostic algorithm for HFpEF. Evidence of high LVFP may be demonstrated by physical examination, radiography, echocardiography, and natriuretic peptide testing, or directly at cardiac catheterization. The clinical testing that is necessary to confirm (or refute) the diagnosis of HFpEF relies upon evaluation of the pretest probability of disease, based upon the presence or absence of findings associated with HFpEF.

In 2018, Reddy and colleagues developed and then validated a multi-variable logistic model to discriminate HFpEF from non-cardiac dyspnoea termed the H$_2$FPEF score (→ Figure 6.3.6).[34]

	Clinical Variable	Values	Points
H$_2$	**H**eavy	Body mass index >30 kg/m^2	2
	Hypertensive	2 or more antihypertensive medicines	1
F	Atrial **F**ibrillation	Paroxysmal or Persistent	3
P	**P**ulmonary Hypertension	Doppler Echocardiographic estimated Pulmonary Artery Systolic Pressure >35 mmHg	1
E	**E**lder	Age >60 years	1
F	**F**illing Pressure	Doppler Echocardiographic E/e' >9	1
	H$_2$FPEF score		Sum (0–9)

(b)

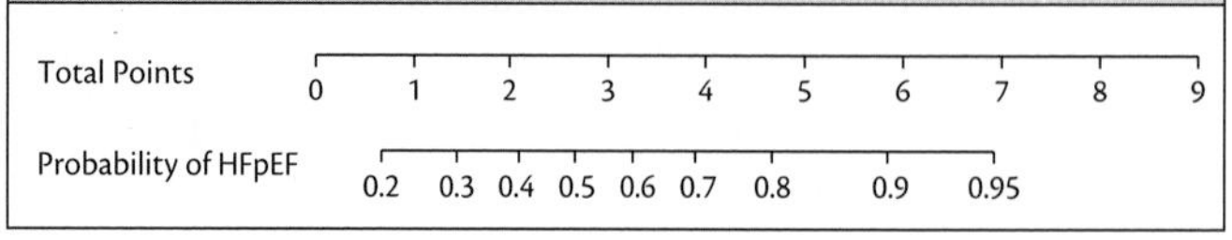

Total Points: 0 1 2 3 4 5 6 7 8 9

Probability of HFpEF: 0.2 0.3 0.4 0.5 0.6 0.7 0.8 0.9 0.95

Figure 6.3.6 Description of the H$_2$FPEF score and point allocations for each clinical characteristic (a), with associated probability of having HFpEF based on the total score as estimated from the model (b).

Reproduced from Reddy YNV, Carter RE, Obokata M, et al. A Simple, Evidence-Based Approach to Help Guide Diagnosis of Heart Failure With Preserved Ejection Fraction. *Circulation*. 2018 Aug 28;138(9):861–870. doi: 10.1161/CIRCULATIONAHA.118.034646 with permission from Wolters Kluwer.

The patient receives a score based upon the presence or absence of characteristics strongly associated with HFpEF, including obesity (BMI >30 kg/m^2, 2 points), treatment with two or more antihypertensives (1 point), history of AF (3 points), elevated PA pressure on echocardiography (>35 mmHg, 1 point), age >60 years (1 point), and elevated LVFP on echocardiography (E/e' >9, 1 point). Using the sum of these score components, one can then estimate the probability that HFpEF is present. Scores of 0–1 point have a probability of <25% of HFpEF, making the diagnosis unlikely, whereas scores of >5 points have >90% probability, making the diagnosis of HFpEF almost a certainty. Patients with scores of 2–5 points have intermediate probability and require more testing. The H$_2$FPEF score was shown to robustly discriminate HFpEF from non-cardiac dyspnoea in the derivation cohort (area under the curve (AUC) 0.84; $P < 0.0001$) and this was confirmed in a separate validation cohort (AUC 0.89; $P < 0.0001$).[34]

A year later, a separate expert consensus diagnostic algorithm was established by the Heart Failure Association (HFA) of the ESC, termed the HFA-PEFF score.[33] The approach is very much the same, wherein indicators of HF are used to estimate the pretest probability that HFpEF is present, but unlike the H$_2$FPEF score, clinical characteristics are not included in the HFA-PEFF score. The latter is based upon characteristic structural and functional changes observed on echocardiography, along with the results of natriuretic peptide testing, with up to 2 points allocated to each domain (→ Figure 6.3.7).[33] Scores of 0–1 points are deemed to be unlikely for a diagnosis of HFpEF, whereas scores of 5–6 points are deemed to be of sufficient evidence to reach a diagnosis of HFpEF without further testing. Intermediate scores of 2–4 points require further testing, including stress testing.

Several studies have been conducted or are under way that prospectively evaluate the algorithms.[37,38,39] Elevations in the H$_2$FPEF and HFA-PEFF scores have both been associated with increased rates of HF hospitalization or CV death, supporting their utility.[40] As would be expected by the inclusion of differing inputs, the two scores do not always agree. Thus, at the current time, our approach is to proceed with further testing if either the HFA-PEFF score or the H$_2$FPEF score falls in the intermediate range. If both are low risk, HFpEF is unlikely, and if both are high risk, then the diagnosis can be confidently made.

In patients with intermediate probability, diastolic exercise stress testing is necessary, which may consist of invasive or non-invasive (echocardiographic) modalities. The gold standard for diagnosis of HFpEF is invasive haemodynamic exercise testing.[33] Patients with elevation in the pulmonary capillary wedge pressure (PCWP) at rest (≥15 mmHg) and/or with exercise (≥25 mmHg) meet the diagnostic criteria for HFpEF.[33] However, invasive testing carries greater cost and is not as widely available as exercise echocardiography. When high-quality images can be obtained, echocardiographic exercise stress testing provides strong diagnostic discrimination,[36] but imaging may be inadequate in 20–30% of patients, in which case referral for the more definitive invasive test is most appropriate.

The most recent ESC guidelines from 2021 present a simplified approach to diagnosing HFpEF, although the elements of the diagnostic algorithms are identical to those of the HFA-PEFF score.[1]

Treatment of heart failure with preserved ejection fraction

A large number of trials have been conducted. However, until recently, no treatment had been shown to convincingly improve

	Functional	Morphological	Biomarker (SR)	Biomarker (AF)
Major	septal e' <7 cm/s or lateral e' <10 cm/s or Average E/e' ≥15 or TR velocity >2.8 m/s (PASP >35 mmHg)	LAVI >34 ml/m^2 or LVMI ≥149/122 g/m^2 (m/w) and RWT >0,42 #	NT-proBNP >220 pg/ml or BNP >80 pg/ml	NT-proBNP >660 pg/ml or BNP >240 pg/ml
Minor	Average E/e' 9–14 or GLS <16%	LAVI 29–34 ml/m^2 or LVMI >115/95 g/m^2 (m/w) or RWT >0,42 or LV wall thickness ≥12 mm	NT-proBNP 125–220 pg/ml or BNP 35–80 pg/ml	NT-proBNP 365–660 pg/ml or BNP 105–240 pg/ml
Major Criteria: 2 points	**>5 points; HFpEF**			
Minor Criteria: 1 point	**2–4 points: Diastolic Stress Test or Invasive Haemodynamic Measurements**			

Figure 6.3.7 Description of the HFA-PEFF score: echocardiographic and natriuretic peptide measurements. Major (2 points) and minor (1 point) criteria are defined from these measures. A score of ≥5 points implies definite HFpEF. An intermediate score (2–4 points) implies diagnostic uncertainty, in which case additional testing is recommend. In all patients, it is recommended to search for the aetiology.

Reproduced from Pieske B, Tschöpe C, de Boer RA, et al. How to diagnose heart failure with preserved ejection fraction: the HFA-PEFF diagnostic algorithm: a consensus recommendation from the Heart Failure Association (HFA) of the European Society of Cardiology (ESC). Eur Heart J. 2019 Oct 21;40(40):3297–3317. doi: 10.1093/eurheartj/ehz641 with permission from Oxford University Press.

HFpEF outcomes. Specifically, HF drugs that have been proven to exert positive effects in HFrEF have generated neutral or borderline significant effects in HFpEF. Among the classes of drugs that have been tested are angiotensin-converting enzyme (ACE) inhibitors, perindopril (PEP-CHF study),[41] angiotensin receptor blockers (ARBs), candesartan (CHARM-Preserved trial),[42] and irbesartan (I-PRESERVE study),[43] mineralocorticoid receptor antagonists (MRAs), spironolactone (TOPCAT trial),[44] inhibition of the sodium–potassium adenosine triphosphatase (Na$^+$/K$^+$ ATPase) with digoxin (DIG-PEF trial),[45] and most recently angiotensin receptor–neprilysin (ARNI) inhibition with sacubitril/valsartan (PARAGON-HF and PARAMOUNT trials).[46,47] An overview of the main trials is provided in ◉ Table 6.3.3. Some trials clearly showed trends towards better outcomes—for example,

hospitalization for HF was reduced in CHARM (candesartan), TOPCAT (spironolactone), and PARAGON-HF (sacubitril/valsartan). But these trials had combined mortality and morbidity endpoints that were not met, and therefore, efficacy of these compounds has not been proven beyond doubt.

Smaller recent trials explored the possibility that nitric oxide (NO) release would be beneficial in HFpEF. Specifically, targeting the NO–cyclic guanosine monophosphate pathway failed to improve exercise capacity or quality of life in HFpEF (RELAX,[6] NEAT-HFpEF,[48] INDIE-HFpEF,[49] VITALITY,[50] and CAPACITY-HFpEF[51] (praliciguat)).

It was in August 2021 that, for the first time, the EMPEROR-Preserved trial demonstrated meaningful benefit from the SGLT2 inhibitor empagliflozin in patients with HFpEF.[52] This

Table 6.3.3 Major outcome trials in HFpEF, evaluating various classes of HF drugs

Trial acronym	Intervention	Major inclusion criteria	Mean FU	Primary endpoint	Drug effect on symptoms
PEP-CHF	Perindopril vs placebo	LV motion index ≥1.4 (LVEF approximately ≥40%), symptomatic HF, treated with diuretic, diastolic dysfunction on ECHO, age ≥70 y	2.1 y	No difference in combined all-cause mortality or CV hospitalization (36% vs 37%; $P = 0.35$)	Perindopril—improvement in functional class and 6MWT
I-PRESERVE	Irbesartan vs placebo	LVEF ≥45%, NYHA classes III and IV with evidence of HF, NYHA class II with HF hospitalization <6 months, age ≥60 y	4.1 y	No difference in combined all-cause mortality or HF hospitalization (24% vs 25%; $P = 0.54$)	Irbesartan—no improvement in MLHFQ
CHARM-Preserved	Candesartan vs placebo	LVEF >40%, NYHA classes II–IV, history of CV hospitalization	3.0 y	Trend towards reduction in combined CV mortality or HF hospitalization by 11% (22% vs 24%; adjusted $P = 0.051$)	Candesartan—not reported
TOPCAT	Spironolactone vs placebo	LVEF ≥45%, ≥1 HF sign, ≥1 HF symptom, HF hospitalization <12 months, or BNP ≥100 pg/mL or NT-proBNP ≥360 pg/mL, age ≥50 y	3.3 y	No difference in combined CV mortality, aborted cardiac arrest, or HF hospitalization (19% vs 20%; $P = 0.14$). Strong differences in outcomes in patients from different geographies	Spironolactone—not reported
DIG-PEF	Digoxin vs placebo	HF with LVEF ≥45%, sinus rhythm	3.1 y	No difference in combined HF mortality or HF hospitalization (21% vs 24%; $P = 0.14$)	Digoxin—not reported
PARAMOUNT	Sacubitril/valsartan vs placebo	HF with LVEF ≥45%, NYHA classes II and III, NT-proBNP >400 pg/mL	12 w	Reduction in NT-proBNP; ratio of change sacubitril/valsartan 0.77 (95% CI 0.64–0.92); $P = 0.005$	Sacubitril/valsartan—improvement in QoL-KCCQ
RELAX	Sildenafil vs placebo	HF with LVEF ≥45%, NYHA classes II–IV, peak VO$_2$ <60% of reference values, NT-proBNP >400 pg/mL, or high LV filling pressures	24 w	No change in peak VO$_2$ ($P = 0.90$)	Sildenafil—no improvement
PARAGON-HF	Sacubitril/valsartan vs placebo	HF with LVEF ≥45%, NYHA classes II–IV, LA enlargement OR LVH and elevated BNP (≥300 pg/mL) or NT-proBNP (≥900 pg/mL), OR HF hospitalization <9 m	35 m (median)	Trend towards reduction in total HF hospitalizations or CV mortality by 13% (95% CI 0.75–1.01); $P = 0.056$	Sacubitril/valsartan—no improvement in QoL-KCCQ
EMPEROR-PRESERVED	Empagliflozine vs placebo	HF with LVEF ≥40%, NYHA classes II–IV, LA enlargement OR LVH and elevated NT-proBNP (≥300 pg/mL; ≥900 pg/mL if AF), OR HF hospitalization <12 m	26 m (median)	Reduction in combined CV mortality or HF hospitalization by 21% (17.1% vs 13.8%, HR 0.79, CI 0.69–0.90; $P < 0.001$)	Empagliflozin improved KCCQ with 1.32 (0.45–2.19), compared to placebo

6MWT, 6-minute walking test; AF, atrial fibrillation; BNP, B-type natriuretic peptide; CI, confidence interval; CV, cardiovascular; ECHO, echocardiography; FU, follow-up; HF, heart failure; HFrEF, heart failure with reduced ejection fraction; HR, hazard ratio; LA, left atrial; LV, left ventricular; LVEF, left ventricular ejection fraction; LVH, left ventricular hypertrophy; m, months; NT-proBNP, N-terminal pro-B-type natriuretic peptide; NYHA, New York Heart Association; w, weeks; y, years.

trial enrolled 5988 HF patients with an LVEF of >40% who were randomized to empagliflozin 10 mg once daily or placebo. The primary efficacy endpoint was a composite of CV mortality and HF hospitalization. After a mean follow-up of 26 months, the primary endpoint was reduced by 21% (hazard ratio (HR) 0.79, 95% confidence interval (CI) 0.69–0.90; P < 0.001). This effect was mainly related to a lower risk of hospitalization for HF in the empagliflozin group, as the effects on CV mortality were small and non-significant (HR 0.91, CI 0.76–1.09). Both secondary endpoints, that is, total number of HF hospitalizations (including repeated) and decline in eGFR slope, were both significantly improved (P < 0.001). Importantly, there appeared to be more benefit in patients with lower LVEF than in those with high LVEF. For instance, for total HF hospitalizations, the subgroup of patients with HFmrEF (LVEF 40–49%) had the strongest effect (HR 0.57, CI 0.42–0.79), with less strong effects in the subgroup with LVEF of 51–60% (HR 0.66, CI 0.48–0.91) and no effects in the subgroup with LVEF of >60% (HR 1.07, CI 0.76–1.46). So for HFpEF, characterized by an LVEF of >50%, the effects are less striking than in the HFmrEF group, although still meaningful.

With SGLT2 inhibition still having to be implemented, currently, treatment is still mostly aimed at reducing symptoms of congestion with diuretics. Furthermore, body weight reduction in obese patients and increasing exercise may further improve symptoms and exercise capacity, and should therefore be considered in appropriate patients.[53,54]

Better phenotyping HFpEF patients with specific aetiologies may improve outcomes in selected patients. For instance, cardiac amyloidosis may present as HFpEF, and recently, tafamidis (ATTR-CM) has been shown to improve outcomes in patients with amyloid heart disease.[55] Furthermore, common underlying aetiologies, such as hypertension and AF, can effectively be treated and this arguably will also improve HF-related outcomes.

Aetiologies and special forms

Primary HFpEF is the most frequent form of HFpEF and typically evolves from a combination of risk factors and comorbidities, including advanced age, female sex, obesity, systemic arterial hypertension, diabetes mellitus, renal dysfunction, anaemia, iron deficiency, sleep disorders, and COPD (➔ Table 6.3.1). HFpEF 'masqueraders', such as heart valve disease, arrhythmias, and pericardial constriction, need to be excluded. Similarly, a patient with a normal LVEF and HF-like symptoms caused by significant CAD is also not considered to have HFpEF.[33]

Secondary HFpEF results from specific causes of HFpEF. Amyloid cardiomyopathy, in particular wild-type transthyretin cardiac amyloidosis (ATTRwt), resulting from myocardial deposition of misfolded transthyretin (TTR) or pre-albumin, has been identified as a relevant cause for secondary HFpEF. Characteristic patterns of echocardiography and cardiac magnetic resonance can strongly suggest the disease. The diagnosis can be made by using non-invasive nuclear imaging when there is no evidence of a monoclonal protein.[56] Associated features, including carpal tunnel syndrome and lumbar spinal stenosis, raise suspicion and may afford a means for early diagnosis.[57] In a prospective single-centre registry, (99m)Tc-DPD scintigraphy demonstrated a moderate to high cardiac tracer uptake in 13.3% of all HFpEF patients.[58] The high prevalence of ATTRwt cardiac amyloidosis in HFpEF was corroborated by other studies. The clinical spectrum of cardiac HFpEF ATTRwt is heterogeneous and differs from the classic phenotype: a significant proportion of women are affected; asymmetric LV hypertrophy and impaired LVEF are not rare, and only a minority have low QRS voltages. Contemporary treatment strategies that suppress expression[58,59] or stabilize TTR[60] have been reported recently to slow or halt disease progression in ATTR polyneuropathy and cardiomyopathy. In consequence, workup for cardiac amyloidosis should be considered in patients with unexplained HFpEF.

Additional specific causes for secondary HFpEF include genetic hypertrophic cardiomyopathies, select forms of myocarditis and inflammatory cardiomyopathies, non-infiltrative and infiltrative cardiomyopathies, and other rare forms.[32]

Gaps in knowledge and future directions

Gaps in knowledge encompass the fields of pathophysiology, diagnosis, and management. LVEF cut-offs are questioned based on recent trial results, and may not be identical for men and women. Also, whether the LVEF is a suitable diagnostic measure at all is challenged repeatedly. Whether other non-invasive parameters, such as global longitudinal strain or LA strain, may result as better diagnostic parameters remains to be demonstrated. Interactions with LVEF from multiple treatments have been observed: for the ARB candesartan (CHARM), the MRA spironolactone (TOPCAT), the ARNI sacubitril/valsartan (PARAGON-HF), and recently the SGLT2 inhibitor empagliflozin (EMPEROR-Preserved). As in these trials, the 'nadir' of LVEF was around 55–60%, above which the drugs were no longer efficacious, and some have suggested that an LVEF of <60% should be regarded as signifying HFmrEF and that HF with an LVEF of >60% needs further study. Also, natriuretic peptides are of limited value in HFpEF, as normal levels do not exclude HFpEF and increased levels may be related to AF that is frequently present. Therefore, new and better biomarkers for HFpEF are needed. Phenomapping and deep molecular phenotyping have recently emerged in order to lay the ground for stratified therapies tailored to specific subsets of patients.[61,62] Clinical phenotypes, such as the obese, pro-fibrotic, or renal dysfunction phenotype, have been discussed. Diagnosing HFpEF is still hampered by the lack of a uniformly applicable diagnostic gold standard, which may consist of invasive haemodynamics with exercise.

Summary

HFpEF is an important and prevalent health problem, for which currently no evidence-based therapies exist that effectively reduce morbidity and mortality. The diagnosis of HFpEF is complex, and likely a number of diagnoses are hidden in the HFpEF phenotype. Future attempts should be made to better phenotype HFpEF and put more targeted treatments to the test. With the advent of

SGLT2 inhibitors, a first evidence-based treatment of HFpEF has entered the clinical arena, which likely will change the face of HFpEF treatment.

Key messages

- HFpEF is a common form of HF that is predominantly seen in patients of advanced age and female sex, and with AF and obesity.
- Diagnosis and clinical workup of HFpEF are complex and requires a staged approach.
- Few evidence-based therapies for HFpEF are available, with only one class of drugs (SGLT2 inhibitors) with convincing results from a well-powered RCT.
- In the last 5 years, we have seen the introduction of targeted therapies for niche indications.

References

1. McDonagh TA, Metra M, Adamo M, et al. 2021 ESC Guidelines for the diagnosis and treatment of acute and chronic heart failure. Eur Heart J 2021;**42**:3599–726.
2. Dunlay SM, Roger VL, Redfield MM. Epidemiology of heart failure with preserved ejection fraction. Nat Rev Cardiol 2017;**14**:591–602.
3. Senni M, Tribouilloy CM, Rodeheffer RJ, et al. Congestive heart failure in the community: a study of all incident cases in Olmsted county, Minnesota, in 1991. Circulation 1998;**98**:2282–9.
4. Groenewegen A, Rutten FH, Mosterd A, Hoes AW. Epidemiology of heart failure. Eur J Heart Fail 2020;**22**:1342–56.
5. Conrad N, Judge A, Tran J, et al. Temporal trends and patterns in heart failure incidence: a population-based study of 4 million individuals. Lancet 2018;**391**:572–80.
6. Redfield MM, Chen HH, Borlaug BA, et al. Effect of phosphodiesterase-5 inhibition on exercise capacity and clinical status in heart failure with preserved ejection fraction: a randomized clinical trial. JAMA 2013;**309**:1268–77.
7. Vergaro G, Ghionzoli N, Innocenti L, et al. Noncardiac versus cardiac mortality in heart failure with preserved, midrange, and reduced ejection fraction. J Am Heart Assoc 2019;**8**:10.
8. Chan MMY, Lam CSP. How do patients with heart failure with preserved ejection fraction die? Eur J Heart Fail 2013;**15**:604–13.
9. Lee MP, Glynn RJ, Schneeweiss S, et al. Risk factors for heart failure with preserved or reduced ejection fraction among Medicare beneficiaries: application of competing risks analysis and gradient boosted model. Clin Epidemiol 2020;**12**:607–16.
10. Ho JE, Enserro D, Brouwers FP, et al. Predicting heart failure with preserved and reduced ejection fraction: the International Collaboration on Heart Failure Subtypes. Circ Heart Fail 2016;**9**:e003116.
11. Savji N, Meijers WC, Bartz TM, et al. The association of obesity and cardiometabolic traits with incident HFpEF and HFrEF. JACC Heart Fail 2018;**6**:701–9.
12. De Boer RA, Nayor M, DeFilippi CR, et al. Association of cardiovascular biomarkers with incident heart failure with preserved and reduced ejection fraction. JAMA Cardiol 2018;**3**:215–24.
13. Trippel TD, Mende M, Düngen H, et al. The diagnostic and prognostic value of galectin-3 in patients at risk for heart failure with preserved ejection fraction: results from the DIAST-CHF study. ESC Heart Fail 2021;**8**:829–41.
14. Brouwers FP, de Boer RA, van der Harst P, et al. Incidence and epidemiology of new onset heart failure with preserved vs. reduced ejection fraction in a community-based cohort: 11-year follow-up of PREVEND. Eur Heart J 2013;**34**:1424–31.
15. Pfeffer MA, Shah AM, Borlaug BA. Heart failure with preserved ejection fraction in perspective. Circ Res 2019;**124**:1598–617.
16. Shah SJ, Borlaug BA, Kitzman DW, et al. Research priorities for heart failure with preserved ejection fraction: National Heart, Lung, and Blood Institute Working Group Summary. Circulation 2020;**141**:1001–26.
17. Reddy YNV, Obokata M, Wiley B, et al. The haemodynamic basis of lung congestion during exercise in heart failure with preserved ejection fraction. Eur Heart J 2019;**40**:3721–30.
18. Kosmala W, Rojek A, Przewlocka-Kosmala M, Mysiak A, Karolko B, Marwick TH. Contributions of nondiastolic factors to exercise intolerance in heart failure with preserved ejection fraction. J Am Coll Cardiol 2016;**67**:659–70.
19. Borlaug BA, Kane GC, Melenovsky V, Olson TP. Abnormal right ventricular–pulmonary artery coupling with exercise in heart failure with preserved ejection fraction. Eur Heart J 2016;**37**:3294–302.
20. Reddy YNV, Obokata M, Verbrugge FH, Lin G, Borlaug BA. Atrial dysfunction in patients with heart failure with preserved ejection fraction and atrial fibrillation. J Am Coll Cardiol 2020;**76**:1051–64.
21. Tamargo M, Obokata M, Reddy YNV, et al. Functional mitral regurgitation and left atrial myopathy in heart failure with preserved ejection fraction. Eur J Heart Fail 2020;**22**:489–98.
22. Gorter TM, Obokata M, Reddy YNV, Melenovsky V, Borlaug BA. Exercise unmasks distinct pathophysiologic features in heart failure with preserved ejection fraction and pulmonary vascular disease. Eur Heart J 2018;**39**:2825–35.
23. Vanderpool RR, Saul M, Nouraie M, Gladwin MT, Simon MA. Association between hemodynamic markers of pulmonary hypertension and outcomes in heart failure with preserved ejection fraction. JAMA Cardiol 2018;**3**:298–306.
24. Gorter TM, van Veldhuisen DJ, Bauersachs J, et al. Right heart dysfunction and failure in heart failure with preserved ejection fraction: mechanisms and management. Position statement on behalf of the Heart Failure Association of the European Society of Cardiology. Eur J Heart Fail 2018;**20**:16–37.
25. Obokata M, Reddy YNV, Melenovsky V, Pislaru S, Borlaug BA. Deterioration in right ventricular structure and function over time in patients with heart failure and preserved ejection fraction. Eur Heart J 2019;**40**:689–98.
26. Verbrugge FH, Guazzi M, Testani JM, Borlaug BA. Altered hemodynamics and end-organ damage in heart failure: impact on the lung and kidney. Circulation 2020;**142**:998–1012.
27. Borlaug BA, Reddy YNV. The role of the pericardium in heart failure: implications for pathophysiology and treatment. JACC Heart Fail 2019;**7**:574–85.
28. Obokata M, Reddy YNV, Pislaru SV, Melenovsky V, Borlaug BA. Evidence supporting the existence of a distinct obese phenotype of heart failure with preserved ejection fraction. Circulation 2017;**136**:6–19.
29. Reddy YNV, Andersen MJ, Obokata M, et al. Arterial stiffening with exercise in patients with heart failure and preserved ejection fraction. J Am Coll Cardiol 2017;**70**:136–48.
30. Chirinos JA, Segers P, Hughes T, Townsend R. Large-artery stiffness in health and disease: JACC state-of-the-art review. J Am Coll Cardiol 2019;**74**:1237–63.
31. Shah SJ, Lam CSP, Svedlund S, et al. Prevalence and correlates of coronary microvascular dysfunction in heart failure with preserved ejection fraction: PROMIS-HFpEF. Eur Heart J 2018;**39**:3439–50.
32. Ter Maaten JM, Damman K, Verhaar MC, et al. Connecting heart failure with preserved ejection fraction and renal dysfunction: the

role of endothelial dysfunction and inflammation. *Eur J Heart Fail* 2016;**18**:588–98.

33. Pieske B, Tschöpe C, De Boer RA, *et al*. How to diagnose heart failure with preserved ejection fraction: the HFA-PEFF diagnostic algorithm: a consensus recommendation from the Heart Failure Association (HFA) of the European Society of Cardiology (ESC). *Eur Heart J* 2019;**40**:3297–17.

34. Reddy YNV, Carter RE, Obokata M, Redfield MM, Borlaug BA. A simple, evidence-based approach to help guide diagnosis of heart failure with preserved ejection fraction. *Circulation* 2018;**138**:861–70.

35. Borlaug BA. Evaluation and management of heart failure with preserved ejection fraction. *Nat Rev Cardiol* 2020;**17**:559–73.

36. Obokata M, Kane GC, Reddy YNV, Olson TP, Melenovsky V, Borlaug BA. Role of diastolic stress testing in the evaluation for heart failure with preserved ejection fraction: a simultaneous invasive-echocardiographic study. *Circulation* 2017;**135**:825–38.

37. Ljung-Faxen U, Venkateshvaran A, Shah SJ, *et al*. Generalizability of HFA-PEFF and H$_2$FPEF diagnostic algorithms and associations with heart failure indices and proteomic biomarkers: insights from PROMIS-HFpEF. *J Card Fail* 2021;**27**:756–65.

38. Sanders-van Wijk S, Barandiarán Aizpurua A, Brunner-La Rocca H-P, *et al*. The HFA-PEFF and H$_2$FPEF scores largely disagree in classifying patients with suspected heart failure with preserved ejection fraction. *Eur J Heart Fail* 2021;**23**:838–40

39. Churchill TW, Li SX, Curreri L, *et al*. Evaluation of 2 existing diagnostic scores for heart failure with preserved ejection fraction against a comprehensively phenotyped cohort. *Circulation* 2021;**143**: 289–91.

40. Selvaraj S, Myhre PL, Vaduganathan M, *et al*. Application of diagnostic algorithms for heart failure with preserved ejection fraction to the community. *JACC Heart Fail* 2020;**8**:640–53.

41. Cleland JGF, Tendera M, Adamus J, Freemantle N, Polonski L, Taylor J. The perindopril in elderly people with chronic heart failure (PEP-CHF) study. *Eur Heart J* 2006;**27**:2338–45.

42. Yusuf S, Pfeffer MA, Swedberg K, *et al*. Effects of candesartan in patients with chronic heart failure and preserved left-ventricular ejection fraction: the CHARM-Preserved trial. *Lancet* 2003;**362**:777–81.

43. Massie BM, Carson PE, McMurray JJ, *et al*. Irbesartan in patients with heart failure and preserved ejection fraction. *N Engl J Med* 2008;**359**:2456–67.

44. Pitt B, Pfeffer MA, Assmann SF, *et al*. Spironolactone for heart failure with preserved ejection fraction. *N Engl J Med* 2014;**370**:1383–92.

45. Ahmed A, Rich MW, Fleg JL, *et al*. Effects of digoxin on morbidity and mortality in diastolic heart failure: the Ancillary Digitalis Investigation Group Trial. *Circulation* 2006;**114**:397–403.

46. Solomon SD, Zile M, Pieske B, *et al*. The angiotensin receptor neprilysin inhibitor LCZ696 in heart failure with preserved ejection fraction: a phase 2 double-blind randomised controlled trial. *Lancet* 2012;**380**:1387–95.

47. Solomon SD, McMurray JJV, Anand IS, *et al*. Angiotensin–neprilysin inhibition in heart failure with preserved ejection fraction. *N Engl J Med* 2019;**381**:1609–20.

48. Redfield MM, Anstrom KJ, Levine JA, *et al*. Isosorbide mononitrate in heart failure with preserved ejection fraction. *N Engl J Med* 2015;**373**:2314–24.

49. Borlaug BA, Anstrom KJ, Lewis GD, *et al*. Effect of inorganic nitrite vs placebo on exercise capacity among patients with heart failure with preserved ejection fraction: the INDIE-HFpEF randomized clinical trial. *JAMA* 2018;**320**:1764–73.

50. Armstrong PW, Lam CSP, Anstrom KJ, *et al*. Effect of vericiguat vs placebo on quality of life in patients with heart failure and preserved ejection fraction: the VITALITY-HFpEF randomized clinical trial. *JAMA* 2020;**324**:1512–21.

51. Udelson JE, Lewis GD, Shah SJ, *et al*. Effect of praliciguat on peak rate of oxygen consumption in patients with heart failure with preserved ejection fraction: the CAPACITY HFpEF randomized clinical trial. *JAMA* 2020;**324**:1522–31.

52. Anker SD, Butler J, Filippatos G, *et al*.; EMPEROR-Preserved Trial Investigators. Empagliflozin in heart failure with a preserved ejection fraction. *N Engl J Med* 2021;**385**:1451–61.

53. Edelmann F, Gelbrich G, Dngen HD, *et al*. Exercise training improves exercise capacity and diastolic function in patients with heart failure with preserved ejection fraction: results of the Ex-DHF (Exercise training in Diastolic Heart Failure) pilot study. *J Am Coll Cardiol* 2011;**58**:1780–91.

54. Kitzman DW, Brubaker PH, Morgan TM, Stewart KP, Little WC. Exercise training in older patients with heart failure and preserved ejection fraction: a randomized, controlled, single-blind trial. *Circ Heart Fail* 2010;**3**:659–67.

55. Maurer MS, Schwartz JH, Gundapaneni B, *et al*. Tafamidis treatment for patients with transthyretin amyloid cardiomyopathy. *N Engl J Med* 2018;**379**:1007–16.

56. Ruberg FL, Grogan M, Hanna M, Kelly JW, Maurer MS. Transthyretin amyloid cardiomyopathy: JACC state-of-the-art review. *J Am Coll Cardiol* 2019;**73**:2872–91.

57. Aus dem Siepen F, Hein S, Prestel S, *et al*. Carpal tunnel syndrome and spinal canal stenosis: harbingers of transthyretin amyloid cardiomyopathy? *Clin Res Cardiol* 2019;**108**:1324–30.

58. Adams D, Gonzalez-Duarte A, O'Riordan WD, *et al*. Patisiran, an RNAi therapeutic, for hereditary transthyretin amyloidosis. *N Engl J Med* 2018;**379**:11–21.

59. Benson MD, Waddington-Cruz M, Berk JL, *et al*. Inotersen treatment for patients with hereditary transthyretin amyloidosis. *N Engl J Med* 2018;**379**:22–31.

60. Maurer MS, Schwartz JH, Gundapaneni B, *et al*. Tafamidis treatment for patients with transthyretin amyloid cardiomyopathy. *N Engl J Med* 2018;**379**:1007–16.

61. Tromp J, Khan MAF, Klip IT, *et al*. Biomarker profiles in heart failure patients with preserved and reduced ejection fraction. *J Am Heart Assoc* 2017;**6**:e003989.

62. Sanders-Van Wijk S, Tromp J, Beussink-Nelson L, *et al*. Proteomic evaluation of the comorbidity–inflammation paradigm in heart failure with preserved ejection fraction: results from the PROMIS-HFpEF study. *Circulation* 2020;**142**:2029–44.

CHAPTER 6.4

Right heart failure

Thomas F Lüscher, Thomas M Gorter,
Susanna Price, Anneline Riele, and
Michael A Gatzoulis

Contents

Introduction

The right ventricle is the Cinderella of heart failure. Indeed, although William Withering's patients suffered from what he called 'dropsy', most likely all had not only left heart failure (HF), but also right HF; modern clinical research has almost exclusively focused on the left ventricle (LV) and its function. Moreover, the success of the Fontan procedure suggested that the right ventricle (RV) may not be absolutely necessary to provide blood into the pulmonary circulation and eventually the left heart.[1] However, we almost forgot William Harvey's seminal discovery that the circulation is a closed circuit and can only properly function if all parts of it serve their purpose. More recently, the RV attracted more attention due to increasing interest in adult congenital heart disease (ACHD), and pulmonary hypertension (PH) and its impact on the RV, as well as in arrhythmogenic cardiomyopathy that affects primarily the RV,[2] among other aspects. Today, there is widespread consensus that a properly functioning RV is essential in almost in all cardiopulmonary diseases.

Right ventricular dysfunction (RVD) has many causes, ranging from intra-atrial shunts, tricuspid valvular heart disease, arrhythmogenic right ventricular cardiomyopathy (ARVC), pulmonary stenosis and/or regurgitation, PH, mitral stenosis and/or regurgitation and left HF, be it with reduced ejection fraction (HFrEF) or with preserved ejection fraction (HFpEF), and other types of CHD (➲ Table 6.4.1).[3]

This chapter reviews the most important conditions leading to RV dysfunction and failure, and their diagnosis and management.

The normal right ventricle

The RV differs substantially from the LV in structure, function, and susceptibility to disease. Indeed, its shape is triangular and extends from the tricuspid valve in the right atrium to near the apex of the heart. Its wall is thickest at the apex and thins towards its base at the atrium, being typically trabeculated towards the apex.

Furthermore, the RV is a low-pressure chamber with an end-diastolic pressure of around 4 mmHg (vs 8 mmHg for the LV) and a peak systolic pressure of around 25 mmHg (vs approximately 130 mmHg for the LV). Thus, while coronary blood flow almost subsides in the LV, this is not the case in the RV and the RV myocardium receives coronary blood flow during both systole and diastole. Importantly, pulmonary vascular resistance (PVR) is much lower (70 dyne/s/cm⁵).[4] Consequently, in a normal circulation, RV workload expends only one-sixth of the amount of energy that is needed for the LV to produce the same amount of stroke volume. This difference between the LV and RV can be illustrated in pressure–volume curves, in which there is a lower peak systolic pressure and there are no distinct isovolumetric contraction and

Table 6.4.1 Causes of right heart failure

	Decreased RV contractility	RV volume overload	RV pressure overload
Acute	Sepsis		Pulmonary embolism
	LVAD support		Acidosis
	RV myocardial infarction	Excessive transfusion Excessive fluid management	Hypoxia
	Myocarditis		ARDS
	Perioperative injury or ischaemia (post-cardiotomy syndrome)		Positive pressure ventilation
Chronic	RV cardiomyopathy	Atrial septal defect	Left heart disease
	Arrhythmogenic cardiomyopathy	Pulmonary regurgitation	Left-sided valve disease
		Tricuspid regurgitation	Chronic pulmonary disease
			Obstructive sleep apnoea
		AV malformations, shunts (ASD, VSD)	RVOT obstruction
			Pericardial disease
			Chronic thromboembolic pulmonary hypertension
			Pulmonary arterial hypertension
	Ebstein anomaly		Restrictive cardiomyopathy
		Extreme obesity	
		Transposition of great arteries (atrial repair)	
		Single ventricle (Fontan palliation)	

ARDS, acute respiratory distress syndrome; ASD, atrial septal defect; AV, atrioventricular; LVAD, left ventricular assist device; RV, right ventricular; RVOT, right ventricular outflow tract; VSD, ventricular septal defect.

relaxation phases in the normal pressure–volume relationship of the RV, which contrasts with the LV and RV output, which starts immediately when RV myocardial contraction begins (◆ Figure 6.4.1). Accordingly, the muscle mass of the RV is much smaller than the LV, which makes it more prone to myocardial dysfunction and failure in the context of pressure or volume overload. On the contrary, given its lower myocardial workload, and thus lower oxygen consumption, the RV is less susceptible to ischaemia than the LV, resulting in low likelihood in RV infarction.[4]

Whereas the bullet-shaped LV has a more radial contraction pattern, with both twisting and rotation movements more suited to overcome the high systemic resistance, the contraction pattern of the RV is different and is characterized by three separate mechanisms: (1) inward movement of the RV free wall from the inlet towards the outflow tract, causing a bellows-like effect; (2) longitudinal shortening of myocardial muscle fibres pulling the tricuspid valve towards the apex; and (3) traction of the RV free wall towards the septum, secondary to LV contraction.

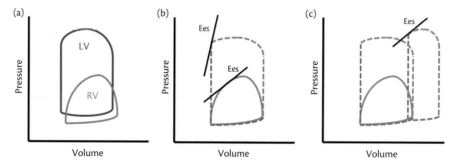

Figure 6.4.1 Conceptual representation of the pressure–volume (PV) relationship of the pressure-loaded right ventricle (RV). (a) PV loops under normal haemodynamic conditions: rectangular PV loop of the left ventricle (LV) (red) illustrating isovolumetric relaxation and contraction phases, and triangular-shaped PV loop of the RV (blue) with absence of clear isovolumetric phases and output starting immediately during systole. (b) In the setting of increased afterload, PV relation of the RV shifts to a more rectangular shape, similar to that for the LV. The diagonal line, representing the end-systolic elastance (Ees), shifts to the left, meaning that contractility of the RV is initially enhanced. (c) With chronically increased pressure load, eventually the RV dilates, leading to increased wall tension and inability of the RV to maintain its contractility, visualized by a rightward shift of the Ees.

Reproduced from TM Gorter *et al. The Right Ventricle in Heart Failure with Preserved Ejection Fraction* (2018) Thesis. With permission from the author. Copyright 2018.

Table 6.4.2 Clinical evidence of right heart failure

Symptoms
Exertional dyspnoea
Fatigue
Orthopnoea
Dizziness
Ankle swelling
Epigastric fullness
Right upper abdominal discomfort
Signs
Jugular venous distension
Peripheral oedema
Hepatosplenomegaly
Ascites
Third heart sound

Source data from Gorter TM, van Veldhuisen DJ, Bauersachs J, et al. Right heart dysfunction and failure in heart failure with preserved ejection fraction: mechanisms and management. Position statement on behalf of the Heart Failure Association of the European Society of Cardiology. Eur J Heart Fail. 2018 Jan;20(1):16–37. doi: 10.1002/ejhf.1029.

This contraction pattern with a high surface-to-volume ratio is more suited to the ability of significantly increasing the stroke volume through the low resistant pulmonary circulation, for instance to meet with increased demand during exercise.[4] Yet, it is also prone to failing in the setting of abnormal loading.

Right ventricular dysfunction

Symptoms

The clinical signs and symptoms of RVD are summarized in ➲ Table 6.4.2.[5,6]

Epidemiology

RVD has many causes and hence, depending on the underlying diseases and their distribution in a given population, the prevalence might differ. Overall, the most common underlying cause of RVD is left-sided HF, be it HFpEF, HFmrEF or HFrEF.[7] Accordingly, reporting exact prevalence rates of RVD is challenging, particularly since the prevalence of RVD depends on the echocardiographic criteria used. For instance, in HFpEF, the prevalence of RVD has been estimated to be between 20% and 30%, depending on whether RV fractional area change (FAC), tricuspid annular plane systolic excursion (TAPSE), or tricuspid annular systolic velocity (RV S′) is used.[8] More recently, also cardiac magnetic resonance (CMR) imaging has been used, which probably relies on more precise measures as it truly assesses changes in volume of a ventricle that is difficult to assess using echocardiography due to its shape and retrosternal position. Using CMR, RVD has been estimated to occur in around 20% of patients with HFpEF.[9]

Besides the imaging criteria used, the stage of left ventricular dysfunction (LVD) obviously is an important determinant of the prevalence of RVD. For instance, with increasing decreases in left ventricular ejection fraction (LVEF), progressive LV myocardial stiffening, and reduced left atrial compliance, left-sided filling pressures are transferred backward to the pulmonary circulation, leading to pulmonary artery pressure (PAP) increases, and hence the pressure load to the RV, which will lead to adverse RV remodelling and eventually RVD. This is even more pronounced as mitral regurgitation (MR) develops with the enlarging LV in more severe HFrEF (➲ Figure 6.4.2).

Furthermore, different exclusion criteria among individual studies in left-sided HF may also affect the prevalence of RVD. For instance, renal dysfunction is associated with PH and, in turn, an increased prevalence of RVD. As such, the prevalence of RVD in left-sided HF may be lower in trials where exclusion criteria led to a selection of patients who are generally healthier than those in real-world registries.

Estimations of the prevalence of RVD in HFpEF is even more challenging, as in the literature, the criteria used to define HFpEF differ, and hence data are not always easy to compare.[8]

Natural history and outcomes

RVD is throughout all cardiac and circulatory conditions associated with bad outcomes and increased mortality. Obviously, as in any cardiac disease, clinical outcomes of RVD depend on the stage and severity of the dysfunction (➲ Table 6.4.3). In patients with severe RVD, mortality is very high and averages at around 40% at 1 year but is dependent on the aetiology of RVD.[7] In a large series of almost 65,000 patients undergoing echocardiography, the combined prevalence of mild, moderate, or severe RVD was 21%. In patients with severe RVD (4% total prevalence), the most common causes were left-sided heart disease in 46%, pulmonary thromboembolic disease in 18%, chronic lung disease in 17%, and pulmonary arterial hypertension (PAH) in 11% of the cases (➲ Figure 6.4.3a). The 1- and 5-year survival rates were: 61% and 33%, respectively, in left-sided heart disease; 76% and 50%, respectively, in PAH; 71% and 49%, respectively, in thromboembolic diseases; but 42% and 8%, respectively, in chronic lung disease (➲ Figure 6.4.3b). Progressive tricuspid regurgitation (TR) and RV–pulmonary artery uncoupling (e.g. reduced TAPSE/systolic pulmonary artery pressure (SPAP) ratio) are associated with much worse survival in severe RVD.[7]

Pathophysiology of right ventricular dysfunction and failure

In a normally unstressed RV, acute pulmonary embolism (PE) leads to acute and severe pressure overload that the thinned-wall RV is not able to cope with. The acute increase in workload leads rapidly to right HF. On the contrary, chronically increased pulmonary pressure in the setting of PAH first leads to adaptive remodelling of the RV, with a leftward shift of the end-systolic pressure–volume relationship and a more rectangular-shaped pressure–volume curve similar to that of the LV, meaning that initially RV contractility is enhanced (➲ Figure 6.4.1a) and the

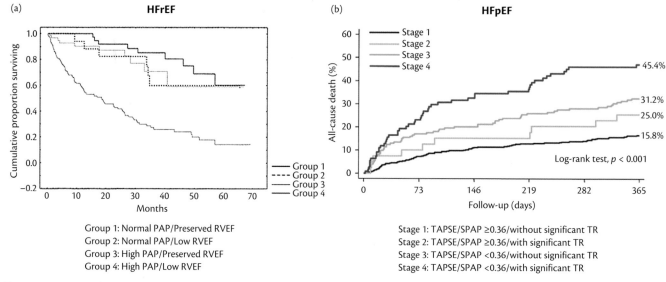

Group 1: Normal PAP/Preserved RVEF
Group 2: Normal PAP/Low RVEF
Group 3: High PAP/Preserved RVEF
Group 4: High PAP/Low RVEF

Stage 1: TAPSE/SPAP ≥0.36/without significant TR
Stage 2: TAPSE/SPAP ≥0.36/with significant TR
Stage 3: TAPSE/SPAP <0.36/without significant TR
Stage 4: TAPSE/SPAP <0.36/with significant TR

Figure 6.4.2 Stages of right heart failure and outcome in left-sided heart failure. PAP, pulmonary artery pressure; RVEF, right ventricular ejection fraction; SPAP, systolic pulmonary artery pressure; TAPSE, tricuspid annular plane systolic excursion; TR, tricuspid regurgitation.

Reproduced from Daubert C, Gold MR, Abraham WT, *et al*; REVERSE Study Group. Prevention of disease progression by cardiac resynchronization therapy in patients with asymptomatic or mildly symptomatic left ventricular dysfunction: insights from the European cohort of the REVERSE (Resynchronization Reverses Remodeling in Systolic Left Ventricular Dysfunction) trial. *J Am Coll Cardiol*. 2009 Nov 10;54(20):1837–46. doi: 10.1016/j.jacc.2009.08.011 with permission from Elsevier. AND Santas E, De la Espriella R, Chorro FJ, *et al*. Right Ventricular Dysfunction Staging System for Mortality Risk Stratification in Heart Failure With Preserved Ejection Fraction. *J Clin Med*. 2020 Mar 18;9(3):831. doi: 10.3390/jcm9030831 with permission from MDPI (http://creativecommons.org/licenses/by/4.0/).

Table 6.4.3 Clinical stages of right ventricular dysfunction and failure

	Stage A	Stage B	Stage C	Stage D
Definition	At risk of RVD without structural or functional abnormalities of the RV (➲ Figure 6.4.6)	RVD without signs or symptoms of RHF (➲ Table 6.4.2)	RVD with prior or current signs or symptoms of RHF (➲ Table 6.4.2)	Refractory RHF requiring specialized interventions
Clinical phenotype	Patients with, for example: ◆ Early stage of PH or exercise PH ◆ LV heart disease or left valve disease ◆ Family history of cardiomyopathy or ARVC ◆ Chronic pulmonary disease ◆ Atherosclerotic disease ◆ Cardiotoxin use ◆ Severe obesity	Patients with structural and/or functional RV disease, irrespective of underlying cause (see stage A), who are normovolaemic and not requiring diuretics	Patients with structural and/or functional RV disease, irrespective of underlying cause (see stage A), who are congested and require loop diuretics	Patients with marked symptoms at rest despite maximal medical, interventional, or surgical therapy or with refractory life-threatening arrhythmias or cardiogenic shock
Echocardiographic features	◆ No RV structural or functional abnormalities ◆ No TR or TR grade 0 with normal PASP (<35 mmHg) ◆ Normal VCI size, with >50% collapsibility	◆ Mild RVD (e.g. TAPSE 14–17 mm) ◆ Concentric remodelling: increased RV mass without RV dilatation ◆ Grade 1 or 2 TR ◆ Mildly increased PASP (35–45 mmHg) ◆ TAPSE/SPAP ratio ≥0.36 ◆ Normal VCI size, with >50% collapsibility	◆ Moderate to severe RVD (e.g. TAPSE <14 mm) ◆ Eccentric remodelling: RV dilatation without septal shift ◆ Grade 3 or 4 TR ◆ Moderately increased PASP (46–60 mmHg) ◆ TAPSE/SPAP ratio <0.36 ◆ Dilated VCI and/or <50% collapsibility	◆ Severely reduced RV systolic function without contractile reserve on inotropes ◆ RV dilatation with septal shift ◆ Grade 3 or 4 TR ◆ Severely increased PASP (>60 mmHg) or low PASP in combination with low-output RV ◆ TAPSE/SPAP ratio <0.36 ◆ Dilated VCI and <50% collapsibility

ARVC, arrhythmogenic right ventricular cardiomyopathy; LV, left ventricular; PASP, pulmonary artery systolic pressure; PH, pulmonary hypertension; RV, right ventricular; RVD, right ventricular dysfunction; SPAP, systolic pulmonary artery pressure; TAPSE, tricuspid annular plane systolic excursion; TR, tricuspid regurgitation; VCI, inferior vena cava.

Source data from Haddad F, Doyle R, Murphy DJ, Hunt SA. Right ventricular function in cardiovascular disease, part II: pathophysiology, clinical importance, and management of right ventricular failure. *Circulation* 2008;117(13):1717–31.

(a) Aetiology of severe RV dysfunction

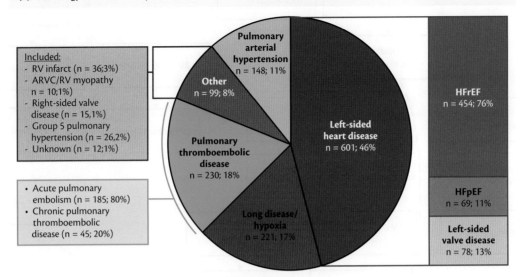

(b) Kaplan–Meier survival based on aetiology of severe RV dysfunction

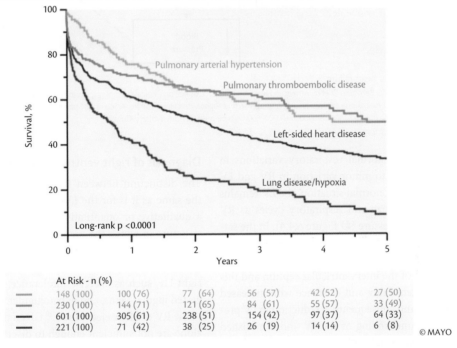

Figure 6.4.3 Aetiology and outcome of severe right ventricular dysfunction. ARVC, arrhythmogenic right ventricular cardiomyopathy; HFpEF, heart failure with preserved ejection fraction; HFrEF, heart failure with reduced ejection fraction; RV, right ventricular.

Reproduced from Padang R, Chandrashekar N, Indrabhinduwat M, *et al.* Aetiology and outcomes of severe right ventricular dysfunction. *Eur Heart J.* 2020 Mar 21;41(12):1273–1282. doi: 10.1093/eurheartj/ehaa037 with permission from Oxford University Press.

increased afterload is well tolerated in the early stages of the disease. However, after long-standing pressure overload, with increased oxygen demand, RV ischaemia, and maladaptive remodelling, the RV dilates and the end-systolic pressure–volume relationship shifts to the right, meaning that RV contractility is reduced, leading to reduced RV stroke volume and ultimately to right HF (➔ Figure 6.4.1c). Consequently, the tricuspid valve annulus also dilates, leading to leaflet malcoaptation and progressive TR, with additional volume overload, increased

central venous pressure, and overt peripheral congestion (➔ Figure 6.4.4).

Because both ventricles are coupled in series and share the interventricular septum and surrounding pericardium, changes in the size, shape, and function of one ventricle have a direct mechanical effect on the size, shape, and pressure–volume relationship of the other ventricle.[10] This phenomenon is termed ventricular interdependence, and both systolic and diastolic ventricular interdependence are involved. Physiological ventricular

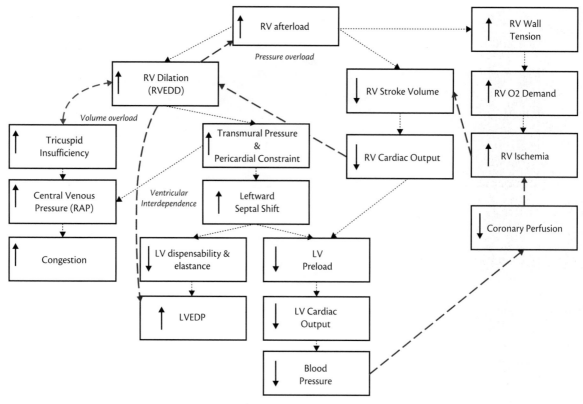

Figure 6.4.4 Pathophysiology of right heart failure.

Reproduced from Konstam MA, Kiernan MS, Bernstein D, *et al*; American Heart Association Council on Clinical Cardiology; Council on Cardiovascular Disease in the Young; and Council on Cardiovascular Surgery and Anesthesia. Evaluation and Management of Right-Sided Heart Failure: A Scientific Statement From the American Heart Association. *Circulation.* 2018 May 15;137(20):e578–e622. doi: 10.1161/CIR.0000000000000560 with permission from Wolters Kluwer.

interdependence is caused by normal respiratory variations in intrathoracic pressures leading to minor variation in RV and LV preload and afterload. In such a normal situation, the LV remains O-shaped throughout the cardiac and respiratory cycles as RV pressure does not exceed LV pressure (➲ Figure 6.4.4). In the setting of increased RV pressure and/or volume overload, RV dilatation and increased transmural pressure within a closed pericardial sac lead to a leftward shift of the interventricular septum and this results in reduced LV distensibility and elastance with increased LV end-diastolic pressure and consequently a reduction in LV preload, leading to effective underfilling of the LV and diminished Frank–Starling recruitment, which ultimately results in reduced cardiac output (➲ Figure 6.4.4).[3] Ventricular interdependence with RV dilatation and leftward septal shift is typically seen in PAH leading to pressure overload and in patients with severe pulmonary regurgitation leading to volume overload. Furthermore, because both ventricles share the interventricular septum and common myocardial muscle fibres, approximately 20–40% of RV systolic pressure and stroke work directly result from LV contraction, because the driving pressure is passed on from the left to the right, via the interventricular septum, and there is traction of the RV free wall near the septal insertion points, secondary to LV contractions.[10] The significance of LV systolic contribution to RV stroke volume is lost when there is severe RV dilatation. In addition, RV systolic function is proportionally reduced when LVEF is reduced and this finding is present in both HFrEF and HFpEF.

Diagnosis of right ventricular dysfunction and failure

The distinction between RV dysfunction and failure is largely the same as it is for the LV—namely, that the former represents a qualitative or quantitative assessment of RV function and/or structure in which the parameter of interest falls outside the recommended range of normal. On the contrary, the latter constitutes a clinical syndrome with typical signs and/or symptoms of right HF, such as exercise intolerance, peripheral oedema, congested jugular veins, and hepatojugular reflux, caused by inability of the RV to fill or eject blood.[10] Given that these signs/symptoms alone are not sufficient enough to discriminate between left- and right-sided HF, cardiac imaging is essential in this context and relies mainly on echocardiography, but more recently also on CMR imaging. Right heart catheterization (RHC) is only performed in selected patients, although it provides precise pressure measurements and this, combined with impedance catheters, provides the most precise information about RV function in relation to afterload.

Echocardiography

Echocardiography is commonly used as the first-line modality in patients with suspected RVD.[11] RV structure and function can be assessed using several methods and parameters (➲ Figure 6.4.5).[8,12,13] Tricuspid annular plane systolic excursion is the most frequently applied parameter in this context and indeed provides prognostic information, independently of

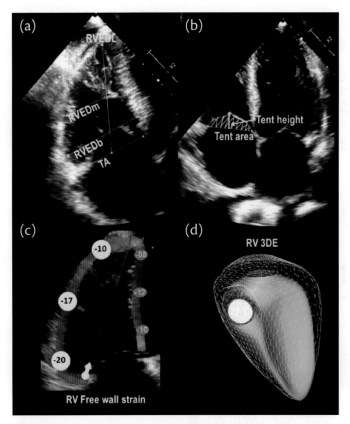

Figure 6.4.5 Echocardiographic assessment of the right ventricle (RV), including: (a) two-dimensional echocardiographic (2DE) RV and tricuspid annulus (TA) dimensions in the RV-focused view at end-diastole; (b) tricuspid valve tenting height and area in the apical four-chamber view during mid systole; (c) RV longitudinal strain of the free wall; and (d) three-dimensional echocardiographic (3DE) endocardial surface reconstruction of the RV in systole (solid) and diastole (mesh). RVEDb, right ventricular end-diastolic base; RVEDm, right ventricular end-diastolic mid; RVEDL, right ventricular end-diastolic length.

Reproduced from Kebed KY, Addetia K, Henry M, Yamat M, Weinert L, Besser SA, Mor-Avi V, Lang RM. Refining Severe Tricuspid Regurgitation Definition by Echocardiography with a New Outcomes-Based 'Massive' Grade. *J Am Soc Echocardiogr.* 2020 Sep;33(9):1087–1094. doi: 10.1016/j.echo.2020.05.007 with permission from Elsevier.

the underlying cause of RVD. The most commonly used cut-off for TAPSE is <17 mm, but some studies have used <16 mm as well. The FAC (RV fractional change or difference between end-diastolic and end-systolic areas measured through an ideally RF-focused apical view) is also used commonly and here the lower limit of normal has been defined as <35%. Of note, the FAC is also predictive of all-cause mortality and HF hospitalization in RVD. Further echocardiographic indices for RVD are RV S' and RV longitudinal strain (➲ Figure 6.4.6).[8]

Finally, three-dimensional echocardiography is increasingly applied for assessment of RV function. Using this technique, an RV ejection fraction (RVEF) of <45% is considered the cut-off for RVD. Further measures to assess primarily RV diastolic function may be pulsed wave Doppler tricuspid inflow patterns (i.e. tricuspid E/A ratio) or hepatic vein diastolic flow, as well as tissue Doppler for lateral tricuspid annular diastolic velocity (e') and right atrial size, commonly reflecting systolic or diastolic dysfunction. Unfortunately, most diastolic indices are also influenced by

age, as the right heart also stiffens, as well as by respiration, heart rate, pulmonary pressure, and other variables, and they have not been widely validated and used in clinical practice, in contrast to LV diastolic indices.

As PH is a major cause of RVD, assessment of PAP during echocardiographic examination is crucial. This includes estimation of pulmonary artery systolic pressure (PASP) by using the TR jet velocity envelope, with addition of the estimated central venous pressure.

It is suggested that RV function cannot be evaluated independently of its load, especially in PH.[14] Therefore, non-invasive parameters for RV–pulmonary artery coupling, such as TASPE/SPAP ratio, in particular, yield important prognostic information in patients with left-sided HF.[7,15]

Further assessments of RVD include RV end-diastolic diameter (normal range <41 mm), RV hypertrophy (normal wall thickness <5 mm), right atrial dilatation (normal right atrial end-diastolic area <18 mm²), RV/LV ratio and septal bowing, and septal bowing and inferior vena cava size and collapsibility for estimation of right atrial pressure (RAP) (➲ Figure 6.4.5). Another informative parameter is RV outflow tract notching on the pulsed wave Doppler profile and peak TR velocity/RV outflow tract velocity.

Cardiac magnetic resonance imaging

The right heart is characterized by a complex geometry, which makes assessment of its function, by using echocardiography, challenging.[9,16] Therefore, CMR is being used increasingly to assess RVD (➲ Figure 6.4.7). Indeed, CMR is able to precisely calculate RV volumes, and hence RVEF. A normal RVEF on CMR imaging is considered to be 45% or higher. An RVEF of <45%, on the other hand, is associated with worse outcomes in a variety of cardiac conditions.

In patients with complex CHD, CMR imaging is often mandatory in follow-up of patients, for prognostic purposes, and for decisions, timing, and evaluation or reinterventions. For instance, phase-contrast imaging of pulmonary flow is the gold standard for correct quantification of pulmonary regurgitation, which is an important item for the timing of pulmonary valve replacement in repaired tetralogy of Fallot, among other parameters.[17]

Furthermore, CMR provides high precision in assessing RV hypertrophy, as well as focal and diffuse myocardial fibrosis using late gadolinium enhancement, T1 time, and extracellular matrix fraction. Lower LV myocardial post-contrast T1 time is associated with higher extracellular matrix and collagen content, and predicts poor prognosis in many cardiac conditions. Late gadolinium enhancement may occur in many cardiac conditions associated with RVD; its location in the septal insertion points of the RV is particularly typical for PH and hypertrophic cardiomyopathy, as well as in LV dysfunction of various types.

Right heart catheterization

The most important threat for the RV is increased pressure load in the setting of PH. For the diagnosis of PH, invasive RHC is mandatory and may provide important information on patients with suspected PH based on echocardiographic signs (e.g. peak TR velocity >2.8 m/s, RV acceleration time <105 ms and /or

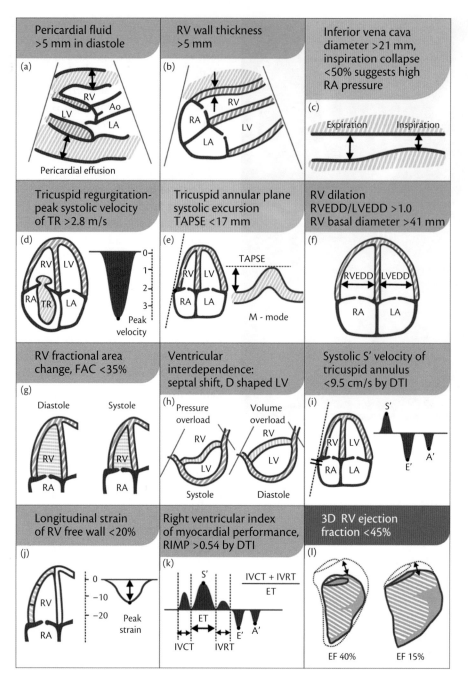

Figure 6.4.6 Echocardiographic assessment of right ventricular dysfunction.
Reproduced from Harjola VP, Mebazaa A, Čelutkienė J, et al. Contemporary management of acute right ventricular failure: a statement from the Heart Failure Association and the Working Group on Pulmonary Circulation and Right Ventricular Function of the European Society of Cardiology. *Eur J Heart Fail*. 2016 Mar;18(3):226–41. doi: 10.1002/ejhf.478. with permission from John Wiley and Sons. AND Reproduced from Gorter TM, Hoendermis ES, van Veldhuisen DJ, et al. Right ventricular dysfunction in heart failure with preserved ejection fraction: a systematic review and meta-analysis. *Eur J Heart Fail*. 2016 Dec;18(12):1472–1487. doi: 10.1002/ejhf.630. with permission from John Wiley and Sons.

mid-systolic notching, RV/LV ratio >1.0, or flattening/bowing of the interventricular septum)[18] or in whom the diagnosis of HFpEF is uncertain based on non-invasive criteria.[19] Conventional measures of RHC that have clinical implications include RAP, RV end-diastolic pressure (RVEDP), PAP, pulmonary capillary wedge pressure (PCWP), cardiac output (CO), and PVR. In the 2022 ESC Guidelines for PH, the definition of PH is mean PAP of >20 mmHg,[18] in line with the 6th World Symposium on PH.[20] The

conventional measures of mean PAP, PCWP, and PVR are further used for the haemodynamic classification of the main PH groups (➲ Table 6.4.4).[21] Furthermore, the 2022 ESC Guidelines, an increase PVR of >2 Wood Units (WU), suggesting the presence of true pulmonary vascular disease, is now also mandatory for the definition of pre-capillary PH.[20] Not surprisingly, the lower mean PAP cut-off of 20 mmHg in combination with a PVR of >2 Wood units used for the definition of isolated post-capillary PH will

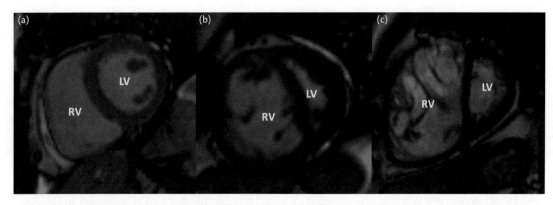

Figure 6.4.7 Cardiac magnetic resonance (CMR) imaging of a normal heart and with right ventricular pressure and volume overload. (a) Normal CMR short-axis image in the end-diastolic phase at the level of the mitral valve papillary muscle, demonstrating thin-walled right ventricular (RV) and normally thickened left ventricular (LV) myocardium that is O-shaped throughout the cardiac cycle. (b) CMR short-axis image of a patient with idiopathic pulmonary arterial hypertension in the end-systolic phase at the level of the mitral valve papillary muscle, showing RV hypertrophy and dilatation and typical end-systolic septal bowing towards the LV. (c) CMR short-axis image in the end-diastolic phase of a patient with repaired tetralogy of Fallot with severe residual pulmonary regurgitation (regurgitation fraction 55%, volume 98 mL, respectively), demonstrating a severely dilated RV, with typical end-diastolic flattening of the interventricular septum, which leads to a D-shaped LV and resulting in underfilling of the LV.

automatically result in a higher prevalence of PH secondary to left heart disease than when the former criteria are used, especially in patients who are not normovolaemic.

The discrimination between PAH and PH secondary to left-sided HF, especially HFpEF, is challenging when there is borderline normal PCWP, since PCWP may be low at rest in patients with early HFpEF who are on optimal diuretic therapy. Furthermore, both elderly patients with 'atypical' PAH and patients with HFpEF may have LV diastolic dysfunction in combination with a preserved LVEF. Therefore, a correct assessment of PCWP is crucial and it should be measured ideally at end-expiration and mid A-wave in a normovolaemic state.[8] In those patients with borderline

normal PCWP where discrimination between PAH and left-sided HF is uncertain, haemodynamic exercise testing or preload augmentation with a fluid challenge or passive leg raise may be useful to better discriminate between isolated pre-capillary PH and combined post- and pre-capillary PH secondary to left-sided HF. This is especially important because for patients with 'true' PAH, PH-specific drugs, such as endothelin receptor antagonists, prostacyclin analogues, and phosphodiesterase type 5 inhibitors, are recommended, but not in HFpEF.[18] Moreover, these PH-specific drugs such as macitentan and prostacyclin are even contraindicated in left-sided HF, because they may result in acute pulmonary oedema and fluid retention.[22]

For selected patients with PAH, pulmonary vasoreactivity testing with inhaled nitric oxide is additionally recommended, to evaluate whether these patients are suitable for treatment with high-dose calcium channel blockers.[18]

For selected cases, more specific invasive measurements can be performed such as for evaluation of intracardiac shunts (e.g. oximetry run in the right atrium and RV and Qp/Qs ratio), and simultaneous RHC and left heart catheterization for evaluation of constrictive pericarditis (e.g. Kussmaul sign, square root sign in the RV and ventricular interdependence).

Right heart failure due to left heart failure

The most important cause of RVD is LVD, be it HFrEF, HFmrHF or HFpEF. Indeed, left HF begets right HF, and hence in patients with RVD, meticulous evaluation of the left heart, the aortic and mitral valves, and pulmonary pressures are essential. HFrEF has been defined by the 2021 ESC Guidelines on the diagnosis and treatment of acute and chronic heart failure[23] as LVEF of <40% with symptoms of HF such as dyspnoea, bendopnoea, and reduced exercise tolerance (except in patients already treated with diuretics or other HF treatments). Also in the intermediate form, heart failure with mid-range ejection fraction (HFmrEF) with an LVEF range of 40–49% has been introduced, but more recent

Table 6.4.4 Haemodynamic classification of pulmonary hypertension subgroups

Definition	Characteristics*	Clinical group(s)
PH	mPAP >20 mmHg	All
Pre-capillary PH	mPAP >20 mmHg PCWP ≤15 mmHg PVR ≥2 WU	1. Pulmonary arterial hypertension 3. PH due to lung diseases 4. Chronic thromboembolic PH 5. PH with unclear and/or multifactorial mechanisms
Isolated post-capillary PH (IpcPH) Combined post-capillary PH (CpcPH)	mPAP >20 mmHg PCWP >15 mmHg PVR <2 WU mPAP >20 mmHg PCWP >15 mmHg PVR ≥2 WU	2. PH due to left heart disease 5. PH with unclear and/or multifactorial mechanisms

DPG, diastolic pressure gradient (diastolic PAP – mean PCWP); mPAP, mean pulmonary artery pressure; PCWP, pulmonary capillary wedge pressure; PH, pulmonary hypertension; PVR, pulmonary vascular resistance; WU, Wood units.

* According to the 6th World Symposium on Pulmonary Hypertension recommendations.[21]

Source data from Galiè N, McLaughlin VV, Rubin LJ, Simonneau G. An overview of the 6th World Symposium on Pulmonary Hypertension. *Eur Respir J* 2019;53(1).

evidence suggests that such patients truly suffer from a milder form of HFrEF as they respond to the same treatment modalities used for HFrEF.[24] HFpEF has been defined as LVEF of >50%, mild to moderate elevations of natriuretic peptide levels, and symptoms of HF. The mechanisms of RVD in the context of HFpEF are essentially the same as those in the setting of HFrEF (see also ⮕ Chapter 6.1).

RV systolic function is often more depressed in HFrEF than in HFpEF,[25] mainly because LV contribution to RV contraction is lost with lower LVEF (see earlier). Furthermore, the RV may be equally involved in the same ischaemic event or intrinsic myocardial disease as the LV (⮕ Acute right ventricular myocardial infarction, p. 340). Hence, RV systolic function and LVEF are closely linked to each other. In HFrEF, RVD may be present in up to 67% of the patients,[25] whereas these prevalence rates are, on average, lower in HFpEF, and dependent on the method used, the prevalence rates in HFpEF are at least 20–30%, but potentially up to 30–50% of the patients.[8] The most important cause of RVD in patients with left-sided HF is PH. Patients with LVD complicated by PH typically have features of more advanced HF, including higher age, longer HF duration, higher prevalence of atrial fibrillation (AF), higher New York Heart Association (NYHA) class, more frequent hospitalization for HF, more diuretic usage, and higher N-terminal pro-B-type natriuretic pepdide (NT-proBNP) levels. Left HF leads to PH via backward transmission of left-sided filling pressures, primarily as a consequence of progressive LV diastolic dysfunction and loss of left atrial compliance and, additionally, by the presence of functional MR (see earlier and ⮕ Chapter 3.3). The majority of patients have isolated post-capillary PH, with only a component of pulmonary venous congestion. However, long-standing pulmonary congestion may result in pulmonary vascular remodelling, leading to a superimposed form of combined post- and pre-capillary PH with higher PVR, higher RV afterload, and more profound RV failure. Currently, this form of PH is diagnosed by both an increased PCWP and an increased PVR (⮕ Table 6.4.4). However, in the setting of left-sided HF, even a high PVR does not automatically indicate irreversible pulmonary vascular disease, because in selected patients with end-stage HF, in combination with high PVR, who received a left ventricular assist device (LVAD), a progressive decrease in PVR and normalization of pulmonary pressures were observed after LVAD implantation.[26]

Some of the drugs approved for PAH (e.g.PDE5-inbitiors: sildenafil, tadalafil; sGC-stimulators: vericiguat, riociguat,; ET-anatgonsist: ambrisentan, bosentan, macitentan; Prostacyclin analogues: i.v. epoprostenol) have been widely tested in PH due to left heart disease (PH-LHD) in both HFrEF and HFpEF, and yet they have either demonstrated no beneficial effect on the primary outcomes or been shown to be even harmful, because pulmonary vasodilatation caused by these drugs in the setting of left heart disease may lead to (acute) pulmonary oedema or peripheral fluid retention.[22] These trials were performed in either various HF patients with no definite PH diagnosis or in cohorts with primarily isolated post-capillary PH. It should be noted that further trials

in patients with PH-LHD should be restricted to those with combined post- and pre-capillary PH, which display true pulmonary vascular disease.[22]

For HFrEF, the primary goal remains treatment of left-sided heart disease using guideline-recommended drugs (see 2021 ESC Heart Failure Guidelines). Improvement in LVEF after initiation and uptitration of guideline-recommended drugs is also accompanied by improvement in RV systolic function.[27] In HFpEF, proper decongestion appears particularly important and SGLT2 inhibitors have been shown to lower pulmonary artery pressure (e.g. EMBRACE-HF trial), albeit there are also no specific therapies recommended for PH secondary to HFpEF.

Irrespective of the type of left heart disease, it remains important that patients are normovolaemic and pulmonary and systemic congestion needs to be treated with adequate diuretic therapy. Intensive management of a patient's volume status is important to prevent development or progression of pulmonary vascular disease, to lower pulmonary pressures and RV afterload, and to prevent the onset and progression of RV remodelling with RV dilatation, progressive TR, and ultimately the development of right HF.[8] Continuous monitoring of pulmonary pressures using an implantable PAP sensor (CardioMEMS™) may be recommended to timely lower pulmonary pressures, primarily using loop diuretics, and to reduce the number of recurrent HF hospitalization, both for HFrEF and HFpEF.[28,29,30]

Besides PH, other factors are also associated with RVD in left-sided HF, including atrial fibrillation (AF), chronic obstructive pulmonary disease (COPD), coronary artery disease (CAD), hypertension, and obesity.[8,25,31] Therefore, modification of relevant comorbidities, such as adequate rate and rhythm control for AF, adequate treatment of significant CAD, systemic hypertension, treatment of COPD and chronic oxygen therapy for severe hypoxaemia, and weight reduction and lifestyle changes for patient obesity and the metabolic syndrome, is recommended.

Valvular heart disease

Tricuspid valve

The tricuspid valve has, as its name reflects, three leaflets that open and close to allow for blood flow from the right atrium into the RV. While tricuspid stenosis is rare, TR of various degrees is seen in at least two-thirds of the general population. Accordingly, mild TR is considered physiological, whereas higher degrees of TR are usually associated with leaflet abnormalities, RVD, and annular dilatation, and are thus considered pathological. Primary or organic TR is caused by congenital or acquired abnormalities (i.e. trauma, pacemaker leads, repeated myocardial biopsies, infective endocarditis, rheumatic fever, or myxomatous degeneration) and accounts for about 8–10% of all TR cases. In contrast, the far more common secondary TR is related to deformation of the tricuspid apparatus due to RVD and RV dilatation. With increasing RV dilatation, the TV annulus dilates initially at the free wall and later in the septal and lateral parts, which leads to increasingly severe TR.

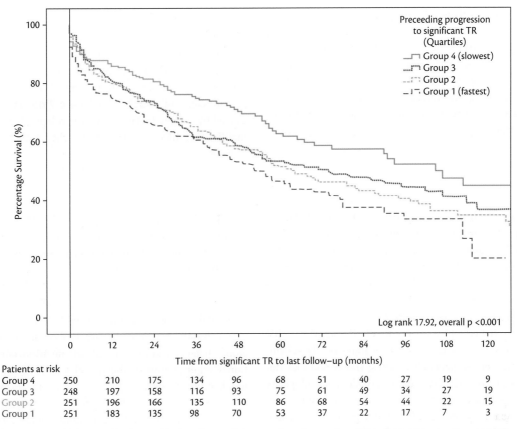

Patients at risk

Group 4	250	210	175	134	96	68	51	40	27	19	9
Group 3	248	197	158	116	93	75	61	49	34	27	19
Group 2	251	196	166	135	110	86	68	54	44	22	15
Group 1	251	183	135	98	70	53	37	22	17	7	3

Figure 6.4.8 Kaplan–Meier survival curve of patients with slow- (group 4), intermediate- (groups 2 and 3), or fast-progressing (group 1) tricuspid regurgitation.
Reproduced from Prihadi EA, van der Bijl P, Gursoy E, *et al*. Development of significant tricuspid regurgitation over time and prognostic implications: new insights into natural history. *Eur Heart J*. 2018 Oct 14;39(39):3574–3581. doi: 10.1093/eurheartj/ehy352 with permission from Oxford University.

The natural history of TR is determined by its severity. In patients without CHD, the major independent determinants of progression are age, pacemaker leads, mild TR at baseline, reduced TAPSE, and annular dilatation.[32] Mortality at follow-up is high and reaches 40% in those with progression to significant TR, particularly in those with fast progression (➲ Figure 6.4.8).

The diagnosis is made clinically and by using echocardiography (➲ Figure 6.4.9).[13] Management of TR has so far been mainly medical, although its effects are rather limited. Diuretics decrease RV overload and, in turn, volume and size, and are thus beneficial initially. In patients with PH, reduction in PVR and pressure by use of endothelin antagonists, prostaglandin analogues, and/ or phosphodiesterase inhibitors might be beneficial (see below).

Surgical repair, or valve replacement, may be considered and is recommended in severe TR by both American and ESC Guidelines.[33] Often, tricuspid annuloplasty and/or repair are simultaneously performed in patients undergoing mitral valve surgery. Indeed, around one-third of patients with MR undergoing surgery have some degree of TR. In some studies, isolated TR surgery has outcomes benefit in those referred early,[34] but guidelines remain more conservative. In those with structural TR, repair may not be possible and valve replacement should be considered, although the results are not convincing. More recently, clipping

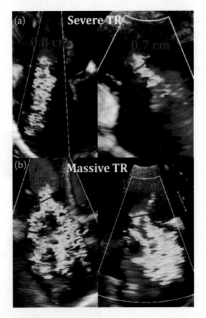

Figure 6.4.9 Colour-flow echocardiography of severe (a) and massive tricuspid regurgitation (b). TR, tricuspid regurgitation.
Reproduced from Kebed KY, Addetia K, Henry M, Yamat M, Weinert L, Besser SA, Mor-Avi V, Lang RM. Refining Severe Tricuspid Regurgitation Definition by Echocardiography with a New Outcomes-Based 'Massive' Grade. *J Am Soc Echocardiogr*. 2020 Sep;33(9):1087–1094. doi: 10.1016/j.echo.2020.05.007 with permission from Elsevier.

has been attempted, with good early results in a small, non-randomized series of highly selected patients[35] and more recently in a randomized trial showing symptomatic but not outcomes benefit.[35a]) Furthermore, the Cardioband®, a percutaneously implantable ring, has been tried, in a smaller, non-randomized series, in patients with mitral valve disease, with reduction in MR and functional improvement,[36] whereas in TR, only few cases have been reported.

Pulmonary valve

Pulmonary stenosis and/or regurgitation, native or post-operative, are common either as an isolated lesion (stenosis) or as part of a congenital heart lesion such as in tetralogy of Fallot.

Congenital pulmonary stenosis is reported in about 7–12% of patients with CHD and may be associated with an atrial septal defect (ASD) or peripheral pulmonary arterial stenosis.[37] Of note, the pulmonary valve is rarely involved in rheumatoid heart disease, endocarditis, or carcinoid syndrome.

Pulmonary stenosis leads to pressure overload of the RV, with modelling and RV hypertrophy, and eventually, if untreated, to RV failure, particularly in patients with severe stenosis. Those with mild to moderate stenosis generally progress slowly and may develop symptoms later on in life. Percutaneous balloon valvuloplasty is the treatment of choice for infants, children, and/or adults, with excellent short- and long-term results.[38] Some patients may come to require either repeat balloon valvuloplasty or pulmonary valve implantation for pulmonary regurgitation, induced at the time or at the index percutaneous intervention, particularly in patients with highly dysplastic pulmonary valves. Balloon valvuloplasty conveys less gratifying results for patients with diffuse pulmonary stenosis such as patients with Noonan syndrome. An extreme, and very rare, variant of pulmonary stenosis is the absent pulmonary valve syndrome, where often the intracardiac anatomy resembles that of tetralogy of Fallot (see below).

Mitral valve

Alterations in mitral valve function, be it stenosis or regurgitation, have profound effects on left atrial structure and function and eventually pulmonary pressures and, as such, is an important cause of RVD. In the Western world, MR is by far the most important cause of mitral valve disease. Primary or organic MR is caused by congenital (mitral valve prolapse)[39] or acquired abnormalities (i.e. infective endocarditis, rheumatic fever, or myxomatous degeneration).

In contrast, the far more common secondary MR is related to remodelling and eventually structural deformation of the mitral apparatus due to, most commonly, LV dilatation in HFrEF associated with premature death.[40] Indeed, with increasing LV dilatation, the mitral valve annulus dilates, leading to increasingly severe MR and, in turn, pulmonary pressures. This eventually leads to pressure overload of the RV, RV hypertrophy, and RVD with TV dilatation and, in the end, TR of increasing degrees. Often such patients also develop AF (➲ Chapter 12.7)) due to remodelling of both the left and right atria.

Commonly, MR and TR are looked at in isolation; yet the global haemodynamic burden arising from concomitant functional regurgitation of the mitral and tricuspid valves appears much more important. As assessed by the proximal flow convergence method, global regurgitant load has significant impact on outcome in HFrEF. The threshold where outcomes of HF are driven by combined valve lesions is a global regurgitant volume of 50 mL, with continuously increasing risk beyond that threshold (➲ Figure 6.4.10).[41]

Management of MR is primarily medical with diuretics, HF drugs, and potentially cardiac resynchronization therapy (CRT) (➲ Chapter 9.2). In more severe forms, surgical reconstruction is the treatment of choice as the technique maintains the subvalvular apparatus, and hence the LV geometry,[42] although not all studies were able to demonstrate superiority as, compared

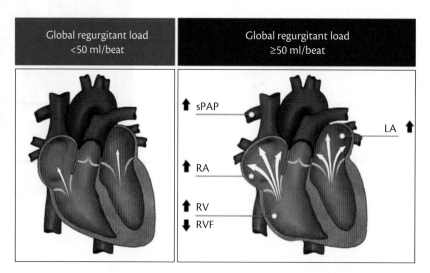

Figure 6.4.10 Global regurgitant volume of mitral and tricuspid regurgitation and haemodynamic consequences. A global regurgitant load of >50 mL/beat is associated with worse outcomes. LA, left atrium; RA, right atrium; RV, right ventricle; RVF, right ventricular function; sPAP, systolic pulmonary artery pressure.
Reproduced from Bartko PE, Arfsten H, Heitzinger G, *et al*. Global regurgitant volume: approaching the critical mass in valvular-driven heart failure. *Eur Heart J Cardiovasc Imaging*. 2020 Feb 1;21(2):168–174. doi: 10.1093/ehjci/jez170 with permission from Oxford University Press.

to valve replacement,[43] RV dysfunction is common after reconstructive mitral surgery. PH, even if reversible after operation, negatively impacted on RV function.[44] In patients with destroyed valves, mitral valve replacement with bioprosthetic or metallic valves is considered. In a substantial percentage of patients undergoing surgery for MR, a TV ring is also implanted due to RVD and TR. Of note, in patients with severe MR, LVEF may be grossly overestimated, and longitudinal strain or, more recently, diffusion tensor imaging with magnetic resonance imaging (MRI) may better reflect true myocardial performance in such patients. Indeed, after surgical repair or valve replacement, LVEF often falls below preoperative values. In patients deemed inoperative or high-risk for surgery, the transcatheter edge-to-edge repair with either the MitraClip[R] or Pascal[R] system is increasingly used, with extremely low operative mortality and excellent symptomatic results.[45] Whether or not outcomes are improved remains controversial, with one trial reporting neutral results[46] and another a reduction in mortality.[47] In contrast to baseline RV function, changes in RV function after MitraClip[R] are independent predictors for survival. Factors associated with decline in RV performance are AF, decrease in LV function, and no reduction in PAP.[48]

Pulmonary arterial hypertension

PH is classified into subgroups based on the haemodynamic characteristics (see earlier) and the underlying aetiology (➲ Table 6.4.4).[22] Around half of patients with PAH have idiopathic, heritable, or drug-induced PAH. Overall, survival of patients with RVD due to PAH is better than that of patients with left heart disease and chronic lung disease leading to RVD.[18] This is mainly the result of better treatment options that are available for PAH patients that directly target the pulmonary vasculature, because reducing RV afterload is the cornerstone in the management of PAH. Currently, three classes of drugs interfering with the endothelin, nitric oxide, and prostacyclin pathways are available in patients with PAH.[49]

Echocardiography, with estimation of PASP, and MRI (➲ Figure 6.4.11) may suggest the diagnosis of PAH, which may be then confirmed with cardiac catheterization and direct measurements of pressures in the LV, pulmonary wedge position, pulmonary artery and RV/RA, and calculation of PVR.

After confirming the diagnosis of PAH, assessing acute vasoreactivity in selected cases, and meticulously ruling out other causes of PH for which PAH drugs are contraindicated (mainly group 2 and 3 PH), the further treatment strategy is based on risk stratification and PAH patients are categorized into low (<5%), intermediate (5–10%), and high risk (>10%), based on a combination of clinical, imaging, and haemodynamic parameters.[18] The basic principle of treatment of PAH is using monotherapy or combination therapy of PAH drugs in order to get, or keep, a patient in the low-risk status with a World Health Organization (WHO) functional class I or II. Most patients with low or intermediate risk initially start with oral combination therapy (e.g. endothelin receptor antagonist plus phosphodiesterase type 5 inhibitor), and patients with high risk preferably start with combination therapy, including an intravenous prostacyclin

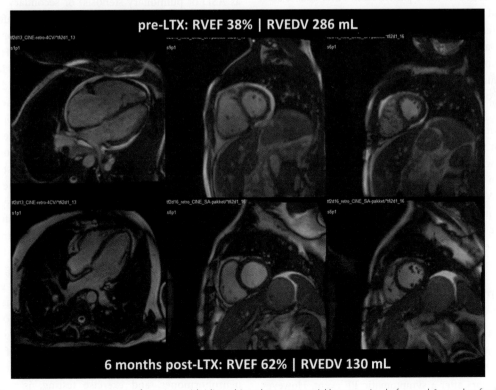

Figure 6.4.11 Cardiac magnetic resonance images of a patient with idiopathic pulmonary arterial hypertension before and 6 months after bilateral lung transplantation. LTX, lung transplantation; RVEDV, right ventricular end-diastolic volume; RVEF, right ventricular ejection fraction.

0analogue.[18,50] When patients remain in intermediate or high risk after 3–6 months, PAH therapy is escalated to combination triple therapy and response to therapy is evaluated every 3–6 months. PAH is a chronic and progressive disease, ultimately leading to severe right HF. In advanced cases that are refractory to maximal medical therapy, bilateral lung transplantation may ultimately be required. When patients survive the perioperative period, almost every RV recovers within weeks to months after bilateral lung transplantation (⊘ Figure 6.4.11).[51,52] Balloon atrial septostomy is available in selected patients as a palliative or bridging procedure to unload the RV.

Chronic lung diseases and/or hypoxia

As described earlier, patients with RVD due to chronic lung disease have the worst prognosis. In patients with COPD, the development of right HF ('cor pulmonale') is associated with a worse prognosis.[53,54] The most important mechanism of RVD in chronic lung disease is chronic hypoxaemia and parenchymal loss and fibrosis leading to pulmonary vascular remodelling, stiffening, and vasoconstriction, resulting in increased PVR, decreased pulmonary compliance, and increased RV afterload. The most prevalent causes of group 3 PH are COPD, interstitial pulmonary fibrosis, and combined pulmonary fibrosis and emphysema. The prevalence of PH in patients with COPD ranges from 30% to 70% in individual studies, whereas the prevalence of PH in other lung diseases is even less clear.[55] The association between the severity of lung disease and the severity of PH is not straightforward and often discrepant; however, these patients with severe PH usually have a low carbon monoxide diffusion capacity. A rigorous diagnostic workup is needed in these patients and other causes such as PH group 2 and 4 need to be ruled out. In addition, it should be clearly evaluated to what extent these patients suffer from PAH. Therefore, patients with chronic lung disease and signs of PH or right HF should be referred to a centre with PH expertise. RHC is also recommended in patients who may qualify for lung transplantation. For patients with isolated group 3 PH, use of PH-specific drugs is not recommended. Treatment is primarily focused on the underlying lung disease, including long-term oxygen therapy in patients with chronic hypoxaemia. RV adaptive remodelling with hypertrophy is common in chronic lung disease, whereas overt RV failure is rare.

Interestingly, RV remodelling and dysfunction may already occur with only minor increases in pulmonary pressures, suggesting that other factors such as hyperinflation, systemic inflammation, and endothelial dysfunction are also potentially involved.[56]

Chronic thromboembolic pulmonary hypertension

In approximately 3.5% of patients with moderate to severe RVD, chronic thromboembolic PH (CTEPH) was the primary underlying cause. CTEPH has a cumulative incidence of 0.1–9.1% within the first 2 years after a symptomatic PE event. However, a significant number of CTEPH patients have no history of a symptomatic PE event. In addition, the symptomatology and clinical signs are often non-specific and resemble those of PAH, and RV function is often preserved in early stages of the disease.[18] Therefore, reaching the correct diagnosis is challenging and takes, on average, 14 months after the first onset of symptoms.[18] The final diagnosis is made after 3 months of anticoagulation treatment, using a combination of RHC (⊘ Table 6.4.4), mismatched perfusion defects on ventilation/perfusion scanning, and specific signs of computed tomography (CT) angiography.[18] After initiation of lifelong anticoagulation, surgical pulmonary endarterectomy is the preferred choice of treatment for all eligible patients, given the relatively low procedural risk and good outcomes with significant symptom relief, near-normalization of haemodynamics, and 3-year survival of 90% after surgery versus 70% for non-operated patients.[18,57] For patients with residual, or recurrent, CTEPH after surgery or those who are inoperable, targeted medical therapy with riociguat is currently recommended, and also the combine ET_A/ET_B-antagonsis Macitentan holds promise in this regard.[18,57] In selected CTEPH patients who are inoperable or have a high risk-to-benefit ratio for pulmonary endarterectomy, balloon pulmonary angioplasty may be considered. However, this option is reserved only for high-volume centres with expertise in this intervention.

Congenital heart disease

Right HF is the end clinical manifestation of many congenital heart conditions, whether operated on or not. Extremely abnormal anatomy such as single ventricle, long-standing volume, and/or pressure overload, as a result of the original lesion (such as ASD or pulmonary stenosis) or secondary to previous intervention (such as pulmonary regurgitation after repair of tetralogy of Fallot, atrial switch procedures for transposition of the great arteries (TGA), and/or ensuing PAH (in a small percentage of patients)), may all contribute to the RV HF phenotype (⊘ Figure 6.4.12). There has been mounting evidence over the past 20 years or so of neuropeptide activation[58] and exercise intolerance[59] in this heterogeneous patient population, which, together with the underlying CHD, suggest the presence of chronic HF.

Although patients with CHD generally respond well to 'rescue' HF therapy, data on elective drug use in most CHD conditions are lacking, with the exception of the extreme end of the spectrum of PAH and CHD, namely Eisenmenger syndrome, whereas practice and patient outlook have been transformed as a result of data on advanced PAH therapy.[60] This is an area that clearly merits attention, and the time is now 'to move from an eminence to evidence-based approach towards managing adult CHD'.[61] For the time being, prevention of right HF in this growing adult patient population is based on early repair, timely reintervention for target haemodynamic lesions, elimination of arrhythmia burden, and optimal lifestyle choices, including diet and exercise. Furthermore, tertiary lifelong surveillance of all patients with CHD with early detection of any decline, incorporating imaging, neurohormones, and exercise testing, is necessary, matched with prompt arrhythmia treatment and timely haemodynamic

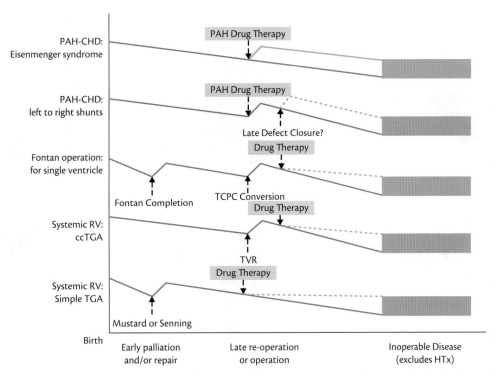

Figure 6.4.12 Adult congenital heart disease subgroups prone to heart failure: drug therapy and potential impact on prognosis. Green box and green line indicate established prognostic benefit. Blue boxes and dotted lines indicate uncertain prognostic benefit. ccTGA, congenitally corrected transposition of the great arteries; CHD, congenital heart disease; HTx, heart transplantation; PAH, pulmonary arterial hypertension; RV, right ventricle; TGA, transposition of the great arteries.
Reproduced from Brida M, Diller GP, Nashat H, Strozzi M, Milicic D, Baumgartner H, Gatzoulis MA. Pharmacological therapy in adult congenital heart disease: growing need, yet limited evidence. *Eur Heart J.* 2019 Apr 1;40(13):1049–1056. doi: 10.1093/eurheartj/ehy480 with permission from Oxford University Press.

intervention/reinterventaion if target lesions are present Mechanical assist device and transplantation are also evolving therapies for this patient cohort and should be considered and discussed with the appropriate patient, in the right setting, before multi-organ failure ensues.[62]

Single ventricle/Fontan palliation

Single ventricle physiology refers to patients with complex CHD who are unsuitable for biventricular repair. This is usually due to a hypoplastic ventricle, and the most common anatomical substrate related to it is tricuspid atresia (with a hypoplastic RV). Francis Fontan from Bordeaux introduced in the early 1970s the radical concept of anastomosing the systemic venous return to the pulmonary arteries, incorporating the right atrium in his early reports, what has since been rightly called the Fontan operation after his name.[1] Following his experiments with dogs, he demonstrated that it is possible to have two separate circulations and a pink patient, without a subpulmonary ventricle, which has since been the standard pathway and direction of travel for most patients with complex CHD and a 'single ventricle physiology'. There have been many modifications of the Fontan operation since, with the latest being the extracardiac total cavo-pulmonary connection (TCPC; ⏩ Figure 6.4.13).

Furthermore, pre-Fontan completion risk factors have been well studied. Thus, patients undergo the Fontan operation with lower perioperative risk and at a younger age, establishing separate pulmonary and systemic circulations, abolishing cyanosis, and offloading the 'single systemic ventricle'. This, is likely to convey better long-term outcomes for contemporary Fontan cohorts than those reported in the literature (85% survival 15 years after the Fontan operation). However, it is unlikely that survival would be normal in patients with single ventricle physiology. Although the concept introduced by Fontan shows that life is possible without a subpulmonary ventricle, there are multiple complications associated with the Fontan physiology, which, in turn, may lead to HF and premature death. With time, central venous hypertension and low CO may result in liver dysfunction, cirrhosis, ascites, varices, hepatorenal syndrome, and the risk of hepatocellular carcinoma. Relatively sluggish pulmonary blood flow increases the risk of thrombus and embolus, especially in the atriopulmonary Fontan (⏩ Figure 6.4.14), which, in turn, increases PVR and central venous pressures. Atrial arrhythmias are common and are the cause and consequence of abnormal Fontan haemodynamics, thus contributing to HF.

Furthermore, any obstruction in the Fontan circuit may have a detrimental effect on haemodynamics and should be actively sought and addressed, if present, in any patient with a failing Fontan circulation. Other complications of the Fontan operation are residual shunts, stroke, protein-losing enteropathy, plastic bronchitis, and systemic ventricular diastolic and systolic dysfunction. The best investment that a patient with a Fontan operation can make after Fontan completion is to remain 'slim and

(a)   (b)   (c)

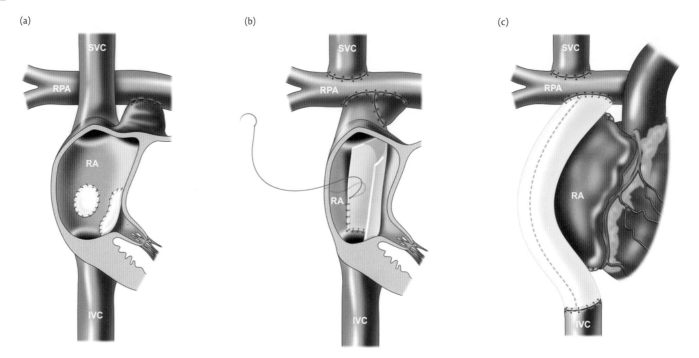

Figure 6.4.13 Fontan modifications. (a) Atriopulmonary Fontan. (b) Total cavo-pulmonary connection (TCPC) with an intra-atrial baffle. (c) Extracardiac TCPC. IVC, inferior vena cava; RA, right atrium; RPA, right pulmonary artery; SVC, superior vena cava.

athletic', the new aspirational mantra for all, particularly relevant to patients with CHD. Female patients at the good end of the Fontan spectrum may have children at relatively low risk, that is, in the right multidisciplinary environment; the best age to have children, in general, is 20–35 years of age, and young age would be an obvious advantage for Fontan patients, reducing pregnancy risks and allowing them to enjoy motherhood.

Systemic right ventricle

There are four types of congenital heart conditions with a systemic right ventricle (SRV), as depicted on ⊃ Figure 6.4.15.[63]

Types C and D are uncommon; they represent a single ventricle physiology and thus abide to the Fontan rules already discussed. Types A and B relate to TGA, with type A in complete TGA following atrial switch procedures (Mustard or Senning

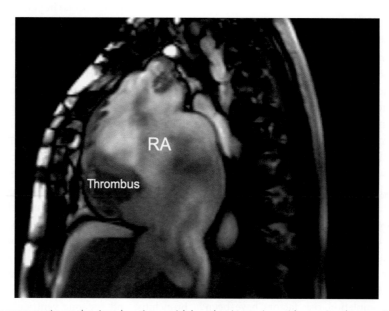

Figure 6.4.14 Cardiac magnetic resonance image showing a large intra-atrial thrombus in a patient with an atriopulmonary Fontan. Note the gigantic right atrium (RA) and 'smoke' in the Fontan flow.
Courtesy of Dr Sonya Babu-Narayan, Royal Brompton Hospital.

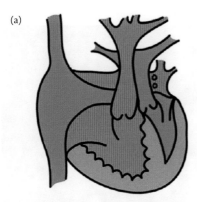

(a)

Complete TGA after Mustard repair
- Systemic RV (hypertrophied and dilated)
- Abnormal AV transport (rigid baffles)
- Sinus node dysfunction, IART, SCD
- SAVV regurgitation secondary to annular dilatation
- Baffle obstructions, leaks, PAH

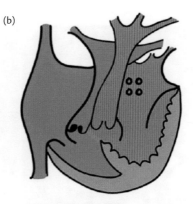

(b)

CCTGA with PS and VSD
- Systemic RV (hypertrophied and dilated)
- "Balanced" circulation (VSD, PS prevents PAH)
- Abnormalities of the conduction system (complete heart block)
- SAVV regurgitation due to intrinsic valve abnormalities

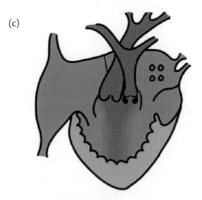

(c)

DIRV, DORV, sub PS
- Systemic RV (hypertrophied and dilated)
- Rudimentary LV located in postero-inferior position
- SubPS prevents PAH, Fontan operation possible
- SAVV regurgitation usually reflects RV disease

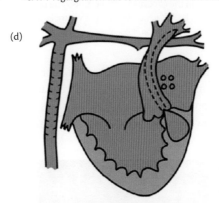

(d)

HLHS – Norwood-Extracardiac Fontan
- Mitral atresia, aortic hypoplasia
- Neo-aorta constructed from pulmonary artery
- RV made systemic (hypertrophied and dilated)
- Extracardiac conduit TCPC Fontan
- Myocardial perfusion insufficiency due to coronary arteries arising from a diminutive aorta

Figure 6.4.15 Basic characteristics of four main congenital heart disease subgroups with a systemic right ventricle. (a) Complete transposition of the great arteries after Mustard repair. (b) Congenitally corrected transposition of the great arteries with pulmonary stenosis and ventricular septal defect. (c) Double-inlet–double-outlet right ventricle with subpulmonary stenosis. (d) Hypoplastic left heart syndrome after Norwood–Fontan operations. AV, atrioventricular; CCTGA, congenitally corrected transposition of the great arteries; DIRV, double-inlet right ventricle; DORV, double-outlet right ventricle; HLHS, hypoplastic left heart syndrome; IART, intra-atrial re-entry tachycardia; LV, left ventricle; PAH, pulmonary arterial hypertension; PS, pulmonary stenosis; RV, right ventricle; SAVV, systemic atrioventricular valve; SCD, sudden cardiac death; TCPC, total cavo-pulmonary connection; TGA, transposition of the great arteries; VSD, ventricular septal defect.

Reproduced from Brida M, Diller GP, Gatzoulis MA. Systemic Right Ventricle in Adults With Congenital Heart Disease: Anatomic and Phenotypic Spectrum and Current Approach to Management. *Circulation*. 2018 Jan 30;137(5):508–518. doi: 10.1161/CIRCULATIONAHA.117.031544. with permission from Wolters Kluwer.

physiological repair) (➲ Figure 6.4.16) and type B in congenitally corrected TGA (ccTGA).

RV dilatation and hypertrophy are universally present as part of SRV remodelling for sustaining the systemic load and circulation. Myocardial perfusion defects are common—maybe, in part, due to demand–supply mismatch through a normal right coronary arterial system—and contribute to RVD. A distinct difference between TGA post-atrial switch and ccTGA is that intrinsic abnormalities of the tricuspid valve (systemic atrioventricular valve) of the Ebstein type are common in the latter and may present as a therapeutic target, namely tricuspid valve replacement (before RV failure ensues). In contrast, TR in simple TGA usually reflects

RVD, and thus tricuspid valve intervention should not be considered in this setting.

Common, time-related complications in patients with an SRV are RVD, HF (➲ Figure 6.4.17), arrhythmias, and sudden cardiac death (SCD). Furthermore, some patients with atrial switch procedures develop atrial baffle obstruction or leak, PAH (≤7%), and clinical deterioration under specific conditions such as pregnancy. SRV dysfunction can develop at any stage, but it is almost uniformly present in older patients, which suggests that the anatomical RV is unable to sustain the systemic load in the long term. Multiple factors have been implicated, including excessive ventricular hypertrophy, SRV remodelling with predominant

(a)   (b)

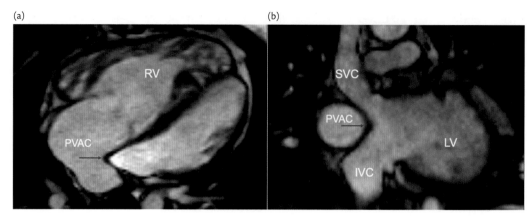

Figure 6.4.16 Cardiac magnetic resonance image showing a patient who underwent a Mustard procedure for complete transposition of the great arteries (TGA). The systemic venous return (SVC and IVC) can be seen directed to the left ventricle via a trousers-like-shaped baffle, with the waist anastomosed at the mitral valve level (a). The remainder of the common atrium (atrial septum is fully excised) allows for the pulmonary venous return to reach the tricuspid valve (PVAC). By creating a second fault in the circulation, patients become pink, albeit they have a systemic right ventricle and the long-term complications associated with it. IVC, inferior vena cava; LV, left ventricle; RV, right ventricle; SVC, superior vena cava.
Figure courtesy of Dr Sonya Babu-Narayan, Royal Brompton Hospital.

circumferential over longitudinal shortening without torsion, as normally found in the systemic LV, impaired atrioventricular transport (rigid atrial baffles), progressive myocardial fibrosis associated with ventricular dysfunction and arrhythmia propensity,

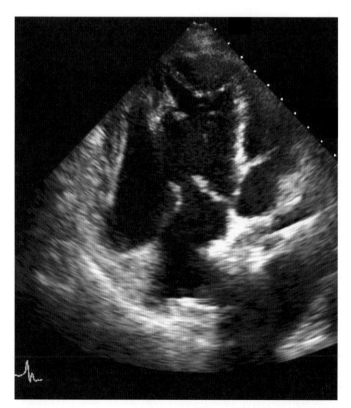

Figure 6.4.17 Two-dimensional echocardiography showing a dilated and hypertrophied right ventricle in a patient who underwent a Mustard procedure for complete transposition of the great arteries. There is right ventricular dysfunction, annular dilatation of the tricuspid valve annulus, with failure of coaptation and thickening of the leaflets, and functional tricuspid regurgitation.
Figure courtesy of Professor Wei Li, Royal Brompton Hospital.

chronotropic incompetence, etc. Furthermore, bradyarrhythmia, tachyarrhythmia, and SCD represent common and potentially devastating late sequelae. Sinus node dysfunction is common in older patients with simple TGA after atrial switch procedures, whereas complete heart block can occur in patients with ccTGA (reported annual risk of 3%) necessitating pacing. The risk of SCD is high among patients with RVD and extensive fibrosis, and primary automatic implantable cardioverter–defibrillator (AICD) implantation should be considered and discussed with the patient.

Management of complications

With regard to management, addressing baffle stenoses with balloon dilatation and/or stenting and occluding shunts or baffle leaks percutaneously have merits. Arrhythmias should be treated promptly; catheter ablation has a role for atrial arrhythmias, most of which have a re-entry mechanism and may relate to the original atrial switch procedure. For patients with ccTGA and intrinsic tricuspid valve abnormalities and moderate to severe TR, as discussed, tricuspid valve replacement should be considered as a prognostic intervention before overt symptoms and advanced RVD ensue. There is some evidence that beta-blockers may play a role, albeit weak, in patients with an SRV. Clearly, more research in this area is needed. Pacing, CRT, and AICDs are all options to consider for the individual patient, together with mechanical assist devices and transplantation for symptomatic patients with recurrent decompensated HF episodes despite optimal therapy.

Tetralogy of Fallot and pulmonary stenosis

Tetralogy (a Greek word meaning 'four things') of Fallot is a condition that was described by Etienne-Louis Arthur Fallot, a French physician, in 1888. He already noticed the four anatomical features of the blue baby syndrome, consisting of: (1) subpulmonary infundibular stenosis; (2) ventricular septal defect (VSD); (3) rightward deviation of the aortic valve, with a biventricular origin of its leaflets; and (4) RV remodelling (i.e. hypertrophy). The diagnosis is invariably made by using echocardiography, often in fetal life nowadays. Patients with tetralogy of Fallot invariably present with cyanosis due to right-to-left shunting at the ventricular level through a large, non-restrictive VSD. Early management consists of intracardiac repair, in some cases after an interim arterial shunt (Blalock–Taussig shunt or Waterston anastomosis), allowing for the infant to grow bigger. Repair of tetralogy of Fallot was first described by Walton Lillehie in Minnesota in the United States in 1955 with cross-circulation. Most patients have a long lifespan, particularly in more contemporary series, whereas repair with VSD closure and relief of RV outflow tract (RVOT) obstruction take place in early life, thus making infants pink and reducing RV pressures to normal or near-normal levels. Aggressive relief of the latter, with liberal use of RVOT or transannular patches and extensive infundibulectomy in early series, leads to severe pulmonary regurgitation, which is well tolerated post-operatively but has detrimental long-term effects.[64] As a result, there has been a change in the management of tetralogy of Fallot, namely: (1) restricting the use of transannular patches and respecting the integrity of the pulmonary valve (as much as possible) during repair in infancy; and (2) employing a proactive pulmonary valve replacement approach in older patients with severe pulmonary regurgitation, before they decompensate, with a view to preserving RV function. A percutaneous pulmonary valve replacement option is also available, particularly suited for patients with a previous conduit type of repair. RV failure is thus uncommon nowadays, with the exception of 'neglected' patients who had repair at an older age, perhaps lost to follow-up, and/or with pulmonary artery hypoplasia and often biventricular involvement. Pulmonary regurgitation and RVOT aneurysm and akinesia are culprit lesions after repair of tetralogy of Fallot, independently associated with RV hypertrophy and dilatation, lower RVEF, and LV systolic dysfunction through an unfavourable ventricular–ventricular interaction.[65] A pilot randomized controlled study of ramipril versus placebo in adults with severe pulmonary regurgitation after repair of tetralogy of Fallot, awaiting surgical pulmonary valve replacement, showed no effect on the RV, but interestingly a beneficial effect on the LV in patients with restrictive RV physiology.[66]

There are variants of tetralogy of Fallot, such as tetralogy with pulmonary atresia or tetralogy with absent pulmonary valve syndrome, which necessitate a conduit type of repair, with the former having more complex and distal diffuse pulmonary artery stenoses and a worse phenotype that merits closer attention. Apart from pulmonary regurgitation, other complications following tetralogy repair are residual RVOT obstruction, residual VSDs, progressive aortic root dilatation with ensuing aortic regurgitation, arrhythmias, and SCD due to myocardial fibrosis (◑ Figure 6.4.18). Haemodynamic targets should be addressed in a timely fashion, whether surgically or percutaneously; optimal timing for pulmonary valve replacement, for example, has evolved and depends on various factors, including severity of pulmonary regurgitation, RV dilatation and RV systolic dysfunction, QRS width, and exercise intolerance.[67] Arrhythmias may be addressed with catheter ablation, whereas AICD implantation as primary or secondary prevention of SCD should be offered, particularly for patients with extensive ventricular fibrosis (◑ Figure 6.4.18).

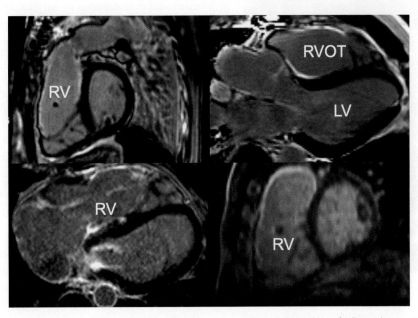

Figure 6.4.18 Cardiac magnetic resonance image with gadolinium enhancement in a patient with tetralogy of Fallot with extensive fibrosis in the right ventricular free wall and the right ventricular aspect of the ventricular septum. The patient was considered for automatic implantable cardioverter–defibrillator (AICD) implantation. LV, left ventricle; RV, right ventricle; RVOT, right ventricular outflow tract.
Figure courtesy of Dr Sonya Babu-Narayan, Royal Brompton Hospital.

Pulmonary stenosis in adulthood

Pulmonary stenosis in adulthood, if native, should be considered for balloon valvuloplasty if moderate to severe (Doppler gradient consistently above 64 mmHg, with signs of RV hypertrophy). For patients with previous intervention, surgical or catheter, the same criteria for reintervention apply as per those in tetralogy of Fallot. Offloading the volume- and/or pressure-loaded RV with pulmonary valve replacement prevents RV failure and improves CO, exercise tolerance, and overall prognosis. Arrhythmias are relatively uncommon but should be addressed promptly. The risk of SCD is lower, compared to that of tetralogy of Fallot, as there is no cyanosis, nor RVOT resection or VSD patching implicated in isolated pulmonary stenosis.

Ebstein anomaly

Ebstein anomaly is a rare malformation of the tricuspid valve and the RV, with quite marked anatomical variability among affected individuals, leading to a wide spectrum of structural alterations, clinical symptoms, and outcomes.[68] Classical and anatomical characteristics of Ebstein anomaly include failure of delamination of the tricuspid valve leaflet from the underlying RV myocardium, apical and downward placement of the functional tricuspid annular hinge points, dilatation of the atrialized portion of the right RV with variable degrees of hypertrophy and thining of the RV wall, anterior leaflet fenestrations and tethering, and finally right atrial ventricular junction dilatation (➲ Figure 6.4.19). As a consequence, different degrees of TR are very common.

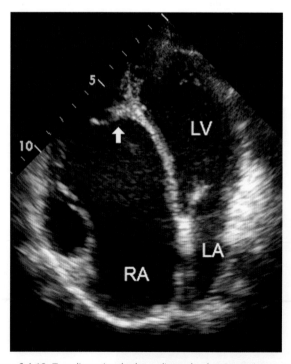

Figure 6.4.19 Two-dimensional echocardiography showing native, severe Ebstein anomaly in a female patient, aged 52, presenting with breathlessness and palpitations. The arrow depicts the grossly displaced tricuspid valve towards the apex. Note the paradoxical position of the ventricular septum, corresponding to the large atrialized portion of the right ventricle. LA, left atrium; LV, left ventricle; RA, right atrium.
Figure courtesy of Professor Wei Li, Royal Brompton Hospital.

The incidence of Ebstein anomaly is around 1 in 200,000 live births. It makes up <1% of all cases of CHD—thus, overall, quite a rare condition.[68] The clinical presentation is quite variable, as the age and presentation of symptoms depend on the anatomical and functional severity of the disease. Arrhythmias, particularly ectopic atrial tachycardia, atrial flutter, and AF, are the most common presenting symptoms in adults. Other clinical features of Ebstein anomaly during adulthood are exercise intolerance, exertional dyspnoea or fatigue, occult cyanosis, and right HF. There is an association of Ebstein anomaly with Wolff–Parkinson–White syndrome, and supraventricular tachycardia related to the latter may be the presenting feature in early life.

Diagnosis is made by imaging, particularly using echocardiography, providing detailed characterization of the tricuspid leaflets, subvalvular apparatus, RV, and right atrium, respectively.[69] However, MRI is also increasingly used. Of note, RV enlargement and RVD result in a paradoxical motion of the intraventricular septum and, less commonly, may lead to LV outflow obstruction. Therefore, LVD may also develop as a result of abnormal intraventricular interaction.

Late presentation of Ebstein anomaly is not uncommon and may be associated with decreased life expectancy due to biventricular failure in severe cases. SCD may also occur due to ventricular arrhythmias. The accumulative overall survival in unoperated adult patients with Ebstein anomaly has been estimated to decrease from 90% at 1 year follow-up to <50% at 20-year follow-up. The clinical phenotype of patients with Ebstein anomaly is very variable; data on operated patients reflect intention-to-treat cohorts. Predictors of unfavourable outcome are extent of tricuspid valve displacement, NYHA classes III and IV, cyanosis, severe TR, and younger age at diagnosis.

As arrhythmias, in particular atrial flutter and AF, are common complications of Ebstein anomaly, electrophysiological assessment and percutaneous or surgical ablation are recommended, beyond operative tricuspid valve repair and plication of the atrialized RV. In general, repair of native Ebstein anomaly in adulthood is only considered for patients with refractory arrhythmia, progressive exercise intolerance, and good TV anatomical substrate. Further, women of reproductive age, willing to have a child maybe considered for surgical repair. Atrial communications, in the form of patent foramen ovale (PFO) or ASD, are common in the setting of Ebstein anomaly and often lead to occult cyanosis, with secondary erythrocytosis. They should not be closed percutaneously, in the presence of severe Ebstein anomaly, as they may address cyanosis but also exaggerate right HF. If deemed necessary, defect closure should take place with tricuspid valve surgery.

Atrial septal defect

ASD is a direct communication between the two atrial chambers that permits shunting of blood normally from left to the right, or right to left, depending on hemodynamic conditions. ASDs are the most common CHD defects presenting in adult hood and are classified into secundum defects (oval fossa, most common ASD type), primum defects (partial atrioventricular septum defect), superior or inferior sinus venosus defects (➲ Figure 6.4.20), coronary sinus defects, and confluent or common atrium.

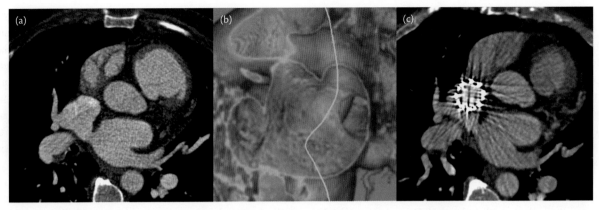

Figure 6.4.20 Computed tomography sequences in a patient with superior sinus venosus atrial septal defect (ASD) undergoing percutaneous repair. (a) Axial CT image demonstrating anomalous drainage of the right middle lobe to the base of the superior vena cava (SVC) at the same level as a superior sinus venosus ASD. (b) Three-dimensional reconstruction demonstrating the superior sinus venosus ASD from the left atrium. The middle lobe pulmonary vein is visible through the defect. The course of the SVC is marked by the green line, and the pink tube is a virtual representation of a covered stent diverting venous flow. (c) Axial CT section at the same level as in (a), demonstrating placement of an SVC stent with a patent pulmonary venous channel posterior to the stent, diverting pulmonary venous flow to the left atrium via the superior sinus venosus ASD.
Figure courtesy of Dr Tom Semple, Royal Brompton Hospital.

The natural history of individuals born with uncorrected ASD is associated with atrial arrhythmias, exercise intolerance and dyspnoea, reduced life expectancy, in particular, starting from the third decade of life due to the development of PH, and, in turn, eventually congestive right HF.[70] However, some patients remain remarkably well and symptom-free throughout adulthood, but with an increased risk of premature death due to progressive RV dilatation, right-sided HF, recurrent pneumonia, PH, atrial flutter, and AF,[71] and paradoxical emboli and stroke later in life. As such, ASD closure is recommended either surgically[72] or increasingly today with catheter-based interventions—remarkably, including for patients with sinus venosus ASDs and partial anomalous pulmonary venous drainage (➲ Figure 6.4.20), in the presence of RV dilatation, irrespective of age.[73] Indeed, ASD closure in adulthood has recently been shown to be associated with normal survival in mid- to longer-term follow-up.[74] There are occasional patients with an ASD who present with PAH that is out of proportion at a relatively young adult age. These patients are the exception to the rule, in that historically PAH and pulmonary vascular disease were very late complications affecting a minority of patients in late adult life. Tertiary expertise in ACHD and PAH are required in managing this so-called grey zone where ASD closure may not be in the interest of the patient in the long term and advanced PAH therapies may have a role instead. There has been interest in a treat-and-repair approach; however, long-term evidence is lacking to support it. Older patients who benefit from late ASD closure remain at risk of arrhythmia, and thromboprophylaxis should be given serious consideration at least for the first 12 months after closure, while reverse remodelling takes place and they are at risk of pulmonary and systemic embolic events.

1. Axial CT image demonstrating anomalous drainage of the right middle lobe to the base of the SVC at the same level as a superior sinus venosus ASD

2. 3D reconstruction demonstrating the superior sinus venosus ASD from the left atrium. The middle lobe pulmonary vein is visible through the defect. The course of the SVC is marked by the green line and the pink tube is a virtual representation of a covered stent diverting venous flow

3. Axial CT section at the same level as in a) demonstrating placement of an SVC stent with a patent pulmonary venous channel posterior to the stent, diverting pulmonary venous flow to the left atrium via the superior sinus venosus ASD

Ventricular septal defect

A VSD can occur as a congenital condition or after acute myocardial infarction.

Congenital ventricular septal defect

A congenital VSD is an opening in the ventricular septum, occurring either in isolation or in the context of another CHD, with a prevalence of 2 in 1000 live births. VSDs are the most common congenital cardiac anomalies in childhood. VSDs are classified into perimembranous (most common), muscular, and doubly committed subarterial defects. VSDs lead to left-to-right and/or right-to-left shunting; the degree and direction of shunting depends on the size of the defect and PVR. Most commonly, VSDs are associated with a left-to-right shunt; in the presence of a large shunt (i.e. Qp/Qs 1.5/1.0), this will lead to increased pulmonary blood flow, increased filling pressures of the RV and LV, and dilatation of the left atrium and LV, and ultimately to RVD.

The diagnosis of VSD is often already made clinically with the presence of a loud systolic murmur and confirmed by echocardiography. Large VSDs should be closed in infancy to prevent the development of PAH. So-called restrictive VSDs, meaning VSDs with low right-sided pressures and large Doppler gradients across them, where the risk of developing early PAH is low, may still allow for a large left-to-right shunt and volume overload of the left atrium and LV, respectively. Such VSDs may be considered for elective closure beyond infancy, particularly if associated complications develop with time (aortic cusp prolapse with early aortic regurgitation, recurrent endocarditis, atrial arrhythmias, and, in some, double-chambered RV (discussed further below). Patients from a different era, where early diagnosis was not the norm, with a moderate-sized or large unoperated VSD presenting in adulthood used to have a reduced life expectancy, with 25-year survival of 86% and 62%, respectively. Such patients develop LV failure and pulmonary vascular disease, with some eventually progressing to Eisenmenger syndrome.

VSDs have been closed traditionally surgically, but today more and more catheter-based closure devices have been used, with excellent results in those with isolated VSDs and normal right-sided pressures, leading to improved functional class and a likely normal life expectancy. Thus, such patients may not need tertiary, lifelong follow-up. However, RV dilatation and hypertrophy with RVD have been reported in some patients with uncomplicated VSD late after successful closure, with an associated abnormal ventilatory response to exercise,[75,76] suggesting an individualized approach and follow-up arrangements by physicians taking care of ACHD patients.

Post-infarction ventricular septal defect

A specific form of VSD occurs after acute myocardial infarction and is associated with markedly worse outcomes. Post-/peri-infarction VSDs were relatively common in the pre-thrombolysis area, while with reperfusion therapies, first with thrombolysis and now with primary percutaneous coronary intervention (PCI), have become very rare except in late presenters, mainly in those with STEM of the left anterior descending coronary artery. If patients develop this mechanical complication, associated mortality remains extremely high.[77] A peri- or post-infarction VSD leads to an acute volume and pressure overload of the RV, with an increase in RV volume and eventually—if untreated—RV failure, cardiogenic shock, and death.

The preferred treatment is still surgical with closure of the defect with a patch.[78] Percutaneous device closure of post-myocardial infarction VSD is an alternative to surgical repair, with the advantage of immediate shunt reduction, thereby unloading the RV and preventing haemodynamic deterioration of the RV. Although the procedure is often technically successful, mortality remains high, especially in cardiogenic shock patients.[79] The 2017 European Society of Cardiology (ESC) Guidelines for the management of acute myocardial infarction in patients presenting with ST-segment elevation (STEMI)[80] recommend to consider implantation of an intra-aortic counterpulsation balloon pump.

Double-chambered right ventricle

A double-chambered RV is characterized by anomalous or hypertrophied muscle bundles, which cause subvalvular RVOT obstruction dividing the RV into a high-pressure proximal and a low-pressure distal chamber.[81,82] As such, the RV is a tripartite structure consisting of the inlet (i.e. the sinus portion), the trabeculous apex (i.e. the body of the chamber), and the outlet (the cornus or infundibulum). The mechanisms of obstruction in this condition may be due to anomalous muscle bands, hypertrophied endogenous trabecular tissue, or, in some cases, a moderator band. The majority of patients with a double-chambered RV have a coexisting restrictive VSD, and this is a recognized complication of the latter and indeed one of the reasons for long-term follow-up.

Double-chambered RV is a progressive condition, and gradients across the obstruction are not always easy to ascertain; if there is moderate stenosis with any signs of RV hypertrophy, elective surgical relief should be offered. The risk of recurrence is very small, and the pulmonary valve is not implicated; thus, there is no need for further intervention for the majority of patients (contrary to pulmonary valve stenosis or tetralogy of Fallot). Adult patients with undiagnosed, neglected, or unrepaired double-chambered RV can present with symptoms such as angina pectoris, syncope, dizziness, dyspnoea on exertion or even at rest, or lower extremity swelling. With further severity of obstruction, there may be right-to-left shunting across the VSD, leading to cyanosis and clubbing. A diagnosis relies primarily on echocardiography and other imaging modalities such as cardiac MRI, but also cardiac catheterization may be helpful in this context.

Arrhythmogenic right ventricular cardiomyopathy

ARVC has recently been renamed arrhythmogenic cardiomyopathy (ACM), as it also may involve the LV, and not only the RV.[2] ACM is a polygenic myocardial disease, with a predominantly autosomal dominant inheritance, leading to progressive ventricular myocyte loss and replacement by fibrous and adipose tissue (➲ Figure 6.4.21). Whereas initially the RV is affected, at later stages, the LV can also be involved. Fibrous and fatty remodelling of the RV leads to a typical ECG pattern with negative T-waves in the precordial leads, with ventricular tachcardia or even ventricular fibrillation being often the first clinical manifestation and eventually leading to RVD and RV failure and sudden death.

Epidemiology

The prevalence of ACM is estimated to range from 1 in 5000 persons in the general population to 1 in 2000 in some European countries such as Italy and Germany[83] where it seems more prevalent. About half of the affected patients have a family history of the disease, but both incomplete penetrance and limited phenotypic expression are common and may account for an underestimation of its prevalence as a familial disease.

Genetics

Causative genetic mutations, mainly affecting proteins of the intercalated disc, particularly the desmosome, a large intercellular junctional protein complex responsible for mechanical coupling of myocytes, have been identified in patients with ACM. Thus, most likely up to 60% of ACM cases are familial, but disease penetrance is incomplete and seem to become more pronounced in males and with advancing age (using in the thirties and forties) and excessive physical exercise. The most common mutations

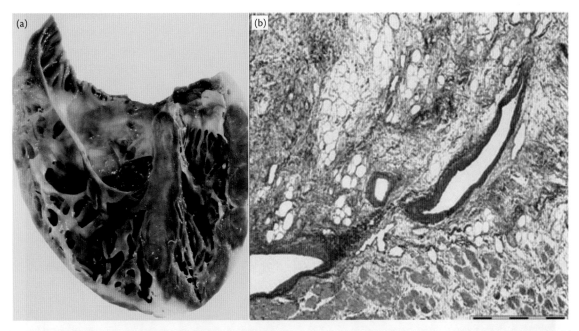

Figure 6.4.21 Macroscopic appearance (a) and histology (b) of the right ventricle in a patient with arrhythmogenic cardiomyopathy. Note the right ventricular myocardium is thinned out and in part substituted by fibrous fatty tissue.

Reproduced from Saguner, A., Brunckhorst, C., and Duru, F., Die arrhythmogene rechtsventrikuläre Dysplasie/Kardiomyopathie, *Cardiovascular Medicine* 2011;14(11):303–314; https://doi.org/10.4414/cvm.2011.01623 https://creativecommons.org/licenses/by-nc-nd/4.0/.

involve desmosomal genes such as *PKP2* (10–45%), followed by *DSP* (10–15%), *DSG2* (7–10%), and *DSC2* (2%). Non-desmosomal genes, such as *TMEM43* p.P358L and *PLN* p.R14del are much less common but can be prevalent in certain populations because of a founder effect.

Diagnosis

The diagnosis of ACM involves ECG patterns, endomyocardial biopsy (EMB), RV endocardial voltage mapping (EVM), and imaging using echocardiography and cardiac MRI. In the 12-lead ECG, ACM typically displays negative T-waves in leads V1–V3 (→ Figure 6.4.22). EMB is not considered routine and should be reserved for special cases. Echocardiography is the first choice,

but increasingly contrast-enhanced cardiac MRI is more often used, as it provides the best tissue characterization (→ Figure 6.4.23).[84] Tissue characterization documenting both fibrous and fatty remodelling of the RV with RVD is essential to distinguish ACM from other conditions affecting RV function.

Management

Management of patients with ACM involves family screening, lifestyle counselling, and implantable cardioverter–defibrillator (ICD) implantation, if required. The phenotypic expression of ARC may be accelerated in individuals taking up excessive physical activities, particularly competitive sports. Indeed, competitive sports is associated with a 2-fold increased risk of ventricular

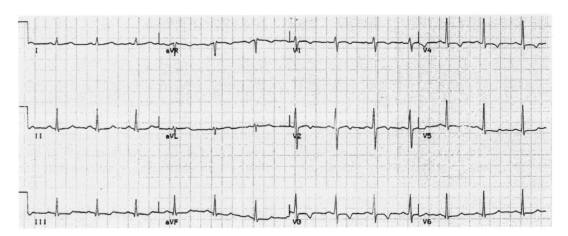

Figure 6.4.22 Electrocardiogram of a patient with arrhythmogenic cardiomyopathy and typical negative T-waves in leads V1 to V4.

Reproduced from Corrado D, van Tintelen PJ, McKenna WJ, *et al*; International Experts. Arrhythmogenic right ventricular cardiomyopathy: evaluation of the current diagnostic criteria and differential diagnosis. *Eur Heart J*. 2020 Apr 7;41(14):1414–1429. doi: 10.1093/eurheartj/ehz669. with permission from Oxford University Press.

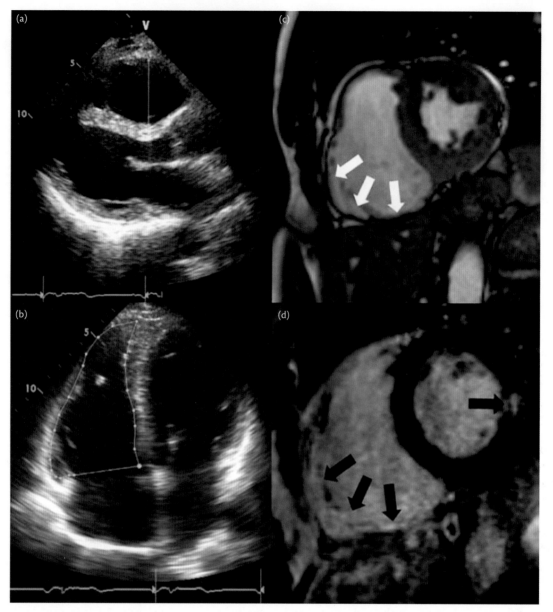

Figure 6.4.23 (a) Transthoracic echocardiography (TTE) (parasternal long axis) demonstrating dilatation of the right ventricular (RV) outflow tract (end-diastolic diameter 22.4 mm/m²). (b) TTE (apical four-chamber view) revealing dilatation of the right ventricle (38 cm²) and akinesis of the RV apex and subtricuspid area, a major criterion for arrhythmogenic right ventricular cardiomyopathy, according to the Revised 2010 Task Force Criteria. (c) Cardiac magnetic resonance (CMR) imaging confirming RV dilatation (end-diastolic volume index 130 mL/m²), with globally reduced RV ejection fraction (34%), wall thinning, and akinesis/dyskinesis of the RV apex and inferior and subtricuspid wall (white arrows). (d) Contrast-enhanced CMR imaging showing late gadolinium enhancement within the RV and left ventricular (LV) lateral wall (black arrows), indicating LV involvement.

arrhythmias and sudden death, as well as an earlier presentation of symptoms, when compared to physically inactive individuals and those who participate only in recreational exercise.[85]

Pharmacological management of ACM may involve HF drugs (➲ Section 8), but there are no randomized trials providing evidence for the effectiveness and safety of such an approach. Thus, use of angiotensin-converting enzyme (ACE) inhibitors, beta-blockers, and/or mineralocorticoid receptor antagonists remains largely empirical. Antiarrhythmics should only be used in patients with ICDs, if required, to reduce the arrhythmia burden.

Catheter ablation has a role in symptomatic management of patients with documented ventricular tachycardia or fibrillation,

with syncope and potentially SCD, and the only effective preventive strategy is implantation of an ICD. The major criteria for use of ICD are: (1) aborted SCD; (2) sustained ventricular tachycardia lasting over 30 seconds; (3) a history of syncope; and (4) marked RVD with FAC of <24% or RVEF of <40% or LVEF of <45%. In highly selected patients with severe RVD and LV involvement, heart transplantation may be considered (➲ Chapter 11.4).

Right ventricular remodelling and Covid-19

It is well established by now that cardiovascular injury occurs in the setting of coronavirus disease 2019 (Covid-19) infection; indeed, cardiac injury, as reflected by increased troponin levels, is present in a significant number of patients with Covid-19 and they are particularly elevated in those with an unfavourable outcome, including mortality. Given the fact that Covid-19 is associated with a high risk of lung involvement, a key focus area is therefore adverse RV remodelling. In a large study involving 510 patients, RV dilatation and RVD were present in 35% and 15% of patients, respectively. Of note, RVD increased stepwise in relation to RV chamber size. The presence of RVD increased the mortality risk, with a hazard ratio of 2.6, and indeed patients without adverse RV remodelling were more likely to survive to hospital discharge, with a hazard ratio of 1.4. In an adjusted analysis, adverse RV remodelling provided a more than 2-fold increase in mortality risk.[86]

Pulmonary embolism

When thrombi within the leg veins, and particularly in veins of the pelvis and the vena cava, dislodge and embolize in the pulmonary circulation, PVR rises acutely, leading to pressure overload of the RV, with initial increases in RV volume, D-shape of the RV, and increases in biomarkers, and eventually RVD and RV failure.[87] Accordingly, patient outcomes in the acute phase of PE is determined by the presence and severity of RVD.[88] An easy and highly predictive variable of mortality is systolic blood pressure at presentation (➲ Figure 6.4.24).[89]

Diagnosis

CT pulmonary angiography (CTPA) is the imaging modality of choice for confirming or ruling out acute PE.[90] However, the diagnostic strategy depends on whether the patient is haemodynamically stable or not. In the unstable patient, the pretest probability of PE is high, but other conditions such as cardiac tamponade, acute coronary syndromes, aortic dissection, acute valvular dysfunction, and hypovolaemia have to be excluded.

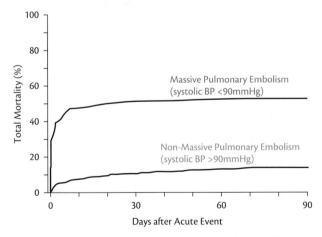

Figure 6.4.24 Total mortality in patients with massive (systolic blood pressure <90 mmHg at presentation) and non-massive pulmonary embolism. BP, blood pressure.
Reproduced from Kucher N, Rossi E, De Rosa M, Goldhaber SZ. Massive pulmonary embolism. *Circulation.* 2006 Jan 31;113(4):577–82. doi: 10.1161/CIRCULATIONAHA.105.592592 with permission from Wolters Kluwer.

Transthoracic echocardiography (TTE) is essential in assessing RVD. Indeed, if acute PE is the cause of haemodynamic decompensation in a highly unstable patient, RVD may provide enough certainty of PE to enable proceeding to immediate reperfusion without further testing. Cardiac MRI is also a very useful diagnostic tool for stable patients with PE but is not readily available in the emergency setting.

In the haemodynamically stable patient, plasma levels of D-dimer should be obtained, with a negative D-dimer allowing for PE to be ruled out. On the other hand, D-dimer levels are not very useful in patients with a high clinical probability of PE, due to its low negative predictive value in such patients.[87]

Risk assessment

Initial risk stratification of acute PE is based on clinical symptoms and signs of haemodynamic instability. In haemodynamically unstable patients with PE, outcomes depend on clinical examination, imaging, and laboratory signs of PE such as D-dimer levels,[91] with severity of RVD on TTE or CTPA being most important. The *Pulmonary Embolism Severity Index* (PESI) involves age, sex (with males doing worse), and heart rate >110 bpm, as well as a history of cancer, HF, or COPD. In addition, elevated cardiac biomarker levels (i.e. troponins, brain natriuretic peptide) are useful to further assess the risk in haemodynamically stable PE patients.[92]

Anticoagulation

Unfractionated heparin (UFH), given as an intravenous infusion, is the recommended initial anticoagulant in haemodynamically unstable patients and those with serious renal impairment (creatinine clearance (CrCl) ≤30 mL/min); dosing is adjusted based on the activated partial thromboplastin time.

High-risk pulmonary embolism

In acute high-risk PE, correction of hypoxaemia and haemodynamic support of the failing RV are important. Emergency reperfusion treatment with systemic intravenous thrombolysis is the treatment of choice in this population.[93] Surgical pulmonary embolectomy[94] or percutaneous treatment with ultrasound catheters, commonly with i.a. low-dose thrombolysis,[95] can be considered in those with contraindications to thrombolysis and/or a high bleeding risk in centres with appropriate experience and resources.

Intermediate- and low-risk pulmonary embolism

For most haemodynamically stable patients with acute PE, parenteral or oral anticoagulation without thrombolysis is appropriate.

If anticoagulation is initiated parenterally, low-molecular weight heparin (LMWH) or fondaparinux are preferred over UFH.[96] Normotensive patients with at least one indicator of elevated PE-related risk, or with aggravating conditions or comorbidity, should be hospitalized. Due to the risk of early haemodynamic decompensation, initially stable patients with signs of RVD and elevated troponin levels should be hospitalized and monitored for several days, whereas systemic thrombolysis is not recommended due to increased bleeding risk and limited expected benefits. Rescue thrombolytic therapy, surgical embolectomy, or percutaneous catheter-directed treatment[95] should be reserved for those with haemodynamic decompensation.

Selected patients with low-risk PE, based on clinical criteria and no RVD, may be considered for early discharge and outpatient anticoagulation.[97]

Follow-up

PE patients should be seen 3–6 months after an acute episode. Any dyspnoea or functional limitation and signs of recurrent venous thromboembolism (VTE), cancer, or bleeding should be assessed for carefully. Extended anticoagulation should be considered in those at increased risk of recurrence (i.e. history of PE, cancer, or comorbidities), according to guidelines.[87]

Post-cardiotomy syndrome

The post-cardiotomy syndrome is defined as a worsening or new development of a pericardial or pleural effusion, commonly weeks after cardiac surgery, as a result of an autoimmune reaction with the pleural and/or pericardial space.[98] The incidence of the post-pericardiotomy syndrome varies widely and may occur in around any cardiac, valvular, or aortic surgery. The syndrome is often associated with some fever, increases in C-reactive protein level, and urgent, rather than elective, procedures and post-operative antibiotic use. In general, corticosteroid therapy resolves the problem, while pericardial or pleural drainage is necessary in only a minority of patients. In a small minority, constrictive pericarditis may develop with dyspnoea and RV HF.

Myocarditis

Background

Myocarditis is an inflammatory response within the myocardium due to a variety of causes, including viruses and, rarely, bacterial or parasitic infections, as well as autoimmune responses (see also ➲ Chapter 12.9). As to the mechanism, several lines of evidence suggest that susceptible individuals mimic peptides from commensal bacteria that can promote the generation of a pool of potentially heart-reactive T-cells.[99] Consequently, viral or, less commonly, bacterial infection damage the heart with the resultant immune reaction that promotes heart-reactive T-cells, rather than direct effects of the agents themselves. Similarly, also medications, vaccines, trauma, and ischaemia can cause tissue damage and promote heart-reactive T-cell responses and antibodies specifically directed against the heart muscle. In genetically predisposed individuals, myocarditis may be also the presentation of a systemic autoimmune disease with myocardial involvement.

Clinical presentation

In the Western world, acute myocarditis typically develops shortly after a viral infection, presenting with malaise, chest pain, palpitations, and signs and symptoms of HF. Less frequently, myocarditis presents with tachy- or bradycardia arrhythmia and rarely with SCD.[100] The clinical course of myocarditis differs vastly. Full-blown myocarditis is defined as myocarditis that leads to severe HF within 4 weeks of symptom onset, requiring medial and/or mechanical LV support. The most common aetiology appears to be viral or autoimmune in nature. Less frequent causes are hypersensitivity and toxic reactions to drugs, as well as giant cell myocarditis—a rare, but particularly aggressive, form of myocarditis that is commonly associated with autoimmune reactions. Giant cells (i.e. confluent macrophages) are pathognomonic for this disease entity upon histological examination of biopsies.

Diagnosis

Proper diagnosis of myocarditis requires EMB, which continues to be the gold standard but does not achieve 100% sensitivity due to sampling errors when the tissue is obtained (as the RV may not be homogenously affected). Therefore, multiple samples should be obtained and immunohistochemistry should be performed to detect CD3-expressing T-cells or CD68-expressing monocytes. The diagnosis of inflammatory cardiomyopathy requires at least seven CD3-positive T-cells for at least 14 CD68-positive monocytes per high-power field during microscopy.

Since myocarditis, in most cases, is transient in nature within days to a few weeks with standard HF therapy, or even resolves spontaneously, EMBs are not warranted in the majority of cases. However, a myocardial biopsy is required in fulminant myocarditis, unexplained and malignant arrhythmias with suspected myocarditis, and HF in spite of optimal therapy.

The ECG provides variable features such as concave ST-segment elevations, commonly less pronounced than in ST-segment elevation infarction without reciprocal changes, prolonged atrioventricular conduction, premature ventricular contractions, or ventricular tachycardia. To detect RV involvement, besides clinical signs of jugular vein congestion and peripheral oedema, echocardiography is required. Typical findings are reduced RVEF, RV dilatation, and regional wall motion abnormalities. Cardiac MRI is particularly useful, with late gadolinium enhancement, due to myocardial necrosis being common and rather specific, as well as oedema formation based on T2 algorithms.[101] As mentioned earlier, MRI is particularly suitable for detecting RV involvement, compared to echocardiography.

Management

Management of myocarditis also involving the RV is similar to HF, in general with beta-blockers, ACE inhibitors, and diuretics, although not really evidence-based. Patients with fulminant myocarditis may require inotropes and mechanical support up to extracorporeal membrane oxygenation (ECMO; ➲ Mechanical circulatory support and extracorporeal membrane oxygenation, p. 340) and ventricular assist devices (VADs), primarily in tertiary centres where such equipment is available.

Ventricular arrhythmias may be treated with intravenous amiodarone, and a LifeVest® may be considered for a few weeks to months before a final decision for implantation of an ICD can be made. Indeed, the latter should be avoided as much as possible, as ventricular arrhythmias recover in most instances. The same applies for RV pacing if bradyarrhythmias occur. Steroids and immunosuppressive agents may be considered in sarcoid myocarditis or vasculitis.

Chronic inflammatory cardiomyopathy is defined as markedly reduced ejection fraction after an acute episode of myocarditis beyond 6 months. In these patients, prednisone, potentially in combination with azathioprine, mycophenolate, or ciclosporin, can be considered, although, convincing evidence is lacking. With pericardial involvement, usually chest pain occurs that is currently treated with non-steroidal anti-inflammatory drugs (NSAIDs). Of note, RV myocarditis may mimic ACM (⊃ Arrhythmogenic right ventricular cardiomyopathy, p. 332), which may be differently diagnosed using three-dimensional electro-anatomical mapping-guided EMB.[102]

Acute right ventricular failure and intensive care management

Acute RV failure is a rapidly progressive syndrome, evidenced by systemic congestion and an acute reduction in CO. The overall prevalence of acute RV failure is unknown, but it accounts for 3–9% of all acute HF (AHF) admissions and is associated with in-hospital mortality of 5–17%, depending on the underlying aetiology. In critical care, acute RVD occurs in up to 58% of patients with severe acute respiratory failure (SARF), and in those with acute respiratory distress syndrome (ARDS), the incidence of acute RV failure is 35–50%, depending on the severity of the underlying disease and the mechanical ventilatory settings.[12,103,104]

The RV is highly vulnerable in the acute and critical care settings, as numerous factors associated with critical illness either worsen RV failure and/or acute RV failure is compounded by interventions intended to support the acutely critically ill patient. The effects of acute RV failure are twofold: (1) reduction in CO; and (2) increase in venous pressure, with consequent effects on all organ systems, including renal congestion and failure. RV failure must be addressed rapidly, and all potentially reversible contributing factors rapidly reversed.

When considering an approach to managing acute RV failure, a number of factors must be considered:

1. The anatomical position of the RV and structural cardiac abnormalities (i.e. sub-systemic, subpulmonary, univentricular, intracardiac communication or shunts, pulmonary stenosis or regurgitation, among others; ⊃ Congenital heart disease, p. 324)

2. Preceding pathological status of the RV (normal or volume or pressure overload, i.e. PH; ⊃ Pulmonary arterial hypertension, p. 323)

3. Current pathological insult

4. Any ongoing interventions or situations that might exacerbate RV failure.

This section will address acute failure of the subpulmonary ventricle in a structurally normal heart, and detail management options in the most critical settings, including monitoring, preload/afterload management, pharmacological support, optimal ventilatory strategies and use of percutaneous mechanical support.

How the right ventricle adapts to acute illness

Certain physiological principles must be regarded when considering acute RV failure. First, although chronic adaptation to afterload increase is heterometric (Starling's law), an acute increase in afterload results in homeometric/systolic functional adaptation (Anrep's law) within minutes. If there is insufficient adaptation, there is resultant limitation of CO, leading to hypotension and shock, and RV dilatation results in sarcomere damage, diastolic dysfunction, and further systemic congestion. The duration of systole increases and may impact not only right, but also left, heart filling.

This acute increase in afterload leads to a number of downstream molecular changes which are only just beginning to be understood (⊃ Table 6.4.5).[105]

Second, although under normal conditions, the RV has a lower oxygen requirement than the LV due to its lower myocardial mass and pre- and afterload acutely and during stress, its oxygen extraction reserve is greater. Normally the RV is perfused in both systole and diastole, but as afterload (and PASP) increases, the tendency for ischaemia increases due to restriction of perfusion to diastole alone and, if it occurs on the basis of chronic elevation of afterload, increased RV myocardial mass.

It is the combination of acute afterload increase plus ischaemia (either type I or II insult) that has been shown to critically compromise CO in acute RV failure. The heart will usually respond by appropriately developing relative tachycardia.

All interventions to treat acute RV failure aim to address the physiological basics of preload, afterload, contractility, optimizing the heart rate to maintain the coronary perfusion pressure, and most importantly rapidly intervening to treat the underlying cause.

Table 6.4.5 Anrep's law of the heart: molecular mechanisms underlying myocardial stretch

◆ Release of angiotensin II

◆ Release of endothelin

◆ Activation of mineralocorticoid receptors

◆ Transactivation of epidermal growth factor receptors

◆ Increased formation of mitochondrial reactive oxygen species

◆ Activation of redox-sensitive kinases upstream of myocardial Na^+/H^+ exchanger (NHE1)

◆ Increase in intracellular Na^+ concentration

◆ Increase in Ca^{2+} transient amplitude through the Na^+/Ca^{2+} exchanger

Source data from Cingolani HE, Pérez NG, Cingolani OH, Ennis IL. The Anrep effect: 100 years later. *Am J Physiol Heart Circ Physiol* 2013;304(2):H175–82.

A systematic approach to right ventricular support in acute/critical illness

As acute RV failure is complex and must be rapidly addressed, a systematic approach is required with repeated re-evaluation and reassessment to determine the effects (beneficial or detrimental) of any intervention. Numerous algorithms have been suggested that are intended to simplify assessment and management (➲ Figure 6.4.25).[12] All include the following measures to be considered:

1. Optimize the volume status: avoid overfilling/diuresing.

2. Reduce the afterload (i.e. PVR):
   a. Use pulmonary vasodilators (preferably inhaled such as nitric oxide).
   b. Treat reversible causes (e.g. low oxygen, low pH, high carbon dioxide, sepsis).

3. Improve RV systolic function:
   a. Treat reversible causes (e.g. ischaemia, arrhythmia, valvular disease).
   b. Maintain right coronary artery perfusion.
   c. Inotropy.

4. Treat any coexisting/contributing factors that may contribute:
   a. PE (➲ Pulmonary embolism, p. 335), dysrhythmias (including ensuring relative tachycardia where required), LV dysfunction, optimizing ventilation, optimizing cardiac electromechanics (including maintaining relative tachycardia—up to 110–120 bpm in some cases).

5. Consider temporary (usually percutaneous) mechanical circulatory support (MCS).

Standard monitoring will depend upon critical illness severity and determined by local/regional guidance informed by national/international guidelines.[106] Factors that are relevant to guiding management of acute RV failure include heart rate, blood pressure, central venous pressure (CVP) (number and waveform), ECG, echocardiography, pulmonary artery catheterization, arterial blood gases (including degree of acidaemia), chest radiography and lung ultrasound, and importantly ventilatory parameters (where used).

Volume status/preload optimization

Initial studies aiming to determine the optimal preload status for the right heart in the context of acute myocardial infarction (see also ➲ Acute right ventricular myocardial infarction, p. 340)

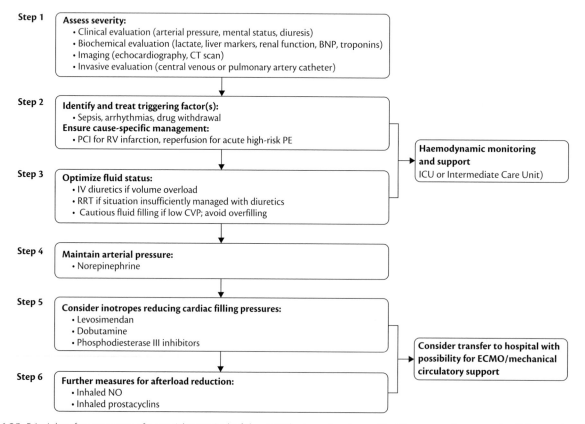

Figure 6.4.25 Principles of management of acute right ventricular failure. BNP, brain natriuretic peptide; CT, computed tomography; CVP, central venous pressure; ECMO, extracorporeal membrane oxygenation; ICU, intensive care unit; IV, intravenous; NO, nitric oxide; PCI, percutaneous coronary intervention; PE, pulmonary embolism; RRT, renal replacement therapy; RV, right ventricular.

Reproduced from Harjola VP, Mebazaa A, Čelutkienė J, *et al.* Contemporary management of acute right ventricular failure: a statement from the Heart Failure Association and the Working Group on Pulmonary Circulation and Right Ventricular Function of the European Society of Cardiology. *Eur J Heart Fail.* 2016 Mar;18(3):226–41. doi: 10.1002/ejhf.478. with permission from John Wiley and Sons.

suggested that maintaining a CVP of <10 mmHg by using normal saline was considered optimal; however, later studies reported a variable response to filling and suggested an optimal CO could be maintained by aiming for a target PCWP of 18–24 mmHg.[107] More recent studies in RV myocardial infarction (RVMI) have suggested combining echocardiographic and haemodynamic data, and demonstrated that maximal RV stroke work index (RVSWI) was associated with filling pressures of 10–14 mmHg, a mean RAP of >14 mmHg was associated with RV distension, and although the haemodynamic response to filling was variable, optimal PCWP (corresponding to maximum LV stroke work index (LVSWI)) was 16 mmHg.[108] Ideally, a transmural pressure of 8–12 mmHg, adjusted according to CO and central venous oxygen saturation ($ScvO_2$) and systemic organ perfusion, can be used, but these parameters are not generally available outside the research setting.[109]

Critical illness adds a further layer of complexity where the mode and parameters of ventilation, rapidly changing volume status due to sepsis/vascular permeability/insensible losses, and the effects of changing doses of analgesia and sedative agents on systolic blood pressure must additionally be taken into consideration.

Maintenance of aortic root pressure for right ventricular perfusion

Vasopressors should be used to avoid systemic arterial hypotension and maintain aortic root pressure (for RV perfusion). To that end, systemic pressures must be above pulmonary pressures with an optimal PVR/systemic vascular resistance (SVR) ratio. The ideal vasopressor would increase systemic pressure and RV contractility without increasing PVR.[110]

The most commonly used agent is noradrenaline, which, at dosages of <0.5 µg/kg/min, increases SVR while reducing PAP, and hence the PVR/SVR ratio. It also exerts some positive inotropic effects via β1-adrenergic receptors, thereby increasing cardiac index and improving RV–pulmonary coupling. Where noradrenaline doses are increasing (generally with >0.23–0.25 µg/kg/min), low-dose vasopressin (0.01–0.03 U/min) may be used as a pulmonary vasodilator, peripheral constrictor, and potential noradrenaline-sparing agent. If doses are escalating, the overall management strategy of the patient should be reconsidered, and all data re-evaluated.

Inotropes and inodilators

To improve impaired RV contractility, inotropes are the treatment of choice. Inotropes are a diverse collection of pluripotent molecules with differing pharmacological properties and shared activities, only one of which is positive inotropy. They will increase dP/dt, with variable effects on CO and cardiac index, alter myocardial oxygen demand, and are variably pro-arrhythmogenic.

There are no high-quality data to suggest any one inotrope is superior to another. Dobutamine has favourable pulmonary vascular effects at dosages of <5 µg/kg/min, whereas high dosages of >10 µg/kg/min should be avoided as they increase PVR and induce tachycardia and systemic hypotension. In contrast, dopamine and adrenaline are not recommended, as they increase myocardial oxygen consumption and induce tachycardia and arrhythmic events.

Inodilators, including milrinone and levosimendan, may be useful in acute RV failure. Milrinone, a phosphodiesterase type 3 inhibitor, inhibits cyclic adenosine monophosphate (AMP) breakdown, increases calcium influx, and, in turn, improves myocardial contractility. Levosimendan is a calcium sensitizer with positive inotropic and lusitropic effects, thereby increasing RV cardiac contractility and improving RV diastolic function, without increasing oxygen consumption, and also exerts some vasodilatation. Experimental evidence suggests that levosimendan improves RV–arterial coupling and might preserve an adequate ventilation/perfusion ratio. However, two randomized, placebo-controlled trials with levosimendan in patients undergoing cardiac surgery provided no advantage of the compound over conventional inotropic drugs in perioperative low CO syndrome. Use of inodilators usually demands concomitant administration of vasoconstrictors to maintain arterial pressure.

Specific pulmonary vasodilators may be more useful to reduce RV afterload in acute RVD. Inhaled nitric oxide (iNO) is an ideal and potent pulmonary vasodilator at 5–40 ppm, with a rapid onset of action and a very short half-life. It is particularly useful in PH and/or hypoxaemia in critically ill patients in whom lowering PAP and improving RV function are essential. This may be the case in severe PH where right-sided systole becomes prolonged and limits filling time on the right (and potentially left) heart. Where not available, nebulized prostacyclin may be considered.

Oral pulmonary vasodilators, such as endothelin receptor antagonists, soluble guanylyl cyclase stimulators such as Riociguat, or the phosphodiesterase type 5 inhibitor sildenafil are not recommended in the acute setting, largely due to their systemic haemodynamic effects, but may be useful once patients are haemodynamically stable and in the longer term. These agents should be started in conjunction with a PH multidisciplinary team.

Right ventricular-protective ventilatory strategies

Both respiratory disease itself and positive pressure ventilation can result in acute RVD and eventually failure. Echocardiographic parameters that should be evaluated include RV dimensions, alteration in TAPSE, reduction in s′ wave on tissue Doppler imaging (TDI), and induction of restrictive RV physiology (seen in 48% of patients in critical care with SARF[104] and associated with positive end-expiratory pressure (PEEP), plateau pressure (Pplat), and carbon dioxide levels. Further, critical illness is associated with increased PVR, which may be worsened in the presence of hypoxic pulmonary vasoconstriction (due to alveolar, pulmonary arterial/bronchial, and arterial hypoxaemia), which is, in turn, worsened by acidaemia. Here the focus is on reducing pulmonary vascular tone by judicious use of pulmonary vasodilators, minimizing PEEP and Pplat, maintaining normoxia, avoiding acidaemia and normocarbia, and ventilating at/near functional residual capacity (FRC).[111] Bronchodilators and drainage of any pleural infusions should be considered, and patient–ventilator dyssynchrony may require paralysis. These basic manoeuvres should be considered in every patient with acute RV failure who is ventilated.

Mechanical circulatory support and extracorporeal membrane oxidation

In SCAI (Society for Cardiovascular Angiography and Interventions) class C–E patients[112] (INTERMACS 1-2)[113] not responding to, or deteriorating despite, conventional interventions, acute MCS may be indicated.[106,114] Depending on the acuity and underlying aetiology, the RV may exhibit a greater capacity for rapid recovery, compared to the LV. Indeed, >50–75% of patients with acute RV failure with a reversible underlying cause recover after device implantation, allowing for device explantation. Percutaneous MCS (pMCS) for RV support may be used as 'bridge to recovery', 'bridge to decision', or 'bridge to transplantation' in some. A number of devices exist, the choice of which generally depends upon the requirement for concomitant oxygenation, relative contraindications to pMCS, concomitant left-sided dysfunction, the underlying aetiology and likely duration of support required, and tolerance to anticoagulation, as some right-sided devices can be run on no/minimal anticoagulation.[114] A major additional driver is local medical and nursing expertise. The decision to institute pMCS should be in discussion with the shock team, as complication rates are high and there is significant medical and nursing expertise required for optimal outcomes.

Conditions requiring specific interventions

A number of specific conditions requiring particular consideration exist. These include acute RV infarction, post-cardiotomy RVD, and post-transplantation and LVAD dysfunction or failure.

Acute right ventricular myocardial infarction

Due to the much lower pressures in the RV, coronary blood flow occurs during both systole and diastole unless severe RV hypertrophy has occurred. Most commonly, RVMI occurs with occlusion of a dominant right coronary artery, proximal to the marginal branches, which supply the right lateral RV wall. In patients with left dominance, occlusion of the left circumflex, and rarely also the anterior descending coronary artery, may affect the lateral and apex of the RV, respectively.[115]

Prevalence

The incidence of RVMI patients with inferior infarction ranges widely from 20% to 80%, depending on the population, as well as on the criteria and imaging modality used in different studies. The most common form is in combination with an inferior infarction, and very rarely as an isolated form. The presence of RV hypertrophy increases the susceptibility of the RV to ischaemia, leading to pronounced RVD in such patients during an inferior infarction or isolated RVMI.

MRI may be much more sensitive in detecting myocardial infarction using late gadolinium enhancement, compared to echocardiography. In the acute setting in the catheterization laboratory, during primary PCI, RVMI may often be overlooked unless it is very severe.

Clinical presentation

Depending on the size of infarction and the degree of dysfunction, the features of RVMI range from peripheral congestion to cardiogenic shock.[116] The classically described hypotension with clear lung fields, and elevated jugular venous pressure in a patient with inferior infarction is a typical clinical finding of RVMI but only occurs in a minority of patients. Similarly, the Kussmaul's venous sign (i.e. distension of the jugular vein upon inspiration) not only occurs in constrictive pericarditis, but also has been shown to occur in RVMI. Thus, clinical signs are not sufficiently sensitive or specific.

RAP may be markedly elevated and exceed the PCWP, similarly to CVP which may mimic the *dip-and-plateau* pattern of constrictive pericarditis. The most severe complications involve ventricular septal rupture, thrombus formation and embolization, TR, and pericarditis, due to frequent transmurality of RVMI.

Patients with predominant RV shock are younger, have a lower prevalence of previous myocardial infarction, and often have multivessel disease and a shorter median time between the index MI and the diagnosis of shock, in comparison to patients with LV shock. RV infarction, in particular when not revascularized, has a prognosis worse than many malignancies if it requires intensive care unit (ICU) admission. For all patients, in-hospital mortality is high (around 53%), with revascularization being as effective under both conditions. In multi-variant analysis, RV, compared to LV shock, was not an independent predictor of lower in-hospital mortality.[117]

Diagnosis

A 12-lead ECG is not always helpful, and a right precordial lead may be required to show ST-segment elevation or changes.[118] Right bundle branch block and complete heart block may also occur, as may life-threatening ventricular arrhythmias. Echocardiography may demonstrate RV dilatation and wall motion abnormalities of the lateral wall and the interventricular septum. Although CMR is generally considered a better imaging modality for the RV, this technique is usually not available in the acute setting, but most useful in the chronic phase.

Management

Besides pPCI, the treatment strategy for RVMI should include maintenance of RV preload and reduction of RV afterload with intravenous fluids in particular.[107] Careful volume loading guided by pulmonary artery catheterization may be considered to guide management, in particular in those requiring inotropic support. If AV block occurs, transient or permanent pacing may be required. Where conventional therapy is insufficient, pMCS may be considered (➲ Mechanical circulatory support and extracorporeal membrane oxygenation, p. 340).

Right ventricular dysfunction post-cardiac surgery

RVD is common post-cardiac surgery where the combination of cardiopulmonary bypass (CPB) and pericardiotomy leads to a reduction in long axis function and longitudinal strain, together with an increase in radial function.[119] By contrast, acute RV failure can occur post-cardiac surgery, resulting from a number of potential factors, including ischaemia, microemboli, air emboli, and/or volume loading, and may be severe, resulting in cardiogenic shock. Acutely (in the operation room), this may be due to elevation in PVR from a protamine reaction.

Post-operative acute RV failure is associated with increased mortality, morbidity, and prolonged length of stay. Management relies on the principles of critical care management of acute RV failure. However, two specific options should be considered. First, where there is any chance the right coronary artery might have been compromised (i.e. coronary implantation or coronary anatomy unknown prior to dissection repair), coronary angiography should be undertaken as a matter of urgency. Second, where severe RV failure occurs, a tight pericardium should be considered, and consideration given to stenting the chest open, even in the absence of a pericardial collection. Finally, where CO is borderline, other measures to consider are reducing enteral feed to trophic levels only (reduces the risk of ileus and further impairment of venous return) and, if the patient is pyrexial, active or passive cooling.

Right ventricular failure post-left ventricular assist device implantation and heart transplantation

RVD and RV failure are relatively frequent complications following LVAD implantation, occurring in up to half of patients, and represent a major cause of post-operative morbidity and mortality.[120] For a haemodynamically successful LVAD implantation, the output of the RV has to match the work of the support device. Thus, initially, this is associated with an increase in RV preload, and to allow for appropriate accommodation of the RV, PVR has to be decreased in order to improve compliance and maintain RV performance, and eventually TR may increase. Preoperative risk factors for post-operative RV failure after LVAD implantation may include female sex,[121] preoperative circulatory failure, presence of end-organ dysfunction (e.g. liver, kidney), haematological alterations, severe RV systolic dysfunction, pulmonary vascular disease, and presence of severe TR. By contrast, certain haemodynamic parameters indicate a lower likelihood to develop acute RV failure, including CVP ≤8 mmHg, PCWP ≤18 mmHg, PVR <2 Wood units, and RVSWI ≤400 mmHg mL/m^2. A scoring system for prediction of RV failure after long-term LVAD implantation has been developed and validated.[122] However, there are no validated predictors of acute RV failure after implantation of short-term percutaneous LVADs. Where acute RV failure occurs, scrupulous attention to good ICU management of the RV is mandated.[121]

Primary graft dysfunction affects ≥7% of patients post-heart transplantation and is the leading cause of early mortality.[123] It may affect either or both ventricles, and diagnosis of RV involvement alone requires a number of parameters to be present: RAP >15 mmHg; PCWP >15 mmHg; CI <2.0:/min/m^2; transpulmonary gradient <15 mmHg; and PASP <50 mmHg (or the need for RV MCS). This complication is most likely related to a combination of insults to the RV, including those related to brain death of the donor, cardioplegia, intermittent and prolonged ischaemia of the donor organ, and reperfusion injury, as well as persistently raised PVR in the recipient. This significantly contributes to early death after heart transplantation. Here, in the event that acute RV failure develops post-transplant and does not respond to standard right heart interventions, a decision should be made early regarding MCS.[3]

References

1. Fontan F, Baudet E. Surgical repair of tricuspid atresia. Thorax 1971;**26**(3):240–8.
2. Corrado D, van Tintelen PJ, McKenna WJ, *et al.* Arrhythmogenic right ventricular cardiomyopathy: evaluation of the current diagnostic criteria and differential diagnosis. Eur Heart J 2020;**41**(14):1414–29.
3. Konstam MA, Kiernan MS, Bernstein D, *et al.* Evaluation and management of right-sided heart failure: a scientific statement from the American Heart Association. Circulation 2018;**137**(20):e578–622.
4. Haddad F, Hunt SA, Rosenthal DN, Murphy DJ. Right ventricular function in cardiovascular disease, part I: anatomy, physiology, aging, and functional assessment of the right ventricle. Circulation 2008;**117**(11):1436–48.
5. Daubert C, Gold MR, Abraham WT, *et al.* Prevention of disease progression by cardiac resynchronization therapy in patients with asymptomatic or mildly symptomatic left ventricular dysfunction: insights from the European cohort of the REVERSE (Resynchronization Reverses Remodeling in Systolic Left Ventricular Dysfunction) trial. J Am Coll Cardiol 2009;**54**(20):1837–46.
6. Santas E, De la Espriella R, Chorro FJ, *et al.* Right ventricular dysfunction staging system for mortality risk stratification in heart failure with preserved ejection fraction. J Clin Med 2020;**9**(3):831.
7. Padang R, Chandrashekar N, Indrabhinduwat M, *et al.* Aetiology and outcomes of severe right ventricular dysfunction. Eur Heart J 2020;**41**(12):1273–82.
8. Gorter TM, van Veldhuisen DJ, Bauersachs J, *et al.* Right heart dysfunction and failure in heart failure with preserved ejection fraction: mechanisms and management. Position statement on behalf of the Heart Failure Association of the European Society of Cardiology. Eur J Heart Fail 2018;**20**(1):16–37.
9. Aschauer S, Kammerlander AA, Zotter-Tufaro C, *et al.* The right heart in heart failure with preserved ejection fraction: insights from cardiac magnetic resonance imaging and invasive haemodynamics. Eur J Heart Fail 2016;**18**(1):71–80.
10. Haddad F, Doyle R, Murphy DJ, Hunt SA. Right ventricular function in cardiovascular disease, part II: pathophysiology, clinical importance, and management of right ventricular failure. Circulation 2008;**117**(13):1717–31.
11. Wu VC, Takeuchi M. Echocardiographic assessment of right ventricular systolic function. Cardiovasc Diagn Ther 2018;**8**(1):70–9.
12. Harjola VP, Mebazaa A, Čelutkienė J, *et al.* Contemporary management of acute right ventricular failure: a statement from the Heart Failure Association and the Working Group on Pulmonary Circulation and Right Ventricular Function of the European Society of Cardiology. Eur J Heart Fail 2016;**18**(3):226–41.
13. Kebed KY, Addetia K, Henry M, *et al.* Refining severe tricuspid regurgitation definition by echocardiography with a new outcomes-based 'massive' grade. J Am Soc Echocardiogr 2020;**33**(9):1087–94.
14. Vonk Noordegraaf A, Westerhof BE, Westerhof N. The relationship between the right ventricle and its load in pulmonary hypertension. J Am Coll Cardiol 2017;**69**(2):236–43.
15. Guazzi M, Bandera F, Pelissero G, *et al.* Tricuspid annular plane systolic excursion and pulmonary arterial systolic pressure relationship in heart failure: an index of right ventricular contractile function and prognosis. Am J Physiol Heart Circ Physiol 2013;**305**(9):H1373–81.
16. Focardi M, Cameli M, Carbone SF, *et al.* Traditional and innovative echocardiographic parameters for the analysis of right ventricular performance in comparison with cardiac magnetic resonance. Eur Heart J Cardiovasc Imaging 2015;**16**(1):47–52.
17. Geva T. Repaired tetralogy of Fallot: the roles of cardiovascular magnetic resonance in evaluating pathophysiology and for pulmonary

valve replacement decision support. J Cardiovasc Magn Reson 2011;**13**(1):9.

18. Humbert M, Kovacs G, Hoeper MM et la. 2022 ESC/ERS Guidelines for the diagnosis and treatment of pulmonary hypertension: Developed by the task force for the diagnosis and treatment of pulmonary hypertension of the European Society of Cardiology (ESC) and the European Respiratory Society (ERS). Endorsed by the International Society for Heart and Lung Transplantation (ISHLT) and the European Reference Networkon rare respiratory diseases (ERN-LUNG). European Heart Journal (2022; 43: 3618–3731.

19. Reddy YNV, Carter RE, Obokata M, Redfield MM, Borlaug BA. A simple, evidence-based approach to help guide diagnosis of heart failure with preserved ejection fraction. Circulation 2018;**138**(9):861–70.

20. Simonneau G, Montani D, Celermajer DS, et al. Haemodynamic definitions and updated clinical classification of pulmonary hypertension. Eur Respir J 2019;**53**(1):1801913.

21. Galiè N, McLaughlin VV, Rubin LJ, Simonneau G. An overview of the 6th World Symposium on Pulmonary Hypertension. Eur Respir J 2019;**53**(1):1802148.

22. Vachiéry JL, Tedford RJ, Rosenkranz S, et al. Pulmonary hypertension due to left heart disease. Eur Respir J 2019;**53**(1):1801897.

23. Ponikowski P, Voors AA, Anker SD, et al. 2016 ESC Guidelines for the diagnosis and treatment of acute and chronic heart failure: the Task Force for the diagnosis and treatment of acute and chronic heart failure of the European Society of Cardiology (ESC). Developed with the special contribution of the Heart Failure Association (HFA) of the ESC. Eur Heart J 2016;**37**(27):2129–200.

24. Lüscher TF. Lumpers and splitters: the bumpy road to precision medicine. Eur Heart J 2019;**40**(40):3292–6.

25. Bosch L, Lam CSP, Gong L, et al. Right ventricular dysfunction in left-sided heart failure with preserved versus reduced ejection fraction. Eur J Heart Fail 2017;**19**(12):1664–71.

26. Salzberg SP, Lachat ML, von Harbou K, Zünd G, Turina MI. Normalization of high pulmonary vascular resistance with LVAD support in heart transplantation candidates. Eur J Cardiothorac Surg 2005;**27**(2):222–5.

27. Santiago-Vacas E, Lupón J, Gavidia-Bovadilla G, et al. Pulmonary hypertension and right ventricular dysfunction in heart failure: prognosis and 15-year prospective longitudinal trajectories in survivors. Eur J Heart Fail 2020;**22**(7):1214–25.

28. Abraham WT, Adamson PB, Bourge RC, et al. Wireless pulmonary artery haemodynamic monitoring in chronic heart failure: a randomised controlled trial. Lancet 2011;**377**(9766):658–66.

29. Desai AS, Bhimaraj A, Bharmi R, et al. Ambulatory hemodynamic monitoring reduces heart failure hospitalizations in 'real-world' clinical practice. J Am Coll Cardiol 2017;**69**(19):2357–65.

30. Adamson PB, Abraham WT, Bourge RC, et al. Wireless pulmonary artery pressure monitoring guides management to reduce decompensation in heart failure with preserved ejection fraction. Circ Heart Fail 2014;**7**(6):935–44.

31. Gorter TM, Hoendermis ES, van Veldhuisen DJ, et al. Right ventricular dysfunction in heart failure with preserved ejection fraction: a systematic review and meta-analysis. Eur J Heart Fail 2016;**18**(12):1472–87.

32. Prihadi EA, van der Bijl P, Gursoy E, et al. Development of significant tricuspid regurgitation over time and prognostic implications: new insights into natural history. Eur Heart J 2018;**39**(39):3574–81.

33. Baumgartner H, Falk V, Bax JJ, et al. 2017 ESC/EACTS Guidelines for the management of valvular heart disease. Eur Heart J 2017;**38**(36):2739–91.

34. Topilsky Y, Khanna AD, Oh JK, et al. Preoperative factors associated with adverse outcome after tricuspid valve replacement. Circulation 2011;**123**(18):1929–39.

35. Nickenig G, Kowalski M, Hausleiter J, et al. Transcatheter treatment of severe tricuspid regurgitation with the edge-to-edge MitraClip technique. Circulation 2017;**135**(19):1802–14.

35a Sorajja P, Whisenant B, Hamid N et al. Transcatheter repair for patients with tricuspid regurgitation. N Engl J Med 2023;388:1833–42.

36. Messika-Zeitoun D, Nickenig G, Latib A, et al. Transcatheter mitral valve repair for functional mitral regurgitation using the Cardioband system: 1 year outcomes. Eur Heart J 2019;**40**(5):466–72.

37. Greene DG, Baldwin ED, et al. Pure congenital pulmonary stenosis and idiopathic congenital dilatation of the pulmonary artery. Am J Med 1949;**6**(1):24–40.

38. Devanagondi R, Peck D, Sagi J, et al. Long-term outcomes of balloon valvuloplasty for isolated pulmonary valve stenosis. Pediatr Cardiol 2017;**38**(2):247–54.

39. Barlow JB, Bosman CK. Aneurysmal protrusion of the posterior leaflet of the mitral valve. An auscultatory–electrocardiographic syndrome. Am Heart J 1966;**71**(2):166–78.

40. Enriquez-Sarano M, Avierinos JF, Messika-Zeitoun D, et al. Quantitative determinants of the outcome of asymptomatic mitral regurgitation. N Engl J Med 2005;**352**(9):875–83.

41. Bartko PE, Arfsten H, Heitzinger G, et al. Global regurgitant volume: approaching the critical mass in valvular-driven heart failure. Eur Heart J Cardiovasc Imaging 2020;**21**(2):168–74.

42. Tuladhar SM, Punjabi PP. Surgical reconstruction of the mitral valve. Heart 2006;**92**(10):1373–7.

43. Acker MA, Parides MK, Perrault LP, et al. Mitral-valve repair versus replacement for severe ischemic mitral regurgitation. N Engl J Med 2014;**370**(1):23–32.

44. Hyllén S, Nozohoor S, Ingvarsson A, Meurling C, Wierup P, Sjögren J. Right ventricular performance after valve repair for chronic degenerative mitral regurgitation. Ann Thorac Surg 2014;**98**(6):2023–30.

45. Maisano F, Franzen O, Baldus S, et al. Percutaneous mitral valve interventions in the real world: early and 1-year results from the ACCESS-EU, a prospective, multicenter, nonrandomized postapproval study of the MitraClip therapy in Europe. J Am Coll Cardiol 2013;**62**(12):1052–61.

46. Obadia JF, Messika-Zeitoun D, Leurent G, et al. Percutaneous repair or medical treatment for secondary mitral regurgitation. N Engl J Med 2018;**379**(24):2297–306.

47. Stone GW, Lindenfeld J, Abraham WT, et al. Transcatheter mitral-valve repair in patients with heart failure. N Engl J Med 2018;**379**(24):2307–18.

48. Ledwoch J, Fellner C, Hoppmann P, et al. Impact of transcatheter mitral valve repair using MitraClip on right ventricular remodeling. Int J Cardiovasc Imaging 2020;**36**(5):811–19.

49. Humbert M, Sitbon O, Simonneau G. Treatment of pulmonary arterial hypertension. N Engl J Med 2004;**351**(14):1425–36.

50. 6th World Symposium on Pulmonary Hypertension, 2018..

51. Hoeper MM, Benza RL, Corris P, et al. Intensive care, right ventricular support and lung transplantation in patients with pulmonary hypertension. Eur Respir J 2019;**53**(1):1801906.

52. 6th World Symposium on Pulmonary Hypertension, 2018.

53. Almagro P, Barreiro B, Ochoa de Echaguen A, et al. Risk factors for hospital readmission in patients with chronic obstructive pulmonary disease. Respiration 2006;**73**(3):311–17.

54. Marti S, Muñoz X, Rios J, Morell F, Ferrer J. Body weight and comorbidity predict mortality in COPD patients treated with oxygen therapy. Eur Respir J 2006;**27**(4):689–96.

55. Kolb TM, Hassoun PM. Right ventricular dysfunction in chronic lung disease. Cardiol Clin 2012;**30**(2):243–56.

56. Hilde JM, Skjørten I, Grøtta OJ, et al. Right ventricular dysfunction and remodeling in chronic obstructive pulmonary disease without pulmonary hypertension. J Am Coll Cardiol 2013;**62**(12):1103–111.

57. Kim NH, Delcroix M, Jais X, et al. Chronic thromboembolic pulmonary hypertension. Eur Respir J 2019;**53**(1):1801915.

58. Bolger AP, Sharma R, Li W, et al. Neurohormonal activation and the chronic heart failure syndrome in adults with congenital heart disease. Circulation 2002;**106**(1):92–9.

59. Diller GP, Dimopoulos K, Okonko D, et al. Exercise intolerance in adult congenital heart disease: comparative severity, correlates, and prognostic implication. Circulation 2005;**112**(6):828–35.

60. Brida M, Diller GP, Nashat H, et al. Pharmacological therapy in adult congenital heart disease: growing need, yet limited evidence. Eur Heart J 2019;**40**(13):1049–56.

61. Lüscher TF. The secret of success of heart failure therapy: a lesson for ACHD? International Journal of Cardiology Congenital Heart Disease 2020;**1**:100003.

62. Budts W, Roos-Hesselink J, Rädle-Hurst T, et al. Treatment of heart failure in adult congenital heart disease: a position paper of the Working Group of Grown-Up Congenital Heart Disease and the Heart Failure Association of the European Society of Cardiology. Eur Heart J 2016;**37**(18):1419–27.

63. Brida M, Diller GP, Gatzoulis MA. Systemic right ventricle in adults with congenital heart disease: anatomic and phenotypic spectrum and current approach to management. Circulation 2018;**137**(5):508–18.

64. Gatzoulis MA, Balaji S, Webber SA, et al. Risk factors for arrhythmia and sudden cardiac death late after repair of tetralogy of Fallot: a multicentre study. Lancet 2000;**356**(9234):975–81.

65. Davlouros PA, Kilner PJ, Hornung TS, et al. Right ventricular function in adults with repaired tetralogy of Fallot assessed with cardiovascular magnetic resonance imaging: detrimental role of right ventricular outflow aneurysms or akinesia and adverse right-to-left ventricular interaction. J Am Coll Cardiol 2002;**40**(11):2044–52.

66. Babu-Narayan SV, Uebing A, Davlouros PA, et al. Randomised trial of ramipril in repaired tetralogy of Fallot and pulmonary regurgitation: the APPROPRIATE study (Ace inhibitors for Potential PRevention Of the deleterious effects of Pulmonary Regurgitation In Adults with repaired TEtralogy of Fallot). Int J Cardiol 2012;**154**(3):299–305.

67. Baumgartner H, De Backer J, Babu-Narayan SV, et al. 2020 ESC Guidelines for the management of adult congenital heart disease. Eur Heart J 2021;**42**(6):563–645.

68. Attenhofer Jost CH, Connolly HM, Dearani JA, Edwards WD, Danielson GK. Ebstein's anomaly. Circulation 2007;**115**(2):277–85.

69. González C, Devesa M, Boada M, Coroleu B, Veiga A, Barri PN. Combined strategy for fertility preservation in an oncologic patient: vitrification of in vitro matured oocytes and ovarian tissue freezing. J Assist Reprod Genet 2011;**28**(12):1147–9.

70. Campbell M. Natural history of atrial septal defect. Br Heart J 1970;**32**(6):820–6.

71. Gatzoulis MA, Freeman MA, Siu SC, Webb GD, Harris L. Atrial arrhythmia after surgical closure of atrial septal defects in adults. N Engl J Med 1999;**340**(11):839–46.

72. Roos-Hesselink JW, Meijboom FJ, Spitaels SE, et al. Excellent survival and low incidence of arrhythmias, stroke and heart failure long-term after surgical ASD closure at young age. A prospective follow-up study of 21–33 years. Eur Heart J 2003;**24**(2):190–7.

73. Hijazi Z, Wang Z, Cao Q, Koenig P, Waight D, Lang R. Transcatheter closure of atrial septal defects and patent foramen ovale under intracardiac echocardiographic guidance: feasibility and comparison with transesophageal echocardiography. Catheter Cardiovasc Interv 2001;**52**(2):194–9.

74. Brida M, Diller GP, Kempny A, et al. Atrial septal defect closure in adulthood is associated with normal survival in the mid to longer term. Heart 2019;**105**(13):1014–19.

75. Heiberg J, Ringgaard S, Schmidt MR, Redington A, Hjortdal VE. Structural and functional alterations of the right ventricle are common in adults operated for ventricular septal defect as toddlers. Eur Heart J Cardiovasc Imaging 2015;**16**(5):483–9.

76. Heiberg J, Redington A, Hjortdal VE. Exercise capacity and cardiac function after surgical closure of ventricular septal defect. Is there unrecognized long-term morbidity? Int J Cardiol 2015;**201**:590–4.

77. Crenshaw BS, Granger CB, Birnbaum Y, et al. Risk factors, angiographic patterns, and outcomes in patients with ventricular septal defect complicating acute myocardial infarction. GUSTO-I (Global Utilization of Streptokinase and TPA for Occluded Coronary Arteries) Trial Investigators. Circulation 2000;**101**(1):27–32.

78. Arnaoutakis GJ, Zhao Y, George TJ, Sciortino CM, McCarthy PM, Conte JV. Surgical repair of ventricular septal defect after myocardial infarction: outcomes from the Society of Thoracic Surgeons National Database. Ann Thorac Surg 2012;**94**(2):436–43; discussion 443–4.

79. Schlotter F, de Waha S, Eitel I, Desch S, Fuernau G, Thiele H. Interventional post-myocardial infarction ventricular septal defect closure: a systematic review of current evidence. EuroIntervention 2016;**12**(1):94–102.

80. Ibanez B, James S, Agewall S, et al. 2017 ESC Guidelines for the management of acute myocardial infarction in patients presenting with ST-segment elevation: the Task Force for the management of acute myocardial infarction in patients presenting with ST-segment elevation of the European Society of Cardiology (ESC). Eur Heart J 2018;**39**(2):119–77.

81. Lucas RV Jr, Varco RL, Lillehei CW, Adams P Jr, Anderson RC, Edwards JE. Anomalous muscle bundle of the right ventricle. Hemodynamic consequences and surgical considerations. Circulation 1962;**25**:443–55.

82. Nakata T, Hattori A, Shimamoto K. Double chambered right ventricle. Lancet 2004;**363**(9415):1137.

83. Peters S, Trümmel M, Meyners W. Prevalence of right ventricular dysplasia-cardiomyopathy in a non-referral hospital. Int J Cardiol 2004;**97**(3):499–501.

84. Saguner AM, Duru F, Brunckhorst CB. Arrhythmogenic right ventricular cardiomyopathy: a challenging disease of the intercalated disc. Circulation 2013;**128**(12):1381–6.

85. Ruwald AC, Marcus F, Estes NA, 3rd, et al. Association of competitive and recreational sport participation with cardiac events in patients with arrhythmogenic right ventricular cardiomyopathy: results from the North American multidisciplinary study of arrhythmogenic right ventricular cardiomyopathy. Eur Heart J 2015;**36**(27):1735–43.

86. Kim J, Volodarskiy A, Sultana R, et al. Prognostic utility of right ventricular remodeling over conventional risk stratification in patients with COVID-19. J Am Coll Cardiol 2020;**76**(17):1965–77.

87. Konstantinides SV, Meyer G, Becattini C, et al. 2019 ESC Guidelines for the diagnosis and management of acute pulmonary embolism developed in collaboration with the European Respiratory Society (ERS). Eur Heart J 2020;**41**(4):543–603.

88. Grifoni S, Olivotto I, Cecchini P, et al. Short-term clinical outcome of patients with acute pulmonary embolism, normal blood pressure, and echocardiographic right ventricular dysfunction. Circulation 2000;**101**(24):2817–22.

89. Kucher N, Rossi E, De Rosa M, Goldhaber SZ. Massive pulmonary embolism. Circulation 2006;**113**(4):577–82.

90. Dronkers CEA, van der Hulle T, Le Gal G, *et al.* Towards a tailored diagnostic standard for future diagnostic studies in pulmonary embolism: communication from the SSC of the ISTH. J Thromb Haemost 2017;**15**(5):1040–3.

91. Van der Hulle T, Cheung WY, Kooij S, *et al.* Simplified diagnostic management of suspected pulmonary embolism (the YEARS study): a prospective, multicentre, cohort study. Lancet 2017;**390**(10091):289–97.

92. Aujesky D, Obrosky DS, Stone RA, *et al.* Derivation and validation of a prognostic model for pulmonary embolism. Am J Respir Crit Care Med 2005;**172**(8):1041–6.

93. Steering Committee. Single-bolus tenecteplase plus heparin compared with heparin alone for normotensive patients with acute pulmonary embolism who have evidence of right ventricular dysfunction and myocardial injury: rationale and design of the Pulmonary Embolism Thrombolysis (PEITHO) trial. Am Heart J 2012;**163**(1):33–8.e1.

94. Keeling WB, Sundt T, Leacche M, *et al.* Outcomes after surgical pulmonary embolectomy for acute pulmonary embolus: a multi-institutional study. Ann Thorac Surg 2016;**102**(5):1498–502.

95. Engelberger RP, Kucher N. Ultrasound-assisted thrombolysis for acute pulmonary embolism: a systematic review. Eur Heart J 2014;**35**(12):758–64.

96. Robertson L, Jones LE. Fixed dose subcutaneous low molecular weight heparins versus adjusted dose unfractionated heparin for the initial treatment of venous thromboembolism. Cochrane Database Syst Rev 2017;**2**(2):CD001100.

97. Barco S, Schmidtmann I, Ageno W, *et al.* Early discharge and home treatment of patients with low-risk pulmonary embolism with the oral factor Xa inhibitor rivaroxaban: an international multicentre single-arm clinical trial. Eur Heart J 2020;**41**(4):509–18.

98. Ramaswamy NK, Nair PM. Pathway for the biosynthesis of delta-aminolevulinic acid in greening potatoes. Indian J Biochem Biophys 1976;**13**(4):394–7.

99. Gil-Cruz C, Perez-Shibayama C, De Martin A, *et al.* Microbiota-derived peptide mimics drive lethal inflammatory cardiomyopathy. Science 2019;**366**(6467):881–6.

100. Cooper LT Jr. Myocarditis. N Engl J Med 2009;**360**(15):1526–38.

101. Friedrich MG, Strohm O, Schulz-Menger J, Marciniak H, Luft FC, Dietz R. Contrast media-enhanced magnetic resonance imaging visualizes myocardial changes in the course of viral myocarditis. Circulation 1998;**97**(18):1802–9.

102. Pieroni M, Dello Russo A, Marzo F, *et al.* High prevalence of myocarditis mimicking arrhythmogenic right ventricular cardiomyopathy differential diagnosis by electroanatomic mapping-guided endomyocardial biopsy. J Am Coll Cardiol 2009;**53**(8):681–9.

103. Boissier F, Katsahian S, Razazi K, *et al.* Prevalence and prognosis of cor pulmonale during protective ventilation for acute respiratory distress syndrome. Intensive Care Med 2013;**39**(10):1725–33.

104. Tavazzi G, Bergsland N, Alcada J, Price S. Early signs of right ventricular systolic and diastolic dysfunction in acute severe respiratory failure: the importance of diastolic restrictive pattern. Eur Heart J Acute Cardiovasc Care 2020;**9**(6):649–56.

105. Cingolani HE, Pérez NG, Cingolani OH, Ennis IL. The Anrep effect: 100 years later. Am J Physiol Heart Circ Physiol 2013;**304**(2):H175–82.

106. Chioncel O, Parissis J, Mebazaa A, *et al.* Epidemiology, pathophysiology and contemporary management of cardiogenic shock: a position statement from the Heart Failure Association of the European Society of Cardiology. Eur J Heart Fail 2020;**22**(8):1315–41.

107. Inohara T, Kohsaka S, Fukuda K, Menon V. The challenges in the management of right ventricular infarction. Eur Heart J Acute Cardiovasc Care 2013;**2**(3):226–34.

108. Berisha S, Kastrati A, Goda A, Popa Y. Optimal value of filling pressure in the right side of the heart in acute right ventricular infarction. Br Heart J 1990;**63**(2):98–102.

109. Pazur JH, Kelly-Delcourt SA, Miskiel FJ, Burdett L, Docherty JJ. The isolation of anti-gum arabic antibodies by affinity chromatography. J Immunol Methods 1986;**89**(1):19–25.

110. Price LC, Wort SJ, Finney SJ, Marino PS, Brett SJ. Pulmonary vascular and right ventricular dysfunction in adult critical care: current and emerging options for management: a systematic literature review. Crit Care 2010;**14**(5):R169.

111. Ventetuolo CE, Klinger JR. Management of acute right ventricular failure in the intensive care unit. Ann Am Thorac Soc 2014;**11**(5):811–22.

112. Baran DA, Grines CL, Bailey S, *et al.* SCAI clinical expert consensus statement on the classification of cardiogenic shock. This document was endorsed by the American College of Cardiology (ACC), the American Heart Association (AHA), the Society of Critical Care Medicine (SCCM), and the Society of Thoracic Surgeons (STS) in April 2019. Catheter Cardiovasc Interv 2019;**94**(1):29–37.

113. Stevenson LW, Pagani FD, Young JB, *et al.* INTERMACS profiles of advanced heart failure: the current picture. J Heart Lung Transplant 2009;**28**(6):535–41.

114. Combes A, Price S, Slutsky AS, Brodie D. Temporary circulatory support for cardiogenic shock. Lancet 2020;**396**(10245):199–212.

115. Kinch JW, Ryan TJ. Right ventricular infarction. N Engl J Med 1994;**330**(17):1211–17.

116. Cohn JN, Guiha NH, Broder MI, Limas CJ. Right ventricular infarction. Clinical and hemodynamic features. Am J Cardiol 1974;**33**(2):209–14.

117. Jacobs AK, Leopold JA, Bates E, *et al.* Cardiogenic shock caused by right ventricular infarction: a report from the SHOCK registry. J Am Coll Cardiol 2003;**41**(8):1273–9.

118. Zehender M, Kasper W, Kauder E, *et al.* Right ventricular infarction as an independent predictor of prognosis after acute inferior myocardial infarction. N Engl J Med 1993;**328**(14):981–8.

119. Diller GP, Wasan BS, Kyriacou A, *et al.* Effect of coronary artery bypass surgery on myocardial function as assessed by tissue Doppler echocardiography. Eur J Cardiothorac Surg 2008;**34**(5):995–9.

120. Sim HT, Beom MS, Kim SR, Ryu SW. Acute thrombotic occlusion of left internal jugular vein compressed by bypass graft for thoracic endovascular aortic repair debranching procedure. Korean J Thorac Cardiovasc Surg 2014;**47**(6):552–5.

121. Dang NC, Topkara VK, Mercando M, *et al.* Right heart failure after left ventricular assist device implantation in patients with chronic congestive heart failure. J Heart Lung Transplant 2006;**25**(1):1–6.

122. Sert DE, Karahan M, Aygun E, Kocabeyoglu SS, Akdi M, Kervan U. Prediction of right ventricular failure after continuous flow left ventricular assist device implantation. J Card Surg 2020;**35**(11):2965–73.

123. Kobashigawa J, Zuckermann A, Macdonald P, *et al.* Report from a consensus conference on primary graft dysfunction after cardiac transplantation. J Heart Lung Transplant 2014;**33**(4):327–40.

SECTION 7

Chronic heart failure: diagnostic and prognostic assessment

CHAPTER 7.1

Heart failure clinical assessment

Michel Komajda, Piotr Ponikowski, and
Evgeny Shlyakhtho

Definitions

There are several definitions of heart failure (HF). According to current European Society of Cardiology (ESC) Guidelines, HF is a clinical syndrome characterized by typical symptoms and signs caused by a structural and functional cardiac abnormality, resulting in reduced cardiac output and/or elevated intracardiac pressures at rest or during stress.[1] Previous definitions characterized HF as inability of the heart to provide adequate blood delivery to meet the requirements of metabolizing tissues or as a pattern of haemodynamic, renal, and neurohormonal response or predominant signs/symptoms.

It can be preceded by a latency period, during which patients are asymptomatic, although an underlying cardiac abnormality is present (asymptomatic cardiac dysfunction). Identification of risk factors for developing HF, particularly hypertension or diabetes mellitus, in asymptomatic patients is critical in order to take preventive measures and start treatment at the precursor stage to prevent the development of signs and symptoms and to improve clinical outcomes.[2,3]

Clinical assessment of HF should use a stepwise approach (⯈ Figure 7.1.1):

1. Assessing symptom severity and limitation of activities

2. Performing a comprehensive clinical examination in order to identify signs suggestive of HF

3. Identifying factors suggestive of an underlying aetiology in order to plan subsequent investigations

4. Assessing the risk of poor clinical outcomes, including death and HF-related hospitalizations.

Different terminologies and descriptive terms for HF based on the clinical severity, pathophysiology, predominant signs/symptoms, and time course of HF are commonly used:

◆ *Chronic* versus *acute/acutely decompensated* HF. Acute HF (AHF) is a life-threatening condition which can be the first manifestation of HF ('*de novo HF*') or a result of the deterioration of a previously diagnosed chronic HF ('*acute-on-chronic HF or decompensated HF*'). It describes the rapid onset of, or change in, symptoms and signs of HF, requires immediate therapeutic measures, and usually leads to urgent hospitalization.

◆ *Advanced HF* alludes to severe symptoms, recurrent hospitalizations, and marked cardiac dysfunction.

◆ *End-stage HF* is observed in bedridden patients and is often refractory to any therapeutic measure, leading to palliative care in order to alleviate symptoms and improve end-of-life quality.

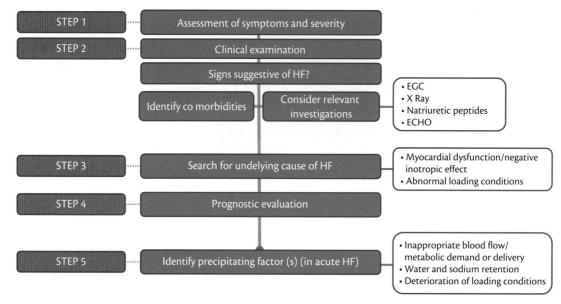

Figure 7.1.1 Stepwise clinical assessment of heart failure.

- *Right-sided HF* and *left-sided HF* are based on the predominance of symptoms and signs suggestive of dysfunction of the right or left ventricle.
- *Congestive HF* alludes to conditions where fluid retention in the body is predominant.
- *HF with reduced* (previously called systolic HF), *preserved* (previously called 'diastolic HF'), or *mildly reduced ejection fraction* (HFrEF, HFpEF, HFmrEF, respectively) is a classification based on the measurement of left ventricular ejection fraction by echocardiography (➲ Chapter 7.3). HFrEF is defined by an ejection fraction of <40%, HFpEF by an EF of ≥50%, and HFmrEF by intermediate values.[1]

Although based on somewhat arbitrary thresholds, this classification allows to identify subgroups of HF patients with distinct phenotypes and with different responsiveness to HF treatments. In brief, patients with HFpEF are more often female, with advanced age and metabolic disorders (obesity and metabolic syndrome), hypertension, kidney dysfunction, and chronic obstructive pulmonary disease, and are less likely to have a history of coronary heart disease than patients with HFrEF. Patients with HFmrEF tend to have a clinical profile close to those with HFrEF, and current guidelines recommend a similar pharmacological approach to that applied to HFrEF, although most data are derived from registries and no specific trial has been conducted in this subgroup. Moreover, in many circumstances, HFmrEF reflects a transitional stage to recovery from, or deterioration to, HFrEF.

Assessment of symptom severity

The cardinal symptoms of HF are *dyspnoea* and *fatigue* which limit exercise tolerance, but none of these symptoms are specific to HF as they may be observed in other conditions, including lung disease or obesity. Breathlessness usually occurs first on exercise and then at rest when the disease progresses. It may aggravate in the resting position, requiring patients to stay sitting (orthopnoea), or can occur abruptly at night (paroxysmal nocturnal dyspnoea). Sometimes patients complain of nocturnal cough or describe wheezing.

Fatigue usually manifests first during exercise and is characterized by a progressive decline in exercise tolerance and prolonged time to recovery after exercise. Patients can also report tiredness.

Other symptoms are less suggestive of HF. These include bloated feeling in relation to volume overload, bendopnoea, depression, loss of appetite, confusion which may affect particularly elderly people, dizziness or syncope related to low cardiac output, and palpitations which may reflect tachycardia or a coexisting arrhythmia.

The most commonly used classification for assessment of symptom severity is the New York Heart Association (NYHA) functional classification, which describes the severity of symptoms and exercise tolerance (➲ Box 7.1.1).[4] This classification is simple and universally used in clinical practice, as well as in

---

Box 7.1.1 New York Heart Association functional classification

Class I: no limitation of physical activity. Ordinary activity does not cause breathlessness or fatigue.

Class II: slight limitation of physical activity. Comfortable at rest, but ordinary physical activity results in undue breathlessness, fatigue, or palpitations.

Class III: marked limitation of physical activity. Comfortable at rest, but less-than-ordinary activity results in undue breathlessness, fatigue, or palpitations.

Class IV: inability to carry out a physical activity without discomfort. Symptoms at rest can be present.

Source data from The Criteria Committee of the New York Heart Association *nomenclature and criteria for diseases of the heart and great vessels*. 9th Ed. Boston, Little and Brown, 1994.

Box 7.1.2 American College of Cardiology Foundation/American Heart Association stages of heart failure

Stage A: at high risk of HF, but without structural heart disease or symptoms of HF

Stage B: structural heart disease, but without signs or symptoms of HF

Stage C: structural heart disease, with prior or current signs or symptoms of HF

Stage D: refractory HF requiring specialized interventions

Source data from Yancy CW, Jessup M, Bozkurt B, *et al.* 2013 ACCF/AHA guideline for the management of heart failure: executive summary: a report of the American College of Cardiology Foundation/American Heart Association Task Force on practice guidelines. *Circulation* 2013;128(16):1810–52.

---

clinical trials, but it has several limitations, including subjectivity and poor interobserver reproducibility, particularly between class II and III patients, and it is poorly correlated with measures of left ventricular function, including ejection fraction, or with exercise capacity.[5,6] However, the severity of symptoms assessed based on the NYHA class is correlated with the risk of death and HF hospitalization.[7] Limitation of exercise capacity is often measured by the 6-minute walk test, which is easy to perform in a corridor and proved to be reproducible and predictive of clinical outcomes.[8,9]

The American College of Cardiology Foundation (ACCF)/ American Heart Association (AHA) have proposed a different classification based on the development and progression of disease (⮑ Box 7.1.2).[10]

Clinical examination

Clinical signs are not specific to HF and can be observed in noncardiac conditions. Therefore, clinical evaluation is not sufficient to diagnose HF but is needed in order to guide additional investigations, including electrocardiogram, chest X-ray, measurement of plasma levels of natriuretic peptides, and imaging, most often with transthoracic echocardiography (⮑ Chapter 7.3).

HF is typically characterized by volume retention with the following associated clinical signs: peripheral oedema (ankle, scrotal, sacral), ascites, anasarca, elevated jugular venous pressure, hepatomegaly with hepatojugular reflux, rapid weight gain (>2 kg/week), pulmonary crepitations, and pleural effusion.

Other signs are related to the activation of the sympathetic nervous system (tachycardia), left ventricular dilatation (laterally displaced apical impulse or S3 gallop, which is highly suggestive of HF, but inconstantly observed), low cardiac output with peripheral hypoperfusion (oliguria, cold extremities, low systolic blood pressure), or an underlying valvular defect (murmur) or arrhythmia (irregular pulse). Pulmonary congestion may be manifested by tachypnoea and result in acute pulmonary oedema, an emergency where the patient is often cyanotic with suffocation and white foamy sputum. Finally, HF can be accompanied by cardiac cachexia and an abnormal respiratory pattern (Cheyne–Stokes respiration).

Overall, the clinical diagnosis of HF remains challenging due to the lack of specificity of signs and symptoms, poor reproducibility between observers, and overlapping profile of other conditions which may be associated with HF as comorbidities: lung, renal, and liver diseases or obesity. In particular, it may be difficult to distinguish between chronic obstructive pulmonary disease and HF.

Another important step in clinical evaluation is to identify comorbidities. They are common, particularly in elderly HF patients, and their presence may interfere with the diagnostic process, increase the risk of death or hospitalization, and influence treatment modalities due to contraindications or intolerance.[11,12] In this regard, it is important to check for chronic obstructive pulmonary disease, asthma, renal dysfunction, diabetes mellitus, cognitive disorders, malignancy, and frailty.

At this stage, after initial assessment, the ESC HF Guidelines propose to apply an algorithm for the diagnosis of HF. It is based on the following steps:

1. Assessment of HF probability using (any of the below increases the risk of HF):
   a. Patient's prior clinical history (history of coronary artery disease, arterial hypertension, diabetes mellitus, exposure to cardiotoxic drugs/radiation, use of diuretics, orthopnoea, paroxysmal nocturnal dyspnoea)
   b. Physical examination (rales, bilateral ankle oedema, heart murmur, jugular venous dilatation, laterally displaced/ broadened apical beat)
   c. Abnormality of the electrocardiogram.

2. Assessment of blood natriuretic peptide levels (only low values below predefined cut-off levels exclude HF) (⮑ Chapter 7.2).

3. Assessment of cardiac function with transthoracic echocardiography (⮑ Chapter 7.3).

Clinical assessment of aetiology

Detailed history taking and a comprehensive clinical examination are essential in order to guide investigations and identify a potentially treatable cause of HF. Certain features, such as arterial hypertension, a history of coronary artery disease/acute coronary syndrome, and exposure to cardiotoxic drugs, increase markedly the likelihood of HF in the presence of suggestive symptoms and signs (see earlier).

Most disorders affecting the heart and circulation, together with a number of non-cardiovascular diseases, may be associated with HF. They can be grouped schematically as:

- diseases of the myocardium
- abnormal loading conditions.

Diseases of the myocardium

Among diseases of the myocardium, ischaemic heart disease is the predominant cause of HF. HF can be a consequence of acute coronary syndrome via a myocardial scar or hibernating or stunned myocardium, or the result of chronic myocardial hypoperfusion due to significant epicardial coronary stenoses or abnormal microcirculation, including endothelial dysfunction.

Specific myocardial diseases are another common cause of HF—these include inherited or non-inherited dilated cardiomyopathy, hypertrophic cardiomyopathy, arrhythmogenic right ventricular cardiomyopathy, restrictive cardiomyopathies, left ventricular non-compaction, and cardiac involvement in muscular dystrophies and laminopathies.

Immune-related, infectious, and inflammatory causes may result from various bacterial agents, fungi, parasites (such as *Trypanosoma cruzi* causing Chagas disease, a common cause of HF in South America), and viruses. Viral infections, including coronavirus disease 2019 (Covid-19), may induce AHF through acute myocarditis.[13] Infectious causes are more frequent in patients with depressed immunity as a result of acquired immune deficiency syndrome or immunosuppressive therapies.

Non-infectious immune cardiac diseases are observed in autoimmune diseases and connective tissue disorders, particularly systemic lupus erythematosus. Less frequently, HF may result from hypersensitivity eosinophilic myocarditis or giant cell myocarditis.

Infiltration of the myocardium is another cause of HF. It may result from haemochromatosis (iron), glycogen storage disorders (Pompe disease), lysosomal storage diseases (Fabry disease), and sarcoidosis. A growing cause of infiltration-related HF is cardiac amyloidosis, which is predominantly observed in elderly patients and can be the result of transthyretin abnormalities or light chain myocardial deposition in myeloma. Malignancy, either by direct infiltration (lymphoma) or from metastases, may also cause HF.

Hormonal and metabolic disorders are often associated with cardiac involvement. Patients with hyperthyroidism, hypothyroidism, acromegaly, Conn's disease, phaeochromocytoma, and Addison's disease can develop HF.

Peripartum cardiomyopathy occurring during the last period of pregnancy or in the first months after delivery is a frequent cause of HF in some geographical areas, including Africa. Diabetes mellitus is a frequent cause of HF, either through the development of accelerated coronary artery disease or through abnormalities of the microcirculation and cardiac metabolism, resulting in '*diabetic cardiomyopathy*'. Obesity is another growing cause of HF worldwide.

Thiamine deficiency, which is commonly observed in alcohol abuse, may result in high-output HF, whereas various deficiencies (such as L-carnitine, selenium, iron, and phosphates) have been associated with the development of HF.

Toxic causes of HF are related to recreational substance abuse (alcohol, cocaine, amphetamines, anabolic steroids), radiation of the precordial area, and cardiotoxic drugs used mainly in oncology. The latter include anthracyclines, monoclonal antibodies, and check-point inhibitors, which may result in fulminant myocarditis.

Heavy metal intoxication with lead, cobalt, or copper is an uncommon cause of HF.

Abnormal loading conditions

The two predominant causes are arterial hypertension and valvular heart disease (mitral, aortic, tricuspid, and pulmonary) in adults, whereas congenital heart diseases remain a major cause of HF during infancy. The presence of HF signs or symptoms in a patient with valvular heart disease is an important finding which should lead to discussing the correction of the valvular defect by surgery or interventional cardiology.

Pericardial causes include constrictive cardiomyopathy, late complication of tuberculosis, and significant pericardial effusion of any cause (malignancy, infection).

Endomyocardial fibrosis and endocardial fibroelastosis are rare causes of HF. Signs and symptoms usually result from an increase in left ventricular filling pressure due to reduced compliance of the left ventricle.

Prognostic evaluation

HF is associated with a high risk of recurrent hospitalization and death. It is therefore important to assess the risk of death or rehospitalization in every individual patient in order to take appropriate therapeutic measures. A number of clinical variables predicting death and/or HF hospitalization have been identified, and several risk scores which include demographic and clinical factors, comorbidities, biomarkers, and imaging data have been developed in the setting of chronic HF and AHF. Box 7.1.3 provides a list of clinical variables associated with poor prognosis.[7,9,11,12,14,15] However, these multivariate prognostic risk scores overall have limited accuracy in predicting mortality, and prediction of the combined endpoint of death or hospitalization or hospitalization alone is even poorer, making the use of these risk scores limited in daily practice.[14,15]

Box 7.1.3 Clinical factors associated with poor outcomes in heart failure

Age
Sex
Advanced NYHA class
Longer heart failure duration
Low systolic blood pressure
High resting heart rate
Signs of fluid overload
Peripheral hypoperfusion
Body weight
Frailty
Diabetes mellitus
Other comorbidities
Depression
Abnormal 6-minute walk test

Acute heart failure

AHF is a life-threatening situation with rapid onset or worsening of symptoms and signs of HF. It can occur *de novo*, but in most instances, it results from deterioration of the condition in a patient with a previous diagnosis of chronic HF ('acute-on-chronic or decompensated HF'). In the latter situation, identification of a precipitating factor is important (see further). In acute-on-chronic HF, deterioration can be progressive, with increasing dyspnoea and/or peripheral oedema or rapid weight increase over a period of days or weeks, or may be abrupt in the setting of acute myocardial dysfunction (such as acute coronary syndrome, acute myocarditis, or arrhythmia with a rapid ventricular rate) or of rapid volume overload as observed in hypertension crisis or rupture of the mitral chordae in Barlow's disease.

The most common clinical profile of AHF is volume overload with signs of peripheral fluid retention. By contrast, cardiogenic shock with low systolic blood pressure, peripheral vasoconstriction, and oliguria is less frequent and associated with a poor prognosis.

Several clinical classifications have been proposed, and the most widely used is the classification at bedside based on the presence or absence of signs of hypoperfusion (cold vs warm if present vs absent) and congestion (wet vs dry if present vs absent).[16] This classification allows to identify four groups: warm and wet, the most common mode of presentation, if the patient is well perfused and congested; cold and wet (both hypoperfused and congested); warm and dry (well perfused without congestion); and cold and dry (hypoperfused without congestion). This classification into four different clinical profiles has important implications for early management of patients in emergency units or hospitals, and also provides useful prognostic information.

The Killip classification is another classification used in the specific setting of AHF complicating acute myocardial infarction. It describes four stages: class I, no clinical signs of HF; class II, HF with rales and S3 gallop; class III, overt pulmonary oedema; and class IV, cardiogenic shock with low systolic blood pressure and evidence of peripheral vasoconstriction, which is associated with a poor prognosis.[17]

Precipitating factors

Identification of factors leading to acute or progressive deterioration of HF is an important step, as appropriate therapeutic measures may result in rapid improvement of symptoms and signs. Schematically, these factors can aggravate underlying silent or mildly symptomatic cardiac dysfunction through four distinct mechanisms, as described in the following sections.

Inappropriate blood flow/oxygen/metabolic demand or delivery to the body

This is typically observed in the presence of infections, particularly pulmonary infections in which both fever (and increased metabolic demand) and inadequate pulmonary gas exchanges occur, severe anaemia, and excessive tachycardia or bradycardia. Tachyarrhythmia, such as atrial fibrillation, is a common precipitating factor where both the increase in heart rate and the loss of atrial contraction together reduce the cardiac output. Thyrotoxicosis, pregnancy, arteriovenous fistulae, and Paget's disease increase markedly the cardiac output and, as such, may trigger HF.

Water and sodium retention

Non-adherence to medications and to sodium restriction measures is a major cause of HF decompensation. Patient education is therefore key in order to reduce the role of this trigger, targeting in particular information on food rich in sodium.

Coexistence of renal failure may alter the sodium–water balance and promote HF. Non-steroid anti-inflammatory drugs, thiazolidinediones, corticosteroid therapy, and some contrast agents may also induce water and sodium retention.

Deterioration of loading conditions

This is observed when an excessive rise in blood pressure occurs ('hypertensive crisis') or in the presence of pulmonary embolism.

Myocardial damage: negative inotropic effect

Acute coronary syndrome or takotsubo syndrome may trigger AHF. Class I antiarrhythmic agents and verapamil are negative inotropic agents and can precipitate HF.

Alcohol and drug abuse can further deteriorate cardiac function by a direct myocardial toxic effect or through coronary vasospasm (cocaine).

Finally, perioperative HF may result from many of the factors mentioned above, together with acute mechanical causes such as ventricular septal defect or free wall rupture after acute coronary syndrome, acute or prosthetic valve incompetence due to infection, or thrombosis.

The ESC has proposed a stepwise approach to the diagnosis of AHF (➲ Figure 7.1.2):[2]

♦ Urgent phase after medical contact in order to confirm/rule out cardiogenic shock or respiratory failure requiring immediate resuscitation measures

♦ Immediate phase during the initial 60–120 minutes after medical contact and transfer to an intensive care unit—this phase should identify potentially treatable causes of AHF

♦ Diagnostic workup to confirm AHF with relevant investigations and initiate appropriate therapy.

Conclusions

Clinical assessment of chronic HF and AHF remains a fundamental step in the diagnostic workup for these conditions. Although symptoms and signs of HF are non-specific, clinical evaluation provides important information on the likelihood of this condition, its severity, and the underlying cause and prognosis.

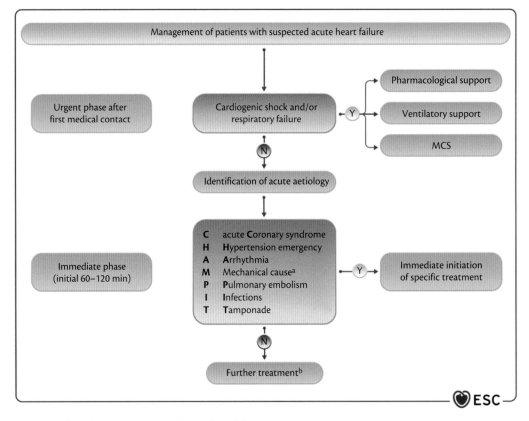

Figure 7.1.2 Stepwise approach to clinical management of acute heart failure.

McDonagh TA, Metra M, Adamo M, *et al*.; ESC Scientific Document Group. 2021 ESC Guidelines for the diagnosis and treatment of acute and chronic heart failure. *Eur Heart J.* 2021 Sep 21;42(36):3599–3726. doi: 10.1093/eurheartj/ehab368. © The European Society of Cardiology. Reprinted by permission of Oxford University Press.

References

1. McDonagh TA, Metra M, Adamo M, *et al*.; ESC Scientific Document Group. 2021 ESC Guidelines for the diagnosis and treatment of acute and chronic heart failure: developed by the Task Force for the diagnosis and treatment of acute and chronic heart failure of the European Society of Cardiology (ESC) With the special contribution of the Heart Failure Association (HFA) of the ESC. *Eur Heart J* 2021;**42**(36):3599–726.

2. Sciarretta S, Palano F, Tocci G, Baldini R, Volpe M. Antihypertensive treatment and development of heart failure in hypertension: a Bayesian network meta-analysis of studies in patients with hypertension and high cardiovascular risk. *Arch Intern Med* 2011;**171**(5):384–94.

3. Zinman B, Wanner C, Lachin JM, *et al*.; EMPA-REG OUTCOME Investigators. Empagliflozin, cardiovascular outcomes, and mortality in type 2 diabetes. *N Engl J Med* 2015;**373**(22):2117–28.

4. The Criteria Committee of the New York Heart Association. *Nomenclature and Criteria for Diagnosis of Diseases of the Heart and Great Vessels*, 9th edition. Boston, MA: Little, Brown, and Co; 1994.

5. Rostagno C, Galanti G, Comeglio M, Boddi V, Olivo G, Gastone Neri Serneri G. Comparison of different methods of functional evaluation in patients with chronic heart failure. *Eur J Heart Fail* 2000;**2**(3):273–80.

6. Goldman L, Hashimoto B, Cook EF, Loscalzo A. Comparative reproducibility and validity of systems for assessing cardiovascular functional class: advantages of a new specific activity scale. *Circulation* 1981;**64**(6):1227–34.

7. Tavazzi L, Tavazzi L, Franzosi MG, *et al*.; GISSI-HF Investigators. Predictors of mortality in 6975 patients with chronic heart failure in the Gruppo Italiano per lo Studio della Streptochinasi nell'Infarto Miocardico-Heart Failure trial: proposal for a nomogram. *Circ Heart Fail* 2013;**6**(1):31–9.

8. Guyatt GH, Sullivan MJ, Thompson PJ, *et al*. The 6-minute walk: a new measure of exercise capacity in patients with chronic heart failure. *Can Med Assoc J* 1985;**132**(8):919–23.

9. Bittner V, Weiner DH, Yusuf S, *et al*. Prediction of mortality and morbidity with a 6-minute walk test in patients with left ventricular dysfunction. SOLVD Investigators. *JAMA* 1993;**270**(14):1702–7.

10. Yancy CW, Jessup M, Bozkurt B, *et al*. 2013 ACCF/AHA guideline for the management of heart failure: executive summary: a report of the American College of Cardiology Foundation/American Heart Association Task Force on practice guidelines. *Circulation* 2013;**128**(16):1810–52.

11. Braunstein JB, Anderson GF, Gerstenblith G, *et al*. Noncardiac comorbidity increases preventable hospitalizations and mortality among Medicare beneficiaries with chronic heart failure. *J Am Coll Cardiol*. 2003;**42**(7):1226–33.

12. Muzzarelli S, Leibundgut G, Maeder MT, *et al*.; TIME-CHF Investigators. Predictors of early readmission or death in elderly patients with heart failure. *Am Heart J*. 2010;**160**(2):308–14.

13. Clerkin KJ, Fried JA, Raikhelkar J, *et al*. COVID-19 and cardiovascular disease. *Circulation* 2020;**141**(20):1648–55.

14. Pocock SJ, Ariti CA, McMurray JJ, *et al.*; Meta-Analysis Global Group in Chronic Heart Failure. Predicting survival in heart failure: a risk score based on 39 372 patients from 30 studies. *Eur Heart J.* 2013;**34**(19):1404–13.

15. Wouter Ouwerkerk W, Adriaan A, Voors AA, Zwinderman AH. Factors influencing the predictive power of models for predicting mortality and/or heart failure hospitalization in patients with heart failure. *JACC Heart Fail* 2014;**2**(5):429–36.

16. Nohria A, Tsang SW, Fang JC, *et al.* Clinical assessment identifies hemodynamic profiles that predict outcomes in patients admitted with heart failure. *J Am Coll Cardiol.* 2003;**41**(10):1797–804.

17. Killip T 3rd, Kimball JT. Treatment of myocardial infarction in a coronary care unit. A two year experience with 250 patients. *Am J Cardiol* 1967;**20**(4):457–64.

CHAPTER 7.2

Biomarkers in diagnostic and prognostic assessment

Rudolf A de Boer, Antoni Bayes-Genis, and James L Januzzi

Contents

Introduction

Biomarkers usually refer to circulating proteins, peptides, metabolites, oligonucleotides, or other molecules that can be measured in blood plasma or serum. Technically, biomarkers may also refer to other physiological parameters or markers, such as blood pressure and body weight, or parameters of cardiac imaging. However, in this chapter, only circulating blood biomarkers are discussed.

In the last decades, a role for biomarkers in the diagnosis and prognosis of heart failure (HF) has been increasingly acknowledged. Ideally, cardiac biomarkers assess in a non-invasive manner the status of a patient with HF, allowing to monitor both changes in the pathophysiology and changes caused in disease management. A wide array of biomarkers have been developed that have an association with changes in cardiomyocytes, the extracellular matrix, and other cardiac structures, whereas several newer biomarkers reflect changes in various tissues relevant to HF, that is, not only the heart, but also the lungs, liver, kidneys, and blood vessels.

Despite the wealth of data supporting their use, biomarkers have only made their way into specific parts of the diagnosis of HF and clinical decision-making, and very few of the thousands of identified markers are even clinically available. Whereas measuring biomarkers is easy, interpreting them properly may be challenging and the necessary studies to expand the role(s) played by biomarkers are lacking. As a result, current use of biomarkers in HF workup and management is limited. In this chapter, we will discuss the most important biomarkers and issues that are important for proper interpretation in HF management.

Different biomarkers and analytical considerations

Different biomarkers

Cardiac-specific biomarkers have certain advantages, as changes in these biomarkers are associated with changes in the cardiac muscle. In the current era, cardiologists and emergency department physicians use natriuretic peptides (NPs) and cardiac troponins (cTns) for various indications.

1. NPs are produced by cardiomyocytes in response to stretch, and are released into the circulation.[1,2] In principle, the NP system is an endogenous neurohormonal system that counteracts the renin–angiotensin system (RAS) and exerts beneficial effects, including vasodilatation, diuresis, and anti-fibrotic effects.[2,3] NPs are thus biologically active proteins that exert their effects via receptors in the vessel wall, kidney, and heart. However, as their levels correlate directly with the extent of myocardial stretch, their role as biomarkers has been studied extensively. There are several NPs used as

biomarkers. Atrial (ANP) and B-type natriuretic peptide (BNP) are the main biologically active NPs. However, they are relatively unstable and therefore, their use is associated with pre-analytical issues and high variability.[4] These limitations have been overcome by assays that measure stable components or metabolites of NPs, most specifically N-terminal proBNP (NT-proBNP) and mid-regional proANP (MR-proANP).

2. cTns are proteins that are part of the sarcomere and interact with actinins to induce myocardial contraction. If the cardiomyocyte membrane is damaged or destroyed, typically when cardiomyocytes die in response to tissue ischaemia and necrosis, troponins leak out of the cells into the circulation. With use of biochemical assays, cTns can be measured reliably and an increase in cTn level inevitably hints towards acute or chronic myocardial disease, and is associated with worse outcomes.[5,6] In the setting of HF, there has been increasing interest in elevations in cTn level, as many patients with acute and chronic HF present with raised cTn levels.

3. There is a wealth of other biomarkers,[7] the use of none of which, however, is currently strongly advocated according to the European Society of Cardiology (ESC) or American Heart Association (AHA)/American College of Cardiology (ACC) guidelines. In a separate paragraph, we will discuss some of the newer markers that have particular potential to enter the clinical arena, with diagnostic, prognostic, or treatment value established in current or future trials.

Analytical considerations

There are important requirements if one wishes to use biomarker levels in clinical decision-making.

First, there needs to be a basic understanding of the biomarker: how it behaves under physiological and pathophysiological circumstances and what organs produce the biomarker (→ Figure 7.2.1).

Furthermore, the dynamics of the biomarker should be known, for example, the typical rise-and-fall pattern of cTn levels in acute ischaemia. Third, one needs to be informed about normal values and about what rise can be considered significant or clinically meaningful.[8] Finally, one needs to know about confounders (see below).

Clearly, a robust assay for biomarker measurement is crucial. An ideal assay should be easy to obtain for clinical laboratories, and have a fast turnaround time to inform results in a timely fashion and low imprecision. Further, one needs to distinguish between variability that normally presents in healthy patients and variability which could signify disease.[8]

Confounders of biomarker results

Circulating levels of biomarkers may differ or fluctuate in relation to other parameters, which may have relevance to the HF phenotype. For NPs and cTns, several confounders have been identified, and evidence is accumulating that factoring in these confounders in the interpretation of biomarker results may fine-tune the message they convey. We will discuss a few general and common confounders.

Age

With increasing age, both NP and cTn levels increase.[1,4,5,9] Minor increases in (very) young patients may already signify clear abnormalities, whereas the same increases in the elderly are very common and may not directly cause alarm. In some cases, higher

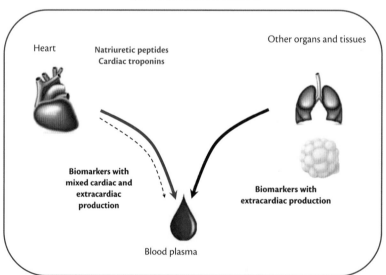

Origin of heart failure biomarkers

Heart — Natriuretic peptides / Cardiac troponins

Other organs and tissues

Biomarkers with mixed cardiac and extracardiac production

Biomarkers with extracardiac production

Blood plasma

Figure 7.2.1 To interpret plasma biomarker levels accurately, it is important to be aware of the origin of the biomarker. For cardiospecific biomarkers, the majority of the plasma pool originates from cardiac production, whereas for non-cardiospecific markers, their plasma levels are a reflection of extracardiac organs.

Source data from Du W, Piek A, Schouten EM, van de Kolk CWA, *et al.* Plasma levels of heart failure biomarkers are primarily a reflection of extracardiac production. *Theranostics.* 2018;8(15):4155–4169.

biomarker values in older subjects may relate to a reduction in renal clearance, but in most, it is thought this finding reflects subtle underlying cardiovascular diseases (e.g. diastolic abnormalities) that accumulate with age.

Sex

NP levels in healthy males are up to 50% lower than in females,[10] which likely reflects the effects of androgens on *NPPB* expression. However, it is uncertain if sex-based differences in NP levels should translate into differential sex-specific cut points for excluding non-acute HF where the lower cut points for NP levels are used. Most studies indicate this to be unlikely to be necessary. In prevalent HF, NP levels generally are elevated to similarly high levels in both men and women, and this increase 'overrides' the baseline differences. In contrast to NPs, cTn levels are generally lower in women than in men.[10] A majority of women have no detectable cTnT and much lower cTnI levels, compared to men. Troponin remains independently prognostic in HF, regardless of sex or cut point used.[5,9,10]

Body mass index

It has been long recognized that higher body mass index is associated with lower levels of BNP and NT-proBNP.[1] Although increased BNP clearance via adipose tissue (which secretes neprilysin and has NP receptors) was originally hypothesized as the cause of this finding, this clearly cannot explain the reduction in NT-proBNP, which is not cleared by either pathway. More recent data have implicated the secretion by adipose tissue of hormones, such as androgens, which suppress *NPPB* expression. Notably, obesity may result in falsely negative results for both BNP and NT-proBNP in up to 20% of obese patients with acute HF.

Renal function

Renal function is, in part, dependent on age and sex. However, renal function itself has profound effects on NP and cTn levels.[1,4,5,9] A lower estimated glomerular filtration rate (eGFR) is associated with higher levels of NPs and cTns. Furthermore, the normal dynamics time curves of biomarker production and release, plateau, and washout are fundamentally changed with worsening renal function. However, within patient strata with a given eGFR (e.g. eGFR 30–50 mL/min), specific NP or cTn levels will still be associated with worse outcomes. Patients with severe renal impairment with cTn levels below the detection limit have a far better course of disease than those with elevated cTn levels.

Concomitant cardiac conditions

Almost all concomitant cardiac conditions can also cause elevated NP and cTn levels.[1,4,5,9] A notorious confounder for NP is atrial fibrillation (AF), which by itself can easily increase NP levels by 2- to 5-fold, depending on the duration of AF paroxysms and the time between the event and blood sampling. Interim acute coronary syndromes and myocardial infarction (MI) are, of course, associated with cTn release, which occurs on top of a 'basal' increase in cTn level. Various other interim events, such as ventricular tachycardia, myocarditis, pulmonary embolism, and cardiac interventions, may also cause an increase in biomarker levels that must be interpreted cautiously, and in totality with all conditions presenting within an individual patient.

Biomarkers in heart failure diagnosis

Diagnosis of HF in a patient presenting with breathlessness for the first time is often difficult, but biomarkers and other investigations can contribute to making the diagnosis. Traditionally, clinical presentation, electrocardiography (ECG), and chest X-ray have been used to diagnose HF, but studies have repeatedly shown a low sensitivity and specificity for making a clinical diagnosis of HF.

NPs are the gold standard biomarkers for HF diagnosis and constitute the bulk of this section.[11,12] They have an indication IA for HF diagnosis according to both ESC and AHA/American College of Cardiology Foundation (ACCF) guidelines.[11,12] More detail on the value of NPs is found in the recently published practical guidance from the Heart Failure Association of the ESC (HFA) on the use of NP levels.[1]

Overall, BNP and NT-proBNP have comparable diagnostic and prognostic accuracy.[13] Other NPs, such as ANP (or MR-proANP), are also comparable, but not as well documented. The recently introduced angiotensin receptor–neprilysin inhibitor sacubitril/valsartan affects the level of NPs that are cleared by neprilysin, such as BNP and ANP, and therefore, NT-proBNP may be the preferred biomarker for quantifying HF severity in patients receiving the drug.[14] Other biomarkers, such as troponins, ST2, galectin-3, and pro-adrenomedullin, are also increased in patients with HF, but they are not currently recommended for HF diagnosis and are discussed later.

Two important principles should be applied to the clinical use of NPs. First, NP measurements should never be a stand-alone test; it is always of greatest value when it complements the physician's clinical skills, along with other available diagnostic tools. Results should always be interpreted while considering the renal function and body mass index, the two most powerful confounders of NP levels.[15,16] Second, NP levels should be interpreted and used as continuous variables to make full use of the biological information provided by the measurement. Cut-off levels may still be useful to make the application of NPs easier for physicians without extensive experience in NP testing.[1]

Acute heart failure

The current recommendation is that NPs should be measured in all patients presenting with symptoms suggestive of new-onset or worsening HF, such as dyspnoea and/or fatigue, as their use facilitates both early diagnosis or early exclusion of HF.[1,11,12]

Optimum NP cut-off levels for the diagnosis of acute HF in patients presenting with acute dyspnoea to the emergency department are higher than those used in the diagnosis of chronic HF in patients with dyspnoea on exertion. ➲ Table 7.2.1 outlines the currently recommended NP cut-offs for the diagnosis of acute HF.[1]

In patients with suspected acute HF, a BNP cut-off level of 100 pg/mL provides an excellent negative predictive value to

Table 7.2.1 Recommended natriuretic peptide cut-offs for acute and non-acute heart failure diagnosis

	Cut-off levels (pg/mL)[a]					
	NT-proBNP			BNP		
	Age <50	Age 50–75	Age >75	Age<50	Age 50–75	Age>75
Acute setting, patients with acute dyspnoea						
HF unlikely	<300			<100		
Grey zone	300–450	300–900	300–1800	100–400		
HF likely	>450	>900	>1800	>400		
Non-acute setting, patients with mild symptoms						
HF unlikely	<125			<35		
Grey zone	125–600			35–150		
HF likely	>60			>150		

[a] Consider reducing cut-off levels by 50% in obese patients.

Source data from Mueller C, McDonald K, de Boer RA, *et al*; Heart Failure Association of the European Society of Cardiology. Heart Failure Association of the European Society of Cardiology practical guidance on the use of natriuretic peptide concentrations. *Eur J Heart Fail*. 2019;21(6):715–731.

exclude the presence of HF, whereas higher values (>400 pg/mL) deliver an excellent positive predictive value.[17] As the NT-proBNP level correlates more strongly with age, age-dependent rule-in cut-offs are preferred for NT-proBNP (450/900/1800 pg/mL; ➲ Table 7.2.1).[18] however, independent of age, an NT-proBNP level of <300 pg/mL provides a very high negative predictive value for HF.[19]

Knowledge of each patient's individual NP level when stable (the so-called dry NP level) helps to interpret marker levels when these patients present with acute symptoms; a change of 100% or more from the stable level suggests a change in clinical state such as decompensation.

Chronic heart failure

In the setting of chronic HF, there is less evidence than in studies performed in the emergency department. However, most of the concepts discussed regarding the use of NPs for diagnostic evaluation of HF in the emergency department also apply in outpatient testing. Nonetheless, current evidence strongly supports the use of NP testing in primary care for accurate evaluation of HF, either as point-of-care testing or in central laboratories.[1,2,3,20,21]

In general, due to their lower levels in the outpatient setting, the main application of NPs has focused on their sensitivity and negative predictive value; lower levels (e.g. BNP <35 pg/mL; NT-proBNP <125 pg/mL; MR-proANP <85 pmol/L) exclude HF with high confidence, whereas higher levels require further evaluation.[22] Currently, the ESC guidelines recommend a cut-off level of 35 and 125 pg/mL for BNP and NT-proBNP, respectively, a strategy that favours minimizing false-negative results. For NT-proBNP, a stratified approach of 50/75/250 pg/mL for ages of <50/50–75/>75 years, respectively, may be considered an alternative.[11,23]

In both the acute and chronic settings, patients with levels in the grey zone require extra physician attention and ancillary testing. Although the final diagnosis is often mild to moderate HF, or HF with preserved ejection fraction (HFpEF),[24,25] rather than HF with reduced ejection fraction (HFrEF), other causes for a modest increase in the NP level should be considered, including primary non-cardiac pathology that causes myocardial stress (e.g. pulmonary hypertension, right ventricular dysfunction secondary to pulmonary embolism, pneumonia, cor pulmonale).

Prognostic monitoring

Besides a proven role to support clinical judgement for HF diagnosis, BNP and NT-proBNP levels also provide substantial prognostic information: across all stages of HF, elevation in the level of either peptide identifies patients at higher risk of development of symptomatic HF or death, compared to matched patients without elevated biomarker levels.[1] Furthermore, addition of serial prognostic assessment via repeated measurement of either peptide—also known as 'monitoring'—has been established as a useful tool not only to predict change in risk, but also to support clinical decision-making.

Among those without prevalent HF, NPs add to clinical variables to predict incident HF. For example, in the Atherosclerosis Risk in Communities study, over a 9.6-year follow-up period, levels of NT-proBNP added substantially to a base model to predict incident HF; compared to a parsimonious base model of clinical variables, addition of NT-proBNP raised the c-statistic for prediction of incident HF by the largest amount of all variables in the model (from 0.77 to 0.80), improved calibration, and reclassified 13% of patients. Addition of NT-proBNP also recalibrated other risk scores for population-incident HF such as the Framingham and Health ABC models.[26] Similar results were reported from the Framingham Heart, Cardiovascular Health, MESA, and PREVEND studies.[27] Notably, for this application, *serial* NP monitoring of ambulatory patients free of HF adds even more prognostic value. For example, in the Cardiovascular Health Study of older patients, baseline NT-proBNP levels in the highest quintile (>267.7 pg/mL) were independently associated with a greater risk of HF (hazard ratio (HR) 3.05, 95% confidence interval (CI) 2.46–3.78) and cardiovascular death (HR 3.02, 95% CI 2.36–3.86), compared to the lowest quintile (<47.5 pg/mL). Adding a second measurement 2–3 years later provided further substantial information: those with increasing levels were at greater adjusted risk of HF (HR 2.13, 95% CI 1.68–2.71) and cardiovascular death (HR 1.91, 95% CI 1.43–2.53), whereas those with decreasing levels were at lower risk of HF (HR 0.58, 95% CI 0.36–0.93) and cardiovascular death (HR 0.57, 95% CI 0.32–1.01), compared to those with unchanged elevated levels.[28] The role of BNP or NT-proBNP measurement as a tool to identify at-risk patients and intensify treatment to prevent incident HF is currently actively explored.

In those with established HF, NP monitoring takes on an even greater importance, as serial levels of each peptide may support clinical decision-making, informing response to therapy in both acute and chronic HF, and may add important information regarding myocardial remodelling in chronic HF.

Across all forms of guideline-directed therapy for HF, BNP and NT-proBNP tend to be reduced after treatment, with the post-therapy 'response' of BNP or NT-proBNP more predictive of prognosis than the baseline value for either peptide. Some treatments (such as angiotensin receptor–neprilysin inhibition and cardiac resynchronization therapy) may result in proportionally greater reductions in NT-proBNP levels.[29,30] Clinicians should remember that changes in BNP level following angiotensin receptor–neprilysin inhibition may be much less predictable,[31] with occasional increases, due to the fact that neprilysin inhibition decreases the degradation of this peptide.

With the knowledge that serial biomarker measurement may inform post-treatment prognosis in HF, the role of such monitoring has been explored.

In chronic HFrEF, where BNP/NT-proBNP levels are driven by congestion, but also by ventricular remodelling status, at 90 days after intensified ambulatory HF therapy, achievement of an NT-proBNP level of <1000 pg/mL was associated with lower adjusted hazard of HF hospitalization/cardiovascular death (HR 0.26, 95% CI 0.15–0.46; $P<0.001$; ➲ Figure 7.2.2a) and all-cause mortality (HR 0.34, 95% CI 0.15–0.77; $P=0.009$; ➲ Figure 7.2.2b), regardless of baseline NT-proBNP level. Importantly, even among those receiving more intensive HFrEF therapy, higher NT-proBNP levels were associated with worse outcome than in those receiving less intensive therapy but with lower NT-proBNP levels, implying 'optimal' medical care in HFrEF might be viewed as achieving both target doses of therapy plus reduction in NT-proBNP level.[32] Mechanistically, this may relate to the fact that reduction in NT-proBNP levels over time is linked to reverse cardiac remodelling with improved left ventricular (LV) size and function, particularly noteworthy when the NT-proBNP level is <1000 pg/mL.[33] Thus, clinicians might serially monitor patients undergoing HFrEF treatment to better understand response to therapy, ventricular remodelling status, and risk of progressive HF complications. Current consensus recommendations suggest measurement of BNP or NT-proBNP levels every 3–6 months if used in this manner.[1]

In acute HF syndromes, much as in chronic states, serial BNP or NT-proBNP measurement provides added information, but gives prognostic information with measurements separated by a much shorter period of time. This is because increased levels of BNP or NT-proBNP in acute HF are predominantly driven by volume overload; with rapid lowering of filling pressures due to decongestive strategies, it is not unusual to see substantial lowering of BNP or NT-proBNP levels over a period of days. These short-term trends in BNP or NT-proBNP levels prior to discharge predict short-term (e.g. up to 180 days) prognosis after discharge.[34,35] For example, Logeart and colleagues reported a pre-discharge BNP level of <350 pg/mL was associated with superior prognosis, compared to higher values.[36] In a more recent European multicentre analysis, Salah and colleagues reported that both a lower absolute discharge NT-proBNP level as well as a reduction in NT-proBNP level of >30% from admission to discharge were associated with superior 180-day prognosis (mortality or mortality/readmission).[35] Taken together, these findings suggest parsimonious sampling of BNP or NT-proBNP (with only admission and post-treatment measurements) for in-hospital monitoring of patients with acute HF might provide clinicians useful information regarding discharge readiness.

Newer biomarkers

Driven by rapid advances in omics, the constellation of candidate biomarkers for measurement in HF is large and continues to grow.[7,37] Though far more numerous than can be enumerated in a single document, as detailed previously, many biomarkers may be fitted into discrete categories focused on myocardial biology (e.g. stretch, injury, remodelling), external stressors (e.g. oxidation, inflammation, neurohormonal activation), and comorbidities (e.g. renal dysfunction) (➲ Figure 7.2.3).[38] In this regard, thousands of new biomarkers have been proposed for measurement to better understand the biology and progression of HF.

Despite rapid gains in biomarker science, the bigger challenge has been to translate such discoveries into actionable clinical knowledge. This is, in part, due to the lack of mechanistic depth into how single or serial measurement of a biomarker may add to the results of BNP or NT-proBNP, and how such information might change diagnostic impressions or be leveraged for better HF treatment. Pre-analytical and analytical challenges may also undermine promising biomarkers due to difficulties with their measurement (e.g. rapid degradation of ANP) and/or interference in their interpretation from common comorbidities (e.g. renal dysfunction and galectin-3).

Examples of biomarkers that may provide added clinical information to NPs and whose importance appears significant/enduring include soluble (s)ST2, insulin-like growth factor binding protein 7 (IGFBP7), and high-sensitivity cTn (hs-cTn).

sST2 is an interleukin 1 receptor family member, whose concentrations are linked to both cardiomyocyte stretch and pulmonary epithelial cell irritation.[39] Elevated concentrations of sST2 interfere with binding of interleukin 33 to its receptor through competitive inhibition; in doing so, favourable anti-remodelling effects of interleukin 33 are lost, with a propensity for myocardial fibrosis, remodelling, and a rising risk of HF hospitalization and both sudden and pump failure death. Concentrations of sST2 are strongly prognostic for HF onset in population-based subjects, as well as predicting worse outcomes in acute and chronic HF. In each case, sST2 typically adds to information from BNP/NT-proBNP; notably, sST2 is not affected by certain pre-analytical

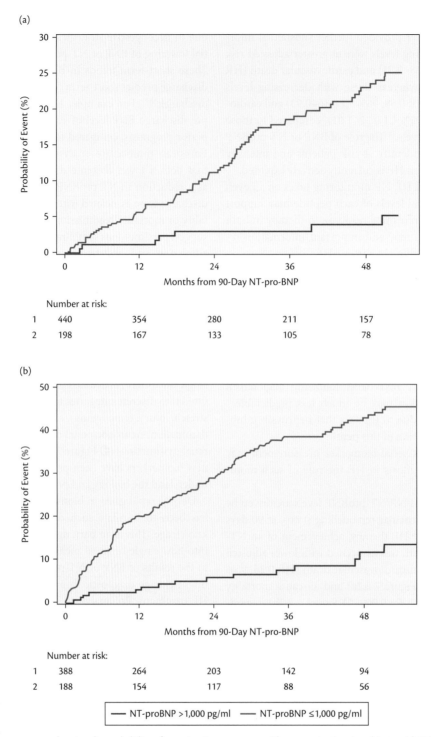

Figure 7.2.2 Cumulative event curves showing the probability of experiencing outcomes with respect to time in subjects with NT-proBNP levels of <1000 pg/mL and those with NT-proBNP levels of >1000 pg/mL at 90 days.

Reproduced from Januzzi JL Jr, Ahmad T, Mulder H, et al. Natriuretic Peptide Response and Outcomes in Chronic Heart Failure With Reduced Ejection Fraction. J Am Coll Cardiol. 2019 Sep 3;74(9):1205–1217. doi: 10.1016/j.jacc.2019.06.055 with permission from Elsevier.

issues that complicate the interpretation of NPs such as obesity or renal failure. Numerous guideline-directed therapies for HF may lower the concentrations of sST2.

IGFBP7 is a member of a large family of insulin-like growth factor binding peptides. However, its main role *in vivo* is as a member of the senescence secretome; higher concentrations of IGFBP7 result in

cell cycle arrest, tissue ageing, and fibrosis. In patients with chronic HF, IGFBP7 is strongly linked to impaired myocardial relaxation, along with obesity and dysglycaemia, a provocative finding that raises a potential role to better phenotype patients with HFpEF.[40] Interestingly, in patients with acute dyspnoea, IGFBP7 measurement adds significantly to NT-proBNP for a more accurate diagnosis

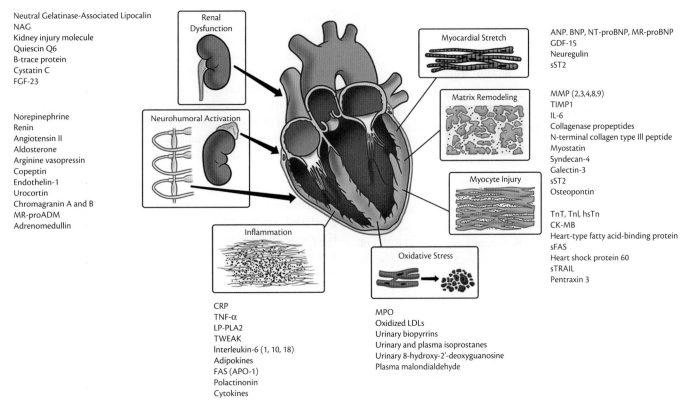

Figure 7.2.3 Various pathophysiological pathways contributing to the development and progression of heart failure and biomarkers representative of the various pathways. ANP, atrial natriuretic peptide; APO, apolipoprotein; BNP, B-type natriuretic peptide; CK-MB, creatinine kinase-muscle/brain; CRP, C-reactive protein; FAS, Fas cell surface death receptor; GDF, growth differentiation factor; hsTn, high-sensitivity troponin; IL, interleukin; LDL, low-density lipoprotein; LP-PLA2, lipoprotein-associated phospholipase A2; MMP, matrix metalloproteinase; MPO, myeloperoxidase; MR-proADM, mid-regional pro-adrenomedullin; MR-proBNP, mid-regional pro-B-type natriuretic peptide; NT-proBNP, N-terminal pro-B-type natriuretic peptide; sFAS, soluble Fas cell surface death receptor; sST2, soluble ST2; sTRAIL, soluble TNF-related apoptosis-inducing ligand; TIMP, tissue inhibitor of metalloproteinases; TNF, tumour necrosis factor; TnI, troponin I; TnT, troponin T.

Reproduced from Ibrahim NE, Januzzi JL Jr. Established and Emerging Roles of Biomarkers in Heart Failure. *Circ Res*. 2018 Aug 17;123(5):614–629. doi: 10.1161/CIRCRESAHA.118.312706. PMID: 30355136 with permission from Wolters Kluwer.

of acute HF, increasing the area under the receiver operating curve for the diagnosis of acute HF (from 0.91 to 0.94; *P*<0.001 for differences), improving model calibration, and significantly reclassifying diagnoses (net reclassification index: +0.25).[41] In both acute and chronic HF, IGFBP7 also supplements NT-proBNP for prognostication of HF events and death. Angiotensin receptor–neprilysin inhibition may lower IGFBP7 concentrations.

Although hs-cTnI and hs-cTnT are well established as biomarkers of myocardial necrosis, with a role in the diagnosis of acute MI, concentrations of hs-cTn are routinely associated with worse prognosis when measured in both acute and chronic HF states.[5,6,7] This is true even when measured together with an NP and even among patients without coronary artery disease. It is reasonable to assume the prognostic information gained from hs-cTn measurement reflects a mixture of pathophysiological triggers for myocyte injury, including coronary- and non-coronary-mediated ischaemia, direct cell death from neurohormonal activation, and exocytosis of cytosolic troponin from stressed cardiomyocytes. Regardless of the cause, higher concentrations of hs-cTn are associated with progressive myocardial remodelling and a heightened risk of HF events, including death.

Emerging biomarkers, such as collagen peptides (which may inform ventricular remodelling), pro-adrenomedullin or CA-125 (proposed as biomarkers of congestion), and growth differentiation factor 15 (suggested as a biomarker of tissue frailty), require more data before their use may be advocated.

Future directions and gaps in knowledge
Multi-biomarker strategies

Seven major classes of biomarkers contributing to the biomarker profile in HF have been postulated: myocardial stretch, myocyte injury, matrix remodelling, inflammation, renal dysfunction, neurohormonal activation, and oxidative stress.[42] A single biomarker is unlikely to reflect all of the facets of HF syndrome, and a multi-marker strategy may characterize better the complexity of HF. In ambulatory HF, the Barcelona Bio-HF Calculator (BCN Bio-HF calculator; available from: www.bcnbiohfcalculator.org) was developed to refine risk stratification, allowing for quick and easy interactive calculations of prognosis and life expectancy at the individual patient level, incorporating multi-markers reflective of different pathophysiological pathways in HF (NT-proBNP, ST2, hsTnT).[43] In acute HF, beyond NT-proBNP, additional indicators may include inflammatory biomarkers, such as interleukin 6 and growth differentiation factor 15, to improve prognosis and establish pathways of activation.[37]

Heart failure with preserved ejection fraction

HFpEF has been placed centre stage in HF research, as the proportion of HF patients with HFpEF is increasing. In HFpEF, we are faced with a multifactorial syndrome with an imperfectly understood pathophysiology that does not respond to therapies that are effective in HFrEF.[44] Part of the challenge is the broad phenotypic variation in those with HFpEF; studies suggest 'clusters' of certain clinical phenotypes could be identified in HFpEF, but it remains unclear if biomarkers can be used to lend further understanding to these phenotypes.[25,45] New biomarker strategies, making use of senescence/cardiometabolic biomarkers such as IGFBP7, collagen biosynthesis remodelling markers such as PIIINP, and the matrix modulator mimecan, may add novel insights and offer additional diagnostic improvement for patients with HFpEF.[45]

Cardiogenic shock

Risk stratification of cardiogenic shock (CS) relies on predictive variables that have been available for decades and proven to be of little help in improving outcomes. A new molecular score has been developed using proteomic technology and validated using enzyme-linked immunosorbent assay (ELISA) in an external cohort. The new CS4P score, which includes liver fatty acid-binding protein (L-FABP), beta-2-microglobulin (B2M), fructose-bisphosphate aldolase B (ALDOB), and SERPING1 (IC1), outperforms the available CardShock and IABP-SHOCK clinical risk scores.[46]

Another biomarker-only score—the cystatin C, lactate, interleukin 6, and NT-proBNP (CLIP) score—outperformed other clinical scores and may be useful as an early decision tool in CS for 30-day mortality risk stratification in infarct-related CS.[47]

Ongoing studies hopefully will confirm that the CS4P and CLIP scores are of value in identifying CS patients and their possible candidacy for early extracorporeal membrane oxygenation (ECMO) therapy.

Incident heart failure

NPs and cTn have the strongest predictive value for incident HF in community-dwelling cohorts.[26,27,28] Recent data suggest that novel biomarkers, including those involved in apoptosis, inflammation, matrix remodelling, and fibrosis, may be helpful in improving prediction of HF onset in elderly patients.[37]

Biomarkers to facilitate drug development

From a clinical trial perspective, biomarkers are a pivotal component of HF clinical trials, and the use of biomarkers in trial design triples the clinical trial success rate. Biomarkers may contribute to a better understanding of pharmacological aspects of candidate drugs, as well as improved characterization of subtypes of disease to aid in the selection of specific therapeutic interventions.[48] Furthermore, some biomarkers such as galectin-3 are, in fact, biotargets and, as such, have attracted considerable attention.[49]

Summary

Biomarkers are widely used in the diagnosis, prognosis assessment, and management of HF. Cardiospecific biomarkers, particularly NPs and cTns, are most often used. Despite decades of research, we only have started to design adequate randomized controlled trials to help us understand how we optimally use the information that comes from (serial) biomarker testing.

In the coming decade, studies should address how biomarkers can complement and optimize currently used clinical models and management. Furthermore, the widespread use of NPs, e.g. in trial design,[50] should be translated into practice guidelines. There are numerous new biomarkers and panels of biomarkers being developed, often with substantial extracardiac production. In HF, a disease characterized by comorbidities, this should not be a problem, but the origin and dynamics of these newer markers have imposed challenges to those using them and many are not ready for prime time.[51]

Key messages

◆ HF biomarkers, especially NPs and cTns, provide powerful and incremental information for accurate diagnosis, prognosis, and treatment choices.

◆ The exact value of biomarkers largely depends on the setting: acute versus chronic HF; HFrEF versus HFpEF; young versus the elderly; and the presence or absence of confounding factors.

◆ Several newer biomarkers are under development and involve newer non-classical analytes and combinations of markers:

• Cardiovascular death or HF hospitalization; and

• All-cause mortality as a function of NT-proBNP levels— those with NT-proBNP levels of <1000 pg/mL at 90 days were found to have lower rates of subsequent events.

References

1. Mueller C, McDonald K, de Boer RA, et al.; Heart Failure Association of the European Society of Cardiology. Heart Failure Association of the European Society of Cardiology practical guidance on the use of natriuretic peptide concentrations. Eur J Heart Fail. 2019;21(6):715–31.

2. Goetze JP, Bruneau BG, Ramos HR, Ogawa T, de Bold MK, de Bold AJ. Cardiac natriuretic peptides. Nat Rev Cardiol. 2020;17(11):698–717.

3. Martinez-Rumayor A, Richards AM, Burnett JC, Januzzi JL Jr. Biology of the natriuretic peptides. Am J Cardiol. 2008;101(3A):3–8.

4. Vasile VC, Jaffe AS. Natriuretic peptides and analytical barriers. Clin Chem. 2017;63(1):50–8.

5. Apple FS, Sandoval Y, Jaffe AS, Ordonez-Llanos J; IFCC Task Force on Clinical Applications of Cardiac Bio-Markers. Cardiac troponin assays: guide to understanding analytical characteristics and their impact on clinical care. Clin Chem. 2017;63(1):73–81.

6. Mair J, Lindahl B, Hammarsten O, et al. How is cardiac troponin released from injured myocardium? Eur Heart J Acute Cardiovasc Care. 2018;7(6):553–60.

7. de Boer RA, Daniels LB, Maisel AS, Januzzi JL Jr. State of the art: newer biomarkers in heart failure. Eur J Heart Fail. 2015;17(6):559–69.

8. Meijers WC, van der Velde AR, Muller Kobold AC, *et al.* Variability of biomarkers in patients with chronic heart failure and healthy controls. Eur J Heart Fail. 2017;19(3):357–65.

9. Chow SL, Maisel AS, Anand I, *et al.*; American Heart Association Clinical Pharmacology Committee of the Council on Clinical Cardiology; Council on Basic Cardiovascular Sciences; Council on Cardiovascular Disease in the Young; Council on Cardiovascular and Stroke Nursing; Council on Cardiopulmonary, Critical Care, Perioperative and Resuscitation; Council on Epidemiology and Prevention; Council on Functional Genomics and Translational Biology; Council on Quality of Care and Outcomes Research. Role of biomarkers for the prevention, assessment, and management of heart failure: a scientific statement from the American Heart Association. Circulation. 2017;135(22):e1054–91.

10. Suthahar N, Meems LMG, Ho JE, de Boer RA. Sex-related differences in contemporary biomarkers for heart failure: a review. Eur J Heart Fail. 2020;22(5):775–88.

11. Ponikowski P, Voors AA, Anker SD, *et al.* 2016 ESC Guidelines for the diagnosis and treatment of acute and chronic heart failure: the Task Force for the diagnosis and treatment of acute and chronic heart failure of the European Society of Cardiology (ESC). Developed with the special contribution of the Heart Failure Association (HFA) of the ESC. Eur J Heart Fail. 2016; 18: 891–975.

12. Yancy CW, Jessup M, Bozkurt B, *et al.* 2013 ACCF/AHA Guideline for the management of heart failure: a report of the American College of Cardiology Foundation/American Heart Association Task Force on practice guidelines. Circulation. 2013; 128: e240–327.

13. Lainchbury JG, Campbell E, Frampton CM, Yandle TG, Nicholls MGG, Richards AM. Brain natriuretic peptide and N-terminal brain natriuretic peptide in the diagnosis of heart failure in patients with acute shortness of breath. J Am Coll Cardiol. 2003;42:728–35.

14. Bayes-Genis A, Barallat J, Richards AM. A test in context: neprilysin: function, inhibition, and biomarker. J Am Coll Cardiol. 2016;68(6):639–53.

15. van Kimmenade RR, Januzzi JL, Bakker JA, *et al.* Renal clearance of B-type natriuretic peptide and amino terminal pro-B-type natriuretic peptide. J Am Coll Cardiol. 2009;53:884–90.

16. Bayés-Genis A, Lloyd-Jones DM, van Kimmenade RRJ, *et al.* Effect of body mass index on diagnostic and prognostic usefulness of amino-terminal pro-brain natriuretic peptide in patients with acute dyspnea. Arch Intern Med. 2007;167:400–7.

17. Maisel AS, Krishnaswamy P, Nowak RM, *et al.*; Breathing Not Properly Multinational Study Investigators. Rapid measurement of B-type natriuretic peptide in the emergency diagnosis of heart failure. N Engl J Med. 2002;347:161–7.

18. Januzzi JL, van Kimmenade R, Lainchbury J, *et al.* NT-proBNP testing for diagnosis and short-term prognosis in acute destabilized heart failure: an international pooled analysis of 1256 patients: the international collaborative of NT-proBNP Study. Eur Heart J. 2006;27:330–7.

19. Januzzi JL, Chen-Tournoux AA, Christenson RH, *et al.* N-terminal pro-B-type natriuretic peptide in the emergency department: the ICON-RELOADED Study. J Am Coll Cardiol. 2018;71:1191–200.

20. Burri E, Hochholzer K, Arenja N, *et al.* B-type natriuretic peptide in the evaluation and management of dyspnoea in primary care. J Intern Med. 2012;272:504–13.

21. Wright SP, Doughty RN, Pearl A, *et al.* Plasma amino-terminal pro-brain natriuretic peptide and accuracy of heart-failure diagnosis in primary care. J Am Coll Cardiol. 2003;42:1793–800.

22. Zaphiriou A, Robb S, Murray-Thomas T, *et al.* The diagnostic accuracy of plasma BNP and NTproBNP in patients referred from primary care with suspected heart failure: results of the UK natriuretic peptide study. Eur J Heart Fail. 2005;7:537–41.

23. Hildebrandt P, Collinson PO, Doughty RN, *et al.* Age-dependent values of N-terminal pro-B-type natriuretic peptide are superior to a single cut-point for ruling out suspected systolic dysfunction in primary care. Eur Heart J. 2010;31:1881–9.

24. Pieske B, Tschöpe C, de Boer RA, *et al.* How to diagnose heart failure with preserved ejection fraction: the HFA-PEFF diagnostic algorithm: a consensus recommendation from the Heart Failure Association (HFA) of the European Society of Cardiology (ESC). Eur Heart J. 2019;40(40):3297–317.

25. Meijers WC, van der Velde AR, de Boer RA. Biomarkers in heart failure with preserved ejection fraction. Neth Heart J. 2016;24(4):252–8.

26. Agarwal SK, Chambless LE, Ballantyne CM, *et al.* Prediction of incident heart failure in general practice: the Atherosclerosis Risk in Communities (ARIC) Study. Circ Heart Fail. 2012;5(4):422–9.

27. de Boer RA, Nayor M, deFilippi CR, *et al.* Association of cardiovascular biomarkers with incident heart failure with preserved and reduced ejection fraction. JAMA Cardiol. 2018;3(3):215–24.

28. deFilippi CR, Christenson RH, Gottdiener JS, Kop WJ, Seliger SL. Dynamic cardiovascular risk assessment in elderly people. The role of repeated N-terminal pro-B-type natriuretic peptide testing. J Am Coll Cardiol. 2010;55(5):441–50.

29. Yu CM, Fung JW, Zhang Q, *et al.* Improvement of serum NT-proBNP predicts improvement in cardiac function and favorable prognosis after cardiac resynchronization therapy for heart failure. J Card Fail. 2005;11(5 Suppl):S42–6.

30. Zile MR, Claggett BL, Prescott MF, *et al.* Prognostic implications of changes in N-terminal pro-B-type natriuretic peptide in patients with heart failure. J Am Coll Cardiol. 2016;68(22):2425–36.

31. Myhre PL, Vaduganathan M, Claggett B, *et al.* B-type natriuretic peptide during treatment with sacubitril/valsartan: the PARADIGM-HF trial. J Am Coll Cardiol. 2019;73(11):1264–72.

32. Januzzi JL Jr, Ahmad T, Mulder H, *et al.* Natriuretic peptide response and outcomes in chronic heart failure with reduced ejection fraction. J Am Coll Cardiol. 2019;74(9):1205–17.

33. Daubert MA, Adams K, Yow E, *et al.* NT-proBNP goal achievement is associated with significant reverse remodeling and improved clinical outcomes in HFrEF. JACC Heart Fail. 2019;7(2):158–68.

34. Kociol RD, Horton JR, Fonarow GC, *et al.* Admission, discharge, or change in B-type natriuretic peptide and long-term outcomes: data from Organized Program to Initiate Lifesaving Treatment in Hospitalized Patients with Heart Failure (OPTIMIZE-HF) linked to Medicare claims. Circ Heart Fail. 2011;4(5):628–36.

35. Salah K, Kok WE, Eurlings LW, *et al.* A novel discharge risk model for patients hospitalised for acute decompensated heart failure incorporating N-terminal pro-B-type natriuretic peptide levels: a European coLlaboration on Acute decompeNsated Heart Failure: ELAN-HF Score. Heart. 2014;100(2):115–25.

36. Logeart D, Thabut G, Jourdain P, *et al.* Predischarge B-type natriuretic peptide assay for identifying patients at high risk of readmission after decompensated heart failure. J Am Coll Cardiol. 2004;43(4):635–41.

37. Bayes-Genis A, Liu PP, Lanfear DE, *et al.* Omics phenotyping in heart failure: the next frontier. Eur Heart J. 2020;41(36):3477–84.

38. Ibrahim NE, Januzzi JL Jr. Established and emerging roles of biomarkers in heart failure. Circ Res. 2018;123(5):614–29.

39. McCarthy CP, Januzzi JL Jr. Soluble ST2 in heart failure. Heart Fail Clin. 2018;14(1):41–8.

40. Gandhi PU, Gaggin HK, Redfield MM, *et al.* Insulin-like growth factor-binding protein-7 as a biomarker of diastolic dysfunction and functional capacity in heart failure with preserved ejection fraction: results from the RELAX trial. JACC Heart Fail. 2016;4(11):860–9.

41. Ibrahim NE, Afilalo M, Chen-Tournoux A, *et al*. Diagnostic and prognostic utilities of insulin-like growth factor binding protein-7 in patients with dyspnea. JACC Heart Fail. 2020;8(5):415–22.

42. Braunwald E. Heart failure. JACC Heart Fail. 2013;1:1–20.

43. Lupon J, de Antonio M, Vila J, *et al*. Development of a novel heart failure risk tool: the Barcelona bioheart failure risk calculator (BCN bio-HF calculator). PLoS One. 2014;9:e85466.

44. Bayes-Genis A, Liu PP, Lanfear DE, *et al*. Omics phenotyping in heart failure: the next frontier. Eur Heart J. 2020;41(36):3477–84.

45. Lam CSP, Voors AA, de Boer RA, Solomon SD, van Veldhuisen DJ. Heart failure with preserved ejection fraction: from mechanisms to therapies. Eur Heart J. 2018;39(30):2780–92.

46. Rueda F, Borràs E, García-García C, *et al*. Protein-based cardiogenic shock patient classifier. Eur Heart J. 2019;40(32):2684–94.

47. Ceglarek U, Schellong P, Rosolowski M, *et al*. The novel cystatin C, lactate, interleukin-6, and N-terminal pro-B-type natriuretic peptide (CLIP)-based mortality risk score in cardiogenic shock after acute myocardial infarction. Eur Heart J. 2021;42(24):2344–52.

48. Bayes-Genis A, Voors AA, Zannad F, Januzzi JL, Mark Richards A, Díez J. Transitioning from usual care to biomarker-based personalized and precision medicine in heart failure: call for action. Eur Heart J. 2018;39(30):2793–9.

49. Suthahar N, Meijers WC, Silljé HHW, Ho JE, Liu FT, de Boer RA. Galectin-3 activation and inhibition in heart failure and cardiovascular disease: an update. Theranostics. 2018;8(3):593–609.

50. Ibrahim NE, Burnett JC Jr, Butler J, *et al*. Natriuretic peptides as inclusion criteria in clinical trials: a JACC: heart failure position paper. JACC Heart Fail. 2020;8(5):347–58.

51. Piek A, Du W, de Boer RA, Silljé HHW. Novel heart failure biomarkers: why do we fail to exploit their potential? Crit Rev Clin Lab Sci. 2018;55(4):246–63.

CHAPTER 7.3

Imaging in heart failure

Contents

7.3.1 Echocardiography

Philippe Debonnaire, Victoria Delgado, Thor Edvardsen, Bogdan A Popescu, and Jeroen J Bax

Introduction

Heart failure is a major public health problem associated with high diagnostic and therapeutic expenses and poor survival. Coronary artery disease (CAD) remains the leading cause of heart failure with reduced left ventricular (LV) ejection fraction (HFrEF), followed by hypertension and diabetes.[1] Ageing and metabolic syndrome increase the prevalence of heart failure with preserved LV ejection fraction (HFpEF).[2,3] The epidemiology, pathophysiology, and natural course of these two entities differ significantly, with superior survival of patients with HFpEF as compared to their counterparts with HFrEF.[4,5] Current guidelines also include the category of heart failure with mildly reduced LV ejection fraction (HFmrEF),[5] which is associated with better outcomes as compared to HFrEF.[6,7,8] However, in terms of demographic and clinical characteristics and response to conventional heart failure therapy, HFmrEF and HFrEF are rather similar.

Therefore, the major questions to be addressed during the evaluation of patients with heart failure symptoms are, first, what causes heart failure symptoms and, second, whether the LV ejection fraction (LVEF) is reduced or not, as this functional parameter is the most frequently used to decide the clinical management of heart failure patients.

Non-invasive cardiac imaging plays a central role in the clinical management of heart failure patients, as it is key to diagnosis, therapeutic decision-making, and prognosis assessment. Currently, four main non-invasive imaging modalities are available: echocardiography; multidetector computed tomography (MDCT); cardiac magnetic resonance (CMR) imaging; and nuclear imaging, including single-photon emission computed tomography (SPECT) and positron emission tomography (PET). The choice of which imaging modality to use in heart failure patients depends on the clinical question to be answered and on the availability, local expertise, contraindications, and associated risks of each imaging technique (➲ Table 7.3.1.1).

In general, due to widespread availability, safety, accuracy, portability, and relatively low cost, echocardiography remains the imaging technique of first choice to evaluate heart failure patients. Following improvements in probe technology and computer software, three-dimensional echocardiography has permitted more accurate and reproducible assessment of cardiac chamber dimensions and ventricular function, compared

Table 7.3.1.1 Value of different non-invasive imaging modalities in the evaluation of heart failure patients in clinical practice

		ECHO	CMR	MDCT	SPECT	PET
Remodelling/dysfunction						
LV	EDV	++	+++	++	++	++
	ESV	++	+++	++	++	++
	EF	++	+++	++	++	++
	Mass	++	+++	++	−	−
RV	EDV	++	+++	++	−	−
	ESV	++	+++	++	−	−
	EF	++	+++	++	−	−
	Mass	++	+++	++	−	−
LV diastolic function		+++	+	−	−	−
Dyssynchrony		++	+	−	+	−
Aetiology						
CAD	Ischaemia	+++	+++	−	+++	+++
	Hibernation	+++	+++	−	+++	+++
	Scar	++	+++	−	++	++
	Coronary anatomy	−	−	+++	−	−
Valvular	Stenosis	+++	+	++	−	−
	Regurgitation	+++	++	−	−	−
Myocarditis		+	+++	−	−	−
Sarcoidosis		+	+++	−	−	++
Hypertrophic CMP	HCM	+++	++	−	−	−
	Amyloidosis	++	+++	−	−	−
Dilated CMP	Myocarditis	+	+++	−	−	−
	Eosinophilic syndromes	+	+++	−	−	−
	Iron: haemochromatosis	+	+++	−	−	−
	Iron: thalassaemia	+	+++	−	−	−
ARVC		++	+++	+	−	−
Restrictive CMP	Pericarditis	++	++	++	−	−
	Amyloidosis	++	+++	+++	−	−
	Endomyocardial fibrosis	+	+++	−	−	−
	Anderson−Fabry	+	+	−	−	−
Unclassified CMP	Takotsubo CMP	++	++	−	−	−
Main advantages/disadvantages						
Availability		High	Low	Reasonable	High	Low
Portability		Yes	No	No	No	No
Cost		Low	High	Moderate	High	High
Image quality		Variable	Good*	High*	Reasonable	High
Radiation		No	No	Yes	Yes	Yes

* Unless presence of arrhythmia.

ARVC, arrhythmogenic right ventricular cardiomyopathy; CAD, coronary artery disease; CMP, cardiomyopathy; CMR, cardiac magnetic resonance; ECHO, echocardiography; EF, ejection fraction; EDV, end-diastolic volume; ESV, end-systolic volume; HCM, hypertrophic cardiomyopathy; LV, left ventricle/ventricular; MDCT, multidetector computed tomography; PET, positron emission tomography; RV, right ventricle; SPECT, single-photon emission computed tomography.

McDonagh TA, Metra M, Adamo M, *et al*; ESC Scientific Document Group. 2021 ESC Guidelines for the diagnosis and treatment of acute and chronic heart failure. *Eur Heart J*. 2021 Sep 21;42(36):3599–3726. doi: 10.1093/eurheartj/ehab368. © The European Society of Cardiology. Reprinted by permission of Oxford University Press.

to two-dimensional echocardiography. In addition, three-dimensional echocardiography has proved its superiority for morphological valve analysis, in particular of the mitral valve.[9] The introduction of cardiac ultrasound contrast agents also has been an important breakthrough. Contrast echocardiography significantly enhances endocardial border delineation in patients with poor acoustic window, increasing diagnostic performance to identify functional disease (chamber volumes, ejection fraction, wall motion abnormalities) and detect structural abnormalities (including hypertrophy, crypts, aneurysms, and cardiac mass). In addition, it permits non-invasive myocardial perfusion imaging.

Furthermore, use of point-of-care ultrasound (POCUS) or focused cardiac ultrasound (FoCUS) has helped in the management of patients with acute heart failure. Miniaturized (pocket-sized) ultrasound systems allow fast evaluation of the haemodynamic condition of the patient and can guide in the differential diagnosis of the heart failure aetiology.

Heart failure diagnosis

The clinical heart failure syndrome is defined as the presence of heart failure symptoms and signs, together with cardiac functional or structural abnormalities.[5] Approximately half of heart failure patients present with HFpEF, formerly called diastolic heart failure, whereas the other half is characterized by HFrEF, referred to as systolic heart failure.[5] Echocardiography remains the first-line recommended imaging modality to detect these abnormalities and establish a heart failure diagnosis.

Heart failure with preserved ejection fraction

The exact definition of HFpEF is an ongoing matter of debate. Recent meta-analyses have shown that HFpEF patients are frequently older women with hypertension, diabetes mellitus, obesity (metabolic syndrome), and/or atrial fibrillation.[4,10] In addition, up to 13% of older patients presenting with HFpEF and thickened LV wall have cardiac amyloidosis.[11] Accordingly, HFpEF is characterized by: (1) preserved (near-normal) LVEF without LV dilatation; and (2) relevant structural heart disease (LV hypertrophy, left atrial enlargement) and/or diastolic dysfunction (Table 7.3.1.2).[5]

Conventional transthoracic echocardiography is the imaging modality of first choice to evaluate patients with HFpEF. Preserved systolic function, defined as LVEF ≥50%, impaired LV relaxation, and an enlarged left atrium are commonly observed. In addition, use of tissue Doppler imaging to assess LV diastolic dysfunction is included in routine evaluation of patients with HFpEF. This echocardiographic technique often demonstrates reduced early diastolic myocardial velocities at the mitral annulus (e′ average <9 cm/s) and/or an increased early mitral inflow-to-e′ ratio (E/e′ >15), at rest or during exercise, reflecting increased LV filling pressure.[5] Current advances in echocardiographic techniques have provided more sensitive tools to detect subtle abnormalities in LV mechanics. Myocardial deformation imaging with tissue Doppler or speckle tracking is able to detect systolic dysfunction even before LV decline (➲ Figure 7.3.1.1).[12] Global and segmental myocardial thickening and shortening can be evaluated, and myocardial segments with active contraction can be differentiated from those (scarred or fibrotic) segments that are passively moved by the surrounding functionally preserved myocardial segments. A significant proportion of patients with HFpEF show impaired LV longitudinal deformation (strain), reflecting subtle systolic dysfunction.[13,14] In addition, characteristic relative apical sparing of longitudinal function relative to the basal and mid portions has high sensitivity and specificity for detection of cardiac amyloidosis.[15] These novel echocardiographic techniques may help to develop effective therapies to reverse or halt the progression of the underlying disease towards overt HFrEF. Ongoing research focuses on standardization of these techniques to evaluate patients who have an increased risk of heart failure but do not yet show structural heart disease based on conventional echocardiography.

Heart failure with mildly reduced ejection fraction

Patients presenting with heart failure symptoms and mildly reduced LV systolic function, defined by LVEF of between 41% to 49%, are referred to as having HFmrEF.[5] The clinical phenotype of these patients resembles more that of HFrEF, with patients more likely to be younger and male, and is commonly associated with CAD. In addition, atrial fibrillation and the presence of multiple comorbidities are less common than in HFpEF

Table 7.3.1.2 Diagnostic criteria for heart failure with reduced (HFrEF), mildly reduced (HFmrEF), and preserved (HFpEF) left ventricular ejection fraction

Heart failure type criteria	HFrEF	HFmrEF	HFpEF
1	Signs and/or symptoms		
2	LVEF ≤40%	LVEF 41–49%	LVEF ≥50%
3	–	–	◆ Structural abnormality: LV hypertrophy or LA dilatation _And/or_ ◆ Diastolic dysfunction: e′ average <9 cm/s or E/e′ ≥15

e′ average, average early diastolic myocardial tissue Doppler velocity of the septal and lateral mitral annulus; E/e′, early pulsed-wave Doppler mitral inflow over e; HFmrEF, heart failure with mildly reduced ejection fraction; HFpEF, heart failure with preserved ejection fraction; HFrEF, heart failure with reduced ejection fraction; LA, left atrial; LV, left ventricular; LVEF, left ventricular ejection fraction.

Based on European Society of Cardiology guideline recommendations.

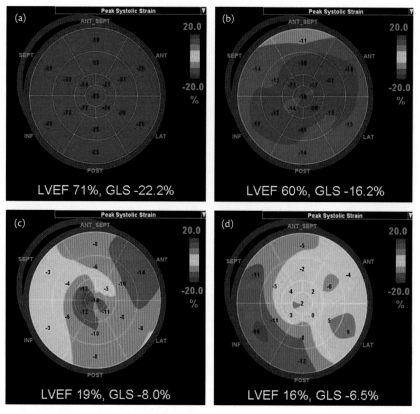

Figure 7.3.1.1 Global longitudinal strain (GLS) assessed by two-dimensional speckle tracking echocardiography to assess left ventricular systolic function. Speckle tracking of myocardial segments throughout cardiac cycle in four-, three-, and two-chamber apical views is performed to assess longitudinal strain. A colour-coded 17-segment bull`s eye plot displays segmental strain values (red is more negative and thus reflects normal deformation; blue reflects reduced deformation). GLS, a sensitive parameter of systolic left ventricular function, is calculated as the mean peak systolic segmental strain value out of 17 segments. (a) Normal volunteer with GLS <−18%. (b) Patient with cardiovascular risk factors (diabetes and hypertension), non-significant coronary artery disease, and preserved left ventricular ejection fraction, showing modestly impaired GLS (>−18%). (c) Severe dilated cardiomyopathy with diffuse segmental dysfunction. (d) Patient with anterolateral myocardial infarction. Note apicolateral dyskinesia.

patients. Mortality, however, of ambulatory HFmrEF patients is lower, compared to patients with HFrEF, and more in line with that of HFpEF patients.[5] Of note, the HFmrEF category also includes patients who have improved LVEF from ≤40% or declined from ≥50%.

Heart failure with reduced left ventricular ejection fraction

Impairment of systolic function, defined as LVEF of <50%, establishes the diagnosis of HFrEF when typical heart failure signs and symptoms coincide. Although initial echocardiographic screening for LV systolic dysfunction is performed by 'eyeballing', extensive experience is mandatory for accurate interpretation. Absolute quantification of LV function by assessment of LVEF, by using the modified Simpson's biplane method (summation of discs), is recommended in daily practice and can be performed by semi-automated applications.[5] Three-dimensional echocardiography provides a novel technique for a more accurate estimation of LV volumes and ejection fraction, more in line with CMR, the gold standard for volumetric chamber assessment (➲ Figure 7.3.1.2).[16] In particular, it (partly) overcomes volume underestimation due to apical foreshortening and geometrical assumptions, inherent

to two-dimensional echocardiography. To increase endocardial border delineation, contrast agents can be administered.

Apart from medical therapy, cardiac resynchronization therapy (CRT), implantable cardioverter–defibrillator (ICD) implantation, coronary artery revascularization, and surgery, including LV reconstruction, valve repair, LV assist devices, and heart transplantation, complete the therapeutic armamentarium for HFrEF patients. Quantification of LVEF is crucial to clinical management of these patients and is a criterion to decide on CRT or implantation of ICD devices. Additional information on CAD, myocardial tissue characteristics, LV geometry, and valvular heart disease (particularly functional mitral regurgitation (MR)) will provide tailored clinical management of heart failure patients. To answer each of these questions, stepwise use of cardiovascular imaging, knowing the strengths and limitations of each imaging technique, is desirable to avoid unnecessary imaging and increased healthcare costs.

Stepwise clinical approach

A series of questions of interest need to be asked after a heart failure diagnosis has been established: (1) whether CAD is present; (2) whether revascularization is indicated; (3) what the LV

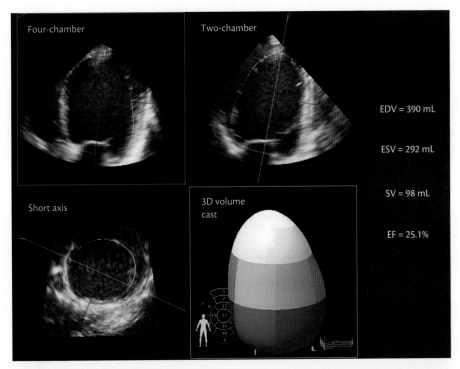

Four-chamber

Two-chamber

EDV = 390 mL

ESV = 292 mL

SV = 98 mL

EF = 25.1%

Short axis

3D volume cast

Figure 7.3.1.2 Three-dimensional (3D) echocardiography left ventricular function assessment in a patient with severe dilated cardiomyopathy. After 3D full volume acquisition of the left ventricle, anatomical landmarks are indicated on reformation planes using post-processing software to allow automated tracing of the endocardial border throughout the cardiac cycle (yellow lines). Manual adjustments to the tracing can be performed. A 3D volume cast of the left ventricle is built and colour-coded per segment. The end-systolic volume (ESV) and end-diastolic volume (EDV), stroke volume (SV), and ejection fraction (EF) are displayed.

geometry is (in terms of volumes and shape); (4) whether MR is present; and (5) whether the patient is a candidate for device therapy. Echocardiography plays an important role in answering each of these questions.

Coronary artery disease

CAD is the main cause of heart failure, with a high prevalence among patients with HFrEF (65%) and those with HFpEF (50%).[1,3] Therefore, an ischaemic aetiology needs to be assessed for in the diagnostic workup of heart failure patients. The various imaging techniques to diagnose the presence of CAD can be grouped into: (1) anatomical tests (invasive coronary angiography, coronary computed tomography angiography, and magnetic resonance angiography) that provide information on the presence, location, severity, and extent of coronary artery lesions; and (2) functional tests (stress echocardiography, nuclear imaging, stress CMR, and perfusion computed tomography) that provide information on the haemodynamic consequences of coronary artery lesions (ischaemia) (➲ Figure 7.3.1.3).

Ischaemia detection by different imaging modalities is mainly based on comparative study of systolic function and/or perfusion at rest and during stress. The latter can be performed pharmacologically using vasodilators (including adenosine and dipyridamole) and inotropes (dobutamine) or by physical exercise. Stress echocardiography identifies ischaemia when deterioration in regional (or global in cases of severe ischaemia) wall motion

thickening occurs during peak stress. Addition of contrast to enhance endocardial border delineation and use of longitudinal strain (rate), largely reflecting subendocardial myocardial layers that are most sensitive to ischaemia, enhance diagnostic accuracy.[17] In addition, assessment of stress-induced perfusion defects and absolute quantification of myocardial blood flow can also be performed by using contrast perfusion echocardiography (➲ Figure 7.3.1.4). Once CAD has been excluded, alternative non-ischaemic cardiomyopathy aetiologies need consideration in the diagnostic workup of heart failure patients. Integration of clinical symptoms, electrocardiography, additional laboratory testing, and alternative non-invasive imaging is crucial. In this regard, echocardiography and particularly CMR are valuable to detect additional functional or structural cardiac abnormalities.[18] Both imaging modalities can provide critical information on left and right chamber dimensions and volumes, right ventricular and LV systolic and diastolic function, and haemodynamics, including filling pressure, shunting, and outflow obstruction. In addition, systematic screening for valvular, myocardial, or pericardial abnormalities (including pericardial effusion) can be performed. Administration of intravenous contrast during echocardiography may be particularly helpful to detect apical forms of hypertrophic cardiomyopathy, myocardial trabeculations and crypts in LV non-compaction cardiomyopathy, and right ventricular aneurysms in arrhythmogenic right ventricular cardiomyopathy (➲ Figure 7.3.1.5). Evaluation of pericardial thickness,

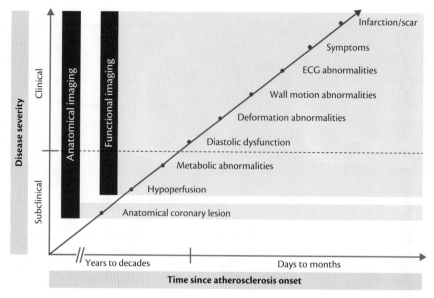

Figure 7.3.1.3 Non-invasive imaging applications to study coronary artery disease targeting different steps in the ischaemic cascade. Modalities and techniques visualizing earlier stages of the ischaemic cascade are more sensitive and specificity is higher when late stages are explored.

interventricular dependence, and significant respiratory variation of filling patterns can be performed accurately by echocardiography or CMR to differentiate between constrictive pericarditis and restrictive cardiomyopathy.

Revascularization

Once the presence of CAD has been diagnosed in heart failure patients, revascularization needs consideration. The presence of ischaemia, assessed by using functional tests, indicates the need for percutaneous or surgical revascularization. However, the peri-procedural mortality risk from surgical or percutaneous revascularization in heart failure patients ranges between 5% (in young patients) and >30% (in elderly patients).[19] Consequently, evaluation of myocardial viability, reflecting potential recovery of

myocardial dysfunction after restoration of coronary blood flow and present in nearly 60% of heart failure patients, has been advocated to identify those patients who will benefit from these procedures.[20] Indeed, improvement in regional and global LV systolic function, heart failure symptoms, and prognosis has been reported after revascularization in patients with viable myocardium. A meta-analysis of non-randomized studies including >3000 patients with CAD and LV dysfunction showed that assessment of myocardial viability prior to revascularization has important prognostic implications.[21] Patients with viable myocardium who were revascularized showed significantly lower annual mortality rate than patients who were medically treated (3.2% vs 16%). In contrast, in patients without myocardial viability, revascularization was not associated with prognostic benefit.[21] A recent substudy

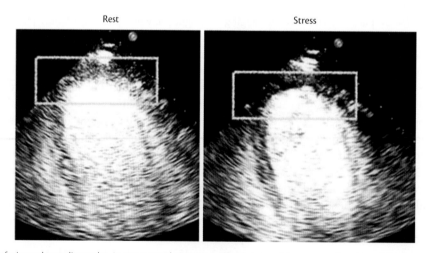

Figure 7.3.1.4 Contrast perfusion echocardiography. At rest, normal contrast replenishment of the myocardium is seen due to normal perfusion. During dobutamine stress, myocardial ischaemia is diagnosed with reduced perfusion in the apical zone.

Reproduced from Nihoyannopoulos P and Vanoverschelde JL. Myocardial ischaemia and viability: the pivotal role of echocardiography. *European Heart Journal.* 2011;32:810–9 with permission from Oxford University Press.

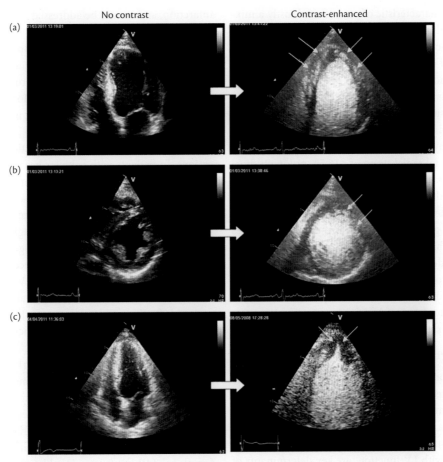

Figure 7.3.1.5 Improved diagnostic accuracy using contrast echocardiography. A 55-year-old patient with symptomatic left ventricular dysfunction is referred for evaluation. Mild hypertrophy is seen on apical four-chamber (a) and short-axis (b) views. Addition of contrast indicates crypts and recesses in the apical and anteroseptal regions (arrows), indicative of left ventricular non-compaction cardiomyopathy. (c) shows the echocardiographic images of a 50-year-old patient with ventricular arrhythmias. On contrast echocardiography, apical hypertrophy is observed on the four-chamber apical view (arrows).

of the randomized controlled trial STICH evaluated the impact of myocardial viability assessment (with SPECT or dobutamine stress echocardiography) and treatment (revascularization vs medical therapy) on long-term outcome in 601 ischaemic heart failure patients.[22] Patients with myocardial viability had superior survival than those without viability (hazard ratio 0.64, 95% confidence interval 0.48–0.86; $P = 0.003$). However, there were no significant differences in survival benefit between revascularization and medical therapy in patients with myocardial viability, compared to those without viability. Besides the selection bias (viability imaging was left to the discretion of the treating physicians in the study protocol), other factors included in the multivariate

analysis and that are also influenced by the presence of myocardial viability, such as LV volumes, shape, and ejection fraction, may have more relevant influence on long-term survival.

The hallmark of myocardial viability assessment is detection of dysfunctional myocardium that will recover after revascularization. Two different dysfunctional viable myocardial states have been defined: (1) 'stunned' myocardium resulting from transient ischaemia which is followed by reperfusion; (2) 'hibernating' myocardium resulting from persistent low coronary blood flow (⊃ Table 7.3.1.3).[23] Functional recovery may take up to 14 months after revascularization and, in general, takes longer for hibernating, compared to stunned, myocardium.[24] Irreversible

Table 7.3.1.3 Left ventricular (dys)function in ischaemic cardiomyopathy

Condition	Resting contractility	Contractile reserve	Resting perfusion	Perfusion reserve	FDG metabolic activity	Recovery after revascularization
Normal	N	++	N	N	N	
Stunning	↓	++	N	↓	N or ↑	++
Hibernation	↓	±	↓	↓	N or ↑	±
Scar	↓	−	↓	↓	↓	−

FDG, 18-fluorodeoxyglucose; N, normal.

myocardial damage is characteristic of scar tissue. Mostly a mixture of scarred, stunned, and hibernating myocardium is present, and viability of dysfunctional myocardium is determined by the relative contribution of each.

Different imaging modalities can assess viability based on the study of (combinations of) different pathophysiological characteristics such as perfusion and/or metabolism, systolic function, contractile reserve, and/or scar (⊕ Table 7.3.1.4).

On echocardiography at rest, an LV end-diastolic wall thickness of ≤6 mm, segmental radial strain of ≤16.5% or longitudinal strain of ≥ −4.5%, global longitudinal LV strain of ≥ −13.7%, or a contrast perfusion defect (damaged microvasculature) have been reported to reflect non-viable myocardial tissue.[25,26,27,28] With stress echocardiography, mainly performed with inotropes (dobutamine), a biphasic response, referring to improved wall motion at low dose and decreased motion (due to ischaemia) at high inotropic dose, is characteristic of viable tissue (⊕ Figure 7.3.1.6). Addition of contrast for optimal endocardial border delineation and strain (rate) assessment further improves diagnostic accuracy of stress echocardiography.[29]

Left ventricular function, size, and shape

Apart from LV functional changes, structural LV alterations are characteristic when heart disease progresses to clinical heart failure. Ventricular remodelling includes increased LV size and mass, development of a more spherical LV geometry, and occurrence of fibrosis. LV size and shape, two parameters reflecting remodelling, together with LV function, are key determinants of prognosis in heart failure patients, particularly after myocardial

infarction, and should be addressed when individual therapeutic strategies are planned.

Severity of LV dysfunction has a major prognostic impact in heart failure patients and is therefore implemented in the Seattle Heart Failure Model that calculates projected survival at baseline and after heart failure treatment.[30] Moreover, depressed LVEF is a major determinant of mortality risk in patients undergoing cardiac surgery.[31]

In addition to prognosis, LV function has therapeutic implications. In patients with valvular heart disease, LV function and dimensions are assessed to guide optimal timing and indication of valvular intervention.[32] Indication for ICD implantation in primary prevention or CRT device therapy relies on LVEF.[33] Echocardiography is the first-line imaging modality to determine LV systolic function, and given its prognostic and therapeutic importance, quantification of LVEF is recommended.

LV size, reflecting the extent of LV remodelling and cardiac damage, may even be a more important prognostic determinant and guide for therapeutic decision-making. Indeed, several studies indicated that LV dimensions offer incremental prognostic value over LVEF in heart failure patients.[34,35] LV end-systolic diameter is an independent prognostic risk marker in patients with significant mitral valve disease and is implemented in guidelines for mitral valve disease management.[36] A too large left ventricle (LV) (end-diastolic diameter >65 mm) in heart failure patients has been reported to jeopardize success after revascularization (despite the presence of viability) and outcome after surgery for organic or functional MR.[37,38] Severe LV dilatation therefore may warrant additional therapeutic measures such as ventricular restoration.[38]

Altered LV shape further decreases LV systolic function by reducing pump efficiency and is associated with the development of functional MR. The LV sphericity index (maximal length-to-width ratio), interpapillary muscle distance, apical papillary muscle displacement (increased papillary muscle-to-mitral annulus length), and increased posterolateral angle (between the posterior leaflet and the mitral annulus) have been used as parameters of the LV shape (remodelling) and strongly relate to success of mitral leaflet repair for (functional) MR.[39] These parameters can be assessed easily by echocardiography. LV shape also impacts ventricular restoration or remodelling surgery, including aneurysmectomy, in heart failure patients.

Mitral regurgitation

As mentioned previously, global or local LV remodelling in heart failure patients can cause functional MR due to mitral leaflet tethering and coaptation failure. Organic MR reflects valvular dysfunction due to primary structural leaflet disease. Functional MR is frequent, occurring in 30–50% of dilated cardiomyopathy patients and in about 12% of patients within 1 month after acute myocardial infarction (ischaemic MR).[40,41] Moderate to severe functional MR has an independent negative prognostic impact in these patients and warrants additional therapeutic measures.[40,41,42] Determining the presence, severity, aetiology, and mechanism of MR in heart failure patients is therefore mandatory, influencing subsequent clinical

Table 7.3.1.4 Current clinical non-invasive imaging modalities and techniques to assess viability

Systolic function and/or contractile reserve
Dobutamine stress echocardiography
Dobutamine stress CMR
Dobutamine gated SPECT
Deformation imaging (tissue Doppler, speckle tracking)
Perfusion and/or metabolism
PET (^{82}Rb, ^{13}NH$_3$, and/or ^{18}FDG)
SPECT (201-thallium, ^{99m}Tc-sestamibi, or ^{99m}Tc-tetrofosmin)
Contrast echocardiography
First-pass perfusion CMR
Scar
Echocardiography and CMR (wall thickness)
Deformation imaging (tissue Doppler, speckle tracking)
CMR delayed enhancement
MDCT delayed enhancement

CMR, cardiac magnetic resonance; FDG, 18-fluorodeoxyglucose; MDCT, multidetector computed tomography; NH$_3$, ammonia; PET, positron emission tomography; Rb, rubidium; SPECT, single-photon emission computed tomography; Tc: technetium.

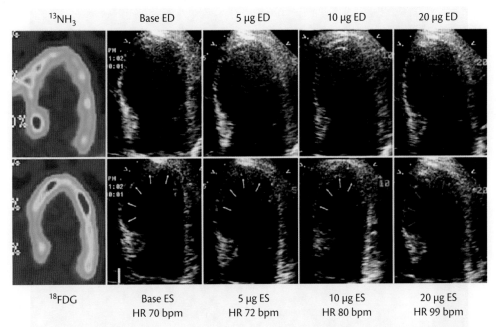

Figure 7.3.1.6 Dobutamine stress echocardiography to assess myocardial viability. Regional myocardial dysfunction (white arrows) is present on apical four-chamber left ventricular view during echocardiography at rest when end-diastolic (ED) and end-systolic (ES) frames are compared at baseline (Base). Preserved (restored) perfusion on $^{13}NH_3$-PET imaging and normal glucose uptake on ^{18}fluorodeoxyglucose-PET imaging at rest indicates myocardial stunning. Revascularization is indicated as regional myocardial dysfunction improves (yellow arrows) at low-dose dobutamine (10 µg) and deteriorates at peak dose (20 µg), the so-called biphasic response, indicating viability with superimposed ischaemia.
Reproduced from Nihoyannopoulos P and Vanoverschelde JL. Myocardial ischaemia and viability: the pivotal role of echocardiography. *European Heart Journal.* 2011;32:810–9 with permission from Oxford University Press.

decision-making. Echocardiography is the first-line modality for this evaluation. Colour Doppler echocardiography identifies the presence of MR and is used for initial appreciation of MR severity. An integrative approach using qualitative and quantitative parameters, including vena contracta width, pulsed-wave pulmonary venous flow, regurgitant jet characteristics, early mitral inflow dominance, stroke volumes, and proximal isovelocity surface area (PISA), is recommended.[39] The latter allows for exact quantification of MR severity by measuring the effective regurgitant orifice area (EROA) and regurgitant volume. Of note, different cut-off values for organic and functional MR severity are reported. To tackle current discrepancies across guidelines for quantitative functional MR assessment, a unifying concept was recently proposed, based on prognostic outcome data.[42] Significant functional MR that further drives heart failure outcome, and is therefore potentially amenable to valve-oriented therapies, was identified by an EROA of ≥30 mm² and a regurgitant volume of ≥45 mL. In addition, when the EROA is between 20 and 29 mm² and the regurgitant volume 30–44 mL, a calculated regurgitant fraction of ≥50% equally implies a high risk. As the EROA in functional MR is rather non-circular, three-dimensional echocardiography may further improve accuracy to quantify MR severity assessment, allowing its direct visualization (➲ Figure 7.3.1.7).[43] Alternatively, CMR also allows quantification of MR severity. MR severity is further appreciated by documentation of the effects of volume loading on left atrial and LV size and pulmonary artery pressures, implemented in treatment criteria.[36]

Subsequent identification of the MR aetiology and mechanism is performed based on morphological and geometrical evaluation of the mitral valve and LV. Organic MR usually presents with excess leaflet mobility due to prolapse or flail (as seen in Barlow's disease and fibroelastic deficiency) or, less frequently, with leaflet restriction throughout the cardiac cycle (as in rheumatic or degenerative disease). Systolic (posterior) leaflet restriction is characteristic of functional MR. Annulus dilatation can be involved in both organic and functional MR.[39] Transoesophageal echocardiography improves accuracy of morphological mitral valve analysis, when transthoracic echocardiography is not conclusive. Three-dimensional echocardiography, however, may offer superior diagnostic performance, allowing an 'en face' mitral view and construction of infinite two-dimensional reformation planes to identify the type, location, and extent of mitral valve lesions (➲ Figure 7.3.1.8). Moreover, it provides a common communication platform with cardiac surgeons. In addition to mitral morphology, geometrical mitral indices, such as coaptation length and distance, annulus diameter, tenting area, and posterior mitral leaflet angle, provide valuable information to evaluate therapeutic options and interventional success prediction, in particular in functional MR. These indices can be addressed by two- and three-dimensional echocardiography.[44]

Therapeutic options in heart failure patients with significant functional MR include optimization of medical therapy, CRT, and percutaneous or surgical intervention such as annuloplasty or mitral valve repair, with or without revascularization. As many heart failure patients with functional MR are at high surgical

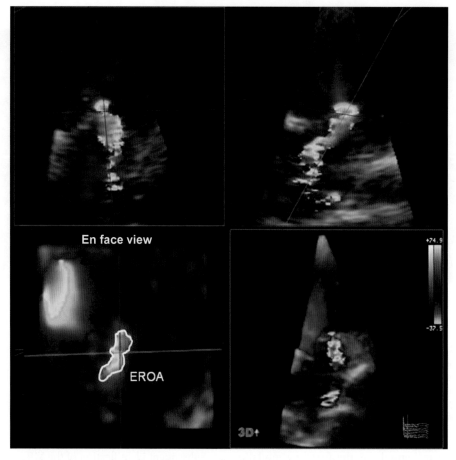

Figure 7.3.1.7 Three-dimensional transthoracic echocardiography to assess the effective regurgitant orifice area in a patient with functional mitral regurgitation. Manual cropping in imaging planes perpendicular to the regurgitant jet direction is performed to obtain the smallest possible effective regurgitant cross-sectional orifice area (EROA). The EROA is subsequently quantified by planimetry in the 'en face' mitral view. Moderate to severe functional mitral regurgitation with an ellipsoid elongated three-dimensional EROA (0.19 cm^2) is noted.

risk, interest in percutaneous techniques, such as (in)direct annuloplasty and leaflet clipping, is growing. Candidate selection, procedural guidance, and follow-up all rely on non-invasive imaging. Two recent randomized controlled trials evaluated the addition of mitral leaflet clipping to optimal medical therapy to treat functional MR. The MITRA-FR trial was neutral, but the COAPT trial showed reduced mortality and heart failure hospitalization with a mitral clip-based strategy.[45,46] Subsequent analysis revealed the importance of baseline MR severity, as well as LV remodelling (function, size, and shape), to (partly) explain the

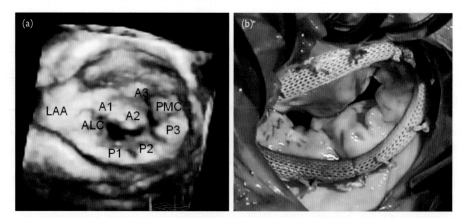

Figure 7.3.1.8 Three-dimensional transoesophageal echocardiography assessment of mitral valve morphology. (a) Superior morphology detection based on three-dimensional acquisition of the mitral valve in the surgical view is noted. The left atrial appendage (LAA), anterolateral (ALC) and posteromedial commissures (PMC), and anterior (A) and posterior (P) mitral leaflet scallops are easily recognized. (b) Real-life mitral valve morphology of the same patient shown in (a) after annuloplasty ring for functional mitral regurgitation showing high accordance with the non-invasive morphology depicted in (a).

differing trial results, highlighting the importance of stringent patient selection, using echocardiography.[47]

Tricuspid valve regurgitation and aortic valve disease related to heart failure are addressed in other chapters of this book.

Cardiac device therapy

Selected heart failure patients may benefit from ICD, CRT, or combined devices (CRT-D). For both ICD and CRT devices, reduced LV systolic function thresholds have been advocated as a main criterion for implantation.[33] In clinical practice, three-dimensional echocardiography may be the future standard for accurate and reproducible assessment of LVEF. In addition to LVEF assessment, non-invasive imaging modalities may have a role in the selection of appropriate candidates, procedural guidance, and/or follow-up of these patients.

Implantable cardioverter–defibrillator

Current primary prevention ICD indications are any cardiomyopathy with an LVEF of ≤35% and New York Heart Association (NYHA) class II and III symptoms, extended to an LVEF of ≤30% for ischaemic cardiomyopathy patients with NYHA class I symptoms.[33] Based on these criteria, however, a significant proportion of patients never experience appropriate therapy and are exposed to an increased risk of early and late complications, including inappropriate ICD shocks that increase all-cause mortality.[48] These issues have fuelled interest in strategies to optimize timing and selection criteria for ICD implantation. In this regard, tissue characterization (scar) techniques and cardiac innervation imaging have shown interesting findings (➲ Figure 7.3.1.9).

Cardiac resynchronization therapy

An LVEF of ≤35%, a QRS width of ≥130 ms, and NYHA class II (ambulatory) to IV symptoms despite optimal medical therapy currently represent the main indication for CRT in heart failure patients.[5] Despite application of these criteria, 30–40% of heart failure patients do not show clinical or echocardiographic response (usually defined as improvement in LV end-systolic volume of ≥15%). Non-invasive imaging may be useful to guide optimization strategies to increase CRT response (➲ Figure 7.3.1.10).[49]

Large non-randomized, single-centre registries consistently showed that patients with left intraventricular mechanical dyssynchrony, referring to significant time delay between contraction of myocardial segments within the LV, have a higher likelihood of CRT response in terms of improvement in symptoms, functional capacity, and LV reverse remodelling. A multitude of techniques using different imaging modalities, such as M-mode, pulsed-wave, tissue Doppler, speckle tracking, and three-dimensional echocardiography, as well as CMR and nuclear imaging, have been applied to assess LV dyssynchrony. To date, however, no consensus exists on which modality or technique to use in clinical practice. Furthermore, the first large multicentre trial (PROSPECT) showed modest accuracy for various echocardiographic indices of LV dyssynchrony to predict response to CRT.[50] Significant inter- and intraobserver variability in echocardiographic measurements was shown, and the need for better

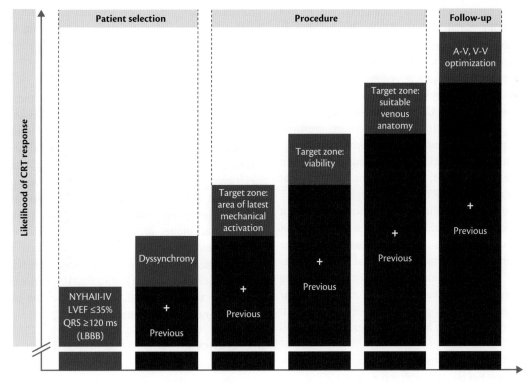

Figure 7.3.1.9 Potential model using non-invasive imaging modalities to optimize benefit from cardiac resynchronization therapy. CRT, cardiac resynchronization therapy; LBBB, left bundle branch block; LVEF, left ventricular ejection fraction; NYHA, New York Heart Association class symptoms.

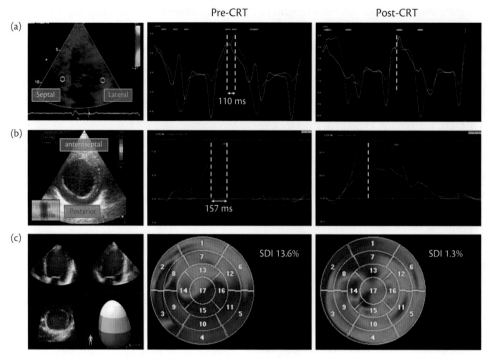

Figure 7.3.1.10 Echocardiographic techniques to assess left intraventricular dyssynchrony. Several imaging techniques can be used to assess left ventricular (LV) dyssynchrony prior to cardiac resynchronization therapy (pre-CRT) and to evaluate the echocardiographic response 6 months after CRT (post-CRT). (a) Tissue Doppler imaging pre-CRT indicating a significant time difference between the peak systolic septal (yellow) and lateral (green) wall in the four-chamber view of ≥65 ms pre-CRT. (b) Semi-automated radial speckle tracking strain at mid-papillary level showing significant time delay of ≥130 ms between the anteroseptal (yellow) and the posterior (pink) wall pre-CRT, indicating significant LV dyssynchrony. The posterior wall is the site with latest activation. (c) Semi-automated parametric three-dimensional imaging of the left ventricle showing significant delay in time to peak minimal volume on colour-coded timing bull's eye plot, with the inferoposterior wall being activated the latest (red), indicating the target zone for LV lead positioning. The standard deviation of the time to reach the minimal volume of all segments comprises the systolic dyssynchrony index (SDI) and represents a marker of LV dyssynchrony.

training and more accurate techniques was emphasized. In this regard, speckle tracking radial strain or LV mechanical dispersion (time dispersion to reach peak systolic deformation in the various LV segments, reflecting mechanical heterogeneity) and three-dimensional echocardiography, providing more automated LV dyssynchrony assessment, may hold great promise for the future and have shown to predict CRT response in single-centre studies.[51,52,53,54] (⊙ Figure 7.3.1.10) Moreover, more impaired baseline global LV myocardial work efficiency, which can be assessed by using simultaneous speckle tracking longitudinal strain and blood pressure measurement, may represent a subgroup of patients who better respond to CRT.[55]

In addition, these techniques allow identification of the site of latest mechanical activation, considered to be the optimal target site for LV lead positioning. Viability of the target zone and the global LV scar extent were reported as additional important determinants of CRT response.[56] Integrated evaluation, including LV dyssynchrony and site of latest activation and myocardial scar with speckle tracking echocardiography, delayed-enhancement CMR, or nuclear techniques, may help to select patients who will benefit from CRT.[49]

Finally, in cases of CRT non-response during follow-up, optimization of atrioventricular and interventricular CRT device timing settings can be attempted. Several echocardiographic protocols, mainly based on Doppler echocardiography, may be helpful, but firm scientific evidence justifying this approach is lacking.

Summary

Non-invasive cardiac imaging modalities are indispensible to enhance our diagnostic and therapeutic performance in managing heart failure patients. At present, the four main non-invasive imaging modalities available are echocardiography, CMR, MDCT, and nuclear imaging, including SPECT and PET. In daily practice, application of these modalities can be integrated to diagnose heart failure, identify heart failure aetiology, be a stepwise guide to therapeutic management, and assess prognosis. Several imaging techniques provide similar information and integrate simultaneous assessment of different aspects of interest to individual patient management. The clinical question, local availability, inherent risks, and institutional expertise therefore mainly determine the choice and timing of the non-invasive imaging technique or modality to use.

References

1. Gheorghiade M, Sopko G, De Luca L, *et al.* Navigating the crossroads of coronary artery disease and heart failure. *Circulation.* 2006;114:1202–13.

2. Lam CS, Donal E, Kraigher-Krainer E, Vasan RS. Epidemiology and clinical course of heart failure with preserved ejection fraction. *Eur J Heart Fail*. 2011;13:18–28.

3. Hogg K, Swedberg K, McMurray J. Heart failure with preserved left ventricular systolic function: epidemiology, clinical characteristics, and prognosis. *J Am Coll Cardiol*. 2004;43:317–27.

4. Meta-analysis Global Group in Chronic Heart Failure (MAGGIC). The survival of patients with heart failure with preserved or reduced left ventricular ejection fraction: an individual patient data meta-analysis. *Eur Heart J*. 2012;33:1750–7.

5. McDonagh TA, Metra M, Adamo M, *et al*.; ESC Scientific Document Group. 2021 ESC Guidelines for the diagnosis and treatment of acute and chronic heart failure. *Eur Heart J*. 2021;42:3599–726.

6. Lund LH, Claggett B, Liu J, *et al*. Heart failure with mid-range ejection fraction in CHARM: characteristics, outcomes and effect of candesartan across the entire ejection fraction spectrum. *Eur Heart J Fail*. 2018;20:1230–9.

7. Koh AS, Tay WT, Teng THK, *et al*. A comprehensive population-based characterization of heart failure with mid-range ejection fraction. *Eur Heart J Fail*. 2017;19:1624–34.

8. Chioncel O, Lainscak M, Seferovic PM, *et al*. Epidemiology and one-year outcomes in patients with chronic heart failure and preserved, mid-range and reduced ejection fraction: an analysis of the ESC Heart Failure Long-Term Registry. *Eur Heart J Fail*. 2017;19:1574–85.

9. Lang RM, Badano LP, Tsang W, *et al*.; American Society of Echocardiography; European Association of Echocardiography. EAE/ASE recommendations for image acquisition and display using three-dimensional echocardiography. *J Am Soc Echocardiogr*. 2012;25:3–46.

10. Borlaug BA, Paulus WJ. Heart failure with preserved ejection fraction: pathophysiology, diagnosis, and treatment. *Eur Heart J*. 2011;32:670–9.

11. González-López E, Gallego-Delgado M, Guzzo-Merello G, *et al*. Wild-type transthyretin amyloidosis as a cause of heart failure with preserved ejection fraction. *Eur Heart J*. 2015;36(38):2585–94.

12. Shah AM, Solomon SD. Myocardial deformation imaging: current status and future directions. *Circulation*. 2012;125:e244–8.

13. Wang J, Khoury DS, Yue Y, Torre-Amione G, Nagueh SF. Preserved left ventricular twist and circumferential deformation, but depressed longitudinal and radial deformation in patients with diastolic heart failure. *Eur Heart J*. 2008;29:1283–9.

14. Wang J, Nagueh SF. Current perspectives on cardiac function in patients with diastolic heart failure. *Circulation*. 2009;119:1146–57.

15. Phelan D, Collier P, Thavendiranathan P, *et al*. Relative apical sparing of longitudinal strain using two-dimensional speckle-tracking echocardiography is both sensitive and specific for the diagnosis of cardiac amyloidosis. *Heart*. 2012;98:1442–8.

16. Mor-Avi V, Jenkins C, Kuhl HP, *et al*. Real-time 3-dimensional echocardiographic quantification of left ventricular volumes: multicenter study for validation with magnetic resonance imaging and investigation of sources of error. *JACC Cardiovasc Imaging*. 2008;1:413–23.

17. Hoit BD. Strain and strain rate echocardiography and coronary artery disease. *Circ Cardiovasc Imaging*. 2011;4:179–90.

18. Karamitsos TD, Francis JM, Myerson S, Selvanayagam JB, Neubauer S. The role of cardiovascular magnetic resonance imaging in heart failure. *J Am Coll Cardiol*. 2009;54:1407–24.

19. Baker DW, Jones R, Hodges J, Massie BM, Konstam MA, Rose EA. Management of heart failure. III. The role of revascularization in the treatment of patients with moderate or severe left ventricular systolic dysfunction. *JAMA*. 1994;272:1528–34.

20. Task Force on Myocardial Revascularization of the European Society of Cardiology (ESC) and the European Association for Cardio-Thoracic Surgery (EACTS), European Association for Percutaneous Cardiovascular Interventions (EAPCI); Wijns W, Kolh P, Danchin N, *et al*. Guidelines on myocardial revascularization. *Eur Heart J*. 2010;31:2501–55.

21. Allman KC, Shaw LJ, Hachamovitch R, Udelson JE. Myocardial viability testing and impact of revascularization on prognosis in patients with coronary artery disease and left ventricular dysfunction: a meta-analysis. *J Am Coll Cardiol*. 2002;39:1151–8.

22. Bonow RO, Maurer G, Lee KL, *et al*. Myocardial viability and survival in ischemic left ventricular dysfunction. *N Engl J Med*. 2011;364:1617–25.

23. Camici PG, Prasad SK, Rimoldi OE. Stunning, hibernation, and assessment of myocardial viability. *Circulation*. 2008;117:103–14.

24. Bax JJ, Visser FC, Poldermans D, *et al*. Time course of functional recovery of stunned and hibernating segments after surgical revascularization. *Circulation*. 2001;104:1314–18.

25. Nihoyannopoulos P, Vanoverschelde JL. Myocardial ischaemia and viability: the pivotal role of echocardiography. *Eur Heart J*. 2011;32:810–19.

26. Roes SD, Mollema SA, Lamb HJ, van der Wall EE, de Roos A, Bax JJ. Validation of echocardiographic two-dimensional speckle tracking longitudinal strain imaging for viability assessment in patients with chronic ischemic left ventricular dysfunction and comparison with contrast-enhanced magnetic resonance imaging. *Am J Cardiol*. 2009;104:312–17.

27. Becker M, Hoffmann R, Kuhl HP, *et al*. Analysis of myocardial deformation based on ultrasonic pixel tracking to determine transmurality in chronic myocardial infarction. *Eur Heart J*. 2006;27:2560–6.

28. Mollema SA, Delgado V, Bertini M, *et al*. Viability assessment with global left ventricular longitudinal strain predicts recovery of left ventricular function after acute myocardial infarction. *Circ Cardiovasc Imaging*. 2010;3:15–23.

29. Plana JC, Mikati IA, Dokainish H, *et al*. A randomized cross-over study for evaluation of the effect of image optimization with contrast on the diagnostic accuracy of dobutamine echocardiography in coronary artery disease. The OPTIMIZE trial. *JACC Cardiovasc Imaging*. 2008;1:145–52.

30. Levy WC, Mozaffarian D, Linker DT, *et al*. The Seattle Heart Failure Model: prediction of survival in heart failure. *Circulation*. 2006;113:1424–33.

31. Roques F, Nashef SA, Michel P, *et al*. Risk factors and outcome in European cardiac surgery: analysis of the EuroSCORE multinational database of 19030 patients. *Eur J Cardiothorac Surg*. 1999;15:816–22; discussion 822–3.

32. Bonow RO, Carabello BA, Chatterjee K, *et al*.; Writing Committee Members; American College of Cardiology/American Heart Association Task Force. 2008 Focused update incorporated into the ACC/AHA 2006 guidelines for the management of patients with valvular heart disease: a report of the American College of Cardiology/American Heart Association Task Force on Practice Guidelines (Writing Committee to Revise the 1998 Guidelines for the Management of Patients With Valvular Heart Disease): endorsed by the Society of Cardiovascular Anesthesiologists, Society for Cardiovascular Angiography and Interventions, and Society of Thoracic Surgeons. *Circulation*. 2008;118:e523–661.

33. Epstein AE, DiMarco JP, Ellenbogen KA, *et al*.; American College of Cardiology/American Heart Association Task Force on Practice Guidelines, American Association for Thoracic Surgery; Society of Thoracic Surgeons. ACC/AHA/HRS 2008 Guidelines for device-based therapy of cardiac rhythm abnormalities: a report of the American College of Cardiology/American Heart Association Task Force on Practice Guidelines (Writing Committee to Revise

the ACC/AHA/NASPE 2002 Guideline Update for Implantation of Cardiac Pacemakers and Antiarrhythmia Devices) developed in collaboration with the American Association for Thoracic Surgery and Society of Thoracic Surgeons. *J Am Coll Cardiol.* 2008;51:e1–62.

34. Agha SA, Kalogeropoulos AP, Shih J, *et al.* Echocardiography and risk prediction in advanced heart failure: incremental value over clinical markers. *J Card Fail.* 2009;15:586–92.

35. Lee TH, Hamilton MA, Stevenson LW, *et al.* Impact of left ventricular cavity size on survival in advanced heart failure. *Am J Cardiol.* 1993;72:672–6.

36. Vahanian A, Beyersdorf F, Praz F, *et al.*; ESC/EACTS Scientific Document Group. 2021 ESC/EACTS Guidelines for the management of valvular heart disease. *Eur Heart J.* 2021;42:4207–8.

37. Rahimtoola SH, Dilsizian V, Kramer CM, Marwick TH, Vanoverschelde JL. Chronic ischemic left ventricular dysfunction: from pathophysiology to imaging and its integration into clinical practice. *JACC Cardiovasc Imaging.* 2008;1:536–55.

38. Braun J, van de Veire NR, Klautz RJ, *et al.* Restrictive mitral annuloplasty cures ischemic mitral regurgitation and heart failure. *Ann Thorac Surg.* 2008;85:430–6; discussion 436–7.

39. Lancellotti P, Moura L, Pierard LA, *et al.*; European Association of Echocardiography. European Association of Echocardiography recommendations for the assessment of valvular regurgitation. Part 2: mitral and tricuspid regurgitation (native valve disease). *Eur J Echocardiogr.* 2010;11:307–32.

40. Bursi F, Enriquez-Sarano M, Nkomo VT, *et al.* Heart failure and death after myocardial infarction in the community: the emerging role of mitral regurgitation. *Circulation.* 2005;111:295–301.

41. Trichon BH, Felker GM, Shaw LK, Cabell CH, O'Connor CM. Relation of frequency and severity of mitral regurgitation to survival among patients with left ventricular systolic dysfunction and heart failure. *Am J Cardiol.* 2003;91:538–43.

42. Bartko PE, Arfsten H, Heitzinger G, *et al.* A unifying concept for the quantitative assessment of secondary mitral regurgitation. *J Am Coll Cardiol.* 2019;73:2506–17.

43. Marsan NA, Westenberg JJ, Ypenburg C, *et al.* Quantification of functional mitral regurgitation by real-time 3D echocardiography: comparison with 3D velocity-encoded cardiac magnetic resonance. *JACC Cardiovasc Imaging.* 2009;2:1245–52.

44. Shanks M, Delgado V, Ng AC, *et al.* Mitral valve morphology assessment: three-dimensional transesophageal echocardiography versus computed tomography. *Ann Thorac Surg.* 2010;90:1922–9.

45. Stone GW, Weissman NJ, Mack MJ; COAPT Investigators. Transcatheter mitral-valve repair in patients with heart failure. Reply. *N Engl J Med.* 2019;380:1980–1.

46. Obadia JF, Messika-Zeitoun D, Leurent G, *et al.*; MITRA-FR Investigators. Percutaneous repair or medical treatment for secondary mitral regurgitation. *N Engl J Med.* 2018;379:2297–306.

47. Pibarot P, Delgado V, Bax JJ. MITRA-FR vs. COAPT: lessons from two trials with diametrically opposed results. *Eur Heart J Cardiovasc Imaging.* 2019;20:620–4.

48. Daubert JP, Zareba W, Cannom DS, *et al.*; MADIT II Investigators. Inappropriate implantable cardioverter–defibrillator shocks in MADIT II: frequency, mechanisms, predictors, and survival impact. *J Am Coll Cardiol.* 2008;51:1357–65.

49. Delgado V, van Bommel RJ, Bertini M, *et al.* Relative merits of left ventricular dyssynchrony, left ventricular lead position, and myocardial scar to predict long-term survival of ischemic heart failure patients undergoing cardiac resynchronization therapy. *Circulation.* 2011;123:70–8.

50. Chung ES, Leon AR, Tavazzi L, *et al.* Results of the Predictors of Response to CRT (PROSPECT) trial. *Circulation.* 2008;117:2608–16.

51. Kapetanakis S, Kearney MT, Siva A, Gall N, Cooklin M, Monaghan MJ. Real-time three-dimensional echocardiography: a novel technique to quantify global left ventricular mechanical dyssynchrony. *Circulation.* 2005;112:992–1000.

52. Marsan NA, Bleeker GB, Ypenburg C, *et al.* Real-time three-dimensional echocardiography as a novel approach to assess left ventricular and left atrium reverse remodeling and to predict response to cardiac resynchronization therapy. *Heart Rhythm.* 2008;5:1257–64.

53. Tanaka H, Nesser HJ, Buck T, *et al.* Dyssynchrony by speckle-tracking echocardiography and response to cardiac resynchronization therapy: results of the Speckle Tracking and Resynchronization (STAR) study. *Eur Heart J.* 2010;31:1690–700.

54. Van der Bijl P, Khidir MJH, Leung M, *et al.* Reduced left ventricular mechanical dispersion at 6 months follow-up after cardiac resynchronization therapy is associated with superior long-term outcome. *Heart Rhythm.* 2018;15:1683–9.

55. Van der Bijl P, Bootsma M, Hiemstra YL, Marsan NA, Bax JJ, Delgado V. Left ventricular 2D speckle tracking echocardiography for detection of systolic dysfunction in genetic, dilated cardiomyopathies. *Eur Heart J Cardiovasc Imaging.* 2019;20:694–9.

56. Bleeker GB, Kaandorp TA, Lamb HJ, *et al.* Effect of posterolateral scar tissue on clinical and echocardiographic improvement after cardiac resynchronization therapy. *Circulation.* 2006;113:969–76.

7.3.2 **Nuclear medicine**

Danilo Neglia and Alessia Gimelli

Introduction

Heart failure (HF) is a clinical syndrome characterized by cardinal symptoms, which may be accompanied by signs, and is most commonly due to myocardial dysfunction, either systolic or diastolic, or both. Myocardial dysfunction may recognize an ischaemic (obstructive and/or functional/microvascular coronary disease) or a non-ischaemic aetiology (i.e. primary/genetic, inflammatory, infiltrative myocardial disease). Abnormalities of the valves, pericardium, or endocardium, and abnormalities of heart rhythm or conduction can also cause or contribute to HF. In practice guidelines from the European Society of Cardiology (ESC)[1] and the American College of Cardiology/American Heart Association (ACC/AHA),[2] the diagnosis, characterization of the cardiac causes, and management of HF rely heavily on cardiac imaging, and appropriate criteria have been developed to assist clinicians with the choice of imaging modalities in different clinical scenarios.[3] In this chapter, we will focus on the specific information which can be gathered from nuclear imaging, starting with a brief description of the relevant modalities and then discussing their applications in different clinical scenarios.

Nuclear modalities

The clinical applications of nuclear imaging in patients with HF, besides evaluation of biventricular function, are mainly based on single-photon computed tomography (SPECT) and positron emission tomography (PET). They are used to assess myocardial perfusion, measuring myocardial blood flow (MBF), and evaluate myocardial viability. The same modalities also allow molecular imaging, with specific tracers capable of labelling relevant processes in HF such as myocardial inflammation, infiltration, and innervation.

Equilibrium radionuclide ventriculography

Equilibrium radionuclide ventriculography, performed after ^{99m}Tc-labelling of red blood cells, is an established method for quantification of both systolic and diastolic left ventricular (LV) and right ventricular (RV) function, with high accuracy and reproducibility. It can substitute echocardiography for monitoring response to treatment in patients with HF or cardiotoxicity in patients on anticancer therapy.[4]

SPECT myocardial perfusion scintigraphy

Myocardial perfusion scintigraphy (MPS) with SPECT is frequently performed to evaluate patients with HF and suspected or known coronary artery disease (CAD) (➲ Figure 7.3.2.1). In the 2021 ESC Guidelines,[1] together with other non-invasive imaging modalities, it has received a Class IIb indication for assessing the presence of myocardial ischaemia and viability in patients with heart failure with reduced ejection fraction (HFrEF) and either intermediate-high pretest probability (PTP) of CAD or known disease. MPS with SPECT may use thallium-201 (^{201}Tl), but more recently technetium-99m labelled tracers (sestamibi and tetrofosmin) are preferred due to better image quality and reduced radiation dose to the patient.[5] Stress–rest or stress-only protocols can be used to assess for the presence of inducible myocardial ischaemia. Rest examination after nitrate administration is advocated to improve the assessment of myocardial viability and avoid underestimation in areas with reduced resting perfusion (➲ Figure 7.3.2.2).[6] Assessment of ventricular function is also feasible through electrocardiogram (ECG)-gated perfusion SPECT acquisitions. Integrating the evaluation of the presence and extent of ischaemia with post-ischaemic LV functional impairment improves stratification of patient risk of cardiac death.[7]

SPECT molecular imaging

Myocardial inflammation

Nuclear imaging with gallium-67 citrate SPECT can be used to diagnose myocardial inflammation. It has a lower sensitivity

(a)   (b)

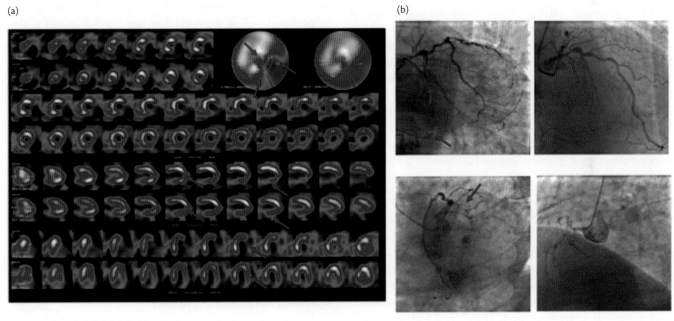

Figure 7.3.2.1 Stress single-photon emission computed tomography (SPECT) for the diagnosis of ischaemic heart failure (HF). This is a 68-year-old male patient with a recent onset of mild dyspnoea on exertion. He is a previous smoker and has cardiovascular risk factors, including hypertension, dyslipidaemia, and obesity. He has a history of previous coronary artery disease (CAD) treated with percutaneous coronary intervention (PCI) and stenting of the left circumflex (LCX) and right coronary artery (RCA). He is on antihypertensives, nitrates, and lipid-lowering and antiplatelet therapy. Two-dimensional echocardiography showed moderate reduction of global left ventricular (LV) systolic function (LV ejection fraction 44%) and inferolateral hypokinesia that was previously unknown. The figure shows SPECT perfusion images by ^{99m}Tc-tetrofosmine as a perfusion tracer (a) obtained after exercise stress (upper rows) and at rest (lower rows) in short-axis and vertical and horizontal long-axis views. The nuclear test demonstrates partially reversible myocardial perfusion defects in the lateral, apical, and inferior walls, that is, in all three coronary myocardial territories (red arrows). Invasive coronary angiography (b) documented the presence of obstructive CAD in the three main vessels (left anterior descending artery (LAD) 75% stenosis, and intrastent occlusion of the LCX and RCA) as the underlying cause of inducible myocardial ischaemia and LV dysfunction. The patient was revascularized by coronary artery bypass grafting (left internal mammary artery (LIMA) > LAD and saphenous vein (SAF) > M1).

Courtesy of Dr A Gimelli, Nuclear medicine department Fondazione Toscana G. Monasterio, Pisa.

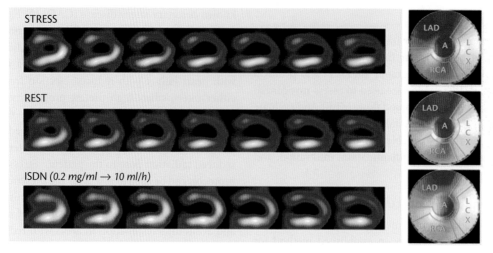

Figure 7.3.2.2 Stress single-photon emission computed tomography (SPECT) for viability imaging. An example of the use of intravenous nitrates to improve detection of viability during stress/rest perfusion SPECT examinations. In this example, stress SPECT images (upper row) demonstrate an evident myocardial perfusion defect in the left anterior descending (LAD) territory, persisting in the resting SPECT images (middle row), thus apparently suggesting previous myocardial infarction. However, after intravenous injection of nitrates followed by a new administration of the tracer (lower row), perfusion in the LAD territory completely normalizes, suggesting the presence of inducible ischaemia with preserved viability.
Courtesy of Dr A Giorgetti, Nuclear medicine department Fondazione Toscana G. Monasterio, Pisa.

and a poorer spatial resolution than PET,[8] so its use is limited to centres without access to fluorodeoxyglucose (FDG)-PET.

Myocardial innervation

Molecular imaging with SPECT using iodine-123 meta-iodobenzylguanidine (MIBG) allows functional assessment of myocardial sympathetic innervation in patients with HF and/or malignant ventricular arrhythmias.[9,10] Assessment of myocardial uptake and washout of ^{123}I-MIBG reflects the tracer uptake into neuronal vesicles through the uptake-1 mechanism of noradrenaline. Impaired cardiac adrenergic innervation, as assessed by ^{123}I-MIBG imaging, is strongly related to major adverse cardiovascular events (MACE) in patients with HF, independently of its cause.[9] In patients with ventricular arrhythmias, ^{123}I-MIBG uptake defects may identify myocardial regions amenable to ablation (➲ Figure 7.3.2.3).[11]

Amyloidosis

SPECT imaging is gaining increasing relevance in the diagnosis of cardiac amyloidosis (CA) using bone-seeking radiolabelled phosphate derivatives which bind specifically to amyloid fibres probably via a calcium-mediated mechanism (➲ Figure 7.3.2.4).[12] Their superior specificity for transthyretin amyloidosis (ATTR) allows the differential diagnosis with light chain amyloidosis (AL), with relevant prognostic and therapeutic implications.[12] A positive ^{99m}Tc-pyrophosphate (PYP), ^{99m}Tc-3,3-diphosphono-1,2-propanodicarboxylic acid (DPD), or ^{99m}Tc-hydroxymethylene diphosphonate (HMDP) study in patients with heart failure with preserved ejection fraction (HFpEF) and suggestive cardiac morphology, after exclusion of a clonal plasma cell process, allows for a clinical diagnosis of cardiac ATTR with nearly 100% specificity, obviating the need for biopsy.[1,13]

PET myocardial perfusion scintigraphy

MPS with PET allows specifically the absolute measurement of MBF in mL/min/g. Even if this is now feasible also with SPECT

and other imaging modalities, PET is still the reference modality to quantitate MBF. Three perfusion tracers are currently used: ^{15}O-water; ^{13}N-ammonia; and rubidium-82.[14] Both ^{15}O-water and ^{13}N-ammonia require an on-site cyclotron to be produced. ^{15}O-water is a diffusible tracer and its uptake in the myocardium is proportional to flow at a wide flow range, which makes it ideal for MBF quantitation. ^{13}N-ammonia is metabolically extracted in the myocardium and its uptake has a non-linear relationship with flow at higher flow values. Rubidium-82, which is produced by a generator, shows a more prominent non-linear myocardial uptake with increasing blood flow. Using appropriate modelling, both ^{13}N-ammonia and rubidium-82 provide accurate measurements of MBF, as compared to ^{15}O-water, and offer a better quality of static images. In patients with HF, the detection of regional perfusion defects by PET is strongly suggestive of the presence of underlying obstructive CAD. Globally impaired MBF and MBF reserve, possibly caused by diffuse coronary atherosclerotic[15,16] or functional disease, are strong independent predictors of adverse outcome in HF patients with an underlying ischaemic[17] or non-ischaemic aetiology.[18,19,20]

PET molecular imaging

Myocardial metabolism and viability

In patients with myocardial dysfunction and HF (HFrEF), molecular PET imaging can be used to assess myocardial glucose metabolism as a marker of ischaemia and viability.[21,22] ^{18}F-FDG is transported into the myocyte by the same trans-sarcolemmal carriers as glucose and is then phosphorylated by hexokinase to FDG-6-phosphate, which is no longer metabolized. Myocardial uptake of FDG is increased by mild to moderate ischaemia, may be decreased in severe ischaemia, and is abolished in scarred myocardium. In patients with ischaemic HF, the combination of MPS by PET or SPECT and metabolic imaging by FDG-PET

(a)

(b)

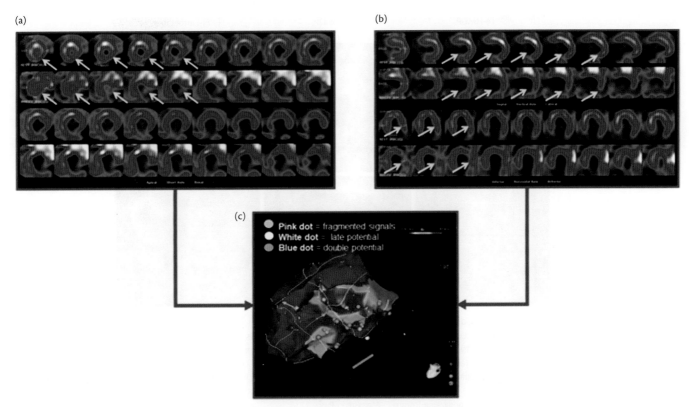

(c)

● **Pink dot** = fragmented signals
● **White dot** = late potential
● **Blue dot** = double potential

Figure 7.3.2.3 Stress single-photon emission computed tomography (SPECT) for innervation imaging. SPECT scans obtained before an ablation procedure in a patient with ventricular arrhythmias. SPECT was performed by ^{99m}Tc-tetrofosmine to assess myocardial perfusion (upper rows) and by [123]I- MIBG to assess cardiac adrenergic innervation (lower rows). Short-axis (a), and vertical and horizontal axis (b) slices showed a 'mismatch' area (relatively preserved perfusion with abnormal innervation) in the inferolateral and inferoapical walls of the left ventricle (arrows), corresponding to abnormal potentials on electroanatomic mapping where the ablation procedure was performed (c).
Courtesy of Dr A Gimelli, Nuclear medicine department Fondazione Toscana G. Monasterio, Pisa.

allows to distinguish ischaemic, viable myocardium (mismatched areas with decreased perfusion and enhanced FDG uptake) from necrotic, non-viable tissue (matched areas with both decreased or absent perfusion and FDG uptake) (➲ Figure 7.3.2.5).

Myocardial inflammation

FDG-PET imaging can also identify inflammatory processes involving the myocardium. In fasting conditions and after a fat-enriched diet, glucose metabolism and FDG uptake in the myocytes are suppressed, whereas it may be increased in activated macrophages and in CD4+ T lymphocytes infiltrating the myocardium. This allows the use of PET for the diagnosis and risk assessment of cardiac inflammatory processes, such as myocarditis and sarcoidosis,[1] which may cause acute or progressive myocardial damage and HF.[23,24] Based on the same principle, FDG-PET in co-registration with CT angiography, can be used for the detection of other active inflammatory/infective conditions involving the large vessels,[25] which may be relevant as additional causes of cardiac dysfunction.

Myocardial innervation

As an alternative to SPECT-MIBG, different PET tracers have been used to assess the autonomic innervation of the heart, providing prognostic and therapeutic information in patients with HF and/or arrhythmias.[10] Adrenergic presynaptic sympathetic nerve function has been assessed, in particular with ^{11}C-labelled hydroxyephedrine (^{11}C-HED), which competes with endogenous noradrenaline for the uptake-1 mechanism, whereas postsynaptic β-adrenoceptors have been tested by ^{11}C-labelled beta-blocking drugs in hypertrophic and dilated cardiomyopathies.[26,27]

Amyloidosis

Thioflavin-T derivative PET radiotracers have been established for imaging beta-amyloid in Alzheimer's disease. Several studies have successfully demonstrated higher myocardial uptake of ^{11}C-PiB, ^{18}F-florbetapir, and ^{18}F-florbetaben in CA,[13,28] clearly distinguishing amyloidosis patients from controls (➲ Figure 7.3.2.4).

Ischaemic heart failure

In patients presenting with LV systolic dysfunction, the primary objective is to document or exclude obstructive CAD as the main cause of HF. In the presence of anginal symptoms despite pharmacological therapy, clinical guidelines recommend invasive coronary angiography (ICA) (Class I).[1,29] In HFrEF patients with an intermediate-high PTP of CAD, stress imaging may be considered as the first diagnostic procedure (Class IIb), and ICA indicated when ischaemia is documented and coronary revascularization is a viable option. On the other hand, in patients with HFrEF and a

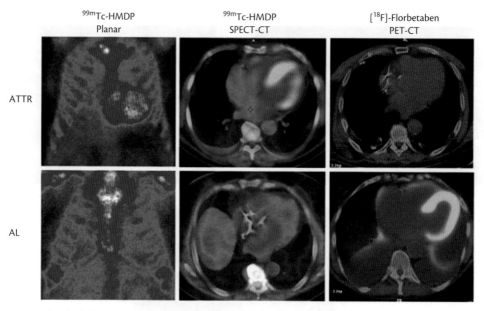

Figure 7.3.2.4 Nuclear imaging for the differential diagnosis between ATTR and AL cardiac amyloidosis. In the case of ATTR cardiac amyloidosis (upper row), scintigraphy with an osteophilic radiopharmaceutical agent (such as ^{99m}Tc-HMDP) frequently shows intense myocardial uptake of the tracer, which can be evidenced in both planar and single-photon emission computed tomography (SPECT) images. Positron emission tomography (PET) scans with specific tracers for the amyloid substance (such as ^{18}F-florbetaben) is frequently negative. By contrast, in the case of AL cardiac amyloidosis (lower row), scintigraphy with an osteophilic radiopharmaceutical agent is negative or rarely weakly positive, whereas PET shows a marked myocardial uptake of the tracer for amyloid (lower row).

Courtesy of Dr D Genovesi, Nuclear medicine department Fondazione Toscana G. Monasterio, Pisa.

low-intermediate PTP, CT coronary angiography (CTCA) should be considered first to rule out CAD (Class IIa), and stress imaging performed to document ischaemia and viability in the presence of obstructive disease (Class IIb).[1,2,29] These recommendations are based on the concept that functional stress tests are required for the diagnosis of an ischaemic aetiology of LV dysfunction and to guide management. In fact, once ischaemic HF is recognized, coronary revascularization, when feasible, is a Class I indication by current ESC guidelines.[30] SPECT or PET are particularly helpful in this context. They are able to accurately detect the presence of moderate-to-severe (>10% of LV myocardium) inducible ischaemia[29,30] and to assess for the presence of sufficient myocardial viability (>50% of LV myocardium)—both helpful to indicate coronary revascularization[1] and to predict LV function recovery.[31] The prognostic benefit of revascularization guided by nuclear viability imaging was suggested, but not fully demonstrated by controlled trials in patients with ischaemic HF.[32,33,34] Coronary revascularization showed a prognostic benefit in those patients

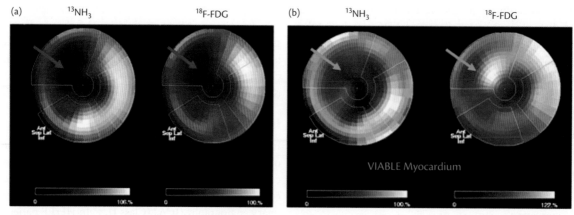

Figure 7.3.2.5 Positron emission tomography (PET) for viability imaging. Two examples of cardiac PET with [13]NH₃ as a flow tracer and ^{18}F-FDG as a metabolic tracer performed to assess myocardial viability in two patients with left ventricular dysfunction who are candidates for coronary revascularization. The examination shown in (a) documents a large area with 'matching' flow and metabolism myocardial abnormalities involving the left anterior descending (LAD) and partially the right coronary artery (RCA) myocardial territories, indicating non-viable scarred myocardium. The examination shown in (b), by contrast, shows an area of flow–metabolism 'mismatch', indicating viable myocardium in the LAD territory.

These exams were performed at Fondazione Toscana G. Monasterio in Pisa, Italy.

with a more extensive viable myocardium and those whose final management was adherent to PET results,[33] in particular when receiving surgical revascularization.[34]

Dilated cardiomyopathy

Dilated cardiomyopathy (DCM) is defined by the presence of LV or biventricular systolic dysfunction (LV ejection fraction <45%), with or without dilatation, in the absence of abnormal loading conditions (hypertension and valve disease) or CAD, sufficient to cause global systolic impairment.[35] The natural history may be characterized by a long preclinical phase possibly evolving into an overt phase of ventricular dilatation and systolic dysfunction, associated with HF symptoms. Nuclear imaging may be used in the diagnostic process of DCM and in prediction of risk.[35] Gated radionuclide imaging may provide an accurate alternative to echocardiography or cardiac magnetic resonance (CMR) imaging to assess biventricular systolic and diastolic function in early diagnosis and follow-up. SPECT and PET rest/stress perfusion and FDG-PET metabolic studies may be clinically relevant to exclude an ischaemic cause of HF (see previous paragraph) and also may provide prognostic stratification of DCM patients. DCM

patients with normal or non-obstructed coronary arteries may show abnormal myocardial perfusion and an ischaemic myocardial metabolic pattern caused by multiple factors, including coronary microvascular/endothelial dysfunction.[36,37] Even if DCM is considered a non-ischaemic myocardial disease, the severity of abnormalities in MBF and flow reserve by quantitative PET is associated with worse clinical outcomes.[18,20] Atherosclerosis risk factors and non-obstructive CAD may coexist, with apparently primitive myocardial dysfunction being an additional cause of impaired MBF reserve.[38,15] Accordingly, use of CTCA in patients with unexplained LV systolic dysfunction, coupled with PET perfusion imaging, could provide additional insights into the aetiology of HF (➲ Figure 7.3.2.6).

Myocarditis

Inflammatory myocardial diseases may present acutely or chronically and may evolve to DCM or a hypokinetic non-DCM.[39] Myocarditis may present with cardiac signs and symptoms of ischaemic disease and thus should be considered in the differential diagnosis of myocardial infarction with non-obstructive coronary arteries. CMR is the advanced imaging of choice,[23] but FDG-PET

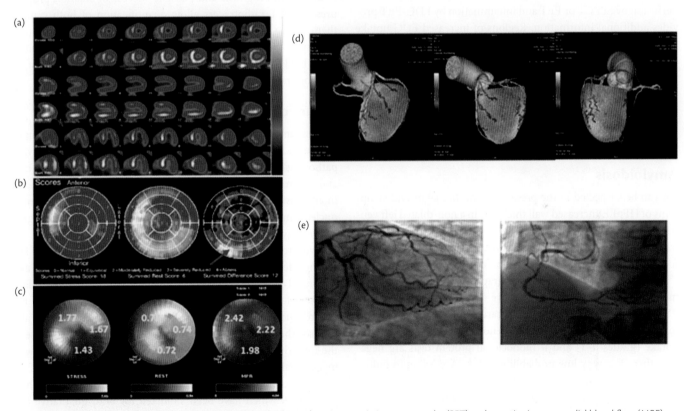

Figure 7.3.2.6 Computed tomography coronary angiography (CTCA) positron emission tomography (PET) and quantitative myocardial blood flow (MBF) to guide management in heart failure with reduced ejection fraction (HFrEF) and multivessel coronary artery disease (CAD). This is a 64-year-old male patient with mild dyspnoea on exertion. He has multiple cardiovascular risk factors, including a family history of premature CAD and familial hypercholesterolaemia, and is under treatment with statins and aspirin. Two-dimensional echocardiography shows mild systolic left ventricular (LV) dysfunction (LV ejection fraction 45%). The figure shows PET perfusion images obtained with $^{13}NH_3$ as a flow tracer (a) during pharmacological stress with intravenous dipyridamole (upper rows) and at rest (lower rows) in short-axis, and vertical and horizontal long-axis views. The semi-quantitative analysis (b) shows a reversible perfusion defect mainly in the inferior wall of the left ventricle (arrow). However, quantitative myocardial blood flow (MBF) (c) demonstrates reduced maximal MBF during stress (<2 mL/min/g) and impaired MBF reserve (<2.5) in all three coronary territories, as also observed in fusion CTCA/PET images (d). Invasive coronary angiography (e) confirmed the presence of three-vessel obstructive CAD, and the patient was referred for surgery for complete revascularization.
These exams were performed at Fondazione Toscana G. Monasterio in Pisa, Italy.

is a potential complementary modality for the diagnosis of suspected myocarditis.[1,40] Using adequate patient preparation, carbohydrate metabolism of the non-inflamed myocardium is suppressed and FDG uptake generally indicates the presence of inflammatory cell infiltrates. Combining this information with CMR imaging has been shown to be potentially clinically relevant in patients with suspected myocarditis.[41]

Sarcoidosis

Cardiac sarcoidosis is characterized by focal myocardial granulomas and may cause conduction disturbances, ventricular arrhythmias, sudden death, and progressive HF. The diagnosis of cardiac involvement in systemic sarcoidosis is challenging and is reported in 5% of cases, but is relevant for risk assessment and management.[24] FDG-PET is a well-established tool for the diagnosis of extracardiac sarcoidosis but has also an emerging role for management of patients with known or suspected cardiac sarcoidosis.[1,24] Whole-body FDG imaging is obtained for the assessment of extracardiac disease activity and to identify potential sites amenable to biopsy, whereas cardiac FDG-PET images showing 'focal' or 'focal on diffuse' myocardial tracer uptake is consistent with cardiac involvement. Combined assessment of myocardial perfusion by SPECT or PET and inflammation by FDG-PET provides additional information. Regions of increased FDG uptake with normal or decreased perfusion represent active myocardial disease in an earlier or more advanced stage, whereas areas with normal/decreased FDG uptake and decreased perfusion represent scarred segments.[42] There is some evidence that patients with a combination of increased focal myocardial uptake of FDG and resting perfusion defects are at high risk of death or ventricular arrhythmias.[43]

Amyloidosis

CA can be suspected in the presence of cardiac signs and symptoms of HFpEF. Increased wall thickness in a non-dilated left ventricle is a prominent echocardiographic characteristic and should trigger further evaluation. The diagnostic algorithm, which is also focused on identifying cardiac amyloidosis subtypes, may include ^{99m}Tc-PYP, DPD, or HMDP scintigraphy, coupled with assessment for monoclonal proteins in the serum and/or urine.[1,44] In PYP, DPD, or HMDP scintigraphy, cardiac uptake can be graded into four levels. If scintigraphy does not show significant cardiac uptake (grades 0–1) and if monoclonal protein tests are negative, there is a very low probability of CA. According to guidelines,[1] if scintigraphy shows significant cardiac uptake (grades 2–3) and if monoclonal protein tests are negative, ATTR CA can be diagnosed without further testing. When at least one of the monoclonal protein tests is abnormal and CMR confirms cardiac involvement, isolated AL (scintigraphy negative) or coexisting AL and ATTR CA (scintigraphy positive) should be diagnosed by histological demonstration and typing of amyloid deposits, usually via endomyocardial biopsy. PET radiotracers have also been proposed for the diagnostic process of CA.[13] ^{18}F-florbetapir has been shown to differentiate patients affected by either subtype

of CA from healthy control subjects.[45] ^{18}F-florbetaben has been tested in patients with histology-proven AL or ATTR CA using a semi-quantitative analysis of PET imaging at different time points, showing that late scans obtained at least 30 minutes after radiotracer injection can reliably discriminate cardiac involvement due to AL amyloidosis from ATTR amyloidosis and non-amyloidotic cardiomyopathy.[46]

Ventricular arrhythmias and innervation imaging

A relevant clinical aspect in both ischaemic and non-ischaemic HF is the risk associated with ventricular arrhythmias, of which cardiac sympathetic tone is considered a potential trigger. Nuclear innervation imaging with ^{123}I-MIBG uses planar and SPECT images, obtained early after tracer injection and 3–5 hours later, to assess the functionality of myocardial sympathetic nerve endings.[10] Impairment of cardiac adrenergic innervation assessed by ^{123}I-MIBG predisposes to the development of malignant ventricular arrhythmias, predicting the need for implantable cardioverter–defibrillators.[47] Regional alterations of cardiac adrenergic tone are better detected by SPECT images and predict both patient prognosis and possible success of ablation procedures.[10,11] PET radiotracers allow quantification of both sympathetic nerve terminals by ^{11}C-HED and post-synaptic receptor density by ^{11}C-CGP. Cardiac sympathetic denervation assessed by ^{11}C-HED PET predicts sudden cardiac death independently of LV ejection fraction in ischaemic HF.[48]

Future directions

Nuclear imaging is still an expanding field with relevant implications in HF. New molecular tracers targeting the most relevant pathophysiological processes involved in myocardial dysfunction and its progression will help both in the diagnostic process and in addressing treatment.[49] Technology developments will benefit nuclear imaging, in particular with diffusion of hybrid imaging technology.

Myocardial ischaemia is one of the more frequent causes of HF. Further development and a more widespread use of hybrid and fusion CT/PET and CT/SPECT imaging, with or without quantitation of MBF and MBF reserve, will help to discriminate between functionally significant obstructive coronary disease and diffuse atherosclerotic and/or microvascular coronary disease as the underlying aetiology of impaired perfusion in patients with myocardial dysfunction, and help to risk-stratify patients.[50,51] The development of ^{18}F-labelled PET perfusion tracers, such as flurpiridaz, which have been validated for both qualitative and quantitative assessment of MBF, will bring potential advantages for routine clinical use.[52]

Abnormalities in myocardial innervation are robust predictors of adverse events in both ischaemic and non-ischaemic HF. The use of new solid-state cardiac cameras with cadmium–zinc–telluride detectors, characterized by higher photon sensitivity and spatial resolution compared to standard cameras, will allow a comprehensive assessment of myocardial innervation and perfusion in a single imaging session and with a limited radiation burden.[10,11] PET tracers labelled with carbon-11 have a short half-life and require an on-site cyclotron for production, which limits their widespread use in the clinical setting. Neuronal tracers labelled with the positron emitter fluorine-18 have been introduced recently, with similar kinetics to the SPECT tracer MIBG, providing myocardial images of high quality and the possibility of reproducible quantification of intraneuronal retention.[10] Fusion of scintigraphic images with electroanatomical maps will provide a useful guide in ablation procedures of ventricular arrhythmias. More data will be needed to confirm the role of innervation imaging in clinical routine.

Cardiovascular device infection, inflammatory myocardium damage, and infiltrative cardiomyopathies are emerging conditions in HF patients where the development of nuclear imaging may have an increasing clinical role for specific diagnosis and addressing specific therapy.[49] In these areas, molecular radionuclide-based imaging has been growing rapidly. For example, there is an expanding use of FDG-PET for imaging infection of LV assist devices where early diagnosis and site of infection may be crucial, and PET may also effectively guide surgical options.[53] In inflammatory myocardial conditions, such as sarcoidosis, FDG-PET molecular imaging not only is useful for diagnosis, but also holds promise to address the need for anti-inflammatory therapies and to predict and monitor response.[54] CA is an emerging cause of HFpEF, and both SPECT and PET amyloid tracers hold promise for more widespread clinical use. Prospective assessments of the efficacy of PET/CT, coupled with use of amyloid-specific radiotracers, in identifying cardiac involvement from ATTR or AL in a multicentre trial are awaited.[13]

Finally, novel targets for nuclear molecular imaging of potential interest in HF are emerging.[49] Novel agents targeting specific components of the immune system, such as chemokine receptors, monocytes, and macrophages, hold promise for a more precise assessment of beneficial versus adverse effects of the inflammatory response to tissue injury. Various mechanisms of myocardial remodelling in response to myocardial injury reparative, angiogenic, and fibrotic factors have also emerged as nuclear imaging targets. It is hoped that these innovative imaging compounds will help not only towards a better assessment of the individual risk of disease progression, but also towards personalized treatment.

Key messages

- Most patients presenting with HFrEF will undergo coronary angiography due to the need to recognize the presence of obstructive CAD. Nuclear modalities (SPECT and PET) are relevant to determine the presence and extent of inducible myocardial ischaemia and viability, both to confirm the diagnosis of ischaemic HF and to help guide management.
- In the European Association of Cardiovascular Imaging (EACVI) appropriateness criteria for the use of cardiovascular imaging in HF derived from European National Imaging Societies voting,[3] SPECT and PET use has been deemed as 'appropriate' for the detection of inducible ischaemia and viability in HFrEF, either before or after coronary angiography, and has received a Class IIb indication in the 2021 ESC Guidelines for the diagnosis and treatment of acute and chronic HF.
- In patients with unexplained LV systolic dysfunction, CTCA/PET hybrid evaluation could evidence the association of non-obstructive coronary atherosclerosis with significantly impaired MBF reserve, with both carrying an unfavourable prognosis and potentially responsive to aggressive medical treatments.
- In patients with both ischaemic and non-ischaemic HF, in particular in its early stages, absolute measurements of MBF and flow reserve by quantitative PET can identify patients with worse clinical prognosis.
- FDG-PET is a potential complementary imaging modality to CMR for the diagnosis of suspected myocarditis.
- Similarly, FDG-PET is not included in the diagnostic criteria but is considered as a valuable tool for the management of patients with suspected cardiac sarcoidosis.
- In patients with HFpEF and suspected CA on the basis of clinical and echocardiographic/CMR findings, the ATTR form can be diagnosed by ^{99m}Tc-PYP, ^{99m}Tc-DPD, or ^{99m}Tc-HMDP scintigraphy, avoiding the need for myocardial biopsy, according to 2021 ESC Guidelines.
- PET with specific tracers for amyloid is promising for distinguishing cardiac involvement from either ATTR or AL.
- Cardiac innervation imaging with ^{123}I-MIBG SPECT or ^{11}C-HED PET can independently predict malignant ventricular arrhythmias and adverse prognosis in patients with HF.

References

1. McDonagh TA, Metra M, Adamo M, et al.; ESC Scientific Document Group. 2021 ESC Guidelines for the diagnosis and treatment of acute and chronic heart failure. Eur Heart J 2021;42:3599–726.
2. Van der Meer P, Gaggin HK, Dec GW. ACC/AHA versus ESC Guidelines on heart failure: JACC guideline comparison. J Am Coll Cardiol 2019;73:2756–68.
3. Garbi M, Edvardsen T, Bax J, et al. EACVI appropriateness criteria for the use of cardiovascular imaging in heart failure derived from European National Imaging Societies voting. Eur Heart J Cardiovasc Imaging 2016;17:711–21.
4. Hesse B, Lindhardt TB, Acampa W, et al. EANM/ESC guidelines for radionuclide imaging of cardiac function. Eur J Nucl Med Mol Imaging 2008;35:851–85.
5. Verberne HJ, Acampa W, Anagnostopoulos C, et al. EANM procedural guidelines for radionuclide myocardial perfusion imaging with SPECT and SPECT/CT: 2015 revision. Eur J Nucl Med Mol Imaging 2015;42:1929–40.
6. Giorgetti A, Pingitore A, Favilli B, et al. Baseline/postnitrate tetrofosmin SPECT for myocardial viability assessment in patients with postischemic severe left ventricular dysfunction: new evidence from MRI. J Nucl Med 2005;46:1285–93.
7. Sharir T, Germano G, Kang X, et al. Prediction of myocardial infarction versus cardiac death by gated myocardial perfusion SPECT: risk stratification by the amount of stress-induced ischemia and the poststress ejection fraction. J Nucl Med 2001;42:831–7.
8. Nishiyama Y, Yamamoto Y, Fukunaga K, et al. Comparative evaluation of 18F-FDG PET and ^{67}Ga scintigraphy in patients with sarcoidosis. J Nucl Med 2006;47:1571–6.

9. Jacobson AF, Senior R, Cerqueira MD, *et al.* Myocardial iodine-123 meta-iodobenzylguanidine imaging and cardiac events in heart failure. Results of the prospective ADMIRE-HF (AdreView Myocardial Imaging for Risk Evaluation in Heart Failure) study. J Am Coll Cardiol 2010;55:2212–21.

10. Gimelli A, Liga R, Agostini D, *et al.* The role of myocardial innervation imaging in different clinical scenarios: an expert document of the European Association of Cardiovascular Imaging and Cardiovascular Committee of the European Association of Nuclear Medicine. Eur Heart J Cardiovasc Imaging. 2021;22:480–90.

11. Gimelli A, Menichetti F, Soldati E, *et al.* Predictors of ventricular ablation's success: viability, innervation, or mismatch? J Nucl Cardiol. 2021;28:175–83.

12. Singh V, Falk R, Di Carli MF, *et al.* State-of-the-art radionuclide imaging in cardiac transthyretin amyloidosis. J Nucl Cardiol 2019;26:158–73.

13. Khor YM, Cuddy S, Falk RH, *et al.* Multimodality imaging in the evaluation and management of cardiac amyloidosis. Semin Nucl Med 2020;50:295–310.

14. Sciagrà R, Lubberink M, Hyafil F, *et al.* Cardiovascular Committee of the European Association of Nuclear Medicine (EANM). EANM procedural guidelines for PET/CT quantitative myocardial perfusion imaging. Eur J Nucl Med Mol Imaging 2021;48:1040–69.

15. Liga R, Marini C, Coceani M, *et al.* Structural abnormalities of the coronary arterial wall—in addition to luminal narrowing—affect myocardial blood flow reserve. J Nucl Med 2011;52:1704–12.

16. Driessen RS, Stuijfzand WJ, Raijmakers PG, *et al.* Effect of plaque burden and morphology on myocardial blood flow and fractional flow reserve. J Am Coll Cardiol 2018;71:499–509.

17. Gupta A, Taqueti VR, van de Hoef TP, *et al.* Integrated noninvasive physiological assessment of coronary circulatory function and impact on cardiovascular mortality in patients with stable coronary artery disease. Circulation 2017;136:2325–36.

18. Neglia D, Michelassi C, Trivieri MG, *et al.* Prognostic role of myocardial blood flow impairment in idiopathic left ventricular dysfunction. Circulation 2002;105:186–93.

19. Cecchi F, Olivotto I, Gistri R, *et al.* Coronary microvascular dysfunction and prognosis in hypertrophic cardiomyopathy. N Engl J Med 2003;349:1027–35.

20. Neglia D, Liga R. Absolute myocardial blood flow in dilated cardiomyopathy: does it matter? JACC Cardiovasc Imaging 2019;12:1709–11.

21. Anagnostopoulos C, Georgakopoulos A, Pianou N, *et al.* Assessment of myocardial perfusion and viability by positron emission tomography. Int J Cardiol 2013;167:1737–49.

22. Allman KC. Noninvasive assessment myocardial viability: current status and future directions. J Nucl Cardiol 2013;20:618–37.

23. Agewall S, Beltrame JF, Reynolds HR, *et al.*; WG on Cardiovascular Pharmacotherapy. ESC working group position paper on myocardial infarction with non-obstructive coronary arteries. Eur Heart J 2017;38:143–53.

24. Writing Group; Document Reading Group; EACVI Reviewers. A joint procedural position statement on imaging in cardiac sarcoidosis: from the Cardiovascular and Inflammation & Infection Committees of the European Association of Nuclear Medicine, the European Association of Cardiovascular Imaging, and the American Society of Nuclear Cardiology. Eur Heart J Cardiovasc Imaging 2017;18:1073–89.

25. Lee SW, Kim SJ, Seo Y, *et al.* F-18 FDG PET for assessment of disease activity of large vessel vasculitis: a systematic review and meta-analysis. J Nucl Cardiol 2019;26:59–67.

26. Schafers M, Dutka D, Rhodes CG, *et al.* Myocardial presynaptic and postsynaptic autonomic dysfunction in hypertrophic cardiomyopathy. Circ Res 1998;82:57–62.

27. Merlet P, Delforge J, Syrota A, *et al.* Positron emission tomography with 11C CGP-12177 to assess beta-adrenergic receptor concentration in idiopathic dilated cardiomyopathy. Circulation 1993;87:1169–78.

28. Zhao L, Fang Q. Recent advances in the noninvasive strategies of cardiac amyloidosis. Heart Fail Rev 2016;21:703–21.

29. Knuuti J, Wijns W, Saraste A, *et al.*; ESC Scientific Document Group. 2019 ESC Guidelines for the diagnosis and management of chronic coronary syndromes. Eur Heart J 2020;41:407–77.

30. Neumann FJ, Sousa-Uva M, Ahlsson A, *et al.* 2018 ESC/EACTS Guidelines on myocardial revascularization. Eur Heart J 2019;40:87–165.

31. Ling LF, Marwick TH, Flores DR, *et al.* Identification of therapeutic benefit from revascularization in patients with left ventricular systolic dysfunction: inducible ischemia versus hibernating myocardium. Circ Cardiovasc Imaging 2013;6:363–72.

32. Beanlands RS, Nichol G, Huszti E, *et al.* F-18-fluorodeoxyglucose positron emission tomography imaging-assisted management of patients with severe left ventricular dysfunction and suspected coronary disease: a randomized, controlled trial (PARR-2). J Am Coll Cardiology 2007;50:2002–12.

33. Mc Ardle B, Shukla T, Nichol G, *et al.* Long-term follow-up of outcomes with F-18-fluorodeoxyglucose positron emission tomography imaging-assisted management of patients with severe left ventricular dysfunction secondary to coronary disease. Circ Cardiovasc Imaging 2016;9:e004331.

34. Velazquez EJ, Lee KL, Jones RH, *et al.* Coronary-artery bypass surgery in patients with ischemic cardiomyopathy. N Engl J Med 2016;374:1511–20.

35. Donal E, Delgado V, Bucciarelli-Ducci C, *et al.*; 2016–18 EACVI Scientific Documents Committee. Multimodality imaging in the diagnosis, risk stratification, and management of patients with dilated cardiomyopathies: an expert consensus document from the European Association of Cardiovascular Imaging. Eur Heart J Cardiovasc Imaging 2019;20:1075–93.

36. Neglia D, De Caterina A, Marraccini P, *et al.* Impaired myocardial metabolic reserve and substrate selection flexibility during stress in patients with idiopathic dilated cardiomyopathy. Am J Physiol Heart Circ Physiol 2007;293:H3270–8.

37. Crea F, Camici PG, Bairey Merz CN. Coronary microvascular dysfunction: an update. Eur Heart J 2014;35:1101–11.

38. Bajaj NS, Osborne MT, Gupta A, *et al.* Coronary microvascular dysfunction and cardiovascular risk in obese patients. J Am Coll Cardiol 2018;72:707–17.

39. Caforio ALP, Adler Y, Agostini C, *et al.* Diagnosis and management of myocardial involvement in systemic immune-mediated diseases: a position statement of the European Society of Cardiology Working Group on Myocardial and Pericardial Disease. Eur Heart J 2017;38:2649–62.

40. Rischpler C, Woodard PK. PET/MR imaging in cardiovascular imaging. PET Clin 2019;14:233–44.

41. Nensa F, Kloth J, Tezgah E, *et al.* Feasibility of FDG-PET in myocarditis: comparison to CMR using integrated PET/MRI. J Nucl Cardiol 2018;25:785–94.

42. Berman JS, Govender P, Ruberg FL, *et al.* Scadding revisited: a proposed staging system for cardiac sarcoidosis. Sarcoidosis Vasc Diffuse Lung Dis 2014;31:2–5.

43. Blankstein R, Osborne M, Naya M, *et al.* Cardiac positron emission tomography enhances prognostic assessments of patients with suspected cardiac sarcoidosis. J Am Coll Cardiol 2014;63:329–36.

44. Garcia-Pavia P, Rapezzi C, Adler Y, *et al.* Diagnosis and treatment of cardiac amyloidosis: a position statement of the ESC Working

Group on Myocardial and Pericardial Diseases. Eur Heart J 2021;42:1554–68.

45. Dorbala S, Vangala D, Semer J, et al. Imaging cardiac amyloidosis: a pilot study using 18F-florbetapir positron emission tomography. Eur J Nucl Med Mol Imaging 2014;41:1652–62.

46. Genovesi D, Vergaro G, Giorgetti A, et al. [18F]-florbetaben PET/CT for differential diagnosis among cardiac immunoglobulin light chain, transthyretin amyloidosis, and mimicking conditions. JACC Cardiovasc Imaging 2021;14:246–55.

47. Hachamovitch R, Nutter B, Menon V, et al. Predicting risk versus predicting potential survival benefit using 123I-mIBG imaging in patients with systolic dysfunction eligible for implantable cardiac defibrillator implantation: analysis of data from the prospective ADMIRE-HF study. Circ Cardiovasc Imaging 2015;8:e003110.

48. Fallavollita JA, Heavey BM, Luisi AJ Jr, et al. Regional myocardial sympathetic denervation predicts the risk of sudden cardiac arrest in ischemic cardiomyopathy. J Am Coll Cardiol 2014;63:141–9.

49. Werner RA, Thackeray JT, Diekmann J, Weiberg D, Bauersachs J, Bengel FM. The changing face of nuclear cardiology: guiding cardiovascular care toward molecular medicine. J Nucl Med 2020;61(7):951–61.

50. Pazhenkottil AP, Benz DC, Grani C, et al. Hybrid SPECT perfusion imaging and coronary CT angiography: long-term prognostic value for cardiovascular outcomes. Radiology 2018;288:694–702.

51. Neglia D, Liga R, Caselli C, et al.; EVINCI Study Investigators. Anatomical and functional coronary imaging to predict long-term outcome in patients with suspected coronary artery disease: the EVINCI-outcome study. Eur Heart J Cardiovasc Imaging 2020;21(11):1273–82.

52. Berman DS, Maddahi J, Tamarappoo BK, et al. Phase II safety and clinical comparison with single-photon emission computed tomography myocardial perfusion imaging for detection of coronary artery disease: flurpiridaz F18 positron emission tomography. J Am Coll Cardiol 2013;61:469–77.

53. Sommerlath Sohns J, Kroehn H, Schoede A, et al. 18F-fluorodeoxyglucose positron emission tomography/computed tomography in left-ventricular assist device infection: initial results supporting the usefulness of image-guided therapy. J Nucl Med 2020;61:971–6.

54. Bravo PE, Singh A, Di Carli MF, Blankstein R. Advanced cardiovascular imaging for the evaluation of cardiac sarcoidosis. J Nucl Cardiol 2019;26:188–99.

7.3.3 Computed tomography in heart failure

Stephan Achenbach and Amina G Rakisheva

Introduction

Computed tomography (CT) offers high-resolution cross-sectional medical imaging and is essential for numerous diagnostic applications. However, visualization of the heart had been, for a long time, limited due to artefacts caused by motion. Modern CT systems unite a number of technical improvements which, over the past two decades, have led to a substantially improved ability to visualize the heart: motion artefacts are reduced as a result of fast gantry rotation times and image reconstruction algorithms that use only parts of one rotation; multidetector row systems acquire several hundred sub-millimetre slices simultaneously, which allows to cover the entire volume of the heart within one short breath-hold; and finally, techniques for electrocardiogram (ECG) synchronization enable visualization of the entire heart in the same cardiac phase, as well as 'cine' imaging in order to depict cardiac motion.

The main clinical application of cardiac CT is coronary artery visualization. Detection and quantification of coronary calcium imaging are used for risk stratification,[1] and contrast-enhanced coronary CT angiography (CTA) is a guideline-endorsed modality for the workup of patients with suspected coronary artery disease (CAD).[2] However, modern applications of cardiac CT extend well beyond the coronary arteries. They make use of the particularly high spatial resolution of CT, and in certain areas, CT has become an indispensable imaging modality to complement echocardiography and cardiac magnetic resonance (CMR).

With its ability to visualize the coronary arteries and provide isotropic, high-resolution imaging of cardiac anatomy and function, without some constraints that affect echocardiography or magnetic resonance imaging, such as poor acoustic windows or the presence of metallic implants, CT can play an important role in selected patients who require imaging in the setting of heart failure management. This chapter describes the potential applications of cardiac CT in this context, with emphasis on specific advantages and limitations.

Cardiac CT technology

Computed tomography was introduced in 1972, but early CT generations did not allow cardiac imaging due to their limited temporal resolution.[3] Modern CT scanners, on the other hand, provide a temporal resolution of 100 ms or better. This is achieved through a combination of very fast rotation speeds and reconstruction algorithms that use only a fraction of one rotation to reconstruct cross-sectional images. While this temporal resolution is generally sufficient for the visualization of cardiac structures, there are exceptions: Particularly high heart rates or arrhythmias may pose a significant challenge, and small structures with very rapid an irregular motion, such as heart valve vegetations, may escape visualization by CT.

When using CT for cardiac imaging, heart rate has a substantial influence. In order to minimize motion artefact, which is particularly important for coronary artery imaging, low heart rates are desirable (below 60 beats/min) and patients will often receive medication specifically to lower heart rate in preparation for the scan. Mid-diastole is the preferred time instant for image reconstruction in low heart rates. However, the diastolic resting period progressively shortens with increasing heart rates so that end-systole (isovolumetric relaxation) may be better suited in patients with higher heart rates or arrhythmias.

Spatial resolution in cardiac CT depends on in-plane resolution and slice thickness. The in-plane resolution of modern CT systems is approximately 0.4–0.5 mm. Since slice thickness is also in the range of 0.5–0.6 mm, CT can be assumed to provide 'isotropic' spatial resolution (equal in all directions of space, see ◆ Figure 7.3.3.1), which is a substantial difference to echocardiography and CMR, which do not provide isotropic resolution.

Synchronization of image acquisition or image reconstruction with the cardiac cycle is another important technical aspect of cardiac CT.[4] Available options comprise spiral acquisition with retrospectively ECG-gated image reconstruction, prospectively ECG-triggered axial acquisition and the so-called prospectively ECG-triggered high-pitch 'flash' mode (◆ Table 7.3.3.1).[5]

Retrospectively ECG-gated image reconstruction is the most robust way of cardiac visualization by CT. It uses data sets acquired during slow, continuous table motion with parallel registration of the patient's ECG. There is substantial oversampling of data through all phases of the cardiac cycle. At the price of relatively high radiation exposure, this allows to freely select the time instant(s) within the cardiac cycle at which images are reconstructed—on one hand permitting the rendering of 'cine' reconstructions to display the heart throughout the entire cardiac cycle, on the other hand allowing to very accurately select the reconstruction time point with minimal motion artefact.

In prospectively ECG-triggered axial acquisition, X-rays will only be emitted during pre-specified segments of the cardiac cycle which are intended to be used for image reconstruction.[10,17] The patient table remains still during these acquisitions and is moved stepwise to the subsequent position while the X-ray tube is switched off. Hence, this acquisition mode is associated with a relatively low radiation dose. However, as opposed to the retrospectively ECG-gated technique described above, prospectively ECG trigged acquisition provides no functional data and is

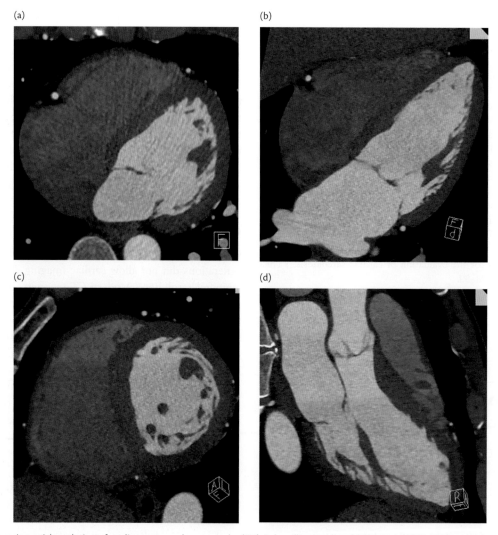

Figure 7.3.3.1 Isotropic spatial resolution of cardiac computed tomography (CT). Sub-millimetre slice thickness and ECG synchronization permit the acquisition of data sets with near-isotropic spatial resolution. (a) Contrast-enhanced axial cross-sectional image as acquired by the CT system. (b, c, d) Multiplanar reconstructions in typical cardiac planes which, owing to the thin slice collimation and gapless spacing, preserve high spatial resolution in all orientations.

Table 7.3.3.1 Methods of ECG synchronization in cardiac computed tomography

	Advantages	Disadvantages
Spiral acquisition with retrospectively ECG-gated image reconstruction	Allows to reconstruct images at any desired time within the cardiac cycle Individual selection of optimal phase for image reconstruction allows to minimize motion artefact 'Cine' reconstructions for assessment of function are possible	High radiation exposure Long duration of data acquisition Long breath-holding Large volume of contrast agent
Prospectively ECG-triggered axial acquisition	Low radiation exposure	'Cine' reconstructions for functional imaging are not possible Limited ability to correct for motion artefact by reconstructing data sets at different time points in the cardiac cycle Duration of image acquisition depends on the number of simultaneous acquired slices and can be long
Prospectively ECG-triggered high-pitch 'flash' mode	Very low radiation exposure Very rapid volume coverage (with one single beat)	Unless the heart rate is low and very stable, motion artefacts may occur Available only for selected scanners

ECG, electrocardiogram.

more vulnerable to artefacts caused by rapid heart motion and arrhythmia.[6]

A further image acquisition mode, the high-pitch 'flash' scan, is available only in selected scanners. It combines prospectively ECG-triggered acquisition with continuous table motion at very high speed. The volume of the heart can be covered in less than one second and radiation exposure is particularly low. With this scan mode, a low and stable heart rate (well below 60/min) is of paramount importance in order to avoid motion artefact, particularly when coronary artery imaging is intended.[7]

Clinical applications of cardiac CT

Coronary CT angiography

Coronary CTA is increasingly used in clinical settings to work up patients with suspected CAD. It is not quite as reliable as invasive coronary angiography, and its robustness depends on the CT technology that is used. Current recommendations include the use of CT systems that allow the acquisition of at least 64 slices simultaneously, slice collimation of no more than 0.625 mm, and a rotation time of 350 ms or less.[3]

The radiation exposure of coronary CTA is sometimes considered a limiting factor. It varies widely and ranges from <1 to 30 mSv.[8,9] Several techniques are available to reduce the radiation dose, and their use depends on available technology, the patient heart rate, and the experience of the operator. Some powerful measures to reduce the dose include use of low tube potential,[23] use of low tube current in combination with iterative image reconstruction, limitation of the scan range, and use of prospectively ECG-triggered image acquisition protocols (which may be hampered by high or irregular heart rates). By applying these measures where appropriate, the German Cardiac CT Registry reported a median effective dose of 2.5 mSv.[10]

The accuracy of coronary CTA for detection of coronary stenosis is high (➲ Figure 7.3.3.2). A meta-analysis of 30 studies with 3722 patients showed a sensitivity of 91% and a specificity of 82% for coronary CTA, in comparison to invasive angiography.[11] Likelihood ratios are important for diagnostic purposes, and the positive and negative likelihood ratios in this meta-analysis (8.9 and 0.022, respectively) indicate that CT is extremely reliable to rule out significant stenoses.

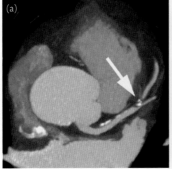 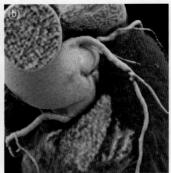 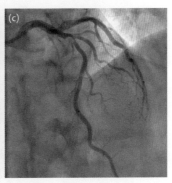

Figure 7.3.3.2 Coronary computed tomography (CT) angiography. High-grade, partly calcified stenosis of the left anterior descending coronary artery. (a) Two-dimensional coronary CT angiography (arrow, stenosis). (b) Three-dimensional volume rendering. Note that the calcifications cannot be separated from the contrast-enhanced lumen, which is a downside of three-dimensional reconstructions. (c) Invasive coronary angiogram in RA cranial projection (arrow, stenosis).

CT is known to perform best in patients with a low pretest likelihood of disease. However, if carefully performed, diagnostic accuracy holds up in patients with a higher pretest risk. In a cohort of 1023 patients with acute symptoms and a high pretest probability of disease, coronary CTA displayed positive and negative likelihood ratios of 3.49 (2.93–4.16) and 0.05 (0.03–0.07), with a sensitivity and specificity of 96.5% and 72.4%, respectively.[12] The recent ISCHEMIA trial confirmed an excellent concordance of coronary CTA and invasive angiography.[13]

Numerous registries have consistently shown that prognosis is excellent following a normal coronary CTA. As an example, in a cohort of 10,037 patients after clinically indicated coronary CTA, the event rate of patients without stenosis on CT was only 0.8%.[14] In the PROMISE trial, which randomized 10,003 patients with suspected CAD to having either coronary CTA or myocardial perfusion imaging as the first diagnostic test, subsequent event rates were equally low in both arms.[15] In some cohorts, the use of coronary CTA as a diagnostic test in suspected CAD has even been shown to significantly reduce—albeit to a small extent—the rate of downstream myocardial infarction.[16,17] It is assumed that this results from the fact that coronary CTA as an initial diagnostic step triggers a more frequent use of statins, owing to the fact that CT not only can visualize stenosis, but also can detect non-stenotic coronary atherosclerotic plaque (⊃ Figure 7.3.3.3).

Current European guidelines recommend the use of coronary CTA as one of the first-line tests in suspected CAD but wisely qualify that CTA should only be chosen when patient characteristics promise high image quality and when adequate technology and expertise are available.[2]

Cardiac morphology

In the practice of cardiology, echocardiography is the method of choice to evaluate cardiac structure and function. This includes the workup of patients with heart failure. CMR is an alternative.

While CT is also able to visualize cardiac anatomy and function, radiation exposure and the requirement for contrast injection are its downsides. In current clinical practice, the use of CT to visualize cardiac morphology is recommended mainly in the context of infective endocarditis and transcatheter aortic valve implantation (TAVI).[18,19] For the latter, cardiac CT imaging is an essential component, due to its ability to visualize the aortic valve, sinuses of Valsalva, and coronary ostia, as a highly accurate basis for prosthetic size selection (⊃ Figure 7.3.3.4).[18]

Systolic and diastolic function

Cardiac CT has the ability to assess left and right ventricular (RV) function based on 'cine' reconstructions showing the heart at different time points in the cardiac cycle (⊃ Figures 7.3.3.5 and 7.3.3.6). Numerous studies have evaluated CT for the assessment of left ventricular (LV) and RV volumes and function. In 2017, Kaniewska *et al.* published a meta-analysis of 53 studies and a total of 1814 patients to compare the diagnostic accuracy of global and regional LV function, and found a mean difference between left ventricular ejection fraction (LVEF) in CT and CMR of only −0.56%.[20] Limits of agreement for LVEF in this meta-analysis were ± 11.0%, which is less than previously reported for comparisons between echocardiography and CMR[21,22,23] but emphasizes that there will always be a certain degree of variability between methods.

For the assessment of RV function, a meta-analysis of 19 studies (including 749 patients) also found close agreement between cardiac CT and CMR, with correlation coefficients of 0.98 for RV end-diastolic volume, 0.98 for RV ejection fraction, and 0.97 for stroke volume.[24]

Direct comparisons of cardiac CT to echocardiography also demonstrate good correlation between these two methods. A recent study compared 320-row CT to echocardiography in 114 patients and demonstrated excellent correlation between

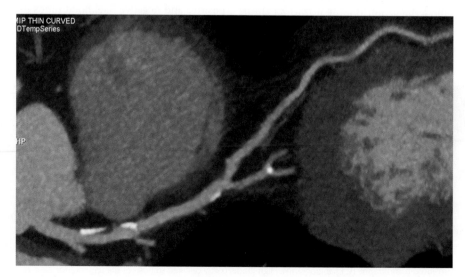

Figure 7.3.3.3 Coronary computed tomography angiography showing the left main and left anterior descending coronary artery with substantial non-obstructive coronary atherosclerotic plaque, but absence of significant stenosis.

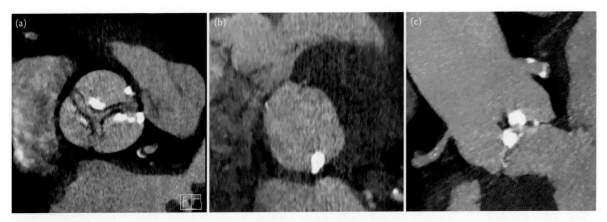

Figure 7.3.3.4 Visualization of the aortic valve at the level of the commissures (a), aortic annulus (b), and aortic root with coronary ostia (c) in a patient under evaluation for transcatheter aortic valve implantation.

CT and two-dimensional echocardiography for end-diastolic volume (EDV) ($r^2 = 0.91$; $P < 0.001$) and end-systolic volume (ESV) ($r^2 = 0.94$; $P < 0.001$), with a small overestimation for ESV and particularly EDV (1.8 and 7.3 mL, respectively). LVEF correlated closely ($r^2 = 0.87$; $P < 0.001$; mean difference $= 0.9\%$).[25]

Assessment of diastolic function by CT is not as straightforward as analysis of systolic function, because in CT, flow velocities need to be derived from volume changes.[26] Nevertheless, Boogers *et al.* reported a 70% accuracy of CT in identifying patients with diastolic dysfunction, on comparing CT to two-dimensional echocardiography and tissue Doppler imaging (TDI), in a cohort of 70 individuals.[27] Finally, the analysis of atrial function may contribute to the refined analysis of heart failure patients and has been shown possible by CT.[28]

Specific advantages and disadvantages of cardiac CT

Advantages of cardiac CT

The most important advantage of cardiac CT over other imaging modalities is its very high spatial resolution and the fact that this spatial resolution is, for all practical purposes, isotropic. Hence, reconstructions in all imaging spatial orientations are possible and anatomical/morphological information is extremely high. This is particularly true for high-contrast resolution, whereas low-contrast resolution and tissue differentiation by CT are poor.

A specific advantage of CT is also the fact that neither calcium nor metal interferes with image quality (outside the coronary arteries). A relevant number of patients with cardiovascular disease—including heart failure—carry metallic implanted

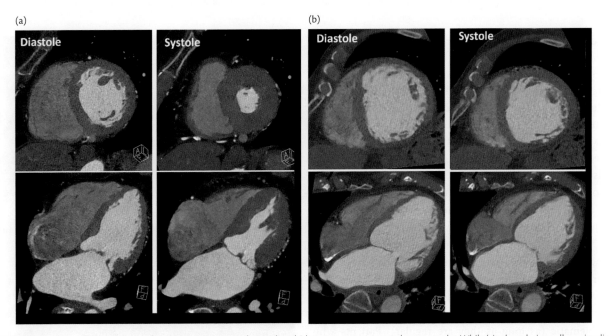

Figure 7.3.3.5 Analysis of left ventricular function in contrast-enhanced multidetector row computed tomography. While 'cine' renderings allow visualization of the heart in motion during the entire cardiac cycle, the frames shown here represent diastole and systole. (a) Patient with normal left ventricular ejection fraction. (b) Patient with severely reduced left ventricular ejection fraction.

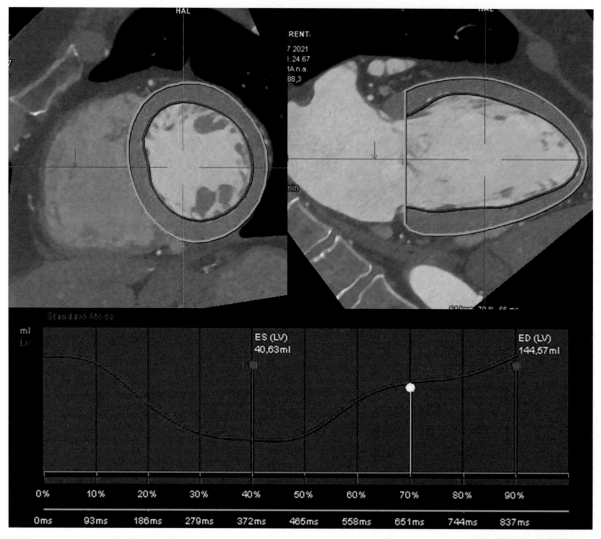

Figure 7.3.3.6 Automated analysis of left ventricular volumes and function in contrast-enhanced cardiac computed tomography without manual input.

cardiac devices. These can cause severe artefacts in echocardiography and CMR, or may prevent CMR imaging completely. In CT, on the other hand, metallic implants usually do not cause relevant artefacts. Cardiac CT can, in fact, be particularly useful for the evaluation of prosthetic valves and the paravalvular territory (➲ Figure 7.3.3.7). Similarly, CT can identify and visualize calcifications of cardiac structures such as the pericardium, the valves, or (infrequently) the myocardium.

A disadvantage that CT shares with CMR—when compared to echocardiography—is the relationship between heart rhythm and image quality. High heart rates are detrimental to image quality of coronary CTA. They are usually not problematic for visualization of non-coronary cardiac morphology or assessment of function. Arrhythmias during data acquisition, however, can cause severe artefacts and may render the data set unevaluable. These include rapid atrial fibrillation, ectopic beats, and complete atrioventricular block. Paced rhythms are not problematic (as long as they are regular). Patients who cannot follow breath-holding commands are usually not well suited for CT imaging.

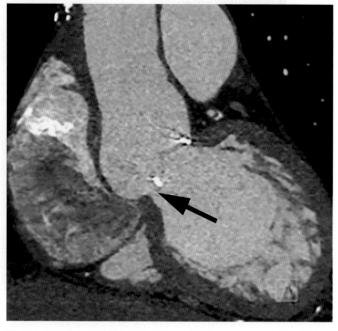

Figure 7.3.3.7 Paravalvular leak of an aortic valve bioprosthesis (arrow).

Table 7.3.3.2 Diagnostic accuracy of coronary CT angiography in patients with HFrEF

	CT system	Number of patients	Mean LVEF (%)	Number of evaluated segments	Diagnostic performance in comparison to invasive angiography (threshold 50% diameter stenosis)			
					Sensitivity (%)	Specificity (%)	NPV (%)	PPV (%)
Andreini, 2007[29]	16 slice	61	34 ± 9	870	99	96.2	99.8	81
Ghostine, 2008[30]	64 slice	93	37 ± 7	1352	73	99	92	97
Andreini, 2009[31]	64 slice	130	34 ± 10	1902	98.1	99.9	98.7	99.8

CT, computed tomography; HFrEF, heart failure with reduced ejection fraction; LVEF, left ventricular ejection fraction; NPV, negative predictive value; PPV, positive predictive value.

Further disadvantages of cardiac CT that need to be taken into consideration when selecting the most appropriate test for an individual patient include the requirement for iodinated contrast injection for most clinical applications, as well as potentially negative effects of radiation exposure.

Use of cardiac CT in heart failure

Ruling out ischaemic cardiomyopathy

Several studies performed in patients with heart failure with reduced ejection fraction (HFrEF) (LVEF <40%) have confirmed that coronary CTA may be useful to rule out obstructive CAD in patients with newly diagnosed heart failure (➔ Table 7.3.3.2).[29,30,31] All studies showed very high sensitivity and specificity, and negative and positive predictive values of coronary CTA. Hence, CT can be used as an alternative to invasive coronary angiography to reliably exclude an ischaemic aetiology of heart failure. Further, heart failure guidelines include cardiac CT as a non-invasive modality for visualization of the coronary anatomy in patients with low-to-intermediate pretest probability of CAD or those with equivocal non-invasive stress tests.[32]

Assessment of the pericardium

Pericardial disease may be an underlying reason for heart failure. CT permits comprehensive evaluation of the pericardium (➔ Figure 7.3.3.8), including identification of pericardial effusion, pericardial thickening, and particularly visualization of calcification. It should be noted that the ability of CT to differentiate small pericardial effusions from pericardial thickening is limited.[33] The diagnosis of constrictive pericarditis in CT should not only be based on pericardial thickness (considered 'increased' above 4 mm) and calcification, but also include morphological changes such as atrial enlargement, narrowing of the left and right ventricles (typically at their base), and potentially the typical 'septal bounce' in functional data sets. In clinical practice, suspicion of constrictive pericarditis will usually be raised based on other diagnostic modalities, and pericardial visualization by CT may serve to strengthen the degree of diagnostic certainty.

Left ventricular assist devices

In patients with terminal heart failure, left ventricular assist devices (LVADs) can be associated with various complications, including

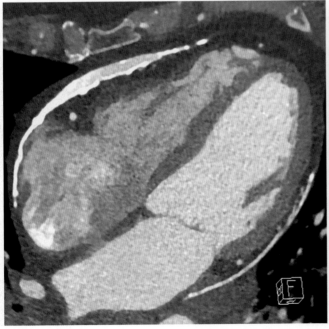
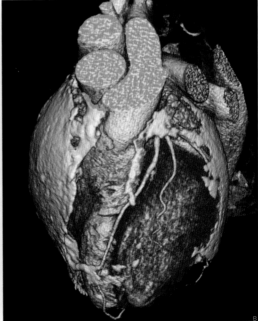

Figure 7.3.3.8 Severe pericardial calcification in a patient with constrictive pericarditis.

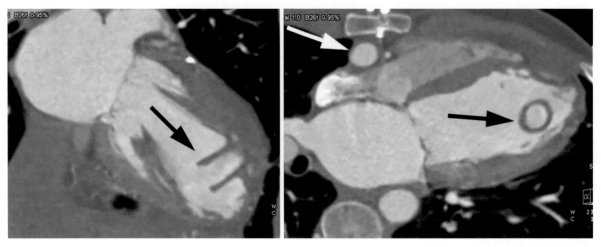

Figure 7.3.3.9 Contrast-enhanced cardiac computed tomography in a patient with a left ventricular assist device (Excor®). Arrows indicate the inflow cannula (black arrows) and outflow cannula (white arrow).

thrombosis of the device and inflow or outflow cannula, as well as inflow cannula obstruction. In general, echocardiography will be the standard imaging tool in LVAD patients. However, a series of 58 LVAD patients with suspected LVAD complications showed that the combined use of CT and echocardiography substantially improved the identification of pathologies leading to device malfunction (with sensitivity increasing from 22% to 67% by adding CT to transthoracic echocardiography).[34] CT will be particularly useful when limitations of the acoustic window may render assessment of ventricular function in LVAD patients difficult or occasionally impossible (➲ Figure 7.3.3.9). Also, a specific advantage of CT is its ability to analyse suspected cannula obstruction.[35,36,37] Overall, the combination of CT with echocardiography should therefore be considered as the imaging approach of choice for LVAD patients unless echocardiography can clearly establish a diagnosis.[38]

Cardiac resynchronization therapy

Through visualization of LV contraction patterns in 'cine' reconstructions, contrast-enhanced CT can identify and quantify dyssynchrony in a robust and reliable fashion. The time from R-wave to maximal wall thickness across six standardized segments (dyssynchrony index, DI) has been shown to be most reproducible and it correlates with two- ($r=0.65$; $P=0.012$) and three-dimensional ($r=0.68$; $P=0.008$) echocardiographic dyssynchrony.[39] In fact, CT-based measures of dyssynchrony have been shown to be associated with lower interobserver variability, compared to echocardiographic parameters.[40] Large clinical trials that have used CT-based assessment of dyssynchrony, however, do not exist and CT should, at best, be considered a fallback solution when echocardiography cannot be performed.

Future directions

It can be confidently predicted that the technology of CT imaging will evolve further. New types of detectors, for example 'photon count detectors', will allow a substantially increased spatial resolution,[41] which will contribute towards making coronary CTA more robust and accurate. These detectors will furthermore allow spectral imaging (analysis of X-ray absorption across various photon energies), which holds potential for improved assessment of myocardial perfusion and viability.

Next to the development of CT technology, artificial intelligence algorithms are likely to be integrated in image evaluation, making diagnosis more accurate and potentially identifying features which escape the human eye. In combination, these developments will lead to a certain increase in clinical applications of cardiac CT. Additionally, the growth of interventional procedures in cardiovascular medicine will be accompanied by a growing volume of CT imaging to plan structural interventions.

Summary

CT with modern multidetector row technology provides robust and very high-resolution imaging of the heart, with accurate and detailed assessment of cardiac structures and function. In patients with known or suspected heart failure, it will usually be an imaging technique of secondary importance, following echocardiography and CMR. CT may be a first-line tool to rule out obstructive CAD, and a backup method to visualize cardiac anatomy and function if poor acoustic windows, metallic artefacts, or other factors limit the diagnostic utility of echocardiography and magnetic resonance. Heart failure specialists should therefore be aware of the potential applications, strengths, and weaknesses of CT for cardiac imaging.

References

1. Piepoli MF, Hoes AW, Agewall S, *et al.*; ESC Scientific Document Group. 2016 European Guidelines on cardiovascular disease prevention in clinical practice. Eur Heart J 2016;37(29): 2315–81.
2. Knuuti J, Wijns W, Saraste A, *et al.* 2019 ESC Guidelines for the diagnosis and management of chronic coronary syndromes. Eur Heart J 2020;41(3):407–77.
3. Abbara S, Blanke P, Maroules CD, *et al.* SCCT guidelines for the performance and acquisition of coronary computed tomographic angiography: a report of the society of Cardiovascular Computed Tomography Guidelines Committee: Endorsed by the North American Society for Cardiovascular Imaging (NASCI). J Cardiovasc Comput Tomogr 2016;10:435–49.

4. Achenbach S. Technology of cardiac computer tomography. In: Camm AJ, Lüscher TF, Maurer G, Serruys PW, eds. *ESC CardioMed*, 3rd edition. Oxford: Oxford University Press; 2018, pp. 538–42. Available from: http://doi.org/10.1093/med/9780198784906.003.0112.

5. Weigold WG, Abbara S, Achenbach S. Standardized medical terminology for cardiac computed tomography: a report of the Society of Cardiovascular Computed Tomography. J Cardiovasc Comput Tomogr 2011;5(3):136–44.

6. Horiguchi J, Yamamoto H, Kihara Y, et al. Prospective ECG-triggered sequential versus retrospective ECG-gated spiral CT: pros and cons. Curr Cardiovasc Imaging Rep 2009;2:447.

7. Flohr TG, McCollough CH, Bruder H, et al. First performance evaluation of a dual-source CT (DSCT) system. Eur Radiol 2006;16(2):256–68.

8. Hausleiter J, Meyer T, Hermann F, et al. Estimated radiation dose associated with cardiac CT angiography. JAMA 2009;301(5):500–7.

9. Stocker TJ, Nühlen N, Schmermund A, et al. Impact of dose reduction strategies on image quality of coronary CTA in real world clinical practice: a subanalysis of PROTECTION VI Registry Data. AJR Am J Roentgenol 2021;217:1344–52.

10. Marwan M, Achenbach S, Korosoglou G, et al. German cardiac CT registry: indications, procedural data and clinical consequences in 7061 patients undergoing cardiac computed tomography. Int J Cardiovasc Imaging 2018;34:807–19.

11. Menke J, Kowalski J. Diagnostic accuracy and utility of coronary CT angiography with consideration of unevaluable results: a systematic review and multivariate Bayesian random-effects meta-analysis with intention to diagnose. Eur Radiol 2016;26:451–8.

12. Linde JJ, Kelbæk H, Hansen TF, et al. Coronary CT angiography in patients with non-ST-segment elevation acute coronary syndrome. J Am Coll Cardiol 2020;75(5):453–63.

13. Mancini GBJ, Leipsic J, Budoff MJ, et al. CT angiography followed by invasive angiography in patients with moderate or severe ischemia: insights from the ISCHEMIA Trial. JACC Cardiovasc Imaging 2021;14(7):1384–93.

14. Villines TC, Hulten EA, Shaw LJ, et al. Prevalence and severity of coronary artery disease and adverse events among symptomatic patients with coronary artery calcification scores of zero undergoing coronary computed tomography angiography J Am Coll Cardiol 2011;58(24):2533–40.

15. Douglas PS, Hoffmann U, Patel MR, et al.; PROMISE Investigators. Outcomes of anatomical versus functional testing for coronary artery disease. N Engl J Med 2015;372:1291–300.

16. Sharma A, Coles A, Sekaran NK, et al. Stress testing versus CT angiography in patients with diabetes and suspected coronary artery disease. J Am Coll Cardiol 2019;73(8):893–902.

18. Blanke P, Weir-McCall JR, Achenbach S, et al. Computed tomography imaging in the context of transcatheter aortic valve implantation (TAVI)/transcatheter aortic valve replacement (TAVR): an expert consensus document of the Society of Cardiovascular Computed Tomography. JACC Cardiovasc Imaging 2019;12(1):1–24.

19. Habib G, Lancelloti P, Antunes M, et al. Guidelines for the management of infective endocarditis. Eur Heart J 2015;36(44):3075–123.

20. Kaniewska M, Schuetz GM, Willun S, et al. Noninvasive evaluation of global and regional left ventricular function using computed tomography and magnetic resonance imaging: a meta-analysis. Eur Radiol 2017;27:1640–59.

21. Van der Vleuten PA, de Jonge GJ, Lubbers DD, et al. Evaluation of global left ventricular function assessment by dual-source computed tomography compared with MRI. Eur Radiol 2009;19:271–7.

22. Asferg C, Usinger L, Kristensen TS, Abdulla J. Accuracy of multi-slice computed tomography for measurement of left ventricular ejection fraction compared with cardiac magnetic resonance imaging and two-dimensional transthoracic echocardiography: a systematic review and meta-analysis. Eur J Radiol 2012;81:e757–62.

23. Sharma A, Einstein AJ, Vallakati A, Arbab-Zadeh A, Mukherjee D, Lichstein E. Meta-analysis of global left ventricular function comparing multidetector computed tomography with cardiac magnetic resonance imaging. Am J Cardiol 2014;113(4):731–8.

24. Fu H, Wang X, Diao K, et al. CT compared to MRI for functional evaluation of the right ventricle: a systematic review and meta-analysis. Eur Radiol 2019;29:6816–28.

25. De Graaf FR, Schuijf JD, van Velzen JE, et al. Incremental prognostic value of left ventricular function analysis over non-invasive coronary angiography with multidetector computed tomography. J Nucl Cardiol 2019;17:225–31.

26. Van der Veen HA, Lessick J, Abadi S, Mutlak D. Accuracy of diastolic function by cardiac computed tomography relative to echo-Doppler: additive clinical and prognostic value. J Comput Assist Tomogr 2021;45(2):242–7.

27. Boogers MJ, van Werkhoven JM, Schuijf JD, et al. Feasibility of diastolic function assessment with cardiac CT: feasibility study in comparison with tissue Doppler imaging. JACC Cardiovasc Imaging 2011;4:246–56.

28. Kataoka A, Funabashi N, Takahashi A, et al. Quantitative evaluation of left atrial volumes and ejection fraction by 320-slice computed-tomography in comparison with three- and two-dimensional echocardiography: a single-center retrospective-study in 22 subjects. Int J Cardiol 2011;153(1):47–54.

29. Andreini D, Pontone G, Pepi M, et al. Diagnostic accuracy of multidetector computed tomography coronary angiography in patients with dilated cardiomyopathy. J Am Coll Cardiol 2007;49(20):2044–50.

30. Ghostine S, Caussin C, Habis M, et al. Non-invasive diagnosis of ischaemic heart failure using 64-slice computed tomography. Eur Heart J 2008;29:2133–40.

31. Andreini D, Pontone G, Bartorelli AL, et al. Sixty-four-slice multidetector computed tomography: an accurate imaging modality for the evaluation of coronary arteries in dilated cardiomyopathy of unknown etiology. Circ Cardiovasc Imaging 2009;2:199–205.

32. McDonagh TA, Metra M, Adamo M, et al. 2021 ESC Guidelines for the diagnosis and treatment of acute and chronic heart failure. Eur Heart J 2021;42(36):3599–726.

33. Wang ZJ, Reddy GP, Gotway MB, et al. CT and MR imaging of pericardial disease. RadioGraphics 2003;23:S167–80.

34. Patel PA, Green CL, Lokhnygina Y, et al. Cardiac computed tomography improves the identification of cardiomechanical complications among patients with suspected left ventricular assist device malfunction. J Cardiovasc Comput Tomogr 2021;15(3):260–7.

35. Raman SV, Sahu A, Merchant AZ, Louis LB 4th, Firstenberg MS, Sun B. Noninvasive assessment of left ventricular assist devices with cardiovascular computed tomography and impact on management. J Heart Lung Transplant 2010;29(1):79–85.

36. Raman SV, Tran T, Simonetti OP, Sun B. Dynamic computed tomography to determine cardiac output in patients with left ventricular assist devices. J Thorac Cardiovasc Surg 2009;137:1213–17.

37. Garcia-Alvarez A, Fernandez-Friera L, Lau JF, et al. Evaluation of right ventricular function and post-operative findings using cardiac computed tomography in patients with left ventricular assist devices. J Heart Lung Transplantation 2011;30(8):896–903.

38. Carr CM, Jacob J, Park SJ, et al. CT of left ventricular assist devices. RadioGraphics 2010;30:429–44.

39. Truong QA, Singh JP, Cannon CP, et al. Quantitative analysis of intraventricular dyssynchrony using wall thickness by multidetector computed tomography. JACC Cardiovasc Imaging 2008;1(6):772–81.

40. Buss SJ, Schulz F, Wolf D, *et al.* Quantitative analysis of left ventricular dyssynchrony using cardiac computed tomography versus three-dimensional echocardiography. Eur Radiol 2012;22:1303–9.

41. Rajendran K, Petersilka M, Henning A, *et al.* Full field-of-view, high-resolution, photon-counting detector CT: technical assessment and initial patient experience. Phys Med Biol 2021;66:10.1088/1361-6560/ac155e.

7.3.4 Cardiac magnetic resonance in heart failure: diagnostic and prognostic assessment

Anna Baritussio, Noor Sharrack, Sven Plein, and Chiara Bucciarelli-Ducci

Introduction

CMR is the reference standard for the assessment of biventricular volumes and function. It is proven to be superior to two- (2D) and three-dimensional (3D) echocardiography,[1] and is independent of geometric assumption and highly reproducible.[1] According to the 2021 European Society of Cardiology (ESC) guidelines for the diagnosis and treatment of acute and chronic HF,[2] CMR is the recommended alternative test to echocardiography for the assessment of biventricular volumes and function in patients with suboptimal or poor acoustic windows (e.g. patients with pulmonary disease, obesity), while being the preferred imaging modality in patients with complex congenital heart disease.[3,4] The unique non-invasive myocardial tissue characterization capabilities of CMR allow the identification of the presence and extent of myocardial fibrosis, myocardial oedema, infiltration, and iron overload.[1] The presence and extent of functional tissue abnormalities inform the differential diagnosis of cardiac dysfunction and guide tailored management and treatment.[2] The 2021 ESC Guidelines recommend the use of CMR to distinguish between ischaemic and non-ischaemic aetiologies of dilated cardiomyopathy (DCM), especially in cases of equivocal clinical or imaging findings (Class of recommendation IIa, Level of evidence C).[2] The role of CMR in the identification of HF aetiology is recognized in a range of cardiomyopathic processes, such as amyloidosis, sarcoidosis, myocarditis, Fabry disease, and non-compaction cardiomyopathy, where it has a Class I recommendation. Additional use of parametric mapping facilitates the differential diagnosis in restrictive cardiomyopathies with similar phenotypes such as in left ventricular (LV) hypertrophy.[5] According to both the 2016 ESC Heart Failure Guidelines and the 2017 ESC Consensus Document on restrictive cardiomyopathies, CMR is the imaging modality of choice to detect and quantify myocardial iron load and to guide subsequent chelation therapy.[2,5] Finally, the use of CMR stress imaging is suggested for the assessment of myocardial ischaemia and viability to guide revascularization decisions in patients with HF and coronary artery disease (CAD) (Class of recommendation IIb, Level of evidence B).[2]

CMR principles and methods

Magnetic resonance imaging (MRI) utilizes the magnetic properties of atomic nuclei—in standard imaging, the hydrogen atom. By exposing tissue to a strong external magnetic field and using a series of radiofrequency pulses, magnetic gradient field switches, and timed data acquisitions, an image is generated that represents the magnetic properties of tissue in the imaging field. Images that highlight different tissue properties can be acquired by varying the order, timing, magnitude, and shape of the radiofrequency pulses.[6,7] The most common tissue properties are the constants T1 and T2 where, in general terms, T1-weighted images display high signal from fat and T2-weighted images show high signal in areas of myocardial oedema or inflammation. In addition, MRI contrast agents can be used to further enhance specific tissue properties and the identification of myocardial fibrosis or infiltration. The so-called 'spin echo sequences' are mainly used for anatomical imaging and tissue characterization. Gradient echo (GRE) sequences, including steady-state free precession (SSFP) imaging, are much faster and routinely used for imaging of cardiac function. On GRE images, blood appears bright, whereas on spin echo images, it is usually dark.

Cine imaging and assessment of left and right ventricular function

Assessment of LV and right ventricular (RV) volumes, mass and ejection fraction (EF) by CMR is usually based on contiguous stacks of cine images covering the whole heart in either the LV short axis or the axial plane, with a slice thickness of around 8–10 mm and an in-plane resolution of at least 2×2 mm. Data are acquired in multiple phases of the cardiac cycle (typically at least 30) and reconstructed into cine images. Images are typically acquired using a series of short (few seconds) breath-holds, with an overall scan time of around 5 minutes for a whole-heart stack.[8,9] SSFP sequences provide excellent delineation of the blood–myocardium interface and allow accurate identification of regional wall motion abnormalities. From these images, volumetric and functional indices, including biventricular end-diastolic and end-systolic volumes, stroke volume, EF, and LV mass, are calculated using the Simpson's method of multiple disc-derived measurements. Due to whole-heart coverage of the acquisition, CMR analysis does not rely on geometric assumptions, making CMR particularly well suited to studying diseased hearts and the right ventricle (RV). Cardiac arrhythmias, particularly ectopy or atrial fibrillation, can lead to suboptimal imaging, but techniques such as arrhythmia detection and real-time imaging can be employed to overcome these challenges.

Flow and valvular disease

Although valve morphology is generally well assessed by echocardiography, CMR can be an alternative, particularly in patients with poor acoustic windows. For flow assessment, velocity-encoding

CMR sequences are used, which enable accurate quantitative measurements for stenotic (peak velocity and peak gradient by applying the Bernoulli equation) and regurgitant valvular lesions (regurgitant volume and fraction).[8] Furthermore, when a shunt is suspected, the pulmonary-to-systemic flow ratio (Qp/Qs) can be determined by measuring flow in the main pulmonary artery and ascending aorta.

Diastolic function

Nearly half of HF patients have abnormalities in diastolic function in the context of preserved EF. CMR can assess diastolic function in several ways. Similarly to echocardiography, flow velocity-encoded CMR can measure early diastolic (E) and atrial systolic (A) peak flow velocities and E/A ratios of the mitral inflow.[10] Furthermore, time–volume curves generated from retrospectively gated cine images can provide indices of global diastolic function such as peak filling rate and time to peak filling rate.

Magnetic resonance tagging is used for quantitative analysis of regional systolic and diastolic function. Selective saturation prepulses are used to superimpose a grid across the field of view. The grid lines are deformed by myocardial contraction, strain, and torsion, allowing direct quantification of myocardial deformation and strain.[8] CMR feature tracking (CMR-FT) is an alternative post-processing method for strain analysis by CMR. In the same way as speckle tracking in echocardiography, it is based on pattern-matching techniques from standard cine images. By defining an area in a pixel in one frame, this can be tracked through successive frames, allowing the measurement of longitudinal, radial, and circumferential strain.

Myocardial perfusion imaging and ischaemia detection

For myocardial perfusion CMR, the dynamic passage of a gadolinium-based contrast bolus is followed through the cardiac chambers and myocardium.[8,9] Gadolinium-based contrast agents shorten the T1 of surrounding tissue and thus increase the signal on T1-weighted pulse sequences. Pharmacological vasodilatation (with adenosine, dipyridamole, regadenoson, or adenosine triphosphate (ATP)) induces a 3- to 5-fold increase in blood flow in myocardial areas perfused by normal coronary arteries, with lower increase in areas perfused by coronary arteries with flow-limiting obstruction. Therefore, contrast arrival in these areas is delayed and reduced, compared to the myocardium with normal coronary supply, and they appear relatively hypointense (dark) on visual inspection. In addition, quantitative perfusion methodology allows myocardial blood flow to be quantified in mL/g/min and presented in pixel-wise perfusion maps. Advantages of quantitative perfusion include removal of subjectivity in the interpretation of perfusion CMR and detection of microvascular disease, as well as providing quantitative assessment for follow-up.[9] Quantitative perfusion mapping is currently transitioning from research to clinical application.

Tissue characterization

A range of CMR methods can be used to interrogate several myocardial tissue properties. The most common methods are T1- and T2-weighted imaging and parametric T1, T2, and T2* mapping, as well as late gadolinium enhancement (LGE) following contrast administration.

T1-weighted imaging, and T1 and ECV mapping

The T1 relaxation time is a constant specific to the field strength of the MRI scanner and tissue composition. In T1-weighted images, fat (which has a short T1) is bright and the myocardium is of intermediate signal. T1 mapping expresses the T1 relaxation time of tissue as absolute values in a pixel-wise map, which can then be displayed using colour or threshold scales to allow quantitative visual interpretation.[8,9] The most used method for T1 mapping is the modified look-locker inversion recovery (MOLLI) pulse sequence, which performs a series of acquisitions over successive heartbeats to generate T1 relaxation curves, but other methods are also available.[8] The most important biological causes of an increase in native myocardial T1 include an increase in interstitial space due to the presence of oedema (e.g. in acute infarction or inflammation) and/or fibrosis and infiltrative processes such as in amyloid deposition. Native T1 myocardial values can be lowered by water–protein interaction and fat or iron content (e.g. in Fabry disease). As gadolinium-based contrast agents are extravascular and extracellular, post-contrast T1 values are lower in tissues with expansion of the extracellular space. In combination with haematocrit levels, native and post-contrast T1 mapping can be used to quantify the extracellular volume (ECV) of tissue. The ECV of normal myocardium has been reported to be in the range of 24–28%.[11] ECV expansion has been demonstrated in a range of cardiac conditions and is most commonly due to excessive collagen deposition or infiltrative processes (fat, protein), therefore serving as a measure of myocardial fibrosis or, more generally, pathologically expanded interstitial space. Low ECV values occur in fat and lipomatous metaplasia.[12]

T2-weighted imaging and T2 mapping

T2-weighted imaging is used for qualitative or semi-quantitative detection of myocardial oedema and inflammation, which prolong T2 relaxation times, making oedematous tissues appear brighter than normal remote myocardium. Standard T2-weighted imaging of myocardial oedema typically utilizes turbo spin echo (TSE), with or without fat saturation pulses, mostly combined with dark-blood preparations.[8,9,13] The most used sequence is short T1 triple inversion recovery prepared fast spin echo sequence (STIR). Here the signal from fat and blood is suppressed to improve the contrast between oedema, normal myocardium, and the LV cavity. A T2 mapping sequence measures the T2 transverse relaxation time in each voxel and then creates a parametric image in which intensity reflects the measured T2 value. The T2 values can be portrayed visually on colour scales and then quantified further within areas of interest.

T2* mapping

T2* is a relaxation parameter arising principally from local magnetic field inhomogeneities, which are increased with iron deposition. With T2* mapping, the T2* relaxation of myocardial tissue is measured from GRE sequences, allowing quantification of tissue iron content.[8,9] T2* mapping is mostly used in the management of patients with beta-thalassaemia major worldwide.

Early and late gadolinium enhancement

Post-contrast T1-weighted imaging allows further tissue characterization. Early after injection of gadolinium-based contrast agents, severely hypovascular regions will not enhance. Early gadolinium-enhanced imaging is typically performed a few minutes after contrast administration to detect thrombus or microvascular obstruction in acute MI. With longer delays from contrast injection, an equilibrium between contrast uptake, distribution, and washout evolves. Areas of infarction or focal fibrosis have slower contrast kinetics and a greater volume of distribution in extracellular water associated with collagen. Using T1-sensitive inversion recovery methods, LGE CMR is usually acquired around 10 minutes after contrast injection and provides high-resolution images of scar or fibrosis. Conventionally, in LGE, the signal from normal myocardium is 'nulled', and thus dark, whereas areas of myocardial injury/fibrosis appear bright.[8,9] LGE images can be assessed either visually or quantitatively based on relative enhancement, compared to the background. The extent and pattern of LGE vary according to the underlying disease process, and is frequently of prognostic significance and can be diagnostic of the underlying aetiology.

Practical clinical issues

CMR does not expose patients to ionizing radiation and there are no known detrimental biological side effects if safety guidelines are followed. Except for intravascular clips, most medical metallic implants are safe in the MRI environment, including nearly all prosthetic cardiac valves, coronary and vascular stents, and orthopaedic implants.[8] However, whenever there is uncertainty regarding a particular device or implant, its safety status should be checked by referring to information provided by the manufacturer and other resources. Many older-generation intracardiac devices, such as pacemakers and implantable cardioverter–defibrillators (ICDs), have traditionally been considered unsafe in MRI, with a risk of malfunction and heating of the pacemaker leads. Today, specialist centres offer MRI for such devices with use of strict safety protocols.[8] In addition, almost all newer implanted cardiac devices are MRI-conditional (generator and leads), which means that patients with these devices can undergo CMR scans under certain conditions, including safety checks and programming of the device into an 'MR-safe' mode. An important limitation of CMR in patients with any implantable cardiac device, particularly generators in the left pectoral position, is distortion of images from metal artefact. Such artefacts can be minimized by using fast gradient echo (FGE) rather than SSFP cine imaging and wide-band LGE methods.

CMR needs to overcome both cardiac and respiratory motion. Most CMR scans are timed with respect to the ECG (ECG-gated) to minimize cardiac motion artefact. In order to minimize respiratory motion artefact, short breath-holds are used (5–10 seconds), or the acquisition is linked to the respiratory cycle with use of diaphragmatic monitoring techniques (respiratory-gated) or retrospective respiratory motion compensation allowing subjects to breathe normally (free breathing).[8] Cardiac and respiratory motion is particularly relevant to HF patients who are frequently breathless and arrhythmic and find it difficult to lie flat in the scanner for longer periods of time. ⊃ Table 7.3.4.1 illustrates possible solutions to overcome these challenges.

In the recent past, early-generation gadolinium-based contrast agents with a linear molecular structure have been linked with a rare multisystemic fibrosing disorder of unknown aetiology called nephrogenic systemic fibrosis (NSF). NSF occurs almost exclusively in patients with acute or chronic severe renal insufficiency (glomerular filtration rate (GFR) <30 mL/min/1.73 m^2)[8] or renal dysfunction caused by the hepatorenal syndrome or in the perioperative liver transplantation period. Linear gadolinium-based contrast agents have also been associated with gadolinium deposition in the brain, although no adverse health effects of this observation are known. For new-generation, macro-cyclic gadolinium-based contrast agents, there are almost no reported cases of NSF. Considering these observations, the European Medicines Agency (EMA) suspended the use of linear gadolinium-based contrast agents for most indications in 2010 and confirmed this decision in 2017. The risk associated with the use of macro-cyclic agents was considered low and their licence was maintained.

CMR protocols for the assessment of heart failure

A typical CMR protocol in HF with optional additions is illustrated in ⊃ Figure 7.3.4.1. A basic protocol can be completed in less than 20 minutes, with more comprehensive protocols lasting 30–60 minutes. Most CMR protocols start with a multi-slice set of low-resolution localizer images in orthogonal planes (transaxial, sagittal, and coronal); this is often followed by the acquisition of a stack of static black blood or bright blood anatomical images.[8] These initial images give an overview of the main cardiovascular structures. These images are also used to plan a series of cine images to define the main cardiac orientations, such as vertical long

Table 7.3.4.1 Solutions to overcome challenges in CMR for heart failure patients

Challenge	Solution
Breathlessness	Use rapid protocols, free breathing acquisition, pillows to elevate the chest and head
Implanted device	Use wide-band LGE, spoiled GRE imaging
Claustrophobia	Use rapid protocols, feet first, prone position, sedation
Erratic heart rhythm (e.g. AF)	Use real-time ungated cine imaging, arrhythmia rejection sequences, single-shot LGE sequences

AF atrial fibrillation; GRE, gradient echo; LGE, late gadolinium enhancement.

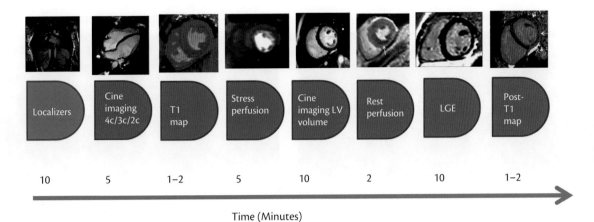

Figure 7.3.4.1 A typical CMR protocol showing the time taken for each acquisition. 4c, four-chamber view; 3c, three-chamber view; 2c, two-chamber view; LV, left ventricular; LGE, late gadolinium enhancement.

axis and horizontal long axis, from which a cine stack in LV short axis covering the heart from the mitral annulus to the LV apex is planned and acquired. Additional multi-slice cine stacks (e.g. in the transaxial plane) provide further information on morphology, relations, and movement (e.g. of muscle, valves, or jets). Tissue characterization sequences may then follow, in particular T2-weighted images for oedema assessment and native T1 and T2 mapping. Vasodilator stress perfusion may be undertaken if an ischaemic aetiology is suspected, followed by early and late gadolinium enhancement to identify focal fibrosis, scar, or infarction. Depending on the suspected aetiology of HF and the referral request, additional sequences can be used, including myocardial blood velocities/flow (e.g. for detecting shunts, valve disease), cardiac iron quantification (iron overload), tagging (pericardial disease, diastology), and real-time imaging during respiration (pericardial constriction).[8]

Differential diagnosis in heart failure

CMR is increasingly used in the diagnosis and risk stratification of patients with HF with reduced, mid-range, and preserved EF.[1]

Although CMR is more commonly performed in the chronic HF setting, its ability to identify myocardial oedema (using T2-weighted imaging and T2 mapping) allows the identification of acute processes leading to HF such as acute myocarditis and acute graft rejection following heart transplantation. A CMR protocol, consisting of T2-weighted (for myocardial oedema) and T1-weighted (LGE) (for myocardial fibrosis) sequences, has been shown to have a high negative predictive value (96%) for excluding a diagnosis of graft rejection, but with low specificity (56%) and low positive predictive value (23%).[14] Indeed, a positive correlation between prolonged T2 relaxation times and severity of graft rejection has been demonstrated by histology and *ex vivo* myocardial water content.[14]

In the current 2021 ESC Heart Failure Guidelines, CMR with LGE is recommended to identify the underlying aetiology of DCM (Class of recommendation IIa, Level of evidence C).[2,15] The presence and distribution pattern of LGE allow the differentiation

between ischaemic and non-ischaemic aetiologies. Moreover, the patterns of LGE (subendocardial, transmural, mid-wall, epicardial, circumferential) reflect the pathophysiological process of the underlying disease. Ischaemic LGE, for example, is always subendocardial and can be partial or full thickness (transmural); this pattern follows the ischaemic necrotic wavefront phenomenon, in which myocardial damage first occurs in the subendocardium, becoming transmural in cases of prolonged ischaemic time. Generally, the LGE patterns observed in non-ischaemic pathologies are distinct and include mid-wall, epicardial, or circumferential patterns in both hypertrophic and dilated hearts (➲ Figure 7.3.4.2).[16]

In patients with HF and ischaemic heart disease, CMR is recommended for the assessment of both myocardial ischaemia and viability to target myocardial revascularization (Class of recommendation IIb, Level of evidence B).[2] Myocardial viability is assessed by LGE, in which areas of myocardial enhancement represent necrotic myocardium and viability is inferred in spared myocardium. The extent of LGE transmurality is inversely proportional to the likelihood of functional recovery of a dysfunctional segment following revascularization.[17] Traditionally, a cut-off value of LGE of <50% transmurality is used to define a viable segment, including when dysfunctional (reversible myocardial dysfunction). Regional wall thinning with limited scar burden (LGE <50%) can represent myocardial hibernation and can be associated with improved wall thickness and thickening after successful revascularization.[18]

The MR-INFORM study has demonstrated that stress CMR is non-inferior to fractional flow reserve (FFR) in patients with stable angina with respect to major adverse cardiac events (MACE),[19] whereas the CE-MARC and CE-MARC2 studies demonstrated that CMR has high diagnostic accuracy, compared to single-photon emission computed tomography, to detect CAD and reduces unnecessary angiography.[20,21]

CMR is the preferred imaging modality to identify the aetiology of non-ischaemic cardiomyopathies and can differentiate between suspected myocarditis, amyloidosis, sarcoidosis, Chagas disease, Fabry disease, non-compaction cardiomyopathy, and

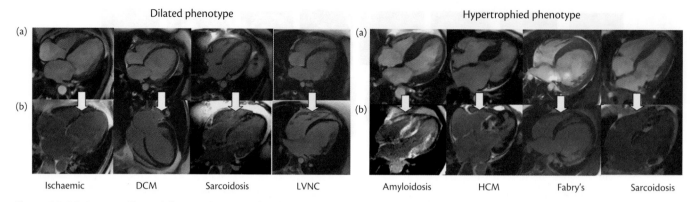

Figure 7.3.4.2 Patterns of late gadolinium enhancement (LGE) in dilated and hypertrophied phenotypes. Panel (a) shows four-chamber cine views of different dilated and hypertrophied phenotypes with their respective LGE patterns in panel (b). DCM, dilated cardiomyopathy; HCM, hypertrophic cardiomyopathy; LVNC, left ventricular non-compaction.

haemochromatosis (Class of recommendation I, Level of evidence C in 2021 ESC Heart Failure guidelines).[2]

The diagnosis of myocarditis in CMR was initially based on the Lake Louise criteria where '2 of 3' diagnostic criteria (myocardial oedema, early gadolinium enhancement (marker of hyperaemia), and LGE) need to be met. The pattern of LGE in myocarditis is typically subepicardial or mid-wall (not following a coronary distribution), except for eosinophilic myocarditis where it is circumferentially subendocardial. The recently revised Lake Louise criteria suggest a '2 out of 2' approach, with one positive T2-based criterion and one positive T1-based criterion. Although based on only two published studies, the combination of T2 mapping (T2-based criterion) and LGE (T1-based criterion) shows excellent accuracy for the detection of acute myocarditis (area under the curve 0.90, total range 0.83–0.97).[22]

Cardiac amyloidosis shows typical features on CMR: LGE can have different distribution patterns, depending on the severity of amyloid deposition,[5] but is typically subendocardial, with a circumferential distribution. Other patients show a so-called 'zebra pattern' (subendocardial enhancement with a dark mid wall) or a transmural extent in more advanced stages of the disease. RV and atrial LGE are also commonly observed. One of the more specific CMR features in cardiac amyloidosis is abnormal myocardial and blood pool contrast kinetics, characterized by early myocardial nulling (before the blood pool) and longer contrast washout, not observed in any other cardiomyopathic processes. Myocardial T1 mapping complements the use of LGE in the diagnosis of cardiac amyloidosis. In addition, it can be used to monitor and track myocardial amyloid infiltration. In contrast to LGE, native myocardial T1 provides an objective quantitative measurement and can be used as a tool to monitor disease severity.[23] Native T1 is frequently found to be elevated in the early stages of cardiac amyloidosis prior to the development of biventricular thickening or detectable LGE. Whereas T1 mapping is a composite signal of both the extra and intracellular space, ECV exclusively measures the extracellular volume and is now the standard measurement used for quantifying the myocardial amyloid burden and disease severity and for monitoring response to treatment in AL cardiac amyloidosis.[24]

Hypertrophic cardiomyopathy (HCM) is characterized by LV hypertrophy (wall thickness >15 mm, or >13 mm in familial cases), which can be symmetrical or asymmetrical. LGE is found in half to two-thirds of patients, and can be limited to the RV insertion points or can involve the hypertrophied areas with a non-ischaemic pattern.[15] Native T1 values are significantly higher in HCM patients, compared to patients with hypertensive heart disease, irrespective of the presence of LGE, and also in genotype-positive, phenotype-negative subjects (i.e. family members of HCM patients) compared to healthy controls.[25]

Fabry disease is characterized by symmetrical LV hypertrophy and non-ischaemic LGE, generally involving the basal–mid inferolateral segments. Native T1 mapping is the most reliable CMR biomarker that allows the distinction of Fabry disease from other hypertrophic phenotypes:[5] native T1 values are generally low in the affected myocardial segments, secondary to typical fat infiltration that characterizes the disease.

CMR is also recommended in the diagnosis of cardiac sarcoidosis. Cardiac involvement is found in up to 20% of patients with sarcoidosis, and CMR may be more sensitive than current clinical criteria in its detection.[5,25] Cardiac sarcoidosis may present as areas of increased wall thickness, due to the presence of granulomas, or as aneurysmal fibrotic myocardial segments. Although no LGE pattern is specific to cardiac sarcoidosis, the most typical patterns include subepicardial and mid-wall LGE along the basal septum and/or inferolateral wall,[5] often associated with mediastinal lymphadenopathy. Myocardial oedema/inflammation and pericardial effusion can also be detected in the acute phase of the disease.

HF due to LV dysfunction is one of the most concerning complications of anticancer therapy, not only because it may lead to interruption of cancer treatment, but also because it carries an adverse prognosis, particularly when detected late. CMR provides unparalleled diagnostic information on acute and late cardiotoxicity, from measuring the left ventricular ejection fraction (LVEF) and strain to the assessment of focal or diffuse oedema and fibrosis.[26] Elevated T2 values have been observed early after initiating cancer therapy (<3 months), compared to controls.

In patients with cancer treatment-related cardiac dysfunction, ECV is generally elevated on completion of treatment.[27,28]

Prognostic value of CMR

Multi-variable prognostic risk scores can help estimate the risk of death and, to a lesser extent, hospitalization in patients with HF. In many forms of HF, accurate measurements of LV and RV size and function and identification and quantification of scar contribute to prognostication. In addition, parametric mapping has major prognostic relevance. In iron overload cardiomyopathy (cardiac siderosis), T2* mapping is a strong predictive marker of HF and arrhythmias and is used to directly guide chelation therapy, obviating the need for myocardial biopsy; this has resulted in an 80% reduction in mortality for this condition in the UK and worldwide.[29] In iron overload cardiomyopathy, reduced T2* relaxation times (<10 ms), found in thalassaemia patients with new-onset HF, defines severe cardiac iron overload and relates to decreased LVEF. Below we will discuss the impact of CMR on the prognosis of more conditions causing HF.

Hypertrophic cardiomyopathy

HF is a common complication in patients with HCM. Because of variability of the phenotypic and clinical presentation of HCM, prognosis is variable and decisions on the need for ICD are challenging. Several studies have shown that the presence and extent of LGE correlate with an increased risk of arrhythmias and sudden cardiac death and may thus influence clinical decision-making. In an international prospective multicentre study of almost 1300 HCM patients, LGE of >15% of the LV myocardial mass doubled the risk of sudden cardiac death for relatively young, asymptomatic patients without conventional risk markers.[30] A meta-analysis of seven studies involving 2993 patients suggested that each 10% increase in LGE represents a 36% increased risk of sudden cardiac death.[31] A similar correlation was seen with the degree of LGE and HF deaths. It has been suggested that CMR should be used as the gold standard technique in the measurement of maximal left ventricular wall thickness (LVWT) due to limitations of echocardiography, particularly in myocardial delineation, inclusion and exclusion of RV trabeculation, and failure to visualize areas of maximal LV hypertrophy.[32] Moreover, artificial intelligence (AI)-based methods to measure LVWT by CMR have proven to be superior to human experts, with potential implications for diagnosis and risk stratification.[33] Routine use of CMR helps reduce the risk of misdiagnosis and sudden cardiac death risk classification.

Dilated cardiomyopathy

DCM is the second most common cause of HF and the most common reason for heart transplantation. CMR allows precise and reproducible calculation of LV and RV volumes, which, according to emerging evidence, may be a better guide to ICD implantation than other imaging modalities.[34] LGE in DCM shows a typical mid-wall pattern in around a third of cases. This allows the exclusion of other causes of DCM such as ischaemic cardiomyopathy, which has obvious prognostic significance. Furthermore, the presence of LGE on CMR has been shown to be an independent

marker of all-cause mortality and hospitalization, as well as of an increased risk of ventricular arrhythmia and sudden cardiac death.[35,36] A recent systematic review and meta-analysis of eight studies including 1242 patients showed the important role of T1-mapping techniques and the calculation of ECV in the risk stratification of DCM.[37]

Ischaemic cardiomyopathy

In addition to identifying CAD as the underlying cause of HF, CMR also serves an important role in the assessment of myocardial viability and the selection of patients for revascularization; this has important prognostic relevance in patients with known or suspected CAD. In screening for stable CAD, the absence of myocardial ischaemia or scar on CMR confers excellent prognosis,[38] and quantitative stress perfusion CMR has independent prognostic relevance in patients with suspected CAD.[39] Furthermore, the presence and amount of LGE seen on CMR are prognostically important. A study of 195 patients found that the presence of any LGE was associated with a hazard ratio of 8.3 for MACE and 10.9 for cardiac mortality.[40] A subsequent meta-analysis and systematic review of 20 studies including 1707 patients with ischaemic cardiomyopathy showed that quantification of the peri-infarct zone predicts long-term mortality and appropriate ICD therapy.[41]

Infiltrative cardiomyopathies

Myocardial involvement in systemic conditions, such as amyloidosis, sarcoidosis, and myocarditis, confers important prognostic markers of disease and influences treatment options. Transmurality of LGE and elevation in native T1 and ECV all correlate with amyloid burden and provide incremental information on outcome.[42] Furthermore, myocardial oedema has been found to be present in cardiac amyloidosis both histologically and with use of T2 mapping with CMR. Elevated T2 values have been shown to be associated with an increased risk of death and remain an independent predictor of adverse prognosis.[43]

In cardiac sarcoidosis, the presence of LGE has been shown to be associated with a 9-fold increased risk of adverse events, including cardiac death,[44] as well as a higher rate of diastolic dysfunction, reduced right ventricular ejection fraction (RVEF), and non-sustained ventricular arrhythmia.[45] Moreover, the presence of LGE in cardiac sarcoidosis has been used to guide endomyocardial biopsy and monitor the efficacy of therapy.[46]

In patients with unexplained cardiomyopathy, CMR has shown features of myocarditis in up to 10% of patients.[47] Additionally, increased LGE at 4 weeks after clinical onset of myocarditis has been inversely correlated with 3-year follow-up LVEF.[48]

CMR to guide heart failure management

Management of patients with HF can be complex, and use of CMR helps guide difficult management decisions.[49] In a prospective study of 150 consecutive HF patients, the use of CMR was found to make a significant impact on clinical management, decision-making, and diagnosis in 65% of patients despite universal use of prior echocardiography in this group.[50] Cardiac resynchronization therapy (CRT), which is recommended in patients with symptomatic chronic HF on optimal medical therapy, severely reduced LVEF (≤35%), and complete left bundle branch block,[51] has revolutionized the treatment of patients with HF. CMR is a valuable alternative to echocardiography for the assessment of LV mechanical dyssynchrony, by identification of the typical septal bounce and apical rocking.[15] For a long time, mechanical dyssynchrony has been considered the predominant mechanism determining CRT response. The presence of myocardial scar, particularly in the lateral wall (which is the area most often paced), has been shown to reduce the response to CRT, irrespective of the presence of mechanical dyssynchrony. LV posterolateral scar is associated with an increased risk of hospitalization for HF and cardiovascular mortality, and is responsible for reduced CRT response; moreover, pacing over LV posterolateral scars is associated with an increased arrhythmic risk.[52] Bilchick et al. studied 75 patients and demonstrated that the absence of posterolateral scar was an important predictor of CRT response.[53] Since the presence, extent, and transmurality of myocardial scar has been shown to predict CRT response,[52] CMR plays a pivotal role in the assessment of myocardial scar prior to cardiac resynchronization.

Future directions

The development of AI is expected to improve image acquisition, interpretation, and availability of CMR. Remote scanning using AI has been implemented and tested in clinical practice. This has the potential to introduce CMR to less experienced centres where local expertise may be limited, increasing accessibility of CMR to the wider HF community.

Current parametric mapping techniques require separate acquisitions for T1 and T2 and have many dependent variables that can affect values such as sequence type, cardiac physiology, and others. CMR fingerprinting is an innovative tool that can achieve simultaneous and reproducible measurements of T1 and T2 maps in a single scan. The potential benefits of this technique include faster acquisition times, more consistency in values due to the lack of dependent variables, and absolving the need for exogenous contrast agents.

Emergence of the use of four-dimensional (4D) flow in CMR allows 3D assessment of blood flow in the time domain. This can be applied both to the great vessels (intravascular), but also to the LV and RV (intramyocardial). Multiple novel haemodynamic imaging biomarkers can be derived from this data set, including flow vortices and LV blood flow kinetic energy that may be reduced in the presence of LV dysfunction. However, the diagnostic role and incremental prognostic impact of these novel biomarkers over established markers, such as EF and scar burden, are yet to be demonstrated.

References

1. Hoffmann R, Barletta G, von Bardeleben S, et al. Analysis of left ventricular volumes and function: a multicenter comparison of cardiac magnetic resonance imaging, cine ventriculography, and unenhanced and contrast-enhanced two-dimensional and three-dimensional echocardiography. J Am Soc Echocardiogr 2014; 27: 292–301.

2. McDonagh TA, Metra M, Adamo M, et al.; ESC Scientific Document Group. 2021 ESC Guidelines for the diagnosis and treatment of acute and chronic heart failure. Eur Heart J 2021; 42(36): 3599–726.

3. Petersen SE, Khanji MY, Plein S, Lancellotti P, Bucciarelli-Ducci C. European Association of Cardiovascular Imaging expert consensus paper: a comprehensive review of cardiovascular magnetic resonance normal values of cardiac chamber size and aortic root in adults and recommendations for grading severity. Eur Heart J Cardiovasc Imaging 2019; 20: 1321–31.

4. Gimelli A, Lancellotti P, Badano LP, et al. Non-invasive cardiac imaging evaluation of patients with chronic systolic heart failure: a report from the European Association of Cardiovascular Imaging (EACVI). Eur Heart J 2014; 35: 3417–25.

5. Habib G, Bucciarelli-Ducci C, Caforio ALP, et al. Multimodality imaging in restrictive cardiomyopathies: an EACVI expert consensus document in collaboration with the 'Working Group on myocardial and pericardial diseases' of the European Society of Cardiology Endorsed by The Indian Academy of Echocardiography. Eur Heart J Cardiovasc Imaging 2017; 18: 1090–1.

6. Ridgway JP. Cardiovascular magnetic resonance physics for clinicians: part I. J Cardiovasc Magn Reson 2010; 12: 71.

7. Biglands JD, Radjenovic A, Ridgway JP. Cardiovascular magnetic resonance physics for clinicians: part II. J Cardiovasc Magn Reson 2021; 14: 66.

8. Kramer CM, Barkhausen J, Bucciarelli-Ducci C, Scott DF, Raymon JK, Nagel E. Standardized cardiovascular magnetic resonance imaging (CMR) protocols: 2020 update. J Cardiovasc Magn Reson 2020; 202; 22: 17.

9. Schulz-Menger J, Bluemke DA, Bremerich J, et al. Standardized image interpretation and post-processing in cardiovascular magnetic resonance—2020 update: Society for Cardiovascular Magnetic Resonance (SCMR): Board of Trustees Task Force on Standardized Post-Processing. J Cardiovasc Magn Reson 2020; 22: 19.

10. Rathi VK, Doyle M, Yamrozik J, et al. Routine evaluation of left ventricular diastolic fu nction by cardiovascular magnetic resonance: a practical approach. J Cardiovasc Magn Reson 2008; 10: 36.

11. Sado DM, Flett AS, Banypersad SM, et al. Cardiovascular magnetic resonance measurement of myocardial extracellular volume in health and disease. Heart. 2012; 98: 1436–41.

12. Haaf P, Garg P, Messroghli, DR, et al. Cardiac T1 mapping and extracellular volume (ECV) in clinical practice: a comprehensive review. J Cardiovasc Magn Reson 2016; 18: 89.

13. Ferreira V, Piechnik S, Robson Matthew D, et al. Tissue characterization by magnetic resonance imaging: novel applications of T1 and T2 mapping, J Thorac Imaging 2014; 29: 147–54.

14. Badano LP, Miglioranza MH, Edvardsen T, et al. European Association of Cardiovascular Imaging/Cardiovascular Imaging Department of the Brazilian Society of Cardiology recommendations for the use of cardiac imaging to assess and follow patients after heart transplantation. Eur Heart J Cardiovasc Imaging 2015; 16: 919–48.

15. Donal E, Delgado V, Bucciarelli-Ducci C, et al. Multimodality imaging in the diagnosis, risk stratification, and management of patients with dilated cardiomyopathies: an expert consensus document from the European Association of Cardiovascular Imaging. Eur Heart J Cardiovasc Imaging 2019; 20: 1075–93.

16. Mahrholdt H, Wagner A, Judd RM, Sechtem U, Kim RJ. Delayed enhancement cardiovascular magnetic resonance assessment of non-ischaemic cardiomyopathies. Eur Heart J 2005; 26: 1461–74.

17. Kim RJ, Fieno DS, Parrish TB, et al. Relationship of MRI delayed contrast enhancement to irreversible injury, infarct age, and contractile function. Circulation 1999; 100: 1992–2002.

18. Shah DJ, Kim HW, James O, *et al*. Prevalence of regional myocardial thinning and relationship with myocardial scarring in patients with coronary artery disease. JAMA 2013; 309: 909–18.

19. Nagel E, Greenwood JP, McCann GP, *et al*. Magnetic resonance perfusion or fractional flow reserve in coronary disease. N Engl J Med 2019; 380: 2418–28.

20. Greenwood JP, Maredia N, Younger JF, *et al*. Cardiovascular magnetic resonance and single-photon emission computed tomography for diagnosis of coronary heart disease (CE-MARC): a prospective trial. Lancet 2012; 379: 453–60.

21. Greenwood JP, Ripley DP, Berry C, *et al*.; CE-MARC 2 Investigators. Effect of care guided by cardiovascular magnetic resonance, myocardial perfusion scintigraphy, or NICE guidelines on subsequent unnecessary angiography rates: the CE-MARC 2 randomized clinical trial. JAMA 2016; 316: 1051–60.

22. Ferreira VM, Schulz-Menger J, Holmvang G, *et al*. Cardiovascular magnetic resonance in nonischemic myocardial inflammation expert recommendations. J Am Coll Cardiol 2018; 72: 3158–76.

23. Fontana M, Martinez-Naharro A, Hawkins PN. Staging cardiac amyloidosis with CMR: understanding the different phenotypes. JACC Cardiovasc Imaging 2016; 9: 1278–9.

24. Fontana M, Banypersad SM, Treibel TA, *et al*. Native T1 mapping in transthyretin amyloidosis. JACC Cardiovasc Imaging 2014; 7: 157–65.

25. Hinojar R, Varma N, Child N, *et al*. T1 mapping in discrimination of hypertrophic phenotypes: hypertensive heart disease and hypertrophic cardiomyopathy findings from the international T1 multicenter cardiovascular magnetic resonance study. Circ Cardiovasc Imaging 2015; 8: e003285.

26. Harries I, Liang K, Williams M, *et al*. Magnetic resonance imaging to detect cardiovascular effects of cancer therapy: JACC cardiooncology state-of-the-art review. JACC CardioOncol 2020; 2(2): 270–92.

27. Haslbauer JD, Lindner S, Valbuena-Lopez S, *et al*. CMR imaging biosignature of cardiac involvement due to cancer-related treatment by T1 and T2 mapping. Int J Cardiol 2019; 275: 179–86.

28. Meléndez GC, Jordan JH, D'Agostino RB, Vasu S, Hamilton CA, Hundley WG. Progressive 3-month increase in LV myocardial ECV after anthracycline-based chemotherapy. JACC Cardiovasc Imaging 2017; 10: 708–9.

29. Daar S, Al Khabori M, Al Rahbi S, Hassan M, El Tigani A, Pennell DJ. Cardiac T2* MR in patients with thalassemia major: a 10-year long-term follow-up. Ann Hematol 2020; 99(9): 2009–17.

30. Chan RH, Maron BJ, Olivotto I, *et al*. Prognostic value of quantitative contrast-enhanced cardiovascular magnetic resonance for the evaluation of sudden death risk in patients with hypertrophic cardiomyopathy. Circulation 2014; 130: 484–95.

31. Weng Z, Yao J, Chan RH, *et al*. Prognostic value of LGE-CMR in HCM: a meta-analysis. JACC Cardiovasc Imaging 2016; 9: 1392–402.

32. Hindieh W, Weissler-Snir A, Hammer H, *et al*. Discrepant measurements of maximal left ventricular wall thickness between cardiac magnetic resonance imaging and echocardiography in patients with hypertrophic cardiomyopathy. Circ Cardiovasc Imaging 2017; 10: e006309.

33. Augusto JB, Davies RH, Bhuva AN, *et al*. Diagnosis and risk stratification in hypertrophic cardiomyopathy using machine learning wall thickness measurement: a comparison with human test–retest performance. Lancet Digit Health 2021; 3: e20–8.

34. Champ-Rigot L, Gay P, Seita F, *et al*. Clinical outcomes after primary prevention defibrillator implantation are better predicted when the left ventricular ejection fraction is assessed by cardiovascular magnetic resonance. Cardiovasc Magn Reson 2020; 22: 48.

35. Halliday BP, Gulati A, Ali A, *et al*. Association between mid-wall late gadolinium enhancement and sudden cardiac death in patients with dilated cardiomyopathy and mild and moderate left ventricular systolic dysfunction. Circulation 2017; 135: 2106–15.

36. Becker MAJ, Cornel JH, van de Ven PM, *et al*. The prognostic value of late gadolinium-enhanced cardiac magnetic resonance imaging in non-ischemic dilated cardiomyopathy: a review and meta-analysis. JACC Cardiovasc Imaging 2018; 11: 1274–84.

37. Kiaos A, Antonakaki D, Bazmpani MA, *et al*. Prognostic value of cardiovascular magnetic resonance T1 mapping techniques in non-ischemic dilated cardiomyopathy: a systematic review and meta-analysis. Int J Cardiol 2020; 312: 110–16.

38. Lipinski MJ, McVey CM, Berger JS, *et al*. Prognostic value of stress cardiac magnetic resonance imaging in patients with known or suspected coronary artery disease: a systematic review and meta-analysis. J Am Coll Cardiol 2013; 62: 826–38.

39. Sammut EC, Villa ADM, Di Giovine G, *et al*. Prognostic value of quantitative stress perfusion cardiac magnetic resonance. JACC Cardiovasc Imaging 2018; 11: 686–94.

40. Kwong RY, Chan AK, Brown KA, *et al*. Impact of unrecognized myocardial scar detected by cardiac magnetic resonance imaging on event-free survival in patients presenting with signs or symptoms of coronary artery disease. Circulation 2006; 113: 2733–43.

41. Haghbayan H, Lougheed N, Deva DP, *et al*. Peri-infarct quantification by cardiac magnetic resonance to predict outcomes in ischemic cardiomyopathy: prognostic systematic review and meta-analysis. Circ Cardiovasc Imaging 2019; 12(11): e009156.

42. Fontana M, Pica S, Reant P, *et al*. Prognostic value of late gadolinium enhancement cardiovascular magnetic resonance in cardiac amyloidosis. Circulation 2015; 132: 1570–9.

43. Kotecha T, Martinez-Naharro A, Treibel TA, *et al*. Myocardial edema and prognosis in amyloidosis. J Am Coll Cardiol 2018; 71: 2919–31.

44. Patel MR, Cawley PJ, Heitner JF, *et al*. Detection of myocardial damage in patients with sarcoidosis. Circulation 2009; 120:1969–77.

45. Patel AR, Klein MR, Chandra S, *et al*. Myocardial damage in patients with sarcoidosis and preserved left ventricular systolic function: an observational study. Eur J Heart Fail 2011; 13: 1231–7.

46. Shimada T, Shimada K, Sakane T, *et al*. Diagnosis of cardiac sarcoidosis and evaluation of the effects of steroid therapy by gadolinium-DTPA-enhanced magnetic resonance imaging. Am J Med 2001; 110: 520–7.

47. Abdel-Aty H, Boye P, Zagrosek A, *et al*. Diagnostic performance of cardiovascular magnetic resonance in patients with suspected acute myocarditis: comparison of different approaches. J Am Coll Cardiol 2005; 45: 1815–22.

48. Wagner A, Schulz-Menger J, Dietz R, *et al*. Long-term follow-up of patients with acute myocarditis by magnetic resonance imaging. MAGMA 2003; 16: 17–20.

49. Garbi M, Edvardsen T, Bax J, *et al*. EACVI appropriateness criteria for the use of cardiovascular imaging in heart failure derived from European National Imaging Societies voting. Eur Heart J Cardiovasc Imaging 2016; 17: 711–21.

50. Abbasi SA, Ertel A, Shah RV, *et al*. Impact of cardiovascular magnetic resonance on management and clinical decision-making in heart failure patients. J Cardiovasc Magn Reson 2013; 15: 89.

51. Brignole M, Auricchio A, Baron-Esquivias G, *et al*. 2013 ESC Guidelines on cardiac pacing and cardiac resynchronization therapy. Eur Heart J 2013; 34: 2281–839.

52. Chalil S, Foley PW, Muyhaldeen SA, *et al*. Late gadolinium enhancement-cardiovascular magnetic resonance as a predictor of response to cardiac resynchronization therapy in patients with ischaemic cardiomyopathy. Europace 2007; 9: 1031–7.

53. Bilchick KC, Kuruvilla S, Hamirani YS, *et al*. Impact of mechanical activation, scar, and electrical timing on cardiac resynchronization therapy response and clinical outcomes. J Am Coll Cardiol 2014; 63: 1657–66.

7.3.5 Cardiopulmonary exercise testing

Luca Moderato, Davide Lazzeroni, Stamatis Adamopoulos, Alain Cohen-Solal, and Massimo Piepoli

Introduction

Cardiopulmonary exercise testing (CPET) was first described by Weber in 1982[1] as a non-invasive method to assess cardiopulmonary system behaviour during physical stress through analysis of exhaled gases to measure minute ventilation, oxygen uptake, and carbon dioxide (CO_2) production. CPET provides a reproducible global assessment of the cardiovascular, ventilatory, and metabolic responses to exercise, thereby giving diagnostic and prognostic information. This tool enables the clinician to evaluate the reasons for dyspnoea and fatigue, as well as to differentiate between pulmonary and cardiac disorders; CPET also allows to optimize the decision-making process and outcome prediction, and objectively determine targets for pharmacological and non-pharmacological therapies,[2] especially in heart failure (HF) patients.[3] Indications for CPET are listed in ➲ Table 7.3.5.1.

Physiology of exercise

Peak exercise capacity is defined as 'the maximum ability of the cardiovascular system to deliver oxygen to muscles and of the muscles to extract oxygen from the blood'. The terms *functional capacity*, *exercise capacity*, *cardiorespiratory fitness*, and *exercise tolerance* are generally considered synonymous and imply that a maximal exercise test has been performed and maximal effort has been given by the individual. Exercise tolerance is therefore determined mainly by three factors: cardiovascular performance, including endothelial function of the peripheral arteries; pulmonary gas exchange; and skeletal muscle metabolism.

During exercise, the large increase in oxygen (O_2) utilization by muscles is achieved by increased extraction of O_2 from the blood perfusing the muscles, by dilatation of selected peripheral vascular beds, increase in cardiac output (CO) (stroke volume (SV) and heart rate (HR)) and pulmonary blood flow, and finally increase in ventilation (➲ Figure 7.3.5.1). From this biochemical viewpoint, muscles, rather than lungs, '*breathe*' during physical activity and the complex mechanisms that coordinate all changes induced by exercise are primarily driven by muscle oxygen needs. In healthy individuals, exercise usually leads to an increase in HR and contractility; ventilation gradually increases, led by the rise of respiratory rate (RR) and alveolar perfusion and ventilation (alveolar recruitment). The rise in HR and contractility will achieve a plateau when maximal exercise capacity is reached. Respiratory capacity far exceeds the demands of peak exercise (pulmonary reserve). This is the reason why in healthy individuals, exercise capacity is rarely affected by respiratory limitation.[1,4]

Table 7.3.5.1 General indications for cardiopulmonary exercise testing

Evaluation of exercise tolerance
Determination of functional impairment or capacity (peak VO_2)
Determination of exercise-limiting factors and pathophysiological mechanisms

Evaluation of undiagnosed exercise intolerance
Assessing the contribution of cardiac and pulmonary aetiology in coexisting disease
Symptoms disproportionate to resting pulmonary and cardiac tests
Unexplained dyspnoea when initial cardiopulmonary testing is non-diagnostic (or standard pulmonary function test is not diagnostic)

Evaluation of patients with cardiovascular disease
Functional evaluation and prognosis in patients with heart failure
Selection for cardiac transplantation
Exercise prescription and monitoring response to exercise training for cardiac rehabilitation (special circumstances, i.e. pacemakers)

Evaluation of patients with respiratory disease
Functional impairment assessment
Chronic obstructive pulmonary disease
Establishing exercise limitation(s) and assessing other potential contributing factors, especially occult heart disease (ischaemia)
Determination of magnitude of hypoxaemia and for oxygen prescription
When objective determination of therapeutic intervention is necessary and not adequately addressed by standard pulmonary function testing
Interstitial lung diseases
Detection of early (occult) gas exchange abnormalities
Overall assessment/monitoring of pulmonary gas exchange
Determination of magnitude of hypoxaemia and for oxygen prescription
Determination of potential exercise-limiting factors
Documentation of therapeutic response to potentially toxic therapy
Pulmonary vascular disease (careful risk–benefit analysis required)
Cystic fibrosis
Exercise-induced bronchospasm

Specific clinical applications
Preoperative evaluation
Clinically relevant research purpose
Lung resection surgery
Elderly patients undergoing major abdominal surgery
Lung volume resection surgery for emphysema (currently investigational)

Exercise evaluation and prescription for pulmonary rehabilitation

Evaluation for impairment–disability

Evaluation for lung and heart–lung transplantation

The Fick equation

The Fick equation is of key importance for evaluation of the utility of functional exercise testing with gas exchange measurement. According to the Fick equation, oxygen uptake (VO_2) equals CO multiplied by the arterial minus mixed venous oxygen content: $VO_2 = (SV \times HR) \times (CaO_2 - CvO_2)$, where SV is stroke volume, HR is heart rate, CaO_2 is the arterial oxygen content, and CvO_2 is the mixed venous oxygen content. Oxygen uptake is usually normalized for body weight and expressed in units of mL O_2/kg/min. One metabolic equivalent (MET) is defined as the resting oxygen uptake and is equal to 3.5 mL/kg/min. At maximal exercise, the Fick equation is expressed as: $VO_2max = (SVmax \times HRmax) \times (CaO_2max - CvO_2max)$; this reflects the

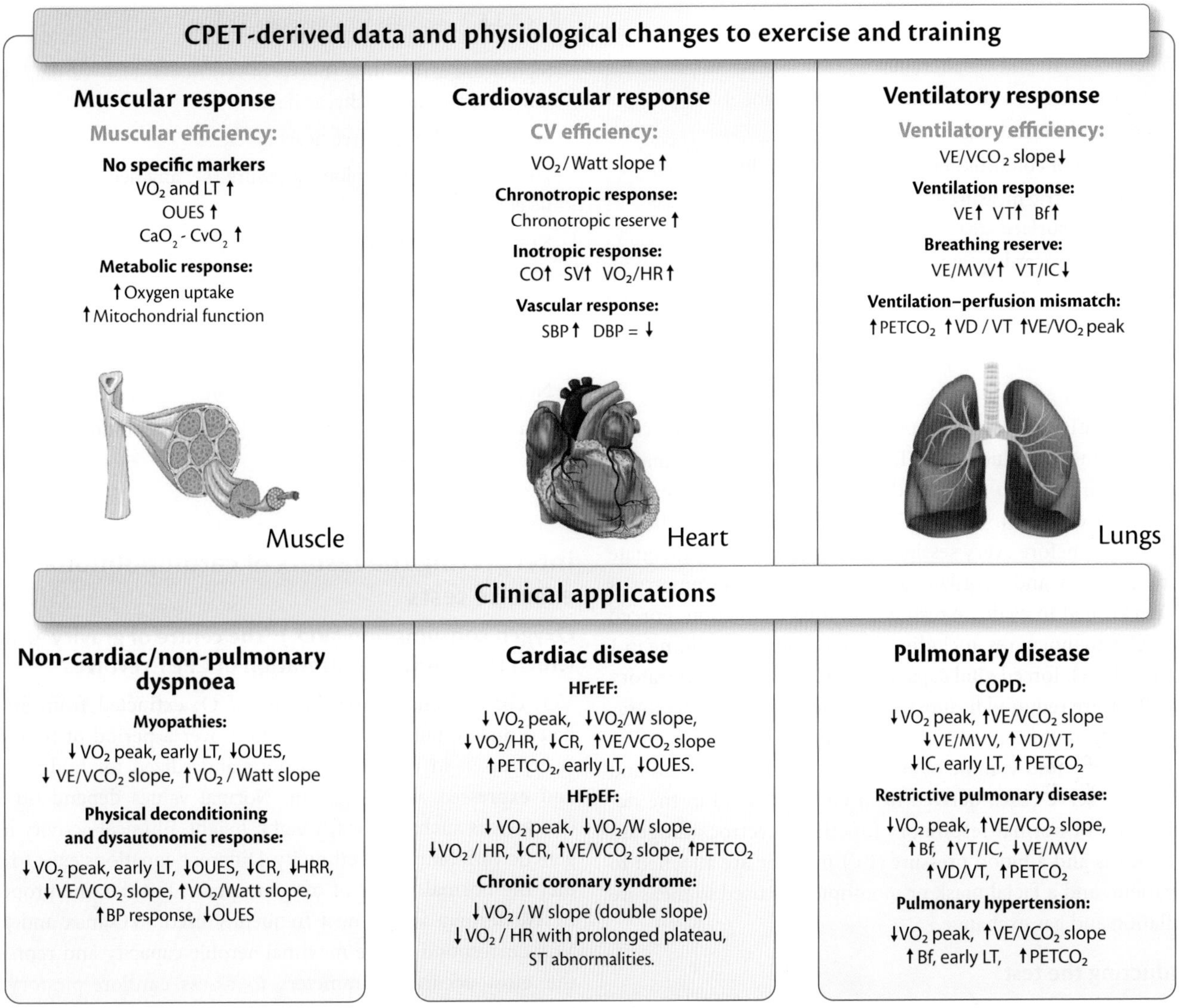

Figure 7.3.5.1 CPET-derived data, pathophysiological implications, and clinical application.

maximal ability of uptake, transport, and use of oxygen, and defines the patient's functional aerobic capacity. In healthy people, a plateau of VO_2 occurs at near-maximal exercise. This plateau has traditionally been used as the best evidence for VO_2max.[4,5] However, in the clinical setting, a clear plateau is often not reached, due to the occurrence of symptoms limiting exercise capacity; consequently, peak VO_2 is often used as a surrogate for VO_2max. VO_2max has become the preferred measure of cardiorespiratory fitness and is the most important measurement in functional exercise testing.[6]

How to perform cardiopulmonary exercise testing

Pretest considerations

Several methods exist for measuring ventilation and respiratory gas during exercise. Most clinical systems rely on breath-by-breath analysis techniques: a non-rebreathing valve is connected to a mouthpiece to prevent mixing of inspired and expired air;

oxygen and CO_2 gas analysers are usually incorporated in a metabolic cart designed for functional testing.

Respiratory volumes are measured by integrating the airflow over time of inspiration and expiration. Average minute volumes are derived from the breath-by-breath data multiplied by RR. The exercise is performed on a bicycle or a treadmill (note: due to non-weight-bearing exercise during cycling, peak oxygen uptake is systematically 10–20% lower than during treadmill exercise); cycle ergometry has become more popular for obese patients and patients with orthopaedic limitations or balance instability. Furthermore, data recorded during a bicycle test are less prone to movement artefacts and allow a more accurate analysis in the case of a ramp protocol. Many different protocols are used for functional testing. The purpose of the test and the fitness level, age, and body surface of the patient determine the choice of protocol. The rate of workload progression can be chosen arbitrarily, although it is recommended to prefer a less steep ramp to optimize gas recording and avoid premature exhaustion; the optimal exercise duration is considered to be between 8 and 12

Box 7.3.5.1 Pretest considerations

- Patient consent and collaboration
- Protocol selection and explanation of test protocol
- History and clinical examination
- Assessment of comorbidities (e.g. orthopaedic limitations)
- Anthropometric measurements: weight, height, body mass index, body surface area
- Resting electrocardiogram, blood pressure, and oxygen saturations
- Pretest spirometry

Box 7.3.5.2 Reasons for stopping CPET

Significant arrhythmia (bursts of ventricular tachycardia, sustained ventricular tachycardia)

Second- or third-degree heart block

Decrease of systolic blood pressure (i.e. any decrease) during heavy exercise

ST-segment depression >2 mm

Patient distress

Chest pain suggestive of cardiac ischaemia

Loss of coordination

Near-syncope, dizziness, or confusion

Symptomatic severe hypoxaemia (oxygen saturation <80%)

---

minutes.[7,8] Patient collaboration is essential to optimize the clinical and diagnostic value of CPET. Patients have to be adequately instructed, in order to perform the best effort possible in relation to their condition (➲ Box 7.3.5.1). Cart calibration has to be performed before every session in order to maintain adequate accuracy of gas and ventilation measurements. Spirometry is then performed to evaluate resting pulmonary function. Forced spirometry manoeuvres, including forced expiratory volume in 1 second (FEV1), forced vital capacity (FVC), and peak expiratory flow (PEF), are required to substantiate the extent of any respiratory limitation during exercise. Maximum voluntary ventilation (the maximum volume of air ventilated in 60 seconds) and breathing reserve (BR), derived from CPET, can aid in the determination of normal respiratory function. Electrocardiogram (ECG) leads and a blood pressure (BP) monitor are attached to the patient, and a facial mask or mouthpiece is used to measure ventilation and gas exchange.

Conducting the test

The test should be started with 1–2 minutes of recording during rest, followed by 2–3 minutes of warm-up (pedalling or walking without resistance). The pedalling rate should be 60–70 rpm throughout the test. The test should be stopped, if 60 rpm can no longer be maintained.

BP should be recorded at rest and every 2 minutes thereafter or during the last minute of each exercise stage in non-ramp protocols; perceived ratings of dyspnoea and fatigue (Borg scale) should be recorded at the end of the test in order to differentiate between dyspnoea and muscular fatigue as the reason for exercise termination. The ECG should be carefully monitored to check for signs of ischaemia or the occurrence arrhythmias.

CPET should be performed as a symptom-limited test, that is, it should be stopped when the patient is unable to maintain a minimal rate of pedalling or if an indication to stop the examination occurs (➲ Box 7.3.5.2).

When the exercise protocol is stopped, the patient is asked to continue pedalling or walking slowly for 1 minute; then 4–5 minutes of further recording is usually performed. It is important to ask the patient at the end of the test which symptom limited their effort the most: leg fatigue, dyspnoea, or chest pain.

Interpreting the results of cardiopulmonary exercise tests

Oxygen consumption (VO_2): 'the centre of gravity around which the whole interpretation of CPET revolves'

VO_2 corresponds to the volume of O_2 extracted from air inhaled during pulmonary ventilation over a period of time, and is expressed in mL/min, usually standardized for body weight and expressed as mL/kg/min. Normal values depend on several factors such age, sex, weight, height, physical activity level, genetic variability, and ethnicity. Different equations exist to predict the normal values of oxygen uptake, but the one proposed by Wasserman is the most frequently used.[5] VO_2max and peak VO_2 correspond to the maximal aerobic capacity and represent the most accurate parameters to assess cardiorespiratory fitness.[4,9] VO_2 represents the first parameter to be considered in CPET evaluation, and all further data collected during exercise should be hierarchically carefully and systematically interpreted in relation to peak VO_2. For that reason, after VO_2 evaluation, the cardiovascular, ventilatory, and metabolic responses during activities should be separately analysed in order to interpret different specific causes of functional capacity limitation.

In fact, VO_2 at peak exercise is the most important parameter to evaluate disease severity in patients with HF, pulmonary hypertension, hypertrophic cardiomyopathy (HCM), chronic obstructive pulmonary disease (COPD), and restrictive pulmonary disease, in addition to physical fitness level.[10,11,12] A normal value for O_2 uptake is considered to be >18–20 mL/kg/min, whereas values of <10 mL/kg/min predict poor prognosis,[6,9] with lower values if the patient is on beta-blocker therapy. Peak VO_2 and O_2 uptake at the metabolic threshold (MT) are also influenced by genetic predisposition, diseases, amount of exercise, and aerobic training types. A normal VO_2 at MT for adults corresponds to around 40–65% of predicted VO_2.[9] The MT value is important for individualized prescription of exercise, as well as for diagnosis of anaemia, physical fitness, myopathies, and cardiomyopathies.[10]

$\Delta VO_2/\Delta WR$ relationship (VO_2/Watt slope): a reliable marker of 'cardiovascular efficiency'

Under physiological conditions, there is a linearity in the increase in VO_2 over the rate of increase in work rate (WR). Therefore, the slope of this relationship is a function of the ability of exercising muscle to extract O_2 and to provide aerobically generated adenosine triphosphate. From a physiological viewpoint, the VO_2/Watt slope represents a marker of cardiovascular efficiency during exercise. The VO_2/Watt slope represents the relationship between VO_2 in mL/min and the workload slope during a ramp protocol. Since there is a linear increase in CO (SV × HR) with workload, a low $\Delta VO_2/\Delta WR$ relationship reflects a decrease in SV, assuming that the chronotropic response is adequate. It is therefore useful in the diagnosis of left ventricular (LV) dysfunction during exertion, similarly to O_2 pulse. Its normal value for adults is considered to be >9–11 mL/min/watt.[1,9] In cardiac patients, a shallow exercise VO_2/WR may be associated with the development of myocardial ischaemia and an increased risk of death.[13]

Oxygen pulse (VO_2/HR): a 'window' to observe stroke volume response to exercise

Oxygen pulse indicates how much O_2 is taken up for heartbeat (= VO_2/HR).[14] It reflects the amount of O_2 extracted per heartbeat and has been used as an estimator of SV during exercise. The O_2 pulse normally increases with incremental exercise because of increases in both SV and O_2 extraction, and then reaches a plateau. According to Fick's law, peak VO_2 corresponds to CO time of the arteriovenous O_2 difference ($CaO_2 - CvO_2$); in turn, CO depends on SV and HR, so that the O_2 pulse can be expressed as $SV*(CaO_2 - CvO_2)$. Commonly, the O_2 pulse is used as a surrogate measurement of SV, although this is only justified when ($CaO_2 - CvO_2$) can be reasonably assumed. Because ($CaO_2 - CvO_2$) increases as WR increases to the subject's maximum exercise level, both in healthy subjects and in HF patients,[14] O_2 pulse represents a surrogate reliable measurement of SV during exercise. Nevertheless, in HF patients, a relevant interpatient variability has been reported in ($CaO_2 - CvO_2$) at peak,[9] mainly due to three major factors: capillary O_2, O_2 diffusion from capillaries into mitochondria, and muscle aerobic capacity. A low, flat O_2 pulse increase may be interpreted as resulting from reduced SV and/or as failure of further skeletal muscle O_2 extraction. The decrease in O_2 pulse during stress testing is a sign of exercise-induced ischaemia (decrease of SV due to wall motion abnormalities in relation to ischaemia but also to mitral regurgitation or decrease in contractilty).[15] A low O_2 pulse therefore may reflect deconditioning, increasing mitral regurgitation during exercise, or ischaemia.[10,16]

Chronotropic response to exercise

During maximal aerobic exercise in healthy humans, VO_2 increases approximately 4-fold; this is achieved by a 2.2-fold increase in HR, up to 1.0-fold increase in SV, and a 1.5-fold increase in arteriovenous O_2 difference.[10] Thus, the increase in HR is the strongest contributor to the ability to perform sustained aerobic exercise.[17] In healthy subjects, HR increases nearly linearly with increasing VO_2. This is mediated initially by a decrease in parasympathetic tone (vagal withdrawal) and, subsequently, by sympathetic activation. Dynamic exercise increases HR more than either isometric or resistance exercise. A normal increase in HR during exercise is ≈10 bpm per MET. Achievement of age-predicted values for maximal HR during exercise is often used as a reflection of maximal or near-maximal effort. However, it should not be misunderstood as an indication for stress test termination.

Furthermore, the variation of HRmax compared to theoretical age-predicted values is huge (± 20 beats) and can be influenced furthermore by medication and sympathetic desensitization in HF. The traditional equation to predict maximal HR (220 bpm − age) was developed based on studies primarily in middle-aged men, some of whom had known coronary artery disease and were taking beta-blockers.[17] This equation has been associated with large intersubject variability. Consequently, an alternative formula from Tanaka et al.[18] (208 − 0.7 × age) is becoming more accepted for determining age-predicted maximal HR. Use of a beta-blocking drug lowers both the incremental rise in HR and the maximal HR obtained during exercise, thus limiting the physiological interpretation of cardiac response to exercise. Other factors that can influence HR include body position, the type of dynamic exercise, certain physical conditions, the state of health, blood volume, sinus node function, medications, and the environment. Chronotropic incompetence represents a powerful CPET prognostic marker for increased cardiac and all-cause mortality.[17] Moreover, the value of HR at MT is of utmost importance for aerobic exercise prescription.[9]

Finally, the change in HR immediately after termination of an exercise test, termed HR recovery (HRR), has received an increasing amount of attention in recent years. The decline in HR after exercise generally exhibits a rapid fall during the first minute after exercise, followed by a slower return to the pre-exercise level.[19] The rapid decline in HR is due to vagal reactivation and a blunted HRR has demonstrated significant and prognostic value, with a strong inverse linear correlation between a reduction in HRR and an increase in all-cause and cardiovascular mortality.[20]

Blood pressure response to exercise

As exercise intensity increases, flow-mediated vasodilatation and the initial decrease in systolic BP are soon overcome by continuously increasing CO and systolic BP until the end of stress testing. The average rise in systolic BP during a progressive exercise test is about 10 mmHg per MET. Diastolic BP typically remains constant or may decline slightly if left heart function keeps up with the increases in CO. Abnormal patterns of BP response include excessive rise (dysregulation of BP control), reduced rise (decreased LV function), or a fall (ischaemia, outflow tract obstruction, or aortic stenosis). A fall in BP despite increasing workload is an important indication for exercise termination.[5,9] Hypertensive individuals often have an exaggerated BP response to exercise, even if resting levels are controlled. A systolic BP of >250 mmHg or a diastolic BP of >115 mmHg during exercise is often an indication for test termination. Hypertensive response to exercise has been associated with a future risk of hypertension in normotensive individuals.[21] Several studies have associated impaired diastolic function with reduced aerobic capacity in people with hypertension and normal systolic LV function.[22] Moreover, a BP of >180/90 mmHg during stage 2 of the Bruce exercise protocol was found to be associated with a greater risk of cardiovascular death in normotensive individuals, but not in those with hypertension.[21]

Pulmonary ventilation (VE)

Ventilation is expressed in L/min. It is determined as the product of RR and the volume of air exhaled in every cycle (tidal volume). At rest, 7–9 L/min are ventilated, but in athletes, this value can reach 200 L/min on maximal exertion.[1] Ventilation increases continuously during progressive effort on CPET, until the respiratory compensation point (RCP) when the body increases the CO_2 output in order to compensate for the accumulation of lactic acid (second lactate threshold).

Oscillatory ventilation

Exertional oscillatory ventilation (EOV) is an abnormal ventilatory phenomenon, consisting of cyclic fluctuation of minute ventilation (VE) and expired gas kinetics, that occurs during exercise.[23] EOV is frequent in HF with reduced, preserved, or mid-range ejection fraction and bears a strong negative prognostic role.[23,24] The most frequently adopted definition is the one recommended by the American Heart Association that defines EOV as persistence of an oscillatory ventilation pattern for at least 60% of exercise duration at an amplitude higher than 15% of the average value of ventilation at rest.[24] Circulatory delay, increased chemosensitivity, pulmonary congestion, and increased ergoreflex signalling have been proposed as mechanisms underlying the generation of EOV in HF patients (⮕ Figure 7.3.5.2).[25]

VE/VCO$_2$ slope (ventilatory efficiency)

The slope obtained from the relationship between VE and VCO_2 (VE/VCO$_2$ slope) quantifies the amount of ventilation required to eliminate 1 L of CO_2. The VE/VCO$_2$ slope can be determined up to the RCP or to the maximal value.

The VE/VCO$_2$ slope is a very sensitive, although non-specific, marker of gas exchange and can be altered by pre- or post-capillary changes, as well as by disorders affecting gas diffusion. It is a major exercise-related risk marker in chronic heart failure, even more powerful than peak VO_2—in fact, an elevation of the VE/VCO$_2$ slope is frequently observed in patients with chronic HF,[26] and can be used to evaluate effectiveness of several treatments, including exercise training, cardiac resynchronization therapy, and heart transplantation.[6,26,27] The normal value should be <30.0, whereas values of between 36 and 44 and >45.0 are, respectively, moderately and severely elevated and are predictive of poor prognosis in HF patients (⮕ Figure 7.3.5.3).[9]

Respiratory exchange ratio

The respiratory exchange ratio (RER) expresses the ratio between CO_2 production and O_2 consumption (VCO_2/VO_2). It is the best non-invasive indicator of exercise; normal people reach a RER > 1.20 at peak exercise, but achieving a RERmax > 1.10 has been generally accepted as a criterion of near maximal, valid exercise.[9,28]

End-tidal carbon dioxide partial pressure

End-tidal partial pressure of CO_2 ($PETCO_2$) is used for non-invasive estimation of alveolar CO_2, and is determined by muscle metabolism (amount of CO_2 production) and influenced by the RR and CO_2 chemoreceptor set point. This reflects ventilation–perfusion mismatch within the pulmonary system, and indirectly cardiac function. Its value ranges from 36 to 42 mmHg, with 3- to 8-mmHg elevations during moderate-intensity exercise, reaching a maximal value with a subsequent drop due to VE increase, characterizing the RCP. Abnormal values may represent disease severity in patients with HF, HCM, pulmonary hypertension, COPD, and restrictive pulmonary disease.[3,21,27]

Breathing reserve (VE/MVV)

BR is the difference between maximal ventilation during exercise (VE) and maximal voluntary ventilation (MVV) at rest. Since direct measurement of MVV is difficult (even during only 15 s), it is most often calculated on the basis of the FEV1: MVV = FEV1 × 40. Normal values are considered to be BR >0.20 or >10 L. It is useful in the differential diagnosis of dyspnoea.[4]

Oxygen uptake efficiency slope

The oxygen uptake efficiency slope (OUES) represents the rate of VO_2 increase in response to a given VE during exercise, and reflects how effectively O_2 is extracted and taken into the body.[29,30] The OUES is mainly influenced by the onset of lactic acidosis, and consequently by blood distribution to the muscles, muscle mass, and O_2 extraction and utilization, but also by lung perfusion and ventilation. It incorporates cardiovascular, musculoskeletal, and respiratory function, and is reduced in proportion to disease severity[30,31] and linked to adverse outcome.[32,33]

Metabolic threshold

It represents the theoretical point during incremental exercise when muscle tissue switches over to anaerobic metabolism as an additional source. Lactic acid begins to accumulate and is buffered in the serum by the bicarbonate system, resulting in increased CO_2 excretion, which causes reflex hyperventilation.

Several methods to calculate the MT are available (⮕ Figure 7.3.5.4A, B):

- Ventilatory equivalents: the ventilatory equivalents method involves simultaneous analysis of multiple variables (VE/VO_2, VE/VCO_2, $PETO_2$, and $PETCO_2$); the MT is defined as the VO_2 value at which VE/VO_2 and $PETO_2$ reach a nadir and thereafter begin to rise consistently, coinciding with unchanged VE/VCO_2 and $PETCO_2$.

- V-slope: the MT is identified as the VO_2 at which the change in slope of the relationship of VCO_2 to VO_2 occurs.

- Modified V-slope: this method determines the point of change in the slope of the relationship of VCO_2 versus VO_2, and defines the VO_2 above which VCO_2 increases faster than VO_2 without hyperventilation.

The MT demarcates the upper limit of a range of exercise intensities that can be accomplished almost entirely aerobically,

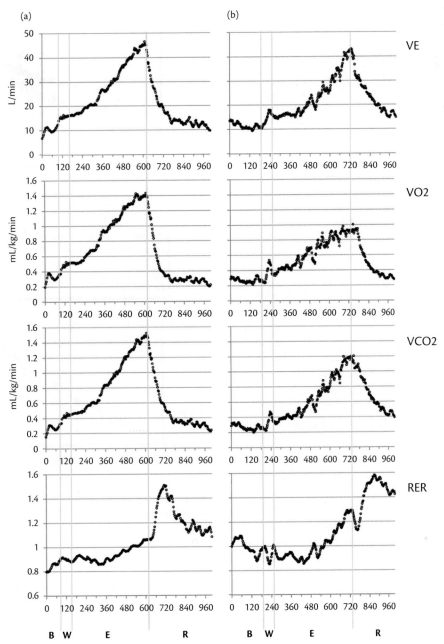

(a) (b)

VE

VO2

VCO2

RER

B W E R   B W E R

Figure 7.3.5.2 An example of symptom-limited cardiopulmonary exercise testing in a healthy subject (a) and a systolic heart failure (SHF) patient (b). Both tests were limited by muscular fatigue. Horizontal axis: time in seconds. B, baseline: resting phase in the setting position; W, warm-up: pedalling phase at 0 W; E, incremental exercise phase; R, recovery phase; the first 2 minutes is a pedalling phase, at 50% of peak workload. Vertical axis: (from upper to lower graph) VE, ventilation (L/min); VO$_2$, oxygen consumption (mL/kg/min); VCO$_2$, carbon dioxide production (mL/kg/min); RER, respiratory exchange ratio.
Healthy subject: age 63 years; weight 70 kg; no pharmacological treatment. Peak heart rate (HR) 150 bpm; peak systolic blood pressure (SBP), 210 mmHg; VO$_2$ at the ventilatory anaerobic threshold (VAT), 13 mL/kg/min; peak VO$_2$, 19.6 mL/kg/min; ventilatory response (VE/VCO$_2$ slope), 27.9; oxygen uptake efficiency slope (OUES), 2072; circulatory power (SBP × peak VO$_2$), 4116 mmHg/mL/kg/min; ventilatory power (VE/VCO$_2$ slope/peak SBP), 7.52 mmHg.
SHF patient: age 56 years; weight, 63 kg. Heart failure due to ischaemic heart disease, in NYHA class II, with implanted cardiac defibrillator and left ventricular ejection fraction (LVEF) of 16%. Medical therapy: carvedilol 6.25 mg twice daily, enalapril 10 mg twice daily, furosemide 75 mg daily, aspirin 100 mg daily, digitalis 0.125 mg daily. Peak HR, 134 bpm; peak SBP, 145 mmHg; VO$_2$ at VAT, 11 mL/kg/min; peak VO$_2$, 14.3 mL/kg/min; VE/VCO$_2$ slope, 30.6; OUES, 1357.27; circulatory power, 2073 mmHg/mL/kg/min; ventilatory power, 4.73 mmHg.
Reproduced from Corrà U, Piepoli MF, Adamopoulos S, *et al.* Cardiopulmonary exercise testing in systolic heart failure in 2014: the evolving prognostic role: a position paper from the committee on exercise physiology and training of the heart failure association of the ESC. *Eur J Heart Fail.* 2014 Sep;16(9):929–41. doi: 10.1002/ejhf.156 with permission from John Wiley and Sons.

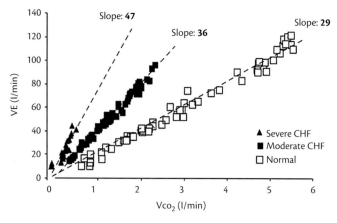

Figure 7.3.5.3 Relationship between ventilation (VE) and carbon dioxide production (VE/VCO$_2$ slope). CHF, chronic heart failure.

Reproduced from Task Force of the Italian Working Group on Cardiac Rehabilitation Prevention; Working Group on Cardiac Rehabilitation and Exercise Physiology of the European Society of Cardiology, Piepoli MF, Corrà U, Agostoni PG, Belardinelli R, Cohen-Solal A, Hambrecht R, Vanhees L. Statement on cardiopulmonary exercise testing in chronic heart failure due to left ventricular dysfunction: recommendations for performance and interpretation. Part I: definition of cardiopulmonary exercise testing parameters for appropriate use in chronic heart failure. *Eur J Cardiovasc Prev Rehabil.* 2006 Apr;13(2):150–64. doi: 10.1097/01.hjr.0000209812.05573.04 with permission from Oxford University Press. © European Society of Cardiology.

whereas WRs below the MT can be sustained essentially indefinitely, and a progressive increase in WR above the MT is associated with a progressive decrease in exercise tolerance.[34] In normal sedentary individuals, the MT occurs at about 50–60% of VO$_2$max predicted values, with a wide range of normal values extending from 35% to 80%.[35]

MT determination is helpful as an indicator of the level of fitness, for exercise prescription, and to monitor the effect of physical training.[36] When the MT is not reached, as in some patients with severe chronic obstructive airway disease,[37] or cannot be determined from the ventilatory response, as in the presence of an oscillatory pattern, an exercise prescription can still be established by using as reference a percentage of peak WR, VO$_2$max, or HR.

A reduction in MT, as in VO$_2$peak, is non-specific—it occurs in a wide spectrum of clinical conditions/diseases and, as such, has limited discriminatory ability in distinguishing between different clinical entities. Values below 40% of predicted VO$_2$max may indicate a cardiac, pulmonary (desaturation), or other limitation in O$_2$ supply to the tissues, or an underlying mitochondrial abnormality (e.g. muscle dysfunction in cardiopulmonary disease, mitochondrial myopathies).

Clinical application in heart failure

Heart failure with reduced ejection fraction

As reported by Balady *et al.*,[38] reduced exercise capacity is the cardinal symptom of chronic HF; exercise capacity traditionally has been assessed in HF by using the New York Heart Association (NYHA) criteria, but this assessment is both subjective and insensitive. Determination of VO$_2$max during a maximal symptom-limited treadmill or bicycle CPET is the most objective method to

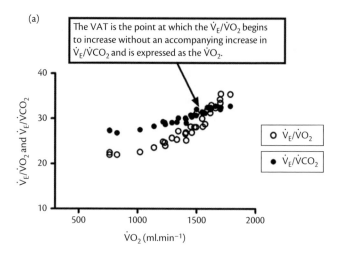

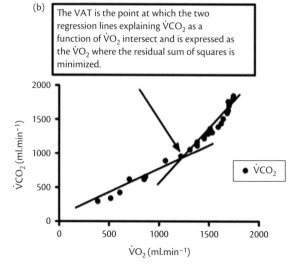

Figure 7.3.5.4 (a) Ventilatory anaerobic threshold determined using the ventilatory equivalents method. (b) Ventilatory anaerobic threshold determined using the V-slope method.

Reproduced from Task Force of the Italian Working Group on Cardiac Rehabilitation Prevention; Working Group on Cardiac Rehabilitation and Exercise Physiology of the European Society of Cardiology, Piepoli MF, Corrà U, Agostoni PG, Belardinelli R, Cohen-Solal A, Hambrecht R, Vanhees L. Statement on cardiopulmonary exercise testing in chronic heart failure due to left ventricular dysfunction: recommendations for performance and interpretation. Part I: definition of cardiopulmonary exercise testing parameters for appropriate use in chronic heart failure. *Eur J Cardiovasc Prev Rehabil.* 2006 Apr;13(2):150–64. doi: 10.1097/01.hjr.0000209812.05573.04 with permission from Oxford University Press. © European Society of Cardiology.

assess exercise capacity in HF patients. By determining the MT, the physician can assess how close the patient is to achieving his or her maximal effort. Thus, CPET has gained widespread application in the functional assessment of patients with HF. It is indicated to:

1. Determine the severity of the disease and help to determine whether HF is the cause of exercise limitation

2. Provide important prognostic information and identify candidates for cardiac transplantation or other advanced treatments

3. Facilitate the exercise prescription

4. Assess the efficacy of new drugs and devices.

Peak VO$_2$ has been shown to predict prognosis in patients with HF in many studies,[39,40,41] not only patients referred for cardiac transplantation,[40] but also women[42] and the geriatric population.[32,43] Recent data also suggest that reporting peak VO$_2$ as a percentage of that predicted by the Wasserman equation may have additional prognostic importance.[44] During CPET, many variables are collected that also confer prognostic information. The ventilatory response to exercise, most frequently measured by the VE/VCO$_2$ slope, as discussed earlier, has been found by several investigators to be even more predictive of outcome than peak VO$_2$. Unlike peak VO$_2$, the VE/VCO$_2$ relation does not require maximal effort.[31,45] Previous studies found that mortality risk increases progressively as the VE/VCO$_2$ slope increases from normal (i.e. 30) to 40.

An interesting two step-approach has been proposed by Corra et al.[6] (<arrows in circle> Figures 7.3.5.5 and 7.3.5.6) to address risk estimation in HF populations. The first step is to distinguish between conventional and unconventional CPET; the second step is focused on peak VO$_2$ and, depending whether the test has been conducted with or without beta-blocker therapy, on both VE/VCO$_2$ and RER, in order to stratify between low- and high-risk patients.

One of the most-established and well-validated approach is with the prognostic score known as the Metabolic Exercise test data combined with Cardiac and Kidney Indexes (MECKI) score,[46] which can assess the risk of cardiovascular mortality and

the need for urgent heart transplantation. The score takes into account six variables that are independently related to prognosis: haemoglobin (Hb), sodium (Na$^+$), kidney function evaluated by means of the Modification of Diet in Renal Disease (MDRD) equation, LV ejection fraction (LVEF) by echocardiography, the percentage of predicted peak O$_2$ consumption (VO$_2$%), and the minute ventilation/CO$_2$ production (VE/VCO$_2$) relationship slope. This easy-to-use parameter, available also with an online calculator, can be extremely helpful to incorporate CPET findings into a clinical perspective and establish the short-term prognosis in patients with HFrEF.

Heart failure with preserved ejection fraction

Although most of the studies in the literature supporting the value of CPET in patients with HF have been performed in cohorts with systolic dysfunction, initial investigations demonstrate that CPET has promise in the evaluation of patients who have HF with preserved ejection fraction (HFpEF) (diastolic dysfunction). The diagnosis of HFpEF can be challenging, as the pathophysiology is heterogeneous, with different phenotypes and concomitant cardiovascular (e.g. atrial fibrillation, arterial hypertension, coronary artery disease, pulmonary hypertension) and non-cardiovascular pathological conditions (diabetes, chronic kidney disease, anaemia, iron deficiency, COPD, and obesity).

The main symptom is usually dyspnoea or reduced tolerance to exercise; CPET findings include usually a reduced peak VO$_2$ with

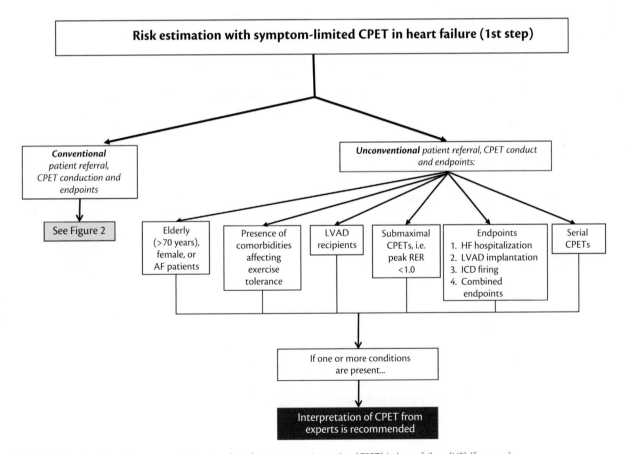

Figure 7.3.5.5 Risk estimation with symptom-limited cardiopulmonary exercise testing (CPET) in heart failure (HF) (first step).

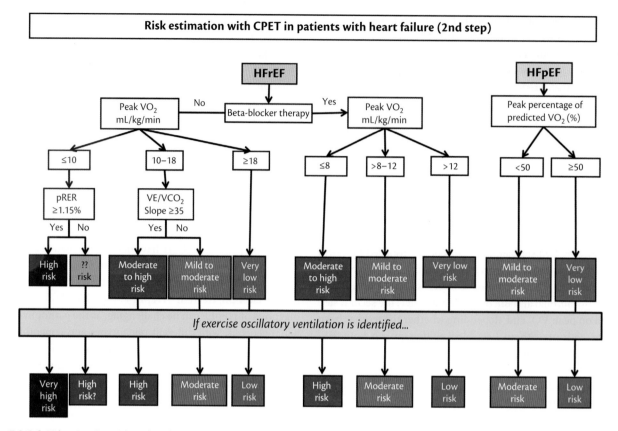

Figure 7.3.5.6 Risk estimation with cardiopulmonary exercise testing (CPET) in patients with heart failure (second step): considering specific prognostic indicators.

impairment in peak CO and a slightly reduced peak VO$_2$; in fact, despite normal systolic contractile function, patients are unable to use the Frank–Starling mechanism adequately to increase SV during exercise due to the presence of increased LV filling pressures.[47] The OUES[44] likewise appears to be comparably reduced in systolic and diastolic dysfunction, and is significantly lower than in healthy subjects. Ventilatory efficiency, expressed as the VE/VCO$_2$ slope, appears to be lower in HF patients with diastolic, compared to systolic, dysfunction.[48,49] In subjects diagnosed with HCM, Arena *et al.*[50] demonstrated that peak VO$_2$ and VE/VCO$_2$ at peak exercise were both significantly correlated with resting pulmonary haemodynamics. An abnormal response effectively identified subjects with pulmonary hypertension. Lastly, initial investigations indicate the VE/VCO$_2$ slope, exercise oscillatory ventilation), and peak VO$_2$ may be significant predictors of adverse events in HF patients with diastolic dysfunction, with the two former CPET variables providing superior prognostic value, compared to the latter.[48,51]

Of note, CPET-derived measures of peak VO$_2$ and ventilatory response (VE/VCO$_2$ slope) have been described to be either similarly reduced[52] or less affected in comparison with HFrEF. However, up to now, the predictive role of CPET-derived parameters has not been standardized for HFpEF and data are still preliminary. Although initial findings are promising, additional research is required before definitive conclusions can be drawn regarding the clinical value of CPET in patients with diastolic dysfunction.

CPET and exercise prescription

Regular aerobic physical activity programmes have been shown to reduce mortality and morbidity in both primary and secondary cardiovascular prevention through synergistic effects of the following mechanisms: anti-atherogenic, anti-ischaemic, antiarrhythmic, and anti-inflammatory effects, improvement in vascular endothelial and autonomic function, and reduced blood clotting and age-related disability.[53] Moreover, the benefit of constant aerobic physical training has been proven to be effective even beyond cardiovascular prevention in terms of reduction of the incidence of both cancer and neurodegenerative diseases.[54]

Since CPET provides direct measurement of both cardiorespiratory fitness and metabolic response to exercise, it represents *the most accurate test for exercise prescription* in several scenarios, including primary and secondary cardiovascular prevention and lung diseases, as well as in optimization of athlete training.

By determining the MT, a precise training WR that includes the VO$_2$ level and specific HR range can be identified. A peak RER of >1.10 is an indicator of maximal effort, and a prescription for exercise can be designated at less than the maximal for the individual patient.[55] Exercise intensity prescriptions are based on the rating of perceived exertion, HR reserve (peak HR minus resting HR), or VO$_2$ reserve (peak VO$_2$ minus resting VO$_2$). Recently, the 2020 European Society of Cardiology (ESC) Guidelines on sports cardiology and exercise in patients with cardiovascular disease have been published by the Task Force on sports cardiology and exercise in patients with cardiovascular disease of the ESC;[56] the Guidelines include the most up-to-date research in exercising individuals with cardiovascular disease, including information regarding risk assessment and management of individuals with cardiovascular disease, to aid physicians in prescribing exercise programmes or providing advice for sports participation. Of all the basic elements of exercise prescription, exercise intensity is generally considered to be the most critical for achieving aerobic fitness and to have the most favourable impact on risk factors. Absolute intensity refers to the rate of energy expenditure during exercise and is usually expressed in kcal/min or METs. Training intensity can be expressed as a percentage of maximal heart rate (HRmax) recorded during an exercise test or predicted on the basis of the equation (HRmax = 220 − age]. However, use of prediction equations for HRmax is not recommended, because there is a large standard deviation around the regression line between age and HRmax.[57] Alternatively, exercise intensity can be expressed relative to the percentage of a person's HRR, which uses a percentage of the difference between HRmax and resting HR and adds it to the resting HR (Karvonen formula).[58]

Although an aerobic training programme based on the target HR can be prescribed on the basis of the exercise test data, *CPET is considered the most accurate and most recommended test in order to prescribe individualized physical activity*, especially in specific populations such as HF patients. Relative exercise intensity refers to a fraction of an individual's maximal power (load) that is maintained during exercise and is usually prescribed as a percentage of maximal aerobic capacity (VO_2max) on the basis of CPET. Different indices of exercise intensity for endurance sports from maximal exercise testing and training zones are reported available.[56] In HF patients, the most commonly evaluated exercise mode is moderate continuous exercise (MCE);[59] in patients in NYHA functional class III, exercise intensity should be maintained at a lower intensity (<40% of VO_2peak), according to perceived symptoms and clinical status during the first 1–2 weeks. This should be followed by a gradual increase in intensity to 50–70% of VO_2peak and, if tolerated, up to 85% of VO_2peak as the primary aim.[60]

Future directions

CPET imaging

CPET imaging is a quite recent and valuable testing modality, which is receiving attention for its potential to combine exercise physiological data with non-invasive recordings of cardiac function by measures of chamber volumes and geometry, valvular status, and systolic and diastolic function.[12] The combination CPET and stress echocardiography can evaluate non-invasively multiple aspects of the cardiovascular system which is otherwise obtainable only with invasive haemodynamic monitoring; for example, in patients with exertional dyspnoea, in particular if hypertensive, the early stages of HFpEF cannot be always detectable by rest echocardiography, whereas the combination of echocardiography and CPET may provide additional information; since patients with normal LV filling pressures or even normal LV diastolic function at rest may reveal

elevated LV filling pressures during effort, diastolic stress testing is indicated and the integration of CPET results, in particular VO_2max and the VE/CO_2 slope with E/e′ ratio at peak stress, may be highly demonstrative of HFpEF.[61,62] Combining CPET with stress echocardiography will also be helpful to reveal the presence of dynamic severe mitral regurgitation, not detectable at rest, and correlate with abnormal VE/VCO_2 and VO_2 peak; this evaluation could also be performed before and after interventional procedures or therapeutic intervention such as cardiac resynchronization therapy or MitraClip to evaluate the clinical benefit.[16]

CPET in the Covid-19 era

Coronavirus disease 2019 (Covid-19) is an emerging infectious disease that has exerted a tremendous impact on public health and worldwide socio-economic development; as are many aspects of the acute disease, the long-term sequelae of Covid-19 are still largely unknown. Chronic fatigue symptoms have been reported in 40% of people recovering from Covid-19. Since CPET plays an important role in several clinical scenarios, including post-acute phase, complications, and disease prognostication (e.g. HF or pulmonary hypertension), it could help physicians to define post-Covid-19 exercise tolerance, dyspnoea assessment and quantification, post-acute respiratory impairment, and post-acute cardiovascular complications, as well as to define the residual risk of post-Covid-19 hospitalization.

Summary

CPET provides an assessment of the cardiovascular, ventilatory, and metabolic responses to exercise. It could be extremely useful in investigating causes of dyspnoea and in assessing prognosis in patients with HF. It could also help the clinician to titrate and evaluate the efficacy of pharmacological and non-pharmacological therapies, in particular for exercise prescription.

The exercise is performed on a bicycle or treadmill, with use of a ramp protocol and wearing a non-rebreathing valve that measures O_2 and CO_2 gas and ventilation.

During the test, ECG, BP, and oxygen saturations are recorded; the test should last 8–12 minutes.

The VO_2 is the most important parameter to evaluate disease severity, whereas other parameters such as VE/VCO_2, VO_2/HR, RER, and VE complete the picture.

CPET is useful in HFrEF, HFmrEF, and HFpEF to determine severity of the disease, provide important prognostic information, facilitate exercise prescription, and assess the efficacy of new drugs and devices.

Key messages

- ◆ CPET provides a full assessment of the cardiovascular, ventilatory, and metabolic responses to exercise.
- ◆ It is indicated to investigate the causes of exercise limitation and dyspnoea and to assess prognosis in HF.
- ◆ It is recommended in screening for heart transplantation indication and exercise prescription.
- ◆ It helps clinicians to titrate and evaluate the efficacy of pharmacological and non-pharmacological therapies.

References

1. Weber KT, Kinasewitz GT, Janicki JS, Fishman AP. Oxygen utilization and ventilation during exercise in patients with chronic cardiac failure. *Circulation* 1982;**65**:1213–23.

2. Guazzi M, Arena R, Halle M, Piepoli MF, Myers J, Lavie CJ. 2016 Focused Update: clinical recommendations for cardiopulmonary exercise testing data assessment in specific patient populations. *Circulation* 2016;**133**:e694–711.

3. Task Force of the Italian Working Group on Cardiac Rehabilitation and Prevention; Working Group on Cardiac Rehabilitation and Exercise Physiology of the European Society of Cardiology; Piepoli MF, Corrà U, Agostoni PG, et al. Statement on cardiopulmonary exercise testing in chronic heart failure due to left ventricular dysfunction: recommendations for performance and interpretation Part I: Definition of cardiopulmonary exercise testing parameters for appropriate use in chronic heart failure. *Eur J Cardiovasc Prev Rehabil* 2006;**13**:150–64.

4. Wasserman K, Whipp BJ. Exercise physiology in health and disease. *Am Rev Respir Dis* 1975;**112**:219–49.

5. Wasserman K, Hansen JE, Sue DY, Stringer WW, Whipp BJ. *Principles of Exercise Testing and Interpretation*, 4th edition. Philadelphia, PA: Lippincott, Williams and Wilkins; 2005.

6. Corrà U, Agostoni PG, Anker SD, et al. Role of cardiopulmonary exercise testing in clinical stratification in heart failure. A position paper from the Committee on Exercise Physiology and Training of the Heart Failure Association of the European Society of Cardiology: cardiopulmonary exercise testing and prognosis in HF. *Eur J Heart Fail* 2018;**20**:3–15.

7. Buchfuhrer MJ, Hansen JE, Robinson TE, Sue DY, Wasserman K, Whipp BJ. Optimizing the exercise protocol for cardiopulmonary assessment. *J Appl Physiol* 1983;**55**:1558–64.

8. Andrew M, Luks Robb W, Glenny H, Robertson T. *Introduction to Cardiopulmonary Exercise Testing*. Springer; 2013.

9. Task Force of the Italian Working Group on Cardiac Rehabilitation and Prevention (Gruppo Italiano di Cardiologia Riabilitativa e Prevenzione, GICR); Working Group on Cardiac Rehabilitation and Exercise Physiology of the European Society of Cardiology. Statement on cardiopulmonary exercise testing in chronic heart failure due to left ventricular dysfunction: recommendations for performance and interpretation Part III: Interpretation of cardiopulmonary exercise testing in chronic heart failure and future applications. *Eur J Cardiovasc Prev Rehabil* 2006;**13**:485–94.

10. Guazzi M, Adams V, Conraads V, et al.; European Association for Cardiovascular Prevention & Rehabilitation; American Heart Association. EACPR/AHA Scientific Statement. Clinical recommendations for cardiopulmonary exercise testing data assessment in specific patient populations. *Circulation* 2012;**126**:2261–74.

11. Sorajja P, Allison T, Hayes C, Nishimura RA, Lam CSP, Ommen SR. Prognostic utility of metabolic exercise testing in minimally symptomatic patients with obstructive hypertrophic cardiomyopathy. *Am J Cardiol* 2012;**109**:1494–8.

12. Guazzi M, Bandera F, Ozemek C, Systrom D, Arena R. Cardiopulmonary exercise testing: what is its value? *J Am Coll Cardiol* 2017;**70**:1618–36.

13. Chaudhry S, Arena R, Wasserman K, et al. Exercise-induced myocardial ischemia detected by cardiopulmonary exercise testing. *Am J Cardiol* 2009;**103**:615–19.

14. Accalai E, Vignati C, Salvioni E, et al. Non-invasive estimation of stroke volume during exercise from oxygen in heart failure patients. *Eur J Prev Cardiol* 2021;**28**:280–6.

15. Belardinelli R, Lacalaprice F, Tiano L, Muçai A, Perna GP. Cardiopulmonary exercise testing is more accurate than ECG-stress testing in diagnosing myocardial ischemia in subjects with chest pain. *Int J Cardiol* 2014;**174**:337–42.

16. Bandera F, Generati G, Pellegrino M, et al. Mitral regurgitation in heart failure: insights from CPET combined with exercise echocardiography. *Eur Heart J Cardiovasc Imaging* 2017;**18**:296–303.

17. Brubaker PH, Kitzman DW. Chronotropic incompetence: causes, consequences, and management. *Circulation* 2011;**123**:1010–20.

18. Tanaka H, Monahan KD, Seals DR. Age-predicted maximal heart rate revisited. *J Am Coll Cardiol* 2001;**37**:153–6.

19. Arena R, Guazzi M, Myers J, Peberdy MA. Prognostic value of heart rate recovery in patients with heart failure. *Am Heart J* 2006;**151**:851. e7–13.

20. Lauer MS. Heart rate recovery: coming back full-circle to the baroreceptor reflex. *Circ Res* 2016;**119**:582–3.

21. Weiss SA, Blumenthal RS, Sharrett AR, Redberg RF, Mora S. Exercise blood pressure and future cardiovascular death in asymptomatic individuals. *Circulation* 2010;**121**:2109–16.

22. Kim H. Determinants of exercise capacity in hypertensive patients: new insights from tissue Doppler echocardiography. *Am J Hypertens* 2003;**16**:564–9.

23. Corrà U. Exercise oscillatory ventilation in heart failure. *Int J Cardiol* 2016;**206**:S13–15.

24. Corrà U, Giordano A, Bosimini E, et al. Oscillatory ventilation during exercise in patients with chronic heart failure. *Chest* 2002;**121**:1572–80.

25. Dhakal BP, Lewis GD. Exercise oscillatory ventilation: mechanisms and prognostic significance. *World J Cardiol* 2016;**8**:258.

26. Poggio R, Arazi HC, Giorgi M, Miriuka SG. Prediction of severe cardiovascular events by VE/VCO2 slope versus peak VO2 in systolic heart failure: a meta-analysis of the published literature. *Am Heart J* 2010;**160**:1004–14.

27. Malfatto G, Facchini M, Branzi G, et al. Reverse ventricular remodeling and improved functional capacity after ventricular resynchronization in advanced heart failure. *Ital Heart J* 2005;**6**:578–83.

28. Guazzi M, Bandera F, Ozemek C, Systrom D, Arena R. Cardiopulmonary exercise testing. *J Am Coll Cardiol* 2017;**70**:1618–36.

29. Torchio R, Guglielmo M, Giardino R, et al. Exercise ventilatory inefficiency and mortality in patients with chronic obstructive pulmonary disease undergoing surgery for non-small-cell lung cancer. *Eur J Cardiothorac Surg* 2010;**38**:14–19.

30. Van Laethem C, Bartunek J, Goethals M, Nellens P, Andries E, Vanderheyden M. Oxygen uptake efficiency slope, a new submaximal parameter in evaluating exercise capacity in chronic heart failure patients. *Am Heart J* 2005;**149**:175–80.

31. Arena R, Myers J, Hsu L, et al. The minute ventilation/carbon dioxide production slope is prognostically superior to the oxygen uptake efficiency slope. *J Card Fail* 2007;**13**:462–9.

32. Davies LC, Wensel R, Georgiadou P, et al. Enhanced prognostic value from cardiopulmonary exercise testing in chronic heart failure by non-linear analysis: oxygen uptake efficiency slope. *Eur Heart J* 2006;**27**:684–90.

33. Task Force of the Italian Working Group on Cardiac Rehabilitation and Prevention; Working Group on Cardiac Rehabilitation and Exercise Physiology of the European Society of Cardiology; Piepoli MF, Corrà U, Agostoni PG, et al. Statement on cardiopulmonary exercise testing in chronic heart failure due to left ventricular dysfunction: recommendations for performance and interpretation Part II: How to perform cardiopulmonary exercise testing in chronic heart failure. *Eur J Cardiovasc Prev Rehabil* 2006;**13**:300–11.

34. Sullivan CS, Casaburi R, Storer TW, Wasserman K. Non-invasive prediction of blood lactate response to constant power outputs

from incremental exercise tests. *Eur J Appl Physiol Occup Physiol* 1995;**71**:349–54.

35. [No authors listed]. Clinical exercise testing with reference to lung diseases: indications, standardization and interpretation strategies. ERS Task Force on Standardization of Clinical Exercise Testing. European Respiratory Society. *Eur Respir J* 1997;**10**:2662–89.

36. Casaburi R, Patessio A, Ioli F, Zanaboni S, Donner CF, Wasserman K. Reductions in exercise lactic acidosis and ventilation as a result of exercise training in patients with obstructive lung disease. *Am Rev Respir Dis* 1991;**143**:9–18.

37. Casaburi R, Porszasz J, Burns MR, Carithers ER, Chang RS, Cooper CB. Physiologic benefits of exercise training in rehabilitation of patients with severe chronic obstructive pulmonary disease. *Am J Respir Crit Care Med* 1997;**155**:1541–51.

38. Balady GJ, Arena R, Sietsema K, et al.; American Heart Association Exercise; Cardiac Rehabilitation, and Prevention Committee of the Council on Clinical Cardiology; Council on Epidemiology and Prevention; Council on Peripheral Vascular Disease; Interdisciplinary Council on Quality of Care and Outcomes Research. Clinician's guide to cardiopulmonary exercise testing in adults: a scientific statement from the American Heart Association. *Circulation* 2010;**122**:191–225.

39. Cohn JN, Johnson GR, Shabetai R, et al. Ejection fraction, peak exercise oxygen consumption, cardiothoracic ratio, ventricular arrhythmias, and plasma norepinephrine as determinants of prognosis in heart failure. The V-HeFT VA Cooperative Studies Group. *Circulation* 1993;**87**(6 Suppl):VI5–16.

40. Mancini DM, Eisen H, Kussmaul W, Mull R, Edmunds Jr LH, Wilson JR. Value of peak exercise oxygen consumption for optimal timing of cardiac transplantation in ambulatory patients with heart failure. *Circulation* 1991;**83**:778–86.

41. Szlachcic J, Masse BM, Kramer BL, Topic N, Tubau J. Correlates and prognostic implication of exercise capacity in chronic congestive heart failure. *Am J Cardiol* 1985;**55**:1037–42.

42. Elmariah S, Goldberg LR, Allen MT, Kao A. Effects of gender on peak oxygen consumption and the timing of cardiac transplantation. *J Am Coll Cardiol* 2006;**47**:2237–42.

43. Parikh MN, Lund LH, Goda A, Mancini D. Usefulness of peak exercise oxygen consumption and the heart failure survival score to predict survival in patients >65 years of age with heart failure. *Am J Cardiol* 2009;**103**:998–1002.

44. Arena R, Myers J, Abella J, et al. Determining the preferred percent-predicted equation for peak oxygen consumption in patients with heart failure. *Circ Heart Fail* 2009;**2**:113–20.

45. Francis DP, Shamim W, Davies LC, et al. Cardiopulmonary exercise testing for prognosis in chronic heart failure: continuous and independent prognostic value from VE/VCO(2)slope and peak VO(2). *Eur Heart J* 2000;**21**:154–61.

46. Agostoni P, Corrà U, Cattadori G, et al. Metabolic exercise test data combined with cardiac and kidney indexes, the MECKI score: a multiparametric approach to heart failure prognosis. *Int J Cardiol* 2013;**167**:2710–18.

47. Farr MJ, Lang CC, Lamanca JJ, et al. Cardiopulmonary exercise variables in diastolic versus systolic heart failure. *Am J Cardiol* 2008;**102**:203–6.

48. Guazzi M, Myers J, Arena R. Cardiopulmonary exercise testing in the clinical and prognostic assessment of diastolic heart failure. *J Am Coll Cardiol* 2005;**46**:1883–90.

49. Moore B, Brubaker PH, Stewart KP, Kitzman DW. VE/VCO2 slope in older heart failure patients with normal versus reduced ejection fraction compared with age-matched healthy controls. *J Card Fail* 2007;**13**:259–62.

50. Arena R, Owens DS, Arevalo J, et al. Ventilatory efficiency and resting hemodynamics in hypertrophic cardiomyopathy. *Med Sci Sports Exerc* 2008;**40**:799–805.

51. Guazzi M, Myers J, Peberdy MA, Bensimhon D, Chase P, Arena R. Exercise oscillatory breathing in diastolic heart failure: prevalence and prognostic insights. *Eur Heart J* 2008;**29**:2751–9.

52. Osman AF, Mehra MR, Lavie CJ, Nunez E, Milani RV. The incremental prognostic importance of body fat adjusted peak oxygen consumption in chronic heart failure. *J Am Coll Cardiol* 2000;**36**:2126–31.

53. Fletcher GF, Ades PA, Kligfield P, et al. Exercise standards for testing and training. *Circulation* 2013;**128**:873–934.

54. Sharma S, Merghani A, Mont L. Exercise and the heart: the good, the bad, and the ugly. *Eur Heart J* 2015;**36**:1445–53.

55. Arena R, Myers J, Guazzi M. The clinical significance of aerobic exercise testing and prescription: from apparently healthy to confirmed cardiovascular disease. *Am J Lifestyle Med* 2008;**2**:519–36.

56. Pelliccia A, Sharma S, Gati S, et al.; ESC Scientific Document Group, 2020 ESC Guidelines on sports cardiology and exercise in patients with cardiovascular disease. *Eur Heart J* 2021;**42**:17–96.

57. Vanhees L, Stevens A. Exercise intensity: a matter of measuring or of talking? *J Cardiopulm Rehabil* 2006;**26**:7879.

58. Myers J, Hadley D, Oswald U, et al. Effects of exercise training on heart rate recovery in patients with chronic heart failure. *Am Heart J* 2007;**153**:1056–63.

59. Balady GJ, Williams MA, Ades PA, et al.; American Heart Association Exercise, Cardiac Rehabilitation, and Prevention Committee, the Council on Clinical Cardiology, American Heart Association Council on Cardiovascular Nursing, American Heart Association Council on Epidemiology and Prevention, American Heart Association Council on Nutrition, Physical Activity, and Metabolism, American Association of Cardiovascular and Pulmonary Rehabilitation. Core components of cardiac rehabilitation/secondary prevention programs: 2007 update: a scientific statement from the American Heart Association Exercise, Cardiac Rehabilitation, and Prevention Committee, the Council on Clinical Cardiology; the Councils on Cardiovascular Nursing, Epidemiology and Prevention, and Nutrition, Physical Activity, and Metabolism; and the American Association of Cardiovascular and Pulmonary Rehabilitation. *Circulation* 2007;**115**:2675–82.

60. Piepoli MF, Conraads V, Corrà U, et al. Exercise training in heart failure: from theory to practice. A consensus document of the Heart Failure Association and the European Association for Cardiovascular Prevention and Rehabilitation. *Eur J Heart Fail* 2011;**13**:347–57.

61. Donal E, Lund LH, Oger E, et al. Value of exercise echocardiography in heart failure with preserved ejection fraction: a substudy from the KaRen study. *Eur Heart J Cardiovasc Imaging*; 2016;**17**:106–13.

62. Kosmala W, Rojek A, Przewlocka-Kosmala M, Mysiak A, Karolko B, Marwick TH. Contributions of nondiastolic factors to exercise intolerance in heart failure with preserved ejection fraction. *J Am Coll Cardiol*; 2016;**67**:659–70.

Cardiac catheterization, invasive imaging, and haemodynamics

Christian W Hamm, Birgit Assmus, and Veselin Mitrovic

Contents

Introduction

Heart failure is a multifactorial, progressive syndrome, with a continuum of symptoms and haemodynamic changes, characterized by reduced effective cardiac output (CO) and elevated ventricular filling pressure. Reduced peripheral muscle perfusion leads to fatigue, and lung congestion leads to dyspnoea (➲ Figure 7.4.1).

The initial oligosymptomatic phase is characterized haemodynamically by normal filling pressures and maintained CO, although echocardiography shows impaired ventricular function. With further progression of the disease, pulmonary capillary wedge pressure (PCWP) becomes elevated, first during exercise and later also at rest, and CO is no longer adequate during exercise. The stage of cardiac decompensation is reached on an individual basis only when PCWP increases and CO decreases to a critical extent.

In this cardiovascular continuum, the heart and lungs form a perfect functional system in which the pulmonary circulation plays a key role. In heart failure, a close cardiorespiratory interaction is observed, and there are pathophysiological consequences of left-sided heart failure on respiratory function, pulmonary gas exchange, pulmonary circulation, and central respiratory regulation.[1,2] The acute, retrograde increase in hydrostatic pressure of the pulmonary capillaries to >20–25 mmHg has several consequences:

1. Increased filtration pressure on alveolar capillary membranes, leading first to interstitial oedema and later to alveolar oedema

2. Extended diffusion distance for pulmonary gas exchange, resulting in hypoxia and reactive vasoconstriction

3. Loss of integrity of alveolar capillary membranes, leading to pulmonary capillary stress rupture and increased permeability for plasma proteins and erythrocytes, as well as increased stiffness of pulmonary vessels and the interstitium. This is accompanied by a decrease in pulmonary compliance and ultimately leads to disturbances in pulmonary circulation, ventilation/perfusion mismatch, and increased dead space ventilation.[3,4,5]

At the end of diastole, pressures of the left ventricle (LV), left atrium (LA), pulmonary veins, and pulmonary capillaries are at the same level, and measurement of PCWP provides indirectly information on left ventricular end-diastolic pressure (LVEDP), which reflects the left ventricular (LV) end-diastolic volume (Figure 7.4.2A).[6]

LVEDP not only is increased as a result of reduced LV contractility and impaired LV compliance, but also can be affected by LV preload and afterload, as well as by the heart rate (➲ Figure 7.4.3). Increased LVEDP and left atrial pressure (LAP), as well as pulmonary venous hypertension, first lead to reversible functional changes and then, as a result of hypoxia and endothelial dysfunction, to active vasoconstriction. These alterations result in irreversible structural vessel changes and pathological remodelling with intimal

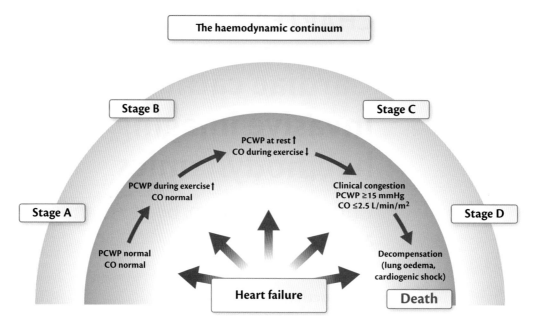

Figure 7.4.1 The haemodynamic continuum in heart failure.

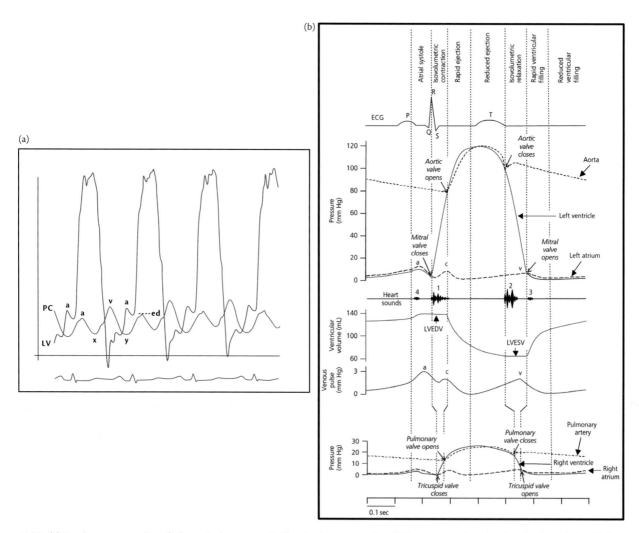

Figure 7.4.2 (a) Simultaneous recording of left ventricular pressure (LVP) and pulmonary capillary (PC) pressure tracings showing the close relationship between the left ventricular end-diastolic pressure (LVEDP) and the pulmonary capillary wedge pressure (PCWP). (b) The Wiggers cycle demonstrating the relationship and timing between cardiac pressure tracings and the electrocardiogram. LVEDV, left ventricular end-diastolic volume; LVESV, left ventricular end-systolic volume.
Reproduced from Stouffer GA, Klein L, McLaughlin DP. *Cardiovascular Hemodynamics for the Clinician*. 2nd ed: Wiley; 2017 with permission from John Wiley and Sons.

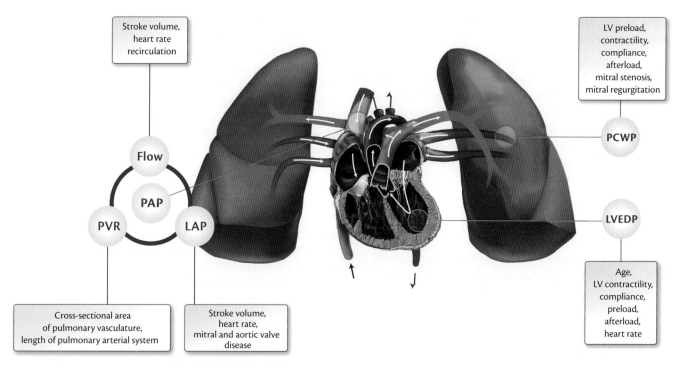

Figure 7.4.3 Influence of different factors on left ventricular (LV) end-diastolic pressure (LVEDP), pulmonary capillary wedge pressure (PCWP), pulmonary artery pressure (PAP), flow, left atrial pressure (LAP), and pulmonary vascular resistance (PVR).

fibrosis and media hypertrophy. Ultimately, there is an increase in pulmonary vascular resistance (PVR), with subsequent right ventricular (RV) dysfunction.

An increase in intravascular volume, along with reduced contractility, first leads to a rise in passive mean pulmonary artery pressure (mPAP), with a transpulmonary gradient (TPG) of <12 mmHg. Should mPAP increase disproportionally above 35–40 mmHg, accompanied by an only slightly increased PCWP of above 22 mmHg, so-called 'out-of-proportion' reactive pulmonary hypertension (PH) occurs.[7]

Lung congestion resulting from left heart failure, with subsequent shear stress and circumferential stretch, triggers several biochemical signals that bring about structural vessel changes, in both the precapillary and capillary regions. The well-known phenomenon of pulmonary capillary stress rupture leads to *de novo* muscularization of the small precapillary vessels. Morphological studies have shown that this is accompanied by pronounced fibrosis of the alveolar walls, an increase in thickness of the basal membranes of the capillary endothelium and alveolar epithelium, and microvascular intima fibrosis.[3] These changes and the aforementioned pulmonary arterial muscularization manifest as increased stiffness of the pulmonary vessels and interstitium, as well as a decrease in pulmonary compliance, all of which translate into an extended diffusion distance for pulmonary gas exchange, and ultimately hypoxia.[8,9]

Chronic lung congestion and, in particular, an acute deterioration lead to ventilation/perfusion mismatch. Alveoli can potentially be perfused, but underventilated, causing effective right-to-left shunting of venous blood through the lungs. Alternatively, the airways can be ventilated, but underperfused, resulting in 'wasted' ventilation, so-called 'dead space'. Increased dead space ventilation is implicated as a potential cause of reduced ventilatory efficiency in patients with congestive heart failure.[8]

Pulmonary alveolar oedema occurs only when the pulmonary capillary pressure rises to values exceeding the plasma colloid osmotic pressure, which is approximately 25–28 mmHg.[4] Interstitial lung oedema will occur in patients without previous increase in pulmonary capillary pressure if it rises to 17–20 mmHg, which, at first, can be fully compensated for by an increase in lymph flow. The lymphatics play a key role in removing liquid from the interstitial space, and if the pumping capacity of the lymphatic channels is exceeded, oedema will occur.[5] Alveolar lung oedema will appear in patients with *de novo* heart failure if the hydrostatic pressure in the capillaries exceeds 25–28 mmHg.[4] The sudden marked increase in pulmonary capillary pressure in acute heart failure has deleterious consequences and can be rapidly fatal in patients not preconditioned by a previous increase in pulmonary capillary pressure.

In contrast, under the same haemodynamic conditions, the situation is totally different in patients with chronic lung congestion and structural changes within the alveolar capillary membrane and small pulmonary vessels due to well-developed compensatory mechanisms.[9,10] Here, an increase in hydrostatic pressure within the capillaries of between 30 and 40 mmHg is well compensated for and lung oedema does not occur. Lymph flow can increase in such a situation to a maximum of 200 mL/hour.[5]

Right heart and pulmonary artery catheterization

Right heart catheterization (RHC) was introduced over 50 years ago, and this semi-invasive diagnostic tool is currently used in critically ill patients. It plays an important role in diagnosing PH and left and right heart disease, as well as in assessing disease severity,[11,12] determining prognosis and response to therapy.[11,13,14] Despite the enduring popularity of pulmonary artery catheterization (PAC), the effects of PAC monitoring on patient outcomes remain somewhat controversial.[15,16,17,18]

Historical background

The first RHC in humans was performed by the German surgeon Werner Forssmann in Berlin-Eberswalde in 1929.[19] Under fluoroscopy, on at least six occasions, he inserted a 65-cm urethral catheter sterilized in hot olive oil into his left cubital vein and guided it into the right atrium (RA), documenting its position by chest X-ray. For his pioneering work, he was awarded the Nobel Prize in medicine in 1956, together with Andre Cournand and Dickinson Richards, who developed catheters that could be placed into the pulmonary arteries.

Flow-guided microcatheterization in cardiopulmonary functional diagnostics was facilitated by Grandjean in 1967 by using the single-lumen 'Pulmocath' microcatheter. In the same year, Swan and Ganz first developed a balloon-tipped, flow-guided, double-lumen catheter, and later a triple-lumen, 7F thermodilution catheter was developed.

Clinical application and controversy surrounding pulmonary artery catheterization

In general, PAC is safe, relatively easy to perform, and mostly well tolerated, and can be undertaken at the bedside. However, training and experience are required for obtaining accurate tracings and proper analysis, as well as for interpretation of pressure curves and haemodynamic data.[11,12] However, PAC is an invasive procedure and can result inevitably in serious complications, including death, as shown in several studies in high-risk surgical patients and those with severe sepsis.[17,18]

Data from clinical studies conducted during the 1980s and 1990s on the use of PAC in critically ill patients were conflicting and led to controversy over the routine use of PAC in these patients.[16,17,20] In the trial on PAC-guided therapy with angiotensin-converting enzyme (ACE) inhibitors conducted by Fonarow et al., it was shown that PCWP, in contrast to the cardiac index (CI), predicts mortality rate in patients with advanced heart failure.[21] In the large, retrospective, non-randomized SUPPORT trial published by Connors et al., which was conducted in patients hospitalized with one or more of nine life-threatening diagnoses, the 30-day mortality rate was significantly higher in the PAC group, although without an excessive risk for patients with heart failure.[20] However, in the large randomized ESCAPE trial in patients hospitalized with severe symptomatic and recurrent heart failure, the cumulative primary endpoint consisting of days alive and out of hospital was reached similarly in both groups.[22] Exercise and quality of life as secondary endpoints improved in both groups, with a consistent trend towards greater improvement within the PAC group and in those sites with the highest patient enrolment. Adverse in-hospital events driven by application of PAC were higher in the PAC group, compared to the clinical assessment group (22% vs 11.5%).[22] The largest prospective PAC trial, with the acronym PAC-MAN, showed neutral results with respect to mortality rate and the primary combined endpoint of death and rehospitalization.[23]

After these studies, doubts were raised regarding the benefits and safety of PAC, leading to several negative and provocative publications in renowned journals.[24,25,26] Nevertheless, applying PAC-guided therapy in critically ill patients did not affect all-cause mortality and hospitalization rate, as was shown in a meta-analysis of 12 randomized trials, including the ESCAPE and PAC-MAN studies.[22,23,27]

These inconsistent results notwithstanding, it appears that when clinically indicated, PAC can be useful for optimizing medical management in critical cases. New studies have shown a significant decrease in mortality rate among patients with advanced heart failure treated with PAC guidance in hospitals with large capacity and teaching programmes.

Importance of data interpretation

A major confounder related to the use of PAC is misinterpretation of the haemodynamic data and inaccurate tracing, which may result in mismanagement of the patient.[28,29] Further sources of error include improperly calibrated or levelled monitors, placement of PAC in the non-3-lung zone, overestimation of PCWP by incomplete wedging of the pulmonary artery (PA) branch, or underestimation of PCWP due to damping of pressure curves. Furthermore, there is wide interobserver variability in the interpretation of haemodynamic data, even among intensive care clinicians and anaesthesiologists.

The technical quality of the PCWP tracing is also an important issue. Several previous studies in the United States and Europe have shown that approximately 30% of PCWP recordings were inadequate and about 50% of cases were misinterpreted. Here, training problems are evident regarding the performance of measurements and their interpretation.[30,31,32]

Indications for pulmonary artery catheterization

Regarding indications for PAC (i.e. the Swan–Ganz catheter), it is important to know that no clinical study thus far has shown that outcomes are improved by use of PAC in critically ill patients. The decision to apply PAC should be based on a clear clinical question that cannot be adequately answered by conventional clinical or imaging assessment.[13,33]

What do guidelines recommend for use of PAC in acute heart failure?[13,33,34]

- Insertion of PAC for the diagnosis of acute decompensated heart failure (ADHF) is usually not necessary.
- PAC can be used to differentiate between cardiogenic and non-cardiogenic mechanisms in complex patients with concurrent cardiac and pulmonary disease.

Box 7.4.1 Potential current indications for use of pulmonary artery catheterization

- Not indicated as routine in high-risk cardiac and non-cardiac patients
- Cardiogenic shock during supportive therapy
- Discordant right and left ventricular failure
- Severe chronic heart failure requiring inotropic, vasopressor, and vasodilator therapy
- Suspected 'pseudosepsis'
- Fulminant myocarditis and peripartum cardiomyopathy
- Haemodynamic differential diagnosis of pulmonary hypertension
- Transplantation workup

Table 7.4.1 Normal haemodynamic values

Pressure measurement	Normal value (mmHg)
Right atrium	
Mean pressure	2–8
a wave	3–7
v wave	3–8
Right ventricle	
Peak systolic pressure	17–32
End-diastolic pressure	2–8
Pulmonary artery	
Mean pressure	10–21
Peak systolic pressure	17–32
End-diastolic pressure	4–15
PAWP mean	6–12
Left atrium	
Mean pressure	6–12
a wave	4–14
v wave	6–16
Left ventricle	
Peak systolic pressure	90–140
End-diastolic pressure	5–12
Aorta	
Mean pressure	70–105

- PAC is frequently used to estimate haemodynamic variables and guide therapy in the presence of severe diffuse pulmonary pathology or ongoing haemodynamic compromise not resolved by initial therapy (Class of recommendation 2B, Level of evidence C).

- In patients on the transplant list, PAC is obligatory prior to surgery (Class of recommendation 2, Level of evidence C).

Further potential current indications for use of PAC are summarized in ➲ Box 7.4.1.[34]

Measured intracardiac pressures and interpretation of haemodynamic waveforms

Each cardiac chamber has distinct waveforms reflecting the RV or LV cardiac cycle. PAC allows measurement of pressures and recording of haemodynamic waves in the RA, right ventricle (RV), and PA, as well as measurement of PCWP and CO by the thermodilution technique or the estimated Fick method. The relationship between pressure curves and the electrocardiogram (ECG) is shown in the Wiggers diagram (➲ Figure 7.4.2b).

Right atrial pressure

In healthy subjects, the normal right atrial pressure (RAP) is 2–8 mmHg (➲ Table 7.4.1). The mean RAP is typically lower than the mean PCWP (mPCWP) in healthy hearts as well as in heart failure. The normal RAP waveform contains three peaks (*a*, *c*, and *v*) and two descents (*x*, *y*) (➲ Figure 7.4.4).[34a] The *a* wave occurs at the end of ventricular diastole and is the result of atrial contraction. The *v* wave occurs as a result of venous filling of the atrium during late ventricular systole. The peak of the *a* wave coincides with the point of maximal filling of the RV and is therefore the value that should be used for measurement of right ventricular end-diastolic pressure (RVEDP) (➲ Figure 7.4.2b).

In clinically relevant tricuspid regurgitation, the *v* wave is prominent, with a steep *y* slope—so-called 'ventricularization' of the RAP curve—mostly associated with right heart failure (➲ Figure 7.4.5a). In patients with tricuspid stenosis, the *a* wave is prominent on the RAP tracing (➲ Figure 7.4.5b), similar to LAP

in mitral stenosis (➲ Figure 7.4.5d), showing higher mean RAP (mRAP) than RVEDP.

During spontaneous respiration, RAP declines during inspiration, as intrathoracic pressure falls to the same degree as the decline in intrapleural pressure (approximately <5 mmHg), and generally reflects intrapericardial pressure. The lack of an inspiratory fall, or even a rise, in RAP with inspiration is known as the Kussmaul sign, indicative of RV diastolic dysfunction and RV overload. RAP rises during expiration as intrathoracic pressure increases. The mRAP should be measured at the end of expiration at the mid portion of the *a* wave. When no clear P-wave is present (atrial fibrillation), the pressure should be read from the waveform at the end of the QRS complex.

Right ventricular pressure

The RV is a low-pressure system in the normal heart. In the absence of pulmonary stenosis, RV systolic pressure (17–32 mmHg) correlates well with systolic pulmonary artery pressure (PAP) despite a small gradient (<5 mmHg) between the RV and the PA (➲ Table 7.4.1). In the absence of relevant tricuspid stenosis or regurgitation, RVEDP (2–8 mmHg) should also correlate significantly with mRAP.

The RV pressure (RVP) waveform is similar in morphology to the LV pressure (LVP) waveform. The durations of systole and isovolumic contraction and relaxation are shorter in the

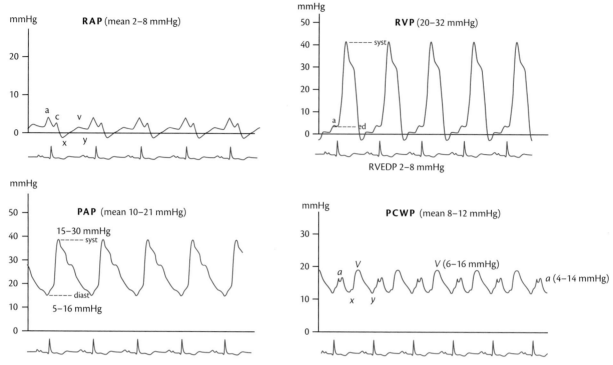

Figure 7.4.4 Normal haemodynamic values and examples of normal pressure waveforms in the right atrium (RAP), right ventricle (RVP), pulmonary artery (PAP), and pulmonary capillary wedge position (PCWP). Note that pressure curves of RAP and RVP illustrate that the position of the pressure transducer is incorrect, above the phlebostatic axis. Diastolic RVP is below the zero line, leading to lower pressure values of a few mmHg. RVEDP, right ventricular end-diastolic pressure.

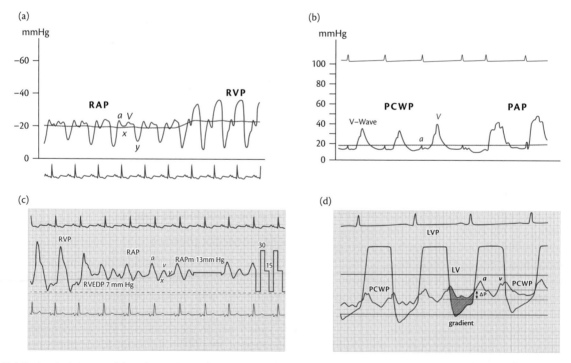

Figure 7.4.5 Ventricularization of the right atrial pressure (RAP) tracing in (a) a patient with severe right ventricular (RV) failure with elevated RV end-diastolic pressure (RVEDP), decreased systolic RV pressure (RVP), and severe tricuspid regurgitation; and (b) a patient with tricuspid stenosis with a transvalvular gradient of about 6 mmHg and prominent *a* wave, *a* > *v*. (c) Prominent *v* wave in mitral regurgitation showing *v* > *a* and mean pulmonary capillary wedge pressure (mPCWP) > pulmonary artery pressure (PAP) diastolic pressure. (d) Prominent *a* wave in mitral stenosis. Simultaneous recording of left ventricular pressure (LVP) and PCWP tracings showing transvalvular pressure gradient between mPCWP and left ventricular end-diastolic pressure (LVEDP).

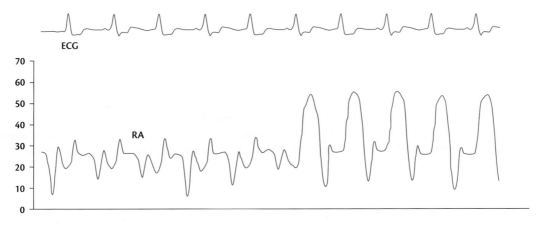

Figure 7.4.6 'Dip plateau' phenomenon in a patient with restrictive cardiomyopathy demonstrating rapid filling in early diastole and abrupt cessation of flow during mid and late diastole.

RV than in the LV. RV diastolic pressure is characterized by an early, rapid-filling wave, followed by a slow-filling phase and the *a* wave at the end of diastole after atrial systolic contraction. RVEDP is generally measured after the *a* wave at the onset of RV isovolumic contraction. The 'dip plateau' phenomenon in RV pressure curves is indicative of early, rapid diastolic filling and abrupt cessation of RV inflow, as commonly found in constrictive pericarditis, restrictive cardiomyopathies, RV infarction, and advanced heart failure with reduced ejection fraction (HFrEF) (➲ Figure 7.4.6).

An elevated systolic RVP usually indicates preserved RV function, whereas a decline in systolic RVP reflects reduced RV contractility. A diagnosis of RV failure should be considered if the systolic RVP is low while the RAP is elevated (>15 mmHg) and the CI is low (<2.0 mL/min/m²).

Pulmonary artery pressure

PAP is influenced by flow, LAP, and PVR, as well as by many additional factors such as stroke volume (SV), heart rate, shunts, cross-sectional area of pulmonary vessels, and pulmonary vessel distensibility (➲ Figure 7.4.3). The normal value for systolic pressure in healthy subjects is 15–30 mmHg, and for diastolic pressure 5–16 mmHg (➲ Table 7.4.1). The peak of the PA wave occurs within the T-wave on a surface ECG (➲ Figure 7.4.2b).

Left heart failure, excessive PVR, or extreme volume overload may yield subsequent PH with elevated PAP. Several studies have shown that normal mPAP at rest is 14 ± 3 mmHg. The upper limit of the normal range is defined as mPAP plus two standard deviations, resulting in a value of 20.6 mmHg.[35] Pulmonary arterial hypertension (PAH) is defined as an increase in mPAP by ≥25 mmHg and mPCWP <15 mmHg, whereas the NIZZA group 2 defined PH as left heart disease with mPAP ≥25 mmHg and PCWP >15 mmHg.[7,36] Up to 60% of patients with severe systolic heart failure and up to 70% with isolated diastolic dysfunction develop PH. Borderline mPAP values are between 21 and 25 mmHg. By definition, mPAP of >21 mmHg is not normal. About 2.5% of a control population have mPAP values in the grey zone between 21 and 25 mmHg without clinical symptoms.[7]

Diastolic PAP is normally 2–3 mmHg higher than mPCWP. When PVR is elevated, the gap between diastolic PAP and mPCWP exceeds 5 mmHg (PAH, acute respiratory distress syndrome, hypoxia, pulmonary embolism).

Pulmonary capillary wedge pressure

The PCWP waveform, with *a* and *v* waves and *x* and *y* descents, is similar to the RAP and LAP waveforms, but it is slightly damped and delayed as a result of transmission through the lungs. PCWP, which is a surrogate for LAP, correlates well with LAP and LVEDP; hence, it represents preload and can be obtained by inflation of the balloon on the tip of the PA catheter. In normal healthy subjects, PCWP is <12 mmHg and 2–7 mmHg below mPAP (➲ Table 7.4.1).

The PCWP is different in patients with acute and chronic heart failure. In acute heart failure, for instance with rupture of papillary muscles or in acute myocardial infarction, a sudden increase in PCWP to 17–20 mmHg can lead to acute lung oedema, whereas patients with chronic heart failure often need an mPCWP of 17–20 mmHg to optimize haemodynamic filling. PCWP must be measured at the end of expiration, negating the effects of alveolar pressure.[37,38] The mPCWP is measured at the mid portion of the *a* wave; in the absence of a P-wave, the pressure should be read from the end of the QRS complex.

The PCWP waveform in heart failure is often characterized by a prominent *v* wave, as can be seen in clinically relevant mitral regurgitation and in states with reduced LV and LA compliance, for example in heart failure with preserved ejection fraction (HFpEF) (➲ Figure 7.4.5c). In this setting, the calculated mPCWP will be elevated and higher than diastolic PAP and may overestimate LVEDP. The presence of a large *v* wave on the PCWP tracing may be misleading and confused with the PA tracing. PAP usually starts at the end of the QRS and peaks at the level of the T-wave, whereas the PCWP *v* wave starts later, after the QRS, and peaks after the T-wave (➲ Figure 7.4.2b).

Left atrial pressure

LAP is usually measured indirectly through balloon occlusion of the distal branch of the PA. The LAP waveforms also can be measured directly by transseptal puncture. Normal LAP values range between 2 and 12 mmHg. Like PCWP and RAP, LAP consists of positive a, c, and v waves and negative x and y descents (➲ Figure 7.4.2b).

Left ventricular pressure

The waveforms of LVP are similar to those of RVP despite higher systolic pressure values. Normal systolic LVP ranges from 90 to 140 mmHg, and 5–12 mmHg during diastole. The mitral valve closes when the LVP exceeds the LAP, and the aortic valve opens when the LVP exceeds the pressure in the aorta during systole. When the LVP declines below the LAP, the mitral valve opens and starts the rapid LV filling phase. LV diastole consists of three phases: an early phase (occurring with opening of the mitral valve); a slow-filling phase (until the onset of LA systole); and an end-diastolic phase after the a wave occurs (the nadir in pressure following the a wave).

The LVEDP reflects the LV preload and is frequently used in the assessment of LV performance. LVEDP does not allow differentiation between systolic and diastolic dysfunction but does give some information about the preload required to obtain an adequate CO. The LVEDP is influenced mainly by myocardial contractility, intravascular status, and LV compliance (➲ Figure 7.4.3).

Calculated or derived haemodynamic parameters

Cardiac output and cardiac index

The two most commonly used methods for measuring CO in clinical practice are the thermodilution method[39] and the Fick principle.[40] Both methods, due to some limitations and physiological assumptions, have advantages and disadvantages that depend on certain haemodynamic situations.

The thermodilution method, known as the indicator dilution method, requires a rapidly administered injection of 10 mL of cold saline at a known temperature (2–5°C) into the proximal port of the catheter in the RA. The subsequent change in temperature of the saline solution is measured by a thermistor at the distal end of the PA catheter. Bolus injection time should be under 4 seconds. The computer-assisted calculation of CO is based on an equation that considers the calibration factor, temperature of the injectate, injected volume, and specific gravity of the blood. The change in temperature over time can be plotted by Fourier analysis. The CO is inversely related to the area under the curve (AUC). A larger AUC reflects a lower CO; vice versa, a smaller AUC is indicative of a higher CO. Normal values for CO are 4–8 L/min, and for CI 2.5–4.5 L/min/m². A CI of <1 L/min/m² is generally incompatible with life.

In new-onset acute heart failure, the CI is low, usually <2.2 L/min/m², which leads to cardiogenic shock. In contrast, in patients with chronic heart failure who are adapted to a low CI by increasing oxygen (O_2) extraction in peripheral tissue, a low CI of 1.0–1.5 L/min/m² is not accompanied by cardiogenic shock. The CO measured by the thermodilution method overestimates flow in patients with low output states; as CO declines, the accuracy of thermodilution CO declines.[41] Thermodilution is most

accurate when used in high-output states. Under ideal conditions, thermodilution can determine CO within an error range of 5–20%. In patients with severe tricuspid regurgitation, the thermodilution technique is not highly accurate,[42,43] but it is useful in this setting and comparable to the Fick principle.[44]

The Fick principle is based on the calculation of oxygen consumption (VO_2) divided by the arteriovenous oxygen saturation difference ($SaO_2 - SvO_2$).[40] While haemoglobin, arterial O_2 saturation, and mixed venous O_2 saturation in the PA are measured directly, most catheterization laboratories assume an average value (e.g. 125 mL/min/m²) as uniform, normalized VO_2 for every patient ('assumed Fick'); others recommend derived empirical formulae to estimate VO_2.[45,46] This is a disadvantage of the Fick method, because corrections for metabolic state, age, and sex are generally not made and errors in VO_2 can be as high as 50%, which leads to falsely elevated CO and CI in patients with severe heart failure. Even under the best conditions, the error using the assumed Fick method is generally 10–15%. Several recent studies have shown a modest, but significant, correlation between Fick and thermodilution measurements of CO. If haemoglobin, venous O_2 saturation (SvO_2), and VO_2 are accurately estimated, the Fick method is more accurate than the thermodilution method in patients with low CO. Accurate measurement of CO is essential for calculation of haemodynamic parameters and optimal pharmacological management.

The CI, PVR, PVR index (PVRi), systemic vascular resistance (SVR), SVR index (SVRi), and TPG can be calculated using the following equations and parameters:

$$\text{Mean arterial pressure, MAP} = SBP + [DBP \times 2])/3 \text{ (mmHg)}$$

$$\text{Body surface area (DuBois formula), BSA} = W^{0.425} \times H^{0.725} \times 0.007184 \text{ (m}^2)$$

$$\text{Pulmonary vascular resistance, PVR} = (80 \times [mPAP - PAWP])/CO \text{ (dyn}\bullet\text{sec}\bullet\text{cm}^{-5})$$

$$\text{PVR index, PVRi} = PVR/BSA \text{ (dyn}\bullet\text{sec}\bullet\text{cm}^{-5}\bullet\text{m}^{-2})$$

$$\text{Systemic vascular resistance, SVR} = (80 \times (MAP - mRAP])/CO \text{ (dyn}\bullet\text{sec}\bullet\text{cm}^{-5})$$

$$\text{SVR index, SVRi} = SVR/BSA \text{ (dyn}\bullet\text{sec}\bullet\text{cm}^{-5}\bullet\text{m}^{-2})$$

$$\text{Fick cardiac output, CO} = (VO_2 \times BSA)/(Hb \times 1.36 \times 10[SaO_2 - SvO_2]) \text{ (L/min)}$$

$$\text{Cardiac index, CI} = CO/BSA \text{ (L/min/m}^2)$$

$$\text{Transpulmonary gradient, TPG} = mPAP - mPAWP \text{ (mmHg)}$$

Mixed venous oxygen saturation

SvO_2 is a marker of adequacy of peripheral organ perfusion and a useful surrogate parameter to monitor disease progression. Pulmonary artery SvO_2 (normal value 75%) decreases when oxygen delivery falls due to reduced CO or tissue O_2 demand increases. In heart failure patients, SvO_2 is usually decreased, depending on disease severity, to values of between 30% and 60%. There is a direct correlation between SvO_2 and CO, haemoglobin, and SaO_2, and an inverse correlation with the metabolic rate.

Transpulmonary gradient and pulmonary vascular resistance

The TPG is the difference between mPAP and mPCWP, whereas PVR is TPG divided by CO.

$$PVR = (mPAP - mPCWP)/CO \text{ (Wood units)}$$

In patients with long-standing post-capillary PH due to left heart failure, a TPG of >15 mmHg or PVR of >3 Wood units reflects pulmonary vascular remodelling, and these patients should undergo vasoreactivity testing if they are on the transplant list. A PVR of >5 Wood units and a negative vasoreactivity test are an absolute contraindication to heart transplantation, due to increased risk of RV failure of the donor heart.

Right ventricular stroke work and right ventricular stroke work index

RV stroke work (RVSW) and RVSW index (RVSWI) are sensitive haemodynamic surrogates of RV function. They are calculated by using mPAP, mRAP, and SV:

$$RVSW = (mPAP - mRAP) \times SV \times 0.0136 \text{ (g/beat)}$$

$$RVSWI = (mPAP - mRAP) \times SVI \times 0.136 \text{ (g•m}^2\text{/beat)}$$

The normal value of RVSWI is 5–10 g•m^2/beat. Values of RVSWI of <5 g•m^2/beat, PCWP of >20 mmHg, and VO$_2$ of <14 mL/kg/min are associated with New York Heart Association (NYHA) classes III and IV, and correlate with elevated mortality, the need for ventricular assist device (VAD) implantation, and heart transplantation at 1 year. Right heart failure is associated with low RVSWI and low PAP, and suggests the need for RV support after left ventricular assist device (LVAD) implantation.

Right heart catheterization

The typical PA catheter is 100–110 cm long (with either three or four lumina) and includes proximal and distal ports. The proximal port is approximately 30 cm from the tip that is placed in the RA. It can be used for measuring pressure or for infusions. The distal end of the catheter has a balloon and a port used to measure PAP and PCWP. The thermistor to measure temperature is located 4 cm proximal to the balloon.

Insertion techniques and approach

The PA catheter is inserted using the Seldinger technique under meticulous sterile conditions. After puncture of the vein, a guidewire is inserted. The dilator and sheath are advanced over the wire through a small skin incision. After removal of the dilator, the catheter can be inserted through the sheath. All lumina of the catheter must be flushed with heparinized saline, and the distal (pulmonary arterial) lumen is connected to a pressure transducer. The balloon should be checked for leaks and proper inflation.

Although current guidelines do not dictate a universal access route for insertion of the PA catheter, the medial antecubital vein in anticoagulated patients should be considered as the ideal access. The use of a fluoroscope is helpful in guiding the tip of the catheter into the PA, and it also minimizes the risk of intravascular or intracardiac knotting with other catheters or leads (e.g. central line, pacemaker, defibrillator) that may be present. If the antecubital vein fails, the right internal jugular approach can be used, although the risk of air embolism must be considered when the internal jugular vein or subclavian vein is chosen. The third option is the femoral approach, which has several major shortcomings: the risk of femoral venous thrombosis or bleeding, disruption of patient mobility, and the need for fluoroscopy and greater expertise to position the catheter. Therefore, it is the least recommended approach. Ultrasound-guided puncture helps to reduce the risk of bleeding due to malpuncture of the artery.[47]

Equipment integrity

The ability to obtain high-quality data and to provide appropriate interpretation for the clinical situation is imperative. This includes ensuring proper assembly and integrity of the haemodynamic equipment.

The two most important procedures during RHC are levelling and zeroing. Key aspects are listed as follows:

1. Levelling

The first step at the beginning of RHC is levelling. According to several publications, the zero point, or zero reference level, is generally recommended to be set at the level of the RA or the tricuspid valve.[48] In practice, the most frequently used zero level in the supine patient is at the mid-thoracic level (recommended by European Society of Cardiology (ESC)/European Respiratory Society (ERS) Guidelines PH 2015)[36] or at one-third of the thoracic diameter below the anterior thoracic surface.[35,49] This is the point (called phlebostatic axis) where the blood will have the lowest pressure.

Appropriate positioning of the transducer is critical. A pressure transducer below the level of the RA will overestimate pressures by 1 mmHg for every 1.4 cm. A transducer above the phlebostatic axis of the RA, on the other hand, will underestimate pressures. According to the computed tomography (CT) study performed by Kovacs et al., one-third of the thoracic diameter primarily represents the RA, whereas the LA is represented best by the mid-thoracic level.[35]

2. Zeroing

The PA catheter must be appropriately zeroed to obtain accurate diagnostic information. Zeroing and referencing are done in one step, but they represent two separate processes. Zeroing involves opening the system to the air to establish an atmospheric pressure of zero. Furthermore, zeroing has to be done before each tracing of the pressure curves in order to prevent pressure measurements from being too low or too high. It is advisable to re-zero the transducer whenever there is a shift in the temperature or transducer level.

Further key aspects include positioning (patients in supine/semi-supine position, with the head elevated from 0° to 45°), tubing (stiff and not too long, tightly locked), presser transducer function (confirmed by frequency response curve), and several patient-specific factors (arrhythmias, anxiety, Cheyne–Stokes respiration, etc.).

Practical aspects of right heart catheterization

The PA catheter is passed through the hub of the introducer and advanced, while the pressure at the tip of the catheter is transduced. Continuous pressure monitoring helps confirm the location of the catheter tip.

To avoid atrial and ventricular arrhythmia and to facilitate the passage of the catheter to the PA, the balloon is filled with approximately 1.0–1.5 cc of air when positioned in the superior vena cava. The risk of arrhythmia is greatest while the catheter tip is in the RV. During placement of the catheter, typical pressure curves can be obtained while the catheter is passing from the RA via the RV into the PA and finally into the wedge position in a medium-sized branch of the PA, ideally in zone 3 of the lung below the level of the LA, where the pulmonary capillary pressure exceeds the mean alveolar pressure, which only occurs in 60% of PA catheter insertions.

If a length of >30 cm of the catheter is introduced and the tracing is still consistent with the RV, the catheter may be coiling within the RV. In this case, the balloon should be deflated, the catheter repositioned until the RA waveform appears, and placement reattempted with reinflation of the balloon.

In the pulmonary capillary wedge position, the balloon should not stay inflated for longer than 1–2 minutes because rupture of the vessel or pulmonary infarction may occur. In patients with PH, 10–14 seconds of wedging should not be exceeded. If the wedge tracing persists although the balloon is deflated, the catheter should be withdrawn until the PA tracing curve appears.

To obtain the wedge pressure, careful and gradual inflation of the balloon should be performed while continuous pressure is monitored. Once the pressure waveform shows a change in amplitude and the pressure drops to approximately the diastolic PAP, no additional inflation of the balloon is needed and should be avoided to prevent vascular damage.

If the tip of the catheter is in the small branch in the distal PA, <1 cc is required to reach the wedge position and further inflation can lead to vessel damage and potentially rupture (➲ Figure 7.4.7a).

Once the final desired position is reached and is stable, the catheter should be secured by locking the introducer hub to prevent migration and vessel damage with infarction or rupture.

Pressure tracings

According to the 2015 ESC/ERS Guidelines on PH, PCWP should be measured at end-expiration, where the effects of swings in intrathoracic pressure are minimal.[36] Pressure recordings should be carried out at rest and in slight apnoeic expiration, with the mouth kept open during the measurement to avoid Valsalva pressing (➲ Figure 7.4.7b). The intracardiac pressures should be measured at end-expiration, because at this point pleural and intrathoracic pressures are equal to the atmospheric pressure regardless of the mode of ventilation.

Most intensive care units (ICUs) use electronic pressure monitors that are designed to measure pressure in time intervals of 4 seconds and to display systolic, diastolic, and mean pressure. However, the computer-generated wedge pressure measurement results are consistently and significantly lower than results obtained by measuring PCWP at the end of expiration, with about 30% risk of misclassification of PH.[50]

Inaccurate bedside monitor interpretation frequently occurs in cases with catheter whip (or fling) and underdamping (pressures overestimated), as well as in overdamped curves (pressures underestimated, absence of bounces in square wave test; obstruction, leak, air, long tube). Here the so-called 'square wave test' (or fast flush test) is recommended. A square wave produced by fast flush should quickly return to baseline with one or two bounces after the square wave.[51] A whip artefact, regardless of the source, causes a falsely elevated systolic pressure and a falsely lowered diastolic pressure on the tracing. Many ICU monitors allow manual selection of the PCWP via a cursor to avoid inaccurate monitor reading.

Complications

RHC is a relatively safe diagnostic method but carries a potential risk of minor and major complications related to the access site (introducer-induced bleeding, malpuncture of an artery, infection) and cardiac (arrhythmia and pericardial tamponade) and pulmonary vascular (rupture or severe bleeding, haemothorax) considerations.[52,53]

The most common complications are unsustained atrial and ventricular arrhythmias (in up to 3%) during passage of the catheter through the RA and RV to the PA. Emergency procedures and a defibrillator should be readily available. Right bundle branch block develops in up to 5%, with an increased risk of transient complete atrioventricular (AV) block in patients with pre-existing left bundle branch block.[53,54] In this setting, fluoroscopic guidance is recommended. Knotting of the catheter can occur in patients with a large LA and LV and severe tricuspid regurgitation. In such cases, the catheter can be usually removed transvenously under fluoroscopic guidance, mostly without venotomy.[55]

Major complications are infrequent. The most feared complications are RV and PA rupture,[56] as well as pulmonary infarction requiring surgical management. In some cases of bleeding, direct coil embolization of the lesion is possible. These complications can be avoided by the combined use of fluoroscopic guidance and careful evaluation of the pressure waveform.[57] Risk factors for PA rupture are advanced age, PH, mitral valve disease, and anticoagulation. Pulmonary infarction is caused by migration of the catheter tip or by a balloon left inflated in the wedge position for an extended period.

Minor complications that have been observed include thrombophlebitis (approximately 3%), venous spasm (2%), reversible left or right bundle branch block, atrial fibrillation, and AV block (first-/second-degree; <0.5%).

Despite these complications, flow-guided catheterization remains a valuable tool for individual haemodynamic assessment in selected patients with a diagnostic and therapeutic indication.

(a)

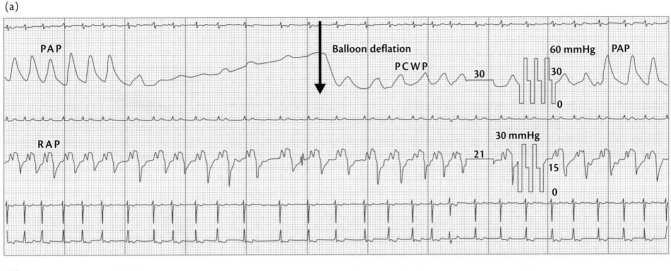

(b)

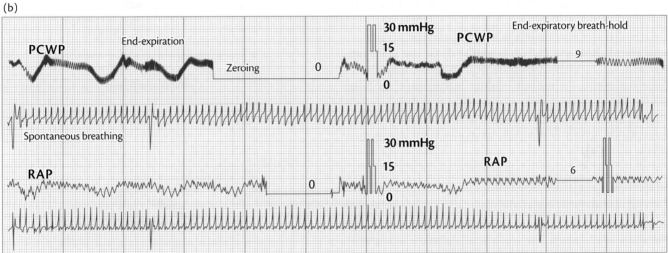

Figure 7.4.7 (a) Example of overwedging. The balloon should not be overinflated in a small branch of the pulmonary artery. Patient with post-capillary pulmonary hypertension, mitral regurgitation (prominent *v* wave), and tricuspid regurgitation (ventricularization of atrial pressure curve). PCWP, post-capillary wedge pressure. (b) Effects of respiratory variations on pulmonary capillary wedge pressure (PCWP) and right atrial pressure (RAP). Measurements of PCWP should performed at end-expiration with slight apnoea.

Exercise right heart catheterization and volume challenge

As the traditional measurement of haemodynamics at rest is of limited benefit in the diagnostic workup of patients with left heart failure, a stress test (exercise or with administration of medication) is used to improve the impact of RHC measurements. In patients with normal resting haemodynamics, but with exertional intolerance or dyspnoea, RHC with exercise or volume challenge plays a key diagnostic role, particularly in the differentiation between primary and secondary PH, HFrEF, and HFpEF. Exercise RHC can unmask PH in patients with heart failure.

Exercise haemodynamics are usually determined in the supine or semi-supine position using a standard bicycle ergometer, with incremental increases in workload by 25 W every 2–3 minutes. Haemodynamics, including PAP, PCWP, and CO, are assessed at rest and at the end of each workload, immediately after exercise, and 6 minutes after the end of exercise. Submaximal exercise

protocols can be used for the diagnosis of HFpEF (e.g. hand grip exercise).

Alternatively, LV diastolic dysfunction at rest can be unmasked with a volume challenge. Infusion of isotonic saline, up to 1–2 L at 100–200 mL/min, can lead to a profound increase in PCWP (up to 10–20 mmHg). Alternatively, volume loading by leg raising provides 250–500 mL of blood volume to the chest within seconds. In general, however, exercise haemodynamic measurements seem to be more sensitive than volume loading for detecting early stages of HFpEF.

Due to a lack of sufficient studies and standardization of exercise protocols, previous guidelines do not address how haemodynamic measurements during exercise should be performed and give no recommendations for the interpretation of exercise haemodynamic data.[36] However, there is a current consensus recommendation on how to diagnose HFpEF, which classifies peak exercise PCWP of >25 mmHg as definite evidence of HFpEF.[58]

In heart failure patients, PVR was shown to decrease during exercise in some studies, but in other studies, PVR remained unchanged or even increased during exercise, particularly in the supine position and when exercise was performed at high workload.[59,60] However, the supine position and mild/moderate exercise allow complete pulmonary vascular recruitment in heart failure patients. In general, PVR declines only slightly.

In normal individuals, PCWP increases during exercise modestly by <20–25 mmHg, and mPAP by <30 mmHg.[61] However, recent studies showed that the rise in PCWP and PAP during exercise increases with age,[62] and 30% of a healthy cohort aged ≥60 years showed an increase in mPCWP values of ≥25 mmHg. When the mPAP rises during exercise above 30 mmHg and PCWP remains below 20 mmHg, exercise-induced PAH should considered.[63] A normal PCWP is frequently measured in patients with HFpEF, especially if the patient is on diuretic therapy, but during exercise, PCWP increases by ≥25 mmHg, unmasking LV diastolic dysfunction.[64]

Recent studies have shown that during exercise, in patients with HFrEF, PAP and PCWP, as well as TPG, rise more rapidly and with a blunted increase in CO, when compared to these parameters in normal, healthy individuals.[65] In heart failure patients, there was a steep increase in PCWP and PAP, with a plateau pattern that demonstrated an inability to augment RVSW, which is indicative of dynamic RV dysfunction (➲ Figure 7.4.8).[65]

Left heart catheterization

Left heart catheterization, including coronary angiography, should be performed as part of the diagnostic workup in patients with suspected heart failure. The objective of coronary angiography is to detect and localize significant coronary artery obstructions as a cause of LV dysfunction, that is, hibernating myocardium. LV angiograms are not routinely necessary, particularly when LV dysfunction is clearly established by magnetic resonance imaging (MRI) or echocardiography. However, LVP measurements may provide valuable additional information on the haemodynamic status and may be an important diagnostic finding in conditions such as constrictive pericarditis.

Indications for coronary angiography

Before patients undergo LV biopsy, the coronary anatomy should be known and may require coronary angiography in the same setting. In younger patients (<60 years) and patients with a low likelihood of CAD, coronary CT may be used to exclude an ischaemic aetiology of LV dysfunction.[66]

Special considerations of left heart catheterization

Left heart catheterization should only be performed when the patient is widely stabilized and recompensated and is able to maintain a supine position for at least 30 minutes. The sterile setting in the catheterization laboratory may be used to extend the procedure to right heart and pulmonary haemodynamic measurements. In special cases of heart failure (e.g. constrictive

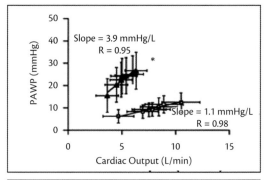

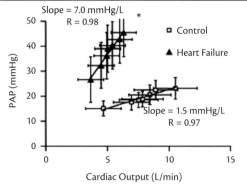

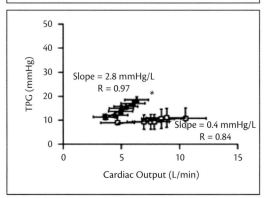

Figure 7.4.8 Relationship between pulmonary capillary wedge pressure (PCWP), mean pulmonary artery pressure (PAP), transpulmonary gradient (TPG), and cardiac output in patients with heart failure and normal controls during incremental exercise.

Reproduced from Lewis GD, Murphy RM, Shah RV, P *et al*. Pulmonary vascular response patterns during exercise in left ventricular systolic dysfunction predict exercise capacity and outcomes. *Circulation Heart Failure*. 2011;4(3):276–85 with permission from Wolters Kluwer.

pericarditis), simultaneous right and left heart catheterization may be decisive for therapeutic management or at least supplementary to echocardiographic findings.

The radial route is the preferred arterial access for catheterization. The amount of contrast medium should be reduced to a minimum (<40 mL) to avoid volume overload and reduce renal toxicity. Many patients with heart failure present with some degree of renal dysfunction, which requires prior hydration therapy to avoid contrast-induced nephropathy. However, in patients with congestive heart failure, intravenous infusions before and after contrast application have to be closely monitored to avoid pulmonary oedema due to acute volume overload. If the glomerular filtration rate is <30 mL/min, the indication and potential information benefit of a coronary angiogram should be critically evaluated, and other less nephrotoxic imaging modalities should be considered (e.g. scintigraphy, MRI).

An LV angiogram is, in most cases, dispensable when a good-quality echocardiogram or MRI is available. MRI provides valuable information on myocardial function and structure. However, it may be useful to measure the LV filling pressure through a pigtail catheter, which gives insights into LV haemodynamics (➲ Figure 7.4.3).

Left heart catheterization under special conditions

In special phenotypes of heart failure, coronary angiography and LVP measurements provide unique diagnostic information.

Aortic stenosis

The assessment of aortic stenosis can usually be performed reliably by echocardiography. Retrograde passage of the aortic valve for diagnostic reasons is not routinely necessary and should be performed by experienced operators.

Aortic regurgitation

Non-invasive imaging is usually sufficient for evaluation. If results are conflicting, aortography can be useful to assess the grade of regurgitation.

Mitral valve stenosis

Simultaneous measurements of PCWP and LVEDP may be obtained to invasively calculate the valve area when echocardiography findings are inconclusive (➲ Figure 7.4.5d).

Mitral regurgitation

Transoesophageal echocardiography is the gold standard method for assessing and localizing mitral regurgitation. An LV angiogram is usually not necessary. PCWP measurements may be helpful to confirm major valve insufficiency in terms of a prominent *v* wave (➲ Figure 7.4.5a).

Hypertrophic obstructive cardiomyopathy

Intraventricular pressure gradients may be assessed by simultaneous pressure measurements in the aorta and LV apex at rest and after extrasystoles (➲ Figure 7.4.9).

Shunt measurements

If a shunt (congenital or post-infarction) is considered to cause heart failure, staged O_2 saturation measurements and haemodynamics play a pivotal role in the assessment and for developing a therapeutic strategy.

Left ventricular pressure–volume loops

The most elegant method to study ventricular contractility, which is represented by the relationship between LV volume and pressure changes during the cardiac cycle, is the analysis of pressure–volume (PV) loops. Ranging from the very early experimental description of the cardiac cycle by Otto Frank in 1985,[67] to the first real-time measurements in *ex vivo* perfused hearts by Suga and Sagawa,[68] to the development of the conductance catheter for (human) *in vivo* studies by Baan *et al.*,[69] the PV loop analysis is the best direct method to assess myocardial contractility for *in vivo* situations.[70,71] In addition, the conductance catheter allows acquisition of segmental PV loops from the LV apex to the base.[72] By summation of the segmental loops, it is possible to obtain a total

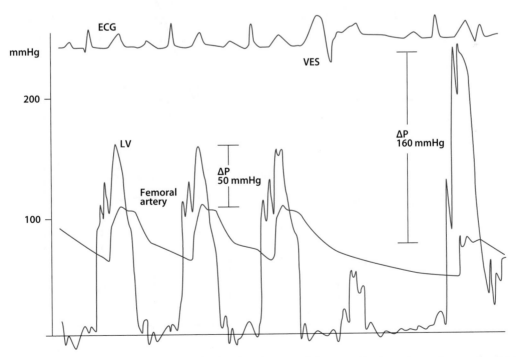

Figure 7.4.9 Simultaneous recording of left ventricular pressure (LVP) and aortic pressure in hypertrophic obstructive cardiomyopathy demonstrating delta P increase from 50 mmHg at rest to 160 mmHg after ventricular extrasystole (VES) (Brockenbrough phenomenon).

volume calculation over the entire cardiac cycle. PV loops depend on changes in preload, afterload, and LV contractility.

Most recently, advanced algorithms allow for a more convenient readout of PV studies, including single-beat acquisition for the determination of end-systolic and end-diastolic PV relationships. This has resulted in more frequent use of the conductance catheter in the catheterization laboratory to study cardiac haemodynamics in the clinical scenario of heart failure, in different types of mechanical circulatory support, in relation to (catheter-based) valve repair or replacement, and for the assessment of LV dyssynchrony. In addition, PV loop analysis is used for assessment of load-independent contractility.[70,73,74]

The schematic of a PV loop in a normal heart is depicted in ⊃ Figure 7.4.10. Following mitral opening, the LV fills and increases its volume, with only a minor increase in LVP. Systole begins with isovolumetric contraction, followed by aortic valve opening, marking the beginning of the ejection period with a decline in volume, while the pressure further increases. After closure of the aortic valve, isovolumetric relaxation occurs, characterized by a rapid decline in pressure with stable volume.

Left ventricular end-systolic pressure–volume relationship

The end-systolic pressure–volume relationship (ESPVR) characterizes the inotropic property of the LV during systole. It is almost linear within the physiological range of end-systolic pressure and volumes. The slope of the ESPVR, that is, the end-systolic elastance (Ees), represents the peak chamber elastance during a

heartbeat and reflects ventricular chamber mechanical properties when there is a maximum number of actin–myosin bonds. Ees decreases in response to negative inotropic drugs, such as beta-blockers or calcium channel blockers, and also with myocardial ischaemia or infarction or intraventricular dyssynchrony. On the other hand, Ees increases with sympathetic activation or in response to inotropes such as dobutamine or levosimendan. Ees, as a measure of LV contractility, is relatively load-independent (⊃ Figure 7.4.10).

Left ventricular end-diastolic pressure–volume relationship

The end-diastolic pressure–volume relationship (EDPVR) is a non-linear relationship that characterizes the diastolic properties of the LV when all actin–myosin bonds have been severed. Thus, the EDPVR is determined by a combination of cardiomyocyte size and extracellular matrix. Ischaemia, oedema, fibrosis, and remodelling processes affect the relaxation characteristics of the LV that are characterized by the EDPVR. The slope of the EDPVR (dp/dV) is an index of chamber stiffness, and compliance is the inverse of stiffness (dV/dp). Thus, with increasing stiffness, there is a leftward shift of the EDPVR (⊃ Figure 7.4.10).

The rate of the relaxation process is also an important parameter of LV performance. During isovolumetric relaxation, the rate of pressure decline is characterized by an exponential time constant of decay (τ), which is the time required for the pressure to fall by 50%. A normal value of τ is 20–30 ms, whereas in the

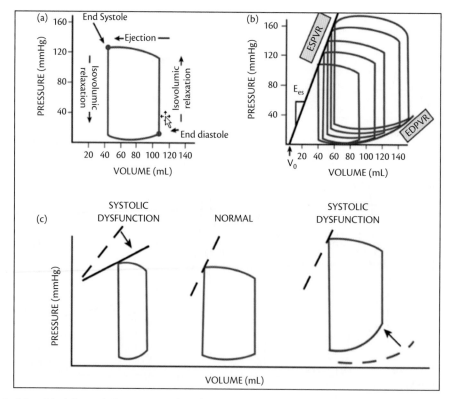

Figure 7.4.10 General principles of the left ventricular pressure–volume loop.
Reproduced from Felker G, Mann D. *Heart Failure: A Companion to Braunwald's Heart Disease.* 4th ed. Philadelphia: Elsevier; 2020 with permission from Elsevier.

setting of LV hypertrophy, τ is prolonged to 70–100 ms. This leads to impaired filling, especially at higher heart rates.

Ventricular–arterial coupling

Ventricular–arterial coupling (VAC) describes the matching between ventricular and vascular properties. The effective arterial elastance (Ea) is the ratio between the end-systolic pressure and the SV, which is determined by the total peripheral resistance and the heart rate. Thus, Ea is the slope of the line connecting V_{ED} on the volume axis to the end-systolic point on the PV loop. The ratio between Ea and Ees is known as the index of VAC and has a normal value of approximately 0.6.

In HFrEF, Ea increases and Ees decreases, so that Ea/Ees increases, reflecting ventricular–arterial mismatch. On the other hand, age and hypertension lead to an increase in Ea and Ees, resulting in normal or only slightly elevated Ea/Ees. Finally, with exercise in healthy individuals, Ees increases, but Ea decreases, thus leading to a decrease in Ea/Ees that may suggest more efficient energy transfer from the LV to the peripheral circulation.[75,76,77]

Interpretation of pressure–volume loop tracings

By changing the preload (e.g. by using transient inferior vena cava occlusion) or the afterload (e.g. by administration of phenylephrine), a family of loops is obtained (➲ Figure 7.4.10). The EDPVR, which is constructed by connecting the end-diastolic PV points of each loop, is non-linear and defines the passive physical properties of the chamber, with the myocardium in its most relaxed state. The ESPVR, constructed by connecting the end-systolic PV points of each loop, defines a reasonably linear relationship that characterizes properties of the chamber, with the myocardium in a state of maximal activation at a given contractile state.

An important difference between HFrEF and HFpEF patients can be found within these PV loops: HFrEF is characterized by decreased contractility and downward and rightward displacement of the ESPVR, whereas HFpEF is characterized by preserved global contractility, but impaired LV relaxation, elevated filling pressures, and increased stiffness, with an upward and leftward shift of the EDPVR, representing raised LVEDP at any given LV end-diastolic volume. This steep EDPVR in patients with HFpEF seems to be the most important determinant for impaired exercise tolerance, with deficient early diastolic recoil, blunted lusitropic or chronotropic response, vasodilator incompetence, and disturbed ventricular–vascular coupling serving contributory roles. Elevated LV filling pressures constitute the hallmark of diastolic LV dysfunction, and filling pressures are considered elevated when the mPCWP is >12 mmHg or when the LVEDP is >16 mmHg.

Technical issues of left ventricular pressure–volume loop measurement

The most important step in PV loop analysis is accurate volume calibration of the catheter prior to the investigation. This can be done usually by using standard pre-procedure measurements of LV end-diastolic volume, together with either SV or ejection fraction determination by echocardiography, CT, or MRI. Since this pre-procedural imaging assumes that cardiac chamber dimensions remain constant between the time of imaging and invasive measurements, these procedures should be closely coordinated. A different method is the combination of hypertonic saline infusion into the PA or RA to determine parallel conductance and thermodilution SV. Importantly, volume calibration has to be repeated in the event of significant bleeding (i.e. a change in haematocrit). In addition, repeated pressure calibration is essential in order to avoid a pressure drift between the beginning and the end of the procedure.

Exercise haemodynamic measurements obtained during PV loop assessment do not differ from exercise haemodynamics assessed during RHC assessment (see earlier). They are usually obtained in the supine position; some academic laboratories have the technical expertise to perform upright studies and concomitant measurement of O_2 consumption (e.g. metabolic cart). It is reasonable to: (1) start at a low level of exercise; (2) titrate upwards at fixed intervals until symptoms appear; and (3) measure haemodynamics at rest, peak exercise, and, if possible, after each stage. During exercise, there can be dramatic fluctuations in intracardiac pressures secondary to wide swings in intrathoracic pressures. Thus, measurements should be made at end-expiration. Heart rate response should also be noted since chronotropic incompetence may be more relevant than the haemodynamic response as an explanation for exertional intolerance.

Volume challenge can also be used to assess diastolic compliance and may unmask occult pulmonary venous hypertension when PH is present. Selective volume loading of the LV can also be accomplished by administering selective pulmonary vasodilators (e.g. inhaled nitric oxide) if there is increased PVR and normal PCWP or LVEDP.

Percutaneous coronary intervention and coronary artery bypass grafting in patients with reduced left ventricular function

If significant CAD of major vessels is documented by the coronary angiogram and LV dysfunction can be attributed, at least in part, to hibernation of viable myocardium, revascularization is indicated. LV function may improve considerably after revascularization.[78]

Future directions

Further development of algorithm-supported interpretation of pressure tracings is likely to allow faster, and sometimes more reliable, assessment of haemodynamic values.

Key messages

- Most information derived from PAC or RHC cannot be predicted by clinical examination.
- Invasive haemodynamic evaluation by flow-guided PAC is indicated when clinical assessment and imaging do not sufficiently explain the aetiology of heart failure.
- It is critical to interpret values with an understanding of the underlying pathophysiology.

- Monitoring without an effective treatment plan will not improve survival.
- PV loop analysis can help to dissect VAC, stiffness, and indices of contractility.
- Left heart catheterization and coronary and structural interventions provide direct treatment approaches.

References

1. Chakko S, Woska D, Martinez H, et al. Clinical, radiographic, and hemodynamic correlations in chronic congestive heart failure: conflicting results may lead to inappropriate care. Am J Med. 1991;90(3):353–9.

2. Ware LB, Matthay MA. Clinical practice. Acute pulmonary edema. N Engl J Med. 2005;353(26):2788–96.

3. Harris P, Heath D. Pulmonary edema. In: Harris P, Heath D. *The Human Pulmonary Circulation*, 3rd edition. New York, NY: Churchill Livingstone; 1986, pp. 373–83.

4. Guyton AC. *Textbook of Medical Physiology*, 7th edition. Philadelphia, PA: Saunders; 1986.

5. Staub NC. Pulmonary edema. Physiol Rev. 1974;54(3):678–811.

6. Flores ED, Lange RA, Hillis LD. Relation of mean pulmonary arterial wedge pressure and left ventricular end-diastolic pressure. Am J Cardiol. 1990;66(20):1532–3.

7. Rosenkranz S, Gibbs JS, Wachter R, De Marco T, Vonk-Noordegraaf A, Vachiéry JL. Left ventricular heart failure and pulmonary hypertension. Eur Heart J. 2016;37(12):942–54.

8. Dixon DL, Mayne GC, Griggs KM, De Pasquale CG, Bersten AD. Chronic elevation of pulmonary microvascular pressure in chronic heart failure reduces bi-directional pulmonary fluid flux. Eur J Heart Fail. 2013;15(4):368–75.

9. Huang W, Kingsbury MP, Turner MA, Donnelly JL, Flores NA, Sheridan DJ. Capillary filtration is reduced in lungs adapted to chronic heart failure: morphological and haemodynamic correlates. Cardiovasc Res. 2001;49(1):207–17.

10. Townsley MI, Fu Z, Mathieu-Costello O, West JB. Pulmonary microvascular permeability. Responses to high vascular pressure after induction of pacing-induced heart failure in dogs. Circ Res. 1995;77(2):317–25.

11. Chatterjee K, Swan HJ, Ganz W, et al. Use of a balloon-tipped flotation electrode catheter for cardiac mounting. Am J Cardiol. 1975;36(1):56–61.

12. Gheorghiade M, Follath F, Ponikowski P, et al. Assessing and grading congestion in acute heart failure: a scientific statement from the Acute Heart Failure Committee of the Heart Failure Association of the European Society of Cardiology and endorsed by the European Society of Intensive Care Medicine. Eur J Heart Fail. 2010;12(5):423–33.

13. Mueller HS, Chatterjee K, Davis KB, et al. ACC expert consensus document. Present use of bedside right heart catheterization in patients with cardiac disease. American College of Cardiology. J Am Coll Cardiol. 1998;32(3):840–64.

14. Swan HJ, Ganz W, Forrester J, Marcus H, Diamond G, Chonette D. Catheterization of the heart in man with use of a flow-directed balloon-tipped catheter. N Engl J Med. 1970;283(9):447–51.

15. Connors AF Jr, McCaffree DR, Gray BA. Evaluation of right-heart catheterization in the critically ill patient without acute myocardial infarction. N Engl J Med. 1983;308(5):263–7.

16. Ivanov R, Allen J, Calvin JE. The incidence of major morbidity in critically ill patients managed with pulmonary artery catheters: a meta-analysis. Crit Care Med. 2000;28(3):615–19.

17. Sandham JD, Hull RD, Brant RF, et al. A randomized, controlled trial of the use of pulmonary-artery catheters in high-risk surgical patients. N Engl J Med. 2003;348(1):5–14.

18. Yu DT, Platt R, Lanken PN, et al. Relationship of pulmonary artery catheter use to mortality and resource utilization in patients with severe sepsis. Crit Care Med. 2003;31(12):2734–41.

19. Forssmann W. Die Sondierung des rechten Herzens. Klin Wochenschr. 1929;8:2085.

20. Connors AF Jr, Speroff T, Dawson NV, et al. The effectiveness of right heart catheterization in the initial care of critically ill patients. SUPPORT Investigators. JAMA. 1996;276(11):889–97.

21. Fonarow G, Stevenson L, Steimle A, et al. Persistently high left-ventricular filling pressures predict mortality despite angiotensin-converting enzyme-inhibition in advanced heart-failure. Circulation. 1994;90:1–488.

22. Binanay C, Califf RM, Hasselblad V, et al. Evaluation study of congestive heart failure and pulmonary artery catheterization effectiveness: the ESCAPE trial. JAMA. 2005;294(13):1625–33.

23. Harvey S, Harrison DA, Singer M, et al. Assessment of the clinical effectiveness of pulmonary artery catheters in management of patients in intensive care (PAC-Man): a randomised controlled trial. Lancet. 2005;366(9484):472–7.

24. Dalen JE, Bone RC. Is it time to pull the pulmonary artery catheter? JAMA. 1996;276(11):916–18.

25. Robin ED. Death by pulmonary artery flow-directed catheter. Time for a moratorium? Chest. 1987;92(4):727–31.

26. Rose H, Venn R. Recently published papers: dying swans and other stories. Crit Care. 2006;10(4):152.

27. Shah MR, Hasselblad V, Stevenson LW, et al. Impact of the pulmonary artery catheter in critically ill patients: meta-analysis of randomized clinical trials. JAMA. 2005;294(13):1664–70.

28. Komadina KH, Schenk DA, LaVeau P, Duncan CA, Chambers SL. Interobserver variability in the interpretation of pulmonary artery catheter pressure tracings. Chest. 1991;100(6):1647–54.

29. Squara P, Bennett D, Perret C. Pulmonary artery catheter: does the problem lie in the users? Chest. 2002;121(6):2009–15.

30. Beller GA, Bonow RO, Fuster V. ACCF 2008 Recommendations for Training in Adult Cardiovascular Medicine Core Cardiology Training (COCATS 3) (revision of the 2002 COCATS Training Statement). J Am Coll Cardiol. 2008;51(3):335–8.

31. Iberti TJ, Fischer EP, Leibowitz AB, Panacek EA, Silverstein JH, Albertson TE. A multicenter study of physicians' knowledge of the pulmonary artery catheter. Pulmonary Artery Catheter Study Group. JAMA. 1990;264(22):2928–32.

32. Papadakos PJ, Vender JS. Training requirements for pulmonary artery catheter utilization in adult patients. New Horiz. 1997;5(3):287–91.

33. [No authors listed]. Pulmonary Artery Catheter Consensus conference: consensus statement. Crit Care Med. 1997;25(6):910–25.

34. Chatterjee K. The Swan–Ganz catheters: past, present, and future. A viewpoint. Circulation. 2009;119(1):147–52.

34a. Stouffer GA, Klein L, McLaughlin DP. *Cardiovascular Hemodynamics for the Clinician*, 2nd edition. Wiley; 2017.

35. Kovacs G, Avian A, Olschewski A, Olschewski H. Zero reference level for right heart catheterisation. Eur Respir J. 2013;42(6):1586–94.

36. Galiè N, Humbert M, Vachiery JL, et al. 2015 ESC/ERS Guidelines for the diagnosis and treatment of pulmonary hypertension: the Joint Task Force for the Diagnosis and Treatment of Pulmonary Hypertension of the European Society of Cardiology (ESC) and the European Respiratory Society (ERS): Endorsed by: Association for European Paediatric and Congenital Cardiology (AEPC), International Society for Heart and Lung Transplantation (ISHLT). Eur Heart J. 2016;37(1):67–119.

37. Berryhill RE, Benumof JL, Rauscher LA. Pulmonary vascular pressure reading at the end of exhalation. Anesthesiology. 1978;49(5):365–8.

38. O'Quin R, Marini JJ. Pulmonary artery occlusion pressure: clinical physiology, measurement, and interpretation. Am Rev Respir Dis. 1983;128(2):319–26.

39. Forrester JS, Ganz W, Diamond G, McHugh T, Chonette DW, Swan HJ. Thermodilution cardiac output determination with a single flow-directed catheter. Am Heart J. 1972;83(3):306–11.

40. Fagard R, Conway J. Measurement of cardiac output: Fick principle using catheterization. Eur Heart J. 1990;11 Suppl I:1–5.

41. Van Grondelle A, Ditchey RV, Groves BM, Wagner WW Jr, Reeves JT. Thermodilution method overestimates low cardiac output in humans. Am J Physiol. 1983;245(4):H690–2.

42. Cigarroa RG, Lange RA, Williams RH, Bedotto JB, Hillis LD. Underestimation of cardiac output by thermodilution in patients with tricuspid regurgitation. Am J Med. 1989;86(4):417–20.

43. Konishi T, Nakamura Y, Morii I, Himura Y, Kumada T, Kawai C. Comparison of thermodilution and Fick methods for measurement of cardiac output in tricuspid regurgitation. Am J Cardiol. 1992;70(4):538–9.

44. Hoeper MM, Maier R, Tongers J, et al. Determination of cardiac output by the Fick method, thermodilution, and acetylene rebreathing in pulmonary hypertension. Am J Respir Crit Care Med. 1999;160(2):535–41.

45. Bergstra A, van Dijk RB, Hillege HL, Lie KI, Mook GA. Assumed oxygen consumption based on calculation from dye dilution cardiac output: an improved formula. Eur Heart J. 1995;16(5):698–703.

46. LaFarge CG, Miettinen OS. The estimation of oxygen consumption. Cardiovasc Res. 1970;4(1):23–30.

47. Ortega R, Song M, Hansen CJ, Barash P. Videos in clinical medicine. Ultrasound-guided internal jugular vein cannulation. N Engl J Med. 2010;362(16):e57.

48. Summerhill EM, Baram M. Principles of pulmonary artery catheterization in the critically ill. Lung. 2005;183(3):209–19.

49. Bridges EJ, Woods SL. Pulmonary artery pressure measurement: state of the art. Heart Lung. 1993;22(2):99–111.

50. Ryan JJ, Rich JD, Thiruvoipati T, Swamy R, Kim GH, Rich S. Current practice for determining pulmonary capillary wedge pressure predisposes to serious errors in the classification of patients with pulmonary hypertension. Am Heart J. 2012;163(4):589–94.

51. Kleinman B, Powell S, Kumar P, Gardner RM. The fast flush test measures the dynamic response of the entire blood pressure monitoring system. Anesthesiology. 1992;77(6):1215–20.

52. Coulter TD, Wiedemann HP. Complications of hemodynamic monitoring. Clin Chest Med. 1999;20(2):249–67, vii.

53. Sprung CL, Elser B, Schein RM, Marcial EH, Schrager BR. Risk of right bundle-branch block and complete heart block during pulmonary artery catheterization. Crit Care Med. 1989;17(1):1–3.

54. Morris D, Mulvihill D, Lew WY. Risk of developing complete heart block during bedside pulmonary artery catheterization in patients with left bundle-branch block. Arch Intern Med. 1987;147(11):2005–10.

55. Mond HG, Clark DW, Nesbitt SJ, Schlant RC. A technique for unknotting an intracardiac flow-directed balloon catheter. Chest. 1975;67(6):731–3.

56. Kearney TJ, Shabot MM. Pulmonary artery rupture associated with the Swan–Ganz catheter. Chest. 1995;108(5):1349–52.

57. Abreu AR, Campos MA, Krieger BP. Pulmonary artery rupture induced by a pulmonary artery catheter: a case report and review of the literature. J Intensive Care Med. 2004;19(5):291–6.

58. Pieske B, Tschöpe C, de Boer RA, et al. How to diagnose heart failure with preserved ejection fraction: the HFA-PEFF diagnostic algorithm: a consensus recommendation from the Heart Failure Association (HFA) of the European Society of Cardiology (ESC). Eur Heart J. 2019;40(40):3297–317.

59. Naeije R, Vanderpool R, Dhakal BP, et al. Exercise-induced pulmonary hypertension: physiological basis and methodological concerns. Am J Respir Crit Care Med. 2013;187(6):576–83.

60. Kovacs G, Berghold A, Scheidl S, Olschewski H. Pulmonary arterial pressure during rest and exercise in healthy subjects: a systematic review. Eur Respir J. 2009;34(4):888–94.

61. Wolsk E, Bakkestrøm R, Thomsen JH, et al. The influence of age on hemodynamic parameters during rest and exercise in healthy individuals. JACC Heart Fail. 2017;5(5):337–46.

62. Lam CS, Borlaug BA, Kane GC, Enders FT, Rodeheffer RJ, Redfield MM. Age-associated increases in pulmonary artery systolic pressure in the general population. Circulation. 2009;119(20):2663–70.

63. Tolle JJ, Waxman AB, van Horn TL, Pappagianopoulos PP, Systrom DM. Exercise-induced pulmonary arterial hypertension. Circulation. 2008;118(21):2183–9.

64. Parker JO, Thadani U. Cardiac performance at rest and during exercise in normal subjects. Bull Eur Physiopathol Respir. 1979;15(5):935–49.

65. Lewis GD, Murphy RM, Shah RV, et al. Pulmonary vascular response patterns during exercise in left ventricular systolic dysfunction predict exercise capacity and outcomes. Circ Heart Fail. 2011;4(3):276–85.

66. Andreini D, Pontone G, Pepi M, et al. Diagnostic accuracy of multidetector computed tomography coronary angiography in patients with dilated cardiomyopathy. J Am Coll Cardiol. 2007;49(20):2044–50.

67. Kuhtz-Buschbeck JP, Drake-Holland A, Noble MIM, Lohff B, Schaefer J. Rediscovery of Otto Frank's contribution to science. J Mol Cell Cardiol. 2018;119:96–103.

68. Suga H. Ventricular energetics. Physiol Rev. 1990;70(2):247–77.

69. Baan J, van der Velde ET, Steendijk P. Ventricular pressure–volume relations in vivo. Eur Heart J. 1992;13 Suppl E:2–6.

70. Bastos MB, Burkhoff D, Maly J, et al. Invasive left ventricle pressure–volume analysis: overview and practical clinical implications. Eur Heart J. 2020;41(12):1286–97.

71. Burkhoff D, Mirsky I, Suga H. Assessment of systolic and diastolic ventricular properties via pressure–volume analysis: a guide for clinical, translational, and basic researchers. Am J Physiol Heart Circ Physiol. 2005;289(2):H501–12.

72. van der Velde ET, van Dijk AD, Steendijk P, et al. Left ventricular segmental volume by conductance catheter and Cine-CT. Eur Heart J. 1992;13 Suppl E:15–21.

73. Borlaug BA, Kass DA. Invasive hemodynamic assessment in heart failure. Cardiol Clin. 2011;29(2):269–80.

74. Felker G, Mann D. Heart Failure: A Companion to Braunwald's Heart Disease, 4th edition. Philadelphia, PA: Elsevier; 2020.

75. Kawaguchi M, Hay I, Fetics B, Kass DA. Combined ventricular systolic and arterial stiffening in patients with heart failure and preserved ejection fraction: implications for systolic and diastolic reserve limitations. Circulation. 2003;107(5):714–20.

76. Paulus WJ. Culprit mechanism(s) for exercise intolerance in heart failure with normal ejection fraction. J Am Coll Cardiol. 2010;56(11):864–6.

77. Penicka M, Bartunek J, Trakalova H, et al. Heart failure with preserved ejection fraction in outpatients with unexplained dyspnea: a pressure–volume loop analysis. J Am Coll Cardiol. 2010;55(16):1701–10.

78. Ryan M, Morgan H, Petrie MC, Perera D. Coronary revascularisation in patients with ischaemic cardiomyopathy. Heart. 2021;107(8):612–18.

SECTION 8

Chronic heart failure: pharmacological management

CHAPTER 8.1

Angiotensin-converting enzyme inhibitors

Roberto Ferrari, Gabriele Guardigli, and Biykem Bozkurt

Introduction

In the 1970s, a series of observations reported that angiotensin II (Ang II) had deleterious effects on the heart, vessels, and kidney. Then came the discovery and development of drugs blocking the renin–angiotensin system (RAS), which clarified the role of this system in several pathological conditions and led to the widespread use of angiotensin-converting enzyme (ACE) inhibitors in the treatment of cardiovascular and renal disease. Originally, these drugs were developed as therapeutic agents targeted to treat hypertension, but several clinical conditions were subsequently identified, such as congestive heart failure (CHF) and acute myocardial infarction (AMI), where ACE inhibitors were also found to be effective. More recently, ACE inhibitors have been shown to be able to treat and prevent ischaemic heart disease and progression towards CHF.

The main purpose of this chapter is to review the clinical data that support the role of ACE inhibitors in the treatment of CHF, as well as their underlying mechanism of action. A short section is dedicated to the discovery of these drugs, to the difference between them, and to their use in the context of the recent coronavirus disease 2019 (Covid-19) pandemic.

How ACE inhibitors came to be

The development of ACE inhibitors is a classical story of university basic research, chance, serendipity, and lack of industry research. Knowledge and discovery of the molecular target of these drugs started about 60 years before the synthesis of the first ACE inhibitor, with the finding and eventually understanding of renin,[1] angiotensin,[2] and ACE.[3] All started with the pioneering work of Robert Tigerstedt from the Karolinska Institute who ground up rabbit kidneys and isolated an extract (renin) that caused the blood pressure to shoot up.[1] After a dark age of uncertainty, in 1940, Eduardo Braun-Menendez (Buenos Aires, Argentina) and Irvine Page (Indianapolis, USA) had independently demonstrated that a large circulating protein (angiotensinogen) was enzymatically cleaved to a smaller peptide (angiotensin).[2] A few years later, the enzyme able to convert angiotensin I in Ang II was discovered.[3] The discovery of ACE inhibitors owes a great deal to the role of bradykinin and to a particular Brazilian snake called *Bothrops jararaca* (➲ Figure 8.1.1).[4] A drastic drop in blood pressure with circulatory collapse would follow the bite of the viper. Seeking to understand the reason for this decrease, the group of Ferreira took venom extracts which they injected into dogs, and discovered that the snake venom, when added to human blood plasma, produced a new potent hypotensive and spasmogenic substance—bradykinin.[5] Later, it was appreciated that the same venom contained a potent small peptide able to act as a bradykinin potentiator factor which, in turn, was associated with inhibition of kinin degradation enzymes.[5] The same enzyme

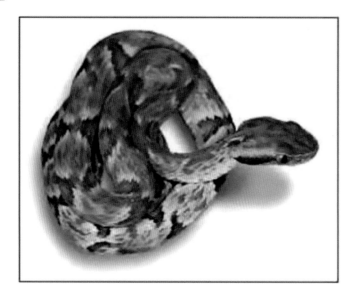

Figure 8.1.1 *Bothrops jararaea* (Brazilian pit viper).
© Mark Moffett/Minden Pictures/corbis.

was also identified as the enzyme responsible for the conversion of angiotensin I to Ang II, which, in contrast to bradykinin, is a potent vasoconstrictor. Therefore, ACE has a double effect: it catalyses, on the one hand, the synthesis of Ang II, and on the other hand, the breakdown of bradykinin (→ Figure 8.1.2). In 1968, John Vane, the Nobel Prize winner, showed that peptides from the Brazilian snake's venom inhibited the activity of ACE from dog lung and proposed to ER Squibb & Sons, an American company, today part of Bristol-Myers Squibb, to start an ACE inhibitor programme with the aim of treating hypertension.[6] Although with scepticism, Squibb began to test more than 2000 chemical structures with ACE inhibition activity but could not find any molecule worth to further development. It was then decided to consider a newly published research on an exopeptidase, also active on ACE.[6] Eighteen months later, after consideration of at least 60 compounds, captopril came about. Its discovery was reported at a cardiovascular hypertension congress in Sao Paulo, Brazil, with images of the viper with its fast zigzag movements and protruding tongue (→ Figure 8.1.1). Delegates were even given the opportunity to visit the snake farm and see the *Bothrops jararaca*, and early clinical trials established its antihypertensive action.[7] The launch of captopril was not as glorious as one can think. Actually, it caused Squibb much headache, as severe hypotensive effects were reported at the high doses (400–1000 mg/day) of captopril that were initially recommended. As a consequence, the doses were drastically reduced, and even with the suggested regime of a starting dose of 25 mg/day and a maintenance dose of 50 mg/day, some patients reported first-dose hypotension. This issue needed to be resolved, as over the years, it became obvious that ACE inhibitors could have an important role in heart failure (HF) when the RAS is highly activated. Under these circumstances, ACE inhibitors are likely to produce much greater hypotensive effects than in hypertensive patients and the combination of low blood pressure, increased potassium level, and renal dysfunction could be a problem for HF patients, potentially causing arrhythmias and eventually death.

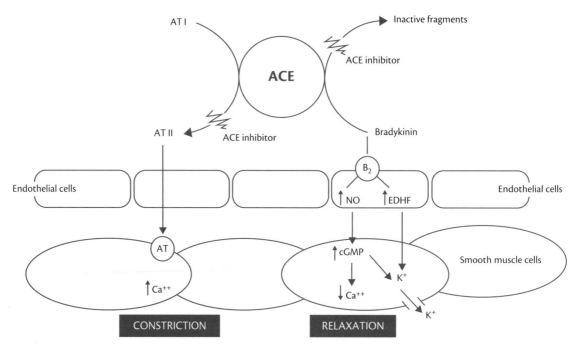

Figure 8.1.2 Activity of angiotensin-converting enzyme (ACE)/kininase. The same enzyme catalyses the synthesis of angiotensin II (AT II) from angiotensin I (AT I), and the breakdown of bradykinin into inactive fragments. AT II interacts with AT receptors on smooth muscle cells, causing calcium-dependent vasoconstriction. Bradykinin acts on endothelial bradykinin receptors, causing the release of nitric oxide (NO) and endothelium-derived hyperpolarizing factor (EDHF), leading to vasorelaxation. ACE inhibitors have a double mechanism of action: (1) inhibition of the ACE-dependent synthesis of AT II; and (2) inhibition of the kininase-dependent breakdown of bradykinin. cGMP, cyclic guanosine monophosphate.

The problem of hypotension was shared also by the rival of captopril: Merck's longer-acting ACE inhibitor enalapril, which had a better side effect profile and an easier dosing schedule. The 'hangover' of Squibb continued for Merck, as the launch dose of enalapril was too high and also caused severe hypotension, particularly in HF patients, leading to the recommendation that initiation with ACE inhibitor therapy in HF should be made under strict medical supervision.[8] Today all this is just 'history'. ACE inhibitors are indicated as first-line therapy in patients with heart failure with reduced ejection fraction (HFrEF). They can be started not necessarily by cardiologists, on a reasonably low dose, with doubling of the dose every 1–2 weeks to reach the target.

ACE inhibitors in patients with congestive heart failure

The outlook of ACE inhibitors shifted from hypertension to HFrEF with the publication of the Cooperative North Scandinavian Enalapril Survival (CONSENSUS) trial, which enrolled patients with advanced HF symptoms (New York Heart Association (NYHA) functional class IV).[9] The study showed 37% less mortality after 1 year of treatment with enalapril. The trial was stopped early, and when the results were shown to the triallists, there was a spellbound silence. There had never been such reduction in mortality in any CHF study (➲ Figure 8.1.3). Further trials produced confirmatory results. The Studies of Left Ventricular Dysfunction (SOLVD) programme showed that, compared to placebo, treatment of enalapril over 3 years prevented 50 premature deaths and 350 admissions per 1000 patients.[10] Taken together, these trials suggest that enalapril, in addition to other drugs, provides mortality and morbidity benefits in HFrEF. These findings are further supported by the results of a systematic overview of 32 trials of

symptomatic HFrEF patients revealing a 23% reduction in total mortality and a 35% reduction in the combined endpoint of mortality or hospitalization for CHF in the ACE inhibitor group.[11] The benefits were observed with different ACE inhibitors and independently of age, gender, aetiology of HF, and NYHA class.[12]

Since established as the first-line treatment for symptomatic HFrEF, ACE inhibitors have been tested for treatment of asymptomatic left ventricular dysfunction (LVD) patients. Actually these patients were already studied in the SOLVD Prevention Trials, with a trend towards lower mortality.[13] Other studies in patients with recent myocardial infarction and LVD, with or without clinical manifestation of HF, including Trandolapril Cardiac Evaluation (TRACE),[14] Acute Infarction Ramipril Efficacy (AIRE),[15] and Survival and Ventricular Enlargement (SAVE) trials,[16] also showed mortality benefits (➲ Figure 8.1.4). A meta-analysis of 12,500 individual data from all these and other studies showed that over a follow-up period of about 4–5 years, there is a 26% risk reduction in total mortality and 20% in myocardial infarction, but no impact on stroke.[17] Benefits were greatest among patients with more severe impairment of left ventricular function, and presumably with higher neuroendocrine activation, precisely defining the phenotype for ACE inhibition treatment: patients with compromised left ventricular function with or without clinical manifestation of HF.

Adverse effects include reversible increase of serum creatinine level, symptomatic hypotension, and angio-oedema. An increase of serum creatinine level of up to 30% is tolerated and does not warrant stopping ACE inhibitor therapy.[12] A small, but significant, increase of serum potassium level has also been reported. Thus, caution is needed for those patients with hyperkalaemia (potassium level >5 mEq/L), receiving potassium supplements or

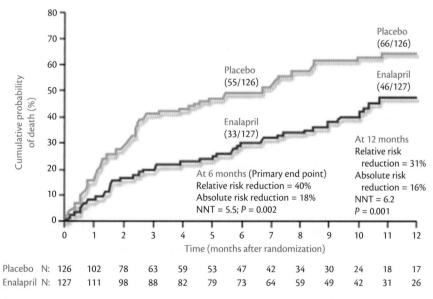

Figure 8.1.3 Kaplan–Meyer mortality curves from the CONSENSUS I study published in *New England Journal of Medicine* in 1987. CONSENSUS I, COoperative North Scandinavian ENalapril SUrvival Study.
Reproduced from CONSENSUS Trial Study Group. Effects of enalapril on mortality in severe congestive heart failure. Results of the Cooperative North Scandinavian Enalapril Survival Study (CONSENSUS). *N Engl J Med.* 1987 Jun 4;316(23):1429–35. doi: 10.1056/NEJM198706043162301 with permission from Massachusetts Medical Society.

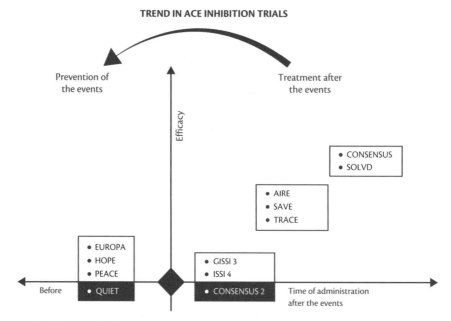

Figure 8.1.4 Diagram showing the efficacy profile of clinical trials on angiotensin-converting enzyme (ACE) inhibitors given as either therapeutic or preventive treatment.

potassium-sparing diuretics or with pre-existing hypotension.[12] Less serious adverse events include cough, diarrhoea, fatigue, and dizziness.

From treatment to prevention of heart failure

A number of large-scale trials have demonstrated better survival with ACE inhibitors provided to unselected patients early after AMI. These trials were: the 4th International Study of Infarct Survival (ISIS-4) and the 3 Gruppo Italiano per lo Studio della Soprovvivenza nell'Infarto Miocardico (GISSI-3).[18,19] A systematic overview of more than 100,000 patients from trials on ACE inhibitors started in the initial phase of AMI showed a modest, but statistically significant (7%), risk reduction in mortality, with a trend towards preventing the development of HF.[20] Thus, over the years, the use of ACE inhibitors in HF has expanded and shifted not only to treat HF, but also to prevent its development. As indicated in ➲ Figure 8.1.4, ACE inhibitors have been systematically studied and used in increasingly less symptomatic patients with HF.

A possible preventive role of ACE inhibitors against AMI, and eventually HF, was tested, but not proven in the Quinapril Ischemic Event Trial (QUIET).[21] Thereafter, the Heart Outcomes Prevention Evaluation (HOPE) and the EURopean trial On reduction of cardiac events with Perindopril in stable coronary Artery disease (EUROPA) trials clearly showed that both ramipril and perindopril in asymptomatic cardiovascular disease (CVD) patients with different risks significantly reduced the progression of the cardiovascular continuum, leading to a reduction in the occurrence of AMI and eventually in HF mortality.[22,23]

These later trials were conducted in patients with preserved ejection fraction without symptoms of HF. However, when tested in patients with HF with preserved (HFpEF) or mid-range ejection fraction (HFmrEF), a real benefit could not be found, probably in relation to the heterogeneity of the underlying pathologies in this group of patients without a specific phenotype.[24]

Mechanism underlying the beneficial effects of ACE inhibitors

The ACE or kinase II is a bivalent zinc metalloproteinase enzyme which regulates the balance between the vasodilator and natriuretic properties of bradykinin and the vasoconstrictive and salt-retention properties of Ang II (➲ Figure 8.1.5). ACE cleaves the C-terminal dipeptide from angiotensin I and bradykinin, thus interacting with RAS and the kallikrein system simultaneously. It follows that ACE is strategically located to control the delicate water/pressure balance in the body.[25]

ACE is present in plasma and a number of tissues such as blood vessels and the heart, brain, kidneys, and adrenal glands. Biochemical measurements show that it is essentially

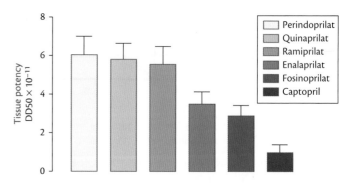

Figure 8.1.5 Differences in relative tissue affinity of various angiotensin-converting enzyme inhibitors.

a tissue-based enzyme present in the heart where it is located mainly in the right atrium, ventricles, and vessels.[26] Strongest immunohistochemical ACE staining is found in the endothelium of large and small arteries, whereas only half of the coronary capillaries are immunoreactive. This explains why ACE inhibitors cause only weak coronary dilatation.[27]

After the initial observation of ACE upregulation in pressure-overloaded, hypertrophied hearts, marked ACE activation has been reported basically in every condition of cardiac injury, with HF being the most relevant.[28,29] Increased ACE activity in HF is not limited to myocytes or endothelial cells; fibroblasts and macrophages also show high ACE activity in HF, leading to ventricular remodelling.[30]

It follows that the main mechanism of action of ACE inhibitors in HF is to counteract the increase in tissue and circulating ACE activity and the consequent neuroendocrine effects, resulting in favourable haemodynamics. ACE inhibitors in HF reduce afterload, preload, and systolic wall stress, such that cardiac output increases without an increase in the heart rate. In addition to this pharmacological effect, ACE inhibitors in the long term exert an important biological effect—preventing further cardiac remodelling, the pivotal mechanism underlying both the onset and the progression of HF.[31] It follows that the beneficial effects of ACE inhibitors in HF are complex and related to several components which can be ascribed both to the reduction of neuroendocrine activation and to the biological effects, leading to: (1) a reduction in systemic vascular resistance without changes in the heart rate;[27] in contrast with other vasodilators (calcium channel antagonists or nitrates), no reflex tachycardia is observed after ACE inhibitor administration, possibly due to vagal stimulation, reduction of sympathetic activity, or reduced baroreceptor sensitivity;[31] (2) increased renal plasma flow, with salt and water secretion consequent to a reduction in aldosterone and antidiuretic hormone production;[27] (3) improved energy supply to the myocardium via peripheral and coronary dilatation;[27] (4) an anti-remodelling effect by altering the balance between the pro-apoptotic effect of Ang II and the anti-apoptotic action of bradykinin;[32,33,34] (5) improvement of endothelial dysfunction via attenuation of Ang II vasoconstriction and bradykinin-mediated upregulation of constitutive nitric oxide synthase (CNOS);[35,36] (6) attenuation of disproportionate excess ventricular hypertrophy to compensate for the lost myocardium (either as a result of AMI or due to muscle damage seen in non-ischaemic cardiomyopathy), and reduction of wall stress which continues to promote left ventricular (LV) dilatation beyond that necessary to maintain cardiac output. When this happens, a vicious circle starts: LV dilatation progressively increases wall stress, the balance between ventricular dilatation and maintenance of cardiac function is altered, neuroendocrine activation is further stimulated, and eventually LV dilatation becomes a pathological, progressive process called remodelling;[37,38] and (7) modulation of Ang II-induced activation of the sympathetic system.

All these effects are independent of age, gender, and aetiology of HF.[39,40]

ACE inhibitors are not all the same

Although the effects of ACE inhibitors in HFrEF can be considered a class effect, there are differences between the various drugs.[41] ACE inhibitors differ in chemical structure, potency, bioavailability, plasma half-life, distribution, elimination, and, more importantly, the affinity for tissue-bound ACE, as shown in ➲ Figure 8.1.4.[27,31] Some contain a sulfhydryl group, with captopril being the prototype. Others include zofenopril, aleceptril, and pilalopril. The sulfhydryl group may have additional properties such as free radical scavenging and effects on prostaglandins, but without clear clinical relevance. The majority of other ACE inhibitors, such as lisinopril, enalapril, and perindopril, contain a carboxyl moiety.

Almost all ACE inhibitors are administered as prodrugs, which have enhanced oral bioavailability, compared to the active drugs. Relative tissue affinity differs among ACE inhibitors: perindoprilat and ramiprilat have the highest affinity for heart homogenates (➲ Figure 8.1.6). This is important, as several investigations have shown that the effects of ACE inhibitors are better correlated with tissue ACE levels than with circulating ACE levels.[27] The relative potency of ACE inhibitors in enhancing bradykinin levels versus reducing Ang II levels may also be important. Perindopril, for example, increases bradykinin levels at doses much lower than those required to reduce Ang II levels. Bradykinin has a powerful anti-apoptotic biological effect and is central to the pharmacological vasodilatation induced by ACE inhibitors. Bradykinin has a short half-life and is thus difficult to measure. It has been reported as either increased or unchanged in patients treated with ACE inhibitors. However, the recent availability of specific bradykinin (B_2) icatibant receptor antagonists with bradykinin antagonists attenuates their antihypertensive effect as well as their beneficial action on endothelial dysfunction, both in animal model and in humans. Increased bradykinin levels induced by ACE inhibitors enhance the expression of endothelial constitutive nitric oxide synthase (ecNOS), the enzyme responsible for nitric oxide (NO) synthesis, with a parallel increase in its enzymatic activity, suggesting an increased production of NO. These effects are abolished by icatibant, suggesting that bradykinin plays an essential role in the ACE inhibitor-induced modulation of the NO pathway (➲ Figure 8.1.5). Thus, ACE inhibitors that are particularly effective in blocking bradykinin degradation, including perindopril, are more likely to influence the rate of NO synthesis and restore endothelium-dependent vasodilatation and to exert powerful anti-apoptotic effects.

How ACE inhibitors compare with angiotensin II receptor blockers in the treatment of heart failure

ACE inhibition causes an increase in angiotensin I, which can lead to the formation of Ang II via non-ACE-mediated pathways. This phenomenon is known as Ang II and aldosterone escape. This and other considerations, such as a lack of bradykinin increase which could be responsible for cough, opened

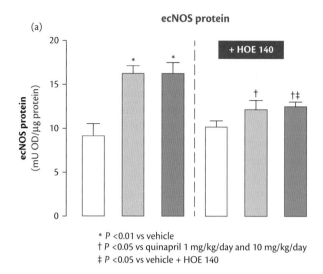

(a)

ecNOS protein

* $P < 0.01$ vs vehicle
† $P < 0.05$ vs quinapril 1 mg/kg/day and 10 mg/kg/day
‡ $P < 0.05$ vs vehicle + HOE 140

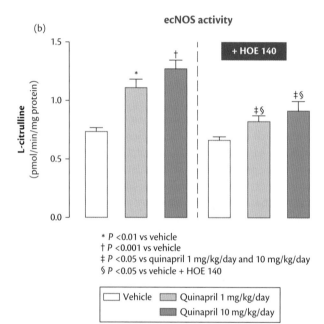

(b)

ecNOS activity

* $P < 0.01$ vs vehicle
† $P < 0.001$ vs vehicle
‡ $P < 0.05$ vs quinapril 1 mg/kg/day and 10 mg/kg/day
§ $P < 0.05$ vs vehicle + HOE 140

☐ Vehicle   ▨ Quinapril 1 mg/kg/day
▨ Quinapril 10 mg/kg/day

Figure 8.1.6 Endothelial constitutive nitric oxide synthase (ecNOS) protein expression (a) and activity (b), measured as L-citrulline production, in the rat aorta. Animals were treated with saline and quinapril, in combination with HOE 140 (icatibant), a bradykinin receptor antagonist. An increase in both ecNOS protein expression and activity was observed after 7 days of quinapril treatment. This effect was partially reversed by co-treatment with quinapril and HOE 140, suggesting that bradykinin plays an essential role in ACE inhibitor-induced modulation of nitric oxide (NO) production. OD, optical density.

the prospect of acting directly on RAS by blocking Ang II receptors, more specifically the Ang II type 1 (AT_1) receptor which causes vasoconstriction (➲ Figure 8.1.7). So the angiotensin receptor blockers (ARBs) were synthetized with the conviction that they could be at least as efficacious as ACE inhibitors, if not more, but with a better tolerability profile.[42] In the Evaluation of Losartan in the Elderly (ELITE) I trial, one of the secondary endpoints (combined mortality and hospitalization for CHF) was surprisingly lower in the losartan versus the captopril group.[42] Interestingly, in ELITE I, no difference was

found in the incidence of renal dysfunction between elderly patients receiving losartan and those treated with captopril. This was the primary endpoint for which the sample size of the study was determined. Despite this negative outcome, attention of the scientific community focused on the positive data obtained in the secondary endpoint and an adequately sized study was then started: the ELITE II. Unfortunately, the preliminary positive results were not confirmed. ELITE II showed that losartan was not superior to captopril in reducing mortality and morbidity.[43] Losartan had fewer side effects than captopril. Similar results were found in the Valsartan Heart Failure Trial (Val-HeFT), which showed that addition of valsartan to standard treatment for CHF, with or without ACE inhibition, did not improve mortality.[44] Thereafter, the effects of candesartan in CHF were investigated in the CHARM programme that consisted of the following parallel-design trials. The first, CHARM-Alternative, compared the effect of candesartan versus placebo in patients with CHF due to systolic dysfunction who were intolerant of ACE inhibitors.[45] Not surprisingly, the ARB did better than the placebo. The second study, CHARM-Added, compared the combination of candesartan and ACE inhibition with ACE inhibition alone in patients with left ventricular systolic dysfunction and CHF.[46] In this study, the combination proved superior to ACE inhibition alone. The third arm, CHARM-Preserved, studied the effect of candesartan in patients with CHF and preserved systolic cardiac function. Here, no significant effect was observed.[47]

It follows that in patients with CHF, there is no evidence that AT_1 receptor blockers are superior to ACE inhibitors, and there is a gap between evidence-based findings favouring the use of ACE inhibitors and those favouring the use of ARBs over ACE inhibitors. The same applies to the prevention or treatment of ischaemic heart disease.

Therefore, ACE inhibitors should currently be considered as the first-line choice in all these indications, with ARBs as an appropriate substitute in cases of intolerance to ACE inhibitors. After CHARM-Added, the value of ACE inhibitor/AT_1 receptor blocker combination therapy has been assessed in several trials. However, whether results were clear or conflicting, the main limitation was that full-dosing ranges of both classes of drugs were not explored. Thus, one cannot ascertain whether the same effect observed in combination would have been obtained with a higher dosage of one drug alone.

Whatever the case, the one 'lucky strike' for both cardiologists and, above all, their patients is the fact that blocking the RAS appears to be a very important strategy in almost all cardiological conditions. This can be achieved by using two different classes of drugs: ACE inhibitors, which have been much more intensively studied than the other, and ARBs.

However, ACE inhibitors remain the first and best choice to block the RAS in HF. Probably the effect of bradykinin compensates for the incomplete blockade of Ang II and explains their superiority over ARBs. The anti-apoptotic effect of bradykinin on apoptosis also makes the difference, as ARBs may even induce apoptosis as a result of a receptor shift, with Ang II preferably binding to the Ang II type 2 (AT_2) receptor as the AT_1 receptor

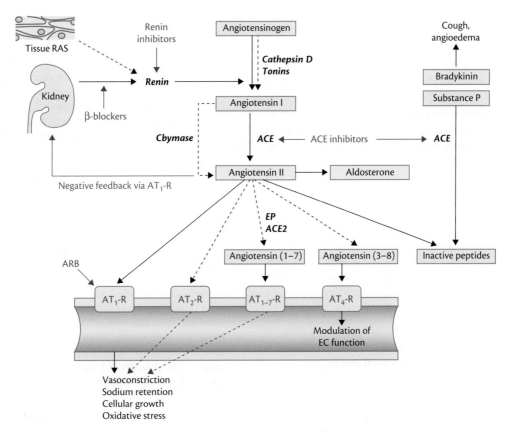

Figure 8.1.7 The renin–angiotensin–aldosterone system. Black arrows show inhibition. Dotted lines show alternative pathways, mainly documented in experimental studies. The RAAS activity is reduced by beta-blockers, direct renin inhibitors, ACE inhibitors, and angiotensin II type 1 receptor blockers. ACE inhibitor, angiotensin-converting enzyme inhibitor; ARB, angiotensin receptor blocker; ATR, angiotensin receptor; EC, endothelial cell; EP, endopeptidase; RAS, renin–angiotensin system; RAAS, renin–angiotensin–aldosterone system.
Reproduced from Staessen JA, Li Y, Richart T. Oral renin inhibitors. *Lancet*. 2006 Oct 21;368(9545):1449–56. doi: 10.1016/S0140-6736(06)69442-7 with permission from Elsevier.

is blocked (➲ Figure 8.1.8). This results in increased apoptosis, which is not useful in counteracting remodelling.[32,33]

Use of ACE inhibitors in the context of the Covid-19 pandemic

In December 2019, an outbreak of pneumonia caused by a novel coronavirus occurred in Wuhan, Hubei Province, China and rapidly spread worldwide.[48]

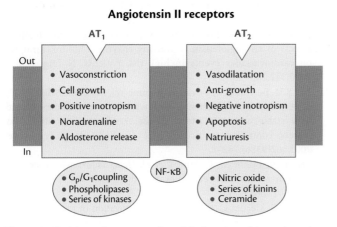

Figure 8.1.8 Schematic representation of the function of the angiotensin II receptors. AT_1, angiotensin II type 1 receptor; AT_2, angiotensin II type 2 receptor; NF-κB, nuclear factor kappa B.

Today, almost 4 years later, thanks to vaccines that seem to have defeated the pandemic, Europe is celebrating the first 'V DAY' were V means vaccine, as the first Pfizer-produced vaccine (already in use in the UK and the USA) began to be distributed and administered in all European Union countries, hoping that in 6 months' time, the pandemic will be under control.

But … what ACE inhibitors has to do with the pandemic?

In the early days, it was suggested that ACE inhibitors (and ARBs) should be carefully considered in Covid-19 patients with hypertension and cardiovascular disease, including HF, and when possible switched to other drugs.[48] This is because ACE2 (not ACE1!) has been identified as a functional receptor for coronavirus, including severe acute respiratory syndrome coronavirus 2 (SARS-CoV-2). Infection starts with binding of the virus spike protein to ACE2, thus allowing penetration of the virus into targeted cells. ACE2, which does the opposite of ACE1, converting Ang II back to angiotensin I, is highly expressed in the lung and heart, the two organs which can be more frequently infected.

Actually, this worry was not supported by a logical pathophysiological background, and the suggestion of not using ACE inhibitors in Covid-19 patients proved to be without serious foundation for a number of reasons[49] and today it has been proved that ACE inhibitors are safe and beneficial even in Covid-19 patients.[50]

Recommendation from the recent ESC Guideline on heart failure

At the meeting of the Heart Failure Association in Florence (29 June to 1 July 2021), and later in London at the European Society of Cardiology (ESC) meeting, the new guidelines on HF were released.[51] ACE inhibitors are recommended in all patients with HFrEF, unless contraindicated or not tolerated (Class I, Level A). They should be uptitrated to the maximum recommended doses indicated in the relevant trials.

There are no specific trials (nor will there be) on use of ACE inhibitors in patients with HFmrEF. However, as the majority of patients with HFmrEF will have systolic dysfunction due to ischaemic heart disease or hypertension, they will be already treated with an ACE inhibitor.

Like for HFmrEF, there are no convincing data on how to treat HFpEF. In particular, PEP-CHF (with perindopril),[52] CHARM-Preserved (with candesartan),[53] and I-PRESERVE (with irbesartan)[54] did not result in a specific disease modification. Thus, ACE inhibitors, in this very heterogeneous set of patients, should be used to treat the underlying pathologies (hypertension, myocardial infarction, angina, etc.), as for HFmrEF.

Conclusions

ACE inhibitors are the gold standard RAS blocker. Not only have their safety and efficacy been extensively documented, but they confer benefits that are at the same time biological, structural, and pharmacological across diseases as clinically diverse as hypertension, CHF, AMI, and ischaemic heart disease, including diabetes. More specifically, ACE inhibitors have been shown to reduce the risk of death, worsening HF in patients with left ventricular systolic dysfunction, and HF. They have also been shown to reduce mortality in AMI and to reduce the risk of major cardiovascular events eventually leading to HF.

References

1. Tigerstedt R, Bergman PG. Niere und krieslau skand. Arch Physiol 1898;8:225–71.
2. Braun-Menendez E, Page IH. Suggested revision of nomenclature: angiotensin. Science 1958;127:242.
3. Fasciolo JC, Houssay BA, Tarquini AC. The blood pressure raising secretion of the ischemic kidney. J Physiol 1938;94:281–90.
4. Erdös EG. The ACE and I: how ACE inhibitors came to be. FASEB J 2006;20:1034–8.
5. Ferreira SH. A bradykinin-potentiating factor (BPF) present in the venom of Bothrops jararaca. Br J Pharmacol 1965;24:163–9.
6. Smith CG, Vane JR. The discovery of captopril. FASEB J 2003;17:788–9.
7. Gavras H, Bruneer HR, Turini GA, et al. Antihypertensive effect of the oral angiotensin converting enzyme inhibitor SQ 14225 in man. N Engl Med 1978;298:991–5.
8. Cleland JGF, Dargie HJ, McAlpine H, et al. Severe hypotension after first dose of enalapril in heart failure. BMJ 1985;291:1309–12.
9. CONSENSUS Trial Study Group. Effects of enalapril on mortality in severe congestive heart failure. Results of the Cooperative North Scandinavian Enalapril Survival Study (CONSENSUS). N Engl J Med 1987;316:1429–35.
10. SOLVD Investigators. Effects of enalapril on survival in patients with reduced left ventricular ejection fractions and congestive heart failure. N Engl J Med 1991;325:293–302.
11. Garg R, Yusuf S. Overview of randomized trials on angiotensin-converting enzyme inhibitors on mortality and morbidity in patients with heart failure. JAMA 1995;18:1450–6.
12. R Ferrari, C Balla, and A Fucili. Heart failure: an historical perspective. Eur Heart J Supplements. 2016; 18 (Supplement G), G3–10. The Heart of the Matter. https://doi.org/10.1093/eurheartj/suw042.
13. SOLVD Investigators. Effect of enalapril on mortality and the development of heart failure in asymptomatic patients with reduced left ventricular ejection fractions. N Engl J Med 1992;327:685–91.
14. Kober L, Torp-Pedersen C, Carlsen JE, et al. A clinical trial of the angiotensin-converting-enzyme inhibitor trandolapril in patients with left ventricular dysfunction after myocardial infarction. Trandolapril Cardiac Evaluation (TRACE) Study Group. N Engl J Med 1995;333:1670–6.
15. [No author listed]. Effect of ramipril on mortality and morbidity of survivors of acute myocardial infarction with clinical evidence of heart failure. The Acute Infarction Ramipril Efficacy (AIRE) Study Investigators. Lancet 1993;342:821–8.
16. Pfefer NA, Braunwald E, Moye LA, et al. Effect of enalapril on survival in patients with reduced left ventricular ejection fractions and congestive heart failure. N Engl J Med 1992;327:669–77.
17. Flather M, Kober L, Pfeffer MA, et al. Meta-analysis of individual patient data from trials of long-term ACE-inhibitors treatment after acute myocardial infarction (SAVE, AIRE, and TRACE studies). Circulation 1997;96(Suppl 1):1–706.
18. [No author listed]. ISIS-4: a randomised factorial trial assessing early oral captopril, oral mononitrate, and intravenous magnesium sulphate in 58,050 patients with suspected acute myocardial infarction. ISIS-4 (Fourth International Study of Infarct Survival) Collaborative Group. Lancet 1995;345:669–85.
19. [No author listed]. GISSI-3: effects of lisinopril and transdermal glyceryl trinitrate singly and together on 6-week mortality and ventricular function after acute myocardial infarction. Gruppo Italiano per lo Studio della Sopravvivenza nell'infarto Miocardico. Lancet 1994;343:1115–22.
20. [No author listed]. Indications for ACE inhibitors in the early treatment of acute myocardial infarction: systematic overview of individual data from 100,000 patients in randomized trials. ACE Inhibitor Myocardial Infarction Collaborative Group. Circulation 1998;97:2202–12.
21. Lees RS, Pitt B, Chan RC, et al. Baseline clinical and angiographic data in the Quinapril Ischemic Event (QUIET) trial. Am J Cardiol 1996;78:1011–16.
22. Heart Outcomes Prevention Evaluation Study Investigators. Effects of an angiotensin-converting-enzyme inhibitor, ramipril, on cardiovascular events in high-risk patients. N Engl J Med 2000;342:145–53.
23. Fox KM, Bertrand M, Ferrari R, Remme WJ, Simmons ML. Efficacy of perindopril in reduction of cardiovascular events among patients with stable coronary artery disease: randomised, double-blind, placebo-controlled, multicentre trial (The EUROPA study). Lancet 2003;362(9386):782–8.
24. Ferrari R, Bohm M, Cleland J, et al. Heart failure with preserved ejection fraction: uncertainties and dilemmas. Eur J Heart Fail 2015;17(7):665–71.
25. Ferrari R, Ceconi C, Curello S, et al. Activation of the neuroendocrine response in heart failure: adaptive or maladaptive process? Cardiovasc Drugs Ther 1996;10:639–47.

26. Dzau VJ, Bernstein K, Celermajer D, et al. Pathophysiologic and therapeutic importance of tissue ACE: a consensus report. Cardiovasc Drugs Ther 2002;16(2):149–60.

27. Ferrari R. Preserving bradykinin or blocking angiotensin II: the cardiovascular dilemma. Dialogues Cardiovasc Med 2004;9:71–89.

28. Pleruzzi F, Abassi ZA, Kelser HR. Expression of renin–angiotensin system components in the heart, kidneys, and lungs of rats with experimental heart failure. Circulation 1993;92:3105–12.

29. [No author listed]. The treatment of heart failure. The Task Force of the Working Group on Heart Failure of the European Society of Cardiology. Eur Heart J 1997;18:736–53.

30. Hokimoto S, Yassue H, Fujimoto K, et al. Expression of angiotensin-converting enzyme in remaining viable myocytes of human ventricles after myocardial infarction. Circulation 1996;94:1513–18.

31. Brown NJ, Vaughan DE. Angiotensin-converting enzyme inhibitors. Circulation 1998;97:1411–20.

32. Ferrari R, Ceconi C, Curello S, Pepi P, Mazzoletti A, Visioli O. Cardioprotective effect of angiotensin-converting enzyme inhibitors in patients with coronary artery disease. Cardiovasc Drugs Ther 1996;10:639–47.

33. Scientific Committee of the PERTINENT Sub-Study, EUROPA-PERTINENT Investigators. PERTINENT: perindropil–thrombosis, inflammation, endothelial dysfunction and neurohormal activation trial: a sub-study of the EUROPA study. Cardiovasc Drugs Ther 2003;17:83–91.

34. [No author listed]. PREAMI: Perindopril and Remodelling in Elderly with Acute Myocardial Infarction: study rationale and design. Cardiovasc Drugs Ther 2000;14:671–9.

35. Ferrari R, Gaurdigli G, Cicchitelli G, Valgimigli M, Soukhomovskaia O, Ceconi C. Cardioprotection with ACE inhibitors: non-angiotensin II-related mechanism. Eur Heart J 2000;2(Suppl I):I22–8.

36. Campbell DJ, Kladis A, Duncan AM. Effects of converting enzyme inhibitors on angiotensin and bradykinin peptides. Hypertension 1994;23:439–49.

37. Ferrari R, Ceconi C, Campo G, et al. Mechanism of remodelling: a question of life (stem cell production) and death (myocyte apoptosis). Circ J 2009;73:1973–82.

38. Cohn JN, Ferrari R, Sharpe N. Cardiac remodelling: concepts and clinical implications: a consensus paper from an international forum on cardiac remodelling. J Am Coll Cardiol 2000;35:569–82.

39. Nicolosi GL, Golcea S, Ceconi C, et al.; PREAMI Investigators. Effects of perindropil on cardiac remodelling and prognostic value of pre-discharge quantitative echocardiographic parameters in elderly patients after acute myocardial infarction: the PREAMI echo sub-study. Eur Heart J 2009;30:1656–65.

40. Cleland JG. ACE inhibitors for myocardial infarction: how should they be used? Eur Heart J 1995;16:153–9.

41. Ferrari R. Effect of ACE inhibition on myocardial ischaemia. Eur Heart J 1998;19(Suppl J):J30–5.

42. Pitt B, Segal R, Martinez FA, et al. Randomised trial of losartan versus captopril in patients over 65 with heart failure (Evaluation of Losartan in the Elderly study, ELITE). Lancet 1997;349:747–52.

43. Pitt B, Poole-Wilson PA, Segal R, et al. Effect of losartan compared with captopril on mortality in patients with symptomatic heart failure: randomised trial: the Losartan Heart Failure Survival Study ELITE II. Lancet 2000;255:1582–7.

44. Cohn JN, Tognoni G; Valsartan Heart Failure Trial Investigators. A randomized trial of the angiotensin-receptor blocker valsartan in chronic heart failure. N Engl J Med 2001;345:1667–75.

45. Pfeffer MA, Swedberg K, Granger CB, et al.; CHARM Investigators and Committees. Effects of candesartan on mortality and morbidity in patients with chronic heart failure: the CHARM-Overall programme. Lancet 2003;362:759–66.

46. Pfeffer MA, McMurray JV, Velazquez EJ, et al. Valsartan, captopril, or both in myocardial infarction complicated by heart failure, left ventricular dysfunction of both. N Engl J Med 2003;349:1893–906.

47. Yusuf S, Pfeffer MA, Swedberg K, et al. Effect of candesartan in patients with chronic heart failure and preserved left ventricular ejection fraction: the CHARM-preserved trial. Lancet 2003;326:777–81.

48. Zheng YY, Ma YT, Zhang JY, Xie X. COVID-19 and the cardiovascular system. Nat Rev Cardiol 2020;17:259–60.

49. Ferrari R, Di Pasquale G, Rapezzi C. Commentary: what is the relationship between Covid-19 and cardiovascular disease? Int J Cardiol 2020;310:167–8.

50. Ferrari R, Di Pasquale G, Rapezzi C. 2019 coronarvirus: what are the implications for cardiology? Eur J Prev Cardiol 2020;27(8):793–6.

51. McDonagh TA, Metra M, Adamo M, et al.; ESC Scientific Document Group. 2021 ESC Guidelines for the diagnosis and treatment of acute and chronic heart failure. Eur Heart J 2021;42(36):3599–726.

52. Cleland JG, Tendera M, Adamus J, et al. Perindopril for elderly people with chronic heart failure: the PEP-CHF study. The PEP Investigators. Eur J Heart Fail 1999;1:211–17.

53. Massie BM, Carson PE, McMurray JJ, et al.; I-PRESERVE Investigators. Irbesartan in patients with heart failure and preserved ejection fraction. N Engl J Med 2008;359:2456–67.

54. Ahmed A, Rich MW, Fleg JL, et al. Effects of digoxin on morbidity and mortality in diastolic heart failure: the ancillary digitalis investigation group trial. Circulation 2006;114:397–403.

CHAPTER 8.2

Angiotensin receptor blockers in heart failure

Ileana L Piña and Magdy Abdelhamid

Contents

Introduction

Angiotensin receptor antagonists (blockers) have become one of the highly recommended interventions for treatment of the pathophysiology of the renin–angiotensin–aldosterone system (RAAS) in patients with heart failure (HF). This chapter will review the discovery of the angiotensin II (AII) receptor and the development of AII antagonists, as well as outline the current recommendations from various practice guidelines.

History

In 1898, the Finnish physiologist Robert Tigerstedt and his student/trainee Per Bergman identified a substance that had pressor qualities when injecting renal cortical extracts into the jugular vein of rabbits and noting an increase in blood pressure. Dr Tigerstedt was, at that time, a professor of physiology at the Karolinska Institute in Stockholm, Sweden. While experimenting with renal medullary and cortical extracts, they found that it was the cortical extracts that consistently resulted in the pressor effects (➔ Figures 8.2.1 and 8.2.2).[1] Published in *Scandinavian Archives of Physiology*, they named the renal extract 'renin'.[2] This discovery initiated the next 100 years of discovery that led to understanding the role of the kidney in hypertension. However, although this was the beginning of the discovery of the renin–angiotensin system (RAS), their discovery laid quiescent for over 40 years.

Interestingly, in 1909, A. Bingel and E. Strauss from Frankfurt not only confirmed the results of Tigerstedt and Bergman, but also extended the work to include extracts of other animals which also caused increases in blood pressure.[3] Their discovery also was dormant until Goldblatt's work, but also showed that renin was equally effective if extracted from the pig and other animals. Unfortunately, their work was also forgotten. It was not until Goldblatt showed persistent elevation of blood pressure in renal ischaemia that interest turned once again to 'renin'.

After noting that there was narrowing of the renal bed in patients who had died of hypertension, Harry Goldblatt tested the hypothesis that clamping the renal arteries would produce ischaemia and could trigger hypertension (➔ Figure 8.2.3),[4] hence the birth of the silver-clamped Goldblatt kidney still used today in research. These results were published in 1934 in *Journal of Experimental Medicine*.[5] The internal secretor of Goldblatt was identified years later as renin.

Simultaneously, work to better define renin had become the focus of two separate group investigators. In 1939, Page, Helmer, and Kohlstaedt in Indianapolis and Braun-Menéndez, Fasciola, and Leloir in Argentina independently reported that renin was not the pressor itself but acted as an enzyme for a substrate.[6,7] By 1939, the two groups had worked out that renin was not by itself a pressor substance, but the specific enzyme for

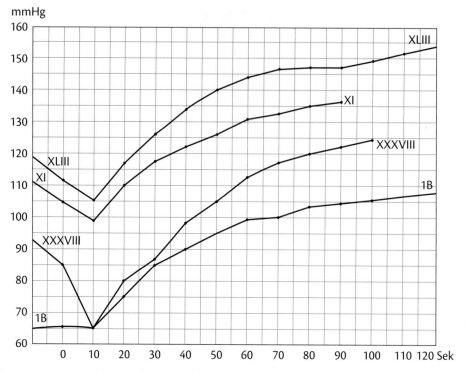

Figure 8.2.1 Effects of injecting renal extracts in the jugular vein on blood pressure. Initial decrease in blood pressure was thought to be an effect on the heart because it was absent after femoral injections.

Reproduced from Phillips MI, Schmidt-Ott KM. The Discovery of Renin 100 Years Ago. *News Physiol Sci.* 1999 Dec;14:271–274. doi: 10.1152/physiologyonline.1999.14.6.271 with permission from the American Physiological Society.

a substrate whose end-products were angiotensin I (AI) and AII. Each group had given a different name to the peptide that resulted in the blood pressure increase, that is, 'angiotonin' by the Page group and 'hipertensina' by the Braun-Menéndez team, but compromised to 'angiotensin' and its precursor 'angiotensinogen'.[8]

Leonard Skeggs and his team found two forms of angiotensin, I and II, and with the discovery of the angiotensin-converting enzyme (ACE), angiotensin II (Ang II) was labelled as the direct causation of hypertension.[9] Today Ang II, a peptide, is recognized as a regulator of blood volume and peripheral vascular resistance.

Periods of 10 s	Blood pressure			Number of heart beats per 10 s	Comments
	Maximal	Minimal	Mean		
34	70	64	67	30	
35	70	64	67	30	
36	66	58	62	30	
37	66	56	61	29	
38	70	62	66	29	Injection of 5 ccm of extract
39	70	60	65	30	
40	84	68	76	30	
41	88	82	85	30	
42	94	86	90	32	
43	98	92	95	32	
44	102	96	99	32	
45	102	98	100	33	
46	106	100	103	33	
50	110	106	108	34	

Figure 8.2.2 Experiment 1B, 8 November 1896. A kidney was pulverized in 21 mL of cold water and injection into the jugular vein. Within approximately 80 seconds, there was a rise in mean blood pressure from 62–67 mmHg to 100 mmHg, that is, an increase by approximately 50%. It was obvious that the injected volume (5 mL) was not responsible for this rise.

Reproduced from Phillips MI, Schmidt-Ott KM. The Discovery of Renin 100 Years Ago. *News Physiol Sci.* 1999 Dec;14:271–274. doi: 10.1152/physiologyonline.1999.14.6.271 with permission from the American Physiological Society.

Ang II is produced in multiple tissues beyond the heart, including the brain, kidney, and vascular tissue. Targets include the adrenals, kidney, brain, vascular smooth muscle, and sympathetic nervous system. Thus, Ang II may be paracrine and autocrine, including remodelling of the myocardium and extracellular matrix.[10]

The angiotensin II receptor

AT1

It was postulated that the Ang II receptor would be located on the plasma membrane of target tissues and stimulate a cellular response. In fact, the Ang II receptors were proposed and cloned as transmembrane helices, and are G protein-coupled (➲ Figure 8.2.3).[11] The best-studied Ang II receptors are AT1 and AT2. There are additional receptors that have been identified, but AT1 and AT2 are the best known and described. Like other known receptors, AT1 and AT2 can be up- or downregulated in various organs. AT1 receptors are found in the heart, adrenals, brain, liver, and kidneys.

The AT1 receptor (a G protein-coupled receptor) is responsible for the majority of the known physiological actions of Ang II on target tissues such as blood pressure regulation, electrolyte and water balance (aldosterone and vasopressin secretion), and renal function. Cellular responses to AT1 receptor signalling include smooth muscle contraction, aldosterone secretion, neuronal

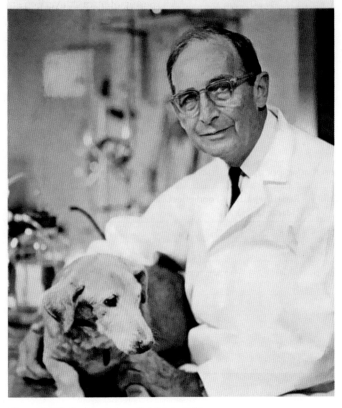

Figure 8.2.3 Professor Harry Goldblatt, 1964.
Image provided by the National Library of Medicine. http://resource.nlm.nih.gov/101416615.

activation, and cell growth and proliferation, among others (shown in ➲ Figure 8.2.4).[11,12,13]

AT2

The Ang II AT2 receptor is clearly distinct from AT1 in structure and function. Initially it is present in high concentrations in fetal tissue, downregulating in the adult human. Research continues into the signalling functions of the AT2 receptor but may suppress tissue and cell growth (remodelling), have a hypotensive effect (opposite to AT1), and support apoptosis.[14]

AII antagonists

Saralasin was the first AII antagonist, and with the discovery of captopril as the first ACE inhibitor (ACEI), the AT1 receptor was forecasted to be favourable, initially for hypertension treatment, but ultimately for HF. Due to saralasin's poor oral absorption, short duration of action, and partial agonist activity, it was not an effective drug.[15] Non-peptides seemed attractive, and after manipulation of the drug structure, losartan was, in 1986, the first successful AII antagonist and approved in 1995. Others then followed.

Losartan

Losartan, marketed as an alternative, in patients with intolerance to ACEIs, has a metabolite that is more potent than the original parent compound. Losartan and its metabolite set the stage for other AII antagonists to be developed.[16]

Valsartan is very similar to losartan. Irbesartan is a noncompetitive inhibitor of the AII receptor, whereas candesartan is a prodrug rapidly converted to a more potent metabolite. Due to its strong binding to the AT1 receptor, candesartan is a more powerful agent than losartan and one of the best studied in HF. Candesartan and olmesartan have the highest affinity for the AT1 receptor. Valsartan and telmisartan have 10-fold less affinity than candesartan. Losartan has the lowest affinity for the receptor. A low affinity for the AT2 receptor allows these drugs to have a physiological impact on all the ramifications of a high AII load. Further elaboration of the chemical structure of the AII antagonists is beyond the scope of this chapter and the reader is referred to other publications. Valsartan and candesartan are the best-studied AII antagonists in chronic HF—initially for heart failure with reduced ejection fraction (HFrEF) (valsartan and candesartan) and heart failure with preserved ejection fraction (HFpEF) (candesartan), and more recently for HFpEF (valsartan).[17,18,19] ➲ Table 8.2.1 lists the pharmacokinetics of approved AII receptor blockers, with bioavailability and dosing for comparison.[13,20,21]

Rationale behind use of angiotensin receptor blockers in treatment of heart failure

Chronic HF is a serious condition associated with high morbidity and mortality rates. Therefore, the goal of any pharmacological therapy is to lower the risk of adverse clinical outcomes associated with this chronic disease.[22]

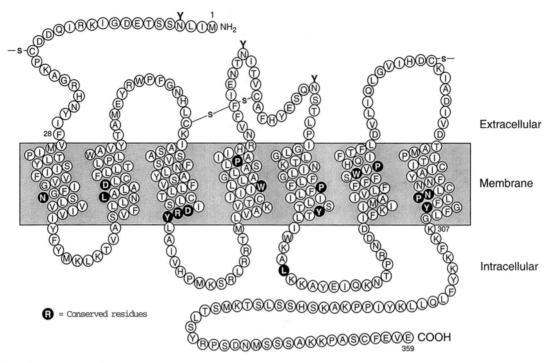

Figure 8.2.4 Secondary structure and consensus sequence of the mammalian angiotensin AT1 receptor. The amino acid sequence shown is based on the derived sequences of five individual cloned mammalian AT1 receptors. The amino acid residues that are highly conserved among G protein-coupled receptors are indicated by bold letters. The positions of the three extracellular carbohydrate chains and of the two extracellular disulfide bonds are also indicated. Reproduced from de Gasparo M, Catt KJ, Inagami T, Wright JW, Unger T. International union of pharmacology. XXIII. The angiotensin II receptors. *Pharmacol Rev.* 2000 Sep;52(3):415–72. with permission from the American Society for Pharmacology and Experimental Therapeutics.

It is a well-known fact that excess activation of the RAS contributes to the pathophysiology of HF. As noted earlier, activation of the RAS results in increased production of AI, which is converted to AII by ACE. AII is a potent vasoconstrictor and also stimulates aldosterone secretion, which increases sodium and water retention. AII and aldosterone are also implicated in other potentially deleterious effects on the cardiovascular system, including endothelial damage, sympathetic activation, collagen formation, and decreased nitric oxide production (➲ Figure 8.2.5).[12] Together, these effects, which initially are compensatory, overshoot and lead to the syndrome known as HF. It is understood that many of these responses may take months or years to develop, and can occur during a time of few symptoms. With the understanding that the RAS plays such a vital role in the progression of HF, two drug classes, namely ACEIs and angiotensin receptor blockers (ARBs), were developed to inhibit the RAS and thus provide a potentially beneficial therapeutic approach for the treatment of HF (➲ Figure 8.2.6).[23,24]

Table 8.2.1 Comparison of angiotensin receptor blockers on market pharmacokinetics

Drug	Biological half-life (hours)	Protein binding (%)	Bioavailability (%)	Renal/hepatic clearance (%)	Food effect	Daily dosage (mg)
Losartan	2	98.7	33	10/90	Minimal	50–100
Candesartan	9	>99	15	60/40	No	4–32
Valsartan	6	95	25	30/70	Decreased by 40–50%	80–320
Irbesartan	11–15	90–95	70	1/99	No	150–300
Telmisartan	24	>99	42–58	1/99	No	40–80
Eprosartan	5	98	13	30/70	No	400–800
Olmesartan	14–16	>99	29	40/60	No	10–40

Source data from de Gasparo M, Catt KJ, Inagami T, Wright JW, Unger T. International Union of Pharmacology. XXIII. The angiotensin II receptors. *Pharmacol Rev.* 2000;52(3):415–72; Cohn JN, Tognoni G. A randomized trial of the angiotensin-receptor blocker valsartan in chronic heart failure. *N Engl J Med.* 2001;345(23):1667–75; and Granger CB, McMurray JJ, Yusuf S, *et al.* Effects of candesartan in patients with chronic heart failure and reduced left-ventricular systolic function intolerant to angiotensin-converting-enzyme inhibitors: the CHARM-Alternative trial. *Lancet.* 2003;362(9386):772–6.

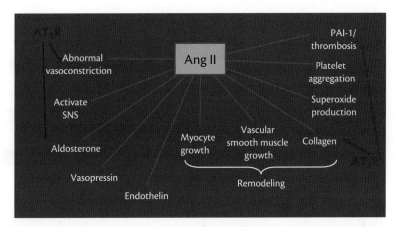

Figure 8.2.5 The deleterious effects of angiotensin II are via stimulation of the AT1 receptors and are due to abnormal vasoconstriction, stimulation of various neurohormones, growth-promoting properties, effects on the vasculature, and activation of prothrombotic pathways. PAI-1, plasminogen activator inhibitor 1; SNS, sympathetic nervous system.
Source data from Brown NJ, Vaughan DE. Prothrombotic effects of angiotensin. *Adv Intern Med.* 2000;45:419–29.

Mechanism of action: targeting the AII receptor

RAS blockade with ARBs is achieved by inhibiting the binding of AII to the AT1 receptor, which is believed to mediate the harmful cardiovascular effects of AII (➲ Figure 8.2.7).[25,26] ARBs are believed to provide a more effective means of blockade of the RAS than is possible with ACEIs, because this blockade at the receptor level is independent of the pathway for AII formation. In addition, this drug class allows the displaced AII to continue to bind to the AT2 receptors that are not blocked by ARBs. Since the AT2 receptors

are believed to mediate favourable vasodilatory and anti-trophic effects, this unopposed stimulation of the AT2 receptors may confer a theoretical advantage with ARBs over ACEIs.[27] Furthermore, ARBs may be better tolerated, as they do not interfere with the degradation of bradykinin that is responsible for cough and possibly other side effects of ACEIs such as angio-oedema.[28] ➲ Table 8.2.2 shows the doses of the most commonly prescribed Ang II receptor antagonists and their doses used in clinical trials.[18,19,29,30,31,32]

➲ Tables 8.2.3, 8.2.4, and 8.2.5 list the clinical trials with AII antagonists for HFrEF, HFpEF, and post-myocardial infarction, respectively.[17,18,19,29,30,31,32,33,34,35,36,37]

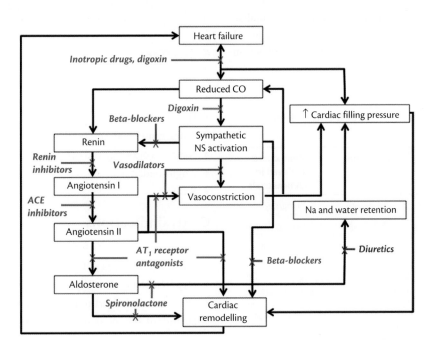

Figure 8.2.6 Neurohormonal changes in heart failure, including pharmacotherapy involved at each mechanism. ACE, angiotensin-converting enzyme; CO, cardiac output; Na, sodium; NS, nervous system.
Source data from Maron BA, and Thomas P. Rocco, Pharmacotherapy of congestive heart failure. *Goodman & Gilman's: The Pharmacological Basis of Therapeutics.* 12th ed. New York: McGraw-Hill 2011. p. 789–813.

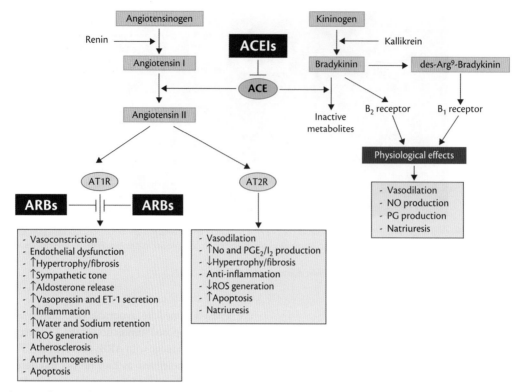

Figure 8.2.7 Mechanism of action of angiotensin-converting enzyme inhibitors (ACEIs) and angiotensin AT1 receptor blockers (ARBs). AT1R, angiotensin AT1 receptor; AT2R, angiotensin AT2 receptor; B1/B2, bradykinin receptor B1 and B2; ET-1, endothelin-1; gK, potassium conductance; NO, nitric oxide; PG, prostaglandin; ROS, reactive oxygen species.
Reproduced from Tamargo J CR, Delpón E. The Renin–Angiotensin System and Bone. *Clinical Reviews in Bone and Mineral Metabolism* volume 2015;13:125–48 (2015) with permission from Springer.

Indications and dosage

♦ An ARB is recommended to reduce the risk of HF hospitalization and cardiovascular death in symptomatic patients unable to tolerate an ACEI or an angiotensin receptor–neprilysin inhibitor (ARNI).

Table 8.2.2 Recommended doses for the best-tested AII receptor blockers in heart failure

Drug	Initial daily dose(s)	Maximum dose(s)	Mean doses achieved in clinical trials
Candesartan	4–8 mg once	32 mg once	24 mg/day
Losartan	25–50 mg once	50–150 mg once	129 mg/day
Valsartan	20–40 mg twice	160 mg twice	254 mg/day

Source data from Aulakh GK, Sodhi RK, Singh M. An update on non-peptide angiotensin receptor antagonists and related RAAS modulators. *Life Sci.* 2007;81(8):615–39; Yusuf S, Pfeffer MA, Swedberg K, *et al.* Effects of candesartan in patients with chronic heart failure and preserved left-ventricular ejection fraction: the CHARM-Preserved Trial. *Lancet.* 2003;362(9386):777–81; Tamargo J, Caballero R, Delpón E. The renin–angiotensin system and bone. *Clin Rev Bone Min Metab* 2015;13:125–48; Kaschina E, Unger T. Angiotensin AT1/AT2 receptors: regulation, signalling and function. *Blood Press.* 2003;12(2):70–88; Hornig B, Kohler C, Drexler H. Role of bradykinin in mediating vascular effects of angiotensin-converting enzyme inhibitors in humans. *Circulation.* 1997;95(5):1115–18; and Pitt B, Poole-Wilson PA, Segal R, *et al.* Effect of losartan compared with captopril on mortality in patients with symptomatic heart failure: randomised trial—the Losartan Heart Failure Survival Study ELITE II. *Lancet.* 2000;355(9215):1582–7.

♦ An ARB may be considered for patients with mildly reduced ejection fraction (HFmrEF) to reduce the risk of HF hospitalization and death.[38]

Side effects

♦ Hypotension

♦ Dizziness and headache

♦ Hyperkalaemia

♦ Worsening renal function

♦ Nausea, vomiting, and diarrhoea

♦ Angio-oedema

♦ Rash.

Contraindications

♦ Pregnancy and breastfeeding

♦ Bilateral renal artery stenosis

♦ Hypotension and/or hypoperfusion

♦ Hyperkalaemia (serum potassium >5 mmol/L)

♦ History of allergy or angio-oedema.

Combined therapy (ARBs and ACEIs) versus ACEIs alone in patients with heart failure

Several small studies have shown that ARB–ACEI combination therapy produces beneficial effects in HF patients. In

Table 8.2.3 Heart failure with reduced ejection fraction trials

Drug	Major inclusion criteria	Mean follow-up	Impact of treatment on primary endpoint
ELITE[30]			
Losartan (n = 352) vs captopril (n = 370)	LVEF ≤40%, NYHA classes II–IV	48 weeks	The 1ry EP (the frequency of persistent increase in serum creatinine level) was not significant; however, the 2ndry EP (reduction in all-cause mortality) was statistically significant (4.8% vs 8.7%; risk reduction 46% (95% CI 5%, 69%); P = 0.035)
ELITE II[29]			
Losartan (n = 1578) vs captopril (n = 1574)	LVEF ≤40%, NYHA classes II–IV	1.5 years	No significant differences in all-cause mortality (average annual mortality rate 11.7 vs 10.4%; P = 0.16) or sudden death or resuscitated arrests (9.0 vs 7.3%; P = 0.08)
CHARM-Added[35]			
Candesartan (n = 1276) vs placebo (n = 1272)	LVEF ≤40%, NYHA classes II–IV, treatment with ACEI	3.4 years	Combined cardiovascular mortality or HF hospitalization rate reduced by 15% (38% vs 42%; P = 0.01)
CHARM-Alternative[19]			
Candesartan (n = 1013) vs placebo (n = 1015)	LVEF ≤40%, NYHA classes II–IV, intolerant to ACEIs	2.8 years	Combined cardiovascular mortality or HF hospitalization rate reduced by 23% (33% vs 40%; P <0.001)
Val-HeFT[18]			
Valsartan (n = 2511) vs placebo (n = 2499)	LVEF <40%, NYHA classes II–IV, treatment with ACEI, LVID >2.9 m/BSA	1.9 years	All-cause mortality was similar in both groups (19.7% vs 19.4%; P = 0.80). Reduction in a co-primary combined EP of all-cause death, cardiac arrest with resuscitation, HF hospitalization, or IV administration of inotropic or vasodilator drugs for ≥4 hours without hospitalization by 13% (29% vs 32%; P = 0.009)

1ry, primary; 2ndry, secondary; ACEI, angiotensin-converting enzyme inhibitor; BSA, body surface area; CI, confidence interval; EP, endpoint; HF, heart failure; LVEF, left ventricular ejection fraction; LVID, left ventricular internal diameter; NYHA, New York Heart Association.

Source data from Tamargo J, Caballero R, Delpón E. The renin–angiotensin system and bone. *Clin Rev Bone Min Metab* 2015;13:125–48; Kaschina E, Unger T. Angiotensin AT1/AT2 receptors: regulation, signalling and function. *Blood Press.* 2003;12(2):70–88; Pfeffer MA, Swedberg K, Granger CB, *et al.* Effects of candesartan on mortality and morbidity in patients with chronic heart failure: the CHARM-Overall programme. *Lancet.* 2003;362(9386):759–66; Yusuf S, Pfeffer MA, Swedberg K, *et al.* Effects of candesartan in patients with chronic heart failure and preserved left-ventricular ejection fraction: the CHARM-Preserved Trial. *Lancet.* 2003;362(9386):777–81; and Aulakh GK, Sodhi RK, Singh M. An update on non-peptide angiotensin receptor antagonists and related RAAS modulators. *Life Sci.* 2007;81(8):615–39.

Table 8.2.4 Heart failure with preserved ejection fraction trials

Drug	Major inclusion criteria	Mean follow-up	Impact of treatment on primary endpoint
CHARM-Preserved[17]			
Candesartan (n = 1514) vs placebo (n = 1509)	LVEF >40%, NYHA classes II–IV, history of cardiac hospitalization	3.0 years	Trend towards a reduction in combined cardiovascular mortality or HF hospitalization by 11% (22% vs 24%; unadjusted P = 0.12, adjusted P = 0.051)
I-PRESERVE[33]			
Irbesartan (n = 2067) vs placebo (n = 2061)	LVEF ≥45%, NYHA classes III–IV with corroborative evidence or NYHA class II with HF hospitalization in recent 6 months, age ≥60 years	4.1 years	No difference in combined all-cause mortality or HF hospitalization (24% vs 25%; P = 0.54)
PARAGON-HF[34]			
Sacubitril/valsartan (n = 2407) vs valsartan (n = 2389)	LVEF ≥45%, NYHA classes II–IV, elevated level of natriuretic peptides, evidence of structural heart disease, diuretic therapy	2.9 years	No difference in total hospitalizations for HF and death from cardiovascular causes (RR 0.87 (0.75–1.01))

HF, heart failure; LVEF, left ventricular ejection fraction; NYHA, New York Heart Association.

Source data from Adam M. Integrating research and development: the emergence of rational drug design in the pharmaceutical industry. *Stud Hist Philos Biol Biomed Sci.* 2005;36(3):513–37; Pitt B, Segal R, Martinez FA, *et al.* Randomised trial of losartan versus captopril in patients over 65 with heart failure (Evaluation of Losartan in the Elderly Study, ELITE). *Lancet.* 1997;349(9054):747–52; and McMurray J, Cohen-Solal A, Dietz R, *et al.* Practical recommendations for the use of ACE inhibitors, beta-blockers, aldosterone antagonists and angiotensin receptor blockers in heart failure: putting guidelines into practice. *Eur J Heart Fail.* 2005;7(5):710–21.

Table 8.2.5 Post-myocardial infarction heart failure trials

Drug	Major inclusion criteria	Mean follow-up	Impact of treatment on primary endpoint
VALIANT[36]			
Valsartan (*n* = 4909) vs **captopril** (*n* = 4909) vs **both** (*n* = 4885)	Acute myocardial infarction (between 0.5 and 10 days previously) complicated by clinical or radiological signs of heart failure, an EF ≤35% on echocardiography, or ≤40% on radionuclide ventriculography	2.1 years	Mortality from any cause and cause-specific mortality were similar in the three treatment groups. A total of 979 patients in the valsartan group (19.9%) died, as did 941 in the valsartan and captopril group (19.3%) and 958 in the captopril group (19.5%)
OPTIMAAL[37]			
Losartan vs captopril	Confirmed acute myocardial infarction and heart failure during acute phase or new Q-wave anterior infarction or reinfarction	2.7 years	Mortality was 18% in the losartan group and 16% in the captopril group (*P* = 0·07)

EF, ejection fraction.

Source data from Massie BM, Carson PE, McMurray JJ, *et al.* Irbesartan in patients with heart failure and preserved ejection fraction. *N Engl J Med.* 2008;359(23):2456–67 and Solomon SD, McMurray JJV, Anand IS, *et al.* Angiotensin–neprilysin inhibition in heart failure with preserved ejection fraction. *N Engl J Med.* 2019;381(17):1609–20.

the Randomized Evaluation of Strategies for Left Ventricular Dysfunction (RESOLVD) Pilot Study,[39] 768 patients received candesartan 4, 8, or 16 mg, candesartan 4 or 8 mg plus enalapril 20 mg, or enalapril 20 mg alone for 43 weeks. Patients in the combination group showed less increase in end-systolic volume (ESV) and end-diastolic volume (EDV), with a trend towards increased ejection fraction, compared to either monotherapy.[40] A meta-analysis of eight trials including a total of 18,061 patients with HF compares the outcome of ARBs and ACEIs versus ACEI therapy alone in patients with HF. In this meta-analysis, combination therapy of an ARB and an ACEI, as compared to ACEI therapy alone, did not reduce important cardiovascular outcomes such as overall mortality or non-fatal myocardial infarction in patients with left ventricular dysfunction or congestive HF. Combination therapy was associated with a reduction in hospital admission for HF, but the risk of hospitalization for any reason was not affected. Combination therapy was associated with increased side effects, such as worsening of renal function, hypotension, and a tendency towards hyperkalaemia, in those trials where information was available.[41]

Guidelines

⮕ Table 8.2.6 lists the recommendations for AII blockers from various guidelines for treatment of chronic HF, including the European Society of Cardiology (ESC),[42] American Heart Association/American College of Cardiology,[43] and National Institute for Health and Care Excellence (NICE),[44] as well as an addition to the ESC Guidelines in 2021 giving a Class IIb recommendation for AII receptor blockers in patients with HFmrEF.[45] Practical guidance is provided in the ESC Guidelines.[42,46]

The future of AII antagonists

The future of AII antagonists may lie in the discovery of newer agents that may impact lipid and glucose metabolism. Losartan's ability to lower uric acid levels also merits further work. The most needed interventions include how to increase the use of these and all other guideline-directed medical therapy that, at this time, are not being used at the appropriate doses, if at all. Patients deserve to receive these survival-improving and hospitalization-reducing agents.[47]

Summary and key messages

- The RAS plays a critical role in the pathophysiology and progression of HF.
- ARBs only block the Ang II effects via the type 1 receptor, which leads to blocking the deleterious effects of Ang II, including vasoconstriction, salt and water retention, left ventricular hypertrophy, increased sympathetic activity, increased aldosterone secretion, cell growth, and fibrosis.
- Long-term therapy with ARBs produces haemodynamic, neurohormonal, and clinical effects consistent with those expected after interference with the RAS, and has been shown in randomized controlled trials to reduce morbidity and mortality.
- ARBs are considered a Class IB indication in patients with HFrEF who are unable to tolerate ACEIs or ARNIs, and a Class IIB indication in patients with HFmrEF (ESC 2021 HF guidelines).
- The risks of treatment with ARBs include hypotension, renal dysfunction, and hyperkalaemia. The risks are greater in diabetic patients, those with lower baseline renal function, and elderly patients or when combined with ACEIs or aldosterone receptor antagonists.
- ARBs should be started at low doses and titrated upward, with an attempt to use doses shown to reduce the risk of cardiovascular events in clinical trials.
- ARBs should be given with caution to patients with low systemic blood pressure, renal insufficiency, or elevated serum potassium levels (>5.0 mEq/L).

Table 8.2.6 Professional societies guidelines[39,40,41,42,43,44,45,46]

ACC/AHA/HFSA guidelines 2022[43]

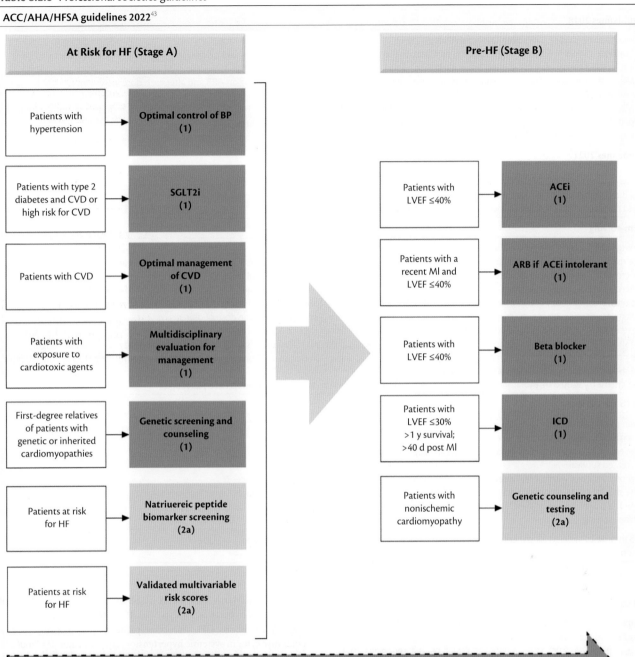

Recommendations for renin–angiotensin system inhibition with ACEI or ARB or ARNI in HFrEF

COR	LOE	
1	A	In patients with previous or current symptoms of chronic HFrEF who are intolerant of ACEIs because of cough or angio-oedema and when use of ARNI is not feasible, the use of *ARBs* is recommended to reduce morbidity and mortality
1	A	In patients with previous or current symptoms of chronic HFrEF, in whom use of ARNI is not feasible, treatment with an ACEI or *ARB* provides high economic value
Value statement: high value (A)		In patients with previous or current symptoms of chronic HFrEF, in whom use of ARNI is not feasible, treatment with an ACEI or *ARB* provides high economic value
1	B–R	In patients with chronic symptomatic HFrEF NYHA class II or III who tolerate an ACEI or *ARB*, replacement by an ARNI is recommended to further reduce morbidity and mortality

(continued)

Table 8.2.6   Continued

NICE guidelines 2018[44]

Alternative treatments if ACE inhibitors are not tolerated

1.4.7   Consider an ARB licensed for heart failure as an alternative to an ACE inhibitor for people who have heart failure with reduced ejection fraction and intolerable side effects with ACE inhibitors [2010]

1.4.8   Measure serum sodium and potassium level, and assess renal function, before and after starting an ARB and after each dose increment [2010, amended 2018]

1.4.9   Measure blood pressure after each dose increment of an ARB. Follow the recommendations on measuring blood pressure, including measurement in people with symptoms of postural hypotension in the NICE guideline on hypertension in adults [2018]

1.4.10   Once that target or maximum tolerated dose of an ARB is reached, monitor the time the person becomes acutely unwell [2010, amended 2018]

ESC guidelines 2021[45]

ARB		
An ARB is recommended to reduce the risk of HF hospitalization and CV death in symptomatic patients unable to tolerate an ACEI or ARNI (patients should also receive a beta-blocker and an MRA)	I	B

Problem-solving

Worsening renal function and hyperkalaemia:

- Some rise in urea (BUN), creatinine, and potassium levels is to be expected after an ACEI: if the increase is small and asymptomatic, no action is necessary.
- An increase in creatinine level of up to 50% above baseline, or 266 μmol/L (3 mg/dL)/eGFR <25 mL/min/1.73 m², whichever is the smaller, is acceptable.
- An increase in potassium level to ≤5.5 mmol/L is acceptable.
- If the urea, creatinine, or potassium levels rise excessively, consider stopping concomitant nephrotoxic drugs (e.g. NSAIDs) and other potassium supplements or retaining agents (triamterene, amiloride) and, if no signs of congestion, reducing the dose of diuretic.
- If greater rises in creatinine or potassium levels than those outlined above persist despite adjustment of concomitant medications, the dose of the ACEI (or ARB) should be halved and blood chemistry rechecked within 1–2 weeks; if there is still an unsatisfactory response, specialist advice should be sought.
- If the potassium level rises to >5.5 mmol/L or the creatinine level increases by >100% or to >310 μmol/L (3.5 mg/dL)/eGFR <20 mL/min/1.73 m², the ACEI (or ARB) should be stopped and a specialist consulted
- Blood chemistry should be monitored frequently and serially until the potassium and creatinine levels have plateaued.

Advice to the patient

- Explain the expected benefits:
  o Improved symptoms and exercise capacity
  o Prevention of worsening of heart failure leading to hospital admission
  o Increased survival.
- Symptoms improve within a few weeks to a few months after starting treatment.
- Advise the patient to report principal adverse effects (i.e. dizziness/symptomatic hypotension, cough)—see 'Problem-solving'.
- Advise the patient to avoid NSAIDs not prescribed by a physician (i.e. purchased over-the-counter) and salt substitutes high in potassium— see 'Problem-solving'.

An ARB may be considered for patients with HFmrEF to reduce the risk of heart failure hospitalization and death	IIb	C

References

1. Phillips MI, Schmidt-Ott KM. The discovery of renin 100 years ago. News Physiol Sci. 1999;14:271–4.

2. Tigerstedt R, Bergman PG. Niere und Kreislauf. Arch Physiol. 1898;8:223–71.

3. Bingel A, Strauss E. Uber die blutdrucksteigernde Substanz der Niere. Dtsch Arch Klin Med. 1909;96:476–92.

4. National Library of Medicine. Dr. Harry Goldblatt. 1964.

5. Goldblatt H, Lynch J, Hanzal RF, Summerville WW. Studies of elevation of systolic blood pressure by means of renal ischaemia. J Exp Med. 1934;59:347–79.

6. Page IH, Helmer OM. A crystalline pressor substance (angiotonin) resulting from the reaction between renin and renin-activator. J Exp Med. 1940;71(1):29–42.

7. Braun-Menéndez E, Fasciolo JC. Mecanismo de la acción hipotensora de la sangre venosa del riñón en isquemia incompleta aguda. Rev Soc Arg Biol. 1939;15:401–10.

8. Braun-Menéndez E, Page IH. Suggested revision of nomenclature: angiotensin. Science. 1958;127(3292):242.

9. Skeggs LT Jr, Marsh WH, Kahn JR, Shumway NP. The existence of two forms of hypertensin. J Exp Med. 1954;99(3):275–82.

10. Dzau VJ, Gibbons GH. Autocrine-paracrine mechanisms of vascular myocytes in systemic hypertension. Am J Cardiol. 1987;60(17):991–1031.

11. de Gasparo M, Catt KJ, Inagami T, Wright JW, Unger T. International Union of Pharmacology. XXIII. The angiotensin II receptors. Pharmacol Rev. 2000;52(3):415–72.

12. Brown NJ, Vaughan DE. Prothrombotic effects of angiotensin. Adv Intern Med. 2000;45:419–29.

13. Burnier M, Brunner HR. Angiotensin II receptor antagonists. Lancet. 2000;355(9204):637–45.

14. Nakajima M, Hutchinson HG, Fujinaga M, et al. The angiotensin II type 2 (AT2) receptor antagonizes the growth effects of the AT1 receptor: gain-of-function study using gene transfer. Proc Natl Acad Sci U S A. 1995;92(23):10663–7.

15. Adam M. Integrating research and development: the emergence of rational drug design in the pharmaceutical industry. Stud Hist Philos Biol Biomed Sci. 2005;36(3):513–37.

16. Aulakh GK, Sodhi RK, Singh M. An update on non-peptide angiotensin receptor antagonists and related RAAS modulators. Life Sci. 2007;81(8):615–39.

17. Yusuf S, Pfeffer MA, Swedberg K, et al. Effects of candesartan in patients with chronic heart failure and preserved left-ventricular ejection fraction: the CHARM-Preserved Trial. Lancet. 2003;362(9386):777–81.

18. Cohn JN, Tognoni G. A randomized trial of the angiotensin-receptor blocker valsartan in chronic heart failure. N Engl J Med. 2001;345(23):1667–75.

19. Granger CB, McMurray JJ, Yusuf S, et al. Effects of candesartan in patients with chronic heart failure and reduced left-ventricular systolic function intolerant to angiotensin-converting-enzyme inhibitors: the CHARM-Alternative trial. Lancet. 2003;362(9386):772–6.

20. Brousil JA, Burke JM. Olmesartan medoxomil: an angiotensin II-receptor blocker. Clin Ther. 2003;25(4):1041–55.

21. Zusman RM. Are there differences among angiotensin receptor blockers? Am J Hypertens. 1999;12(12 Pt 3):231S–5S.

22. Levy D, Kenchaiah S, Larson MG, et al. Long-term trends in the incidence of and survival with heart failure. N Engl J Med. 2002;347(18):1397–402.

23. Erhardt LR. A review of the current evidence for the use of angiotensin-receptor blockers in chronic heart failure. Int J Clin Pract. 2005;59(5):571–8.

24. Maron BA, Rocco TP. Pharmacotherapy of congestive heart failure. In: Brunton L, Chabner BA, Knollman B, eds. Goodman & Gilman's: The Pharmacological Basis of Therapeutics, 12th edition. New York, NY: McGraw-Hill; 2011, pp. 789–813.

25. McMurray JJ. Angiotensin receptor blockers for chronic heart failure and acute myocardial infarction. Heart. 2001;86(1):97–103.

26. Tamargo J, Caballero R, Delpón E. The renin–angiotensin system and bone. Clin Rev Bone Min Metab 2015;13:125–48.

27. Kaschina E, Unger T. Angiotensin AT1/AT2 receptors: regulation, signalling and function. Blood Press. 2003;12(2):70–88.

28. Hornig B, Kohler C, Drexler H. Role of bradykinin in mediating vascular effects of angiotensin-converting enzyme inhibitors in humans. Circulation. 1997;95(5):1115–18.

29. Pitt B, Poole-Wilson PA, Segal R, et al. Effect of losartan compared with captopril on mortality in patients with symptomatic heart failure: randomised trial—the Losartan Heart Failure Survival Study ELITE II. Lancet. 2000;355(9215):1582–7.

30. Pitt B, Segal R, Martinez FA, et al. Randomised trial of losartan versus captopril in patients over 65 with heart failure (Evaluation of Losartan in the Elderly Study, ELITE). Lancet. 1997;349(9054):747–52.

31. McMurray J, Cohen-Solal A, Dietz R, et al. Practical recommendations for the use of ACE inhibitors, beta-blockers, aldosterone antagonists and angiotensin receptor blockers in heart failure: putting guidelines into practice. Eur J Heart Fail. 2005;7(5):710–21.

32. Pfeffer MA, Swedberg K, Granger CB, et al. Effects of candesartan on mortality and morbidity in patients with chronic heart failure: the CHARM-Overall programme. Lancet. 2003;362(9386):759–66.

33. Massie BM, Carson PE, McMurray JJ, et al. Irbesartan in patients with heart failure and preserved ejection fraction. N Engl J Med. 2008;359(23):2456–67.

34. Solomon SD, McMurray JJV, Anand IS, et al. Angiotensin–neprilysin inhibition in heart failure with preserved ejection fraction. N Engl J Med. 2019;381(17):1609–20.

35. McMurray JJ, Ostergren J, Swedberg K, et al. Effects of candesartan in patients with chronic heart failure and reduced left-ventricular systolic function taking angiotensin-converting-enzyme inhibitors: the CHARM-Added trial. Lancet. 2003;362(9386):767–71.

36. Velazquez EJ, Pfeffer MA, McMurray JV, et al. VALsartan In Acute myocardial iNfarcTion (VALIANT) trial: baseline characteristics in context. Eur J Heart Fail. 2003;5(4):537–44.

37. Dickstein K, Kjekshus J; OPTIMAAL Steering Committee of the OPTIMAAL Study Group. Effects of losartan and captopril on mortality and morbidity in high-risk patients after acute myocardial infarction: the OPTIMAAL randomised trial. Optimal Trial in Myocardial Infarction with Angiotensin II Antagonist Losartan. Lancet. 2002;360(9335):752–60.

38. Hill RD, Vaidya PN. Angiotensin II receptor blockers (ARB). Treasure Island, FL: StatPearls Publishing; 2022.

39. McKelvie RS, Yusuf S, Pericak D, et al. Comparison of candesartan, enalapril, and their combination in congestive heart failure: randomized evaluation of strategies for left ventricular dysfunction (RESOLVD) pilot study. The RESOLVD Pilot Study Investigators. Circulation. 1999;100(10):1056–64.

40. Hamroff G, Katz SD, Mancini D, et al. Addition of angiotensin II receptor blockade to maximal angiotensin-converting enzyme inhibition improves exercise capacity in patients with severe congestive heart failure. Circulation. 1999;99(8):990–2.

41. Kuenzli A, Bucher HC, Anand I, et al. Meta-analysis of combined therapy with angiotensin receptor antagonists versus ACE inhibitors alone in patients with heart failure. PLoS One. 2010;5(4):e9946.

42. Ponikowski P, Voors AA, Anker SD, et al. 2016 ESC Guidelines for the diagnosis and treatment of acute and chronic heart failure. Rev Esp Cardiol. 2016;69(12):1167.

43. Heidenreich PA, Bozkurt B, Aguilar D, et al. 2022 AHA/ACC/HFSA guideline for the management of heart failure: a report of the American College of Cardiology/American Heart Association Joint Committee on Clinical Practice Guidelines. J Am Coll Cardiol. 2022;79(17):1757–80.

44. Taylor CJ, Moore J, O'Flynn N. Diagnosis and management of chronic heart failure: NICE guideline update 2018. Br J Gen Pract. 2019;69(682):265–6.

45. McDonagh T, Metra M, Adamo M, et al. ESC Guidelines for the diagnosis and treatment of acute and chronic heart failure. Eur Heart J. 2021;42:3599–726.

46. Ponikowski P, Voors AA, Anker SD, et al. 2016 ESC Guidelines for the diagnosis and treatment of acute and chronic heart failure: The Task Force for the Diagnosis and Treatment of Acute and Chronic Heart Failure of the European Society of Cardiology (ESC) Developed with the special contribution of the Heart Failure Association (HFA) of the ESC. Eur Heart J. 2016;37(27):2129–200.

47. Greene SJ, Fonarow GC, DeVore AD, et al. Titration of medical therapy for heart failure with reduced ejection fraction. J Am Coll Cardiol. 2019;73(19):2365–83.

CHAPTER 8.3

Angiotensin II receptor–neprilysin inhibitor

Petar M Seferović, Michele Senni, Marija Polovina, and Andrew JS Coats

Contents

Introduction

Sacubitril/valsartan is the first-in-class angiotensin receptor–neprilysin inhibitor (ARNI). Its two components act in concert to potentiate the favourable cardiovascular effects of the natriuretic peptide (NP) system, while simultaneously counteracting the increased activity of angiotensin II. Sacubitril/valsartan has been proven to be more effective in reducing the risk of cardiovascular mortality and hospitalization for heart failure (HF), compared to the angiotensin-converting enzyme (ACE) inhibitor enalapril in patients with HF with reduced ejection fraction (HFrEF). Hence, sacubitril/valsartan is now considered as one of the foundational treatment modalities of HFrEF recommended for all HFrEF patients, with a favourable impact on clinical outcomes, symptoms, and quality of life. The beneficial effects of sacubitril/valsartan seem to extend to patients with HF with mildly reduced ejection fraction (HFmrEF) and possibly even to some patients with HF with preserved ejection fraction (HFpEF). This chapter provides a summary of the most relevant aspects in the development and pharmacodynamic and pharmacokinetic properties of sacubitril/valsartan. It also provides a review of the clinical trial data that support the role of ARNIs in contemporary treatment of HF.

Development and mechanism of action

HF is associated with the activation of the three neurohormonal axes, namely, the renin–angiotensin–aldosterone system (RAAS), sympathetic nervous system (SNS), and NP system. Activation of the RAAS and SNS leads to vasoconstriction, water and sodium retention, and increased cardiac contractility, which help to maintain cardiac output in the short term. However, in the long run, activation of the RAAS and SNS have detrimental consequences, as they promote left ventricular (LV) hypertrophy, remodelling, and fibrosis that eventually lead to deterioration in LV function. Indeed, randomized controlled trials have demonstrated that inhibition of both the RAAS and the SNS confers substantial improvement in survival and reduction in HF hospitalization in patients with HFrEF. However, despite neurohormonal inhibition of the RAAS and SNS, with the use of multiple agents (i.e. ACE inhibitors or angiotensin receptor blockers (ARBs), mineralocorticoid receptor antagonists (MRAs), and beta-blockers), residual mortality has remained high, which provided a rationale for targeting modulation of NP activity as a novel strategy to improve outcomes in patients with HFrEF.

The NP system acts in opposition to the effects of RAAS and SNS activation. It exerts protective effects on the cardiovascular system by increasing renal natriuresis and diuresis, promoting vasodilatation, and decreasing the activity of the RAAS and SNS. There are three types on NPs, namely, atrial natriuretic peptide (ANP), B-type natriuretic peptide (BNP), and C-type natriuretic peptide (CNP). ANP and BNP are predominantly produced by the atria and ventricles, respectively, in response to elevated wall stress, and exert their actions systemically, whereas CNP is produced by the vascular endothelium where it acts in a paracrine manner.[1] Increased levels of angiotensin II and endothelin can also promote NP secretion from the ventricles.[2] NPs are produced in an inactive pre-pro form, which is then cleaved into an active NP and an inactive N-terminal (NT) pro-NP fragment. They are inactivated by three mechanisms: excretion in body fluids (e.g. via renal and liver elimination); NP receptor C-mediated internalization; and neprilysin-mediated proteolysis. Neprilysin (a neutral endopeptidase) is a membrane-bound enzyme predominantly expressed in the kidney where it plays a major role in NP clearance. In addition to NPs, neprilysin catalyses the degradation of other vasodilator peptides, including bradykinin, aminopeptidase P, and adrenomedullin to varying degrees, as well as vasoconstrictor peptides, including endothelin 1 and angiotensin II. Thus, the net effect of neprilysin inhibition on vascular tone will depend on whether the predominant substrates degraded are vasodilators or vasoconstrictors. Consequently, a benefit obtained from enhancing the NPs may be offset by increased angiotensin II.[3]

Early strategies of increasing NP activity by directly inhibiting neprilysin failed to provide sustained treatment benefits, probably due to the opposing effect of elevated angiotensin II and endothelin levels. This led to the strategy of simultaneous inhibition of the RAAS and NP system. The first such strategy included omapatrilat, a combination of an ACE inhibitor and a neprilysin inhibitor. When compared with enalapril, omapatrilat was no more effective in reducing the risk of the combined primary endpoint of all-cause mortality or HF hospitalization in HFrEF patients in the Omapatrilat Versus Enalapril Randomized Trial of Utility in Reducing events (OVERTURE), but there was a small reduction in the secondary outcome of all-cause mortality or cardiovascular hospitalization by 9%,[4] However, the rate of angio-oedema in the omapatrilat group significantly exceeded that in the enalapril group, likely due to unintended accumulation of bradykinin resulting from inhibition of its key breakdown enzymes by omapatrilat (in rank order for degrading bradykinin: ACE > aminopeptidase P ≥ neprilysin).[5] A higher risk of serious angio-oedema was also observed in hypertensive patients receiving omapatrilat, compared to those who received enalapril,

in the Omapatrilat Cardiovascular Treatment Versus Enalapril (OCTAVE) trial, a finding which led to the termination of further development of omapatrilat.[6]

The next strategy to explore was to exert further downstream inhibition of the RAAS by an ARB, notably valsartan, in combination with the neprilysin inhibitor sacubitril. This strategy gave rise to the first-in-class ARNI sacubitril/valsartan (➲ Figure 8.3.1).

Sacubitril/valsartan has been proven to exert multiple beneficial effects of dual RAAS and neprilysin inhibition, while the risk of angio-oedema remains low. The low risk of angio-oedema is the result of preserved activity of two of the three enzymes responsible for bradykinin breakdown (i.e. ACE and aminopeptidase P, which are not substrates for sacubitrilat, the active metabolite of sacubitril). The ARNI class represents a potential shift in the treatment of HF from partial neurohormonal system inhibition to integrated composite neurohormonal system modulation (➲ Figure 8.3.2).

Pharmacokinetic properties and dosing of sacubitril/valsartan

Following oral administration, sacubitril/valsartan is rapidly absorbed (unaffected by food intake) and dissociates into valsartan and sacubitril, which is converted into sacubitrilat. Valsartan in sacubitril/valsartan has higher bioavailability, compared to valsartan used as monotherapy, corresponding to a 40% higher systemic exposure to valsartan (i.e. 97/103 mg of sacubitril/valsartan is equivalent to 160 mg of valsartan).[7] With twice-daily dosing, a steady-state drug concentration is reached in 3 days.[5] Serum levels of both sacubitril and valsartan can increase in patients with significant renal and/or hepatic impairment, as well as in older individuals due to impaired metabolism and excretion.

Sacubitril/valsartan in chronic heart failure with reduced ejection fraction

The efficacy and safety of sacubitril/valsartan for cardiovascular outcomes in patients with HFrEF was evaluated in the Prospective comparison of ARNI with ACEI to Determine Impact on Global Mortality and morbidity in Heart Failure (PARADIGM-HF) trial.[8] The trial assessed whether sacubitril/valsartan was superior to enalapril in reducing the primary endpoint of cardiovascular

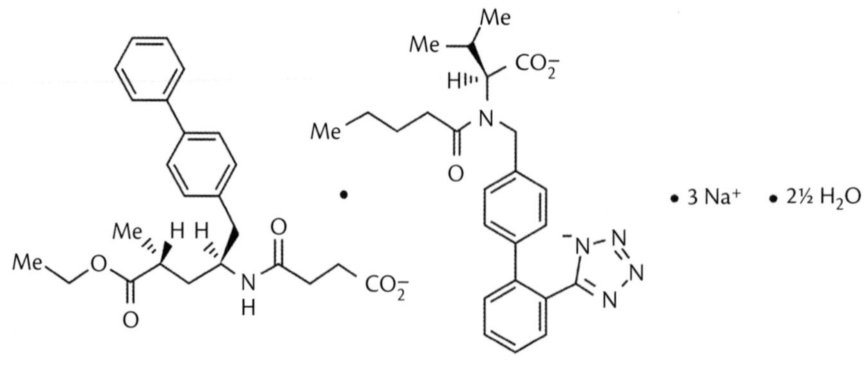

Figure 8.3.1 Sacubitril/valsartan molecule.

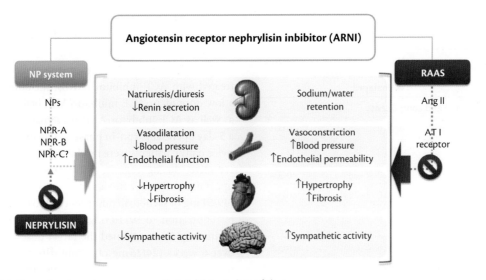

Figure 8.3.2 Beneficial effects of angiotensin receptor–neprilysin inhibitor in heart failure.
Reproduced from Volpe M. Natriuretic peptides and cardio-renal disease. *Int J Cardiol*. 2014 Oct 20;176(3):630–9. doi: 10.1016/j.ijcard.2014.08.032 with permission from Elsevier.

death or HF hospitalization. The study included stable ambulatory patients with HFrEF (→ Table 8.3.1).

Prior to randomization in the PARADIGM trial, all patients completed a 6- to 8-week run-in period, during which it was required that the target doses of both drugs were attained and

tolerated. The trial was prematurely terminated after a median follow-up of 27 months because of the highly significant reduction in the primary composite endpoint, as well as in cardiovascular mortality, with sacubitril/valsartan than with enalapril. Treatment with sacubitril/valsartan resulted in a 20% lower

Table 8.3.1 Major inclusion and exclusion criteria and main patient characteristics in clinical trials of sacubitril/valsartan in heart failure with reduced ejection fraction

	PARADIGM-HF	TITRATION
Study drug (target dose)	Sacubitril/valsartan (107/97 mg BD)	Sacubitril/valsartan (107/97 mg BD)
Comparator (target dose)	Enalapril (10 mg BD)	NA
Number of patients	8399	498*
Inclusion criteria		
LVEF	≤40% (changed to ≤35% later in the trial)	≤35%
NYHA class	II–IV (outpatients)	II–IV (outpatients/inpatients)
BNP/NT-proBNP	BNP ≥150 pg/mL (or NT-proBNP ≥600 pg/mL) If hospitalized within the previous 12 months, ≥100 pg/mL (or NT-proBNP ≥400 pg/mL)	NA
ACE inhibitor/ARB-naïve	No	Yes
Exclusion criteria	Symptomatic hypotension Systolic BP <100 mg (screening); <95 mmHg (randomization) eGFR <30 mL/min History of angio-oedema	Previous intolerance of recommended doses of ACE inhibitor/ARB Symptomatic hypotension Systolic BP <100 mg or >180 mmHg History of angio-oedema
Patient characteristics		
Mean age (years)	~64	~64
Female sex (%)	21–22	20–22
Baseline LVEF (%)	29–30 (mean)	~30 (mean)

* Number of patients randomized.

ACE, angiotensin-converting enzyme; ARB, angiotensin receptor blocker; BD, twice daily; BNP, B-type natriuretic peptide; BP, blood pressure; eGFR, estimated glomerular filtration rate; HFrEF, heart failure with reduced ejection fraction; LVEF, left ventricular ejection fraction; NA, not applicable; NT-proBNP, N-terminal pro-B-type natriuretic peptide; NYHA, New York Heart Association.

Source data from McMurray JJ, Packer M, Desai AS, Gong J, Lefkowitz MP, Rizkala AR, *et al*. Angiotensin-neprilysin inhibition versus enalapril in heart failure. *N Engl J Med*. 2014;371(11):993–1004.

Table 8.3.2 Primary and secondary outcomes in the PARADIGM-HF trial

PARADIGM-HF	HR (95% CI) Sacubitril/valsartan vs enalapril	P-value
Primary composite outcome and components		
Death from cardiovascular causes or first hospitalization for worsening heart failure	0.80 (0.73–0.87)	<0.001
Death from cardiovascular causes	0.80 (0.71–0.89	<0.001
First hospitalization for worsening heart failure	0.79 (0.71–0.89)	<0.001
Secondary outcomes		
Death from any cause	0.84 (0.76–0.93)	<0.001
Change in KCCQ clinical summary score at 8 months	1.64 (0.63–2.65)	0.001
New-onset atrial fibrillation	0.97 (0.72–1.31)	0.83
Decline in renal function*	0.86 (0.65–1.13)	0.28

* Defined as end-stage renal disease or a decrease of ≥50% in the estimated glomerular filtration rate (eGFR) from randomization or a decrease in the eGFR of >30% relative to a baseline of <60 mL/min/1.73 m².

CI, confidence interval; HR, hazard ratio; KCCQ, Kansas City Cardiomyopathy Questionnaire.

Source data from McMurray JJ, Packer M, Desai AS, Gong J, Lefkowitz MP, Rizkala AR, et al. Angiotensin-neprilysin inhibition versus enalapril in heart failure. N Engl J Med. 2014;371(11):993–1004. AND Senni M, McMurray JJ, Wachter R, McIntyre HF, Reyes A, Majercak I, et al. Initiating sacubitril/valsartan (LCZ696) in heart failure: results of TITRATION, a double-blind, randomized comparison of two uptitration regimens. Eur J Heart Fail. 2016;18(9):1193–202.

risk of cardiovascular death or HF hospitalization, compared to enalapril, with a significant reduction in both components of the primary endpoint (⮕ Table 8.3.2).

The treatment effect was consistent, regardless of age, sex, race, and a number of clinical characteristics according to a predefined subgroup analysis plan. There was a significant 16% reduction in all-cause mortality, as well as in death due to pump failure and sudden cardiac death.[9] Patients in the sacubitril/valsartan group had a lower risk of first and total (first and recurrent) hospitalizations for worsening HF (by 21% and 23%, respectively) and were less likely to require admission to intensive care units or to need inotropic agents and mechanical circulatory support or heart transplantation, compared to those receiving enalapril.[10] The reduction in HF hospitalization with sacubitril/valsartan occurred quickly, with an effect evident within the first 30 days after randomization. There was an improvement in patient-reported functional status (as measured with use of the Kansas City Cardiomyopathy Questionnaire clinical summary score). In general, the drug was safe and well tolerated. Although patients in the sacubitril/valsartan group experienced symptomatic hypotension more frequently than those in the enalapril group, more participants assigned to enalapril discontinued the study medication due to adverse effects. The rates of worsening renal function and severe hyperkalaemia were lower with sacubitril/valsartan than with enalapril, whereas the rate of angio-oedema was comparable.

The TITRATION study provided an insight into the tolerability of initiating and uptitrating sacubitril/valsartan by using two different dosing regimens in a broader population of HFrEF patients (⮕ Table 8.3.1). The study enrolled patients previously treated with ACE inhibitors/ARBs, including patients receiving a low dose of an ACE inhibitor/ARB before enrolment (50.4%), as well as ACE inhibitor/ARB-naïve patients (6.6%).[11] Following a 5-day open-label run-in phase (24/26 mg of sacubitril/valsartan twice daily), patients were randomized to a 'condensed' or a 'conservative' dosing regimen. The 'condensed' regimen included uptitration of sacubitril/valsartan to the target dose over 3 weeks (49/51 mg of sacubitril/valsartan twice daily for 2 weeks, followed by uptitration to 97/103 mg twice daily). In the 'conservative' regimen, patients attained the target dose in a stepwise manner over 6 weeks (24/26 mg of sacubitril/valsartan twice daily for 2 weeks, followed by uptitration to 49/51 mg twice daily for 3 weeks, and then to 97/103 mg twice daily until the end of the study). Furthermore, patients were stratified according to the pre-study dose of the ACE inhibitor/ARB into a low-dose stratum (i.e. pre-study low dose of ACE inhibitor/ARB and ACE inhibitor/ARB-naïve patients) and a high-dose stratum. The study demonstrated that patients in the 'condensed' arm had an increased frequency of predefined adverse events, including hypotension, renal dysfunction, hyperkalaemia, and angio-oedema, compared to the 'conservative' arm, but the difference was not statistically significant. Overall, 76% of the study participants achieved the target dose of sacubitril/valsartan over 12 weeks, without a significant difference between the two dosing regimens. However, patients in the low-dose stratum, as well as those with lower blood pressure, were more likely to attain the target dose without adverse effects if they were uptitrated 'conservatively'. These observations bear important practical implications, given that the ability to attain the target dose can be improved by starting with a low dose and allowing a more gradual uptitration of sacubitril/valsartan.[12]

Several mechanistic studies have demonstrated that the beneficial effects of sacubitril/valsartan in HFrEF include LV reverse remodelling, improvement in systolic and diastolic function, and reduction in functional mitral regurgitation and arterial stiffness.[13,14,15] In the Prospective Study of Biomarkers, Symptom Improvement, and Ventricular Remodeling During Sacubitril/Valsartan Therapy for HF (PROVE-HF), the median LV ejection fraction (LVEF) increased from approximately 28% to approximately 38% during 12 months of treatment with sacubitril/valsartan, whereas both end-diastolic and end-systolic volume indices decreased significantly.[13] There was also a significant decrease in the left atrial volume index and an improvement in parameters of diastolic function. These findings were further substantiated by the Effects of Sacubitril/Valsartan vs. Enalapril on Aortic Stiffness in Patients With Mild to Moderate HF With Reduced Ejection Fraction (EVALUATE-HF) trial, in which signs of LV reverse remodelling became apparent as early as 12 weeks of sacubitril/valsartan treatment, compared to treatment with enalapril.[16] In the Pharmacological Reduction of Functional, Ischemic Mitral Regurgitation (PRIME) study of patients with LVEF of 25–50% and severe functional mitral regurgitation, 12 months of sacubitril/valsartan treatment conferred a significant reduction in the LV end-diastolic volume index, a decrease in the regurgitant orifice area, and an improvement in mitral regurgitation.[14]

In addition, a post hoc analysis of the PARADIGM-HF trial suggested long-term beneficial effects on renal function.[17] There was also an improvement in glycaemic control in patients with diabetes or elevated glycated haemoglobin (HbA1c) (i.e. greater reduction in HbA1c and lower rate of insulin initiation with sacubitril/valsartan than with enalapril).[18]

Sacubitril/valsartan in acute heart failure with reduced ejection fraction

The PIONEER trial (Comparison of Sacubitril-Valsartan versus Enalapril on Effect on NT-proBNP in Patients Stabilized from an Acute Heart Failure Episode) assessed the efficacy and safety of treatment with sacubitril/valsartan for 8 weeks in patients hospitalized for acute HF.[19] Briefly, the study randomized patients hospitalized with HFrEF and elevated NP levels to receiving either sacubitril/valsartan or enalapril following haemodynamic stabilization and decongestion (➲ Table 8.3.3).

Approximately 50% of enrolled patients in the PIONEER-HF trial had no previous exposure to ACE inhibitors/ARBs; the median duration of hospital stay was approximately 5 days, and only approximately 11% of the patients required admission to intensive care units. The primary endpoint of the trial was to compare the time-averaged proportional change in N-terminal pro-B-type natriuretic peptide (NT-proBNP) levels between the two treatment arms. It was demonstrated that patients receiving sacubitril/valsartan achieved a greater reduction in NT-proBNP level, compared to those in the enalapril group, and the beneficial effect of sacubitril/valsartan became evident in the first week of treatment. Moreover, an exploratory analysis demonstrated a 46% risk reduction in the composite of death, rehospitalization for HF, implantation of an LV assist device, or listing for heart transplantation.[20] There was also a 42% risk reduction in the composite of cardiovascular death and HF rehospitalization, primarily driven by a 36% lower risk of rehospitalization for HF.[20] The beneficial effects were consistent in ACE inhibitor/ARB-naïve patients and were observed across all doses of sacubitril/valsartan.[21] The risk

Table 8.3.3 Major inclusion and exclusion criteria and main patient characteristics in clinical trials of sacubitril/valsartan in patients with acute heart failure

	PIONEER-HF	TRANSITION
Study drug (target dose)	Sacubitril/valsartan (107/97 mg BD)	Sacubitril/valsartan (107/97 mg BD)
Comparator (target dose)	Enalapril (10 mg BD)	NA
Number of patients	881	1002
Inclusion criteria		
LVEF	≤40%	≤40%, NYHA classes II–IV, systolic BP ≥100 mmHg
BNP/NT-proBNP	NT-proBNP level ≥1600 pg/mL or BNP level ≥400 pg/mL	NA
ACE inhibitor/ARB-naïve	Yes	Yes
Time of randomization	>24 hours up to 10 days after admission	≥12 hours pre-discharge or between days 1 and 14 post-discharge
Haemodynamic stability	Systolic BP ≥100 mmHg for at least 6 hours, with no increase in the dose of intravenous diuretics and no use of intravenous vasodilators during the preceding 6 hours and no use of intravenous inotropes during the preceding 24 hours	NA
Exclusion criteria	History of hypersensitivity or intolerance of sacubitril/valsartan ACE inhibitors/ARBs; eGFR <30 mL/min/1.73 m²	Symptomatic hypotension Systolic BP <100 mg or >180 mmHg History of angio-oedema Severe hepatic impairment, biliary cirrhosis, and cholestasis
Patient characteristics		
Age (years)	61–63 (median)	~67
Female sex (%)	26–30	~24
Baseline LVEF (%)	24–25 (median)	~29 (mean)

ACE, angiotensin-converting enzyme; ARB, angiotensin receptor blocker; BD, twice daily; BNP, B-type natriuretic peptide; BP, blood pressure; eGFR, estimated glomerular filtration rate; LVEF, left ventricular ejection fraction; NA, not applicable; NT-proBNP< N-terminal pro-B-type natriuretic peptide; NYHA, New York Heart Association.

Source data from Velazquez EJ, Morrow DA, DeVore AD, Duffy CI, Ambrosy AP, McCague K, *et al*. Angiotensin-Neprilysin Inhibition in Acute Decompensated Heart Failure. *N Engl J Med*. 2019;380(6):539–48 AND Wachter R, Senni M, Belohlavek J, Straburzynska-Migaj E, Witte KK, Kobalava Z, *et al*. Initiation of sacubitril/valsartan in haemodynamically stabilised heart failure patients in hospital or early after discharge: primary results of the randomised TRANSITION study. *Eur J Heart Fail*. 2019;21(8):998–1007.

of serious adverse effects, including worsening renal function, hyperkalaemia, symptomatic hypotension, and angio-oedema, was comparable between the two treatment arms.

An open-label extension of the PIONEER-HF trial indicated that early in-hospital initiation of sacubitril/valsartan and continuation of treatment for 12 weeks conferred a more significant reduction in NP levels, compared to initial enalapril treatment for 8 weeks followed by a switch to sacubitril/valsartan for 4 weeks.[22] Furthermore, patients with early in-hospital initiation of sacubitril/valsartan had a 31% lower risk of cardiovascular death or HF rehospitalization during 12 weeks of follow-up, compared to those patients who were initially treated with enalapril in hospital and later (after 8 weeks) switched to sacubitril/valsartan. This observation points to the importance of early initiation of sacubitril/valsartan in vulnerable hospitalized patients in order to achieve greater improvement in outcomes.

The TRANSITION trial assessed the tolerability and safety of initiating sacubitril/valsartan during hospitalization for acute HFrEF (>12 hours pre-discharge), compared to drug initiation within 14 days post-discharge (➲ Table 8.3.3).[23] Most patients (88.4% in the pre-discharge group and 84.5% in the post-discharge group) were started on the lowest dose of sacubitril/valsartan (24/26 mg twice daily) and the target dose (103/97 mg twice daily) was attained in approximately 50% of the patients, regardless of the time of drug initiation. However, patients with a higher baseline systolic blood pressure (>120 mmHg) and better renal function and those with *de novo* acute HFrEF were more likely to achieve and maintain the target dose of sacubitril/valsartan.[24]

From a practical standpoint, appropriate timing of in-hospital initiation of sacubitril/valsartan in patients with acute HF should be based on two important criteria:

1. Patients should be haemodynamically stabilized. This means that all of the following criteria need to be met:
   a. Stable systolic blood pressure of ≥100 mmHg for at least 6 hours
   b. No use of inotropes/vasopressors for at least 24 hours
   c. No use of intravenous vasodilators for at least 6 hours
   d. Unchanged dose of intravenous (or preferably oral) diuretics.
2. Patients should be euvolaemic.

Patients with residual volume overload (hypervolaemia) require further decongestive therapy and may deteriorate clinically, which imposes a relative contraindication to the use of sacubitril/valsartan. Furthermore, patients with hypovolaemia, characterized by borderline low blood pressure, a propensity for orthostatic hypotension, decreased skin turgor, significant increase in haematocrit, and worsening renal function, can be at high risk of deterioration and should not be considered for in-hospital sacubitril/valsartan initiation.

Sacubitril/valsartan in heart failure with preserved ejection fraction

The Prospective comparison of ARNI with ARB on the Management Of heart failUre with preserved ejection fraction (PARAMOUNT) trial was the first to evaluate potential treatment benefits with sacubitril/valsartan in patients with HFpEF.[25] The

trial assessed the effect of sacubitril/valsartan versus valsartan on the change in NT-proBNP levels (primary outcome) at 12 weeks in patients with HFpEF (➲ Table 8.3.4). The results demonstrated a significantly greater reduction in NT-proBNP levels with sacubitril/valsartan, compared to treatment with valsartan. This encouraging result called for a prospective evaluation of the effect of ARNIs on clinical outcomes in patients with HFpEF.

The Prospective Comparison of ARNI with ARB Global Outcomes in HF With Preserved Ejection Fraction (PARAGON-HF) trial was a randomized, double-blind, event-driven trial that assessed the long-term efficacy and safety of sacubitril/valsartan versus valsartan in patients with HFpEF (➲ Table 8.3.4).[26] Before randomization, all patients entered a run-in period to ensure tolerability of both drugs at half the target doses. The primary endpoint was a composite of cardiovascular death and total (first and recurrent) HF hospitalizations. After a median follow-up of 35 months, the incidence of the primary endpoint was lower in the sacubitril/valsartan group, but the difference failed to meet statistical significance (➲ Table 8.3.5). Neither of the two components of the primary endpoint were significantly reduced with sacubitril/valsartan, compared to treatment with valsartan. There were more cases of symptomatic hypotension and angio-oedema, and fewer cases of hyperkalaemia, in the sacubitril/valsartan arm.

A prespecified sub-analysis indicated heterogeneity in risk reduction according to sex and baseline LVEF, suggesting a possible favourable effect of sacubitril/valsartan in women and patients with below-median LVEF (≤57%). Indeed, there was a significant reduction in the primary endpoint in women, even after adjustment for baseline differences between the sexes, that was primarily driven by a reduction in HF hospitalization. Several mechanisms were proposed to explain this effect (e.g. sex-related differences in cardiac remodelling whereby women tend to have higher normal LVEF and may have had more LV systolic dysfunction at any given LVEF; sex differences in NP peptide biology whereby sacubitril/valsartan-mediated potentiation of the NP system might have been beneficial in terms of post-menopausal loss of oestrogen-dependent stimulation of this system in females, etc.), but the true explanation awaits further studies. However, the reduction in HF hospitalization rates was not associated with improvements in functional status or quality of life in women. Moreover, changes in NT-proBNP levels and increases in the urinary cyclic guanosine monophosphate (cGMP)-to-creatinine ratio were similar in both women and men.[27] The PARAGLIDE-HF (Prospective comparison of ARNI with ARB Given following stabiLization In DEcompensated HFpEF) demonstrated that among patients with EF >40% stabilized after an episode of worsening HF, sacubitril/valsartan led to a greater reduction in NT-proBNP levels compared with valsartan (ratio of change: 0.85; 95%CI: 0.73–0.999; P = 0.049) and was associated with clinical benefit, albeit at a cost of more symptomatic hypotension.[27a] Furthermore, in the pooled analyses of the PARAGLIDE-HF and PARAGON-HF trials, treatment with sacubitril/valsartan was associated with a significant reduction in cardiovascular and renal events in patients with HFmrEF and HFpEF.[27b]

A post hoc analysis of the pooled PARADIGM-HF and PARAGON-HF data indicated that the effect of sacubitril/

Table 8.3.4 Major inclusion and exclusion criteria and main patient characteristics in clinical trials of sacubitril/valsartan in heart failure with preserved ejection fraction

	PARAMOUNT	PARAGON-HF	PARALLAX
Study drug (target dose)	Sacubitril/valsartan (107/97 mg BD)	Sacubitril/valsartan (107/97 mg BD)	Sacubitril/valsartan (107/97 mg BD)
Comparator (target dose)	Valsartan (160 mg BD)	Valsartan (160 mg BD)	Standard medical treatment: Enalapril (10 mg BD) or valsartan (160 mg BD) daily) in patients with hypertension OR Placebo in patients without hypertension
Number of patients	301	4822	2566
Inclusion criteria			
LVEF	≥45%	≥45%	≥40%
NYHA class	II–IV	II–IV	II–IV
BNP/NT-proBNP	NT-proBNP levels >400 pg/mL	HF hospitalization within 9 months prior to screening visit and NT-proBNP levels >200 pg/mL (>600 pg/mL for patients in AF at screening) or NT-proBNP levels >300 pg/mL (>900 pg/mL for patients in AF at screening)	NT-proBNP >220 pg/mL for patients with no AF, or >600 pg/mL for patients with AF
ACE inhibitor/ARB-naïve	Yes	Yes	Yes
Exclusion criteria	Prior LVEF <45% at any time Acute decompensated heart failure Uncontrolled hypertension eGFR <30 mL/min/1.73 m² Isolated right heart failure Haemodynamically significant VHD Hypertrophic cardiomyopathy	Prior LVEF <40% at any time Acute coronary syndrome Acute decompensated heart failure Uncontrolled hypertension Life-threatening/uncontrolled cardiac arrhythmia Isolated right heart failure Haemodynamically significant VHD or CHD History of angio-oedema	Prior LVEF <40% at any time Acute coronary syndrome Acute decompensated heart failure Uncontrolled hypertension eGFR <30 mL/min/1.73 m² History of angio-oedema
Patient characteristics			
Mean age (years)	~71	~73	~73
Female sex (%)	56–57	52	~50–51
Baseline LVEF (%)	58 (mean)	~57 (median)	57–58

ACE, angiotensin-converting enzyme; AF, atrial fibrillation; ARB, angiotensin receptor blocker; BD, twice daily; BNP, B-type natriuretic peptide; CHD, congenital heart disease; eGFR, estimated glomerular filtration rate; LVEF, left ventricular ejection fraction; NT-proBNP, N-terminal pro-B-type natriuretic peptide; NYHA, New York Heart Association; VHD, valvular heart disease.

Source data from Solomon SD, Zile M, Pieske B, Voors A, Shah A, Kraigher-Krainer E, et al. The angiotensin receptor neprilysin inhibitor LCZ696 in heart failure with preserved ejection fraction: a phase 2 double-blind randomised controlled trial. *Lancet.* 2012;380(9851):1387–95 AND Solomon SD, McMurray JJV, Anand IS, Ge J, Lam CSP, Maggioni AP, et al. Angiotensin–Neprilysin Inhibition in Heart Failure with Preserved Ejection Fraction. *New England Journal of Medicine.* 2019;381(17):1609–20 AND Pieske B, Wachter R, Shah SJ, Baldridge A, Szeczoedy P, Ibram G, et al. Effect of Sacubitril/Valsartan vs Standard Medical Therapies on Plasma NT-proBNP Concentration and Submaximal Exercise Capacity in Patients With Heart Failure and Preserved Ejection Fraction: The PARALLAX Randomized Clinical Trial. *JAMA.* 2021;326(19):1919–29.

valsartan on the risk of cardiovascular mortality and HF hospitalization appeared to be modified by LVEF, with treatment benefits primarily observed in individuals with LVEF below the normal range.[28] The modification of treatment effects by LVEF appeared to be present in both men and women, although women tended to derive benefit to higher LVEFs.[28] Moreover, another post hoc analysis of the PARAGON-HF trial suggested a gradient in the relative and absolute treatment effects with sacubitril/valsartan, ranging from patients with a recent (<30 days) HF hospitalization (in whom there was approximately 25–30% relative risk reduction) to patients never hospitalized (in whom there was no significant risk reduction).[29] This observation points to a possibility for improving outcomes with sacubitril/valsartan in high-risk HFpEF patients with recent hospitalization for worsening HF that merits further validation.

The PARALLAX trial (Effect of Sacubitril/Valsartan vs Standard Medical Therapies on Plasma NT-proBNP Concentration and Submaximal Exercise Capacity in Patients With Heart Failure and Preserved Ejection Fraction) randomized patients with HFpEF to sacubitril/valsartan versus standard medical treatment (➲ Table 8.3.4).[30] The primary endpoints were change in NT-proBNP levels at 12 weeks and change in the 6-minute walking test distance at 24 weeks. Compared to standard treatment, sacubitril/valsartan provided a greater reduction in NP levels at 12 weeks but failed to improve exercise tolerance at 24 weeks. However, a prespecified secondary analysis indicated a significant clinical benefit with sacubitril/valsartan in terms of a reduction in HF hospitalizations and a composite of cardiovascular death or HF hospitalization. In addition, significant renal protection was observed,

Table 8.3.5 Primary and secondary outcomes in the PARAGON-HF trial

PARAGON-HF	Ratio of difference (CI) Sacubitril/valsartan vs valsartan	P-value
Primary composite outcome and components		
Total (first and recurrent) hospitalizations for heart failure and death from cardiovascular causes	RR 0.87 (0.75–1.01)	0.06
Total number (first and recurrent) of hospitalizations for heart failure	RR 0.85 (0.72–1.00)	–
Death from cardiovascular causes	HR 0.95 (0.79–1.16)	–
Secondary outcomes		
Change in NYHA class from baseline to 8 months (% of patients)	15.0 vs 12.6	–
Improved	76.3 vs 77.8	–
Unchanged	8.7 vs 9.6	–
Worsened		
Change in KCCQ clinical summary score at 8 months	Difference 1.0 (0.0–2.1)	–
Renal composite outcome*	HR 0.50 (0.33–0.77)	0.83
Death from any cause	HR 0.97 (0.84–1.13)	–

* Defined as death from renal failure, end-stage renal disease, or a decrease in the estimated glomerular filtration rate of 50% or more from baseline.
CI, confidence interval; HR, hazard ratio; KCCQ, Kansas City Cardiomyopathy Questionnaire; NYHA, New York Heart Association; RR, risk ratio.
Source data from Solomon SD, McMurray JJV, Anand IS, Ge J, Lam CSP, Maggioni AP, *et al.* Angiotensin–Neprilysin Inhibition in Heart Failure with Preserved Ejection Fraction. *New England Journal of Medicine.* 2019;381(17):1609–20.

Table 8.3.6 Major inclusion and exclusion criteria and main patient characteristics in the PARADISE-MI trial

PARADISE-MI	
Study drug (target dose)	Sacubitril/valsartan (107/97 mg BD)
Comparator (target dose)	Ramipril (5 mg BD)
Number of patients	5661
Inclusion criteria	◆ Acute myocardial infarction (STEMI or NSTEMI) AND ◆ LVEF ≤40% AND/OR ◆ Pulmonary congestion requiring intravenous diuretics
Additional criteria	At least one of the prespecified risk-augmenting factors: ◆ Age ≥70 years ◆ Diabetes mellitus ◆ Previous myocardial infarction ◆ eGFR <60 mL/min/1.73 m^2 ◆ AF ◆ LVEF <30% ◆ Killip class III or IV ◆ STEMI without reperfusion within the first 24 hours
Exclusion criteria	◆ History of HF prior to randomization ◆ Cardiogenic shock ◆ Persistent clinical heart failure ◆ eGFR <30 mL/min/1.73 m^2 ◆ Hypersensitivity to ACE inhibitors or sacubitril/valsartan or history of angio-oedema
Patient characteristics	
Age (years)	~64 (median)
Female sex (%)	23–25
Baseline LVEF (%)	36–37 (mean)

ACE, angiotensin-converting enzyme; ARB, angiotensin receptor blocker; BD, twice daily; BNP, B-type natriuretic peptide; BP, blood pressure; eGFR, estimated glomerular filtration rate; LVEF, left ventricular ejection fraction; NT-proBNP, N-terminal pro-B-type natriuretic peptide; NSTEMI, non-ST-segment elevation myocardial infarction; NYHA, New York Heart Association; STEMI, ST-segment elevation myocardial infarction.
Source data from Pfeffer MA, Claggett B, Lewis EF, Granger CB, Køber L, Maggioni AP, *et al.* Angiotensin Receptor-Neprilysin Inhibition in Acute Myocardial Infarction. *N Engl J Med.* 2021;385(20):1845–55.

as evidenced by a slower deterioration in the estimated glomerular filtration rate (eGFR) at 6 months.

Sacubitril/valsartan in acute myocardial infarction

The PARADISE-MI trial (Angiotensin Receptor–Neprilysin Inhibition in Acute Myocardial Infarction) assessed the efficacy and safety of early introduction of sacubitril/valsartan in patients with acute myocardial infraction complicated by reduced LVEF of ≤40% and/or pulmonary congestion (➲ Table 8.3.6).[31] Patients with a history of HF before an index myocardial infarction and those with haemodynamic instability and/or an eGFR of <30 mL/min were excluded.

Eligible patients were randomized to receiving sacubitril/valsartan or ramipril within a median of approximately 4 days after an index myocardial infarction. The study population comprised mostly patients with ST-segment elevation myocardial infarction (approximately 75%) and coronary reperfusion (mostly primary percutaneous intervention) was performed in approximately 89% of the patients. The primary endpoint was a composite of cardiovascular mortality or incident HF (i.e. HF hospitalization or an outpatient episode of symptomatic HF). Despite a numerically lower incidence of the primary endpoint in the sacubitril/valsartan group, compared to the ramipril group, the difference failed to reach statistical significance and there

was no significant risk reduction in either cardiovascular death or HF events. Nevertheless, sacubitril/valsartan treatment was associated with a lower risk of the composite of total HF hospitalizations, outpatient HF events, and cardiovascular mortality. Patients in the sacubitril/valsartan group were more likely to have hypotension, compared to those receiving ramipril who were more likely to experience cough-related adverse events.

Sacubitril/valsartan in advanced heart failure with reduced ejection fraction

The effects of sacubitril/valsartan versus valsartan on the reduction of NT-proBNP levels and clinical outcomes in patients with advanced HFrEF were assessed in the LIFE trial (Entresto (LCZ696) In Advanced Heart Failure) (➲ Table 8.3.7).[32]

Table 8.3.7 Major inclusion and exclusion criteria and main patient characteristics in the LIFE trial

	LIFE trial
Study drug (target dose)	Sacubitril/valsartan (103/97 mg BD)
Comparator (target dose)	Valsartan (160 mg BD)
Number of randomized patients	335
Inclusion criteria	◆ NYHA class IV in previous 3 months ◆ Receiving GDMT for HF for ≥3 months and/or intolerant of GDMT ◆ LVEF ≤35% ◆ BNP ≥250 pg/mL or NT-proBNP ≥800 pg/mL ◆ Systolic BP ≥90 mmHg
Additional criteria	At least one additional objective finding of advanced HF: ◆ Current inotropic therapy/use of inotropes within 6 months ◆ ≥1 HF hospitalization within 6 months ◆ LVEF ≤25% within 12 months ◆ Decreased peak VO$_2$ within 12 months ◆ 6-minute walking test distance <300 m within 3 months
Exclusion criteria	◆ eGFR <20 mL/min/1.73 m^2 ◆ Symptomatic hypotension at randomization or systolic BP <90 mmHg ◆ Severe liver dysfunction ◆ Acute coronary syndrome, planned or recent coronary revascularization (PCI or CABG), or biventricular pacing ◆ Currently hospitalized and listed status for heart transplant ◆ Current or scheduled for LVAD implantation within 30 days of study enrolment ◆ Comorbid conditions that may interfere with completing the study protocol or cause death within 1 year ◆ Hypersensitivity to ARNIs, ACE inhibitors, and ARBs or history of angio-oedema
Patient characteristics	
Age (years)	~60 (mean)
Female sex (%)	~27%
Baseline LVEF (%)	~20% (mean)

ACE, angiotensin-converting enzyme; ARB, angiotensin receptor blocker; ARNI, angiotensin receptor–neprilysin inhibitor; BD, twice daily; BNP, B-type natriuretic peptide; BP, blood pressure; CABG, coronary artery bypass surgery; eGFR, estimated glomerular filtration rate; GDMT, guideline-directed medical therapy; LVAD, left ventricular assist device; LVEF, left ventricular ejection fraction; NT-proBNP, N-terminal pro-B-type natriuretic peptide; NYHA, New York Heart Association; PCI, percutaneous coronary intervention; VO$_2$, oxygen consumption.
Source data from Mann DL, Givertz MM, Vader JM, Starling RC, Shah P, McNulty SE, *et al.* Effect of Treatment With Sacubitril/Valsartan in Patients With Advanced Heart Failure and Reduced Ejection Fraction: A Randomized Clinical Trial. *JAMA Cardiology.* 2021.

The primary endpoint was a change in the area under the curve of NT-proBNP relative to baseline, measured over 24 weeks of therapy.[32] The trial was prematurely stopped in March 2020 and the study protocol and statistical analysis were modified, so that none of the clinical endpoints would be affected by coronavirus disease 2019 (Covid-19). The results demonstrated that neither sacubitril/ valsartan nor valsartan reduced the median NT-proBNP level below the baseline, and the difference in the proportional change in the ratio of NT-proBNP-to-baseline for sacubitril/valsartan versus valsartan was non-significant. Likewise, there was no difference between sacubitril/valsartan and valsartan for the secondary clinical endpoint of the number of days alive, out of hospital, or free from HF events (HF hospitalization, LV assist device implantation, heart transplantation, or continuous inotropic infusion). There was also no improvement with sacubitril/valsartan, compared to treatment with valsartan, in cardiovascular mortality or HF hospitalization or in cardiovascular death or all-cause death (hazard ratio 1.32; *P*-value = 0.20).

With regard to the tolerability and safety aspects, the average daily dose of study medications was 195 mg and 154 mg for sacubitril/valsartan and valsartan, respectively (48% of the target dose), and there was a statistically significant higher rate of hyperkalaemia with sacubitril/valsartan. Although hypotension occurred more frequently in the sacubitril/valsartan group, the difference was not statistically significant and there was no difference in worsening renal function.

The results of the LIFE trial suggest that improvement in outcomes observed in patients with less severe HFrEF could not be translated to the advanced HF population, possibly because profound shifts in neurohormonal activation, severe myocardial dysfunction, and end-organ damage limit the ability to respond favourably to treatment with sacubitril/valsartan.

Safety and tolerability

According to clinical trial data, treatment with sacubitril/valsartan is generally safe and well tolerated, albeit associated with a greater risk of hypotension, compared to treatment with ACE inhibitors or ARBs. A meta-analysis of clinical trials enrolling patients receiving sacubitril/valsartan for either HF or hypertension (*n* = 22,510), compared with standard therapy or placebo, indicated that the risk of adverse events and serious adverse events was comparable between sacubitril/valsartan and an active control (ACE inhibitor or ARB), as well as between sacubitril/valsartan and placebo.[33] However, the risk of hypotension was significantly higher with sacubitril/valsartan, compared to treatment with an ACE inhibitor/ARB, and the risk of angio-oedema appeared to increase with longer follow-up. Similarly, a meta-analysis of clinical trials focusing on patients with HF (*n* = 14,959 patients) indicated a greater risk of symptomatic hypotension with sacubitril/valsartan, compared to treatment with an ACE inhibitor/ARB, despite the fact that most trials required a run-in period to ensure drug tolerability and excluded patients with systolic blood pressure of ≤100 mmHg.[34] Nevertheless, the risk of worsening renal function (i.e. decline in eGFR) and serious hyperkalaemia was lower with sacubitril/valsartan and there was no evidence of a significant difference between sacubitril/ valsartan and active comparators with respect to angio-oedema.

Data from observational studies provide further insight into the tolerability and safety of sacubitril/valsartan in real-world practice where patient characteristics and quality of management (i.e. uptitration and adherence) may differ from clinical trials. This is underlined in a systematic review and meta-analysis indicating differences between real-world patients receiving sacubitril/

valsartan ($n = 16,952$) and those enrolled in the PARADIGM-HF trial, in terms of older age, fewer cases of ischaemic aetiology, and less frequent comorbidities (i.e. hypertension and diabetes) among real-world patients.[35] Moreover, sacubitril/valsartan was uptitrated to the target dose in only 35% of patients and it was discontinued in approximately 13%.[35] Another analysis of the real-world effectiveness and safety of sacubitril/valsartan suggested superior efficacy of sacubitril/valsartan in improving clinical outcomes, functional class, and NP levels, compared to standard therapy, in the majority of studies.[36] The most frequent adverse effects were hypotension and hyperkalaemia, with mixed results on the reported frequency between patients receiving sacubitril/valsartan and those on standard therapy.[36]

Given that neprilysin acts as one of the enzymes responsible for the clearance of amyloid-β peptides from the brain, there has been some concern about potential long-term implications of treatment with ARNIs in cognitive function. Although experimental data suggest that neprilysin inhibition may be associated with cognitive dysfunction, available clinical evidence does not support an increased risk of dementia with sacubitril/valsartan.[37] However, a prospective follow-up and a more sensitive assessment may be necessary to determine the long-term safety of ARNIs with respect to cognitive function.

Sacubitril/valsartan: current guideline recommendations

Sacubitril/valsartan was approved for treatment of symptomatic patients with HFrEF by both the United States Food and Drug Administration (FDA) and the European Medicines Agency in 2015. The approval was extended by the FDA in 2021 to patients with HF in general, with a note that the effect was more evident in patients with LVEF below normal.

The 2021 Update to the 2017 American College of Cardiology Expert Consensus Decision Pathway for Optimization of Heart Failure Treatment recommended the use of sacubitril/valsartan in patients with HFrEF in preference to ACE inhibitors/ARBs, as part of guideline-directed medical therapies.[38]

In the 2021 European Society of Cardiology (ESC)/Heart Failure Association (HFA) Guidelines for diagnosis and treatment of acute and chronic HF, sacubitril/valsartan is recommended as replacement for an ACE inhibitor in patients with HFrEF to reduce the risk of HF hospitalization and death, with a Class I recommendation, Level of evidence B.[39] Sacubitril/valsartan may be considered as the first-line therapy in ACE inhibitor-naïve patients with HFrEF (Class IIb, Level of evidence B).[39] In addition, sacubitril/valsartan may be considered in patients with HFmrEF to reduce the risk of HF hospitalization and death, based on pooled PARADIGM-HF and PARAGON-HF data (Class IIb, Level of evidence C).[39]

The 2021 ESC/HFA Guidelines and an expert consensus document also suggest that, instead of a sequential introduction, a simultaneous introduction of the four classes of evidence-based therapies for HFrEF—ARNI/ACE inhibitor/ARB (if ARNI/ACE inhibitor-intolerant), beta-blocker, MRA, and sodium–glucose cotransporter 2 inhibitor—should be commenced, taking into account the individual patient's profile (i.e. clinical characteristics such as blood pressure, heart rate, renal function, serum potassium levels, etc.).[39,40] Within a short period of time (e.g. 1 month), the four classes of medications should be added (in the order most appropriate to individual patient characteristics) and then drug doses should be uptitrated to the target doses used in clinical trials or to the maximum tolerated dose.[40] Considering that sacubitril/valsartan is associated with a lower risk of worsening renal function and severe hyperkalaemia, initiation and uptitration of medications such as MRAs may be facilitated with its use, instead of ACE inhibitors/ARBs. Following initiation of sacubitril/valsartan, the dose of loop diuretics may be decreased in patients without signs of congestion, in particular, if simultaneously taking sodium–glucose cotransporter 2 inhibitors and/or having borderline low blood pressure (100–110 mmHg). The use of a contemporary, comprehensive treatment of HFrEF (i.e. sacubitril/valsartan, beta-blocker, MRA, and sodium–glucose cotransporter 2 inhibitor) appears to provide complementary therapeutic benefits and better prognosis, compared to earlier standard treatment (ACE inhibitor/ARB and beta-blocker).[41] Current evidence supports an early introduction of sacubitril/valsartan as the first-line therapy in haemodynamically stabilized patients admitted to hospital for acute HFrEF, alongside initiation of other HF therapies, including in patients with *de novo* HFrEF and/or without previous exposure to ACE inhibitors/ARBs.[23,42] Not only is this strategy safe and feasible, but it is also associated with greater improvement in clinical outcomes and a better risk/benefit profile, compared to first initiating ACE inhibitors/ARBs.[23,24]

Practical considerations of sacubitril/valsartan use

Sacubitril/valsartan should be initiated in symptomatic ambulatory patients with HF or in those hospitalized for HF, after achieving haemodynamic stabilization, relieving congestion, and restoring 'euvolaemia'.[39] The usual starting dose of sacubitril/valsartan is 49/51 mg twice daily (or 24/26 mg twice daily in selected patients) and the target dose is 97/103 mg twice daily.[39] The list of cautions and contraindications, and practical advice on dosing and addressing side effects and tolerability issues are provided in ◗ Box 8.3.1.

Future directions

Clinical research on ARNIs continues along several avenues. First, there are two ongoing randomized controlled trials, namely the PANORAMA-HF study and the PERSPECTIVE trial. The PANORAMA-HF study (ClinicalTrials.gov identifier: NCT02678312) will be the largest trial to date to assess the safety and efficacy of sacubitril/valsartan versus enalapril in paediatric patients with HFrEF.[43] The PERSPECTIVE trial (ClinicalTrials.gov identifier: NCT02884206) aims to evaluate long-term effects of sacubitril/valsartan, compared to valsartan, on cognitive function as assessed by the CogState Global Cognitive Composite Score. The study will enrol symptomatic patients with HF and

---

Box 8.3.1 Practical aspects on the use of sacubitril/valsartan

Cautions

- A washout period of ≥36 hours after cessation of an ACE inhibitor is necessary to avoid angio-oedema.
- Hyperkalaemia may be worsened by sacubitril/valsartan therapy, especially in patients taking mineralocorticoid receptor antagonists, K^+ supplements, or K^+-sparing diuretics.
- There is limited clinical experience in patients with moderate hepatic impairment (Child–Pugh B classification).

Contraindications

- Concomitant use of an ACE inhibitor or ARB
- Concomitant use with aliskiren-containing medicinal products in patients with diabetes mellitus or those with renal impairment (eGFR <60 mL/min/1.73 m^2)
- A history of angio-oedema (including angio-oedema associated with earlier ACE inhibitor use or hereditary/idiopathic angio-oedema)
- Bilateral renal artery stenosis
- Hypersensitivity/allergic reaction
- eGFR <30 mL/min/1.73 m^2*
- Serum K^+ level >5.4 mmol/L
- Severe hepatic impairment, biliary cirrhosis, or cholestasis (Child–Pugh C classification)
- Symptomatic hypotension or systolic BP <90 mmHg**
- Significant hypovolaemia
- Pregnancy/lactation

Drug initiation and uptitration**

- The usual starting dose is 49/51 mg BD.
- A starting dose of 24/26 mg BD is indicated in selected patients:
  - ACE inhibitor/ARB-naïve
  - Previously on low-dose ACE inhibitor/ARB
  - Borderline low systolic BP (100–110 mmHg)
  - eGFR 30–60 mL/min/1.73 m^2** (also eGFR 15–30 mL/min/1.73 m^2)*
  - Hepatic impairment (Child–Pugh B classification)
  - Elderly (in accordance with eGFR).
- Check serum electrolyte, urea, and creatinine levels at drug initiation and 1–2 weeks afterwards.
- Double the dose in 2- to 4-weekly intervals, and recheck serum electrolyte, urea, and creatinine levels 1–2 weeks later.
- Aim for the target dose (97/103 mg BD) or the maximum tolerated dose.

Side effects and tolerability issues

Hypotension

- Asymptomatic low BP or mild dizziness/light-headedness are frequent after drug initiation and usually spontaneously resolve with time.
- Symptomatic hypotension:
  - Consider reducing the dose of loop diuretics (if no signs of congestion).
  - Consider discontinuation of vasodilators (if not necessary).

Worsening renal function

- A small and transitory rise in serum urea and creatinine levels is expected after drug initiation and resolves spontaneously.
- In patients with a greater increase in serum urea and creatinine levels, stop concomitant use of medications with a nephrotoxic effect (e.g. non-steroidal anti-inflammatory drugs) and consider reducing the dose of loop diuretics (if no signs of congestion).
- If serum urea and creatinine levels remain elevated, reduce the dose of sacubitril/valsartan and recheck blood biochemistry after 1–2 weeks.
- In patients with persistent decrease of eGFR <30 mL/min/1.73 m^2, discontinue sacubitril/valsartan and consult a nephrologist.

Hyperkalaemia

- The risk of hyperkalaemia is generally lower with sacubitril/valsartan, compared to treatment with ACE inhibitors/ARBs.
- A small increase (serum K^+ ≤5.5 mmol/L) can occur, which is of no concern.
- In patients with elevated serum K^+ levels of >5.5 mmol/L, consider stopping K^+-sparing drugs (e.g. amiloride, triamterene) and/or K^+ supplements.
- If the serum K^+ level remains elevated (>5.5 mmol/L), reduce the dose of sacubitril/valsartan and recheck blood biochemistry after 1–2 weeks.
- In patients with persistently elevated K^+ levels of >5.5 mmol/L, consider potassium-binding medications.

* The United States Federal Drug Administration and European Medicines Agency drug labelling allows cautious use of sacubitril/valsartan with a starting dose of 24/26 mg twice daily in patients with eGFR of 15–30 mL/min/1.73 m^2.
** According to the 2021 European Society of Cardiology/Heart Failure Association Guidelines for the diagnosis and treatment of acute and chronic heart failure.[39]
ACE, angiotensin-converting enzyme; ARB, angiotensin receptor blocker; BD, twice daily; BP, blood pressure; eGFR, estimated glomerular filtration rate; K^+, potassium.

LVEF of >40%, who will receive the study medications for 3 years. Second, the ongoing ENVAD-HF (Sacubitril/Valsartan in Left Ventricular Assist Device Recipients) phase 4 open-label study aims to assess the safety and tolerability of sacubitril/valsartan, compared to standard of care, for the treatment of blood pressure in patients with implanted HeartMate 3 LV assist devices.

The primary outcome of the study is freedom from all-cause death, deterioration in renal function, hyperkalaemia, or symptomatic hypotension after 3 months of treatment. Finally, there is a mounting body of real-world evidence that will provide a more nuanced insight into the safety, tolerability, and most clinically relevant practical issues about the use of sacubitril/valsartan.

Key messages

◆ Compared with enalapril, sacubitril/valsartan demonstrated a significant reduction in cardiovascular mortality or HF hospitalization (by 20%) and all-cause mortality (by 16%), and an improvement in functional capacity in ambulatory patients with symptomatic HFrEF (PARADIGM-HF trial). Sacubitril/valsartan was associated with significant attenuation of both death due to pump failure and sudden cardiac death.

◆ In patients hospitalized with acute HFrEF, sacubitril/valsartan (initiated in hospital after achieving haemodynamic stabilization, or within 10 days post-discharge), compared to enalapril, provided a 46% lower risk of mortality, rehospitalization, or HF progression, without a significant difference in major adverse events (PIONEER-HF trial). Early in-hospital introduction of sacubitril/valsartan provided an additional lower risk of mortality and rehospitalization (by 31%), compared to in-hospital treatment with ACE inhibitors and a post-discharge switch to sacubitril/valsartan.

◆ Sacubitril/valsartan was not superior, compared to valsartan, in reducing the risk of death and hospitalizations for HF in ambulatory patients with HF and LVEF of ≥45% (PARAGON-HF trial). However, a prespecified analysis suggested that there may be a therapeutic benefit in individuals with lower LVEF (≤57%) and in women.

◆ There is evidence that the therapeutic benefits of sacubitril/valsartan in HFrEF are mediated by mechanisms including (but not limited to) LV reverse remodelling, improvement in LV systolic and diastolic function, reduction in left atrial volume, and functional mitral regurgitation. There is also evidence of a reno-protective effect and improvement in glycaemic control in patients with diabetes mellitus.

◆ Sacubitril/valsartan is generally safe and well tolerated, but the risk of symptomatic hypotension is higher, compared to treatment with ACE inhibitors/ARBs. Patients with lower blood pressure or those tolerating low doses of ACE inhibitors/ARBs are more likely to attain the target dose of sacubitril/valsartan by starting with a low dose (24/26 mg) and gradually uptitrating to the target/maximum tolerated dose.

◆ Worsening renal function and hyperkalaemia occur less frequently with sacubitril/valsartan, compared to treatment with ACE inhibitors/ARBs, which may allow for easier optimization of other evidence-based therapies, including MRAs.

◆ Current guidelines recommend ARNIs as the mainstay treatment of symptomatic patients with HFrEF. Available evidence suggests that therapeutic benefits extend to patients with HFmrEF and perhaps even to selected patients with HFpEF (e.g. women, patients with recent HF hospitalization).

References

1. Daniels LB, Maisel AS. Natriuretic peptides. J Am Coll Cardiol. 2007;50(25):2357–68.

2. Rademaker MT, Charles CJ, Espiner EA, Frampton CM, Nicholls MG, Richards AM. Combined inhibition of angiotensin II and endothelin suppresses the brain natriuretic peptide response to developing heart failure. Clin Sci (Lond). 2004;106(6):569–76.

3. Rossi F, Mascolo A, Mollace V. The pathophysiological role of natriuretic peptide-RAAS cross talk in heart failure. Int J Cardiol. 2017;226:121–5.

4. Packer M, Califf RM, Konstam MA, et al. Comparison of omapatrilat and enalapril in patients with chronic heart failure: the Omapatrilat Versus Enalapril Randomized Trial of Utility in Reducing Events (OVERTURE). Circulation. 2002;106(8):920–6.

5. McCormack PL. Sacubitril/valsartan: a review in chronic heart failure with reduced ejection fraction. Drugs. 2016;76(3):387–96.

6. Kostis JB, Packer M, Black HR, Schmieder R, Henry D, Levy E. Omapatrilat and enalapril in patients with hypertension: the Omapatrilat Cardiovascular Treatment vs. Enalapril (OCTAVE) trial. Am J Hypertens. 2004;17(2):103–11.

7. Katsi V, Skalis G, Pavlidis AN, et al. Angiotensin receptor neprilysin inhibitor LCZ696: a novel targeted therapy for arterial hypertension? Eur Heart J Cardiovasc Pharmacother. 2015;1(4):260–4.

8. McMurray JJ, Packer M, Desai AS, et al. Angiotensin-neprilysin inhibition versus enalapril in heart failure. N Engl J Med. 2014;371(11):993–1004.

9. Desai AS, McMurray JJ, Packer M, et al. Effect of the angiotensin-receptor-neprilysin inhibitor LCZ696 compared with enalapril on mode of death in heart failure patients. Eur Heart J. 2015;36(30):1990–7.

10. Packer M, McMurray JJ, Desai AS, et al. Angiotensin receptor neprilysin inhibition compared with enalapril on the risk of clinical progression in surviving patients with heart failure. Circulation. 2015;131(1):54–61.

11. Senni M, McMurray JJ, Wachter R, et al. Initiating sacubitril/valsartan (LCZ696) in heart failure: results of TITRATION, a double-blind, randomized comparison of two uptitration regimens. Eur J Heart Fail. 2016;18(9):1193–202.

12. Senni M, McMurray JJV, Wachter R, et al. Impact of systolic blood pressure on the safety and tolerability of initiating and up-titrating sacubitril/valsartan in patients with heart failure and reduced ejection fraction: insights from the TITRATION study. Eur J Heart Fail. 2018;20(3):491–500.

13. Januzzi JL Jr, Prescott MF, Butler J, et al. Association of change in N-terminal pro-B-type natriuretic peptide following initiation of sacubitril-valsartan treatment with cardiac structure and function in patients with heart failure with reduced ejection fraction. JAMA. 2019;322(11):1085–95.

14. Kang DH, Park SJ, Shin SH, et al. Angiotensin receptor neprilysin inhibitor for functional mitral regurgitation. Circulation. 2019;139(11):1354–65.

15. Williams B, Cockcroft JR, Kario K, et al. Effects of sacubitril/valsartan versus olmesartan on central hemodynamics in the elderly with systolic hypertension: the PARAMETER Study. Hypertension. 2017;69(3):411–20.

16. Desai AS, Solomon SD, Shah AM, et al. Effect of sacubitril-valsartan vs enalapril on aortic stiffness in patients with heart failure and reduced ejection fraction: a randomized clinical trial. JAMA. 2019;322(11):1077–84.

17. Damman K, Gori M, Claggett B, et al. Renal effects and associated outcomes during angiotensin-neprilysin inhibition in heart failure. JACC Heart Fail. 2018;6(6):489–98.

18. Seferovic JP, Claggett B, Seidelmann SB, et al. Effect of sacubitril/valsartan versus enalapril on glycaemic control in patients with heart failure and diabetes: a post-hoc analysis from the PARADIGM-HF trial. Lancet Diabetes Endocrinol. 2017;5(5):333–40.

19. Velazquez EJ, Morrow DA, DeVore AD, et al. Angiotensin-neprilysin inhibition in acute decompensated heart failure. N Engl J Med. 2019;380(6):539–48.

20. Morrow DA, Velazquez EJ, DeVore AD, et al. Clinical outcomes in patients with acute decompensated heart failure randomly assigned to sacubitril/valsartan or enalapril in the PIONEER-HF trial. Circulation. 2019;139(19):2285–8.

21. Berg DD, Braunwald E, DeVore AD, *et al.* Efficacy and safety of sacubitril/valsartan by dose level achieved in the PIONEER-HF trial. JACC Heart Fail. 2020;8(10):834–43.

22. DeVore AD, Braunwald E, Morrow DA, *et al.* Initiation of angiotensin-neprilysin inhibition after acute decompensated heart failure: secondary analysis of the open-label extension of the PIONEER-HF trial. JAMA Cardiol. 2020;5(2):202–7.

23. Wachter R, Senni M, Belohlavek J, *et al.* Initiation of sacubitril/valsartan in haemodynamically stabilised heart failure patients in hospital or early after discharge: primary results of the randomised TRANSITION study. Eur J Heart Fail. 2019;21(8):998–1007.

24. Senni M, Wachter R, Witte KK, *et al.* Initiation of sacubitril/valsartan shortly after hospitalisation for acutely decompensated heart failure in patients with newly diagnosed (*de novo*) heart failure: a subgroup analysis of the TRANSITION study. Eur J Heart Fail. 2020;22(2):303–12.

25. Solomon SD, Zile M, Pieske B, *et al.* The angiotensin receptor neprilysin inhibitor LCZ696 in heart failure with preserved ejection fraction: a phase 2 double-blind randomised controlled trial. Lancet. 2012;380(9851):1387–95.

26. Solomon SD, McMurray JJV, Anand IS, *et al.* Angiotensin–neprilysin inhibition in heart failure with preserved ejection fraction. N Engl J Med. 2019;381(17):1609–20.

27. McMurray JJV, Jackson AM, Lam CSP, *et al.* Effects of sacubitril-valsartan versus valsartan in women compared with men with heart failure and preserved ejection fraction. Circulation. 2020;141(5):338–51.

27a. Mentz RJ, Ward JH, Hernandez AF, *et al.* Angiotensin-neprilysin inhibition in patients with mildly reduced or preserved ejection fraction and worsening heart failure. J Am Coll Cardiol. 2023;82(1):1–12.

27b. Vaduganathan M, Mentz RJ, Claggett BL, *et al.* Sacubitril/valsartan in heart failure with mildly reduced or preserved ejection fraction: a pre-specified participant-level pooled analysis of PARAGLIDE-HF and PARAGON-HF. Eur Heart J. 2023. doi: 10.1093/eurheartj/ehad344. Online ahead of print.

28. Solomon SD, Vaduganathan M, Claggett BL, *et al.* Sacubitril/valsartan across the spectrum of ejection fraction in heart failure. Circulation. 2020;141(5):352–61.

29. Vaduganathan M, Claggett BL, Desai AS, *et al.* Prior heart failure hospitalization, clinical outcomes, and response to sacubitril/valsartan compared with valsartan in HFpEF. J Am Coll Cardiol. 2020;75(3):245–54.

30. Pieske B, Wachter R, Shah SJ, *et al.* Effect of sacubitril/valsartan vs standard medical therapies on plasma NT-proBNP concentration and submaximal exercise capacity in patients with heart failure and preserved ejection fraction: the PARALLAX randomized clinical trial. JAMA. 2021;326(19):1919–29.

31. Pfeffer MA, Claggett B, Lewis EF, *et al.* Angiotensin receptor-neprilysin inhibition in acute myocardial infarction. N Engl J Med. 2021;385(20):1845–55.

32. Mann DL, Givertz MM, Vader JM, *et al.* Effect of treatment with sacubitril/valsartan in patients with advanced heart failure and reduced ejection fraction: a randomized clinical trial. JAMA Cardiol. 2022;7(1):17–25.

33. Pereira GME, Duarte GS, Katerenchuk V, *et al.* Safety and tolerability of sacubitril-valsartan: a systematic review and meta-analysis. Expert Opin Drug Saf. 2021;20(5):577–88.

34. Zhang H, Huang T, Shen W, *et al.* Efficacy and safety of sacubitril-valsartan in heart failure: a meta-analysis of randomized controlled trials. ESC Heart Fail. 2020;7(6):3841–50.

35. Giovinazzo S, Carmisciano L, Toma M, *et al.* Sacubitril/valsartan in real-life European patients with heart failure and reduced ejection fraction: a systematic review and meta-analysis. ESC Heart Fail. 2021;8(5):3547–56.

36. Proudfoot C, Studer R, Rajput T, *et al.* Real-world effectiveness and safety of sacubitril/valsartan in heart failure: a systematic review. Int J Cardiol. 2021;331:164–71.

37. Cannon JA, Shen L, Jhund PS, *et al.* Dementia-related adverse events in PARADIGM-HF and other trials in heart failure with reduced ejection fraction. Eur J Heart Fail. 2017;19(1):129–37.

38. Maddox TM, Januzzi JL Jr, Allen LA, *et al.* 2021 update to the 2017 ACC expert consensus decision pathway for optimization of heart failure treatment: answers to 10 pivotal issues about heart failure with reduced ejection fraction: a report of the American College of Cardiology Solution Set Oversight Committee. J Am Coll Cardiol. 2021;77(6):772–810.

39. McDonagh TA, Metra M, Adamo M, *et al.* 2021 ESC Guidelines for the diagnosis and treatment of acute and chronic heart failure: developed by the Task Force for the diagnosis and treatment of acute and chronic heart failure of the European Society of Cardiology (ESC) With the special contribution of the Heart Failure Association (HFA) of the ESC. Eur Heart J. 2022;24(1):4–131.

40. Rosano GMC, Moura B, Metra M, *et al.* Patient profiling in heart failure for tailoring medical therapy. A consensus document of the Heart Failure Association of the European Society of Cardiology. Eur J Heart Fail. 2021;23(6):872–81.

41. Vaduganathan M, Claggett BL, Jhund PS, *et al.* Estimating lifetime benefits of comprehensive disease-modifying pharmacological therapies in patients with heart failure with reduced ejection fraction: a comparative analysis of three randomised controlled trials. Lancet. 2020;396(10244):121–8.

42. Ambrosy AP, Braunwald E, Morrow DA, *et al.* Angiotensin receptor–neprilysin inhibition based on history of heart failure and use of renin–angiotensin system antagonists. J Am Coll Cardiol. 2020;76(9):1034–48.

43. Shaddy R, Canter C, Halnon N, *et al.* Design for the sacubitril/valsartan (LCZ696) compared with enalapril study of pediatric patients with heart failure due to systemic left ventricle systolic dysfunction (PANORAMA-HF study). Am Heart J. 2017;193:23–34.

CHAPTER 8.4

Beta-blocker therapy

Daniela Tomasoni, Marianna Adamo, Hiroyuki Tsutsui, and Marco Metra

Contents

Introduction

The history of beta-blocker therapy in heart failure (HF) is among the most fascinating in cardiology. HF is characterized by symptoms and signs due to myocardial failure and insufficient cardiac output. Thus, beta-blockers were initially contraindicated in patients with HF, given their acute negative inotropic effects. However, since 1975, relatively small studies started showing the beneficial effects of administration of beta-blockers in patients with severe refractory HF. Then, controlled clinical trials performed in thousands of patients with chronic HF with reduced ejection fraction (HFrEF) have consistently shown that long-term administration of beta-blockers is associated with a significant improvement in left ventricular (LV) function, clinical course, and survival. Thus, the results of relatively small studies have led to large controlled trials confirming the beneficial effects of a class of agents initially contraindicated, and beta-blockers are now the mainstay of medical treatment of HFrEF.

Historical notes

Beta-blockers were initially contraindicated in patients with HF. Indeed, serious untoward effects and worsening HF were observed when standard large doses of beta-blockers, typically given to treat other cardiovascular (CV) diseases, were administered to patients with HF. Single groups, however, started small studies showing the benefits of beta-blockers in patients with advanced HF and tachycardia. The first study was issued in 1975 and included seven patients with cardiomyopathy and showed an improvement in cardiac function assessed by phonocardiography, carotid pulse curve tracings, apexcardiography, and echocardiography.[1] The aim of this initial study was to reduce heart rate, prolong diastole, and decrease myocardial energy consumption. Further small studies confirmed these results, and also showed an improvement in LV function and reverse remodelling with long-term beta-blocker therapy, possible after early deterioration related to the loss of adrenergic support to myocardial function.[2,3,4] The first study showing a favourable impact on outcome was also conducted in a small cohort. It was a non-randomized, retrospective study, including only 37 patients (beta-blocker, $n = 24$; placebo, $n = 13$) and showing an improvement in survival with beta-blocker therapy, compared to historical controls on digoxin and diuretic treatment.[5] This study anticipated the outcome of large-scale trials that were concluded almost 20 years later. Consistent results also came from analyses of major post-infarction trials, showing that beta-blockade had beneficial effects on outcome and these effects were more evident in patients with signs of HF and/or LV dysfunction.[6,7]

In the same years, chronic adrenergic activation was shown to be a major independent determinant of the clinical course and poor prognosis of patients with HF (⮂ Figure 8.4.1).[8,9,10,11] However, this hypothesis needed to be confirmed by trials where blockade of

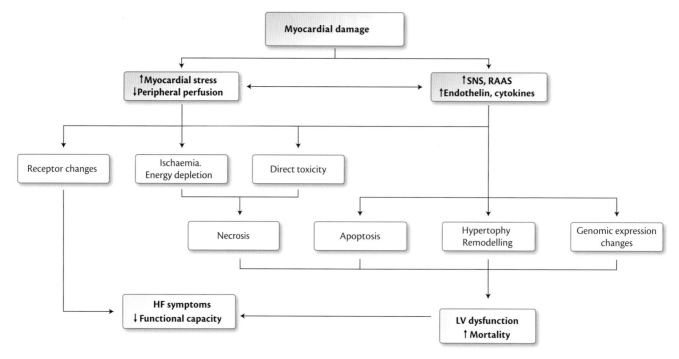

Figure 8.4.1 Mechanisms of untoward effects of neurohormonal activation in heart failure. HF, heart failure; LV, left ventricular; RAAS, renin–angiotensin–aldosterone system, SNS, sympathetic nervous system.

Reproduced from Metra M, Nodari S, D'Aloia A, Bontempi L, Boldi E, Cas LD. A rationale for the use of beta-blockers as standard treatment for heart failure. *Am Heart J*. 2000 Mar;139(3):511–21. doi: 10.1016/s0002-8703(00)90096-6 with permission from Elsevier.

the adrenergic drive could improve outcomes. The first trials with metoprolol and bisoprolol were underpowered and did not show significant results. Investigators were, however, persistent to pursue their hypothesis, and a significant reduction in mortality of up to 34–35% with bisoprolol, carvedilol, and metoprolol succinate, compared to placebo, could be shown in major outcome trials.[12,13,14] Further studies then showed differences between beta-blockers, focused on specific subgroups such as elderly patients or patients with mildly reduced ejection fraction.[15,16,17] Lastly, new issues were raised, such as that of the role of heart rate reduction versus protection from other effects of adrenergic drive and efficacy in patients with HFrEF and atrial fibrillation (AF).[18,19,20,21,22]

Mechanisms of action

The untoward effects of sympathetic stimulation are mainly mediated by β1-adrenergic receptors (ARs). These receptors belong to the G-coupled receptor family, exerting their action through the conversion of adenosine triphosphate (ATP) into cyclic adenosine monophosphate (cAMP), which acts via protein kinase A to exert its positive inotropic, positive chronotropic, and growth-promoting effects.[23,24] β1-ARs represent approximately 80% of all ARs in cardiac myocytes of healthy subjects. HF leads to downregulation and reduced sensitivity of β1-ARs, with a concomitant increase in the proportion of β2-ARs of up to 35–40% and of α1-ARs.[23,25,26] Such changes cause a decrease in cardiac response to the adrenergic drive and contribute to reduced exercise tolerance but, at the same time, protect the heart from the untoward effects of heightened adrenergic drive.

Patients with HF have increased sympathetic activity and this occurs almost selectively in the heart and kidneys, where noradrenaline spillover is increased by 540% and 206%, respectively, but not in other organs such as the lungs.[27,28] Noradrenaline, at concentrations similar to those found in the failing heart, causes direct toxicity and induces apoptosis and fibrosis. These effects are mainly mediated by β1-AR stimulation.[23,24,29,30] Despite the fact that, in the end-stage failing heart, 50–60% of the total signal-transducing potential is lost through β1-AR downregulation and reduced sensitivity, substantial signalling capacity remains, leading to LV structural remodelling with eccentric myocardial hypertrophy and fibrosis, loss of myocardial cells, and changes in gene expression ($\circleddash$ Figure 8.4.1).[24,31] These untoward effects of the adrenergic drive are blocked by beta-blockers. Consistently, long-term administration of beta-blockers has been associated with LV reverse remodelling, improvement in LV ejection fraction (LVEF), a decline in LV volumes, reduced severity of mitral regurgitation, and a less spherical LV shape.[3,24,32]

Although blockade of the untoward effects of heightened adrenergic drive on myocardial cells is the most likely explanation for the beneficial effects of beta-blockers in patients with HFrEF, the heart rate also has direct untoward effects on the myocardium and may favour HF progression.[33] Some of the beneficial effects of beta-blockade in HFrEF are likely mediated by heart rate reduction. The relative importance of this mechanism remains unsettled, as it would require a comparison between a beta-blocker and pure heart rate reduction such as with ivabradine. However, this effect may have a major role, more than with the beta-blocker dose itself.[21,22]

Pharmacological characteristics

Beta-blockers are a heterogeneous group of agents. Several beta-blockers are available, but only four have been shown to be effective in the treatment of HFrEF and are recommended by guidelines: bisoprolol, carvedilol, metoprolol succinate (controlled release (CR)/extended release (XL)), and nebivolol.[34,35]

Pharmacokinetic and chemical differences include metabolism, plasma half-life, and lipid solubility, whereas pharmacodynamic differences include intrinsic sympathomimetic activity, selectivity for β1-ARs, characteristics of binding to β1-ARs, inverse agonism, and ancillary properties. All beta-blockers used for treatment of HF are lipophilic, with extensive liver metabolism. Lipid solubility allows these compounds to reside longer and at higher concentrations in cell membranes.[36] Beta-blockers with intrinsic sympathomimetic activity have been associated with increased mortality in placebo-controlled trials.

On the basis of their selectivity for β1-ARs and the presence of ancillary properties, beta-blockers are subdivided into three classes (➲ Table 8.4.1). First-generation, non-selective beta-blockers include propranolol and timolol, which are not used in the treatment of HF. They block both β-ARs with similar affinity. Inhibition of β2-ARs can cause bronchospasm, hyperglycaemia, and peripheral vasoconstriction, with reduced tolerance both in patients with a failing heart and in those with comorbidities. Second-generation, cardioselective beta-blockers include compounds that selectively block β1-ARs, with greater affinity, compared to β2-ARs. These beta-blockers are better tolerated in patients with concomitant comorbidities. Metoprolol belongs to this family and is 74-fold more selective for β1-ARs than for β2-ARs, whereas bisoprolol presents an even higher affinity (119-fold). The third-generation agents have ancillary properties. They include β1-AR selective (nebivolol), mildly selective (carvedilol), or non-selective (bucindolol) agents. Nebivolol is a β1-AR selective agent (352-fold), with associated β3 agonism and additional vasodilatory properties mediated by nitric oxide release. The nitric oxide-generating properties of nebivolol may improve endothelial function, decrease peripheral vascular resistance, and decrease aortic central pressure and aortic stiffness. Carvedilol blocks also β2- and α1-ARs, and has additional antioxidant and antiproliferative properties. Alpha-1 adrenergic receptors cause peripheral and renal vasoconstriction and myocardial hypertrophy, and β2-ARs may mediate untoward effects on myocardial cells. These characteristics of carvedilol may explain, at least partly, its beneficial effects, compared to metoprolol tartrate, on LV function and outcomes.[15,16,22]

Clinical results

Cardiac function

Beta-blockade has short-term untoward haemodynamic effects that are overcome by favourable effects on the biology of the myocyte in the long term. Beta-blockers may halt or, at least temporarily, reverse the progressive decline in LV function, which is a hallmark of HFrEF. The effects of beta-blockers on LV function are biphasic. Studies with serial echocardiography have shown a decrease from baseline in LVEF in the first few days of treatment, followed by a return to baseline values after 1 month and an increase in LVEF from baseline that becomes significant after at least 3 months of treatment.[3] A decrease in LV volumes and a less spherical LV shape are described at 3 and 12 months.[3,37] LV diastolic function and right ventricular function are also improved by long-term beta-blockade.[38]

In the only prospective, placebo-controlled trial testing different doses of carvedilol, the highest dose was associated with a greater improvement in LVEF and a better prognosis.[39] Besides higher beta-blocker doses, other predictors of a greater improvement in LVEF were a non-ischaemic aetiology of HF, higher baseline blood pressure, higher baseline heart rate, and demonstration of contractile reserve by dobutamine echocardiography.[40,41]

Functional capacity and symptoms

Impairment in exercise capacity in patients with HF is due to both myocardial dysfunction and abnormalities in β-AR signalling, resulting in reduced cardiac sensitivity to sympathetic stimulation. Beta-blocker treatment improves myocardial function; thus, it

Table 8.4.1 Pharmacological characteristics of beta-blockers

Generation/class	Agent	β1/β2 selectivity	β1/α1 selectivity	Inverse agonism	Ancillary properties
First/non-selective	Propranolol	2.1	–	Moderate	None
Second/selective for β1	Metoprolol succinate	74	–	Strong	None
	Bisoprolol	119	–	Moderate to weak	None
Third/selective or non-selective, with favourable ancillary properties	Nebivolol	352	–	Moderate	Vasodilatation Nitric oxide release β3 agonist
	Carvedilol	7.3	2.4	Moderate to weak	Vasodilatation (α1 blockade) Antioxidant
	Bucindolol	1.4	66	Weak	Vasodilatation Sympatholysis

would be expected to improve exercise capacity. However, beta-blocker treatment may further desensitize the heart to the adrenergic drive, if β-ARs are blocked and not upregulated. Despite improvement in cardiac function and stroke volume, both at rest and during exercise, the chronotropic response is inadequate and the cardiac output may fail to rise sufficiently during exercise to allow improvement in maximal functional capacity.[2] In multicentre trials, carvedilol also failed to improve submaximal exercise performance, which is less dependent on the maximal heart rate.[39]

Major outcomes

Bisoprolol, carvedilol, and metoprolol succinate reduced mortality by 34–35% in randomized, placebo-controlled clinical trials.[12,13,14] Nebivolol reduced the primary endpoint of death or CV hospitalization in a trial enrolling patients aged ≥70 years who had previous HF hospitalization or an LVEF of ≤35%.[17] The results of the main randomized clinical trials are summarized at ❱ Table 8.4.2.[12,13,14,17,42,43] Both sudden cardiac death and worsening HF death were reduced in these trials. Sudden cardiac death was reduced by 44% in the Cardiac Insufficiency Bisoprolol Study II (CIBIS II) (hazard ratio (HR) 0.56, 95% confidence interval (CI) 0.39–0.80; $P=0.0011$), and by 41% in the Metoprolol CR/XL Randomised Intervention Trial in Congestive Heart Failure (MERIT-HF) (HR 0.59, 95% CI 0.45–0.78; $P=0.0002$).[12,13] The Carvedilol Prospective Randomized Cumulative Survival (COPERNICUS) trial was aimed at the enrolment of patients with more severe HF, compared to previous trials, as defined by an LVEF of ≤25% and symptoms at rest or on minimal exertion. The benefits of beta-blocker therapy were confirmed with a 35% reduction in the risk of death, and a 24% reduction in the risk of death or all-cause hospitalization in patients assigned to carvedilol.[14]

The Study of the Effects of Nebivolol Intervention on Outcomes and Rehospitalisation in Seniors with Heart Failure (SENIORS) enrolled 2128 patients with HF aged ≥70 years who had a history of hospital admission for HF within the previous year or an LVEF of ≤35%. Thus, patients with mildly reduced or preserved LVEF also could be enrolled,[17] and randomly assigned to nebivolol (titrated from 1.25 mg once daily to 10 mg once daily) or placebo. The study showed a reduction in the primary composite endpoint of all-cause mortality or CV hospitalization in the nebivolol group (HR 0.86, 95% CI 0.74–0.99; $P=0.039$).[17] Results from the SENIORS trial were less significant than those from previous trials. However, when a similar population of patients was considered (younger patients with LVEF ≤35%), nebivolol was as effective as other beta-blockers.[17]

All beta-blockers that have been studied in large trials showed beneficial effects on patient outcomes. The impact on outcome of differences between beta-blockers was tested in small studies and in the Carvedilol Or Metoprolol European Trial (COMET), which compared carvedilol to metoprolol tartrate.[15,16] All-cause mortality was 34% for carvedilol, and 40% for metoprolol (HR 0.83, 95% CI 0.74–0.93; $P=0.0017$).[15] Of note, metoprolol tartrate, and not metoprolol succinate, was administered in this trial. Differences between metoprolol tartrate and metoprolol succinate, as well as between carvedilol and β1-AR selective compounds, may explain the findings of this trial.[22]

Practical recommendations

The indications and practical recommendations for the use of beta-blockers are outlined in guidelines for the management

Table 8.4.2 Randomized controlled outcome trials on beta-blockers in patients with heart failure

Trial	Agent	Main inclusion criteria	Number of patients	Mean follow-up	Primary endpoint	HR (95% CI) with beta-blocker versus placebo; P-value
CIBIS-II[12]	Bisoprolol	LVEF ≤0.35, NYHA classes III/IV	2647	1.3 years	All-cause mortality	0.66 (0.54–0.81); P <0.0001
MERIT-HF[13]	Metoprolol succinate	LVEF ≤0.40, NYHA classes II–IV	3991	1.0 year	All-cause mortality	0.66 (0.53–0.81); P = 0.00009
COPERNICUS[14]	Carvedilol	LVEF ≤0.25, symptoms at rest or on mild exertion, euvolaemia	2289	10.4 months	All-cause mortality	0.65 (0.52–0.81); P = 0.00013
CAPRICORN[43]	Carvedilol	Post-myocardial infarction, LVEF ≤0.40; mild or no symptoms of HF	1959	1.3 years	All-cause mortality or cardiovascular hospitalization	0.92 (0.80–1.07)
BEST[42]	Bucindolol	LVEF ≤0.35, NYHA classes III/IV	2708	2 years	All-cause mortality	0.90 (0.78–1.02); P = 0.10
SENIORS[17]	Nebivolol	Aged ≥70 years, HF hospitalization in previous year or LVEF ≤0.35%	2128	21 months	All-cause mortality or cardiovascular hospitalization	0.86 (0.74–0.99); P = 0.039

All-cause mortality alone was reduced in CAPRICORN (HR 0.77, 95% CI 0.60–0.98; P = 0.03). Cardiovascular mortality was reduced in BEST (HR 0.86; 95% CI 0.74–0.99). P-values for COPERNICUS and BEST are unadjusted.

BEST, Beta-Blocker Evaluation of Survival Trial; CAPRICORN, Carvedilol Post-Infarct Survival Control in Left Ventricular Dysfunction; CI, confidence interval; CIBIS-II, Cardiac Insufficiency Bisoprolol Study; COPERNICUS, CarvedilOl ProspEctive RaNdomIzed CUmulative Survival; HR, hazard ratio; LVEF, left ventricular ejection fraction; MERIT-HF, Metoprolol CR/XL Randomised Intervention Trial in Congestive Heart Failure; NYHA, New York Heart Association; SENIORS, Study of the Effects of Nebivolol Intervention on Outcomes and Rehospitalisation in Seniors with Heart Failure.

and treatment of HF.[34] Only beta-blockers shown to be effective in outcomes trials—bisoprolol, carvedilol, metoprolol succinate (CR/XL), and nebivolol—are recommended. Beta-blockers, along with other evidence-based treatment, should be initiated as soon as possible in clinically stable patients with HFrEF, starting at a low dose with gradual uptitration every 1–2 weeks up to bradycardia of 50–60 bpm, other side effects, or the target dose administered in clinical trials and recommended in guidelines. Ivabradine should be administered in patients who have a heart rate of ≥70 bpm in sinus rhythm and who do not tolerate beta-blockade.[34]

The modality of initiation of beta-blocker therapy with regard to concomitant therapy with an angiotensin-converting enzyme inhibitor (ACEI) has been a practical issue. In the CIBIS-III trial, initiating treatment with a beta-blocker (bisoprolol) followed by administration of an ACEI (enalapril) was compared to the opposite sequence in patients who had not been treated previously with these agents. No difference in efficacy and safety was observed between the two treatment regimens.[44] Current European Society of Cardiology (ESC) guidelines do not make specific recommendations regarding which drug should be started first.[34] Generally, an individualized approach, taking into consideration patients' clinical characteristics (fluid status, symptoms, blood pressure, heart rate, comorbidities), should always be preferred with regard to both the sequence of drug initiation and drug doses.[45]

It may be necessary to withdraw ongoing beta-blocker therapy in patients with severe haemodynamic impairment and signs of low cardiac output. However, multiple studies have shown that discontinuation of beta-blocker therapy is associated with an increased risk of death and this remains significant after adjustment for baseline variables related to HF severity.[46,47,48]

Use in clinical practice

Beta-blockers remain underused, underdosed, and discontinued in a meaningful proportion of patients with HFrEF.[49,50,51,52] This may be due to the presence of contraindications, including severe bradycardia, second- or third-degree atrioventricular block, hypotension, low cardiac output, bronchial wheezing, and peripheral vascular disease.[51] However, clinical inertia remains a major cause in a meaningful proportion of cases.[49,50,51]

Specific patient groups

Patients with heart failure and mildly reduced or preserved ejection fraction

There is a lack of evidence supporting the use of beta-blockers in patients with heart failure with preserved ejection fraction (HFpEF). The only prospective trial that included such patients was SENIORS. No interaction between LVEF and the effects of nebivolol on the primary outcome was shown, with HR (95% CI) for patients with LVEF ≤35% and >35% of 0.87 (0.73–1.05) and 0.82 (0.63–1.05), respectively.[17,53] However, the SENIORS trial was not designed and powered to assess the efficacy of nebivolol in patients with HFpEF. Moreover, the LVEF cut-off used for defining a low LVEF (35%) was too low in this trial, compared to the current cut-off for HFpEF.[34]

In an individual patient data meta-analysis of 11 trials, stratified according to baseline LVEF and heart rhythm, beta-blockers was found to reduce all-cause and CV mortality and to improve LVEF, compared to placebo, in patients in sinus rhythm with an LVEF of ≥50%.[19] Based on these data on outcomes, beta-blockers are now recommended also in patients with mildly reduced LVEF (HFmrEF), that is, with an LVEF of 41–49%.[34] In contrast, no benefit has been shown in patients with HFpEF, that is, with an LVEF of ≥50%, and this drug cannot be recommended in these patients unless for treatment of comorbidities such as AF with a high ventricular rate or hypertension.[34]

Patients with atrial fibrillation

AF and HF often coexist, with up to 50% of patients with HF developing AF over the course of their disease. Both conditions facilitate the occurrence, and aggravate the prognosis, of each other. The efficacy of beta-blockers in patients with HFrEF and concomitant AF is uncertain in the absence of randomized trials investigating the issue. A large individual patient data meta-analysis of all major beta-blocker trials in HFrEF, including 18,254 patients, with 13,946 (76%) patients in sinus rhythm and 3066 (17%) with AF at baseline, showed a significant reduction in all-cause mortality in patients in sinus rhythm (HR 0.73, 0.67–0.80; $P < 0.001$), but not in patients with AF (HR 0.97, 0.83–1.14; $P = 0.73$), with a significant P-value for interaction of baseline rhythm ($P = 0.002$). The lack of efficacy for the primary endpoint was consistent in all subgroups of AF, including age, sex, LVEF, New York Heart Association (NYHA) class, heart rate, and baseline medical therapy.[18] Lack of efficacy in patients with AF was confirmed in a more recent analysis.[19]

The AF-CHF trial randomized 1376 patients with AF and HFrEF (LVEF ≤35% with symptomatic congestive HF or LVEF <25% regardless of symptom status) to rhythm control versus a rate control strategy. A propensity-matched analysis of the AF-CHF trial showed that use of beta-blockers was significantly associated with lower mortality, but not with lower hospitalization rates, in HFrEF patients with AF.[54] In a meta-analysis of harmonized individual patient data from 11 double-blind randomized controlled trials ($n = 17,200$), a higher heart rate at baseline was associated with greater all-cause mortality for HFrEF patients in sinus rhythm (HR 1.11 per 10 bpm, 95% CI 1.07–1.15; $P < 0.0001$), but not those with AF (HR 1.03 per 10 bpm; 95% CI 0.97–1.08; $P = 0.38$). Beta-blockers improved survival only in patients in sinus rhythm, and a lower achieved resting heart rate, irrespective of treatment, was associated with better prognosis only for patients in sinus rhythm.[20] The recent Rate Control Therapy Evaluation in Permanent Atrial Fibrillation (RATE-AF) trial compared use of digoxin to bisoprolol in patients with HF, persistent AF, and NYHA class II–IV symptoms. Compared to bisoprolol, digoxin had the same effect on quality of life at 6 months (primary endpoint) and a better effect on symptoms, as assessed by the European Heart Rhythm Association (EHRA) and NYHA functional class. Only 19% of the patients had LVEF <50%, so that most of the patients could be considered as having HFmrEF or HFpEF.[55]

In conclusion, as data regarding the effects of beta-blockers on outcomes in patients with AF and HF are based on retrospective analyses, no prospective study to date has addressed the clinical efficacy of beta-blockers in patients with HF and AF, and beta-blockers had similar safety in patients with AF, compared to those in sinus rhythm, guidelines have maintained an indication for beta-blockers in all patients with HFrEF, and now also in those with HFmrEF, independently of their cardiac rhythm, to reduce mortality and HF hospitalization.[34] On the other hand, when used as part of a rate control strategy in patients with AF, beta-blockers should be considered, although with no higher priority compared to other drugs such as digoxin or amiodarone.[34]

Future directions

Despite its proven efficacy, beta-blockade as treatment for chronic HFrEF still has some limitations. First, there is the heterogeneity of response, with a small number of patients who do not respond, have potential harm, and cannot tolerate beta-blockade. Improvements in clinical pharmacological activity of these agents and a better understanding of the role of different pharmacokinetic and pharmacodynamic characteristics could help to improve both the heterogeneity of response and tolerability. Also genetic biomarker identification of patients who respond differentially, either better or worse, or not at all, may be useful. AR polymorphisms could theoretically be responsible for different responses. DNA data banks were obtained from major trials to assess the clinical implications of such polymorphisms. Significant interactions were found only with bucindolol, leading to the proposal of a fourth generation of beta-blockers, that is, those selective for specific AR polymorphisms and with pharmacogenetic indications.[56]

Beyond different genetic profiles, an individualized approach to beta-blockade treatment should be encouraged. A recent post hoc analysis of the BIOSTAT-CHF trial investigated sex differences in the optimal dose of ACEIs/ARBs and beta-blockers in patients with HFrEF. In men, the lowest HRs of death or hospitalization for HF occurred at 100% of the recommended dose of ACEIs or ARBs and beta-blockers, but women showed approximately 30% lower risk once beta-blocker doses reached 50–60% of the guideline-recommended target dose, with no further decrease in risk at higher doses. These sex differences were still present after adjusting for clinical covariates, including age and body surface area, and were confirmed in the ASIAN-HF cohort.[57]

Summary and key messages

Guideline-directed medical therapy in patients with HFrEF includes use of beta-blockers, ACEIs/ARBs or ARNIs, mineralocorticoid receptor antagonists, and, more recently, sodium–glucose cotransporter 2 inhibitors. Beta-blockers counteract the main mechanisms causing progression of HF and poor outcomes, hyperadrenergic activation, and tachycardia. Favourable effects occur in the long term, whereas initial worsening of cardiac function can be expected because of their acute negative impact on myocardial contractility. Clinical trials demonstrated that bisoprolol, carvedilol, metoprolol succinate, and nebivolol reduced the risk of mortality and HF hospitalization, compared to placebo, and only these agents are indicated for patients with HFrEF.[34,35] Beta-blockers should be initiated in stable patients as soon as possible, at low doses and then uptitrated up to the target dose or to the maximum tolerated dose. Based on retrospective analyses of clinical trials, beta-blockers may be considered also in patients with HFmrEF, but not in those with HFpEF, to reduce the risk of HF hospitalization and death.[34] Patients with HFpEF, as well as those with HFrEF and concomitant AF, showed a lack of benefits that require further investigations. Further improvement in beta-blocker therapy is needed with new compounds and/or a more personalized approach to patient selection. Prospective trials are needed that address patients with HFpEF and possibly specific subgroups of patients with HFpEF, as well as those with concomitant AF.

References

1. Waagstein F, Hjalmarson A, Varnauskas E, Wallentin I. Effect of chronic beta-adrenergic receptor blockade in congestive cardiomyopathy. Br Heart J. 1975;37(10):1022–36.
2. Metra M, Nardi M, Giubbini R, Dei Cas L. Effects of short- and long-term carvedilol administration on rest and exercise hemodynamic variables, exercise capacity and clinical conditions in patients with idiopathic dilated cardiomyopathy. J Am Coll Cardiol. 1994;24(7):1678–87.
3. Hall SA, Cigarroa CG, Marcoux L, Risser RC, Grayburn PA, Eichhorn EJ. Time course of improvement in left ventricular function, mass and geometry in patients with congestive heart failure treated with beta-adrenergic blockade. J Am Coll Cardiol. 1995;25(5):1154–61.
4. Waagstein F, Caidahl K, Wallentin I, Bergh CH, Hjalmarson A. Long-term beta-blockade in dilated cardiomyopathy. Effects of short- and long-term metoprolol treatment followed by withdrawal and readministration of metoprolol. Circulation. 1989;80(3):551–63.
5. Swedberg K, Hjalmarson A, Waagstein F, Wallentin I. Prolongation of survival in congestive cardiomyopathy by beta-receptor blockade. Lancet. 1979;1(8131):1374–6.
6. Norwegian Multicenter Study Group. Timolol-induced reduction in mortality and reinfarction in patients surviving acute myocardial infarction. N Engl J Med. 1981;304(14):801–7.
7. Chadda K, Goldstein S, Byington R, Curb JD. Effect of propranolol after acute myocardial infarction in patients with congestive heart failure. Circulation. 1986;73(3):503–10.
8. Cohn JN. Plasma norepinephrine and mortality. Clin Cardiol. 1995;18(3 Suppl I):I9–12.
9. Cohn JN, Levine TB, Olivari MT, et al. Plasma norepinephrine as a guide to prognosis in patients with chronic congestive heart failure. N Engl J Med. 1984;311(13):819–23.
10. Swedberg K, Eneroth P, Kjekshus J, Wilhelmsen L. Hormones regulating cardiovascular function in patients with severe congestive heart failure and their relation to mortality. CONSENSUS Trial Study Group. Circulation. 1990;82(5):1730–6.
11. Francis GS, Benedict C, Johnstone DE, et al. Comparison of neuroendocrine activation in patients with left ventricular dysfunction with and without congestive heart failure. A substudy of the Studies of Left Ventricular Dysfunction (SOLVD). Circulation. 1990;82(5):1724–9.
12. [No authors listed]. The Cardiac Insufficiency Bisoprolol Study II (CIBIS-II): a randomised trial. Lancet. 1999;353(9146):9–13.

13. [No authors listed]. Effect of metoprolol CR/XL in chronic heart failure: Metoprolol CR/XL Randomised Intervention Trial in Congestive Heart Failure (MERIT-HF). Lancet. 1999;353(9169):2001–7.

14. Packer M, Coats AJ, Fowler MB, et al. Effect of carvedilol on survival in severe chronic heart failure. N Engl J Med. 2001;344(22):1651–8.

15. Poole-Wilson PA, Swedberg K, Cleland JG, et al. Comparison of carvedilol and metoprolol on clinical outcomes in patients with chronic heart failure in the Carvedilol Or Metoprolol European Trial (COMET): randomised controlled trial. Lancet. 2003;362(9377):7–13.

16. Metra M, Giubbini R, Nodari S, Boldi E, Modena MG, Dei Cas L. Differential effects of beta-blockers in patients with heart failure: a prospective, randomized, double-blind comparison of the long-term effects of metoprolol versus carvedilol. Circulation. 2000;102(5):546–51.

17. Flather MD, Shibata MC, Coats AJ, et al. Randomized trial to determine the effect of nebivolol on mortality and cardiovascular hospital admission in elderly patients with heart failure (SENIORS). Eur Heart J. 2005;26(3):215–25.

18. Kotecha D, Holmes J, Krum H, et al. Efficacy of beta blockers in patients with heart failure plus atrial fibrillation: an individual-patient data meta-analysis. Lancet. 2014;384(9961):2235–43.

19. Cleland JGF, Bunting KV, Flather MD, et al. Beta-blockers for heart failure with reduced, mid-range, and preserved ejection fraction: an individual patient-level analysis of double-blind randomized trials. Eur Heart J. 2018;39(1):26–35.

20. Kotecha D, Flather MD, Altman DG, et al. Heart rate and rhythm and the benefit of beta-blockers in patients with heart failure. J Am Coll Cardiol. 2017;69(24):2885–96.

21. McAlister FA, Wiebe N, Ezekowitz JA, Leung AA, Armstrong PW. Meta-analysis: beta-blocker dose, heart rate reduction, and death in patients with heart failure. Ann Intern Med. 2009;150(11):784–94.

22. Metra M, Torp-Pedersen C, Swedberg K, et al. Influence of heart rate, blood pressure, and beta-blocker dose on outcome and the differences in outcome between carvedilol and metoprolol tartrate in patients with chronic heart failure: results from the COMET trial. Eur Heart J. 2005;26(21):2259–68.

23. Bristow MR. Beta-adrenergic receptor blockade in chronic heart failure. Circulation. 2000;101(5):558–69.

24. Metra M, Nodari S, D'Aloia A, Bontempi L, Boldi E, Cas LD. A rationale for the use of beta-blockers as standard treatment for heart failure. Am Heart J. 2000;139(3):511–21.

25. Bristow MR, Ginsburg R, Umans V, et al. Beta 1- and beta 2-adrenergic-receptor subpopulations in nonfailing and failing human ventricular myocardium: coupling of both receptor subtypes to muscle contraction and selective beta 1-receptor down-regulation in heart failure. Circ Res. 1986;59(3):297–309.

26. Fowler MB, Laser JA, Hopkins GL, Minobe W, Bristow MR. Assessment of the beta-adrenergic receptor pathway in the intact failing human heart: progressive receptor down-regulation and subsensitivity to agonist response. Circulation. 1986;74(6):1290–302.

27. Hasking GJ, Esler MD, Jennings GL, Burton D, Johns JA, Korner PI. Norepinephrine spillover to plasma in patients with congestive heart failure: evidence of increased overall and cardiorenal sympathetic nervous activity. Circulation. 1986;73(4):615–21.

28. Swedberg K, Viquerat C, Rouleau JL, et al. Comparison of myocardial catecholamine balance in chronic congestive heart failure and in angina pectoris without failure. Am J Cardiol. 1984;54(7):783–6.

29. Mann DL, Kent RL, Parsons B, Cooper GT. Adrenergic effects on the biology of the adult mammalian cardiocyte. Circulation. 1992;85(2):790–804.

30. Communal C, Singh K, Pimentel DR, Colucci WS. Norepinephrine stimulates apoptosis in adult rat ventricular myocytes by activation of the beta-adrenergic pathway. Circulation. 1998;98(13):1329–34.

31. Lowes BD, Gilbert EM, Abraham WT, et al. Myocardial gene expression in dilated cardiomyopathy treated with beta-blocking agents. N Engl J Med. 2002;346(18):1357–65.

32. Lowes BD, Gill EA, Abraham WT, et al. Effects of carvedilol on left ventricular mass, chamber geometry, and mitral regurgitation in chronic heart failure. Am J Cardiol. 1999;83(8):1201–5.

33. Swedberg K, Komajda M, Bohm M, et al. Ivabradine and outcomes in chronic heart failure (SHIFT): a randomised placebo-controlled study. Lancet. 2010;376(9744):875–85.

34. McDonagh TA, Metra M, Adamo M, et al. 2021 ESC Guidelines for the diagnosis and treatment of acute and chronic heart failure. Eur Heart J. 2021;42(36):3599–726.

35. Yancy CW, Jessup M, Bozkurt B, et al. 2017 ACC/AHA/HFSA Focused Update of the 2013 ACCF/AHA Guideline for the Management of Heart Failure: a report of the American College of Cardiology/American Heart Association Task Force on Clinical Practice Guidelines and the Heart Failure Society of America. Circulation. 2017;136(6):e137–61.

36. Lopez-Sendon J, Swedberg K, McMurray J, et al. Expert consensus document on beta-adrenergic receptor blockers. Eur Heart J. 2004;25(15):1341–62.

37. Doughty RN, Whalley GA, Gamble G, MacMahon S, Sharpe N. Left ventricular remodeling with carvedilol in patients with congestive heart failure due to ischemic heart disease. Australia-New Zealand Heart Failure Research Collaborative Group. J Am Coll Cardiol. 1997;29(5):1060–6.

38. Quaife RA, Christian PE, Gilbert EM, Datz FL, Volkman K, Bristow MR. Effects of carvedilol on right ventricular function in chronic heart failure. Am J Cardiol. 1998;81(2):247–50.

39. Bristow MR, Gilbert EM, Abraham WT, et al. Carvedilol produces dose-related improvements in left ventricular function and survival in subjects with chronic heart failure. MOCHA Investigators. Circulation. 1996;94(11):2807–16.

40. Metra M, Nodari S, Parrinello G, Giubbini R, Manca C, Dei Cas L. Marked improvement in left ventricular ejection fraction during long-term beta-blockade in patients with chronic heart failure: clinical correlates and prognostic significance. Am Heart J. 2003;145(2):292–9.

41. de Groote P, Delour P, Mouquet F, et al. The effects of beta-blockers in patients with stable chronic heart failure. Predictors of left ventricular ejection fraction improvement and impact on prognosis. Am Heart J. 2007;154(3):589–95.

42. Beta-Blocker Evaluation of Survival Trial Investigators; Eichhorn EJ, Domanski MJ, Krause-Steinrauf H, Bristow MR, Lavori PW. A trial of the beta-blocker bucindolol in patients with advanced chronic heart failure. N Engl J Med. 2001;344(22):1659–67.

43. Dargie HJ. Effect of carvedilol on outcome after myocardial infarction in patients with left-ventricular dysfunction: the CAPRICORN randomised trial. Lancet. 2001;357(9266):1385–90.

44. Willenheimer R, Erdmann E, Follath F, et al. Comparison of treatment initiation with bisoprolol vs. enalapril in chronic heart failure patients: rationale and design of CIBIS-III. Eur J Heart Fail. 2004;6(4):493–500.

45. Rosano GMC, Moura B, Metra M, et al. Patient profiling in heart failure for tailoring medical therapy. A consensus document of the Heart Failure Association of the European Society of Cardiology. Eur J Heart Fail. 2021;23(6):872–81.

46. Metra M, Torp-Pedersen C, Cleland JG, et al. Should beta-blocker therapy be reduced or withdrawn after an episode of decompensated heart failure? Results from COMET. Eur J Heart Fail. 2007;9(9):901–9.

47. Jondeau G, Neuder Y, Eicher JC, et al. B-CONVINCED: Beta-blocker CONtinuation Vs. INterruption in patients with Congestive

heart failure hospitalizED for a decompensation episode. Eur Heart J. 2009;30(18):2186–92.

48. Prins KW, Neill JM, Tyler JO, Eckman PM, Duval S. Effects of beta-blocker withdrawal in acute decompensated heart failure: a systematic review and meta-analysis. JACC Heart Fail. 2015;3(8):647–53.

49. Greene SJ, Butler J, Albert NM, et al. Medical therapy for heart failure with reduced ejection fraction: the CHAMP-HF Registry. J Am Coll Cardiol. 2018;72(4):351–66.

50. Greene SJ, Fonarow GC, DeVore AD, et al. Titration of medical therapy for heart failure with reduced ejection fraction. J Am Coll Cardiol. 2019;73(19):2365–83.

51. Maggioni AP, Anker SD, Dahlstrom U, et al. Are hospitalized or ambulatory patients with heart failure treated in accordance with European Society of Cardiology guidelines? Evidence from 12,440 patients of the ESC Heart Failure Long-Term Registry. Eur J Heart Fail. 2013;15(10):1173–84.

52. Savarese G, Bodegard J, Norhammar A, et al. Heart failure drug titration, discontinuation, mortality and heart failure hospitalization risk: a multinational observational study (US, UK and Sweden). Eur J Heart Fail. 2021;23(9):1499–511.

53. Van Veldhuisen DJ, Cohen-Solal A, Bohm M, et al. Beta-blockade with nebivolol in elderly heart failure patients with impaired and preserved left ventricular ejection fraction: data from SENIORS (Study of Effects of Nebivolol Intervention on Outcomes and Rehospitalization in Seniors With Heart Failure). J Am Coll Cardiol. 2009;53(23):2150–8.

54. Cadrin-Tourigny J, Shohoudi A, Roy D, et al. Decreased mortality with beta-blockers in patients with heart failure and coexisting atrial fibrillation: an AF-CHF substudy. JACC Heart Fail. 2017;5(2):99–106.

55. Kotecha D, Bunting KV, Gill SK, et al. Effect of digoxin vs bisoprolol for heart rate control in atrial fibrillation on patient-reported quality of life: the RATE-AF randomized clinical trial. JAMA. 2020;324(24):2497–508.

56. Bristow MR, Murphy GA, Krause-Steinrauf H, et al. An alpha2C-adrenergic receptor polymorphism alters the norepinephrine-lowering effects and therapeutic response of the beta-blocker bucindolol in chronic heart failure. Circ Heart Fail. 2010;3(1):21–8.

57. Santema BT, Ouwerkerk W, Tromp J, et al. Identifying optimal doses of heart failure medications in men compared with women: a prospective, observational, cohort study. Lancet. 2019;394(10205):1254–63.

CHAPTER 8.5

Mineralocorticoid receptor antagonists

Bertram Pitt, João Pedro Ferreira, and
Faiez Zannad

Contents

Introduction

Hypertension, heart failure, post-myocardial infarction complicated with heart failure or systolic dysfunction, and albuminuric chronic kidney disease are the cardiovascular clinical syndromes where mineralocorticoid receptor antagonists (MRAs) have shown a beneficial effect. The treatment goals for these patients are to improve clinical status, functional capacity, and quality of life, and prevent hospital admissions and reduce mortality.[1]

MRAs have been shown to improve survival in patients with heart failure with reduced ejection fraction (HFrEF).[1] In patients with heart failure with preserved ejection fraction (HFpEF), MRA therapy is less well established.[1,2] In acute heart failure, MRAs have not been tested yet in a randomized controlled trial targeting morbidity and mortality.[3] In the post-myocardial infarction setting, MRAs have been shown to improve morbidity and mortality in patients with heart failure or systolic dysfunction.[4] In patients with hypertension, the MRA spironolactone has been shown to be the most effective add-on drug for the treatment of resistant hypertension.[5]

The mechanisms by which MRAs improve outcomes in these settings are likely related to the fact that mineralocorticoid receptors are present not only in the epithelial cells of the renal tubule, but also in the myocardium, vascular wall, endothelium, macrophages, and intestines, as well as the eye, and aldosterone has a multitude of effects beyond sodium and potassium homeostasis (➲ Figure 8.5.1).[6]

This chapter will provide an appraisal of the different types of MRA drugs and their pharmacological differences with respect to their mechanism of action, pharmacokinetics, monitoring, adverse effects, and drug interactions in patients with heart failure.

Mineralocorticoid receptor antagonists: a pharmacological and clinical perspective

Two MRAs are commonly used in clinical practice: spironolactone and eplerenone. Eplerenone has less affinity for progesterone and androgen receptors than spironolactone, and consequently has fewer gynaecological and andrological side effects. Moreover, spironolactone can increase cortisol and glycated haemoglobin levels more than eplerenone; therefore, eplerenone potentially has a more favourable profile for patients with diabetes mellitus.[7]

Finerenone is an MRA with potentially higher affinity for mineralocorticoid receptors present in the myocardium.

Potassium canrenoate is a spironolactone metabolite soluble in aqueous fluids that can be used in intravenous formulations. However, its use in clinical practice is still very limited.

These MRA formulations will be discussed in the following sections.

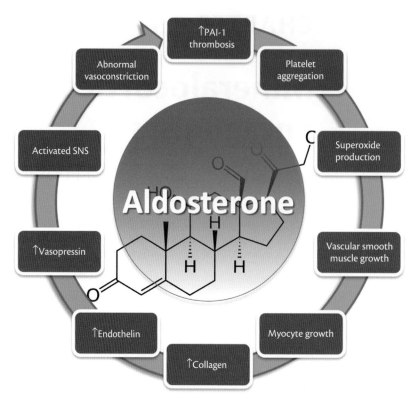

Figure 8.5.1 The mechanisms via which mineralocorticoid receptor antagonists (MRAs) improve outcomes remain speculative but likely include the fact that mineralocorticoid receptors are present not only in epithelial cells of the renal tubule, but also in the myocardium, vascular wall, endothelium, macrophages, and intestines, as well as the eye, and aldosterone has a multitude of effects beyond sodium and potassium homeostasis. PAI-1, plasminogen activator inhibitor 1; SNS, sympathetic nervous system.

Spironolactone

Spironolactone (17-hydroxy-7α-mercapto-3-oxo-17α-pregn-4-ene-21-carboxylic acid γ-lactone acetate) was developed in the 1950s and is a non-selective MRA with moderate affinity for both progesterone and androgen receptors. Spironolactone is poorly soluble in aqueous fluids, and an intravenous formulation is not available for routine clinical use.[8]

Mechanism of action

Spironolactone is a specific pharmacological antagonist of aldosterone, acting primarily through competitive binding of receptors at the aldosterone-dependent sodium–potassium exchange site in the distal convoluted renal tubule. By this mechanism, spironolactone can increase, in a dose-dependent fashion, the amount of excreted sodium and water, while retaining potassium.[9] Therefore, in this way, spironolactone can act both as a diuretic and as an antihypertensive drug, which is useful in cardiovascular conditions where secondary aldosteronism is usually involved, including heart failure and hypertension. However, many other spironolactone actions are not explained by these mechanisms, and are possibly due to its 'genomic' (e.g. anti-fibrotic) effects which are attained at lower doses and that can explain the positive results in several conditions, including heart failure.[10] The doses and main findings of spironolactone and eplerenone in heart failure and myocardial infarction with systolic dysfunction or heart failure are described in ➲ Table 8.5.1.

Pharmacokinetics and pharmacodynamics

Spironolactone has extensive and complex metabolism in humans. Its absorption can reach 80–90% and it is not affected by food.[11,12] However, it undergoes extensive hepatic metabolism into active metabolites, that is, canrenone and sulfur-containing metabolites, with prolonged half-lives ranging from 14 to 17 hours.[13] Following a single dose of oral spironolactone, peak serum concentrations of the drug and its metabolites occur at 1–2 and 2–4 hours, respectively. This relatively slow peak of action has been related to the time active metabolites take to reach steady-state plasma levels. The natriuretic effect of spironolactone only occurs at dosages of above 25 mg/day, peaking at 12–24 hours and declining over a period of 48–72 hours.[8]

Monitoring, adverse effects, and frequent drug interactions

Spironolactone and eplerenone (➲ Eplerenone, p. 483) are generally safe and well tolerated. Despite the fact that the rates of mild to moderate hyperkalaemia and elevations in creatinine levels occur more frequently in patients treated with MRAs, the incidence of life-threatening hyperkalaemia or renal injury, or both, does not differ between MRA and placebo groups in large randomized clinical trials.[2,4,14,15] Nevertheless, clinical guidelines recommend close monitoring of renal function and electrolyte levels throughout the course of MRA therapy. Some authors define appropriate testing as a laboratory panel including creatinine and

Table 8.5.1 Main findings of mineralocorticoid receptor antagonist trials

Variable	RALES	EMPHASIS	EPHESUS	TOPCAT
Population	HFrEF Severe symptoms	HFrEF Mild symptoms	HFrEF Post-myocardial infarction	HFpEF Symptomatic
Drug (vs placebo)	Spironolactone	Eplerenone	Eplerenone	Spironolactone
Dose	~25 mg/day	~50 mg/day	~50 mg/day	15–45 mg/day
Primary endpoint	ACM	CO	CO	CO
HR (95% CI) for TTx	0.70 (0.60–0.82)	0.63 (0.54–0.74)	0.87 (0.79–0.95)	0.89 (0.77–1.04)

~, approximately; ACM, all-cause mortality; CI, confidence interval; CO, composite outcome of death from cardiovascular causes or hospitalization for heart failure in EMPHASIS and TOPCAT, and death from cardiovascular causes or hospitalization for cardiovascular events in EPHESUS; HFpEF, heart failure with preserved ejection fraction; HFrEF, heart failure with reduced ejection fraction; HR, hazard ratio; TTx, treatment.

potassium levels within 120 days before initiation, two or more measurements during the early post-initiation period (days 1–10), and three or more measurements during the extended post-initiation period (days 11–90). These recommendations are rarely followed in clinical practice and their association with better outcomes is yet to be determined.[16]

Spironolactone is contraindicated in patients with an estimated glomerular filtration rate (eGFR) of below 30 mL/min/1.73 m^2, plasma creatinine level of above 2.5 mg/dL, and/or serum potassium level of above 5.5 mmol/L. Frequent adverse effects include mild hyperkalaemia, worsening renal function, and gynaecomastia. These adverse effects are rarely severe and commonly reversible after stopping the drug. A full list of possible adverse effects and drug interactions is presented in ⊃ Box 8.5.1 and ⊃ Box 8.5.2, respectively.

Box 8.5.1 Possible side effects of mineralocorticoid receptor antagonists

All patients receiving mineralocorticoid receptor antagonists (MRAs) should be observed for evidence of fluid or electrolyte imbalance (e.g. hyperkalaemia, hyponatraemia, hypomagnesaemia, hypochloraemic alkalosis).

The most common side effects of MRAs include the following.

Hyperkalaemia

Patients at higher risk of hyperkalaemia include those aged over 75 years, with impaired renal function, diabetes, and/or a previous history of hyperkalaemia.

Hyponatraemia

Hyponatraemia may be caused or aggravated by MRAs, especially when these drugs are administered in combination with other diuretics.

Worsening renal function

Renal function may be aggravated by MRA administration. However, it is not associated with poor prognosis.

Gynaecomastia

Gynaecomastia may develop in association with the use of spironolactone. The development of gynaecomastia appears to be related to both the dosage level and the duration of therapy, and is normally reversible when spironolactone is discontinued or replaced by other non-steroidal MRAs such as eplerenone or finerenone.

Eplerenone

Eplerenone (pregn-4-ene-7,21-dicarboxylic acid, 9,11-epoxy-17-hydroxy-3-oxo, γ-lactone, methyl ester) was derived from spironolactone by the introduction of a 9,11-epoxy bridge and by substitution of the 17α-thioacetyl group of spironolactone with a carbomethoxy group. *In vitro*, eplerenone has 10- to 20-fold lower affinity for the mineralocorticoid receptor relative to spironolactone. However, the *in vivo* dosage of eplerenone required to inhibit aldosterone receptors by 50% is approximately half that of spironolactone.[17] In contrast to spironolactone, eplerenone has little affinity for the androgen, progesterone, and glucocorticoid receptors (100–1000 times lower than spironolactone), and consequently has fewer 'sexual' side effects.[18] Eplerenone also has a shorter half-life and fewer inactive metabolites, as compared to spironolactone.[19]

Differences in the study populations and a lack of head-to-head outcome trials do not allow a recommendation of one agent over the other. However, in the presence of 'sexual' adverse effects (e.g. gynaecomastia), a strategy of switching spironolactone for eplerenone should be preferred over stopping the drug. Furthermore, eplerenone (and not spironolactone) was tested and proved to be beneficial in patients with HFrEF and mild symptoms (in the EMPHASIS-HF trial) and in patients with myocardial infarction complicated by systolic dysfunction or heart failure or diabetes (in the EPHESUS trial). Smaller mechanistic

---

Box 8.5.2 Possible treatment interactions of mineralocorticoid receptor antagonists

Concomitant administration of MRAs with the following drugs or potassium sources may lead to severe hyperkalaemia and/or renal dysfunction and should be avoided:

- Other potassium-sparing diuretics
- Angiotensin-converting enzyme inhibitors
- Angiotensin II receptor blockers
- Other aldosterone antagonists
- Non-steroidal anti-inflammatory drugs (e.g. indomethacin)
- Heparin and low-molecular-weight heparin
- Potassium supplements and potassium-rich diet

studies also suggest that eplerenone may have a more favourable metabolic profile than spironolactone, as eplerenone does not induce elevations in cortisol level or glycated haemoglobin, whereas spironolactone does.[20] This may be of particular interest for patients with concomitant heart failure and diabetes.

Mechanism of action

Eplerenone is also a specific pharmacological antagonist of aldosterone; hence it also has the same diuretic and potassium-sparing properties of spironolactone. However, many other eplerenone actions are also not explained by these 'non-genomic' mechanisms and are possibly due to its 'genomic' effects.[19,21] Recommended dosages and the main cardiovascular indications of eplerenone are described in ⊃ Table 8.5.1.

Pharmacokinetics and pharmacodynamics

Compared to spironolactone, eplerenone is rapidly absorbed in the gastrointestinal tract; its peak maximum concentration is within 1.5 hours, its metabolites are inactive, and its elimination half-life is only 4–6 hours.[22] Moreover, eplerenone has approximately 50% less protein-binding capacity, potentially explaining the difference in receptor affinity and potency.[23]

Monitoring, adverse effects, and frequent drug interactions

'Sexual'-related side effects are less frequent with eplerenone. Monitoring and contraindications are similar to those of spironolactone. A full list of possible adverse effects and drug interactions is presented in ⊃ Box 8.5.1 and Box 8.5.2, respectively.

Potassium canrenoate

Potassium canrenoate is a spironolactone metabolite that is soluble in aqueous fluids. A single intravenous dose of potassium canrenoate immediately (i.e. in <30 minutes) blocks the aldosterone receptors and has demonstrated a rapid natriuretic effect within 6 hours after administration.[24] Intravenous potassium canrenoate at 200 mg immediately reaches plasma concentrations approximately 10-fold greater than those obtained with 200 mg of oral spironolactone. The half-life of canrenoate ranges from 3 to 6 hours; however, at 24 hours, the plasma concentrations after an intravenous infusion of 200 mg of potassium canrenoate remain higher than those achieved with 200 mg of spironolactone.[25,26]

The properties described for potassium canrenoate make this drug very attractive for acute oedematous states in which aldosterone blockade may be important (e.g. acute heart failure).

This drug has been prospectively studied in the Early Aldosterone Blockade in Acute Myocardial Infarction (ALBATROSS) trial, with a remarkable safety profile. In this trial, 1603 patients were randomized to receive an MRA regimen with a single intravenous bolus of potassium canrenoate (200 mg), followed by oral spironolactone (25 mg once daily) for 6 months in addition to standard therapy, or to standard therapy alone. The primary outcome of the study was the composite of death, resuscitated cardiac arrest,

significant ventricular arrhythmia, indication for implantable defibrillator, or new or worsening heart failure at 6-month follow-up. The primary outcome rates were low, that is, they occurred in 95 (11.8%) and 98 (12.2%) patients in the treatment and control groups, respectively, and the study was underpowered to detect a significant between-group difference (hazard ratio 0.97, 95% confidence interval 0.73–1.28). However, the safety profile was remarkable, with hyperkalaemia of above 5.5 mmol/L occurring in only 3% and 0.2% of patients in the treatment and standard therapy groups, respectively ($P < 0.0001$), with no death or hospitalization associated with hyperkalaemia.[27]

Finerenone

While both spironolactone and eplerenone have been shown to be effective in various settings, they may be underused or inconsistently prescribed due to their relatively frequent incidence of mild hyperkalaemia. Furthermore, patients with common conditions, such as diabetes mellitus or chronic kidney disease, are at particular risk of developing hyperkalaemia and may be even less likely to receive currently available MRA therapy due to safety concerns.[28]

Finerenone is a non-steroidal MRA, with higher selectivity for the mineralocorticoid receptor, compared to spironolactone, and stronger receptor-binding affinity than eplerenone. This preclinical combination of potency and selectivity towards the mineralocorticoid receptor could potentially reduce the side effects commonly attributed to MRAs. Moreover, in preclinical studies, equinatriuretic doses of finerenone provided a greater reduction in proteinuria than eplerenone.[29]

Mechanism of action

Finerenone is a potent, highly selective non-steroidal MRA. The selectivity of finerenone for the heart and kidney is approximately 500-fold greater than that for the glucocorticoid, androgen, and progesterone receptors (in cellular transactivation assays).[30]

Pharmacokinetics and pharmacodynamics

Finerenone has a pharmacokinetic profile characterized by low blood clearance, long half-life (approximately 8.5 hours), and high oral bioavailability (94% in rats).[31]

Monitoring, adverse effects, and frequent drug interactions

In a direct comparison, finerenone is associated with lower rates of hyperkalaemia and worsening renal function, as compared to those of spironolactone or in an indirect comparison with eplerenone.[32]

Finerenone improved cardiovascular and renal outcomes in patients with type 2 diabetes and albuminuric chronic kidney disease.[33,34] Nonetheless, experience with finerenone is much more scarce than that with steroidal MRAs; hence its safety profile requires additional studies and post-marketing surveillance. A full list of possible adverse effects and drug interactions is presented in ⊃ Box 8.5.1 and Box 8.5.2, respectively.

Other non-steroidal mineralocorticoid receptor antagonists

Many other non-steroidal MRAs are under development and/or human testing. A detailed description of these agents is given by Kolkhof and colleagues.[30]

Main heart failure clinical studies in humans

Heart failure with reduced ejection fraction and post-myocardial infarction complicated with systolic dysfunction or heart failure

In HFrEF (and post-myocardial infarction with systolic dysfunction), MRA therapy has been evaluated in three large randomized controlled trials: (1) the Randomized Aldactone Evaluation Study—RALES;[14] (2) the Eplerenone in Patients with Systolic Heart Failure and Mild Symptoms—EMPHASIS;[15] and (3) the Eplerenone Post-Myocardial Infarction—EPHESUS.[14] These trials showed that MRAs, in addition to standard therapy, substantially reduced the risk of both morbidity and mortality among patients with severe and mild HFrEF and those with post-myocardial infarction with systolic dysfunction. Therefore, MRAs should be provided to all HFrEF patients unless contraindicated (IA indication).[1] In the case of intolerance (e.g. gynaecomastia, hyperkalaemia, worsening renal function, sexual dysfunction), clinicians should assess all possible causes, including medication interactions, and consider other agents in the MRA class before stopping treatment (➲ Figure 8.5.2).

Post-myocardial infarction without systolic dysfunction

The role of MRAs in post-myocardial infarction without systolic dysfunction has been evaluated in two randomized controlled trials (i.e. the ALBATROSS[27] and the REMINDER[35] trials), which demonstrated safety of MRA therapy in this setting, but not reduced morbidity and mortality because these trials were largely underpowered to these outcomes. Consequently, until larger and adequately powered trials are conducted, MRA therapy cannot be routinely advised in myocardial infarction patients without systolic dysfunction or heart failure.

Heart failure with preserved ejection fraction

In HFpEF, MRA therapy may be considered in selected patients, particularly those with an ejection fraction of <55%.[1]

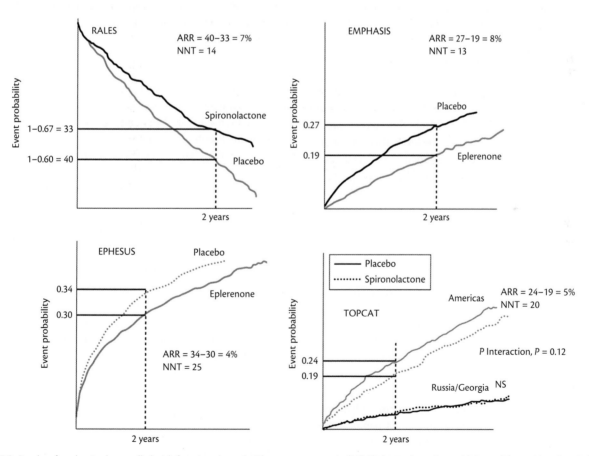

Figure 8.5.2 Results of randomized controlled trials for mineralocorticoid receptor antagonist (MRA) therapy in patients with heart failure with reduced ejection fraction (HFrEF) (RALES, EMPHASIS, and EPHESUS) and heart failure with preserved ejection fraction (HFpEF) (TOPCAT). ARR, absolute risk reduction; EMPHASIS, Eplerenone in Patients with Systolic Heart Failure and Mild Symptoms; EPHESUS, Eplerenone post-Myocardial Infarction; NNT, number needed to treat; NS, not significant; RALES, Randomized Aldactone Evaluation Study; TOPCAT, Treatment of Preserved Cardiac Function Heart Failure With an Aldosterone Antagonist.

Reproduced from Ferreira JP, Mentz RJ, Pizard A, Pitt B, Zannad F. Tailoring mineralocorticoid receptor antagonist therapy in heart failure patients: are we moving towards a personalized approach? *Eur J Heart Fail*. 2017 Aug;19(8):974–986. doi: 10.1002/ejhf.814 with permission from John Wiley and Sons.

However, several aspects must be considered to provide clinicians with practical guidance to tailor MRA therapy in such patients. It is our opinion that, unless contraindicated, spironolactone should be provided to HFpEF patients with overlapping clinical profiles of those randomized from 'the Americas' in the TOPCAT trial (➲ Figure 8.5.2).[36] In TOPCAT, a high proportion of patients enrolled in Eastern Europe (Russia and Georgia) had low or indetectable levels of spironolactone (and its active metabolites) in their blood; consequently, these patients did not experience the therapeutic effects of the drug.[37] Moreover, patients from Eastern Europe had an overall low risk profile and event rates compatible with the age-matched population from those countries. Given all these factors, the TOPCAT trial can only be analysed in the light of findings from patients enrolled in 'the Americas' where spironolactone did reduce hospitalization for heart failure and cardiovascular death.

Acute heart failure

In acute heart failure, the evidence is much more scarce, and MRAs have not been evaluated in an adequately powered morbidity and mortality trial in this context. Notwithstanding, the 'Efficacy and Safety of Spironolactone in Acute Heart Failure: The ATHENA-HF Randomized Clinical Trial' tested whether high-dose spironolactone could be more efficient than placebo for reducing N-terminal pro-B-type natriuretic peptide (NT-proBNP) levels.[3] The primary hypothesis of ATHENA-HF was that treatment with spironolactone (100 mg/day) versus placebo would lead to greater NT-proBNP level reductions at 96 hours. NT-proBNP levels did not differ between the two groups, nor did the other prespecified endpoints (dyspnoea, congestion, urine output, weight loss, and events). Of note, changes in potassium and creatinine levels also did not differ between the groups. The 360 patients included in the ATHENA-HF trial had relatively mild acute heart failure. Their median age was 65 years; the median eGFR was 57 mL/min/1.73 m^2, and both sodium and urea levels were within normal range. The 30-day death rate was low (<4%). It is therefore unlikely that these patients had 'diuretic resistance'. More importantly, as described earlier, spironolactone might have been an inappropriate drug choice for the planned 96-hour endpoint. Oral spironolactone has a slow onset of action: it is a pro-drug that needs to be metabolized to the main active metabolite potassium canrenoate, a process that may take up to 24–48 hours, which makes it inappropriate for acute states. It is also possible that gastrointestinal congestion might have limited spironolactone absorption. Therefore, it was unlikely that significant pharmacodynamic effects could be observed within the short study observation time. Consistently, the change in potassium level, a strong biochemical surrogate of the pharmacodynamic effect of spironolactone, was very marginal and not significantly different between the groups. This hypothesis was confirmed by the measurement of plasma canrenoate levels, showing lower-than-expected levels at 96 hours.[38]

Hypertension and heart failure prevention

Many patients, particularly those with established HFpEF and those at high risk of developing heart failure, have high blood pressure. MRAs can be a drug of choice for these patients. In a double-blind, placebo-controlled crossover trial, 335 patients with systolic blood pressure of at least 140 mmHg (or ≥135 mmHg in those with diabetes) rotated through 3 months of therapy with spironolactone, bisoprolol, doxazosin, and placebo, in addition to their baseline antihypertensive drugs. Spironolactone achieved greater blood pressure reduction and hence represents the most effective add-on drug for the treatment of resistant hypertension.[5] Based on these findings, spironolactone should be the preferred add-on treatment for patients with resistant hypertension.

In 527 patients at high risk of developing heart failure, enrolled in the Heart Omics in Ageing (HOMAGE) trial, spironolactone (compared to control) reduced the circulating levels of procollagen type I carboxy-terminal propeptide (PICP) a direct marker of collagen synthesis, and reduced NT-proBNP levels, blood pressure, and left atrial volume.[39]

Together, these findings support the role of MRAs in heart failure prevention, but further and larger studies are needed.

Other settings

In a randomized controlled trial including 823 patients with diabetes and albuminuria who were receiving an angiotensin-converting enzyme inhibitor or an angiotensin receptor blocker, participants were randomly assigned to receiving several doses of finerenone or a matching placebo for 3 months. The primary outcome was the ratio of urinary albumin-to-creatinine. Finerenone demonstrated a dose-dependent reduction in urinary albumin:creatinine ratio, without increased severe hyperkalaemia or worsening renal dysfunction.[32]

In the FIDELIO-DKD (Finerenone in Reducing Kidney Failure and Disease Progression in Diabetic Kidney Disease; ClinicalTrials.gov identifier: NCT02540993) trial, finerenone (compared to placebo) significantly reduced the combined risk of time to first occurrence of kidney failure, sustained decrease in eGFR of ≥40%, or renal death in patients with type 2 diabetes and diabetic kidney disease.[33] These findings were expanded in the FIGARO-DKD (Efficacy and Safety of Finerenone in Subjects With Type 2 Diabetes Mellitus and the Clinical Diagnosis of Diabetic Kidney Disease; ClinicalTrials.gov identifier: NCT02545049) trial.[34]

Together, findings support the benefit of eplerenone and non-steroidal MRAs in patients with diabetes.

A growing body of literature suggests that the use of MRAs in end-stage renal disease patients is beneficial.[40] The ALCHEMIST trial will test the effects of spironolactone on major cardiovascular events in chronic haemodialysis patients in a large, double-blind randomized controlled trial (NCT01848639).

Potassium-binding therapies

The advent of potassium-binding therapies may reassure clinicians to prescribe MRAs to subgroups of patients with a high risk of hyperkalaemia. Additionally, well-conducted investigations should continue to provide quality evidence in high-risk patients, and well-powered prospective randomized controlled trials will be required to determine the effect of these agents on cardiovascular outcomes.[41]

Future directions

Newer non-steroidal MRAs should be compared to steroidal MRAs to test their superiority and better tolerability in patients with heart failure.

The combination of MRAs and sodium–glucose cotransporter 2 inhibitors should be tested in selected populations, including those with heart failure.

Newer potassium binders may be used to enable MRA therapy.

Conclusions

This chapter describes the pharmacological basis of MRAs from a clinical point of view, providing the background for understanding the efficacy of these agents in heart failure and related conditions. Further evidence is required in special populations such as acute heart failure or dialysis patients. MRAs are generally safe. However, the advent of novel MRAs (e.g. finerenone) and potassium-binding therapies can potentially increase MRA treatment rates in populations at high risk of MRA intolerance and side effects.

Summary

Hypertension, post-myocardial infarction, and heart failure are the cardiovascular clinical syndromes in which MRAs have shown a beneficial effect. Most guidelines, while recommending MRAs, do not make a clear recommendation as to which MRAs should be used, how doses should be titrated, or what monitoring is indicated. This chapter provides an appraisal of the different types of MRA drugs and their pharmacological differences with respect to their mechanism of action, pharmacokinetics, monitoring, adverse effects, and drug interactions.

Key messages

- MRAs are beneficial to patients with hypertension, heart failure, and albuminuric chronic kidney disease, and those who had myocardial infarction complicated with heart failure or systolic dysfunction.

- MRAs are still underused in these conditions, and optimal implementation of these therapies is required.

- Newer non-steroidal MRAs (e.g. finerenone) are better tolerated than older steroidal MRAs (e.g. spironolactone) and may help for better implementation of these therapies.

References

1. McDonagh TA, Metra M, Adamo M, et al. 2021 ESC Guidelines for the diagnosis and treatment of acute and chronic heart failure. Eur Heart J. 2021;42(36):3599–726.
2. Pitt B, Pfeffer MA, Assmann SF, et al. Spironolactone for heart failure with preserved ejection fraction. N Engl J Med. 2014;370(15):1383–92.
3. Butler J, Anstrom KJ, Felker GM, et al. Efficacy and safety of spironolactone in acute heart failure: the ATHENA-HF randomized clinical trial. JAMA Cardiol. 2017;2(9):950–8.
4. Pitt B, Williams G, Remme W, et al. The EPHESUS trial: eplerenone in patients with heart failure due to systolic dysfunction complicating acute myocardial infarction. Eplerenone Post-AMI Heart Failure Efficacy and Survival Study. Cardiovasc Drugs Ther. 2001;15(1):79–87.
5. Williams B, MacDonald TM, Morant S, et al. Spironolactone versus placebo, bisoprolol, and doxazosin to determine the optimal treatment for drug-resistant hypertension (PATHWAY-2): a randomised, double-blind, crossover trial. Lancet. 2015;386(10008):2059–68.
6. Vecchiola A, Lagos CF, Carvajal CA, Baudrand R, Fardella CE. Aldosterone production and signaling dysregulation in obesity. Curr Hypertens Rep. 2016;18(3):20.
7. Yamaji M, Tsutamoto T, Kawahara C, et al. Effect of eplerenone versus spironolactone on cortisol and hemoglobin A(1)(c) levels in patients with chronic heart failure. Am Heart J. 2010;160(5):915–21.
8. Sica DA. Pharmacokinetics and pharmacodynamics of mineralocorticoid blocking agents and their effects on potassium homeostasis. Heart Fail Rev. 2005;10(1):23–9.
9. Karim A. Spironolactone: disposition, metabolism, pharmacodynamics, and bioavailability. Drug Metab Rev. 1978;8(1):151–88.
10. Zannad F, Alla F, Dousset B, Perez A, Pitt B. Limitation of excessive extracellular matrix turnover may contribute to survival benefit of spironolactone therapy in patients with congestive heart failure: insights from the randomized aldactone evaluation study (RALES). Rales Investigators. Circulation. 2000;102(22):2700–6.
11. Overdiek HW, Hermens WA, Merkus FW. New insights into the pharmacokinetics of spironolactone. Clin Pharmacol Ther. 1985;38(4):469–74.
12. Overdiek HW, Merkus FW. Influence of food on the bioavailability of spironolactone. Clin Pharmacol Ther. 1986;40(5):531–6.
13. Gardiner P, Schrode K, Quinlan D, et al. Spironolactone metabolism: steady-state serum levels of the sulfur-containing metabolites. J Clin Pharmacol. 1989;29(4):342–7.
14. Pitt B, Zannad F, Remme WJ, et al. The effect of spironolactone on morbidity and mortality in patients with severe heart failure. Randomized Aldactone Evaluation Study Investigators. N Engl J Med. 1999;341(10):709–17.
15. Zannad F, McMurray JJ, Krum H, et al. Eplerenone in patients with systolic heart failure and mild symptoms. N Engl J Med. 2011;364(1):11–21.
16. Cooper LB, Hammill BG, Peterson ED, et al. Consistency of laboratory monitoring during initiation of mineralocorticoid receptor antagonist therapy in patients with heart failure. JAMA. 2015;314(18):1973–5.
17. Delyani JA. Mineralocorticoid receptor antagonists: the evolution of utility and pharmacology. Kidney Int. 2000;57(4):1408–11.
18. Garthwaite SM, McMahon EG. The evolution of aldosterone antagonists. Mol Cell Endocrinol. 2004;217(1–2):27–31.
19. Struthers A, Krum H, Williams GH. A comparison of the aldosterone-blocking agents eplerenone and spironolactone. Clin Cardiol. 2008;31(4):153–8.
20. Yamaji M, Tsutamoto T, Kawahara C, et al. Effect of eplerenone versus spironolactone on cortisol and hemoglobin A1(c) levels in patients with chronic heart failure. Am Heart J. 2010;160(5):915–21.
21. Struthers AD. Aldosterone: cardiovascular assault. Am Heart J. 2002;144(5 Suppl):S2–7.
22. Cook CS, Berry LM, Bible RH, Hribar JD, Hajdu E, Liu NW. Pharmacokinetics and metabolism of [14C]eplerenone after oral administration to humans. Drug Metab Dispos. 2003;31(11):1448–55.
23. Mantero F, Lucarelli G. Aldosterone antagonists in hypertension and heart failure. Ann Endocrinol. 2000;61(1):52–60.
24. Ceremuzynski L, Budaj A, Michorowski B. Single-dose i.v. aldactone for congestive heart failure: a preliminary observation. Int J Clin Pharmacol Ther Toxicol. 1983;21(8):417–21.
25. Krause W, Karras J, Seifert W. Pharmacokinetics of canrenone after oral administration of spironolactone and intravenous injection of canrenoate-K in healthy man. Eur J Clin Pharmacol. 1983;25(4):449–53.

26. Osore H, Harrow TA. Cardiovascular and renal properties of potassium-sparing diuretics of the spirolactone group—I: effects of SC-14266/371 (potassium canrenoate) on renal transport Na$^+$, K$^+$-ATPase activity. Biochem Pharmacol. 1982;31(24):4068–71.

27. Beygui F, Cayla G, Roule V, et al. Early aldosterone blockade in acute myocardial infarction: the ALBATROSS randomized clinical trial. J Am Coll Cardiol. 2016;67(16):1917–27.

28. Juurlink DN, Mamdani MM, Lee DS, et al. Rates of hyperkalemia after publication of the Randomized Aldactone Evaluation Study. N Engl J Med. 2004;351(6):543–51.

29. Kolkhof P, Delbeck M, Kretschmer A, et al. Finerenone, a novel selective nonsteroidal mineralocorticoid receptor antagonist protects from rat cardiorenal injury. J Cardiovasc Pharmacol. 2014;64(1):69–78.

30. Kolkhof P, Nowack C, Eitner F. Nonsteroidal antagonists of the mineralocorticoid receptor. Curr Opin Nephrol Hypertens. 2015;24(5):417–24.

31. Barfacker L, Kuhl A, Hillisch A, et al. Discovery of BAY 94-8862: a nonsteroidal antagonist of the mineralocorticoid receptor for the treatment of cardiorenal diseases. ChemMedChem. 2012;7(8):1385–403.

32. Pitt B, Kober L, Ponikowski P, et al. Safety and tolerability of the novel non-steroidal mineralocorticoid receptor antagonist BAY 94-8862 in patients with chronic heart failure and mild or moderate chronic kidney disease: a randomized, double-blind trial. Eur Heart J. 2013;34(31):2453–63.

33. Bakris GL, Agarwal R, Anker SD, et al. Effect of finerenone on chronic kidney disease outcomes in type 2 diabetes. N Engl J Med. 2020;383(23):2219–29.

34. Pitt B, Filippatos G, Agarwal R, et al. Cardiovascular events with finerenone in kidney disease and type 2 diabetes. N Engl J Med. 2021;385(24):2252–63.

35. Montalescot G, Pitt B, Lopez de Sa E, et al. Early eplerenone treatment in patients with acute ST-elevation myocardial infarction without heart failure: the Randomized Double-Blind Reminder Study. Eur Heart J. 2014;35(34):2295–302.

36. Pfeffer MA, Claggett B, Assmann SF, et al. Regional variation in patients and outcomes in the treatment of preserved cardiac function heart failure with an Aldosterone Antagonist (TOPCAT) Trial. Circulation. 2015;131(1):34–42.

37. de Denus S, O'Meara E, Desai AS, et al. Spironolactone metabolites in TOPCAT: new insights into regional variation. N Engl J Med. 2017;376(17):1690–2.

38. De Denus S, Leclair G, Dubé MP, et al. Spironolactone metabolite concentrations in decompensated heart failure: insights from the ATHENA-HF trial. Eur J Heart Fail. 2020;22(8):1451–61.

39. Cleland JGF, Ferreira JP, Mariottoni B, et al. The effect of spironolactone on cardiovascular function and markers of fibrosis in people at increased risk of developing heart failure: the heart 'OMics' in AGEing (HOMAGE) randomized clinical trial. Eur Heart J. 2021;42(6):684–96.

40. Pitt B, Rossignol P. Mineralocorticoid receptor antagonists in patients with end-stage renal disease on chronic hemodialysis. J Am Coll Cardiol. 2014;63(6):537–8.

41. Pitt B, Bakris GL, Bushinsky DA, et al. Effect of patiromer on reducing serum potassium and preventing recurrent hyperkalaemia in patients with heart failure and chronic kidney disease on RAAS inhibitors. Eur J Heart Fail. 2015;17(10):1057–65.

CHAPTER 8.6

Heart rate reduction with ivabradine in heart failure

Michael Böhm and Michel Komajda

Heart rate and cardiovascular disease risk

Elevated resting heart rate (RHR) is associated with cardiovascular risk in the general population,[1] and cardiovascular risk factors such as obesity[2] and diabetes,[3] hypertension,[4] coronary heart disease,[5] coronary heart disease with impaired left ventricular function,[6] and chronic heart failure.[7] Thus, it has an impact on prognosis throughout the cardiovascular continuum. Although the association of the RHR with morbidity and mortality, generally at a threshold of above 70 bpm, is convincing, effective RHR reduction with beta-blockers or ivabradine have not always shown significant risk reductions such as in stable coronary artery disease[8] and coronary artery disease with impaired left ventricular function.[9] However, a reduction in the RHR with ivabradine was associated with a reduction in cardiovascular death and heart failure hospitalization in chronic heart failure in the Systolic Heart Failure Treatment with the I_f Inhibitor Ivabradine Trial (SHIFT).[10] Therefore, the RHR represents a significantly modifiable risk factor in heart failure.[11] This concept is summarized in ◐ Figure 8.6.1.[11]

Heart rate effects of ivabradine

Ivabradine inhibits hyperpolarization-activated cyclic nucleotide-gated (HCN) channels expressed exclusively in sinus nodal cells[12] and was the first clinically available drug to reduce the RHR without other known effects on the cardiovascular system. Ivabradine binds the inner side of the HCN channel when it is in its open state.[12] Therefore, ivabradine has the highest binding capacity when a large number of channels are in the open state, which is usually the case when the RHR is high.[12,13] Therefore, the binding capacity and negative chronotropic effect are most pronounced at high RHR, and only small RHR reductions are achieved when the RHR is low.[14] This phenomenon might be referred to as 'use dependence' and might have important implications for cardiovascular safety,[14] as at low baseline heart rate (HR), HR reductions are smaller than at high HR.

Association between heart rate and clinical outcomes

Elevated RHR has been associated with incident heart failure in the general population (Rotterdam Study),[15] in patients following myocardial infarction and heart failure (DIAMOND),[16] and in chronic stable heart failure (SHIFT)[17] (◐ Figure 8.6.2). Interestingly, high RHR at discharge (>84 bpm) after hospitalization for worsening heart failure was associated with cardiovascular death within the following year.[18] Beta-blockers are negative chronotropic drugs which have been shown to reduce morbidity and mortality in large outcome trials, and are a guideline-recommended heart failure treatment.[19,20,21] In a meta-analysis of beta-blocker trials, the number of heartbeats reduced with beta-blocker treatment was closely associated with improvement in

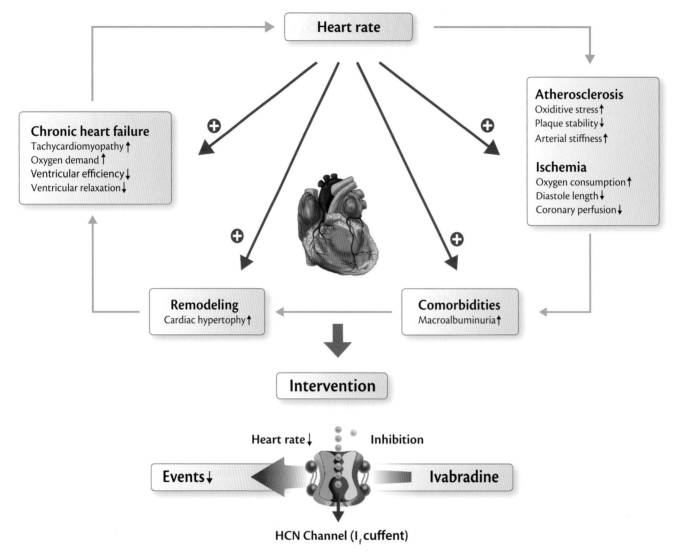

Figure 8.6.1 Heart rate in the cardiovascular continuum and the potential influence of ivabradine. The heart rate is a risk indicator in all cardiovascular conditions, but a modifiable risk factor only in chronic heart failure. Ivabradine binds to the HCN channel, inhibiting I_f currents, thereby reducing phase IV depolarization of the action potential, leading to heart rate reduction.

Reproduced from Nikolovska Vukadinović A, Vukadinović D, Borer J, *et al*. Heart rate and its reduction in chronic heart failure and beyond. *Eur J Heart Fail*. 2017 Oct;19(10):1230–1241. doi: 10.1002/ejhf.902 with permission from John Wiley and Sons.

ejection fraction and risk reduction of all-cause death.[22] The HR achieved on beta-blockers was associated with a reduction in annualized mortality rate.[22] However, at baseline, the lowest RHR achieved with treatment in beta-blocker trials was only 70 bpm.[22] Interestingly, the RHR achieved with treatment was associated with a risk reduction, but not the dose of the beta-blockers applied.[23] These findings point towards a significant role of the RHR and RHR reduction in patients with heart failure to improve outcomes beyond beta-blocker dose.

Results of the SHIFT trial

Results from the SHIFT trial demonstrated that ivabradine safely lowers the RHR in patients in sinus rhythm with a HR of above 70 bpm.[10] Treatment with ivabradine at a starting dose of 5 mg twice daily and uptitrated to 7.5 mg twice daily or downtitrated to 2.5 mg twice daily, according to RHR changes below 50 bpm,

resulted in placebo-controlled RHR reductions of 10.9 bpm at 28 days, 9.1 bpm at 1 year, and 8.1 bpm at the end of the study (⊙ Figure 8.6.3).[10] Treatment with ivabradine was associated with a reduction of the composite primary endpoint of cardiovascular death or hospital admission for worsening of heart failure, compared to placebo.[10] This result was primarily driven by hospital admission for heart failure.[7,10] In patients with a RHR above the median (RHR of 75 bpm), not only the composite primary endpoint and heart failure hospitalization were significantly reduced, but also all-cause death, cardiovascular death, and death from heart failure (⊙ Figure 8.6.4).[24] Patients with the highest RHR showed a greater reduction in HR, and ivabradine provided a greater treatment effect to reduce outcomes.[7] A RHR achieved of between 50 and 60 bpm after 28 days of treatment since initiation and forced drug dose uptitration resulted in 50% lower number of cardiovascular outcomes, compared to patients who remained at

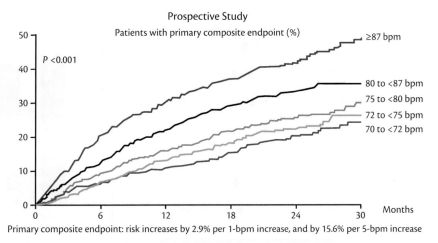

Figure 8.6.2 Kaplan–Meier cumulative event curves for the primary composite endpoint (cardiovascular death or heart failure hospitalization) according to patient groups defined by quintiles of heart rate at 28 days on placebo. Log rank P-values show the difference between the groups.

Reproduced from Böhm M, Swedberg K, Komajda M, *et al*.; SHIFT Investigators. Heart rate as a risk factor in chronic heart failure (SHIFT): the association between heart rate and outcomes in a randomised placebo-controlled trial. *Lancet*. 2010 Sep 11;376(9744):886–94. doi: 10.1016/S0140-6736(10)61259-7 with permission Elsevier.

a RHR of >75 bpm with treatment.[7] In general, the treatment was safe. More symptomatic bradycardia (5% with ivabradine, compared to 1% with placebo) requiring dose reductions (5% vs 1%, respectively) was observed. A small, albeit significant, increase by 1% in incident atrial fibrillation was observed.[10]

In these patients, shortly after previous hospitalization for worsening heart failure, where the risk is particularly high (the so-called 'vulnerable phase'), early rehospitalization after an index hospitalization markedly increased the risk of death in the following year, regardless of whether the cause of hospitalization was due to heart failure or myocardial infarction.[25] The treatment effect

of ivabradine was similar in this high-risk population to that in the overall population of the SHIFT trial,[26] and the relative risk reduction was similar in patients with severe impairment of left ventricular function,[27] resulting in a large absolute reduction of events prevented as the absolute risk was higher. In addition, the nominal effect of risk reduction was independent from the beta-blocker dose applied but depended on the RHR at baseline before treatment.[28]

Ivabradine effects according to risk indicators

A low systolic blood pressure (SBP) (<120 mmHg) is prevalent in 15–25% of heart failure patients and is associated with a

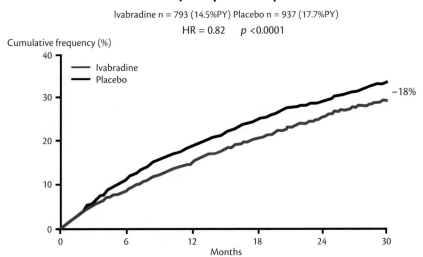

Figure 8.6.3 Kaplan–Meier cumulative event curves for the primary composite endpoint (cardiovascular death or heart failure hospitalization) for ivabradine or placebo. Primary results of the SHIFT study.

Reproduced from Swedberg K, Komajda M, Böhm M, *et al*.; SHIFT Investigators. Ivabradine and outcomes in chronic heart failure (SHIFT): a randomised placebo-controlled study. *Lancet*. 2010 Sep 11;376(9744):875–85. doi: 10.1016/S0140-6736(10)61198-1 with permission from Elsevier.

Effect of Ivabradine on Outcomes

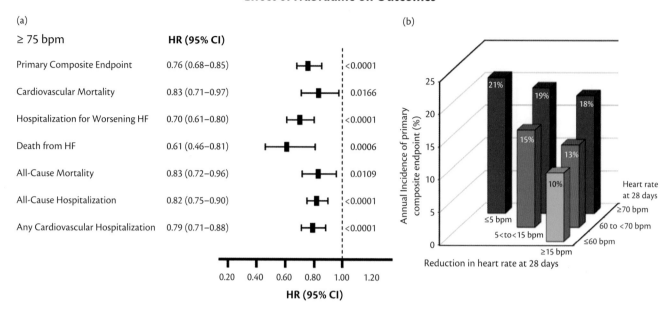

Figure 8.6.4 Forest plots (a) demonstrating the hazard ratio (with 95% confidence intervals) for the primary composite endpoint (cardiovascular death or heart failure hospitalization), cardiovascular mortality, hospitalization for worsening heart failure, death from heart failure, all-cause mortality, all-cause hospitalization, and any cardiovascular hospitalization for ivabradine compared to placebo. Panel (b) shows the annual incidence of the primary composite endpoint according to the heart rate achieved after uptitration of ivabradine at 28 days or a reduction in the heart rate at 28 days. Of note, all endpoints were significantly reduced and this reduction was closely associated with the heart rate achieved and the heart rate reduction in patients with chronic heart failure at a heart rate of ≥75 bpm.

Reproduced from Böhm M, Borer J, Ford I, *et al*. Heart rate at baseline influences the effect of ivabradine on cardiovascular outcomes in chronic heart failure: analysis from the SHIFT study. *Clin Res Cardiol*. 2013 Jan;102(1):11–22. doi: 10.1007/s00392-012-0467-8 with permission from Springer.

greater risk of post-discharge and in-hospital mortality, as well as worsening heart failure.[29,30] Some physicians are afraid of further reducing blood pressure with guideline-recommended treatments, leading to undertreatment of this high-risk population. Ivabradine is devoid of any vascular effect and therefore does not lower blood pressure, unlike many other guideline-recommended heart failure drugs. In patients with low blood pressure, ivabradine had a similar treatment effect to that in patients with higher blood pressure,[31] and importantly treatment with ivabradine was associated with a nominal increase of 2 mmHg rather than a blood pressure drop on treatment.[10] In patients at advanced age, undertreatment with beta-blockers and mineralocorticoid receptor antagonists has been reported,[32] even though the risk of hospitalization is higher in this population and these drugs have shown efficacy on mortality and morbidity across different risk profiles in heart failure patients.[33] In patients aged above 75 years, the treatment effect of ivabradine was maintained and not different over the whole spectrum of age groups.[34] There are concerns that left bundle branch block (LBBB) might select patients with conduction disorders, making them more prone to bradyarrhythmic complications after I_f inhibition with ivabradine. However, no deleterious signals in Holter studies was detected.[35] In patients with LBBB, the treatment effect was also maintained,[36] and as the absolute risk was higher with a similar magnitude of treatment effect, this resulted in a lower number needed to treat.

In patients with diabetes, cardiovascular death and hospitalizations were higher than in patients without diabetes.[37] In a post hoc analysis of SHIFT, the treatment effect of ivabradine in diabetes was not affected and was similar to that observed in patients without diabetes.[38] Similar findings were observed in patients with impaired renal function.[39] While higher RHR is a significant predictor of worsening renal function,[39,40] an effect of RHR reduction on renal function decline was not shown.[39] Pulmonary diseases, in particular chronic obstructive pulmonary disease (COPD), are highly prevalent in the heart failure population.[41] In the SHIFT population, there was no significant difference in treatment effect with ivabradine, compared to patients without COPD.[42] Finally, the cumulative comorbidity load according to the number of comorbidities was studied in SHIFT.[43] There was increasing mortality and morbidity with increasing numbers of up to four or more comorbidities. However, the relative treatment effect of ivabradine was maintained (➲ Figure 8.6.5).[43] Taking all these results together, ivabradine appears to be safe and efficacious in patients with heart failure and significant comorbidities.

Practical considerations, clinical perspectives, and future directions

In the failing heart, there is a negative force–frequency relationship (➲ Figure 8.6.6).[44,45] The positive force–frequency relationship (so-called 'Treppe') was first discovered by Bowditch in

Outcomes in SHIFT According to Comorbidity Load

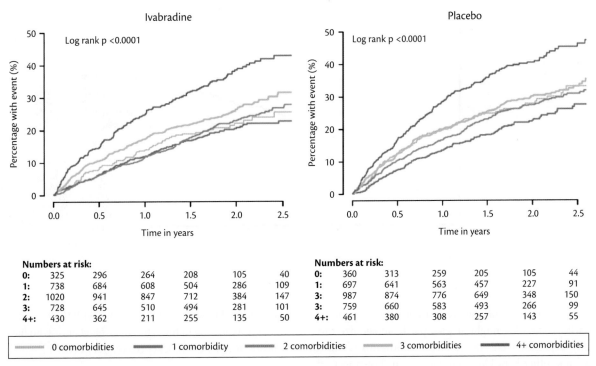

Figure 8.6.5 Outcomes according to comorbidities (≥4) on the primary outcome (cardiovascular death or heart failure hospitalization) with ivabradine (left) or placebo (right). Data from the SHIFT study.

Reproduced from Böhm M, Robertson M, Ford I, *et al*. Influence of Cardiovascular and Noncardiovascular Co-morbidities on Outcomes and Treatment Effect of Heart Rate Reduction With Ivabradine in Stable Heart Failure (from the SHIFT Trial). *Am J Cardiol*. 2015 Dec 15;116(12):1890–7. doi: 10.1016/j.amjcard.2015.09.029 with permission from Elsevier.

1871.[46] On exercise, maximal oxygen uptake is achieved at a HR of approximately 80 bpm in heart failure patients, whereas that in patients without heart failure is achieved at around 160 bpm.[47] Therefore, a reduction in the RHR and exercise HR might be associated with an increase in contractility. In line with this suggestion are results from clinical experiments in patients with severe heart failure (New York Heart Association class III). In these patients, intravenous administration of ivabradine was associated with a HR reduction without any change in cardiac index resulting from an increase in stroke volume.[48] Given the negative inotropic effect of beta-blockers with a drop in left ventricular ejection fraction and an increase in filling pressures after

Pathophysiology

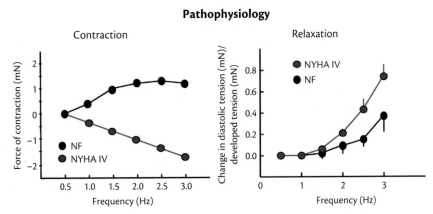

Figure 8.6.6 Isometric force of contraction (left) and change in diastolic tension (right) in isolated, electrically driven cardiac preparations *in vitro* from patients with severe heart failure (New York Heart Association (NYHA) class IV) or non-failing hearts (NF). Of note, the heart failure force of contraction declined (negative force–frequency relationship, on negative 'Treppe'), with a relaxation deficit, in patients with NYHA class IV.

Reproduced from Böhm M, La Rosée K, Schmidt U, *et al*. Force–frequency relationship and inotropic stimulation in the nonfailing and failing human myocardium: implications for the medical treatment of heart failure. *Clin Investig*. 1992 May;70(5):421–5. doi: 10.1007/BF00235525 with permission from Springer.

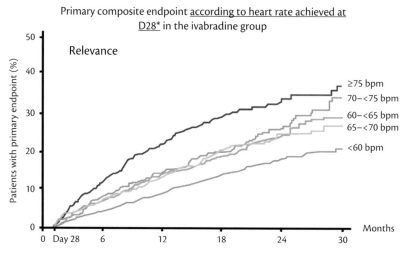

What Can We Achieve to Target Heart Rate?

Figure 8.6.7 Incidence event curves for the primary composite endpoint according to heart rate achieved at 4 weeks after dose uptitration of ivabradine. Note that the optimal heart rate associated with the lowest event rates is between 50 and 60 bpm.

treatment initiation in heart failure patients,[49] a reduction in the RHR with ivabradine might at least partly antagonize these contractility-depressant effects. Indeed, co-administration of carvedilol[49] and other beta-blockers[50] have been shown to facilitate uptitration of beta-blockers, with more rapid RHR reduction and greater increase in ejection fraction after co-administration of these drugs.[49,50] Therefore, a new concept might be concomitant application of beta-blockers and ivabradine. This should be scrutinized in large controlled trials.

RHR reduction with ivabradine remains an important component of heart failure therapy for patients in sinus rhythm with a RHR of above 70 bpm. It was shown to reduce the cardiovascular death and heart failure hospitalization composite, which was primarily driven by heart failure hospitalization, and has been classified with a Class IIa recommendation in the European Society of Cardiology (ESC) Heart Failure Guidelines.[51] Since the RHR is an important modifiable risk factor, with a doubling risk from a RHR of 87 bpm compared to 70–72 bpm, it should be pharmacologically adjusted with ivabradine on top of maximally tolerated doses of beta-blockers, as suggested by the SHIFT trial.[7,10] Physicians should achieve an optimal RHR of 50–60 bpm on treatment at which the RHR-associated risk is maximally reduced (➲ Figure 8.6.7).[7] Since a high RHR remains a risk marker also in other cardiovascular and non-cardiovascular conditions, it might be the future direction and worthwhile to initiate randomized controlled trials in conditions other than chronic heart failure, including cancer, chronic disease such as COPD, and critical illness, as well as neurological disease, as an adjunctive therapy.[52] According to the data described above, the 2021 ESC Guidelines for the diagnosis and treatment of acute and chronic heart failure recommend ivabradine for symptomatic patients in sinus rhythm with a left ventricular ejection fraction of ≤35% and a RHR of ≥70 bpm, together with an evidence-based dose of beta-blocker, or the maximum tolerated dose below that, and guideline-directed therapies with a Class IIa, Level B recommendation. Ivabradine should also

be considered in symptomatic patients with the same characteristics who are unable to tolerate a beta-blocker or who have contraindications to a beta-blocker (Class IIa, Level C).[53]

Key messages

- Elevated RHR is associated with cardiovascular risk in numerous conditions and is therefore a valuable risk marker.

- In chronic heart failure, the RHR is a modifiable risk factor, as the SHIFT study has shown a risk reduction in patients in sinus rhythm with a heart rate of >70 bpm and an ejection fraction of <35%.

- For these patients, the new ESC Guidelines recommend the use of ivabradine (Class IIa, Level B), as well as for patients who do not tolerate a beta-blocker (Class IIa, Level C). The HR might also be relevant in other conditions, such as renal failure, COPD, cancer, and critical illness, but outcome data are lacking so far.

References

1. Kannel WB, Kannel C, Paffenbarger RS Jr, Cupples LA. Heart rate and cardiovascular mortality: the Framingham Study. Am Heart J 1987;113:1489–94.
2. Shigetoh Y, Adachi H, Yamagishi S, et al. Higher heart rate may predispose to obesity and diabetes mellitus: 20-year prospective study in a general population. Am J Hypertens 2009;22:151–5.
3. Carnethon MR, Yan L, Greenland P, et al. Resting heart rate in middle age and diabetes development in older age. Diabetes Care 2008;31:335–9.
4. Paul L, Hastie CE, Li WS, et al. Resting heart rate pattern during follow-up and mortality in hypertensive patients. Hypertension 2010;55:567–74.
5. Gillum RF, Makuc DM, Feldman J. Pulse rate, coronary heart disease, and death: the NHANES I Epidemiologic Follow-up Study. Am Heart J 1991;121:172–7.
6. Fox K, Ford I, Steg PG, Tendera M, Robertson M, Ferrari R. Heart rate as a prognostic risk factor in patients with coronary artery disease and left-ventricular systolic dysfunction (BEAUTIFUL): a subgroup analyses of a randomized controlled trial. Lancet 2008;372:817–21.

7. Böhm M, Swedberg K, Komajda M, et al.; SHIFT Investigators. Heart rate as a risk factor in chronic heart failure (SHIFT): the association between heart rate and outcomes in a randomised placebo-controlled trial. Lancet 2010;376:886–94.

8. Fox K, Ford I, Steg PG, Tendera M, Ferrari R. Ivabradine for patients with stable coronary artery disease and left-ventricular systolic dysfunction (BEAUTIFUL): a randomised, double-blind, placebo-controlled trial. Lancet 2008;372:807–16.

9. Fox K, Ford I, Steg PG, Tardif JC, Tendera M, Ferrari R; SIGNIFY Investigators. Ivabradine in stable coronary artery disease without clinical heart failure. N Engl J Med 2014;371:1091–9.

10. Swedberg K, Komajda M, Böhm M, et al. Ivabradine and outcomes in chronic heart failure (SHIFT): a randomised placebo-controlled study. Lancet 2010;376:875–85.

11. Nikolovska-Vukadinović A, Vukadinović D, Borer J, et al. Heart rate and its reduction in chronic heart failure and beyond. Eur J Heart Fail 2017;19:1230–41.

12. DiFrancesco D, Camm JA. Heart rate lowering by specific and selective I(f) current inhibition with ivabradine: a new therapeutic perspective in cardiovascular disease. Drugs 2004;64:1757–65.

13. Dobre D, Borer JS, Fox K, et al. Heart rate: a prognostic factor and therapeutic target in chronic heart failure. The distinct roles of drugs with heart rate-lowering properties. Eur J Heart Fail 2014;16:76–85.

14. Ragueneau I, Laveille C, Jochemsen R, Resplandy G, Funck-Brentano C, Jaillon P. Pharmacokinetic–pharmacodynamic modeling of the effects of ivabradine, a direct sinus node inhibitor, on heart rate in healthy volunteers. Clin Pharmacol Ther 1998;64:192–203.

15. Nanchen D, Leening MJ, Locatelli I, et al. Resting heart rate and the risk of heart failure in healthy adults: the Rotterdam Study. Circ Heart Fail 2013;6:403–10.

16. Fosbøl EL, Seibaek M, Brendorp B, et al.; Danish Investigations and Arrhythmia ON Dofetilide Study Group. Long-term prognostic importance of resting heart rate in patients with left ventricular dysfunction in connection with either heart failure or myocardial infarction: the DIAMOND study. Int J Cardiol 2010;140:279–86.

17. Borer JS, Deedwania PC, Kim JB, Böhm M. Benefits of heart rate slowing with ivabradine in patients with systolic heart failure and coronary artery disease. Am J Cardiol 2016;118:1948–53.

18. Greene SJ, Vaduganathan M, Wilcox JE, et al.; EVEREST Trial Investigators. The prognostic significance of heart rate in patients hospitalized for heart failure with reduced ejection fraction in sinus rhythm: insights from the EVEREST (Efficacy of Vasopressin Antagonism in Heart Failure: Outcome Study With Tolvaptan) trial. JACC Heart Fail 2013;1:488–96.

19. Lechat P, Hulot JS, Escolano S, et al. Heart rate and cardiac rhythm relationship with bisoprolol benefit in chronic heart failure in CIBIS II Trial. Circulation 2001;103:1428–33.

20. Hjalmarson A, Goldstein S, Fagerberg B, et al. Effects of controlled-release metoprolol on total mortality, hospitalizations, and well-being in patients with heart failure: the Metoprolol CR/XL Randomized Intervention Trial in congestive heart failure (MERIT-HF). MERIT-HF Study Group. JAMA 2000;283:1295–302.

21. Packer M, Fowler MB, Roecker EB, et al.; Carvedilol Prospective Randomized Cumulative Survival (COPERNICUS) Study Group. Effect of carvedilol on the morbidity of patients with severe chronic heart failure: results of the carvedilol prospective randomized cumulative survival (COPERNICUS) study. Circulation 2002;106:2194–9.

22. Flannery G, Gehrig-Mills R, Billah B, Krum H. Analysis of randomized controlled trials on the effect of magnitude of heart rate reduction on clinical outcomes in patients with systolic chronic heart failure receiving beta-blockers. Am J Cardiol 2008;101:865–9.

23. McAlister FA, Wiebe N, Ezekowitz JA, Leung AA, Armstrong PW. Meta-analysis: beta-blocker dose, heart rate reduction, and death in patients with heart failure. Ann Intern Med 2009;150:784–94.

24. Böhm M, Borer J, Ford I, et al. Heart rate as baseline influences the effect of ivabradine on cardiovascular outcomes in chronic heart failure: analyses from SHIFT study. Clin Res Cardiol 2013;102:11–22.

25. Abrahamsson P, Swedberg K, Borer JS, et al. Risk following hospitalization in stable chronic systolic heart failure. Eur J Heart Fail 2013;15:885–91.

26. Komajda M, Tavazzi L, Swedberg K, et al.; SHIFT Investigators. Chronic exposure to ivabradine reduces readmissions in the vulnerable phase after hospitalization for worsening systolic heart failure: a post-hoc analysis of SHIFT. Eur J Heart Fail 2016;18:1182–9.

27. Borer JS, Böhm M, Ford I, et al. Efficacy and safety of ivabradine in patients with severe chronic systolic heart failure (from the SHIFT Study). Am J Cardiol 2014;113:497–503.

28. Swedberg K, Komajda M, Böhm M, et al.; SHIFT Investigators. Effects on outcomes of heart rate reduction by ivabradine in patients with congestive heart failure: is there an influence of beta-blocker dose? Findings from the SHIFT (Systolic Heart failure treatment with the I(f) inhibitor ivabradine Trial) study. J Am Coll Cardiol 2012;59:1938–45.

29. Gheorghiade M, Vaduganathan M, Ambrosy A, et al. Current management and future directions for the treatment of patients hospitalized for heart failure with low blood pressure. Heart Fail Rev 2013;18:107–22.

30. Ambrosy AP, Vaduganathan M, Mentz RJ, et al. Clinical profile and prognostic value of low systolic blood pressure in patients hospitalized for heart failure with reduced ejection fraction: insights from the efficacy of vasopressin antagonism in heart failure: outcome study with tolvaptan (EVEREST) trial. Am Heart J 2013;165:216–25.

31. Komajda M, Böhm M, Borer JS, et al.; SHIFT Investigators. Efficacy and safety of ivabradine in patients with chronic systolic heart failure according to blood pressure level in SHIFT. Eur J Heart Fail 2014;16:810–16.

32. Muntwyler J, Cohen-Solal A, Freemantle N, Eastaugh J, Cleland JG, Follath F. Relation of sex, age and concomitant diseases to drug prescription for heart failure in primary care in Europe. Eur Heart J Fail 2004;6:663–8.

33. Maison P, Cunin P, Hemery F, et al. Utilisation of medications recommended for chronic heart failure and the relationship with annual hospitalisation duration in patients over 75 years of age. A pharmacoepidemiological study. Eur J Clin Pharmacol 2005;61:445–51.

34. Tavazzi L, Swedberg K, Komajda M, et al.; SHIFT Investigators. Efficacy and safety of ivabradine in chronic heart failure across the age spectrum: insights from the SHIFT study. Eur J Heart Fail 2013;15:1296–303.

35. Böhm M, Borer JS, Camm J, et al. Twenty-four-hour heart lowering with ivabradine in chronic heart failure: insights from the SHIFT Holter substudy. Eur J Heart Fail 2015;17:518–26.

36. Reil JC, Robertson M, Ford I, et al. Impact of left bundle branch block on heart rate and its relationship to treatment with ivabradine in chronic heart failure. Eur J Heart Fail 2013;15:1044–52.

37. Van Deursen VM, Urso R, Laroche C, et al. Co-morbidities in patients with heart failure: an analysis of the European Heart Failure Pilot Survey. Eur J Heart Fail 2014;16:103–11.

38. Komajda M, Tavazzi L, Francq BG, et al.; SHIFT Investigators. Efficacy and safety of ivabradine in patients with chronic systolic heart failure and diabetes: an analysis from the SHIFT trial. Eur J Heart Fail 2015;17:1294–301.

39. Voors AA, van Veldhuisen DJ, Robertson M, et al. The effect of heart rate reduction with ivabradine on renal function in patients

with chronic heart failure: an analysis from SHIFT. Eur J Heart Fail 2014;16:426–34.

40. Böhm M, Schumacher H, Schmieder RE, *et al.* Resting heart rate is associated with renal disease outcomes in patients with vascular disease: results of the ONTARGET and TRANSCEND studies. J Intern Med 2015;278:38–49.

41. Jencen MT, Marott JL, Lange P, *et al.* Resting heart rate is a predictor of mortality on COPD. Eur Respir J 2013;42:341–9.

42. Tavazzi L, Swedberg K, Komajda M, *et al.*; SHIFT Investigators. Clinical profiles and outcomes in patients with chronic heart failure and chronic obstructive pulmonary disease: an efficacy and safety analysis of SHIFT study. Int J Cardiol 2013;170:182–8.

43. Böhm M, Robertson M, Ford I, *et al.* Influence of cardiovascular and noncardiovascular co-morbidities on outcomes and treatment effect of heart rate reduction with ivabradine in stable heart failure (from the SHIFT Trial). Am J Cardiol 2015;116:1890–7.

44. Mulieri LA, Hasenfuss G, Leavitt B, Allen PD, Alpert NR. Altered myocardial force–frequency relation in human heart failure. Circulation 1992;85:1743–50.

45. Böhm M, La Rosée K, Schmidt U, Schulz C, Schwinger RH, Erdmann E. Force–frequency relationship and inotropic stimulation in the nonfailing and failing human myocardium: implications for the medical treatment of heart failure. Clin Investig 1992;70:421–5.

46. Bowditch HP. Über die Eigenthümlichkeiten der Reizbarkeit, welche die Muskelfasern des Herzens zeigen. Berichte über die Verhandlungen der Königlich Sächsischen Gesellschaft der Wissenschaften zu Leipzig: Mathematisch-Physische Klasse 1871;23:652–89.

47. Kindermann M, Schwaab B, Finkler N, Schaller S, Böhm M, Fröhlig G. Defining the optimum upper heart rate limit during exercise: a study in pacemaker patients with heart failure. Eur Heart J 2002;23:1301–8.

48. De Ferrari GM, Mazzuero A, Agnesina L, *et al.* Favourable effects of heart rate reduction with intravenous administration of ivabradine in patients with advanced heart failure. Eur J Heart Fail 2008;10:550–5.

49. Bagriy AE, Schukina EV, Samoilova OV, *et al.* Addition of ivabradine to β-blocker improves exercise capacity in systolic heart failure patients in a prospective, open-label study. Adv Ther 2015;32:108–19.

50. Hidalgo FJ, Anguita M, Castillo JC, *et al.* Effect of early treatment with ivabradine combined with beta-blockers versus beta-blockers alone in patients hospitalised with heart failure and reduced left ventricular ejection fraction (ETHIC-AHF): a randomised study. Int J Cardiol 2016;217:7–11.

51. Ponikowski P, Voors AA, Anker SD, *et al.*; Authors/Task Force Members; Document Reviewers. 2016 ESC Guidelines for the diagnosis and treatment of acute and chronic heart failure: The Task Force for the diagnosis and treatment of acute and chronic heart failure of the European Society of Cardiology (ESC). Developed with the special contribution of the Heart Failure Association (HFA) of the ESC. Eur J Heart Fail 2016;18:891–975.

52. Böhm M. Heart rate: from heart failure to chronic diseases and cancer. Is there a role for supportive care by heart rate reduction? Eur J Heart Fail 2017;19:250–2.

53. McDonagh TA, Metra M, Adamo M, *et al.*; ESC Scientific Document Group. 2021 ESC Guidelines for the diagnosis and treatment of acute and chronic heart failure. Eur Heart J 2021;42:3599–726.

CHAPTER 8.7

Vasodilators in heart failure

Eftihia Polyzogopoulou, Maria Nikolaou, John Parissis, and Alexandre Mebazaa

Contents

Introduction

The management of acute heart failure (AHF) requires, almost by definition, urgent evaluation and in-hospital treatment. Evaluation is based primarily on the presence and extent of congestion and hypoperfusion, and treatment should start immediately as time is synonymous with cardiac muscle loss. Initial management targets the restoration of haemodynamic imbalance by modifying preload (diuretics, venodilators), afterload (arterial dilators, vasopressors), and contractility (inotropes). Unfortunately, the observations and trials on AHF treatment have only been consistent with symptom relief and have not been translated to survival benefit of one class over another. By contrast, the use of inotropes and vasopressors has raised concerns about their short- and long-term safety, especially if used in inappropriate populations.[1,2] Consequently, the role of 'safer' classes of medication has been prioritized. Traditionally, diuretics are the mainstay treatment for decongestion, but vasodilators have also a pivotal role in managing preload, afterload, and secondarily contractility, acting variously in the cardiac pressure–volume loops, without increasing oxygen demands.

Historical perspective: the trajectory behind current heart failure treatment

The approach to heart failure (HF) patients has dramatically changed in the last 50 years. Up to the mid-seventies, management targeted water retention and cardiac contractility, and was limited to bed rest, fluid restriction, and pharmacological treatment with diuretics and digitalis.[3] A favourable response to afterload reduction in congestive HF was first demonstrated in the early seventies, when a couple of small, but remarkable, haemodynamic studies were published.[4,5,6] The innovative theory drew further attention from scientists and demonstrated the role of arterial impedance in cardiac performance.[7,8] It became gradually apparent that outflow resistance (afterload) was severely impaired in cases of congestive HF and inversely related to stroke volume, forwarding the management towards a 'haemodynamic' concept.[9,10]

The primary use of parenteral vasodilators, such as nitroprusside and phentolamine, showed promising results in the acute setting. Short-term intravenous infusion produced rapid reductions in left ventricular filling pressures and increases in cardiac output, with minor effects on the heart rate and mean arterial pressure, whereas clinical improvement in congested patients was almost immediate.[5,6] Following the general enthusiasm, a large number of vasodilating drugs, with different mechanisms and sites of action, were clinically tested in various settings.[11,12,13,14,15,16] These short-term studies concluded that regardless of the vasodilator used, arterial and venous dilatation produced considerable haemodynamic improvement in patients.[17]

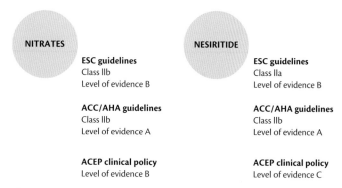

Figure 8.7.1 Recommendations for use of vasodilators in acute heart failure. ACC, American College of Cardiology; ACEP, American College of Emergency Physicians; AHA, American Heart Association; ESC, European Society of Cardiology.
Source data from McDonagh TA, Metra M, Adamo M, *et al*; ESC Scientific Document Group. 2021 ESC Guidelines for the diagnosis and treatment of acute and chronic heart failure. *Eur Heart J*. 2021 Sep 21;42(36):3599–3726.

This impressive response to short-term vasodilator administration led to the assumption that long-term use may also be efficacious in the management of HF patients.[18,19,20,21,22] In the mid-eighties, current knowledge summarized that predominant venodilators, such as nitrates, lowered ventricular filling pressures and relieved pulmonary congestion, whereas primarily arterial vasodilators, such as hydralazine or minoxidil, were subsequently shown to raise cardiac output (CO) significantly while only slightly reducing ventricular filling pressures.[23] Regimens with balanced arterial and venodilating properties were also assessed. Nitrates, in combination with hydralazine or prazosin, were thought to be useful, and at the time novel agents, such as angiotensin-converting enzyme inhibitors (ACEIs), were also tested.[24] This wide spectrum of available vasodilators revealed contradictory effects in the long term and raised questions about the pathophysiological explanation for each outcome, as well as the impact of long-term use on mortality.[25]

In 1986, the first large randomized trial on the effect of vasodilators on mortality in chronic HF was published. The Veterans Administration Cooperative Study on Vasodilator Therapy of Heart Failure (V-HeFT) group compared the effect of prazosin (20 mg/day) versus the combination of hydralazine (300 mg/day) and isosorbide dinitrate (160 mg/day) versus placebo in chronic HF patients.[26] This landmark trial showed for the first time that a medical intervention may alter long-term clinical outcomes in HF patients, since the combination of hydralazine and isosorbide dinitrate reduced the 3-year mortality risk by 36%, compared to placebo or prazosin. The results of this study were received with enthusiasm but also reinforced the speculation that the role of vasodilators differs significantly because of their different mechanism of action. ACEIs, as novel vasodilators, have in parallel drawn researchers' attention.[27,28] A few years later, in 1991, direct comparison of the combination of hydralazine and isosorbide dinitrate to enalapril (20 mg/day) in patients with mild to moderate HF symptoms showed superiority of enalapril in terms of mortality.[26] The 18% risk reduction in the enalapril group was attributed to a reduction in sudden cardiac death, mostly in patients

with less severe symptoms. These remarkable observations led to the current concept of HF treatment, based on neurohormonal modification (such as renin–angiotensin–aldosterone system (RAAS) inhibition and beta-blockade), rather than on haemodynamic adaptation.

Consequently, during the last 30 years, interest in the use of vasodilators has been redirected to treatment of AHF. Their use is quite common in the management of AHF, representing the second most frequently used class of medication, after diuretics.[29] It is worth mentioning though that the use of vasodilators exhibits substantial geographical variation and appears less prominent in North America than in other regions of the world.[29,30]

This discrepancy though is currently no longer reflected in the American College of Cardiology (ACC)/American Heart Association (AHA) and European Society of Cardiology (ESC) guidelines, which have been harmonized with indication IIb, as shown in ➔ Figure 8.7.1.[31,32]

Sites and mechanisms of action

Vasodilators may be classified according to the mechanism of action, as presented in ➔ Figure 8.7.2, or according to the site of action in the circulation, into predominantly arterial dilators (afterload reduction), predominantly venodilators (preload reduction), and combined balanced dilators.[33]

Selective arterial dilators, such as hydralazine, reduce systemic vascular resistance and left ventricular (LV) afterload.[34] As a result, sympathetic stimulation, due to a baroreceptor reflex in response to the fall in arterial pressure, increases heart rate and inotropy. The net haemodynamic response is an increase in CO, with a small increase in right atrial pressure (RAP). The effect of reducing afterload on enhancing CO is even greater in failing hearts because stroke volume is more sensitive to the influence of elevated afterload in a heart with impaired contractility. By unloading the heart, the cardiac function curve shifts up and to the left.

Selective venodilators, such as nitrates, increase venous capacitance and reduce venous pressure and concomitant proximal capillary hydrostatic pressure, alleviating symptoms of pulmonary oedema.[34] By reducing RAP, right ventricular preload decreases, followed by a decrease in stroke volume and CO. Reduced CO causes a fall in arterial pressure, which reduces afterload on the left ventricle and leads to baroreceptor reflex responses, both of which can shift the cardiac function curve up and to the left.[34] The cardiac effects (decreased CO) of venous dilatation are more pronounced in a normal heart than in a failing heart because of where the heart is operating on the Frank–Starling curve.

Concerning the effects of mixed vasodilators, such as nitroprusside, in general, they decrease systemic vascular resistance and arterial pressure, with relatively little change in right atrial (or central venous) pressure (i.e. little change in cardiac preload), and they have relatively little effect on CO.

Intravenous vasodilators

Vasodilators, due to their vasoconstriction reversal effect, by reducing preload and afterload, are the main 'symptom relief' agents available as an acute vasodilator intervention upon presentation

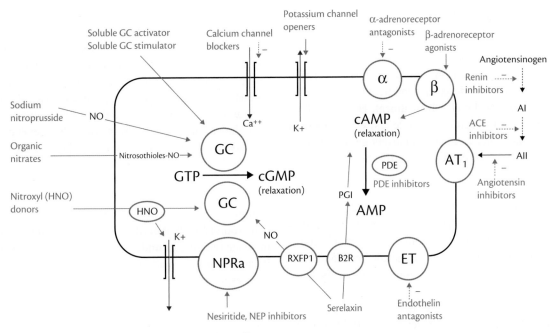

Figure 8.7.2 Molecular mechanism of action of a wide range of vasodilators.

in the emergency department.[35] Even though there is extensive experience with the use of vasodilators, and based on studies, they have well-established short-term beneficial effects, robust data regarding long-term favourable outcomes are still lacking.[32]

According to current guidelines and bibliography, vasodilators are considered as a supplementary therapeutic agent, in addition to diuretics, for the management of patients with AHF, primarily those with elevated or normal blood pressure. Particularly, as stated by the ESC guidelines, the use of vasodilators in AHF is classified as Class IIb, which indicates that their use may be considered in AHF as evidence and expert opinion support their usefulness and efficacy. The Level B recommendation derives from single randomized clinical trials or large, non-randomized studies. The ACC/AHA and American College of Emergency Physicians (ACEP) recommendations are in line with the European guidelines, as shown in ➔ Figure 8.7.1. The European and American guidelines do not distinguish among the three approved vasodilator agents (nitrates, sodium nitroprusside, and nesiritide). The Level A recommendation is based on studies of nesiritide, which is the only new vasodilator approved in the last 20 years.[30]

Whereas intravenous diuretics are the cornerstone of AHF therapy, the main clinical indication for vasodilator use is hypertensive AHF as initial therapy for symptom and congestion improvement. Also, they should be considered in symptomatic patients with systolic blood pressure (SBP) of above 110 mmHg and if symptomatic hypotension is absent. Dose titration and close monitoring should be applied in order to avoid abrupt blood pressure reduction or hypotension, and should be used with caution in patients with underlying mitral or aortic valve stenosis.[31]

Intravenous vasodilator therapy is a time-sensitive intervention. Data from the Registry Focused on Very Early Presentation and Treatment in Emergency Department of Acute Heart Failure

(REALITY-AHF) have shown that early vasodilator administration (within the first 6 hours) with an SBP reduction of <25% has beneficial effect on diuretic response and reduced mortality in hospitalized patients with AHF.[36] Another large-scale registry, the Acute Decompensated Heart Failure National Registry (ADHERE), studied the association of mortality and time to treatment with vasoactive agents, including vasodilators, within 48 hours of hospitalization. Early use (<6 hours) of vasodilators was associated with lower initial in-hospital mortality, compared to late administration, in patients admitted with a diagnosis of AHF.[37]

The incorporation of vasodilators in the initial management algorithm of AHF based on clinical phenotypes is shown in ➔ Figure 8.7.3.

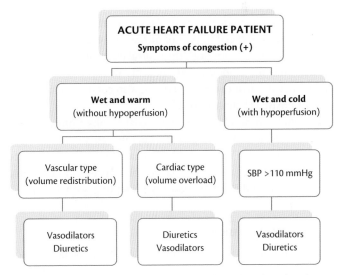

Figure 8.7.3 Use of vasodilators in acute heart failure based on clinical phenotypes. SBP, systolic blood pressure.

Currently used vasodilators

Nitrates

Nitrates are potent vasodilators, one of the oldest used agents in the treatment of chronic angina, and in New York Heart Association (NHYA) classes II–IV and reduced ejection fraction, they are recommended as Class IIa, Level A/B treatment. However, study results are controversial regarding the role and effectiveness of nitrates in AHF; therefore, according to current guidelines, they are classified as 'may be considered' (Class IIb) because data are derived from single randomized or large-non-randomized clinical trials (Level B).[31] Nitrates remain the cornerstone treatment in patients with hypertensive AHF as a result of their confirmed haemodynamic and microvascular beneficial actions. Regardless of their general safety, there are cautions and contraindications to their use. The main contraindications include low blood pressure (<110 mmHg), LV outflow obstruction, and use of phosphodiesterase inhibitors.[38]

However, even though nitrates are frequently used in hypertensive HF, due to a lack of strong evidence of mortality in non-hypotensive, acute decompensated HF, underutilization has been reported and restricted to approximately one-third of those patients.[39]

Based on Wakai et al.'s and Farag et al.'s reviews,[40,41] there is no clear short-term benefit from nitrate vasodilatation in AHF. In agreement are the results of the NITRO-EAHFE study, which have shown no positive effect on short-term prognosis,[42] and whereas the GALACTIC randomized clinical trial on the use of vasodilators (including nitrates) in patients presenting with AHF reported no improvement in all-cause mortality and rehospitalization.[43] Conversely, post hoc analysis of the ALARM-HF study revealed improved in-hospital outcome in patients with AHF who received nitrates in combination with diuretics.[2] Positive effects of high-dose nitrate therapy in hypertensive AHF, in terms of reduced intubation rate, reduced length of stay, and fewer admissions to the intensive care unit, have been shown also in Wang et al.'s recent review analysis.[44] Additionally, a few years ago, a systematic review by Alexander et al. demonstrated a short-term beneficial impact of nitrate use, even though there was no impact on mortality.[45] The neutral effect of nitrates on the 30-day outcome among elderly patients who presented to the emergency department with AHF was also confirmed in the recent ELISABETH clinical trial.[46]

In summary, despite the controversial results from previous studies and the lack of large-scale randomized studies, nitrates should be included in the standard of care in the acute care setting. Nitrates, because of their favourable short-term outcomes, are primarily indicated in patients presenting with hypertensive AHF.

Sodium nitroprusside

Sodium nitroprusside is one of the oldest intravenous vasodilators used in the treatment of AHF, and it is classified as a Class IIb, Level B recommendation according to the latest ESC guidelines.[32] Due to its vascular relaxation effect, it is a practical choice for severely congested patients with hypertensive AHF, especially when aortic or mitral regurgitation is present. Of special consideration should be the need for close haemodynamic monitoring for potential side effects (myocardial ischaemia due to coronary steal, light sensitivity, cyanide toxicity, abrupt hypotension, and rebound hypertension).[47,48] Although previous studies have shown that sodium nitroprusside has beneficial effects on all-cause mortality, compared to placebo or diuretics, more recent studies, especially on AHF without myocardial ischaemia, are lacking.[49] Of special note is that the UK's National Institute for Health and Care Excellence recommends against the use of sodium nitroprusside in AHF patients.[50]

In summary, in everyday common practice, sodium nitroprusside remains an underutilized, but efficacious, vasodilator. It can be used as an adjunct to diuretics, or as an alternative to nitrates, in selected congested patients presenting with hypertensive AHF, while taking into consideration its side effect profile.

Nesiritide

Nesiritide, a synthetic form of B-type natriuretic peptide (BNP), has dual actions: vasodilatation and natriuresis. Its use is suggested as a supplementary therapy for dyspnoea relief in volume-overloaded patients under appropriate diuretic treatment.[50] Based on the results of Vasodilatation in the Management of Acute Congestive Heart Failure (VMAC) study, which showed superiority of nesiritide compared to nitrates, it was a highly promising agent in the management of AHF, especially in patients with renal failure, on beta-blocker therapy, and with coronary artery disease.[51] Nowadays, after publication of data from the Acute Study of Clinical Effectiveness of Nesiritide in Decompensated Heart Failure (ASCEND-HF) which showed no impact of nesiritide on death or HF hospitalization and non-significant dyspnoea improvement, nesiritide is not recommended as first-line treatment for the management of AHF.[52]

Other intravenous vasodilators

Bradycardic calcium channel blockers

The non-dihydropyridine calcium channel blockers (NDCCs) verapamil and diltiazem are well-established rate control agents that provide rapid symptom relief in patients with atrial fibrillation. Due to their beneficial effects on myocardial relaxation and diastolic filling, according to the latest ESC guidelines, in the setting of HF with preserved ejection fraction (≥40%), diltiazem and verapamil are recommended as first-line drugs (Class I, Level B) for rate control in patients with atrial fibrillation.[53]

Non-bradycardic calcium channel blockers

Clevedipine is a late-generation dihydropyridine calcium channel blocker (CCB) approved by the Food and Drug Administration (FDA) for the management of AHF with hypertension. It is a safe and rapid-acting antihypertensive agent through arteriolar vasodilatation and peripheral vascular resistance reduction, which provides direct symptom relief in hypertensive AHF. Although results from the PRONTO study have shown that clevedipine is more effective in the management of AHF with elevated blood pressure, compared to standard of care treatment, PRONTO II was withdrawn. Further well-designed randomized studies focusing on short-term and morbidity and mortality endpoints are needed.[54]

Failed vasodilators

Serelaxin

Serelaxin is a recombinant form of endogenous human relaxin-2 and is a hormone with vasodilatory and end-organ protective effects. According to results from RELAX-AHF, it was a promising, safe agent which has shown beneficial effects in worsening AHF during hospitalization, but the later RELAX-AHF-2 trial failed to meet the primary endpoint of cardiovascular mortality at day 180 or worsening HF after 5 days.[55] Even though a recent meta-analysis has shown that serelaxin is safe and associated with lower all-cause mortality, its use is not recommended in the AHF setting.[56]

Ularitide

Ularitide is the synthetic form of the natriuretic peptide urodilatin and induces vasodilatation and natriuresis. It has favourable haemodynamic and clinical effects such as significant blood pressure reduction and dyspnoea relief. However, according to the results of Trial of Ularitide Efficacy and Safety in Acute Heart Failure (TRUE-AHF), early administration of ularitide did not reveal a positive impact on clinical progression and the cardiovascular mortality endpoint.[57]

Future agents

Nitroxyl donors

Nitroxyl (HNO) donors are a promising agent with arteriolar and venous dilatory action. The most recent study is the Study Assessing Nitroxyl Donor Upon Presentation with Acute Heart Failure (STAND-UP AHF) trial, a phase 2 randomized, double-blind, placebo-controlled clinical trial of HNO donors (cimlanod) in patients hospitalized for AHF. The study has shown beneficial effects regarding congestion, which were not sustained after discontinuation of the drug.[58] Previous studies with second-generation nitroxyl donors (BMS-986231) had shown promising haemodynamic positive effects.[59]

Oral vasodilators

Nitrates/hydralazine

After the introduction of chronic HF modification treatment with lifesaving therapies, the role of traditional oral vasodilators, although historically meaningful, has been limited. Undoubtedly, the favourable haemodynamic alteration via preload/afterload reduction promotes a beneficial long-term effect on cardiovascular remodelling. On top of this haemodynamic action, several drug classes demonstrate clear neurohormonal effects that modify the vicious cycles of HF (RAAS inhibitors, beta-blockers with vasodilatory properties, angiotensin receptor–neprilysin inhibitors). The landmark V-HeFT study showed that the combination of hydralazine (300 mg/day) and isosorbide dinitrate (160 mg/day) reduced the 3-year mortality risk by 36%, compared to prazosin (20 mg/day) or placebo, in patients with chronic congestive HF treated with digoxin and diuretics.[26] However, the publication of the V-HeFT II trial a few years later demonstrated that enalapril (20 mg/day) was associated with a clear survival benefit of 28% over the combination of hydralazine and isosorbide dinitrate.[60] Additionally, since population-based analyses have been consistent with variations in renin–angiotensin activity and nitric oxide bioavailability, the African-American Heart Failure Trial (A-HeFT) was designed. This double-blind, placebo-controlled trial randomized patients self-identified as being of African descent, who had an LVEF of <35%, in NYHA class III or IV, to an escalating dose of hydralazine hydrochloride and isosorbide dinitrate or placebo, on top of established treatment with RAAS inhibitors and beta-blockers. The A-HeFT trial was halted prematurely due to a significant 43% reduction in mortality in the combination arm, after a mean follow-up of 10 months.[61]

Thus, according to the above observations, as well as 2021 ESC HF guidelines,[32] hydralazine and isosorbide dinitrate may be considered in symptomatic patients with HF with reduced ejection fraction (HFrEF) who can tolerate neither an ACEI nor an angiotensin receptor blocker (ARB) (or in whom these drugs are contraindicated) to reduce the risk of death (Class IIb, Level of evidence B). Finally, hydralazine and isosorbide dinitrate should be considered in self-identified black patients with an LVEF of ≤35% or with an LVEF of <45% combined with a dilated left ventricle in NYHA class III or IV despite treatment with an ACEI, a beta-blocker, and a mineralocorticoid receptor antagonist (MRA), to reduce the risk of HF hospitalization and death (Class IIa, Level of evidence B).

Calcium channel blockers

Oral NDCCs are not recommended for the treatment of patients with HFrEF. Bradycardic CCBs (diltiazem and verapamil) have been demonstrated to be unsafe in patients with HFrEF. Thus, these agents are not recommended for reducing blood pressure in patients with HFrEF because of their negative inotropic action and risk of worsening HF. On the other hand, there are various dihydropyridine CCBs; some are known to increase sympathetic tone and may have a negative safety profile in HFrEF. There is evidence on safety only for amlodipine and felodipine in patients with HFrEF, and they can be used only if there is a compelling indication in patients with HFrEF. Thus, amlodipine and felodipine should be considered to reduce blood pressure when hypertension persists despite treatment with a combination of an ACEI (or alternatively an ARB), a beta-blocker, an MRA, and a diuretic. Furthermore, amlodipine may be considered in patients unable to tolerate a beta-blocker to relieve angina (effective antianginal treatment, safe in HF) (Class IIb, Level of evidence B).[32]

Table 8.7.1 Main characteristics of intravenous vasodilators

Agent	Mechanism of action	Initial dose	Maximum dose	Adverse effects	Contraindications
Nitrates	Vasodilatation, soluble guanylyl cyclase activation ↓ intracellular calcium ↓ biventricular filling pressure ↓ pulmonary capillary wedge pressure ↓ systemic arterial blood pressure	10–20 µg/min	200 µg/min	Hypotension, flushing, tachycardia, resistance, tolerance	Hypotension, LV outflow tract obstruction, co-administration with phosphodiesterase inhibitors
Nitroprusside	↓ vascular smooth muscle relaxation ↓ systemic arterial blood pressure ↓ right atrial pressure	0.3 µg/kg/min	5 µg/kg/min	Hypotension, cyanide toxicity	Hypotension, active ischaemia (coronary steal)
Nesiritide	Mimics biological effects of BNP ↓ pulmonary capillary wedge pressure ↓ diuresis/natriuresis	Bolus 2 µg/kg	0.01 µg/kg/min	Hypotension	Hypotension

BNP, B-type natriuretic peptide; LV, left ventricular.

Summary

The main characteristics and practical information (doses, side effects, mechanism of action) of the most commonly used intravenous vasodilators are shown in ➲ Table 8.7.1.[32,39,48,49]

For clinicians' everyday practice, a simple decision-making algorithm/questionnaire is proposed, as shown in ➲ Figure 8.7.4.

In conclusion, despite lack of evidence regarding long-term efficacy of vasodilators, according to current literature and guidelines, these drugs are recommended as first-line agents for the management of patients with AHF. These agents should be used in a pathophysiological manner, so as to achieve the maximum effect. The clinical phenotype that will clearly benefit from vasodilatation treatment is hypertensive AHF with intravascular volume redistribution in order to rapidly decrease ventricular preload and afterload. In volume-overloaded patients, usually with a normotensive clinical phenotype, vasodilators have a supplementary role, after adequate diuretic therapy, in order to reverse persistent congestion.

Finally, oral vasodilators (like hydralazine and nitrates) have limited use in chronic HFrEF and should be used mainly in patients with intolerance or contraindications to ACEIs or ARBs.

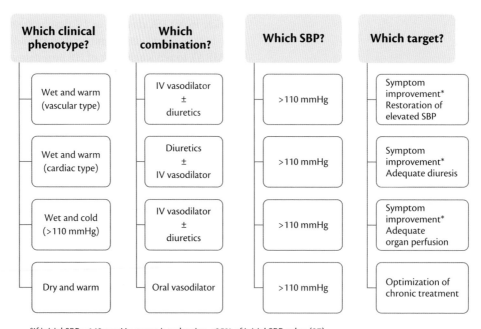

*If initial SBP >140 mmHg, target is reduction <25% of initial SBP value (37)
SBP: systolic blood pressure, IV: intravenous

Figure 8.7.4 Decision-making algorithm/questionnaire.

References

1. Mebazaa A, Motiejunaite J, Gayat E, *et al.*; ESC Heart Failure Long-Term Registry Investigators. Long-term safety of intravenous cardiovascular agents in acute heart failure: results from the European Society of Cardiology Heart Failure Long-Term Registry. Eur J Heart Fail 2018;20(2):332–41.

2. Mebazaa A, Parissis J, Porcher R, *et al.* Short-term survival by treatment among patients hospitalized with acute heart failure: the global ALARM-HF registry using propensity scoring methods. Intensive Care Med 2011;37:290–301.

3. Ferrari R, Balla C, Fucili A. Heart failure: an historical perspective. Eur Heart J Supplements 2016;18(Suppl G):G3–10.

4. Franciosa JA, Guiha NH, Limas CJ, *et al.* Improved left ventricular function during nitroprusside infusion in acute myocardial infarction. Lancet 1972;1:650–4.

5. Guiha NH, Cohn JN, Mikulic E, *et al.* Treatment of refractory heart failure with infusion of nitroprusside. N Engl J Med 1974;291:587.

6. Majid PA, Siabma B, Taylor SH. Phentolamine for vasodilator treatment of severe heart failure. Lancet 1971;2:719.

7. Cohn JN. Vasodilator therapy for heart failure. The influence of impedance on left ventricular performance. Circulation 1973;48(1):5–8.

8. Mason DT. Afterload reduction and cardiac performance. Physiologic basis of systemic vasodilators as a new approach in treatment of congestive heart failure. Am J Med 1978;65(1):106–25.

9. Cohn JN, Franciosa JA. Vasodilator therapy of cardiac failure (first of two parts). N Engl J Med 1977;297(1):27–31.

10. Cohn JN, Franciosa JA. Vasodilator therapy of cardiac failure (second of two parts). N Engl J Med 1977;297(5):254–8.

11. Pouleur H, Covell JW, Ross J Jr. Effects of nitroprusside on venous return and central blood volume in the absence and presence of acute heart failure. Circulation 1980;61(2):328–37.

12. Miller RR, Awan NA, Joye JA, *et al.* Combined dopamine and nitroprusside therapy in congestive heart failure. Greater augmentation of cardiac performance by addition of inotropic stimulation to afterload reduction. Circulation 1977;55(6):881–4.

13. Henning RJ, Shubin H, Weil MH. Afterload reduction with phentolamine in patients with acute pulmonary edema. Am J Med 1977;63(4):568–73.

14. Chatterjee K, Parmley WW, Massie B, *et al.* Oral hydralazine therapy for chronic refractory heart failure. Circulation 1976;54(6):879–83.

15. Franciosa JA, Mikulic E, Cohn JN, *et al.* Hemodynamic effects of orally administered isosorbide dinitrate in patients with congestive heart failure. Circulation 1974;50(5):1020–4.

16. Miller RR, Awan NA, Maxwell KS, *et al.* Sustained reduction of cardiac impedance and preload in congestive heart failure with the antihypertensive vasodilator prazosin. N Engl J Med 1977;297(6):303–7.

17. Levine TB. Role of vasodilators in the treatment of congestive heart failure. Am J Cardiol 1985;55(2):32A–5A.

18. Franciosa JA, Jordan RA, Wilen MM, *et al.* Minoxidil in patients with chronic left heart failure: contrasting hemodynamic and clinical effects in a controlled trial. Circulation 1984;70(1):63–8.

19. Franciosa JA, Weber KT, Levine TB, *et al.* Hydralazine in the long-term treatment of chronic heart failure: lack of difference from placebo. Am Heart J 1982;104(3):587–94.

20. Franciosa JA, Goldsmith SR, Cohn JN. Contrasting immediate and long-term effects of isosorbide dinitrate on exercise capacity in congestive heart failure. Am J Med 1980;69(4):559–66.

21. Awan NA, Miller RR, DeMaria AN, *et al.* Efficacy of ambulatory systemic vasodilator therapy with oral prazosin in chronic refractory heart failure. Concomitant relief of pulmonary congestion and elevation of pump output demonstrated by improvements in symptomatology, exercise tolerance, hemodynamics and echocardiography. Circulation 1977;56(3):346–54.

22. Bellocci F, Ansalone G, Santarelli P, *et al.* Oral nifedipine in the long-term management of severe chronic heart failure. J Cardiovasc Pharmacol 1982;4(5):847–55.

23. Franciosa JA. Long-term vasodilator therapy of chronic left ventricular failure: does it work? Int J Cardiol 1984;5(4):433–9.

24. Franciosa JA, Pierpont G. Cardiovascular clinical pharmacology of impedance reducing agents. J Chron Dis 1981;34:341–52.

25. Furberg CD, Yusuf S. Effect of vasodilators on survival in chronic congestive heart failure. Am J Cardiol 1985;55(8):1110–13.

26. Cohn JN, Archibald DG, Ziesche S, *et al.* Effect of vasodilator therapy on mortality in chronic congestive heart failure. Results of a Veterans Administration Cooperative Study. N Engl J Med 1986;314(24):1547–52.

27. [No authors listed]. A placebo-controlled trial of captopril in refractory chronic congestive heart failure. Captopril Multicenter Research Group. J Am Coll Cardiol 1983;2(4):755–63.

28. CONSENSUS Trial Study Group. Effects of enalapril on mortality in severe congestive heart failure. Results of the Cooperative North Scandinavian Enalapril Survival Study (CONSENSUS). N Engl J Med 1987;316(23):1429–35.

29. Singh A, Laribi S, Teerlink JR, Mebazaa A. Agents with vasodilator properties in acute heart failure. Eur Heart J 2017;38(5):317–25.

30. Holt DB, Pang PS. Vasodilator therapies in the treatment of acute heart failure. Curr Heart Fail Rep 2019;16(1):32–7.

31. McDonagh TA, Metra M, Adamo M, *et al.*; ESC Scientific Document Group. 2021 ESC Guidelines for the diagnosis and treatment of acute and chronic heart failure. Eur Heart J 2021;42(36):3599–726.

32. Yancy CW, Jessup M, Bozkurt B, *et al.* American College of Cardiology Foundation; American Heart Association Task Force on Practice Guidelines. 2013 ACCF/AHA guideline for the management of heart failure: a report of the American College of Cardiology Foundation/American Heart Association Task Force on Practice Guidelines. J Am Coll Cardiol 2013;62(16):e147–239.

33. Opie LH, Gersh BJ. *Drugs for the Heart*, 8th edition. Philadelphia, PA: Elsevier Saunders; 2013.

34. Klabunde RE. Vasodilator drugs. In: Klabunde RE. *Cardiovascular Pharmacology Concepts*, 2nd edition. Philadelphia, PA: Lippincott, Williams and Wilkins; 2012, pp. 101–10.

35. Metra M, Teerlink J, Voors A, *et al.* Vasodilators in the treatment of acute heart failure: what we know, what we don't. Heart Fail Rev 2009;14:299–307.

36. Kitai T, Tang W, Xanthopoulos A, *et al.* Impact of early treatment with intravenous vasodilators and blood pressure reduction in acute heart failure. Open Heart 2018;5:e000845.

37. Peacock W, Emerman C, Constanzo M, *et al.* Early vasoactive drugs improve heart failure outcomes. Congest Heart Fail 2009;15:256–64.

38. Alzahri M, Rohra A, Peacock F. Nitrates as the treatment of acute heart failure. Card Fail Rev 2016;2(1):51–5.

39. Tarvasmäki T, Harjola V-P, Tolonen J, *et al.* Management of acute heart failure and the effect of systolic blood pressure on the use of intravenous therapies. Eur Heart J Acute Cardiovasc Care 2013;2(3):219–25.

40. Wakai A, McCabe A, Kidney R, *et al.* Nitrates for acute heart failure syndromes. Cochrane Database Syst Rev 2013;8:CD005151.

41. Farag M, Shoaib A, Gorog D. Nitrates for the management of acute heart failure syndromes, a systematic review. J Cardiovasc Pharmacol Ther 2017;22(1):20–7.

42. Herrero-Puente P, Jacob J, Martin-Sanchez F, *et al*. Influence of intravenous nitrate treatment on early mortality among patients with acute heart failure. NITRO-EAHFE Study. Rev Esp Cardiol 2015;68(11):959–67.

43. Kozhuharov N, Goudev A, Flores D, *et al*. Effect of a strategy of comprehensive vasodilation vs usual care on mortality and heart failure rehospitalization among patients with acute heart failure. The GALACTIC randomized clinical trial. JAMA 2019;322(23):2292–302.

44. Wang K, Samai K. Role of high-dose intravenous nitrates in hypertensive acute heart failure. Am J Emerg Med 2020;38(1):132–7.

45. Alexander P, Alkhawam L, Curry J, *et al*. Lack of evidence for intravenous vasodilators in ED patients with acute heart failure: a systematic review. Am J Emerg Med 2015;33(2):133–41.

46. Freund Y, Cachanado M, Delannoy Q, *et al*. Effect of an emergency department care bundle on 30-day hospital discharge and survival among elderly patients with acute heart failure: the ELISABETH randomized clinical trial. JAMA 2020;324(19):1948–56.

47. Opasish C, Cioffi G, Gualco A. Nitroprusside in decompensated heart failure: what should a clinician really know? Curr Heart Fail Rep 2009;6:182–90.

48. Piper S, McDonagh T. The role of intravenous vasodilators in acute heart failure management. Eur J Heart Fail 2014;16:827–34.

49. Carlson M, Eckman P. Review of vasodilators in acute decompensated heart failure: the old and the new. J Cardiac Fail 2013;19:478e493.

50. National Institute for Health and Care Excellence. Acute heart failure: diagnosis and management. Clinical guideline [CG187]. London: National Institute for Health and Care Excellence; 2014.

51. Publication Committee for the VMAC Investigators (Vasodilatation in the Management of Acute CHF). Intravenous nesiritide vs nitroglycerin for treatment of decompensated congestive heart failure: a randomized controlled trial. JAMA 2002;287(12):1531–40.

52. O'Connor CM, Starling RC, Hernandez AF, *et al*. Effect of nesiritide in patients with acute decompensated heart failure. N Engl J Med 2011;365(1):32–43.

53. Hindricks G, Potpara T, Dagres N, *et al*. 2020 ESC Guidelines for the diagnosis and management of atrial fibrillation developed in collaboration with the European Association for Cardio-Thoracic Surgery (EACTS): The Task Force for the diagnosis and management of atrial fibrillation of the European Society of Cardiology (ESC) Developed with the special contribution of the European Heart Rhythm Association (EHRA) of the ESC. Eur Heart J 2020;42:373–498.

54. Levy P, Laribi S, Mebazaa A. Vasodilators in acute heart failure: review of the latest studies. Curr Emerg Hosp Med Rep 2014;2(2):126–32.

55. Metra M, Teerlink JR, Cotter G, *et al*. Effects of serelaxin in patients with acute heart failure. N Engl J Med 2019;381:716–26.

56. Teerlink J, Davison B, Cotter G, *et al*. Effects of serelaxin in patients admitted for acute heart failure: a meta-analysis. Eur J Heart Fail 2020;22:315–29.

57. Packer M, O'Connor C, McMurray JJV, *et al*. Effect of ularitide on cardiovascular mortality in acute heart failure. N Engl J Med 2017;376:1956–64.

58. Felker M, McMurray J, Cleland J, *et al*. Effects of a novel nitroxyl donor in acute heart failure: the STAND-UP AHF Study. JACC Heart Fail 2021;9(2):146–57.

59. Tita C, Gilbert E, van Bakel A, *et al*. A phase 2a dose-escalation study of the safety, tolerability, pharmacokinetics and haemodynamic effects of BMS-986231 in hospitalized patients with heart failure with reduced ejection fraction. Eur J Heart Fail 2017;19(10):1321–32.

60. Cohn JN, Johnson G, Ziesche S, *et al*. A comparison of enalapril with hydralazine–isosorbide dinitrate in the treatment of chronic congestive heart failure. N Engl J Med 1991;325:303–10.

61. Taylor AL, Ziesche S, Yancy C, *et al*.; African-American Heart Failure Trial Investigators. Combination of isosorbide dinitrate and hydralazine in blacks with heart failure. N Engl J Med 2004;351(20):2049–57.

CHAPTER 8.8

Digitalis glycosides

Udo Bavendiek and Johann Bauersachs

Contents

Introduction

Digitalis glycosides have been known as potential medical therapy for heart failure for several centuries,[1] and in 1785, Withering described its systematic use for the first time.[2] Despite newer drugs with excellent, well-proven efficacy in patients with heart failure with reduced ejection fraction (HFrEF), such as beta-blockers, angiotensin-converting enzyme (ACE) inhibitors, and mineralocorticoid receptor antagonists (MRAs), digitalis glycosides are still frequently used worldwide.[3,4] Digitalis glycosides are widely available, very cheap, and often part of heart failure treatment, particularly in patients with advanced HFrEF and/or atrial fibrillation. However, the value of digitalis glycosides for current HFrEF therapy is uncertain, as there are only a few randomized clinical trials with digoxin that had been performed before current standard HFrEF medical treatment was established. In addition, the dosages of digitalis glycosides used traditionally appear to be too high, as the therapeutic window of digitalis is narrow, with a risk of serious side effects. Thus, the dosages have to be carefully selected and adapted according to comorbidities, especially in worsening kidney function.

In this chapter, we will summarize current knowledge on pharmacodynamics and pharmacokinetics of digitalis glycosides, particularly digoxin and digitoxin, adverse effects, and toxicity, as well as the evidence for clinical use in patients with heart failure. We put in perspective the equivocal results of retrospective analyses of digitalis use in non-randomized settings that have led to considerable uncertainty about the safe use of digitalis glycosides. Finally, we provide recommendations for use of digitalis glycosides in current clinical practice for patients with heart failure and/or atrial fibrillation.

Digitalis glycosides

The digitalis glycosides with relevant clinical use are digoxin and digitoxin.[5] These agents derive from naturally occurring precursor glycosides of the leaves of the foxglove species *Digitalis purpurea* (digitoxin) and *Digitalis lanata* (digoxin and digitoxin). Digoxin and digitoxin are still extracted from dried foxglove leaves, because full synthesis is difficult and very costly. Derived from digoxin, the half-synthetic digitalis glycosides beta-acetyldigoxin and metildigoxin are also available. All cardiac glycosides consist of combinations of a non-sugar moiety, an aglycone (or genin), with 1–4 sugar residues attached. The pharmacological properties reside in the genin, whereas the nature of the sugar residues attached to the genin influences the pharmacokinetic properties, for example, water solubility, enteral resorption, plasma protein binding, and biotransformation. Whereas the pharmacodynamics of digoxin and digitoxin are similar, marked differences in their pharmacokinetic properties have to be considered in clinical use and are essential to the choice of digoxin or digitoxin for the individual patient.[5,6]

Mechanisms of action/pharmacodynamics

Digitalis glycosides mediate their pharmacological action by inhibition of plasma membrane-bound sodium (Na^+)/potassium (K^+)-ATPase. The Na^+/K^+-ATPase is a ubiquitously expressed ATPase, consisting of α-, β-, and γ-subunits. The α-subunit compromises the catalytic subunit and a highly conserved digitalis glycoside binding site. The Na^+/K^+-ATPase exchanges intracellular Na^+ with extracellular K^+ in a 3:2 ratio. Specific binding of digitalis glycosides inhibits Na^+/K^+-ATPase activity. This changes intracellular Na^+, K^+, and calcium (Ca^{2+}) concentrations and results in different modes of digitalis actions, depending on the Na^+/K^+-ATPase density and expression of subunit isoforms in target cells/tissue (➲ Figure 8.8.1). Digitalis glycoside binding and action on the Na^+/K^+-ATPase are inhibited by K^+ and magnesium (Mg^{2+}) ions.[5,7,8,9]

Myocardial effects

Increased intracellular Na^+ concentrations resulting from inhibition of Na^+/K^+-ATPase by digitalis glycosides promote the exchange of intracellular Na^+ with extracellular Ca^{2+} by the Na^+/Ca^{2+} exchanger. As consequence, intracellular Ca^{2+} concentrations and filling of Ca^{2+} stores in the sarcoplasmic reticulum are increased. During the next cycle of excitation–contraction coupling, Ca^{2+} release from the sarcoplasmic reticulum is augmented and higher amounts of Ca^{2+} bind to contractile proteins, resulting in an increased force of myocardial contraction (positive inotrope) and stroke volume. These effects usually require higher dosages of digitalis glycosides.

Neurohormonal effects

At lower dosages, digitalis glycosides increase the sensitivity of carotid sinus baroreceptors and activate central vagal nuclei. The resulting increase in parasympathetic tone inhibits the sympathetic tone and the release of adrenergic neurohormones, for example, noradrenaline, reducing the peripheral vascular resistance and heart rate. At higher dosages, digitalis glycosides increase sympathetic nervous system activity and the sympathetic tone, promoting vasoconstriction and electrophysiological disturbances (see below).

Electrophysiological effects

Direct effects of digitalis glycosides on the sinoatrial and atrioventricular (AV) node conduction system are related to actions on diastolic potential and depolarization by changes of intracellular ion homeostasis. Observed inhibition of automaticity, prolongation of conduction times (negative dromotropy), and reduction in heart rate (negative chronotropy) by digitalis glycosides presumably do not result from direct cellular actions of digitalis glycosides at the conduction system, but rather indirectly through the above-described parasympathomimetic and sympathicoinhibitory effects, as they could not be observed in patients after cardiac transplantation. Marked changes in intracellular Na^+, K^+, and Ca^{2+} concentrations or increased sympathetic nervous system activity and sympathetic tone may be the reason for significant alterations in diastolic potentials, spontaneous depolarizations, automaticity, and conduction observed with high doses of digitalis glycosides or under conditions enhancing sensitivity

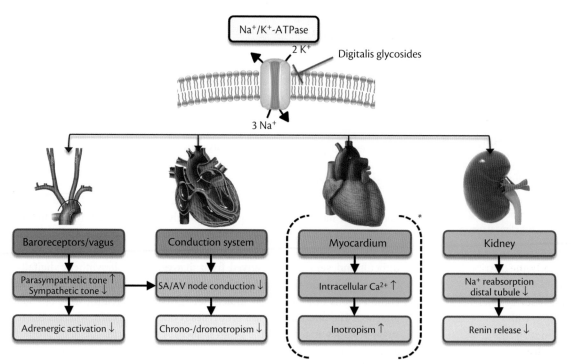

*minor importance, because higher doses and digitalis serum concentrations are necessary

Figure 8.8.1 Digitalis glycosides: mechanisms of action and pharmacodynamics. AV, atrioventricular; Na^+/K^+-ATPase, sodium/potassium ATPase; SA, sinoatrial.

to pharmacological actions of digitalis glycosides (e.g. hypokalaemia, hypomagnesaemia).

Extracardiac effects

Inhibition of Na^+/K^+-ATPase in non-myocardial cells/tissue may also mediate potential clinically relevant pharmacological effects of digitalis glycosides. For example, diuretic effects of digitalis glycosides already described by Withering may be a result of inhibition of Na^+ reabsorption in the distal tubule (highly expressed Na^+/K^+-ATPase), accompanied by suppression of renin secretion.

Initially, beneficial effects of digitalis glycosides on symptoms of HFrEF were primarily assigned to their positive inotropic actions. Because inotropic actions are observed at higher serum concentrations of digitalis glycosides (although in the former 'therapeutic' range), this was accompanied by adverse or toxic side effects. With better understanding of heart failure pathophysiology, sustained and overshooting activation of neurohormonal systems was identified as a key underlying mechanism. Favourable effects of digitalis glycosides on neurohormonal systems especially occur if these are disturbed and overactivated in HFrEF, but not in patients without heart failure. Thus, actions on neurohormonal, and probably other extracardiac, systems observed with lower doses and serum concentrations of digitalis glycosides seem to be of particular importance for beneficial effects of digitalis glycosides in heart failure.

Pharmacokinetics

(See ⮞ Table 8.8.1.)[6,10]

Absorption

Intestinal absorption of digoxin and digitoxin is a passive process. The polarity or lipid solubility determines the rate and extent of absorption. Because digoxin is less lipophilic and more polar than digitoxin, enteral resorption, and therefore bioavailability, is reduced to 60–80% after oral administration and serum protein binding is 20–40%. Lipophilic digitoxin shows almost complete enteral absorption, with a high bioavailability in the range of 95–100% after oral administration and high plasma protein binding of about 90–97%. These properties of digitoxin are not significantly changed in patients with renal and hepatic dysfunction or in the elderly.

Distribution

The skeletal muscle, myocardium, kidney, and liver represent the main compartments of distribution, similar for digoxin and digitoxin. In the elderly, the distribution volume is considerably lower due to reduced skeletal muscle mass (up to 40%), which represents the major tissue compartment. Digoxin has a fairly prompt tissue distribution, with a half-life of 30–60 minutes after oral or intravenous administration. Due to high protein binding, after oral intake, the distribution of digitoxin takes longer than that of digoxin (4–10 hours). Because digoxin is primarily eliminated renally by passive glomerular filtration and tubular secretion, total clearance is significantly reduced with impaired renal function,

Table 8.8.1 Properties of digoxin and digitoxin

	Digoxin	Digitoxin
Bioavailability (%) (oral administration)	60–80	95–100
Plasma protein binding (%)	20–40	90–97
Tissue distribution	High	Low
Distribution volume (L/kg)	High (4–7)	Low (0.4–0.7)
Half-life (days)	1–2 (dependent on renal function, 5 days in terminal renal failure)	6–7 (independent of renal function)
Steady-state blood levels after initiation of maintenance dose (days)	5–10	20–30
Metabolism (%)	<30 (10% hepatic)	50–75 (hepatic)
Elimination (%)	70–80 renal 20–30, extrarenal	60, renal 40, extrarenal
Daily decay (%)	20–30	7–10
Dose reduction with reduced kidney function	Necessary	Not necessary
Target serum concentrations	0.5–0.9 ng/mL (0.65–1.15 nmol/L)	8–18 ng/mL (10.5–23.6 nmol/L)
Toxic serum concentrations (ng/mL)	>2	>30
Loading dose (PO, IV) (mg) (distributed over 3 days)	0.75–1.5	0.5–1.0
Daily maintenance dose (PO) (mg)	0.0625–0.25	0.035–0.1

IV, intravenous; PO, oral.

although extrarenal clearance is unaffected. Compensatory excretion of digoxin in the faeces is not sufficient for compensation of impaired renal clearance, causing accumulation of digoxin. In contrast, impaired renal function does not influence elimination of digitoxin because the reduced renal clearance is fully compensated by extrarenal (enterohepatic) clearance, keeping total clearance constant. In patients with cirrhosis of the liver and advanced renal dysfunction, total clearance of digitoxin is also impaired, with relevant elevations in serum concentrations of digitoxin.

Metabolism

Renal excretion of unchanged digoxin is the predominant mode of elimination, and metabolism to digoxin reduction products is not of relevance in most patients. In about 10% of patients, significant metabolism to reduction products accounts for 30–40% of total urinary excretion of digoxin. As digoxin reduction products are formed by the bacterial flora of the gastrointestinal tract, antibiotic therapy may significantly affect metabolism of digoxin to cardio-inactive products, which might be of relevance to digoxin treatment in patients with significant metabolism of digoxin to reduction products. Renal clearance of unchanged digitoxin is of minor relevance, compared to that of digoxin.

Extensive metabolism of digitoxin occurs in the liver, and metabolic biotransformation is the major route of elimination. Pharmacodynamic effects of digitoxin and its half-life are mainly mediated by unmetabolized digitoxin.

Elimination/excretion

Elimination of digoxin and its derivatives mainly depends on renal excretion (70–80% renal; 20–30% extrarenal). The excretory half-life of digoxin is 1–2 days in patients with normal renal function and is prolonged in impaired renal function, being up to 5 days in terminal renal failure. The half-life of digitoxin is 6–7 days, irrespective of renal function. With normal liver and renal function, 60% of digitoxin is eliminated via the urine and 40% is excreted via enteral secretion into the bile or directly through the mucosal wall. A significant part of secreted digitoxin (6–7% per day) recirculates enterohepatically. If renal elimination is reduced due to impaired renal function, compensation occurs through increased metabolism and excretion via the faeces. Although renal excretion is diminished in the elderly, this is compensated by increased enterohepatic elimination and therefore, the elimination half-life of digitoxin is unchanged.

Dosage and serum concentrations

Routes of administration and dosage

Digoxin and digitoxin can be administered orally and intravenously. Treatment may be started with a loading or maintenance dose. Oral administration of a maintenance dose for initiation of treatment should be preferred as this avoids overdosing and side effects, and is usually sufficient in stable patients. By administration of a maintenance dose, stable target serum concentrations of digoxin and digitoxin are achieved after 5–10 and 20–30 days, respectively.[5,6,10] Daily oral maintenance dosages of digoxin are 0.125 and 0.25 mg, but even have to be reduced to 0.0625 mg, especially with impaired renal function. Daily oral maintenance dosages of digitoxin are 0.05, 0.07, and 0.1 mg, but even have to be reduced to 0.035 mg (➲ Table 8.8.1). Doses of digoxin and digitoxin also have to be reduced in the very elderly with low body weight (reduced skeletal muscle compartment). Use of a loading dose (three times maintenance dose daily for 3 days) for faster achievement of therapeutic blood levels should be limited to the treatment of tachycardic atrial fibrillation if concerns or presence of haemodynamic instability exist. Oral administration of the loading dose is preferred over intravenous administration to avoid side effects due to fast accumulation and overdosing. Intravenous administration should be limited to situations of acute decompensation or haemodynamic instability due to atrial fibrillation.

Serum concentrations

Significant variance of interindividual serum concentrations of digitalis glycosides has been described, which often cannot be explained, even if individual patient data influencing serum concentrations are available (e.g. age, body weight, digitalis dose, renal function). Therefore, at initiation of therapy, serum concentrations have to be determined and titrated for the individual patient until stable target concentrations are achieved.[5,6,10] Therapeutic serum concentrations of digoxin should be in the range of 0.5–0.9 ng/mL (0.65–1.15 nmol/L),[11,12,13,14] and for digitoxin between 10 and 18 ng/mL (10.5–23.6 nmol/L).[15] Blood concentrations should be determined no earlier than 6 hours after the last intake, to ensure that equilibration between blood and tissue is stable. In contrast to digoxin, serum concentrations of digitoxin do not increase with impaired renal function and therefore, dose reductions are not necessary. In the elderly, digoxin and digitoxin doses have to be reduced because of lower muscle mass and volume of distribution.[5,6,10]

Drug interactions

Drug interactions involving digitalis glycosides are of pharmacodynamic or pharmacokinetic type. Because the pharmacokinetics of digoxin and digitoxin markedly differ, it is important to differentiate drug interactions between these digitalis glycosides. Relevant drug interactions are summarized in ➲ Table 8.8.2.[5,10]

Adverse effects and toxicity

Adverse effects and toxicity of digitalis glycosides are rare at serum concentrations in the recommended therapeutic range (digoxin 0.5–0.9 ng/mL; digitoxin 8–18 ng/mL).[11,12,13,14,15] Toxic effects mainly result from overdosing of digitalis glycosides with serum concentrations of >2.0 ng/mL of digoxin and >30 ng/mL of digitoxin. Signs of overdosing and toxicity include different cardiac arrhythmias (90%, e.g. sinus bradycardia, sinus arrest, high-grade AV block, (supra)ventricular arrhythmias), gastrointestinal (50–60%, e.g. nausea, vomiting, diarrhoea, loss of appetite and weight), and neurological (10–15%, e.g. disturbance of colour vision, confusion, hallucination). To avoid toxicity, early detection of adverse effects or signs of toxicity is important. Serum concentrations and responsiveness to digitalis glycosides not only are dependent on the administered dose, but also are related to concurrent conditions and medications (➲ Table 8.8.2).[5,6,10] For instance, in the presence of hypokalaemia, hypomagnesaemia, hypercalcaemia, and hypothyroidism, adverse effects and symptoms may occur even at serum concentrations in the therapeutic range, due to increased sensitivity to digitalis glycosides.

Therapy of adverse effects and intoxication

If signs of potential adverse effects or toxicity occur, administration of digitalis glycosides should be stopped and serum concentrations determined. If adverse effects are not severe and serum concentrations are close to the therapeutic range, interruption of digitalis treatment temporarily usually is sufficient. Conditions which increase digitalis glycoside sensitivity and serum concentrations or potentiate digitalis glycoside actions (e.g. hypokalaemia, treatment with AV conduction inhibitors) should be corrected or discontinued. In cases of severe adverse effects or signs of toxicity (e.g. high-grade conduction disturbances, arrhythmias), hypo- or hyperkalaemia should be corrected and Mg^{2+} should be substituted. Bradyarrhythmias can be treated with atropine intravenously or, if necessary, by temporary ventricular

Table 8.8.2 Pharmacokinetic and pharmacodynamic interactions with digoxin and digitoxin

Mechanism of interaction	SDC	Interacting Drugs	Digoxin	Digitoxin
Pharmacokinetic				
Gastrointestinal absorption				
Decreased	↓	Antacids	+	+
		Neomycin	+	
		Cholestyramine	+	+
		Colestipol	+	+
		Metoclopramide	+	
		Phenytoin	+	
Increased	↑	Atropine	+	
Trapping of glycosides in enterohepatic circulation (faecal excretion ↑)	↑	Cholestyramine		+
		Colestipol		+
Metabolism of glycoside				
Increased	↓	Phenobarbital		+
		Phenytoin		+
		Phenylbutazone		+
		Isoniazid		+
		Ethambutol		+
		Rifampin		+
		Spironolactone		+
		Hyperthyroidism		+
Decreased	↑	Antibiotic therapy	+	
		Amiodarone	+	+
		Mexiletine		+
		Propafenone		+
Volume of distribution				
Decreased	↑	Quinidine	+	
Clearance				
Decreased	↑	Quinidine	+	+
		Spironolactone	+	+
Pharmacodynamic				
Alteration of serum electrolytes				
Hypokalaemia		Diet	+	+
Digitalis efficacy/side effects ↑		Corticosteroids	+	+
		Non-potassium-sparing diuretics	+	+
Hyperkalaemia		Potassium salts	+	+
Digitalis efficacy/side effects ↓		Potassium-sparing diuretics	+	+
Hypercalcaemia		Calcium salts (IV)	+	+
Digitalis efficacy/side effects ↑				
Arrhythmogenic		Beta-adrenergic agonists	+	+
		Class I and III antiarrhythmics	+	+
		Reserpine	+	+
		Theophylline	+	+
		Succinylcholine	+	+
Inhibition of SA/AV node conduction		Beta-adrenergic blockers	+	+
		Non-dihydropyridine CCB**	+	+
		Class I and III antiarrhythmics	+	+

AV, atrioventricular; CCB, calcium channel blocker; IV, intravenous; SA, sinoatrial. SDC, serum digitalis concentration.

pacing. Amiodarone or lidocaine may be used for ventricular arrhythmias. Electrical cardioversion has an increased risk of inducing severe rhythm disturbances in patients with severe digitalis toxicity and should be used with caution or only if ventricular fibrillation occurs. Digitalis antibodies (purified Fab fragments of immunoglobulin G (IgG) class) can be given for elimination of cardiac glycosides in severe toxicity. In cases of digitoxin overdosing/toxicity, the enterohepatic circulation should be interrupted by administration of activated charcoal or an anion exchanger, for example, cholestyramine. Forced diuresis, peritoneal dialysis, and haemodialysis are inefficient for elimination of digoxin and digitoxin. Haemoperfusion, in particular with surface-bound digitalis antibodies (alternatively, but less effective with activated charcoal or plasmapheresis), is effective in reducing the digoxin or digitoxin body content.[5,16]

Contraindications

Substantial contraindications to use of digitalis glycosides are related to their pharmacodynamic and pharmacokinetic properties: ventricular tachyarrhythmias, second- and third-degree AV block, bradycardia due to sick sinus or carotid sinus syndrome without pacemaker, accessory conduction disease (Wolff–Parkinson–White syndrome), acute myocardial infarction, hypertrophic obstructive cardiomyopathy, relevant hypokalaemia (<3.2 mmol/L), and hypercalcaemia (e.g. hyperparathyroidism).

Clinical trials with digitalis in heart failure

Heart failure with reduced ejection fraction

Before the first randomized clinical trials demonstrated better outcomes with ACE inhibitors and beta-blockers in patients with HFrEF, only small controlled studies investigated the effects of digitalis in these patients. Initial studies of very small size demonstrated that digoxin improved symptoms and exercise capacity in patients with impaired ventricular function.[17,18] The ensuing placebo-controlled clinical studies PROVED and RADIANCE with higher, but still rather small, patient numbers investigated the effect of digoxin withdrawal in patients with HFrEF in sinus rhythm. In patients with background heart failure therapy consisting of only diuretics (PROVED) or diuretics plus ACE inhibitors (RADIANCE), withdrawal of digoxin worsened heart failure, exercise capacity, and parameters of quality of life.[19,20]

The DIG trial

Until now, the DIG trial is the only prospective, placebo-controlled, randomized clinical trial providing data of the effect of digitalis glycosides on outcomes in patients with heart failure. The DIG trial included 6800 patients in New York Heart Association (NYHA) classes I–IV, a left ventricular ejection fraction (LVEF) <45%, and a background heart failure therapy, which were equally randomized to placebo or digoxin. Patients with atrial fibrillation were excluded. Patients received a background therapy with ACE inhibitors and diuretics but not beta-blockers, because results of beta-blocker trials were not available before start of the DIG trial. Digoxin had a neutral effect on the primary endpoint of overall

mortality as well as on the predefined secondary endpoints cardiovascular mortality and mortality due to worsening of heart failure. Digoxin significantly reduced the predefined secondary endpoint cardiovascular hospitalizations which was driven by a 28% reduction of hospitalizations for worsening heart failure within a median study follow-up of 37 month (❍ Figure 8.8.2).[11]

DIG trial: gender and digoxin serum concentrations

Because of known differences in women and men with respect to risk, causes, and prognosis of heart failure, as well as a proportion of only 20% of women in the DIG trial population, any differences in the effect of digoxin in women could have been subsumed by the effect of digoxin in men. Therefore, a post hoc analysis of the DIG trial investigated the effects of digoxin therapy according to gender. In this analysis, digoxin therapy was associated with an increased risk of death from any cause in women, but not in men.[21] Further analysis of the male trial population (1171 patients with available digoxin serum concentrations measured 1 month after randomization to digoxin and 2611 patients randomized to placebo) demonstrated an association of digoxin serum concentrations of <0.9 ng/mL with reduced mortality, a neutral effect on mortality at serum concentrations of 0.9–1.1 ng/mL, but increased mortality at serum concentrations of >1.2 ng/mL.[12]

As the latter caused concerns about digoxin therapy in heart failure, more detailed analyses of the DIG trial population followed. Analysis of a patient population containing both genders (n = 3366 randomized to placebo; n = 1578 randomized to digoxin, with available digoxin serum concentrations) demonstrated a significant linear relationship between digoxin serum concentrations and mortality in both women and men, with no significant difference between genders. Digoxin serum concentrations of <0.9 ng/mL were significantly associated with reduced mortality in men, whereas there was a neutral effect in women. In contrast, digoxin serum concentrations of >1.2 ng/mL were associated with increased mortality in women, driving increased mortality in the population including women and men, as there was a neutral effect observed in men alone. Digoxin serum concentrations of <0.9 ng/mL were associated with a reduced rate of heart failure hospitalization in both genders.[13]

An even more detailed analysis included patients from the DIG trial with an LVEF of ≤45%, as well as patients from the ancillary DIG trial with an LVEF of >45% (❍ Heart failure with mid-range and preserved ejection fraction, p. 511). A total of 1687 patients randomized to digoxin, with available digoxin serum concentrations, and 3861 patients randomized to placebo were analysed. In this population, patients with high digoxin serum concentrations (≥1.0 ng/mL) were older and had worse renal function and more indicators of heart failure, compared to those who received placebo, and therefore represented per se a higher-risk population. After multivariate adjustment for covariates and also after propensity score matching, digoxin serum concentrations of <1.0 ng/mL, compared to placebo, were associated with significantly reduced overall, cardiovascular-, and heart failure-related mortality, whereas a neutral effect was obtained for these endpoints at digoxin serum concentrations of >1.0 ng/mL versus placebo. In addition, heart failure-related hospitalization was significantly reduced by digoxin at serum concentrations of <1.0 mg/mL, as well as ≥1.0 ng/mL, compared to placebo. Strong predictors of high digoxin serum concentrations were age, female sex, impaired renal function, use of diuretics, pulmonary congestion, and digoxin doses of ≥0.25 mg/day.[14]

Overall, data from the DIG trial suggest that digoxin treatment in HFrEF should target serum concentrations of 0.5–0.9 ng/mL. In patients with one or several risk factors for high serum digoxin concentrations, treatment should be started at low doses of 0.125 or even 0.0625 mg/day, respectively, instead of 0.25 mg/day. Digoxin serum concentrations should be monitored around 4 weeks after start of treatment and repeated, if necessary, to guide therapy.

DIG trial: NYHA class and LVEF

In a protocol-prespecified subgroup analysis of 2-year outcomes in the DIG trial, digoxin significantly reduced all-cause and heart failure-related mortality, as well as all-cause and heart failure-related hospitalizations in a high-risk patient population (NYHA classes III and IV or LVEF <25%).[22] In contrast, in the low-risk patient population, digoxin did not reduce the combined endpoint all-cause-mortality and all-cause-related hospitalizations, but significantly reduced heart failure-related mortality and hospitalization. A further analysis of the entire DIG trial population including patients of the ancillary trial representing an LVEF range of 3–85% demonstrated an LVEF inflection point of around 35%, below which the composite endpoint of cardiovascular death and HF hospitalization in this specific analysis linearly increased in placebo-treated patients.[23] In addition, this analysis showed a clear benefit of digoxin on the primary composite endpoint of this analysis below an LVEF of around 35%, with a smaller, if any, effect above that value.

Heart failure with mid-range and preserved ejection fraction

DIG main and ancillary trials

The ancillary part of the DIG trial included 998 patients randomized to digoxin or placebo with an LVEF of >45%. In this patient population, digoxin, compared to placebo, had no effect on the primary endpoint of heart failure hospitalization or heart failure mortality, and on other outcomes such as overall, cardiovascular-, or heart failure-related mortality during a mean follow-up of 37 months.[24] For heart failure hospitalizations, there was a trend of a statistical significance within the overall median follow-up and a significant reduction in a prespecified analysis at 2 years after randomization. However, these results have to be interpreted with caution because digoxin had no effect on the overall study endpoints. The lack of statistical significance of digoxin effects in the ancillary DIG trial has been suggested to be due to the small sample size, as well as the high proportion of patients included within NYHA classes I and II (approximately 75% of all patients), explaining the low event rates in the trial. Analysis of the entire DIG population, including that in the ancillary trial, enabled analysis of patient populations within LVEF ranges representing HFrEF (LVEF <40%), heart failure with mid-range ejection fraction (HFmrEF; LVEF 40–49%), and heart failure with preserved ejection fraction (HFpEF; LVEF ≥50%).[23] In line with results of the DIG main trial, digoxin had neutral effects on mortality

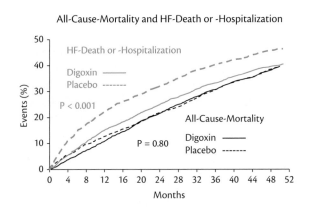

Mortality

	DIGOXIN (N = 3397)	PLACEBO (N = 3403)	RISK RATIO (95% CI)	P VALUE
	no. of patients (%)			
All-Cause	1181 (34.8)	1194 (35.1)	0.99 (0.91–1.07)	0.80
Cardiovascular	1016 (29.9)	1004 (29.5)	1.01 (0.93–1.10)	0.78
Worsening heart failure	394 (11.6)	449 (13.2)	0.88 (0.77–1.01)	0.06

Hospitalization

	DIGOXIN (N = 3397)	PLACEBO (N = 3403)	RISK RATIO (95% CI)	P VALUE
	no. of patients (%)			
Cardiovascular	1694 (49.9)	1850 (54.4)	0.87 (0.81–0.93)	<0.001
Worsening heart failure	910 (26.8)	1180 (34.7)	0.72 (0.66–0.79)	<0.001

Figure 8.8.2 Effects of digoxin on mortality and hospitalization in heart failure patients in the DIG trial.
Source data from Digitalis Investigation G. The effect of digoxin on mortality and morbidity in patients with heart failure. *N Engl J Med* 1997;336(8):525–33.

endpoints but significantly reduced heart failure hospitalization in HFrEF. In contrast, digoxin had no effect on either mortality or heart failure hospitalization in HFmrEF and HFpEF.

Heart failure and atrial fibrillation

Randomized controlled outcome trials of reasonable size investigating the impact of digitalis glycosides on mortality and morbidity in patients with atrial fibrillation are not available. Only few clinical studies have investigated the effects of digitalis glycosides in atrial fibrillation with and without heart failure. All prospective randomized clinical trials described earlier included patients pretreated with digoxin. This was necessary to achieve the required recruitment numbers because at the time the majority of patients were treated with digitalis glycosides. Potential withdrawal of digoxin by randomization to placebo within these trials does not allow inclusion of patients with atrial fibrillation because of endangering patients receiving digitalis for rate control of atrial fibrillation. Therefore, only patients in sinus rhythm were included in randomized trials such as RADIANCE, PROVED, and the DIG trial.

Prospective studies with low patient numbers performing open-label or placebo-controlled digoxin treatment demonstrated effective overall heart rate control with digoxin at rest and on exertion in patients with atrial fibrillation with and without HFrEF. Rate control with digoxin was comparable to that with beta-blocker and better than with calcium channel blocker monotherapy. The most effective rate control was achieved by combination therapy with beta-blocker and digoxin.[25,26] Similar results were obtained in a post hoc analysis of 2027 patients randomized to rate control in the AFFIRM trial, which primarily compared rate control therapy to rhythm control therapy in atrial fibrillation.[27]

Recently, the RATE-AF trial compared the effects of digoxin to those of bisoprolol in permanent atrial fibrillation within an open-label, randomized trial design. Around 20% of the 160 patients included had an LVEF of <50%. Digoxin was equally effective, compared to bisoprolol, in heart rate control (at rest and on exertion) and there were no significant differences in the primary endpoint of patient-reported quality of life survey (SF-36 questionnaire) and most secondary outcomes. Digoxin was significantly better than bisoprolol in secondary outcomes, including surrogate parameters of heart failure (N-terminal pro-B-type natriuretic peptide (NT-proBNP), NYHA class), but these results should only be considered as hypothesis-generating.[28]

Assumption versus evidence from clinical trials

Numerous studies retrospectively investigated the treatment effects of digoxin on mortality and morbidity in heart failure and/ or atrial fibrillation. Observational studies, analyses of registries, secondary analyses of randomized clinical trials primarily performed for other purposes, or meta-analyses reported conflicting results: whereas some studies reported an association of digoxin treatment with increased mortality, others indicated a neutral effect or reduced mortality with digoxin treatment[29] (sometimes even based on analyses of the same data by different investigators).[30,31,32] A comprehensive meta-analysis including a very large number of all available observational and experimental studies demonstrated that increases in mortality in patients treated with digoxin are most likely driven by prescription bias: clinical deterioration leads the treating physician to prescribe an additional drug (e.g. digoxin) and consequently sicker patients are more likely treated with digoxin than healthier patients.[33]

The existence of significant prescription bias for digoxin treatment was proven by further analysis of the DIG trial. Forty-four per cent of patients in the DIG trial were pretreated with digoxin. Consistent with the overall trial results described above, independently of pretreatment with digoxin, randomization to digoxin had a neutral effect on mortality and significantly reduced heart failure hospitalization (⊃ Figure 8.8.3a). In contrast, 'observational' non-randomized pretreatment with digoxin before randomization was associated with increased mortality and hospitalization in the trial populations, independent of randomization to placebo or to digoxin, even after adjustment for baseline population differences (⊃ Figure 8.8.3b). The higher risk of both outcomes in those who had previously received digoxin persisted even if they received placebo during the trial.[34] Overall, based on available data from placebo-controlled clinical trials investigating the effect of randomized digoxin treatment, there is no evidence that digoxin increases mortality but rather reduces heart failure hospitalization in HFrEF. The prescription of digoxin is an indicator of disease severity and worse prognosis, which cannot be fully accounted for by statistical adjustments of non-randomized data retrospectively analysed.[34,35]

Ongoing clinical trials with digitalis in heart failure (and atrial fibrillation)

Heart failure with reduced ejection fraction

Despite the evidence for a potential benefit of digitalis treatment in HFrEF, an open question still remains of whether digitalis glycosides improve outcomes in those patients treated with contemporary guideline-directed heart failure therapy. This is important, because after completion of the DIG trial, different pharmacological (beta-blockers, MRAs, angiotensin receptor-neprilysin inhibitors (ARNIs), sodium–glucose cotransporter 2 (SGLT2) inhibitors) and device (cardiac resynchronization therapy, implantable cardioverter–defibrillator) therapies demonstrated improved outcomes in HFrEF. In particular, the lack of mortality-reducing beta-blocker therapy in the DIG trial was criticized. However, digitalis is a very cheap market-authorized drug in many countries and still might be an important option, especially if use of contemporary state-of-the-art heart failure therapy is limited due to cost reasons.

A significant number of patients with heart failure suffer from atrial fibrillation. Compared to patients in sinus rhythm, these patients have a worse prognosis, morbidity, and quality of life.[36] Importantly, individual-patient data analyses from randomized beta-blocker trials in HFrEF revealed a significant reduction in mortality and hospitalization for heart failure only in patients in sinus rhythm and a neutral effect on these endpoints in patients with atrial fibrillation.[37] Thus, there is high need to find medications improving outcomes in patients with HFrEF and atrial fibrillation.[38] Results from the RATE-AF trial are promising, demonstrating safe use and potential beneficial effects of digoxin, compared to bisoprolol, on surrogate parameters of quality of life and heart failure in patients with permanent atrial fibrillation and heart failure symptoms.[28]

In sum, potential beneficial effects of digitalis at low serum concentrations in HFrEF have to be confirmed in prospective, randomized trials including patients in sinus rhythm as well as those with atrial fibrillation. Two of these trials, both funded by public organizations, are ongoing, as described below.

The DIGitoxin to Improve ouTcomes in patients with advanced chronic Heart Failure (DIGIT-HF) trial is a pragmatic, multicentre, randomized, double-blind, parallel-group, placebo-controlled phase 4 trial. The objective is to demonstrate that digitoxin at serum concentrations of 8–18 ng/mL, on top of contemporary guideline-directed heart failure therapy, reduces the composite endpoint of all-cause mortality or first hospital admission for worsening HF in patients with advanced chronic HFrEF (NYHA classes III and IV and LVEF ≤40%, or NYHA class II and LVEF ≤30%).[39] Investigators of the DIGIT-HF trial chose digitoxin for two reasons. First, digitoxin displays advantageous pharmacological properties, compared to digoxin, ensuring more stable serum concentrations, even in patients with advanced renal failure. Second, prospective trials on heart failure outcomes with digitoxin are missing.

Similarly, the Digoxin Evaluation in Chronic heart failure: Investigational Study In Outpatients in the Netherlands (DECISION) trial using digoxin was initiated. This trial examines whether low serum concentrations of digoxin (0.5–0.9 ng/mL) reduces the primary composite endpoint of (repeated) heart failure hospitalization and cardiovascular mortality in heart failure patients (NYHA class II—ambulatory IV) with reduced or mid-range ejection fractions (LVEF <50%) (ClinicalTrials.gov identifier: NCT03783429).

Although DIGIT-HF includes patients with more advanced chronic HFrEF and DECISION includes heart failure patients with an LVEF of up to 49%, both trials will independently provide important evidence of whether the cardiac glycosides digitoxin and digoxin have beneficial effects on outcomes in patients with HFrEF. Notably, both trials include patients in sinus rhythm and those with atrial fibrillation.

Heart failure with preserved ejection fraction

Results from the DIG ancillary trial indicate neutral effects of digitalis on outcomes in patients suffering from HFpEF in sinus rhythm.[24] Keeping in mind that the ancillary DIG trial represented a low-risk population (approximately 75% in NYHA classes I and II) with low event rates and digoxin serum concentrations were available only in a minority of patients, the question remains as to whether HFpEF patients with advanced stages of heart failure and in sinus rhythm might benefit from digitalis treatment with low serum concentrations.

Patients with permanent atrial fibrillation included in the RATE-AF trial predominantly represented a HFpEF patient population. Improvement in some surrogate parameters of heart failure and atrial fibrillation by digoxin within low serum concentrations in RATE-AF[28] might indicate a potential benefit on more robust outcomes in patients suffering from HFpEF and atrial fibrillation. Therefore, clinical trials investigating digoxin effects in HFpEF, which are still lacking, should focus on populations with advanced heart failure and/or atrial fibrillation and target low digitalis serum concentrations.

Recommendations for clinical use of digitalis

Outcome data regarding the effects of digitalis glycosides in heart failure patients treated with contemporary guideline-directed pharmacotherapy and/or device therapy are missing. Nevertheless, available data from randomized clinical trials on digitalis glycosides provide good evidence that use of digitalis glycosides in patients with heart failure, but also in those with atrial fibrillation, is safe within low serum concentrations. Serum concentrations exceeding ranges provided in ➲ Dose and target serum concentrations should be avoided to prevent side effects and adverse outcomes. Randomized trial data indicate favourable effects of digitalis glycosides within low serum concentrations on outcomes in patients with HFrEF and in sinus rhythm. Of these, in particular high-risk patients (LVEF <25%, NYHA class ≥ III) seem to benefit. Especially if initiation or continuation of modern pharmacological and device therapy in HFrEF is limited due to comorbidities or advanced disease (e.g. hypotension, advanced renal dysfunction), digitalis treatment still represents one of the few remaining therapeutic options to improve symptoms, exercise capacity, and quality of life, and importantly even may attenuate repeated heart failure hospitalizations.

The following recommendations for safe use of digitalis glycosides in clinical practice are provided for different clinical indications (➲ Figure 8.8.4):

- Sinus rhythm:
  - *HFrEF*: in patients treated with ACE inhibitor (or angiotensin receptor blocker/ARNI), beta-blocker, MRA, SGLT2 inhibitor, and device therapy (cardiac resynchronization therapy) and, *in particular, if use of these therapies is limited*:
    - NYHA classes II–IV: digitalis glycosides may be considered to reduce the risk of hospitalization (all-cause and heart failure-related).[40]
    - NYHA classes III and IV or LVEF <25%: digitalis glycosides should be considered to improve symptoms and exercise capacity, and to reduce the risk of hospitalization (all-cause and heart failure-related), according to a subanalysis of the DIG trial[22] (in our view).
  - *HFmrEF/HFpEF*: digitalis glycosides are not recommended.
- Atrial fibrillation: sufficient rate control with beta-blocker.
  - *HFrEF*: in patients with contemporary guideline-directed pharmacological or device therapy (see earlier) and, in particular, if use of these therapies is limited and:
    - NYHA classes III and IV: digitalis glycosides may be considered to improve symptoms, haemodynamics, and

(a) Randomization

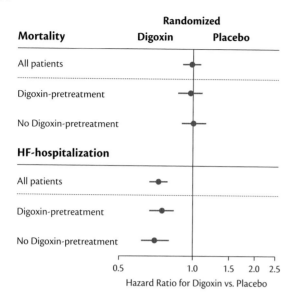

Table 8.2.3 Digoxin dosage and serum concentration

	Daily dose	Target serum concentration	
Digoxin	0.0625–0.25 mg	0.5–0.9 ng/mL	(0.65–1.15 mmol/L)
Digitoxin	0.035–0.1 mg	8–18 ng/mL	(10.5–23.6 mmol/L)

exercise. Optimal rate control should be guided by symptoms (NYHA class, European Heart Rhythm Association (EHRA) score), LVEF impairment, and haemodynamics (blood pressure) for the individual patient.[40]

- NYHA class IV/acute heart failure: digitalis glycosides are recommended for rapid rate control, preferably initiated by administration of an intravenous loading dose followed by an oral maintenance dose.[40]

Dose and target serum concentrations

Importantly, treatment of heart failure patients with digitalis glycosides for the clinical scenarios described above has to target low serum concentrations (➲ Table 8.2.3).

- *Initiation of treatment*: treatment is started *per os* with a maintenance dose. Initiation of treatment with a loading dose (orally or intravenously, depending on haemodynamic stability) should only be used in the setting of acute heart failure or decompensation due to tachycardic atrial fibrillation.
- *HFrEF, sinus rhythm, and eGFR ≥60 mL/min*: due to available evidence from clinical trials, digoxin use should be the first choice.
- *eGFR <60 mL/min*: digitoxin may be the first choice; digoxin has to be used with caution because of an increased risk of elevated serum concentrations due to its primarily renal elimination.

Future directions

We need more data on digitalis glycosides for patients with heart failure and/or atrial fibrillation who are treated with current standard therapies. Two ongoing large trials including HFrEF patients with and without atrial fibrillation will define the role of digitalis glycosides on top of modern HFrEF treatment: DECISION and DIGIT-HF. Also specific patient groups such as those with acute decompensated heart failure are in need of more efficient treatments. Digitalis glycosides may also be of value in this population that is almost devoid of any evidence-based therapy.

(b) Observational study

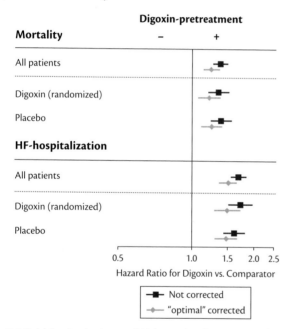

Figure 8.8.3 (a) Randomized versus (b) 'observational' comparison of digoxin effects on mortality and heart failure (HF) hospitalizations in the DIG trial.
Reproduced from Aguirre Dávila L, Weber K, Bavendiek U, Bauersachs J, Wittes J, Yusuf S, Koch A. Digoxin-mortality: randomized vs. observational comparison in the DIG trial. *Eur Heart J.* 2019 Oct 21;40(40):3336–3341. doi: 10.1093/eurheartj/ehz395 with permission Oxford University Press.

Summary and key messages

Digitalis glycosides have still their role as second-line drugs for heart failure, especially for advanced HFrEF when first-line treatments are maximized or not tolerated, and for atrial fibrillation with high heart rate despite beta-blocker treatment. Digitalis glycosides should be given with caution, as the therapeutic window is narrow and serious side effects may occur. Determination of target serum concentrations is recommended 3–4 weeks after start of treatment, with adaptation of the dosage accordingly. Especially for digoxin that is almost exclusively

exercise capacity (in our view, although there is no evidence from clinical trials).

- *HFmrEF/HFpEF*: digitalis glycosides are not recommended.
- Atrial fibrillation: insufficient rate-control with beta-blocker use.
- *HFpEF/HFmrEF/HFrEF*:
  - NYHA classes I–III: digitalis glycosides are recommended to achieve sufficient rate control at rest and on

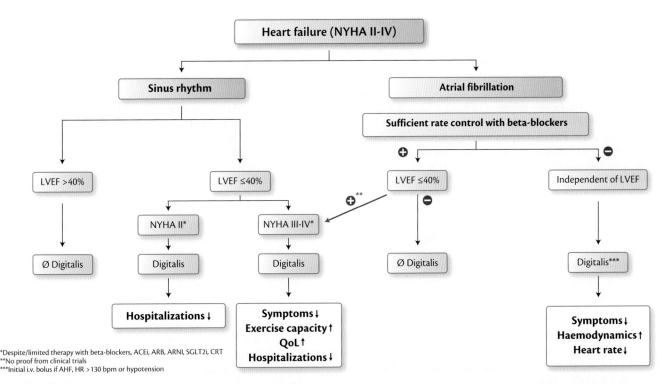

Figure 8.8.4 Recommendations for use of digitalis glycosides in heart failure. ACE, angiotensin-converting enzyme inhibitor; AF, atrial fibrillation; AHF, acute heart failure; ARB, angiotensin receptor blocker; ARNI, angiotensin receptor–neprylisin inhibitor; BB, beta-blocker; CRT, cardiac resynchronisation therapy; HR, heart rate; LVEF, left ventricular ejection fraction; QoL, quality of life; SGLT2i, sodium–glucose cotransporter 2 inhibitor; SR, sinus rhythm.

cleared by the kidney, reduction of the daily dose and repeated determination of the serum concentration are necessary when renal function deteriorates.

References

1. Packer M. Why is the use of digitalis withering? Another reason that we need medical heart failure specialists. Eur J Heart Fail 2018;**20**(5):851–52.

2. Withering W. *An Account of the Foxglove and Some of Its Medical Uses with Practical Remarks on Dropsy and Other Diseases.* London: G. G. J. and J. Robinson; 1785.

3. Crespo-Leiro MG, Anker SD, Maggioni AP, *et al.*; Heart Failure Association (HFA) of the European Society of Cardiology (ESC). European Society of Cardiology Heart Failure Long-Term Registry (ESC-HF-LT): 1-year follow-up outcomes and differences across regions. Eur J Heart Fail 2016;**18**(6):613–25.

4. Patel N, Ju C, Macon C, *et al.* Temporal trends of digoxin use in patients hospitalized with heart failure: analysis from the American Heart Association Get with the Guidelines-Heart Failure Registry. JACC Heart Fail 2016;**4**(5):348–56.

5. Smith TW, Antman EM, Friedman PL, Blatt CM, Marsh JD. Digitalis glycosides: mechanisms and manifestations of toxicity. Part I. Prog Cardiovasc Dis 1984;**26**(5):413–58.

6. Smith TW. Pharmacokinetics, bioavailability and serum levels of cardiac glycosides. J Am Coll Cardiol 1985;**5**(5 Suppl A):43A–50A.

7. Smith TW, Antman EM, Friedman PL, Blatt CM, Marsh JD. Digitalis glycosides: mechanisms and manifestations of toxicity. Part II. Prog Cardiovasc Dis 1984;**26**(6):495–540.

8. Hauptman PJ, Kelly RA. Digitalis. Circulation 1999;**99**(9):1265–70.

9. Gheorghiade M, Ferguson D. Digoxin. A neurohormonal modulator in heart failure? Circulation 1991;**84**(5):2181–6.

10. Belz GG, Breithaupt-Grogler K, Osowski U. Treatment of congestive heart failure: current status of use of digitoxin. Eur J Clin Invest 2001;**31**(Suppl 2):10–17.

11. Digitalis Investigation Group. The effect of digoxin on mortality and morbidity in patients with heart failure. N Engl J Med 1997;**336**(8):525–33.

12. Rathore SS, Curtis JP, Wang Y, Bristow MR, Krumholz HM. Association of serum digoxin concentration and outcomes in patients with heart failure. JAMA 2003;**289**(7):871–8.

13. Adams KF Jr, Patterson JH, Gattis WA, *et al.* Relationship of serum digoxin concentration to mortality and morbidity in women in the Digitalis Investigation Group trial: a retrospective analysis. J Am Coll Cardiol 2005;**46**(3):497–504.

14. Ahmed A, Rich MW, Love TE, *et al.* Digoxin and reduction in mortality and hospitalization in heart failure: a comprehensive post hoc analysis of the DIG trial. Eur Heart J 2006;**27**(2):178–86.

15. Bavendiek U, Aguirre Davila L, Schwab J, *et al.*; DIGIT-HF Study Group. Digitoxin serum concentrations affecting patient safety and potential outcome in patients with HFrEF—analyses of the ongoing DIGIT-HF-trial. Eur Heart J 2017;**38**:P6168.

16. Smith TW, Antman EM, Friedman PL, Blatt CM, Marsh JD. Digitalis glycosides: mechanisms and manifestations of toxicity. Part III. Prog Cardiovasc Dis 1984;**27**(1):21–56.

17. Guyatt GH, Sullivan MJ, Fallen EL, *et al.* A controlled trial of digoxin in congestive heart failure. Am J Cardiol 1988;**61**(4):371–5.

18. Bussey HI, Hawkins DW, Gaspard JJ, Walsh RA. A comparative trial of digoxin and digitoxin in the treatment of congestive heart failure. Pharmacotherapy 1988;**8**(4):235–40.

19. Packer M, Gheorghiade M, Young JB, *et al.* Withdrawal of digoxin from patients with chronic heart failure treated with angiotensin-converting-enzyme inhibitors. RADIANCE Study. N Engl J Med 1993;**329**(1):1–7.

20. Uretsky BF, Young JB, Shahidi FE, Yellen LG, Harrison MC, Jolly MK. Randomized study assessing the effect of digoxin withdrawal in patients with mild to moderate chronic congestive heart failure: results of the PROVED trial. PROVED Investigative Group. J Am Coll Cardiol 1993;**22**(4):955–62.

21. Rathore SS, Wang Y, Krumholz HM. Sex-based differences in the effect of digoxin for the treatment of heart failure. N Engl J Med 2002;**347**(18):1403–11.

22. Gheorghiade M, Patel K, Filippatos G, et al. Effect of oral digoxin in high-risk heart failure patients: a pre-specified subgroup analysis of the DIG trial. Eur J Heart Fail 2013;**15**(5):551–9.

23. Abdul-Rahim AH, Shen L, Rush CJ, Jhund PS, Lees KR, McMurray JJV; VICCTA-Heart Failure Collaborators. Effect of digoxin in patients with heart failure and mid-range (borderline) left ventricular ejection fraction. Eur J Heart Fail 2018;**20**(7):1139–45.

24. Ahmed A, Rich MW, Fleg JL, et al. Effects of digoxin on morbidity and mortality in diastolic heart failure: the Ancillary Digitalis Investigation Group trial. Circulation 2006;**114**(5):397–403.

25. Farshi R, Kistner D, Sarma JS, Longmate JA, Singh BN. Ventricular rate control in chronic atrial fibrillation during daily activity and programmed exercise: a crossover open-label study of five drug regimens. J Am Coll Cardiol 1999;**33**(2):304–10.

26. Khand AU, Rankin AC, Martin W, Taylor J, Gemmell I, Cleland JG. Carvedilol alone or in combination with digoxin for the management of atrial fibrillation in patients with heart failure? J Am Coll Cardiol 2003;**42**(11):1944–51.

27. Olshansky B, Rosenfeld LE, Warner AL, et al.; AFFIRM Investigators. The Atrial Fibrillation Follow-up Investigation of Rhythm Management (AFFIRM) study: approaches to control rate in atrial fibrillation. J Am Coll Cardiol 2004;**43**(7):1201–8.

28. Kotecha D, Bunting KV, Gill SK, et al.; Rate Control Therapy Evaluation in Permanent Atrial Fibrillation (RATE-AF) Team. Effect of digoxin vs bisoprolol for heart rate control in atrial fibrillation on patient-reported quality of life: the RATE-AF randomized clinical trial. JAMA 2020;**324**(24):2497–508.

29. Bavendiek U, Aguirre Davila L, Koch A, Bauersachs J. Assumption versus evidence: the case of digoxin in atrial fibrillation and heart failure. Eur Heart J 2017;**38**(27):2095–9.

30. Whitbeck MG, Charnigo RJ, Khairy P, et al. Increased mortality among patients taking digoxin: analysis from the AFFIRM study. Eur Heart J 2013;**34**(20):1481–8.

31. Gheorghiade M, Fonarow GC, van Veldhuisen DJ, et al. Lack of evidence of increased mortality among patients with atrial fibrillation taking digoxin: findings from post hoc propensity-matched analysis of the AFFIRM trial. Eur Heart J 2013;**34**(20):1489–97.

32. Patel NJ, Hoosien M, Deshmukh A, et al. Digoxin significantly improves all-cause mortality in atrial fibrillation patients with severely reduced left ventricular systolic function. Int J Cardiol 2013;**169**(5):e84–6.

33. Ziff OJ, Lane DA, Samra M, et al. Safety and efficacy of digoxin: systematic review and meta-analysis of observational and controlled trial data. BMJ 2015;**351**:h4451.

34. Aguirre Davila L, Weber K, Bavendiek U, et al. Digoxin-mortality: randomized vs. observational comparison in the DIG trial. Eur Heart J 2019;**40**(40):3336–41.

35. Rush CJ, Campbell RT, Jhund PS, Petrie MC, McMurray JJV. Association is not causation: treatment effects cannot be estimated from observational data in heart failure. Eur Heart J 2018;**39**(37):3417–38.

36. Kotecha D, Piccini JP. Atrial fibrillation in heart failure: what should we do? Eur Heart J 2015;**36**(46):3250–7.

37. Kotecha D, Holmes J, Krum H, et al.; Beta-Blockers in Heart Failure Collaborative Group. Efficacy of beta blockers in patients with heart failure plus atrial fibrillation: an individual-patient data meta-analysis. Lancet 2014;**384**(9961):2235–43.

38. Bauersachs J, Veltmann C. Heart rate control in heart failure with reduced ejection fraction: the bright and the dark side of the moon. Eur J Heart Fail 2020;**22**(3):539–42.

39. Bavendiek U, Berliner D, Davila LA, et al.; DIGIT-HF Investigators and Committees. Rationale and design of the DIGIT-HF trial (DIGitoxin to Improve ouTcomes in patients with advanced chronic Heart Failure): a randomized, double-blind, placebo-controlled study. Eur J Heart Fail 2019;**21**(5):676–84.

40. McDonagh TA, Metra M, Adamo M, et al.; ESC Scientific Document Group. 2021 ESC Guidelines for the diagnosis and treatment of acute and chronic heart failure. Eur Heart J 2021;**42**(36):3599–726.

CHAPTER 8.9

Diuretics

Jeroen Dauw, Stephen Gottlieb,
and Wilfried Mullens

Contents

Introduction: a historical perspective on diuretic therapy

Fluid overload, called 'dropsy', has been recognized as a disease entity since ancient history, treated with a variety of measures, including emetics, induced excessive sweating, and evacuating fluids from the lower legs and body cavities by puncturing. It took until the second half of the past century before the modern diuretic classes were introduced.[1] Mercurials were used up to the 1960s to treat fluid overload in heart failure, but they came with a cost of potential serious toxicity. Acetazolamide became the first available oral diuretic in 1954, increasing renal sodium (Na^+) excretion in combination with bicarbonate. However, its efficacy was reduced after only 5 days due to compensatory mechanisms,[2] and the acidifying effect limited its chronic use in patients. Chlorothiazide was developed a year later. Thiazides had the advantage of inducing a diuretic effect that was sustained longer than that of acetazolamide, and it thus had rapid uptake in clinical practice.[3] A decade later, a new potent diuretic was discovered and called 'frusemide'; it was much more powerful than thiazides in increasing urine output and renal Na^+ excretion.[4] Shortly thereafter, potassium-sparing diuretics, such as spironolactone and triamterene, became available and provided a solution for the potassium loss caused by the other diuretic agents. Since then, increasing insights into renal physiology have led to a better understanding of the pharmacokinetics of diuretics. In this chapter, the pharmacokinetics and pharmacodynamics of the different diuretic classes are explored and attention is given to their use in an integrative approach in the treatment of heart failure.

Renal sodium handling and alterations in heart failure

As most diuretics are aimed at increasing renal Na^+ excretion, it is important to understand normal renal Na^+ handling and alterations which occur due to heart failure. The amount of Na^+ that is freely filtered at the glomerulus depends on the glomerular filtration rate (GFR). Under normal circumstances, the kidney manages to keep the GFR stable despite changes in mean arterial pressure. Different mechanisms regulate the vascular tone of the afferent and efferent arterioles, and these maintain renal blood flow and intraglomerular capillary pressures. In states of decreased renal blood flow, such as heart failure, the GFR is also maintained by increased filtration fraction. Slower flow through the glomerulus allows for longer filtration time and thus increases the fraction of plasma that is filtered in Bowman's space. As a consequence, the blood leaving the intraglomerular capillaries and flowing towards the peritubular capillary network is more concentrated and has a higher oncotic pressure.

At the proximal convoluted tubule, the majority (65%) of Na^+ is reabsorbed via exchange with H^+ or in conjunction with phosphate, organic solutes, amino acids, and glucose. Carbonic anhydrase plays a key role, as it drives the Na^+/H^+ exchange by catalysing the formation of water (H_2O) and carbon dioxide (CO_2) intraluminally and the opposite reaction intracellularly, resulting in net Na^+ and bicarbonate reabsorption (➲ Figure 8.9.1). Of note, the sodium–glucose cotransporter 2 (SGLT2) is situated in this segment. In heart failure, Na^+ reabsorption at the proximal tubule is increased (up to 75%) for various reasons.[5] First, an increased filtration fraction increases the capillary oncotic pressure, promoting Na^+ reabsorption. Second, angiotensin II directly stimulates the Na^+/H^+ exchanger. Third, lymphatic flow increases and washes out interstitial proteins, with a lower interstitial colloid oncotic pressure and higher Na^+ reabsorption as a result.

The thick ascending part of the loop of Henle reabsorbs approximately 25% of Na^+ via the $Na^+–K^+–2Cl^-$ cotransporter 2 (NKCC2). Importantly, the macula densa is situated at this site, playing a central role in the tubuloglomerular feedback. Decreased chloride (Cl^-) uptake via NKCC2 through macula densa cells serves as a signal of decreased GFR and leads to secretion of prostaglandin E2 and nitric oxide. This relaxes the afferent arteriole and subsequently increases renal blood flow, intraglomerular pressure, and GFR. In addition, juxtaglomerular cells release renin, activating the renin–angiotensin–aldosterone axis. Angiotensin II increases the efferent arteriolar tone, further increasing the intraglomerular pressure and GFR. In patients with heart failure, higher reabsorption of ions at the proximal tubule leads to lower delivery of Na^+ and Cl^- to the loop of Henle. As a consequence, the already high renin secretion and neurohormonal activation are further increased. In addition, loop diuretics interfere with Cl^- uptake by blocking NKCC2, also aggravating neurohormonal activation.

The distal convoluted tubule (5%) and collecting duct (5%) are both responsible for the remaining Na^+ reabsorption. The Na^+/Cl^- cotransporter (NCC) reabsorbs Na^+ at the distal convoluted tubule. In heart failure, their activity is enhanced due to neurohormonal activation. In the case of chronic loop diuretic use, hypertrophy of distal tubular cells can occur,[6] leading to increased Na^+ reabsorption and diminished efficacy of loop diuretics (➲ Diuretic resistance, p. 526). At the collecting duct, the epithelial Na^+ channel (eNAC) allows the reabsorption of the remaining Na^+. As its activity is upregulated by aldosterone, heart failure also increases Na^+ reabsorption in this segment. Last, the collecting tubules also contain specific aquaporin channels, allowing for water reabsorption as the distal convoluted tubule and collecting ducts are otherwise impermeable to water (in contrast to other segments). The number of aquaporin channels is regulated by arginine–vasopressin (AVP), with higher levels leading to more water reabsorption. As heart failure is associated with elevated AVP levels, water reabsorption is increased. In general, reabsorption at the distal tubule and collecting duct are an important process in the dilution of urine and water homeostasis. Dysregulation of these segments due to heart failure not only leads to increased Na^+ reabsorption, but also can impair regulation of osmolality leading to hyponatraemia.

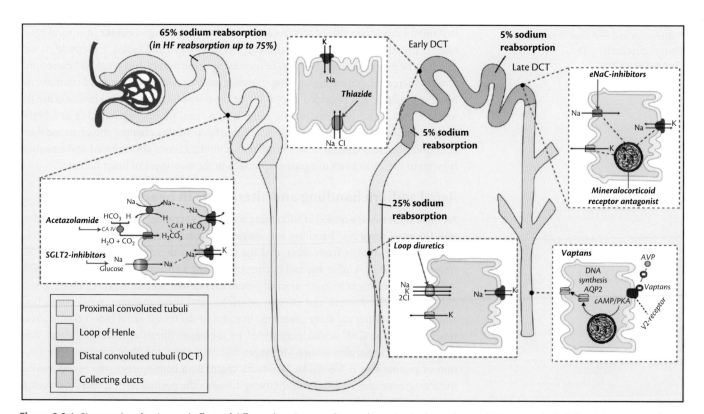

Figure 8.9.1 Sites, modes of action, and effects of different diuretics on sodium reabsorption in the nephron. AQP2, aquaporin 2; AVP, arginine vasopressin; cAMP, cyclic adenosine monophosphate; eNAC, epithelial sodium channel; HF, heart failure; PKA, protein kinase A; SGLT2, sodium–glucose cotransporter 2.
Reproduced from Mullens W, Damman K, Harjola VP, *et al*. The use of diuretics in heart failure with congestion — a position statement from the Heart Failure Association of the European Society of Cardiology. *Eur J Heart Fail*. 2019 Feb;21(2):137–155. doi: 10.1002/ejhf.1369 with permission from John Wiley and Sons.

In conclusion, even in healthy individuals, almost all filtered Na^+ is reabsorbed along the tubule, leading to a loss of only 1–2% of the filtered Na^+ (also called fractional sodium excretion). In heart failure, the discussed alterations further increase Na^+ reabsorption and can lead to a fractional sodium excretion of <1%.

Diuretic classes

Different diuretic classes are now available for treatment of volume overload. Despite their name, most act primarily by increasing renal Na^+ excretion and are actually 'natriuretics'. The only exceptions are vasopressin antagonists (and osmotic diuretics). The pharmacological properties of the most potent diuretic classes are displayed in ➲ Table 8.9.1 and further discussed below.

Loop diuretics

Loop diuretics are the most potent diuretic class and can augment fractional sodium excretion by up to 25%. They are the mainstay treatment for volume overload in heart failure. Furosemide, bumetanide, and torsemide are the three loop diuretics currently available. They all work by blocking Na^+ reabsorption via the NKCC2 at the ascending loop of Henle. As a consequence, they also increase renal potassium, Cl^-, and magnesium excretion. Furosemide and bumetanide are both short-working agents (4–6 hours), whereas torsemide has a longer duration of action (up to 18 hours). In addition, the bioavailability after oral intake is highly variable for furosemide and diminishes with simultaneous food intake. In contrast, bumetanide and torsemide have high bioavailability and absorption of torsemide is not influenced by food. Although loop diuretics are highly protein-bound (>90%), hypoalbuminaemia has no relevant effect on pharmacokinetics as long as it is >20 g/L (2 g/dL). Loop diuretics are not filtered at the glomerulus but are actively secreted at the proximal tubule. Organic anion transporters (OATs) on the basolateral side are responsible for uptake, whereas intraluminal secretion is performed by the multidrug resistance protein 4 (Mrp4). Other organic anions such as urate, as well as drugs such as statins, angiotensin-converting enzyme (ACE) inhibitors and β-lactam antibiotics, are secreted via the same mechanism, and high plasma levels of these agents might reduce the tubular levels of loop diuretics.[7] This is especially important in the case of chronic kidney disease (CKD), as this is associated with higher circulating levels of organic anions and urate, as well as acidosis, all interfering with uptake and luminal secretion of loop diuretics; higher loop diuretic dosing is needed in these patients. However, furosemide is metabolized in the kidney, which is responsible for 90% of its elimination, and thus furosemide can accumulate and lead to toxicity in CKD. In contrast, bumetanide and torsemide are both dependent on hepatic and renal clearance and are thus safer in CKD.

Because intestinal congestion could interfere with loop diuretic reabsorption in acute heart failure, guidelines recommend administering loop diuretics intravenously (Class I, Level of evidence B). The dose–response curve of loop diuretics shows a

Table 8.9.1 Pharmacology of the most potent diuretic classes

Site of action	Proximal tubule	Loop diuretics Ascending loop of Henle			Thiazides Distal convoluted tubule			
Drugs	Acetazolamide	Furosemide	Bumetanide	Torsemide	Hydrochlorothiazide	Metolazone	Chlortalidone	Indapamide
Dose equivalents within class (mg)	–	40	1	20	50	2.5	25	1.25
Oral bioavailability (%)	Unknown	10–100	80–100	80–100	65–75	40–65	60–70	~90
Absorption affected by food	No	Yes (worse)	Yes (worse)	No	Unknown	Unknown	Unknown	Unknown
Half-life (hours)	2.5–5.4	1.5–3	1–1.5	3–6	6–15	14–20	40–60	14–24
Onset of action Oral (hours) Intravenous (min)	1 2	1–2 5	1–2 2–3	1–2 10	2 –	1 –	2–3 –	1–2 –
Duration of action (hours)	8–12	4–6	4–6	6–8	6–12	12–24	24–72	24–36
Renal elimination (%)	90	50	50% (hepatic)	20	95	80	65	70
Dosing (mg), oral: Start Maintenance Maximal total daily dose	250 250–375 500*	20–40 40–240 600	0.5–1 1–5 10	5–10 10–20 200	25 25–100 200	2.5 2.5–10 20	25 25–100 200	1.25 1.25–5 5
Potency (FENa%)	4	20–25			5–8			

* The standard intravenous dosing for acetazolamide is 500 mg.

FENa, fractional excretion of sodium.

Source data from Mullens W, Damman K, Harjola VP, *et al.* The use of diuretics in heart failure with congestion — a position statement from the Heart Failure Association of the European Society of Cardiology. *Eur J Heart Fail.* 2019 Feb;21(2):137–155. doi: 10.1002/ejhf.1369.

sigmoidal logarithmic relationship (➲ Figure 8.9.2), which has several implications for correct dosing. First, a certain threshold level has to be reached before the diuretic exerts its effect. In patients with heart failure, this threshold is higher due to the above-mentioned renal alterations. In CKD, the threshold is higher and the curve is shifted to the right. Second, as the scale is logarithmic, the dose should be multiplied in a stepwise manner, instead of linearly increased. This is why it is reasonable to double the dose when the diuretic response is insufficient. Third, there is a ceiling dose above which no additional natriuresis is achieved. However, higher dosing could prolong the time at ceiling levels. The ceiling is decreased in patients with heart failure, as well as in those with CKD.

Repeated dosing can be a solution to tackle the lower peak response in these patients, as both bumetanide and furosemide are short-acting. However, despite inducing a similar urine output, natriuresis decreases with repeated loop diuretic administration (the braking phenomenon).[8] If administered once daily, furosemide induces a diuretic response over 6 hours, followed by a post-diuretic Na^+ retention phase through the rest of the day.[9] Depending on the dietary salt intake, this retention phase could compensate for the diuretic-induced Na^+ loss. Sufficient salt restriction tackles this in healthy individuals, but severe salt restriction in acute heart failure is debated. Moreover, hypertonic saline infusions have been associated with better natriuresis, although data are too limited to support its use. If

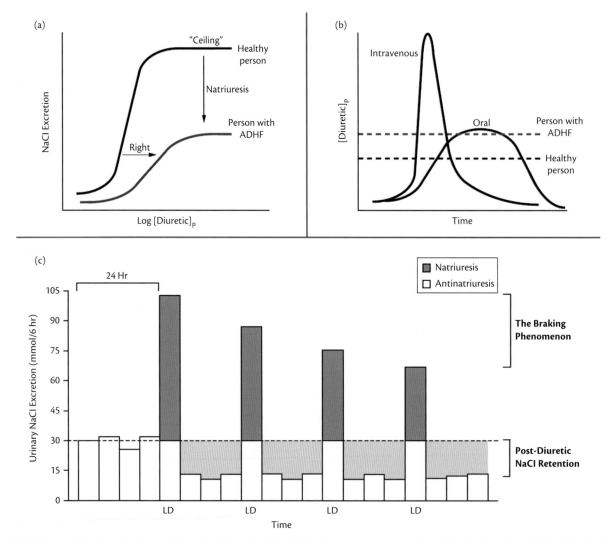

Figure 8.9.2 Pharmacokinetics and pharmacodynamics of loop diuretics. (a) The dose–response curve of loop diuretics has a sigmoidal logarithmic shape in healthy volunteers, as well as in patients with acute decompensated heart failure (ADHF). The curve shows a rightward shift for ADHF, with a higher threshold necessary to get a diuretic effect and a lower 'ceiling', meaning lower maximal natriuresis can be achieved. (b) Plasma concentration curves over time for an oral loop diuretic dose and an equivalent intravenous bolus dose are displayed, with an indicated threshold concentration for healthy persons and patients with ADHF. An intravenous bolus dose easily surpasses the diuretic threshold in ADHF, whereas an oral dose might rise to just only a little above the threshold. (c) Panel showing repeated loop diuretic doses (LD) once daily on consecutive days, with bars indicating sodium chloride (NaCl) excretion in a 6-hour collection. Diuretic administrations are followed by post-diuretic sodium retention during the rest of the day. Repeated dosing leads to lower response to every new administration (braking phenomenon).

Reproduced from Ellison DH, Felker GM. Diuretic Treatment in Heart Failure. *N Engl J Med*. 2017 Nov 16;377(20):1964–1975. doi: 10.1056/NEJMra1703100. Erratum in: *N Engl J Med*. 2018 Feb 1;378(5):492. with permission from Massachusetts Medical Society.

the same loop diuretic dose is repeated the following day, a new loop diuretic response phase is induced over 6 hours, but total natriuresis is lower than the day before. This braking phenomenon might be explained by neurohormonal activation by loop diuretics (➲ Renal sodium handling and alterations in heart failure, p. 517), intravascular depletion due to slow plasma refilling, or depletion of extracellular fluid volume itself. In addition, long-term loop diuretic therapy can induce adaptations at the distal convoluting tubule, with hypertrophy and increased Na$^+$ reabsorption, which hamper diuretic response. Dosing in acute and chronic heart failure are discussed in ➲ Practical use of diuretics, p. 522.

Thiazides

Thiazides block the NCC at the distal convoluted tubule and are used primarily as treatment for hypertension and also for heart failure. Most thiazides also elicit some carbonic anhydrase inhibition, but this does not seem to significantly contribute to their diuretic effect. Thiazides not only lead to higher Na$^+$ and Cl$^-$ excretion, but also increase loss of potassium and magnesium. The thiazide class of diuretics consists of 'true' thiazides (e.g. hydrochlorothiazide) and 'thiazide-like' agents (e.g. metolazone, chlortalidone, indapamide). Although these drugs have a longer duration of action than loop diuretics, their potency is significantly lower, increasing fractional sodium excretion by 5–8%. Except for chlorothiazide, all other thiazides are only available as oral formulations. They have steady bioavailability (>50% in general). Metolazone and chlortalidone have slow absorption, reaching peak levels only after around 8 hours. Thiazides are transported highly protein-bound (75–99%), except for hydrochlorothiazide (40%). Just like loop diuretics, thiazides are not filtered, but secreted at the proximal tubule via OATs and Mrp4. They are thus prone to the same interactions with other inorganic anions and drugs. Most thiazides are renally cleared and can accumulate in CKD. In addition, thiazides are considered ineffective as monotherapy if the GFR is <30 mL/min/1.73 m^2, because both the lower filtration rates and the increased filtration fraction, with higher proximal Na$^+$ reabsorption, lead to less Na$^+$ delivery in the distal tubule. In heart failure, the main role of thiazides is as add-on therapy in cases of insufficient response to loop diuretics alone. Especially in chronic loop diuretic therapy, renal adaptations with distal tubular hypertrophy and increased Na$^+$ reabsorption at this segment might contribute to a decreased diuretic response and these can be overcome by adding a thiazide diuretic. Although metolazone is often considered as the best choice, there is currently no evidence to choose one thiazide over another.[10] Whereas clearly synergistic with loop diuretics, the (sometimes) profound hypokalaemia make these medications risky and mandate close monitoring of electrolytes.

Potassium-sparing diuretics

This class of diuretics inhibit Na$^+$ reabsorption by eNACs at the collecting ducts and consists of direct eNAC inhibitors (triamterene and amiloride) and mineralocorticoid receptor antagonists (MRAs) that regulate eNAC activity by inhibiting the nuclear aldosterone receptor. In general, they are weak diuretics, only increasing fractional sodium excretion by 2%. As this diuretic class does not lead to potassium loss, but rather inhibits potassium secretion at the collecting ducts, they are called 'potassium-sparing diuretics'. In addition, MRAs exhibit other pleiotropic effects in heart failure related to aldosterone inhibition such as reverse cardiac remodelling, inhibition of collagen synthesis, and reduction of malignant arrhythmias. Triamterene is a prodrug that is easily absorbed and rapidly metabolized to active compounds, whereas amiloride is directly active. Protein binding is high (67%) for triamterene, but low (23%) for amiloride. Both are secreted at the proximal tubule via the same mechanisms as loop diuretics and thiazides. These agents have a duration of action of 12–24 hours. Triamterene and amiloride have a limited role in heart failure because there is hardly any evidence for their use and because of their rather weak potency.

In contrast, MRAs are widely used in heart failure, as they have a Class I indication as disease-modifying drugs in heart failure with reduced ejection fraction (HFrEF).[11] Spironolactone is a prodrug that is metabolized into its active form canrenone, whereas eplerenone exerts its effects on the mineralocorticoid receptor directly. As nuclear processing is involved, these drugs have a slow onset of action and might take up to 48 hours to become maximally effective. Both drugs are well absorbed, with a bioavailability of 90% for spironolactone and 69% for eplerenone, and are transported protein-bound. They are not secreted but can pass directly through the basolateral membrane of the collecting duct cells due to their lipid solubility. The half-life of eplerenone is significantly shorter (3–6 hours) than that of canrenone (16.5 hours). In contrast to spironolactone, eplerenone has weaker anti-androgenic effects due to its lower affinity for the steroidal hormone receptor. Although a low dose (25–50 mg) already has important disease-modifying properties in HFrEF, the natriuretic effect is more important at higher doses (≥100 mg). They are primarily used in patients with heart failure as part of guideline-directed medical therapy for their direct cardiac effects and as a preventive measure to avoid hypokalaemia during loop diuretic use.

Proximal tubule diuretics

As most Na$^+$ reabsorption occurs in the proximal tubule and the fraction of reabsorbed Na$^+$ is even increased in heart failure, the proximal tubule seems a good target for diuretic therapy. In addition, blocking sodium chloride reabsorption in the proximal tubule increases Cl$^-$ delivery to the macula densa and could reduce neurohormonal activation. Currently, two agents that block proximal Na$^+$ reabsorption are available: acetazolamide and SGLT2 inhibitors. Acetazolamide inhibits carbonic anhydrase, leading to loss of Na$^+$ and bicarbonate. It has a variable uptake if doses go above 10 mg/kg. It is highly protein-bound (70–90%); it is not metabolized and is mainly eliminated unchanged in the urine. The duration of action of the drug is longer than that of loop diuretics and is up to 24 hours if extended-release formulations are used. In chronic use, the diuretic effects wean off because of compensatory distal Na^+ uptake and acidosis decreasing the available bicarbonate. Its potency is limited with an increase in fractional sodium excretion of 4%, but this is higher than that of potassium-sparing diuretics. Side effects include peripheral neuropathy. Observational studies[12,13] and one small clinical trial[14] indicated that acetazolamide, in conjunction with loop diuretics, can boost diuretic response, resulting in increased natriuresis. The ongoing Acetazolamide in Decompensated Heart Failure With Volume OveRload (ADVOR) trial (ClinicalTrials.gov identifier: NCT03505788) is investigating whether adding intravenous acetazolamide to loop diuretics improves decongestion in acute heart failure.[15]

SGLT2 inhibitors are a new class of heart failure drugs. By blocking the sodium-glucose cotransporter in the proximal tubule, they inhibit Na^+ and glucose reabsorption. SGLT2 inhibitors exert pleiotropic effects beyond increased renal Na^+ excretion and glucosuria. In recent large clinical trials, they reduced heart failure hospitalization and cardiovascular death by 25% in HFrEF,[16,17] although the mechanism underlying the benefit is controversial. The diuretic properties of SGLT2 inhibitors are currently insufficiently understood, with conflicting results regarding the effects on renal Na^+ excretion.[18,19] In a small randomized study, combination of SGLT2 inhibitors with loop diuretics did not result in improved decongestion or natriuresis. In contrast, urine output was higher, probably explained by glucosuria-induced osmotic diuresis.[20] The use of SGLT2 inhibitors and their diuretic properties are the subject of ongoing research in heart failure.

Vasopressin receptor antagonists

Vasopressin receptor antagonists (vaptans) are the only 'true diuretics', as they inhibit aquaporin-mediated water reabsorption at the collecting duct. Vaptans are antagonists of AVP and inhibit their receptor (V_2R) at the collecting duct. As a result, the number of aquaporin channels at the luminal membrane is decreased, leading to less water reabsorption. In addition, some vasopressin antagonists also inhibit $V_{1a}R$, which is localized in vascular smooth muscle cells, leading to vasodilatation. Tolvaptan is an orally administered selective V_2R antagonist and is the only well-studied vasopressin antagonist in heart failure. It has a bioavailability of 56%, and is transported highly protein-bound (>98%) and primarily eliminated by hepatic metabolization. After 2–4 hours, there is onset of action that remains for around 24 hours. In the Efficacy of Vasopressin Antagonism in Heart Failure Outcome Study With Tolvaptan (EVEREST) trial on the addition of tolvaptan in standard 4133 acute heart failure patients, tolvaptan did not improve heart failure rehospitalization or mortality when given for 60 days.[21] In addition, although tolvaptan improved diuresis and weight loss in acute heart failure, it did not improve dyspnoea in two independent recent trials.[22,23] As the primary driver of volume overload in heart failure is Na^+ retention and given the lack of evidence, routine use of vaptans is not indicated. Their potential role in advanced heart failure stages, which is associated with high AVP levels and secondary dilutional hyponatraemia, has to be elucidated in future studies.

Practical use of diuretics

Acute heart failure

Goal of therapy and measurement of diuretic response

Before starting diuretic therapy, good haemodynamic phenotyping of patients is essential to set adequate treatment goals and to determine the need for inotropic/vasodilatory therapy and/or mechanical circulatory support (➲ Chapter 10). In patients with congestion, two distinct types can be recognized: volume overload and volume redistribution. In patients with volume redistribution, splanchnic vasoconstriction and reduced venous capacitance lead to mobilization of pooled blood, increasing preload and filling pressures and resulting in pulmonary oedema.[24] These patients typically only have mild peripheral oedema and tend to present acutely, often associated with hypertension. The main treatment goal should be to increase venous capacitance, which can be targeted with vasodilators. In contrast, patients with volume overload have gained weight, with clear clinical signs of volume overload (peripheral oedema, pleural effusion, and/or ascites). For these patients, the primary treatment goal is to remove the extra fluid, for which diuretics are the first-line treatment.

Different measures of diuretic response have been proposed (➲ Table 8.9.2). Both weight and urine output (and intake) are prone to measurement errors and these measurements are often not congruent.[25] Weight loss and urine output, while clearly of benefit in many patients, have not been associated with improved outcomes, but weight gain is associated with a worse prognosis.[26,27] Urine output can be used as a more direct measure of diuretic response, but collection can be cumbersome without the use of a bladder catheter. Furthermore, urine output does not distinguish between renal Na^+ and water loss. Despite their disadvantages, both urine output and weight loss remain valuable tools to assess diuretic efficacy, with a urine output of >100–150 mL/hour indicating a good response. Recently, urinary Na^+ measurements have

Table 8.9.2 Strengths and weaknesses of different measures of diuretic response

Metric	Reproducibility	Convenience	Plausibility
Weight loss	++	++++	+
Urine output	++++/++*	+++	++
Net fluid loss	+	++	+
Renal sodium excretion	++++/++*	++	+++
Fractional sodium excretion	++++	++	+++
Urinary sodium/ furosemide concentration	++++	+	++++

High reproducibility indicates a low measurement error. Convenience represents the ease of use in clinical practice. Plausibility indicates how much the measurement is related to the direct effect of diuretics.

* With/without bladder catheter.

Source data from Verbrugge FH. Editor's Choice—Diuretic resistance in acute heart failure. *Eur Heart Journal Acute Cardiovasc Care.* 2018;7(4):379–89.

gained interest in assessing diuretic response. High renal Na[+] excretion has been associated with improved outcomes in multiple observational studies[28] and is a better prognosticator than fluid loss.[27] A spot urine sample taken 1–2 hours after loop diuretic administration has a good correlation with total renal Na[+] excretion after 6 hours[29] and allows for early assessment of diuretic response. A urinary Na[+] concentration of >50–70 mmol/L can be considered as a good response. Importantly, for all measurements of diuretic response, the loop diuretic dose, renal function, body composition, and the degree of volume overload should be taken into account when interpreting the results.

Definition of euvolaemia

The final goal of diuretic therapy is to restore extracellular and plasma volume to an 'ideal' euvolaemic state that is adequate to meet metabolic demands without increased filling pressures. This is of great importance as patients who are still congested at discharge have a very poor prognosis.[30] In addition, the European Society of Cardiology (ESC) Guidelines recommend to exclude persistent congestion prior to discharge.[11] However, defining euvolaemia and when it is achieved is subjective and extremely challenging. Clinical signs and relief of dyspnoea as markers of euvolaemia might miss subclinical, but haemodynamically relevant, congestion. A reference weight, based on the patient's weight prior to the acute heart failure event, is often used. Although setting a weight goal might seem reasonable, this does not necessarily represent adequate decongestion.[25] Moreover, heart failure is associated with muscle wasting and cachexia, so that a patient's 'euvolaemic weight' can change over time.

Natriuretic peptides are markers of myocardial wall tension and their levels rise in response to increased filling pressures and drop during diuretic therapy. However, due to their rather slow changes in response to changes in filling pressures and the absence of benefit of N-terminal pro-B-type natriuretic peptide (NT-proBNP)-guided decongestion in a recent trial,[31] the current role of natriuretic peptides as treatment goal is limited. Other biomarkers, such as adrenomedullin, CA-125, and soluble CD146, are being investigated.

Haemoconcentration, measured as a rise in the haematocrit, is a surrogate marker for a reduction in plasma volume and has been proposed as a sign of euvolaemia. However, the haematocrit is defined not only by plasma volume, but also by red blood cell count. As a consequence, anaemia and all its causes influence the haematocrit. In addition, the patient's 'reference haematocrit' is mostly unknown and changes are often small, making it difficult to interpret. Of note, only late haemoconcentration has been associated with improved outcomes. Direct plasma volume measurement using an iodine-131-labelled human serum albumin indicator dilution technique allows setting specific haematocrit treatment goals and might improve heart failure readmissions and mortality,[32] but is prone to the same flaws in case of changes in red blood cell volume.

Importantly, the creatinine level often rises during decongestive treatment and might lead to stopping diuretic treatment because of concerns about kidney injury. This worsening renal function is a common phenomenon but is not necessarily associated with worse prognosis. In particular, patients who respond well to diuretic therapy have a better prognosis than those without worsening renal function but with ongoing congestion at discharge.[33] In addition, often there are no markers of tubular injury present in cases of worsening renal function.[34] Thus, in cases of good diuretic response, worsening renal function should not hamper diuretic treatment. In contrast, in cases of worsening renal function with a poor diuretic response, other approaches to symptomatic improvement may be needed.[35]

Different imaging techniques allow to assess congestion and might be useful to guide treatment.[36] With echocardiography, left- and right-sided filling pressures can be estimated, but there are no data to support its use to guide decongestive treatment. Lung ultrasound is a recently introduced technique, which can directly visualize pulmonary oedema and has a higher sensitivity and specificity than chest X-ray for diagnosing acute heart failure.[37] In a small trial, tailoring of diuretic therapy, based upon lung ultrasound after acute heart failure admission, reduced worsening heart failure and mortality,[38] but more data are necessary to support its use as a tool to guide decongestion.

In conclusion, no single parameter can be used to determine euvolaemia. Probably an integrative approach using clinical signs, biomarkers, and imaging techniques is the best method (➲ Figure 8.9.3).

Treatment regimen and dosing

A flow chart on the use of diuretics and assessment of diuretic response, as proposed by the Heart Failure Association and endorsed by the ESC Guidelines, is displayed in ➲ Figure 8.9.4.[11,39a] Loop diuretics are the first-line agents to treat volume overload, as they are the most potent diuretics. In acute heart failure, high central venous pressures lead to intestinal oedema, with reduced perfusion, which can interfere with normal absorption of diuretics. Moreover, renal congestion can also decrease renal blood flow and, in combination with increased neurohormonal activity, can lead to a higher diuretic threshold. Therefore, guidelines advise to administer loop diuretics intravenously (Class I, Level of evidence C),[11] bypassing intestinal absorption and ensuring a high peak concentration to overcome the diuretic threshold level (➲ Figure 8.9.2).[39b] Further, loop diuretics should be given as fast as possible because delay is associated with worse prognosis.[40]

The first dose given should be based on the chronic home dose if patients are taking loop diuretics chronically. According to current guidelines, if patients are diuretic-naïve, an initial bolus of 20–40 mg of furosemide is advised, while at least an equivalent dose to the home dose is indicated in the case of chronic loop diuretic use.[11] The Diuretic Strategies in Patients with Acute Decompensated Heart Failure (DOSE) trial randomized 308 patients with acute heart failure in a 2 × 2 factorial design to 1 time the oral home dose versus 2.5 times the oral home dose and to continuous infusion versus bolus therapy.[41] After 72 hours, there was no difference in patients' global assessment of symptoms for dosing or route of administration, but higher doses led to better dyspnoea relief, more weight loss, and more net fluid loss. Despite

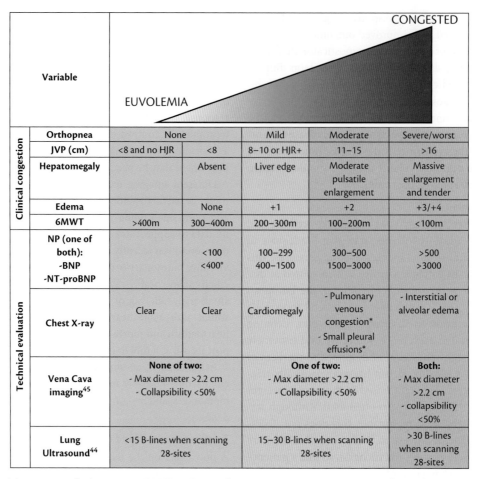

Variable					
Clinical congestion	**Orthopnea**	None		Mild	Moderate	Severe/worst
	JVP (cm)	<8 and no HJR	<8	8–10 or HJR+	11–15	>16
	Hepatomegaly		Absent	Liver edge	Moderate pulsatile enlargement	Massive enlargement and tender
	Edema		None	+1	+2	+3/+4
	6MWT	>400m	300–400m	200–300m	100–200m	<100m
Technical evaluation	**NP (one of both):** -BNP -NT-proBNP		<100 <400°	100–299 400–1500	300–500 1500–3000	>500 >3000
	Chest X-ray	Clear	Clear	Cardiomegaly	- Pulmonary venous congestion* - Small pleural effusions*	- Interstitial or alveolar edema
	Vena Cava imaging[45]	**None of two:** - Max diameter >2.2 cm - Collapsibility <50%		**One of two:** - Max diameter >2.2 cm - Collapsibility <50%		**Both:** - Max diameter >2.2 cm - collapsibility <50%
	Lung Ultrasound[44]	<15 B-lines when scanning 28-sites		15–30 B-lines when scanning 28-sites		>30 B-lines when scanning 28-sites

Figure 8.9.3 Multimodal assessment of volume status. 6MWT, 6-minute walking test; BNP, B-type natriuretic peptide; HJR, hepatojugular reflux; JVP, jugular venous pressure; NP, natriuretic peptide; NT-proBNP, N-terminal pro-B-type natriuretic peptide. * The chest X-ray can be clear, but the presence of abnormalities suggests a higher degree of congestion.
Reproduced from Mullens W, Damman K, Harjola VP, et al. The use of diuretics in heart failure with congestion — a position statement from the Heart Failure Association of the European Society of Cardiology. *Eur J Heart Fail.* 2019 Feb;21(2):137–155. doi: 10.1002/ejhf.1369 with permission from John Wiley and Sons.

more worsening renal function in the high-dose group, this was not associated with worse outcome.[42] The HFA Cardio-Renal Dysfunction Study Group advised starting with 1–2 times the oral home dose in acute heart failure patients. Up to 200 mg of furosemide can be administered as a bolus, as this is generally considered as a maximal ceiling dose, with a maximum total daily dose of 400–600 mg. Given the short duration of action of loop diuretics, a bolus should be given at least twice daily (up to four times daily) to maximize the diuretic effect and to tackle post-diuretic Na$^+$ retention. Alternatively, a continuous infusion can be used, but this should always be preceded by a loop diuretic bolus to have plasma levels above the threshold from the start. There is often concern about possible ototoxicity, but this occurs with extremely high concentrations, and thus when boluses are given over 5 minutes, ototoxicity is rarely, if ever, seen.

As diuretic response will already be apparent within 6 hours, early reassessment is possible, in addition to evaluation of daily weights, vital signs, and signs of congestion. Urine output and urinary Na$^+$ are the two preferred methods for early evaluation of diuretic response. A urine output >100–150 mL/hour indicates a good response but needs to be averaged over the 6 hours of diuretic

action. In contrast, urinary Na$^+$ allows for early assessment of diuretic response that can already be measured after 2 hours, with a value of >50–70 mmol/L indicating a good response.[28] Although there is a good overall correlation between urine output and renal Na$^+$ excretion, urinary Na$^+$ offers independent prognostic information, especially in patients at the lower end of urine output. Importantly, urine collection should start immediately after the loop diuretic has been administered, but equally important is that the patient should empty their bladder first prior to starting the collection to ensure proper measurements. If the diuretic response is sufficient, the same loop diuretic dose can be continued twice daily. If not, the dose should be doubled and the response should again be reassessed. On the second day of admission, the total urine output can be evaluated and is advised to be >3–4 L over 24 hours. Currently, there are no data to support urinary Na$^+$ assessment during consecutive days of diuretic therapy.

In cases where the diuretic response is still not satisfactory after maximal loop diuretic doses, a second diuretic can be added. The Cardiorenal Rescue Study in Acute Decompensated Heart Failure (CARRESS-HF) compared stepped pharmacological care versus ultrafiltration in 188 acute heart failure patients with worsening renal function and ongoing congestion. In the protocol, urine output was assessed on a daily basis and loop diuretic doses were doubled if urine output was insufficient. If a maximum dose of 500 mg of furosemide was reached, adding a thiazide was the next step. There was no difference in the primary endpoint of change in serum creatinine level and body weight after 4 days.[43] Given this evidence and the renal adaptations that occur during loop diuretic treatment with increased Na+ reabsorption in the distal tubule, thiazides are considered as the first-choice add-on therapy. Of

note, combining thiazides and loop diuretics increases the risk of electrolyte disturbances with hypokalaemia and hyponatraemia. Thus, it is considered safer to first maximize the dose of loop diuretics before instituting thiazides. As a second-line agent, acetazolamide or amiloride can be considered. MRAs are not advised as acute add-on diuretic therapy, as their onset of action is slow, and in the Aldosterone Targeted Neurohormonal Combined with Natriuresis Therapy in Heart Failure (ATHENA-HF) trial, using a natriuretic dose of 100 mg of spironolactone combined

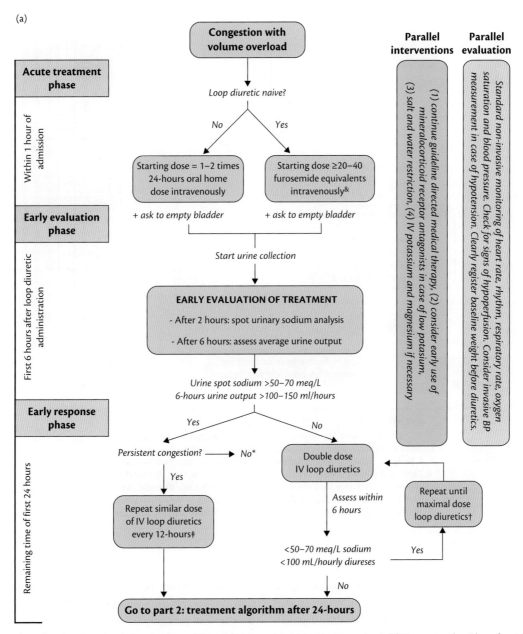

Figure 8.9.4 Flow chart showing diuretic use in acute heart failure. (a) Congestion with volume overload. (b) Treatment algorithm after 24 hours. Total loop diuretic dose can be administered either as a continuous infusion or as a bolus infusion. BP, blood pressure; HF, heart failure; IV, intravenous; SGLT2-I, sodium–glucose cotransporter 2 inhibitor; UF, ultrafiltration; UO, urine output. Higher doses should be considered in patients with reduced glomerular filtration rate. * Consider other reasons for dyspnoea, given the quick resolution of congestion. † The maximal dose for IV loop diuretics is generally considered furosemide 400–600 mg or 10–15 mg bumetanide. ‡ In patients with good diuresis following a single loop diuretic administration, once-daily dosing can be considered.

Reproduced from Mullens W, Damman K, Harjola VP, et al. The use of diuretics in heart failure with congestion — a position statement from the Heart Failure Association of the European Society of Cardiology. Eur J Heart Fail. 2019 Feb;21(2):137–155. doi: 10.1002/ejhf.1369 with permission from John Wiley and Sons.

(b)

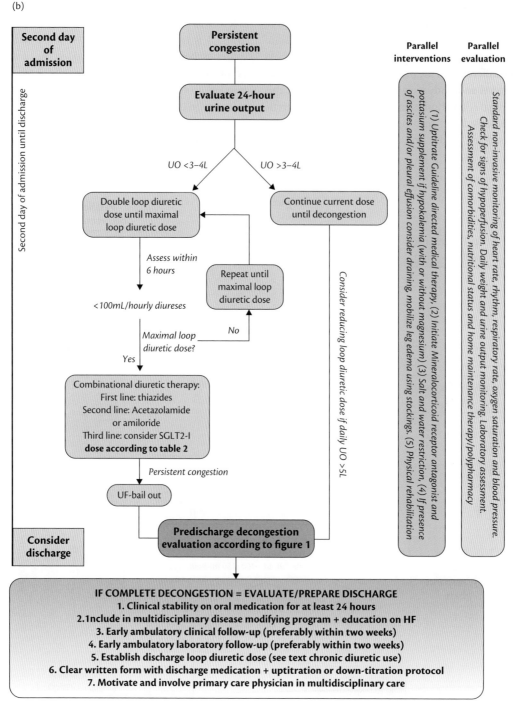

Figure 8.9.4 Continued

with loop diuretics was not superior to 25 mg of spironolactone or placebo with loop diuretics in reducing NT-proBNP levels after 96 hours.[44] However, MRAs can be useful in preventing hypokalaemia, and starting MRAs during decongestive treatment might enhance their use as they are a Class I indication in patients with HFrEF as part of disease-modifying therapy.

Diuretic resistance

In general, diuretic resistance is defined as persistent congestion despite adequate diuretic therapy.[45] However, this qualitative definition depends on what is considered as 'adequate'. A more quantitative approach is to use diuretic response, as suggested in the previous paragraph, with diuretic resistance being an insufficient diuretic response. Using a stepped pharmacological protocol allows to already tackle several mechanisms that contribute to diuretic resistance (➲ Table 8.9.3). In addition, vasodilatory therapy can help in relieving renal congestion and improving renal blood flow. Neurohormonal blockers are preferably continued, as loop diuretics can increase neurohormonal activation by blocking Cl⁻ reabsorption in the macula densa. If stepped pharmacological

Table 8.9.3 Most important aetiologies of diuretic resistance and possible solutions

Problem	Mechanism	Solution
Insufficient absorption	Bowel oedema	Intravenous administration, change to torsemide or bumetamide
Impaired renal blood flow	Venous congestion Increased intra-abdominal pressure	Vasodilatory therapy Paracentesis of ascites
Reduced GFR	Increased organic anions with competititve binding to OATs, limiting loop diuretic secretion	High loop diuretic dosing
Increased sodium reabsorption in proximal tubule	High filtration fraction Neurohormonal activation	Acetazolamide Continue neurohormonal blockers
Neurohormonal activation	Loop diuretics blocking macula densa	Continue neurohormonal blockers
Increased sodium reabsorption in distal tubule	Hypertrophy of distal tubule due to chronic loop diuretic use	Thiazide diuretics

GFR, glomerular filtration rate; OAT, organic anion transporter.

care and other measures fail, ultrafiltration can be considered (➲ Chapter 10.2). Currently, there is little evidence to support ultrafiltration as a first-line therapy.

Chronic heart failure

Diuretics are recommended by current guidelines to be used to alleviate symptoms, improve exercise capacity, and reduce HF hospitalization in patients with congestion (Class I, Level of evidence C).[11] However, there have been no randomized trials evaluating the effect of loop diuretics on outcomes in heart failure. The CardioMEMS Heart Sensor Allows Monitoring of Pressure to Improve Outcomes in Class III Heart Failure (CHAMPION) trial evaluated the outcome of tailored therapy according to continuous pulmonary arterial pressure measurements via an implanted sensor in 550 heart failure patients with a heart failure hospitalization in the preceding 12 months. Pulmonary sensor-guided therapy reduced heart failure hospitalizations by 28% and this was mainly due to changes in diuretic therapy.[46] This study supports the use of diuretic therapy in high-risk patients and also emphasizes the importance of tailoring the diuretic therapy according to patient congestion status. In addition, recent data from the Organized Program to Initiate Lifesaving Treatment in Hospitalized Patients with Heart Failure (OPTIMIZE-HF) registry suggested that HF patients receiving a loop diuretic prescription after heart failure hospitalization had lower 30-day all-cause mortality.[47] However, chronic loop diuretic use is also associated with important disadvantages: (1) faster decline of GFR; (2) electrolyte disturbances; (3) orthostatic hypotension, especially due to the combination with neurohormonal blockers; (4) neurohormonal activation; and (5) patient discomfort due to periods of high urine output after loop diuretic intake. In addition, in stable and low-risk patients on low-dose loop diuretic therapy, trying to stop the diuretic did not result in more congestive episodes in a recent randomized trial.[48] Further, loop diuretics might hamper uptitration of neurohormonal blockers due to hypotension.[49] In contrast to loop diuretics, these neurohormonal blockers have robust evidence of improving outcome in HFrEF and maximal uptitration might facilitate loop diuretic withdrawal.

In patients who require chronic loop diuretic therapy, the lowest possible dose is recommended, but it is often challenging to define the optimal dose, even with contemporary resources. In addition, there are no good predictors to determine loop diuretic downtitration success.[50] After an episode of acute heart failure, it might be necessary to prescribe a higher loop diuretic dose at discharge than what the patient was taking before. Alternatively, if the patient was on furosemide, switching to bumetanide or torsemide may be sufficient, given their better and more predictable bioavailability. Of note, combination diuretic therapy should be avoided in outpatient care because of the increased risk of electrolyte disturbances. A short period of combination therapy can be considered in the case of persisting congestion, but should be performed with close monitoring of electrolytes. Whether one loop diuretic should be preferred over another in chronic oral treatment is currently unknown, but given its longer duration of action and good bioavailability, torsemide is attractive. The ToRsemide compArisoN With furoSemide FORManagement of Heart Failure (TRANSFORM-HF) trial (ClinicalTrials.gov identifier: NCT03296813) is an ongoing 6000-patient randomized trial comparing the effects of outpatient treatment with furosemide to torsemide on 12-month all-cause mortality.

Electrolyte and acid–base disturbances

A practical approach to common electrolyte and acid–base disturbances is given in ➲ Table 8.9.4.

Future directions

Although use of urinary Na$^+$ is promising in early evolution of diuretic response, no trials have shown improved outcomes if urinary Na$^+$ is used as a target to tailor treatment. In addition, there are insufficient data to guide the use of urinary Na$^+$ during consecutive days of diuretic therapy. Further research aimed at resolving these issues is necessary. Moreover, urinary Na$^+$ measures might become of value to tailor outpatient therapy and to improve self-management of congestion by heart failure patients. Indeed, urinary Na$^+$ has recently been shown to drop a week before heart failure admission.[51] In the future, this could

Table 8.9.4 Common electrolyte and acid–base disturbances in diuretic therapy

	Hypokalaemia	Hyponatraemia	Hypomagnesaemia	Metabolic alkalosis
Definition	K$^+$ <3.5 mmol/L	Na$^+$ <135 mmol/L	Mg^{2+} <0.7 mmol/L	pH >7.45 and ↑ HCO$_3^-$
Pathophysiology	Diuretic use results in hypokalaemia Predisposing factors in HF can play a role, e.g. cachexia with low K$^+$ intake and chronic hypomagnesaemia	Dilution: impaired free water excretion. Clinical picture of volume overload with inappropriate high Uosm (≥100 mOsm/L). Typical in the setting of ADHF Depletion: true body deficit of Na$^+$. Typical in the setting of chronic excessive diuretic use (and strict Na$^+$ intake) Clinical picture of volume depletion with low Uosm (<100 mOsm/L) and UNa (<50 mEq/L)	Diuretic use results in hypomagnesaemia	Potassium loss shifts H$^+$ into the cells Decrease in intravascular volume leads to higher filtration fraction in the kidney, increasing proximal sodium chloride reabsorption. In the collecting duct, therefore, decreased activity of the Cl$^-$/HCO$_3^-$ exchanger pendrin and less HCO$_3^-$ reabsorption
Clinical significance	Can lead to severe arrhythmias Increases NCC-mediated Na$^+$ reabsorption in the distal tubule	Can lead to altered consciousness and cerebral oedema	Can lead to hypokalaemia and hypocalcaemia Can cause altered mental status, muscle weakness, and tetany if severe	Decreases diuretic response Can cause altered sensations and neuromuscular irritability
Treatment	Consider discontinuation of thiazide diuretics Upfront use of MRA during decongestion Increase the dose of RAAS-blocking agent IV substitution of K$^+$ and Mg^{2+}: peripheral or central, depending on severity of K$^+$ deficit	Dilution: temporarily stop distal-acting diuretics, limit water intake, promote distal nephron flow (loop diuretics, hypertonic saline, acetazolamide/SGLT2 inhibitor) or vaptans, correction of K$^+$ and Mg^{2+} deficiencies Depletion: stop distal-acting diuretics*, calculate Na$^+$ deficit and administer IV Na$^+$, correction of K$^+$ and Mg^{2+} deficiencies	Consider discontinuation of thiazide diuretics IV substitution of Mg^{2+}	Consider administration of acetazolamide if still volume-overloaded Upfront use of MRA during decongestion IV administration of KCl

* Distal-acting diuretics include thiazide-like diuretics, MRAs, and amiloride.
ADHF, acute decompensated heart failure; Cl$^-$, chloride; HCO$_3^-$, bicarbonate; HF, heart failure; IV, intravenous; K$^+$, potassium; KCl, potassium chloride; Mg^{2+}, magnesium; MRA, mineralocorticoid receptor antagonist; Na$^+$, sodium; NCC, Na$^+$/Cl$^-$ cotransporter; RAAS, renin–angiotensin–aldosterone system; SGLT2, sodium–glucose cotransporter 2; Uosm, urine osmolality; UNa, urine sodium.
Source data from Mullens W, Damman K, Harjola VP, *et al.* The use of diuretics in heart failure with congestion — a position statement from the Heart Failure Association of the European Society of Cardiology. *Eur J Heart Fail.* 2019 Feb;21(2):137–155. doi: 10.1002/ejhf.1369.

become an alternative to pulmonary sensor-guided management, but more evidence is needed first. Lastly, SGLT2 inhibitors are a new class of heart failure drugs with diuretic properties. Their diuretic properties and role in acute heart failure need to be elucidated.

Summary

Diuretic therapy is a cornerstone treatment of heart failure. Good knowledge of pharmacological properties of the different diuretics can enhance their proper and tailored use in the acute heart failure setting. Loop diuretics remain the backbone of diuretic therapy and should be correctly dosed before adding other diuretics. Implementing a diuretic protocol with early diuretic response evaluation might lead to better and faster decongestion. In chronic outpatient treatment, tailoring of the loop diuretic dose remains challenging, with no good tools to predict the lowest necessary dose. In stable, low-risk patients, it is worthwhile and safe to try to stop diuretics to allow for maximal uptitration of neurohormonal blockers.

References

1. Eknoyan G. A history of edema and its management. Kidney Int Suppl. 1997;59:S118–26.
2. Ford RV, Spurr CL, Moyer JH. The problem of bioassay and comparative potency of diuretics. II. Carbonic anhydrase inhibitors as oral diuretics. Circulation. 1957;16(3):394–8.
3. Matheson NA, Morgan TN. Diuretic action of chlorothiazide. Lancet. 1958;271(7032):1195–9.
4. Robson AO, Ashcroft R, Kerr DNS, Teasdale G. The diuretic response to frusemide. Lancet. 1964;284(7369):1085–8.
5. Mullens W, Verbrugge FH, Nijst P, Tang WHW. Renal sodium avidity in heart failure: from pathophysiology to treatment strategies. Eur Heart J. 2017;38(24):1872–82.
6. Kaissling B, Bachmann S, Kriz W. Structural adaptation of the distal convoluted tubule to prolonged furosemide treatment. Am J Physiol. 1985;17(3):374–81.

7. Burckhardt G. Drug transport by organic anion transporters (OATs). Pharmacol Ther. 2012;136(1):106–30.

8. Verbrugge FH, Nijst P, Dupont M, Penders J, Tang WHW, Mullens W. Urinary composition during decongestive treatment in heart failure with reduced ejection fraction. Circ Hear Fail. 2014;7(5):766–72.

9. Wilcox CS, Mitch WE, Kelly RA, et al. Response of the kidney to furosemide. I. Effects of salt intake and renal compensation. J Lab Clin Med. 1983;102(3):450–8.

10. Jentzer JC, Dewald TA, Hernandez AF. Combination of loop diuretics with thiazide-type diuretics in heart failure. J Am Coll Cardiol. 2010;56(19):1527–34.

11. McDonagh TA, Metra M, Adamo M, Gardner RS, Baumbach A, Böhm M, et al. 2021 ESC Guidelines for the diagnosis and treatment of acute and chronic heart failure. Eur Heart J. 2021;42(36):3599–726.

12. Knauf H, Mutschler E. Sequential nephron blockade breaks resistance to diuretics in edematous states. J Cardiovasc Pharmacol. 1997;29(3):367–72.

13. Verbrugge FH, Dupont M, Bertrand PB, et al. Determinants and impact of the natriuretic response to diuretic therapy in heart failure with reduced ejection fraction and volume overload. Acta Cardiol. 2015;70(3):265–73.

14. Verbrugge FH, Martens P, Ameloot K, et al. Acetazolamide to increase natriuresis in congestive heart failure at high risk for diuretic resistance. Eur J Heart Fail. 2019;21(11):1415–22.

15. Mullens W, Verbrugge FH, Nijst P, et al. Rationale and design of the ADVOR (Acetazolamide in Decompensated Heart Failure with Volume Overload) trial. Eur J Heart Fail. 2018;20(11):1591–600.

16. McMurray JJV, Solomon SD, Inzucchi SE, et al. Dapagliflozin in patients with heart failure and reduced ejection fraction. N Engl J Med. 2019;381(21):1995–2008.

17. Packer M, Anker SD, Butler J, et al. Cardiovascular and renal outcomes with empagliflozin in heart failure. N Engl J Med. 2020;383(15):1413–24.

18. Griffin M, Rao VS, Ivey-Miranda J, et al. Empagliflozin in heart failure: diuretic and cardiorenal effects. Circulation. 2020;142(11):1028–39.

19. Mordi NA, Mordi IR, Singh JS, Mccrimmon RJ, Struthers AD, Lang CC. Renal and cardiovascular effects of SGLT2 inhibition in combination with loop diuretics in patients with type 2 diabetes and chronic heart failure: the RECEDE-CHF trial. Circulation. 2020;142(18):1713–24.

20. Boorsma EM, Beusekamp JC, Maaten JM, et al. Effects of empagliflozin on renal sodium and glucose handling in patients with acute heart failure. Eur J Heart Fail. 2021;23(1):68–78.

21. Konstam MA, Gheorghiade M, Burnett JC, et al. Effects of oral tolvaptan in patients hospitalized for worsening heart failure: the EVEREST outcome trial. J Am Med Assoc. 2007;297(12):1319–31.

22. Felker GM, Mentz RJ, Cole RT, et al. Efficacy and safety of tolvaptan in patients hospitalized with acute heart failure. J Am Coll Cardiol. 2017;69(11):1399–406.

23. Konstam MA, Kiernan M, Chandler A, et al. Short-term effects of tolvaptan in patients with acute heart failure and volume overload. J Am Coll Cardiol. 2017;69(11):1409–19.

24. Fallick C, Sobotka PA, Dunlap ME. Sympathetically mediated changes in capacitance redistribution of the venous reservoir as a cause of decompensation. Circ Heart Fail. 2011;4(5):669–75.

25. Testani JM, Brisco MA, Kociol RD, et al. Substantial discrepancy between fluid and weight loss during acute decompensated heart failure treatment. Am J Med. 2015;128(7):776–83.e4.

26. Ambrosy AP, Cerbin LP, Armstrong PW, et al. Body weight change during and after hospitalization for acute heart failure: patient characteristics, markers of congestion, and outcomes: findings from the ASCEND-HF trial. JACC Heart Fail. 2017;5(1):1–13.

27. Hodson DZ, Griffin M, Mahoney D, et al. Natriuretic response is highly variable and associated with 6-month survival: insights from the ROSE-AHF trial. JACC Heart Fail. 2019;7(5):383–91.

28. Tersalvi G, Dauw J, Gasperetti A, et al. The value of urinary sodium assessment in acute heart failure. Eur Heart J Acute Cardiovasc Care. 2021;10(2):216–23.

29. Testani JM, Hanberg JS, Cheng S, et al. Rapid and highly accurate prediction of poor loop diuretic natriuretic response in patients with heart failure. Circ Heart Fail. 2016;9(1):1–8.

30. Rubio-Gracia J, Demissei BG, ter Maaten JM, et al. Prevalence, predictors and clinical outcome of residual congestion in acute decompensated heart failure. Int J Cardiol. 2018;258:185–91.

31. Stienen S, Salah K, Moons AH, et al. NT-proBNP (N-terminal pro-B-type natriuretic peptide)-guided therapy in acute decompensated heart failure PRIMA II randomized controlled trial (Can NT-proBNP-guided therapy during hospital admission for acute decompensated heart failure reduce mortality and readmissions?). Circulation. 2018;137(16):1671–83.

32. Strobeck JE, Feldschuh J, Miller WL. Heart failure outcomes with volume-guided management. JACC Heart Fail. 2018;6(11):940–8.

33. Metra M, Davison B, Bettari L, et al. Is worsening renal function an ominous prognostic sign in patients with acute heart failure? The role of congestion and its interaction with renal function. Circ Heart Fail. 2012;5(1):54–62.

34. Ahmad T, Jackson K, Rao VS, et al. Worsening renal function in patients with acute heart failure undergoing aggressive diuresis is not associated with tubular injury. Circulation. 2018;137(19):2016–28.

35. Mullens W, Damman K, Testani JM, et al. Evaluation of kidney function throughout the heart failure trajectory: a position statement from the Heart Failure Association of the European Society of Cardiology. Eur J Heart Fail. 2020;22(4):584–603.

36. Pellicori P, Platz E, Dauw J, et al. Ultrasound imaging of congestion in heart failure: examinations beyond the heart. Eur J Heart Fail. 2021;23(5):703–12.

37. Price S, Platz E, Cullen L, et al. Expert consensus document: echocardiography and lung ultrasonography for the assessment and management of acute heart failure. Nat Rev Cardiol. 2017;14(7):427–40.

38. Rivas-Lasarte M, Álvarez-García J, Fernández-Martínez J, et al. Lung ultrasound-guided treatment in ambulatory patients with heart failure: a randomized controlled clinical trial (LUS-HF study). Eur J Heart Fail. 2019;21(12):1605–13.

39a. Mullens W, Damman K, Harjola VP, et al. The use of diuretics in heart failure with congestion: a position statement from the Heart Failure Association of the European Society of Cardiology. Eur J Heart Fail. 2019;21(2):137–55.

39b. Ellison DH, Felker GM. Diuretic treatment in heart failure. N Engl J Med. 2017;377(20):1964–75.

40. Matsue Y, Damman K, Voors AA, et al. Time-to-furosemide treatment and mortality in patients hospitalized with acute heart failure. J Am Coll Cardiol. 2017;69(25):3042–51.

41. Felker GM, Lee KL, Bull DA, et al. Diuretic strategies in patients with acute decompensated heart failure. N Engl J Med. 2011;364(9):797–805.

42. Brisco MA, Zile MR, Hanberg JS, et al. Relevance of changes in serum creatinine during a heart failure trial of decongestive strategies: insights from the DOSE trial. J Card Fail. 2016;22(10):753–60.

43. Bart BA, Goldsmith SR, Lee KL, et al. Ultrafiltration in decompensated heart failure with cardiorenal syndrome. N Engl J Med. 2012;367(24):2296–304.

44. Butler J, Anstrom KJ, Felker GM, et al. Efficacy and safety of spironolactone in acute heart failure: the ATHENA-HF randomized clinical trial. JAMA Cardiol. 2017;2(9):950–8.

45. Verbrugge FH. Editor's choice: diuretic resistance in acute heart failure. Eur Heart J Acute Cardiovasc Care. 2018;7(4):379–89.

46. Abraham WT, Adamson PB, Bourge RC, *et al.* Wireless pulmonary artery haemodynamic monitoring in chronic heart failure: a randomised controlled trial. Lancet. 2011;377(9766):658–66.

47. Faselis C, Arundel C, Patel S, *et al.* Loop diuretic prescription and 30-day outcomes in older patients with heart failure. J Am Coll Cardiol. 2020;76(6):669–79.

48. Rohde LE, Rover MM, Neto JAF, *et al.* Short-term diuretic withdrawal in stable outpatients with mild heart failure and no fluid retention receiving optimal therapy: a double-blind, multicentre, randomized trial. Eur Heart J. 2019;40(44):3605–12.

49. Dauw J, Mullens W. Diuretics after heart failure hospitalization, not for all! J Am Coll Cardiol. 2020 Nov 17;76(20):2418.

50. Martens P, Verbrugge FH, Boonen L, Nijst P, Dupont M, Mullens W. Value of routine investigations to predict loop diuretic down-titration success in stable heart failure. Int J Cardiol. 2018;250:171–5.

51. Martens P, Dupont M, Verbrugge FH, *et al.* Urinary sodium profiling in chronic heart failure to detect development of acute decompensated heart failure. JACC Heart Fail. 2019;7(5):404–14.

CHAPTER 8.10

Inotropes and inodilators

Jan Biegus, Piotr Ponikowski, and
Christoph Maack

Contents

Introduction

Acute decompensation of heart failure (HF) (i.e. acute HF (AHF)) is the most frequent cause of hospitalization in patients aged >65 years in Europe. It portends a high risk of mortality and, even after haemodynamic stabilization, predicts adverse outcomes in the following year(s).[1,2] In most cases, early identification of patients requiring inotropic support is based on the presence of clinical signs and symptoms of hypoperfusion (⊃ Tables 8.10.1 and 8.10.2). First, it is essential to consider whether the patient is 'dry' or 'wet', with the latter typically associated with signs of congestion (oedema) which can be treated with diuretics,[2] and second, whether the patient is 'warm' or 'cold', with cold and sweaty skin being a typical sign of cardiogenic shock. When blood pressure (BP) drops, sympathetic activation increases the resistance of peripheral arteries (i.e. in the skin) in an attempt to centralize blood flow towards the vital organs, such as the heart and brain, where vasodilatation then predominates. Together with decreased cardiac output, this net increase in systemic vascular resistance (SVR) compromises peripheral perfusion. In addition, oliguria, mental confusion, dizziness, and narrow pulse pressure are typical clinical signs (⊃ Tables 8.10.1).[2] In the blood, hypoperfusion can manifest with elevated levels of serum creatinine, metabolic acidosis, and elevated serum lactate level, reflecting tissue hypoxia (⊃ Table 8.10.1).[2] In general, use of intravenous inotropes and vasopressors should be restricted to patients with left ventricular (LV) systolic dysfunction, low cardiac output, and low systolic BP (e.g. <90 mmHg) resulting in poor vital organ perfusion.[2]

Pathophysiology of contractile dysfunction in heart failure

To better understand the modes of action of inotropes, it is essential to comprehend the process of excitation–contraction (EC) coupling in cardiac myocytes. During each cardiac action potential, calcium (Ca^{2+}) enters cardiac myocytes via L-type Ca^{2+} channels (LTCCs), triggering an even greater release of Ca^{2+} from the sarcoplasmic reticulum (SR), the Ca^{2+} store in the cell (⊃ Figure 8.10.1).[3,4] This Ca^{2+} release via ryanodine receptors (RyRs) accounts for approximately 70% of the total Ca^{2+} that activates the myofilaments during contraction. During diastole, Ca^{2+} is taken back into the SR via the SR Ca^{2+}-ATPase (SERCA), while Ca^{2+} that entered the myocyte via LTCCs is exported by sodium (Na$^+$)/Ca^{2+} exchanger (NCX) (⊃ Figure 8.10.1).[3,4] In HF with reduced ejection fraction (HFrEF), a main defect that accounts for systolic and diastolic dysfunction is downregulation of SERCA expression and activity, which slows the uptake of Ca^{2+} during diastole and lowers the SR Ca^{2+} load, and thereby SR Ca^{2+} release, during systole.[3,5] These defects slow relaxation, decrease contractile force, and surface in particular at higher heart rates when the mere frequency-dependent increase in net Ca^{2+} influx via

Table 8.10.1 Signs and symptoms of hypoperfusion

Cold, sweaty extremities
Pale skin
Fatigue, even at rest
Dyspnoea (not related to pulmonary congestion)
Oliguria or anuria
Mental confusion
Dizziness
Narrow pulse pressure
Metabolic acidosis
Elevated serum lactate levels
Elevated serum creatinine levels
Elevated aminotransferase levels

LTCCs can be handled neither by the slowed SERCA nor by the notoriously slow NCX, resulting in an increase in diastolic Ca^{2+} and tension and depletion of SR Ca^{2+}. As a result, the normally positive force–frequency relationship as one critical mechanism of the healthy heart to increase inotropy reverses and becomes negative.[6]

Under physiological conditions, noradrenaline is released from sympathetic nerve endings during sympathetic activation and stimulates β-adrenergic receptors (ARs) on cardiac myocytes, which couple with the stimulatory G protein (G_s) and activate adenylyl cyclase (AC) to produce cyclic adenosine monophosphate (cAMP).[7] cAMP activates protein kinase A (PKA), which phosphorylates, and thereby activates, LTCCs, accelerates SERCA, increases SR Ca^{2+} release via RyRs, and decreases myofilament Ca^{2+} affinity (⮕ Figure 8.10.1).[7] In patients with HFrEF, chronic activation of the sympathetic nervous system desensitizes and downregulates β-ARs, which decreases the inotropic, chronotropic, and lusitropic response of the heart to adrenergic stimulation.[8,9]

Classification of inotropes

Inotropes are a heterogeneous group of drugs used to increase cardiac contractility in patients with HFrEF. Intravenous inotropes are used especially to maintain or rescue tissue perfusion by

Table 8.10.2 The most common populations of patients receiving intravenous inotropes

Patient populations
Any type of shock (cardiogenic, septic, mixed)
Acute heart failure with overt hypoperfusion
Advanced heart failure as a bridge to left ventricular assist device or transplant
Advanced heart failure for symptom relief or palliation
Low haemodynamic reserve requiring administration of cardio-depressive drugs (i.e. anaesthetics)

increasing cardiac output and/or modifying vascular resistance in patients with AHF and hypoperfusion via distinct pathways.[3] Recently, a new classification of inotropes based on differences in their modes of action has been proposed. Accordingly, inotropes are divided into three classes: calcitropes, myotropes, and mitotropes (⮕ Table 8.10.3).[10] Calcitropes are the largest group of agents, including catecholamines, phosphodiesterase 3 (PDE3) inhibitors, and cardiac glycosides. They increase inotropy by increasing the amplitude of intracellular Ca^{2+} transients via different mechanisms. In contrast, myotropes are drugs that directly target sarcomeres without affecting cytosolic Ca^{2+} concentrations. Mitotropes are compounds that improve inotropy indirectly by improving mitochondrial function. However, whereas some mitotropes, such as the mitochondria-targeted peptide elamipretide,[11] indeed improved mitochondrial function and myocardial performance in *preclinical* studies,[12] this inotropic effect did not translate into humans with HFrEF.[13] Therefore, we refer to previous reviews on mitotropes[10,14] and instead will focus on calcitropes and myotropes in this chapter. Nevertheless, it is important to point out that the interplay between EC coupling and mitochondrial energetics, mostly mediated by adenosine diphosphate (ADP) and Ca^{2+}, plays an important role when considering the energetic effects of different inotropes, the details of which were reviewed previously[3,15] but would be beyond the scope of this chapter.

Calcitropes

Catecholamines

Catecholamines are the most commonly used drugs within the class of calcitropes. There are three endogenous (i.e. adrenaline, noradrenaline, and dopamine) and two synthetic catecholamines (i.e. dobutamine and isoproterenol) available for clinical use (⮕ Table 8.10.4).[16,17] The different catecholamines stimulate $β_1$-, $β_2$-, $α_1$-, D_1-, and D_2-ARs with different affinities (⮕ Table 8.10.4).[16] Thus, their haemodynamic actions not only are limited to increasing cardiac contractility via $β_1$-ARs, but also regulate the vascular tone. This differential pattern of receptor activation is a rationale for tailoring their use towards specific clinical situations. The recommended doses of catecholamines used in acute heart failure are presented in ⮕ Table 8.10.5.

Dobutamine

The most commonly used drug to treat cardiogenic shock is the synthetic compound dobutamine. It acts primarily on $β_1$-ARs on cardiac myocytes, inducing a positive inotropic effect. On the vasculature, less potent and efficient stimulation of vasodilating $β_2$-ARs and vasoconstricting $α_1$-ARs results in a rather neutral *direct* effect on the SVR.[3,17,18] However, the positive inotropic (and moderate chronotropic) effect of dobutamine increases the cardiac output and BP, which leads to relief from endogenous sympathetic activation, resulting in an *indirect* decrease of SVR (⮕ Figure 8.10.2).[18,19] This profile is haemodynamically attractive for patients with advanced HF. The favourable haemodynamic effect comes at the cost of elevated myocardial oxygen (O_2) consumption (+15% at 10 μg/kg per minute), although this increase is less

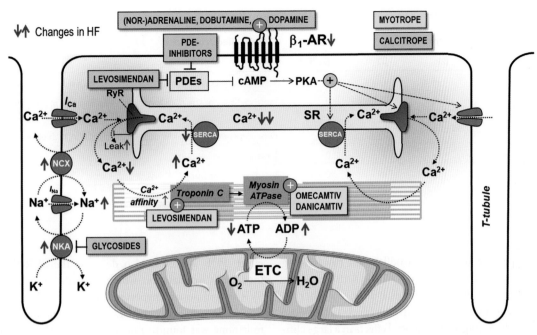

Figure 8.10.1 Defects in excitation–contraction coupling in heart failure and mode of action of inotropes. AR, adrenergic receptor; PDE, phosphodiesterase; cAMP, cyclic adenosine monophosphate; PKA, protein kinase A; SR, sarcoplasmic reticulum; SERCA, SR Ca^{2+} ATPase; RyR, ryanodine receptor; I_{Ca} and I_{Na}, Ca^{2+} and Na^{+} currents; NCX, Na^{+}/Ca^{2+} exchanger; NKA, Na^{+}/K^{+}-ATPase; ETC, electron transport chain; T-tubule, transverse tubule. Red arrows ($\uparrow\downarrow$) indicate the direction of change in heart failure. Green: calcitropes; yellow: myotropes. Levosimendan is a hybrid of a myotrope and a calcitrope.

Reproduced from Maack C, Eschenhagen T, Hamdani N, *et al.* Treatments targeting inotropy. *Eur Heart J.* 2019 Nov 21;40(44):3626–3644. doi: 10.1093/eurheartj/ehy600 with permission from Oxford University Press.

pronounced than the increase in cardiac output at the same dose (+43%) (➲ Figure 8.10.2),[18] with a higher risk of arrhythmias.

Adrenaline and noradrenaline

The endogenous catecholamines adrenaline and noradrenaline, which, besides β_1- and β_2-ARs, activate primarily α_1-ARs, promote vasoconstriction that is useful in patients with septic shock in whom vasodilatation underlies hypotension (➲ Table 8.10.4). Noradrenaline may also be considered in patients with cardiogenic shock despite treatment with another inotrope, to

increase BP and perfusion of the vital organs if required. The combination of adrenaline with dobutamine, however, appears to portend a particular risk of life-threatening adverse events, likely through a more pronounced increase in heart rate, which, together with vasoconstriction, result in tissue ischaemia and increased lactate formation.[20,21,22]

Dopamine

The haemodynamic profile of dopamine is wide and dose-dependent, as it activates different receptors at various doses.

Table 8.10.3 Inotropes and their classification

Class	Type	Mechanism of action	Drugs
Calcitropes	Catecholamines	$\uparrow$ cAMP, $\uparrow$ Ca^{2+}	Adrenaline Noradrenaline Dopamine Dobutamine Isoproterenol Phenylephrine
	PDE inhibitors	$\downarrow$ PDE3, $\uparrow$ cAMP, $\uparrow$ Ca^{2+}	Milrinone, enoximone, inamrinon
	Cardiac glycosides	$\downarrow$ Na^{+}-K^{+} ATPase, $\uparrow$ Ca^{2+}	Digoxin
	Istaroxime	$\downarrow$ Na^{+}-K^{+} ATPase, $\uparrow$ Ca^{2+}	Istaroxime
Mixed myotrope/ calcitrope	Ca^{2+} sensitizer/PDE3 inhibitor	$\uparrow$ Ca^{2+} sensitivity of myosin-binding protein C, $\downarrow$ PDE3, $\uparrow$ cAMP, $\uparrow$ Ca^{2+}	Levosimendan
Myotropes	Myosin activator	$\uparrow$ time of actin/myosin interaction (power stroke)	Omecamtiv mecarbil, danicamtiv

Ca^{2+}, calcium; cAMP, cyclic adenosine monophosphate; Na^{+}, sodium; PDE3, phosphodiesterase 3.

Table 8.10.4 Receptor binding profiles of catecholamines and their clinical effects

Catecholamine	Adrenergic receptors				Clinical effect/comments
	α1	β1	β2	D1/D2	
Adrenaline	++++	+++	++++	0	Inotropy/vasoconstriction (increased SVR), high risk of arrhythmia
Noradrenaline	++++	+++	+	0	Inotropy/vasoconstriction (increased SVR), high risk of arrhythmia
Dopamine	+++	++	+++	++++	Inotropy Dose-dependent effect: low dose—vasodilatation; high dose—vasoconstriction
Dobutamine	++	+++	+	0	Inotropy/vasodilatation
Isoproterenol	0	++++	++++	0	Inotropy/chronotropy/high risk of arrhythmia
Phenylephrine	++++	+	+	0	Vasoconstriction (increased SVR)

+ to ++++, increasing degree of positive effect; 0, neutral effect.
SVR, systemic vascular resistance.

At low doses, dopamine promotes vasodilatation (by binding to dopaminergic D_1 and D_2 receptors) (⤳ Table 8.10.4) and increases blood flow to the heart, lungs, brain, kidney, and other organs. However, renal (diuretic and natriuretic) effects of low-dose dopamine are now discouraged after neutral effects in a large clinical trial.[23] At higher doses, dopamine increases BP by increasing the SVR via α_1-ARs and exert positive inotropic and chronotropic effects via β-ARs (⤳ Figure 8.10.1), respectively.

Phosphodiesterase 3 inhibitors

In human cardiomyocytes, the breakdown of cAMP is mediated primarily by PDE3. Inhibitors of PDE3 (i.e. milrinone, enoximone, inamrinone, and levosimendan) inhibit degradation of cAMP and thereby increase intracellular Ca^{2+} transients (⤳ Figures 8.10.1 and 8.10.3). PDE3 inhibition potentiates β-AR-mediated positive inotropic effects without direct interaction with the receptors.[24] As PDE inhibitors act downstream of β-ARs, they circumvent desensitization and downregulation of β-ARs, as well as their blockade through β-blockers, both common in patients with HF. In fact, in contrast to catecholamines, the efficacy and potency of PDE inhibitors are maintained in patients with HFrEF treated with β-blockers.[25] Apart from their inotropic

effect, PDE inhibitors also decrease the SVR through cAMP-mediated vasodilatation, which is beneficial in patients with high SVR or pulmonary hypertension, but this limits their application in patients with low BP. However, the oral PDE3 inhibitor milrinone was found to be associated with increased mortality, when compared to placebo, in patients with advanced HF.[26]

Adverse effects of catecholamines and PDE inhibitors

A major downside of β_1-AR activation and PDE3 inhibition, especially upon chronic administration, is that they induce maladaptive signal transduction in cardiac myocytes, leading to

Table 8.10.5 Doses of inotropes used in acute heart failure

Inotrope	Dose
Dobutamine	Infusion 2–20 μg/kg/min (β+)
Dopamine	Infusion 3–5 μg/kg/min; inotropic (β+) >5 μg/kg/min (β+), vasopressor (α+)
Milrinone	Bolus 25–75 μg/kg over 10–20 minutes; infusion 0.375–0.75 μg/kg/min
Enoximone	Bolus 0.5–1.0 mg/kg over 5–10 minutes; infusion 5–20 μg/kg/min
Levosimendan	Bolus 12 μg/kg over 10 minutes (optional); infusion 0.1 μg/kg/min, which can be decreased to 0.05 μg/kg/min or increased to 0.2 μg/kg/min
Noradrenaline	Infusion 0.2–1.0 μg/kg/min
Adrenaline	Infusion 0.05–0.5 μg/kg/min 1 mg intravenously during resuscitation, repeated every 3–5 minutes

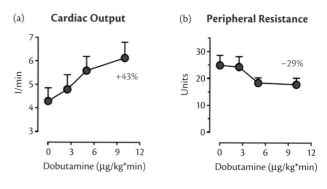

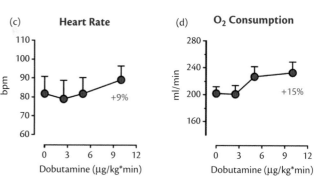

Figure 8.10.2 Haemodynamic effects of dobutamine in n = 10 patients with cardiovascular disease, including two patients with congestive heart failure and seven with coronary artery disease. Dose-dependent effects on cardiac output (a), systemic vascular resistance (b), heart rate (c), and oxygen (O_2) consumption (d) are shown.

Reproduced from Jewitt D, Birkhead J, Mitchell A, Dollery C. Clinical cardiovascular pharmacology of dobutamine. A selective inotropic catecholamine. *Lancet*. 1974 Aug 17;2(7877):363–7. doi: 10.1016/s0140-6736(74)91754-1 with permission from Elsevier.

arrhythmias, hypertrophy, and programmed cell death, with the latter two resulting in maladaptive cardiac remodelling (⮞ Figure 8.10.3). This is illustrated by the fact that mice that overexpress β_1-ARs develop HFrEF.[27] β-ARs increase the synthesis of cAMP, which activates PKA, and thereby Ca^{2+}-transporting channels and pumps. In addition to this canonical action, cAMP also activates the *exchange protein directly activated by cAMP* (Epac), further activating Ca^{2+}/calmodulin-dependent protein kinase II (CaMKII), which phosphorylates various Na^+- and Ca^{2+}-transporting proteins, mostly synergistic with PKA-mediated actions (⮞ Figure 8.10.3).[5] The net result is an increase and acceleration of force generation and relaxation (positive *inotropic* and *lusitropic* effects), maintaining the refilling of the ventricles at elevated heart rates (positive *chronotropic* effect).[13] CaMKII activation, however, induces arrhythmias (through phosphorylation of RyRs, but also through activation of the late Na^+ current), and also triggers cardiac hypertrophy and programmed cell death.[3] It is widely perceived that these adverse events account for the excess mortality observed in patients with HF treated with dobutamine. In addition, chronic sympathetic stimulation in advanced HF desensitizes and downregulates β-ARs via PKA, GRK2 (also known as β-ARK1), and β-arrestin (⮞ Figure 8.10.3), reducing the inotropic reserve in these patients.

Cardiac glycosides

Cardiac glycosides (i.e. digoxin and digitoxin) inhibit the Na^+/K^+-ATPase (NKA), which increases intracellular Na^+ concentrations. This hampers diastolic Ca^{2+} extrusion via the NCX and supports Ca^{2+} influx via the reverse-mode NCX during systole, thereby increasing diastolic $[Ca^{2+}]$, Ca^{2+} transient amplitudes, and consequently inotropy (⮞ Figures 8.10.1 and 8.10.4). On the other hand, elevated $[Na^+]_i$ accelerates mitochondrial Ca^{2+} efflux via the mitochondrial NCX, reducing Ca^{2+} activation of the Krebs cycle and its regeneration of NADH required for adenosine triphosphate (ATP) production, and NADPH required for antioxidation (⮞ Figure 8.10.4).[15,28] In fact, cardiac glycosides induce oxidation of NADPH and the emission of reactive O_2 species from mitochondria that account for digitalis-induced arrhythmias.[28] Use of digoxin in patients with chronic (stable) HFrEF improves hospitalization for HF, but not total mortality.[29] Therefore, digoxin may be considered for patients with chronic HFrEF.

Myotropes

Myotropes are drugs that directly target sarcomeres without affecting cytosolic Ca^{2+} concentrations. We here discuss levosimendan as a Ca^{2+} sensitizer and omecamtiv mecarbil (OM) and danicamtiv as myosin activators.

Ca^{2+} sensitizer: levosimendan

Calcium sensitizers shift the relationship between $[Ca^{2+}]_c$ and force development of sarcomeres to the left, increasing force at any given $[Ca^{2+}]_c$. The disadvantage of Ca^{2+} sensitization at the cellular level is that it impedes relaxation following the decrease in $[Ca^{2+}]_c$. In contrast to pure Ca^{2+} sensitizers, levosimendan, which increases the affinity of troponin C to bind Ca^{2+}, neither prolongs relaxation time nor compromises diastolic relaxation, because levosimendan is also a PDE3 inhibitor that increases cAMP with similar potency as it increases force (⮞ Figure 8.10.1).[30,31]

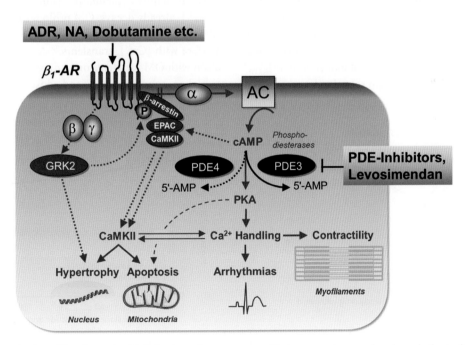

Figure 8.10.3 Signal transduction of β1-adrenergic stimulation in cardiac myocytes and its impact on inotropy, but also arrhythmias, hypertrophy, and apoptosis. ADR, adrenaline; NA, noradrenaline; AR, adrenergic receptor; AC, adenylyl cyclase; cAMP, cyclic adenosine monophosphate; PDE, phosphodiesterase; PKA, protein kinase A; EPAC, exchange protein directly activated by cAMP; 5′-AMP, 5′-adenosine monophosphate; CaMKII, Ca^{2+}/calmodulin-dependent protein kinase II; GRK2, G protein-coupled receptor kinase 2; α, β, γ, α-, β- and γ-subunits of the stimulatory G protein, respectively.

Reproduced from Maack C, Eschenhagen T, Hamdani N, *et al.* Treatments targeting inotropy. *Eur Heart J.* 2019 Nov 21;40(44):3626–3644. doi: 10.1093/eurheartj/ehy600 with permission from Oxford University Press.

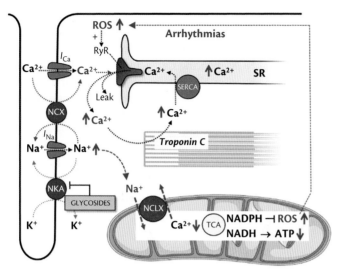

Figure 8.10.4 Mode of action of cardiac glycosides. ROS, reactive oxygen species; SR, sarcoplasmic reticulum; SERCA, SR Ca^{2+}-ATPase; RyR, ryanodine receptor; I_{Ca} and I_{Na}, Ca^{2+} and Na^+ currents; NCX; Na^+/Ca^{2+} exchanger; NKA, Na^+/K^+-ATPase; NCLX, mitochondrial Na^+/Ca^{2+} exchanger; TCA, tricarboxylic acid (Krebs) cycle. Red arrows ($\uparrow \downarrow$) indicate the direction of change in response to cardiac glycosides.
Reproduced from Maack C, Eschenhagen T, Hamdani N, *et al.* Treatments targeting inotropy. *Eur Heart J.* 2019 Nov 21;40(44):3626–3644. doi: 10.1093/eurheartj/ehy600 with permission from Oxford University Press.

Clinical activity of levosimendan during long-term treatment is mainly determined by its active metabolite OR-1896, which has a much longer half-life (81 vs 1 hour).[32] OR-1896 has a roughly similar potency to levosimendan, and PDE3 inhibition also contributes to the inotropic effect of the metabolite.[33] Besides its effects on EC coupling, levosimendan also activates sarcomeric ATP-dependent potassium (K^+) currents (I_{KATP}), which may add to its vasodilating activity and potentially provide cardioprotection through activation of mitochondrial I_{KATP}.[3] Altogether, these data indicate that with regard to levosimendan,

PDE3 inhibition synergizes with Ca^{2+} sensitization for its inotropic action (➲ Figure 8.10.1), which may be particularly relevant to the failing myocardium in humans where PDE3 plays a dominant role in controlling intracellular cAMP.[24,34,35,36]

Several clinical trials tested the effects of levosimendan in patients with HF, comparing it either to placebo or to dobutamine. In the SURVIVE trial, 1327 patients hospitalized with AHF who required inotropic support were randomized to levosimendan or dobutamine.[37] Although levosimendan led to more sustained reductions in B-type natriuretic peptide (BNP) levels in the first 5 days after randomization, mortality after 180 days (the primary endpoint) was not different between dobutamine and levosimendan (➲ Figure 8.10.5).[37] Several lines of evidence suggest that patients treated with β-blockers have a more favourable outcome when treated with levosimendan,[38,39] indicating that this may protect from excessive adrenergic activation mediated by PDE3 inhibition.[3] Although levosimendan did not improve outcome of AHF patients in single head-to-head comparisons,[37,40] meta-analyses suggest benefits of levosimendan over placebo or dobutamine as a comparator, respectively.[30,41]

Myosin activators: omecamtiv mecarbil and danicamtiv

OM is a selective cardiac myosin activator that binds to the catalytic domain of cardiac myosin and increases the transition rate of myosin into the strongly actin-bound force-generating state.[42,43,44] The (short- and long-term) pharmacodynamic effect of the drug is an increase in systolic ejection time (SET), and thereby stroke volume (➲ Figure 8.10.6a,b). This is a consequence of an increase in the number of myosin heads interacting with actin filaments, facilitating a longer duration of systole, even as $[Ca^{2+}]_c$ already decays. OM prolongs the time and amplitude, but not the rate, of cell shortening and contraction and does not interfere with $[Ca^{2+}]_c$ transients.[43] As a downside, myosin activation with OM can deteriorate diastolic function, in particular at higher concentrations and doses.[3,43] Through increased

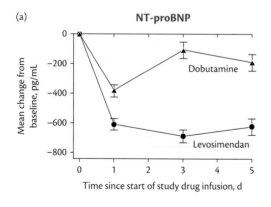

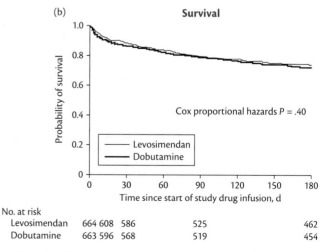

No. at risk					
Levosimendan	664	608	586	525	462
Dobutamine	663	596	568	519	454

Figure 8.10.5 Effects of levosimendan and dobutamine on NT-proBNP level in the first 5 days after randomization (a) and on survival in the first 180 days after randomization (b) in patients with acute heart failure.
Source data from Mebazaa A, Nieminen MS, Packer M, Cohen-Solal A, Kleber FX, Pocock SJ, Thakkar R, Padley RJ, Põder P, Kivikko M; SURVIVE Investigators. Levosimendan vs dobutamine for patients with acute decompensated heart failure: the SURVIVE Randomized Trial. *JAMA.* 2007 May 2;297(17):1883–91. doi: 10.1001/jama.297.17.1883.

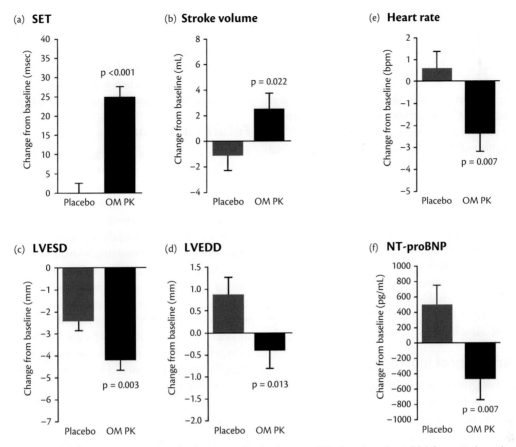

Figure 8.10.6 Effects of omecamtiv mecarbil (OM PK) or placebo on systolic ejection time (SET; a), stroke volume (b), left ventricular end-systolic diameter (LVESD; c), left ventricular end-diastolic diameter (LVEDD; d), heart rate (e), and NT-proBNP (f) in $n = 427$ patients with chronic heart failure with reduced ejection fraction (HFrEF) after 180 days of treatment.

Reproduced from Teerlink JR, Diaz R, Felker GM, *et al.* Omecamtiv Mecarbil in Chronic Heart Failure With Reduced Ejection Fraction: Rationale and Design of GALACTIC-HF. *JACC Heart Fail.* 2020 Apr;8(4):329–340. doi: 10.1016/j.jchf.2019.12.001 with permission from Elsevier.

stroke volume, cardiac output increases, likely lowering the endogenous sympathetic tone, as indicated by a modest lowering in the heart rate in patients with HF treated with OM (➲ Figure 8.10.6e).[3] In a large animal model of HF, OM increased stroke volume and cardiac output without an increase in O_2 consumption,[45] indicating that OM improves the mechanical efficiency of the heart.

OM dose-dependently improved symptoms (dyspnoea) in patients with AHF, induced reverse remodelling of the left ventricle, and reduced N-terminal pro-B-type natriuretic peptide (NT-proBNP) levels in patients with chronic HFrEF (➲ Figure 8.10.6).[46,47] In the GALACTIC-HF trial on patients with chronic HFrEF, of whom 25% were hospitalized for AHF, OM reduced the combined primary endpoint of cardiovascular death and hospitalization for HF by 8%, without reducing the individual components of the primary endpoint alone.[48] The benefit provided by OM increases with decreasing LVEF (➲ Figure 8.10.7).[49] Furthermore, in patients with *severe* HF, OM reduced the primary endpoint by 20%, whereas there was no reduction in patients with less severe HF.[50] If the compound gets approved by regulatory agencies, its use may be considered, in addition to standard therapy, for HFrEF patients to reduce the risk of cardiovascular mortality and hospitalization for HF.[8] In light of the subgroup analyses, patients

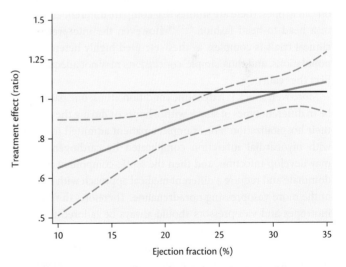

Figure 8.10.7 Estimates from Poisson regression models with the ejection fraction expressed as restricted cubic spline (solid line) (dashed line, 95% confidence interval) demonstrated the increasing beneficial relative treatment effect of OM with decreasing ejection fraction for the primary composite end point of time-to-first heart failure or cardiovascular death event (interaction $P = 0.004$ by ejection fraction as continuous variable).

Reproduced from Teerlink JR, Diaz R, Felker GM, *et al*; GALACTIC-HF Investigators. Effect of Ejection Fraction on Clinical Outcomes in Patients Treated With Omecamtiv Mecarbil in GALACTIC-HF. *J Am Coll Cardiol.* 2021 Jul 13;78(2):97–108. doi: 10.1016/j.jacc.2021.04.065 with permission from Elsevier.

with advanced HFrEF[50] and low LVEF (🡒 Figure 8.10.7),[49] in particular, should benefit in terms of morbidity.

A second myosin activator in advanced development is danicamtiv, which has overall comparable effects on EC coupling and cardiac haemodynamics as OM. In the LV and atrial myocardium from dogs with HFrEF, danicamtiv increased myosin ATPase activity and Ca^{2+} sensitivity in vitro, and improved LV stroke volume and left atrial emptying fraction in vivo.[51] The positive inotropic effect of danicamtiv occurred also in the atrial myocardium, which may contribute to LV filling during diastole, and which may explain why OM was found to be more effective in patients in sinus rhythm than in patients with atrial fibrillation.[48] Also in patients with HFrEF, danicamtiv improved LV stroke volume and longitudinal and circumferential strain, as well as left atrial function index.[51] In engineered heart tissue generated from inducible pluripotent stem cell-derived cardiomyocytes of patients with HF, danicamtiv caused a slightly smaller increase in diastolic tension, with comparable increases in systolic tension, compared to OM.[52] Larger-scale clinical trials are required to test the clinical effects of danicamtiv in patients with HFrEF.

Clinical applicability of inotropes

In most in-hospital use, intravenous calcitropes are administered to preserve function of the vital organs in critically ill patients. By rescuing perfusion, the short-term outcome (in terms of critical hours/days) should be improved. However, the impact of calcitropes in the long term is rather unfavourable.[3] In contrast, although not suitable for use in cardiogenic shock, myotropes are safe and improve morbidity in patients with HFrEF, even when initiated in acute decompensated patients (who are not in shock).[48] Although there are limited placebo-controlled studies on calcitropes, there are studies that compare different calcitropes in a head-to-head fashion.[37,53,54] However, the interpretation of clinical trials is complex, as they recruited highly heterogeneous populations, and thus 'simple' conclusions may not adequately reflect the reality.

Moreover, shock is a dynamic condition. Thus, one patient may be in different types of shock within hours or during the course of their hospitalization. For example, a patient admitted to hospital with myocardial infarction complicated by cardiogenic shock may develop infection, and then the septic component may predominate and require a different medical approach with inclusion of the more vasopressing noradrenaline. Therefore, the choice of inotropes and vasopressors should always be tailored to the individual clinical and haemodynamic situation of the patient. An understanding of the modes of action and clinical effects of these compounds will help the clinician to make the right choices.

Guideline recommendations

According to the current European Society of Cardiology (ESC)'s HF Guidelines, use of inotropes should be limited to patients with systolic HF and hypotension (systolic BP <90 mmHg) and signs/symptoms of hypoperfusion who do not respond to standard treatment to improve peripheral perfusion and maintain end-organ function (IIb, C).[2] Inotropes should be used with caution,

starting at low doses and uptitrating them with close monitoring. Routine use of inotropes is not recommended.[2] Noradrenaline, rather than adrenaline, may be considered to increase BP and tissue perfusion in patients with cardiogenic shock despite the use of inotropes (IIb, B), whereas PDE inhibitors and levosimendan, due to their vasodilatory effects, can cause hypotension.[2]

Future directions

Developing inotropes that improve haemodynamics in patients with HFrEF without a negative impact on prognosis is a particular challenge. Whereas compounds that interfere with adrenergic signalling have a negative impact on long-term cardiac myocyte biology and patient outcome, the development of drugs that bypass this axis is likely a promising concept. With regard to the positive, but quantitatively small, effects of OM in patients with chronic HFrEF, future research should be directed at optimizing the selection of patients for whom this compound provides the most benefit, such as those in sinus rhythm and those with low LVEF and high NT-proBNP levels. Furthermore, additional concepts to specifically fix the defects in EC coupling, such as improving SERCA function with use of antisense oligonucleotides,[55] could be a promising avenue to improve inotropy without adverse effects on cardiac energetics.

Key messages

- Inotropes target ARs, Ca^{2+} handling, or sarcomeres in cardiac myocytes, or a combination of these.

- The most commonly used inotropes to treat patients with AHF are the β1-adrenergic agonist dobutamine and the Ca^{2+} sensitizer and PDE inhibitor levosimendan.

- Use of catecholamines, PDE inhibitors, and levosimendan should be limited to patients with systolic HF and hypotension (systolic BP <90 mmHg) and/or signs/symptoms of hypoperfusion to increase cardiac output and BP, improve peripheral perfusion, and maintain end-organ function.

- Noradrenaline, rather than adrenaline, may be considered to increase BP and vital organ perfusion in patients with cardiogenic shock despite the use of inotropes, whereas PDE inhibitors and levosimendan can cause hypotension due to vasodilatory actions.

- Drugs that exclusively target adrenergic signalling (catecholamines and PDE inhibitors) are associated with adverse outcome.

- Levosimendan, with its hybrid Ca^{2+} sensitization and PDE3 inhibition, could be useful in selected patient populations, which may include patients treated with β-blockers.

- The novel myosin activator OM targets sarcomeres without affecting cytosolic Ca^{2+} handling, prolongs SET, and reduces hospitalization for HF or cardiovascular mortality in patients with chronic HF, especially those with strongly reduced systolic function.

- Future research should be directed towards developing a personalized approach to optimally tailoring the use of myosin activators for patients with HF who will best benefit from these compounds.

References

1. Chioncel O, Mebazaa A, Harjola V-P, et al.; ESC Heart Failure Long-Term Registry. Clinical phenotypes and outcome of patients hospitalized for acute heart failure: the ESC Heart Failure Long-Term Registry. *Eur J Heart Fail*. 2017;19:1242–54.

2. McDonagh TA, Metra M, Adamo M, et al. 2021 ESC Guidelines for the diagnosis and treatment of acute and chronic heart failure: developed by the Task Force for the diagnosis and treatment of acute and chronic heart failure of the European Society of Cardiology (ESC). With the special contribution of the Heart Failure Association (HFA) of the ESC. *Eur J Heart Fail*. 2022;24:4–131.

3. Maack C, Eschenhagen T, Hamdani N, et al. Treatments targeting inotropy. *Eur Heart J*. 2019;40:3626–44.

4. Bers DM. Excitation–Contraction Coupling and Cardiac Contractile Force, 2nd edition. Dordrecht: Kluwer Academic Publisher; 2001.

5. Bers DM. Altered cardiac myocyte Ca regulation in heart failure. *Physiology (Bethesda)*. 2006;21:380–7.

6. Hasenfuss G, Schillinger W, Lehnart SE, et al. Relationship between Na^+-Ca^{2+}-exchanger protein levels and diastolic function of failing human myocardium. *Circulation*. 1999;99:641–8.

7. Tilley DG. G protein-dependent and G protein-independent signaling pathways and their impact on cardiac function. *Circ Res*. 2011;109:217–30.

8. Bristow MR. Treatment of chronic heart failure with beta-adrenergic receptor antagonists: a convergence of receptor pharmacology and clinical cardiology. *Circ Res*. 2011;109:1176–94.

9. Lohse MJ, Engelhardt S, Eschenhagen T. What is the role of beta-adrenergic signaling in heart failure? *Circ Res*. 2003;93:896–906.

10. Psotka MA, Gottlieb SS, Francis GS, et al. Cardiac calcitropes, myotropes, and mitotropes: JACC review topic of the week. *J Am Coll Cardiol*. 2019;73:2345–53.

11. Szeto HH. First-in-class cardiolipin-protective compound as a therapeutic agent to restore mitochondrial bioenergetics. *Br J Pharmacol*. 2014;171:2029–50.

12. Sabbah HN, Gupta RC, Kohli S, Wang M, Hachem S, Zhang K. Chronic therapy with elamipretide (MTP-131), a novel mitochondria-targeting peptide, improves feft ventricular and mitochondrial function in dogs with advanced heart failure. *Circ Heart Fail*. 2016;9:e002206.

13. Butler J, Khan MS, Anker SD, et al. Effects of elamipretide on left ventricular function in patients with heart failure with reduced ejection fraction: the PROGRESS-HF phase 2 trial. *J Card Fail*. 2020;26:429–37.

14. von Hardenberg A, Maack C. Mitochondrial therapies in heart failure. *Handb Exp Pharmacol*. 2017;243:491–514.

15. Bertero E, Maack C. Calcium signaling and reactive oxygen species in mitochondria. *Circ Res*. 2018;122:1460–78.

16. Overgaard CB, Dzavik V. Inotropes and vasopressors: review of physiology and clinical use in cardiovascular disease. *Circulation*. 2008;118:1047–56.

17. Tuttle RR, Mills J. Dobutamine: development of a new catecholamine to selectively increase cardiac contractility. *Circ Res*. 1975;36:185–96.

18. Jewitt D, Birkhead J, Mitchell A, Dollery C. Clinical cardiovascular pharmacology of dobutamine. A selective inotropic catecholamine. *Lancet*. 1974;2:363–7.

19. Williams RS, Bishop T. Selectivity of dobutamine for adrenergic receptor subtypes: *in vitro* analysis by radioligand binding. *J Clin Invest*. 1981;67:1703–11.

20. Léopold V, Gayat E, Pirracchio R, et al. Epinephrine and short-term survival in cardiogenic shock: an individual data meta-analysis of 2583 patients. *Intensive Care Med*. 2018;44:847–56.

21. Levy B, Clere-Jehl R, Legras A, et al. Epinephrine versus norepinephrine for cardiogenic shock after acute myocardial infarction. *J Am Coll Cardiol*. 2018;72:173–82.

22. Tarvasmäki T, Lassus J, Varpula M, et al. Current real-life use of vasopressors and inotropes in cardiogenic shock: adrenaline use is associated with excess organ injury and mortality. *Crit Care*. 2016;20:208.

23. Bellomo R, Chapman M, Finfer S, Hickling K, Myburgh J. Low-dose dopamine in patients with early renal dysfunction: a placebo-controlled randomised trial. Australian and New Zealand Intensive Care Society (ANZICS) Clinical Trials Group. *Lancet*. 2000;356:2139–43.

24. Molenaar P, Christ T, Hussain RI, et al. PDE3, but not PDE4, reduces beta(1)- and beta(2)-adrenoceptor-mediated inotropic and lusitropic effects in failing ventricle from metoprolol-treated patients. *Br J Pharmacol*. 2013;169:528–38.

25. Metra M, Nodari S, D'Aloia A, et al. Beta-blocker therapy influences the hemodynamic response to inotropic agents in patients with heart failure: a randomized comparison of dobutamine and enoximone before and after chronic treatment with metoprolol or carvedilol. *J Am Coll Cardiol*. 2002;40:1248–58.

26. Packer M, Carver JR, Rodeheffer RJ, et al. Effect of oral milrinone on mortality in severe chronic heart failure. The PROMISE Study Research Group. *N Engl J Med*. 1991;325:1468–75.

27. Engelhardt S, Hein L, Wiesmann F, Lohse MJ. Progressive hypertrophy and heart failure in beta1-adrenergic receptor transgenic mice. *Proc Natl Acad Sci U S A*. 1999;96:7059–64.

28. Liu T, Brown DA, O'Rourke B. Role of mitochondrial dysfunction in cardiac glycoside toxicity. *J Mol Cell Cardiol*. 2010;49:728–36.

29. Digitalis Investigation Group. The effect of digoxin on mortality and morbidity in patients with heart failure. *N Engl J Med*. 1997;336:525–33.

30. Pollesello P, Parissis J, Kivikko M, Harjola VP. Levosimendan meta-analyses: is there a pattern in the effect on mortality? *Int J Cardiol*. 2016;209:77–83.

31. Szilagyi S, Pollesello P, Levijoki J, et al. The effects of levosimendan and OR-1896 on isolated hearts, myocyte-sized preparations and phosphodiesterase enzymes of the guinea pig. *Eur J Pharmacol*. 2004;486:67–74.

32. Antila S, Kivikko M, Lehtonen L, et al. Pharmacokinetics of levosimendan and its circulating metabolites in patients with heart failure after an extended continuous infusion of levosimendan. *Br J Clin Pharmacol*. 2004;57:412–15.

33. Orstavik O, Manfra O, Andressen KW, et al. The inotropic effect of the active metabolite of levosimendan, OR-1896, is mediated through inhibition of PDE3 in rat ventricular myocardium. *PLoS One*. 2015;10:e0115547.

34. Eschenhagen T. PDE4 in the human heart: major player or little helper? *Br J Pharmacol*. 2013;169:524–7.

35. Nikolaev VO, Bunemann M, Schmitteckert E, Lohse MJ, Engelhardt S. Cyclic AMP imaging in adult cardiac myocytes reveals far-reaching beta1-adrenergic but locally confined beta2-adrenergic receptor-mediated signaling. *Circ Res*. 2006;99:1084–91.

36. Kajimoto K, Hagiwara N, Kasanuki H, Hosoda S. Contribution of phosphodiesterase isozymes to the regulation of the L-type calcium current in human cardiac myocytes. *Br J Pharmacol*. 1997;121:1549–56.

37. Mebazaa A, Nieminen MS, Packer M, et al.; SURVIVE Investigators. Levosimendan vs dobutamine for patients with acute decompensated heart failure: the SURVIVE randomized trial. *JAMA*. 2007;297:1883–91.

38. Mebazaa A, Nieminen MS, Filippatos GS, et al. Levosimendan vs. dobutamine: outcomes for acute heart failure patients on β-blockers in SURVIVE. *Eur J Heart Fail*. 2009;11:304–11.

39. Kivikko M, Pollesello P, Tarvasmäki T, Sarapohja T, Nieminen MS, Harjola V-P. Effect of baseline characteristics on mortality in the SURVIVE trial on the effect of levosimendan vs dobutamine in acute heart failure: sub-analysis of the Finnish patients. *Int J Cardiol.* 2016;215:26–31.

40. Packer M, Colucci W, Fisher L, *et al.*; REVIVE Heart Failure Study Group. Effect of levosimendan on the short-term clinical course of patients with acutely decompensated heart failure. *JACC Heart Fail.* 2013;1:103–11.

41. Landoni G, Biondi-Zoccai G, Greco M, *et al.* Effects of levosimendan on mortality and hospitalization. A meta-analysis of randomized controlled studies. *Crit Care Med.* 2012;40:634–46.

42. Morgan BP, Muci A, Lu PP, *et al.* Discovery of omecamtiv mecarbil the first, selective, small molecule activator of cardiac myosin. *ACS Med Chem Lett.* 2010;1:472–7.

43. Malik FI, Hartman JJ, Elias KA, *et al.* Cardiac myosin activation: a potential therapeutic approach for systolic heart failure. *Science.* 2011;331:1439–43.

44. Teerlink JR, Diaz R, Felker GM, *et al.* Omecamtiv mecarbil in chronic heart failure with reduced ejection fraction: rationale and design of GALACTIC-HF. *JACC Heart Fail.* 2020;8:329–40.

45. Shen YT, Malik FI, Zhao X, *et al.* Improvement of cardiac function by a cardiac myosin activator in conscious dogs with systolic heart failure. *Circ Heart Fail.* 2010;3:522–7.

46. Teerlink JR, Felker GM, McMurray JJV, *et al.* Chronic Oral Study of Myosin Activation to Increase Contractility in Heart Failure (COSMIC-HF): a phase 2, pharmacokinetic, randomised, placebo-controlled trial. *Lancet.* 2016;388:2895–903.

47. Teerlink JR, Felker GM, McMurray JJ, *et al.*; ATOMIC-AHF Investigators. Acute treatment with omecamtiv mecarbil to increase contractility in acute heart failure: the ATOMIC-AHF study. *J Am Coll Cardiol.* 2016;67:1444–55.

48. Teerlink JR, Diaz R, Felker GM, *et al.*; GALACTIC-HF Investigators. Cardiac myosin activation with omecamtiv mecarbil in systolic heart failure. *N Engl J Med.* 2021;384:105–16.

49. Teerlink JR, Diaz R, Felker GM, *et al.* Effect of ejection fraction on clinical Outcomes in patients treated with omecamtiv mecarbil in GALACTIC-HF. *J Am Coll Cardiol.* 2021;78:97–108.

50. Felker GM, Solomon SD, Claggett B, *et al.* Assessment of omecamtiv mecarbil for the treatment of patients with severe heart failure: a post hoc analysis of data from the GALACTIC-HF randomized clinical trial. *JAMA Cardiol.* 2022;7:26–34.

51. Voors AA, Tamby JF, Cleland JG, *et al.* Effects of danicamtiv, a novel cardiac myosin activator, in heart failure with reduced ejection fraction: experimental data and clinical results from a phase 2a trial. *Eur J Heart Fail.* 2020;22:1649–58.

52. Shen S, Sewanan LR, Jacoby DL, Campbell SG. Danicamtiv Enhances systolic function and Frank–Starling behavior at minimal diastolic cost in engineered human myocardium. *J Am Heart Assoc.* 2021;10:e020860.

53. Chen HH, Anstrom KJ, Givertz MM, *et al.*; NHLBI Heart Failure Clinical Research Network. Low-dose dopamine or low-dose nesiritide in acute heart failure with renal dysfunction: the ROSE acute heart failure randomized trial. *JAMA.* 2013;310:2533–43.

54. Leopold V, Gayat E, Pirracchio R, *et al.* Epinephrine and short-term survival in cardiogenic shock: an individual data meta-analysis of 2583 patients. *Intensive Care Med.* 2018;44:847–56.

55. Grote Beverborg N, Später D, Knöll R, *et al.* Phospholamban anti-sense oligonucleotides improve cardiac function in murine cardio-myopathy. *Nat Commun.* 2021;12:5180.

CHAPTER 8.11

Sodium–glucose cotransporter 2 inhibitors

Petar M Seferović, Francesco Cosentino, Giuseppe Rosano, and James Januzzi

Contents

Introduction

The rise in use of sodium–glucose cotransporter 2 (SGLT2) inhibitors in cardiovascular care is a major achievement in early twenty-first century healthcare. Because of their glucosuric effects in patients with hyperglycaemia, drugs from this class were initially developed as a novel therapy for treatment of type 2 diabetes mellitus (T2DM). However, in the course of their study, SGLT2 inhibitors were found to reduce cardiovascular and kidney events in patients with T2DM.[1,2,3,4,5,6] Subsequent trials revealed that treatment with SGLT2 inhibitors also improves outcomes in patients with chronic heart failure with reduced ejection fraction (HFrEF), even without T2DM,[7,8] with lower rates of heart failure (HF) decompensation, fewer hospitalization, lower rates of death, and improved health status. SGLT2 inhibitors are also being explored for treatment of HF with preserved ejection fraction (HFpEF), and results from studies supporting a possible role for SGLT1/2 inhibitors have been reported recently.[6,9]

The path leading to use of SGLT2 inhibitors as cardiac therapeutics is fascinating. The role of the kidney as a major organ for excretion of glucose in the setting of hyperglycaemia has been recognized for thousands of years—the first known mention of symptoms from T2DM dates back to >1500 years BC when Egyptian physicians first described a diagnosis accompanied by polyuria and wasting. Many thousands of years later, recognition that spillage of glucose into the urine resulted in polyuria led to the naming of the diagnosis diabetes (meaning 'pump' to reflect the increased urine output) and mellitus (meaning 'honey' to describe the sweetness of the urine). Physicians whose role was to diagnose the presence of T2DM on the basis of their tasting urine soon became more commonplace, one of the first examples of a medical condition diagnosed through detection of a biological marker in bodily fluids.

Subsequently, in the nineteenth century, high doses of phlorizin (a flavonoid found in the bark of the apple tree) were recognized to cause glucosuria when administered in high doses. Because of its high affinity for SGLT1, use of phlorizin never developed as a treatment for hyperglycaemia; ultimately, congeners with greater affinity for SGLT2 were developed in the 1990s, leading to a new candidate therapy for treatment of T2DM.

It was at that time that a fortuitous twist of fate led to the discovery of the cardiovascular benefits of SGLT2 inhibitors—as a consequence of unexpectedly elevated cardiovascular risk associated with thiazolidinedione therapy for T2DM, the United States Food and Drug Administration issued *Guidance for Industry* on cardiovascular outcomes trials (CVOTs) of new antidiabetic therapies.[10] In this guidance document, it was recommended that prospective safety studies for new therapies for T2DM should include blinded adjudication and a statistical strategy to demonstrate acceptable risk–benefit balance. While these CVOTs were really safety studies and never designed to demonstrate the significant benefits of SGLT2 inhibitors that were ultimately revealed, they nonetheless led to a recognition of a new cardiovascular disease therapeutic.

Mechanism of action

The glucose-lowering effects of SGLT2 inhibitors do not explain their cardiovascular benefits, as a reduction in cardiovascular events is seen across the spectrum of haemoglobin A1c and preserved in those without T2DM. Nonetheless, a review of how SGLT2 inhibitors lower blood glucose is worthwhile.

A scientific understanding of how glycaemia results in glucosuria played a large part in the development of SGLT2 inhibitors for treatment of T2DM. In individuals without T2DM, between 100 and 200 g of glucose are filtered into the urine; a large majority of this glucose is reabsorbed in the proximal convoluted tubule by SGLT2 (a low-affinity, high-capacity pump), whereas the remaining glucose is subsequently retained by SGLT1 (a high-affinity, low-capacity pump) more distally. Both SGLT1 and SGLT2 are located in the apical membrane of the proximal tubular cells and absorb glucose across an electrochemical gradient created via first-stage binding of sodium; in turn, this creates a glucose concentration gradient between the cell and plasma, leading to passive exit of glucose through the glucose transporter 2 (GLUT2) uniporter located in the basolateral membrane of the tubular cell.

In states of normoglycaemia, little to no glucose is lost in the urine. However, when the plasma glucose level rises, proximal convoluted tubular reabsorption of urinary glucose increases until it reaches its maximum resorptive capacity: at higher urinary concentrations, the ability to reabsorb glucose begins to fall and glucosuria increases. This renal threshold for glucose reabsorption appears to be around 220 mg/min; clinically, this corresponds to a blood glucose concentration of >130 mg/dL. By inhibiting SGLT2, the renal threshold for tubular reabsorption is shifted, such that greater amounts of glucose are released via the urine (thus lowering plasma concentrations), but when the circulating glucose level is lower (and hence less is filtered into the urine), SGLT2 inhibitors carry a negligible risk of hypoglycaemia. It is for this reason that treatment with SGLT2 inhibitors may be used safely in patients without T2DM.

When used as a therapy for T2DM, besides their hypoglycaemic effects, SGLT2 inhibitors cause mild (and usually transient) diuretic and natriuretic effects, modest weight loss, and a small degree of blood pressure lowering.[11] In addition, haemoconcentration occurs, which has been associated with the cardiovascular benefit of the drug class.[11] Of course, in considering the cardiovascular benefits of SGLT2 inhibitors, it is necessary to concede that there is overlap between these effects related to glucose lowering (particularly as a large percentage of cardiac patients have T2DM) and whichever mechanisms underlying their cardiac benefits. Nonetheless, a large and growing list of mechanisms have been proposed to explain the non-hypoglycaemic cardiovascular beneficial effects of SGLT2 inhibitors (➲ Box 8.11.1).[12,13] The extent of the proposed mechanisms is substantial and exceeds the scope of this chapter, but was recently reviewed.[12,13] Each proposed

---

Box 8.11.1 Proposed mechanisms of SGLT inhibition to explain cardiovascular and renal benefits

Heart failure

1. Osmotic diuresis and natriuresis
2. Direct cardiac effects:
   a. Sodium/hydrogen cotransporter blockade
   b. Reduction in CaMKII (reduces sarcoplasmic Ca^{2+} leak → improves contractility)
   c. Increased phosphorylation levels of myofilament regulatory proteins
   d. Epigenetic modification
3. Reduction of sympathetic nervous system overdrive
4. Possible improvement in myocardial efficiency
5. Improved oxygen delivery through stimulation of renal EPO secretion
6. Reduction of inflammation (→ activation of adenosine monophosphate-activated protein kinase)
7. Reduction of oxidative stress (improving mitochondrial function)
8. Metabolic: lowering of HbA1c, blood pressure, body weight, and vascular stiffness

Atherosclerosis

1. Reduction of inflammation
2. Reduction of epicardial fat and noxious signals, including leptin and RAAS
3. Reduction of oxidative stress
4. Improved endothelial function
5. Shift of circulating vascular progenitor cells towards M2 polarization
6. Reduction in uric acid levels
7. Improvement of fatty liver disease

Kidney disease

1. Metabolic: lowering of HbA1c and body weight
2. Reduction in blood pressure and vascular stiffness
3. Restoration of the tubuloglomerular feedback
4. Reduction in workload regarding ATP production
5. Anti-inflammatory and anti-fibrotic effects, reduction of oxidative stress
6. Reduction in uric acid levels

ATP, adenosine triphosphate; Ca^{2+}, calcium; CaMKII, Ca^{2+}/calmodulin-dependent kinase; EPO, erythropoietin; HbA1c, glycated haemoglobin; RAAS, renin–angiotensin–aldosterone system; SGLT, sodium–glucose cotransporter. Reproduced from Zelniker TA, Braunwald E. Mechanisms of Cardiorenal Effects of Sodium-Glucose Cotransporter 2 Inhibitors: JACC State-of-the-Art Review. *J Am Coll Cardiol*. 2020 Feb 4;75(4):422–434. doi: 10.1016/j.jacc.2019.11.031. Erratum in: *J Am Coll Cardiol*. 2020 Sep 22;76(12):1505 with permission from Elsevier.

---

mechanism of benefit remains speculative and in need of confirmation, but some bear specific commenting ➲ Figure 8.11.1.

SGLT2 inhibitors have weak diuretic and natriuretic effects beyond those caused by glucosuria. This may be partially due to the

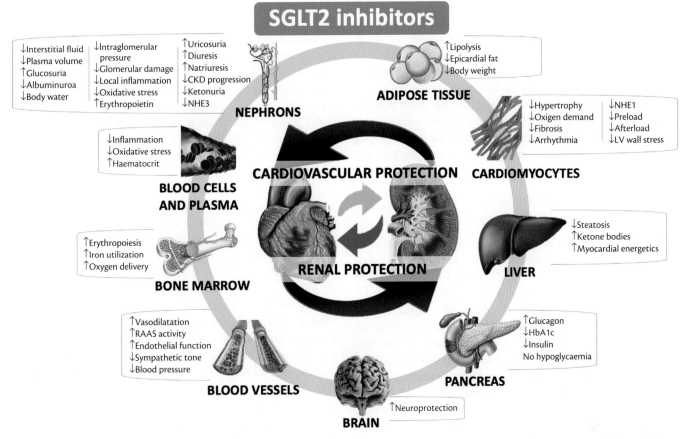

Figure 8.11.1 Beneficial effects of sodium–glucose cotransporter 2 (SGLT2) inhibitors. CKD, chronic kidney disease; HbA1c, glycated haemoglobin; LV, left ventricular; NHE, sodium–hydrogen exchanger; RAAS, renin–angiotensin–aldosterone system.

fact that SGLT2, but not SGLT1, co-localizes with the renal sodium/hydrogen exchanger (NHE) and SGLT2 inhibitors appear to also block the NHE and augment natriuresis. Despite the putative value of decongestion in the face of a diagnosis of HF, the diuretic and natriuretic effects of SGLT2 inhibitors appear somewhat transient. Furthermore, a recent randomized trial of patients chronically treated with empagliflozin did not demonstrate compelling reduction in filling pressures at rest or with exercise.[14]

Much attention has focused on potential improvement in heart muscle function where SGLT2 inhibition has been shown to have pleiotropic effects. Experimentally, inhibition of SGLT2 results in a shift to more efficient, fatty acid-based myocardial metabolism and improves energetics.[15] Additionally, SGLT2 inhibitors have many other direct effects on myocardial biology, including improved calcium handling, reduction in heart muscle inflammation, downregulation of the renin–angiotensin–aldosterone system, and minimization of oxidative stress through impact on mitochondrial function.[13] In addition, inhibition of the NHE may be associated with enhanced myocardial resistance to injury, creating a 'cardioprotective' milieu.[13] Lending credence to a direct impact on myocardial function, treatment of patients with HFrEF with SGLT2 inhibitors resulted in significant reverse cardiac remodelling, reduction in left ventricular and left atrial volumes, and improvement in ejection fraction.[15,16,17]

Given the role of progressive kidney disease on the risk of HF complications, a significant benefit of SGLT2 inhibition is likely conferred through their favourable impact on kidney function.[18] From patients with diabetes, with or without proteinuric chronic kidney disease (CKD), to those with HF, treatment with SGLT1/ 2 or SGLT2 inhibitors has consistently been shown to reduce progression of renal dysfunction.[1,2,6,8,18] Numerous mechanisms have been invoked to explain how SGLT2 inhibition may slow progression of renal dysfunction.[11,13] A prime mechanism is activation of the tubuloglomerular feedback, triggered by increased sodium concentration in the macula densa, and resulting in vasoconstriction of the afferent glomerular arterioles and reduction in intraglomerular pressure. This effect reduces hyperfiltration, mitigates shear stress, and thus contains further nephron damage.

Lastly, while most of the focus has been placed on how SGLT2 inhibition leads to cardiovascular risk prevention, targeting SGLT1 may also cause reduction in cardiac events.[6,9] Although SGLT1 is responsible for only a fraction of renal glucose reabsorption, this cotransporter plays an important role in glucose, galactose, and lactose absorption in the intestines. Inhibition of SGLT1 results in an upregulation of glucagon-like peptide 1 (GLP1); whether this would be expected to result in reductions in atherothrombotic events seen in the trials of GLP1 receptor agonists is speculative. However, a recent trial of an SGLT1/2 inhibitor for treatment of patients with T2DM and CKD reported a reduction in vascular events, including myocardial infarction and stroke.[6] This finding is divergent from most studies of SGLT2 inhibitors where impact on vascular events was less noteworthy.

In summary, although SGLT2 inhibition has revolutionized the treatment of patients with T2DM, CKD, and HF, much remains unclear about the mechanism(s) that explain the reduced incidence of major adverse cardiovascular and renal events among patients treated with these agents. Well-performed mechanistic/translational studies parsing these benefits are needed.

Role of SGLT2 inhibitors in preventing heart failure in patients with type 2 diabetes

T2DM increases the risk of HF and is associated with higher mortality rates and a greater burden of HF hospitalization, compared to individuals without T2DM.[2,3,4,5,6,7,8] T2DM can compromise the heart via several mechanisms. First, diabetic macrovascular disease leads to coronary artery disease (CAD), myocardial ischaemia, and ischaemic cardiomyopathy. In addition, T2DM can directly cause injury to myocardial structure, function, and metabolism, potentially leading to HF. Four different SGLT2 inhibitors (empagliflozin, canagliflozin, dapagliflozin, and ertugliflozin) have been evaluated in CVOTs in individuals with T2DM across different stages of the cardiovascular continuum. All four SGLT2 inhibitors have been shown to cause a consistent reduction in the risk of HF hospitalization, regardless of the baseline cardiovascular risk or history of HF.

The EMPA-REG OUTCOME (Empagliflozin, Cardiovascular Outcomes, and Mortality in Type 2 Diabetes) trial provided the first evidence that SGLT2 inhibition reduced HF-related hospitalization in patients with T2DM.[5] This study randomized individuals with prior atherosclerotic cardiovascular disease and T2DM to empagliflozin or placebo. Empagliflozin reduced the risk of HF hospitalization by 35%,[5] with similar benefits in people with or without a history of HF at recruitment.[19] In addition, the effect of empagliflozin on the composite outcome of cardiovascular death or hospitalization for HF was reduced by 34%.[9] The favourable effects on HF events occurred within the first 6 months after treatment initiation, with an even earlier divergence of the Kaplan–Meier curves. The CANagliflozin cardioVascular Assessment Study (CANVAS Program), enrolling T2DM patients with established atherosclerotic cardiovascular disease (66%) or at high cardiovascular risk (34%),[11] also showed a substantial 33% reduction in the risk of HF hospitalization. This finding was not considered statistically significant based on the prespecified sequence of hypothesis testing.[11]

Further support to the therapeutic benefit of canagliflozin comes from the Canagliflozin and Renal Events in Diabetes with Established Nephropathy Clinical Evaluation (CREDENCE) trial, showing a 34% relative risk reduction in cardiorenal outcomes, compared to placebo, in patients with T2DM and kidney dysfunction (albuminuria and eGFR 30 to <90 mL/min/1.73 m^2) who were already on optimal doses of angiotensin-converting enzyme

(ACE) inhibitors or angiotensin receptor blockers (ARBs).[13] Importantly, this trial has confirmed a robust attenuation of 31% in the composite risk of cardiovascular death or HF hospitalization, including a significant risk reduction in HF hospitalization.

The DECLARE TIMI-58 trial (Dapagliflozin and Cardiovascular Outcomes in Type 2 Diabetes) assessed the effects of dapagliflozin versus placebo on cardiovascular outcomes in a predominantly (59%) primary prevention population of patients with T2DM. Despite a neutral effect on the 3-point major adverse cardiovascular events (MACE) outcome, dapagliflozin significantly reduced a composite of cardiovascular death or HF hospitalization by 17%.[14] This effect was due to a significant 27% risk reduction in HF hospitalization. In the VERTIS CV (Cardiovascular Outcomes with Ertugliflozin in Type 2 Diabetes) trial, ertugliflozin was non-inferior to placebo with respect to its key secondary outcome of cardiovascular death or hospitalization for HF.[20] There was, however, a 30% reduction in the risk of hospitalization for HF alone, consistent with the effects of other SGLT2 inhibitors on this outcome.[21] These benefits appeared similar across most baseline subgroups, whereas larger effects have been identified among participants with reduced kidney function (i.e estimated glomerular filtration rate (eGFR) <60 mL/min/1.73 m^2),[22] albuminuria, or on prescribed diuretics).[23] Data from the SCORED (Sotagliflozin in Patients with Diabetes and Chronic Kidney Disease) trial on the combined SGLT1/2 inhibitor sotagliflozin in patients with T2DM and CKD (median eGFR 45 mL/min/1.73 m^2) and from the DAPA-CKD (Dapagliflozin in Patients with Chronic Kidney Disease) trial in patients with albuminuric CKD confirmed the benefit on HF in patients with reduced eGFR.[18,21] Indeed, sotagliflozin and dapagliflozin reduced the risk of cardiovascular death or hospitalization for HF by 33% and 29%, respectively, with similar effects observed across the spectrum of kidney function.[24]

Clinical trial evidence supports the use of SGLT2 inhibitors for the prevention of HF in patients with T2DM and established cardiovascular disease or multiple risk factors. On that basis, the 2019 European Society of Cardiology Guidelines on the management of diabetes and pre-diabetes and cardiovascular diseases stipulate that SGLT2 inhibitors are recommended to lower the risk of HF hospitalization in patients with T2DM.[25]

Role of SGLT2 inhibitors in treating heart failure

Given the consistent beneficial effects of SGLT2 inhibitors in improving cardiorenal outcomes and attenuating the risk of HF hospitalization in patients with T2DM, the most recent trials aimed to evaluate the impact of these medications on cardiovascular outcomes in individuals with established HF, regardless of T2DM status.

The first trial to provide evidence for the therapeutic benefits of SGLT2 inhibition in patients with HF and HFrEF was DAPA-HF (Dapagliflozin and Prevention of Adverse Outcomes in Heart Failure).[26] This trial assessed the impact of dapagliflozin (10 mg once daily) versus placebo, in addition to standard therapy,

Table 8.11.1 Major inclusion and exclusion criteria in clinical trials of SGLT2 inhibitors in heart failure

	DAPA-HF	EMPEROR-Reduced	SOLOIST-WHF	EMPEROR-Preserved
Treatment	Dapagliflozin 10 mg OD vs placebo	Empagliflozin 10 mg OD vs placebo	200 mg OD (with a dose increase to 400 mg OD, depending on side effects) vs placebo	Empagliflozin 10 mg OD vs placebo
Patients	With or without T2DM	With or without T2DM	T2DM	With or without T2DM
Key inclusion criteria	◆ LVEF ≤40% ◆ NYHA classes II–IV ◆ NT-proBNP ≥600 pg/mL (or ≥400 pg/mL if the patient had been hospitalized for HF within the previous 12 months) ◆ NT-proBNP ≥900 pg/mL in patients with AF, regardless HF hospitalization	◆ LVEF ≤40% ◆ HF hospitalization within 12 months ◆ NYHA classes II–IV ◆ NT-proBNP ≥600 pg/mL if LVEF ≤30% ◆ NT-proBNP ≥1000 pg/mL if LVEF 31–35% ◆ NT-proBNP ≥2500 pg/mL if LVEF 36–40% ◆ NT-proBNP thresholds doubled in patients with AF	◆ HF hospitalization or urgent visit for worsening HF ◆ HF diagnosis >3 months ◆ Randomized when haemodynamically stable, prior to hospital discharge, or within 3 days of discharge ◆ BNP ≥150 pg/mL (≥450 pg/mL for patients with AF) or NT-proBNP ≥600 pg/mL (≥1800 pg/mL for patients with AF)	◆ LVEF >40% ◆ NYHA classes II–IV. ◆ NT-proBNP >300 pg/mL for patients without AF ◆ NT-proBNP >900 pg/ml for patients with AF ◆ Structural heart disease within 6 months prior to inclusion or documented hospitalization for HF within 12 months prior to inclusion
Concomitant HF therapy	◆ Standard therapy for HFrEF and according to locally recognized guidelines	◆ Appropriate dose of medical therapy for HF consistent with prevailing local and international cardiovascular guidelines	◆ Patients with LVEF of <40% should be on beta-blockers and renin–angiotensin–aldosterone system inhibitors, as per local guidelines, unless contraindicated	◆ Stable dose of diuretics (if prescribed) ◆ Standard of care therapy mostly for comorbidities (hypertension, coronary artery disease), as per discretion of the treating physician
Key exclusion criteria	◆ Current or recent (past 4 weeks) acute decompensated HF or hospitalization due to decompensated HF ◆ Recent (past 12 weeks) myocardial infarction, unstable angina, coronary artery bypass surgery, stroke, or transient ischaemic attack ◆ Symptomatic hypotension or SBP <95 mmHg ◆ eGFR <30 mL/min/1.73 m² ◆ Heart transplant recipient or listed for heart transplant	◆ Acute decompensated HF ◆ Recent (past 90 days) acute coronary syndrome, major cardiovascular surgery, stroke, or transient ischaemic attack ◆ Symptomatic hypotension and/or SBP <100 mmHg ◆ Symptomatic hypotension or SBP <95 mmHg ◆ eGFR <20 mL/min/1.73 m² ◆ Heart transplant recipient or listed for heart transplant	◆ Recent (past 3 months) acute coronary syndrome ◆ Recent cardiac surgery or coronary procedure within 1 month or planned during the study ◆ Recent (past month) stroke ◆ End-stage heart failure ◆ eGFR <30 mL/min/1.73 m²	◆ Acute decompensated HF ◆ Recent (past 90 days) acute coronary syndrome, major cardiovascular surgery, stroke, or transient ischaemic attack ◆ Symptomatic hypotension and/or SBP <100 mmHg ◆ eGFR <20 mL/min/1.73 m² ◆ Heart transplant recipient or listed for heart transplant

AF, atrial fibrillation; eGFR, estimated glomerular filtration rate; HF, heart failure; HFrEF, heart failure with reduced ejection fraction; LVEF, left ventricular ejection fraction; NYHA, New York Heart Association; OD, once daily; SBP, systolic blood pressure; SGLT2, sodium–glucose cotransporter 2; T2DM, type 2 diabetes mellitus.

on cardiovascular mortality or worsening HF in patients with symptomatic HFrEF, with or without T2DM. Key inclusion and exclusion criteria are presented in ⦿ Table 8.11.1. During a median follow-up of 18.2 months, dapagliflozin treatment resulted in 26% lower risk of the primary composite endpoint of cardiovascular mortality or worsening HF (defined as either unplanned HF hospitalization or urgent visit resulting in intravenous therapy for HF). The beneficial effects of dapagliflozin occurred early, with a statistically significant risk reduction evident by 28 days after randomization.[27] Both components of the primary outcome were reduced, including an 18% reduction in cardiovascular mortality and a 30% reduction in hospitalization or urgent visit for HF. Dapagliflozin was also associated with an improvement in key secondary outcomes, namely a 17%

reduction in all-cause mortality and an improvement in functional status at 8 months. There was no significant difference in composite renal outcomes. The observed benefits were consistent across a spectrum of predefined subgroups, most importantly one including study participants with or without T2DM. A post hoc analysis indicated that among approximately 11% of patients receiving sacubitril/valsartan, there was no difference in the efficacy of dapagliflozin. A further subanalysis confirmed that the beneficial effects of dapagliflozin were similar, irrespective of the type or doses of background HF medications.[28] Furthermore, dapagliflozin appeared safe and effective in vulnerable subgroups of patients, including those with recent HF hospitalization (<12 months), the elderly, and those with impaired renal function.[27,29,30]

Further evidence for the favourable effects of SGLT2 inhibition in HFrEF came from the EMPEROR-Reduced (Cardiovascular and Renal Outcomes with Empagliflozin in Heart Failure) trial, which assessed the impact of empagliflozin (10 mg once daily) versus placebo on cardiovascular outcomes in symptomatic individuals with HFrEF, with and without T2DM.[31] The major inclusion and exclusion criteria are presented in ➲ Table 8.11.1. After a median follow-up of 16 months, there was a 25% risk reduction with empagliflozin, compared to placebo, in the composite primary outcome of cardiovascular mortality or HF hospitalization, driven by a 31% risk reduction in HF hospitalization.[31] Empagliflozin treatment also reduced key secondary outcomes, including total number of HF hospitalizations, and the annual rate of decline in the eGFR was slower in the empagliflozin group than in the placebo group. All-cause mortality was not significantly reduced. There was a 24% lower risk of mortality, hospitalization, or emergent visit requiring intravenous therapy for HF, that became statistically significant at only 12 days after randomization.[32] There was no heterogeneity in treatment effects according to T2DM status, age, sex, or background therapy, including sacubitril/valsartan (approximately 20% of the trial population). There was also a significant improvement in functional status with empagliflozin that was sustained at 8 and 12 months of follow-up.[33] Treatment with empagliflozin proved to be effective in a subset of high-risk patients with clinically identified signs of volume overload in the 4 weeks prior to randomization.[34] In those patients, risk reduction in the primary endpoint and prevention of decline in renal function occurred to a similar extent as in euvolaemic patients, even though risk reduction in first and repeated hospitalization for HF was less compelling. Also, patients receiving empagliflozin were less likely to require intensification of diuretic treatment, regardless of their volume status. Empagliflozin also granted similar improvement in functional status and functional class in patients with and without volume overload. Interestingly, changes in body weight, haematocrit, and natriuretic peptides did not track each other in their time course nor in individual patients, casting doubt on a diuretic effect being a significant mechanism underlying the therapeutic action.[34]

The SOLOIST-WHF (Sotagliflozin in Patients with Diabetes and Recent Worsening Heart Failure) trial was designed to evaluate the effect of sotagliflozin (SGTL2/1 inhibitor) on cardiovascular outcomes in patients with T2DM who were recently hospitalized for worsening HF.[35] However, enrolment was terminated prematurely due to financial reasons and the coronavirus disease 2019 (Covid-19) pandemic. Participants were randomized to sotagliflozin 200–400 mg once daily or placebo. Key eligibility criteria are shown in ➲ Table 8.11.1. This trial enrolled T2DM patients with mildly reduced or reduced left ventricular ejection fraction (LVEF) (approximately 79%), as well as diabetic patients with HF and preserved LVEF of ≥50% (HFpEF). Sotagliflozin, compared to placebo, was associated with a 33% lower risk of the primary outcome of the total number of cardiovascular deaths, hospitalizations, and urgent visits for HF treatment (first and recurrent).[35] The treatment effect was consistent in prespecified subgroups, including stratification according to the timing of the

first dose of sotagliflozin or placebo (i.e. before or 3 days after hospital discharge), as well as in patients with LVEF of <50% and ≥50%. The key secondary endpoint of the total number of HF hospitalizations was reduced by 36% with sotagliflozin, whereas the rates of cardiovascular and total mortality were similar in both treatment arms.

The available data suggest consistent and substantial cardiovascular benefits of SGLT2 inhibition in patients with HFrEF, irrespective of T2DM status. This was confirmed in a meta-analysis of the DAPA-HF and EMPEROR-Reduced trials that demonstrated a 26% risk reduction in the combined endpoint of cardiovascular mortality or HF hospitalization, as well as a risk reduction in cardiovascular deaths, all-cause mortality, and renal events, with SGLT2 inhibition.[36a] The observed benefits occurred in addition to the recommended HF medications used in a large proportion of patients in both trials, suggesting that SGLT2 inhibitors have a complementary role to standard treatment in improving cardiovascular outcomes in HFrEF. Results of the SOLOIST-WHF trial provide evidence for safety of early introduction of SGLT2 inhibitors following haemodynamic stabilization in patients hospitalized for HF. This was confirmed by the EMPULSE (Empagliflozin in Patients Hospitalized for Acute Heart Failure) trial, which randomized patients hospitalized for acute HF (regardless of LVEF) to receiving empagliflozin or placebo. The median time to randomization was 3 days from hospital admission. Patients treated with empagliflozin were 36% more likely to experience a clinical benefit (a composite of death, number of HF events, time to first HF event, and change in the Kansas City Cardiomyopathy Questionnaire Total Symptom Score from baseline to 90 days), compared those receiving placebo, without heterogeneity in treatment effects between patients with and those without T2DM.[36b]

The EMPEROR-Preserved (Empagliflozin in Heart Failure with a Preserved Ejection Fraction) trial is the first study to provide evidence for a significant risk reduction in cardiovascular outcomes in ambulatory patients with HFpEF or HF with mildly reduced ejection fraction.[37] In this trial, patients with symptomatic HF (with or without T2DM) and LVEF of >40% were randomized to empagliflozin or placebo. Major eligibility criteria are presented in ➲ Table 8.11.1. The primary composite outcome of cardiovascular death or hospitalization for HF was reduced significantly by 21% with empagliflozin, compared to placebo.[37] Secondary endpoint analysis demonstrated a reduction in the total number (first and recurrent) of hospitalizations for HF by 27%, as well as a slower decline in eGFR with empagliflozin, compared to placebo. Predefined subgroup analyses indicated that treatment benefits of empagliflozin were consistent, regardless of diabetes status, age, sex, comorbidities, and LVEF category (<50%, ≥50% to <60%, and ≥60%). Treatment was safe and well tolerated, with a similar rate of serious adverse events in both study arms. Hypotension and uncomplicated genital or urinary tract infections were more commonly observed in patients receiving empagliflozin than in those receiving placebo.[37]

Evidence in support of the favourable effects of SGLT2 inhibition in HFpEF has come from the DELIVER trial with dapagliflozin.[37a] This trial randomized 6263 patients with HF, left ventricular ejection fraction ≥40% and elevated natriuretic peptide levels to receive either dapagliflozin 10 mg or placebo. In addition to ambulatory outpatients, the trial population included hospitalized and recently hospitalized patients as well as patients with HF and improved EF (defined as patients whose EF improved from ≤40% to >40% by the time of enrolment). After a median of 2.3 years, a statistically significant 18% reduction in the primary composite endpoint of cardiovascular death or worsening HF was observed with dapagliflozin, driven by a 21% risk reduction in worsening HF events (defined as an unplanned hospitalization for HF or an urgent visit for HF). Consistent results were observed in patients with a left ventricular ejection fraction ≥60% and those with a left ventricular ejection fraction of <60%, as well as patients with recent hospitalization[37b] or those with HF and improved EF.[37c] The incidence of adverse events was similar between dapagliflozin and placebo.

Furthermore, a meta-analysis using data from the EMPEROR-Preserved and DELIVER trials demonstrated that treatment with an SGLT2 inhibitor provided a 20% risk reduction in cardiovascular death or first HF hospitalization (HR, 0.80; 95% CI 0.73–0.87) with consistent reductions in both components of the primary outcome: cardiovascular death (HR, 0.88; 95% CI 0.77–1.00) and first HF hospitalization (HR, 0.74; 95% CI, 0·67–0·83).[37d]

The impact of SGLT2 inhibitors on measures of functional status has also been explored in several smaller-scale trials. In the DEFINE-HF (Dapagliflozin Effects on Biomarkers, Symptoms, and Functional Status in Patients With Heart Failure With Reduced Ejection Fraction) trial including patients with HFrEF with and without T2DM, dapagliflozin had a neutral effect on the reduction of natriuretic peptide levels over 12 weeks of treatment, but increased the proportion of patients achieving a combined endpoint of improved functional status or ≥20% reduction in natriuretic peptide level.[38] Similarly, in the EMPERIAL (Effect of EMPagliflozin on ExeRcise ability and heart failure symptoms In patients with chronic heart failure)-Reduced and EMPERIAL-Preserved trials, empagliflozin had a neutral effect on the change in 6-minute walk distance in patients with HFrEF and those with HFpEF, respectively, after 12 weeks of treatment.[39] These results stand in contrast to an improvement in measures of functional status observed in the larger-scale DAPA-HF and EMPEROR-Reduced trials and might reflect the shorter follow-up duration and smaller scale of these studies.

Based on the available clinical trial data, the 2021 Update to the 2017 American College Cardiology Expert Consensus Decision Pathway for Optimization of Heart Failure Treatment recommends the use of SGLT2 inhibitors (dapagliflozin and empagliflozin) for treatment of symptomatic (New York Heart Association (NYHA) classes II and IV) patients with HFrEF (LVEF ≤40%), with or without diabetes, in conjunction with a background standard therapy for HF (ACE inhibitor, ARB, or angiotensin receptor–neprilysin inhibitor (ARNI) (preferred), beta-blocker, and diuretic (if required)).[40] Before initiating an SGLT2 inhibitor, it is recommended to ensure an eGFR of ≥30 mL/min/1.73 m^2 for dapagliflozin or ≥20 mL/min/1.73 m^2 for empagliflozin.[40]

The 2021 European Society of Cardiology/Heart Failure Association Guidelines for the diagnosis and treatment of acute and chronic HF recommend the use of an SGLT2 inhibitor (dapagliflozin or empagliflozin) in patients with HFrEF to reduce cardiovascular mortality and the risk of HF hospitalization (Class I, Level of evidence A).[41] In addition to ACE inhibitors or sacubitril/valsartan (or an ARB in patients intolerant of ACE inhibitors or sacubitril/valsartan), beta-blockers, and mineralocorticoid receptor antagonists, SGLT2 inhibitors constitute the four pillars of HFrEF treatment. They should be used in all patients with HFrEF (who are already receiving an ACE inhibitor or sacubitril/valsartan, beta-blockers, and mineralocorticoid receptor antagonists), regardless of their T2DM status. Use of SGLT2 inhibitors is facilitated by the fact that there is no requirement for dose intensification/modification or the risk of hypotension or electrolyte disturbances (e.g. hyperkalaemia). Caution is stipulated regarding a risk of genital mycotic infections and a reversible small reduction in eGFR that can be expected upon treatment initiation.[41]

Safety aspects of treatment with SGLT2 inhibitors

Early clinical trials of SGLT2 inhibitors in patients with T2DM have raised concerns about their potential association with serious adverse effects, including urinary tract infections, bone fractures, limb amputations, diabetic ketoacidosis, and acute kidney injury. Fortunately, for most adverse events, early signals of harm have not been supported by later data. A meta-analysis including 110 controlled trials in patients with T2DM has indicated that SGLT2 inhibitors, as a class, do not increase the risk of urinary tract infections, despite their pharmacological glucosuric effect. Conversely, SGLT2 inhibitors do increase the risk of genital mycotic infections by 3- to 4-fold, with an even greater risk observed in women. Optimizing T2DM care and improving personal hygiene may help to prevent infection and, in most cases, oral antifungals (i.e. a single dose of oral fluconazole) or topical antifungal creams (i.e. miconazole or clotrimazole for 1–3 days) can be used to successfully treat the infection.[42] A safety analysis of the CANVAS Program has suggested an increased risk of bone fractures and lower limb amputations with canagliflozin. This risk has not been reported with canagliflozin in the CREDENCE trial, and a meta-analysis of 63 trials with different SGLT2 inhibitors has not provided support to a greater risk of bone fractures with SGLT2 inhibitors, compared to placebo or active comparators.[43] Thus far, research evidence on the risk of lower limb amputations is limited to the few described cases receiving canagliflozin in the CANVAS Program, and more data are needed to establish whether there may be a true risk and whether the risk applies to all or select SGLT2 inhibitors.[43] Furthermore, a meta-analysis of eight placebo-controlled trials has provided reassuring results with regard to the risk of acute kidney injury, which was, in fact, lower with use of SGLT2 inhibitors (or neutral after exclusion of the EMPA-REG Outcome results which heavily favoured a lower risk).[43] Nevertheless, situations where the risk of acute kidney injury may be exacerbated include states of volume depletion (e.g. due to excessive use of diuretics), excessive intraglomerular pressure decrease (e.g. concomitant introduction of SGLT2 inhibitors and renin–angiotensin–aldosterone system blockers), and renal medullary hypoxic injury (e.g. concomitant use of non-steroidal anti-inflammatory drugs and iodine contrast dyes).[44] Acute kidney injury needs to be distinguished from a functional, transient drop in eGFR seen early after initiation of SGLT2 inhibitors, with subsequent stabilization of eGFR or return to baseline levels with continued treatment. This effect is likely the result of NHE inhibition in the renal proximal tubule and increased delivery of sodium and chloride to the macula densa, which, in turn, triggers the tubuloglomerular feedback, resulting in vasoconstriction of the proximal afferent arteriole and a drop in intraglomerular pressure. In the long run, this effect plays an important role in slowing the decline in eGFR, an effect confirmed in clinical trials. Lastly, rare cases of 'euglycaemic' diabetic ketoacidosis (characterized by lower-than-expected glucose levels) have been described in diabetic patients, possibly due to increased glucagon release and decreased renal ketone body excretion with SGTL2 inhibitor treatment. The risk of ketoacidosis may be exacerbated by acute illness or critical injury, especially in insulin-dependent patients, and if ketoacidosis does occur, permanent discontinuation of use of SGLT2 inhibitors is advised.[45] Reassuringly, a meta-analysis of 26 clinical trials including 18 placebo-controlled trials indicated a similar risk in both patients treated with SGLT2 inhibitors as well as those receiving placebo or incretin-based glucose-lowering medications.[43]

Safety analysis of randomized clinical trials of SGLT2 inhibitors in the treatment of patients with HF have confirmed their overall favourable safety profile. In the DAPA-HF and EMPEROR-Reduced trials, serious adverse events were infrequent and occurred at similar rates in both intervention and placebo arms of the respective trials. Even further, in DAPA-HF, serious renal adverse events were less frequently observed with dapagliflozin. In the SOLOIST-WHF trial, severe hypoglycaemia (1.5% vs 0.3%) and diarrhoea (6.1% vs 3.4%) occurred more frequently with sotagliflozin, likely due to SGLT1 inhibition, whereas the rates of other serious adverse events were comparable between the two study arms. A meta-analysis of DAPA-HF and EMPEROR-Reduced trial data suggested no excess risk in serious adverse events, compared to placebo.[36]

Future directions

Ongoing trials of SGLT2 inhibitors in patients with HF (with and without T2DM) are expected to provide answers to the currently unresolved questions on the mechanisms and clinical scope of these medications in the treatment of HF. Of note, promising results from the SOLOIST-WHF trial in a subset of diabetic HF patients with LVEF of ≥50% have strengthened the rationale for assessing the effects of SGLT2 inhibitors in the treatment of HFpEF. Further data on the impact of SGLT2 inhibition on cardiovascular outcomes are expected from EMPACT-MI (A Study to Test Whether Empagliflozin Can Lower the Risk of Heart Failure and Death in People Who Had a Heart Attack (ClinicalTrials.gov identifier: NCT04509674). EMPACT-MI is expected to provide insight into the safety and efficacy of introducing empagliflozin within 2 weeks of an acute myocardial infarction in patients

with a high risk of developing HF. The primary endpoint of this study is a composite of all-cause mortality or HF hospitalization. Furthermore, several other ongoing studies are evaluating the effects of SGLT2 inhibition on different domains of health status and exploring the impact on cardiac physiology and metabolism, as assessed by modern comprehensive imaging modalities.

Key messages

♦ SGLT2 inhibitors (canagliflozin, dapagliflozin, empagliflozin, ertugliflozin, and sotagliflozin) provide significant cardiovascular and renal protection and reduce the risk of HF hospitalization in individuals with T2DM, including those with CKD. These medications can be considered as an essential treatment for the prevention of HF in T2DM.

♦ In patients with HFrEF, dapagliflozin and empagliflozin have proven beneficial in reducing the risk of cardiovascular mortality or hospitalization for HF, regardless of sex, age, T2DM status, baseline LVEF, or background medical therapy. Therefore, dapagliflozin and empagliflozin are recommended in the treatment of all patients with HFrEF, in addition to standard HF medications, and should be introduced early in the treatment course. Their use is facilitated by the lack of requirement for uptitration or the risk of hypotension or electrolyte disturbances.

♦ Sotagliflozin has been shown to provide favourable effects in reducing HF events and cardiovascular mortality in individuals with T2DM and recent hospitalization for worsening HF, suggesting that SGLT2 inhibition can be safe and beneficial even in vulnerable patients soon after stabilization of decompensated HF. The role of SGLT2 inhibitors in the treatment of acute HF is being explored in ongoing trials.

♦ In patients with HFpEF and those with HF with mildly reduced ejection fraction, empagliflozin has been shown to cause attenuation in cardiovascular death or HF hospitalization, regardless of T2DM status. These results suggest that SGLT2 inhibitors may be drugs with significant cardiovascular protection in patients with HFpEF, but this remains to be confirmed.

♦ SGLT2 inhibitors have a generally favourable safety profile. In randomized controlled trials of patients with HF, serious adverse events were infrequent and occurred at similar rates in both intervention and placebo arms.

References

1. Heerspink HJL, Stefansson BV, Correa-Rotter R, et al. Dapagliflozin in patients with chronic kidney disease. N Engl J Med. 2020;383(15):1436–46.
2. Neal B, Perkovic V, Mahaffey KW, et al. Canagliflozin and cardiovascular and renal events in type 2 diabetes. N Engl J Med. 2017;377(7):644–57.
3. Perkovic V, Jardine MJ, Neal B, et al. Canagliflozin and renal outcomes in type 2 diabetes and nephropathy. N Engl J Med. 2019;380(24):2295–306.
4. Wiviott SD, Raz I, Bonaca MP, et al. Dapagliflozin and cardiovascular outcomes in type 2 diabetes. N Engl J Med. 2019;380(4):347–57.
5. Zinman B, Wanner C, Lachin JM, et al. Empagliflozin, cardiovascular outcomes, and mortality in type 2 diabetes. N Engl J Med. 2015;373(22):2117–28.

6. Bhatt DL, Szarek M, Pitt B, *et al.* Sotagliflozin in patients with diabetes and chronic kidney disease. N Engl J Med. 2021;384(2):129–39.

7. McMurray JJV, Solomon SD, Inzucchi SE, *et al.* Dapagliflozin in patients with heart failure and reduced ejection fraction. N Engl J Med. 2019;381(21):1995–2008.

8. Packer M, Anker SD, Butler J, *et al.* Cardiovascular and renal outcomes with empagliflozin in heart failure. N Engl J Med. 2020;383(15):1413–24.

9. Bhatt DL, Szarek M, Steg PG, *et al.* Sotagliflozin in patients with diabetes and recent worsening heart failure. N Engl J Med. 2021;384(2):117–28.

10. US Food and Drug Administration. Guidance for industry on diabetes mellitus—evaluating cardiovascular risk in new antidiabetic therapies to treat type 2 diabetes. 2008. Available from: www.federalregister.gov/documents/2008/12/19/E8-30086/guidance-for-industry-on-diabetes-mellitus-evaluating-cardiovascular-risk-in-new-antidiabetic.

11. Zelniker TA, Braunwald E. Cardiac and renal effects of sodium–glucose co-transporter 2 inhibitors in diabetes: JACC state-of-the-art review. J Am Coll Cardiol. 2018;72(15):1845–55.

12. Zelniker TA, Braunwald E. Clinical benefit of cardiorenal effects of sodium–glucose cotransporter 2 inhibitors: JACC state-of-the-art review. J Am Coll Cardiol. 2020;75(4):435–47.

13. Zelniker TA, Braunwald E. Mechanisms of cardiorenal effects of sodium–glucose cotransporter 2 inhibitors: JACC state-of-the-art review. J Am Coll Cardiol. 2020;75(4):422–34.

14. Omar M, Jensen J, Frederiksen PH, *et al.* Effect of empagliflozin on hemodynamics in patients with heart failure and reduced ejection fraction. J Am Coll Cardiol. 2020;76(23):2740–51.

15. Santos-Gallego CG, Requena-Ibanez JA, San Antonio R, *et al.* Empagliflozin ameliorates adverse left ventricular remodeling in nondiabetic heart failure by enhancing myocardial energetics. J Am Coll Cardiol. 2019;73(15):1931–44.

16. Lee MMY, Brooksbank KJM, Wetherall K, *et al.* Effect of empagliflozin on left ventricular volumes in patients with type 2 diabetes, or prediabetes, and heart Failure with reduced ejection fraction (SUGAR-DM-HF). Circulation. 2021;143(6):516–25.

17. Santos-Gallego CG, Vargas-Delgado AP, Requena-Ibanez JA, *et al.* Randomized trial of empagliflozin in nondiabetic patients with heart failure and reduced ejection fraction. J Am Coll Cardiol. 2021;77(3):243–55.

18. Neuen BL, Young T, Heerspink HJL, *et al.* SGLT2 inhibitors for the prevention of kidney failure in patients with type 2 diabetes: a systematic review and meta-analysis. Lancet Diabetes Endocrinol. 2019;7(11):845–54.

19. Fitchett D, Zinman B, Wanner C, *et al.* Heart failure outcomes with empagliflozin in patients with type 2 diabetes at high cardiovascular risk: results of the EMPA-REG OUTCOME(R) trial. Eur Heart J. 2016;37(19):1526–34.

20. Cannon CP, Pratley R, Dagogo-Jack S, *et al.* Cardiovascular outcomes with ertugliflozin in type 2 diabetes. N Engl J Med. 2020;383(15):1425–35.

21. McGuire DK, Shih WJ, Cosentino F, *et al.* Association of SGLT2 inhibitors with cardiovascular and kidney outcomes in patients with type 2 diabetes: a meta-analysis. JAMA Cardiol. 2021;6(2):148–58.

22. Morales A, Painter T, Li R, *et al.* Rare variant mutations in pregnancy-associated or peripartum cardiomyopathy. Circulation. 2010;121(20):2176–82.

23. Cosentino F, Cannon CP, Cherney DZI, *et al.* Efficacy of ertugliflozin on heart failure-related events in patients with type 2 diabetes mellitus and established atherosclerotic cardiovascular disease: results of the VERTIS CV Trial. Circulation. 2020;142(23):2205–15.

24. Bhatt DL, Szarek M, Pitt B, *et al.* Sotagliflozin in patients with diabetes and chronic kidney disease. N Engl J Med. 2021;384(2):129–39.

25. Cosentino F, Grant PJ, Aboyans V, *et al.* 2019 ESC Guidelines on diabetes, pre-diabetes, and cardiovascular diseases developed in collaboration with the EASD. Eur Heart J. 2020;41(2):255–323.

26. McMurray JJV, Solomon SD, Inzucchi SE, *et al.* Dapagliflozin in patients with heart failure and reduced ejection fraction. N Engl J Med. 2019;381(21):1995–2008.

27. Berg DD, Jhund PS, Docherty KF, *et al.* Time to clinical benefit of dapagliflozin and significance of prior heart failure hospitalization in patients with heart failure with reduced ejection fraction. JAMA Cardiol. 2021;6(5):499–507.

28. Docherty KF, Jhund PS, Inzucchi SE, *et al.* Effects of dapagliflozin in DAPA-HF according to background heart failure therapy. Eur Heart J. 2020;41(25):2379–92.

29. Martinez FA, Serenelli M, Nicolau JC, *et al.* Efficacy and safety of dapagliflozin in heart failure with reduced ejection fraction according to age: insights from DAPA-HF. Circulation. 2020;141(2):100–11.

30. Lainščak M, Milinković I, Polovina M, *et al.* Sex- and age-related differences in the management and outcomes of chronic heart failure: an analysis of patients from the ESC HFA EORP Heart Failure Long-Term Registry. Eur J Heart Fail. 2020;22(1):92–102.

31. Packer M, Anker SD, Butler J, *et al.* Cardiovascular and renal outcomes with empagliflozin in heart failure. N Engl J Med. 2020;383(15):1413–24.

32. Packer M, Anker SD, Butler J, *et al.* Effect of empagliflozin on the clinical stability of patients with heart failure and a reduced ejection fraction: the EMPEROR-Reduced trial. Circulation. 2021;143(4):326–36.

33. Butler J, Anker SD, Filippatos G, *et al.* Empagliflozin and health-related quality of life outcomes in patients with heart failure with reduced ejection fraction: the EMPEROR-Reduced trial. Eur Heart J. 2021;42(13):1203–12.

34. Packer M, Anker SD, Butler J, *et al.* Empagliflozin in patients with heart failure, reduced ejection fraction, and volume overload: EMPEROR-Reduced trial. J Am Coll Cardiol. 2021;77(11):1381–92.

35. Bhatt DL, Szarek M, Steg PG, *et al.* Sotagliflozin in patients with diabetes and recent worsening heart failure. N Engl J Med. 2020;384(2):117–28.

36a. Zannad F, Ferreira JP, Pocock SJ, *et al.* SGLT2 inhibitors in patients with heart failure with reduced ejection fraction: a meta-analysis of the EMPEROR-Reduced and DAPA-HF trials. Lancet. 2020;396(10254):819–29.

36b. Voors AA, Angermann CE, Teerlink JR, *et al.* The SGLT2 inhibitor empagliflozin in patients hospitalized for acute heart failure: a multinational randomized trial. Nat Med. 2022;28(3):568–74.

37. Anker SD, Butler J, Filippatos G, *et al.* Empagliflozin in heart failure with a preserved ejection fraction. N Engl J Med. 2021;385(16):1451–61.

37a. Solomon SD, McMurray JJV, Claggett B, *et al.* Dapagliflozin in heart failure with mildly reduced or preserved ejection fraction. N Engl J Med. 2022;387:1089–98.

37b. Cunningham JW, Vaduganathan M, Claggett BL, *et al.* Dapagliflozin in patients recently hospitalized with heart failure and mildly reduced or preserved ejection fraction. J Am Coll Cardiol. 2022;80(14):1302–10.

37c. Vardeny O, Fang JC, Desai AS, *et al.* Dapagliflozin in heart failure with improved ejection fraction: a prespecified analysis of the DELIVER trial. Nature Medicine. 2022;28(12):2504–11.

37d. Vaduganathan M, Docherty KF, Claggett BL, *et al.* SGLT-2 inhibitors in patients with heart failure: a comprehensive meta-analysis of five randomised controlled trials. Lancet. 2022;400(10354):757–67.

38. Nassif ME, Windsor SL, Tang F, *et al.* Dapagliflozin effects on biomarkers, symptoms, and functional status in patients with heart failure with reduced ejection fraction: the DEFINE-HF trial. Circulation. 2019;140(18):1463–76.

39. Abraham WT, Lindenfeld J, Ponikowski P, *et al.* Effect of empagliflozin on exercise ability and symptoms in heart failure patients with reduced and preserved ejection fraction, with and without type 2 diabetes. Eur Heart J. 2021;42(6):700–10.

40. Maddox TM, Januzzi JL Jr, Allen LA, *et al.* 2021 Update to the 2017 ACC expert consensus decision pathway for optimization of heart failure treatment: answers to 10 pivotal issues about heart failure with reduced ejection fraction: a report of the American College of Cardiology Solution Set Oversight Committee. J Am Coll Cardiol. 2021;77(6):772–810.

41. McDonagh TA, Metra M, Adamo M, *et al.* 2021 ESC Guidelines for the diagnosis and treatment of acute and chronic heart failure: developed by the Task Force for the diagnosis and treatment of acute and chronic heart failure of the European Society of Cardiology (ESC) With the special contribution of the Heart Failure Association (HFA) of the ESC. Eur Heart J. 2021;42(36):3599–726.

42. Engelhardt K, Ferguson M, Rosselli JL. Prevention and management of genital mycotic infections in the setting of sodium–glucose cotransporter 2 inhibitors. Ann Pharmacother. 2021;55(4):543–8.

43. Donnan JR, Grandy CA, Chibrikov E, *et al.* Comparative safety of the sodium glucose co-transporter 2 (SGLT2) inhibitors: a systematic review and meta-analysis. BMJ Open. 2019;9(1): e022577.

44. Szalat A, Perlman A, Muszkat M, Khamaisi M, Abassi Z, Heyman SN. Can SGLT2 inhibitors cause acute renal failure? Plausible role for altered glomerular hemodynamics and medullary hypoxia. Drug Saf. 2018;41(3):239–52.

45. Seferovic PM, Coats AJS, Ponikowski P, *et al.* European Society of Cardiology/Heart Failure Association position paper on the role and safety of new glucose-lowering drugs in patients with heart failure. Eur J Heart Fail. 2020;22(2):196–213.

CHAPTER 8.12

Ancillary pharmacological treatment options

Stefan Agewall, Isabelle C van Gelder, and Irina Savelieva

Contents

Introduction

Heart failure (HF) is a common condition and is often associated with a poor prognosis. Management of HF remains a significant challenge. Furthermore, many of the patients with HF have multiple comorbidities. The most recent European Society of Cardiology (ESC) Guidelines and American College of Cardiology (ACC)/American Heart Association (AHA) Guidelines on pharmacological treatment of patients with HF with reduced ejection fraction (HFrEF) are quite clear. Still there are areas of much controversy within HF treatment. These patients often suffer from coronary artery disease (CAD) and arrhythmias that may be associated with a high risk of complications and might be lethal.

In this chapter, we discuss ancillary pharmacological treatment options such as anticoagulant treatment, statin treatment, and treatment with antiarrhythmic drugs.

Anticoagulants

HF is a complex syndrome with many interactions between the failing myocardium and cerebral dysfunction, including stroke. Stroke is the most common cause of disability in adult life and a major cause of death. A strong interaction between HF and ischaemic stroke is well established. Stroke contributes significantly to morbidity and mortality in HF patients.[1] The mechanisms involved in the occurrence of stroke in HF patients are heterogeneous and include atrial fibrillation (AF) in the setting of comorbidities, decreased blood flow velocity in the dilated hypokinetic or akinetic chambers of the heart with rheological alterations, increased aggregation of thrombocytes, reduced fibrinolysis, endothelial dysfunction, inflammatory activation, and malfunctioning of cerebral autoregulation, which are factors contributing to the risk of thromboembolism related to HF.[2,3,4] In addition, stroke may be associated with concomitant factors such as small-vessel occlusion and large-artery atherosclerosis, especially in those with ischaemic HF.[2] Studies in patients with HFrEF and those with HF with preserved ejection fraction (HFpEF) have shown higher rates of stroke and systemic embolic events, as compared to the general population, ranging between 7% and 10%, with no difference between HFpEF and HFrEF.[3] Thus, in HF, not only the syndrome of HF, but also, and probably differentially, associated comorbidities such as hypertension, vascular disease, CAD, and diabetes mellitus contribute to the occurrence of stroke.

In patients with documented AF and HF, it is recommended to start long-term treatment with oral anticoagulation if the CHA_2DS_2-VASc score is ≥ 2 in men or ≥ 3 in women. Long-term anticoagulation should be considered in patients with AF and HF and a CHA_2DS_2-VASc score of 1 in men or 2 in women.[5,6] Until now, however, the debate is ongoing on whether or not to start antithrombotic strategies in patients with HF and sinus rhythm.[7] Several trials investigated the possible benefit of anticoagulation in patients with HF and sinus rhythm. In the Warfarin versus Aspirin in Reduced Cardiac Ejection Fraction (WARCEF) trial, a reduced risk of ischaemic stroke with warfarin, as compared to aspirin, was offset by more major bleeding events. There was no difference between the primary endpoint of ischaemic stroke, intracerebral haemorrhage, and death, which was comparable between the two groups (7.47 events per 100 patient-years in the warfarin group and 7.93 in the aspirin group, hazard ratio 0.93, 95% confidence interval 0.79–1.10; $P = 0.40$).[8] Meta-analyses have confirmed an increased risk of bleeding outweighing the prevention of ischaemic stroke.[9]

Direct oral anticoagulants are now recommended in preference to vitamin K antagonists, except in those with moderate or severe mitral stenosis or mechanical prosthetic heart valves.[5,6] In the COMMANDER HF trial (a study to assess the effectiveness and safety of rivaroxaban in reducing the risk of death, myocardial infarction (MI), or stroke in participants with HF and CAD following an episode of decompensated HF), patients with HFrEF, CAD, and elevated plasma concentrations of natriuretic peptides without documented AF were randomly assigned to low-dose rivaroxaban (2.5 mg twice daily) or to placebo. COMMANDER HF showed that rivaroxaban 2.5 mg twice daily did not improve the composite outcome of all-cause mortality, MI, or stroke, nor HF-related deaths or HF hospitalization.[10] One of the reasons why rivaroxaban 2.5 mg twice daily did not improve cardiovascular (CV) outcomes in these HFrEF patients may be that, except for the too low dosage, thrombin-mediated events are not the major driver of HF-related events in HF patients. This again emphasizes that the mechanism of stroke is much more complex than previously anticipated, as also demonstrated in patients with embolic stroke of unknown source.[11,12] Thus, anticoagulation should not routinely be instituted in patients with HFrEF who are in sinus rhythm and do not have documented AF.

However, of interest, some HFrEF patients without AF may benefit from start of anticoagulation. In a non-prespecified subgroup analysis of the Cardiovascular Outcomes for People Using Anticoagulation Strategies (COMPASS) trial, low-dose rivaroxaban, on top of aspirin, was associated with a reduction in ischaemic events in patients with HF, mainly HF with mildly reduced ejection fraction (HFmrEF) or HFpEF (patients with New York Heart Association (NYHA) functional class III or IV HF or left ventricular ejection fraction (LVEF) of <30% were excluded).[12] Based on the above, low-dose rivaroxaban may be considered in patients with concomitant CAD or peripheral artery disease, a high risk of stroke, and no major haemorrhagic risk.[13] Additionally, patients with an intraventricular thrombus or with a high thrombotic risk (e.g. after a peripheral embolism or those with known peripartum or left ventricular (LV) non-compaction cardiomyopathy) should be considered for anticoagulation.[6]

Statins

There has been a large discussion on the role of lipid-lowering therapy in HF patients. The issue of whether or not to use statins in patients with HF remains controversial. It is well established that hydroxymethylglutaryl coenzyme A (HMG-CoA) reductase inhibitors (statins) reduce CAD events in patients with and without CV disease. Thus, it may be logical to suppose that statins prevent MI and consequent cardiac damage, and so reduce the risk of patients developing HFrEF. However, in many of the major lipid-lowering trials on the effects of statin therapy, HF patients were excluded,[14,15] and patients with severely symptomatic HF were excluded in other trials.[16,17] In a meta-analysis of 17 major primary and secondary prevention randomized trials with 132,538 participants conducted over 4.3 years, statins modestly reduced the risks of non-fatal hospitalization for HF, but not HF death.[18] The authors found no difference in risk reduction between those who suffered an incident MI and those did not and therefore, this benefit did not seem to be due to prevention of MI preceding HF. Thus, a noteworthy finding from this study concerns the mechanisms by which statin therapy reduced the risk of HF hospitalization. Interestingly, neither a reduced risk of non-fatal MI nor a decrease in low-density lipoprotein cholesterol (LDL-C) level correlated with the risk of HF hospitalization. These results may raise the possibility that statins might have exerted beneficial effects on HF hospitalization through their pleiotropic properties. In the WOSCOPS trial, pravastatin therapy led to a 35% reduction in the long-term risk of hospitalization for HF.[19] HF events subsequent to MI were significantly reduced by pravastatin treatment, compared to placebo, and incident HF not preceded by MI was also less common in pravastatin-treated patients, although the difference was not significant. This is consistent with the finding in the meta-analysis above[18] that statins reduce HF risk through mechanisms additional to prevention of acute MI. It is also in line with the hypothesis that statins may prevent HF. These results raise the possibility that statins might have exerted beneficial effects on HF hospitalization through their pleiotropic properties. In contrast, treatment with statins has not decreased the risk of morbidity and mortality in two large-scale placebo-controlled trials of patients with established HF (CORONA and GISSI-HF).[20,21] CORONA and GISSI-HF were large-scale placebo-controlled trials of statin treatment in subjects with NYHA class II–IV HF. CORONA recruited 5011 ischaemic systolic HF patients aged ≥60 years, whereas GISSI-HF included 4574 patients with HF of any aetiology aged ≥18 years. The active treatment arm used 10 mg/day of rosuvastatin in both trials, and median follow-up was 46.8 months in GISSI-HF and 32.8 months in CORONA. In GISSI-HF, the co-primary endpoints were time to death, and time to death or CV hospitalization. In CORONA, the primary endpoint was the composite of CV death, non-fatal MI, or non-fatal stroke. No significant decrease in the primary composite mortality/morbidity endpoint was seen in actively treated subjects in either trial. However, CORONA did show that rosuvastatin therapy led to fewer CV hospitalizations.[20]

Some criticisms on the CORONA trial have been raised; the patients were quite old (mean age 73 years) and a large majority were in advanced HF stages.[20] In the CORONA trial, patients in the lowest N-terminal pro-B-type natriuretic peptide tertile did actually benefit from rosuvastatin therapy, with a significant reduction in the primary outcome.[22] Thus, it has been suggested that in patients with less advanced HF, statin therapy might be beneficial in reduction of coronary events, whereas in severe HF, it would be too late for the potential benefits from statin therapy due to progressive loss of pump function. The CORONA trial was a randomized controlled trial (RCT), whereas the Evaluation of Losartan In The Elderly 2 (ELITE 2) study reported that patients who received statin therapy at baseline had lower mortality, compared to non-statin users.[23] The authors suggested that in chronic HF, treatment with statins may be related to lower mortality, independent of cholesterol level, disease aetiology, and clinical status.

Patients with dyslipidaemia, obesity, and type 2 diabetes are at heightened risk of developing HF, but the most common phenotype in these individuals is HFpEF.[24,25] In a registry study of 9140 patients with HF and LVEF of ≥50%, the patients were divided into those treated with ($n = 3427$) and those not treated with statins ($n = 5713$). Statins were associated with better 1-year survival, reduced CV death, and composite all-cause mortality or CV hospitalization.[26] In a meta-analysis, Fukuta et al.[27] examined the effect of statin therapy on mortality in patients with HF with LVEF of ≥45% with use of propensity score analysis. The authors suggested that statin therapy was associated with reduced mortality. Another meta-analysis included 11 eligible studies with 17,985 patients with HF and LVEF of >45%. Statin use was associated with a 40% lower risk of mortality.[28] These results may suggest statin therapy is associated with improved survival rates in patients with HFpEF. However, RCTs are needed to confirm the efficacy of statins in HFpEF.

Cholesterol paradox and pleiotropic effects

Raised plasma cholesterol level is a causal risk factor for CAD. However, low serum total cholesterol level is associated with poor prognosis in patients with established HF (in contrast to patients without HF); thus, there is a recognized 'cholesterol paradox' in this cardiac condition. Notably, cholesterol level has an inverse correlation with disease severity markers in other diseases which have a strong inflammatory component (e.g. chronic kidney disease, severe rheumatoid arthritis). Thus, possible reasons for the inverse association of cholesterol level with HF may be linked, in part, to greater systemic inflammation in certain groups of patients. Statins have multiple biological effects. These pleiotropic effects of statins may potentially influence the course of HF. Statins may decrease vascular and myocardial oxidative stress[29] and may possess anti-inflammatory properties.[30] It has also been suggested that statins might reduce muscle strength[31] and alter energy metabolism during aerobic exercise, but some available data indicate that statins may even have beneficial effects by preserving or even increasing lean mass and exercise performance.[31]

In conclusion, treatment with statins is recommended in patients at high risk of CV disease or with CV disease. Based on current evidence, routine administration of statins in patients with HF without other indications for their use (e.g. CAD) is not recommended. Because there is no evidence of harm in patients on statin treatment after the occurrence of HF, there is no need for statin discontinuation for patients already on treatment.

Antiarrhythmic drugs

Antiarrhythmic drugs are classified using the Singh–Vaughan Williams classification (◐ Table 8.12.1), which is based on the mechanisms of action of antiarrhythmic drugs, most of which target cardiac myocyte transmembrane ion currents altering the channel structure, dynamics, or gating process, with resultant effects on cardiac excitability, effective refractory periods, conduction, or abnormal automaticity.[32,33] There are four classes of antiarrhythmic drugs: sodium channel blockers (class I), β-adrenoceptor antagonists (class II), drugs that predominantly block potassium channels and prolong action potential duration (APD) without affecting intracardiac conduction (class III), and non-dihydropyridine L-type calcium channel blockers (class IV). Class I drugs are further divided into those with intermediate- (IA), fast- (IB), and slow- (IC) offset kinetics of sodium channel blockade.

Modernized Singh–Vaughan Williams classification

In 2018, a revised classification based on that by Singh–Vaughan Williams, but significantly modified and advanced to incorporate contemporary knowledge on the existing drugs and their physiological sequelae and agents with novel mechanisms of action to new targets/mechanisms that may be developed in the future, was proposed.[34] It includes agents such as the If current (hyperpolarization-activated cyclic nucleotide-gated channel) inhibitor ivabradine (class 0), acknowledges the existence of sodium current components and subspecies of potassium channels, and expands class II to include β-adrenergic receptor blockers and activators, M2 receptor activators (digoxin) and inhibitors (atropine), and A1 receptor activators (adenosine, tecadenosone) under the umbrella of autonomic inhibitors and activators. Class III contains potassium channel blockers and openers. The revised classification incorporates new classes with additional targets, including channels involved in automaticity, mechanically sensitive ion channels, connexins controlling electrotonic cell coupling, and molecules underlying longer-term signalling processes affecting structural remodelling.

Antiarrhythmic drugs used to treat arrhythmias in heart failure

One of the core goals of the antiarrhythmic drug classification is guidance in selection of an effective agent for a specific type of arrhythmia, with minimal off-target action. The main concerns and caveats of antiarrhythmic drug therapy in HF are a potential adverse impact on ventricular function and the risk of proarrhythmia, particularly during decompensation of HF.

Table 8.12.1 Classification and pharmacological properties of antiarrhythmic drugs

Class	Drugs	Channel blockade			Receptor blockade			Other MOA	APD	ECG
		Na⁺	Ca²⁺	K⁺	α	β	M2			
IA: intermediate offset kinetics	Ajmaline	● A							↑	0/↑ PR, ↑ QRS, QT and JT
	Cibenzoline	● A	○	⊘			○		↑	↑ PR, QRS and QT
	Disopyramide*	● A		⊘			○		↑	↓/↑ PR, ↑ QRS, QT and JT
	Pilsicainide	● A							↑	↑ PR, QRS and QT
	Procainamide*	● I		⊘					↑	0/↑ PR, ↑ QRS, QT and JT
	Quinidine*	● A		⊘	○		⊘		↑	↓/↑ PR, ↑ QRS, QT and JT
IB: fast offset kinetics	Lidocaine*	○I							↓	0/↓ QT, ↓ JT
	Mexiletine	○I							↓	0/↓ QT, ↓ JT
	Phenytoin	○I							↓	0
IC: slow offset kinetics	Flecainide	● A							0/↑	↑ PR, QRS and QT
	Propafenone*	● A	⊘			⊘			0/↑	↑ PR, QRS and QT
II	Atenolol, Carvedilol								0/↓	↑ PR, 0/↓ QT
	Esmolol, Metoprolol									
	Nadolol, Propranolol					●				
III	Amiodarone*	○	⊘	⊘	⊘	⊘			↑	↑PR, QRS, QT and JT
	Dronedarone	○	⊘	⊘	⊘	⊘			↑	↑PR, QRS, QT and JT
	Dofetilide			● IKur					↑	0 PR, ↑QT and JT
	Ibutilide	INaL		○IKur					↑	0/↓ PR, ↑QT and JT
	Sotalol			● IKur		●			↑	↑PR, QT and JT
IV	Diltiazem		⊘						↓	↑PR
	Verapamil*		●						↓	↑PR
V	Adenosine							IKAdo	↑	↑PR
	Atropine						●			
	Digoxin							● Na⁺/K⁺-ATPase		↑PR, ↓JT
	Ivabradine							● If		
								Antianginal drug		
	Ranolazine	○		○IKur				Antianginal drug	↑	↑QT and JT
		● INaL								
	Vernakalant	○I		⊘		⊘				

↑Antiarrhythmic drugs are subdivided using the Singh-Vaughan Williams system and their effects on targets (channels, receptors, or pumps), and clinical effects are presented following the Sicilian Gambit classification system. Class I AADs are subdivided in three groups [fast (IB), intermediate (IA) and slow (IC)] according to the time constants for recovery from block (offset kinetics) and the affinity for the open (○) or inactivated (I) states of the Na⁺ channels is shown. The relative potency of blockade of ion channels and receptors and their extracardiac side effects observed at therapeutic plasma levels are classified as low (open circles), moderate (striped circles), or high (black circles).

□ indicates agonist, ↑ indicates increase or prolong; ↓ indicates decrease or shorten.

0, minimal effect; α/β, α- and β-adrenoceptors; A, activated state Na⁺ channel blocker; APD, action potential duration; ECE, # extracardiac effects; HR, heart rate; I, inactivated state Na⁺ channel blocker; Kr, rapid component of the delayed rectifier outward K⁺ current; LVF, left ventricular function/contractility; M2, muscarinic receptor subtype 2; MOA, mechanism of action.

*Active metabolites.

With the advent of cardiac implantable electronic devices (CIEDs) for management of life-threatening ventricular arrhythmias, and left atrial ablation for management of AF, antiarrhythmic drugs have relatively limited indications: for symptom relief; to control tachyarrhythmias that may cause deterioration of LV systolic function (e.g. AF with fast ventricular rates irresponsive to atrioventricular (AV) blockade, frequent ventricular premature beats); and as an add-on to device and/or ablation intervention (e.g. to reduce the frequency of shockable tachyarrhythmias or electrical storm, or to deter recurrent AF).

Class IB antiarrhythmic drugs: lidocaine and mexiletine

Among class I (agents with principal action on the sodium channels), only *mexiletine* and *lidocaine* (class IIb) can be used for treating ventricular arrhythmias in patients with HF, whereas classes IA (*disopyramide*) and IC (*flecainide* and *propafenone*) are not recommended in these patients because of their negative inotropic effect and the risk of ventricular proarrhythmias.[35]

For treatment of significant ventricular arrhythmias, mexiletine is given at 200–300 mg three times daily; a loading dose of 400 mg can be used, followed by 200 mg three times daily, but the maximum dose should not exceed 1200 mg/day. An 8- to 24-hour infusion of lidocaine at 1–4 mg/min is administered after the first loading bolus, in order to reach a steady state. Mexiletine and lidocaine are predominantly metabolized by the liver, and drug elimination may be delayed in HF and other causes of hepatic insufficiency.

Beta-blockers

The class II drugs *beta-blockers* are widely used in the management of HF, but their efficacy as antiarrhythmics is modest, largely due to their beneficial effect on the underlying pathology and LV function; in AF, beta-blockers are useful to control ventricular rates.

Class III agents: sotalol and dofetilide

The class III (HERG channel-mediated rapid potassium current blockers) agent *d,l-sotalol* is generally avoided in the setting of HF but may be used in selected patients, more commonly for ventricular arrhythmias, if certain provision is followed such as QT interval monitoring and ensuring there is no significant LV hypertrophy. Sotalol also exerts non-selective competitive β1-adrenoceptor antagonism (predominantly confined to the levo-isomer l-sotalol), devoid of intrinsic sympathomimetic or membrane-stabilizing activity.[36] Of note, d-sotalol, a potassium channel blocker with no beta-blocking activity, has been associated with increased mortality in patients with recent MI and LV dysfunction.[37] Oral sotalol dosages range from 160 to 480 mg/day on a twice-daily regimen. Hypotension and bradycardia are the most frequent CV adverse effects of sotalol, with an incidence of 6–10%, whereas ventricular proarrhythmias associated with prolongation of the QT interval occur in 1–4.3% of patients and are dose-related. The incidence of torsades de pointes was reported at 1.9%. Aggravation of HF necessitated treatment withdrawal in 1.5% of patients. Sotalol is eliminated predominantly via the renal route, with renal impairment accounting for the reduced plasma sotalol clearance in patients with chronic kidney disease and older patients.[35]

Another pure rapid potassium current blocker *dofetilide* has been proven to have a neutral effect on all-cause mortality, cardiac and arrhythmic deaths, and hospitalization for HF in the Danish Investigations of Arrhythmia and Mortality on Dofetilide (DIAMOND) trials, including DIAMOND-CHF (LVEF ≤35%, 60% of patients with NYHA class III–IV HF) and DIAMOND-MI (2–7 days post-MI, LVEF ≤35%, 40% with NYHA class III–IV HF),[38,39] and is recommended for treatment of both AF and ventricular arrhythmias. The dose depends on renal function (the drug is contraindicated if creatinine clearance is <20 mL/min), and in-hospital initiation and 3-day continuous electrocardiogram (ECG) monitoring in a facility that can provide cardiac resuscitation is mandatory because of the risk of QT prolongation and proarrhythmia (the drug is not recommended if QTc is >440 ms or >500 ms in the presence of ventricular conduction abnormalities).

The major safety concern about dofetilide is its torsadogenic potential, which is dose-related; in RCTs, the incidence of polymorphic ventricular tachycardia (VT) or torsades de pointes varied between 0.6% and 3.3%, with more than three-quarters of episodes occurring during the first 3–4 days of drug initiation. If, on treatment, the QT interval is prolonged to >500 ms or by >15%, compared to the baseline, the dose should be reduced. Dofetilide is used in the United States but is not available in many European countries and the rest of the world.

Multichannel blockers: amiodarone and dronedarone

The multichannel blocker *amiodarone* is the most commonly employed drug in HFrEF because of its cardiac safety. Amiodarone exhibits the effects of all four classes of Singh–Vaughan Williams classification affecting several cardiac ion currents (sodium, potassium, and L-type calcium), as well as α- and β-adrenoceptors. This unique combination of electrophysiological effects makes amiodarone the most potent antiarrhythmic with a relatively low proarrhythmic potential.

Oral amiodarone reaches steady-state plasma levels after several weeks, unless large loading doses are used, as a result of a multi-compartmental distribution, including intravascular and tissue compartments, and adipose tissue which serves as drug reservoir. Amiodarone slows AV conduction and thus offers an additional benefit of ventricular rate control during recurrences of AF, but is not commonly employed for long-term rate control because of the risk of adverse effects. Co-administration with digoxin, beta-blockers, or non-dihydropyridine calcium channel blockers increases the risk of bradycardia and AV block, as well as hypotension; thus, ECG and blood pressure should be monitored. High lipophilic affinity and iodine moieties contribute to significant extracardiac toxicity, including thyroid dysfunction and pulmonary fibrosis.

The derivative of amiodarone *dronedarone*, which is devoid of the iodine group, with reduced lipophilic properties and a shorter half-life, has been associated with a 2.29-fold increase in CV death and major adverse events in the Permanent Atrial fibriLLAtion outcome Study using dronedarone on top of standard therapy (PALLAS) in patients with permanent AF,[40] and a 2.3-fold increase in all-cause mortality in the ANtiarrhythmic trial with DROnedarone in Moderate to severe congestive heart failure Evaluating morbidity DecreAse (ANDROMEDA) study in patients with HF (LVEF <35%) and NYHA functional classes III–IV.[41] Both studies were halted prematurely. Dronedarone is not recommended in patients with HF and those with permanent AF.

Atrial arrhythmias

Atrial premature beats and non-sustained atrial tachycardia

Atrial premature beats (APBs) and non-sustained atrial tachycardia (NSAT) are a common finding in older individuals, and frequent APBs are considered a marker of atrial electrical vulnerability and a predictor of incident AF. There is no consensus on whether pharmacological suppression of APBs and runs of NSAT reduces the risk of AF and cardiovascular morbidity and mortality, nor on what the threshold is for intervention. Amiodarone and beta-blockers are the preferred option in HFrEF if antiarrhythmic drug therapy is indicated. But, importantly, optimization of medical therapy for underlying heart disease may reduce the arrhythmia burden and deter the development of arrhythmia-induced cardiomyopathy.

Atrial fibrillation

HF and AF are increasingly prevalent conditions, with a multifaceted inter-relationship, acting as a risk factor and a trigger for each other and affecting each other's prognosis. AF, which is both a cause and a consequence of HF, confers a threefold increased risk of incident HF, whereas structural, neurohormonal, and electrophysiological remodelling associated with HF creates a background for the initiation and perpetuation of AF.[42] Thus, tachycardia-induced cardiomyopathy is a long-recognized complication of AF, affecting 3–25% of patients with atrial tachyarrhythmias. In HFrEF, the prevalence of AF increases with worsening LV systolic function and NYHA functional class, reaching 50–60% in very advanced disease.[42] AF is also a common comorbidity in older patients with HFpEF and diastolic dysfunction, which is often associated with increased left atrial pressure, dilatation, fibrosis, and resultant atrial remodelling forming the substrate for AF, with a 5.26-fold higher risk. In epidemiological surveys, just over half of patients with permanent AF also have HF; the corresponding values for paroxysmal and persistent varieties are 33% and 44%, respectively.[43]

Rhythm and rate control

There are two primary clinical approaches to the arrhythmia.

Rate control

In rate control, the ventricular rate is slowed to a level which is physiologically appropriate. Advantages of the rate control approach include ease and simplicity with avoiding potential toxicity of antiarrhythmic drugs or the risks and discomfort associated with electrical cardioversion or invasive left atrial ablation for recurrences of AF.

It is not clear exactly what this rate should be, and two approaches have been debated: (1) *strict rate control* (with a target ventricular rate response of <80 bpm at rest and <110 bpm on moderate exercise), usually achieved by a combination of two drugs with an AV-blocking effect and repeatedly assessed by different means.

These definitions are largely based on the results of the RACE (RAte Control Efficacy in permanent AF) II study in permanent AF.[44] In a post hoc analysis of this study, in a subgroup of 287 patients with a history of predominantly HFpEF (32.4% had an LVEF of 40% or lower), the cumulative incidence of the primary outcome did not differ significantly between the strict control and

the lenient control groups.[45] Likewise, post hoc analyses of trials of beta-blockers in HFrEF patients (MERIT-HF and CIBIS)[46,47] and in older patients with HFpEF (SENIORS)[48] have shown that a lower heart rate (usually <80 bpm) in patients with AF had no impact on prognosis. A subsequent meta-analysis of 11 studies exposed the reduced benefit of beta-blockers on mortality or hospital admissions in patients with AF.[49]

While lenient rate control with a resting heart rate of <110 bpm can be employed as the initial target, it should not lead to the assumption that lenient rate control remains an acceptable, or a preferable, option to a more aggressive rate control approach in the long term.

Beta-blockers, which are part of the mainstream therapy of HF, remain first line for acute and long-term rate control, particularly in patients with HFrEF and HfmrEF, not in the least due to their efficacy at high sympathetic drive, and can be used either alone or in combination with digoxin; a non-dihydropyridine calcium channel blocker can be considered in stable patients with HfpEF (➲ Tables 8.12.2 and 8.12.3). Digoxin (62.5–250 μg daily), which has an anti-adrenergic effect, increases the AV node refractory period, and inhibits the sodium–potassium adenosine triphosphatase pump, with resultant improvement in ventricular contractility, may be considered as first line for rate control in patients with permanent AF who are intolerant of beta-blockers, particularly older patients who lead a sedentary lifestyle, or as second-line remedy for those with a suboptimal response to AV blockade by beta-blockers (or calcium channel blockers). In a small randomized, open-label study in older patients, the majority of whom had HFpEF, digoxin favoured better than bisoprolol in respect of symptom relief and quality of life scores, and was associated with greater adherence to treatment at 6 months.[50] Digitoxin is a potential alternative to digoxin and is currently being evaluated in a randomized, placebo-controlled trial (ClinicalTrials.gov identifier: NCT03783429).

Amiodarone is advocated as a last resort, especially in patients with HFrEF—it is a powerful and effective rate-limiting agent, but it has an extensive catalogue of adverse side effects. There is no firm agreement on its use, mainly because of extracardiac side effects (the 2021 ESC Guidelines on management of HF assign it a Class IIa indication, whereas the 2020 ESC Guidelines on management of AF consider it a Class IIb indication).

Rate control remains an essential component of therapy, even if the primary strategy is rhythm control (e.g. in the case of a recurrent arrhythmia).

Rhythm control

Rhythm control consists of restoration and long-term maintenance of sinus rhythm. Antiarrhythmic drugs (ion channel blockers) are predominantly used, but occasionally autonomic manipulation, for example, with beta blockers, may prove valuable.

The Atrial Fibrillation in Congestive Heart Failure (AF-CHF) trial compared rate and rhythm control strategies in 1376 patients with HFrEF (LVEF ≤35%, NYHA classes II–IV), who were followed for a mean of 37 months.[51] The study showed no benefit of

Table 8.12.2 Drugs for acute rate control in atrial fibrillation

Drug	Route of administration	Dose	Onset	Recommendation (Class)	Level of evidence
Esmolol	Intravenous	0.5 mg/kg over 1 min, followed by 0.05-0.2 mg/kg/min infusion	5 min	I	C*
Metoprolol	Intravenous	2.5-5 mg over 2 min followed by repeat doses if necessary	5 min	I	C*
Propranolol	Intravenous	0.15 mg/kg	5 min	I	C*
Diltiazem	Intravenous	0.25 mg/kg over 2 min followed by 5-15 mg/h infusion	2-7 min	I	B
Verapamil	Intravenous	0.075-0.15 mg/kg over 2 min	3-5 min	I	B
Digoxin	Intravenous	0.25 mg each 2 h, max 1.5 mg	2 h	IIb[†]	B
Amiodarone	Intravenous	As for cardioversion[†]	6-8 h	IIb[†]	C
Sotalol	Intravenous	1-1.5 mg/kg over 5-10 min	15-30 min	III	B

* For all beta-blockers.

[†] A Class I indication for patients with poor ventricular function and moderately fast ventricular rates (Level of evidence B).

[‡] A Class IIa indication for patients with poor ventricular function and moderately fast ventricular rates (Level of evidence C).

Source data from Camm AJ, Lip GY, De Caterina R, *et al.*; ESC Committee for Practice Guidelines-CPG; Document Reviewers. 2012 focused update of the ESC Guidelines for the management of atrial fibrillation: an update of the 2010 ESC Guidelines for the management of atrial fibrillation--developed with the special contribution of the European Heart Rhythm Association. *Europace.* 2012 Oct;14(10):1385–413. doi: 10.1093/europace/eus305.

rhythm control on top of optimal HF therapy with regard to the primary endpoint of CV death (26.7% vs 25.2% in the rhythm vs rate control groups, hazard ratio 1.058, 95% CI 0.86–1.30; $P = 0.59$), as well as prespecified secondary endpoints, including total mortality, worsening HF, stroke, and hospitalization.

While older clinical trials comparing mainly traditional (antiarrhythmic drugs) rhythm control to rate control have shown no major differences in outcomes between the two treatment strategies for AF,[51,52] recent trials in HF that employed a more effective means of rhythm control (ablation)[53] or

Table 8.12.3 Drugs for long-term rate control in atrial fibrillation

Drug	Dose	Type of recommendation	Level of evidence	Potential adverse effects
Digoxin	Loading dose: 250 μg every 2 hours; up to 1500 μg; maintenance dose 125–250 μg daily	I	B	Bradycardia, atrioventricular block, atrial arrhythmias, ventricular tachycardia
Diltiazem	120–360 mg daily	I	B	Hypotension, atrioventricular block, heart failure
Verapamil	120–360 mg daily	I	B	Hypotension, atrioventricular block, heart failure
Atenolol	50–100 mg daily	I	C*	Hypotension, bradycardia, heart failure, deterioration of chronic obstructive pulmonary disease or asthma
Metoprolol	50–200 mg daily	I	C*	
Propranolol	80–240 mg daily	I	C*	
Bisoprolol	5–10 mg daily	I	C*	
Carvedilol	25–100 mg daily	I	C*	
Sotalol	80–320 mg	IIb[†]	C	Bradycardia, QT prolongation, torsades de pointes (risk <1%), photosensitivity, pulmonary toxicity, polyneuropathy, hepatic toxicity, thyroid dysfunction, gastrointestinal upset
Amiodarone	800 mg daily for 1 week, then 600 mg daily for 1 week, then 400 mg daily for 4–6 weeks; maintenance dose 200 mg daily	IIb[†]	C	Bradycardia, QT prolongation, torsades de pointes (risk <1%), photosensitivity, pulmonary toxicity, polyneuropathy, hepatic toxicity, thyroid dysfunction, gastrointestinal upset

* For all beta-blockers.

[†] Useful during recurrence of atrial fibrillation.

Source data from Camm AJ, Lip GY, De Caterina R, *et al.*; ESC Committee for Practice Guidelines-CPG; Document Reviewers. 2012 focused update of the ESC Guidelines for the management of atrial fibrillation: an update of the 2010 ESC Guidelines for the management of atrial fibrillation--developed with the special contribution of the European Heart Rhythm Association. *Europace.* 2012 Oct;14(10):1385–413. doi: 10.1093/europace/eus305.

intervening early in the course of AF[54] have consistently demonstrated a greater freedom from AF, with ensuing improvement in symptoms, NYHA functional class, and LVEF, compared to pharmacological rate (and rhythm) control. Rhythm control is the preferable treatment in many patients with recent-onset AF, in those who are highly symptomatic with AF or whose symptoms of HF are worsened by the arrhythmia, including tachycardia-induced cardiomyopathy, and in younger and active individuals with limited left atrial remodelling.[55] Early rhythm control intervention with antiarrhythmic drugs has yielded improvement in maintenance of sinus rhythm and HF functional class in patients with AF and stable moderate HF enrolled in the RACE (Routine vs. Aggressive risk factor-driven upstream rhythm Control for prevention of Early AF in HF) 3 trial, in which antiarrhythmic drug therapy was combined with optimization of medical therapy for underlying heart disease and lifestyle modifications.[56] Antiarrhythmic drugs were effective in nearly 50% of the patients and were mainly limited by reversible non-serious adverse effects. There is a strong drive towards implementation of rhythm control by means of pulmonary vein isolation, with or without substrate modification, early in the course of AF, especially in patients with HFrEF, due to accumulating evidence of symptom relief, ventricular function improvement, and overall prognostic benefit, including mortality,[55] although the favourable effect of ablation may be less substantial in unselected patients outside controlled clinical trials.[57]

Pharmacological cardioversion

Pharmacological cardioversion is undertaken in haemodynamically stable patients, mainly those with a recent-onset (usually no longer than 1 week) episode of AF, as its success rate decreases significantly as AF persists beyond this limit.[58] In patients with known sick sinus syndrome or AV conduction disturbances without pacemaker backup, or those with prolonged QTc (>500 ms), pharmacological cardioversion should be considered only after an adequate risk assessment has been carried out.

Intravenous *amiodarone, ibutilide,* and *vernakalant* (◗ Table 8.12.4) can be used for pharmacological cardioversion of AF in patients with HF. *Intravenous amiodarone* is the only agent which is recommended in patients with HFrEF. Cardioversion with intravenous amiodarone is delayed by 8–24 hours, but it has the benefit of AV blockade and slowing the ventricular response rate, thus providing symptomatic relief before sinus rhythm has been restored.[59,60]

Ibutilide is modestly effective for conversion of AF and may be used in patients with HFpEF (with no significant LV hypertrophy), with caution in selected patients with HFmrEF and NYHA functional classes I and II, but its use is limited by a sizeable risk of polymorphic VT or torsades de pointes (incidence of torsades de pointes requiring electrical cardioversion, 0.5–1.7%; self-terminating polymorphic VT, 2.6–6.7%).[61] The overall conversion rates for atrial flutter are almost twofold higher than for AF (56–70% vs 31–44%, respectively).[62]

Vernakalant may be considered with caution for cardioversion in patients with HFpEF and selected HFmrEF with NYHA class I

Table 8.12.4 Pharmacological cardioversion of atrial fibrillation in heart failure

Drug	Dose	Efficacy	Time to conversion	Can be used*	Acute side effects
Amiodarone	150 mg IV bolus, or 5–7 mg/kg IV infusion over 1–2 hours; if necessary, continue infusion at 50 mg/hour; maximum dose up to 1200 mg over 24 hours	34–69% (bolus) 55–95% (bolus plus infusion)	6–24 hours	HFrEF, HFmrEF, HFpEF	Hypotension, bradycardia, QT interval prolongation (low risk of torsades de pointes), phlebitis
Ibutilide	1 mg IV over 10 minutes, repeat if necessary 0.01 mg/kg if body weight < 60 kg	44–58%	90 minutes	HFpEF, HFmrEF (with caution, in NYHA class I–II patients)	QT interval prolongation, torsades de pointes, bradycardia
Vernakalant	3 mg/kg IV over 10 minutes, repeat 2 mg/kg IV if necessary	47–61%	90 minutes (median 8–14 minutes)	HFpEF, HFmrEF (with caution, in NYHA class I–II patients)	Hypotension and non-sustained ventricular tachycardia, QT prolongation (but low risk of torsades de pointes), sinus bradycardia
Dofetilide	125, 250, 500 µg PO twice daily†	6, 10, 30%, respectively	24–36 hours (70% of patients)	HFpEF, HFmEF, HFrEF	QT interval prolongation, torsades de pointes

* If heart failure history and ventricular function are established; otherwise, IV amiodarone or electrical cardioversion is indicated.

† Determined by creatinine clearance (CrCl); contraindicated if CrCl is <20 mL/min. If CrCl is >60 mL/min, the dose is 500 µg twice daily. If CrCl is 40–60 mL/min, the dose is 250 µg twice daily. If CrCl is 20 to <40 mL/min, the dose is 125 µg twice daily.

HFmrEF, heart failure with mildly reduced ejection fraction; HFpEF, heart failure with preserved ejection fraction; HFrEF, heart failure with reduced ejection fraction; IV, intravenous; NYHA, New York Heart Association; PO, *per os.*

Reproduced from Savelieva I, Graydon R, Camm AJ. Pharmacological cardioversion of atrial fibrillation with vernakalant: evidence in support of the ESC Guidelines. *Europace.* 2014 Feb;16(2):162–73. doi: 10.1093/europace/eut274 with permission from Oxford University Press.

and II (who should be haemodynamically stable, with no signs of decompensation), being mindful of the risk of hypotension and non-sustained ventricular arrhythmias in these patients (7.3% vs 1.6% on placebo at 2 hours).[58] It is contraindicated in NYHA classes III and IV and HFrEF, hypotension <100 mmHg, recent (<30 days) acute coronary syndrome, severe aortic stenosis, QT interval prolongation (uncorrected QT at baseline >440 ms), slow ventricular rates, and a history of second- or third-degree AV block in the absence of a pacemaker.

Antiarrhythmic drugs for maintenance of sinus rhythm

Prophylactic antiarrhythmic drug therapy is recommended for the vast majority of patients with paroxysmal AF when paroxysms occur frequently and are associated with significant symptoms or lead to worsening LV function, and for patients with persistent AF following cardioversion when the likelihood of maintenance of sinus rhythm is uncertain, especially in the presence of risk factors for recurrence such as left atrial enlargement, evidence for depressed atrial function, reduced LVEF, or long duration of the arrhythmia. Antiarrhythmic drugs may be required after ablation for AF if intervention alone does not eliminate the arrhythmia. Amiodarone has been reported to be most commonly prescribed because of its anti-fibrillatory, as well as AV conduction-slowing, properties.

Sotalol

Sotalol has relatively low efficacy and is associated with a risk of QT interval prolongation and proarrhythmia, which may be poorly predictable in patients with HF, particularly HFrEF. Therefore, sotalol is not commonly used for AF management in the HF setting.

Dofetilide

Unlike sotalol, dofetilide is considered safer to use in patients with advanced HF. In the DIAMOND AF substudy of DIAMOND-CHF and DIAMOND-MI trials in patients with LVEF of ≤35% and NYHA functional classes III and IV, 506 patients with AF at baseline were more likely to remain in sinus rhythm on treatment with dofetilide 500 µg twice daily, compared to those on placebo (79% vs 42%).[63] Dofetilide had no effect on mortality in patients in whom AF persisted during the study, but restoration and maintenance of sinus rhythm were associated with a 56% reduction in death. In the dose-ranging SAFIRE-D study of 325 patients with persistent AF or flutter for 2–26 weeks, dofetilide exhibited a dose-related effect: 40%, 37%, and 58% of patients receiving 250, 500, and 1000 µg of dofetilide, respectively, were in sinus rhythm after 1 year, compared to 25% in the placebo group.[64] The QT-prolonging effect and torsadogenic potential, as well as its dependence on renal clearance necessitating in-hospital initiation and monitoring, limit the use and availability of dofetilide.

Amiodarone

The potential of amiodarone to maintain sinus rhythm in patients with AF and a relative cardiac safety in patients with significant structural heart disease has been shown repeatedly in observational and prospective, randomized controlled studies. In the CTAF trial, amiodarone administered at 10 mg/kg for 2 weeks, followed by 300 mg/day for 4 weeks and a maintenance dose of 200 mg, reduced the incidence of recurrent AF by 57%.[65]

Despite prolonging cardiac repolarization, amiodarone has a low torsadogenic potential. The incidence of torsades de pointes was only 0.7% in 2878 patients treated with amiodarone in 17 uncontrolled studies, whereas no proarrhythmic effects were described among 1464 patients treated in seven controlled studies.[66] The residual risk of torsades de pointes with amiodarone occurs mainly in patients with other risk factors such as bradycardia or hypokalaemia.

Given its neutral effect on all-cause mortality, amiodarone should be considered a drug of choice for management of AF in patients with HF, including HFrEF and HFpEF, on a background of hypertensive heart disease with significant LV hypertrophy.

Amiodarone may cause multiple non-target effects, which range from transient and relatively trivial (e.g. gastrointestinal disturbances) to partially preventable (e.g. skin toxicity) and medically correctable (e.g. underactive thyroid) to serious such as pulmonary toxicity, liver damage, hyperthyroidism, bradycardia, significant or irreversible neurological symptoms (e.g. peripheral neuropathy), and visual disturbances (e.g. optic neuritis). The adverse effects of amiodarone seem to occur less frequently at low doses (100–200 mg daily) than at higher maintenance doses (300–400 mg daily), but idiosyncratic reactions can arise.

Dronedarone

Dronedarone does not significantly prolong the QT interval and has a low potential for causing torsades de pointes.

The antiarrhythmic potential of dronedarone and the effects on mortality and morbidity have been extensively studied. The EURopean trial In atrial fibrillation or flutter patients receiving Dronedarone for the maintenance of Sinus rhythm (EURIDIS) and its American-Australian-African equivalent ADONIS have shown that dronedarone 400 mg twice daily was superior to placebo in the prevention of recurrent AF and was also effective in controlling ventricular rates.[67] Subsequently, ATHENA (A placebo-controlled, double-blind Trial to assess the efficacy of dronedarone for the prevention of cardiovascular Hospitalization or death from any cause in patients with Atrial fibrillation and flutter) has demonstrated that dronedarone prolonged the time to first CV hospitalization or death from any cause (the composite primary endpoint) by 24% (P <0.001), compared to placebo, in high-risk patients.[68] This effect was driven by the reduction in CV hospitalization (25%), particularly hospitalization for AF (37%). All-cause mortality was similar in the dronedarone and placebo groups (5% and 6%, respectively); however, dronedarone significantly reduced death from CV causes.

However, following premature termination of the ANDROMEDA study in HF patients with LVEF of <36% and NYHA functional classes III and IV,[41] and the PALLAS study in high-risk patients with permanent AF,[40] due to excess death and other adverse outcomes, the use of dronedarone has been restricted and the drug is not indicated in patients with HF.

Ventricular arrhythmias

Ventricular premature beats and non-sustained ventricular tachycardia

The initial management of ventricular arrhythmias in HF should start with correction of potential precipitating factors such as electrolyte abnormalities (particularly hypo- or hyperkalaemia and hypomagnesaemia) and optimization of HF drug therapy. Beta-blockers are the first-line treatment, followed by more potent antiarrhythmic drugs in symptomatic patients with a high burden of ventricular ectopics, but their efficacy is lower than that of non-pharmacological therapy such as ablation.

Mexiletine and lidocaine are effective in suppression of ectopic ventricular automaticity and triggered activity caused by delayed afterdepolarizations, and they also may interfere with the re-entrant mechanism of arrhythmias by converting unidirectional to bidirectional block in partially depolarized myocardium observed during ischaemia. The efficacy of mexiletine as monotherapy was assessed in small studies and during programmed electrical stimulation, and ranged between 20% and 30% in suppressing induced VT and 75% in reducing the number of non-sustained VT (NSVT) runs.[69]

The ability of amiodarone to suppress ventricular premature complexes (VPCs) and NSVT runs has been proven in several RCTs. Thus, in Canadian Amiodarone Myocardial Infarction Trial (CAMIAT), which enrolled patients with recent MI and LV systolic dysfunction, amiodarone almost completely abolished frequent VPCs or repetitive ventricular forms in 84% of patients, compared to 35% in the placebo group.[70] Similarly, in the CHF-STAT study, after 3 months of therapy, the proportion of patients with NSVT decreased from 77% to 33%.[71] However, there has been no well-established link between suppression of VPCs and NSVT and the effect on sudden death and all-cause mortality.

The drug d,l-sotalol may be used for control of ventricular arrhythmias, particularly those associated with stable ischaemic heart disease. It is effective in suppressing complex forms of ventricular ectopy, displaying superior anti-ectopic activity to beta-blockers, but is not suitable for patients with HF on a background of hypertensive heart disease and LV hypertrophy and significant LV systolic impairment. Sotalol at doses of 160–640 mg/day reduced ventricular ectopy, most notably higher-grade ventricular arrhythmias (polymorphic and repetitive premature ventricular complexes, couplets and runs of NSVT); this action was maintained in the presence of mild LV dysfunction and was sustained in the long term (approximately 2–6 years).[36]

Because of its cardiac safety, amiodarone is usually recommended in patients with HFrEF and high ventricular premature beat burden when beta-blockers alone are ineffective.[68]

Ventricular tachycardia

Acute management of VT includes intravenous beta-blockers, amiodarone (150–300 mg intravenous bolus), lidocaine, and mexiletine, which may also prevent immediate recurrence of VT and the occurrence of ventricular fibrillation (VF). Amiodarone remains the only antiarrhythmic drug that can be used in patients with an advanced NYHA functional class, based on the older CHF-STAT and GESICA (Grupo de Estudio de la Sobrevida en la Insuficiencia Cardiaca en Argentina) trials (mean LVEF 25% and 20%, respectively; NYHA functional class III or IV 43% vs 79%, respectively).[71,72] In the GESICA trial, all-cause mortality and sudden death were reduced by 28% ($P<0.03$) and 27% ($P=0.056$), respectively, as was death from progressive HF (by 23%).[72] In the CHF-STAT study of 674 patients with NYHA classes II to IV, therapy with amiodarone did not affect sudden death or all-cause death rates, but caused a substantial increase in LVEF, with a significant reduction in the combined endpoint of cardiac death and HF hospitalization observed in the non-ischaemic group, suggesting a greater benefit in these patients.[71]

Long-term management of VT involves the use of implantable cardioverter–defibrillators (ICDs).[73] Antiarrhythmic drugs are reserved as adjunctive treatment to devices. In patients with resistant recurrent VT and/or electrical storm, catheter ablation is preferred.

Ancillary antiarrhythmic drug therapy in patients with cardiac implantable electronic devices

Combined *amiodarone and beta-blocker* therapy, and *sotalol* (240 mg/day) monotherapy, were both superior to beta-blockade in the Optimal Pharmacological Therapy in Cardioverter Defibrillator Patients (OPTIC) trial in reducing ICD shocks in patients with LVEF of ≤40%.[74] Amiodarone has been shown to reduce ICD interventions when used for secondary prevention.

Mexiletine used in combination with amiodarone in the Ventricular Tachycardia Ablation or Escalated aNtiarrhythmic Drugs in Ischemic Heart Disease (VANISH) trial in ICD patients with ischaemic heart disease has not been found effective for preventing recurrence of ventricular arrhythmias.[75]

Beta-blockers and optimizing HF therapy are associated with reduced arrhythmias in CIED recipients.[76]

Ranolazine, an antianginal drug, which inhibits the late sodium current and the ultrarapid potassium current, has its antiarrhythmic effect in ventricular arrhythmias tested in the Ranolazine Implantable Cardioverter–Defibrillator (RAID) study in 1012 high-risk ICD recipients who were randomized to ranolazine 1000 mg twice daily or to placebo.[77] There was no difference in the primary endpoint of VT or VF requiring appropriate ICD therapy or death; the study was underpowered due to high rates of discontinuation. In prespecified secondary endpoint analyses, ranolazine administration was associated with a significant reduction in recurrent VT or VF requiring ICD therapy (hazard ratio 0.70, 95% confidence interval 0.51–0.96; $P=0.028$), without evidence for increased mortality.

Where to initiate, and how to monitor, antiarrhythmic drug therapy

In-hospital initiation under monitored conditions conveys benefits of accurate assessment of the efficacy and prompt recognition of adverse effects such as bradycardia, conduction abnormalities, excessive QT interval prolongation, proarrhythmia, and intolerance or idiosyncrasy. For some antiarrhythmic agents, e.g. dofetilide, there is a formal mandate for in-hospital initiation.

If an antiarrhythmic drug is initiated on an outpatient basis (e.g. common for amiodarone), an ECG control or trans-telephonic ECG monitoring should be arranged to provide the surveillance of heart rate, PR and QT interval durations, QRS width, and assessment of the efficacy of treatment. Assessment of drug level concentration is appropriate if the drug has a narrow therapeutic window, marked pharmacokinetic variability exists, and there is no appropriate direct measure of the desired therapeutic effect but a suitable and accessible laboratory assay.

Appropriate follow-up should be planned in the long term: ECG, renal, and, in the case of agents with known hepatic toxicity, liver function tests after initiation of antiarrhythmic drugs, the frequency of which is determined by the specific drug properties (e.g. a detailed dronedarone protocol) and the severity of the underlying heart disease and concomitant conditions. Renal function tests should be carried out every 6 months in patients with preserved renal function, every 3 months in those with chronic kidney disease, and more frequently in those with advanced renal dysfunction. Patient education on the goals of therapy and potential adverse effects should be part of the initiation and follow-up of treatment.

Treating proarrhythmias

Effective treatment requires accurate recognition and confirmation of drug-induced proarrhythmia and prompt discontinuation of the implicated agent. Important also are the identification and modification (whenever possible) of risk factors potentially associated with arrhythmia onset or worsening (e.g. female gender, advanced age, renal or liver dysfunction, hypokalaemia, hypomagnesaemia, high drug doses/concentrations, rapid intravenous administration, bradycardia, QT prolongation).

In the case of drug-related proarrhythmia, the first line of management is to stop the offending drug. However, in selected cases, implantation of an ICD needs to be considered, based on the individual characteristics of the patient and the future risk of life-threatening ventricular tachyarrhythmias.

The offending drug should be stopped, and intravenous administration of magnesium sulfate, irrespective of serum magnesium levels, should be administered (e.g. 2000-mg bolus, followed by a second bolus and by continuous infusion if the proarrhythmia persists). Bradycardia and pauses that may trigger torsades de pointes should be reversed by either pacing at >70 bpm or isoproterenol infusion. Hypokalaemia should be corrected, aiming at replenishing the serum potassium concentration to the high-normal range (i.e. 4.5–5.0 mEq/L).

Beta-blockers may be used in some circumstances.

In milder cases, arrhythmias due to digitalis toxicity can be managed by discontinuation of the drug, potassium supplementation, and observation. For digitalis-induced life-threatening arrhythmias, several antiarrhythmic drugs have been proposed in the past (e.g. phenytoin, lidocaine, beta-blockade). More recently, digitalis-specific antibodies have proven effective in reversing digitalis toxicity by rapidly binding to, and acutely lowering, serum digitalis. Isoproterenol infusion or cardiac pacing is usually effective when symptomatic bradyarrhythmias secondary to conduction abnormalities occur.

Future directions

At present, the role of oral anticoagulants (OACs) and statins in HF patients remains controversial. The mechanisms involved in the occurrence of stroke in HF are heterogeneous and probably differ from those in AF patients. That may be a reason why until now all trials have been negative. On the other hand, the lower dose used (2×2.5 mg rivaroxaban instead of 15–20 mg) may also have contributed to the fact that the COMMANDER HF study did not improve the composite outcome of all-cause mortality, MI, or stroke, nor HF-related deaths or HF hospitalization.[9] Interestingly, and in line with the HF data, also no benefit was observed from routine OAC use in patients with acute ischaemic stroke of undetermined source with no documented AF.[10,11] The latter highlights the fact that the mechanisms involved in stroke are much more complex than previously anticipated. For the future, data on the role of hypercoagulability in well-phenotyped HF patients may contribute to identification of those who may benefit from OACs. In addition, higher dosages of OACs may be an option, although the bleeding risk profile in HF patients also should be carefully taken into account.

The mechanisms explaining why statins could act beneficially in HF patients may differ from those involved in patients with CAD. Interestingly, there is also evidence for a 'cholesterol paradox' in HF patients. Further, the pleiotropic effects of statins are incompletely resolved. Studies in extensively phenotyped HF patients may help to identify those patients who may benefit from statins.

Finally, arrhythmias often occur in patients with HF. The first treatment step always should be identification of triggers for these arrhythmias, for example, exacerbation of HF, significant ischaemia, or severe valve disease. These should be adequately resolved first. Only thereafter should antiarrhythmic drugs be instituted, unless haemodynamic instability warrants an earlier start. The number of antiarrhythmic drugs that can be safely and effectively instituted in HF patients is limited. Nowadays, ablation has become a major player for treatment of arrhythmias, also in HF.[74] Future studies must focus on outcome improvement of ablation of atrial and ventricular arrhythmias in HF patients.

Key messages

- In patients with documented AF and HF, it is recommended to start long-term treatment with oral anticoagulation if the CHA_2DS_2-VASc score is ≥2 in men and ≥3 in women. Long-term anticoagulation should be considered in patients with AF and HF and a CHA_2DS_2-VASc score of 1 in men and 2 in women.

- Anticoagulation should not be instituted routinely in patients with HFrEF who are in sinus rhythm and do not have documented AF.

- Low-dose rivaroxaban may be considered in patients with concomitant CAD or peripheral artery disease, a high risk of stroke, and no major haemorrhagic risk. Additionally, patients with an intraventricular thrombus or with a high thrombotic risk (e.g. after a peripheral embolism or those known with a peripartum or LV non-compaction cardiomyopathy) should be considered for anticoagulation.

♦ Treatment with statins is recommended in patients at high risk of CV disease or with CV disease. Based on current evidence, routine administration of statins in patients with HF without other indications for their use (e.g. CAD) is not recommended. Because there is no evidence of harm in patients on statin treatment after the occurrence of HF, there is no need for statin discontinuation for patients already on treatment.

♦ Arrhythmias often occur in patients with HF. The first treatment step always should be identification of triggers for these arrhythmias (e.g. exacerbation of HF, significant ischaemia, severe valve disease). These should be adequately resolved first. Only thereafter should antiarrhythmic drugs be instituted, unless haemodynamic instability warrants an earlier start. The number of antiarrhythmic drugs that can be safely and effectively instituted in HF patients is limited. Nowadays, ablation has become a major player for treatment of arrhythmias, also in HF.

References

1. Kristensen SL, Jhund PS, Kober L, et al. Comparison of outcomes after hospitalization for worsening heart failure, myocardial infarction, and stroke in patients with heart failure and reduced and preserved ejection fraction. Eur J Heart Fail 2015;17:169–76.

2. Haeusler KG, Laufs U, Endres M. Chronic heart failure and ischemic stroke. Stroke 2011;42:2977–82.

3. Watson T, Shantsila E, Lip GY. Mechanisms of thrombogenesis in atrial fibrillation: Virchow's triad revisited. Lancet 2009;373:155–66.

4. Doehner W, Ural D, Haeusler KG, et al. Heart and brain interaction in patients with heart failure: overview and proposal for a taxonomy. A position paper from the Study Group on Heart and Brain Interaction of the Heart Failure Association. Eur J Heart Fail 2018;20:199.

5. Hindricks G, Potpara T, Dagres N, et al. 2020 ESC Guidelines for the diagnosis and management of atrial fibrillation developed in collaboration with the European Association for Cardio-Thoracic Surgery (EACTS). Eur Heart J 2021;42(5):373–498.

6. McDonagh TA, Metra M, Adamo M, et al. 2021 ESC Guidelines for the diagnosis and treatment of acute and chronic heart failure. Eur Heart J 2021;42(36):3599–726.

7. Homma S, Thompson JL, Pullicino PM, et al.; WARCEF Investigators. Warfarin and aspirin in patients with heart failure and sinus rhythm. N Engl J Med 2012;366:1859–69.

8. Hopper I, Skiba M, Krum H. Updated meta-analysis on antithrombotic therapy in patients with heart failure and sinus rhythm. Eur J Heart Fail 2013;15:69–78.

9. Zannad F, Anker SD, Byra WM, et al.; COMMANDER HF Investigators. Rivaroxaban in patients with heart failure, sinus rhythm, and coronary disease. N Engl J Med 2018;379:1332–42.

10. Diener HC, Sacco RL, Easton JD, et al. Dabigatran for prevention of stroke after embolic stroke of undetermined source. N Engl J Med 2019;380:1906–17.

11. Hart RG, Sharma M, Mundl H, et al.; NAVIGATE ESUS Investigators. Rivaroxaban for stroke prevention after embolic stroke of undetermined source. N Engl J Med 2018;378:2191–201.

12. Branch KR, Probstfield JL, Eikelboom JW, et al. Rivaroxaban with or without aspirin in patients with heart failure and chronic coronary or peripheral artery disease. Circulation 2019;140:529–37.

13. Visseren FLJ, Mach F, Smulders YM, et al. 2021 ESC guidelines on cardiovascular disease prevention in clinical practice. Eur Heart J 2021;42:3227–337.

14. Scandinavian Simvastatin Survival Study Group. Randomised trial of cholesterol lowering in 4444 patients with coronary heart disease: the Scandinavian Simvastatin Survival Study (4S). Lancet 1994;344:1383–9.

15. Long-Term Intervention with Pravastatin in Ischaemic Disease (LIPID) Study Group. Prevention of cardiovascular events and death with pravastatin in patients with coronary heart disease and a broad range of initial cholesterol levels. N Engl J Med 1998;339:1349–57.

16. Sacks FM, Pfeffer MA, Moye LA, et al. The effect of pravastatin on coronary events after myocardial infarction in patients with average cholesterol levels. N Engl J Med 1996;335:1001–9.

17. Heart Protection Study Collaborative Group. MRC/BHF Heart Protection Study of cholesterol lowering with simvastatin in 20,536 high-risk individuals: a randomised placebo-controlled trial. Lancet 2002;360:7–22.

18. Preiss D, Campbell RT, Murray HM, et al. The effect of statin therapy on heart failure events: a collaborative meta-analysis of unpublished data from major randomized trials. Eur Heart J 2015;36:1536–46.

19. Ford I, Murray H, McCowan C, Packard CJ. Long-term safety and efficacy of lowering low-density lipoprotein cholesterol with statin therapy: 20-year follow-up of West of Scotland Coronary Prevention Study. Circulation 2016;133:1073–80.

20. Kjekshus J, Apetrei E, Barrios V, et al.; CORONA Group. Rosuvastatin in older patients with systolic heart failure. N Engl J Med 2007;357:2248–61.

21. Tavazzi L, Maggioni AP, Marchioli R, et al.; GISSI-HF Investigators. Effect of rosuvastatin in patients with chronic heart failure (the GISSI-HF trial): a randomised, double-blind, placebo-controlled trial. Lancet 2008;372:1231–9.

22. Cleland JGF, McMurray JJV, Kjekshus J, et al. Plasma concentration of amino-terminal pro-brain natriuretic peptide in chronic heart failure: prediction of cardiovascular events and interaction with the effects of rosuvastatin: a report from CORONA (Controlled Rosuvastatin Multinational Trial in Heart). J Am Coll Cardiol 2009;54:1850–9.

23. Anker SD, Clark AL, Winkler R, et al. Statin use and survival in patients with failure hospitalizations: the CORONA trial (controlled rosuvastatin multinational trial in heart failure). JACC Heart Fail 2014;2:289–97.

24. Obokata M, Reddy YN, Pislaru SV, Melenovsky V, Borlaug BA. Evidence supporting the existence of a distinct obese phenotype of heart failure with preserved ejection fraction. Circulation 2017;136:6–19.

25. Kitzman DW, Shah SJ. The HFpEF obesity phenotype: the elephant in the room. Am Coll Cardiol 2016;68:200–3.

26. Alehagen U, Benson L, Edner M, Dahlström U, Lund LH. Association between use of statins and mortality in patients with heart failure and ejection fraction of ≥50. Inhibitors of 3-hydroxy-3-methylglutaryl-coenzyme A (HMG-CoA) reductase occasionally cause myopathy characterized by weakness, pain, and elevated serum creatine phosphokinase (CK). Circ Heart Fail 2015;8(5):862–70.

27. Fukuta H, Goto T, Wakami K, Ohte N. The effect of statins on mortality in heart failure with preserved ejection fraction: a meta-analysis of propensity score analyses. Int J Cardiol 2016;214:301–6.

28. Liu G, Zheng XX, Xu YL, Ru J, Hui RT, Huang XH. Meta-analysis of the effect of statins on mortality in patients with preserved ejection fraction. Am J Cardiol 2014;113:1198–204.

29. Wang CY, Liao JK. Current advances in statin treatment: from molecular mechanisms to clinical practice. Arch Med Sci 2007;3:S91–6.

30. Ray KK, Cannon CP, Cairns R, et al.; PROVE IT-TIMI 22 Investigators. Relationship between uncontrolled risk factors and C-reactive protein levels in patients receiving standard or intensive statin therapy for acute coronary syndromes in the PROVE IT-TIMI 22 trial. J Am Coll Cardiol 2005;46:1417–24.

31. Bielecka-Dabrowa A, Fabis J, Mikhailidis DP, et al. Prosarcopenic effects of statins may limit their effectiveness in patients with heart failure. Trends Pharmacol Sci 2018;39:331–53.

32. Vaughan Williams EM. Classification of anti-arrhythmic drugs. In: Sandoe E, Flensted-Jansen E, Olesen KH, eds. Symposium on Cardiac Arrhythmias. Sodertalje: AB Astra; 1970, pp. 449–72.

33. Singh BN, Vaughan Williams EM. A fourth class of antiarrhythmic action? Effect of verapamil on ouabain toxicity, on atrial and ventricular intracellular potentials, and on other features of cardiac function. Cardiovasc Res 1972;6:109–19.

34. Lei M, Wu L, Terrar DA, Huang CL. Modernized classification of cardiac antiarrhythmic drugs. Circulation 2018;138:1879–96.

35. Dan GA, Martinez-Rubio A, Agewall S, et al.; ESC Scientific Document Group. Antiarrhythmic drugs—clinical use and clinical decision making: a consensus document from the European Heart Rhythm Association (EHRA) and European Society of Cardiology (ESC) Working Group on Cardiovascular Pharmacology, endorsed by the Heart Rhythm Society (HRS), Asia-Pacific Heart Rhythm Society (APHRS) and International Society of Cardiovascular Pharmacotherapy (ISCP). Europace 2018;20:731–2an.

36. Waldo AL, Camm AJ, deRuyter H, et al. Effect of d-sotalol on mortality in patients with left ventricular dysfunction after recent and remote myocardial infarction. The SWORD Investigators. Survival With Oral d-Sotalol. Lancet 1996;348:7–12.

37. Fitton A, Sorkin EM. Sotalol. An updated review of its pharmacological properties and therapeutic use in cardiac arrhythmias. Drugs 1993;46:678–719.

38. Torp-Pedersen C, Møller M, Bloch-Thomsen PE, et al.; Danish Investigations of Arrhythmia and Mortality on Dofetilide Study Group. Dofetilide in patients with congestive heart failure and left ventricular dysfunction. N Engl J Med 1999;341:857–65.

39. Køber L, Bloch Thomsen PE, Møller M, et al.; Danish Investigations of Arrhythmia and Mortality on Dofetilide (DIAMOND) Study Group. Effect of dofetilide in patients with recent myocardial infarction and left-ventricular dysfunction: a randomised trial. Lancet 2000;356:2052–8.

40. Connolly SJ, Camm AJ, Halperin JL, et al. Dronedarone in high-risk permanent atrial fibrillation. N Engl J Med 2011;365:2268–76.

41. Køber L, Torp-Pedersen C, McMurray JJ, et al.; Dronedarone Study Group. Increased mortality after dronedarone therapy for severe heart failure. N Engl J Med 2008;358:2678–87.

42. Savelieva I, Camm AJ. Atrial fibrillation and heart failure: natural history and pharmacological treatment. Europace 2004;5 Suppl 1:S5–19.

43. Chiang CE, Naditch-Brule L, Murin J, et al. Distribution and risk profile of paroxysmal, persistent, and permanent atrial fibrillation in routine clinical practice: insight from the real-life global survey evaluating patients with atrial fibrillation international registry. Circ Arrhythm Electrophysiol 2012;5:632–9.

44. Van Gelder IC, Groenveld HF, Crijns HJ, et al. Lenient versus strict rate control in patients with atrial fibrillation. N Engl J Med 2010;362:1363–73.

45. Mulder BA, van Veldhuisen DJ, Crijns HJ, et al.; RACE II investigators. Lenient vs. strict rate control in patients with atrial fibrillation and heart failure: a post-hoc analysis of the RACE II study. Eur J Heart Fail 2013;15:1311–18.

46. Lechat P, Hulot JS, Escolano S, et al. Heart rate and cardiac rhythm relationships with bisoprolol benefit in chronic heart failure in CIBIS II Trial. Circulation 2001;103:1428–33.

47. Van Veldhuisen DJ, Aass H, El Allaf D, et al. Presence and development of atrial fibrillation in chronic heart failure. Experiences from the MERIT-HF Study. Eur J Heart Fail 2006;8:539–46.

48. Mulder BA, van Veldhuisen DJ, Crijns HJ, et al. Effect of nebivolol on outcome in elderly patients with heart failure and atrial fibrillation: insights from SENIORS. Eur J Heart Fail 2012;14:1171–8.

49. Kotecha D, Holmes J, Krum H, et al.; Beta-Blockers in Heart Failure Collaborative Group. Efficacy of beta blockers in patients with heart failure plus atrial fibrillation: an individual-patient data meta-analysis. Lancet 2014;384:2235–43.

50. Kotecha D, Bunting KV, Gill SK, et al.; Rate Control Therapy Evaluation in Permanent Atrial Fibrillation (RATE-AF) Team. Effect of digoxin vs bisoprolol for heart rate control in atrial fibrillation on patient-reported quality of life: the RATE-AF randomized clinical trial. JAMA 2020;324:2497–508.

51. Roy D, Talajic M, Nattel S, et al.; Atrial Fibrillation and Congestive Heart Failure Investigators. Rhythm control versus rate control for atrial fibrillation and heart failure. N Engl J Med 2008;358:2667–77.

52. Caldeira D, David C, Sampaio C. Rate vs rhythm control in patients with atrial fibrillation and heart failure: a systematic review and meta-analysis of randomised controlled trials. Eur J Intern Med 2011;22:448–55.

53. Chen S, Pürerfellner H, Meyer C, et al. Rhythm control for patients with atrial fibrillation complicated with heart failure in the contemporary era of catheter ablation: a stratified pooled analysis of randomized data. Eur Heart J 2020;41:2863–73.

54. Rillig A, Magnussen C, Ozga AK, et al. Early rhythm control therapy in patients with atrial fibrillation and heart failure. Circulation 2021;144:845–58.

55. Camm AJ, Savelieva I. Atrial fibrillation: the rate versus rhythm management controversy. J R Coll Physicians Edinb 2012;42(Suppl 18):23–34.

56. Al-Jazairi MIH, Nguyen BO, De With RR, et al.; RACE 3 Investigators. Antiarrhythmic drugs in patients with early persistent atrial fibrillation and heart failure: results of the RACE 3 study. Europace 2021;23:1359–68.

57. Noseworthy PA, van Houten HK, Gersh BJ, et al. Generalizability of the CASTLE-AF trial: catheter ablation for patients with atrial fibrillation and heart failure in routine practice. Heart Rhythm 2020;17:1057–65.

58. Savelieva I, Graydon R, Camm AJ. Pharmacological cardioversion of atrial fibrillation with vernakalant: evidence in support of the ESC Guidelines. Europace 2014;16:162–73.

59. Hilleman DE, Spinler SA. Conversion of recent-onset atrial fibrillation with intravenous amiodarone: a meta-analysis of randomized controlled trials. Pharmacotherapy 2002;22:66–74.

60. Khan IA, Mehta NJ, Gowda RM. Amiodarone for pharmacological cardioversion of recent-onset atrial fibrillation. Int J Cardiol 2003;89:239–48.

61. Kowey PR, Vanderlught JT, Luderer JR. Safety and risk/benefit analysis of ibutilide for acute conversion of atrial fibrillation/flutter. Am J Cardiol 1996;78:46A–52A.

62. Stambler BS, Wood MA, Ellenbogen KA, Perry KT, Wakefield LK, VanderLugt JT; Ibutilide Repeat Dose Investigators. Efficacy and safety of repeated intravenous doses of ibutilide for rapid conversion of atrial flutter or fibrillation. Circulation 1996;94:1613–2621.

63. Pedersen OD, Bagger H, Keller N, Marchant B, Kober L, Torp-Pedersen C; Danish Investigation of Arrhythmia and Mortality ON Dofetilide Study Group. Efficacy of dofetilide in the treatment of atrial fibrillation-flutter in patients with reduced left ventricular

function. A Danish Investigations of Arrhythmia and Mortality ON Dofetilide (DIAMOND) Substudy. Circulation 1001;104:292–6.

64. Singh S, Zoble RG, Yellen L, *et al.*; Dofetilide Atrial Fibrillation Investigators. Efficacy and safety of oral dofetilide in converting to and maintaining sinus rhythm in patients with chronic atrial fibrillation or atrial flutter: the Symptomatic Atrial Fibrillation Investigative Research on Dofetilide (SAFIRE-D) Study. Circulation 2000;102:2385–90.

65. Roy D, Talajic M, Dorian P, *et al.*; Canadian Trial of Atrial Fibrillation Investigators. Amiodarone to prevent recurrence of atrial fibrillation. N Engl J Med 2000;342:913–20.

66. Hohnloser SH, Klingenheben T, Singh BN. Amiodarone-associated proarrhythmic effects. A review with special reference to torsade de pointes tachycardia. Ann Intern Med 1994;121:529–35.

67. Singh BN, Connolly SJ, Crijns HJ, *et al.*; EURIDIS and ADONIS Investigators. Dronedarone for maintenance of sinus rhythm in atrial fibrillation or flutter. N Engl J Med 2007;357:987–99.

68. Hohnloser SH, Crijns H, Eickels M, *et al.* Effect of dronedarone on cardiovascular events in atrial fibrillation. N Engl J Med 2009;360:668–78.

69. Manolis AS, Deering TF, Cameron J, Estes NA 3rd. Mexiletine: pharmacology and therapeutic use. Clin Cardiol 1990;13:349–59.

70. Cairns JA, Connolly SJ, Roberts R, Gent M. Randomised trial of outcome after myocardial infarction in patients with frequent or repetitive ventricular premature depolarisations: CAMIAT. Canadian Amiodarone Myocardial Infarction Arrhythmia Trial Investigators. Lancet 1997;349:675–82.

71. Singh SN, Fletcher RD, Fisher SG, *et al.* Amiodarone in patients with congestive heart failure and asymptomatic ventricular arrhythmia. N Engl J Med.1995; 333:77–82.

72. Doval HC, Nul DR, Grancelli HO, Perrone SV, Bortman GR, Curiel R. Randomised trial of low-dose amiodarone in severe congestive heart failure. Grupo de Estudio de la Sobrevida en la Insuficiencia Cardiaca en Argentina (GESICA). Lancet 1994;344:493–8.

73. Priori SG, Blomström-Lundqvist C, Mazzanti A, *et al.* 2015 ESC Guidelines for the management of patients with ventricular arrhythmias and the prevention of sudden cardiac death. Europace 2015;17:1601–87.

74. Hohnloser SH, Dorian P, Roberts R, *et al.* Effect of amiodarone and sotalol on ventricular defibrillation threshold: the optimal pharmacological therapy in cardioverter defibrillator patients (OPTIC) trial. Circulation 2006;114:104–9.

75. Sapp JL, Wells GA, Parkash R, *et al.* Ventricular tachycardia ablation versus escalation of antiarrhythmic drugs. N Engl J Med 2016;375:111–21.

76. Tseng AS, Kunze KL, Lee JZ, *et al.* Efficacy of pharmacologic and cardiac implantable electronic device therapies in patients with heart failure and reduced ejection fraction: a systematic review and network meta-analysis. Circ Arrhythm Electrophysiol 2019;12:e006951.

77. Zareba W, Daubert JP, Beck CA, *et al.*; RAID Trial Investigators. Ranolazine in high-risk patients with implanted cardioverter-defibrillators: the RAID trial. J Am Coll Cardiol 2018;72:636–45.

CHAPTER 8.13

New and emerging therapies in heart failure

Giuseppe Rosano, Gerasimos Filippatos, and Randall Starling

Introduction

Over the last three decades, treatment of heart failure has substantially changed, due to the introduction of drug classes that have progressively reduced cardiovascular mortality and morbidity,[1] especially in patients with heart failure with reduced ejection fraction (HFrEF).[2]

This change of paradigm mirrors the advanced understanding of the pathophysiology of heart failure. Treatment of HFrEF in the eighties was limited to digoxin and diuretics that were only effective for the relief of symptoms, without efficacy in reducing mortality.[3] These drug therapies targeted volume overload (congestion) and myocardial dysfunction (pump failure). At the end of the eighties, the understanding of heart failure as a disorder of circulatory haemodynamics, neurohormonal imbalance, pathological cardiac remodelling, and increased arrhythmogenic instability led to the development of novel treatments with efficacy in reducing morbidity and mortality.[4] These treatments included vasodilator therapy with hydralazine/isosorbide dinitrate combination and the ushering of drugs correcting the neurohormonal imbalance (angiotensin-converting enzyme (ACE) inhibitors, beta-blockers, angiotensin T1 receptor blockers, mineralocorticoid receptor antagonists (MRAs), ivabradine, and the angiotensin receptor blocker/neprilysin inhibitor combination). After the withdrawal of flosequinan in the early 1990s, because of an increased risk of mortality and fatal arrhythmias, the bar for approval of new drugs in heart failure has been raised and regulatory agencies have requested evidence for the efficacy of new treatments on mortality and morbidity endpoints.[5]

Drugs targeting vascular and endothelial dysfunction in heart failure

Vascular reactivity is impaired in heart failure and associated with decreased exercise tolerance and poor clinical outcome.[6] There is consistent evidence that the xanthine oxidase (XO) metabolic pathway plays a role in the pathophysiology of chronic heart failure.[7] As such, XO blockage generating oxygen radical accumulation has emerged as an intriguing novel treatment option to prevent oxygen radical accumulation and its detrimental effects. Allopurinol (300 mg/day) has been shown to improve peripheral arterial vasodilatation and blood flow in hyperuricaemic patients with HFrEF,[8] as well as New York Heart Association (NYHA) functional class in patients with HFrEF. Direct myocardial effects for allopurinol, and hence a reduction of radical load and uric acid production, have been demonstrated in HFrEF.[7] Whether this effect translates into a prognostic benefit remains to be elucidated.

The nitric oxide (NO)–soluble guanylate cyclase (sGC)–cyclic guanosine monophosphate (cGMP) pathway plays a key role in vascular tissues, such as in the regulation of myocardial function through normal vascular smooth muscle cell relaxation.[9] Further, endothelial dysfunction resulting in reduced NO availability has been identified as a central mechanism in cardiovascular disease. This pathway is impaired in heart failure patients, leading to decreased protection against myocardial injury, ventricular remodelling, and the cardiorenal syndrome.[9] Among sGC stimulators, cinaciguat was found in a placebo-controlled phase 2b trial[10] to decrease pulmonary and systemic vascular resistance, as well as arterial pressure, and to increase the cardiac index in patients with acute heart failure. However, the trial was stopped early due to an increased rate of hypotension at doses of ≥200 μg/hour.

The phase 2b COMPOSE trials (COMPOSE 1 and 2, and COMPOSE early) investigated the safety and efficacy of different doses of cinaciguat, compared to placebo, in patients with acute heart failure. The three trials were terminated prematurely because of hypotensive events observed even with low doses.[11] The sGC activator ataciguat is currently being studied in ongoing clinical trials.

Since the presence of pulmonary hypertension aggravates the clinical course of heart failure, the sGC stimulator riociguat has been studied in patients with pulmonary hypertension secondary to systolic left ventricular dysfunction, showing an improvement in pulmonary vascular resistance, stroke volume, and cardiac index without concomitant increase in heart rate.[12] Riociguat improved exploratory haemodynamic and echocardiographic parameters, and ameliorated the quality of life, with a good safety profile.[12]

The sGC stimulator vericiguat has been studied in HFrEF (SOCRATES reduced) and heart failure with preserved ejection fraction (HFpEF) (SOCRATES preserved), and is currently moving into phase 3 for HFrEF.

The SOCRATES preserved trial[13] demonstrated that vericiguat was well tolerated and did not change N-terminal pro-B-type natriuretic peptide (NT-proBNP) levels and left atrial volume, but was associated with an improvement in the quality of life in patients with HFpEF. The VICTORIA trial[14] in HFrEF patients found that the incidence of death from cardiovascular causes or hospitalization for heart failure was lower among those who received vericiguat, compared to those who received placebo.

Thus, clinical evidence supports that sGC stimulators are promising candidates for a potential role in the future heart failure treatment strategy.

Omecamtiv mecarbil

The selective cardiac myosin activator omecamtiv mecarbil has been shown to improve cardiac function in patients with HFrEF. The GALACTIC-HF trial[15] found a lower incidence of heart failure event or death from cardiovascular causes in patients who received omecamtiv mecarbil, compared to those who received placebo. In a post hoc analysis of the GALACTIC-HF clinical trial,[16] treatment with omecamtiv mecarbil reduced the composite endpoint of time to first heart failure event or cardiovascular death among patients with severe heart failure. These data suggest the efficacy of omecamtiv mecarbil in patients for whom current treatment options are limited.

Adenosine A1 agonists

Adenosine A1 agonists modulate ischaemic cardiac injury and tissue injury and promote repair in response to stress. Partial adenosine A1 receptor (A1R) agonists protect and improve cardiac function at doses that do not result in adverse effects on the heart rate, atrioventricular conduction, and blood pressure, suggesting that these compounds may constitute a valuable new therapy for chronic heart failure.[17] Among A1R agonists, neladenoson bialanate is currently being studied for the treatment of heart failure. In patients with chronic HFrEF, treatment with neladenoson bialanate was not associated with dose-dependent favourable effects on cardiac structure and function, cardiac risk markers, or clinical outcome, but was associated with a dose-dependent decrease in renal function.[18] In patients with HFpEF, there was no significant dose–response effect of neladenoson on exercise performance.[19]

Beta-3 agonists

There is evidence from clinical and animal studies that beta-3 adrenergic receptor (beta3AR) activation is beneficial in severe heart failure. As such, beta3AR agonists are a promising therapeutic option for the treatment of this disease.[20] Recently, mirabegron has been studied as an add-on therapy, on top of standard care, to prevent or delay myocardial remodelling in patients at high risk of developing HFpEF. The BEAT-HF trial[21] suggested that beta-3 AR stimulation with mirabegron increased left ventricular ejection fraction in patients with severe heart failure, with a good safety profile. The ongoing BEAT-HF II (NCT03926754) is assessing the structural and functional cardiac effects of treatment with mirabegron in patients with moderate to severe chronic heart failure.

Mineralocorticoid receptor antagonists

MRAs have been demonstrated to be lifesaving therapies for patients with HFrEF. Clinical trials have demonstrated the effectiveness of MRAs in reducing mortality and hospitalizations in patients with chronic HFrEF. Indeed, RALES,[22] EPHESUS,[23] and EMPHASIS-HF[24] trials found that MRAs consistently reduced morbidity and mortality in this population. As such, guidelines recommend MRAs as standard therapy in all symptomatic HFrEF patients, that is, NYHA functional classes II–IV, who are already receiving an ACE inhibitor and a beta-blocker.[1] However, steroidal MRAs have a number of contraindications that limit their use in clinical practice such as the risk of hyperkalaemia and/or worsening renal function.[2]

With regard to hyperkalaemia, it is more frequently observed with spironolactone in at-risk patients. For MRAs, the optimal dose and frequency of dosing should be defined by taking into account the pre-therapy serum potassium levels.[2] In the future, MRA therapy could be more liberal with simultaneous use of potassium-binding agents.[25]

The ARTS-HF study[26] in patients hospitalized for worsening chronic HFrEF with type 2 diabetes mellitus and/or chronic kidney disease showed that the proportion of patients with a relative decrease in NT-proBNP level of >30% from baseline to day 90 was similar in the eplerenone and finerenone groups. The incidence of the clinical composite endpoint (all-cause death, cardiovascular hospitalization, or emergency presentation for worsening chronic heart failure) at day 90 was lower with all finerenone doses (except 2.5–5 mg), compared to eplerenone, with the lowest incidence observed in the finerenone 10–20 mg dose group.

The FIGARO-DKD trial showed that finerenone had beneficial effects in reducing hospitalization for heart failure, the risk of cardiovascular death, and the incidence of new-onset heart failure in patients with type 2 diabetes mellitus and chronic kidney disease who were on a background of maximal renin–angiotensin system (RAS) blockade therapy.[27,28]

Future directions

In the last decades, there has been a marked increase in the understanding of the pathophysiological mechanisms underlying heart failure. Genetic-, cellular-, and organ-level molecular changes in the heart have been elucidated.

Pharmacotherapies in heart failure, such as ACE inhibitors, β-adrenergic receptor blockade, calcium channel blockers, diuretics, and inhibition of the renin–angiotensin–aldosterone system, have provided benefit in terms of decreased morbidity and mortality. However, this approach is symptom-oriented and cannot stop disease progression and reversal from heart failure to a healthy state, thus increasing the value of a gene therapy approach targeting the underlying mechanisms.

RNA-based therapy in heart failure

Especially during the current coronavirus disease 2019 (Covid-19) pandemic, we have seen the tremendous power of ribonucleic acid (RNA) modulation that has become a promising approach for next-generation vaccines. However, there is multiple evidence for RNA therapy to serve as a powerful treatment of several types of disease, including cardiovascular disease and heart failure.[29] This is the case for both coding as well as non-coding RNAs. In particular, the field of non-coding RNA-based therapies has now come to the attention of cardiovascular research. Multiple non-coding RNA-based studies have been conducted in large-animal models, including pigs, rabbits, dogs, and non-human primates, and recently even in patients with heart failure.[29] A few, but increasing, number of antisense oligonucleotide drugs have already been approved by the Food and Drug Administration for targeting messenger RNAs (mRNAs). Recently, the first therapeutic microRNA (miRNA)-based inhibitory strategies have been tested in heart failure patients, as well as in healthy volunteers, to study the effects on wound healing (NCT04045405; NCT03603431). A combination of novel therapeutic RNA targets, large-animal models, *ex vivo* studies with human cells/tissues, and new delivery techniques will likely lead to significant progress in the development of non-coding RNA-based next-generation therapeutics for cardiovascular disease.

Preclinical large-animal studies of non-coding RNA therapeutics

Indeed, large-animal models, such as pigs or non-human primates, have been used as a model for mimicking human heart disease.[30] An initial study that investigated miRNA therapeutics in large-animal models targeted the miRNA miR-92a. This miRNA is ubiquitously expressed and has multiple functions in the body, including modulation of angiogenic pathways,[31] but also in cancer.[32] In an ischaemia–reperfusion injury pig model, miR-92 inhibition led to a reduction in infarct size, decreased cardiomyocyte apoptosis, and better myocardial function after inhibition of miR-92a expression.[33] Likewise, applied locked nucleic acid (LNA)-modified anti-miR-15b we applied in another myocardial infarction pig model restored porcine cardiac function.[34] Another miRNA, miR-132, was investigated in the, so far, largest pig study. Previously miR-132 was identified to be crucially involved in cardiac function.[35] miR-132 is both necessary and sufficient for driving pathological cardiomyocyte growth, a hallmark of adverse cardiac remodelling. The safety, tolerability, favourable pharmacokinetics, dose-dependent pharmacokinetic/pharmacodynamic (PK/PD) relationships, and the high clinical potential of an anti-miR-132 treatment in pigs following myocardial infarction have been documented.[36] These have been validated in two further large-animal models; first, miR-132 inhibition also showed strong cardiac improvement for both systolic and diastolic parameters, together with transformative tissue effects such as anti-hypertrophic and anti-fibrotic effects, in a chronic model of heart failure in pigs.[37] Very recently, miR-132 inhibition was also shown to result in positive cardiac effects in a non-ischaemic model of hypertrophic cardiomyopathy, showing promising potential of miR-132 in general heart failure treatment.[38]

Clinical evidence for non-coding RNA therapeutics

Next to pig studies, an miR-92a inhibitor was tested in two phase 1 clinical trials and was named MRG-110 (miRagen Therapeutics Inc., NCT03603431 and NCT03494712).[39] MRG-110 was expected to accelerate wound healing by improving blood flow via its pro-angiogenic properties. This was evidenced in a pig model where administration of anti-miR-92a inhibitors significantly increased blood flow and revascularization in peri-wound areas. Recently, a clinical dose ascending and dose repetition phase 1b study was initiated to assess the safety, pharmacokinetics, and pharmacodynamic parameters of an anti-miR-132 inhibitor in stable heart failure patients (NCT04045405).[40] Indeed, this study was the first clinical trial of an antisense drug in heart failure patients, and the miR-132 inhibitor CDR132L was shown to be safe and well tolerated, confirmed linear plasma pharmacokinetics with no signs of accumulation, and already suggested cardiac functional improvements such as >20% reduction in NT-proBNP level, on top of heart failure general treatment. Although this study is limited by the small patient numbers, the indicative efficacy of this drug is very encouraging, justifying additional clinical studies to confirm the beneficial pharmacodynamic effects of CDR132L in the treatment of heart failure.

References

1. McDonagh TA, Metra M, Adamo M, et al. 2021 ESC Guidelines for the diagnosis and treatment of acute and chronic heart failure. Eur Heart J. 2021;42(36):3599–726.

2. Rosano GMC, Moura B, Metra M, et al. Patient profiling in heart failure for tailoring medical therapy. A consensus document of the Heart Failure Association of the European Society of Cardiology. Eur J Heart Fail. 2021;23(6):872–81.

3. Hinder M, Yi BA, Langenickel TH. Developing drugs for heart failure with reduced ejection fraction: what have we learned from clinical trials? Clin Pharmacol Ther. 2018;103(5):802–14.

4. Seferovic PM, Ponikowski P, Anker SD, et al. Clinical practice update on heart failure 2019: pharmacotherapy, procedures, devices and patient management. An expert consensus meeting report of the Heart Failure Association of the European Society of Cardiology. Eur J Heart Fail. 2019;21(10):1169–86.

5. Loudon BL, Noordali H, Gollop ND, Frenneaux MP, Madhani M. Present and future pharmacotherapeutic agents in heart failure: an evolving paradigm. Br J Pharmacol. 2016;173(12):1911–24.

6. Varin R, Mulder P, Tamion F, et al. Improvement of endothelial function by chronic angiotensin-converting enzyme inhibition in heart failure: role of nitric oxide, prostanoids, oxidant stress, and bradykinin. Circulation. 2000;102(3):351–6.

7. Doehner W, Anker SD. Xanthine oxidase inhibition for chronic heart failure: is allopurinol the next therapeutic advance in heart failure? Heart. 2005;91(6):707–9.

8. Doehner W, Schoene N, Rauchhaus M, et al. Effects of xanthine oxidase inhibition with allopurinol on endothelial function and peripheral blood flow in hyperuricemic patients with chronic heart failure: results from 2 placebo-controlled studies. Circulation. 2002;105(22):2619–24.

9. Gheorghiade M, Marti CN, Sabbah HN, et al. Soluble guanylate cyclase: a potential therapeutic target for heart failure. Heart Fail Rev. 2013;18(2):123–34.

10. Erdmann E, Semigran MJ, Nieminen MS, et al. Cinaciguat, a soluble guanylate cyclase activator, unloads the heart but also causes hypotension in acute decompensated heart failure. Eur Heart J. 2013;34(1):57–67.

11. Gheorghiade M, Greene SJ, Filippatos G, et al. Cinaciguat, a soluble guanylate cyclase activator: results from the randomized, controlled, phase IIb COMPOSE programme in acute heart failure syndromes. Eur J Heart Fail. 2012;14(9):1056–66.

12. Bonderman D, Ghio S, Felix SB, et al. Riociguat for patients with pulmonary hypertension caused by systolic left ventricular dysfunction: a phase IIb double-blind, randomized, placebo-controlled, dose-ranging hemodynamic study. Circulation. 2013;128(5):502–11.

13. Pieske B, Maggioni AP, Lam CSP, et al. Vericiguat in patients with worsening chronic heart failure and preserved ejection fraction: results of the SOluble guanylate Cyclase stimulatoR in heArT failurE patientS with PRESERVED EF (SOCRATES-PRESERVED) study. Eur Heart J. 2017;38(15):1119–27.

14. Armstrong PW, Pieske B, Anstrom KJ, et al. Vericiguat in patients with heart failure and reduced ejection fraction. N Engl J Med. 2020;382(20):1883–93.

15. Teerlink JR, Diaz R, Felker GM, et al. Cardiac myosin activation with omecamtiv mecarbil in systolic heart failure. N Engl J Med. 2021;384(2):105–16.

16. Felker GM, Solomon SD, Claggett B, et al. Assessment of omecamtiv mecarbil for the treatment of patients with severe heart failure: a post hoc analysis of data from the GALACTIC-HF randomized clinical trial. JAMA Cardiol. 2022;7(1):26–34.

17. Dinh W, Albrecht-Küpper B, Gheorghiade M, Voors AA, van der Laan M, Sabbah HN. Partial adenosine A1 agonist in heart failure. Handb Exp Pharmacol. 2017;243:177–203.

18. Voors AA, Bax JJ, Hernandez AF, et al. Safety and efficacy of the partial adenosine A1 receptor agonist neladenoson bialanate in patients with chronic heart failure with reduced ejection fraction: a phase IIb, randomized, double-blind, placebo-controlled trial. Eur J Heart Fail. 2019;21(11):1426–33.

19. Shah SJ, Voors AA, McMurray JJV, et al. Effect of neladenoson bialanate on exercise capacity among patients with heart failure with preserved ejection fraction: a randomized clinical trial. JAMA. 2019;321(21):2101–12.

20. Rasmussen HH, Figtree GA, Krum H, Bundgaard H. The use of beta3-adrenergic receptor agonists in the treatment of heart failure. Curr Opin Investig Drugs. 2009;10(9):955–62.

21. Bundgaard H, Axelsson A, Hartvig Thomsen J, et al. The first-in-man randomized trial of a beta3 adrenoceptor agonist in chronic heart failure: the BEAT-HF trial. Eur J Heart Fail. 2017;19(4):566–75.

22. Pitt B, Zannad F, Remme WJ, et al. The effect of spironolactone on morbidity and mortality in patients with severe heart failure. Randomized Aldactone Evaluation Study Investigators. N Engl J Med. 1999;341(10):709–17.

23. Pitt B, Remme W, Zannad F, et al. Eplerenone, a selective aldosterone blocker, in patients with left ventricular dysfunction after myocardial infarction. N Engl J Med. 2003;348(14):1309–21.

24. Zannad F, McMurray JJ, Krum H, et al. Eplerenone in patients with systolic heart failure and mild symptoms. N Engl J Med. 2011;364(1):11–21.

25. Lainscak M, Vitale C, Seferovic P, Spoletini I, Cvan Trobec K, Rosano GM. Pharmacokinetics and pharmacodynamics of cardiovascular drugs in chronic heart failure. Int J Cardiol. 2016;224:191–8.

26. Filippatos G, Anker SD, Böhm M, et al. A randomized controlled study of finerenone vs. eplerenone in patients with worsening chronic heart failure and diabetes mellitus and/or chronic kidney disease. Eur Heart J. 2016;37(27):2105–14.

27. Filippatos G, Anker SD, Agarwal R, et al. Finerenone reduces risk of incident heart failure in patients with chronic kidney disease and type 2 diabetes: analyses from the FIGARO-DKD Trial. Circulation. 2022;145(6):437–47.

28. Pitt B, Filippatos G, Agarwal R, et al. Cardiovascular events with finerenone in kidney disease and type 2 diabetes. N Engl J Med. 2021;385(24):2252–63.

29. Huang CK, Kafert-Kasting S, Thum T. Preclinical and clinical development of noncoding RNA therapeutics for cardiovascular disease. Circ Res. 2020;126(5):663–78.

30. Clauss S, Bleyer C, Schüttler D, et al. Animal models of arrhythmia: classic electrophysiology to genetically modified large animals. Nat Rev Cardiol. 2019;16(8):457–75.

31. Bonauer A, Carmona G, Iwasaki M, et al. MicroRNA-92a controls angiogenesis and functional recovery of ischemic tissues in mice. Science. 2009;324(5935):1710–13.

32. Wu X, Cui X, Yue C, Liu X, Mo Z. Expression of miR-92a in colon cancer tissues and its correlation with clinicopathologic features and prognosis. Am J Transl Res. 2021;13(8):9627–32.

33. Hinkel R, Penzkofer D, Zühlke S, et al. Inhibition of microRNA-92a protects against ischemia/reperfusion injury in a large-animal model. Circulation. 2013;128(10):1066–75.

34. Hullinger TG, Montgomery RL, Seto AG, *et al*. Inhibition of miR-15 protects against cardiac ischemic injury. Circ Res. 2012;110(1):71–81.

35. Ucar A, Gupta SK, Fiedler J, *et al*. The miRNA-212/132 family regulates both cardiac hypertrophy and cardiomyocyte autophagy. Nat Commun. 2012;3:1078.

36. Foinquinos A, Batkai S, Genschel C, *et al*. Preclinical development of a miR-132 inhibitor for heart failure treatment. Nat Commun. 2020;11(1):633.

37. Batkai S, Genschel C, Viereck J, *et al*. CDR132L improves systolic and diastolic function in a large animal model of chronic heart failure. Eur Heart J. 2021;42(2):192–201.

38. Hinkel R, Batkai S, Bähr A, *et al*. AntimiR-132 attenuates myocardial hypertrophy in an animal model of percutaneous aortic constriction. J Am Coll Cardiol. 2021;77(23):2923–35.

39. Gallant-Behm CL, Piper J, Dickinson BA, Dalby CM, Pestano LA, Jackson AL. A synthetic microRNA-92a inhibitor (MRG-110) accelerates angiogenesis and wound healing in diabetic and nondiabetic wounds. Wound Repair Regen. 2018;26(4):311–23.

40. Täubel J, Hauke W, Rump S, *et al*. Novel antisense therapy targeting microRNA-132 in patients with heart failure: results of a first-in-human phase 1b randomized, double-blind, placebo-controlled study. Eur Heart J. 2021;42(2):178–88.

SECTION 9

Chronic heart failure: non-pharmacological management

CHAPTER 9.1

Implantable cardioverter–defibrillators

Gianluigi Savarese, Cecilia Linde, and
Kenneth Dickstein

Contents

Introduction

The first use of an implantable cardioverter–defibrillator (ICD) was reported in 1980, when Dr Michel Mirowski and colleagues implanted the first device in a woman who survived a cardiac arrest after a myocardial infarction (MI) at the Johns Hopkins Hospital.

An ICD is a small battery-powered device made up of three four key parts, including: (1) a pulse generator; (2) one (single-chamber device) or two (dual-chamber device) transvenous leads, which deliver electrical signals from the pulse generator to the heart; and (3) bipolar electrodes, which are used for pacing and sensing (➲ Figure 9.1.1). The ICD generator includes the battery, voltage converters and resistors, capacitors to store charges, microprocessors and integrated circuits to analyse the rhythm and control therapy delivery, memory to store data, and a telemetry module. An ICD is able to identify the type of cardiac rhythm through ventricular sensing of the R wave rate. One or more ventricular tachycardia (VT) and/or ventricular fibrillation (VF) zones are usually programmed. The fastest rate (i.e. the VF zone) is treated with a shock, whereas episodes of tachycardia in the VT zones can be treated with anti-tachycardia pacing (ATP) or low-energy synchronized shocks or they can be monitored through observation. Supraventricular arrhythmias might be detected within the VT zone, and therefore, there are algorithms available that discriminate between supraventricular and ventricular tachycardias for both single- and dual-chamber ICDs. This is simpler in dual-chamber devices, which can include information from the atrial electrogram to distinguish between supraventricular and ventricular tachycardias. ICDs also have pacing functions for bradycardias.[1]

Use of ICDs represents nowadays a key treatment for primary prevention of sudden cardiac death (SCD) and for treating life-threatening ventricular arrhythmias. ICDs also facilitate collection of useful data that may be conducted via remote monitoring. In 2016, >100,000 ICD implantations were performed in the member countries of the European Society of Cardiology (ESC).[2]

Risk of sudden cardiac death in patients with heart failure

SCD is defined as a non-traumatic, unexpected fatal event due to cardiac causes (known or identified at autopsy, or in the absence of obvious extracardiac causes identified postmortem and therefore likely due to an arrhythmic event), occurring within 1 hour from the onset of symptoms in an apparently healthy individual.[3]

The risk of SCD in patients with heart failure with reduced ejection fraction (HFrEF) has been decreasing over the last 20 years, with a 1-year risk of SCD of approximately 7% from the RALES trial published in 1999 and corresponding estimates of approximately 4% from the PARADIGM-HF study in 2014, accounting for a decrease in rates

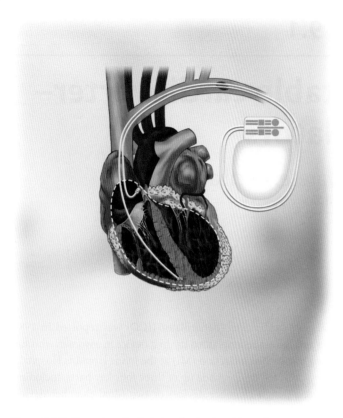

Figure 9.1.1 Illustration of a dual-chamber implantable cardioverter–defibrillator. The pulse generator is usually placed subcutaneously on the fascia of the pectoralis major muscle. The transvenous right ventricular lead contains the shocking coils and pacing electrodes. The transvenous right atrial lead has sensing and pacing functions.

of 44%.[4] The risk of life-threatening ventricular arrhythmias has been shown to be similar in patients with ischaemic and non-ischaemic HF, although those with non-ischaemic HF have a higher risk of non-SCD.[5] Beyond the introduction of the use of ICDs for primary prevention of SCD, which has been only rarely implemented in real-world clinical practice and in pharmacological randomized trials, this reduction in SCD risk can be explained by the use of guideline-directed medical therapy for HFrEF.[6] In a meta-analysis of 30 trials on HFrEF, beta-blockers reduced the risk of SCD by 31%,[7] which potentially could be explained by the effects on circadian catecholamine surges, prevention of further MI in patients with ischaemic heart disease, and reverse remodelling.[6] In a meta-analysis of five randomized controlled trials, mineralocorticoid receptor antagonists (MRAs) have been shown to reduce the risk of SCD by 23%, with potential underlying mechanisms involving beneficial ventricular remodelling, stimulation of the central adrenergic system, and suppression of the proarrhythmic effects of aldosterone at cellular levels.[8]

Although angiotensin-converting enzyme (ACE) inhibitors have not been reported to impact the risk of SCD,[9,10] a reduction in risk was observed with candesartan in the CHARM-Reduced trial.[11] In the PARADIGM-HF trial, sacubitril/valsartan versus enalapril reduced the risk of SCD by 20%, which might be associated with reverse remodelling and attenuation of myocardial fibrosis.[12] Additionally, sacubitril/valsartan has also been reported to reduce the need for ICD implantation. In the PROVE-HF trial, use of sacubitril/valsartan led to an increase in ejection fraction (EF) by 4.8 points at 6 months and by 9.6 points at 12 months, with the consequence that after 6 months of treatment, 32% of patients who were eligible for ICD at baseline improved their EF to >35%, and therefore were no longer eligible, with 62% being ineligible at 1 year.[13] In the DAPA-HF trial, dapagliflozin, a sodium–glucose cotransporter 2 inhibitor, reduced the risk of SCD by 19%, with potential reasons being favourable effects on the autonomic nervous system, left ventricular remodelling, and myocardial metabolism.[14] Finally, cardiac resynchronization therapy (CRT) also has been shown to reduce the substrate for ventricular arrhythmias, and therefore the risk of SCD, not only through favouring left ventricular structural remodelling (i.e. improving preloading, prolonging cell survival, reducing fibrosis, and increasing the EF), but also through favouring electrical remodelling by improving ion (such as calcium, potassium, and sodium) channel currents and beta-adrenergic response, and by abbreviating the action potential duration.[15,16] Consistently, CRT super-responders have shown a lower risk of ventricular arrhythmias and all-cause death, compared to CRT non-responders.[17] Conversely, CRT has been suggested to increase the risk of ventricular arrhythmias in non-responders by facilitating re-entry circuits through initiating activation near or within scar.[18]

Although mortality is high in patients with HF with preserved EF (HFpEF), the risk of SCD has been shown to be lower than in HFrEF.[19] In the TOPCAT trial (EF ≥45%), approximately 20% of all deaths were SCD.[20] In the CHARM-preserved trial (EF >40%), the rates of SCD were 3-fold lower than in the CHARM-Reduced.[11] In the I-PRESERVE trial, 26% of all deaths occurred suddenly.[21] In the PARAGON-HF trial, 22% of all deaths were due to SCD, and the risk of SCD decreased along with increasing EF.[22]

Mechanisms leading to sudden cardiac death in heart failure

In patients with HFrEF, SCD is associated with a high risk of VT. Myocardial fibrosis and scar, associated with systolic dysfunction and ischaemic heart disease, and therefore with both ischaemic and non-ischaemic cardiomyopathy, represent important substrates for ventricular re-entrant arrhythmias.[23,24] However, mechanisms other than myocardial fibrosis and scar can contribute to the increased arrhythmic risk in HF, and therefore to the risk of SCD. Mechanical stretch secondary to acute or chronic loading, which might characterize at least some phases of the HF course, impacts the effective refractory period and the mean action potential duration, potentially leading to ventricular arrhythmias.[25,26] Increased sympathetic activity and an inhomogeneous distribution of sympathetic innervation, which might be secondary to areas of post-MI necrosis or fibrosis, have also been associated with an increased risk of VT.[27,28] High circulatory concentrations of endothelin-1 and noradrenaline due to neurohormonal activation in HF also contribute to the proarrhythmic status.[29] A failing heart is also characterized by altered expression, distribution, and density of specific gap junctions, leading to abnormal propagation of electrical impulse and to altered calcium, sodium, and potassium currents, thus increasing the risk of VT.[30,31] Similar mechanisms as in HFrEF have been advocated to explain the risk of SCD in HFpEF.[32]

Implantable cardioverter–defibrillators for primary prevention of sudden cardiac death

Over the last >20 years, use of ICDs has been the key treatment for prevention of SCD.

The first trial to test the efficacy of ICDs for primary prevention of SCD in HF was the MADIT I trial published in 1996. This study randomized 196 patients to either ICD or conventional medical therapy, who had prior MI, EF of <35%, New York Heart Association (NYHA) classes I–III, a documented episode of asymptomatic non-sustained VT, and inducible non-suppressible VT from electrophysiological studies. Over a mean follow-up of 27 months, ICD reduced the risk of all-cause death by 54%.[33]

The MUSTT trial randomized 704 patients to antiarrhythmic therapy, including drugs or ICD, or to no antiarrhythmic therapy, who had an EF of ≤40%, coronary artery disease, and sustained VT induced by programmed stimulation. Within 5 years of randomization, antiarrhythmic therapy reduced the risk of cardiac arrest or death from arrhythmia by 27% and the risk of all-cause mortality by 20%. The risk of cardiac arrest or death was 76% lower in those who received an ICD, compared to those who had antiarrhythmic therapy with drugs. As many as 53% of patients received digoxin, 58% diuretics, and 75% ACE inhibitors as HF medications. Beta-blocker use was lower in those assigned to the antiarrhythmic therapy arm (29% vs 51%).[34]

The subsequent MADIT II trial randomized 1232 patients with prior MI (≤1 month) and an EF of ≤30% in a 3:2 ratio to receiving an ICD or conventional medical therapy. Over a mean follow-up period of 20 months, ICD reduced the risk of all-cause death by 31%, with consistent effects across several subgroups of patients. In this trial, 70% of patients received a beta-blocker, 70% an ACE inhibitor, 57% digoxin, and 76% a diuretic.[35]

In the DEFINITE trial which enrolled 458 patients with non-ischaemic HF, EF of ≤35%, and ventricular complexes or non-sustained VT, who were mainly treated with ACE inhibitors (86%) and beta-blockers (85%), over a mean follow-up period of 29 months, the ICD treatment group showed only a trend towards a statistically significant reduction in the risk of all-cause death ($P = 0.08$) and significant reduction in the risk of SCD by 80%.[36]

In the SCD-HeFT study, 2521 patients with EF of ≤35% and NYHA classes II and III were randomized to conventional therapy plus placebo, conventional therapy plus amiodarone, or conventional therapy plus a conservatively programmed, shock-only, single-lead ICD. In the trial, 52% of patients had HF with an ischaemic aetiology; use of renin–angiotensin system inhibitors was high (>95%), and 69% of patients received beta-blockers, 70% digoxin, and 82% diuretics. Over a median follow-up period of 46 months, ICD reduced the risk of all-cause death by 23%, compared to control, whereas no risk reduction was observed with amiodarone. Results were consistent regardless of the HF aetiology.[37] An analysis considering an extended follow-up of up to 11 years still showed a 13% reduction of all-cause mortality with ICD. However, a 19% reduction in risk was observed with ICD in patients with ischaemic HF, whereas no benefit was observed in those with non-ischaemic HF, with a statistically significant interaction in this subgroup analysis.[38]

The COMPANION trial randomized 1520 patients with more advanced HF (i.e. NYHA class III or IV, including both ischaemic and non-ischaemic aetiologies, and a QRS interval of at least 120 ms) to receiving, in a 1:2:2 ratio, optimal pharmacological therapy alone, or in combination with a CRT-pacemaker (CRT-P), or in combination with a CRT-defibrillator (CRT-D). Compared to optimal pharmacological therapy alone, CRT-D reduced the primary outcome of HF death or hospitalization by 40% and the risk of all-cause death by 36%, whereas corresponding estimates were 34% and 24%, respectively, for CRT-P. Results were consistent regardless of the HF aetiology.[39]

In the REVERSE trial, patients with mild HFrEF were randomized to CRT (CRT-D or CRT-P) ON versus OFF. At 5-year follow-up, CRT-D use was associated with a 65% lower risk of all-cause mortality, compared to treatment with CRT-P.[40]

The more recent DANISH trial randomized 556 patients with symptomatic non-ischaemic HF to ICD or to usual care. Over a median follow-up period of 68 months, ICD did not reduce the primary outcome of all-cause mortality, whereas it reduced the risk of SCD by 50%.[41] ICD did not affect health-related quality of life, as evaluated by the Minnesota Living with Heart Failure Questionnaire (MLHFQ).[42] However, in patients with a higher risk of SCD, as estimated by higher Seattle Proportional Risk Model (SPRM) scores, ICD reduced the risk of all-cause death by 55%.[43]

A meta-analysis of 11 trials that also included the DANISH trial showed an equal 24% risk reduction in all-cause mortality with ICD in both patients with ischaemic HF and those with non-ischaemic HF (➲ Figure 9.1.2).[44]

More contemporary evidence on ICD for primary prevention of SCD in HFrEF is limited to post hoc analyses of trials and observational studies. In the PARADIGM-HF trial, after propensity matching of eligible patients with versus those without an ICD, use of an ICD was associated with a 56% lower risk of SCD in both patients with and those without ischaemic HF.[45] In an analysis of the Swedish HF Registry which considered data up to 2016, use of ICD in patients with an indication for primary prevention of SCD was associated with 27% and 12% lower risk of all-cause death at 1 and 5 years, respectively, with results being consistent among patients with and those without ischaemic heart disease.[46] Data from the Swedish HF Registry also showed in the same setting a 24% and an 18% lower risk of all-cause death with CRT-D vs CRT-P at 1 and 3 years, respectively.[47] In the prospective EU-CERT-ICD study which enrolled 2327 patients across 15 European countries with a guideline recommendation for prophylactic ICD implantation, use of ICD was associated with a 27% lower risk of all-cause death.[48]

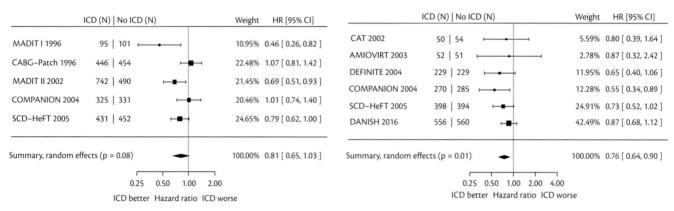

Figure 9.1.2 Meta-analysis of randomized controlled trials on implantable cardioverter–defibrillators for prevention of sudden cardiac death.
Reproduced from Shun-Shin MJ, Zheng SL, Cole GD, Howard JP, Whinnett ZI, Francis DP. Implantable cardioverter defibrillators for primary prevention of death in left ventricular dysfunction with and without ischaemic heart disease: a meta-analysis of 8567 patients in the 11 trials. *Eur Heart J.* 2017 Jun 7;38(22):1738–1746. doi: 10.1093/eurheartj/ehx028 with permission from Oxford University Press.

ICD for primary prevention of SCD has also been tested in the setting of immediate post-MI and in patients in need of coronary revascularization. In the IRIS trial, 898 patients were enrolled 5–31 days after an acute MI if they had evidence of reduced EF (≤40%) and a heart rate of ≥90 bpm on the first electrocardiogram (ECG) within 48 hours after the MI, or evidence of non-sustained VT during Holter monitoring, or both. Although the risk of SCD was reduced by 45% in patients receiving an ICD, there was no difference in risk of all-cause death across the trial arms, and the risk of non-SCD death was 2-fold higher in patients receiving an ICD.[49]

The DINAMIT trial randomized 674 patients 6–40 days after an MI, with reduced EF (≤35%) and impaired cardiac autonomic function defined as depressed heart rate variability or an elevated average 24-hour heart rate. In the study, ICD reduced the risk of SCD by 58% but increased the risk of non-SCD death by 75%.[50]

The CABG-PATCH trial randomized 900 patients with EF of ≤35% and signal-averaged ECG (duration of the filtered QRS complex: >114 ms; root-mean-square voltage in the terminal 40 ms of the QRS complex: <20 μV; or duration of the terminal filtered QRS complex at <40 μV: >38 ms) with coronary artery disease scheduled for elective bypass surgery. Over a mean follow-up period of 32 months, ICD implantation did not affect the risk of all-cause mortality.[51]

Based on the evidence, the 2021 ESC Guidelines on HF provide a class I, Level of evidence A recommendation for use of ICD for primary prevention of SCD and reduction of all-cause mortality in patients with symptomatic HF (NYHA classes III–IV) of an ischaemic aetiology (excluding those with an MI in the prior 40 days) and an EF of ≤35% despite ≥3 months of optimal medical therapy, provided that they are expected to survive >1 year with good functional status. Accordingly, ICD implantation is not indicated within 40 days of an MI and in patients in NYHA class IV who are refractory to pharmacological therapy, unless they are candidates for CRT or ventricular assist device (VAD)

or cardiac transplantation (➲ Table 9.1.1).[52] Conversely, American guidelines provide a Class I, Level of evidence A recommendation for patients in NYHA classes II–III, regardless of ischaemic/non-ischaemic aetiology of HF, whereas they also provide a Class I, Level of evidence A recommendation for ischaemic HF and a Class IIb, Level of evidence B recommendation for non-ischaemic HF in patients in NYHA class I and with EF of ≤30%.[53]

Data supporting the use of ICD for primary prevention of SCD in patients with HF with mildly reduced EF (HFmrEF) and HFpEF are very limited. In the SCD-HeFT trial, approximately 370 patients reported an EF of >35% at a repeated EF assessment. In these patients, ICD, compared to placebo, led to a risk reduction of all-cause death of 38%, which was 36% in patients with a repeated EF of ≤35%, without any interaction between treatment assignment and repeated EF for mortality.[54] However, in an observational cohort study, where 34% of ICD-implanted patients no longer had an indication for ICD at follow-up due to improvement in EF, those without an indication at follow-up reported a significantly lower rate of appropriate ICD therapies, compared to those with a persisting indication (2.8% vs 10.7%, respectively), which raises the question of whether ICD generator explantation, rather than replacement, should be considered in these patients.[55] In the setting of an EF of >35%, the MADIT S-ICD trial, which aimed to randomize post-MI patients with diabetes and EF of 36–50% to subcutaneous ICD (S-ICD) or to control, has been prematurely terminated due to poor enrolment.[56]

Implantable cardioverter–defibrillators for primary prevention of sudden cardiac death in subgroups of patients with HFrEF

Older age is associated with very high competing risk in patients with HFrEF, that is death from non-SCD, with older patients reporting a higher risk of all-cause mortality, but fewer ICD shocks/therapies.[57] This factor might be particularly important in patients

Table 9.1.1 Recommendations for use of implantable cardioverter–defibrillators in patients with heart failure from the 2021 European Society of Cardiology Guidelines on heart failure

Recommendations	Class	Level
Secondary prevention		
An ICD is recommended to reduce the risk of SCD and all-cause mortality in patients who recovered from a ventricular arrhythmia causing haemodynamic instability, and who are expected to survive for >1 year with good functional status, in the absence of reversible causes or unless the ventricular arrhythmia occurred <48 hours after a myocardial infarction	I	A
Primary prevention		
An ICD is recommended to reduce the risk of SCD and all-cause mortality in patients with symptomatic HF (NYHA classes II and III) of an ischaemic aetiology (unless they had a myocardial infarction in the prior 40 days) and an EF of ≤35% despite ≥3 months of optimal medical therapy, provided they are expected to survive substantially longer than 1 year with good functional status	I	A
An ICD should be considered to reduce the risk of SCD and all-cause mortality in patients with symptomatic HF (NYHA classes II and III) of a non-ischaemic aetiology, and an EF of ≤35% despite ≥3 months of optimal medical therapy, provided they are expected to survive substantially longer than 1 year with good functional status	II	A
Patients should be carefully evaluated by an experienced cardiologist before generator replacement, because management goals and the patient's needs and clinical status may have changed	IIa	B
A wearable ICD may be considered for patients with HF who are at risk of SCD, for a limited period as a bridge to an implanted device	IIb	B
ICD implantation is not recommended within 40 days of an MI, as implantation at this time does not improve prognosis	III	A
ICD therapy is not recommended in patients in NYHA class IV with severe symptoms refractory to pharmacological therapy, unless they are candidates for CRT, a ventricular assist device, or cardiac transplantation	III	C

CRT, cardiac resynchronization therapy; EF, ejection fraction; ICD, implantable cardioverter–defibrillator; MI, myocardial infarction; NYHA, New York Heart Association; SCD, sudden cardiac death.

McDonagh TA, Metra M, Adamo M, *et al*; ESC Scientific Document Group. 2021 ESC Guidelines for the diagnosis and treatment of acute and chronic heart failure. *Eur Heart J*. 2021 Sep 21;42(36):3599–3726. doi: 10.1093/eurheartj/ehab368. © The European Society of Cardiology. Reprinted by permission of Oxford University Press.

with non-ischaemic HF where the risk of non-SCD is higher.[5] In the DANISH trial, where use of ICD for primary prevention of SCD reduced the risk of SCD, but not the primary outcome of all-cause death, there was a linear correlation between ICD-associated reduction in risk of all-cause mortality and age, with an optimal cut-off for ICD implantation of ≤70 years. Consistently, although rates of SCD were quite similar in patients aged ≤70 and those aged >70 years (i.e. 1.8 vs 1.6 per 100 patient-years, respectively), the risk of non-SCD was 2-fold lower in the first age group compared to the latter (i.e. 2.7 vs. 5.4 per 100 patient-years, respectively).[58] In the observational EU-CERT-ICD which enrolled both patients with ischaemic and those with non-ischaemic HF, ICD was associated with lower mortality in patients aged <75 years, but not in those aged ≥75 years.[48] However, these findings were not observed in other randomized controlled trials or observational studies.[46]

Another subgroup where the efficacy of ICD for primary prevention of SCD is debated is represented by women. Whereas some studies have reported no survival benefit, others have found improved survival regardless of sex, and other studies still have described better outcome in women compared to men.[46,48,59,60]

In a pooled analysis of MADIT I, MADIT II, DEFINITE, and SCD-HeFT studies, ICD was associated with 44% reduced all-cause mortality in patients without diabetes, but not in those with diabetes.[61] Analysis of the EU-CERT-ICD study consistently showed a lower incidence of appropriate ICD shocks in patients with diabetes, but higher mortality, indicating that non-competing events (i.e. risk of non-SCD death) might limit the need for an ICD in this population.[62] Consistently, the efficacy of ICD has been shown to decrease along with increasing comorbidities.[63]

Prediction of risk of sudden cardiac death

Identifying patients at higher risk of SCD might be relevant for patient selection for ICD. Among others, the SPRM is one of the most used scoring system for estimation of SCD risk.[64] Variables which are incorporated in this score are younger age, male sex, and higher body mass index, which are independently associated with a higher risk of SCD, and diabetes, hyper-/hypotension, higher creatinine level, and hyponatraemia, which are associated with a lower risk of SCD. Its calculation, in combination with use of the Seattle Heart Failure Model (SHFM), which predicts overall mortality,[65] has been shown to significantly contribute to discriminating those patients at high risk of SCD but with a lower risk of competing events, and therefore who are more likely to benefit from ICD for primary prevention of SCD.[43,66] Apart from the SPRM, non-sustained VT has been identified as a predictor of SCD in patients with left ventricular dysfunction.[67] Other factors have been proposed more recently that significantly contribute to risk stratification of SCD. In patients with dilated cardiomyopathy, myocardial scar quantification using late gadolinium enhancement (LGE) on magnetic resonance imaging (MRI) has shown strong and incremental prognostic value in SCD risk stratification beyond EF.[68,69,70,71] In particular, in non-ischaemic cardiomyopathy, the relationship between scar on MRI and the risk of events might be curvilinear, with a plateau at approximately 20–25% of scar size,[70] and a ring-like pattern of scar has been associated with malignant arrhythmic events.[72] Therefore, a new risk score considering both clinical and MRI parameters, which include assessment of fibrosis via LGE, has been released.[73]

Although the risk of SCD is lower in patients with HF with higher EF, some selected patients with a particularly high risk might still benefit from an ICD for primary prevention of SCD. A prediction model from the I-PRESERVE trial considering age, gender, history of diabetes and MI, left bundle branch block on ECG, and the natural logarithm of N-terminal pro-B-type natriuretic peptide (NT-proBNP) has been shown to identify patients with a ≥10% cumulative incidence of SCD over 5 years, while taking into account competing risks, which is similar to observations from the SCD-HeFT trial in HFrEF.[74]

Implantable cardioverter–defibrillators for secondary prevention of life-threatening arrhythmic events and sudden cardiac death in heart failure

ICD implantation has been shown to impact survival also in patients who experienced a prior episode of cardiac arrest—VT or VF. In the AVID trial, 1016 patients who had been resuscitated from near-fatal VF, or who had undergone cardioversion from sustained VT and had syncope or other serious cardiac symptoms together with an EF of ≤40%, were randomized to ICD versus class III antiarrhythmic drugs. ICD led to a reduction in death rates of 39% at 1 year, 27% at 2 years, and 31% at 3 years.[75] In the CIDS trial, where 659 patients with resuscitated VF or VT or with unmonitored syncope were randomized to ICD or amiodarone, ICD non-significantly reduced the risk of all-cause death and arrhythmic mortality.[76] Similarly, in the CASH trial, ICD non-significantly reduced the risk of all-cause mortality, compared to amiodarone and metoprolol.[77] However, in a meta-analysis of these trials, ICD reduced the risk of all-cause death by 28%, and the risk of arrhythmic death by 50%.[78]

Based on this evidence, current 2021 ESC Guidelines on HF provide a Class I, Level of evidence A recommendation for ICD to reduce the risk of SCD and all-cause mortality in patients who have recovered from ventricular arrhythmia causing haemodynamic instability and who are expected to survive for at least 1 year with good functional status, in the absence of reversible causes or unless the ventricular arrhythmia occurred <48 hours after an MI (➲ Table 9.1.1).[52] Similar recommendations are provided in American guidelines.[53]

Complications

Complications might occur during, but also after, implantation of an ICD. In an analysis of the US National Cardiovascular Data Registry (NCDR), the most common in-hospital complications associated with ICD implantation included lead dislodgement (1.0%), haematoma (0.9%), pneumothorax (0.5%), and cardiac arrest (0.3%), which were less frequent in high-volume hospitals.[79] In-hospital mortality has been shown to be 0.2%.[80]

Up to 11% of new implantations might be affected by complications within the early post-discharge period, including haematomas and device and lead malfunction.[81,82] In the US NCDR analysis, 2.6 per 100 patient-years required reoperation for device malfunction or infection, whereas 3.5 per 100-patient years required hospitalization without reoperation, with highest rates associated with mechanical complications rather than with device infection. Highest rates of complications were seen within 90 days post-implantation. Patients receiving an ICD for secondary prevention or a CRT-D were at higher risk of complications.[83] Up to one of four transvenous ICD leads have been reported to have mechanical complication when patients were followed up for up to 10 years.[84] In the NCDR analysis, 1.7% of all ICD implantations were complicated by infections, with generator replacement being associated with a higher risk, compared to an initial implant (1.9% vs 1.6%).[85]

A large meta-analysis of 60 studies reported an average device infection rate of 1–1.3%.[86] Infections might be limited to the pocket, but can also involve the leads and cause infective endocarditis. In a Danish nationwide registry, the incidence of infectious endocarditis following ICD implantation was 3.7 per 1000 patient-years.[87] Antibiotic prophylaxis has been shown to significantly reduce the risk of infection.[88] Lead/device extraction is mandatory to control the infection, together with antimicrobial therapy and long-term suppressive antibiotic therapy in selected cases. Reassessment of the indication for reimplantation is recommended after resolution of infection.[89]

In patients with ICD for primary prevention, receiving a shock for any arrhythmia has been shown to be associated with worse prognosis.[90] Beyond appropriate shocks, inappropriate shocks might also occur, representing a further complication associated with ICD. In a contemporary population of patients with ICD, the rate of inappropriate shocks over a follow-up period of 46.6 months was 6%.[91] Inappropriate therapy was more common in patients with atrial fibrillation and less common among patients aged ≥65 years.[92] The risk of inappropriate shocks does not differ between dual-chamber and single-chamber devices.[93] In the MADIT-CRT trial, use of carvedilol has been associated with a 50% lower risk of inappropriate therapy due to atrial fibrillation, compared to metoprolol.[94] In the MADIT-RIT trial, programming of ICD therapies for tachyarrhythmias of 200 bpm or faster or with a prolonged delay in therapy at 170 bpm or faster reduced the risk of a first inappropriate ATP or shock by 79%, as compared to conventional programming (with a 2.5-s delay at 170–199 bpm and a 1.0-s delay at ≥200 bpm).[95] In the ADVANCE III trial, a long detection interval (30 of 40 intervals), compared to a standard detection interval (18 of 24 intervals), reduced the incidence of inappropriate ATP and shocks by 37%.[96] Repeated shocks, even if appropriate, carry the risk of affecting the psychological well-being of patients. However, it has been shown that the association between receipt of shocks and psychological distress is mediated in >50% of cases by high ICD-related concerns.[97]

In HFrEF patients in need of pacing for atrioventricular block, high percentages of right ventricular apical pacing through an

ICD might worsen left ventricular systolic dysfunction. In this setting, biventricular pacing with a CRT-D is the best therapeutic option. This is supported by trial evidence, as well as by current 2021 ESC Guidelines on HF which provide a Class IIa, Level of evidence B recommendation for an upgrade to CRT for those patients with an EF of ≤35% who received a conventional pacemaker or an ICD and subsequently developed worsening HF despite optimal medical therapy and who have a significant proportion of right ventricular pacing.[52,98]

Follow-up and remote monitoring

ICD requires follow-up interrogation on a regular basis. After a first in-person visit, usually within 3 months after implantation, long-term follow-up is conducted, with at least one in-person visit per year when remote monitoring is available.[99] The instructions for performing remote monitoring should be explained at the time of implantation. Common parameters that should be assessed during an ICD interrogation are the longevity of the battery which is estimated according to the measured voltage, detection of tachycardias and bradycardic events, pacing thresholds, and both sensing and capture algorithms. An in-person clinical visit is important to check the status of the pocket and to assess for potential infections. Evidence on remote monitoring comes from several randomized controlled trials. In a patient-level data meta-analysis of the IN-TIME, ECOST, and TRUST trials, home/remote monitoring with daily verification of transmission was associated with a 38% risk reduction of all-cause death at 1 year and also with reduced risk of all-cause mortality or HF hospitalization, compared to conventional follow-up, suggesting that remote monitoring could contribute to preventing HF exacerbation.[100]

Subcutaneous implantable cardioverter–defibrillator

Selected populations that might not require pacing, CRT, or ATP (i.e. patients needing an ICD for primary prevention of SCD) might be candidates for an S-ICD. The generator is usually implanted in the left lateral region of the thorax and the lead is tunnelled towards the parasternal region. S-ICDs avoid complications associated with implantation of transvenous ICDs, for example, pneumothorax, endocarditis and system infections, tamponade, tricuspid regurgitation. S-ICDs might also be an option for patients who previously underwent explantation of a transvenous ICD. Observational studies suggest similar shock efficacy and short-term complications with both S-ICDs and transvenous ICDs.[101] In the PRAETORIAN trial which randomized 849 patients with an indication for an ICD, but none for pacing, over a median follow-up period of 49 months, non-inferiority for S-ICD versus transvenous ICD was shown, with similar rates of complications and inappropriate shocks,[102] as well as no difference in shock efficacy.[103] In a cohort study assessing the long-term clinical outcomes of S-ICDs versus transvenous ICDs, S-ICDs were associated with lower lead complications (i.e. requiring replacement or repositioning of the lead without elective pulse generator replacement), but higher non-lead complications (pocket erosion, defibrillation threshold testing failure, and device failure).[104]

Future perspectives

A reduction in the risk of SCD over time, together with the findings of the DANISH trial downgrading the role of ICDs for primary prevention of SCD in non-ischaemic HF, has questioned the one-fits-all approach to prophylactic use of ICD in HFrEF. Future research might aim to optimize patient selection for ICD and for CRT-P versus CRT-D, by identifying those phenotypes at higher risk of SCD, and therefore more likely to benefit from this intervention.

Summary and key messages

- HFrEF carries a high risk of SCD, which has decreased over time following the introduction of new pharmacological therapies and CRT.
- Randomized controlled trials showed that ICDs reduce mortality in HFrEF, both as a primary and a secondary prevention intervention.
- The DANISH trial questioned the efficacy of ICDs in patients with non-ischaemic HFrEF by reporting neutral results on all-cause mortality.
- There is debatable evidence on ICD efficacy in younger versus older patients, males versus females, and patients with versus those without diabetes.
- Parameters other than EF, e.g. quantification of myocardial fibrosis and scar size, might better identify patients with a higher risk of SCD, and therefore improve patient selection for primary prevention ICD.
- Better patient selection for ICD and for CRT-P versus CRT-D is needed, which might lead to better implementation of the use of these treatments in clinical practice.
- S-ICD might be a valid therapeutic option for selected populations that might not require pacing, CRT, or ATP (i.e. patients needing an ICD for primary prevention of SCD).

References

1. DiMarco JP. Implantable cardioverter–defibrillators. N Engl J Med. 2003;349(19):1836–47.
2. Raatikainen MJP, Arnar DO, Merkely B, et al. A decade of information on the use of cardiac implantable electronic devices and interventional electrophysiological procedures in the European Society of Cardiology countries: 2017 report from the European Heart Rhythm Association. Europace. 2017;19(suppl 2):ii1–90.
3. Priori SG, Blomstrom-Lundqvist C, Mazzanti A, et al. 2015 ESC Guidelines for the management of patients with ventricular arrhythmias and the prevention of sudden cardiac death: the Task Force for the Management of Patients with Ventricular Arrhythmias and the Prevention of Sudden Cardiac Death of the European Society of Cardiology (ESC). Endorsed by: Association for European Paediatric and Congenital Cardiology (AEPC). Eur Heart J. 2015;36(41):2793–867.
4. Shen L, Jhund PS, Petrie MC, et al. Declining risk of sudden death in heart failure. N Engl J Med. 2017;377(1):41–51.

5. Narins CR, Aktas MK, Chen AY, et al. Arrhythmic and mortality outcomes among ischemic versus nonischemic cardiomyopathy patients receiving primary implantable cardioverter–defibrillator therapy. JACC Clin Electrophysiol. 2022;8(1):1–11.

6. Packer M. Major reduction in the risk of sudden cardiac death in patients with chronic heart failure with the use of drug and device combinations that favourably affect left ventricular structure. Eur J Heart Fail. 2019;21(7):823–6.

7. Al-Gobari M, El Khatib C, Pillon F, Gueyffier F. Beta-blockers for the prevention of sudden cardiac death in heart failure patients: a meta-analysis of randomized controlled trials. BMC Cardiovasc Disord. 2013;13:52.

8. Bapoje SR, Bahia A, Hokanson JE, et al. Effects of mineralocorticoid receptor antagonists on the risk of sudden cardiac death in patients with left ventricular systolic dysfunction: a meta-analysis of randomized controlled trials. Circ Heart Fail. 2013;6(2):166–73.

9. Cleland JG, Erhardt L, Murray G, Hall AS, Ball SG. Effect of ramipril on morbidity and mode of death among survivors of acute myocardial infarction with clinical evidence of heart failure. A report from the AIRE Study Investigators. Eur Heart J. 1997;18(1):41–51.

10. Garg R, Yusuf S. Overview of randomized trials of angiotensin-converting enzyme inhibitors on mortality and morbidity in patients with heart failure. Collaborative Group on ACE Inhibitor Trials. JAMA. 1995;273(18):1450–6.

11. Solomon SD, Wang D, Finn P, et al. Effect of candesartan on cause-specific mortality in heart failure patients: the Candesartan in Heart failure Assessment of Reduction in Mortality and morbidity (CHARM) program. Circulation. 2004;110(15):2180–3.

12. Desai AS, McMurray JJ, Packer M, et al. Effect of the angiotensin-receptor–neprilysin inhibitor LCZ696 compared with enalapril on mode of death in heart failure patients. Eur Heart J. 2015;36(30):1990–7.

13. Felker GM, Butler J, Ibrahim NE, et al. Implantable cardioverter-defibrillator eligibility after initiation of sacubitril/valsartan in chronic heart failure: insights from PROVE-HF. Circulation. 2021;144(2):180–2.

14. Curtain JP, Docherty KF, Jhund PS, et al. Effect of dapagliflozin on ventricular arrhythmias, resuscitated cardiac arrest, or sudden death in DAPA-HF. Eur Heart J. 2021;42(36):3727–38.

15. Barra S, Providencia R, Narayanan K, et al. Time trends in sudden cardiac death risk in heart failure patients with cardiac resynchronization therapy: a systematic review. Eur Heart J. 2020;41(21):1976–86.

16. Aiba T, Tomaselli G. Electrical remodeling in dyssynchrony and resynchronization. J Cardiovasc Transl Res. 2012;5(2):170–9.

17. Yuyun MF, Erqou SA, Peralta AO, et al. Risk of ventricular arrhythmia in cardiac resynchronization therapy responders and super-responders: a systematic review and meta-analysis. Europace. 2021;23(8):1262–74.

18. Deif B, Ballantyne B, Almehmadi F, et al. Cardiac resynchronization is pro-arrhythmic in the absence of reverse ventricular remodelling: a systematic review and meta-analysis. Cardiovasc Res. 2018;114(11):1435–44.

19. Vaduganathan M, Patel RB, Michel A, et al. Mode of death in heart failure with preserved ejection fraction. J Am Coll Cardiol. 2017;69(5):556–69.

20. Vaduganathan M, Claggett BL, Chatterjee NA, et al. Sudden death in heart failure with preserved ejection fraction: a competing risks analysis from the TOPCAT trial. JACC Heart Fail. 2018;6(8):653–61.

21. Zile MR, Gaasch WH, Anand IS, et al. Mode of death in patients with heart failure and a preserved ejection fraction: results from the Irbesartan in Heart Failure With Preserved Ejection Fraction Study (I-Preserve) trial. Circulation. 2010;121(12):1393–405.

22. Desai AS, Vaduganathan M, Cleland JG, et al. Mode of death in patients with heart failure and preserved ejection fraction: insights from PARAGON-HF trial. Circ Heart Fail. 2021;14(12):e008597.

23. Iles L, Pfluger H, Lefkovits L, et al. Myocardial fibrosis predicts appropriate device therapy in patients with implantable cardioverter-defibrillators for primary prevention of sudden cardiac death. J Am Coll Cardiol. 2011;57(7):821–8.

24. Alvarez CK, Cronin E, Baker WL, Kluger J. Heart failure as a substrate and trigger for ventricular tachycardia. J Interv Card Electrophysiol. 2019;56(3):229–47.

25. Zabel M, Portnoy S, Franz MR. Effect of sustained load on dispersion of ventricular repolarization and conduction time in the isolated intact rabbit heart. J Cardiovasc Electrophysiol. 1996;7(1):9–16.

26. Franz MR, Cima R, Wang D, Profitt D, Kurz R. Electrophysiological effects of myocardial stretch and mechanical determinants of stretch-activated arrhythmias. Circulation. 1992;86(3):968–78.

27. Fallavollita JA, Heavey BM, Luisi AJ Jr, et al. Regional myocardial sympathetic denervation predicts the risk of sudden cardiac arrest in ischemic cardiomyopathy. J Am Coll Cardiol. 2014;63(2):141–9.

28. Cao JM, Fishbein MC, Han JB, et al. Relationship between regional cardiac hyperinnervation and ventricular arrhythmia. Circulation. 2000;101(16):1960–9.

29. Dai DZ, Dai Y. Induced ion currents and the endothelin pathway as targets for anti-arrhythmic agents. Curr Opin Investig Drugs. 2008;9(9):1001–8.

30. Poelzing S, Rosenbaum DS. Altered connexin43 expression produces arrhythmia substrate in heart failure. Am J Physiol Heart Circ Physiol. 2004;287(4):H1762–70.

31. Jiang N, Zhou A, Imran H, et al. Cardiac resynchronization and circulating markers of sarcoplasmic reticulum calcium handling and sudden death risk. JACC Clin Electrophysiol. 2021;7(9):1079–83.

32. Manolis AS, Manolis AA, Manolis TA, Melita H. Sudden death in heart failure with preserved ejection fraction and beyond: an elusive target. Heart Fail Rev. 2019;24(6):847–66.

33. Moss AJ, Hall WJ, Cannom DS, et al. Improved survival with an implanted defibrillator in patients with coronary disease at high risk for ventricular arrhythmia. Multicenter Automatic Defibrillator Implantation Trial Investigators. N Engl J Med. 1996;335(26):1933–40.

34. Buxton AE, Lee KL, Fisher JD, Josephson ME, Prystowsky EN, Hafley G. A randomized study of the prevention of sudden death in patients with coronary artery disease. Multicenter Unsustained Tachycardia Trial Investigators. N Engl J Med. 1999;341(25):1882–90.

35. Moss AJ, Zareba W, Hall WJ, et al. Prophylactic implantation of a defibrillator in patients with myocardial infarction and reduced ejection fraction. N Engl J Med. 2002;346(12):877–83.

36. Kadish A, Dyer A, Daubert JP, et al. Prophylactic defibrillator implantation in patients with nonischemic dilated cardiomyopathy. N Engl J Med. 2004;350(21):2151–8.

37. Bardy GH, Lee KL, Mark DB, et al. Amiodarone or an implantable cardioverter–defibrillator for congestive heart failure. N Engl J Med. 2005;352(3):225–37.

38. Poole JE, Olshansky B, Mark DB, et al. Long-term outcomes of implantable cardioverter–defibrillator therapy in the SCD-HeFT. J Am Coll Cardiol. 2020;76(4):405–15.

39. Bristow MR, Saxon LA, Boehmer J, et al. Cardiac-resynchronization therapy with or without an implantable defibrillator in advanced chronic heart failure. N Engl J Med. 2004;350(21):2140–50.

40. Gold MR, Daubert JC, Abraham WT, et al. Implantable defibrillators improve survival in patients with mildly symptomatic heart failure receiving cardiac resynchronization therapy: analysis of the long-term follow-up of remodeling in systolic left ventricular dysfunction (REVERSE). Circ Arrhythm Electrophysiol. 2013;6(6):1163–8.

41. Kober L, Thune JJ, Nielsen JC, *et al*. Defibrillator implantation in patients with nonischemic systolic heart failure. N Engl J Med. 2016;375(13):1221–30.

42. Bundgaard JS, Thune JJ, Nielsen JC, *et al*. The impact of implantable cardioverter–defibrillator implantation on health-related quality of life in the DANISH trial. Europace. 2019;21(6):900–8.

43. Kristensen SL, Levy WC, Shadman R, *et al*. Risk models for prediction of implantable cardioverter–defibrillator benefit: insights from the DANISH trial. JACC Heart Fail. 2019;7(8):717–24.

44. Shun-Shin MJ, Zheng SL, Cole GD, Howard JP, Whinnett ZI, Francis DP. Implantable cardioverter defibrillators for primary prevention of death in left ventricular dysfunction with and without ischaemic heart disease: a meta-analysis of 8567 patients in the 11 trials. Eur Heart J. 2017;38(22):1738–46.

45. Rohde LE, Chatterjee NA, Vaduganathan M, *et al*. Sacubitril/valsartan and sudden cardiac death according to implantable cardioverter–defibrillator use and heart failure cause: a PARADIGM-HF analysis. JACC Heart Fail. 2020;8(10):844–55.

46. Schrage B, Uijl A, Benson L, *et al*. Association between use of primary-prevention implantable cardioverter–defibrillators and mortality in patients with heart failure: a prospective propensity score-matched analysis from the Swedish Heart Failure Registry. Circulation. 2019;140(19):1530–9.

47. Schrage B, Lund LH, Melin M, *et al*. Cardiac resynchronization therapy with or without defibrillator in patients with heart failure. Europace. 2022;24(1):48–57.

48. Zabel M, Willems R, Lubinski A, *et al*. Clinical effectiveness of primary prevention implantable cardioverter–defibrillators: results of the EU-CERT-ICD controlled multicentre cohort study. Eur Heart J. 2020;41(36):3437–47.

49. Steinbeck G, Andresen D, Seidl K, *et al*. Defibrillator implantation early after myocardial infarction. N Engl J Med. 2009;361(15):1427–36.

50. Hohnloser SH, Kuck KH, Dorian P, *et al*. Prophylactic use of an implantable cardioverter–defibrillator after acute myocardial infarction. N Engl J Med. 2004;351(24):2481–8.

51. Bigger JT Jr. Prophylactic use of implanted cardiac defibrillators in patients at high risk for ventricular arrhythmias after coronary-artery bypass graft surgery. Coronary Artery Bypass Graft (CABG) Patch Trial Investigators. N Engl J Med. 1997;337(22):1569–75.

52. McDonagh TA, Metra M, Adamo M, *et al*. 2021 ESC Guidelines for the diagnosis and treatment of acute and chronic heart failure. Eur Heart J. 2021;42(36):3599–726.

53. Al-Khatib SM, Stevenson WG, Ackerman MJ, *et al*. 2017 AHA/ACC/HRS Guideline for management of patients with ventricular arrhythmias and the prevention of sudden cardiac death: executive summary: a report of the American College of Cardiology/American Heart Association Task Force on Clinical Practice Guidelines and the Heart Rhythm Society. J Am Coll Cardiol. 2018;72(14):1677–749.

54. Adabag S, Patton KK, Buxton AE, *et al*. Association of implantable cardioverter defibrillators with survival in patients with and without improved ejection fraction: secondary analysis of the Sudden Cardiac Death in Heart Failure Trial. JAMA Cardiol. 2017;2(7):767–74.

55. Adabag S, Patton KK, Buxton AE, *et al*. Association of implantable cardioverter defibrillators with survival in patients with and without improved ejection fraction: secondary analysis of the Sudden Cardiac Death in Heart Failure Trial. JAMA Cardiol. 2017;2(7):767–74.

56. Kutyifa V, Beck C, Brown MW, *et al*. Multicenter Automatic Defibrillator Implantation Trial-Subcutaneous Implantable Cardioverter Defibrillator (MADIT S-ICD): design and clinical protocol. Am Heart J. 2017;189:158–66.

57. Saba S, Adelstein E, Wold N, Stein K, Jones P. Influence of patients' age at implantation on mortality and defibrillator shocks. Europace. 2017;19(5):802–7.

58. Elming MB, Nielsen JC, Haarbo J, *et al*. Age and outcomes of primary prevention implantable cardioverter–defibrillators in patients with nonischemic systolic heart failure. Circulation. 2017;136(19):1772–80.

59. Sticherling C, Arendacka B, Svendsen JH, *et al*. Sex differences in outcomes of primary prevention implantable cardioverter–defibrillator therapy: combined registry data from eleven European countries. Europace. 2018;20(6):963–70.

60. Ghanbari H, Dalloul G, Hasan R, *et al*. Effectiveness of implantable cardioverter–defibrillators for the primary prevention of sudden cardiac death in women with advanced heart failure: a meta-analysis of randomized controlled trials. Arch Intern Med. 2009;169(16):1500–6.

61. Sharma A, Al-Khatib SM, Ezekowitz JA, *et al*. Implantable cardioverter–defibrillators in heart failure patients with reduced ejection fraction and diabetes. Eur J Heart Fail. 2018;20(6):1031–8.

62. Junttila MJ, Pelli A, Kentta TV, *et al*. Appropriate shocks and mortality in patients with versus without diabetes with prophylactic implantable cardioverter defibrillators. Diabetes Care. 2020;43(1):196–200.

63. Steinberg BA, Al-Khatib SM, Edwards R, *et al*. Outcomes of implantable cardioverter–defibrillator use in patients with comorbidities: results from a combined analysis of 4 randomized clinical trials. JACC Heart Fail. 2014;2(6):623–9.

64. Shadman R, Poole JE, Dardas TF, *et al*. A novel method to predict the proportional risk of sudden cardiac death in heart failure: derivation of the Seattle Proportional Risk Model. Heart Rhythm. 2015;12(10):2069–77.

65. Levy WC, Mozaffarian D, Linker DT, *et al*. The Seattle Heart Failure Model: prediction of survival in heart failure. Circulation. 2006;113(11):1424–33.

66. Bilchick KC, Wang Y, Cheng A, *et al*. Seattle Heart Failure and Proportional Risk Models predict benefit from implantable cardioverter–defibrillators. J Am Coll Cardiol. 2017;69(21):2606–18.

67. de Sousa MR, Morillo CA, Rabelo FT, Nogueira Filho AM, Ribeiro AL. Non-sustained ventricular tachycardia as a predictor of sudden cardiac death in patients with left ventricular dysfunction: a meta-analysis. Eur J Heart Fail. 2008;10(10):1007–14.

68. Di Marco A, Anguera I, Schmitt M, *et al*. Late gadolinium enhancement and the risk for ventricular arrhythmias or sudden death in dilated cardiomyopathy: systematic review and meta-analysis. JACC Heart Fail. 2017;5(1):28–38.

69. Gao P, Yee R, Gula L, *et al*. Prediction of arrhythmic events in ischemic and dilated cardiomyopathy patients referred for implantable cardiac defibrillator: evaluation of multiple scar quantification measures for late gadolinium enhancement magnetic resonance imaging. Circ Cardiovasc Imaging. 2012;5(4):448–56.

70. Klem I, Klein M, Khan M, *et al*. Relationship of LVEF and myocardial scar to long-term mortality risk and mode of death in patients with nonischemic cardiomyopathy. Circulation. 2021;143(14):1343–58.

71. Zegard A, Okafor O, de Bono J, *et al*. Myocardial fibrosis as a predictor of sudden death in patients with coronary artery disease. J Am Coll Cardiol. 2021;77(1):29–41.

72. Muser D, Nucifora G, Muser D, *et al*. Prognostic value of nonischemic ringlike left ventricular scar in patients with apparently idiopathic nonsustained ventricular arrhythmias. Circulation. 2021;143(14):1359–73.

73. Guaricci AI, Masci PG, Muscogiuri G, *et al*. CarDiac magnEtic Resonance for prophylactic Implantable-cardioVerter defibrillAtor ThErapy in Non-Ischaemic dilated CardioMyopathy: an international Registry. Europace. 2021;23(7):1072–83.

74. Adabag S, Rector TS, Anand IS, *et al*. A prediction model for sudden cardiac death in patients with heart failure and preserved ejection fraction. Eur J Heart Fail. 2014;16(11):1175–82.

75. Antiarrhythmics versus Implantable Defibrillators (AVID) Investigators. A comparison of antiarrhythmic-drug therapy with implantable defibrillators in patients resuscitated from near-fatal ventricular arrhythmias. N Engl J Med. 1997;337(22):1576–83.

76. Connolly SJ, Gent M, Roberts RS, et al. Canadian implantable defibrillator study (CIDS): a randomized trial of the implantable cardioverter defibrillator against amiodarone. Circulation. 2000;101(11):1297–302.

77. Kuck KH, Cappato R, Siebels J, Ruppel R. Randomized comparison of antiarrhythmic drug therapy with implantable defibrillators in patients resuscitated from cardiac arrest: the Cardiac Arrest Study Hamburg (CASH). Circulation. 2000;102(7):748–54.

78. Connolly SJ, Hallstrom AP, Cappato R, et al. Meta-analysis of the implantable cardioverter defibrillator secondary prevention trials. AVID, CASH and CIDS studies. Antiarrhythmics vs Implantable Defibrillator study. Cardiac Arrest Study Hamburg. Canadian Implantable Defibrillator Study. Eur Heart J. 2000;21(24):2071–8.

79. Freeman JV, Wang Y, Curtis JP, Heidenreich PA, Hlatky MA. The relation between hospital procedure volume and complications of cardioverter–defibrillator implantation from the implantable cardioverter–defibrillator registry. J Am Coll Cardiol. 2010;56(14):1133–9.

80. Van Rees JB, de Bie MK, Thijssen J, Borleffs CJ, Schalij MJ, van Erven L. Implantation-related complications of implantable cardioverter–defibrillators and cardiac resynchronization therapy devices: a systematic review of randomized clinical trials. J Am Coll Cardiol. 2011;58(10):995–1000.

81. Reynolds MR, Cohen DJ, Kugelmass AD, et al. The frequency and incremental cost of major complications among Medicare beneficiaries receiving implantable cardioverter–defibrillators. J Am Coll Cardiol. 2006;47(12):2493–7.

82. Ezzat VA, Lee V, Ahsan S, et al. A systematic review of ICD complications in randomised controlled trials versus registries: is our 'real-world' data an underestimation? Open Heart. 2015;2(1):e000198.

83. Ranasinghe I, Parzynski CS, Freeman JV, et al. Long-term risk for device-related complications and reoperations after implantable cardioverter–defibrillator implantation: an observational cohort study. Ann Intern Med. 2016;165(1):20–9.

84. Koneru JN, Jones PW, Hammill EF, Wold N, Ellenbogen KA. Risk factors and temporal trends of complications associated with transvenous implantable cardiac defibrillator leads. J Am Heart Assoc. 2018;7(10):e007691.

85. Prutkin JM, Reynolds MR, Bao H, et al. Rates of and factors associated with infection in 200 909 Medicare implantable cardioverter–defibrillator implants: results from the National Cardiovascular Data Registry. Circulation. 2014;130(13):1037–43.

86. Polyzos KA, Konstantelias AA, Falagas ME. Risk factors for cardiac implantable electronic device infection: a systematic review and meta-analysis. Europace. 2015;17(5):767–77.

87. Ozcan C, Raunso J, Lamberts M, et al. Infective endocarditis and risk of death after cardiac implantable electronic device implantation: a nationwide cohort study. Europace. 2017;19(6):1007–14.

88. Klug D, Balde M, Pavin D, et al. Risk factors related to infections of implanted pacemakers and cardioverter–defibrillators: results of a large prospective study. Circulation. 2007;116(12):1349–55.

89. Blomstrom-Lundqvist C, Traykov V, Erba PA, et al. European Heart Rhythm Association (EHRA) international consensus document on how to prevent, diagnose, and treat cardiac implantable electronic device infections—endorsed by the Heart Rhythm Society (HRS), the Asia Pacific Heart Rhythm Society (APHRS), the Latin American Heart Rhythm Society (LAHRS), International Society for Cardiovascular Infectious Diseases (ISCVID), and the European Society of Clinical Microbiology and Infectious Diseases (ESCMID) in collaboration with the European Association for Cardio-Thoracic Surgery (EACTS). Eur Heart J. 2020;41(21):2012–32.

90. Poole JE, Johnson GW, Hellkamp AS, et al. Prognostic importance of defibrillator shocks in patients with heart failure. N Engl J Med. 2008;359(10):1009–17.

91. Briongos-Figuero S, Garcia-Alberola A, Rubio J, et al. Long-term outcomes among a nationwide cohort of patients using an implantable cardioverter–defibrillator: UMBRELLA study final results. J Am Heart Assoc. 2021;10(1):e018108.

92. Greenlee RT, Go AS, Peterson PN, et al. Device therapies among patients receiving primary prevention implantable cardioverter–defibrillators in the Cardiovascular Research Network. J Am Heart Assoc. 2018;7(7):e008292.

93. Peterson PN, Greenlee RT, Go AS, et al. Comparison of inappropriate shocks and other health outcomes between single- and dual-chamber implantable cardioverter–defibrillators for primary prevention of sudden cardiac death: results from the Cardiovascular Research Network longitudinal study of implantable cardioverter–defibrillators. J Am Heart Assoc. 2017;6(11):e006937.

94. Ruwald MH, Abu-Zeitone A, Jons C, et al. Impact of carvedilol and metoprolol on inappropriate implantable cardioverter–defibrillator therapy: the MADIT-CRT trial (Multicenter Automatic Defibrillator Implantation With Cardiac Resynchronization Therapy). J Am Coll Cardiol. 2013;62(15):1343–50.

95. Moss AJ, Schuger C, Beck CA, et al. Reduction in inappropriate therapy and mortality through ICD programming. N Engl J Med. 2012;367(24):2275–83.

96. Gasparini M, Proclemer A, Klersy C, et al. Effect of long-detection interval vs standard-detection interval for implantable cardioverter–defibrillators on antitachycardia pacing and shock delivery: the ADVANCE III randomized clinical trial. JAMA. 2013;309(18):1903–11.

97. Thylen I, Moser DK, Stromberg A, Dekker RA, Chung ML. Concerns about implantable cardioverter–defibrillator shocks mediate the relationship between actual shocks and psychological distress. Europace. 2016;18(6):828–35.

98. Curtis AB, Worley SJ, Adamson PB, et al. Biventricular pacing for atrioventricular block and systolic dysfunction. N Engl J Med. 2013;368(17):1585–93.

99. Slotwiner D, Varma N, Akar JG, et al. HRS Expert Consensus Statement on remote interrogation and monitoring for cardiovascular implantable electronic devices. Heart Rhythm. 2015;12(7):e69–100.

100. Hindricks G, Varma N, Kacet S, et al. Daily remote monitoring of implantable cardioverter–defibrillators: insights from the pooled patient-level data from three randomized controlled trials (INTIME, ECOST, TRUST). Eur Heart J. 2017;38(22):1749–55.

101. Chue CD, Kwok CS, Wong CW, et al. Efficacy and safety of the subcutaneous implantable cardioverter defibrillator: a systematic review. Heart. 2017;103(17):1315–22.

102. Knops RE, Olde Nordkamp LRA, Delnoy PHM, et al. Subcutaneous or transvenous defibrillator therapy. N Engl J Med. 2020;383(6):526–36.

103. Knops RE, van der Stuijt W, Delnoy P, et al. Efficacy and safety of appropriate shocks and antitachycardia pacing in transvenous and subcutaneous implantable defibrillators: an analysis of all appropriate therapy in the PRAETORIAN trial. Circulation. 2022;146(4):e10–11.

104. Brouwer TF, Yilmaz D, Lindeboom R, et al. Long-term clinical outcomes of subcutaneous versus transvenous implantable defibrillator therapy. J Am Coll Cardiol. 2016;68(19):2047–55.

CHAPTER 9.2

Cardiac resynchronization therapy for heart failure

Pieter Martens, Eva Goncalvesova, and Wilfried Mullens

Contents

Introduction

Cardiac resynchronization therapy (CRT) is one of the most successful therapies for patients with heart failure and reduced ejection fraction (HFrEF), demonstrating improvements in quality of life and reduction in heart failure hospitalization, as well as in all-cause mortality. Despite its well-acknowledged clinical benefits and cost-effectiveness, it remains a widely underused treatment option, with only one in three guideline-recommended patients actually receiving a CRT device, underscoring the importance of continued medical education on this topic outside of the field of electrophysiology (◓ Figure 9.2.1). This chapter focuses on the mechanism of action of CRT and trial evidence that has led to current guideline indications, and discusses preimplant and post-implant patient characteristics and decision-making related to CRT relevant to the heart failure specialist.

Mechanisms underlying the benefits of cardiac resynchronization therapy

Contraction of the left ventricle (LV) is neatly coordinated by electrical conduction through the His–Purkinje system, resulting in homogeneous left ventricular (LV) excitation and synchronous muscle fibre shortening, and thereby in an optimized LV contraction pattern with maximized pump efficiency. The presence of conduction abnormalities in heart failure results in marked regional heterogeneity in muscle fibre shortening, further compromising an already impaired LV function.[1] The earlier-contracting segments (typically LV septum) waste part of their regional work through pre-stretching of the quiescent opposing wall, which only contracts during late systole. Additionally, the later-contracting segments are exposed to a higher regional load instigated by the early-contracting zones.[2] In an attempt to overcome regional wall stress, the LV progressively dilates and remodels. The deleterious effects of this dyssynchronous activation are not limited to the macroscopic level, characterized by the typically spherical, dyssynchronous LV with significant mitral regurgitation. At a molecular level, alterations in ion channel signalling, calcium handling, β-adrenergic signalling, myofilament function, redox balance, mitochondrial function, cardiac metabolism, and bioenergetics also occur. Furthermore, altered electromechanical synchronicity during systole also affects mechanical synchronicity during diastole and comprises efficient atrioventricular (AV) coupling.

CRT has the ability to target all the aforementioned pathophysiological alterations. CRT both acutely and chronically improves cardiac function but also efficiently targets a plethora of cellular maladaptations (◓ Figure 9.2.2). Acute invasive haemodynamic studies indicate that CRT harmonizes regional work, resulting in a left and

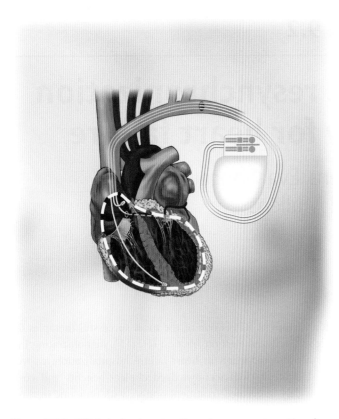

Figure 9.2.1 CRT device implantation. The pulse generator is positioned subcutaneously on the fascia of the pectoralis major muscle. Three leads connect the generator with the right atrium, right ventricle, and left ventricle via the coronary sinus. In the case of CRT-D, the right ventricular lead contains shock coils and pacing electrodes.

upward shift of the end-systolic pressure–volume relation (⮕ Figure 9.2.2a). Importantly, this is achieved without increased myocardial oxygen consumption and sympathetic nerve activity. Furthermore, AV filling is improved and functional mitral regurgitation is diminished, both beneficially reducing pulmonary capillary wedge pressure. More chronically, CRT induces cardiac reverse remodelling (⮕ Figure 9.2.2b), also targeting exercise-related mitral regurgitation, left atrial morphology and function, pulmonary vascular function, right ventricular-to-pulmonary-artery coupling, and ventricular interdependence.[3,4] Interestingly, at a molecular level, these alterations are associated with *contractile remodelling* due to improvement in calcium cycling, intrinsic myofilament force, and sensitivity to calcium and increased beta-adrenergic responsiveness (⮕ Figure 9.2.2c). This enhanced contractility is met by *energetic remodelling*, with improved mitochondrial respiration and adenosine triphosphate (ATP) production, as well as restoration of the metabolic fingerprint. Simultaneously, CRT results in *structural remodelling*, reducing mediators of cellular fibrosis and improving cellular survival by decreasing pro-apoptotic mediators. Finally, CRT results in *electrical remodelling*, improving repolarizing potassium currents and reducing late sodium leakage, which partially explain the antiarrhythmic effects with CRT observed in randomized controlled trials (RCTs).

Evidence for cardiac resynchronization therapy

CRT improves cardiac function and heart failure symptoms and reduces mortality and morbidity in a cost-efficient manner. Numerous trials have established the effects of CRT (⮕ Table 9.2.1). Most evidence for the beneficial effect of CRT lies with HFrEF patients who are symptomatic (New York Heart Association (NYHA) ≥ class II), are in sinus rhythm, and have a left bundle branch block (LBBB) morphology. ⮕ Table 9.2.2 gives an overview of the latest 2021 European Society of Cardiology (ESC) Guidelines for the selection of CRT.[5]

Symptoms

Most evidence for CRT is available for patients who have symptomatic (NYHA ≥ class II) HFrEF. Nevertheless, the Multicenter Automatic Defibrillator Implantation with Cardiac Resynchronization Therapy (MADIT-CRT) trial did include 265 patients (7.8%) functioning in NYHA class I. These patients showed a non-significant (hazard ratio (HR) 0.66, 95% confidence interval (CI) 0.30–1.42; $P = 0.29$) trend towards lower all-cause death. Therefore, guidelines recommend CRT only in patients who are symptomatic (NYHA ≥ class II).

QRS morphology

A large meta-analysis of 33 trials investigating the effect of QRS morphology on the treatment effect of CRT illustrated that patients with an LBBB morphology had a 36% risk reduction in a composite of adverse clinical outcome, whereas such strong effect is less observed in patients with a non-LBBB morphology.[6] Indeed, with a broader QRS width (>150 ms) or after longer follow-up, benefits are also seen in patients with non-LBBB morphology. As a result, guidelines give the strongest evidence for patients with an LBBB morphology. Patients with right bundle branch block (RBBB) do not benefit from CRT, unless they show a so-called masked LBBB on the electrocardiogram (ECG), characterized by a broad, slurred, sometimes notched R-wave on leads I and aVL, together with a left axis deviation.

Baseline left ventricular ejection fraction

Most trials included patients with a baseline left ventricular ejection fraction (LVEF) below 35% (or 30%; ⮕ Table 9.2.1). However, the REsynchronization reVErses Remodeling in Systolic left vEntricular dysfunction (REVERSE) trial enrolled patients with an LVEF of up to 40%. Furthermore, an echo-core laboratory analysis of the MADIT-CRT trial indicated that 38% of patients actually had an LVEF above the entry criteria cut-off, with LVEF of up to 45%.[7] These patients actually had similar benefits in terms of death and heart failure hospitalization, and might actually demonstrate a greater degree of reverse remodelling.

Optimal medical therapy

CRT has been tested in HFrEF patients with residual symptoms and a persistently reduced LVEF despite optimal background treatment with neurohormonal blockers. However, observational studies indicated that patients with an indication for CRT with

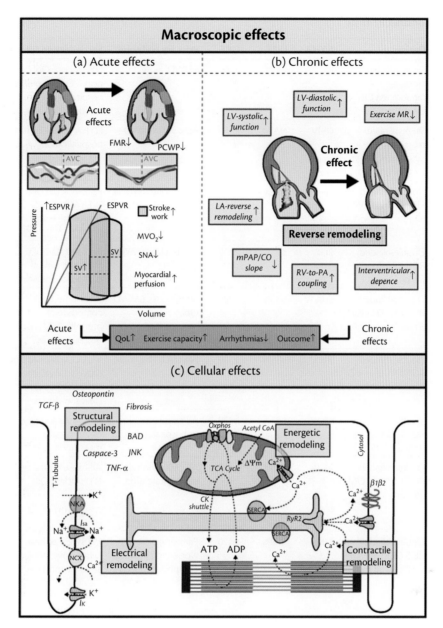

Figure 9.2.2 Mechanisms of CRT action. Panel (a) illustrates the acute effects of CRT. Panel (b) depicts the chronic effects of CRT. Panel (c) shows the cellular effects of CRT. AVC, aortic valve closure; BAD, BCL2-associated agonist of cell death proteins; CK, creatinine kinase; CO, cardiac output; ESPVR, end-systolic pressure volume relation; FMR, functional mitral regurgitation; JNK, c-Jun N-terminal kinase; LA, left atrium; LV, left ventricle; mPAP, mean pulmonary artery pressure; MR, mitral regurgitation; MVO_2, myocardial oxygen consumption; OXPHOS, mitochondrial oxidative phosphorylation system; PA, pulmonary artery; PCWP, pulmonary capillary wedge pressure; QoL, quality of life; RV, right ventricle; SNA, sympathetic nerve activity; SV, stroke volume; TCA, tricarboxylic acid cycle; TNF-α, tumour necrosis factor alpha; $\Delta\Psi_m$, inner mitochondrial membrane potential.

Reproduced from Mullens W, Auricchio A, Martens P, et al. Optimized implementation of cardiac resynchronization therapy: a call for action for referral and optimization of care: A joint position statement from the Heart Failure Association (HFA), European Heart Rhythm Association (EHRA), and European Association of Cardiovascular Imaging (EACVI) of the European Society of Cardiology. Eur J Heart Fail. 2020 Dec;22(12):2349–2369. doi: 10.1002/ejhf.2046 with permission from John Wiley and Sons https://creativecommons.org/licenses/by-nc/4.0/.

electromechanical dyssynchrony seemed to respond less, in terms of reverse remodelling, to the beneficial effects of neurohormonal blockers.[8,9] Indeed, patients with LBBB only experienced 2% LVEF improvement, compared to 8% in patients with a narrow QRS, after 6 months of medical therapy. Additionally, LVEF improvement seems to be less in patients in whom CRT was postponed for longer. Molecular analysis indicates that electromechanical dyssynchrony is associated with lower expression of target receptors of neurohormonal blockers.[10] As a result, evidence to support mandatory use of optimal medical therapy is limited and therefore, guidelines and a joined position paper from the Heart Failure Association (HFA)/European Heart Rhythm Association (EHRA)/European Association of Cardiovascular Imaging (EACVI) indicate that timing of CRT implantation should be considered already simultaneous with optimization of medical therapy, at least in the group of patients with typical LBBB.[11]

Table 9.2.1 Overview of landmark CRT trials

Trial	N	Design	NYHA	LVEF	QRS	Primary endpoint	Secondary endpoint	Main findings
MUSTIC-SR	58	Single-blinded, crossover, randomized CRT vs OMT, 6 mo	III	<35%	≥150	6MWD	NYHA class, QoL, peak VO$_2$, LV volumes, hospitalizations, mortality	CRT-P improved 6MWD, NYHA class, peak VO$_2$, LV volumes, and hospitalization
PATH-CHF	41	Single-blinded, crossover, randomized RV vs LV vs BiV, 12 mo	III–IV	NA	≥150	Peak VO$_2$, 6MWD	NYHA class, QoL, hospitalization	CRT-P improved NYHA class, QoL, and 6MWD and reduced hospitalization
MIRACLE	453	Double-blinded RCT, CRT vs OMT, 6 mo	III–IV	≤35%	≥130	NYHA class, 6MWD, QoL	Peak VO$_2$, LVEDD, LVEF, MR, clinical composite endpoint	CRT-P improved NYHA class, QoL, and 6MWD and reduced LVEDD and hospitalization
MIRACLE ICD	369	Double-blinded RCT, CRT-D vs ICD, 6 mo	III–IV	≤35%	≥130	NYHA class, 6MWD, QoL	Peak VO$_2$, LVEDD, LVEF, MR, clinical composite endpoint	CRT-D improved NYHA class, QoL, and peak VO$_2$
CONTAK-CD	490	Double-blinded RCT, CRT-D vs ICD, 6 mo	II, III, IV	≤35%	≥120	NYHA class, 6MWD, QoL	LV volume, LVEF, composite of mortality, VT/VF, and hospitalizations	CRT-D improved 6MWD, NYHA class, and QoL, reduced LV volume, and increased LVEF
MIRACLE-ICD II	186	Double-blinded RCT, CRT-D vs ICD, 6 mo	II	≤35%	≥130	Peak VO$_2$	VE/VCO$_2$, NYHA, QoL, 6MWD, LV volume, LVEF, composite clinical endpoint	CRT-D improved NYHA, VE/VCO$_2$, reduced LV volume, and improved LVEF
COMPANION	1520	Double-blinded RCT, CRT-D vs CRT-P vs OMT, 15 mo	III–IV	≤35%	≥120	All-cause mortality or hospitalization	All-cause mortality, cardiovascular mortality	CRT-P and CRT-D reduced all-cause mortality or hospitalization
CARE-HF	813	Double-blinded RCT, CRT-P vs OMT, 29.4 mo	III–IV	≤35%	≥120	All-cause mortality or hospitalization	All-cause mortality, NYHA class, QoL	CRT-P reduced all-cause mortality and hospitalization, and improved NYHA class and QoL
REVERSE	610	Double-blinded RCT, CRT-ON vs CRT-OFF, 12 mo	I–II	≤40%	≥120	Percentage worsened by clinical composite endpoint	LVESV index, heart failure hospitalization, all-cause mortality	CRT-P/CRT-D did not change the primary endpoint and did not reduce all-cause mortality, but reduced LVESV index and heart failure hospitalization
MADIT-CRT	1820	Single-blinded, randomized CRT-D vs ICD, 12 mo	I, II	≤30%	≥130	All-cause mortality or heart failure hospitalization	All-cause mortality and LVESV	CRT-D reduced the endpoint of heart failure hospitalization or all-cause mortality and LVESV, but did not reduce all-cause mortality
RAFT	1798	Double-blinded, randomized CRT-D vs ICD, 40 mo	II, III	≤30%	≥120	All-cause mortality or heart failure hospitalization	All-cause mortality and cardiovascular death	CRT-D reduced the endpoint of all-cause mortality or heart failure hospitalization. In NYHA class III, CRT-D only reduced significantly all-cause mortality

BiV, biventricular; CARE-HF, Cardiac Resynchronization-Heart Failure; CONTAK-CD, CONTAK-Cardiac Defibrillator; COMPANION, Comparison of Medical Therapy, Pacing and Defibrillation in Heart Failure; CRT, cardiac resynchronization therapy; CRT-D, cardiac resynchronization therapy with defibrillator; CRT-P, cardiac resynchronization therapy with pacemaker; ICD, implantable cardioverter–defibrillator; LV, left ventricular; LVEDD, left ventricular end-diastolic dimension; LVEF, left ventricular ejection fraction; LVESV, left ventricular end-systolic volume; MADIT-CRT, Multicenter Automatic Defibrillator Implantation Trial with Cardiac Resynchronization Therapy; MIRACLE, Multicenter InSync Randomized Clinical Evaluation; MIRACLE-ICD, Multicenter InSync Implantable Cardioverter Defibrillator trial; mo, months; MR, mitral regurgitation; MUSTIC, Multisite Stimulation in Cardiomyopathies; NYHA, New York Heart Association; OMT, optimal medical therapy; PATH-CHF, Pacing Therapies in Congestive Heart Failure trial; QoL, quality of life; RAFT, Resynchronization-Defibrillation for Ambulatory Heart Failure Trial; RCT, randomized controlled trial; RV, right ventricular; VE/VCO$_2$, minute ventilation/minute volume carbon dioxide production; VF, ventricular fibrillation; VO$_2$, volume of oxygen; VT, ventricular tachycardia; 6MWD, 6-minute walking distance.

Table 9.2.2 2021 guideline indications for cardiac resynchronization therapy

Recommendation	Class
1. Patients in sinus rhythm + LBBB QRS morphology	
CRT is recommended for symptomatic patients with HF in SR with LVEF ≤35%, QRS duration ≥150 ms, and an LBBB QRS morphology despite OMT, in order to improve symptoms and reduce morbidity and mortality	IA
CRT should be considered for symptomatic patients with HF in SR with LVEF ≤35%, QRS duration of 130–149 ms, and an LBBB QRS morphology despite OMT, in order to improve symptoms and reduce morbidity and mortality	IIa
2. Patients in sinus rhythm + non-LBBB QRS morphology	
CRT should be considered for symptomatic patients with HF in SR with LVEF of ≤35%, QRS duration of ≥150 ms, and a non-LBBB QRS morphology despite OMT, in order to improve symptoms and reduce morbidity	IIa
CRT may be considered for symptomatic patients with HF in SR with LVEF ≤35%, QRS duration of 130–149 ms, and a non-LBBB QRS morphology despite OMT, in order to improve symptoms and reduce morbidity	IIb
3. Patients with QRS <130 ms	
CRT is not indicated in patients with HF and QRS duration <130 ms without an indication for RV pacing	III
4. In patients with HF with permanent AF who are candidates for CRT	
CRT should be considered for patients with HF and LVEF ≤35% in NYHA class III or IV despite OMT if they are in AF and have intrinsic QRS ≥130 ms, provided a strategy to ensure biventricular capture is in place, in order to improve symptoms and reduce morbidity and mortality	IIa
AVJ ablation should be added in the case of incomplete biventricular pacing (<90–95%) due to conducted AF	IIa
5. Recommendation for upgrade from RV pacing to cardiac resynchronization therapy	
Patients who have received a conventional pacemaker or an ICD and who subsequently develop symptomatic HF with LVEF ≤35% despite OMT, and who have a significant proportion of RV pacing, should be considered for upgrade to CRT	IIa

AF, atrial fibrillation; AVJ, atrioventricular junction; CRT, cardiac resynchronization therapy; HF, heart failure; ICD, implantable cardioverter–defibrillator; IV, intravenous; LBBB, left bundle branch block; LVEF, left ventricular ejection fraction; OMT, optimal medical therapy; RV, right ventricular; SR, sinus rhythm.
Glikson M, Nielsen JC, Kronborg MB, et al; ESC Scientific Document Group. 2021 ESC Guidelines on cardiac pacing and cardiac resynchronization therapy. Eur Heart J. 2021 Sep 14;42(35):3427–3520. doi: 10.1093/eurheartj/ehab364. © The European Society of Cardiology. Reprinted by permission of Oxford University Press.

Cardiac resynchronization therapy in patients with atrial fibrillation

Guidelines formulate a Class IIa indication for CRT in patients with atrial fibrillation (AF), despite the fact that only 262 patients with AF were randomized in the original CRT trials, provided a strategy to ensure biventricular capture is in place. Despite limited trial evidence, up to 26% of patients had AF at the time of implantation in the EuroCRT survey II.[12] AF might result in inefficient biventricular pacing due to fast and irregular conduction creating spontaneous or (pseudo-)fusion beats. Indeed, observational data indicate that AF with rapid conduction is the number one reason for loss of biventricular pacing. Gasparini et al.[13] demonstrated that patients with AF who underwent AV junctional ablation had a similar benefit from CRT as patients in sinus rhythm, whereas this was not the case for AF patients who underwent pharmacological slowing of AV conduction—a concept which has more recently been supported by the APAF-CRT trial in which patients with fast-conduction AF experienced mortality benefit with AV node ablation and CRT. Importantly, patients included in the APAF-CRT had a QRS duration of ≤110 ms and benefit was observed independent of the baseline LVEF.

Cardiac resynchronization therapy in patients with a pacing indication

Guidelines recommend CRT for HFrEF patients with a classic pacing indication who are expected to receive a high burden of right ventricular (RV) pacing (Class IA recommendation) or patients with a classic pacemaker or implantable cardioverter–defibrillator (ICD) who developed heart failure (Class IIa recommendation for upgrade). In the EuroCRT survey, this cohort represented up to 23% of the entire CRT population. Nevertheless, limited data are available from clinical trials.[12] The ongoing BUDAPEST-CRT trial (ClinicalTrials.gov identifier: NCT02270840) will determine the benefit of upgrade from an ICD to a CRT-defibrillator (CRT-D) in symptomatic HFrEF patients with RV pacing (>20%).

Narrow QRS

The EchoCRT trial further supplemented the data from the RethinQ trial, illustrating that CRT is harmful in patients with a QRS duration of <130 ms, even in the presence of mechanical dyssynchrony assessed by echocardiography. Therefore, CRT is not indicated in patients with a narrow QRS.

Guidelines versus registries

While guidelines offer a strong level of recommendation for selected patients in sinus rhythm and with a long QRS width or LBBB, data from the EuroCRT Survey II indicate that only 67% of patients had a Class I indication, 26% a Class IIa indication, 5% a Class IIb indication, and 2% a Class III indication. Similarly, data from unselected American CRT surveys indicate a rate of >20% off-label use of CRT.[14] While CRT is globally underused (only a third of eligible candidates receive a CRT device), in clinical practice, CRT is frequently offered to patients in whom the level of evidence is less robust than a Class I or IIA indication. A recent joint position paper from the HFA/EHRA/EACVI describes strategies to reduce underutilization of CRT.[11]

Preimplant considerations

While guideline indications help heart failure doctors to identify the right candidates for CRT, other elements are often necessary before CRT. For instance, the role of preimplant imaging and evaluation of comorbidities can help decide between CRT-pacemaker (CRT-P) and CRT-D implantation.

Role of preimplant imaging

It is well acknowledged that the degree of crude preimplant mechanical dyssynchrony (apical rocking, septal flash) is associated with acute haemodynamic improvement and good LV remodelling following CRT.[15,16] However, using mechanical dyssynchrony for selection of CRT has failed to better select patients with improved outcome (outcome is determined by more than just LV remodelling). As such, the absence of preimplant mechanical dyssynchrony should *never* defer the implantation of a CRT device if patients have a guideline indication. One has to bear in mind that RCTs with wide QRS which have all demonstrated mortality and morbidity benefit of CRT only used LVEF as an imaging parameter. Surely, echocardiography goes far beyond LVEF measurements. It should also evaluate the potential presence of other relevant abnormalities, either in terms of treatment priorities or post-implant monitoring (valve diseases, RV function, pulmonary hypertension, structural abnormalities). Other imaging techniques or echocardiographic parameters have not been used to guide studies in RCTs, and therefore should not be used for selection of CRT candidates. Yet, preimplant imaging might help to understand the potential benefit of CRT better and to guide auxiliary therapies. For example, preimplant imaging (especially magnetic resonance imaging to detect scar burden) is useful in the assessment of the risk of sudden cardiac death (SCD) and might therefore be helpful in determining the choice between CRT-P and CRT-D. Additionally, echocardiography remains an indispensable tool to detect disease progression following CRT, and mechanism(s) related to ongoing disease following implantation which might be amenable to auxiliary therapies (e.g. residual secondary mitral regurgitation amenable to percutaneous edge-to-edge mitral valve repair).

Role of comorbidities

Comorbidities are frequent in heart failure and affect functional status and clinical outcome.[17,18] Furthermore, comorbidities might influence the delivery of heart failure therapies and might even influence the benefit of certain therapies.[19] Numerous observational studies indicate that the presence of multiple comorbidities significantly increases all-cause mortality. Due to this competing risk of comorbidity-driven mortality, patients with numerous comorbidities will derive less benefit from an implantable cardioverter–defibrillator (ICD) (➲ CRT-pacemaker versus CRT-defibrillator, p. XXX). Nevertheless, an elegant analysis from the MADIT-CRT trial indicates that the presence of multiple comorbidities does *not* diminish the treatment effect of CRT to reduce morbidity and mortality.[20] Therefore, patients with comorbidities do derive significant benefit from CRT, yet appropriate individualization of when to implant CRT-D versus CRT-P is particularly important in this population.[21] Certain comorbidities are of particular interest in CRT, as they might influence the success of the implantation procedure (e.g. history of valve surgery), choice between CRT-P and CRT-D (comorbidities limiting life expectancy), symptomatic improvement, and reverse remodelling response after implantation.

CRT-pacemaker versus CRT-defibrillator

Importantly, there is a paradox with regard to CRT and SCD. While CRT reduces the need for an ICD, it improves survival and reduces the rate of death due to heart failure, thereby exposing patients to an increased duration of life in which SCD can occur. In order to derive maximal benefit from an ICD, patients need to have a high risk of dying from SCD mediated by ventricular arrhythmias, and need to have a low risk of dying from other causes (non-SCD-mediated death). As such, this ratio should be taken into account during decision-making between CRT-P and CRT-D (➲ Figure 9.2.3). For instance, large areas of scar and an ischaemic aetiology of heart failure are associated with a higher risk of SCD. The burden of non-sustained ventricular tachycardia (NSVT) on Holter evaluation also predicts a higher risk of SCD.[22] In addition, some genetic mutations are associated with a higher risk of SCD. On the other hand, trial data suggest that women have a lower risk of SCD. Furthermore, the DANISH trial illustrates that on top of a contemporary background of disease-modifying therapies for HFrEF, a primary prevention ICD strategy in all patients with a non-ischaemic aetiology of heart failure might not improve long-term survival.[23] Nevertheless, ICDs did reduce SCD efficiently in the DANISH trial; however, with advanced age, a trade-off for non-SCD mortality occurs and thus the benefit in terms of long-term survival diminishes. Indeed, a statistical interaction was observed with age and patients aged younger than 59 years did derive benefit from a primary prevention ICD in non-ischaemic heart failure, because patients are likely to live longer (duration over which they can be exposed to potential SCD death) and have fewer comorbidities (lower non-SCD death). Individualized decision-making of CRT-P versus CRT-D remains important, as no head-to-head powered trials exist comparing CRT-P versus CRT-D and a Bayesian network analysis suggests no proven superiority of CRT-D over CRT-P. Furthermore, CRT-Ds come at significantly higher cost, as well as being associated with a risk of inappropriate therapy and a higher potential of shock coil lead failure. Finally, in balancing the risk of SCD and that of non-SCD, the impact of resynchronization itself, as well as improvements in pharmacological care attained by CRT, cannot be forgotten.[24] Data from the CARE-HF and REVERSE trials indicate that resynchronization therapy, as well as the potential to increase beta-blocking agents, diminishes the risk of ventricular tachycardia (VT)/ventricular fibrillation (VF), especially in patients with extensive LV reverse remodelling. One may consider not to implant a CRT-D, especially in non-ischaemic cardiomyopathy patients who: (1) are elderly; or (2) have advanced symptoms (NYHA classes III/IV); or (3) have life-shortening comorbidity (e.g. severe lung disease or stage IV chronic kidney disease), and hence are likely to die for reasons other than sudden arrhythmic death.

Disease modification instead of response after CRT

No consensus exists on how to measure response to CRT and numerous metrics are used, including functional, event-based,

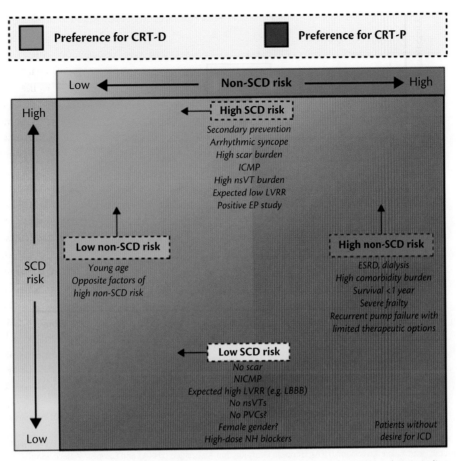

Figure 9.2.3 Conceptual framework for individualizing of CRT-P versus CRT-D. Red indicates preference for CRT-P, and green indicates preference for CRT-D. Balancing of choice is made by evaluating the risk of SCD (depicted in yellow, with dark yellow indicating high SCD risk and light yellow indicating low SCD risk) and the risk of non-SCD (depicted in blue, with dark blue indicating high risk of non-SCD and light blue indicating low risk of non-SCD). CRT-D, cardiac resynchronization therapy with defibrillator; CRT-P, cardiac resynchronization therapy with pacemaker; ICMP, ischaemic cardiomyopathy; SCD, sudden cardiac death; nsVT, non-sustained ventricular tachycardia; EP, electrophysiology; NICMP, non-ischaemic cardiomyopathy; PVC, premature ventricular complex; NH, neurohormonal blocker; ESRD, end-stage renal disease; ICD, implantable cardioverter–defibrillator; LVRR, left ventricular reverse remodelling.

imaging, or composite metrics.[25] The importance of certain metrics might also differ according to the stakeholders (e.g. patients, doctors, payers, industry). Functional metrics, such as NYHA class or the 6-minute walking test, are also influenced by patient bias as, for example, the greatest improvement in functional metrics in the GREATER-EARTH study occurred after implantation during the run-in phase before LV only of CRT pacing was switched on.

Additionally, agreement between metrics on what constitutes response is also poor, as this is most often based upon a binary endpoint (yes or no) and these metrics often are not in line with each other. For instance, LV reverse remodelling does not relate to the degree of functional improvement in many studies. Furthermore, Yu et al. illustrated that LV end-systolic volume (LVESV) changes only had an area under the curve of 0.711. The best LVESV cut-off had a sensitivity and specificity of 70%, indicating that 30% of patients are systematically misclassified when using reverse remodelling parameters. Yet LV reverse remodelling remains a commonly used endpoint, which is based upon the fact that therapies which improve LV structure are associated with better long-term outcomes.[26] However, this is clearly not the same

as stating that patients who do not have significant LV reverse remodelling (e.g. LVESV >15%) derive no benefit from CRT, as the natural history of HFrEF is progressive in nature (⊕ Figure 9.2.4).

Additionally, investigators examined the predictive value of baseline characteristics that were commonly present in CRT trials. For instance, male gender, non-ischaemic aetiology of heart failure, high LV volumes, low glomerular filtration rate, and absence of mechanical dyssynchrony have all been associated with less LV reverse remodelling following CRT implantation in observational studies. Yet, in a post hoc analysis of the major CRT trials powered for mortality and morbidity (CARE-HF, RAFT, COMPANION, and MADIT-CRT), the P-value for statistical interaction between the aforementioned clinical features and the endpoint of mortality or heart failure admission was not statistically significant. Therefore, on hard clinical endpoints, these patients derive an equal benefit, yet often manifest lower degrees of LV reverse remodelling. However, even CRT patients who fail to demonstrate reverse remodelling and have a heart failure admission still derive haemodynamic benefit from their device, as temporarily halting biventricular pacing is associated with acute haemodynamic deterioration.

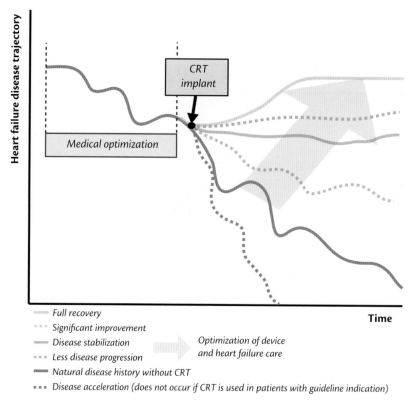

Figure 9.2.4 Role of CRT in disease modification of the heart failure disease trajectory. The grey arrow indicates the role of auxiliary heart failure optimization following CRT implantation.

Reproduced from Mullens W, Auricchio A, Martens P, *et al*. Optimized implementation of cardiac resynchronization therapy: a call for action for referral and optimization of care: A joint position statement from the Heart Failure Association (HFA), European Heart Rhythm Association (EHRA), and European Association of Cardiovascular Imaging (EACVI) of the European Society of Cardiology. *Eur J Heart Fail*. 2020 Dec;22(12):2349–2369. doi: 10.1002/ejhf.2046 with permission from John Wiley and Sons https://creativecommons.org/licenses/by-nc/4.0/.

Finally, labelling patients as responders or non-responders interferes with optimal delivery of care. In the recent ADVANCE-CRT registry study, patients who were labelled as responders were much less likely to have their therapy optimized following CRT implantation.[27] As such, the concept of 'disease modification' will help optimization of care in all patients, irrespective of their individual degree of response (➲ Figure 9.2.4).

Post-implant considerations

Importance of CRT care pathways following CRT implantation

Follow-up of CRT patients is often divided across several cardiology subspecialties and large differences exist across hospitals.[28] Although a comprehensive post-CRT implantation follow-up has not been tested in RCTs, it is possible to identify numerous factors amenable to improvement in the care of CRT patients. Furthermore, such a comprehensive follow-up of CRT patients in a dedicated CRT clinic is endorsed by several cardiac societies and results in improvement of workflow for a typical complex multimorbid patient population. Nevertheless, the care for the CRT patient warrants the training of a cardiologist and allied healthcare professional, with focused training on devices and heart failure-based interventions. Such training has been endorsed by the HFA. ➲ Figure 9.2.5 depicts a flow chart of optimized CRT care, highlighting important elements directly following implantation, before discharge, and at early and longer follow-up.

Optimal device programming

The CRT device should always be programmed with the aim of achieving 100% of biventricular pacing (while avoiding unnecessary atrial pacing) in order to attain the patient's maximal functionality. During device analysis, one has to distinguish between parameters that can be used as diagnostics, parameters that can be measured, and features that can be programmed (➲ Box 9.2.1). The most important programmable features are the pacing mode, lower rate, upper rate, capture output, AV and VV interval, and tachy-programming.

First, the pacing mode depends on the underlying atrial rhythm. In patients in sinus rhythm, a DDD pacing mode is preferred. Rate responsiveness is typically programmed off initially after CRT implantation. The type of rate responsiveness (accelerometer, minute ventilation, closed-loop system, heart sound) depends on the manufacturer. Some might be preferred in patients with known chronotropic incompetence. During ambulatory follow-up (once the beta-blocker dose is maximally uptitrated), exercise testing and device analysis (rate histogram) can be used to detect chronotropic incompetence, with programming of rate

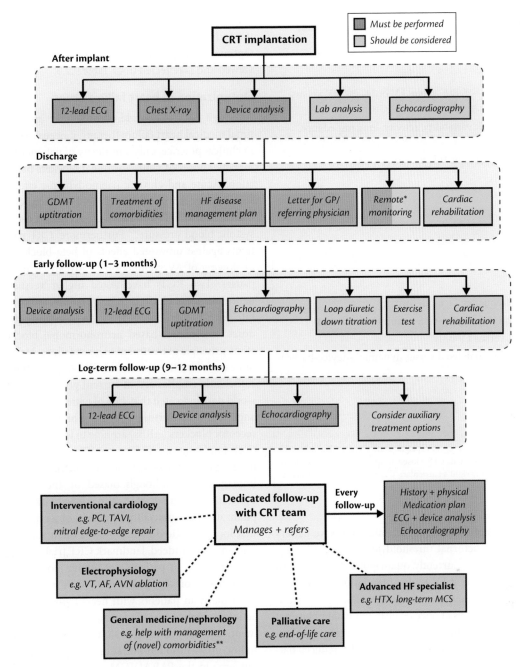

Figure 9.2.5 Flow chart showing essential elements of structured post-implant CRT care. AF, atrial fibrillation; AVN, atrioventricular node; CRT, cardiac resynchronization therapy; ECG, electrocardiogram; GDMT, guideline-directed medical therapy; GP, general practitioner; HF, heart failure; HTX, heart transplant; MCS, mechanical circulatory support; PCI, percutaneous coronary intervention; TAVI, transcatheter aortic valve implant; VT, ventricular tachycardia.

responsiveness if indicated. In patients with permanent AF, an inhibited mode is preferred, which can be DDIR if an atrial lead is present or VVIR if no atrial lead is present. The DDDR mode should be reserved for patients with paroxysmal AF.[25,29]

Second, the lower rate should be programmed low, to allow sensing of intrinsic atrial rhythms and to avoid unnecessary atrial pacing. Landmark CRT trials often used a lower rate of 35–40 bpm, with hysteresis off. Right atrial pacing has been shown to be associated with the development of left atrial dyssynchrony and progressive left atrial remodelling, and is an independent predictor for the development of AF.[3,30,31] In patients with AF

who receive adequate rate control, the lower rate is typically programmed higher (60–75 bpm), with rate responsiveness on. Atrial support pacing (higher lower rate) did not show any benefit in the PEGASUS-CRT trial.

Third, the upper rate should be programmed sufficiently high (e.g. 80% of maximal age-predicted heart rate) to ensure persistent biventricular pacing during exercise. Programming a too low upper rate might result in intrinsic conduction with loss of biventricular capture during exercise.

Fourth, the pacing output should be programmed with sufficient margin to ensure biventricular capture. Modern devices are

Box 9.2.1 Device analysis in cardiac resynchronization therapy

Diagnostics

1. Battery longevity
2. % ASVP—% APVP—% BiV versus LV only—% BiV versus RV sense response—% effective
3. Heart failure log: HR variability, activity, lung impedance, sleep…
4. Arrhythmias (afib, ectopy, VT, Vsense response,…)
5. Impedance trends

Measurements

1. Impedance
2. Sensitivity
3. Thresholds

Programming

1. Lower–upper frequency (+ mode switch)
2. R-response (accelerometer—CLS—minute ventilation)
3. BiV versus RV versus LV only
4. AV–VV times (manual: fixed versus dynamic—device-based)
5. Output leads
6. Sensitivity
7. Biv sense response
8. Tachy settings

APVP, atrial pace ventricular pace; ASVP, atrial sense ventricular pace; AV, atrioventricular; BiV, biventricular; CLS, closed-loop stimulation; HR, heart rate; LV, left ventricular; RV, right ventricular; VT, ventricular tachycardia; VV, interventricular.

equipped with auto-capture features that might improve battery longevity.[32] However, nocturnal threshold testing might be unpleasant for some patients. Currently, quadripolar LV leads allow for programming of different LV lead configurations, with great benefit in reducing phrenic nerve stimulation. Pacing from different LV lead configurations at once (multipoint pacing) has not been demonstrated to significantly improve the degree of LV reverse remodelling following CRT, and significantly reduces battery life.

Fifth, AV and VV delays should be optimally programmed, as observational studies have found suboptimal programming as a factor associated with poor response to CRT. Nevertheless, the role of routine echocardiographic (time-demanding) AV optimization is questionable, in comparison to empirical programming of a 100- to 120 ms sensed AV interval. Most new devices from different vendors have automated algorithms that individualize AV/VV timings, with some algorithms also creating fusion between spontaneous conduction and LV stimulation or using a haemodynamic sensor for optimization. None of these algorithms have proven to be superior to echocardiographic optimization, although a superiority study with LV fusion pacing is ongoing. In the light of the neutral results of optimizing AV and VV interval in all-comers, AV and VV optimization might therefore be reserved for specific patients (e.g. long interatrial delay).

Finally, tachy-programming should be individualized based on the indication for the ICD (primary vs secondary prevention). Optimal tachy-programming of CRT-Ds and ICDs has been reviewed and is reflected in ➲ Table 9.2.3.

Optimization of heart failure drugs

Although CRT is considered only after implementation of optimal medical heart failure therapy, it needs to be emphasized that in clinical practice, only a minority of patients are able to tolerate maximal doses of neurohormonal blockers before CRT implantation. Acute and chronic haemodynamic effects of CRT might significantly change this scenario. Data from the CARE-HF trial indicated that CRT results in, on average, a 6-mmHg increase in systolic blood pressure.[33] Furthermore, CRT pacing protects patients against unwanted effects of beta-blocker uptitration such as slowing of AV conduction, bradycardia, and sinoatrial nodal pauses. Two RCTs have tested higher versus lower doses of neurohormonal blockers in heart failure, indicating a lower event rate with higher doses. Therefore, attaining guideline-directed doses of evidence-based neurohormonal blockers is a cornerstone principle of treatment of heart failure. Medical optimization of heart failure therapies after CRT implantation is a concept insufficiently emphasized in current guidelines. Interestingly, real-world data indicated that 45% of patients on submaximal doses of angiotensin-converting enzyme inhibitors (ACEIs)/angiotensin receptor blockers (ARBs) are able to tolerate uptitration following CRT implantation, and up to 57% of patients on submaximal doses of beta-blockers are able to tolerate higher doses after CRT implantation.[34] Although biased by the observational nature, uptitration was associated with a lower risk of heart failure hospitalization and mortality. Similarly, observational data indicated that loop diuretic downtitration is often feasible following CRT implantation. Indeed, landmark CRT trials indicate that between 73% and 97% of patients are taking loop diuretics at the time of implantation. Loop diuretic downtitration might be possible particularly in patients with heart failure with a non-ischaemic aetiology, higher dose of loop diuretics, significant LVEF improvement, and reduction in systolic pulmonary artery pressures at follow-up.[34] Although initiation of sacubitril/valsartan improved outcome in the PARADIGM-HF trial, only a small minority of patients were treated with CRT. Real-world data indicated that initiation of sacubitril/valsartan in CRT and ICD patients results in incremental reverse remodelling, and a significant reduction in the burden of VT/VF and appropriate ICD therapies.[35] Additionally, due to the reduction in wall stress, the burden of premature ventricular complexes (PVCs) is significantly diminished following CRT implantation.[35] This is important as PVCs are a common reason for loss of biventricular pacing in CRT patients, and therefore, sacubitril/valsartan-mediated reductions in PVCs are associated with improvement in the percentage of biventricular pacing.[35] Although often underappreciated by patients and primary care physicians, physical exercise following CRT or ICD implantation has proven safe in the ACTION-HF trial.[36] Furthermore, observational and randomized data suggested that cardiac rehabilitation following CRT implantation is

Table 9.2.3 2015 guidelines on programming of implantable cardioverter–defibrillators

Recommendation	Class
For *primary prevention* ICD patients, tachyarrhythmia detection duration criteria should be programmed to require the tachycardia to continue for at least 6–12 seconds or for 30 intervals before completing detection, to reduce total therapies	IA
For *primary prevention* ICD patients, the slowest tachycardia therapy zone limit should be programmed between 185 and 200 bpm, to reduce total therapies	IA
For *secondary prevention* ICD patients, tachyarrhythmia detection duration criteria should be programmed to require the tachycardia to continue for at least 6–12 seconds or for 30 intervals before completing detection, to reduce total therapies	IB
Discrimination algorithms to distinguish SVT from VT should be programmed to include rhythms with rates faster than 200 bpm and potentially up to 230 bpm (unless contraindicated), to reduce inappropriate therapies	IB
It is recommended to activate lead failure alerts to detect potential lead problems	IB
For *secondary prevention* ICD patients for whom the clinical VT rate is known, it is reasonable to programme the slowest tachycardia therapy zone at least 10 bpm below the documented tachycardia rate, but not faster than 200 bpm, to reduce total therapies	IIa
It can be useful to programme more than one tachycardia detection zone to allow effective use of tiered therapy and/or SVT–VT discriminators and allow for a shorter delay in time-based detection programming for faster arrhythmias	IIa
When a morphology discriminator is activated, it is reasonable to reacquire the morphology template when the morphology match is unsatisfactory, to improve the accuracy of the morphology discriminator	IIa
It is reasonable to choose single-chamber ICD therapy in preference to dual-chamber ICD therapy if the sole reason for the atrial lead is SVT discrimination, unless a known SVT exists that may enter the VT treatment zone, to reduce both lead-related complications and the cost of ICD therapy	IIa
For S-ICD, it is reasonable to programme two tachycardia detection zones: one zone with tachycardia discrimination algorithms from a rate of r200 bpm, and a second zone without tachycardia discrimination algorithms from a rate of Z230 bpm, to reduce avoidable shocks	IIa
Programming a non-therapy zone for tachycardia monitoring might be considered to alert clinicians to untreated arrhythmias	IIb
It may be reasonable to disable the SVT discriminator timeout function, to reduce inappropriate therapies	IIb
It may be reasonable to activate lead 'noise' algorithms that withhold shocks when detected VT/VF is not confirmed on a shock or other far-field channel, to avoid therapies for non-physiological signals	IIb
It may be reasonable to activate T-wave oversensing algorithms, to reduce inappropriate therapies	IIb
It may be reasonable to programme the sensing vector from bipolar to integrated bipolar in true bipolar leads at risk of failure of the cable to the ring electrode, to reduce inappropriate therapies	IIb

ICD, implantable cardioverter–defibrillator; SVT, supraventricular tachycardia; VF, ventricular fibrillation; VT, ventricular tachycardia.
Reproduced from Wilkoff BL, Fauchier L, Stiles MK, *et al*; Document Reviewers. 2015 HRS/EHRA/APHRS/SOLAECE expert consensus statement on optimal implantable cardioverter–defibrillator programming and testing. *Europace*. 2016 Feb;18(2):159–83. doi: 10.1093/europace/euv411 with permission from Oxford University Press.

associated with a larger degree of functional improvement, LV reserve remodelling, and reduction in heart failure hospitalization and mortality. Finally, screening for the presence of certain comorbidities, such as iron deficiency, might be important following CRT implantation. The IRON-CRT trial showed that treating iron deficiency in patients with persistently reduced LVEF after CRT implantation resulted in incremental reverse remodelling and improved cardiac performance measured by the force–frequency relationship.[37]

Inclusion in remote monitoring

In remote monitoring of CRT devices, a distinction should be made between device-related remote monitoring and monitoring of heart failure status through measurement of physiological parameters. Patients with CRT have heart failure due to ischaemic or non-ischaemic heart disease, and are therefore at increased risk of clinical events such as ventricular or supraventricular arrhythmias, which can interrupt CRT or worsen their heart failure status.[38] Additionally, technical problems related to battery and leads can have an impact on patient prognosis and might warrant detection and appropriate action as early as possible. These parameters can be monitored by the device and remotely transmitted to the treating physician.[39] Early detection of clinical or technical issues was shown to reduce clinical outcome, inclusive of all-cause mortality, in the IN-TIME trial.[40] Remote monitoring should therefore be implemented in patients with CRT.[29] Nevertheless, a well-organized system should be in place to ensure the healthcare provider looks at the remote monitoring results, interpret and decides on therapeutic consequences, and ensures appropriate interventions will be taken. Several trials failed to show benefit of remote monitoring of only physiological parameters to detect worsening heart failure, in order to improve clinical outcome.

Managing arrhythmias in cardiac resynchronization therapy

Arrhythmias are common in heart failure patients, and often have an impact on morbidity, mortality, and functioning of the CRT device. Atrial tachyarrhythmias and frequent PVCs are responsible for 50% and 10%, respectively, of cases with low percentage of biventricular pacing and they can further compromise LV systolic function, which can lead to heart failure decompensation. Suppression of atrial tachyarrhythmias in the presence of HFrEF is challenging, and little consensus exists about the best strategy for maintenance of sinus rhythm.[41,42] Guidelines recommend amiodarone (Class IA), although a large amount of observational and randomized data exist on AF ablation (Class IIA recommendation) in patients with HFrEF. Cumulatively, these data suggest that AF ablation with the goal to reduce AF burden is associated with LVEF improvement, functional capacity, and quality of life in comparison to rate control. At longer follow-up, the CASTLE-AF trial suggests that AF ablation leads to a reduced risk of heart failure admission and all-cause mortality in selected patients. However, even though ablation in the CASTLE-AF trial and other observational data does not seem to lead to sinus rhythm 100% of the time, AF ablation itself seems to benefit HFrEF patients, mainly through reducing the AF burden.[43] While this might be an attractive therapeutic approach in selected HFrEF patients, this is likely insufficient for HFrEF patients with a CRT device, as effectively reaching 100% of biventricular pacing necessitates more than AF burden reduction alone. Therefore, AV nodal ablation should be considered as the preferred treatment strategy. However, patients in whom it is believed that sinus rhythm can be achieved 100% of the time could be considered for AF, rather than AV nodal, ablation.

Frequent PVCs (although less as atrial tachyarrhythmias) can result in a low percentage of biventricular pacing and further worsen LV systolic function.[44] PVCs can occur due to ventricular stretch-activated ion channels. Interestingly, sacubitril/valsartan is associated with both wall stress reduction and a reduction in PVC burden in CRT patients. If despite heart failure therapy optimization, PVCs remain, resulting in poor biventricular pacing, amiodarone or PVC ablation can be considered.[42]

Ventricular arrhythmias often occur in CRT patients and, by nature of selection, mostly in CRT-D patients.[21] Ventricular arrhythmias are associated with the disease severity of HFrEF. Furthermore, after appropriate ICD therapy, the risk of heart failure decompensation is significantly increased, which is not the case after inappropriate ICD therapy. This indicates that the occurrence of ventricular arrhythmias in HFrEF is mostly linked to disease progression. Therefore, heart failure therapy optimization is mandatory not only to treat, but also to prevent, ventricular arrhythmias in HFrEF.[45] Additionally, triggers such as volume overload, ion disturbances, loss of biventricular pacing, and others should be actively determined and treated.

Disease progression after cardiac resynchronization therapy

Heart failure is a progressive disease. While CRT can stabilize the disease trajectory, most heart failure patients remain to have heart failure disease and auxiliary treatment options might be indicated in selected cases. The CRT specialist team should not only manage technical aspects of CRT devices, but also detect and understand the mechanisms of heart failure disease progression (➲ Figure 9.2.5). Imaging plays an essential role in detecting potential disease progression. Persistence of significant functional mitral regurgitation and of mechanical dyssynchrony, and progressive atrial, LV, and RV remodelling all indicate progression of the heart failure syndrome and warrant consideration of appropriate interventions. The MitraClip might improve morbidity and mortality in selected heart failure patients on optimal background medical therapy, inclusive of CRT.[46] Additional data indicate that the MitraClip could lead to incremental reverse remodelling in CRT patients without sufficient LV disease modification. The presence of mechanical dyssynchrony after CRT should prompt re-evaluation of lead integrity and position, as well as attempts for better device programming. As wasted myocardial work increases in patients with residual mechanical dyssynchrony,[47] appropriate selection of suitable candidates for novel heart failure therapies that could reduce afterload (e.g. sacubitril/valsartan, sodium–glucose cotransporter 2 inhibitors, vericiguat) might be important.[48,49] The CRT specialist team should be able to detect the occurrence of new cardiac abnormalities (e.g. ischaemia, arrhythmias, aortic stenosis), and refer for additional therapies such as revascularization, ablation, or transcatheter aortic valve implantation when necessary or determine whether palliative care is more suitable.[50] In a selected group of patients, heart transplantation or LV assist device implantation should be considered.

Disease remission after cardiac resynchronization therapy

A very small subgroup of CRT patients demonstrate overwhelming benefit from CRT to an extent that every aspect of their heart failure disease seems to dissipate (normalization of echocardiogram and N-terminal pro-B-type natriuretic peptide levels, and resolution of symptoms). These patients can be considered as being in full remission. A small prospective randomized pilot trial suggested that closely supervised neurohumoral blocker withdrawal ('CRT-only strategy') is feasible and safe in patients with myocardial recovery after CRT.[51] However, in patients with cardiac comorbidities, such as hypertension, and mainly supraventricular arrhythmias, continuation of beta-blockers, ACEIs, or ARBs is often preferred. These results differ from the 'Withdrawal of pharmacological treatment for heart failure in patients with recovered dilated cardiomyopathy' (TRED-HF) trial because patients in the TRED-HF trial had dilated cardiomyopathy and did not have LBBB cardiomyopathy that was persistently controlled by biventricular pacing.[52] In contrast, data from MUSTIC and MADIT-CRT indicate that turning off biventricular pacing ('medical strategy only') will result in reoccurrence of the heart failure syndrome.

Future directions

Alternative resynchronization strategies have been developed that might also effectively treat electromechanical dyssynchrony, including His bundle and LBBB area pacing, endocardial LV lead pacing, and wireless LV stimulation. Acute haemodynamic and short-term reverse remodelling studies with these novel pacing strategies illustrate similar haemodynamic, functional, and re-modelling improvement as with CRT. Nevertheless, these strategies will have to show at least equal benefit in terms of morbidity and mortality endpoints in RCTs with head-to-head comparison with CRT before they can be implemented in clinical practice as a replacement for CRT.

Summary and key messages

- ♦ CRT results in acute and chronic haemodynamic and structural changes on a macroscopic level and in cellular adaptations on a microscopic level.
- ♦ CRT is a well-established lifesaving therapy for HFrEF patients, especially those in sinus rhythm and with an LBBB morphology.
- ♦ Despite its well-established role from RCTs, CRT remains underutilized in clinical practice, with only a third of eligible patients receiving the device.
- ♦ Response to CRT is a vague and arbitrary concept and should be replaced by disease modification. Certain patients can manifest with less cardiac reverse remodelling despite exhibiting benefit on hard endpoints.
- ♦ CRT is a treatment for heart failure that allows for improvement in functional status and heart failure disease severity. However, auxiliary therapies are often necessary. CRT allows for uptitration of guideline-directed medical therapy after implantation.
- ♦ Structured heart failure care after CRT implantation in a multidisciplinary CRT clinic is associated with improved outcome and excellent patient workflow.

References

1. Prinzen FW, Hunter WC, Wyman BT, McVeigh ER. Mapping of regional myocardial strain and work during ventricular pacing: experimental study using magnetic resonance imaging tagging. J Am Coll Cardiol 1999;33(6):1735–42.
2. Chalil S, Stegemann B, Muhyaldeen S, et al. Intraventricular dyssynchrony predicts mortality and morbidity after cardiac resynchronization therapy: a study using cardiovascular magnetic resonance tissue synchronization imaging. J Am Coll Cardiol 2007;50(3):243–52.
3. Martens P, Deferm S, Bertrand PB, et al. The detrimental effect of RA pacing on LA function and clinical outcome in cardiac resynchronization therapy. JACC Cardiovasc Imaging 2020;13(4):895–906.
4. Martens P, Verbrugge FH, Bertrand PB, et al. Effect of cardiac resynchronization therapy on exercise-induced pulmonary hypertension and right ventricular–arterial coupling. Circ Cardiovasc Imaging 2018;11(9):e007813.
5. Glikson M, Nielsen JC, Kronborg MB, et al. 2021 ESC Guidelines on cardiac pacing and cardiac resynchronization therapy. Eur Heart J 2021;42(35):3427–520.
6. Sipahi I, Carrigan TP, Rowland DY, Stambler BS, Fang JC. Impact of QRS duration on clinical event reduction with cardiac resynchronization therapy: meta-analysis of randomized controlled trials. Arch Intern Med 2011;171(16):1454–62.
7. Kutyifa V, Kloppe A, Zareba W, et al. The influence of left ventricular ejection fraction on the effectiveness of cardiac resynchronization therapy: MADIT-CRT (Multicenter Automatic Defibrillator Implantation Trial With Cardiac Resynchronization Therapy). J Am Coll Cardiol 2013;61(9):936–44.
8. Wang NC, Singh M, Adelstein EC, et al. New-onset left bundle branch block-associated idiopathic nonischemic cardiomyopathy and left ventricular ejection fraction response to guideline-directed therapies: the NEOLITH study. Heart Rhythm 2016;13(4):933–42.
9. Sze E, Samad Z, Dunning A, et al. Impaired recovery of left ventricular function in patients with cardiomyopathy and left bundle branch block. J Am Coll Cardiol 2018;71(3):306–17.
10. Vanderheyden M, Mullens W, Delrue L, et al. Myocardial gene expression in heart failure patients treated with cardiac resynchronization therapy responders versus nonresponders. J Am Coll Cardiol 2008;51(2):129–36.
11. Mullens W, Auricchio A, Martens P, et al. Optimized implementation of cardiac resynchronization therapy: a call for action for referral and optimization of care. Eur J Heart Fail 2020;22(12):2349–69.
12. Dickstein K, Normand C, Auricchio A, et al. CRT Survey II: a European Society of Cardiology survey of cardiac resynchronisation therapy in 11 088 patients: who is doing what to whom and how? Eur J Heart Fail 2018;20(6):1039–51.
13. Gasparini M, Auricchio A, Metra M, et al. Long-term survival in patients undergoing cardiac resynchronization therapy: the importance of performing atrio-ventricular junction ablation in patients with permanent atrial fibrillation. Eur J Heart 2008;29(13):1644–52.
14. Fein AS, Wang Y, Curtis JP, Masoudi FA, Varosy PD, Reynolds MR. Prevalence and predictors of off-label use of cardiac resynchronization therapy in patients enrolled in the National Cardiovascular Data Registry Implantable Cardiac–Defibrillator Registry. J Am Coll Cardiol 2010;56(10):766–73.
15. Breithardt OA, Stellbrink C, Kramer AP, et al. Echocardiographic quantification of left ventricular asynchrony predicts an acute hemodynamic benefit of cardiac resynchronization therapy. J Am Coll Cardiol 2002;40(3):536–45.
16. Verbeek XAAM, Auricchio A, Yu Y, et al. Tailoring cardiac resynchronization therapy using interventricular asynchrony. Validation of a simple model. Am J Physiol Heart Circ Physiol 2006;290(3):H968–H977.
17. Lee CS, Chien CV, Bidwell JT, et al. Comorbidity profiles and inpatient outcomes during hospitalization for heart failure: an analysis of the U.S. nationwide inpatient sample. BMC Cardiovasc Disord 2014;14:73.
18. Martens P, Nijst P, Verbrugge FH, Smeets K, Dupont M, Mullens W. Impact of iron deficiency on exercise capacity and outcome in heart failure with reduced, mid-range and preserved ejection fraction. Acta Cardiol 2018;73(2):115–23.
19. Martens P, Verbrugge F, Nijst P, Dupont M, Tang WH, Mullens W. Impact of iron deficiency on response to and remodeling after cardiac resynchronization therapy. Am J Cardiol 2017;119(1):65–70.
20. Zeitler EP, Friedman DJ, Daubert JP, et al. Multiple comorbidities and response to cardiac resynchronization therapy: MADIT-CRT long-term follow-up. J Am Coll Cardiol 2017;69(19):2369–79.

21. Martens P, Verbrugge FH, Nijst P, et al. Incremental benefit of cardiac resynchronisation therapy with versus without a defibrillator. Heart 2017;103(24):1977–84.

22. Mittal S, Aktas MK, Moss AJ, et al. The impact of nonsustained ventricular tachycardia on reverse remodeling, heart failure, and treated ventricular tachyarrhythmias in MADIT-CRT. J Cardiovasc Electrophysiol 2014;25(10):1082–7.

23. Kober L, Thune JJ, Nielsen JC, et al. Defibrillator implantation in patients with nonischemic systolic heart failure. N Engl J Med 2016;375(13):1221–30.

24. Shen L, Jhund PS, Petrie MC, et al. Declining risk of sudden death in heart failure. N Engl J Med 2017;377(1):41–51.

25. Daubert JC, Saxon L, Adamson PB, et al. 2012 EHRA/HRS expert consensus statement on cardiac resynchronization therapy in heart failure: implant and follow-up recommendations and management. Europace 2012;14(9):1236–86.

26. Kramer DG, Trikalinos TA, Kent DM, Antonopoulos GV, Konstam MA, Udelson JE. Quantitative evaluation of drug or device effects on ventricular remodeling as predictors of therapeutic effects on mortality in patients with heart failure and reduced ejection fraction: a meta-analytic approach. J Am Coll Cardiol 2010;56(5):392–406.

27. Varma N, Boehmer J, Bhargava K, et al. Evaluation, management, and outcomes of patients poorly responsive to cardiac resynchronization device therapy. J Am Coll Cardiol 2019;74(21):2588–603.

28. Gorodeski EZ, Magnelli-Reyes C, Moennich LA, Grimaldi A, Rickard J. Cardiac resynchronization therapy–heart failure (CRT-HF) clinic: a novel model of care. PLoS One 2019;14(9):e0222610.

29. Brignole M, Auricchio A, Baron-Esquivias G, et al. 2013 ESC Guidelines on cardiac pacing and cardiac resynchronization therapy: the Task Force on cardiac pacing and resynchronization therapy of the European Society of Cardiology (ESC). Developed in collaboration with the European Heart Rhythm Association (EHRA). Eur Heart J 2013;34(29):2281–329.

30. Adelstein E, Saba S. Right atrial pacing and the risk of postimplant atrial fibrillation in cardiac resynchronization therapy recipients. Am Heart J 2008;155(1):94–9.

31. Sade LE, Atar I, Ozin B, Yuce D, Muderrisoglu H. Determinants of new-onset atrial fibrillation in patients receiving CRT: mechanistic insights from speckle tracking imaging. JACC Cardiovasc Imaging 2016;9(2):99–111.

32. Boriani G, Rusconi L, Biffi M, et al. Role of ventricular Autocapture function in increasing longevity of DDDR pacemakers: a prospective study. Europace 2006;8(3):216–20.

33. Cleland JG, Daubert JC, Erdmann E, et al. The effect of cardiac resynchronization on morbidity and mortality in heart failure. N Engl J Med 2005;352(15):1539–49.

34. Martens P, Verbrugge FH, Nijst P, et al. Feasibility and association of neurohumoral blocker up-titration after cardiac resynchronization therapy. J Card Fail 2017;23(8):597–605.

35. Martens P, Nuyens D, Rivero-Ayerza M, et al. Sacubitril/valsartan reduces ventricular arrhythmias in parallel with left ventricular reverse remodeling in heart failure with reduced ejection fraction. Clin Res Cardiol 2019;108(10):1074–82.

36. Zeitler EP, Piccini JP, Hellkamp AS, et al. Exercise training and pacing status in patients with heart failure: results from HF-ACTION. J Card Fail 2015;21(1):60–7.

37. Martens P, Dupont M, Dauw J, et al. The effect of intravenous ferric carboxymaltose on cardiac reverse remodelling following cardiac resynchronization therapy: the IRON-CRT trial. Eur Heart J 2021;42(48):4905–14.

38. Ousdigian KT, Borek PP, Koehler JL, Heywood JT, Ziegler PD, Wilkoff BL. The epidemic of inadequate biventricular pacing in patients with persistent or permanent atrial fibrillation and its association with mortality. Circ Arrhythm Electrophysiol 2014;7(3):370–6.

39. Whellan DJ, Ousdigian KT, Al-Khatib SM, et al. Combined heart failure device diagnostics identify patients at higher risk of subsequent heart failure hospitalizations: results from PARTNERS HF (Program to Access and Review Trending Information and Evaluate Correlation to Symptoms in Patients With Heart Failure) study. J Am Coll Cardiol 2010;55(17):1803–10.

40. Hindricks G, Taborsky M, Glikson M, et al. Implant-based multiparameter telemonitoring of patients with heart failure (IN-TIME): a randomised controlled trial. Lancet 2014;384(9943):583–90.

41. Calkins H, Hindricks G, Cappato R, et al. 2017 HRS/EHRA/ECAS/APHRS/SOLAECE expert consensus statement on catheter and surgical ablation of atrial fibrillation: executive summary. J Arrhythm 2017;33(5):369–409.

42. Kirchhof P, Benussi S, Kotecha D, et al. 2016 ESC Guidelines for the management of atrial fibrillation developed in collaboration with EACTS. Eur Heart J 2016;37(38):2893–962.

43. Marrouche NF, Brachmann J, Andresen D, et al. Catheter ablation for atrial fibrillation with heart failure. N Engl J Med 2018;378(5):417–27.

44. Cheng A, Landman SR, Stadler RW. Reasons for loss of cardiac resynchronization therapy pacing: insights from 32 844 patients. Circ Arrhythm Electrophysiol 2012;5(5):884–8.

45. Priori SG, Blomstrom-Lundqvist C, Mazzanti A, et al. 2015 ESC Guidelines for the management of patients with ventricular arrhythmias and the prevention of sudden cardiac death: the Task Force for the Management of Patients with Ventricular Arrhythmias and the Prevention of Sudden Cardiac Death of the European Society of Cardiology (ESC). Endorsed by: Association for European Paediatric and Congenital Cardiology (AEPC). Eur Heart J 2015;36(41):2793–867.

46. Stone GW, Lindenfeld J, Abraham WT, et al. Transcatheter mitral-valve repair in patients with heart failure. N Engl J Med 2018;379(24):2307–18.

47. Aalen J, Storsten P, Remme EW, et al. Afterload hypersensitivity in patients with left bundle branch block. JACC Cardiovasc Imaging 2019;12(6):967–77.

48. McMurray JJV, Solomon SD, Inzucchi SE, et al. Dapagliflozin in patients with heart failure and reduced ejection fraction. N Engl J Med 2019;381(21):1995–2008.

49. McMurray JJ, Packer M, Desai AS, et al. Angiotensin–neprilysin inhibition versus enalapril in heart failure. N Engl J Med 2014;371(11):993–1004.

50. Martens P, Vercammen J, Ceyssens W, et al. Effects of intravenous home dobutamine in palliative end-stage heart failure on quality of life, heart failure hospitalization, and cost expenditure. ESC Heart Fail 2018;5(4):562–9.

51. Nijst P, Martens P, Dauw J, et al. Withdrawal of neurohumoral blockade after cardiac resynchronization therapy. J Am Coll Cardiol 2020;75(12):1426–38.

52. Halliday BP, Wassall R, Lota AS, et al. Withdrawal of pharmacological treatment for heart failure in patients with recovered dilated cardiomyopathy (TRED-HF): an open-label, pilot, randomised trial. Lancet 2019;393(10166):61–73.

CHAPTER 9.3

Cardiac surgery (bypass surgery and remodelling surgery)

Felix Schoenrath, Franz-Josef Neumann, Miguel Sousa Uva, and Volkmar Falk

Contents

Introduction

Estimates of the prevalence of coronary artery disease (CAD) among patients with heart failure vary considerably across studies, reflecting differences in populations and study designs. In the past decade, mortality from acute myocardial infarction has declined in many countries worldwide,[1,2,3] since pathways for prompt revascularization have been established and revascularization modalities have improved. Despite these improvements, 20% of all survivors of myocardial infarction will suffer from heart failure within 5 years after the initial presentation, and ischaemic heart disease (IHD) is the main reason for heart failure in up to 60% of patients.[4]

The diagnosis of IHD not only provides prognostic information in the heart failure population, but also helps to guide a causal therapy, such as revascularization and ventricular reconstruction, which are not an option in dilated cardiomyopathy of non-ischaemic aetiologies.[5] Coronary artery bypass grafting (CABG) is a highly effective treatment in patients with IHD and heart failure, but the indication has to be justified in the light of emerging evidence for interventional approaches and state-of-the-art medical therapy.

Left ventricular (LV) aneurysms are a well-recognized complication after acute myocardial infarction due to transmural ischaemia, with alteration in the ventricular geometry as a response to myocardial injury. Surgical ventricular reconstruction aims to reduce the LV volume and reshape the spherical left ventricle to a more physiological conical shape in order to reduce wall stress and prevent progression of pathological LV remodelling. Decision regarding the best treatment option and method requires a multidisciplinary Heart Team evaluation and patient involvement.[6] Patients with heart failure undergoing surgical revascularization or ventricular reconstruction require tight perioperative management and should be followed in a heart failure clinic.

Preoperative considerations

Indication for revascularization

The joint European Society of Cardiology (ESC)/European Association for Cardio-Thoracic Surgery (EACTS) guidelines on myocardial revascularization and the ESC guidelines for the diagnosis and treatment of acute and chronic heart failure recommend CABG as the first choice in patients with CAD, heart failure, and LVEF of ≤35%, and percutaneous coronary intervention (PCI) as an alternative to CABG.[6,7]

Despite the lack of a randomized trial comparing the two revascularization methods, CABG and PCI are complementary techniques. CABG carries an up-front higher early risk of death and perioperative morbidity, particularly in cases of comorbidities, and in observational studies, PCI has been associated with inferior long-term survival and freedom from major adverse cardiovascular events (MACE), particularly in the case of three-vessel disease or diabetes mellitus. The presence of diabetes is an important feature to consider when discussing the revascularization modality. Patients with CAD, diabetes, and LVEF of ≤49% who are treated with CABG show a significantly lower incidence of major adverse cardiac and cerebrovascular events and better long-term survival, compared to those treated with PCI, without a higher risk of stroke.[8] The Society of Thoracic Surgeons (STS) score and the European System for Cardiac Operative Risk Evaluation II (EuroSCORE II) can support the assessment of operative risk and can guide Heart Team discussions.

Ischaemia and viability

The mechanisms via which CABG, on top of best medical therapy, reduces late all-cause mortality in patients with IHD is unknown. Potential candidates include: (1) ischaemia—angina reversal; (2) improvement in LV function; and (3) recovery from hibernating, but viable, myocardium. Data from the Surgical Treatment for Ischemic Heart Failure (STICH) trial showed no significant interaction between inducible ischaemia and the treatment effect of CABG.[9] Similarly, the effect of CABG was unchanged whether the patient had angina (hazard ratio (HR) 0.89, 95% confidence interval (CI) 0.71–1.13) or not (HR 0.68, 95% CI 0.50–0.94) (P for interaction = 0.14). However, patients assigned to CABG were more likely to report improvement in angina than those assigned to medical therapy alone (odds ratio (OR) 0.70, 95% CI 0.55–0.90; P <0.01).[10] In the STICH trial, improvement in LVEF of ≥10% at 24 months in patients with IHD was uncommon and did not differ between patients assigned to CABG and medical therapy (19%) and those assigned to medical therapy alone (16%).[11] Improved survival with CABG plus medical therapy, compared to medical therapy alone, may be the result of myocardial collateralization, through the grafts, preventing the adverse consequences of plaque rupture and subsequent myocardial infarction, thereby reinforcing the importance of complete revascularization.[12]

Based on retrospective studies, assessment of myocardial viability is considered crucial for identifying patients who would most likely benefit from revascularization.[13,14] Contrary to these findings, the prospective, randomized assessment of myocardial viability in the STICH trial showed no significant interaction between the presence or absence of myocardial viability and the beneficial effect of CABG plus medical therapy over medical therapy alone (P = 0.34 for interaction). An increase in left ventricular ejection fraction (LVEF) was observed only in patients with myocardial viability, irrespective of treatment assignment. This improvement in LVEF at 4 months was not associated with long-term survival.[15] A more recent sub-analysis of the STICH trial, using echocardiographic assessment of LVEF in 618 patients at baseline and 24 months, showed that improvement in LVEF of >10% (HR 0.61, 95% CI 0.44–0.84; P = 0.004) and randomization to CABG (HR 0.72, 95% CI 0.57–0.90; P = 0.004)

were independently associated with a reduced hazard of mortality.[11]

According to myocardial viability testing (using single-photon emission computed tomography (SPECT) or dobutamine echocardiography, or both), 81% of patients in the STICH trial had viable myocardium,[15] and differences compared to the 'non-viable cohort' might simply have been overlooked. Criticism of the STICH trial included potential bias, lack of blinding, the modality, and incompleteness of viability testing.[16] The authors of the viability substudy also stated that the physiological complexity underpinning the potential therapeutic benefit of surgical revascularization cannot be surmised from the results of a single test of myocardial viability, particularly when those results are expressed in a dichotomous fashion (i.e. patients having or not having viability).[15]

In this context, viability assessment should be interpreted in conjunction with the degree of LV dysfunction, the coronary anatomy and the completeness of revascularization, and the surgical or percutaneous ability to supply target vessels and the affected myocardium. Current guidelines state that cardiac magnetic resonance (CMR) imaging, stress echocardiography, SPECT, or positron emission tomography (PET) may be considered for decision-making.[7]

Antithrombotic management

Continuation with acetylsalicylic acid (ASA) results in fewer ischaemic events but is associated with more blood loss. Therefore, current guidelines recommend continuation in the majority of patients, but stopping ASA at least 5 days before cardiac surgery in patients who refuse blood transfusions, who are at high risk of re-exploration for bleeding such as complex and redo operations, severe renal insufficiency, haematological disease, and hereditary platelet function deficiencies.[17]

As dual antiplatelet therapy (DAPT) with ASA and P2Y12 receptor inhibitors (clopidogrel, ticagrelor, and prasugrel) until the operation significantly increases the risk of bleeding, transfusions, and re-exploration for bleeding, P2Y12 receptor inhibitors should be discontinued before CABG whenever possible,[12] or if feasible, elective operations may be postponed until the DAPT treatment period is completed. If the risk of thromboembolic events exceeds that of bleeding events, two strategies are recommended in the current guidelines:[17]

1. Bridging therapy with cangrelor or glycoprotein (GP) IIb/IIIa inhibitors

2. Surgery may be performed without discontinuation of P2Y12 receptor inhibitors.

The optimal time for restarting oral P2Y12 receptor inhibitors after surgery should be as soon as it is deemed safe and in consideration of the risks of bleeding and ischaemia, which is normally between 48 and 96 hours after surgery. Even without stent implantation, DAPT is recommended in all patients with acute coronary syndrome (ACS), independently of the revascularization treatment,[17] and DAPT after CABG has been associated with reduced all-cause mortality[18,19] and better vein graft patency.

Anticoagulation

In patients taking vitamin K antagonists (VKAs), oral anticoagulation should be stopped before surgery and the international normalized ratio (INR) should be below 1.5 on the day of surgery.[17] If direct factor Xa inhibition is used, treatment should be stopped ≥2 days before surgery or according to the factor Xa activity in patients with renal failure. In patients with a high ischaemic risk, for example, those with CHA_2DS_2VASc score of >4, bridging should be performed, preferably with unfractionated heparin (UFH). Restarting anticoagulation is recommended as follows: UFH 12–24 hours after surgery; VKAs >24 hours after surgery; and direct-acting oral anticoagulant (DOACs) >72 hours after surgery.[17]

Post-operative dual-pathway inhibition (DPI) was studied in the COMPASS trial[20] and is a further treatment option to reduce the risk of ischaemic complications in patients with severe CAD at the cost of increased major bleeding. Importantly, the trial excluded patients with severe heart failure (New York Heart Association (NYHA) classes III and IV, LVEF <30%). No head-to-head comparison of DPI versus DAPT has been published; both low-dose rivaroxaban and P2Y12 receptor inhibitors might be reasonable additions to aspirin for patients at high thrombotic risk (atherosclerosis in at least two vascular beds, smokers, and patients with renal failure, diabetes, or moderate heart failure).[20]

Guideline-directed heart failure therapy and statins

Perioperatively, renin–angiotensin–aldosterone system (RAAS) inhibitors should be discontinued, as the risk of perioperative hypotension is increased with a concomitant higher need for vasopressors,[17] and should be restarted as soon as haemodynamic stability is achieved. Trials on sacubitril/valsartan in acute decompensated heart failure,[21] as well as in stable heart failure patients,[22] showed a clinical improvement within weeks, compared to placebo, supporting the idea of early initiation of guideline-directed medical therapy (GDMT) as soon as patients are haemodynamically stable after surgery.

Beta-blockers should be continued during the perioperative period, as should statins. Besides their lipid-lowering activity, statins have pleiotropic properties in the cardiovascular system.[23] According to the pathophysiological consideration that endothelial function is improved, the ACTIVE trial (ClinicalTrials.gov identifier: NCT01528709) will randomize patients to answer the question of whether high-dose statin treatment helps to prevent vein graft disease after CABG. No consensus guidelines for the perioperative use of sodium–glucose cotransporter 2 (SGLT2) inhibitors exist. Discontinuation at least 24 hours prior to major surgery reduces the risk of euglycaemic ketoacidosis, according to the pharmacological characteristics of gliflozins.

Preoperative *prophylactic* administration of the calcium sensitizer and phosphodiesterase 4 (PDE4) inhibitor levosimendan did not improve perioperative outcomes in patients with a reduced LVEF undergoing cardiac surgery, mainly CABG (66%).[24] Levosimendan for *treatment* of acute LV dysfunction (LVEF <25%, inotropic support, intra-aortic balloon pump) in patients undergoing cardiac surgery (19% with isolated CABG) failed to reduce mortality in the CHEETAH trial.[25] A trend ($P = 0.08$) towards shorter intensive care unit (ICU) stays was seen in LEVO CTS and has been reported by others,[26] as well as the effect of improved respiratory muscle function in respirator weaning.[27]

A meta-analysis on inotropic agents and vasodilator strategies for the treatment of cardiogenic shock in cardiac surgery did not support a specific inotropic or vasodilator therapy.[28]

Surgical ventricular reconstruction

Most patients with LV aneurysms are asymptomatic at initial presentation; some will complain of dyspnoea attributed to heart failure or of angina attributed to volume overload of the left ventricle, with increased oxygen consumption and ongoing ischaemia.

According to the current guidelines on myocardial revascularization (ESC/EACTS, 2018), surgical ventricular reconstruction (restoration, repair) (SVR) might be performed in experienced centres in patients with LVEF of ≤35% at the time of CABG in the presence of scarring and moderate LV remodelling.[7] As a stand-alone procedure, there are no guideline-recommended indications for SVR and the decision is usually left to the discretion of the Heart Team, taking into account the patient's functional status and the severity of LV remodelling. According to Castelvecchio and colleagues, SVR should be considered in patients with predominant heart failure symptoms (NYHA class III) in the presence of an enlarged left ventricle (left ventricular end-systolic volume index (LVESVI) >60 mL/m^2) with clear regional akinesia.[29] Cardiovascular imaging, with transthoracic two-dimensional echocardiography, plays a crucial role in preoperative assessment of LV volume and shape, global LV function, and location and extent of scarring, as well as the viability of myocardium remote from the scar. Gadolinium-enhanced CMR imaging is an accurate and reproducible method for quantifying LV volume and systolic function in patients with IHD;[30] it allows clear visualization of LV thrombi and enables differentiation between scar tissue and viable myocardium.[31] Even though no prognostic benefit was demonstrated in the STICH trial with regard to preoperative identification of viable myocardium or visual assessment of regional LV function,[32,33] this approach is widely used in centres specialized in SVR.[29,34] Contrast-enhanced cardiac computed tomography (CCT) can be used for preoperative assessment of patients with LV aneurysms,[35] especially in cases where magnetic resonance imaging (MRI) is not feasible. Use of advanced echocardiographic techniques, such as three-dimensional echocardiography for more precise evaluation of LV volume and shape,[36] assessment of contractility of the remaining LV, and speckle-tracking echocardiography for detecting viable myocardium[37] may improve the preoperative evaluation of patients. It is important to note that two-dimensional echocardiography tends to underestimate the true volume of the left ventricle, in comparison to LV ventriculography[38] and MRI in patients with a dilated left ventricle.[39] LV diastolic function, as assessed by echocardiography, is another important predictor of outcome in these patients,[40] as is right ventricular (RV) dysfunction assessed by tricuspid annular plane systolic excursion (TAPSE).[41] Although LV dilatation and NYHA class ≥3 are prerequisites for performing SVR, worse outcomes have been reported in patients with a severely dilated left ventricle (LVESVI >90 mL/m²) and severely reduced LVEF (<25%), as well as in those in NYHA class IV.[42,43]

Technical aspects

In addition to patient-related factors, the outcome following CABG is related to the long-term patency of grafts. All guideline-relevant technical considerations are displayed in ➲ Figure 9.3.1, according to the 2018 ESC/EACTS Guidelines on myocardial revascularization,[7] and we recommend this chapter in the revascularization guideline from the 2018 ESC/EACTS Guidelines[7] for further reading.

To briefly summarize the technical aspects, arterial grafts, specifically the internal mammary arteries (IMAs), should be used primarily. However, in observational propensity-matched studies, use of two IMAs was either associated with no long-term

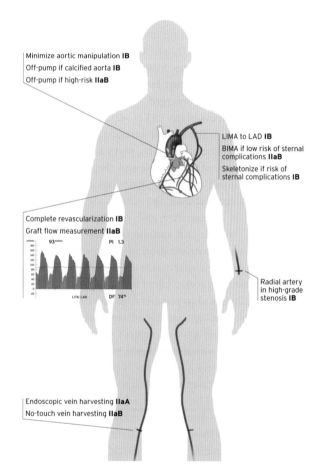

Minimize aortic manipulation **IB**
Off-pump if calcified aorta **IB**
Off-pump if high-risk **IIaB**

LIMA to LAD **IB**
BIMA if low risk of sternal complications **IIaB**
Skeletonize if risk of sternal complications **IB**

Complete revascularization **IB**
Graft flow measurement **IIaB**

93 ml/min   PI 1.3
LITA-LAD   DF 74%

Radial artery in high-grade stenosis **IB**

Endoscopic vein harvesting **IIaA**
No-touch vein harvesting **IIaB**

Figure 9.3.1 Technical aspects of coronary artery bypass grafting. BIMA, bilateral internal mammary artery; CABG, coronary artery bypass grafting; LIMA, left internal mammary artery; LAD, left anterior descending coronary artery.
Neumann FJ, Sousa-Uva M, Ahlsson A, et al.; ESC Scientific Document Group. 2018 ESC/EACTS Guidelines on myocardial revascularization. Eur Heart J. 2019 Jan 7;40(2):87–165. doi: 10.1093/eurheartj/ehy394. © European Society of Cardiology. Reproduced with permission by Oxford University Press.

survival advantage over use of a single IMA or this advantage disappeared in patients with LVEF of <30%.[44,45] The radial artery (RA) constitutes an alternative as a second arterial graft in patients in whom bilateral IMA (BIMA) grafting is not feasible or as a third arterial graft but requires the presence of a tight native coronary artery stenosis.[7] Calcium channel blocker therapy in patients with RA grafts was shown to significantly reduce intermediate-term occlusion rates.[46] Short-term, as well as long-term, graft failure is a limiting factor associated with the use of vein grafts. If used, saphenous vein grafts can be harvested by using an open, minimally invasive or a full endoscopic approach, with fewer surgical site complications after endoscopic harvesting.

Trials on on- and off-pump CABG have shown no difference in clinical outcomes in the general CABG population if performed by experienced surgeons[47,48]. Completeness of revascularization is crucial; it has been shown to be even more important in patients with LV dysfunction and should not be compromised by the use of off-pump CABG. To avoid the deleterious effect of global myocardial ischaemia associated with aortic cross-clamping and cardioplegia, on-pump assisted beating heart revascularization has been used and is associated with favourable early results.[49] When off-pump grafting of the left IMA (LIMA) to the left anterior descending artery (LAD) is combined with PCI to non-LAD vessels, it provides the opportunity to perform hybrid coronary revascularization, which can be used in selected patients with multivessel disease.[50]

Surgical ventricular reconstruction

Several surgical techniques of SVR and variations thereof exist, with two main approaches: linear reconstruction and endoventricular circular plasty with or without a patch. Simple linear reconstruction was first introduced by Cooley et al.[51] and then further modified by several groups. Linear resection combined with septoplasty demonstrated good results with regard to reverse remodelling and survival.[52] The technique of endoventricular circular patch plasty involves exclusion of scarred areas of the interventricular septum and the free wall of the left ventricle, with further application of a Dacron or pericardial patch sutured to the endocardial muscle and scar tissue.[53] After opening the left ventricle parallel to the LAD, careful assessment of the transition zone between scarred and non-scarred myocardium and use of an oval-shaped patch allow for avoiding a critical reduction in LV volume and preserving the elliptical shape of the left ventricle. An alternative technique involving the exclusion of scarred myocardium and the use of endoventricular circular sutures without use of a patch and other modifications for anterior and posterior LV remodelling have subsequently been introduced.[54,55] Regardless of the surgical technique, it is important to achieve a certain degree of reduction in LV volume during SVR. A decrease in the LVESVI by around 30–40%, while maintaining a residual LVESVI of <60–70 mL/m², was associated with longer patient survival and better functional status.[31,56] Overcorrection leading to a critical left ventricular end-diastolic volume index (LVEDVI) may lead to diastolic non-compliance of the left ventricle and progression of heart failure, and must therefore be avoided.[34] Cardiopulmonary bypass[29] is necessary to perform SVR, but surgery can be performed on the beating heart, which also facilitates direct assessment of contractile function in the border zone of the aneurysm.[52] It is generally accepted that CABG should be performed together with SVR when there is a need to achieve complete revascularization and preserve the myocardium remote from the scar.[57] In patients with moderate and severe mitral regurgitation, SVR might also be combined with mitral valve repair or replacement; usually mitral valve annuloplasty with undersized mitral rings is performed.[29,58]

Outcome

Although a number of randomized controlled trials (RCTs) have addressed the comparison of interventional and surgical revascularization, these trials mostly excluded patients with heart failure and impaired LV function; <1% of patients included in RCTs comparing PCI and CABG had reduced LV function.[59] Almost no outcome data are available for patients with heart failure with preserved ejection fraction (HFpEF).[60]

Heart failure with preserved ejection fraction

Data from the SWEDEHEART register[60] showed higher mortality in patients with HFpEF after CABG, compared to those without a history of heart failure and with normal LVEF (6-year mortality: 33.9% vs 13.2%, respectively). Hwang *et al.* were able to demonstrate that overall mortality in HFpEF patients was higher when CAD was evident. Complete revascularization (two-thirds PCI, one-third CABG) was associated with less deterioration in LVEF and lower mortality, compared to incomplete revascularization, independent of other factors in the same cohort. Given the paucity of effective treatments for HFpEF, prospective trials are urgently needed to determine optimal evaluation and management of CAD in HFpEF.[61]

Heart failure with reduced ejection fraction

Patients with heart failure with reduced ejection fraction (HFrEF) are at increased risk of perioperative morbidity and mortality, when compared to those with milder forms of LV dysfunction or normal LVEF.[62] As a result, patients with low LVEF are often advised against surgery. Paradoxically, these patients may benefit most from CABG.[62,63]

The STICH trial compared medical therapy alone to medical therapy plus CABG in 1212 patients with CAD and LV systolic dysfunction (LVSD).[64] Patients with angina Canadian Cardiovascular Society (CCS) class III or IV or left main disease were excluded. At 5 years, there was no difference in all-cause mortality between the two arms, but CABG did improve the rates of cardiovascular death and a composite of all-cause mortality and cardiovascular hospitalization. STICHES extended the follow-up period of the original trial to 10 years and showed that CABG, in addition to medical therapy, significantly improved all-cause mortality, compared to medical therapy alone, with an absolute risk reduction of 8%, an incremental median survival benefit of nearly 18 months, and prevention of one all-cause death for every

14 patients treated.[65] To a large extent, this benefit of CABG was driven by patients with three-vessel disease.[65]

There is no randomized trial comparing outcomes of PCI to those of CABG in patients with ischaemic heart failure and LVSD. In a propensity-matched comparison of 2126 patients with multivessel disease and LVEF of ≤35%, treated by everolimus-eluting stent PCI or CABG, and followed for up to 4 years, with a median of 2.9 years, PCI was associated with a similar risk of death, a higher risk of myocardial infarction (HR 2.16; 95% CI 1.42–3.28; $P=0.0003$), a lower risk of stroke (HR 0.57; 95% CI 0.33–0.97; $P=0.04$), and a higher risk of repeat revascularization (HR 2.54; 95% CI 1.88–3.44; $P<0.0001$).[66] A meta-analysis comparing surgical and percutaneous revascularization strategies to each other and to medical therapy alone in patients with LVSD (LVEF ≤40%) showed that, compared to medical therapy alone, CABG (HR 0.67, 95% CI 0.51–0.86; $P<0.001$) and PCI (HR 0.73, 95% CI 0.62–0.85; $P<0.001$) were associated with a significant mortality reduction.[67] When comparing the two methods of revascularization, CABG was associated with a survival benefit, compared to PCI (HR 0.82, 95% CI 0.75–0.90; $P<0.001$). In a retrospective cohort study of 12,113 patients with multivessel, LAD, or left main CAD and LVEF of <35%, two groups of 2397 propensity-matched patients treated by PCI or CABG were compared and followed up for 5.2 years. Patients who received PCI had significantly higher rates of mortality (HR 1.6, 95% CI 1.3–1.7), death from cardiovascular disease (HR 1.4, 95% CI 1.1–1.6), MACE (HR 2.0, 95% CI 1.9–2.2), subsequent revascularization (HR 3.7, 95% CI 3.2–4.3), hospitalization for myocardial infarction (HR 3.2, 95% CI 2.6–3.8), and heart failure (HR 1.5, 95% CI 1.3–1.6), compared to matched patients who underwent CABG.[68] The extent of CAD, stratified to one-vessel disease with LAD involvement, left main CAD or two-vessel disease, and three-vessel disease, was a significant modifier of treatment effect (P_{int} <0.001). The survival benefit of CABG was large in patients with three-vessel disease, but questionable in those with one-vessel disease and LAD involvement. With respect to cardiovascular mortality, a robust benefit of CABG, as compared to PCI, was only found in patients with three-vessel disease. Three other ground-breaking and extensively discussed trials on the optimal revascularization strategy were published in 2019 and 2020.[69,70,71] Although not powered to answer the question regarding the right revascularization strategy in HFrEF patients, a non-significant increase in the primary endpoint (death, stroke, myocardial infarction) was seen in patients with an LVEF of <50% after PCI, compared to those who received CABG, in the EXCEL trial. For the NOBLE trial, no data were reported for HFrEF. This is also true for the ISCHEMIA trial that included only 4% of the patients in the overall cohort who had a history of heart failure.[69] Since evidence from meta-analyses and retrospective comparisons, even in matched cohorts, has to be interpreted with caution, this topic merits the attention of an RCT in order to provide an irrefutable and truly unbiased answer that will enable clinicians to deliver the highest standard of healthcare to patients with poor LVEF.

Acute heart failure

Early revascularization is crucial in acute cardiogenic shock following acute myocardial infarction. These findings are based on the SHOCK trial, which demonstrated that emergency revascularization with PCI or CABG improved long-term survival in patients with cardiogenic shock complicating ST-segment elevation myocardial infarction (STEMI), when compared to initial intensive medical therapy.[72] All-cause mortality at 6 months was lower in the group assigned to revascularization, compared to the medically treated patients (50.3% vs 63.1%, respectively).[70] A sub-analysis of the SHOCK trial comparing patients treated with CABG or PCI showed similar survival rates between the two subgroups.[73] With no randomized trials available, Mehta and colleagues compared four observational studies, which also suggested similar mortality rates for PCI and CABG in patients with STEMI and multivessel CAD complicated by cardiogenic shock.[74] Despite these findings, and with increased mortality associated with delayed treatment, PCI is obviously the default strategy, performed with rates of over 95%.[75] According to current guidelines, CABG should be considered in patients with ongoing ischaemia and large areas of jeopardized myocardium if PCI of the infarct-related artery cannot be performed.[7]

Surgical ventricular reconstruction

In the STICH trial, CABG accompanied by SVR did not show better survival, compared to CABG alone, in patients with IHD.[64] These results raised a lot of discussion, as the study was restricted by inclusion/exclusion criteria, there was a broad range of baseline LV volumes, and there were questions about the adequacy of LV volume reduction achieved with SVR and whether a target level exists for the LVESVI that should be achieved after SVR.[43] Hospital mortality after SVR ranges between 1% and 8%.[56] Average survival at 5 and 10 years after SVR are 71.5% and 53.9%, respectively, based on pooled data from 47 studies (8571 patients).[76] Severe mitral regurgitation is a prognostic marker for worse survival after SVR,[55] although Athanasuleas et al. showed increased 30-day, but not increased 5-year, mortality rates if concomitant mitral surgery is needed.[42] Overall, there are uncertainties regarding: (a) optimal patient selection (a very large and extensively remodelled left ventricle at baseline and restrictive physiology of the remaining myocardium may prevent any clinical benefit); and (b) the importance of achieving an ideal reduction in post-operative LVESVI (no undercorrection and no overcorrection). Therefore, SVR may be considered in selected patients treated in centres with expertise. ⊃ Figure 9.3.2 summarizes parameters that should be considered when planning SVR to achieve a favourable outcome.

Future perspectives and gaps in evidence

Since the only randomized, prospective data regarding surgical revascularization in heart failure from the STICH trial revealed the above-mentioned shortcomings and represented a cohort that is nearly 20 years old, contemporary data in this field are desperately lacking. In the randomized controlled REVIVED BCIS2 trial, revascularization by PCI plus medical therapy did not result in a lower incidence of death from any cause or hospitalization for heart failure, compared with medical therapy.[77] In this trial no comparison with CABG was performed. Further analysis of the trial data should help to weigh the value of viability testing.

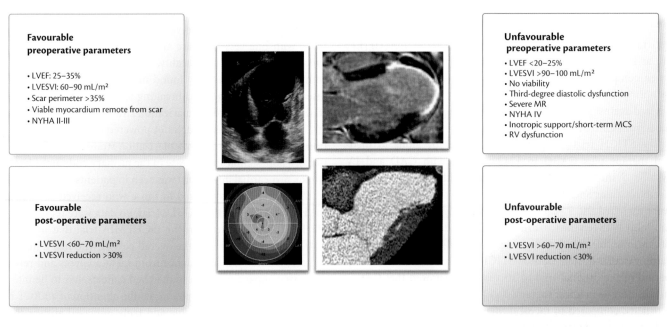

Favourable preoperative parameters

- LVEF: 25–35%
- LVESVI: 60–90 mL/m²
- Scar perimeter >35%
- Viable myocardium remote from scar
- NYHA II–III

Favourable post-operative parameters

- LVESVI <60–70 mL/m²
- LVESVI reduction >30%

Unfavourable preoperative parameters

- LVEF <20–25%
- LVESVI >90–100 mL/m²
- No viability
- Third-degree diastolic dysfunction
- Severe MR
- NYHA IV
- Inotropic support/short-term MCS
- RV dysfunction

Unfavourable post-operative parameters

- LVESVI >60–70 mL/m²
- LVESVI reduction <30%

Figure 9.3.2 Cardiovascular imaging in patients with left ventricular aneurysm for planning of surgical ventricular reconstruction and prognosis of outcome after the surgery. LVEF, left ventricular ejection fraction; LVEDVI, left ventricular end-diastolic volume index; LVESVI, left ventricular end-systolic volume index; MCS, mechanical circulatory support; MR, mitral regurgitation; NYHA, New York Heart Association; RV, right ventricular.

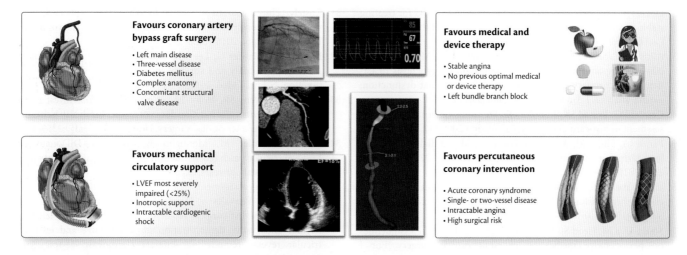

Figure 9.3.3 Perspectives of revascularization in heart failure. LVEF, left ventricular ejection fraction.

The therapeutic spectrum of heart failure approaches has widened. Comparison of CABG to state-of-the-art medical, interventional, and device therapy, on the one hand, and comparison of CABG to rapidly improving outcomes of long-term mechanical circulatory support, on the other hand, should be carried out. A potential outlook is displayed in ⊃ Figure 9.3.3.

The interesting approach of short-term mechanical LV support with rotary blood pumps that showed promising results in patients undergoing high-risk PCI or in reducing toxicity of inotropic support in patients with myocarditis should be evaluated in high-risk CABG procedures in patients with severely impaired LVEF if it bears the potential to improve outcome.

Summary and key messages

- The long-term mortality of ischaemic heart disease is still high.
- Viability testing should be an integral part of the decision-making process in patient evaluation for revascularization.
- ASA, beta-blockers, and statins should not be stopped in the perioperative setting (CABG).
- Arterial grafts, specifically the IMAs, should be used primarily for CABG.
- Percutaneous and surgical revascularization are complementary approaches for symptomatic relief of angina in HFrEF, whereas only CABG has a proven prognostic impact.
- The aims of SVR are to reduce LV volume and reshape a spherical left ventricle to a more physiological conical shape to reduce wall stress and prevent progression of pathological LV remodelling.
- NYHA class ≥3, a severely dilated left ventricle (LVESVI >90 mL/m^2), severely reduced LVEF (<25%), and impaired RV function are associated with impaired outcomes after SVR.
- All decisions should be guided by a specialized heart failure team, with a thorough understanding of the risks and benefits of all available medical, percutaneous, and surgical treatment options.

References

1. Khera S, Kolte D, Aronow WS, *et al*. Non-ST-elevation myocardial infarction in the United States: contemporary trends in incidence, utilization of the early invasive strategy, and in-hospital outcomes. J Am Heart Assoc. 2014;3(4):e000995.
2. Khera S, Kolte D, Palaniswamy C, *et al*. ST-elevation myocardial infarction in the elderly: temporal trends in incidence, utilization of percutaneous coronary intervention and outcomes in the United States. Int J Cardiol. 2013;168(4):3683–90.
3. Kolte D, Khera S, Aronow WS, *et al*. Trends in incidence, management, and outcomes of cardiogenic shock complicating ST-elevation myocardial infarction in the United States. J Am Heart Assoc. 2014;3(1):e000590.
4. Go AS, Mozaffarian D, Roger VL, *et al*.; American Heart Association Statistics Committee and Stroke Statistics Subcommittee. Heart disease and stroke statistics: 2014 update: a report from the American Heart Association. Circulation. 2014;129(3):e28–292.
5. Khera S, Panza JA. Surgical revascularization for ischemic cardiomyopathy in the post-STICH era. Cardiol Rev. 2015;23(4):153–60.
6. McDonagh TA, Metra M, Adamo M, *et al*.; ESC Scientific Document Group. Corrigendum to: 2021 ESC Guidelines for the diagnosis and treatment of acute and chronic heart failure. Eur Heart J. 2021;42:3599–726.
7. Neumann FJ, Sousa-Uva M, Ahlsson A, *et al*.; ESC Scientific Document Group. 2018 ESC/EACTS Guidelines on myocardial revascularization. Eur Heart J. 2019;40(2):87–165.
8. Nagendran J, Bozso SJ, Norris CM, *et al*. Coronary artery bypass surgery improves outcomes in patients with diabetes and left ventricular dysfunction. J Am Coll Cardiol. 2018;71(8):819–27.
9. Petrie MC, Jhund PS, She L, *et al*.; STICH Trial Investigators. Ten-year outcomes after coronary artery bypass grafting according to age in patients with heart Failure and left ventricular systolic dysfunction: an analysis of the extended follow-up of the STICH trial (Surgical Treatment for Ischemic Heart Failure). Circulation. 2016;134(18):1314–24.
10. Jolicœur EM, Dunning A, Castelvecchio S, *et al*. Importance of angina in patients with coronary disease, heart failure, and left ventricular systolic dysfunction: insights from STICH. J Am Coll Cardiol. 2015;66(19):2092–100.
11. Perry AS, Mann DL, Brown DL. Improvement of ejection fraction and mortality in ischaemic heart failure. Heart. 2020;heartjnl–2020–316975.

12. Doenst T, Haverich A, Serruys P, *et al.* PCI and CABG for treating stable coronary artery disease: JACC review topic of the week. J Am Coll Cardiol. 2019;73(8):964–76.

13. Allman KC, Shaw LJ, Hachamovitch R, Udelson JE. Myocardial viability testing and impact of revascularization on prognosis in patients with coronary artery disease and left ventricular dysfunction: a meta-analysis. J Am Coll Cardiol 2002;39:1151–8.

14. Camici PG, Prasad SK, Rimoldi OE. Stunning, hibernation, and assessment of myocardial viability. Circulation 2008;117:103–14.

15. Panza JA, Ellis AM, Al-Khalidi HR, *et al.* Myocardial viability and long-term outcomes in ischemic cardiomyopathy. N Engl J Med. 2019;381(8):739–48.

16. Hassanabad AF, MacQueen KT, Ali I. Surgical treatment for ischemic heart failure (STICH) trial: a review of outcomes. J Card Surg. 2019;34(10):1075–82.

17. Sousa-Uva M, Head SJ, Milojevic M, *et al.* 2017 EACTS Guidelines on perioperative medication in adult cardiac surgery. Eur J Cardiothorac Surg. 2018;53(1):5–33.

18. Verma S, Goodman SG, Mehta SR, *et al.* Should dual antiplatelet therapy be used in patients following coronary artery bypass surgery? A meta-analysis of randomized controlled trials. BMC Surg. 2015;15:112.

19. Deo SV, Dunlay SM, Shah IK, *et al.* Dual anti-platelet therapy after coronary artery bypass grafting: is there any benefit? A systematic review and meta-analysis. J Card Surg. 2013;28:109–16.

20. Eikelboom JW, Connolly SJ, Bosch J, *et al.*; COMPASS Investigators. Rivaroxaban with or without aspirin in stable cardiovascular disease. N Engl J Med. 2017;377(14):1319–30.

21. Velazquez EJ, Morrow DA, DeVore AD, *et al.*; PIONEER-HF Investigators. Angiotensin–neprilysin inhibition in acute decompensated heart failure. N Engl J Med. 2019;380(6):539–48.

22. McMurray JJ, Packer M, Desai AS, *et al.*; PARADIGM-HF Investigators and Committees. Angiotensin–neprilysin inhibition versus enalapril in heart failure. N Engl J Med. 2014;371(11):993–1004.

23. Spadaccio C, Antoniades C, Nenna A, *et al.* Preventing treatment failures in coronary artery disease: what can we learn from the biology of in-stent restenosis, vein graft failure, and internal thoracic arteries? Cardiovasc Res. 2020;116(3):505–19.

24. Mehta RH, Leimberger JD, van Diepen S, *et al.*; LEVO-CTS Investigators. Levosimendan in patients with left ventricular dysfunction undergoing cardiac surgery. N Engl J Med. 2017;376(21):2032–42.

25. Landoni G, Lomivorotov VV, Alvaro G, *et al.*; CHEETAH Study Group. Levosimendan for hemodynamic support after cardiac surgery. N Engl J Med. 2017;376(21):2021–31.

26. Jiménez-Rivera JJ, Álvarez-Castillo A, Ferrer-Rodríguez J, *et al.* Preconditioning with levosimendan reduces postoperative low cardiac output in moderate–severe systolic dysfunction patients who will undergo elective coronary artery bypass graft surgery: a cost-effective strategy. J Cardiothorac Surg. 2020;15(1):108.

27. Roesthuis L, van der Hoeven H, Sinderby C, *et al.* Effects of levosimendan on respiratory muscle function in patients weaning from mechanical ventilation. Intensive Care Med. 2019;45(10):1372–81.

28. Uhlig K, Efremov L, Tongers J, *et al.* Inotropic agents and vasodilator strategies for the treatment of cardiogenic shock or low cardiac output syndrome. Cochrane Database Syst Rev. 2020;11:CD009669.

29. Castelvecchio S, Pappalardo OA, Menicanti L. Myocardial reconstruction in ischaemic cardiomyopathy. Eur J Cardiothorac Surg. 2019;55:i49–56.

30. Karamitsos TD, Francis JM, Myerson S, Selvanayagam JB, Neubauer S. The role of cardiovascular magnetic resonance imaging in heart failure. J Am Coll Cardiol. 2009;54(15):1407–24.

31. Castelvecchio S, Garatti A, Gagliardotto PV, Menicanti L. Surgical ventricular reconstruction for ischaemic heart failure: state of the art. Eur Heart J Suppl. 2016;18:E8–14.

32. Bonow RO, Maurer G, Lee KL, *et al.*; STICH Trial Investigators. Myocardial viability and survival in ischemic left ventricular dysfunction. N Engl J Med. 2011;364(17):1617–25.

33. Prior DL, Stevens SR, Holly TA, *et al.*; STICH Trial Investigators. Regional left ventricular function does not predict survival in ischaemic cardiomyopathy after cardiac surgery. Heart. 2017;103(17):1359–67.

34. Dor V, Sabatier M, Montiglio F, Civaia F, DiDonato M. Endoventricular patch reconstruction of ischemic failing ventricle. a single center with 20 years' experience. advantages of magnetic resonance imaging assessment. Heart Fail Rev. 2004;9(4):269–86.

35. Solowjowa N, Penkalla A, Dandel M, *et al.* Multislice computed tomography-guided surgical repair of acquired posterior left ventricular aneurysms: demonstration of mitral valve and left ventricular reverse remodelling. Interact Cardiovasc Thorac Surg. 2016;23(3):383–90.

36. Politi MT, Vivas MF, Filipini E, *et al.* Three-dimensional echocardiography for predicting postoperative ventricular volumes after surgical ventricular reconstruction of left ventricular aneurysm: a case-based presentation. Echocardiography. 2017;34(8):1250–3.

37. Omar AM, Bansal M, Sengupta PP. Advances in echocardiographic imaging in heart failure with reduced and preserved ejection fraction. Circ Res. 2016; 119(2):357–74.

38. Isomura T, Hoshino J, Fukada Y, *et al.*; RESTORE Group. Volume reduction rate by surgical ventricular restoration determines late outcome in ischaemic cardiomyopathy. Eur J Heart Fail. 2011;13(4):423–31.

39. Rigolli M, Anandabaskaran S, Christiansen JP, Whalley GA. Bias associated with left ventricular quantification by multimodality imaging: a systematic review and meta-analysis. Open Heart. 2016;3(1):e000388.

40. Kim KH, She L, Lee KL, *et al.* Incremental prognostic value of echocardiography of left ventricular remodeling and diastolic function in STICH trial. Cardiovasc Ultrasound. 2020;18(1):17.

41. Garatti A, Castelvecchio S, Di Mauro M, Bandera F, Guazzi M, Menicanti L. Impact of right ventricular dysfunction on the outcome of heart failure patients undergoing surgical ventricular reconstruction. Eur J Cardiothorac Surg. 2015;47(2):333–40.

42. Athanasuleas CL, Buckberg GD, Stanley AW, *et al.*; RESTORE Group. Surgical ventricular restoration in the treatment of congestive heart failure due to post-infarction ventricular dilation. J Am Coll Cardiol. 2004;44(7):1439–45.

43. Michler RE, Rouleau JL, Al-Khalidi HR, *et al.*; STICH Trial Investigators. Insights from the STICH trial: change in left ventricular size after coronary artery bypass grafting with and without surgical ventricular reconstruction. J Thorac Cardiovasc Surg. 2013;146(5):1139–45.e6.

44. Mohammadi S, Kalavrouziotis D, Cresce G, *et al.* Bilateral internal thoracic artery use in patients with low ejection fraction: is there any additional long-term benefit? Eur J Cardiothorac Surg. 2014;46(3):425–31.

45. Galbut DL, Kurlansky PA, Traad EA, Dorman MJ, Zucker M, Ebra G. Bilateral internal thoracic artery grafting improves long-term survival in patients with reduced ejection fraction: a propensity-matched study with 30-year follow-up. J Thorac Cardiovasc Surg. 2012;143(4):844–53.e4.

46. Gaudino M, Benedetto U, Fremes SE, *et al.*; RADIAL Investigators. Effect of calcium-channel blocker therapy on radial artery grafts after coronary bypass surgery. J Am Coll Cardiol. 2019;73(18):2299–306.

47. Diegeler A, Börgermann J, Kappert U, *et al.*; GOPCABE Study Group. Off-pump versus on-pump coronary-artery bypass grafting in elderly patients. N Engl J Med. 2013;368(13):1189–98.

48. Lamy A, Devereaux PJ, Prabhakaran D, *et al.*; CORONARY Investigators. Five-year outcomes after off-pump or on-pump coronary-artery bypass grafting. N Engl J Med. 2016;375(24):2359–68.

49. Xia L, Ji Q, Song K, *et al.* Early clinical outcomes of on-pump beating-heart versus off-pump technique for surgical revascularization in patients with severe left ventricular dysfunction: the experience of a single center. J Cardiothorac Surg. 2017;12(1):11.

50. Gasior M, Zembala MO, Tajstra M, *et al.*; POL-MIDES (HYBRID) Investigators. Hybrid revascularization for multivessel coronary artery disease. JACC Cardiovasc Interv. 2014;7:1277–83.

51. Cooley DA, Collins HA, Morris GC Jr, Chapman DW. Ventricular aneurysm after myocardial infarction; surgical excision with use of temporary cardiopulmonary bypass. J Am Med Assoc. 1958;167(5):557–60.

52. Mickleborough LL, Carson S, Ivanov J. Repair of dyskinetic or akinetic left ventricular aneurysm: results obtained with a modified linear closure. J Thorac Cardiovasc Surg. 2001;121(4):675–82.

53. Dor V, Saab M, Coste P, Kornaszewska M, Montiglio F. Left ventricular aneurysm: a new surgical approach. Thorac Cardiovasc Surg. 1989;37(1):11–19.

54. Caldeira C, McCarthy PM. A simple method of left ventricular reconstruction without patch for ischemic cardiomyopathy. Ann Thorac Surg. 2001;72(6):2148–9.

55. Garatti A, Castelvecchio S, Bandera F, Guazzi M, Menicanti L. Surgical ventricular restoration: is there any difference in outcome between anterior and posterior remodeling? Ann Thorac Surg. 2015;99(2):552–9.

56. Buckberg G, Athanasuleas C, Conte J. Surgical ventricular restoration for the treatment of heart failure. Nat Rev Cardiol. 2012;9(12):703–16.

57. Di Donato M, Castelvecchio S, Menicanti L. Surgical treatment of ischemic heart failure: the Dor procedure. Circ J. 2009;73 Suppl A:A1–5.

58. Suma H, Tanabe H, Uejima T, Isomura T, Horii T. Surgical ventricular restoration combined with mitral valve procedure for endstage ischemic cardiomyopathy. Eur J Cardiothorac Surg. 2009;36(2):280–4.

59. Gaudino M, Hameed I, Khan FM, *et al.* Treatment strategies in ischaemic left ventricular dysfunction: a network meta-analysis. Eur J Cardiothorac Surg. 2020;ezaa319.

60. Dalén M, Lund LH, Ivert T, Holzmann MJ, Sartipy U. Survival after coronary artery bypass grafting in patients with preoperative heart failure and preserved vs reduced ejection fraction. JAMA Cardiol. 2016;1(5):530–8.

61. Hwang SJ, Melenovsky V, Borlaug BA. Implications of coronary artery disease in heart failure with preserved ejection fraction. J Am Coll Cardiol. 2014;63(25 pt A):2817–27.

62. Omer S, Adeseye A, Jimenez E, Cornwell LD, Massarweh NN. Low left ventricular ejection fraction, complication rescue, and long-term survival after coronary artery bypass grafting. J Thorac Cardiovasc Surg. 2022;163(1):111–19.e2.

63. Panza JA, Velazquez EJ, She L, *et al.* Extent of coronary and myocardial disease and benefit from surgical revascularization in ischemic LV dysfunction [Corrected]. J Am Coll Cardiol. 2014;64(6):553–61.

64. Velazquez EJ, Lee KL, Deja MA, *et al.*; STICH Investigators. Coronary-artery bypass surgery in patients with left ventricular dysfunction. N Engl J Med. 2011;364(17):1607–16.

65. Velazquez EJ, Lee KL, Jones RH, *et al.* Coronary-artery bypass surgery in patients with ischemic cardiomyopathy. N Engl J Med. 2016;374(16):1511–20.

66. Bangalore S, Guo Y, Samadashvili Z, Blecker S, Hannan EL. Revascularization in patients with multivessel coronary artery disease and severe left ventricular systolic dysfunction: everolimus-eluting stents versus coronary artery bypass graft surgery. Circulation. 2016;133(22):2132–40.

67. Wolff G, Dimitroulis D, Andreotti F, *et al.* Survival benefits of invasive versus conservative strategies in heart failure in patients with reduced ejection fraction and coronary artery disease: a meta-analysis. Circ Heart Fail. 2017;10(1):e003255.

68. Sun LY, Gaudino M, Chen RJ, Bader Eddeen A, Ruel M. Long-term outcomes in patients with severely reduced left ventricular ejection fraction undergoing percutaneous coronary intervention vs coronary artery bypass grafting. JAMA Cardiol. 2020;5(6):631–41.

69. Maron DJ, Hochman JS, Reynolds HR, *et al.*; ISCHEMIA Research Group. Initial invasive or conservative strategy for stable coronary disease. N Engl J Med. 2020;382(15):1395–407.

70. Holm NR, Mäkikallio T, Lindsay MM, *et al.*; NOBLE Investigators. Percutaneous coronary angioplasty versus coronary artery bypass grafting in the treatment of unprotected left main stenosis: updated 5-year outcomes from the randomised, non-inferiority NOBLE trial. Lancet. 2020;395(10219):191–9.

71. Stone GW, Kappetein AP, Sabik JF, *et al.*; EXCEL Trial Investigators. Five-year outcomes after PCI or CABG for left main coronary disease. N Engl J Med. 2019;381(19):1820–30.

72. Hochman JS, Sleeper LA, Webb JG, *et al.* Early revascularization in acute myocardial infarction complicated by cardiogenic shock. SHOCK Investigators. Should We Emergently Revascularize Occluded Coronaries for Cardiogenic Shock. N Engl J Med. 1999;341:625–34.

73. White HD, Assmann SF, Sanborn TA, *et al.* Comparison of percutaneous coronary intervention and coronary artery bypass grafting after acute myocardial infarction complicated by cardiogenic shock: Results from the Should We Emergently Revascularize Occluded Coronaries for Cardiogenic Shock (SHOCK) trial. Circulation 2005;112:1992–2001.

74. Mehta RH, Lopes RD, Ballotta A, *et al.* Percutaneous coronary intervention or coronary artery bypass surgery for cardiogenic shock and multivessel coronary artery disease? Am Heart J. 2010;159(1):141–7.

75. Thiele H, Zeymer U, Neumann FJ, *et al.*; IABP-SHOCK II Trial Investigators. Intraaortic balloon support for myocardial infarction with cardiogenic shock. N Engl J Med. 2012;367(14):1287–96.

76. Klein P, Bax JJ, Shaw LJ, Feringa HH, Versteegh MI, Dion RA, Klautz RJ. Early and late outcome of left ventricular reconstruction surgery in ischemic heart disease. Eur J Cardiothorac Surg. 2008; 34(6):1149–57.

77. Perera D, Clayton T, O'Kane PD, *et al.* Percutaneous revascularization for ischemic left ventricular dysfunction. N Engl J Med. 2022;387(15):1351–60.

CHAPTER 9.4

Valve interventions

Stefan Orwat, Stefan D Anker, and
Helmut Baumgartner

Introduction

Valvular heart disease (VHD) and heart failure (HF) are closely related.[1,2] Untreated severe primary VHD ultimately ends up in HF being then a main cause of death. Secondary VHD in HF of other causes, on the other hand, is known to aggravate morbidity and mortality.[1,2] Correct distinction between primary and secondary VHD is critical, as treatment strategies differ fundamentally. In primary VHD, valve intervention is indicated early—ideally before HF develops.[1,2] There remain, however, difficult subgroups in whom other HF causes coexist, and the severity of VHD remains challenging to assess.[1,2] Intervention in secondary VHD is currently considered in patients who remain symptomatic despite optimal HF treatment when secondary VHD is assumed to be a relevant driver of HF and its consequences.[1,2] However, the selection of patients with secondary VHD who benefit from valve intervention remains difficult. The evolvement of transcatheter VHD intervention has now dramatically changed treatment options, particularly in secondary VHD. The consideration of valve intervention therefore plays an important role in the non-pharmacological management of HF. In this context, aortic stenosis (AS), mitral regurgitation (MR), and tricuspid regurgitation (TR) deserve close consideration. This chapter primarily focuses on intervention in secondary VHD, while addressing selected aspects for primary VHD related to HF, but otherwise referring to VHD guidelines[1] and related literature. The currently used or investigated technical approaches for transcatheter valve interventions are summarized in ◆ Figure 9.4.1.

Aortic stenosis

AS causes HF by increasing afterload, which results in left ventricular (LV) hypertrophy and LV remodelling.[1] As a single cause, LV pressure overload from AS causes LV systolic dysfunction relatively late in the course of the disease, in most patients after symptom onset. As soon as patients present with HF symptoms, AS has a very poor prognosis and timely valve intervention is recommended.[1]

Diagnosis of severe AS is relatively straightforward in the presence of 'high-gradient AS' defined by a transvalvular flow velocity of ≥4 m/s, a mean pressure gradient (PGmean) of ≥40 mmHg, and an aortic valve area (AVA) of <1.0 cm² calculated using the continuity equation, and intervention is recommended in all these patients with HF symptoms, regardless of the left ventricular ejection fraction (LVEF).[1] It becomes more difficult when the AVA and gradient are discordant. This is typically encountered in the presence of low-flow conditions (stroke volume <35 mL/m² of body surface area)—the so-called 'low-flow, low-gradient AS' (AVA <1.0 cm², peak velocity <4 m/s, PGmean <40 mmHg).[3]

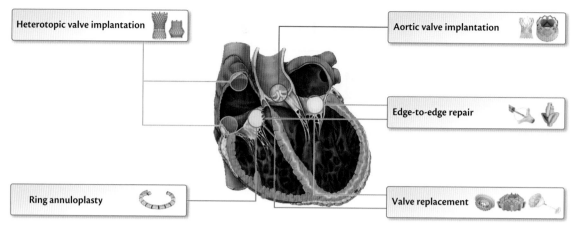

Figure 9.4.1 Overview of current devices for the treatment of valve diseases.

The currently recommended management of patients with HF and suspected severe low-flow, low-gradient AS is summarized in ⮕ Figure 9.4.2. Assessment of the LVEF is here the first step.

Low-flow, low-gradient aortic stenosis with reduced LVEF (<50%)

Low-dose dobutamine echocardiography can help to distinguish between true severe AS and pseudo-severe AS in this situation. While patients with true severe AS (dobutamine-stimulated flow increase resulting in gradient increase with no significant change in AVA) are likely to benefit from valve intervention, patients with pseudo-severe AS (dobutamine-stimulated flow increase resulting in AVA enlargement with little gradient increase) do not.[1] In patients without flow reserve under dobutamine administration (i.e. <20% flow increase), quantification of valve calcification by computed tomography has proven useful (⮕ Figure 9.4.2).[1]

Low-flow, low-gradient aortic stenosis with preserved LVEF (≥50%)

HF patients presenting with low-flow, low-gradient AS and preserved LVEF are the most difficult group. In order to identify patients with severe AS who benefit from intervention, an integrated approach including clinical and imaging criteria—in particular calcium scoring—is recommended (⮕ Figure 9.4.2).[1]

Moderate aortic stenosis and heart failure

Approximately 10% of patients with AS have HF with reduced ejection fraction (HFrEF), but only those with severe stenosis have currently a Class I recommendation for aortic valve replacement.[1,4] Recent studies suggest that patients with HFrEF and moderate AS have a worse outcome than comparable patients without stenosis, and may benefit from catheter intervention if suitable.[5] However, the outcome of randomized trials remains to be awaited before general recommendations can be made for this patient group.[6]

Treatment modalities

For treatment of severe AS, transcatheter aortic valve implantation (TAVI) as an alternative to surgery has gained increasing importance in recent years, particularly in patients with advanced HF. More than 25% of TAVI patients now have HF with LVEF <45%.[7]

The choice between TAVI and surgical aortic valve replacement (SAVR) should be made by the Heart Team according to individual features, including age, surgical risk, clinical, anatomical and procedural aspects, and weighing the risks and benefits of each approach, as well as the preference of the properly informed patient.[1]

TAVI has been shown to be non-inferior to SAVR in reducing clinical events, which include mortality and stroke, in patients at high and intermediate surgical risk. In randomized controlled trials (RCTs) comparing TAVI and SAVR in a low-risk population, the average age was over 70 years. Therefore, the guidelines recommend SAVR in patients younger than 75 years who are at low surgical risk, whereas TAVI is recommended for patients older than 75 years or who are at high surgical risk (STS-PROM score or EuroSCORE II >8%).

In this context, limitations and open questions regarding the use of TAVI, compared to SAVR in younger and low-risk patients need to be kept in mind: the higher rate of pacemaker requirement and left bundle branch block[8] and of paravalvular leakage (even with the latest generation of TAVI devices, at least mild paravalvular leakage is seen in >30%)[9,10] may compromise the long-term outcome after this intervention. In addition, approximately half of TAVI patients have coronary artery disease.[11] Of these, some may require coronary angiography at a later stage. This can be particularly difficult with self-expanding valves and required access to the left coronary artery,[12] as the device may hinder access to the ostia.

Aortic regurgitation

Severe aortic regurgitation (AR) causes LV dilatation and eventually progressive LV dysfunction, HF, and poor outcome. Early surgery is therefore recommended to avoid HF development. Although medical therapy may improve the symptoms of these patients, SAVR is recommended for all symptomatic patients with severe AR, regardless of LVEF.[1] In cases of high surgical risk or other reasons why surgery seems to be unfavourable, the Heart

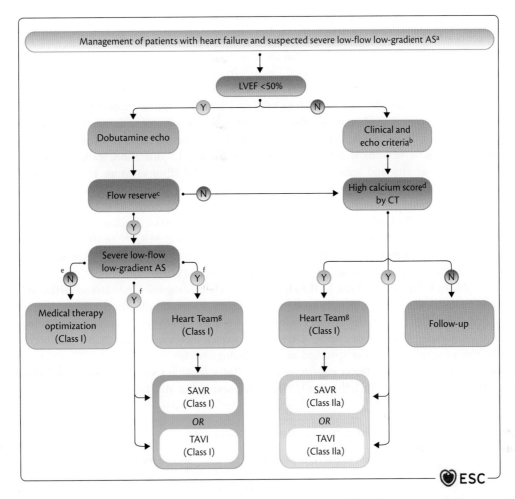

Figure 9.4.2 Management of patients with severe low-flow, low-gradient aortic stenosis and heart failure. AS, aortic stenosis; CT, computed tomography; EuroSCORE II, European System for Cardiac Operative Risk Evaluation II; LVEF, left ventricular ejection fraction; OMT, optimal medical therapy; SAVR, surgical aortic valve replacement; STS-PROM, Society of Thoracic Surgeons Predicted Risk of Mortality; TAVI, transcatheter aortic valve implantation. [a] Valve area <1 cm², peak velocity <4.0 m/s, mean gradient <40, stroke volume index <35 mL/m². [b] Age >70 years, typical symptoms without other explanations, left ventricular hypertrophy or reduced left ventricular longitudinal function, mean gradient 30–40 mmHg, valve area <0.8 cm², stroke volume index <35 mL/m² assessed by techniques other than standard Doppler. [c] Flow reserve is defined as a stroke volume index increase of >20%. [d] Aortic stenosis is very likely if the calcium score is >3000 in men and >1600 in women. Aortic stenosis is likely if the calcium score is >2000 in men and >1200 in women. Aortic stenosis is unlikely if the calcium score is <1600 in men and <800 in women. [e] Increase in valve area to >1.0 cm² in response to flow increase (flow reserve) during dobutamine echo. [f] Increase in mean gradient to at least 40 mmHg without significant change in valve area in response to flow increase (flow reserve) during dobutamine echo. [g] SAVR is recommended in patients aged <75 years and at low surgical risk (STS-PROM score or EuroSCORE II <4%), whereas TAVI is recommended in those aged >75 years or at high/prohibitive surgical risk (STS-PROM score or EuroSCORE II >8%). In all other cases, the choice between TAVI and SAVR is recommended to be decided by the Heart Team, weighing the pros and cons of each procedure, according to age, life expectancy, individual patient preference, and features including clinical and anatomical aspects. Colour code for classes of recommendation: green for Class of recommendation I; yellow for Class of recommendation IIa (see Table 1 in reference (2) for further details on classes of recommendation).

McDonagh TA, Metra M, Adamo M, *et al*; ESC Scientific Document Group. 2021 ESC Guidelines for the diagnosis and treatment of acute and chronic heart failure. *Eur Heart J.* 2021 Sep 21;42(36):3599–3726. doi: 10.1093/eurheartj/ehab368. © The European Society of Cardiology. Reprinted by permission of Oxford University Press.

Team can also discuss the treatment of AR by TAVI.[13,14] Even in non-calcified aortic valves, TAVI may be a treatment option in highly selected patients.[15]

Mitral regurgitation

MR is the most common VHD encountered in patients with HF (approximately 10–20% of all HF patients), and many HF patients experience an increase in regurgitation over time.[16] Patients with severe MR have a very high risk of being hospitalized with HF symptoms.[17]

In the assessment of MR, imaging should answer three key questions:[18]

1. What is the mechanism of MR?

2. What is the severity of MR?

3. What are the consequences of MR on the left ventricle (LV), left atrium (LA), and pulmonary circulation?

Diagnosis of MR is mainly performed by transthoracic and transoesophageal echocardiography but may be supplemented by other modalities such as cardiac magnetic resonance imaging or invasive assessment of haemodynamics, especially if the severity remains uncertain by echocardiography.[19]

For grading of MR severity, current guidelines recommend an integrated approach in which the classification is not based on a single measured value but is derived from the combination of several parameters.[20] Criteria for severe MR are summarized in ➲ Table 9.4.1. Assessment of severity should be made after optimization of drug therapy and, if necessary, cardiac resynchronization therapy (CRT). It is of utmost importance to correctly differentiate between primary and secondary MR, as therapeutic strategies differ fundamentally.

Primary MR is caused by structural abnormalities of the valve apparatus and—if severe—eventually leads to HF because of LV volume overload. Intervention is therefore recommended early to avoid development of HF.[1] Surgery, preferably repair, is currently recommended as the modality of choice. Only if patients are judged inoperable or at high surgical risk by the Heart Team and the valve is anatomically suitable, percutaneous repair may be considered (Class IIb).[1] In the American College of Cardiology (ACC)/American Heart Association (AHA) guidelines, increased risk of surgery is further specified using the STS score. Above a score of 6, a transcatheter edge-to-edge repair (TEER) should be considered (Class IIa indication).[21] The

recommendation is based on the EVEREST II trial, in which patients with primary/organic MR were randomized to TEER or surgery.[22]

In *secondary MR*, the valve leaflets and chordae are structurally normal and MR results from an imbalance between closing and tethering forces secondary to alterations in LV and left atrial (LA) geometry.[1,23] It is frequently a disease of the LV (dilated or ischaemic cardiomyopathy) caused by various mechanisms such as LV dilatation, leaflet restriction, dyssynchrony, or increased LV filling pressure. It can also be caused by LA dilatation or altered atrial/annular dynamics, and elevated LA pressure with enlargement of the mitral annulus in patients with long-standing atrial fibrillation (AF) and is then referred to as atrial functional MR.[24,25] In the latter form, LV function may also be normal or only mildly impaired and the ventricle may be of normal size.[25]

If echocardiography indicates moderate MR, but the symptoms suggest severe insufficiency, echocardiography under physical stress may be helpful.[26] Particularly in secondary regurgitation, a marked increase in regurgitation can occasionally be observed during exercise.

The association with worse outcome has not only been shown for severe, but also for moderate and even mild, secondary MR

Table 9.4.1 Severe mitral regurgitation criteria based on echocardiography

	Primary mitral regurgitation	Secondary mitral regurgitation
Qualitative		
Mitral valve morphology	Flail leaflet, ruptured papillary muscle, severe retraction, large perforation	Normal leaflets, but with severe tenting, poor leaflet coaptation
Colour flow jet area	Large central jet (>50% of LA) or eccentric wall impinging jet of variable size Large throughout systole Holosystolic/dense/triangular	Normal leaflets, but with severe tenting, poor leaflet coaptation Large central jet (>50% of LA) or eccentric wall impinging jet of variable size Large throughout systole Holosystolic/dense/triangular
Semi-quantitative		
Vena contracta width (mm)	≥7 (≥8 mm for biplane)	≥7 (≥8 mm for biplane)
Pulmonary vein flow	Systolic flow reversal	Systolic flow reversal
Mitral inflow	E-wave dominant (>1.2 m/s)	E-wave dominant (>1.25 m/s)
TVI mitral/TVI aortic	>1.4	>1.4
Quantitative		
EROA (2D PISA, mm^2)	≥40 mm^2	≥40 mm^2 (may be ≥30 mm^2 if elliptical regurgitant orifice area)
Regurgitant volume (mL/beat)	≥60 mL	≥60 mL (may be ≥45 mL if low flow conditions)
Regurgitant fraction (%)	≥50%	≥50%
Structural		
Left ventricle	Dilated (ESD ≥40 mm)	Dilated
Left atrium	Dilated (diameter ≥55 mm or volume ≥60 mL/m^2)	Dilated

2D, two-dimensional; ESD, end-systolic diameter; EROA, effective regurgitant orifice area; LA, left atrium; PISA, proximal isovelocity surface area; TVI, time–velocity integral.

Vahanian A, Beyersdorf F, Praz F, *et al*; ESC/EACTS Scientific Document Group. 2021 ESC/EACTS Guidelines for the management of valvular heart disease. *Eur Heart J*. 2022 Feb 12;43(7):561–632. doi: 10.1093/eurheartj/ehab395. © The European Society of Cardiology. Reprinted by permission of Oxford University Press.

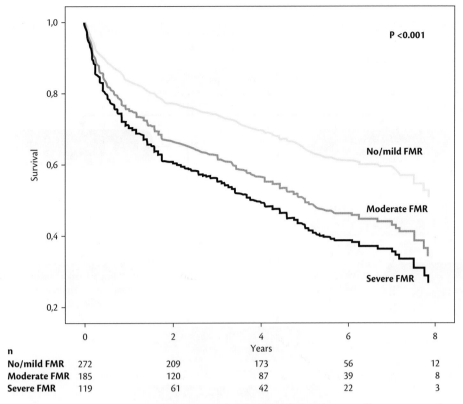

n					
	0	2	4	6	8
No/mild FMR	272	209	173	56	12
Moderate FMR	185	120	87	39	8
Severe FMR	119	61	42	22	3

Figure 9.4.3 Survival according to severity of secondary mitral regurgitation (SMR). Adjusted survival curves of long-term mortality according to severity of MR (P <0.001), adjusted for the clinical confounder model (i.e. age, sex, ischaemic aetiology of heart failure, serum creatinine, and NT-proBNP). FMR, functional mitral regurgitation.

Reproduced from Goliasch G, Bartko PE, Pavo N, *et al.* Refining the prognostic impact of functional mitral regurgitation in chronic heart failure. *Eur Heart J.* 2018 Jan 1;39(1):39–46. doi: 10.1093/eurheartj/ehx402 with permission from Oxford University Press.

(⊃ Figure 9.4.3).[27] The difficult question is when MR is a marker of worse outcome and when it is a cause of increased mortality which can be reversed with its treatment. Since current data suggest that MR intervention does not improve outcome when it is not severe enough (see later), criteria for 'severe secondary MR' were adapted in the recent guidelines and moved back closer to primary MR (⊃ Table 9.4.1).

Current guidelines recommend early referral of patients with HF and moderate or severe MR to a multidisciplinary Heart Team, including HF specialists, for assessment and treatment planning.[2]

In the current European Society of Cardiology (ESC) Guidelines,[1,2] the therapeutic approach in patients with HF and secondary MR has significantly changed.[1,2] After establishing guideline-directed medical treatment (GDMT) with the four standard medications (angiotensin-converting enzyme inhibitor (ACEI)/angiotensin receptor–neprilysin inhibitor (ARNI), beta-blocker, mineralocorticoid receptor antagonist (MRA), sodium–glucose cotransporter 2 inhibitor (SGLT2i)), and increasing to a dosage still tolerated by the patient, patient-specific interventions are recommended to reduce hospitalization and mortality.

Treatment of MR should be considered if HF symptoms and significant secondary MR persist with GDMT, including CRT if indicated. The eventual need for coronary revascularization must also be included into the considerations (⊃ Figure 9.4.4).

In addition, it is recommended that care should be taken to ensure that there is not too much time between the maximum tolerated GDMT and the implementation of valve intervention. Therefore, HF patients undergoing GDMT should be re-evaluated after approximately 3 months regarding valve regurgitation and, if necessary, referred for eventual valve therapy.

Treatment of secondary MR should always be decided within the Heart Team. Surgical treatment should be considered in patients who require revascularization and are not at high surgical risk.[1,2] It may also be considered in patients without the need for revascularization if the surgical risk is low. Otherwise TEER should be considered in carefully selected patients who fulfil the criteria for achieving a reduction in HF hospitalizations. For these, guidelines refer to the population included in the RCT Cardiovascular Outcomes Assessment of the MitraClip Percutaneous Therapy for Heart Failure Patients with Functional Mitral Regurgitation (COAPT; COAPT-like criteria).[28] The main inclusion criteria were:

1. Symptomatic secondary MR (3+ or 4+ by independent echocardiographic core laboratory assessment) due to cardiomyopathy of either ischaemic or non-ischaemic aetiology.

2. The subject has been adequately treated as per applicable standards, including for coronary artery disease, LV dysfunction, MR, and HF.

3. New York Heart Association (NYHA) functional classes II, III, or ambulatory IV.

4. The subject has had at least one hospitalization for HF in the 12 months prior to enrolment and/or a corrected

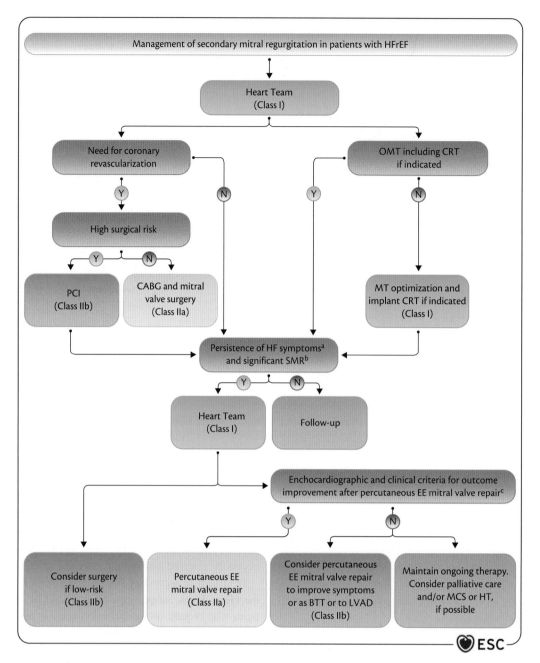

Figure 9.4.4 Management of secondary mitral regurgitation in patients with heart failure with reduced ejection fraction. BTT, bridge to transplantation; CABG, coronary artery bypass graft; CRT, cardiac resynchronization therapy; EE, edge-to-edge; EROA, effective regurgitant orifice area; HF, heart failure; LVAD, left ventricular assist device; LVEF, left ventricular ejection fraction; LVESD, left ventricular end-systolic diameter; MCS, mechanical circulatory support; MT, medical therapy; NYHA, New York Heart Association; OMT, optimal medical therapy; PCI, percutaneous coronary intervention; SMR, secondary mitral regurgitation; TR, tricuspid regurgitation. [a] NYHA classes II–IV. [b] Moderate to severe or severe (EROA >30 mm²). [c] All of the following criteria must be fulfilled: LVEF 20–50%; LVESD <70 mm; systolic pulmonary pressure <70 mmHg; absence of moderate or severe right ventricular dysfunction or severe TR; and absence of haemodynamic instability. Colour code for classes of recommendation: green for Class of recommendation I; yellow for Class of recommendation IIa; orange for Class of recommendation IIb (see Table 1 in reference (2) for further details on classes of recommendation).
McDonagh TA, Metra M, Adamo M, et al; ESC Scientific Document Group. 2021 ESC Guidelines for the diagnosis and treatment of acute and chronic heart failure. *Eur Heart J.* 2021 Sep 21;42(36):3599–3726. doi: 10.1093/eurheartj/ehab368. © The European Society of Cardiology. Reprinted by permission of Oxford University Press.

B-type natriuretic peptide (BNP) level of ≥300 pg/mL or a corrected N-terminal proBNP (NT-proBNP) level of ≥1500 pg/mL.

5. The local Heart Team has determined that mitral valve surgery will not be offered as a treatment option, even if the subject is randomized to the control group.

6. LVEF of ≥20% and ≤50%.

7. LV end-systolic dimension of ≤70 mm.

8. Systolic pulmonary artery pressure of ≤70 mmHg.

9. No moderate or severe right ventricular dysfunction.

8. Anatomy judged suitable for TEER.

This RCT demonstrated a significant benefit of TEER in addition to GDMT, compared to GDMT alone, for the primary endpoint of death or HF rehospitalization at 2 years, as well as for several prespecified secondary endpoints, including all-cause mortality (⮕ Figure 9.4.5a). These results have recently been confirmed over a 3-year period and the improvement was independent of the aetiology—ischaemic (ICM) or non-ischaemic cardiomyopathy.[29]

However, a second RCT studying the effectiveness of TEER versus GDMT in secondary MR—MITRA-FR[30]—failed to demonstrate a significant benefit over a follow-up period of 2 years (⮕ Figure 9.4.5b).[31] The discrepant results of these two trials have been discussed excessively since their publication.[32,33] Differences in trial design, patient selection, definition of MR severity, use of medical therapy, and technical factors may play a role (⮕ Table 9.4.2). The most striking differences between the

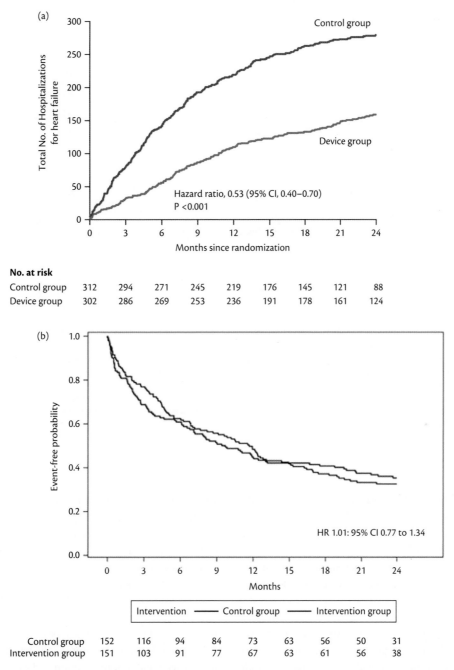

Figure 9.4.5 Impact of transcatheter mitral valve repair on the outcome of patients with heart failure in randomized controlled trials: COAPT (a) and MITRA-FR (b) Trial. (a) Hospitalization for heart failure in the COAPT trial. (b) Kaplan–Meier estimates of survival without a primary outcome event (death from any cause or unplanned hospitalization for heart failure). CI, confidence interval; HR, hazard ratio.

A. Reproduced from Stone GW, Lindenfeld J, Abraham WT, et al; COAPT Investigators. Transcatheter Mitral-Valve Repair in Patients with Heart Failure. *N Engl J Med*. 2018 Dec 13;379(24):2307–2318. doi: 10.1056/NEJMoa1806640 with permission from Massachusetts Medical Society. B. Reproduced from Iung B, Armoiry X, Vahanian A, et al; MITRA-FR Investigators. Percutaneous repair or medical treatment for secondary mitral regurgitation: outcomes at 2 years. *Eur J Heart Fail*. 2019 Dec;21(12):1619–1627. doi: 10.1002/ejhf.1616 with permission from John Wiley and Sons.

Table 9.4.2 Key differences between COAPT and MITRA-FR trials

Primary endpoint		MITRA-FR	COAPT
		All-cause death and hospitalization for CHF at 1 year	**All hospitalizations for CHF within 2 years (including recurrent events)**
Key exclusion criteria	Heart failure severity	NYHA class <II	NYHA class <II ACC/AHA stage D heart failure
	Left ventricular dimensions	No exclusion criteria	LVESD >70 mm
	Coronary artery disease	CABG or PCI performed within 1 month	
	Right ventricle	No exclusion criteria	Right-sided congestive heart failure with moderate or severe right ventricular dysfunction
	Pulmonary disease	No exclusion criteria	COPD with home oxygen therapy or chronic oral steroid use
			Estimated or measured PAP >70 mmHg
Principal baseline	Number of patients screened	452	1576
Characteristics	Number of patients enrolled (ITT)	304	614
	Mean age (years)	70 ± 10	72 ± 12
	Mean LVEF (%)	33 ± 7	31 ± 10
	MR severity (EROA, cm^2)	0.31 ± 0.10	0.41 ± 0.15
	Mean indexed LVEDV (mL/m^2)	135 ± 35	10 ± 34
Safety and efficacy	Complications (%)[a]	14.6	8.5
Endpoints in the intervention arm	Implantation of multiple clips (%)	54	62
	Post-procedural	92	95
	MR grade ≤2 + at 1 year (%)[b]	83	95
	Hospitalization for CHF at 1 year (%)	49	38
	30-day mortality (%)	3.3	2.3
	1-year mortality (%)	24	19

[a] MITRA-FR definition of prespecified serious adverse events: device implant failure, transfusion or vascular complication requiring surgery, atrial septal defect, cardiogenic shock, cardiac embolism/stroke, tamponade, and urgent cardiac surgery.

[b] According to the European Society of Cardiology/European Association for Cardio-Thoracic Surgery guidelines in MITRA-FR, and the AHA/ACC Guidelines in COAPT.

ACC, American College of Cardiology: AHA, American Heart Association; CABG, coronary artery bypass graft; CHF, congestive heart failure; COPD, chronic obstructive pulmonary disease; EROA, effective regurgitant orifice area; ITT, intention to treat; LVEDV, left ventricular end-diastolic volume; LVEF, left ventricular ejection fraction; LVESD, left ventricular end-systolic diameter; MR, mitral regurgitation; NYHA, New York Heart Association; PAP, pulmonary artery pressure; PCI, percutaneous coronary intervention.

Reproduced from Praz F, Grasso C, Taramasso M, *et al*. Mitral regurgitation in heart failure: time for a rethink. *Eur Heart J*. 2019 Jul 14;40(27):2189–2193. doi: 10.1093/eurheartj/ehz222 with permission from Oxford University Press.

study populations are that COAPT patients had more severe MR and less dilated LVs. Because of different definitions used in the two trials, suspected differences in MR reduction and procedural complications are less certain.[34]

The differences in patient characteristics stimulated post hoc analyses. However, even when patients were selected according to COAPT criteria, no clear benefit from TEER was observed in the MITRA-FR trial.[33] Conversely, a subgroup with 'MITRA-FR' characteristics was analysed in the COAPT trial. There was no difference in mortality and hospitalization, but this group of patients showed an improvement in quality of life and 6-minute walking test.[35]

The differences in patient characteristics between trials (more severe MR and less dilated LVs in COAPT) led to the concept of 'disproportionately' severe MR as a criterion to predict benefit from valve intervention.[36] However, even this group of patients

from MITRA-FR were not found to benefit from intervention.[37] In addition, surveys of unselected HF patients in Canada have shown that only a relatively small proportion of patients are true 'COAPT' candidates.[38]

Thus, the discrepant results of the two currently available RCTs as yet could not be entirely resolved, and further research will be required to improve patient selection for valve intervention.

If the aforementioned COAPT inclusion criteria are not met, interventional therapy may still be considered by the Heart Team (Class IIb indication) to improve the patient's symptoms (e.g. reduced exertional dyspnoea, improved walking distance) or to stabilize the patient until possible transplantation or LV assist device (LVAD) therapy according to current guidelines.[1,2]

Technical suitability remains an important issue in decision-making. Unfavourable anatomical conditions for TEER were recently summarized in a consensus document[39] and should be excluded beforehand. For example, in the presence of a very short posterior mitral leaflet or MR mainly caused by a cleft in one leaflet, an inadequate reduction of MR by TEER is to be expected. This is of particular importance as relevant residual MR (grade 2 or higher) has been shown to be associated with poor long-term outcomes.[40,41]

To what extent patients with atrial functional MR benefit from TEER remains a matter of debate. Patients with this type of secondary MR often have preserved LV systolic function, in addition to long-standing AF, and may therefore also be suitable candidates for surgical annuloplasty.[42] If LA dilatation is not advanced, preservation or restoration of sinus rhythm can often also reduce MR.[43]

Current ESC guidelines are based on data for TEER using the MitraClip device (Abbott Vascular, Santa Clara, CA, USA), for which results of randomized trials (EVEREST II, COAPT, MITRA-FR) are available, as well as of large registries (REALISM, TRAMI Registry, European Sentinel Registry, ACCESS-EU, GRASP, MitraSwiss). Further RCT results are expected soon (e.g. RESHAPE-HF II).

Future directions of interventional treatment techniques

In the meantime, the next generation of MitraClip, as well as another TEER device (PASCAL Transcatheter Valve Repair System, Edwards Lifesciences, Irvine, CA, USA), have been introduced to the market.[44] These differ not only in design, but also in function. For example, separate leaflet grasp is possible with the newer devices (▶ Video 9.4.1).

A comparison of the two available TEER systems (MitraClip vs PASCAL) is currently being conducted in the CLASP IID/IIF trial in patients with both primary and secondary MR. Results will be available in the upcoming years (available from: https://clinicaltrials.gov/ct2/show/NCT03706833).

In addition to the largely used TEER devices, other percutaneous mitral valve repair systems have been developed and evaluated in studies in recent years (▶ Figure 9.4.1). Direct annuloplasty as a catheter procedure comes closest to surgical annuloplasty. In this procedure, a band (Cardioband, Edwards Lifesciences) is fixed to the annulus, with multiple anchors, and finally tightened, resulting in a reduction of the annulus size and consequently a reduction in MR.[45] This procedure has the advantage over TEER therapy in that it does not preclude other subsequent catheter-based valve interventions.

Indirect annuloplasty with the Carillon device is introduced via the coronary sinus and thus results in a reduction of the annulus, which, in turn, can lead to a significant reduction in the mitral regurgitant volume.[46]

Another new treatment method is valve replacement via transapical access. Different valve types with different anchoring mechanisms are being tested or are already in the approval process (e.g. Evoque TMVR/Edwards; Intrepid (Medtronic/APOLLO trial); Neovasc Tiara). For the Evoque and Intrepid systems, transseptal delivery has also been evaluated. For the Tendyne system, CE approval was obtained in 2020, but clinical studies are still lacking. Initial results of the feasibility study are promising and show comparable results to patients treated by TEER.[47] Implantation appears to be feasible, even in cases of severe leaflet and ring calcification, and may therefore offer a true adjunct to TEER. However, further studies addressing in particular the risk of LV outflow tract obstruction and the durability of these valves are needed.

Tricuspid regurgitation

TR is most frequently secondary and then caused by pressure and/or volume overload-mediated right ventricular dilatation or right atrium and tricuspid annulus enlargement in association with chronic AF.[1] Secondary TR is mostly associated with left-sided VHD or LV dysfunction (isolated in <10% of subjects) and independently related to mortality.[48] In patients with HF and reduced LVEF, secondary TR is a very frequent finding and has been demonstrated to be an independent predictor of outcomes in these patients (▶ Figure 9.4.6).[49]

Similarly to secondary MR, even mild TR is already associated with worse outcome,[49] and the question of when secondary TR is a marker of worse outcome and when it causes worse outcome that can be approved by valve intervention remains insufficiently resolved.[1] Surgery in isolated TR is associated with high in-hospital mortality of close to 10%[50] and is currently performed in a minority of affected patients. The evolution of catheter interventional treatment options which have been shown to effectively reduce TR severity and improve symptoms with low procedural risk has gained great interest in the interventional treatment of the 'forgotten valve'.[51]

This resulted in new insights in the anatomy of this valve, which is highly variable and determines success of interventional treatment. In most cases, the valve consists of a large anterior and septal leaflet, with a smaller posterior leaflet. However, the leaflets are often fused or can be divided into smaller leaflets by clefts.[52]

Assessment of TR is clinically and echocardiographically even more challenging than that of the mitral valve. This is due to, on one hand, difficult (transoesophageal) echocardiographic visualization and, on the other hand, the different mechanisms leading to regurgitation. Numerous criteria, such as vena contracta, proximal isovelocity surface area (PISA), effective regurgitant orifice area (EROA), contour and density of the continuous wave spectrum, or systolic reflux into the hepatic veins, exist and can be used to classify TR severity.[53] There is no single measured value that allows a precise severity classification, and an integrated approach including multiple signs and parameters is recommended (▶ Table 9.4.3).[20,53]

Recently, especially in device studies, classification of severity into five grades has been introduced. Severe TR is further differentiated into severe, massive, and torrential regurgitation.[54] This allows a more precise classification of TR reduction after valve intervention.

The width of the tricuspid annulus serves as a surrogate for TR severity. In addition to the diameters, the function of the right

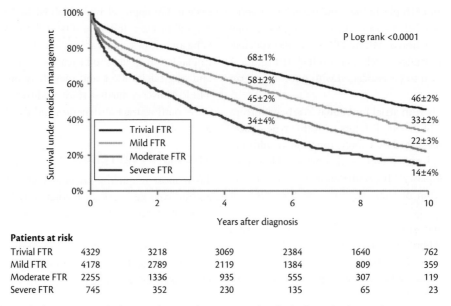

Figure 9.4.6 Survival under medical management by functional tricuspid regurgitation (FTR). The figure displays Kaplan–Meier curves for the various FTR grades (trivial to severe) at long-term follow-up.

Reproduced from Benfari G, Antoine C, Miller WL, *et al*. Excess Mortality Associated With Functional Tricuspid Regurgitation Complicating Heart Failure With Reduced Ejection Fraction. *Circulation*. 2019 Jul 16;140(3):196–206. doi: 10.1161/CIRCULATIONAHA.118.038946 with permission from Wolters Kluwer.

ventricle must be determined, especially in cases of more than mild insufficiency,[20] and three-dimensional volumetric measurements are particularly suitable.

Table 9.4.3 Echocardiographic criteria for grading severity of tricuspid regurgitation

Qualitative	
Tricuspid valve morphology	Abnormal/flail
Colour flow regurgitant jet	Very large central jet or eccentric wall impinging jet[a]
CW signal of regurgitant jet	Dense/triangular with early peaking
Semi-quantitative	
Vena contracta width (mm)	>7[a,b]
PISA radius (mm)	>9[c]
Hepatic vein flow[c]	Systolic flow reversal
Tricuspid inflow	E-wave dominant ≥1 m/s[d]
Quantitative	
EROA (mm²)	≥40
Regurgitant volume (mL/beat)	≥45
Enlargement of cardiac chambers/vessels	RV, RA, inferior vena cava

[a] At a Nyquist limit of 50–60 cm/s.
[b] Preferably biplane.
[c] Baseline Nyquist limit shift of 28 cm/s.
[d] In the absence of other causes of elevated RA pressure.

CW, continuous wave; EROA, effective regurgitant orifice area; PISA, proximal isovelocity surface area; RA, right atrium; RV, right ventricle.

Vahanian A, Beyersdorf F, Praz F, *et al*; ESC/EACTS Scientific Document Group. 2021 ESC/EACTS Guidelines for the management of valvular heart disease. *Eur Heart J*. 2022 Feb 12;43(7):561–632. doi: 10.1093/eurheartj/ehab395. © The European Society of Cardiology. Reprinted by permission of Oxford University Press.

Currently recommended management of TR is summarized in ➲ Figure 9.4.7.[1]

If patients with HF and severe secondary TR remain symptomatic despite medical therapy (especially with diuretics and aldosterone antagonists), evaluation for valve intervention may be considered. As in severe MR, the time to decide on therapy should not be delayed too long to prevent irreversible remodelling of the right ventricle. Similarly to MR, if regurgitation is too severe with extreme annulus dilatation, intervention may no longer achieve symptomatic or clinical improvement. In addition, severe right ventricular dysfunction and pulmonary hypertension—in particularly if pre-capillary—adversely affect post-interventional outcome.[55]

Several catheter-based interventional procedures have been introduced in recent years and may be considered when surgical valve repair is not an option (➲ Figure 9.4.1). These include direct annuloplasty (Cardioband,[56] edge-to-edge repair with TriClip[56] and PASCAL[57]) and heterotopic or orthotopic valve implantation.[58]

⬤ Videos 9.4.2 and 9.4.3 show examples of echocardiograms prior to and after TR treatment with TriClip and Cardioband, respectively.

In the last 3–4 years, numerous studies have demonstrated effective catheter interventional treatment of TR,[51,57] with TEER being the most commonly used technique. In most cases, this involves bicuspidization of the tricuspid valve by coaptation of the leaflet edges of the septal and anterior leaflets.

With the first-generation models, good TR reduction and stable clinical improvement over 1 year were documented in the TRILUMINATE trial.[59] It has also been shown that patients with procedural failure tend to have a worse prognosis at follow-up.[60] Predictors of procedural failure have been shown to be a large

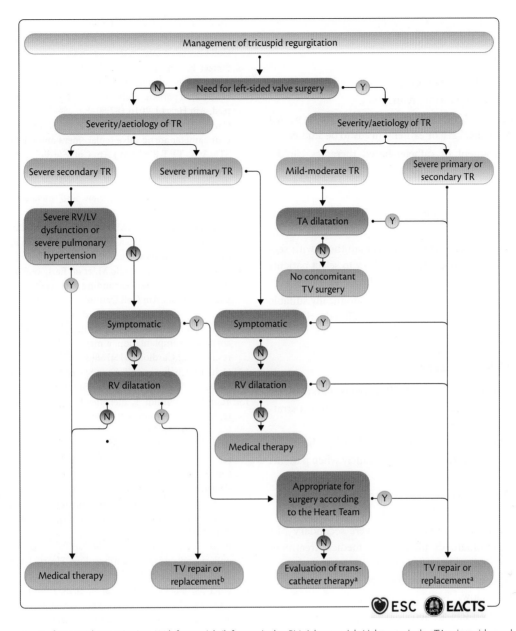

Figure 9.4.7 Management of tricuspid regurgitation. LV, left ventricle/left ventricular; RV, right ventricle/right ventricular; TA, tricuspid annulus; TR, tricuspid regurgitation; TV, tricuspid valve. [a] The Heart Team with expertise in the treatment of tricuspid valve disease evaluates anatomical eligibility for transcatheter therapy, including jet location, coaptation gap, leaflet tethering, and potential interference with pacing lead. [b] Replacement when repair is not feasible.
Vahanian A, Beyersdorf F, Praz F, et al; ESC/EACTS Scientific Document Group. 2021 ESC/EACTS Guidelines for the management of valvular heart disease. *Eur Heart J.* 2022 Feb 12;43(7):561–632. doi: 10.1093/eurheartj/ehab395. © The European Society of Cardiology. Reprinted by permission of Oxford University Press.

gap and an unfavourable location of the main regurgitation in the posteroseptal commissure.[61]

In addition, this method has also been shown to be associated with longer survival and lower HF rehospitalization in a propensity score-matched case-control study, compared to medical therapy alone.[62]

In this regard, there are also several RCTs currently under way that will provide a conclusion on the pros and cons of intervention in the foreseeable future (e.g. CLASP II TR Pivotal; TRISCEND II; TRILUMINATE Pivotal; Tri-FR; TRIC-I-HF; TriValve, D-TRIK German Registry for transcatheter tricuspid valve intervention; TRIC-IT Italian Registry for transcatheter tricuspid valve intervention).

Future directions

Aortic stenosis:

- Optimal timing of intervention to avoid HF development in the long term still requires refinement.
- Improvement of treatment techniques further lowering the risk of intervention and providing optimal early results, as well as durable valves, may further reduce the threshold for intervention.

- Ongoing studies will demonstrate whether HF patients with moderate AS benefit from intervention.

Secondary MR:

- The criteria for selecting patients who are likely to benefit from MR intervention require further refinement.
- Optimal timing of MR intervention—when symptoms persist despite optimal medical HF or earlier—needs to be studied.
- Technical improvement of catheter-based therapies can be expected.

Secondary TR:

- Ongoing RCTs will demonstrate whether TR intervention improves outcome.
- The patient group is more heterogeneous than those with secondary MR, and appropriate criteria for how to select patients for TR intervention need to be established.
- To expand the group of patients who are anatomically suitable for transcatheter interventions with efficient TR reduction, further technical development is required.

Summary and key messages

- It is critical to correctly distinguish HF patients with primary VHD from those with secondary VHD, as the treatment strategies differ fundamentally.
- In primary VHD, intervention should ideally avoid the development HF and is indicated early, and definitely when patients develop HF.
- Patients with HF and secondary VHD require careful evaluation by an interdisciplinary Heart Team.
- In selected patients with moderate to severe secondary MR who remain symptomatic despite optimal medical treatment and CRT if indicated, percutaneous edge-to-edge mitral valve repair should be considered. Surgical intervention may be considered if the risk is low.
- Catheter-based treatment of secondary TR is currently still at an early stage. In patients who remain symptomatic despite medical treatment, intervention may be considered by the Heart Team.

References

1. Vahanian A, Beyersdorf F, Praz F, et al. 2021 ESC/EACTS Guidelines for the management of valvular heart disease. Eur Heart J. 2022;43(7):561–632.
2. McDonagh TA, Metra M, Adamo M, et al. 2021 ESC Guidelines for the diagnosis and treatment of acute and chronic heart failure. Eur Heart J. 2021;42(36):3599–726.
3. Baumgartner H, Hung J, Bermejo J, et al. Recommendations on the echocardiographic assessment of aortic valve stenosis: a focused update from the European Association of Cardiovascular Imaging and the American Society of Echocardiography. J Am Soc Echocardiogr. 2017;30(4):372–92.
4. Clavel MA, Burwash IG, Pibarot P. Cardiac imaging for assessing low-gradient severe aortic stenosis. JACC Cardiovasc Imaging. 2017;10(2):185–202.
5. Jean G, van Mieghem NM, Gegenava T, et al. Moderate aortic stenosis in patients with heart failure and reduced ejection fraction. J Am Coll Cardiol. 2021;77(22):2796–803.
6. Spitzer E, van Mieghem NM, Pibarot P, et al. Rationale and design of the Transcatheter Aortic Valve Replacement to UNload the Left ventricle in patients with ADvanced heart failure (TAVR UNLOAD) trial. Am Heart J. 2016;182:80–8.
7. Carroll JD, Vemulapalli S, Dai D, et al. Procedural experience for transcatheter aortic valve replacement and relation to outcomes: the STS/ACC TVT Registry. J Am Coll Cardiol. 2017;70(1):29–41.
8. Faroux L, Chen S, Muntane-Carol G, et al. Clinical impact of conduction disturbances in transcatheter aortic valve replacement recipients: a systematic review and meta-analysis. Eur Heart J. 2020;41(29):2771–81.
9. Thourani VH, Kodali S, Makkar RR, et al. Transcatheter aortic valve replacement versus surgical valve replacement in intermediate-risk patients: a propensity score analysis. Lancet. 2016;387(10034):2218–25.
10. Williams M, Slater J, Saric M, et al. Early outcomes with the Evolut R repositionable self-expanding transcatheter aortic valve in the United States. J Am Coll Cardiol. 2016;67(13):2172.
11. D'Ascenzo F, Conrotto F, Giordana F, et al. Mid-term prognostic value of coronary artery disease in patients undergoing transcatheter aortic valve implantation: a meta-analysis of adjusted observational results. Int J Cardiol. 2013;168(3):2528–32.
12. Ochiai T, Chakravarty T, Yoon SH, et al. Coronary access after TAVR. JACC Cardiovasc Interv. 2020;13(6):693–705.
13. Yoon SH, Schmidt T, Bleiziffer S, et al. Transcatheter aortic valve replacement in pure native aortic valve regurgitation. J Am Coll Cardiol. 2017;70(22):2752–63.
14. Jiang J, Liu X, He Y, et al. Transcatheter aortic valve replacement for pure native aortic valve regurgitation: a systematic review. Cardiology. 2018;141(3):132–40.
15. Pesarini G, Lunardi M, Piccoli A, et al. Effectiveness and safety of transcatheter aortic valve implantation in patients with pure aortic regurgitation and advanced heart failure. Am J Cardiol. 2018;121(5):642–8.
16. Bartko PE, Pavo N, Perez-Serradilla A, et al. Evolution of secondary mitral regurgitation. Eur Heart J Cardiovasc Imaging. 2018;19(6):622–9.
17. Goel SS, Bajaj N, Aggarwal B, et al. Prevalence and outcomes of unoperated patients with severe symptomatic mitral regurgitation and heart failure: comprehensive analysis to determine the potential role of MitraClip for this unmet need. J Am Coll Cardiol. 2014;63(2):185–6.
18. Grayburn PA, Thomas JD. Basic principles of the echocardiographic evaluation of mitral regurgitation. JACC Cardiovasc Imaging. 2021;14(4):843–53.
19. Myerson SG, d'Arcy J, Christiansen JP, et al. Determination of clinical outcome in mitral regurgitation with cardiovascular magnetic resonance quantification. Circulation. 2016;133(23):2287–96.
20. Lancellotti P, Moura L, Pierard LA, et al. European Association of Echocardiography recommendations for the assessment of valvular regurgitation. Part 2: mitral and tricuspid regurgitation (native valve disease). Eur J Echocardiogr. 2010;11(4):307–32.
21. Otto CM, Nishimura RA, Bonow RO, et al. 2020 ACC/AHA Guideline for the management of patients with valvular heart disease: a report of the American College of Cardiology/American Heart Association Joint Committee on Clinical Practice Guidelines. J Am Coll Cardiol. 2021;77:e25–197.
22. Feldman T, Kar S, Elmariah S, et al. Randomized comparison of percutaneous repair and surgery for mitral regurgitation: 5-year results of EVEREST II. J Am Coll Cardiol. 2015;66(25):2844–54.

23. Asgar AW, Mack MJ, Stone GW. Secondary mitral regurgitation in heart failure: pathophysiology, prognosis, and therapeutic considerations. J Am Coll Cardiol. 2015;65(12):1231–48.

24. Bartko PE, Hulsmann M, Hung J, et al. Secondary valve regurgitation in patients with heart failure with preserved ejection fraction, heart failure with mid-range ejection fraction, and heart failure with reduced ejection fraction. Eur Heart J. 2020;41(29):2799–810.

25. Deferm S, Bertrand PB, Verbrugge FH, et al. Atrial functional mitral regurgitation: JACC review topic of the week. J Am Coll Cardiol. 2019;73(19):2465–76.

26. Bertrand PB, Schwammenthal E, Levine RA, Vandervoort PM. Exercise dynamics in secondary mitral regurgitation: pathophysiology and therapeutic implications. Circulation. 2017;135(3):297–314.

27. Goliasch G, Bartko PE, Pavo N, et al. Refining the prognostic impact of functional mitral regurgitation in chronic heart failure. Eur Heart J. 2018;39(1):39–46.

28. Stone GW, Lindenfeld J, Abraham WT, et al. Transcatheter mitral-valve repair in patients with heart failure. N Engl J Med. 2018;379(24):2307–18.

29. Mack MJ, Lindenfeld J, Abraham WT, et al. 3-year outcomes of transcatheter mitral valve repair in patients with heart failure. J Am Coll Cardiol. 2021;77(8):1029–40.

30. Obadia JF, Messika-Zeitoun D, Leurent G, et al. Percutaneous repair or medical treatment for secondary mitral regurgitation. N Engl J Med. 2018;379(24):2297–306.

31. Iung B, Armoiry X, Vahanian A, et al. Percutaneous repair or medical treatment for secondary mitral regurgitation: outcomes at 2 years. Eur J Heart Fail. 2019;21(12):1619–27.

32. Pibarot P, Delgado V, Bax JJ. MITRA-FR vs. COAPT: lessons from two trials with diametrically opposed results. Eur Heart J Cardiovasc Imaging. 2019;20(6):620–4.

33. Iung B, Messika-Zeitoun D, Boutitie F, et al. Characteristics and outcome of COAPT-eligible patients in the MITRA-FR trial. Circulation. 2020;142(25):2482–4.

34. Praz F, Grasso C, Taramasso M, et al. Mitral regurgitation in heart failure: time for a rethink. Eur Heart J. 2019;40(27):2189–93.

35. Lindenfeld J, Abraham WT, Grayburn PA, et al. Association of effective regurgitation orifice area to left ventricular end-diastolic volume ratio with transcatheter mitral valve repair outcomes: a secondary analysis of the COAPT trial. JAMA Cardiol. 2021;6(4):427–36.

36. Grayburn PA, Sannino A, Packer M. Proportionate and disproportionate functional mitral regurgitation: a new conceptual framework that reconciles the results of the MITRA-FR and COAPT trials. JACC Cardiovasc Imaging. 2019;12(2):353–62.

37. Messika-Zeitoun D, Iung B, Armoiry X, et al. Impact of mitral regurgitation severity and left ventricular remodeling on outcome after MitraClip implantation: results from the Mitra-FR trial. JACC Cardiovasc Imaging. 2021;14(4):742–52.

38. Fine NM, McAlister FA, Howlett JG, Youngson E, Ezekowitz JA. Low prevalence of transcatheter mitral valve repair eligibility in a community heart failure population. Circ Heart Fail. 2020;13(5):e006952.

39. Lim DS, Herrmann HC, Grayburn P, et al. Consensus document on non-suitability for transcatheter mitral valve repair by edge-to-edge therapy. Structural Heart. 2021;5(3):227–33.

40. Kar S, Mack MJ, Lindenfeld J, et al. Relationship between residual mitral regurgitation and clinical and quality-of-life outcomes after transcatheter and medical treatments in heart failure: COAPT trial. Circulation. 2021;144(6):426–37.

41. Reichart D, Kalbacher D, Rubsamen N, et al. The impact of residual mitral regurgitation after MitraClip therapy in functional mitral regurgitation. Eur J Heart Fail. 2020;22(10):1840–8.

42. Carino D, Lapenna E, Ascione G, et al. Is mitral annuloplasty an effective treatment for severe atrial functional mitral regurgitation? J Card Surg. 2021;36(2):596–602.

43. Nishino S, Watanabe N, Ashikaga K, et al. Reverse remodeling of the mitral valve complex after radiofrequency catheter ablation for atrial fibrillation: a serial 3-dimensional echocardiographic study. Circ Cardiovasc Imaging. 2019;12(10):e009317.

44. Szerlip M, Spargias KS, Makkar R, et al. 2-year outcomes for transcatheter repair in patients with mitral regurgitation from the CLASP study. JACC Cardiovasc Interv. 2021;14(14):1538–48.

45. Messika-Zeitoun D, Nickenig G, Latib A, et al. Transcatheter mitral valve repair for functional mitral regurgitation using the Cardioband system: 1-year outcomes. Eur Heart J. 2019;40(5):466–72.

46. Witte KK, Lipiecki J, Siminiak T, et al. The REDUCE FMR trial: a randomized sham-controlled study of percutaneous mitral annuloplasty in functional mitral regurgitation. JACC Heart Fail. 2019;7(11):945–55.

47. Sorajja P, Moat N, Badhwar V, et al. Initial feasibility study of a new transcatheter mitral prosthesis: the first 100 patients. J Am Coll Cardiol. 2019;73(11):1250–60.

48. Topilsky Y, Maltais S, Medina Inojosa J, et al. Burden of tricuspid regurgitation in patients diagnosed in the community setting. JACC Cardiovasc Imaging. 2019;12(3):433–42.

49. Benfari G, Antoine C, Miller WL, et al. Excess mortality associated with functional tricuspid regurgitation complicating heart failure with reduced ejection fraction. Circulation. 2019;140(3):196–206.

50. Zack CJ, Fender EA, Chandrashekar P, et al. National trends and outcomes in isolated tricuspid valve surgery. J Am Coll Cardiol. 2017;70(24):2953–60.

51. Taramasso M, Alessandrini H, Latib A, et al. Outcomes after current transcatheter tricuspid valve intervention: mid-term results from the international TriValve Registry. JACC Cardiovasc Interv. 2019;12(2):155–65.

52. Hahn RT, Weckbach LT, Noack T, et al. Proposal for a standard echocardiographic tricuspid valve nomenclature. JACC Cardiovasc Imaging. 2021;14(7):1299–305.

53. Zoghbi WA, Adams D, Bonow RO, et al. Recommendations for non-invasive evaluation of native valvular regurgitation: a report from the American Society of Echocardiography developed in collaboration with the Society for Cardiovascular Magnetic Resonance. J Am Soc Echocardiogr. 2017;30(4):303–71.

54. Hahn RT, Thomas JD, Khalique OK, Cavalcante JL, Praz F, Zoghbi WA. Imaging assessment of tricuspid regurgitation severity. JACC Cardiovasc Imaging. 2019;12(3):469–90.

55. Stocker TJ, Hertell H, Orban M, et al. Cardiopulmonary hemodynamic profile predicts mortality after transcatheter tricuspid valve repair in chronic heart Failure. JACC Cardiovasc Interv. 2021;14(1):29–38.

56. Nickenig G, Weber M, Schueler R, et al. 6-month outcomes of tricuspid valve reconstruction for patients with severe tricuspid regurgitation. J Am Coll Cardiol. 2019;73(15):1905–15.

57. Kitamura M, Fam NP, Braun D, et al. 12-month outcomes of transcatheter tricuspid valve repair with the PASCAL system for severe tricuspid regurgitation. Catheter Cardiovasc Interv. 2021;97(6):1281–9.

58. Fam NP, von Bardeleben RS, Hensey M, et al. Transfemoral transcatheter tricuspid valve replacement with the EVOQUE system: a multicenter, observational, first-in-human experience. JACC Cardiovasc Interv. 2021;14(5):501–11.

59. Lurz P, von Bardeleben SR, Weber M, *et al.* Transcatheter edge-to-edge repair for treatment of tricuspid regurgitation. J Am Coll Cardiol. 2021;77(3):229–39.

60. Mehr M, Taramasso M, Besler C, *et al.* 1-year outcomes after edge-to-edge valve repair for symptomatic tricuspid regurgitation: results from the TriValve Registry. JACC Cardiovasc Interv. 2019;12(15):1451–61.

61. Besler C, Orban M, Rommel KP, *et al.* Predictors of procedural and clinical outcomes in patients with symptomatic tricuspid regurgitation undergoing transcatheter edge-to-edge repair. JACC Cardiovasc Interv. 2018;11(12):1119–28.

62. Taramasso M, Benfari G, van der Bijl P, *et al.* Transcatheter versus medical treatment of patients with symptomatic severe tricuspid regurgitation. J Am Coll Cardiol. 2019;74(24):2998–3008.

Discover all content online by searching for this book's title or ISBN at academic.oup.com/oxford-medicine-online.

If you do not have access, or are interested in accessing other titles, you can recommend it to your librarian.

CHAPTER 9.5

Ancillary procedures

Andrew JS Coats, Piotr P Ponikowski,
Maria-Rosa Costanzo, and
William T Abraham

Introduction

The other chapters in this section on non-pharmacological treatment for heart failure (HF) cover some very important initiatives in the management of heart failure with reduced ejection fraction (HFrEF) and increasingly also heart failure with preserved ejection fraction (HFpEF). Effective treatments for HF are still an urgent priority because of the large residual mortality and morbidity of this condition. Much recent innovation has been in the field of implantable devices, as well as in other procedures which offer potential benefit. Some of these have recently received approval both in the United States and in Europe, particularly through the new Breakthrough Devices Program of the United States Food and Drug Administration (FDA) (➲ Figure 9.5.1).[1] This program accelerates considerably the time to offer therapy to selected patients, and also allows novel clinical trial methodologies and more achievable interim trial endpoints to be used for initial approval. Early market access and reimbursement possibilities are thus enabled, and early conditional approval allows some revenue to flow to the innovator manufacturers, which, as part of the program, commit to ongoing trial evaluation to allow later generation of evidence to satisfy statutory requirements for efficacy and safety documentation.

This chapter reviews recently approved procedures and devices, and explores what might be on the horizon in this area, with already successful phase 2 trial results. The readers of this chapter are also advised to look at ➲ Chapters 9.4 and 12.6–12.7 on valve interventions and catheter ablation techniques. These will not be covered in this chapter.

Cardiac contractility modulation

Cardiac contractility modulation (CCM) is an FDA-approved device therapy for treatment of symptomatic HFrEF. It is one of the ancillary devices approved by the US FDA (➲ Figure 9.5.2). It utilizes the OPTIMIZER* Smart Implantable Pulse Generator, which is an electrical stimulation device placed adjacent to the ventricular muscle, but designed to stimulate the muscle in the absolute refractory period of the cardiac cycle, thereby showing no pacemaker or resynchronization activity. It was the first therapy approved by the FDA under its Breakthrough Therapy Device scheme. It is indicated to reduce symptoms and improve exercise tolerance in patients with HF, with its main indication being for patients with reduced and moderately reduced LVEF and normal QRS duration who currently do not have other device-based therapeutic alternatives in the United States. When approved, CCM™ was implanted in over 3500 patients and was available in Europe and in more than 40 other countries. Despite improvements in drug and device treatment of HFrEF, survival rates and symptom burden remain poor. Thus, CCM, if proven to be clinically beneficial, could fulfil a significant unmet medical need. CCM has been studied in patients with symptomatic HF on optimal medical therapy (OMT) and

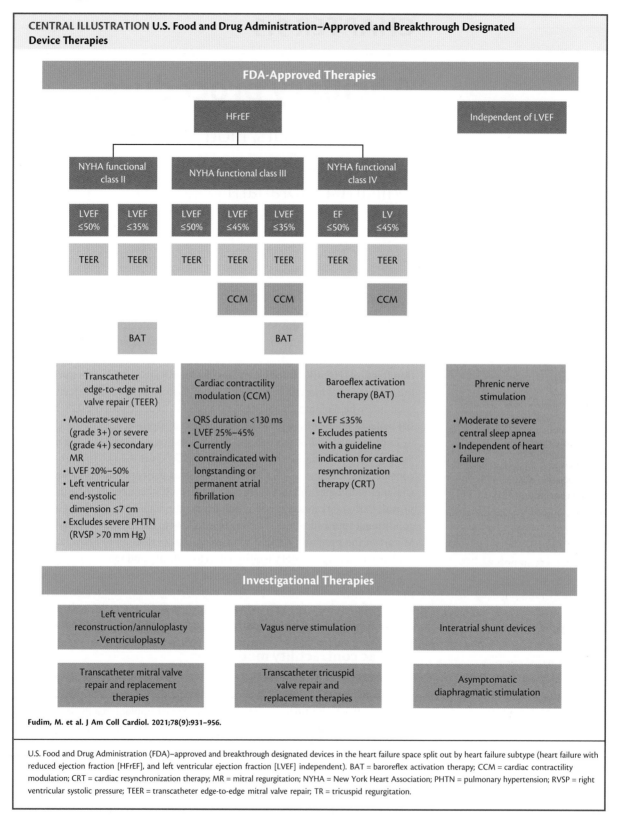

CENTRAL ILLUSTRATION U.S. Food and Drug Administration–Approved and Breakthrough Designated Device Therapies

Fudim, M. et al. J Am Coll Cardiol. 2021;78(9):931–956.

U.S. Food and Drug Administration (FDA)–approved and breakthrough designated devices in the heart failure space split out by heart failure subtype (heart failure with reduced ejection fraction [HFrEF], and left ventricular ejection fraction [LVEF] independent). BAT = baroreflex activation therapy; CCM = cardiac contractility modulation; CRT = cardiac resynchronization therapy; MR = mitral regurgitation; NYHA = New York Heart Association; PHTN = pulmonary hypertension; RVSP = right ventricular systolic pressure; TEER = transcatheter edge-to-edge mitral valve repair; TR = tricuspid regurgitation.

Figure 9.5.1 Heart failure procedure/devices approved or designated eligible through the Breakthrough Device Program by the United States Food and Drug Administration (FDA).

Reproduced from Fudim M, Abraham WT, von Bardeleben RS, Lindenfeld J, et al, Device Therapy in Chronic Heart Failure: JACC State-of-the-Art Review. J Am Coll Cardiol. 2021 Aug 31;78(9):931–956. doi: 10.1016/j.jacc.2021.06.040 with permission from Elsevier .

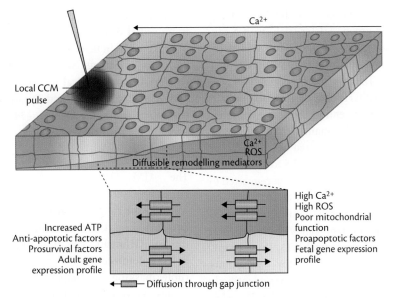

Figure 9.5.2 Conjectured influence of CCM electrical pulses on intact ventricular myocardium. Local application of CCM is thought to induce a molecular and metabolic sink for elevated levels of diastolic calcium and ROS, and other abnormalities associated with the pathophysiology of the failing myocardium. Intercellular gradients lead to the diffusion of various mediators across gap junctions, acting in a source–sink relationship, to ameliorate the harmful milieu of the failing myocardium adjacent to the region of CCM application (inset). Over time, chronic CCM therapy is thought to generate gradients that enable propagation of reverse remodelling throughout the myocardium. ATP, adenosine triphosphate; Ca^{2+}, calcium; CCM, cardiac contractility modulation; ROS, reactive oxygen species.

Source data from Lyon AR, Samara MA, Feldman DS. Cardiac contractility modulation therapy in advanced systolic heart failure. *Nat Rev Cardiol*. 2013 Oct;10(10):584–98. doi: 10.1038/nrcardio.2013.114. Epub 2013 Aug 13. Erratum in: *Nat Rev Cardiol*. 2014 Apr;11(4):188.

with a QRS duration of <130 ms and an ejection fraction (EF) of <45%, and as such, it has been investigated in patients ineligible for cardiac resynchronization therapy (CRT). In such patients, CCM has been shown in three studies of small to medium size to improve quality of life (QoL), left ventricular ejection fraction (LVEF), indices of diastolic function, New York Heart Association (NYHA) classification, 6-minute walking test (6MWT) distance, and peak oxygen consumption (VO_2) during cardiopulmonary stress testing. These findings have recently been confirmed in the Bayesian-designed randomized FIX-HF-5C study, an approved trial design under the Expedited Access Pathway of the FDA. These trial results thus led to the subsequent approval of CCM by the FDA to improve 6-minute hall walk (6MHW) distance, QoL, and functional status of NYHA class III HF patients who remain symptomatic despite guideline-directed medical therapy (GDMT), are in normal sinus rhythm, are not indicated for CRT, and have an LVEF ranging from 25% to 45%. This trial, although not powered as a mortality and morbidity trial, also showed a nominally, but borderline, significant reduction in the 6-month composite rate of cardiac mortality and HF hospitalization, with the composite of cardiovascular death and HF hospitalization reduced from 10.8% to 2.9% ($P = 0.048$). Based on the first three trials, HF treatment guidelines had already suggested CCM could be considered in patients with symptomatic HF despite OMT and with normal or mildly prolonged QRS duration and reduced LVEF. Since interventions targeted at ameliorating exercise intolerance in HFrEF are becoming increasingly important in advanced HF, we performed an updated individual patient systematic review and meta-analysis to evaluate the efficacy of

CCM, with a focus on functional capacity and QoL instruments in HFrEF patients.

Mode of action

CCM is an electrical technique that delivers biphasic pulses of relatively high voltage to the right ventricular septum during the absolute refractory period in the myocardium, via a small implantable pulse generator in a minimally invasive procedure. It has been shown to improve calcium handling, reverse fetal myocyte gene expression, and facilitate reverse remodelling. CCM has been reported to increase inotropic efficacy, with no commensurate increase in myocardial oxygen consumption. The mode of action has been reviewed[2] and includes quick-onset positive inotropy, associated with changes in cardiomyocyte calcium (Ca^{2+}) fluxes and phospholamban phosphorylation. Cardiac reverse remodelling and contractility increases have been described and are hypothesized to be the mechanism underlying an increase in exercise capacity that is a consistent feature of the interventional trials of CCM.

Clinical trial data

CCM has been studied in mild to moderately symptomatic HF patients with a QRS duration of <130 ms and an EF of <45%, and thereby who were ineligible for CRT. In such patients, CCM has been shown in three prospective randomized controlled trials (RCTs) to improve QoL, LVEF, NYHA class, 6MWT distance, and peak VO_2. The first[3] was a small pilot study that randomized 49 NYHA class III–IV HFrEF subjects with a normal QRS duration to either active or inactive devices for 6 months. The

6MWT distance and peak VO_2 were numerically, but not significantly, higher in the active group. A later trial,[4] with a randomized, double-blind, crossover design, randomly assigned 164 NYHA class II–III HFrEF patients to 3 months of sham treatment first or sham treatment second. The co-primary endpoints of peak VO_2 and Minnesota Living with Heart Failure Questionnaire (MLWHFQ) were both better at the end of the active treatment periods, compared to the end of the sham treatment periods (both $P = 0.03$). The FIX-HF5 trial[5] randomized 428 NYHA class II–IV HFrEF (≤35%) patients with a narrow QRS to either CCM plus GDMT or GDMT alone. The primary endpoint requested by the FDA, namely the ventilatory anaerobic threshold (VAT), was an unusual one because VAT is frequently unmeasurable in HF patients. Although the VAT was not significantly improved, there was improvement in the more reliable peak VO_2 (by 0.65 mL/ kg/min; $P = 0.024$), as well as in MLWHFQ (by −9.7 points; $P < 0.0001$). A post hoc hypothesis-generating analysis identified a subgroup (characterized by baseline EF of ≥25% and NYHA class III symptoms) in which all parameters were improved by CCM and this hypothesis was subsequently tested in the FIX-HF-5C study, a Bayesian-designed confirmatory trial. The FIX-HF-5C study confirmed a significant increase in peak VO_2 in this patient cohort, which led to approval under the Expedited Access Pathway of the FDA. The trial results thus led to subsequent approval of CCM by the FDA to improve 6MHW distance, QoL, and functional status of NYHA class III HF patients who remain symptomatic despite GDMT, are in normal sinus rhythm, are not indicated for CRT, and have an LVEF ranging from 25% to 45%. The FIX-HF-5C study was not a mortality and morbidity trial, but it was associated with a nominally significant reduction in the 6-month composite rate of cardiac mortality and HF hospitalization, with the composite of cardiovascular death and HF hospitalization reduced from 10.8% to 2.9% ($P = 0.048$).[6]

A recent individual patient data (IPD) meta-analysis of all non-confounded prospective RCTs of CCM versus control reported on the effects of CCM on functional capacity and/or QoL questionnaires in patients with HF.[7] Five trials were identified, including four randomized studies enrolling 801 participants for all endpoints of interest, and for peak VO_2 alone ($n = 60$). Compared to control, CCM increased peak VO_2 by 0.93 mL/kg/ min (0.56–1.30); $P < 0.00001$), along with improved 6MWT distance of 18 m (5.5–30.5; $P = 0.005$) and improved MLWHFQ QoL estimate, suggesting statistically significant and clinically meaningful improvements. There were insufficient data for any assessment of survival.

Registry data

CCM is approved in CE-mark countries for NYHA classes II, III, and ambulatory IV. Data on 503 patients receiving CCM based on these indications in the European Union, including some patients with atrial fibrillation, were reported in the CCM-REG, a prospective, observational registry study conducted between October 2013 and October 2019 that included 503 patients from 51 European centres.[8] HF hospitalization decreased from 0.74 before to 0.25 after study entry events per patient-year during the

2-year follow-up ($P < 0.0001$). NYHA class and MLWHFQ also improved at 6, 12, 18, and 24 months ($P < 0.0001$), with similar improvements in three LVEF tertiles (≤25%, 26–34%, and ≥35%) and also in patients with atrial fibrillation or those in sinus rhythm. Overall survival was compared to that predicted by the MAGGIC risk score at 1 and 3 years, and was improved in the entire cohort and in the LVEF 26–34% and ≥35% subgroups, compared to the predicted rates.

Ongoing trials

The AIM HIGHer Study (ClinicalTrials.gov identifier: NCT05064709) is designed to assess CCM[*] in HF subjects with LVEF in the range of ≥40% and ≤60%, thus approximating to, and including, the heart failure with mildly reduced ejection fraction (HFmrEF) group. It aims to recruit 1500 participants in a randomized parallel group intervention trial with quadruple masking (participant, care provider, investigator, outcomes assessor), so that the subject, entire site research team, implanting physician, Clinical Events Committee (CEC), and clinical study monitors will all be blinded to treatment assignment. The endpoints are: Part 1, efficacy endpoints—change in 6-minute walk distance (6MWD) from baseline to 6 months and change in Kansas City Cardiomyopathy Questionnaire Clinical Summary Score (KCCQ CSS) at 6 months; and Part 2 endpoint—the hierarchical composite of mortality, morbidity, and health status outcomes (KCCQ CSS) over 18 months. The INTEGRA-D study will assess a hybrid class III medical device that combines CCM[*] therapy and a single-chamber implantable cardiac defibrillator (ICD) in HFrEF patients who are in NYHA class III with an LVEF in the range of 25–35%, with a Class I indication for an ICD according to the current American College of Cardiology Foundation (ACCF)/American Heart Association (AHA)/Heart Rhythm Society (HRS) Guidelines.

Autonomic modulation

Despite improvements in management of HFrEF, many patients remain with NYHA class II or III symptoms, with reduced survival, ongoing risk of frequent HF hospitalization, poor QoL, and limited functional capacity.[9,10] In addition, the majority of HFrEF patients are not eligible for advanced HF treatments with limited availability such as left ventricular assist device (LVAD) and transplantation. Therefore, there remains an ongoing need for effective therapies targeted at symptomatic patients in NYHA classes II and III. Exercise limitation, disabling symptoms, and disease progression in HFrEF patients have all been linked to overactivity of the sympathetic nervous system and underactivity of the parasympathetic nervous system. These changes in autonomic balance are thought to play a major role in their genesis of these abnormalities. Autonomic imbalance also exacerbates myocardial remodelling, peripheral vasoconstriction, and salt and water retention, and is associated with mortality and a risk of HF hospitalization.[11] Much success in the therapy of HF has come from procedures or drugs designed to modify abnormal body responses that are believed to be harmful and frequently occur as a reaction to HF. Such success stories include the realization that neurohormonal overactivity could cause damage to cardiac muscle, peripheral vasculature, and other organs such as the kidney. This led to the investigation of many pharmacological agents that modify receptor responses to such exaggerated and prolonged neurohormonal overactivity. This is the background to the development of many effective treatments for HFrEF, including angiotensin-converting enzyme (ACE) inhibitors, angiotensin receptor blockers (ARBs), beta-blockers, mineralocorticoid receptor antagonists (MRAs), and sacubitril/valsartan. In an analogous way, it is well known that sympathovagal imbalance is common and associated with adverse outcomes in many HF-related syndromes. There has long been interest in ways to modify the sympathovagal balance and other aspects of the autonomic nervous system, particularly as this system is so powerful in controlling aspects of cardiovascular and respiratory function. There is much overlap between autonomic dysfunction and the clinical features of HF, including arrhythmia, hypo- and hypertension, renal dysfunction, abnormal cerebral function, impaired blood volume control, and even general physical symptoms such as dizziness, nausea, and other symptoms.

Device therapies for autonomic modulation have been tested by using a number of different approaches, including direct vagal stimulation, spinal cord stimulation (SCS), renal artery nerve denervation, and baroreflex stimulation.

Vagal stimulation

Results on vagal stimulation have been variable from the three studies of implanted devices in HF that have been published to date. The early encouraging effects seen in the non-randomized ANTHEM-HF trial[12] on LVEF, 6MWT distance, and NYHA class were not confirmed in the later, larger RCTs INOVATE-HF and NECTAR-HF. In INOVATE-HF[13] which included 707 NYHA class III HFrEF patients, the primary efficacy endpoint of death or worsening HF was not improved (30.3% vs 25.8%, hazard ratio 1.14, 95% confidence interval (CI) 0.86–1.53; $P=0.37$) despite favourable effects on NYHA class and 6MHW distance. The NECTAR-HF trial compared randomized 6-month periods of therapy 'on' versus therapy 'off' in 87 HFrEF patients and showed a small reduction in left ventricular end-systolic volume (LVESV), but no difference in left ventricular end-systolic diameter (LVESD) or LVEF. Vagal stimulation is being evaluated in a pivotal trial.[14]

Spinal cord stimulation

SCS, which can modify autonomic balance, has not shown consistent benefits in HFrEF. The DEFEAT-HF trial[15] randomized (on a 3:2 basis) 66 HFrEF patients but failed to show a significant effect on the primary endpoint of change in left ventricular end-systolic volume index (LVESVI) after 6 months of SCS therapy in the treatment arm, compared to the control arm (SCS OFF: −2.2, 95% CI −9.1 to 4.6; SCS ON: 2.1, 95% CI −2.7 to 6.9; $P=0.30$). Secondary endpoints also were not significantly improved. This was despite an earlier non-randomized pilot study showing improved NYHA class, MLWHFQ, peak VO_2, and LVEF.[16]

Renal sympathetic denervation

Renal denervation (RDN) can reduce sympathetic predominance and has been suggested as a treatment for refractory hypertension. Several small trials have investigated its potential in the treatment of HF. The SYMPLICITY-HF study (ClinicalTrials. gov identifier: NCT01392196) was terminated early with apparently no physiological response, according to the entry on ClinicalTrials.org stating 'Terminated (No evidence of a physiological response; no significant safety concerns; post 24-month follow-up; Data Monitoring Committee agreed)'. In another trial, 60 HFrEF patients were randomized to the RDN group or control group, with significant improvement in LVEF, 6MWT distance, NYHA class, and N-terminal pro-B-type natriuretic peptide (NT-proBNP) level.[17] A meta-analysis of studies on RDN in HFrEF patients that included two small controlled studies (80 patients) and two uncontrolled studies (21 patients) suggested an increase in LVEF and a reduction in LV end-diastolic diameter, but clearly larger controlled trials are still required.[18]

Baroreflex stimulation

One novel treatment recently developed to address the unmet needs of patients with HFrEF is that of electrical stimulation to correct the cardiac autonomic modulation characteristic of HF. One implantable device has received approval in both the European Union and the United States: the CVRx® BAROSTIM NEO™ system (CVRx Inc., Minneapolis, MN, USA). This an implantable device capable of modifying cardiac autonomic balance via electrical activation of the baroreflex near the carotid sinus, the main sympatho-inhibitory reflex that regulates cardiovascular function via simultaneous inhibition of sympathetic outflow and activation of the parasympathetic nervous system. This mechanism has been termed baroreflex activation therapy (BAT). In HF, BAT has been examined in two multicentre RCTs (HOPE4HF[19] and BeAT-HF[20]), which have shown that BAT is safe and significantly improves functional status, QoL scores, exercise capacity, and NT-proBNP levels. An individual patient meta-analysis from all patients enrolled in these two prospective trials was presented at the Heart Failure Association (HFA) meeting in June 2021. It reported BAT improved exercise capacity, QoL, and functional capacity in NYHA class II and III HFrEF patients, and was associated with an improvement in NT-proBNP levels in subjects with a lower baseline level of NT-proBNP.

The phase 2 HOPE4HF trial randomized 69 HFrEF patients to control and 76 patients to BAT for 6 months. The primary safety endpoint was system- and procedure-related major adverse neurological and cardiovascular events. The primary efficacy endpoints were improved NYHA functional class ($P=0.002$ for change in distribution), QoL score (−17.4±2.8 points vs 2.1±3.1 points; $P<0.001$), and 6MWT distance (59.6±14 m vs 1.5±13.2 m; $P=0.004$), along with reduced NT-proBNP levels ($P=0.02$) and a trend towards fewer days of hospitalization for HF ($P=0.08$). The phase 3 BeAT-HF trial was also a randomized trial of BAT that included 408 randomized patients divided into four patient strata. Interim results for registration have been presented for 6MHW, MLWHFQ QoL score, and NT-proBNP levels, with an ongoing trial evaluating major clinical outcomes. In a cohort of 245 patients, which more precisely matched the types of patients identified in the FDA-approved instructions for use (enrolment criteria plus NT-proBNP level <1600 pg/mL), BAT improved QoL ($\Delta = -14.1$, 95% CI -19 to -9; $P<0.001$), with an increase in 6MHW distance (+60 m, 95% CI 40–80; $P<0.001$) and a reduction in NT-proBNP levels (-25%, 95% CI -38 to -9; $P=0.004$).

Respiratory rhythm modulation

Types of sleep apnoea

HF affects older patients who frequently have multiple comorbidities, some of which can contribute to the symptom burden and adverse outcomes characteristic of HF. Many common risk factors can cause both cardiovascular disease and other chronic disorders, including chronic lung disease. Smoking, obesity, male gender, and hypertension are all associated with an increased risk of HF, and all are associated with other important chronic lung diseases. One other condition that is associated with similar risk factors to those of HF is that of sleep-disordered breathing, particularly obstructive sleep apnoea (OSA). Sleep apnoea occurs in two main patterns—OSA and central sleep apnoea (CSA)—although some patients may have a mixed pattern. The two types have distinct pathophysiological causes and consequences, and are increasingly recognized as requiring separate therapeutic management strategies.

Obstructive sleep apnoea

OSA affects 2–4% of adults and is particularly frequent in HF, with a third or more of all HF patients having OSA, and this may justify specific treatment in its own right to relieve symptoms such as poor sleep and daytime sleepiness. OSA is mainly an anatomical problem caused by upper airway obstruction, often due to episodes of upper airway collapse. These result in intermittent airway occlusion, accompanied by consequent loss of airflow, arterial deoxygenation and carbon dioxide retention, and reflex arousal secondary to disturbed arterial blood gases. Obstructive apnoea or hypopnoea can occur throughout sleep, and is somewhat irregular and quite distinct from CSA, which is also common in HF. The most commonly recommended treatment for OSA is use of a positive pressure airway mask during sleep. While this treatment can improve OSA-related symptoms, there is no evidence that this alters outcomes or the prognosis. The need for therapy should be discussed with the patient and if the number of apnoea episodes are above 15 per hour, then treatment is indicated to reduce this to below 15. There are three types of positive airway mask treatment: continuous positive airway pressure (CPAP); bilevel positive airway pressure (BiPAP), in which pressure levels decrease during exhalation; and BiPAP-adaptive servo-ventilation (ASV), in which the two pressures are under the control of sensors embedded within the device that measure ventilatory parameters. Mask-based therapy should be combined with lifestyle changes such as weight loss in obese patients, regular exercise, and avoidance of alcohol and other sedatives prior to retiring for the night.

Custom-made oral appliances that push the mandible forward or specially designed mouth guards can assist to a limited extent, and upper airway surgery is occasionally used in severe cases unresponsive to, or intolerant of, mask therapy. There have been few trials on treatment of OSA in HF. The ongoing ADVENT-HF trial (ClinicalTrials.gov identifier: NCT01128816) recruited HF patients with either OSA or CSA and completed recruitment of 732 patients, although it was initially intended to accumulate 540 primary endpoints (death or first cardiovascular hospital admission or new-onset atrial fibrillation/flutter requiring anticoagulation, but not hospitalization or delivery of an appropriate shock from an ICD not resulting in hospitalization), and this seems unlikely to be achieved with only 732 patients recruited. The treatment intervention was ASV in addition to optimal standard therapy for HF versus optimal standard therapy alone for HF. Patients recruited had HFrEF (LVEF ≤45%), with sleep apnoea (either OSA or CSA), with an apnoea–hypopnoea index (AHI) of ≥15. Outside of HF, there was no evidence of clinical benefits in terms of major clinical outcomes (mortality or hospitalization rates) in a meta-analysis of trials on treatment of OSA using CPAP.[21]

Central sleep apnoea

CSA is the more common type of sleep apnoea in severe HF and is partly a complication of HF as a consequence of reflex abnormalities caused by HF—suppressed baroreflex sensitivity and increased chemoreflex sensitivity. CSA has consistently been shown to be associated with a worse prognosis in HF patients.[22] CSA causes similar symptoms to OSA, and the two types can be hard to differentiate without a formal sleep study, but such differentiation is essential in clinical management, due to the fact that the recommended treatment of OSA, that is, ASV mask therapy, is contraindicated in HFrEF if the sleep apnoea pattern is predominantly central. Thus, understanding how to diagnose and treat CSA is of increasing importance in HF practice.

CSA is caused by a fluctuating central respiratory drive that results in rhythmical respiratory activity during sleep due to unopposed oscillations in the respiratory reflex drive, itself a consequence of chemoreflex dominance in cardiopulmonary control. CSA in patients with HF is commonly of the Cheyne–Stokes type, characterized by cycles of deep, rapid crescendo–decrescendo breathing (hyperpnoea), followed by a period of slower, shallower breathing (hypopnoea) or no breathing at all (apnoea).[23,24]

Central to the pathophysiology of CSA is respiratory control system instability associated with rhythmic fluctuations in $PaCO_2$, sympathovagal imbalance, and prolonged circulation time—all of which, when combined with impaired lung gas exchange, can cause periodic breathing, via $PaCO_2$ being driven intermittently below the apnoeic threshold. These regular cycles of apnoea, hypoxia, and arousal increase sympathetic nervous system activation, as well as the risk of arrhythmias, and CSA is thought to contribute to the downward cycle of HF, including an increased risk of recurrent HF hospitalization, ventricular arrhythmias, and mortality.[25]

The optimum treatment for CSA was historically thought to be ASV airway mask therapy, until a large randomized study, namely the SERVE-HF trial, showed a significant increase in cardiovascular mortality in HFrEF patients with CSA when treated in this way.[26] Because of this, ASV is now a Class III contraindication in HFrEF guidelines. An alternative treatment of CSA in HFrEF is available via an implantable phrenic nerve stimulator—the remedē System, which was developed to physiologically correct the respiratory rhythm abnormalities that underlie CSA. The system stimulates the phrenic nerve to prevent apnoea or shallow breathing and is designed to normalize the breathing pattern.[27] The remedē System (Respicardia Inc., Minnetonka, MN, USA) is a transvenous unilateral phrenic nerve stimulator system that is FDA-approved for treatment of moderate to severe CSA. It has been tested in several trials, including a pilot evaluation and a pivotal trial.[28] The pivotal trial for FDA approval showed a significant effect on the primary endpoint, with the proportion of CSA patients in the treatment group having ≥50% reduction in the AHI, compared to the control group, at 6 months. Improvements were also seen in respiratory metrics (AHI, central apnoeas, oxygenation, arousal, and percentage of time in rapid eye movement sleep) and patient-reported outcomes (Patient Global Assessment and the Epworth Sleepiness Scale), with no safety concerns, with 91% freedom from device-related serious adverse events. Although it was not powered to assess major outcomes, there was no difference in either all-cause or cardiovascular mortality.

The remedē System phrenic nerve stimulation therapy has been subject to a pilot trial (n = 57; ClinicalTrials.gov identifier: NCT01124370) and a pivotal study (n = 151; ClinicalTrials.gov identifier: NCT01816776). A recent report combined these in a pooled analysis, by using similar endpoints, and reported on all patients who received the remedē System for treatment of CSA in these two trials, with 141 (68%) having concomitant HF. Of 208 patients so treated, a remedē device implant was successful in 197 (95%). Device treatment reduced AHI at 6 months by a median of −22.6 episodes/hour, with a median 58% reduction from baseline (P <0.001), along with improvement in sleep variables through 12 months of follow-up. In patients with HF and EF of ≤45%, phrenic nerve stimulation was associated with improvement in LVEF from 27.0% to 31.1% at 12 months (P = 0.003). Additional studies on HFrEF with CSA will be needed to evaluate the effect of treatment with phrenic nerve stimulation on major clinical outcomes.

Summary and conclusions

This chapter has reviewed approved but not yet standard device interventions that may benefit selected subsets of patients with HF.

Disclosures

Professor Coats declares no conflicts related to this work. Outside of this work, in the last 3 years, Professor Coats declares having received honoraria and/or lecture fees from: Astra Zeneca, Boehringer Ingelheim, Menarini, Novartis, Servier, Vifor, Abbott, Actimed, Arena, Cardiac Dimensions, Corvia, CVRx, Enopace, ESN Cleer, Faraday, Impulse Dynamics, Respicardia, and Viatris.

References

1. Fudim M, Abraham WT, von Bardeleben RS, et al. Device therapy in chronic heart failure: JACC state-of-the-art review. J Am Coll Cardiol. 2021;78(9):931–56.
2. Lyon AR, Samara MA, Feldman DS. Cardiac contractility modulation therapy in advanced systolic heart failure. Nat Rev Cardiol. 2013;10:584–98.
3. Neelagaru SB, Sanchez JE, Lau SK, et al. Nonexcitatory, cardiac contractility modulation electrical impulses: feasibility study for advanced heart failure in patients with normal QRS duration. Heart Rhythm. 2006;3(10):1140–7.
4. Borggrefe MM, Lawo T, Butter C, et al. Randomized, double-blind study of non-excitatory, cardiac contractility modulation electrical impulses for symptomatic heart failure. Eur Heart J. 2008;29:1019–28.
5. Kadish A, Nademanee K, Volosin K, et al. A randomized controlled trial evaluating the safety and efficacy of cardiac contractility modulation in advanced heart failure. Am Heart J. 2011;161:329–37.e1–2.
6. Abraham WT, Kuck KH, Goldsmith RL, et al. A randomized controlled trial to evaluate the safety and efficacy of cardiac contractility modulation. JACC Heart Fail. 2018;6:874–83.
7. Giallauria F, Cuomo G, Parlato A, Raval NY, Kuschyk J, Stewart Coats AJ. A comprehensive individual patient data meta-analysis of the effects of cardiac contractility modulation on functional capacity and heart failure-related quality of life. ESC Heart Fail. 2020;7(5):2922–32.
8. Kuschyk J, Falk P, Demming T, et al. Long-term clinical experience with cardiac contractility modulation therapy delivered by the optimizer smart system. Eur J Heart Fail. 2021;23:1160–9.
9. McDonagh TA, Metra M, Adamo M, et al. 2021 ESC Guidelines for the diagnosis and treatment of acute and chronic heart failure. Eur Heart J. 2021;42(36):3599–726.
10. Yancy CW, Jessup M, Bozkurt B, et al. 2017 ACC/AHA/HFSA focused update of the 2013 ACCF/AHA guideline for the management of heart failure: a report of the American College of Cardiology/American Heart Association Task Force on Clinical Practice Guidelines and the Heart Failure Society of America. J Am Coll Cardiol. 2017;70:776–803.
11. Ponikowski P, Anker SD, Chua TP, et al. Depressed heart rate variability as an independent predictor of death in chronic congestive heart failure secondary to ischemic or idiopathic dilated cardiomyopathy. Am J Cardiol. 1997;79:1645–50.
12. Premchand RK, Sharma K, Mittal S, et al. Autonomic regulation therapy via left or right cervical vagus nerve stimulation in patients with chronic heart failure: results of the ANTHEM-HF trial. J Card Fail. 2014;20(11):808–16.
13. Gold MR, Van Veldhuisen DJ, Hauptman PJ, et al. Vagus nerve stimulation for the treatment of heart failure: the INOVATE-HF trial. J Am Coll Cardiol. 2016;68(2):149–58.
14. ClinicalTrials.gov. ANTHEM-HFrEF Pivotal Study. ClinicalTrials.gov identifier: NCT03425422. Available from: http://clinicaltrials.gov/ct2/show/NCT03425422.
15. Zipes DP, Neuzil P, Theres H, et al.; DEFEAT-HF Trial Investigators. Determining the feasibility of spinal cord neuromodulation for the treatment of chronic systolic heart failure: the DEFEAT-HF study. JACC Heart Fail. 2016;4(2):129–36.
16. Tse HF, Turner S, Sanders P, et al. Thoracic spinal cord simulation for heart failure as a restorative treatment (SCS HEART study): first-in-man experience Heart Rhythm. 2015;12:588–95.
17. Chen W, Ling Z, Xu Y, et al. Preliminary effects of renal denervation with saline irrigated catheter on cardiac systolic function in patients

with heart failure: a prospective, randomized, controlled, pilot study. *Catheter Cardiovasc Interv*. 2016;89:E153–61.

18. Fukuta H, Goto T, Wakami K, Ohte N. Effects of catheter-based renal denervation on heart failure with reduced ejection fraction: a systematic review and meta-analysis. *Heart Fail Rev*. 2017;22(6):657–64.

19. Abraham WT, Zile MR, Weaver FA, *et al*. Baroreflex activation therapy for the treatment of heart failure with a reduced ejection fraction. *J Am Coll Cardiol*. 2015;3:487–96.

20. Zile MR, Lindenfeld J, Weaver FA, *et al*. Baroreflex activation therapy in patients with heart failure with reduced ejection fraction. *J Am Coll Cardiol*. 2020;76(1):1–13.

21. Patil SP, Ayappa IA, Caples SM, Kimoff RJ, Patel SR, Harrod CG. Treatment of adult obstructive sleep apnea with positive airway pressure: an American Academy of Sleep Medicine systematic review, meta-analysis, and GRADE assessment. *J Clin Sleep Med*. 2019;15:301–34.

22. Javaheri S, Shukla R, Zeigler H, Wexler L. Central sleep apnea, right ventricular dysfunction and low diastolic blood pressure are predictors of mortality in systolic heart failure. *J Am Coll Cardiol*. 2007;49:2028–34.

23. Cheyne J. A case of apoplexy, in which the fleshy part of the heart was converted into fat. *Dublin Hosp Reports*. 1818;2:216–23.

24. Stokes W. Observations on some cases of permanently slow pulse. *Dublin Quarterly Journal of Medical Sciences*. 1846;2:73–85.

25. Jilek C, Krenn M, Sebah D, *et al*. Prognostic impact of sleep disordered breathing and its treatment in heart failure: an observational study. *Eur J Heart Fail*. 2011;13:68–75.

26. Cowie MR, Wegscheider K, Teschler H. Adaptive servo-ventilation for central sleep apnea in heart failure. *N Engl J Med*. 2016;374:690–1.

27. Abraham WT, Jagielski D, Oldenburg O, *et al*.; remedē Pilot Study Investigators. Phrenic nerve stimulation for the treatment of central sleep apnea. *JACC Heart Fail*. 2015;5:360–9.

28. Costanzo MR, Ponikowski P, Javaheri S, *et al*. Transvenous neurostimulation for central sleep apnoea: a randomised controlled trial. *Lancet*. 2016;388(10048):974–82.

CHAPTER 9.6

Cardiovascular rehabilitation and lifestyle modifications

Maurizio Volterrani, Alain Cohen-Solal, Stamatis Adamopulos, Dimitris Miliopoulos, Ferdinando Iellamo, and Massimo Piepoli

Contents

Introduction

Heart failure (HF) is a syndrome characterized by high mortality, frequent hospitalization, poor quality of life (QoL), multiple comorbidities, and a complex therapeutic regimen.

Heart failure with reduced ejection fraction (HFrEF) affects more than an estimated 3 million people in the United States.[1] Despite the availability of multiple treatment options, outcomes remain suboptimal, with high rates of rehospitalization and death.[2] This is, in part, due to inadequate adoption of guideline-directed medical therapy.[3]

Therefore, non-pharmacological management strategies represent an important contribution to HF therapy.

Education and counselling

The goals of education and counselling are to help patients, their families, and caregivers acquire the knowledge, skills, strategies, problem-solving abilities, and motivation necessary for adherence to the treatment plan and effective participation in self-care. Inclusion of family members and other caregivers is especially important, because HF patients often suffer from cognitive impairment, functional disabilities, multiple comorbidities, and other conditions that limit their ability to fully comprehend, appreciate, or enact what they learn.[4,5,6,7,8,9,10,11,12,13]

Self-care

Self-care describes the process whereby a patient participates actively in the management of his or her HF, usually with the help of a family member or caregiver. Self-care includes both maintenance and management.[14,15]

Self-care maintenance refers to healthy lifestyle choices (e.g. exercising, maintaining normal body weight) and treatment adherence behaviours (e.g. monitoring weight changes, limiting dietary sodium intake, taking medications). Self-care management is a cognitive process that includes recognizing signs and symptoms, evaluating their importance, implementing a self-care treatment strategy (e.g. diuretic administration), and evaluating its effectiveness.

Patients should acquire skills which include, for example, the ability to read food labels, adapt preferred foods to low-sodium versions, select low-sodium foods, prepare food with little or no added sodium, and track sodium intake.

Because cognitive impairment and depression are common in HF and can seriously interfere with learning, patients should be screened for these. This can be done with the help of several standardized questionnaires such as the Patient Health Questionnaire-2,[16] Beck Depression Inventory,[17] and Depression Interview and Structured Hamilton (DISH).[18]

Patients found to be cognitively impaired need additional support to manage their HF. Education sessions should address specific issues (e.g. non-adherence to pharmacological therapy) and their causes (e.g. forgetting), and employ strategies that promote behavioural change, including motivational interventions.

Expertise in HF management provides the majority of education and counselling, supplemented by physician input and, when available and needed, input from dieticians and other healthcare providers.

Education and counselling sessions should be performed on a periodical basis, offering to patients a variety of options for learning about HF: videotapes, one-on-one or group discussions, telephone calls, mailed information, and Internet.

Repeated exposure to material is recommended because a single session is never sufficient.

Counselling should test knowledge of the name, dose, and purpose of each medication, sorting foods into high- and low-sodium categories, and the preferred method for tracking medication dosing, and reiterate symptoms of worsening HF, as well as when to call the healthcare provider because of specific symptoms or weight changes.

During acute care hospitalization, only essential education is recommended, with the goal of assisting patients to understand HF, the goals of its treatment, and post-hospitalization medications and follow-up regimen. Education started during hospitalization should be supplemented and reinforced within 1–2 weeks after discharge, continued for 3–6 months, and reassessed periodically.

These programmes focus on multiple aspects of patient care, including optimization of drug therapy, patient and family/caregiver education and counselling, emphasis on self-care, and early attention to signs and symptoms of fluid overload. It is recommended that HF disease management includes integration and coordination of care between the primary care physician and HF care specialists and with other agencies such as home health and cardiac rehabilitation.

It is recommended that patients in a HF disease management programme be followed until they or their family/caregivers demonstrate independence in following the prescribed treatment plan, adequate or improved adherence to treatment guidelines, improved functional capacity, and symptom stability. Higher-risk patients with more advanced HF may need to be followed up permanently. Patients who experience increasing episodes of exacerbation or who demonstrate instability after discharge from a programme should be referred again to the service.

Patients and family should be informed that adequate time (weeks to months) must be given to allow medical therapies to exert a beneficial therapeutic effect. In addition, issues such as access to care, adherence to medications and other self-care behaviours, as well as knowledge about HF, should also be addressed.

Seriously ill patients with HF and their families should be educated to understand that patients with HF are at high risk of death, even while aggressive efforts are made to prolong life.

Patients with HF should be made aware that their disease is potentially life-limiting, but that pharmacological and device therapies and self-management can prolong life.

Essential elements of patient education and target behaviours are as follows: (1) identifying specific signs and symptoms (e.g. increasing fatigue or shortness of breath with usual activities, dyspnoea at rest, nocturnal dyspnoea or orthopnoea, oedema); (2) performing daily weights; (3) developing an action plan for how and when to notify the healthcare provider; (4) changes to make in diet, fluid, and diuretics. Smoking cessation, maintenance of blood pressure within the target range, maintenance of normal HbA1c if diabetic, and maintaining a specific body weight are other fundamental aspects of counselling and educational programmes.

Diet, nutrition, and supplements

Congestion, or fluid overload, is a classic clinical feature of patients presenting with HF. It is a generalized process that usually develops gradually. Peripheral congestion in patients with HF usually develops over weeks or even months, and patients may present 'acutely' having gained over 20 L of excess fluid, and hence over 20 kg of excess weight.

Dietary instruction regarding sodium intake is recommended for all patients with HF, along with restriction of daily fluid intake to <2 L, especially in those with severe hyponatraemia (serum sodium <130 mEq/L) and patients demonstrating fluid retention despite diuretic therapy.

However, the role of sodium restriction is not clear, although it is part of traditional management of HF and recommended in guidelines.[19] In conditions of congestion, the only effect of sodium restriction appears to be to increase the sensation of thirst.[20] In patients with chronic HF, a normal sodium diet is associated with better outcomes, albeit on a background of very high loop diuretic doses.[21] It seems reasonable to suggest to patients that they should not add large quantities of salt to their diet, but excessive restriction has no role.

In HF patients, there is potential harm from increasing salt and fluid intake associated with nutritional support. Currently, several international cardiology guidelines recommend a multidisciplinary approach to preventing malnutrition, including regular monitoring of body weight, as well as avoidance of excessive fluid and/or salt intake.[22,23,24]

Historically, dietary recommendations for HF management focused on sodium and fluid restrictions. More recently, some studies reported associations of these recommendations with higher readmission rates and increased mortality,[25,26] and the usefulness of salt restriction in HF management remains debated.[27] These restrictions may have interfered with patients' normal eating habits, resulting in weight loss and anorexia.[28]

Indeed, attention should be paid to nutrition of patients with HF and unintentional weight loss or muscle wasting, up to cardiac cachexia. Measurement of caloric intake and pre-albumin levels may be useful in determining appropriate nutritional supplementation, and caloric supplementation is highly recommended. Multivitamin and mineral supplementation should also be considered to ensure adequate intake of the recommended daily value of essential nutrients. In this context, supplementation with nutraceuticals may be an option. Patients should avoid using products containing ephedra, ephedrine, or its metabolites because of an increased risk of mortality and morbidity, as well as products that may interfere with the drugs prescribed (e.g. digoxin, vasodilators, beta-blockers, antiarrhythmic drugs, anticoagulants).

Alterations in cardiac energy metabolism and nutritional intake represent a critical component in the evolution of HF disease. Nutrition significantly affects the function and efficiency of myocardial tissue, and adequate ingestion of energy and macronutrients may improve cardiac function and longevity.[29]

In the healthy heart, the myocardium utilizes prevalently fatty acids (FAs) as metabolic substrate,[30] whereas in HF, the primary energetic substrate shifts from FA to glucose for oxidation.[31] Switching from FA to glucose oxidation protects cardiomyocytes from oxidative radical excess and cell damage. However, an excess of glucose availability can be detrimental to cardiac function, favouring cardiac hypertrophy and a less efficient response during stress.[32] It can be assumed that adequate support of carbohydrates with nutrition would maintain an optimal glucose level to guarantee efficient cardiac function. High-fat feeding too does not negatively influence cardiac function,[33] but reduced utilization of free FAs as energy source contributes to cardiovascular deterioration in HF.[32]

Conflicting data exist on the effects of a controlled diet on heart function and clinical outcomes in patients with chronic heart failure.[34] The nutritional approach to HF patients should consider first of all the body mass index (BMI) of any given individual, which can be stratified into low, average, and high ranges. The safety diet in underweight HF patients (i.e. BMI <18 kg/m^2) should be hypercaloric (35–40 kcal/kg/day), with a protein intake of 1.5 g/kg of body weight,[17] a fat intake of 1.0–1.5 g/kg of body weight, and a high carbohydrate intake of almost 4–5 g/kg of body weight.[35] In patients with moderate BMI (between 25 and 29.9 kg/m^2), high adherence to the MedDiet was associated with a lower incidence of HF and mortality[36,37,38] and a hypocaloric diet reduced clinical complications.[39] In overweight HF patients, an average caloric restriction of 20–30% of the daily caloric intake is helpful to improve metabolism. Protein intake should be about 1.5 g/kg of bodyweight, carbohydrate intake 3–4 g/kg of body weight, and fat intake 0.8–1.0 g/kg of body weight, whereas ingestion of saturated and polyunsaturated fats is associated with increased all-cause mortality[40] and should be avoided. Supplementation with nutraceuticals should also be considered, but clear evidence of the beneficial effects of nutraceuticals is still lacking.[41]

A very recent meta-analysis[41] showed that coenzyme Q10 (CoQ10) may have a role in reducing the risk of all-cause mortality in HF patients, while the Mediterranean diet may reduce the risk of incident HF; however, the certainty of evidence for both was low. None of the interventions were associated with a decrease in HF hospitalization. However, thiamine, L-carnitine, and vitamin D were found to have possible beneficial effect on left ventricular ejection fraction (LVEF). Overall, there was suboptimal quality and level of evidence regarding the impact of nutritional supplements and dietary interventions on HF. Only a handful of interventions assessed the risk of all-cause mortality in HF patients and prevention of incident HF in patients without established HF. For the majority of the interventions, including DASH diet, vitamin D, vitamin D plus calcium, caffeine, chocolate, processed meat, eggs, zinc, and intermittent fasting, no randomized controlled trial (RCT) data exist on clinical outcomes.

Although results on the beneficial effect of CoQ10 are mainly driven by one RCT (Q-SYMBIO—Coenzyme Q10 as Adjunctive Treatment of Chronic Heart Failure: A Randomized, Double-blind, Multi-Centre Trial with Focus on Symptoms, Biomarker Status),[42] nevertheless CoQ10 is an attractive option, given that it is readily available at low cost, and has a favourable side effect profile and a strong pathophysiological rationale in HF. No RCT data exist regarding the impact of other dietary interventions in HF such as intermittent fasting, ketogenic diet, and DASH diet.

Overall, there is suboptimal quality and level of evidence regarding the impact of nutritional supplements and dietary interventions in HF.

Alcohol is not forbidden, but patients with HF should be advised to limit alcohol consumption to no more than two standard drinks per day for men or to one standard drink per day for women, whereas patients with alcohol-induced cardiomyopathy should abstain completely from alcohol consumption.

A recent meta-analysis suggested that, for secondary prevention of cardiovascular disease, current drinkers may not need to stop drinking but should be informed that lower levels of intake (up to 105 g/week) may be associated with reduced risks. This meta-analysis confirmed and extended to a larger number of patients those reported by another meta-analysis study conducted 10 years ago.[43]

It should be outlined that most of the studies addressing the issue of nutrition in HF reported nutritional evaluation through self-administered food questionnaires, a methodological approach that is helpful for large populations but that carries a risk of bias.

Muscle wasting and cachexia

Muscle wasting, also known as sarcopenia, and cachexia are generally common comorbidities associated with HF, with significant impact on patients' clinical course.

Muscle wasting or sarcopenia (derived from the Greek words *sarx* meaning flesh, and *penia* meaning loss) is a 'progressive and generalised skeletal muscle disorder that is associated with increased likelihood of adverse outcomes including falls, fractures, physical disability and mortality'.[44]

The etymology of 'cachexia' comes from the Greek words *kakos* (meaning bad) and *hexis* (meaning habit/condition), thus creating the Greek word *kakhexia* which evolved to its final state in the mid-sixth century. It means weakness and wasting of the body due to severe chronic illness. Cachexia is associated with many chronic diseases—most prominently cancer, coeliac disease, and HF where it is more accurately termed cardiac cachexia. This latter term originates from a medical thesis from 1860.[45]

A major challenge lies in whether these conditions are distinct from each other and, if not, which comes first. In most cases, they are both present in varying degrees, especially in advanced HF. In earlier stages, one of them may appear first—usually muscle wasting—although eventually leading to the aforementioned overlapping condition.

Unfortunately, sarcopenia and cachexia are rarely detected by most physicians, only being an afterthought in decision-making and patient management, despite its well-documented effect on patients' QoL and prognosis, as will be described later in this chapter.

Sarcopenia

According to the most recent update of the European Working Group on Sarcopenia in Older People (EWGSOP), sarcopenia can be defined as a skeletal muscle disorder that fulfils at least two of the following criteria: (1) low muscle strength; (2) low muscle quality or quantity; and (3) low physical performance.[44]

The first indicators of development of sarcopenia in patients are symptoms or clinical signs such as falling, weakness, slow walking speed, or difficulty rising from a chair.

The prevalence of sarcopenia in HF is around 20%, as demonstrated by the SICA-HF study which enrolled HF patients (69% with reduced ejection fraction). Patients with sarcopenia had reduced ejection fraction, peak oxygen consumption, and exercise time, as well as weaker grip and quadriceps strength.[46]

It is important to note that muscle wasting usually predates weight loss and cachexia by a significant amount of time, and thus remains undiagnosed.[47] As a result, the aforementioned questionnaires and assessment tools are necessary for uncovering its presence.

Cachexia

Cachexia is defined as a 'complex metabolic syndrome associated with underlying illness and characterized by loss of muscle with or without loss of fat mass', with weight loss being the most prominent clinical feature in adults.[48]

The diagnostic criteria of cachexia in adults (irrespective of the aetiology) consist of the presence of an underlying disease and body weight loss of ≥5% in ≤12 months (or BMI <20 kg/m²), along with at least three of the following: (1) decrease in muscle strength; (2) fatigue; (3) anorexia; (4) low fat-free mass index; and (5) abnormal biochemistry—inflammation, anaemia, low serum albumin levels.

The prevalence of cachexia in HF patients varies between 16% and 42%, depending on the sample population. Specifically, an analysis of the Val-HeFT trial revealed that unintentional weight loss of ≥5% occurred in 15.7% of the enrolled patients,[49] whereas 42% of patients enrolled in the SOLVD trial suffered the same weight loss.[50] As a way to measure the importance of this comorbidity, it is estimated that around 1.2 million HF patients in Europe have cardiac cachexia.[51]

As seen with sarcopenia, the presence of cachexia is associated with worse outcomes in HF patients. Weight loss in the SOLVD, Val-HeFT, and GISSI-HF trials was associated with increased mortality and risk of both cardiovascular and non-cardiovascular events.[49,50]

Mechanisms underlying cachexia and sarcopenia development in heart failure

The development of these conditions in HF is multifactorial. First, there are changes in muscle structure due to continuous exposure of muscles to a state of constant inflammation and low cardiac output. Specifically, a combination of mitochondrial dysfunction, fatty tissue infiltration of muscles, muscle fibre transformation, myocyte apoptosis, and myofibril degeneration gradually leads to sarcopenia and later cachexia, in combination with other factors described in ◗ Figure 9.6.1.[47] In addition, deconditioning of muscles at advanced HF stages due to impaired exercise capacity is also a contributing factor.[52]

Malnutrition also has an important role through either loss of appetite or epigastric discomfort in congested patients. Appetite is regulated by a multitude of mediators such as neuropeptide Y and ghrelin, which are orexigenic, or pro-opiomelanocortin, which is anorexigenic. In particular, ghrelin administration in cachectic New York Heart Association (NYHA) class III HF patients resulted in improvement in LVEF and peak oxygen consumption during exercise, as well as increased muscle strength and lean body mass.[53] Of note, inflammatory cytokines (mainly tumour necrosis factor alpha, which increases in HF) also cause loss of appetite.[54]

Another crucial factor is metabolic imbalance, which promotes predominance of a catabolic state. The main affected hormone is growth hormone. Growth hormone stimulates insulin-like growth factor 1 (IGF-1) production, which has anabolic effects.[55] Cachectic HF patients have increased levels of growth hormone, with a simultaneous decrease of IGF-1 levels—evidence of growth hormone resistance.

Treatment

Treatment of sarcopenia and cachexia is a challenging task due to limited available options, alongside an often already advanced stage of the disease. A prerequisite of the treatment options discussed below is initiation and/or optimization of optimal guideline-directed HF medical and device therapy, given its well-documented benefit in disease prognosis and weight loss.[50,56,57]

Nutritional advice is the first step in managing cachectic HF patients. The PICNIC study demonstrated the beneficial effects of personalized nutritional intervention on diet optimization in malnourished HF patients, as defined by the Mini Nutritional Assessment (MNA) score,[58] with a significant reduction in mortality and HF-related hospitalization. According to a consensus statement from the Heart Failure Society of America Scientific Statements Committee, a goal daily protein intake of ≥1.1 g/kg is

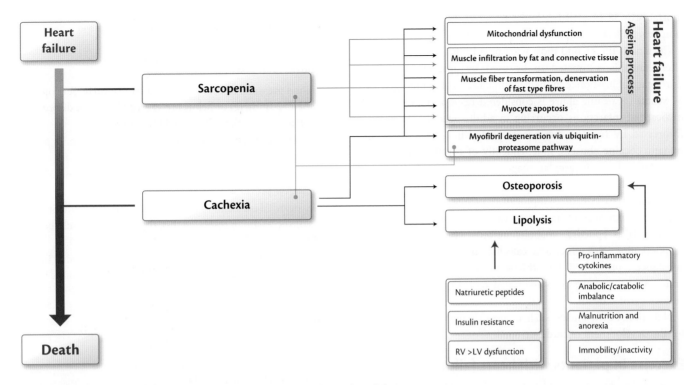

Figure 9.6.1 Mechanism underlying cachexia and sarcopenia development in heart failure.

Reproduced from von Haehling S. The wasting continuum in heart failure: from sarcopenia to cachexia. *Proc Nutr Soc.* 2015 Nov;74(4):367–77. doi: 10.1017/S0029665115002438 with permission from Cambridge University Press.

recommended.[59] In cases of critical illness or planned cardiac surgery, enteral or parenteral support may be required, with goals of albumin of ≥3 g/dL, pre-albumin of ≥16 g/dL, BMI of ≥18.5–20 kg/m², and an iron-replete state.[60]

Exercise training is a crucial part of muscle wasting treatment and HF in general, with proven reduction in mortality, hospitalization, and QoL.[61,62,63] The HF Guidelines of the European Society of Cardiology (ESC) recommend regular aerobic exercise to improve functional capacity and symptoms.[64] Aerobic exercise training has been reported to reverse impairment of skeletal muscle oxidative capacity.[65] However, resistance training is more suitable for reversing muscle wasting; a meta-analysis showed that this modality can improve muscle strength in HF patients.[66] Recently, a combined approach of aerobic, resistance, and inspiratory muscle training (ARIS) in the ARISTOS-HF trial provided the best results in both muscle strength and functional parameters such as the 6-minute walking test.[67]

In conclusion, sarcopenia and cachexia, when present, carry a significant burden on HF patients. Despite initially being distinct entities, they end up as an overlapping clinical presentation, especially in the setting of advanced HF. Due to their multifactorial pathophysiology, there are limited treatment options, with guideline-directed HF treatment and exercise training being the most effective.

Smoking and recreational substance use

Smoking is a strong modifiable risk factor for cardiovascular diseases. In observational studies, smoking has been associated with

a higher risk of developing HFrEF, independently of other lifestyle risk factors.[68,69,70,71] In the Women's Health Initiative study, the adjusted risk of incident HFrEF for never-smokers was 0.43 (95% confidence interval (CI) 0.33–0.55) and 0.47 (95% CI 0.37–0.60) for past smokers, compared to current smokers.[70] In this study, smoking was also associated with HF with preserved ejection fraction (HFpEF) with similar hazard ratios (HRs). Finally, in the Jackson Heart Study, after adjustment for traditional risk factors and incident coronary heart disease, current smoking (HR 2.82, 95% CI 1.71–4.64), smoking intensity among current smokers (≥20 cigarettes/day: HR 3.48, 95% CI 1.65–7.32), and smoking burden among ever-smokers (≥15 pack-years: HR 2.06, 95% CI 1.29–3.3) were significantly associated with incident HF hospitalization, in comparison to never smoking.[72]

Smoking causes HF partly through causing ischaemic heart disease, but studies indicate also a more direct effect of smoking on cardiac structure and function. Large cross-sectional echocardiography studies of mainly healthy individuals compared smokers and non-smokers and reported greater left ventricular (LV) mass, poorer systolic function of the left and right ventricles, and also worse diastolic function as reflected by higher E/e′.[73,74] Subtle changes in cardiac structure and function in smokers have also been reported from magnetic resonance imaging studies.[71,72,73,74,75]

A recent review reported that approximately 16% of HF patients continued smoking after HF diagnosis and persistent smoking was associated with poor health status, ventricular tachycardia, and arterial stiffness. Persistent smoking increased the HR of mortality by 38.4% (HR 1.384, 95% CI 1.139–1.681) and readmission by 44.8% (HR 1.448, 95% CI 1.086–1.930).[76]

Cocaine is the second most widespread illicit drug in Europe, after cannabis, estimated to be used by around 13 million Europeans at least once in their lifetime (3.9% of adults aged 15–64 years).[77] Cocaine abuse is considered responsible for 25% of myocardial infarctions occurring in adults aged 18–45 years.[78] Depressed LV function has been reported in 4–18% of asymptomatic cocaine abusers, independently of coronary artery disease. Several cardiovascular magnetic resonance studies have confirmed the presence of myocardial oedema in up to 47%, and fibrosis in up to 73%, of asymptomatic cocaine users.[79]

Several toxic factors have been associated with HF development such as ephedra, anabolic steroids, chloroquine, cobalt, amphetamine, clozapine, and catecholamines.[80] Some of these substances, prescribed for athletic performance enhancement and weight loss, have been associated with LV dysfunction and sudden cardiac death.

Nutritional deficiencies, such as anorexia nervosa, can account for the development of cardiomyopathy.[80]

Exercise in patients with heart failure

Exercise is highly recommended, regardless of LVEF.[81,82] This recommendation is based on evidence from meta-analyses of RCTs, which have demonstrated significant improvement in exercise tolerance and QoL.[83,84] Studies have also revealed a modest effect on all-cause mortality, HF-specific mortality, all-cause hospitalization, and HF-specific hospitalization. As with any treatment, exercise prescription in patients with HF requires an individualized approach, with careful evaluation of contraindications.[85]

The list of potential contraindications to exercise is long (❯ Box 9.6.1). In contrast, there is even evidence that exercise-induced physical conditioning reduces the overall risk of clinically relevant arrhythmias.[86]

Risk stratification

Key components in risk stratification and primary evaluation before starting an exercise programme and sport participation are a *baseline clinical assessment* (medical history and physical examination), *blood investigations* (full blood count, creatinine, and electrolytes), *assessment of functional capacity* (a maximal exercise test also to evaluate for potential complications during exercise, such as exercise hypertension/hypotension, myocardial ischaemia, or arrhythmias; cardiopulmonary exercise testing better stratifies the risk and additionally provides data for prescription of exercise intensity),[87] *additional examinations* (echocardiography and other tests according to comorbidities such as lung function tests, body plethysmography, oxygen saturation, and arterial blood gases before and after exercise), and *medical therapy optimization* (medication and device techniques, such as cardiac resynchronization therapy and implantable cardioverter–defibrillator, should be considered before starting exercise programmes).[88]

Exercise intervention should be individually tailored and should follow a structured scheme for several weeks that will be

---

Box 9.6.1 Summary of contraindications to exercise in individuals with heart failure

Cardiovascular status

1. Blood pressure: SBP <90 mmHg or >160 mmHg. A drop in SBP (>20 mmHg) or below pre-exercise level or a disproportionate rise (i.e. >200 mmHg for SBP)
2. Heart rate at rest: <40 bpm or >100 bpm (>120 bpm in permanent AF)
3. Progressive worsening of exercise tolerance or dyspnoea at rest over previous 3–5 days
4. Myocardial ischaemia should be excluded; if treatment is unsuccessful in resolving this, then exercise should be limited to its threshold
5. Acute or unstable cardiac status (i.e. acute myocardial infarction, myocarditis, and pericarditis; haemodynamic instability; unstable cardiac rhythm)
6. Severe symptomatic valve disease
7. Severe hypertrophic obstructive cardiomyopathy
8. Intracardiac or pulmonary embolus
9. Acute deep vein thrombosis
10. New-onset AF/atrial flutter

Respiratory status

1. Oxygen saturation (SpO_2): <88% or undetermined cyanosis
2. Respiratory rate: <5 or >40 breaths/minute
3. Uncontrolled asthma or chronic obstructive airway disease

Other conditions

1. Clinical instability (e.g. active bleeding, fever, concomitant comorbidities limiting exercise capacity)
2. Excessive muscle soreness or fatigue (Borg RPE >15/20) that is residual from last exercise or activity session

AF, atrial fibrillation; bpm, beats/minute; RPE, Rating of Perceived Exertion; SBP, systolic blood pressure.
Source data from Piepoli MF, Davos C, Francis DP, Coats AJ; ExTraMATCH Collaborative. Exercise training meta-analysis of trials in patients with chronic heart failure (ExTraMATCH). *BMJ*. 2004 Jan 24;328(7433):189. doi: 10.1136/bmj.37938.645220.EE.

---

regularly adapted according to objective and subjective measures and symptoms. High-risk patients should be counselled more frequently during early phases. Initially supervised exercise should ideally be implemented, and non-supervised home-based sessions should be gradually added.[89] When all these measures are followed, the overall risk from exercise is low, even during higher-intensity exercises and in patients with more severe HF.[90,91]

During the exercise session, patients should monitor symptoms, as well as exercise intensity, according to heart rate response and the power generated (watts on ergometry). In atrial fibrillation (AF), exercise can only be monitored by power or Borg Rating of Perceived Exertion (RPE).

Follow-up examinations for exercise recommendations should be scheduled regularly (i.e. at least every 3–6 months). Intervals

Box 9.6.2 Data collection for appropriate assessment of safety of exercise intervention and sports participation in individuals with heart failure

1. Medical history, current body weight, symptom(s)
2. Barriers to exercise and sports participation (symptom recognition, language, literacy, self-care, knowing when to contact the healthcare provider)
3. Premorbid level of function (e.g. mobility aids), activity and exercise response, and fitness level
4. Primary diagnosis
5. Concomitant illness (e.g. arrhythmias, musculoskeletal or lung disease, diabetes, deconditioning)
6. Medications
7. Blood investigations (e.g. blood chemistry, full blood count and blood glucose, natriuretic peptides)
8. Specific restrictions on mobilization according to acute and post-acute clinical condition
9. Type and level of planned exercise and sports participation

Source data from Piepoli MF, Davos C, Francis DP, Coats AJ; ExTraMATCH Collaborative. Exercise training meta-analysis of trials in patients with chronic heart failure (ExTraMATCH). *BMJ*. 2004 Jan 24;328(7433):189. doi: 10.1136/bmj.37938.645220.EE.

between examinations depend on the disease state, severity of HF and comorbidities, stability of disease, age of the patient, supervision of exercise sessions (supervised vs home-based), and adherence to the programme.

Adherence to exercise can be improved by exploring patient preferences and any potential barriers to its implementation. Adherence may be improved by setting goals for behavioural changes (e.g. weight reduction in the morbidly obese and patients with diabetes). ⮑ Box 9.6.2 lists the data to be collected/verified first in order to assess the safety of exercise intervention in HF.

Exercise prescription

Exercise programmes should be individually prescribed and adjusted in terms of frequency, intensity, duration, modalities, and progression.[92] Based on the risk profile, the level of supervision and monitoring required has to be individually determined.

Although there are still limited data regarding the role of exercise in the management of advanced or acute HF, early mobilization through an individualized programme has been advised, with small muscle strength exercise and respiratory training, alone or in combination.[92,93,94] Each patient affected by recent unstable HF occurrence can benefit from either an inpatient or an outpatient exercise programme.[92,93] In high-risk patients, that is, clinically unstable patients with advanced HF (NYHA classes III and IV, needing intermittent or continuous drug infusion and/or mechanical support), supervised hospital-based exercise programmes should be considered as a transition phase to promote stabilization before starting a longer-term phase of outpatient exercise programmes.

Early outpatient exercise programmes promote long-term adherence to exercise training and sports participation. These programmes are generally delivered within the first 3–6 months after the event and for at least 8–12 weeks, up to 1 year.

Aerobic/endurance exercise

Aerobic exercise is recommended for stable patients with HF (NYHA classes I–III), because of its well-demonstrated efficacy and safety.[17] Recommendations on optimal exercise dose in HF have been previously described in ESC and American Heart Association (AHA) guidelines (⮑ Table 9.6.1).[92,93,95,98] The most evaluated exercise mode is steady-state moderate continuous exercise (MCE), as it has been proven to be safe and well tolerated.[92,93,95,96,97,98] In patients with HF with NYHA functional class III, exercise intensity should be kept at a low level (50% of peak VO_2), according to perceived symptoms and clinical status, during the first 1–2 weeks. A gradual increase in intensity (60–80% of peak VO_2 if tolerated) is the primary aim.[92,93] High-intensity interval training (HIIT) programmes have been considered to be an alternative exercise modality for low-risk patients with HF.[98] A meta-analysis showed that HIIT was superior to MCE in improving peak VO_2 in HFrEF in the short term.[99] However, this superiority disappeared in a subgroup analysis of isocaloric protocols. Moreover, it has been shown that HIIT programmes in HF patients present lower feasibility, compared to MCE. In the largest study in this field by Ellingsen *et al.*,[91] 51% of patients in the HIIT group did not reach the target intensity, whereas 80% of patients in the MCE group trained above the target.

Table 9.6.1 Optimal exercise training dose for patients with chronic heart failure

	Aerobic exercise	Resistance exercise
Frequency	3–5 days/week	2–3 days/week
Intensity	50–80% of peak VO_2	Borg RPE <15 (40–60% of 1RM)
Duration	20–60 minutes	10–15 repetitions in at least one set of 8–10 different upper and lower body exercises
Mode	Interval or continuous	
Progression	A progressive increasing training regimen should be prescribed, with regular follow-up monitoring (at least every 3–6 months) to adjust the duration and level of exercise to the attained level of tolerance	A progressive increasing training regimen should be prescribed, with regular follow-up monitoring (at least every 3–6 months) to adjust the duration and level of exercise to the attained level of tolerance

1RM, one repetition maximum; peak VO_2, peak oxygen consumption; RPE, Rating of Perceived Exertion.

A recent study indicated that it may be safe and effective to start early with moderate-intensity interval exercise also after acute decompensation and in parallel with titrating medication.[100] Data are rare and not yet conclusive, and therefore, further research is needed to define indications for exercise training in this patient group.

Resistance exercise

Guidelines recommend that resistance exercise training can complement, but not substitute, aerobic exercise training in HF patients.[92,98,101] In this regard, resistance exercise reverts skeletal muscle mass loss and deconditioning without excessive stress on the heart. The training intensity can preferably be set at the level of resistance at which the patient can perform 10–15 repetitions at 15 on the Borg RPE scale. It is suggested that exercise training should focus initially on increasing muscle mass by using resistance exercise programmes in patients with combined HF and altered skeletal muscle function and muscle wasting.[102,103] A recent meta-analysis showed that resistance exercise as a single intervention has the capacity to increase muscle strength, aerobic capacity, and QoL in patients with HFrEF who are unable to participate in aerobic exercise programmes.[104] Also, in advanced HF or in patients with very low exercise tolerance, resistance exercise can be safely applied if small muscle groups are trained.[92,94,104]

Respiratory exercise

It is likely that abnormalities of skeletal muscles in patients with HF, in terms of increased ergo reflex, mitochondrial abnormalities, decreased oxidative enzyme activities, and muscle atrophy, also affect respiratory muscles.[105] The benefits of inspiratory muscle training in HFrEF patients are well described and include improvements in peak VO_2, dyspnoea, and muscle strength, for example.[105,106] Typical training protocols involve inspiratory muscle training three, six, or seven times per week, with intensity ranging from 30% to 60% of maximal inspiratory pressure and with duration ranging from 15 to 30 minutes, for an average of 10–12 weeks.[105] This training modality could be recommended to the most severely deconditioned patients with HF as an initial alternative, who may then transition to conventional exercise training and sports participation, to optimize cardiopulmonary benefits.[107]

Combination of aerobic and resistance exercise

When feasible for the individual patient with HF, the guidelines recommend performing resistance exercise in combination with aerobic exercise training.[92,108,109] It has been concluded that most studies have demonstrated superior effects of combined aerobic and resistance exercise training versus aerobic exercise training alone for improving muscle strength, endurance, and QoL in chronic HF.[98,99,100,101,102,103,104,105,106,107,108,109,110] Historically, aquatic exercise has not been recommended for individuals with HF, due to concerns that the increase in central blood volume and cardiac preload as a consequence of hydrostatic pressure may not be tolerated.[111] Lately, a meta-analysis has, however, shown that aquatic exercise training is a safe and effective alternative for HF patients that can improve exercise capacity, muscle strength, and QoL, similarly to land-based exercise training programmes.[112]

Therefore, low-risk patients with HF may currently participate in low- to moderate-intensity aquatic sports.

Heart failure with preserved ejection fraction

Currently, exercise recommendations in HFpEF are based on a few trials[113] involving a limited number of patients (<300, stable patients, ejection fraction ≥45% in exercise training groups overall). Results have shown that exercise intervention for 12–24 weeks increases maximal exercise capacity (mean improvement of peak VO_2 +2.7 mL/kg/min, 95% CI 1.79–3.65) and improves QoL, but has no impact on diastolic dysfunction.[114] Instead primary effects seem to be induced within the periphery by improvement in oxidative energy metabolism within the skeletal muscle and in vascular function.[115]

Exercise should primarily focus on moderate intensities of endurance exercise. MCE (3–5 days/week, 40 minutes per session, 60% peak heart rate) is generally recommended and has been successfully examined in most of the trials that have been conducted so far.

Moderate-intensity dynamic resistance (60% of one repetition maximum, 15 repetitions per exercise) can be added from the start.[114]

Higher-endurance intensities, such as HIIT (4×4 minutes at 85–90% peak heart rate, with 3 minutes of active recovery), have revealed positive effects on myocardial function, but data are still scarce and limited to a small group of patients with diabetes[110] and HFpEF.[116] In the latter trial, HIIT performed over 4 weeks significantly improved peak VO_2 and LV diastolic function, whereas these measures remained unchanged in the continuous exercise group.[116] Thus, higher-intensity exercise should be limited to stable patients and could be gradually introduced after 4 weeks of moderate continuous training.

Exercise sessions should start with short phases of 10 minutes of endurance exercises and 10 minutes of resistance exercises, which should gradually be extended in time over a period of 4 weeks. The final aim should be ≥3 days per week of at least 30–45 minutes. Depending on the patient's symptomatic status and ability, exercise intensity may be increased and intervals of higher intensity may be introduced.

Duration of intervention seems to be important in HFpEF for inducing functional and structural cardiovascular changes. Likewise, interventions over 2 years in healthy individuals reversed early signs of diastolic malfunction.[117,118] In elderly patients with longer metabolic dysfunction, exercise duration of 12–20 weeks[119] may either be too short or the 'therapeutic window' may be too late to reverse structural changes.

Air travel counselling and leisure

The problem of air travelling (or prolonged car travelling) for cardiac patients is frequently discussed because these patients are often concerned by their comfort and safety during these travels. We will not deal here with the problem of airplane pilots, but only with that of passengers, nor that of professional drivers of taxis or of heavy goods vehicles.

Travelling, particularly by air, generates stress problems linked especially to access to the airport, parking problems, difficulty of carrying often heavy luggage for long-distance flights, and delays in queues, but also time differences that may result in fatigue and difficulty of proper timing for taking medication.[120]

Since 2021, air transport has been well secured for people with cardiac diseases. Some flights last >12 hours, which can cause undeniable fatigue. The cabin of an airplane is not a normal space. Temperature is controlled, but humidity is reduced, generally by 10–20%, which can cause drying out of cabin air and patient dehydration. It is therefore important that patients drink water regularly. In addition, there is restriction of patient movements due to the cramped conformation of the cabins.[120]

The pressure inside a cabin varies, although it is supposed to be relatively constant at an altitude equivalent to between 1525 and 2038 m (between 5000 and 8000 ft). As the plane climbs, there is a corresponding decrease in cabin pressure and partial oxygen pressure (PaO_2). The standard barometric pressure at sea level is 760 mmHg, decreases to 1525 m (5000 ft) at 565 mmHg with PaO_2 to 75 mmHg (10 kPa). At 2438 m, or 8000 ft, the PaO_2 in the cabin air drops further to 65 mmHg (8.5 kPa). Fortunately, the haemoglobin dissociation curve usually keeps arterial blood saturation at 90% or higher.[120]

The normal response to hypobaric hypoxia is a moderate increase in heart rate, which increases the oxygen demand of the myocardium. In patients with severe coronary artery disease, this may eventually cause symptoms. Likewise, patients with a pulmonary diffusion disorder, such as pulmonary fibrosis or interstitial oedema, may be more short of breath. However, in the vast majority of cases, if the patient is capable of moderate exertion, this should not be a problem.

Patients should carry their medications with them in their hand luggage and take them at the prescribed times. They must have their prescription and, if possible, a written note from the doctor for customs and the police.

Some specific aspects

Stable coronary artery disease is not a contraindication to flying, provided there is no unstable angina pectoris or a very recent hospitalization for acute coronary syndrome. A patient with unstable angina should not fly within days of hospitalization. After an uncomplicated myocardial infarction, after approval from the airline, repatriation can be considered after a week, even though it is classically recommended to wait 3–4 weeks. The patient should be stable, with no signs of decompensation.

Patients who have had coronary angioplasty can fly after 5 days.

In the event of coronary artery bypass, it is not recommended to fly <15 days after a procedure and air travel is best done after 4–6 weeks. Significant ventricular arrhythmia or AF and HF should also be excluded.

HF in NYHA classes I, II, or III must be stabilized. In the event of NYHA class IV, flying is a priori contraindicated. In cases of hypoxaemia, additional oxygen therapy may be necessary. In the event of pulmonary arterial hypertension (systolic pulmonary artery pressure >60 mmHg), it may be necessary to consider additional oxygen therapy because of the risk of hypoxic pulmonary vasoconstriction.[121]

Patients with cyanotic congenital heart disease generally tolerate cabin PO_2 tension. There is no contraindication to flying with a defibrillator or a single- or triple-chamber pacemaker. The patient with a defibrillator must inform the police at the airport that they wear the device.

Thromboembolic disease (venous thrombosis, pulmonary embolism)

The problem of thromboembolic disease during air travel has been widely evaluated in recent years. What has been mistakenly called 'economy class syndrome' can also be seen in front-of-flight passengers in business class when the flight is long. It is confirmed that the risk of thromboembolic events doubles after a 4-hour flight and increases further with longer or repeated flights. This same risk also applies to travel by coach, bus, and train. The presence of obesity, being very tall, taking oral contraceptives, or pre-existing thrombopathy increases the risk of thromboembolic complications in 1 in 6000 healthy subjects over a 4-hour flight. There are passengers at increased risk of thromboembolic complications. Dehydration and immobility increase the risk and the general recommendation that applies to everyone is to move around during a flight and to avoid alcohol.[120] Venous contention is generally desirable. Use of aspirin is controversial. Low-molecular weight heparins or new non-vitamin K oral anticoagulants (NOACs) can be given to high-risk patients the day before their flight.

In total, in the vast majority of cases, there is no contraindication to air travel for a HF subject. However, it is important during the rehabilitation programme to explain all these elements to patients to reduce their stress and so they can minimize the risk of air travel.

Sexual activity and psychosocial aspects

Cardiovascular events cause significant stress to the patient or their partner regarding sexual activity after the event. There is therefore a great need for information, counselling, and advice on sexuality in the rehabilitation phase.[122]

Before initiating education and possible treatment, it is important to define the patient's sexual activity and level of satisfaction.[123] One should know the possible problems so as not to miss unrevealed or false ideas. Likewise, comorbidities must be known, as well as the presence of symptoms during sexual intercourse (shortness of breath, pain) and the possible need to take nitrates during sexual intercourse. It is important to know if the patient has erectile dysfunction, which may require specific treatment. It should be noted that there are very important cultural and personal differences to take into account when discussing sexual activity with a patient and/or their partner. Indeed, some people may legitimately consider that their sexual function is a private matter and that discussing sexual activity may, in some cultures, seem inadequate or even inappropriate. For men, it is important to determine the risk of sexual activity. A patient's reported functional capacity can be used to estimate cardiovascular risk during sexual activity, but in some cases, a stress test may be required to accurately assess the degree of effort involved in intercourse relative to the patient's physical capacities.[124]

In general, for *low-risk* patients who can perform moderate-intensity exercise without symptoms, sexual activity is generally safe. This is the case for patients who have been effectively revascularized, and who have controlled hypertension, asymptomatic valve disease, or moderate NYHA class I cardiac dysfunction. In these patients, sexual activity is not a problem.

At-risk patients are those with severe cardiovascular disease, who have symptoms for moderate or mild physical activities in whom sexual activity can pose a significant risk and in whom a reduction or cessation of sexual activity, unless or until the situation has stabilized, can be considered. Risk factors are generally unstable angina, uncontrolled hypertension, NYHA class III or IV HF, recent myocardial infarction, high-risk atrial or ventricular rhythm disorders, particularly during exertion, presence of a defibrillator with frequent appropriate shocks or uncontrolled AF, hypertrophic cardiomyopathy, and symptomatic aortic stenosis.

Intermediate-risk patients are those in whom assessment by stress testing is desirable before recommending sexual activity. One can include in these categories patients with angina pectoris, myocardial infarction dating from 2 to 8 weeks, NYHA class II and III HF, peripheral vascular diseases without cardiac involvement such as arteritis of the lower limbs, and a history of stroke or transient ischaemic attack. Patients can be moved to a higher- or lower-risk category based on other investigations, including stress testing.

Role of cardiovascular drugs

Cardiovascular drugs are a well-known cause of sexual dysfunction. Beta-blockers and thiazide diuretics have a recognized effect on erectile dysfunction. The effects of angiotensin-converting enzyme (ACE) inhibitors or angiotensin receptor blockers are a priori very moderate, if not neutral.[125] It is important to remind the patient that they should never suddenly stop their medication if they suspect a side effect on their sexual function related to treatment. Often, reducing the dosage or changing the drug class will improve sexual dysfunction.

It is important to suggest that patients and their partners increase their physical activity together. This not only reduces the risk associated with having sex, but also promotes intimacy. If the patient is able to perform physical activity corresponding to 3–5 metabolic equivalent (METs) without symptoms, such as walking on a treadmill at 5–8 km per hour or climbing two floors fairly quickly, resumption of sexual activity does not pose a problem. In some cases, a stress test is desirable, especially to determine if physical activity triggers a symptom that was not apparent before the heart attack. In difficult cases, one may discuss with the patient and their partner the possibility of having other types of sex that cause less physical stress. Kissing with sexual touching and masturbation may be preferred for a variable period of time.

For patients with angina pectoris or myocardial infarction, once they are stabilized, sexual activity can be resumed about a week after the cardiac event. Patients with a complicated myocardial infarction or HF should only resume sexual activity gradually

after a fairly long period of time and may require a stress test to determine whether or not they are fit for resumption of sexual activity. It is important to reassure patients who are often very worried about the risks accompanying sexual activity.

After coronary artery bypass grafting, it is important to reassure the patient, the essential limit being the alteration of the sternal scar in the event of a sternotomy. In these conditions, it is necessary to suggest modification of positions during sexual intercourse.

For HF patients, resumption of sexual activity is very dependent on the haemodynamic severity and its functional impact. This is usually not a problem for patients in NYHA class I or II. For NYHA class IV patients, it is important to optimize treatment to reduce shortness of breath and fatigue during intercourse. Sildenafil and other PDE5 inhibitors, used for erectile dysfunction, should not be used in cases of symptomatic or severe hypotension, nor should nitrates be used in cases of angina pectoris.

Devices

Having a pacemaker implanted is not a contraindication or a limitation to sexual activity. It is known that when using a defibrillator, there is considerable anxiety and fear of appropriate or inappropriate shock during sexual activity.[124] It is important to educate these patients and to perform a stress test to show the absence of risk of defibrillator shock in moderate physical activities. On the other hand, in the event of repeated shocks or arrhythmias, it is preferable to reconsider the risk of sexual activity. In this case, it may be necessary to change the settings of the defibrillator.

Psychosocial risk factors

There is abundant literature showing that psychosocial risk factors (PSRFs), such as low socio-economic status, social isolation, type D personality, depression, and anxiety, increase the risk of coronary artery disease and contribute to altering the QoL and prognosis of patients with coronary artery disease.[126]

PSRFs also act as barriers to changes in lifestyle and treatment adherence, and may reduce the effects of cardiovascular rehabilitation. In addition, there is a bidirectional interaction between PSRFs and the cardiovascular system. Stress, anxiety, and depression interact with the cardiovascular system via neuroendocrine and behavioural mechanisms. Conversely, coronary artery disease and associated treatments can lead to distress in patients, including anxiety and depression.

In practice, PSRFs can be assessed by using simple screening questionnaires, more standardized questionnaires, or structured clinical interviews. Psychotherapy and treatments can improve symptoms related to any PSRF and QoL.[127,128]

Multimodal behavioural intervention that incorporates counselling for PSRFs and coping with illness should be integrated into a comprehensive cardiac rehabilitation programme. Patients with clinical distress syndromes should be referred for psychological treatment or for psychological and/or psychopharmacological drug interventions.

In summary, the success of cardiac rehabilitation can strongly depend on the connection between brain and body, and this interaction needs to be reflected in the assessment and management of PSRFs, in line with robust scientific evidence, with trained staff integrated into the cardiac rehabilitation team.

Future directions

The pandemic period is changing the approach to management of patients with HF. Thanks to innovative technologies, patients will certainly be able to detect early signs of instability or check vital parameters on a daily basis, through his/her self-monitoring.

The use of customized dedicated apps will empower the patient to follow more adequate and effective gender-oriented exercise programmes, which will combine aerobic and resistance training sessions, due to the use of remote monitoring devices.

Complete cardiac rehabilitation programmes will also be available at home, thanks to the use of digital platforms that deliver class lessons managed by a physiotherapist, as well as individual nutrition and behavioural education sessions which can also be dedicated to psychological aspects.

Key messages

- Non-pharmacological management strategies are an important, non-replaceable contribution to HF therapy.

- Active participation of the patient is required for management of their HF.

- In order to identify signs and symptoms of HF, it is important to train the patient in self-monitoring, with involvement of caregivers.

- Close focus on management of old and new risk factors is required.

- All patients with HF should train with use of gender-specific personalized programmes.

- Implementation of home-based rehabilitation programmes is useful to increase the number of enrolled HF patients.

References

1. Murphy SP, Ibrahim NE, Januzzi JL Jr. Heart failure with reduced ejection fraction: a review. JAMA 2020;**32**:488–504.
2. Shah KS, Xu H, Matsouaka RA, *et al*. Heart failure with preserved, borderline, and reduced ejection fraction: 5-year outcomes. J Am Coll Cardiol 2017;**70**:2476–86.
3. Greene SJ, Butler J, Albert NM, *et al*. Medical therapy for heart failure with reduced ejection fraction: the CHAMP-HF registry. J Am Coll Cardiol 2018;**72**:351–66.
4. Boyd KJ, Murray SA, Kendall M, Worth A, Frederick BT, Clausen H. Living with advanced heart failure: a prospective, community-based study of patients and their carers. Eur J Heart Fail 2004;**6**:585–91.
5. Brostrom A, Stromberg A, Dahlstrom U, Fridlund B. Sleep difficulties, daytime sleepiness, and health-related quality of life in patients with chronic heart failure. J Cardiovasc Nurs 2004;**19**:234–42.
6. Clark JC, Lan VM. Heart failure patient learning needs after hospital discharge. Appl Nurs Res 2004;**17**:150–7.
7. Horowitz CR, Rein SB, Leventhal H. A story of maladies, misconceptions and mishaps: effective management of heart failure. Soc Sci Med 2004;**58**:631–43.
8. Martinez-Selles M, Garcia Robles JA, Munoz R, Serrano JA, Frades E, Dominguez MM. Pharmacological treatment in patients with heart failure: patients knowledge and occurrence of polypharmacy, alternative medicine and immunizations. Eur J Heart Fail 2004;**6**:219–26.
9. Moser DK, Watkins JF. Conceptualizing self-care in heart failure: a life course model of patient characteristics. J Cardiovasc Nurs 2008;**23**:205–18.
10. Rogers AE, Addington-Hall JM, Abery AJ, McCoy AS, Bulpitt C, Coats AJ. Knowledge and communication difficulties for patients with chronic heart failure: qualitative study. BMJ 2000;**321**:605–7.
11. Rollnick S, Mason P, Butler C. *Health Behavior Change: A Guide for Practitioners*. New York, NY: Churchill Livingston; 1999.
12. Fitzgibbon ML, *et al*. Understanding population health from multilevel and community-based models. In: Shumaker S, Schron E, Ockenen J, eds *The Handbook of Health Behavior Change*. New York, NY: Springer Publishing; 2018.
13. Saarmann L, Daugherty J, Riegel B. Patient teaching to promote behavioral change. Nurs Outlook 2000;**48**:281–7.
14. Riegel B, Carlson B, Glaser D. Development and testing of a clinical tool measuring self-management of heart failure. Heart Lung 2000;**29**:4–15.
15. Riegel B, Dickson VV. A situation-specific theory of heart failure self-care. J Cardiovasc Nurs 2008;**23**:190–6.
16. Kroenke K, Spitzer RL, Williams JB. The Patient Health Questionnaire-2: validity of a two-item depression screener. Med Care 2003;**41**:1284–92.
17. Beck A, Steer R, Carbin M. Psychometric properties of the Beck Depression Inventory: twenty-five years of evaluation. Clin Psychol Rev 1988;**8**:77–100.
18. Berkman LF, Blumenthal J, Burg M, *et al*. Effects of treating depression and low perceived social support on clinical events after myocardial infarction: the Enhancing Recovery in Coronary Heart Disease Patients (ENRICHD) randomized trial. JAMA 2003;**289**:3106–16.
19. Murphy SP, Ibrahim NE, Januzzi JL Jr. Heart failure with reduced ejection fraction: a review. JAMA 2020;**324**:488–504.
20. Shah KS, Xu H, Matsouaka RA, *et al*. Heart failure with preserved, borderline, and reduced ejection fraction: 5-year outcomes. J Am Coll Cardiol 2017;**70**:2476–86.
21. Greene SJ, Butler J, Albert NM, *et al*. Medical therapy for heart failure with reduced ejection fraction: the CHAMP-HF registry. J Am Coll Cardiol 2018;**72**:351–66.
22. Lainscak M, Blue L, Clark AL, *et al*. Self-care management of heart failure: practical recommendations from the Patient Care Committee of the Heart Failure Association of the European Society of Cardiology. Eur J Heart Fail 2011;**13**:115–26.
23. McDonagh TA, Blue L, Clark AL, *et al*. European Society of Cardiology Heart Failure Association standards for delivering heart failure care. Eur J Heart Fail 2011;**13**:235–41.
24. Yancy CW, Jessup M, Bozkurt B, *et al*. 2013 ACCF/AHA guideline for the management of heart failure: a report of the American College of Cardiology Foundation/American Heart Association Task Force on Practice Guidelines. J Am Coll Cardiol 2013;**62**:e147–239.
25. Doukky R, Avery E, Mangla A, *et al*. Impact of dietary sodium restriction on heart failure outcomes. JACC Heart Fail 2016;**4**:24–35.
26. Abshire M, Xu J, Baptiste D, *et al*. Nutritional interventions in heart failure: a systematic review of the literature. J Card Fail 2015;**21**:989–99.
27. Hummel SL, Konerman MC. Dietary sodium restriction in heart failure: a recommendation worth its salt? JACC Heart Fail 2016;**4**:36–8.
28. Jefferson K, Ahmed M, Choleva M, *et al*. Effect of a sodium-restricted diet on intake of other nutrients in heart failure: implications for research and clinical practice. J Card Fail 2015;**21**:959–62.

29. Bianchi VE. Nutrition in chronic heart failure patients: a systematic review. Heart Fail Rev 2020;**25**:1017–26

30. Sack MN, Kelly DP. The energy substrate switch during development of heart failure: gene regulatory mechanisms (review). Int J Mol Med 1998;**1**(1):17–24.

31. Taegtmeyer H, Sen S, Vela D. Return to the fetal gene program: a suggested metabolic link to gene expression in the heart. Ann N Y Acad Sci 2010;**1188**:191–8.

32. Neglia D, De Caterina A, Marraccini P, et al. Impaired myocardial metabolic reserve and substrate selection flexibility during stress in patients with idiopathic dilated cardiomyopathy. Am J Physiol Heart Circ Physiol 2007;**293**(6):H3270–8.

33. Chess DJ, Xu W, Khairallah R, et al. The antioxidant tempol attenuates pressure overload-induced cardiac hypertrophy and contractile dysfunction in mice fed a high-fructose diet. Am J Physiol Heart Circ Physiol 2008;**295**(6):H2223–30.

34. Feinberg J, Nielsen EE, Korang SK, et al. Nutrition support in hospitalised adults at nutritional risk. Cochrane Database Syst Rev 2017;**5**:CD011598.

35. Weijs PJM, Wolfe RR. Exploration of the protein requirement during weight loss in obese older adults. Clin Nutr 2016;**35**(2):394–8.

36. Tektonidis TG, Akesson A, Gigante B, Wolk A, Larsson SC. Adherence to a Mediterranean diet is associated with reduced risk of heart failure in men. Eur J Heart Fail 2016;**18**(3):253–9.

37. Wirth J, di Giuseppe R, Boeing H, Weikert C. A Mediterranean-style diet, its components and the risk of heart failure: a prospective population-based study in a non-Mediterranean country. Eur J Clin Nutr 2016;**70**(9):1015–21.

38. Chrysohoou C, Panagiotakos DB, Aggelopoulos P, et al. The Mediterranean diet contributes to the preservation of left ventricular systolic function and to the long-term favorable prognosis of patients who have had an acute coronary event. Am J Clin Nutr 2010;**92**(1):47–54.

39. Colin Ramirez E, Castillo Martinez L, Orea Tejeda A, Rebollar Gonzalez V, Narvaez David R, Asensio Lafuente E. Effects of a nutritional intervention on body composition, clinical status, and quality of life in patients with heart failure. Nutrition 2004;**20**(10):890–5.

40. Colin-Ramirez E, Castillo-Martinez L, Orea-Tejeda A, Zheng Y, Westerhout CM, Ezekowitz JA. Dietary fatty acids intake and mortality in patients with heart failure. Nutrition 2014;**30**(11–12):1366–71.

41. Khan MS, Khan F, Gregg C, et al. Dietary interventions and nutritional supplements for heart failure: a systematic appraisal and evidence map. Eur J Heart Fail 2021;**23**(9):1468–76.

42. Mortensen SA, Rosenfeldt F, Kumar A, et al. The effect of coenzyme Q10 on morbidity and mortality in chronic heart failure: results from Q-SYMBIO: a randomized double-blind trial. JACC Heart Fail 2014;**2**:641–9.

43. Costanzo S, Di Castelnuovo A, Donati MB, Iacoviello L, de Gaetano G. Alcohol consumption and mortality in patients with cardiovascular disease: a meta-analysis. J Am Coll Cardiol. 2010;**55**:1339–47.

44. Cruz-Jentoft AJ, Bahat G, Bauer J, et al.; Writing Group for the European Working Group on Sarcopenia in Older People 2 (EWGSOP2), and the Extended Group for EWGSOP2. Sarcopenia: revised European consensus on definition and diagnosis. Age Ageing 2019;**48**:16–31.

45. Doehner W, Anker SD. Cardiac cachexia in early literature: a review of research prior to Medline. Int J Cardiol 2002;**85**:7–14.

46. Fülster S, Tacke M, Sandek A, et al. Muscle wasting in patients with chronic heart failure: results from the studies investigating co-morbidities aggravating heart failure (SICA-HF). Eur Heart J 2013;**34**:512–19.

47. Von Haehling S. The wasting continuum in heart failure: from sarcopenia to cachexia. Proc Nutr Soc 2015;**74**:367–77.

48. Evans WJ, Morley JE, Argilés J, et al. Cachexia: a new definition. *Clin Nutr* 2008;**27**:793–9.

49. Rossignol P, Masson S, Barlera S, et al.; GISSI-HF and Val-HeFT Investigators. Loss in body weight is an independent prognostic factor for mortality in chronic heart failure: insights from the GISSI-HF and Val-HeFT trials. Eur J Heart Fail 2015;**17**:424–33.

50. Anker SD, Negassa A, Coats AJS, et al. Prognostic importance of weight loss in chronic heart failure and the effect of treatment with angiotensin-converting-enzyme inhibitors: an observational study. Lancet 2003;**361**:1077–83.

51. Von Haehling S, Anker SD. Prevalence, incidence and clinical impact of cachexia: facts and numbers: update 2014. J Cachexia Sarcopenia Muscle 2014;**5**:261–3.

52. Rehn TA, Munkvik M, Lunde PK, Sjaastad I, Sejersted OM. Intrinsic skeletal muscle alterations in chronic heart failure patients: a disease-specific myopathy or a result of deconditioning? Heart Fail Rev 2012;**17**:421–36.

53. Nagaya N, Moriya J, Yasumura Y, et al. Effects of ghrelin administration on left ventricular function, exercise capacity, and muscle wasting in patients with chronic heart failure. Circulation 2004;**110**:3674–9.

54. Landi F, Liperoti R, Russo A, et al. Association of anorexia with sarcopenia in a community-dwelling elderly population: results from the ilSIRENTE study. Eur J Nutr 2013;**52**:1261–8.

55. Blum WF, Alherbish A, Alsagheir A, et al. The growth hormone-insulin-like growth factor-I axis in the diagnosis and treatment of growth disorders. Endocr Connect 2018;7:R212–22.

56. Clark AL, Coats AJS, Krum H, et al. Effect of beta-adrenergic blockade with carvedilol on cachexia in severe chronic heart failure: results from the COPERNICUS trial. J Cachexia Sarcopenia Muscle 2017;**8**:549–56.

57. Springer J, Tschirner A, Haghikia A, et al. Prevention of liver cancer cachexia-induced cardiac wasting and heart failure. Eur Heart J 2014;**35**:932–41.

58. Bonilla-Palomas JL, Gámez-López AL, Castillo-Domínguez JC, et al. Nutritional intervention in malnourished hospitalized patients with heart failure. Arch Med Res 2016;**47**:535–40.

59. Bauer J, Biolo G, Cederholm T, et al. Evidence-based recommendations for optimal dietary protein intake in older people: a position paper from the PROT-AGE Study Group. J Am Med Dir Assoc 2013;**14**:542–59.

60. Vest AR, Chan M, Deswal A, et al. Nutrition, obesity, and cachexia in patients with heart failure: a consensus statement from the Heart Failure Society of America Scientific Statements Committee. J Card Fail 2019;**25**:380–400.

61. Gomes Neto M, Durães AR, Conceição LSR, Saquetto MB, Ellingsen Ø, Carvalho VO. High intensity interval training versus moderate intensity continuous training on exercise capacity and quality of life in patients with heart failure with reduced ejection fraction: a systematic review and meta-analysis. Int J Cardiol 2018;**261**:134–41.

62. Belardinelli R, Georgiou D, Cianci G, Purcaro A. 10-year exercise training in chronic heart failure: a randomized controlled trial. J Am Coll Cardiol 2012;**60**:1521–8.

63. O'Connor CM, Whellan DJ, Lee KL, et al.; HF-ACTION Investigators. Efficacy and safety of exercise training in patients with chronic heart failure: HF-ACTION randomized controlled trial. JAMA 2009;**301**:1439–50.

64. Ponikowski P, Voors AA, Anker SD, et al.; ESC Scientific Document Group. 2016 ESC Guidelines for the diagnosis and treatment of acute and chronic heart failure: the Task Force for the diagnosis and treatment of acute and chronic heart failure of the European

Society of Cardiology (ESC). Developed with the special contribution of the Heart Failure Association (HFA) of the ESC. *Eur Heart J* 2016;**37**:2129–200.

65. Adamopoulos S, Coats AJ, Brunotte F, *et al*. Physical training improves skeletal muscle metabolism in patients with chronic heart failure. J Am Coll Cardiol 1993;**21**:1101–6.

66. Giuliano C, Karahalios A, Neil C, Allen J, Levinger I. The effects of resistance training on muscle strength, quality of life and aerobic capacity in patients with chronic heart failure. A meta-analysis. Int J Cardiol 2017;**227**:413–23.

67. Laoutaris ID, Piotrowicz E, Kallistratos MS, *et al*.; ARISTOS-HF trial (Aerobic R InSpiratory Training OutcomeS in Heart Failure) Investigators. Combined aerobic/resistance/inspiratory muscle training as the 'optimum' exercise programme for patients with chronic heart failure: ARISTOS-HF randomized clinical trial. Eur J Prev Cardiol 2021;**28**:1626–35.

68. Agarwal SK, Chambless LE, Ballantyne CM, *et al*. Prediction of incident heart failure in general practice. Circ Heart Fail 2012;**5**:422–9.

69. Gopal DM, Kalogeropoulos AP, Georgiopoulou VV, *et al*. Cigarette smoking exposure and heart failure risk in older adults: the Health, Aging, and Body Composition Study. Am Heart J 2012;**164**:236–42.

70. Noel CA, LaMonte MJ, Roberts MB, *et al*. Healthy lifestyle and risk of incident heart failure with preserved and reduced ejection fraction among post-menopausal women: the Women's Health Initiative Study. Prev Med 2020;**138**:106155.

71. Kamimura D, Cain LR, Mentz RJ, *et al*. Cigarette smoking and incident heart failure: insights from the Jackson Heart Study. Circulation 2018;**137**:2572–82.

72. Nadruz W, Claggett B, Gonçalves A, *et al*. Smoking and cardiac structure and function in the elderly: the ARIC study (Atherosclerosis Risk in Communities). Circ Cardiovasc Imaging 2016;**9**:1–7.

73. Moreira HT, Armstrong AC, Nwabuo CC, *et al*. Association of smoking and right ventricular function in middle age: CARDIA study. Open Heart 2020;**7**:e001270.

74. Hendriks T, van Dijk R, Alsabaan NA, van der Harst P. Active tobacco smoking impairs cardiac systolic function. Sci Rep 2020;**10**:1–6.

75. Son YJ, Lee HJ. Association between persistent smoking after a diagnosis of heart failure and adverse health outcomes: a systematic review and meta-analysis. Tob Induc Dis 2020;**18**:1–11.

76. European Monitoring Centre for Drugs and Drug Addiction. *Annual Report 2009: The State of the Drugs Problem in Europe*. Luxembourg: Publications Office of the European Union; 2009.

77. Qureshi AI, Suri MF, Guterman LR, Hopkins LN. Cocaine use and the likelihood of nonfatal myocardial infarction and stroke: data from the Third National Health and Nutrition Examination Survey. Circulation 2001;**103**:502–6.

78. Aquaro GD, Gabutti A, Meini M, *et al*. Silent myocardial damage in cocaine addicts. Heart 2011;**97**:2056–62.

79. Figueredo VM. Chemical cardiomyopathies: the negative effects of medications and nonprescribed drugs on the heart. Am J Med 2011;**124**:480–8

80. Becker AE, Grinspoon SK, Klibanski A, Herzog DB. Eating disorders. N Engl J Med 1999;**340**(14):1092–8.

81. Ponikowski P, Voors AA, Anker SD, *et al*. 2016 ESC Guidelines for the diagnosis and treatment of acute and chronic heart failure: the Task Force for the diagnosis and treatment of acute and chronic heart failure of the European Society of Cardiology (ESC). Developed with the special contribution of the Heart Failure Association of the ESC. Eur Heart J 2016;**37**:2129–200.

82. Long L, Mordi IR, Bridges C, *et al*. Exercise-based cardiac rehabilitation for adults with heart failure. Cochrane Database Syst Rev 2019;**1**:CD003331.

83. Rees K, Taylor RS, Singh S, Coats AJS, Ebrahim S. Exercise based rehabilitation for heart failure. Cochrane Database Syst Rev 2004;**3**:CD003331.

84. Sagar VA, Davies EJ, Briscoe S, *et al*. Exercise-based rehabilitation for heart failure: systematic review and meta-analysis. Open Heart 2015;**2**:e000163.

85. Smart NA, Taylor R, Walker S, *et al*. Exercise training for chronic heart failure (ExTraMATCH II): why all data are not equal. Eur J Prev Cardiol 2019;**26**:1229–31.

86. Pandey *et al*. Safety and efficacy of exercise training in patients with an implantable cardioverter–defibrillator: a meta-analysis. JACC Clin Electrophysiol 2017;**3**:117–26.

87. Corra U, Agostoni PG, Anker SD, *et al*. Role of cardiopulmonary exercise testing in clinical stratification in heart failure. A position paper from the Committee on Exercise Physiology and Training of the Heart Failure Association of the European Society of Cardiology. Eur J Heart Fail 2018;**20**:3–15.

88. O'Connor CM, Whellan DJ, Lee KL, *et al*.; HF-ACTION Investigators. Efficacy and safety of exercise training in patients with chronic heart failure: HF-ACTION randomized controlled trial. JAMA 2009;**301**:1439–50.

89. Dalal HM, Taylor RS, Jolly K, *et al*. The effects and costs of home-based rehabilitation for heart failure with reduced ejection fraction: the REACH-HF multicentre randomized controlled trial. Eur J Prev Cardiol 2019;**26**:262–72.

90. Rognmo O, Moholdt T, Bakken H, *et al*. Cardiovascular risk of high-versus moderate-intensity aerobic exercise in coronary heart disease patients. Circulation 2012;**126**:1436–40.

91. Ellingsen O, Halle M, Conraads V, *et al*. High-intensity interval training in patients with heart failure with reduced ejection fraction. Circulation 2017;**135**:839–49.

92. Piepoli MF, Conraads V, Corra U, *et al*. Exercise training in heart failure: from theory to practice. A consensus document of the Heart Failure Association and the European Association for Cardiovascular Prevention and Rehabilitation. Eur J Heart Fail 2011;**13**:347–57.

93. Corra U, Piepoli MF, Carre F, *et al*. Secondary prevention through cardiac rehabilitation: physical activity counselling and exercise training: key components of the position paper from the Cardiac Rehabilitation Section of the European Association of Cardiovascular Prevention and Rehabilitation. Eur Heart J 2010;**31**:1967–74.

94. Alvarez P, Hannawi B, Guha A. Exercise and heart failure: advancing knowledge and improving care. Methodist Debakey Cardiovasc J 2016;**12**:110–15.

95. Balady GJ, Williams MA, Ades PA, *et al*. Core components of cardiac rehabilitation/secondary prevention programs: 2007 update: a scientific statement from the American Heart Association Exercise, Cardiac Rehabilitation, and Prevention Committee, the Council on Clinical Cardiology; the Councils on Cardiovascular Nursing, Epidemiology and Prevention, and Nutrition, Physical Activity, and Metabolism; and the American Association of Cardiovascular and Pulmonary Rehabilitation. Circulation 2007;**115**:2675–82.

96. Piepoli MF, Corra U, Benzer W, *et al*. Secondary prevention through cardiac rehabilitation: from knowledge to implementation. A position paper from the Cardiac Rehabilitation Section of the European Association of Cardiovascular Prevention and Rehabilitation. Eur J Cardiovasc Prev Rehabil 2010;**17**:1–17.

97. Taylor RS, Sagar VA, Davies EJ, *et al*. Exercise-based rehabilitation for heart failure. Cochrane Database Syst Rev 2014;**4**:CD003331.

98. Gayda M, Ribeiro PAB, Juneau M, Nigam A. Comparison of different forms of exercise training in patients with cardiac disease: where does high-intensity interval training fit? Can J Cardiol 2016;**32**:485–94.

99. Gomes Neto M, Duraes AR, Conceicao LSR, Saquetto MB, Ellingsen O, Carvalho VO. High intensity interval training versus moderate intensity continuous training on exercise capacity and quality of life in patients with heart failure with reduced ejection fraction: a systematic review and meta-analysis. Int J Cardiol 2018;**261**:134–41.

100. Doletsky A, Andreev D, Giverts I, *et al.* Interval training early after heart failure decompensation is safe and improves exercise tolerance and quality of life in selected patients. Eur J Prev Cardiol 2017;**25**:9–18.

101. Cornelis J, Beckers P, Taeymans J, Vrints C, Vissers D. Comparing exercise training modalities in heart failure: a systematic review and meta-analysis. Int J Cardiol 2016;**221**:867–76.

102. Conraads VM, Beckers PJ. Exercise training in heart failure: practical guidance. Heart 2010;**96**:2025–31.

103. Williams MA, Haskell WL, Ades PA, *et al.* Resistance exercise in individuals with and without cardiovascular disease: 2007 update: a scientific statement from the American Heart Association Council on Clinical Cardiology and Council on Nutrition, Physical Activity, and Metabolism. Circulation 2007;**116**:572–84.

104. Giuliano C, Karahalios A, Neil C, Allen J, Levinger I. The effects of resistance training on muscle strength, quality of life and aerobic capacity in patients with chronic heart failure: a meta-analysis. Int J Cardiol 2017;**227**:413–23.

105. Sadek Z, Salami A, Joumaa WH, Awada C, Ahmaidi S, Ramadan W. Best mode of inspiratory muscle training in heart failure patients: a systematic review and meta-analysis. Eur J Prev Cardiol 2018;**25**:1691–701.

106. Wu J, Kuang L, Fu L. Effects of inspiratory muscle training in chronic heart failure patients: a systematic review and meta-analysis. Congenit Heart Dis 2018;**13**:194–202.

107. Smart NA, Giallauria F, Dieberg G. Efficacy of inspiratory muscle training in chronic heart failure patients: a systematic review and meta-analysis. Int J Cardiol 2013;**167**:1502–7.

108. Vanhees L, Geladas N, Hansen D, *et al.* Importance of characteristics and modalities of physical activity and exercise in the management of cardiovascular health in individuals with cardiovascular risk factors: recommendations from the EACPR. Part II. Eur J Prev Cardiol 2012;**19**:1005–33.

109. Balady GJ, Williams MA, Ades PA, *et al.* Core components of cardiac rehabilitation/secondary prevention programs: 2007 update: a scientific statement from the American Heart Association Exercise, Cardiac Rehabilitation, and Prevention Committee, the Council on Clinical Cardiology; the Councils on Cardiovascular Nursing, Epidemiology and Prevention, and Nutrition, Physical Activity, and Metabolism; and the American Association of Cardiovascular and Pulmonary Rehabilitation. Circulation 2007;**115**:2672682.

110. Beckers PJ, Denollet J, Possemiers NM, Wuyts FL, Vrints CJ, Conraads VM. Combined endurance-resistance training vs. endurance training in patients with chronic heart failure: a prospective randomized study. Eur Heart J 2008;**29**:1858–66.

111. Tei C, Horikiri Y, Park JC, *et al.* Acute hemodynamic improvement by thermal vasodilation in congestive heart failure. Circulation 1995;**91**:2582–90.

112. Adsett JA, Mudge AM, Morris N, Kuys S, Paratz JD. Aquatic exercise training and stable heart failure: a systematic review and meta-analysis. Int J Cardiol 2015;**186**:22–8.

113. Smart NA, Haluska B, Jeffriess L, Leung D. Exercise training in heart failure with preserved systolic function: a randomized controlled trial of the effects on cardiac function and functional capacity. Congest Heart Fail 2012;**18**:295–301.

114. Pandey A, Garg S, Khunger M, *et al.* Dose–response relationship between physical activity and risk of heart failure: a meta-analysis. Circulation 2015;**132**:1786–94.

115. Adams V, Reich B, Uhlemann M, Niebauer J. Molecular effects of exercise training in patients with cardiovascular disease: focus on skeletal muscle, endothelium, and myocardium. Am J Physiol Heart Circ Physiol 2017;**313**:H72–88.

116. Angadi SS, Mookadam F, Lee CD, Tucker WJ, Haykowsky MJ, Gaesser GA. High-intensity interval training vs. moderate-intensity continuous exercise training in heart failure with preserved ejection fraction: a pilot study. J Appl Physiol 2015;**119**:753–8.

117. Pathak RK, Elliott A, Middeldorp ME, *et al.* Impact of CARDIOrespiratory FITness on arrhythmia recurrence in obese individuals with atrial fibrillation: the CARDIO-FIT study. J Am Coll Cardiol 2015;**66**:985–96.

118. Howden EJ, Sarma S, Lawley JS, *et al.* Reversing the cardiac effects of sedentary aging in middle age: a randomized controlled trial: implications for heart failure prevention. Circulation 2018;**137**:1549–60.

119. Kitzman DW, Brubaker P, Morgan T, *et al.* Effect of caloric restriction or aerobic exercise training on peak oxygen consumption and quality of life in obese older patients with heart failure with preserved ejection fraction: a randomized clinical trial. JAMA 2016;**315**:36–46.

120. Joy M. Cardiovascular disease and airline travel. Heart 2007;**93**:1507–9.

121. Broberg CS, Uebing A, Cuomo L, Thein SL, Papadopoulos MG, Gatzoulis MA. Adult patients with Eisenmenger syndrome report flying on commercial airlines. Heart 2007;**93**;1599–603.

122. Steinke EE, Jaarsma T. Sexual counselling and cardiovascular disease: practical approaches. Asian J Androl 2015;**17**:32–9.

123. Steinke EE, Jaarsma T, Barnason SA, *et al.* Sexual counselling for individuals with cardiovascular disease and their partners: a consensus document from the American Heart Association and the ESC Council on Cardiovascular Nursing and Allied Professions (CCNAP). Circulation 2013;**128**:2075–96.

124. Lange RA, Levine GN. Sexual activity and ischemic heart disease. Curr Cardiol Rep 2014;**16**:445.

125. Baumhakel M, Schlimmer N, Kratz M, Hackett G, Jackson G, Bohm M. Cardiovascular risk, drugs and erectile function: a systematic analysis. Int J Clin Pract 2011;**65**:289–98.

126. Pogosova N, Saner H, Pedersen SS, *et al.* Psychosocial aspects in cardiac rehabilitation: from theory to practice. A position paper from the Cardiac Rehabilitation Section of the European Association of Cardiovascular Prevention and Rehabilitation of the European Society of Cardiology. Eur J Prev Cardiol 2015;**22**:1290–306.

127. Perk J, De Backer G, Gohlke H, *et al.* European Guidelines on cardiovascular disease prevention in clinical practice (version 2012). The Fifth Joint Task Force of the European Society of Cardiology and Other Societies on Cardiovascular Disease Prevention in Clinical Practice (constituted by representatives of nine societies and by invited experts). Eur Heart J 2012;**33**:1635–701.

128. Piepoli MF, Corra U, Benzer W, *et al.* Secondary prevention through cardiac rehabilitation: from knowledge to implementation. A position paper from the Cardiac Rehabilitation Section of the European Association of Cardiovascular Prevention and Rehabilitation. Eur J Cardiovasc Prev Rehabil 2010;**17**:1–17.

SECTION 10

Acute heart failure

CHAPTER 10.1

Acute heart failure: diagnostic and prognostic assessment

Ovidiu Chioncel, Gerasimos Filippatos, Alexandre Mebazaa, Veli-Pekka Harjola, and Josep Masip

Contents

Introduction

There is a large spectrum of acute heart failure (AHF) presentations resulting from the interaction between an acute precipitant and a patient's underlying cardiac and overall medical condition, including previous comorbidities.[1] The heterogeneity of the pathophysiology and clinical presentations of this syndrome as well as the variable relationship between the chronic condition and the episodes of acute decompensation remain major factors hindering a simple and thorough definition of this condition.

AHF refers to rapid or gradual onset or worsening of symptoms and/or signs of HF, reflecting diverse abnormalities of congestion and/or hypoperfusion status, leading to unplanned hospital admission, ED visit or outpatient visit. It is a medical condition, very often life-threatening and requiring urgent evaluation with subsequent initiation/intensification of treatment, including IV therapies or intervention.[1]

AHF is a 'multi-event disease', and any clinical event associated with worsening signs/symptoms should be acknowledged. Including only hospitalizations for AHF, the burden of AHF is largely underestimated, since many patients do present in ED or ambulatory office for worsening signs/symptoms of AHF. Secondly, performance bar measures aimed to decrease hospitalizations may convert into increasing number of ED visits. AHF patients may have comparable risk irrespective of the decision to hospitalize versus administer outpatient intravenous diuretics.[2] In all the cases, the presentation is by definition, unplanned.[1,3,4]

AHF is the leading cause of hospitalizations worldwide, especially in individuals aged 65 years or older, and accounts for 2–10% of all hospitalizations, depending on the type of hospital.[3–5] Patients with AHF have a variety of underlying heart diseases, risk factors, comorbidities, and precipitants leading to acute decompensation.[5]

AHF is associated with high mortality and re-hospitalization rates. Overall, in-hospital mortality ranges from 2.4% to 10%.[5–8] The highest in-hospital mortality rate was seen in patients with cardiogenic shock, and 50% of deaths occurred on the first day of admission suggesting that early identification of hypoperfusion signs, as well as appropriateness of initial therapies, is crucial in this setting.[9]

For post-discharge mortality, the UK-National Heart Failure Audit reported a 1-year mortality of 30%.[10] In the ESC-HF-LT Registry study, 27% of AHF patients died at 1 year, 26% were re-admitted due to HF, and 44% of patients died or have been re-admitted within 1 year following discharge.[9]

AHF may be the first manifestation of HF (new onset), or more frequently (70% of AHF) it is related to an acute decompensation of chronic HF[1,4,11] and regardless of clinical presentation, either *new onset* or decompensation of chronic HF, these patients are evaluated and treated in different clinical settings, outpatient clinic, ED, and in-hospital. Mortality at discharge may be similar for both clinical presentations, but one-year mortality and re-hospitalization rates are higher in patients with acutely decompensated chronic HF.[12,13] AHF episodes may occur in patients with or without previous cardiac dysfunction. Acute loss of myocardial tissue (e.g. acute myocardial infarction (AMI), myocarditis) or mechanical cause (spontaneous rupture of MV chordae, valvular perforation in case of acute endocarditis) lead to AHF especially in patients with previously normal cardiac structure. Usually, these patients have a clear aetiological factor the resolution of which contributes to HF remission. Of patients with known cardiac dysfunction, some have history of HF while others may evolve asymptomatically for variable period of time. In these

patients, interaction between acute precipitants and cardiac substrate leads to destabilization.

Diagnostic workup

The ESC-HF Guidelines recommend that the diagnostic workup must start at the time of the first medical contact, and be continued throughout the initial patient pathway.[1] Although, some diagnostic and therapeutic tools are now available in the prehospital setting before admission to the ED, whether more effective pre-hospital care would alter the clinical outcome remains to be proven in randomized clinical trials.[14] Furthermore, pre-hospital assessment and management should not delay the rapid transfer of AHF patients to the most appropriate medical environment.[14,15]

The initial clinical evaluation of patients suspected of AHF should confirm the diagnosis of AHF, assess severity of AHF, and identify precipitating factors.[16] Initial diagnosis of AHF should be based on clinical judgment to integrate patient history with assessing the symptoms and signs/symptoms of congestion and/or hypoperfusion by physical examination (→ Figure 10.1.1).

A history of heart failure is the most useful historical parameter. Previously documented cardiac dysfunction (myocardial infarction, valvular disease, coronary artery disease) increase probability of heart failure, and its absence decreases the likelihood.[16]

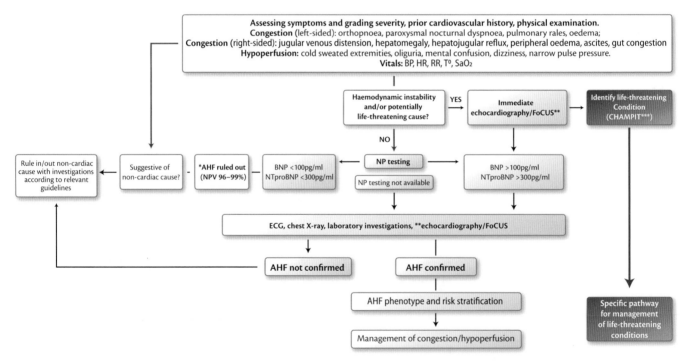

Figure 10.1.1 Diagnostic workup for patients with suspected acute heart failure.

AHF, acute heart failure; BP, blood pressure; HR, heart rate; NP, natriuretic peptide; NPV, negative predictive value; NTproBNP, N-terminal pro-B-type natriuretic peptide; RR, respiratory rate; T, body temperature.

*Unexpectedly low levels of NPs can be detected in some patients with decompensated end-stage HF, flash pulmonary oedema, or right sided AHF.

**Immediate echocardiography is mandatory only in patients with haemodynamic instability (particularly in cardiogenic shock) and in patients suspected of acute life-threatening structural or functional cardiac abnormalities (mechanical complications, acute valvular regurgitation, aortic dissection). Early echocardiography should be considered in all patients with de novo AHF and in those with unknown cardiac function; however, the optimal timing is unknown (preferably within 48 h from admission, if the expertise is available).

***CHAMPIT is the acronym for the following life-threatening causes: acute **C**oronary syndrome, **H**ypertension, **A**rrhythmia, acute **M**echanical cause and **P**ulmonary embolism, **I**nfections and **T**amponade.

Dyspnoea is the most common symptom of AHF. However, the characteristics of dyspnoea should be objectively assessed by evaluating the respiratory rate, intolerance of the supine position, and degree of hypoxia. The presence of paroxysmal nocturnal dyspnoea increases the likelihood of the diagnosis of acute heart failure.[17] A reduced likelihood of AHF as the cause of dyspnoea is suggested by the absence of orthopnoea, paroxysmal nocturnal dyspnoea, and leg oedema.[17]

Typically, symptoms and signs of AHF reflect fluid overload (pulmonary congestion and/or peripheral oedema) or, less often, reduced cardiac output with peripheral hypoperfusion.[1,11] Congestion is a typical feature of AHF, and physical examination should primarily focus on the presence of congestion which would support the diagnosis of AHF. Left-sided congestion may cause dyspnoea, orthopnoea, bendopnoea, paroxysmal nocturnal dyspnoea, cough, tachypnoea, pathological lung auscultation (rales, crackles, wheezing), and hypoxaemia.[17] The absence of rales and a normal chest radiography do not exclude the presence of left-sided congestion. Indeed, 20–30% of patients with elevated pulmonary-artery wedge pressure may have a normal chest radiography.[18]

Right-sided congestion may cause increased body weight, bilateral peripheral oedema, decreased urine output, abdominal pain, nausea, jugular vein distension (JVD), or positive hepato-jugular reflux, ascites, and hepatomegaly.[17] JVD has the best accuracy for the diagnosis of AHF and in the absence of isolated right ventricular systolic dysfunction, JVD reliably predicts pulmonary capillary wedgepressure (PCWP) >15 mm Hg.[19] Although, elevation in right atrial pressure mirrors an elevation in PCWP in most patients with HF, approximately 25% to 30% of patients have discordance between right- and left-sided filling pressures, with an isolated elevation on either side[20–22] (⊃ Figure 10.1.2).

Though rare, in patients with hypovolaemic state, there may not be any evidence of congestion or elevated filling pressures, but rather decreased cardiac output accompanied with low or normal ventricular filling pressures(e.g. in the setting of over-diuresis or other fluid losses in patients with HF). Once the hypovolaemic state is corrected, patients with AHF usually have elevated filling pressures and unveil congestive signs.

Symptoms and signs of hypoperfusion indicate severity[23,24] and may include hypotension, tachycardia, weak pulse, mental confusion, anxiety, fatigue, cold sweated extremities, and decreased urine output. Clinical signs of hypoperfusion may appear in patients with left or right ventricular (LV or RV), or bi-ventricular dysfunctions, as well as in patients with reduced or preserved E.F.[23]

However, no single element from physical examination can accurately diagnose HF, and diagnosis involves integration of multiple physical findings, and diagnosis decisions should be based on comprehensive clinical examination.[25,26]

Since the sensitivity and specificity of symptoms and signs, are modest, diagnosis of AHF should be further confirmed by appropriate additional investigations such as ECG, chest X-ray, lung ultrasound, laboratory assessment (with specific biomarkers, mostly natriuretic peptides), and echocardiography[1,11] (⊃ Figure 10.1.1).

Natriuretic peptides (NPs), such as B-type natriuretic peptide (BNP) and N-terminal pro-B-type natriuretic peptide (NT-proBNP), are an integral component of HF diagnosis workup

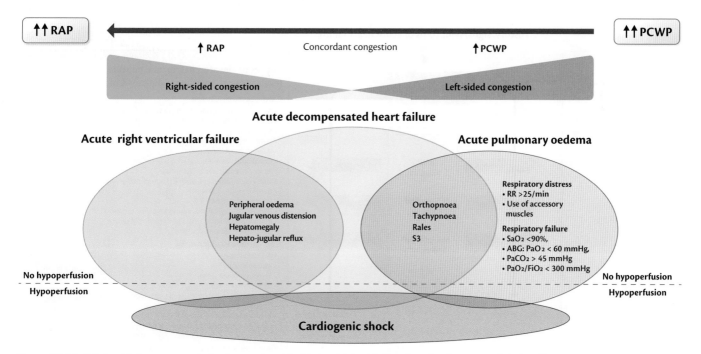

Figure 10.1.2 Relationship between congestion (concordant, left-sided and right-sided), and overlapping among clinical profiles.
ABG, arterial blood gases; ADHF, acute decompensated heart failure; AHF, acute heart failure; APO, acute pulmonary oedema; CS, cardiogenic shock; CT, computed tomography; HJR, hepato-jugular reflux; JVD, jugular venous distension; LUS, lung ultrasound; PaO^2 and PaCo^2, partial pressure of oxygen and carbon dioxide; PCWP, pulmonary capillary wedge pressure; RAP, right atrial pressure; RR, respiratory rate; RVF, right ventricular failure;SpO2, peripheral oxygen saturation.
*All clinical criteria are mandatory for APO diagnosis.

in many clinical settings, especially when the diagnosis is uncertain, based on their high negative predictive value.[1,11] Upon presentation to the ED or CCU/ICU, a plasma NP level (BNP, NT-proBNP, or MR-proANP) should be measured in all patients with acute dyspnoea and suspected AHF to help in the differentiation of AHF from non-cardiac causes of acute dyspnoea.[1,11] The use of these biomarkers has the highest class of recommendation to support exclusion of HF, due to the very high negative predictive value (94–97%) (➲ Figure 10.1.3). However, NPs are largely unspecific for HF diagnosis and several clinical conditions other than HF can result in an increase in NP levels, while other conditions are associated with NPs level lower than expected[27] (➲ Figure 10.1.3). Thus, individualized interpretation of biomarker levels, particularly in special populations and in the setting of competing diagnoses and comorbidities is recommended.[28,29] Furthermore, patient-level changes need to be interpreted according to baseline levels.

When plasma NP levels are not available or are above the cut-offs, additional investigations (i.e. chest X-ray, echocardiography, lung ultrasound) are needed (➲ Figure 10.1.1).

Cardiac imaging is the key step in order to define the underlying cardiac pathology.[1] Along with the initial routine assessment (clinical examination, electrocardiogram) and laboratory parameters (NPs, troponins, D-dimer, inflammation markers), imaging modalities are pivotal for accurate diagnosis of AHF in ED and help to guide initial therapeutic and disposition decisions.[17]

Chest X-ray is helpful in identification of pulmonary congestion (pulmonary venous congestion, pleural effusion, interstitial or alveolar oedema, and cardiomegaly) and to detect the presence and position of intracardiac devices.[1] Chest X-ray is also useful to identify alternative pathology, especially pneumonia, pleural effusion, and pneumothorax. However, clinicians should not rule out AHF in patients with no radiographic signs of congestion, since in about 20–30% patients with AHF, chest X-ray is nearly normal.[30] Also, there is a large inter-observer variability in the interpretation of the radiological signs of pulmonary congestion.[31,32]

ECG can provide useful information about underlying cardiac disease or potential precipitants (e.g. myocardial ischaemia, arrhythmias, pulmonary embolism (PE)), targets for specific therapies (e.g. rate control and anticoagulation for atrial fibrillation, pacing for bradycardia) and may help to select possible candidates for device therapies (cardiac resynchronization therapy, if the patient has left bundle branch block).[1,11,33] Of note, ECG may direct further imaging modalities (i.e. coronary angiography for ST elevation myocardial infarction, CT scan for RV strain, echocardiography for low QRS voltage).

Echocardiography enables prompt detection of essential structural abnormalities and objectively confirm pulmonary and systemic congestion.[32] Current guidelines do not recommend immediate echocardiography in all patients presenting with AHF.[1,11]

Immediate echocardiography is mandatory only in patients with haemodynamic instability (particularly in cardiogenic shock) and in patients suspected of acute life-threatening structural or functional cardiac abnormalities (mechanical complications, acute valvular regurgitation, aortic dissection). Early echocardiography should be considered in all patients with de novo AHF and in those patients with unknown cardiac structure and function or when structure or function have substantially

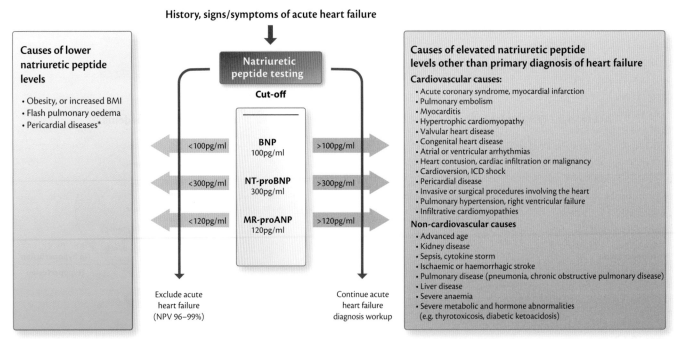

Figure 10.1.3 Utilization of natriuretic peptide testing in diagnosis of acute heart failure.
AHF, acute heart failure; BNP, brain natriuretic peptide; HF, heart failure; MR-pro-ANP, mid regional atrial natriuretic peptide; NT-pro-BNP, N terminal fragment of brain natriuretic peptide; NPV, negative predictive value.

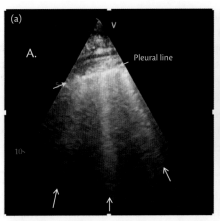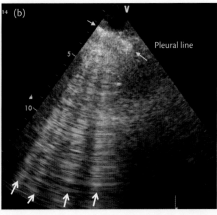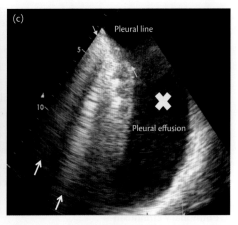

Figure 10.1.4 Pulmonary ultrasound examination as part of FoCUS protocol with detection of B-lines (white arrows in (a–c)). B-lines are 'comet-tail' artefacts arising from the thickened pleural line (yellow arrows) and extending indefinitely. Density of B-lines is increased as result of fluid accumulation due to compression caused by the pleural effusion (white cross in c). B-lines and are associated with extravascular lung water but can also be found in other conditions with increases in lung density (e.g. interstitial lung disease).

changed since previous studies; however, the optimal timing is unknown (preferably within 48 h from admission, if the expertise is available).[11,17]

The diagnostic value of bedside-focused cardiac ultrasound (FoCUS) and lung ultrasound (LUS) provides the shortest path to AHF diagnosis and life-saving therapies during the first 2 h after admission.[1,17,32] FoCUS examination allows quick differentiation of the pathophysiology of the haemodynamic instability through the identification of cardiac tamponade, RV or LV dysfunction, detection of pulmonary (lung B-lines), and right-side congestion (inferior vena cava diameter and respiratory variation) and associated severe valvular dysfunction.[32]

Lung ultrasonography has emerged as a valuable modality to detect pulmonary congestion in patients with AHF[32,34] (➲ Figure 10.1.4). This bedside technique enables the detection of interstitial fluid in the pulmonary parenchyma (visualization of B-lines) in a rapid manner, and its ability to rule in and rule out significant interstitial syndrome is superior compared to chest X-ray.[35]

Also, the number and extent of B-lines increases with the severity of congestion.[35,36] However, any condition that causes fluid build-up in the lymphatic interlobular septae at the pleural surface may produce B-lines, thus limiting the ability of pulmonary ultrasound alone to discriminate between AHF from other causes of pulmonary oedema.[34] Other pathological conditions, such as pleural effusion, pneumonia, and pneumothorax, can be also reliably detected with LUS.

Additional laboratory tests are helpful in the evaluation of patients with AHF. Cardiac troponin may be helpful to exclude myocardial ischaemia as precipitating factor of AHF.[1,37] However, cardiac troponin, in particular when measured with high-sensitive assays, is elevated in 80–90% of patients with AHF, often without obvious myocardial ischaemia or an acute coronary event.[37]

The initial laboratory evaluation should also include a basic assessment of the function of other organ systems (e.g. kidney, liver, blood). Blood urea nitrogen or urea, creatinine, and electrolytes (sodium, potassium) are useful to identify associated non-cardiac comorbidities and may help to guide the treatment.[1]

Liver function tests are often impaired in patients with AHF due to haemodynamic derangements, both reduced output and increased venous congestion,[38,39] and identify patients at risk of poor prognosis.[38-41]

D-dimer should be measured where acute PE is suspected.[1,11]

An infection trigger can be evaluated by measurement of inflammatory markers (e.g. C-reactive protein and procalcitonin).[42]

Since both hypothyroidism and hyperthyroidism may precipitate AHF, thyroid-stimulating hormone should be assessed in newly diagnosed AHF.[1,11]

Arterial blood gas analysis may be useful when a precise measurement of pH and O_2 and CO_2 partial pressure is needed (i.e. patients with respiratory distress).[1] Arterial lactate is a prognostic marker in patients presenting with hypoperfusion or haemodynamic instability and its variations, in addition to overall clinical status, markers of end-organ dysfunction, and echocardiographic parameters, may guide escalation or weaning of pharmacological or mechanical circulatory support. When arterial blood sample is not available, measurement of the venous lactate offers similar decisional information, since there is no arterio-venous gradient of blood lactate and there are no prognostic differences between venous and arterial lactate.[1]

Additional imaging modalities (for example, MRI) are rarely needed during the initial work-up but may be helpful during further investigations.

During the workup of the diagnostic process, careful evaluation of the potential cause or trigger of acute decompensation should be performed (➲ Box 10.1.1) and coexisting life-threatening clinical conditions, and/or precipitants that require urgent treatment/correction need to be immediately identified and managed.[1]

As stated in the 2021 ESC guidelines, known and treatable causes of AHF must be addressed during initial workup of AHF diagnosis.[1] Numerous factors may trigger AHF episodes (➲ Box 10.1.1), but several of these conditions are considered 'life-threatening' causes/aetiologies, follow specific management pathways and triage dispositions, and must be identified and treated before initiation of any other standard HF management algorithm process (➲ Figure 10.1.1). They included acute **c**oronary syndrome, **h**ypertension, **a**rrhythmia, acute **m**echanical cause and **p**ulmonary embolism, **i**nfections and **t**amponade (CHAMPIT).[1] In parallel, alternative causes for the patient's symptoms and signs (e.g. worsening COPD, asthma, pulmonary infection, severe anaemia, acute renal failure)[1], should be identified (➲ Figure 10.1.1).

The diagnostic workup should continue with the identification of clinical phenotypes (Acutely Decompensated HF, Acute Pulmonary Oedema, Acute Right Failure and Cardiogenic Shock) supporting the initiation of the early individualized treatments (➲ Figure 10.1.2).

Acutely decompensated HF

Acutely decompensated HF (ADHF) is the most common form, representing 60–70% of AHF presentations in observational studies.[9] These patients have history of chronic HF and very often previous HF hospitalizations. Typically, they present with symptoms and signs of systemic congestion that worsen gradually. Since the main pathophysiological alteration is progressive fluid retention, signs and symptoms reflect increasing left and right filling pressures, and less often with signs of hypoperfusion. Chest X-ray shows increased cardiothoracic index with pulmonary venous congestion (redistribution and perihilar haze). A large inferior vena cava (IVC) diameter with diminished respiratory variations is a common echo finding.[32]

Acute right failure

Acute right failure (ARF) can be defined as a rapidly progressive syndrome with systemic congestion resulting from impaired RV filling and/or reduced RV output.[39] RV failure is observed in 3–9% of AHF admissions, and the in-hospital mortality of patients with acute RV failure ranges from 5 to 17%.[9,43] The clinical presentation of acute right ventricular failure may vary depending on the underlying cause and presence of comorbidities.[43,44] In general, the predominant clinical features of acute right ventricular failure include: (1) elevated right atrial and central venous pressure displayed as jugular venous distension; (2) signs of systemic venous congestion due to fluid retention manifesting as peripheral oedema, ascites, pleural effusions, congestive hepatomegaly and hepatojugular reflux, and anasarca; (3) low cardiac output leading to peripheral and organ hypoperfusion; and (4) atrial or ventricular arrhythmias.[43,44] The initial triage is based on clinical assessment of vital signs and congestion and clinical history (e.g. knowledge of congenital or acquired heart disease, pre-existing pulmonary hypertension, recurrent episodes of pulmonary embolism). The diagnosis or exclusion of aetiologies requiring specific treatment (such as pulmonary embolism, pulmonary hypertension, or acute right myocardial infarction) should be prioritized.

ECG may reveal arrhythmias, signs suggesting right atrial and/or ventricular overload, or ischaemia. Chest X-ray shows an enlarged right contour and the absence of pulmonary venous congestion. Focused echocardiography provides bedside information on right ventricular size and function, as well as data about right filling pressure (IVC diameter and respiratory variations). Arterial blood gases and blood lactate should be assessed in presence of hypoxemia.[43,44]

Acute pulmonary oedema

Acute pulmonary oedema (APO) is the second most common clinical presentation of AHF (14–38%), though its reported prevalence and in-hospital mortality may vary considerably by geographic region.[45] Methodological differences among the registries, that are representative for distinct AHF populations from different clinical settings (ED, in-hospital, CCU) and variability of the time point of classification at different phase of acuity may contribute to the wide differences in the prevalence of APO. Also, overlapping features among AHF clinical profiles (➲ Figure 10.1.2) and/or the confounding presence of noncardiac comorbidities may lead to incomplete or inaccurate classification. Pathogenesis of this clinical profile is a rapid increase in pulmonary capillary hydrostatic pressure and transvascular fluid filtration that exceeds the lymphatic interstitial drainage capacity.[45–48] APO is a high-acuity presentation and the clinical picture is characterized by pulmonary congestion in the face of an acutely increased afterload.[45] Although clinical signs of pulmonary congestion were also reported in other clinical profiles, such as ADHF, the distinctive feature of APO patients is the severity of pulmonary congestion accompanied by respiratory distress (higher respiratory rate > 25/min or use of accessory muscles) and hypoxemia, both contributing to progressive respiratory failure that may lead to cardiorespiratory collapse in hours or minutes, unless therapeutic action is taken.[46]

Since there are variable definitions and due to poor inter-rater reliability based on the clinical diagnosis, several clinical criteria are necessary for diagnosis that require further confirmation through additional tests.[47] Beside symptoms, key clinical findings are respiratory distress and respiratory failure (➲ Figure 10.1.2). Diagnostic confirmation requires at least two of the following additional criteria, more specific for AHF: clear signs of pulmonary congestion on chest X-ray or CT scan, > three B-lines in two chest zones on each hemithorax on LUS, signs of elevated filling pressures on echo (E/E' > 15), BNP > 400 pg/ml or N-ProBNP > 900 pg/ml (or 1800 pg/ml in > 75 years), elevated pulmonary capillary pressure on catheterization, increased total lung water on pulse contour, and thermodilution analysis system.[47] This diagnosis algorithm highlights the importance of respiratory distress and respiratory failure, which should be treated with oxygen and non-invasive ventilation. In some instances, hypoxemia may be too severe or may not be promptly improved by decongestive therapies. The decision to initiate invasive mechanical ventilation must be anticipated and should be based on clinical judgment, considering the overall clinical picture, but should not be delayed until the patient is in extremis or has an altered level of consciousness.[45,48]

Patients with APO often present hypertension on admission, either as precipitant or as reactive stress response. Low systolic blood pressure (SBP) at presentation or clinical signs of hypoperfusion, even subtle, portend a poor prognosis.[45]

A search for the precipitant and underlying aetiology must be conducted early in the course of hospitalization. It is important to identify those aetiologies that will not respond to conventional intravenous (IV) therapies, such as mechanical complications of AMI, valvular endocarditis, and prosthetic valve dysfunction.[48]

Cardiogenic shock

Cardiogenic shock (CS) represents the most severe form of AHF. The prevalence of CS varies according to the definition of CS, clinical setting care, and era of data collection. CS accounts for 2–5% of AHF presentations, with a prevalence in ICU/ICCU datasets of 14–16%.[39,49] In-hospital mortality varied between 30% and 60%,[9,39,49] with nearly half of in-hospital deaths occurring within the first 24 h of presentation.[9]

CS is a syndrome caused by a primary cardiovascular disorder in which inadequate cardiac output results in a life-threatening state of tissue hypoperfusion associated with impairment of tissue oxygen metabolism and hyperlactataemia. Depending on its severity, CS may result in multi-organ dysfunction and death.[39] CS may arise in advanced chronic HF when acute precipitants trigger decompensation or may manifest as an acute onset, *de novo* presentation, most often caused by an acute coronary syndrome (ACS).[39]

Based on clinical criteria, diagnosis of CS mandates the presence of clinical signs of hypoperfusion, such as cold sweated extremities, oliguria, mental confusion, dizziness, narrow pulse pressure. Of note, hypoperfusion is not always accompanied by hypotension, as blood pressure may be preserved by compensatory vasoconstriction (with/without pressor agents), albeit at the cost of impaired tissue perfusion and oxygenation. In addition, biochemical manifestations of hypoperfusion, elevated creatinine, metabolic acidosis, and elevated serum lactate, are present. The presence of clinical signs of peripheral hypoperfusion even with preserved SBP, is referred as 'pre-shock' and precedes overt CS. Pre-shock may occur in severe AHF presenting with diverse clinical phenotypes and can also be associated with clinical signs of tissue hypoperfusion but without compromising cellular metabolism and having normal lactate.[39] At end spectrum of severity, refractory CS has been defined as CS with ongoing evidence of tissue hypoperfusion despite administration of adequate doses of two vasoactive medications and treatment of the underlying aetiology.[39] The classification proposed by Society for Cardiovascular Angiography and Interventions (SCAI)[50] describes five stages of CS, from A (at risk of CS) to E (extremis) (➲ Figure 10.1.5) including a modifier for cardiac arrest. This classification can be applied rapidly at the bedside upon patient presentation, across all clinical settings. Recently, the SCAI classification has been validated in a large cohort of unselected intensive cardiac care unit (ICCU) patients[51] providing robust mortality risk stratification regardless of CS aetiology, in a manner that was amplified by the presence of CA.[52]

A 12-lead ECG should be performed immediately, and in several instances helps to identify underlying causes (ACS, PE, tamponade).[1,39]

Echocardiography has a central role to identify potential underlying causes and associated pathophysiology, because without identification and treatment of the underlying cause, the outcome is usually fatal. Standard echocardiographic evaluation or FoCUS when available in ED should provide rapidly sufficient information to confirm/exclude tamponade, mechanical complications of AMI, LV outflow tract obstruction, or severe valvular lesions. Concomitant assessment of LV and RV function, and estimation of left and right filling pressures should also be included in echo protocols.[1,32,39,49]

Since acute respiratory failure is present in almost all CS patients, arterial blood gas analysis with determination of blood gases and lactate is recommended in all patients and is highly indicative for the further need of invasive mechanical ventilation.[39]

Prognosis

One of the major goals of AHF risk stratification is to match the risk profile of the patient with the type and intensity of care throughout hospitalization stay. Thus, risk-stratification in AHF

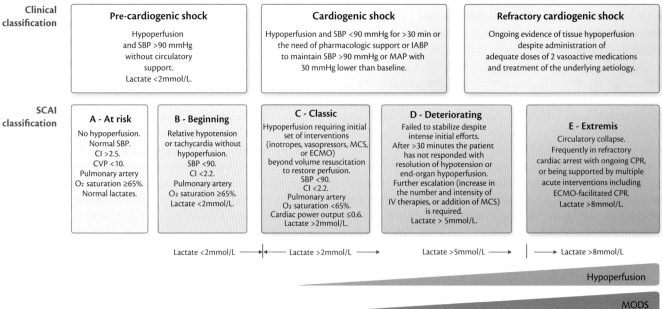

Figure 10.1.5 Cardiogenic shock classification: Clinical classification is based on clinical severity and the response to the treatment. The Society for Cardiovascular Angiography and Interventions (SCAI) classification utilizes bedside clinical assessment of hypoperfusion and vital signs, measurement of lactate level, invasive haemodynamic evaluation, and response to the initial therapies. The two classifications are presented with possible overlapping.

CI, cardiac index; CPR, cardio-pulmonary resuscitation; CVP, central venous pressure; ECMO, extracorporeal membrane oxygenation; IABP, intra-aortic balloon pump; MAP, mean arterial pressure; MCS, mechanical circulatory support; MODS, multi-organ dysfunction syndrome; SBP, systolic blood pressure.

Reproduced from Chioncel O, Parissis J, Mebazaa A, et al. Epidemiology, pathophysiology and contemporary management of cardiogenic shock - a position statement from the Heart Failure Association of the European Society of Cardiology. *Eur J Heart Fail.* 2020 Aug;22(8):1315–1341. doi: 10.1002/ejhf.1922 with permission from John Wiley and Sons.

is a dynamic process.[1,17] At initial presentation in ED, risk stratification may guide the appropriateness of disposition decisions and of initial therapeutic interventions, during hospitalization risk-stratification may identify the candidates for device therapy or surgical interventions, and at discharge may help to identify high-risk patients who require more intense follow-up or to plan elective interventions for selected patients.[53,54]

Once an AHF diagnosis is made and after initial stabilization and management in ED, accurate prognostic information may enhance the physician's ability to predict outcomes, thus informing disposition decisions for patients with AHF.[55] Several disposition options regarding the ultimate placement of the patient should be considered (➲ Figure 10.1.6), including ICU, a cardiology ward, or discharge at home. Because the response to AHF treatment is not immediate, an observation period after initial therapy is useful to define the correct disposition.[56,57]

Patient disposition after complete ED management is one of the most important decisions to be made by emergency physicians.[55] This would allow high-risk patients to receive prompt and aggressive in-hospital therapy, whereas low-risk patients could be safely discharged to home without exposure to potential risk associated to hospitalization and to reduce costly inpatient admissions.[55,58]

In the last decade, several risk scores have been developed for use in EDs with the aim of objectively supporting disposition decision-making process.[59,60] Recently, two of these risk scores,

MESSI and EHMRG, have been prospectively and externally validated for prediction of 30-day mortality, with 0% mortality in low-risk categories.[61,62] In both risk scores, several clinical variables, such as preserved SBP, normal respiratory rate, SpO2 > 95%, low troponin value and no ACS at presentation, creatinine < 1.5 mg/dl, and potassium 3.5–5 mEq/l, identified low risk categories. However, these scores are informative only for disposition decisions and do not guide safe management options. Also, broad generalizability has not yet been shown for any single risk score, and their implementation is not widespread.[63] AHF populations can vary widely in clinical characteristics, and even more powerful risk scores need recalibration to increase its precision for specific populations.[61,62] Recently, the Acute Cardiovascular Care Association proposed a checklist that may be used to ensure safely discharge of AHF patients from the ED, but this checklist may be used only in conjunction with clinical judgment and patients discharged home must be followed up in the first week at the HF clinic or by a nurse call.[63]

Further research, including impact studies followed by broad use of the algorithms may improve care efficiency of those at lower risk and enhance safety by decreasing inappropriate discharge of high-risk patients.[64]

Of note, establishing a risk score guided by the patient risk of adverse events, is only one component of the process of disposition decision making. Many non-medical circumstances, including socio-economic status and adequacy of family support

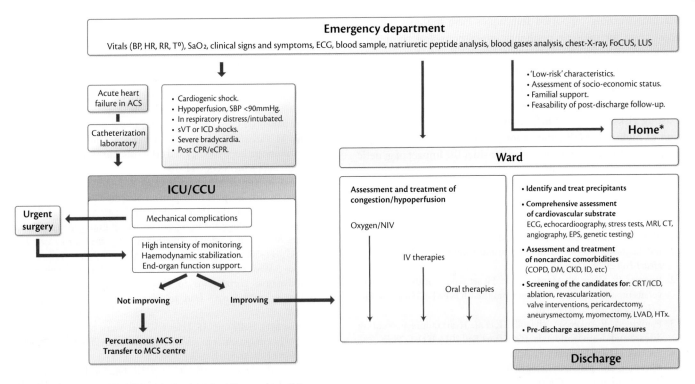

Figure 10.1.6 Disposition decisions in patients with acute heart failure.

ACS, acute coronary syndrome; BP, blood pressure; CCU, coronary care unit; CKD, chronic kidney disease; COPD, chronic obstructive pulmonary disease; CT, computed tomography; DM, diabetes mellitus; CPR, cardiopulmonary resuscitation; CRT, cardiac resynchronization therapy; ECG, electrocardiography; eCPR, extracorporeal membrane oxygenation supported cardiopulmonary resuscitation; EPS, electrophysiological studies; FoCUS, focused cardiac ultrasound; HR, heart rate; HTx, heart transplant; ICD, internal cardiac defibrillator ; ICU, intensive care unit; ID, iron deficiency; IV, intravenous; LVAD, left ventricular assist devices; LUS, lung ultrasound; MCS, mechanical circulatory support; MRI, magnetic resonance imaging; NIV, non-invasive ventilation; RR, respiratory rate; SaO$_2$, oxygen saturation SBP, systolic blood pressure; sVT, sustained ventricular tachycardia; T°, body temperature.

* When available, a short stay in observation unit to assess the response to therapies may be necessary.

must be considered[1,64] ($\circlearrowright$ Figure 10.1.4). Furthermore, once appropriately treated and risk stratified, a reliable mechanism for early outpatient follow-up is mandatory. Thus, risk prediction scores are powerful tools for predicting risk of adverse events but should not be used in isolation from other considerations when making disposition decisions for AHF patients.

AHF hospitalization represents an important opportunity to assess patient prognosis. A better understanding of the mechanisms underlying the poor prognosis of patients hospitalized for AHF may help provide better care and improve post-discharge mortality.[65]

A comprehensive assessment in these patients is necessary to identify multiple prognostic characteristics that may become possible therapeutic targets. Candidate predictors can be obtained from patient demographics, clinical history, physical examination, disease characteristics, laboratory tests, and previous treatment.[53,54]

In general, prognostic studies use a multivariable approach in their design and analysis to determine the important predictors of the studied outcomes and to provide outcome probabilities for different combinations of predictors. The aim is to determine whether an outcome can reliably be attributed to a particular risk factor, with adjustment for other causal factors (confounders) using a multivariable approach. In clinical trials and registries, the predictive factors for post-discharge mortality included age, history of previous hospitalization, congestion, SBP, heart rate,

QRS duration, renal function, markers of organ injury, and non-cardiac comorbidities (such as diabetes, cerebrovascular disease, chronic obstructive pulmonary disease, liver cirrhosis).

Post-hoc analyses derived from observational studies and clinical trials[68–71] have combined various risk markers from multivariable models in risk scores.

Given the complexity and heterogeneity of AHF, risk score modelling have not been easily adapted to clinical practice, and its impact on management has not been adequately established. There are also several other methodological limitations, including modest discriminatory capacity, and absence of prospective validation. Furthermore, studies to evaluate the effect of using of prognostic model on current medical practice are currently missing and only impact analysis can determine whether use of the risk-score model is better than usual care.[53,54]

Future directions

AHF represents a broad spectrum of disease states, and in addition to clinical profile scheme future classifications should include clinical variables designated as therapeutic targets. Risk stratification in AHF is an important component of the initial assessment and its major goal is to match the risk profile of the patient with the type and intensity of care, facilitating disposition decisions and initial management. However, the accuracy of the current algorithms based on several 'risk-variables' is rather poor.

Machine-learning-supported techniques have the advantage of accounting for multiple nonlinear interactions and combining machine learning with more traditional statistical techniques may provide an increased performance to predict the risk of decompensation and post-discharge mortality in AHF. Furthermore, quantitative proteomics analyses, when used in conjunction to existing risk scores may help clinicians in the early identification of high-risk AHF patients for prompt invasive procedures. Future research studies should also consider the impact of genetic polymorphisms on the initial responsiveness of medical therapies and subsequent risk of in-hospital complications.

References

1. McDonagh TA, Metra M, Adamo M, et al. 2021 ESC Guidelines for the diagnosis and treatment of acute and chronic heart failure. *Eur J Heart Fail* 2022; 24:4–131.

2. Ferreira JP, Metra M, Mordi I, et al. Heart failure in the outpatient versus inpatient setting: findings from the BIOSTAT-CHF study. *Eur J Heart Fail*. 2019;21:112–20.

3. Ponikowski P, Anker SD, AlHabib KF, et al.. Heart failure: preventing disease and death worldwide. *ESC Heart Fail* 2014;1(1):4–25.

4. Farmakis D and Filippatos G. Acute heart failure: epidemiology, classification, and pathophysiology. *The ESC Textbook of Intensive and Acute Cardiovascular Care* (3 edn). Edited by Marco Tubaro, Pascal Vranckx, Susanna Price, Christiaan Vrints, and Eric Bonnefoy. Oxford University Press. 2021: pp. 603–616.

5. Filippatos G, Angermann CE, Cleland JGF, et al. Global differences in characteristics, precipitants, and initial management of patients presenting with acute heart failure. *JAMA Cardiol.* 2020;5(4):401–10.

6. Chioncel O, Vinereanu D, Datcu M, et al.. The Romanian Acute Heart Failure Syndromes (RO-AHFS) Registry. *Am Heart J* 2011;162:142–53.

7. Kapłon-Cieslicka A, Benson L, Chioncel O, et al. A comprehensive characterization of acute heart failure with preserved versus mildly reduced versus reduced ejection fraction – insights from the ESC-HFA EORP Heart Failure Long-Term Registry. *Eur J Heart Fail.* 2022;24(2):335–50.

8. Crespo-Leiro MG, Anker SD, Maggioni AP, et al. European Society of Cardiology Heart Failure Long-Term Registry (ESC-HF-LT): 1-year follow-up outcomes and differences across regions. *Eur J Heart Fail.* 2016;18(6):613–25.

9. Chioncel O, Mebazaa A, Harjola VP, et al. Clinical phenotypes and outcome of patients hospitalized for acute heart failure: the ESC Heart Failure Long-Term Registry. *Eur J Heart Fail* 2017;19:1242–54.

10. Donkor A, Cleland J, McDonagh T, Hardman S. National Heart Failure Audit 2016. 2017. National Institute for Cardiovascular Outcomes Research (NICOR), London.

11. Ponikowski P, Voors AA, Anker SD, et al. 2016 ESC guidelines for the diagnosis and treatment of acute and chronic heart failure: The Task Force for the diagnosis and treatment of acute and chronic heart failure of the European Society of Cardiology (ESC). Developed with the special contribution of the Heart Failure Association (HFA) of the ESC. *Eur J Heart Fail* 2016;18:891–975.

12. Butt JH, Fosbol EL, Gerds TA, et al. Readmission and death in patients admitted with new-onset versus worsening of chronic heart failure: insights from a nationwide cohort. *Eur J Heart Fail* 2020;22(10):1777–85.

13. Javaloyes P, Miro O, Gil V, et al. Clinical phenotypes of acute heart failure based on signs and symptoms of perfusion and congestion at emergency department presentation and their relationship with patient management and outcomes. *Eur J Heart Fail* 2019;21(11):1353–65.

14. Harjola P, Miró Ò, Martín-Sánchez FJ, et al.. Pre-hospital management protocols and perceived difficulty in diagnosing acute heart failure. *ESC Heart Fail.* 2020;7(1):289–296.

15. Takahashi M, Kohsaka S, Miyata H, et al. Association between prehospital time interval and short-term outcome in acute heart failure patients. *J Card Fail* 2011;17(9):742–7.

16. Arrigo M, Parissis JT, Akiyama E, Mebazaa A. Understanding acute heart failure: pathophysiology and diagnosis. *Eur Heart J Supplements* 2016;18 (Supplement G), G11–18

17. Mebazaa A, Yilmaz MB, Levy P, et al. Recommendations on pre-hospital & early hospital management of acute heart failure: a consensus paper from the Heart Failure Association of the European Society of Cardiology, the European Society of Emergency Medicine and the Society of Academic Emergency Medicine. *Eur J Heart Fail* 2015;17:544–58.

18. Chakko S, Woska D, Martinez H, et al.. Clinical, radiographic, and hemodynamic correlations in chronic congestive heart failure: conflicting results may lead to inappropriate care. *Am J Med* 1991;90:353–9.

19. Drazner MH, Hellkamp AS, Leier CV, et al. Value of clinician assessment of hemodynamics in advanced heart failure: the ESCAPE trial. *Circ Heart Fail* 2008;1:170–7.

20. Drazner MH, Prasad A, Ayers C, et al. The relationship of right- and left-sided filling pressures in patients with heart failure and a preserved ejection fraction. *Circ Heart Fail* 2010;3:202–6.

21. Drazner MH, Brown RN, Kaiser PA, et al. Relationship of right- and left-sided filling pressures in patients with advanced heart failure: a 14-year multi-institutional analysis. *J Heart Lung Transplant* 2012;31:67–72.

22. Campbell P, Drazner MH, Kato M, et al. Mismatch of right- and left-sided filling pressures in chronic heart failure. *J Card Fail* 2011;17:561–8.

23. Chioncel O, Mebazaa A, Maggioni AP, et al. Acute heart failure congestion and perfusion status – impact of the clinical classification on in-hospital and long-term outcomes; insights from the ESC-EORP-HFA Heart Failure Long-Term Registry. *Eur J Heart Fail.* 2019;21(11):1338–52.

24. Javaloyes P, Miró Ò, Gil V, et al.. Clinical phenotypes of acute heart failure based on signs and symptoms of perfusion and congestion at emergency department presentation and their relationship with patient management and outcomes. *Eur J Heart Fail.* 2019;21(11):1353–65.

25. Girerd N, Seronde MF, Coiro S, et al. Integrative assessment of congestion in Heart Failure throughout the patient journey. *JACC Heart Fail* 2018;6:273–85.

26. Thibodeau JT, Drazner MH. The role of the clinical examination in patients with heart failure. *JACC Heart Fail* 2018;6:543–51

27. Chioncel O, Collins SP, Greene SJ, et al. Natriuretic peptide-guided management in heart failure. *J Cardiovasc Med* 2016;17:556–68.

28. Yancy CW, Jessup M, Bozkurt B, et al.. 2017 ACC/AHA/HFSA focused update of the 2013 ACCF/AHA guideline for the management of heart failure: a report of the American College of Cardiol- ogy/ American Heart Association Task Force on Clinical Practice Guidelines and the Heart Failure Society of America. *Circulation* 2017;136:e137–61.

29. Bozkurt B, Coats AJ, Tsutsui H, et al. Universal definition and classification of heart failure: A report of the Heart Failure Society of America, Heart Failure Association of the European Society of Cardiology, Japanese Heart Failure Society and Writing Committee of the Universal Definition of Heart Failure. *Eur J Heart Fail.* 2021;S1071-9164(21)00050-6.

30. Collins SP, Lindsell CJ, Storrow AB, Abraham WT, ADHERE Scientific Advisory Committee, Investigators and Study Group. Prevalence of negative chest radiography results in the emergency department patient with decompensated heart failure. *Ann Emerg Med* 2006;47:13–18.

31. Alaseri Z. Accuracy of chest radiography interpretation by emergency physicians. *Emerg Radiol* 2009;16:111–114.

32. Čelutkienė J, Lainscak M, Anderson L, et al. Imaging in patients with suspected acute heart failure: timeline approach position statement on behalf of the Heart Failure Association of the European Society of Cardiology. *Eur J Heart Fail* 2020;22:181–95.

33. Adriaan A. Voors and Piotr Ponikowski. Acute heart failure: diagnosis. *ESC CardioMed* (3rd edn) Edited by A. John Camm, Thomas F. Lüscher, Gerald Maurer, and Patrick W. Serruys, 2018. Oxford University Press, Oxford.

34. Ferre RM, Chioncel O, Pang PS, Lang RM, Gheorghiade M, Collins SP. Acute heart failure: the role of focused emergency cardiopulmonary ultrasound in identification and early management. *Eur J Heart Fail.* 2015;17(12):1223–7.

35. Volpicelli G, Elbarbary M, Blaivas M, et al. International evidence-based recommendations for point-of-care lung ultrasound. *Intensive Care Med* 2012;38:577–91.

36. Al Deeb M, Barbic S, Featherstone R, Dankoff J, Barbic D. Point-of-care ultra- sonography for the diagnosis of acute cardiogenic pulmonary edema in patients presenting with acute dyspnea: a systematic review and meta-analysis. *Acad Emerg Med* 2014;21:843–52.

37. Harjola VP, Parissis J, Bauersachs J, et al. Acute coronary syndromes and acute heart failure: a diagnostic dilemma and high-risk combination. A statement from the Acute Heart Failure Committee of the Heart Failure Association of the European Society of Cardiology. *Eur J Heart Fail.* 2020;22(8):1298–314.

38. Ambrosy AP, Gheorghiade M, Bubenek S, et al. The predictive value of transaminases at admission in patients hospitalized for heart failure: findings from the RO-AHFS registry. *Eur Heart J Acute Cardiovasc Care* 2013;2(2):99–108.

39. Chioncel O., Parissis J, Mebazaa A, et al. Epidemiology, pathophysiology and contemporary management of cardiogenic shock – a position statement from the Heart Failure Association of the European Society of Cardiology. *Eur J Heart Fail* 2020;22:1315–41.

40. Biegus J, Hillege HL, Postmus D, et al., Abnormal liver function tests in acute heart failure: relationship with clinical characteristics and outcome in the PROTECT study. *Eur J Heart Fail.* 2016;18:830–9.

41. Nikolaou M, Parissis J, Yilmaz MB, et al. Liver function abnormalities, clinical profile, and outcome in acute decompensated heart failure. *Eur Heart J* 2013;34(10):742–9.

42. Mockel M, de Boer RA, Slagman AC, et al. Improve Management of acute heart failure with ProcAlCiTonin in EUrope: results of the randomized clinical trial IMPACT EU Biomarkers in Cardiology (BIC) 18. *Eur J Heart Fail* 2020; 22(2):267–75.

43. Harjola VP, Mebazaa A, Čelutkienė J, et al.. Contemporary management of acute right ventricular failure: a statement from the Heart Failure Association and the Working Group on Pulmonary Circulation and Right Ventricular Function of the European Society of Cardiology. *Eur J Heart Fail* 2016;18(3):226–41.

44. Konstantinides SV, Meyer G, Becattini C, et al. 2019 ESC Guidelines for the diagnosis and management of acute pulmonary embolism developed in collaboration with the European Respiratory Society (ERS). *Eur Heart J* 2020 21;41(4):543–603.

45. Chioncel O, Ambrosy AP, Bubenek S, et al. Epidemiology, pathophysiology, and in-hospital management of pulmonary edema: data from the Romanian Acute Heart Failure Syndromes registry. *J Cardiovasc Med* 2016;17(2):92–104.

46. Masip J. Noninvasive ventilation in acute heart failure. *Curr Heart Failure Rep* 2019 16:89–97.

47. Masip J, Peacock WF, Price S, et al.Indications and practical approach to non-invasive ventilation in acute heart failure. *Eur Heart J.* 2018:39:17–25.

48. Chioncel O, Collins SP, Ambrosy AP, Gheorghiade M, Filippatos G. Pulmonary oedema-therapeutic targets. *Card Fail Rev* 2015;1(1):38–45.

49. Chioncel O, Collins SP, Ambrosy AP, et al.. Therapeutic advances in the management of cardiogenic shock. *Am J Ther.* 2019;26(2):e234–47.

50. Baran DA, Grines CL, Bailey S, et al.. SCAI Clinical expert consensus statement on the classification of cardiogenic shock: this document was endorsed by the American College of Cardiology (ACC), the American Heart Association (AHA), the Society of Critical Care Medicine (SCCM), and the Society of Thoracic Surgeons (STS) in April 2019. *Catheter Cardiovasc Interv* 2019;94:29–37.

51. Jentzer JC, van Diepen S, Barsness GW, et al. Cardiogenic shock classification to predict mortality in the cardiac intensive care unit. *J Am Coll Cardiol* 2019;74:2117–28.

52. Naidu SS, Baran DA, Jentzer JC, et al. SCAI SHOCK Stage Classification Expert Consensus Update: A Review and Incorporation of Validation Studies: This statement was endorsed by the American College of Cardiology (ACC), American College of Emergency Physicians (ACEP), American Heart Association (AHA), European Society of Cardiology (ESC) Association for Acute Cardiovascular Care (ACVC), International Society for Heart and Lung Transplantation (ISHLT), Society of Critical Care Medicine (SCCM), and Society of Thoracic Surgeons (STS) in December 2021. *J Am Coll Cardiol.* 2022;79(9):933–46.

53. Chioncel O, Collins SP, Greene SJ, et al. Predictors of post-discharge mortality among patients hospitalized for acute heart failure. *Card Fail Rev* 2017;;3(2):122–9.

54. Passantino A, Monitillo F, Iacoviello M, et al. Predicting mortality in patients with acute heart failure: Role of risk scores. *World J Cardiol* 2015;26;7:902–11.

55. Miró O, Levy PD, Möckel M, et al. Disposition of emergency department patients diagnosed with acute heart failure. *Eur J Emerg Med* 2017;24:2–12.

56. Collins SP, Pang PS, Fonarow GC, Yancy CW, Bonow RO, Gheorghiade M. Is hospital admission for heart failure really necessary? The role of the emergency department and observation unit in preventing hospitalization and rehospitalization. *J Am Coll Cardiol.* 2013;61:121–6.

57. Masri A, Althouse AD, McKibben J, et al. Outcomes of heart failure admissions under observation versus short inpatient stay. *J Am Heart Assoc.* 2018;7(3):e007944.

58. Michaud AM, Parker SIA, Ganshorn H, Ezekowitz JA, McRae AD. Prediction of early adverse events in emergency department patients with acute heart failure: a systematic review. *Can J Cardiol.* 2018;34(2):168–79.

59. Miró O, Rossello X, Gil V, et al.. Predicting 30-day mortality for patients with acute heart failure in the emergency department: a cohort study. *Ann Intern Med* 2017;167:698–705.

60. Lee DS, Stitt A, Austin PC, et al. Prediction of heart failure mortality in emergent care: a cohort study. *Ann Intern Med* 2012;156:767–75.

61. Wussler D, Kozhuharov N, Sabti Z, et al. External Validation of the MEESSI Acute Heart Failure Risk Score: A Cohort Study. *Ann Intern Med* 2019;170(4):248–56.

62. Lee DS, Lee JS, Schull MJ, et al. Prospective validation of the emergency heart failure mortality risk grade for acute heart failure. *Circulation* 2019;139(9):1146–56.

63. Masip J, Frank Peacok W, Arrigo M, *et al.* Acute Heart Failure in the 2021 ESC Heart Failure Guidelines: a scientific statement from the Association for Acute CardioVascular Care (ACVC) of the European Society of Cardiology. *Eur Heart J Acute Cardiovasc Care* 2022;11(2):173–85.

64. Collins SP, Pang P. ACUTE Heart failure risk stratification a step closer to the holy grail? *Circulation* 2019;139:1157–61.

65. Cohen-Solal A, Laribi S, Ishihara S, *et al.* Prognostic markers of acute decompensated heart failure: The emerging roles of cardiac biomarkers and prognostic scores. *Arch Cardiovasc Dis* 2015;108: 64–74.

66. O'Connor CM, Abraham WT, Albert NM, *et al.* Predictors of mortality after discharge in patients hospitalized with heart failure: an analysis from the Organized Program to Initiate Lifesaving Treatment in Hospitalized Patients with Heart Failure (OPTIMIZE-HF). *Am Heart J* 2008;156:662–73.

67. Salah K, Kok WE, Eurlings LW, *et al.* A novel discharge risk model for patients hospitalised for acute decompensated heart failure incorporating N-terminal pro-B-type natriuretic peptide levels: a European coLlaboration on Acute decompeNsated Heart Failure: ELAN-HF Score. *Heart* 2014;100:115–25.

68. Lassus J, Gayat E, Mueller C *et al.* Incremental value of biomarkers to clinical variables for mortality prediction in acutely decompensated heart failure: the Multinational Observational Cohort on Acute Heart Failure (MOCA) study. *Int J Cardiol* 2013;168: 2186–94.

69. Felker GM, Leimberger JD, Califf RM, *et al.* Risk stratification after hospitalization for decompensated heart failure. *J Card Fail* 2004;10:460–6..

70. O'Connor C, Hasselblad V, Mehta RH, *et al.* Triage after hospitalization with advanced heart failure: the ESCAPE (Evaluation Study of Congestive Heart Failure and Pulmonary Artery Catheterization Effectiveness) risk model and discharge score. *J Am Coll Cardiol* 2010;55:872–8.

71. Khazanie P, Heizer GM, Hasselblad V, *et al.* Predictors of clinical outcomes in acute decompensated heart failure: acute study of clinical effectiveness of nesiritide in decompensated heart failure outcome models. *Am Heart J* 2015;170:290–7.

CHAPTER 10.2

Acute heart failure: pharmacological and non-pharmacological management

Katerina Fountoulaki, John Parissis, Sean Collins, Mehmet Birhan Yilmaz, and Alexandre Mebazaa

Contents

Introduction

Acute heart failure (AHF) includes a wide spectrum of clinical conditions with varied aetiologies and triggers. AHF may be the first manifestation of heart failure (HF) (new onset) or, more frequently, be due to an acute decompensation of chronic HF. Specific extrinsic factors (e.g. acute coronary syndromes, arrhythmias, excessive hypertension, infection, non-adherence with salt/fluid intake or medications, severe anaemia, drugs and toxic substances) may trigger AHF in patients with pre-existing cardiac dysfunction.[1]

Patients with AHF can present with four major clinical phenotypes with possible overlaps between them: acutely decompensated HF (ADHF), which is the most common form accounting for 50–70% of presentations; acute cardiogenic pulmonary oedema (ACPO); isolated right ventricular (RV) failure; and cardiogenic shock (CS).[1] Clinical presentations are mainly based on bedside evaluation and categorization by clinical signs of congestion ('wet' vs 'dry' if present vs absent) and hypoperfusion ('cold' vs 'warm' if present vs absent), to allow differentiation into four distinct profiles: 'wet-warm' – patients demonstrating congestion and adequate peripheral perfusion; 'wet-cold' – with congestion and hypoperfusion; 'dry-cold' – free of congestion but with hypoperfusion; and 'dry-warm' – free of either congestion or hypoperfusion.[2] Of note, hypoperfusion is often accompanied by hypotension, but is not synonymous with it. Congestion and/or hypoperfusion may lead to injury and dysfunction of target organs (i.e. heart, lungs, kidneys, liver, intestine, brain) with increased risk of mortality.[3]

Consequently, it should be stressed that appropriate therapy requires appropriate identification of the specific AHF clinical phenotype and the underlying pathophysiology. Treatment strategies include apparently paradoxical antagonistic interventions, such as vasodilators vs vasoconstrictors and decongestion vs fluid resuscitation.[4] The aim of this chapter is to give a concise clinical overview of the evidence-based pharmacological and non-pharmacological treatment of AHF, providing a basis for clinical algorithms.

Time-sensitive approach in the management of acute heart failure

Several clinical trials and observational studies have suggested a 'time-sensitive' approach, especially for the management of specific phenotypes such as CS and ACPO that encompass high-morbidity characteristics.[5–7] Acute kidney injury (AKI) and/or multiple organ dysfunction syndrome (MODS) may occur in case of CS or AHF with severe systolic dysfunction, leading to poor outcomes.

Accordingly, early prehospital management is considered a critical component of care.[8,9] In the pre-hospital setting, AHF patients should benefit from:

♦ Noninvasive monitoring, including pulse oximetry, BP, respiratory rate, and a continuous ECG

♦ Oxygen therapy in hypoxaemic patients or noninvasive ventilation (NIV) in patients with respiratory distress

♦ Vasodilators and/or diuretics based on BP and clinical judgment of the degree of congestion. Diagnostic tools, as natriuretic peptides measured using a point-of-care device, are available in the ambulance in some countries and may aid in diagnosis during prolonged transfers.[9]

AHF patients should be transferred without delay to the hospital, preferably to a centre with a cardiology department and/or emergency department (ED) or coronary care unit/intensive care unit (CCU/ICU) with AHF expertise.[1]

The critical first step after first medical contact is determination of the severity of cardiopulmonary instability. CS and respiratory failure must be immediately identified, and patients should be triaged to a location where resuscitation and prompt cardiovascular and respiratory support can be provided.[1] CS is defined as the presence of systolic BP < 90 mmHg for > 30 min (or need of catecholamines to maintain systolic BP > 90mmHg), associated with clinical signs of pulmonary congestion as well as impaired organ perfusion with at least one of the following: (i) altered mental status, (ii) cold and clammy skin and extremities, (iii) serum lactate >2.0 mmol/L, (iv) oliguria with urine output < 30 mL/h (< 0.5 mL/kg/min), caused by a cardiac condition.[10]

The next step within the initial 60–120 min should comprise the evaluation for aetiologies or major precipitants leading to AHF, which have their specific treatments and need to be corrected urgently (➲ Table 10.2.1). The leading causes of AHF are captured by the CHAMPIT acronym – acute Coronary syndrome, Hypertension emergency, Arrhythmia, acute Mechanical cause (e.g. mechanical complication of acute coronary syndrome, acute native or prosthetic valve regurgitation due to endocarditis, aortic dissection), Pulmonary embolism, Infections (viral or bacterial) and Tamponade.[1] Other precipitating factors include noncompliance with medical treatment and diet restrictions, medications (e.g. non-steroidal anti-inflammatory drugs (NSAIDs), steroids), a chronic obstructive pulmonary disease (COPD) exacerbation, worsening renal function, anaemia, and thyroid disorders. If an underlying precipitant of HF is not apparent, it is important to

Table 10.2.1 Major precipitants/causes of acute heart failure and their urgent specific treatments

Major precipitants/causes	Urgent treatment
Acute coronary syndrome	Immediate invasive strategy with intent to perform revascularization
Hypertension	Aggressive BP reduction (in the range of 25% during the first few hours) with iv vasodilators and loop diuretics
Arrhythmia	Medical therapy (rhythm and rate control), electrical cardioversion (atrial or ventricular arrhythmia with haemodynamic compromise), temporary pacing (conducting disturbances)
Acute mechanical cause	Circulatory support with surgical or percutaneous intervention
Pulmonary embolism	Primary reperfusion in case of shock or hypotension by iv thrombolysis (mainly), catheter-based approach or surgical embolectomy
Sepsis	Rapid detection of bacterial infection and initiation of specific antibiotic treatment
Tamponade	Pericardiocentesis

iv, intravenous; BP, blood pressure.

hunt for a cause whilst monitoring is in progress with the aim of trying to identify reversible precipitants and initiate diagnosis-specific therapy.[1]

Finally, clinical presentation mainly based on bedside clinical examination provides personalized care for patients with AHF (➲ Figure 10.2.1).[1]

Disposition decision making

The overwhelming majority of AHF patients presenting to the ED are hospitalized. Studies are ongoing to assess whether short-stay observational units (less than 24–48 hours) or discharge directly from the ED can be implemented effectively and safely for selected patients.[11,12] Clinical scoring criteria have been developed to determine the severity and prognosis of AHF patients and can assist in identifying the patients who need the highest level of in-patient care.[12,13] However, triaging patients with AHF to a level of care is mainly based on clinical judgement.

The criteria for CCU/ICU admission may include any of the following[1]:

♦ need for intubation or already intubated

♦ signs/symptoms of hypoperfusion (oliguria, cold peripheries, altered mental status, lactate > 2mmol/L, metabolic acidosis, SvO_2 < 65%)

♦ heart rate < 40 or > 130 bpm, systolic BP < 90 mmHg.

The remaining patients with AHF are managed on an ordinary ward. Step-down from the CCU/ICU is determined by clinical stabilization and resolution of life-threatening conditions. Further management includes involvement of a multidisciplinary

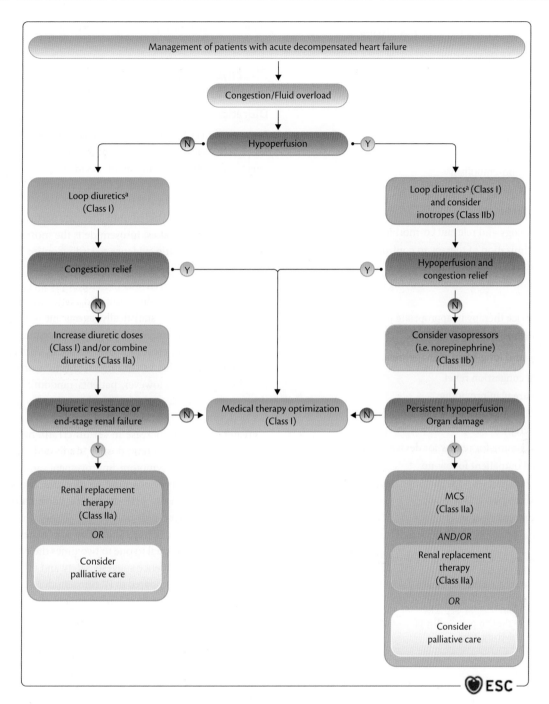

Figure 10.2.1 Management of acute decompensated heart failure.

MCS, mechanical circulatory support.

[a] Adequate diuretic doses to relieve congestion and close monitoring of diuresis is recommended, regardless of perfusion status.

McDonagh TA, Metra M, Adamo M, et al; ESC Scientific Document Group. 2021 ESC Guidelines for the diagnosis and treatment of acute and chronic heart failure. *Eur Heart J.* 2021 Sep 21;42(36):3599–3726. doi: 10.1093/eurheartj/ehab368. © The European Society of Cardiology. Reprinted by permission of Oxford University Press.

team, optimization of medical and device therapies, and development of the discharge plan.[1]

Goals of treatment

During the in-hospital stay of patients with AHF, different stages requiring different therapeutic approaches can be distinguished.[1]

The goals of treatment during the subsequent stages of AHF management are summarized in ⊃ Box 10.2.1.

In most patients hospitalized with ADHF, oral disease-modifying HF therapy should be continued on admission, except in the presence of haemodynamic instability. In particular, discontinuation of beta-blockers in AHF patients has been associated with significantly increased in-hospital mortality, short-term mortality, and the combined endpoint of short-term rehospitalization or mortality. Beta-blockers should be withheld when a patient is hospitalized after recent initiation or increase of the dosage and in cases of CS. Doses of angiotensin-converting enzyme inhibitors (ACEIs), angiotensin receptor blockers (ARBs), mineralocorticoid receptor antagonist (MRAs), sacubitril/valsartan should be reduced or temporarily discontinued in patients with hyperkalaemia and significant worsening of renal function. In de novo AHF, evidence-based oral therapies should be initiated promptly after stabilization.[1,8]

Patients hospitalized for AHF are medically fit for discharge when they are haemodynamically stable, decongested, and on evidence-based oral HF therapy for at least 24 hours before discharge. Patient education and enrollment in a detailed evidence-based management plan is an important part of the discharge phase.[1]

Pharmacological treatment of acute heart failure

Diuretics

Intravenous (IV) loop diuretics are the cornerstone of treatment for patients with AHF and signs of fluid overload.[1] The therapeutic effect of diuretics is a function of loss of body sodium and fluid, resulting in reductions in cardiac filling pressures, decongestion, and symptomatic relief. In AHF patients with signs of hypoperfusion, diuretics should be avoided until adequate perfusion is restored.[1]

Among loop diuretics, furosemide is the most commonly used. However, there is little evidence regarding optimal timing, dosing, and mode of delivery.[1] The Diuretic Optimization Strategies Evaluation (DOSE) trial was the largest prospective double-blind randomized trial to evaluate initial diuretic strategies in AHF patients. There were no statistically significant differences in either of the co-primary endpoints of global assessment of symptoms, or change in serum creatinine over 72 hours, with furosemide administration by bolus vs continuous infusion or in high-dose vs low-dose groups.[14] However, patients randomized to the higher dose strategy had a more favourable outcome with regard to relief of dyspnoea, reduction in weight and net fluid loss, albeit with a greater risk of an increase in serum creatinine.[14] It is therefore recommended that diuretic dosing is adjusted based on diuretic responsiveness and symptom improvement, and the dose modified according to previous dose of diuretics and renal function. Consequently, de novo AHF or diuretic naive patients should receive initial IV furosemide bolus of 20–40 mg, whereas patients on chronic oral diuretic therapy should be administered IV bolus furosemide of at least equal to one to two times their outpatient dose.[1] Moreover, initial evidence suggests safety and efficacy of subcutaneous furosemide compared to IV furosemide, as a first step toward a potentially new home-based management of worsening HF.[15]

Acetazolamide, a carbonic anhydrase inhibitor, inhibits sodium reabsorption in the proximal tubule whereas further beneficial effects may be related to increased delivery of chloride to the macula densa, which decreases renin secretion and neurohormonal activation.[16] The ADVOR (Acetazolamide in Decompensated Heart Failure with Volume Overload) trial has shown that the addition of IV acetazolamide (500 mg once daily) to standardized loop diuretic therapy in patients with AHF resulted in a greater incidence of successful decongestion within 3 days after randomization.[17] Recently, it has been demonstrated that early initiation of the sodium glucose cotransporter-2 (SGLT-2) inhibitor empagliflozin in AHF reduced the incidence of AKI and diuretic dose requirements.[18] SGLT-2 inhibitors act at the level of the proximal tubule, causing natriuresis and glycosuria, with no activation of renin secretion by the macula densa.[13]

The individual response to diuretics is crucial to achieve euvolaemia. Failure to decongest despite adequate and escalating doses of diuretics, also known as 'diuretic resistance', is reported in up to one third of hospitalized HF patients and is associated with a poor prognosis.[19] Several metrics of diuretic response have been suggested, such as weight loss or net fluid output per unit of 40 mg of furosemide, or urinary sodium measurement after the initiation of loop-diuretic therapy.[19,20] Strategies to overcome diuretic resistance include sequential nephron blockade by using a combination of diuretics, such as a thiazide diuretic or oral metolazone, in addition to a loop diuretic. This approach requires careful monitoring to avoid marked electrolyte disturbances, hypotension, dehydration, and worsening renal function.[20,21] Positive inotropes can also be used to improve diuresis in the setting of resistance due to low cardiac output.[20,21] Studies using vasoactive agents like low-dose dopamine and low-dose nesiritide, aquaretics such as tolvaptan, or adenosine antagonists such as rolofylline, to enhance the effect of diuretic therapy in AHF have been disappointing.[22–25] Moreover, the addition of high-dose spironolactone (100 mg daily for 96 hours) to the diuretic regimen in AHF was safe but did not improve clinical congestion and outcomes.[26] Finally, AHF patients with refractory oedema unresponsive to diuretic therapy may be considered for ultrafiltration (➲ Renal replacement therapy, p. 665).

Vasodilators

After diuretics, vasodilators are the most common IV therapy in AHF for symptomatic relief.[1] They have a dual mechanism of action as they act as both arteriodilators, reducing afterload and left and right ventricular pressures, and venodilators, reducing preload and allowing redistribution of fluid away from the pulmonary circulation.[13] Their IV administration may be considered as initial therapy in patients presenting with AHF and systolic BP >110 mmHg to improve symptoms and reduce congestion.[1] However, robust evidence that these agents improve outcomes is lacking.[1] Intravenous vasodilators used in clinical practice are nitrates and nesiritide (➲ Table 10.2.2).[1] Vasodilators should be used with caution in patients with significant mitral or aortic stenosis or predominant RV failure.[1,8]

As a class, nitrates provide exogenous nitric oxide, which binds to soluble guanylate cyclase, producing cyclic GMP (cGMP) and vascular smooth muscle relaxation. At higher doses (≥ 150–250 µg/min) nitrates dilate arteries, including those from the coronary vasculature, while at lower doses, they act predominantly on the venous circulation.[27] Although, there is wide experience in the use of nitrates in the management of hypertensive AHF,

they have been evaluated in surprisingly few large, well-designed trials, and quality data are lacking.[27] A systematic review of treatment with IV nitrates used in ED and ED-like settings suggested that they do improve short-term symptoms and appear safe to administer but with no evidence for longer-term outcomes.[27] The Goal-directed Afterload Reduction in Acute Congestive Cardiac Decompensation (GALACTIC) Study showed that a strategy that emphasized early intensive and sustained vasodilation, compared with usual care, did not significantly improve a composite outcome of all-cause mortality and AHF rehospitalizations at 180 days.[29] However, this trial focused on oral therapy rather than parenteral titration. Among older patients with AHF in the ED, use of a guideline-based comprehensive care bundle that included early intravenous nitrate boluses compared with usual care did not result in a statistically significant difference in the number of days alive and out of the hospital at 30 days.[30]

Nesiritide, a recombinant form of human brain natriuretic peptide (BNP) with arterial and venous vasodilator properties, was shown to have a small and not significant effect on dyspnoea when used in combination with other therapies but did not reduce mortality or HF rehospitalization in the ASCEND-HF trial (Acute Study of Clinical Effectiveness of Nesiritide in Decompensated Heart Failure).[31] Nesiritide is not currently available in many European countries. Symptoms and BP should be monitored frequently when using vasodilators and their dosing should be carefully controlled to avoid hypotension, which is associated with increased incidence of AKI and adverse outcomes.[32,33]

Several newer IV vasodilators have been investigated to assess safety and efficacy in AHF on top of standard of care. The RELAX-AHF-2 trial (Efficacy, Safety and Tolerability of Serelaxin When Added to Standard Therapy in AHF-2) evaluated the effect of serelaxin, a recombinant form of human relaxin-2, a vasodilator hormone that contributes to cardiovascular and renal adaptations during pregnancy.[34] Serelaxin did not impact cardiovascular mortality at 180 days and the trend for a reduction of worsening HF at 5 days was not statistically significant.[34] Ularitide, a chemically synthesized analogue of the naturally occurring vasodilator urodilatin, was tested in the TRUE-AHF (Trial of Ularitide Efficacy and Safety in Acute Heart Failure) and failed to show any significant effect on long-term cardiovascular mortality.[35] Clevidipine, a short-acting dihydropyridine L-type

Table 10.2.2 Intravenous vasodilators used in the management of acute heart failure: dosing, main side effects and limitations

Drug	Dosing	Main side effects	Limitations
Nitroglycerine	Start with 10–20 µg/min, increase up to 200 µg/min	Hypotension, headache	Tolerance is common after 24–48 hours
Isosorbide dinitrate	Start with 1 mg/h, increase up to 10 mg/h	Hypotension, headache	Tolerance is common after 24–48 hours
Nitroprusside	Start with 0.3 µg/kg/min and increase up to 5 µg/kg/min	Hypotension, isocyanate toxicity	Light sensitive Invasive BP monitoring required
Nesiritide	Bolus 2 µg/kg + infusion 0.01 µg/kg/min	Hypotension Worsening in renal function	Not currently available in many European countries

BP, blood pressure.

Source data from McDonagh TA, Metra M, Adamo M, et al; ESC Scientific Document Group. 2021 ESC Guidelines for the diagnosis and treatment of acute and chronic heart failure. *Eur Heart J.* 2021 Sep 21;42(36):3599-3726. doi: 10.1093/eurheartj/ehab368.

calcium channel blocker that mediates the influx of calcium in smooth muscle leading to arterial dilation, is currently approved for the acute management of severe hypertension.[27] A pilot randomized open-label study (PRONTO) of clevidipine vs standard of care IV antihypertensive therapy in ED patients with hypertensive AHF has demonstrated that clevidipine safely and rapidly reduces BP and improves dyspnoea more effectively than standard of care antihypertensive therapy.[36]

Inotropes and vasopressors

Inotropes are the third pharmacological pillar in the treatment of AHF patients.[1] According to AHF registries, IV inotropes are administered to 6% to 12% of patients with AHF, with wide variations in practice.[13] Their use is limited by adverse effects, including arrhythmogenesis, hypotension, and increased myocardial oxygen demand, that contribute to an unfavourable impact on long-term survival.[1] The ESC-HF-LT registry has reported a detrimental association between the use of IV inotropes and/or vasopressors and long-term all-cause mortality, as well as in-hospital mortality.[37] Therefore, inotropes are only indicated when patients have symptoms, signs, and laboratory findings of low cardiac output and end-organ hypoperfusion.[1] Inotropic agents are not recommended in cases of hypotensive AHF where the underlying cause is hypovolaemia or other potentially correctable factors.[1] Thus, a fluid challenge of up to 250 mL is recommended as the first-line treatment in cases of hypoperfusion if there is no sign of overt fluid overload.[8]

Inotropes currently used in clinical practice (➲ Table 10.2.3) are classified as calcitropes, acting through an increase in intracellular calcium concentration.[38] These include beta-adrenergic agonists (dobutamine, dopamine, epinephrine, and norepinephrine) and phosphodiesterase type III (PDE) inhibitors (milrinone and enoximone), both acting through an increase in intracellular cyclic adenosine monophosphate levels, which cause the release of calcium from the sarcoplasmic reticulum and calcium–sodium

exchange at the sarcolemma level.[13] Levosimendan, which enhances cardiac contractility through calcium sensitization of the contractile apparatus, is also classified as a calcitrope.[38]

More specifically, dobutamine enhances cardiac contractility via its stimulatory effect on myocardial beta-1 receptors and also affects the peripheral vasculature due to its combined action on vascular alpha-1 and beta-2 receptors. It is usually started with 2–3 µg/kg/min IV infusion rate and can be gradually up-titrated to 20 µg/kg/min according to the patient's clinical response. In clinical practice, low doses of dobutamine (< 5 µg/kg/min) lead to increased cardiac output through enhanced inotropy, and simultaneously reduce afterload by exerting a vasodilatory effect on the peripheral arterial vasculature. In doses exceeding 10 µg/kg/min, the effect on peripheral vessels shifts towards vasoconstriction.[39,40] It is primarily used in the CCU/ICU setting for short-term improvement of symptoms. However, several studies have linked its use to an increase in mortality rates. It is noteworthy that the effect of dobutamine may be blunted in patients who are receiving chronic beta-blockade therapy. Moreover, tolerance to the inotropic effect may develop even after short administration periods.[1,39]

Dopamine is an endogenous catecholamine. Two trials of dopamine in AHF, the Dopamine in Acute Decompensated Heart Failure II (DAD-HF II) trial and the Renal Optimization Strategies Evaluation – Acute Heart Failure (ROSE-AHF) trial, have demonstrated that there was no added benefit with the addition of dopamine to standard diuretic regimen.[22,23] Moreover, there is evidence that dopamine should not be used routinely in CS patients.[8]

PDE inhibitors, epitomized by milrinone, have both inotropic and vasodilating effects, thus increasing cardiac output and decreasing pulmonary artery pressure, pulmonary wedge pressure, and systemic and pulmonary vascular resistance.[40] Their mechanism of action is independent of the beta-adrenergic pathway, and subsequently their use is suitable for patients with

Table 10.2.3 Inotropes and/or vasopressors used in the management of acute heart failure

Drug	Mechanism of action	Bolus	Infusion rate
Dobutamine	Beta-agonist	No	2–20 µg/kg/min
Dopamine	Beta-agonist	No	3–5 µg/kg/min: inotropic effect > 5 µg/kg/min: vasoconstriction
Milrinone*	PDE inhibitor	25–75 µg/kg over 10–20 min	0.375–0.75 µg/kg/min
Enoximone*	PDE inhibitor	0.5–1.0 mg/kg over 5–10 min	5–20 µg/kg/min
Levosimendan*	Calcium sensitizer	12 µg/kg over 10 min (optional, only in euvolemic and eukalemic state), bolus not recommended in hypotensive patients	0.1 µg/kg/min, which can be decreased to 0.05 or increased to 0.2 µg/kg/min
Norepinephrine	Beta-agonist	No	0.2–1.0 µg/kg/min

* Milrinone, enoximone, and levosimendan are inodilators.

PDE, phosphodiesterase.

Source data from McDonagh TA, Metra M, Adamo M, et al; ESC Scientific Document Group. 2021 ESC Guidelines for the diagnosis and treatment of acute and chronic heart failure. *Eur Heart J.* 2021 Sep 21;42(36):3599-3726. doi: 10.1093/eurheartj/ehab368.

chronic heart failure under beta-blockade who present with AHF or CS.[1] In the large OPTIME-CHF (Outcomes of a Prospective Trial of Intravenous Milrinone for Exacerbations of Chronic Heart Failure) trial on AHF patients, milrinone gave no additional benefit beyond placebo, yet caused more complications, such as hypotensive episodes and arrhythmias.[41] The Prospective Randomized Milrinone Survival Evaluation (PROMISE) trial concluded that the use of milrinone in symptomatic HF patients, despite optimal medical therapy, was associated with increased mortality and readmission rates compared with placebo.[42] In clinical practice, milrinone is used in patients with AHF who maintain adequate systolic BP, unless combined with a vasopressor. Due to its relatively long half-life and renal clearance, milrinone should be used with caution in patients with impaired renal function.[39]

Levosimendan is also an inodilator (it promotes vasodilation through the opening of adenosine triphosphate-dependent potassium channels on vascular smooth muscle cells), and therefore is not suitable for the treatment of patients with hypotension (systolic BP < 85 mmHg) CS, unless in combination with a vasopressor.[1] A particular characteristic of the drug is its prolonged action that lasts several days after discontinuation of the infusion, and is provided by the long elimination half-life of its active metabolite of approximately 80 h. In patients with AHF, levosimendan achieves significant dose-dependent increases in cardiac output and stroke volume and decreases in pulmonary capillary wedge pressure, mean blood pressure, mean pulmonary artery pressure, mean right atrial pressure, and total peripheral resistance.[43] In addition to its haemodynamic effects, levosimendan has been shown to have anti-inflammatory, anti-oxidative and anti-apoptotic properties.[44] However, in the Survival of Patients With Acute Heart Failure in Need of Intravenous Inotropic Support (SURVIVE) trial, levosimendan did not demonstrate a mortality benefit when compared to dobutamine.[45] Levosimendan is currently recommended in the treatment of AHF to reverse the effect of beta-blockade, if the latter is thought to be contributing to hypotension with subsequent hypoperfusion.[1] Recently, areas of its clinical application have expanded to takotsubo cardiomyopathy, RV failure and pulmonary hypertension, cardiorenal syndrome, cardiac surgery, and critical care.[43]

Norepinephrine is a vasoconstrictor through its action on alpha-1 receptors and, in the case of AHF, is usually used in combination with classical inotropes in CS to restore BP or in association with dobutamine or inodilators to avoid hypotension.[1] Epinephrine causes vasodilation at low doses (< 0.01 µg/kg/min) and inotropy along with vasoconstriction at higher doses (0.05–0.5 µg/kg/min). Epinephrine may result in lactic acidosis while its use in CS has been associated with increased mortality and should be avoided.[40] It is used primarily in the setting of cardiac arrest.[1]

Careful choice of the most appropriate inotrope for each individual case is of paramount importance and should be determined by medical history, comorbid conditions, background medications, and haemodynamic condition (➲ Table 10.2.4).[39] Inotropic agents should be used for the shortest amount of time

Table 10.2.4 Choice of the proper inotrope according to clinical profile in acute heart failure patients

Clinical setting	Inotrope of choice
Ischaemic heart failure	Levosimendan Dobutamine
RV failure and/or pulmonary hypertension	Levosimendan Milrinone
Chronic beta-blocker therapy	Levosimendan Milrinone
Persistent hypotension	Norepinephrine
Primary renal failure	Dobutamine*
Acute cardiorenal syndrome	Levosimendan Dopamine Dobutamine
Impaired hepatic function	Dobutamine[†]
Acute cardio-hepatic dysfunction	Levosimendan
Cardiopulmonary bypass surgery	Dobutamine Levosimendan Milrinone
Severe takotsubo	Levosimendan
Sepsis-related acute heart failure	Norepinephrine Dobutamine Levosimendan

* Dobutamine is the drug with the shortest half-life (2 min); caution with milrinone and levosimendan due to their long half-lives.
[†] Levosimendan is predominantly excreted via the liver.

possible and in the lowest effective dose until the therapeutic goal of haemodynamic stabilization and restoration of vital organ perfusion is achieved.[1] During the time of inotropic weaning, standard oral HF treatment should be reinstated with the aim of reaching target doses after the complete withdrawal of inotropic support.[39]

Novel molecules may improve cardiac performance by targeting distinct mechanisms of action.[38] Oral omecamtiv mecarbil, an activator of cardiac myosin has raised interest due to its alternative inotropic mechanism that is less likely to cause side effects, but it failed to demonstrate improvement in dyspnoea in AHF.[46]

Rate control in atrial fibrillation

Before starting rate control in patients with AHF and rapid atrial fibrillation, underlying causes of elevated heat rate (HR), such as ischaemia, infection, anaemia, and pulmonary embolism should be identified and treated. Further, in those with AHF, decongestion with intravenous diuretics should be first-line therapy. Primary rate control in these patients should be approached with extreme caution to avoid precipitation of hypotension. The choice of drug and target HR depend on patient characteristics, symptoms, left ventricular (LV) function, and haemodynamics.[47] In patients with AHF, digoxin, and/or IV beta blockers (esmolol, landiolol) should be considered as the first-line therapy. Amiodarone may be considered in the acute setting of atrial fibrillation, whereas calcium channel blockers (diltiazem, verapamil) could be an option in patients with LV ejection fraction (LVEF) > 40%.[1,47] The optimal HR target for patients with AHF is usually < 110 bpm guided by haemodynamic and symptomatic improvement.[47]

Thromboembolism prophylaxis

Parenteral anticoagulants (e.g. low molecular weight heparin) is recommended in patients who are not already on oral anticoagulants, unless contraindicated, to reduce the risk of deep venous thrombosis and pulmonary embolism.[1]

Aquaretics

Vasopressin 2 receptor antagonists, such as tolvaptan, may promote aquaresis by blocking the action of arginine-vasopressin (AVP) at the V2 receptor in renal tubules, thus blocking the resorption of free water as urine passes through the collecting ducts. In patients with euvolemic or hypervolemic hyponatremia of diverse origin, tolvaptan was effective in increasing serum sodium concentrations, with thirst and dehydration recognized as adverse effects.[48] In the Efficacy of Vasopressin Antagonism in Heart Failure Outcome Study with Tolvaptan (EVEREST) trial, tolvaptan had no effect on long-term mortality or HF-related morbidity in patients hospitalized with HF. However, it did significantly improve hyponatremia in patients with a baseline serum sodium of less than 134 mmol/l and oedema score.[24] Tolvaptan has not been approved for the treatment of hyponatremia in patients with HF in Europe.

Opiates, anxiolytics, and sedatives

Routine use of opiates is not recommended in AHF, and they should only be reserved for patients with severe/intractable pain or anxiety.[1] Dose-dependent side effects include nausea, vomiting and aspiration, hypotension, bradycardia, and hypoventilation. In the Acute Decompensated Heart Failure National Registry (ADHERE), morphine use was associated with higher rates of mechanical ventilation, ICU admission and death.[49]

Anxiolytics and sedatives may be needed in patients with agitation or delirium. Benzodiazepines (lorazepam or diazepam) may be the safest approach. The new α2-adrenergic receptor agonist dexmetomidine causes less central respiratory depression and has shown better results than midazolam in patients with ACPO intolerant to NIV.[50]

Other medical therapy

Glycaemic control is recommended to target a blood glucose concentration between 144 and 180 mg/dl, yet avoiding hypoglycaemia.[10]

Stress ulcers prophylaxis should follow general recommendations for critically ill patients. In CS, no nutrition in the early phase and initial parenteral nutrition may be preferred.[10]

Once haemodynamic stabilization is achieved and before discharge, ferric carboxymaltose should be considered in patients with iron deficiency, defined as serum ferritin <100 ng/mL or serum ferritin 100–299 ng/mL with transferrin saturation <20%, to improve symptoms and reduce rehospitalizations.[51]

Non-pharmacological treatment of acute heart failure

Oxygen therapy, non-invasive and invasive ventilation

Although 90% of AHF patients complain of dyspnoea, fewer than half present with respiratory failure affecting the blood gas analysis, in the form of hypoxaemia, hypercapnia, acidosis, or a combination of them.[50] Significant respiratory failure is essentially seen in patients with ACPO, in CS and in cases associated with other lung pathologies (COPD, pneumonia, large pleural effusion, etc.) which may occur concomitantly in patients with AHF. Moreover, in isolated RV failure, respiratory failure is seen in acute pulmonary embolism or decompensated chronic pulmonary hypertension. In ACPO, respiratory failure occurs when an excess of interstitial and alveoli fluid results in a significant reduction of gas exchange and a concomitant shunting. In CS, the lung hypoperfusion increases the ventilation–perfusion mismatch whereas metabolic (lactic) acidosis increases the compensatory respiratory load.[50]

Routine monitoring of transcutaneous arterial oxygen saturation (SpO_2) is recommended, whereas arterial blood gas should be restricted to patients in whom oxygenation cannot be readily assessed by pulse oximetry.[1] A venous sample might acceptably indicate pH and PCO_2, especially in patients with a previous history of COPD.[1] It is recommended to administer oxygen as early as possible in patients with SpO_2 < 90% or PO_2 < 60mmHg to correct hypoxaemia.[1] However, hyperoxia should be avoided, as in non-hypoxaemic patients oxygen causes vasoconstriction and a reduction in cardiac output. Moreover, in COPD patients, hyperoxygenation may increase ventilation–perfusion mismatch, suppressing ventilation and leading to hypercapnia.[1]

There are two main modalities of NIV: continuous positive airway pressure (CPAP) and pressure support ventilation with positive end-expiratory pressure (NIPPV or BiPAP).[50] CPAP requires minimal training and equipment (can be applied without the aid of a ventilator) and is a feasible technique in the prehospital setting. NIPPV requires a ventilator, experience for setting the ventilator to the changing needs of the patient, and adequate synchrony. Either technique can be used as a first line treatment in ACPO, but it is reasonable to prefer NIPPV in cases of acidosis, hypercapnia, or concomitant COPD.[50] A new modality 'high flow nasal cannula' seems promising in patients with hypoxaemic AHF with less severe respiratory failure.[50] NIV reduces respiratory distress, may decrease intubation rates, and, with lower evidence, reduce mortality in high risk patients.[1] The use of NIV remains limited in hypotensive patients, but it may be cautiously considered in properly selected CS cases without severe haemodynamic instability. In isolated RV failure, positive pressure may be detrimental as the increase in RV afterload may aggravate RV failure.[50]

Before implementing NIV, it is necessary to check for contraindications (→ Box 10.2.2).[50] To ensure the success of NIV, close monitoring of the patient and the device is necessary, with special attention paid to risk factors for failure (→ Box 10.2.3).[50] If NIV is going to be successful, the patient will generally show

---

Box 10.2.2 Contraindications for the use of non-invasive ventilation

Absolute

Cardiac or respiratory arrest
Anatomical abnormality (unable to fit the interface)
Inability to keep patent airway
Refractory hypoxaemia (after application of NIV)
Sustained severe hypotension

Relative

Agitation or poor cooperation
Mild hypotension
Upper gastrointestinal haemorrhage or vomiting
Inability to expectorate copious secretions
Recent frail upper gastrointestinal or airway surgery
Multiple organ failure
Isolated right ventricular failure

Reproduced from Masip J, Peacock WF, Price S, et al; Acute Heart Failure Study Group of the Acute Cardiovascular Care Association and the Committee on Acute Heart Failure of the Heart Failure Association of the European Society of Cardiology. Indications and practical approach to non-invasive ventilation in acute heart failure. *Eur Heart J*. 2018 Jan 1;39(1):17-25. doi: 10.1093/eurheartj/ehx580 with permission from Oxford University Press.

Box 10.2.3 Predictors of failure of non-invasive ventilation therapy

Before initiation

Physician inexperience
Inadequate equipment
ARDS
Altered mental status
Shock
High severity scores
Copious secretions
Extremely high respiratory rate
Severe hypoxaemia in spite of high FiO$_2$

After initiation

Inappropriate ventilator settings
Unfitting interface
Excessive air leakage
Asynchrony with the ventilator
Poor tolerance to NIV
Neurological or underlying disease impairment

After 60–90 min

No reduction in respiratory rate
No reduction in carbon dioxide
No improvement in pH
No improvement in oxygenation
Signs of fatigue

ARDS = acute respiratory distress syndrome; FiO$_2$ = fraction of inspired oxygen; NIV = non-invasive ventilation.
Reproduced from Masip J, Peacock WF, Price S, et al; Acute Heart Failure Study Group of the Acute Cardiovascular Care Association and the Committee on Acute Heart Failure of the Heart Failure Association of the European Society of Cardiology. Indications and practical approach to non-invasive ventilation in acute heart failure. *Eur Heart J*. 2018 Jan 1;39(1):17-25. doi: 10.1093/eurheartj/ehx580 with permission from Oxford University Press..

---

improvement in respiratory and heart rate, work of breathing, and gas exchange in approximately 60 minutes.[50] Mild sedation may be used with caution in patients with poor tolerance of the interface or poor synchrony with the ventilator, only after non-pharmacological approaches (e.g. reassuring the patient, changing the interface, tuning the ventilator, etc.) have failed. Minimal intermittent doses of a single drug may be preferable to continuous infusions or combinations of different agents (➲ Opiates, anxiolytics, and sedatives, p. 664).[50] NIV is usually stopped when a satisfactory recovery has been achieved or conversely, if there are signs of NIV failure, requiring endotracheal intubation (EI) (➲ Table 10.2.5).[50] After mid- or long-term use of NIV (>24 h), a weaning period is often needed by decreasing FiO$_2$ and positive end-expiratory pressure progressively.[50] Fortunately, EI and mechanical ventilation are only required in a minority of AHF patients. If invasive ventilation is required, lung-protected ventilation (tidal volume of 6 mL/kg predicted body weight) should be applied to prevent pulmonary injury.[10]

Renal replacement therapy

Development of AKI with worsening renal function during hospitalization for AHF is increasingly common and has significant impact on patients' outcome. The underlying pathophysiology of worsening renal function in AHF is complex and multifactorial; it results from the haemodynamic and neurohumoral alterations that occur in the setting of low cardiac output and decreased renal blood flow, with venous congestion. Treatment includes optimization of fluid status and haemodynamics, avoidance of nephrotoxic agents, and optimization of HF therapy.[52] Classic indications for initiating renal replacement therapy (RRT) for AKI, independent of its aetiology, are severe hyperkalemia (potassium > 6.5 mmol/L, rapidly increasing, or with ECG changes) and severe metabolic acidosis (pH < 7.15).[1,52] The threshold of uraemia for RRT initiation in order to treat or prevent uraemic complications is less well defined. Moreover, optimal timing for RRT initiation beyond life-threatening situations remains unclear. At the present time, there is no evidence to support RRT over loop diuretics as first-line therapy in AHF patients. RRT may be temporarily needed in

Table 10.2.5 Criteria for endotracheal intubation

Cardiac or respiratory arrest
Progressive worsening of altered mental status
Progressive worsening of pH, PaCO$_2$, or PO$_2$ despite NIV
Progressive signs of fatigue during NIV
Need to protect the airway
Persistent haemodynamic instability
Agitation or intolerance to NIV with progressive respiratory failure

PaCO$_2$, arterial partial carbon dioxide pressure; PaO$_2$, arterial partial oxygen pressure; NIV, non-invasive ventilation.
Reproduced from Masip J, Peacock WF, Price S, et al; Acute Heart Failure Study Group of the Acute Cardiovascular Care Association and the Committee on Acute Heart Failure of the Heart Failure Association of the European Society of Cardiology. Indications and practical approach to non-invasive ventilation in acute heart failure. *Eur Heart J*. 2018 Jan 1;39(1):17-25. doi: 10.1093/eurheartj/ehx580 with permission from Oxford University Press.

patients with refractory pulmonary oedema and diuretic resistant fluid overload.[1]

Several modalities of RRT are available, based on distinct underlying principles of diffusion and convection: isolated or continuous ultrafiltration (UF) with or without a component of solute clearance (haemofiltration or haemodialysis).[52] Haemofiltration is based on a difference in pressure between the two sides of the dialysis membrane leading to convection of water (UF) and dissolved small and middle-sized molecules (< 60 kDa). Molecules, including 'myocardial depressant' cytokines, are dragged through a more permeable membrane by the generated transmembrane pressure together with water into the so-called effluent. Haemodialysis is solute removal by diffusion across a membrane from an area of high concentration to an area of low concentration. During dialysis, blood and dialysate flows are separated by a semipermeable membrane, and the dialysate, an electrolyte solution, flows in the opposite direction to the blood flow. Dialysis is a very efficient modality for the clearance of small molecules (<20 kDa).[52] The best modality in AHF is still controversial. Although continuous techniques have been associated with better haemodynamic tolerance and a greater chance of renal recovery, randomized controlled trials have not shown a difference in recovery or mortality.[52]

The physiological benefits of UF over diuretic treatment could include the rapid and predictable fluid removal and the greater removal of sodium with the same amount of water. UF can remove fluid at rates of up to 500 mL/h, but in practice, 200–300 mL/h is considered adequate. Lower rates may be used if there is significant RV disease or pulmonary arterial hypertension. Individualizing UF rates ('starting low, going slow') is probably an adequate strategy to treat AHF patients with fluid overload and may be translated into greater haemodynamic stability and a less pronounced neurohormonal response. In randomized trials, the typical treatment period has been 24 hours, but ultrafiltration membranes can last up to 72 hours with care. Dosage adaptation of drugs removed by RRT should be taken into account.[1,21,52]

Recently, devices for veno-venous peripheral UF have been developed, which are potentially more user friendly in cardiological practice. Good peripheral access with two venous lines and a minimum blood flow rate of 10-40 mL/minute are necessary to run peripheral UF.[52]

In cases of CS, the filter of a continuous RRT device can easily be included in the extracorporeal membrane oxygenation (ECMO) circuit.[10]

Mechanical circulatory support

Despite advances in medical therapy and coronary revascularization, the mortality of CS has remained nearly unchanged at 40–50% over the last two decades.[10] For a subset of these patients who cannot be stabilized with pharmacological management, temporary or durable mechanical circulatory support (MCS) may be necessary to augment CO and support end-organ perfusion.[1] The most important determinant of success is the correct timing of implantation to avoid significant, potentially irreversible end-organ injury.

The intra-aortic balloon pump (IABP) has traditionally been used to support the circulation until the surgical correction of specific acute mechanical complications (e.g. interventricular septal rupture and acute mitral regurgitation), during severe acute myocarditis and in patients with acute myocardial infarction or ischaemia before, during and after percutaneous or surgical revascularization.[1,10] However, the Intra-aortic Balloon Pump in Cardiogenic Shock II (IABP-Shock II) trial did not demonstrate a mortality benefit with IABP compared to standard therapy, in patients suffering from acute myocardial infarction and CS.[53] Therefore, routine use of an IABP cannot be recommended.[1]

Other forms of MCS, including short-term percutaneous devices (e.g. Impella, TandemHeart) and veno-arterial (VA) ECMO, are being used more frequently at referral centres despite lack of strong evidence on outcome.[1] Of note, severe or life-threatening bleeding and peripheral vascular complications were reported with the Impella device.[10] The complete percutaneous ECMO system generally consists of a centrifugal pump, a heat exchanger, and an oxygenator. Advantages of VA-ECMO include the low cost in comparison to other percutaneous devices, the high flow providing full circulatory support even in resuscitation situations, the ability to provide full oxygenation, and also a combined support of RV and LV.[10] However, it increases LV afterload and that may lead to inadequate LV unloading.[10] Multiple venting manoeuvres have been described to prevent LV volume overload which are beyond the scope of this chapter. Recent developments with user-friendly miniaturized systems have led to a wider adoption of VA-ECMO by interventional cardiologists.[10]

In patients with refractory shock, MCS should be considered as 'bridge' to recovery, decision, or transplant. In this case, patient selection is extremely important and should be based on their overall risk, age, comorbidities, neurological status and end-organ damage. A difficult decision to withdraw MCS may need to be made when the patient has no potential for cardiac recovery and is not eligible for heart transplant.[2]

Other interventions

Although fluid restriction seems reasonable in AHF patients with congestion and is commonly practiced, aggressive sodium and fluid restriction has not been shown to have any significant difference in weight loss, clinical stability, or 30-day rate of readmission, and is associated with significant increase in thirst. Marked fluid restriction should be reserved for patients with significant hyponatremia.[13]

In patients with AHF and pleural effusion and/or ascites, fluid evacuation with paracentesis may be considered in order to alleviate symptoms. Prompt reduction in intra-abdominal pressure through ascitic paracentesis may also improve renal filtration by partially normalizing the transrenal pressure gradient.[2]

For critically ill patients admitted to CCU/ICU, general accepted strategies avoid correction of haemoglobin levels > 7g/dl unless there is a clinical bleeding problem.[10]

Future directions

Compared to chronic HF, management of AHF is largely based on expert consensus documents with less robust evidence to guide diagnosis, risk stratification, and management. There are important areas of uncertainty over the best definition of AHF, the pathophysiologic understanding, the phenotypical variability, the appropriate risk stratification, and the long-term benefits of acute-phase therapies.

The 'time-to-treatment' concept requires further prospective evaluation. More research on the mechanisms causing the poor outcomes of AHF patients is clearly needed. Pharmacologic management will continue to progress with new vasoactive and inotropic agents as well as therapies for co-morbid conditions such as diabetes, renal dysfunction, and anaemia. Additional research is needed to clarify timing and outcomes of mechanical therapies. Strategies to prevent rehospitalization in the vulnerable phase of HF deserve to be addressed. Ultimately, more extensive studies will help define the safety, efficacy, and cost-effectiveness of novel models of care, such as outpatient management with subcutaneous loop diuretics, short stay units, and home hospitalizations.[1]

Key messages

AHF is a major diagnostic and therapeutic challenge in clinical practice and requires a systematic and multidisciplinary approach. Life-saving therapy in patients with CS and severe respiratory failure in the first 'golden hour' is of paramount importance. Accurate patient evaluation according to individual causes and precipitants, fluid status, and haemodynamics is a key to treatment selection for each patient. Current treatment modalities help patient stabilization and symptoms control during the initial phase of hospital admission, but beyond that, there are no therapies effective to reduce the burden of morbidity and mortality of AHF.

References

1. McDonagh TA, Metra M, Adamo M, et al. 2021 ESC Guidelines for the diagnosis and treatment of acute and chronic heart failure: Developed by the Task Force for the diagnosis and treatment of acute and chronic heart failure of the European Society of Cardiology (ESC) with the special contribution of the Heart Failure Association (HFA) of the ESC. Eur Heart J. 2021;42(36):3599–3726.

2. Ponikowski P, Voors AA, Anker SD, et al. ESC Scientific Document Group. 2016 ESC Guidelines for the diagnosis and treatment of acute and chronic heart failure: The Task Force for the diagnosis and treatment of acute and chronic heart failure of the European Society of Cardiology (ESC). Developed with the special contribution of the Heart Failure Association (HFA) of the ESC. Eur Heart J. 2016;37:2129–2200.

3. Harjola VP, Mullens W, Banaszewski M, et al. Organ dysfunction, injury and failure in acute heart failure: from pathophysiology to diagnosis and management. A review on behalf of the Acute Heart Failure Committee of the Heart Failure Association (HFA) of the European Society of Cardiology (ESC). Eur J Heart Fail. 2017;19(7):821–836.

4. Ferreira J. Vascular phenotypes of acute decompensated vs new-onset heart failure: treatment implications. ESC Heart FAIL. 2017; 4(4):679–685.

5. Shiraishi Y, Kawana M, Nakata J, Sato N, Fukuda K, Kohsaka S. Time-sensitive approach in the management of acute heart failure. ESC Heart Fail. 2021;8(1):204–221.

6. Peacock WF, Emerman C, Costanzo MR, et al. Early vaso-active drugs improve heart failure outcomes. Congest Heart Fail. 2009;15(6):256–264.

7. Matsue Y, Damman K, Voors AA, et al. Time-to-furosemide treatment and mortality in patients hospitalized with acute heart failure. J Am Coll Cardiol. 2017;69(25):3042–3051.

8. Čerlinskaitė K, Javanainen T, Cinotti R, Mebazaa A. Global Research on Acute Conditions Team (GREAT) Network. Acute heart failure management. Korean Circ J. 2018;48(6):463–480.

9. Mebazaa A, Yilmaz MB, Levy P, et al. Recommendations on pre-hospital & early hospital management of acute heart failure: a consensus paper from the Heart Failure Association of the European Society of Cardiology, the European Society of Emergency Medicine and the Society of Academic Emergency Medicine. Eur J Heart Fail. 2015;17(6):544–558.

10. Thiele H, Ohman EM, de Waha-Thiele S, et al. Management of cardiogenic shock complicating myocardial infarction: an update 2019. Eur Heart J. 2019;40(32):2671–2683.

11. Collins SP, Storrow AB, Levy PD, et al. Early management of patients with acute heart failure: state of the art and future directions – a consensus document from the SAEM/HFSA acute heart failure working group. Acad Emerg Med. 2015;22(1):94–112.

12. Miró Ò, Peacock FW, McMurray JJ, et al. Acute Cardiovascular Care Association position paper on safe discharge of acute heart failure patients from the emergency department. Eur Heart J Acute Cardiovasc Care. 2017; 6(4):311–320.

13. Gupta AK, Tomasoni D, Sidhu K, et al. Evidence-based management of acute heart failure. Can J Cardiol. 2021;37(4):621–631.

14. Felker GM, Lee KL, Bull DA, et al. Diuretic strategies in patients with acute decompensated heart failure. N Engl J Med. 2011;364(9):797–805.

15. Gilotra NA, Princewill O, Marino B, et al. Efficacy of intravenous furosemide versus a novel, ph-neutral furosemide formulation administered subcutaneously in outpatients with worsening heart failure. JACC Heart Fail. 2018;6(1):65–70.

16. Verbrugge FH, Martens P, Ameloot K, et al. Acetazolamide to increase natriuresis in congestive heart failure at high risk for diuretic resistance. Eur J Heart Fail. 2019;21(11):1415–1422.

17. Mullens W, Dauw J, Martens P, et al. Acetazolamide in acute decompensated heart failure with volume overload. N Engl J Med. 2022;387(13):1185–1195.

18. Kambara T, Shibata R, Osanai H, et al. Importance of sodium-glucose cotransporter 2 inhibitor use in diabetic patients with acute heart failure. Ther Adv Cardiovasc Dis. 2019;13:1753944719894509.

19. Gupta R, Testani J, Collins S. Diuretic resistance in heart failure. Curr Heart Fail Rep. 2019;16(2):57–66.

20. Mullens W, Damman K, Harjola VP, et al. The use of diuretics in heart failure with congestion – a position statement from the Heart Failure Association of the European Society of Cardiology. Eur J Heart Fail. 2019;21(2):137–155.

21. Vazir A, Cowie MR. Decongestion: diuretics and other therapies for hospitalized heart failure. Indian Heart J. 2016;68 Suppl 1(Suppl 1):S61–68.

22. Triposkiadis FK, Butler J, Karayannis G, et al. Efficacy and safety of high dose versus low dose furosemide with or without dopamine infusion: the Dopamine in Acute Decompensated Heart Failure II (DAD-HF II) trial. Int J Cardiol. 2014;172(1):115–121.

23. Wan SH, Stevens SR, Borlaug BA, et al. Differential response to low-dose dopamine or low-dose nesiritide in acute heart failure

with reduced or preserved ejection fraction: results from the ROSE AHF Trial (Renal Optimization Strategies Evaluation in Acute Heart Failure). Circ Heart Fail. 2016;9(8):e002593.

24. Konstam MA, Gheorghiade M, Burnett JC Jr, et al. Effects of oral tolvaptan in patients hospitalized for worsening heart failure: the EVEREST Outcome Trial. JAMA. 2007;297(12):1319–1331.

25. Massie BM, O'Connor CM, Metra M, et al. Rolofylline, an adenosine A1-receptor antagonist, in acute heart failure. N Engl J Med. 2010;363(15):1419–1428.

26. Butler J, Anstrom KJ, Felker GM, et al. Efficacy and safety of spironolactone in acute heart failure: The ATHENA-HF randomized clinical trial. JAMA Cardiol. 2017;2(9):950–958.

27. Singh A, Laribi S, Teerlink JR, Mebazaa A. Agents with vasodilator properties in acute heart failure. Eur Heart J. 2017;38(5): 317–325.

28. Alexander P, Alkhawam L, Curry J, et al. Lack of evidence for intravenous vasodilators in ED patients with acute heart failure: a systematic review. Am J Emerg Med. 2015;33(2):133–141.

29. Kozhuharov N, Goudev A, Flores D, et al. Effect of a strategy of comprehensive vasodilation vs usual care on mortality and heart failure rehospitalization among patients with acute heart failure: the GALACTIC Randomized Clinical Trial. JAMA. 2019;322(23):2292–2302.

30. Freund Y, Cachanado M, Delannoy Q, et al. Effect of an emergency department care bundle on 30-day hospital discharge and survival among elderly patients with acute heart failure: the ELISABETH randomized clinical trial. JAMA. 2020;324(19):1948–1956.

31. O'Connor CM, Starling RC, Hernandez AF, et al. Effect of nesiritide in patients with acute decompensated heart failure. N Engl J Med. 2011;365(1):32–43.

32. Patel PA, Heizer G, O'Connor CM, et al. Hypotension during hospitalization for acute heart failure is independently associated with 30-day mortality: findings from ASCEND-HF. Circ Heart Fail. 2014;7(6):918–925.

33. Arao Y, Sawamura A, Nakatochi M, et al. Early blood pressure reduction by intravenous vasodilators is associated with acute kidney injury in patients with hypertensive acute decompensated heart. Circ J. 2019;83(9):1883–1890.

34. Metra M, Teerlink JR, Cotter G, et al. Effects of serelaxin in patients with acute heart failure. N Engl J Med. 2019;381(8):716–726.

35. Packer M, O'Connor C, McMurray JJV, et al. Effect of ularitide on cardiovascular mortality in acute heart failure. N Engl J Med. 2017;376(20):1956–1964.

36. Peacock WF, Chandra A, Char D, et al. Clevidipine in acute heart failure: Results of the A Study of Blood Pressure Control in Acute Heart Failure – A Pilot Study (PRONTO). Am Heart J. 2014;167(4):529–36.

37. Mebazaa A, Motiejunaite J, Gayat E, et al. Long-term safety of intravenous cardiovascular agents in acute heart failure: results from the European Society of Cardiology Heart Failure Long-Term Registry. Eur J Heart Fail. 2018;20(2):332–341.

38. Psotka MA, Gottlieb SS, Francis GS, et al. Cardiac calcitropes, myotropes, and mitotropes: JACC review topic of the week. J Am Coll Cardiol. 2019;73(18):2345–2353.

39. Bistola V, Arfaras-Melainis A, Polyzogopoulou E, et al. Inotropes in acute heart failure: from guidelines to practical use: therapeutic options and clinical practice. Card Fail Rev. 2019;5(3):133–139.

40. Farmakis D, Agostoni P, Baholli L, et al. A pragmatic approach to the use of inotropes for the management of acute and advanced heart failure: An expert panel consensus. Int J Cardiol. 2019;297:83–90.

41. Felker GM, Benza RL, Chandler AB, et al. Heart failure etiology and response to milrinone in decompensated heart failure: results from the OPTIME-CHF study. J Am Coll Cardiol. 2003;41(6):997–1003.

42. Packer M, Carver JR, Rodeheffer RJ, et al. Effect of oral milrinone on mortality in severe chronic heart failure. The PROMISE Study Research Group. N Engl J Med. 1991;325(21):1468–1475.

43. Papp Z, Agostoni P, Alvarez J, et al. Levosimendan efficacy and safety: 20 years of SIMDAX in clinical use. Card Fail Rev. 2020;6:e19.

44. Farmakis D, Alvarez J, Gal TB, et al. Levosimendan beyond inotropy and acute heart failure: Evidence of pleiotropic effects on the heart and other organs: An expert panel position paper. Int J Cardiol. 2016 Nov 1;222:303–312.

45. Mebazaa A, Nieminen MS, Packer M, et al. Levosimendan vs dobutamine for patients with acute decompensated heart failure: the SURVIVE randomized trial. JAMA. 2007;297(17):1883–1891.

46. Teerlink JR, Felker GM, McMurray JJV, et al. Acute treatment with omecamtiv mecarbil to increase contractility in acute heart failure: The ATOMIC-AHF Study. J Am Coll Cardiol. 2016;67(12):1444–1455.

47. Hindricks G, Potpara T, Dagres N, et al. 2020 ESC Guidelines for the diagnosis and management of atrial fibrillation developed in collaboration with the European Association for Cardio-Thoracic Surgery (EACTS). Eur Heart J. 2021;42(5):373–498.

48. Schrier RW, Gross P, Gheorghiade M, et al; SALT Investigators. Tolvaptan, a selective oral vasopressin V2-receptor antagonist, for hyponatremia. N Engl J Med. 2006;355(20):2099–2112.

49. Peacock WF, Hollander JE, Diercks DB, et al. Morphine and outcomes in acute decompensated heart failure: an ADHERE analysis. Emerg Med J. 2008 Apr;25(4):205–209.

50. Masip J, Peacock WF, Price S, et al. Indications and practical approach to non-invasive ventilation in acute heart failure. Eur Heart J. 2018;39(1):17–25.

51. Ponikowski P, Kirwan BA, Anker SD, et al; AFFIRM – AHF Investigators. Ferric carboxymaltose for iron deficiency at discharge after acute heart failure: a multicentre, double-blind, randomised, controlled trial. Lancet 2020;396:1895–1904.

52. Schaubroeck HA, Gevaert S, Bagshaw SM, et al. Acute cardiorenal syndrome in acute heart failure: focus on renal replacement therapy. Eur Heart J Acute Cardiovasc Care. 2020;9(7):802–811.

53. Thiele H, Zeymer U, Neumann FJ, et al. Intra-aortic balloon counterpulsation in acute myocardial infarction complicated by cardiogenic shock (IABP-SHOCK II): final 12 month results of a randomised, open-label trial. Lancet. 2013;382(9905):1638–1645.

SECTION 11

Advanced heart failure

CHAPTER 11.1

Advanced heart failure: assessment

Tuvia Ben Gal, Mariell Jessup, and Maria-Rosa Costanzo

Contents

Introduction

Heart failure (HF) syndrome is increasingly prevalent throughout the world and is associated with profound morbidity, mortality, and societal economic burden.[1] At any given time, only a small fraction of patients with HF can be designated being at an advanced stage of the disease.[2] Nevertheless, these patients, having failed optimal medical therapy, have an increasingly narrow list of therapeutic options available to them: palliative care, heart transplantation (HTx), or mechanical circulatory support (MCS); some patients receive all three of these options in a short period of time. These advanced HF options are covered in subsequent chapters. The aim of this chapter is to review the appropriate assessment of the patient suspected to have advanced HF.

Summary and key messages

Much has been learned over the past five decades as clinicians have struggled to predict the course of advanced HF syndrome, appropriately choose the best candidates for HTx and MCS, maintain their patients' vital organ function while waiting for a donor heart or for the optimal timing for MCS surgery, and, finally, recognize the futility of these advanced therapies in certain patients with end-stage disease. Two prime lessons learned are worth emphasizing:

1. In patients suspected to have progressive HF symptoms despite treatment, serious consideration should be given to referring the patient, as early as possible, to a centre equipped to deliver advanced HF therapies.[3] All too often, patients are at death's door when they are referred to a tertiary care or specialized HF centre, too late for effective treatment. This late referral pattern continues to be a major gap in HF care everywhere in the world.

2. Clinicians miss the multiple clues that their patient has deteriorated significantly, focusing wrongly only on the value of the left ventricular ejection fraction (LVEF). Indeed, as outlined below, there are now well-recognized patterns and risk scores to aid in the earlier recognition of the deteriorating HF patient.[4]

Epidemiology and prognosis of advanced heart failure

Definition

The defining signs, symptoms, and other diagnostic criteria for advanced HF have been published[5] and are summarized in ➲ Box 11.1.1.

The definition incorporates elements of the patient's course of disease, exertional capacity, laboratory parameters, and measures of organ dysfunction. Other characterization schemes are reviewed below. The American HF guidelines have classified all HF patients into four stages; the assessment outlined in this chapter is for patients defined as

Box 11.1.1 Updated HFA-ESC criteria for defining advanced heart failure

All of the following criteria must be present despite optimal guideline-directed treatment:

1. Severe and persistent symptoms of heart failure [NYHA class Ill (advanced) or IV].

2. Severe cardiac dysfunction defined by a reduced LVEF ≤ 30%. isolated RV failure (e.g., ARVC) or non-operable severe valve abnormalities or congenital abnormalities or persistently high (or increasing) BNP or NT-proBNP values and data of severe diastolic dysfunction or LV structural abnormalities according to the ESC definition of HFpEF and HFmrEF.

3. Episodes of pulmonary or systemic congestion requiring high-dose intravenous diuretics (or diuretic combinations) or episodes of low output requiring inotropes or vasoactive drugs or malignant arrhythmias causing > 1 unplanned visit or hospitalization in the last 12 months.

4. Severe impairment of exercise capacity with inability to exercise or low 6MWTD (<300m) or $pV0_2$ (<12–14 mL/kg/min), estimated to be of cardiac origin.

In addition to the above, extra-cardiac organ dysfunction due to heart failure (e.g. cardiac cachexia, liver, or kidney dysfunction) or type 2 pulmonary hypertension may be present but are not required.

Criteria 1 and 4 can be met in patients who have cardiac dysfunction (as described in criterion #2), but who also have substantial limitation due to other conditions (e.g. severe pulmonary disease, non-cardiac cirrhosis, or most commonly by renal disease with mixed aetiology). These patients still have limited quality of life and survival due to advanced disease and warrant the same intensity of evaluation as someone in whom the only disease is cardiac, but the therapeutic options for these patients are usually more limited.

ARVC, arrhythmogenic right ventricular cardiomyopathy; BNP, B-type natriuretic peptide; ESC, European Society of Cardiology; HFA, Heart Failure Association; HFmrEF, heart failure with mildly reduced ejection fraction; HFpEF, heart failure with preserved ejection fraction; LV, left ventricular; LVEF, left ventricular ejection fraction; NT-proBNP, N-terminal pro B-type natriuretic peptide; NYHA, New York Heart Association; $pV0_2$, peak exercise oxygen consumption; RV, right ventricular; 6MWTD, 6-minute walk test distance.

Reproduced from Crespo-Leiro MG, Metra M, Lund LH, et al. Advanced heart failure: a position statement of the Heart Failure Association of the European Society of Cardiology. *Eur J Heart Fail.* 2018 Nov;20(11):1505-1535. doi: 10.1002/ejhf.1236 with permission.

having Stage D, characterized by refractoriness or intolerance to guideline-directed medical therapy.[6,7]

Prevalence

It is not easy to calculate the prevalence of patients with advanced HF, as existing cohorts have been characterized using various definitions of the syndrome. Mayo Clinic investigators surveyed participants in their Olmsted County cohort and found only 0.2% of the population had Stage D symptoms.[8] Various estimates of the prevalence have ranged widely from 6% to 25% among patients with established HF, influenced by the population studied. Manufacturers of left ventricular assist devices estimate that approximately 250,000 to 500,000 people have advanced disease in the United States, and a similar number is estimated for Europe.

Prognosis

Patients unable to tolerate optimal oral therapy for HF due to hypotension and/or progressive renal and hepatic dysfunction have an ominous prognosis. Life expectancy without extraordinary measures, such as MCS or HTx, is typically measured in months. As outlined below, there are several risk scores consisting of clinical, laboratory, and haemodynamic parameters shown to have prognostic value, aimed at assisting clinicians in the estimate of individual patients' prognosis. The scores help both clinicians and patients during shared decision-making conversations but should be applied cautiously as no risk score is perfect and, in general, risk scores developed in stable HF populations tend to underestimate the risk of individuals with advanced disease.

Profiles of advanced heart failure patients

Patients with HF develop irreversible, advanced signs and symptoms via different clinical pathways. Some may present de novo with a life-threatening myocarditis, for example, while others may have a years-long journey of progressive myocardial failure. For each patient, the clinician must try to determine the aetiology of the HF and the cause of decompensation, while simultaneously administering treatment. It is useful to have a common vocabulary to describe the symptomatic trajectory of each patient to other members of the HF team.

The Interagency Registry for Mechanically Assisted Circulatory Support (INTERMACS) classified advanced HF according to seven clinical profiles, ranging from patients on the brink of death (INTERMACS level 1) to clinically stable patients without current indications for HTx or MCS (INTERMACS level 7), as shown in ➔ Table 11.1.1.[9] The INTERMACS profiles were devised to provide consistent criteria to describe the clinical characteristics of advanced HF patients, clarify the target populations for MCS, and explain the available treatment alternatives. Unquestionably, the INTERMACS classification provides key prognostic information on HF patients undergoing MCS. For example, patients not needing inotropic support before MCS implantation (INTERMACS profiles 4–7) have significantly better survival and shorter hospitalizations than patients requiring high doses of inotropes (INTERMACS profiles 1–3). The INTERMACS profiles are also useful in assessing outcomes after urgent HTx: mortality rates in INTERMACS level 1 patients are significantly higher than among INTERMACS level 2–4 patients during the first year after HTx.

Important aspects of the clinical history in advanced heart failure

The acquisition of an accurate patient history is critically important in advanced HF. The clinician has two goals in eliciting a

Table 11.1.1 Interagency Registry for Mechanically Assisted Circulatory Support Profiles

Profile	NYHA class	Description	Time frame for intervention
INTERMACS 1	IV	Critical cardiogenic shock Patient with life-threatening hypotension despite rapidly escalating inotropic support, critical organ hypoperfusion	Definitive intervention needed within hours
INTERMACS 2	IV	Progressive decline on inotropic support Patient dependent on inotropic support, with progressive deterioration in nutrition, renal function, fluid retention, or other major status indicators	Definitive intervention needed within a few days
INTERMACS 3	IV	Stable but inotrope-dependent Patient with stable blood pressure, organ function, nutrition, and symptoms on continuous intravenous inotropic support, but demonstrating repeated failure to wean from inotropic agents due to symptomatic hypotension, worsening symptoms, or progressive organ dysfunction. Patient can be in the hospital or at home	Definitive elective intervention within a period of weeks/a few months
INTERMACS 4	IV	Resting symptoms in a patient who is at home on oral therapy Patient can be stabilized close to normal volume status but experiences daily symptoms of congestion at rest or during activities of daily living. Some patients may shuttle between 4 and 5	Definitive elective intervention within a period of weeks/a few months
INTERMACS 5	IV	Exertion intolerant Comfortable at rest and with activities of daily living, but unable to engage in any other activity, living predominantly within the house, frequently with moderate water retention and some level of kidney dysfunction. If underlying nutritional status and organ function are marginal, patient may be more at risk than INTERMACS 4 and require definitive intervention	Variable urgency, depends upon maintenance of nutrition, organ function, and activity
INTERMACS 6	IIIB	Exertion limited Comfortable at rest, without evidence of fluid overload, able to engage in activities of daily living and minor activities outside the home, but experiences fatigue within a few minutes of any meaningful exertion	Variable, depends upon maintenance of nutrition, organ function, and activity level
INTERMACS 7	III	Advanced NYHA class III symptoms Clinically stable with a reasonable level of comfortable activity, without current or recent episodes of decompensation	HT or circulatory support may not currently be indicated

Reproduced from Stevenson LW, Pagani FD, Young JB, et al. INTERMACS profiles of advanced heart failure: the current picture. *J Heart Lung Transplant.* 2009 Jun;28(6):535-41. doi: 10.1016/j.healun.2009.02.015 with permission from Elsevier.

careful history: (i) Does the HF syndrome have reversible causes? (ii) Are there therapeutic options for advanced HF that may be contraindicated for a particular patient? Some key examples and considerations for both goals follow.

Does the HF syndrome have reversible causes?

In addition to a review of current medications, it is important to understand why patients may not be receiving a component of guideline-directed medical therapy. Were they unduly hypotensive on angiotensin-converting enzyme -inhibitors to explain the small dose currently prescribed? Did they develop severe hyperkalemia in response to mineralocorticoid receptor antagonists ? Were patients truly unable to tolerate key medicines or did their clinical team have concerns about increasing the doses? Many patients referred to a tertiary centre for advanced care options will respond to an optimized medical regimen and have prolonged clinical stability.

Equally important is the assessment of whether the patient has experienced any of the hallmarks of the advanced HF syndrome.[5] These include recurrent HF hospitalizations, increasing HF signs and symptoms despite optimal medical therapy, recurrent episodes

of ventricular arrhythmias requiring implantable cardioverter-defibrillator (ICD) shocks, diminished response to previously effective diuretic dosages, worsening renal function necessitating a reduction in optimal therapy, onset of sleep disordered breathing, and involuntary weight loss or muscle wasting. Any of these characteristics are often the harbinger of a dire prognosis.

Are there therapeutic options for advanced HF that may be contraindicated for a particular patient?

Heart transplantation and durable MCS are well-established therapies for a select subset of advanced HF patients (see subsequent sections of this chapter). Before these options are discussed, however, the exclusion criteria for both treatments must be considered in the patient's medical history. A major challenge for the success of advanced therapies is a patient's inability to adhere to the medical regimen and/or follow-up clinic visits or lack of social support. The presence of significant renal dysfunction or the need for dialysis, frailty, advanced biological age, poor nutrition, or previous loss of limbs are all barriers in the management of patients with advanced HF. Active cancer or a recent history of malignancy may preclude HTx. Alcohol or illicit drug abuse, including opiate addiction or active smoking, can preclude consideration of advanced HF therapies. Finally, a thorough mental health evaluation should be performed to determine if a psychological/psychiatric disorder can be medically controlled or precludes either HTx and/or MCS.[3]

The physical examination in patients with advanced heart failure

Once history and symptoms have been recorded, the physical examination of the patient with advanced HF supplies crucial information on clinical status, prognosis, and appropriate therapy. The two key parameters to be assessed include volume and perfusion status.

Volume assessment

Helpful measures of volume status include assessment of the jugular venous pressure (JVP), the detection of positive abdominal-jugular reflux (AJR), hepatic enlargement, tenderness and pulsatility, lower extremity oedema, and, in some cases, anasarca. Importantly, before isolated lower extremity oedema is attributed to fluid overload, conditions that include third-spacing from hypoalbuminemia, venous insufficiency, or therapy with calcium channel blockers, must be excluded.

Jugular venous pressure is correlated with direct measurements of central venous pressure (CVP), which, in turn is generally one half of the pulmonary capillary wedge pressure (PCWP). Concomitant orthopnea and elevated JVP may indicate a PCWP >30 mmHg. The JVP should be inspected on both sides of the neck and at various degrees of incline, as jugular venous distention may be missed in the supine position but be apparent when the patient is sitting upright. The contour of the JVP may provide clues to underlying concomitant abnormalities: a prominent V wave may imply right ventricular (RV) failure associated with severe tricuspid regurgitation, or increased RV afterload caused by pulmonary arterial hypertension. Atrial fibrillation usually results in the absence of A waves in the JVP.

Although the presence of pulmonary rales or decreased breath sounds due to pleural effusions are helpful in the diagnosis of pulmonary oedema, these findings may be absent due to enhanced lymphatic drainage and greater storage of blood in compliant pulmonary veins. Likewise, weight changes may be helpful in the assessment of a patient's volume status, although they lack sensitivity and specificity as they may not occur in patients with concomitant cardiac cachexia and fluid overload.

Cardiac examination findings consistent with advanced HF include displacement of the apical impulse due to left ventricular enlargement; the presence of a third heart sound, which, although not specific, is both a sensitive marker of increased filling pressure and a prognostic indicator; the auscultation of a functional mitral regurgitation murmur; and a tricuspid regurgitation murmur indicative of RV volume and/or pressure overload. Accentuation of the pulmonary component of the second heart sound may be present with pulmonary arterial hypertension.

The assessment of perfusion

Assessment of reduced cardiac output (CO) is a critical step in the evaluation for advanced therapies but does not always indicate poor perfusion. Indeed, studies have shown that elevated filling pressures better correlate to survival than CO or cardiac index. [10]

Symptoms of poor perfusion may include excessive sleepiness or fatigue with muscle weakness, lightheadedness, cognitive impairment, difficulty in concentrating, and even syncope. Reduced CO is commonly compensated by an increase in peripheral vascular constriction resulting in cold extremities. Other physical findings include a proportional pulse pressure below 25%, according to the formula (systolic blood pressure – diastolic blood pressure)/systolic blood pressure. Other signs of low CO are perioral or nail bed cyanosis. More recently, new signs of worsening HF have been described. The first, flexo-dyspnoea[11], later named bendopnea, implying shortness of breath while bending forward.[12] The second is a combination of signs and symptoms termed orthodema, a score combining oedema with orthopnea that correlates well with HF rehospitalizations.[13]

Non-invasive imaging in advanced heart failure

Utilization of the functional, haemodynamic, and diagnostic data derived from the echocardiography, cardiac computed tomography (CCT), and cardiac magnetic resonance (CMR) studies in HF patients, discussed in detail, respectively, in ➲ Chapters 7.3.1, 7.3.3, and 7.3.4 of this book, supplies therapeutic guidance and prognostic information. The following section is therefore restricted to the clues provided by these imaging modalities in advanced HF.

Echocardiographic parameters in advanced heart failure

The deteriorating clinical manifestations of advanced HF may often be preceded by subtle echocardiographic changes. Left ventricular (LV) function should be actively assessed, focusing on the dimensions of the left atrium and the left ventricle, worsening functional mitral regurgitation, reduced RV function and/or an increased RV diameter with associated worsening of tricuspid regurgitation, elevated pulmonary pressures, and dilatation of the inferior vena cava with decreased or absent respirophasic diameter changes (➲ Table 11.1.2).[5]

Echocardiography for the selection and management of patients undergoing MCS implantation

Echocardiography is considered the first-line imaging modality in the pre-MCS evaluation process, during the MCS implantation itself, and in the post-operative long-term follow up. Echo is critical for the assessment of post MCS implantation complications, especially concerning the presence of RV dysfunction. At the time of left ventricular assist device (LVAD) implantation, LV output is restored towards normal, and the cardiac physiology changes, with attendant effects on RV function. The subsequent unloading of the LV lowers the pulmonary vasculature pressure, resulting in RV afterload reduction. Depending on the ensuing effect on RV

Table 11.1.2 Clinical, laboratory, echocardiographic (imaging) parameters and risk score data of advanced HF that can be used to trigger referral to an advanced heart failure centre*

Imaging	Risk score data
LVEF ≤ 30%	MAGGIC predicted survival ≤80% at 1 year
Large area of akinesis/dyskinesis or aneurysm	SHFM predicted survival ≤80% at 1 year
Moderate–severe mitral regurgitation†	
RV dysfunction	
sPAP ≥ 50 mmHg	
Moderate–severe tricuspid regurgitation	
Difficult to grade aortic stenosis	
IVC dilated or without respiratory variation	

Clinical	Laboratory
> 1 HF hospitalization in last year	eGFR < 45 mL/min
NYHA class III–IV	SCr ≥ 160 mmol/L
Intolerant of optimal dose of any GDMT HF drug	K > 5.2 or < 3.5 mmol/L
Increasing diuretic requirement	Hyponatremia
SBP ≤ 90 mmHg	Hb ≤ 120 g/L
Inability to perform CPET	NT-proBNP ≥ 1000 pg/mL
6MWT	
CRT non-responder clinically	
Cachexia, unintentional weight loss	

6MWT, 6-min walk test; CPET, cardiopulmonary exercise test; CRT, cardiac resynchronization therapy; eGFR, estimated glomerular filtration rate; GDMT, guideline-directed medical therapy; Hb, haemoglobin; HF, heart failure; IVC, inferior vena cava; K, potassium; KCCQ, Kansas City Cardiomyopathy Questionnaire; LVEF, left ventricular ejection fraction; MAGGIC, Meta-Analysis Global Group in Chronic Heart Failure; MLHFQ, Minnesota Living with Heart Failure Questionnaire; Na, sodium; NT-proBNP, N-terminal pro-B-type natriuretic peptide; NYHA, New York Heart Association; PA, pulmonary artery; RV, right ventricular; SBP, blood pressure; SCr, serum creatinine; SHFM, Seattle Heart Failure Model.

*Note that this table reflects many clinically relevant but sometimes subjective and non-specific criteria. With these criteria, sensitivity has been prioritized over specificity, i.e. many criteria may be present in patients who do not need referral, but by considering these criteria in a comprehensive assessment, there is a lower risk that high-risk patients may be missed or referred too late. While cut-offs exist for transplantation listing or left ventricular assist device implantation, there are no data to support specific cut-offs for referral to a HF centre.

†Moderate mitral regurgitation alone is not sufficient, but is one factor suggesting risk of progression and should be considered together with other variables.

Reproduced from Crespo-Leiro MG, Metra M, Lund LH, et al. Advanced heart failure: a position statement of the Heart Failure Association of the European Society of Cardiology. *Eur J Heart Fail.* 2018 Nov;20(11):1505-1535. doi: 10.1002/ejhf.1236 with permission from John Wiley and Sons.

preload there may be interventricular septum shifting to the left, which reduces the effectiveness of RV systolic contraction.

Echocardiography, combined with the haemodynamic assessment, helps to assess whether the native RV can cope with the new post-LVAD physiology. Severe RV enlargement, elevated pulmonary vascular resistance (PVR), elevated right atrial pressure, RV systolic dysfunction, and significant tricuspid regurgitation are

associated with post LVAD RV failure. RV systolic function is commonly assessed visually but may also be evaluated objectively by quantitative methods, such as right ventricular stroke work index (RVSWI), tricuspid annular plane systolic excursion (TAPSE), fractional area change (FAC), tricuspid annular systolic velocity by TDI, and STE-based longitudinal strain.[14] These echocardiographic measurements of RV function should be recognized and combined with other clinical and haemodynamic parameters to assess the potential need for RV support post LVAD implantation.

Other valuable information provided by echocardiography before LVAD implantation includes determination of the potential placement site of the inflow cannula and the landing zone of the outflow graft, assessment of valvular function to determine the presence and severity of aortic or tricuspid regurgitation and to evaluate the integrity of the interatrial septum. Worsening aortic regurgitation, a known complication of long term MCS support, results in reduced forward flow and may require aortic valve replacement during LVAD implantation if aortic regurgitation is worse than moderate. Patent foramen ovale should be closed during LVAD implantation to prevent the occurrence of 'paradoxical emboli'.

Cardiac computed tomography and other imaging modalities in advanced heart failure

Accurate assessment of the LV and RV dimensions and function is of major importance in the evaluation and decision-making process of patients with advanced HF. Although CCT is neither the most commonly used nor the 'gold standard' imaging technique for assessing bi-ventricular parameters, electrocardiogram (ECG)-gated CCT may be an accurate alternative in specific cases such as suboptimal echocardiographic window or inability to perform CMR due to claustrophobia or presence of MRI-incompatible cardiac implantable electronic devices (CIEDs).[15,16] CMR with its high spatial and temporal resolution is the optimal tool to assess the function and dimensions of the right and left ventricles and for the assessment of viability and composition of the myocardium.[21] Late gadolinium enhancement in CMR images has been shown to predict contractile function after revascularization.[22] Therefore, CMR assessment of myocardial viability can help to determine if the cardiac function of an advanced HF patient can be improved by percutaneous coronary intervention or coronary artery bypass graft before consideration of HTx or MCS. The main indications and applications for each one of the available imaging modalities in the assessment of heart failure patients is presented in ➲ Table 11.1.3.[23]

Haemodynamic assessment in advanced heart failure

The three fundamental indications for invasive haemodynamic assessment in patients with advanced HF are: (i) clarification of an ambiguous haemodynamic picture, (ii) assessment of the presence, severity, and reversibility of pulmonary hypertension, and (iii) consideration of eligibility for advanced therapies.[24] Additional key questions that can be addressed by invasive haemodynamic monitoring include evaluation of intracardiac pressures during exercise, determination of RV afterload mismatch, and inotropic reserve.

Table 11.1.3 Main indications and applications for currently available imaging modalities in the assessment of heart failure patients

Parameter	2D Echo	3D Echo	Strain	CMR	Nuclear	CT
LV/RV volumes	RU	AJ		AJ (GS)		AJ
LV systolic function	RU	AJ	AJ	AJ (GS)		
LV diastolic function	RU (GS)		AJ	AJ		
RV function	RU	AJ	AJ	AJ (GS)		
Ischemia	RU		AJ	AJ (GS)	AJ (GS)	
Viability	RU		AJ	AJ (GS)	AJ (GS)	
Cardiomyopathies Other HF aetiologies	RU		AJ	AJ (GS)		AJ
Risk assessment (arrhythmias)						
Therapy guidance (CRT)						
Follow up	RU					

Mid-grey: best performance of the technique for this indication. Light grey: The technique could provide useful information for this indication. Dark grey: no/little use for this indication. AJ, provides additional information to that obtained with 2D echocardiogram; GS, gold standard. RU, routinely used for this indication; LV, left ventricular; RV, right ventricular.
Reproduced from Melero-Ferrer JL, López-Vilella R, Morillas-Climent H, et al. Novel Imaging Techniques for Heart Failure. *Card Fail Rev.* 2016 May;2(1):27-34. doi: 10.15420/cfr.2015:29:2 with permission from Radcliffe Cardiology.

The latter is essential to predict whether the RV of a transplanted heart will perform normally or whether the native RV will withstand the altered physiology after LVAD surgery. According to the 2016 International Society for Heart and Lung Transplantation (ISHLT) guidelines,[25] a right heart catheterization (Class I, LOE C) is required for all potential HTx candidates to assess eligibility. For listed patients, right heart catheterization is recommended every 3–6 months especially if pulmonary arterial hypertension is present or the clinical condition worsens. A vasodilator challenge is indicated when pulmonary artery (PA) systolic pressure is > 50 mmHg, trans-pulmonary gradient > 15 mmHg, or PVR > 3 Wood units and systolic BP is > 85 mmHg. If vasodilator challenge fails to achieve haemodynamic values acceptable for HTx, these measurements should be reassessed after a period of therapy with diuretics, inotropes, and vasodilators.[25] Nearly 30 years after publication the recommendations regarding haemodynamic responses to vasodilators[26] remain valid to identify patients at highest risk for poor posttransplant outcomes, such as those in whom the PVR cannot be reduced < 2.5 Wood units with vasodilators, or those in whom this value is achieved at the expense of systemic arterial hypotension.

It is important to recognize that PA pressure and PVR have limitations in their ability to predict RV function after LVAD implantation. Neither parameter entirely describes RV performance or effects of afterload on the RV and neither has emerged as a predictor of RV function after LVAD implant in multivariable models. The systolic PA pressure is determined by both vascular resistance and RV function. Indeed, systolic PA pressure can be low in very late stages of RV failure. In addition, PVR is a calculated measure, and it does not account for PA compliance, as shown in ➲ Figure 11.1.1.[27]

Several studies conducted in high-volume MCS centres have attempted to identify the most accurate predictors of RV function after LVAD implantation. These variables are shown in ➲ Table 11.1.4.

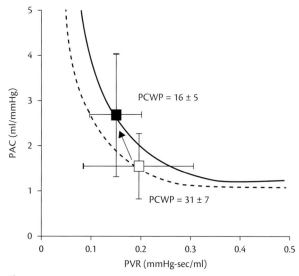

Figure 11.1.1 Pulmonary haemodynamics before and after treatment of acutely decompensated heart failure.
PAC, PVR, and τ before (open box) and after (closed box) treatment for acute decompensated heart failure. Because PCWP decreases, the shift in PVR and PAC does not completely follow the original hyperbola.
PAC, pulmonary arterial capacitance; PVR, pulmonary vascular resistance; PCWP, pulmonary capillary wedge pressure.
Reproduced from Dupont M, Mullens W, Skouri HN, et al. Prognostic role of pulmonary arterial capacitance in advanced heart failure. *Circ Heart Fail.* 2012 Nov;5(6):778–85. doi: 10.1161/CIRCHEARTFAILURE.112.968511 with permission from Wolters Kluwer.

Assessing functional capacity in advanced heart failure

In HF, the heart attempts to pump blood to fulfil end-organ needs at the expense of a progressive increase in filling pressures. In this setting, the ability of the cardiovascular system to accelerate oxygen supply, to initiate and sustain exercise, is a direct measure

Table 11.1.4 Selected haemodynamic parameters proposed as predictors of right ventricular failure after implantation of a left ventricular assist device

Haemodynamic parameter	Definition	Cutoff value for risk
CVP	CVP	Low risk < 12 mmHg Moderate risk > 12 and < 16 High risk > 16 mmHg
CVP/PCW	CVP/PCW	> 0.6
RVSWI	$(mPA - CVP) \times (CI/HR)$	< 350 ml/m^{2*}mmHg
PAPi	$(PA_{syst} - PA_{diast})/RAP$	> 2
PVR	$(mPA - PCW)/CO$	> 3–5 Wood Units
TR	Ventricularization of RA waveform	Present
Kussmaul's sign	Inspiratory increase in CVP	Present

CVP, central venous pressure; PAPi, pulmonary artery pulsatility index; PCW, pulmonary capillary wedge pressure; PVR, pulmonary vascular resistance; RAP, right atrial pressure; RVSWI, right ventricular stroke work index; TR, tricuspid regurgitation.

of HF severity. The cardiopulmonary exercise test (CPET) permits measurement of many variables reflective of metabolic responses to low-level, intermediate, and maximum exercise. It is more precise and reproducible than other measures of physical function, precisely assesses volitional effort, BP, and ventilatory efficiency, provides organ-specific information, and facilitates an assessment of the response to therapies as well as prognosis.[28] For example, in HF with reduced ejection fraction (HFrEF), a 6% decrease in peak VO$_2$ is associated with a 5% higher risk of mortality/cardiovascular hospitalization.[29]

The variables essential for the evaluation of patients with advanced HF include the following: VO$_2$ is the amount of oxygen an individual can utilize in cellular metabolism, and it is measured as the product of CO and the difference between arterial and venous oxygen content. Peak VO$_2$ refers to the highest VO$_2$ achieved during a maximal effort incremental exercise test. It can be indexed to weight, resting metabolic rate (1 MET= 3.5 ml/Kg/min) or expressed as percent predicted, a measure which accounts for age, sex, height, and weight. Since the 1991 landmark study by Mancini et al.[30] showing that peak VO$_2$ is superior to LVEF in predicting outcomes of advanced HF patients, this measurement remains a highly valuable prognostic marker in contemporary patient populations. The 2016 International ISHLT guidelines reaffirm the value of peak VO$_2$ measurement as a guide to list patients for heart transplantation (➲ Table 11.1.5).

Importantly, the ISHLT guidelines state that a maximal CPET is defined as one with a respiratory exchange ratio (RER) > 1.05 and achievement of anaerobic threshold on optimal pharmacologic therapy (Class I, Level of Evidence: B). Notably, the ISHLT guidelines do not mention achievement of > 85% target heart rate (HR) as a measure of maximum effort, because most patients are unable to achieve this goal due to treatment with beta-blockers. The RER is the ratio of ventilatory equivalents for CO$_2$ and O$_2$ (RER = VCO$_2$/VO$_2$). When the RER is < 1.05, peak VO$_2$ does not

Table 11.1.5 International Society for Heart and Lung Transplantation Recommendations on Cardiopulmonary Stress Testing to Guide Listing for Heart Transplantation: 2006 vs 2016

2006 Guideline recommendation	2016 Guideline recommendation
1.1. Cardiopulmonary stress testing to guide transplant listing	1.1. Cardiopulmonary stress testing to guide transplant listing
A maximal cardiopulmonary exercise test is defined as one with a respiratory exchange ratio (RER) > 1.05 and achievement of an anaerobic threshold on optimal pharmacologic therapy (Class I, Level of Evidence: B).	Continuing approval without change.
	The presence of a CRT device does not alter the current peak VO$_2$ cutoff recommendations (Class I, Level of Evidence: B).
In patient's intolerant of a β-blocker, a cutoff for peak oxygen consumption (VO2) of ≤ 14 ml/kg/min should be used to guide listing (Class I, Level of Evidence: B).	Continuing approval without change.
In the presence of a β-blocker, a cutoff for peak VO2 of ≤ 12 ml/kg/min should be used to guide listing (Class I, Level of Evidence: B).	Continuing approval without change.
In young patients (< 50 years) and women, it is reasonable to consider using alternate standards in conjunction with peak VO2 to guide listing, including percent of predicted (≤ 50%) peak VO2 (Class IIa, Level of Evidence: B).	Continuing approval without change.
In the presence of a sub-maximal cardiopulmonary exercise test (RER < 1.05), use of ventilation equivalent of carbon dioxide (VE/VCO2) slope of > 35 as a determinant in listing for transplantation may be considered (Class IIb, Level of Evidence: C).	Continuing approval without change.
In obese (body mass index [BMI] > 30 kg/m2) patients, adjusting peak VO2 to lean body mass may be considered. A lean body mass–adjusted peak VO2 of < 19 ml/kg/min can serve as an optimal threshold to guide prognosis (Class IIb, Level of Evidence: B).	Continuing approval without change.
Listing patients based solely on the criterion of a peak VO2 measurement should not be performed (Class III, Level of Evidence: C).	Continuing approval without change.

Reproduced from Mehra MR, Canter CE, Hannan MM, et al; International Society for Heart Lung Transplantation (ISHLT) Infectious Diseases, Pediatric and Heart Failure and Transplantation Councils. The 2016 International Society for Heart Lung Transplantation listing criteria for heart transplantation: A 10-year update. *J Heart Lung Transplant.* 2016 Jan;35(1):1-23. doi: 10.1016/j.healun.2015.10.023 with permission from Elsevier.

accurately reflect either functional impairment or prognosis. In this case, another variable, the ventilatory equivalents for CO$_2$ (VE/VCO$_2$) can be used to assess HF stage. In normal individuals, < 29 litre of minute ventilation are needed to eliminate 1 litre of CO$_2$. The greater the ventilatory effort required to eliminate a given amount of CO$_2$, the more severe is the HF. VE/VCO$_2$ > 35 is indicative of advanced HF.

Furthermore, VE/VCO_2 closely reflects RV function, PA pressure, and PVR during exercise. Importantly, VE/VCO_2 adds prognostic information to peak VO_2 in patients who have achieved maximal volitional effort. Another value predictive of HF severity is the aerobic work efficiency, or the amount of VO_2 relative to workload ($\Delta VO_2/\Delta WR$). The more the subject relies on anaerobic metabolism, the more depressed this value is in term of amount of VO_2 use per watts of work achieved. Values of aerobic work efficiency below 10 ml O_2/min/W are considered abnormal. The dyspnoea index, which is the ratio of VE to maximal voluntary ventilation (MVV), (which can also be calculated as FEV1 × 35), is essential to determine the relative contribution of pulmonary versus cardiac limitations to exercise. In essence, VE/MVV measures how close a subject gets to the ventilatory ceiling; a value > 80% indicates a pulmonary mechanical limitation to exercise.

Two additional CPET parameters are especially relevant to the advanced HF population.[26] One is the presence of exercise oscillatory ventilation (EOV), the exercise equivalent of Hunter–Cheyne–Stokes periodic breathing at rest. EOV is deemed to be present if the cyclic variation occurs for at least 60% of exercise and the amplitude is ≥ 15% of baseline. In normal individuals VE rises linearly and smoothly during exercise. In contrast, in patients with advanced HF, the VE increase is not only depressed due to the prolonged circulatory time from impaired cardiac systolic performance, but it assumes an undulatory pattern whose cycle length and amplitude depend upon the magnitude of decrease in cardiac index. In multiple studies, the presence of EOV confers a high mortality risk (⊃ Figure 11.1.2).

Additional important CPET values should be considered in the assessment of advanced HF. Heart rate recovery (HRR) is the

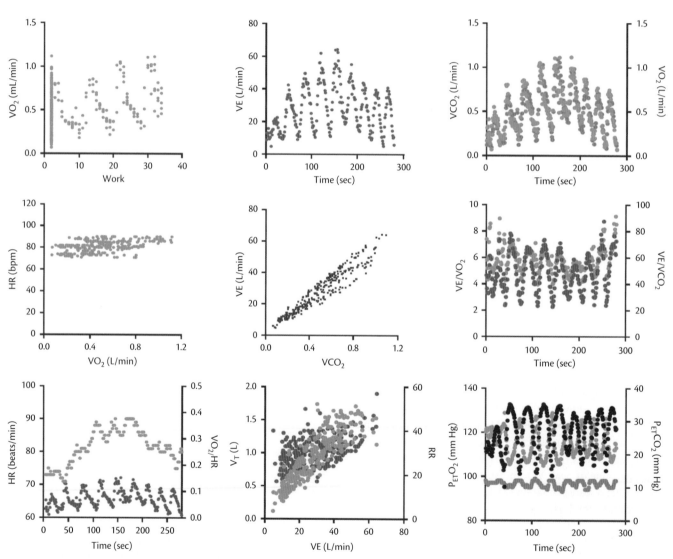

Figure 11.1.2 Plot CPET report from a patient with HFrEF and exercise oscillatory ventilation.
EOV is a specific VE abnormal phenotype occurring in approximately 30% of patients with mid-to-late manifestations of chronic heart failure, characterized by cyclic fluctuation of VE and expired gas kinetics of variable amplitude, frequency, and duration. Because oscillatory manifestations may occur even in normal subjects, criteria for an abnormal definition are an oscillatory pattern at rest that persists for ≥60% of the exercise test at an amplitude of ≥15% of the average resting value.
CPET, cardiopulmonary exercise testing; EOV, exercise oscillatory ventilation; HR, heart rate; $P_{ET}CO_2$, partial pressure of end-tidal carbon dioxide; $P_{ET}O_2$, partial pressure of end-tidal oxygen; RR, respiratory rate; Vco_2, volume of carbon dioxide released; VE, ventilation; Vo_2, peak oxygen consumption; V_T, tidal volume.
Guazzi M, Bandera F, Ozemek C, Systrom D, Arena R. Cardiopulmonary exercise testing: what is its value? *JACC* 2017; 70 1618–36. http://dx.doi.org/10.1016/j.jacc.2017.08.012

rate at which HR decelerates 1 minute into recovery. A HRR < 12 bpm, indicative of delayed vagal reactivation, is an adverse risk factor which maintains its prognostic value even with beta-blocker therapy. Partial pressure of end-tidal CO_2 ($PETCO_2$) which is < 33 at rest or rises < 3 with exercise is associated with a poor prognosis. Notably, dyspnoeic patients with very high VE/VCO_2 (> 60) and very low $PETCO_2$ (< 20) should be evaluated for concomitant pulmonary vascular disease. The oxygen uptake efficiency slope (OUES) is the slope of VO_2/Log VE, indicating the absolute increase in VO_2 associated with a 10-fold rise in

ventilation. Advanced HF is associated with a smaller increase in VO_2 per increase in ventilation resulting in lower OUES. In addition to having a high prognostic value in advanced HF, OUES can discriminate between HF and chronic obstructive pulmonary disease.

Since several CPET variables can help determine the presence of advanced HF, the field is moving toward a multivariable CPET risk assessment for all patients being evaluated as candidates for advanced HF therapies (➲ Figure 11.1.3 and ➲ Table 11.1.6).

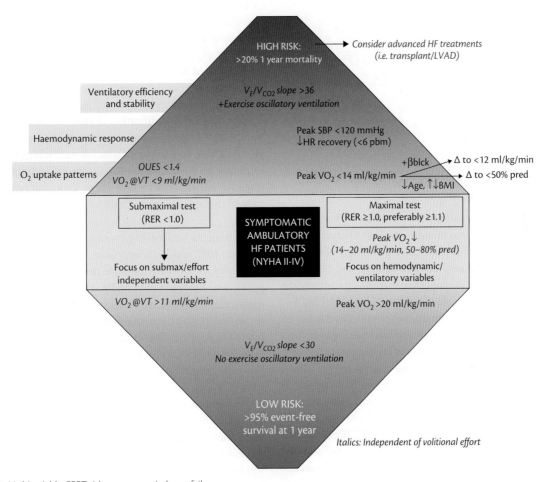

Figure 11.1.3 Multivariable CPET risk assessment in heart failure.

CPET evaluation should start with an assessment of whether there was maximum volitional effort, as indicated by RER >1.0 to 1.1. Heart rate >85% of predicted also signals maximum effort but is often not achieved in patients with HF on nodal agents and/or with chronotropic incompetence. VO_2 responses: peak VO_2 remains the gold standard metric of fitness and should be a focal point of CPET interpretation if maximum effort was achieved. Peak VO_2 <14 ml/kg/min purports poor prognosis, although a lower threshold value of <12 ml/kg/min should be used in patients tolerating beta-blockade. For young patients and those with high or low BMI, peak VO_2 should be interpreted as a % of predicted, with values <50% indicating a poor prognosis. For patients who do not achieve maximum effort, the focus should shift to O_2 uptake variables that are independent of volitional effort (i.e. OUES <1.4 and VO_2 at VT <9 ml/kg/min indicating a poor prognosis). Hemodynamic responses: failure to achieve SBP >120 mm Hg and failure to augment SBP with exercise is associated with poor prognosis, particularly when coupled with a peak VO_2 <14 ml/kg/min or reduced cardiac output augmentation. Both chronotropic incompetence and slow heart rate recovery (<6 beats/min) also purport a poor prognosis. Ventilatory efficiency and stability: Steep VE/VCO_2 slope (indicative of inefficient ventilation) and EOV are among the most potent predictors of poor outcome in HF. The presence of EOV is consistently associated with a 1-year mortality >20%. The combination of high VE/VCO_2 slope and EOV represents a particularly high-risk population, with 1 study indicating 6-month HF hospitalization (40%) and death (15%) in excess of that in the referent group (16% and 1%, respectively).

BMI, body mass index; CPET, cardiopulmonary exercise testing; EOV, exercise oscillatory ventilation; HF, heart failure; LVAD, left ventricular assist device; O_2 oxygen; OUES, oxygen uptake efficiency slope; RER, respiratory exchange ratio; SBP, systolic blood pressure; VCO_2, carbon dioxide output; VE, ventilation; VO_2, oxygen uptake; VT, ventilatory threshold.

Reproduced from Malhotra R, Bakken K, D'Elia E, Lewis GD. Cardiopulmonary Exercise Testing in Heart Failure. *JACC Heart Fail*. 2016 Aug;4(8):607–16. doi: 10.1016/j.jchf.2016.03.022 with permission from Elsevier.

Table 11.1.6 Cardiopulmonary exercise testing for physiologic risk stratification

Rule out/ address first	Rule IN/ consider advanced heart failure therapies
Correctable anaemia/iron deficiency	RER > 1.05
Pulmonary mechanical limit (VE/MVV >0.9)	Peak VO_2 < 12 mL/Kg/min or < 50% predicted
Inadequate pacing (CRT, rate responsive pacing)	VE/VCO_2 slope >36
Severe RV-PV dysfunction > LV dysfunction ◆ High RAP/PCWP ◆ RVEF < 30% that falls with exercise ◆ RV–PA uncoupling	Exercise oscillatory ventilation
	Failure to augment SBP
	Failure to augment CO with elevated left sided filling pressures

CRT, cardiac resynchronization therapy; LV, left ventricle; MVV, maximal voluntary ventilation; PA, pulmonary artery; PCWP, pulmonary arterial wedge pressure; RAP, right atrial pressure; RER, respiratory exchange ratio; RV, right ventricle; RVEF, right ventricular ejection fraction; RV-PV, VE

Evaluating prognosis and need for referral in advanced heart failure

Assessment of risk for poor outcomes in patients with advanced HF should be divided into two broad categories: (1) recognition by general cardiologists and primary care physicians of features that should trigger referral to specialized centres, and (2) evaluation of the candidacy for advanced HF therapies or palliative care for patients at institutions capable of offering HTx and/or MCS.

For general cardiologists or primary care physicians, it is key to recognize when HF is progressing toward advanced stages. This task is challenging. Systematic screening of certain patient groups has been suggested as a way of improving referral to specialized centres. For example, one small study suggested that consistent screening of recipients of cardiac resynchronization therapy (CRT) may identify candidates for HTx or MCS who would have otherwise been deemed as not having advanced HF. The Screening for Advanced Heart Failure Treatment (SEE-HF) study[33] showed that among actively screened CRT or ICD recipients with persistently low LVEF (< 40%) and elevated NYHA class (III–IV), 26% had a previously unrecognized need for advanced HF therapies. Clinical decision supports (CDS) may also help to identify patients potentially eligible for advanced therapies. Evans et al.[34] developed a computer application that, by automatically extracting information from the patient's integrated electronic health record, could monitor HF status and alert the treating physician when the criteria for advanced HF were met. Compared to the year before introduction of CDS, a higher number of patients were referred to specialized centres when CDS was used.

CDS approaches are not widely used, and simpler tools are needed to ensure timely referral. A study from the Swedish Heart Failure Registry showed that patients with NYHA class III-IV, a LVEF < 40%, and ≥ 1 easily identifiable risk factors had lower

1-year survival than similar patients undergoing HTx or MCS. Five risk factors were suggested as triggers for referral to an advanced HF centre. These include a systolic blood pressure (SBP) < 90 mmHg, a serum creatinine level > 160 μmol/l, haemoglobin < 120 g/l, absence of a renin–angiotensin system antagonist, and lack of a beta-blocker. Based on these findings the authors recommend referral to an advanced HF centre when ≥ 1 risk factors are present.[35] The aim of this study was not to achieve optimal biological discrimination but rather to provide simple, memorable, and distinct criteria that can be used by busy clinicians. Other investigators have suggested that referral to a specialized HF centre should be triggered by persistent NYHA class III–IV symptoms or recurrent hospitalization despite optimal medical therapy, or inability to tolerate appropriate treatment due to hypotension, worsening renal function, or hyponatremia. These suggestions do not imply that all patients with these characteristics should be considered for HTx and/or MCS, but rather underscore the appropriateness of an expert assessment by a HF specialist. Importantly, such evaluation may lead to further optimization of medical therapy, identification of patients who may benefit from implantable haemodynamic sensors, and increased appropriate use of CIEDs. In addition, palliative care, which has been shown to reduce re-hospitalizations and improve quality of life of end-stage HF patients not eligible for, or choosing not to pursue, advanced therapies, is more likely to be offered at a specialized HF centre.

For patients undergoing evaluation at specialized HF centres, between 1997 and 2018, approximately 100 risk scores have been developed. It is neither possible nor appropriate to discuss these prediction models individually. However, a few general comments can be made. The risk prediction scores vary according to patient populations analysed, and statistical approaches and modeling applied. The discriminatory ability for predicting all-cause mortality, cardiovascular death, or composite endpoints is generally better than that for HF hospitalizations. Predictors frequently appearing in many of the risk models include age, sex, body mass index, diabetes mellitus, heart rate, LVEF, NYHA class, SBP, natriuretic peptides levels, sodium, and blood urea nitrogen and creatinine (⮞ Figure 11.1.4 and ⮞ Table 11.1.7). Most risk models have a high risk of bias, approximately 45% have internal validation, and only 24% are strengthened by external validation.

Heart Failure Survival Score

The Heart Failure Survival Score (HFSS) was developed in the 1990s by using the data from 268 ambulatory patients referred for consideration of HTx from 1986 to 1991 and was validated in the same study in a group of 199 similar patients from 1993 to 1995.[37] Multivariate analysis revealed independent risk factors that were used to create an invasive and a non-invasive version of the scale. The latter included HF aetiology, peak VO_2, mean arterial blood pressure, resting heart rate, serum sodium, LVEF, and intraventricular conduction delay > 120 ms. The invasive version adds PCWP to the non-invasive variables. Because PCWP did not improve discrimination, the non-invasive version is the most frequently used. According to the HFSS, patients fall in one

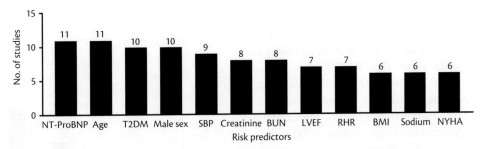

Figure 11.1.4 Most common variables examined in 40 retrieved articles published between 2013 and 2019 on models of HF risk prediction.
BMI, body mass index; BUN, blood urea nitrogen; HF, heart failure; LVEF, left ventricular ejection fraction; NT-Pro BNP, N-terminal pro-B-type natriuretic peptide; NYHA, New York Heart Association; RHR, resting heart rate; SBP, systolic blood pressure; T2DM, type 2 diabetes mellitus.
Reproduced from Di Tanna GL, Wirtz H, Burrows KL, Globe G. Evaluating risk prediction models for adults with heart failure: A systematic literature review. *PLoS One.* 2020 Jan 15;15(1):e0224135. doi: 10.1371/journal.pone.0224135.

of three risk groups: low (≥ 8.10), medium (7.20-8.09), or high (≤ 7.19). The highest risk patients should be promptly evaluated for advanced HF therapies due to their high probability of death over a 1-year follow-up. Although still used, the prognostic value of the HFSS in patients receiving contemporary guideline-directed medical therapy is unknown.

Table 11.1.7 Most common scores used for risk stratification of patients with heart failure

Score	Components	Comments
HFSS	♦ Presence/absence coronary artery disease ♦ Resting heart rate ♦ Left ventricular ejection fraction ♦ Mean arterial blood pressure ♦ Presence/absence of intraventricular conduction delay ♦ Serum sodium ♦ Peak oxygen uptake HFSS = [(0.0216 × resting HR) + (−0.0255 × mean BP) + (−0.0464 × LVEF) + (−0.047 × serum sodium) + (−0.0546 × peak VO$_2$) + (0.608 × presence or absence of IVCD) + (0.6931 × presence or absence of ischaemic heart disease)]	Score is based on a sum of these variables multiplied by defined coefficients Low risk: ≥8.1 Medium risk: HFSS 7.20 to 8.09 High risk: HFSS ≤7.1
SHFM	♦ Demographics ♦ Clinical characteristics ♦ Medications ♦ Laboratory data ♦ Devices www.seattleheartfailuremodel.org	Incorporates impact of interventions (medical and device) and provides estimates of 1, 2, and 5-year survival
MECKI	♦ Percent predicted peak VO$_2$ ♦ VE/VCO$_2$ slope ♦ Haemoglobin ♦ Serum sodium ♦ LVEF ♦ eGFR by MDRD	Incorporates data from the CPET as well as kidney function
MAGGIC	♦ Age ♦ Gender ♦ LVEF ♦ Systolic blood pressure ♦ Body mass index ♦ Serum creatinine ♦ NYHA class ♦ Smoking history ♦ Co-morbidities (e.g., diabetes, COPD) ♦ Length of heart failure diagnosis ♦ Medications www.heartfailurerisk.org	Risk model converted into integer score Generalizable to a broad spectrum of patients

BP, blood pressure; COPD, chronic obstructive pulmonary disease; CPET, cardiopulmonary exercise test; eGFR, estimated glomerular filtration rate; HFSS, Heart Failure Survival Score; HR, heart rate; IVCD, intraventricular conduction defect; LVEF, left ventricular ejection fraction; MAGGIC, Meta-Analysis Global Group in Chronic Heart Failure; MDRD, Modification of Diet in Renal Disease; MECKI, Metabolic Exercise test data combined with Cardiac and Kidney Indexes; NYHA, New York Heart Association; SHFM, Seattle Heart Failure Model; VE/VCO$_2$, minute ventilation–carbon dioxide production relationship; VO$_2$, oxygen consumption.

Seattle Heart Failure Model

The Seattle Heart Failure Model (SHFM)[38] was designed to predict the composite outcome of death, urgent HTx, and MCS in a cohort of 1125 HF patients from the PRAISE I clinical trial database. The SHFM was then prospectively validated in approximately 10,000 patients enrolled in five additional clinical trials. The SHFM consists of 20 variables indicative of the patient's clinical characteristics (age, gender, NYHA class, SBP, ischaemic aetiology, LVEF), laboratory values (serum sodium, haemoglobin, uric acid, total cholesterol, percentage of lymphocytes), medications (beta-blocker, angiotensin-converting enzyme inhibitor or angiotensin receptor blocker, statin, aldosterone antagonist, furosemide-equivalent loop diuretic dose, allopurinol), and CIED therapy. According to the scores obtained from these variables, patients are assigned to a low-, medium- or high-risk category. As first developed, the SHFM provides accurate prediction of the 1-, 2-, and 3-year survival of patients with stable chronic ambulatory HF, but it consistently underestimates the mortality risk of individuals with advanced HF. Accordingly, the SHFM was updated in 2013 with the addition of diabetes mellitus, measures of renal function, natriuretic peptides levels, and the use of inotropes, intra-aortic balloon pump, mechanical ventilation, and ultrafiltration. A calculator for the newer SHFM is available on the internet (http://depts.washington.edu/shfm). Independent studies have confirmed the accuracy of the updated SHFM, but the large number of variables required to accurately estimate the risk of death may challenge its routine use.

The Meta-Analysis Global Group in Chronic Heart Failure (MAGGIC)

The MAGGIC meta-analysis deserves special mention because it includes individual data on 39,372 HF patients with both HFrEF and HFpEF from 30 cohort studies of which 6 were clinical trials. Multivariable methods selected a final model inclusive of 13 independent predictors of mortality in the following order of prognostic strength: age, lower ejection fraction, NYHA class, serum creatinine, diabetes, not prescribed beta-blocker, lower systolic BP, lower body mass, time since diagnosis, current smoker, COPD, male gender, and not prescribed ACE-inhibitor or angiotensin-receptor blockers. Conversion into an easy-to-use integer risk score identified an instructive 3-year mortality risk gradient between six groups, ranging from 10% to 70%.[39] The MAGGIC score calculator is accessible at www.heartfailurerisk.org. Importantly, when the MAGGIC score was externally validated in 51,043 individual patients enrolled in the Swedish Heart Failure Registry, it was found to have good discrimination (C index = 0.741).[40] The difference between the model-predicted and the observed 3-year mortality in the six risk groups varied between 5% and 12%. Calibration assessment demonstrated slight overprediction for the lowest risk patients, and underprediction in high-risk patients (◑ Figure 11.1.5).[41] These findings underscore the complexity of evaluating the true likelihood of poor outcomes in advanced HF patients.

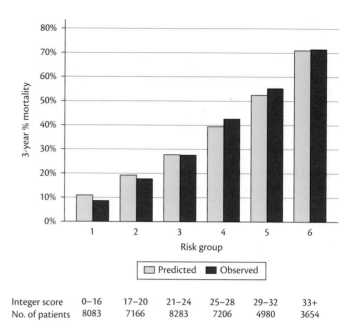

Integer score	0–16	17–20	21–24	25–28	29–32	33+
No. of patients	8083	7166	8283	7206	4980	3654

Figure 11.1.5 Observed versus MAGGIC-predicted 3-year mortality in six risk groups.

Risk groups 1–4 represent the first four quintiles of risk (integer scores 0–16, 17–20, 21–24, and 25–28, respectively). Risk groups 5 and 6 represent the top two deciles of risk (integer scores 29–32 and 33 or more, respectively).

Reproduced from Pocock SJ, Ariti CA, McMurray JJ, et al; Meta-Analysis Global Group in Chronic Heart Failure. Predicting survival in heart failure: a risk score based on 39 372 patients from 30 studies. *Eur Heart J.* 2013 May;34(19):1404-13. doi: 10.1093/eurheartj/ehs337 with permission from Oxford University Press.

Model for end-stage liver disease

The model for end-stage liver disease (MELD) was originally developed to assess short-term prognosis of cirrhotic patients undergoing elective placement of trans-jugular intrahepatic portosystemic shunts (TIPS). The MELD score was later used to prioritize liver allocation according to disease severity. More recently, the MELD score has also been shown to have prognostic value in HF patients.[42] The original MELD score consists of three easily obtainable variables, the international normalized ratio (INR), serum bilirubin, and serum creatinine. The fact that renal and hepatic dysfunction are correlated with unfavourable outcomes in HF patients forms the basis for the use of the MELD scale to improve risk stratification in HF patients, as it has been confirmed in diverse HF populations. However, the principal limitation to the application of the MELD score in HF patients is that it cannot be used in individuals receiving oral anticoagulants, which alter INR values. To overcome this drawback, the modified MELD (modMELD) and the MELD excluding INR (MELD-XI) were developed.[43] In the modMELD the INR is substituted with albumin, whereas the MELD-XI only includes bilirubin and creatinine. Both modifications of the MELD score have shown promise in assessing the risk of poor outcomes in HF patients referred for HTx evaluation or MCS implantation.

Metabolic Exercise Cardiac Kidney Indexes (MECKI) Score

The importance of this score is that it specifically targeted the risk for the composite endpoint of cardiovascular death and urgent HTx. This risk model was derived from a cohort of 2716 HFrEF patients followed for an average of 4 years at 13 centres.[44] Six variables independently predicted the outcome of interest (haemoglobin, sodium, estimated glomerular filtration rate (eGFR) by the Modification of Diet in Renal Disease (MDRD) equation, LVEF, % predicted Peak VO_2 and the VE/VCO_2 slope). Four distinct risk groups emerged according to a MECKI score < 5%, 5–10%, 10–15%, and > 15% and their respective 2-year event free survival was 99%, 95%, 90%, and 75% by Kaplan–Meier analysis (⮕ Figure 11.1.6). The MECKI score identified the risk of study endpoints with AUC values of 0.804 (0.754–0.852) at 1 year, 0.789 (0.750–0.828) at 2 years, 0.762 (0.726–0.799) at 3 years and 0.760 (0.724–0.796) at 4 years. The most obvious limitation of the MECKI score is its development and validation only in a white population from a single country.

A 2018 comparison of the prognostic value of the MECKI score with that of the HFSS and SHFM in 6112 HF patients followed up for a median of 3.67 years, revealed that the MECKI score outperformed the HFSS and SHFM both at 2 and 4 years.[45] However, external validation of these results is lacking.

Ominous co-morbidities and social determinants of health

With the improved overall survival of HF patients, the burden of risk factors, prolonged advanced HF, and advanced age become more frequent. In-depth discussion of individual co-morbidities in the HF patient and their effect on patient's quality of life and prognosis are discussed in ⮕ Chapter 12. The co-morbidities most frequently present in advanced HF patients are briefly discussed below.

Diabetes

Difficulty in achieving diabetic control and end-organ involvement should be assessed. Non-adherence as the cause of poorly controlled diabetes should be carefully investigated as this behaviour may extend to life-saving therapy used after MCS and/or HTx. Uncontrolled diabetes with end-organ involvement is a relative contraindication for HTx but not necessarily for LVAD implantation. Immunosuppression after HTx with tacrolimus and steroids may result in rapid progression of the end-organ dysfunction. Surprisingly, there is increasing data suggesting improved diabetic control post LVAD implantation.

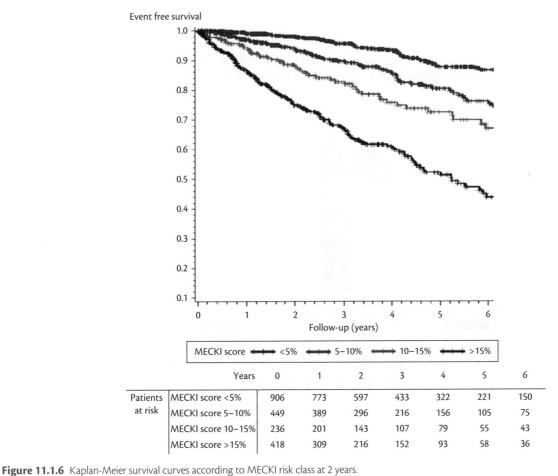

MECKI score	<5%	5–10%	10–15%	>15%

	Years	0	1	2	3	4	5	6
Patients at risk	MECKI score <5%	906	773	597	433	322	221	150
	MECKI score 5–10%	449	389	296	216	156	105	75
	MECKI score 10–15%	236	201	143	107	79	55	43
	MECKI score >15%	418	309	216	152	93	58	36

Figure 11.1.6 Kaplan-Meier survival curves according to MECKI risk class at 2 years.
MECKI score: < 5% (906 cases), 5–10% (449 cases), 10–15% (236 cases), and >15% (418 cases). The curves were arbitrarily ended at 6 years.
Reproduced from Agostoni P, Corrà U, Cattadori G, et al; MECKI Score Research Group. Metabolic exercise test data combined with cardiac and kidney indexes, the MECKI score: a multiparametric approach to heart failure prognosis. *Int J Cardiol*. 2013 Sep 10;167(6):2710-8. doi: 10.1016/j.ijcard.2012.06.113 with permission from Elsevier.

Hypertension

Uncontrolled hypertension is a serious therapeutic challenge in advanced HF patients. Hypertension might cause early graft dysfunction after HTx or reduced efficacy of LVAD support attributed to the increased afterload. Furthermore, after LVAD implantation, hypertension has been associated with an increased risk of haemorrhagic strokes. In addition, uncontrolled hypertension is a common and reversible precipitating factor for acute decompensated heart failure and therefore should be strictly controlled prior to referring a patient for advanced therapies.

Renal function

In advanced HF patients, the combination of longstanding reduction in cardiac output, sustained increase in CVP, and comorbidities, such as diabetes and hypertension, can result in progression of renal disease. Worsening kidney function with or without significant hyperkalemia may require modification of life-saving HF medications.

Smoking

Smoking habits should be clearly assessed due to the reduced survival of actively smoking heart transplanted patients: Typically, active tobacco use precludes HTx because it is a powerful risk factor for development and progression of cardiac allograft vasculopathy.

Pulmonary diseases

Besides the effects of active smoking on the benefits of advanced HF interventions, oxygen dependence due to chronic pulmonary disease attributed to past smoking or any other cause is typically a contraindication for both HTx and MCS. Other pulmonary diseases, such as interstitial lung disease or pulmonary fibrosis, also preclude advanced HF therapies. Severe pulmonary disease exposes the advanced HF patient undergoing any surgical therapy to prolonged ventilation and difficult weaning which is associated with infectious and metabolic complications, as well as de-conditioning.

Vascular diseases

The same factors leading to coronary atherosclerosis often involve other vascular beds. Severe aortic atherosclerosis may be prohibitive both for vascular anastomosis at the time of HTx and for placement of the outflow cannula of a LVAD.

Muscle wasting

Severe muscle wasting and/or cardiac cachexia is frequent in advanced HF patients at all ages. It is driven by systemic inflammation and the release of cytokines, such as tumor necrosis factor alfa similarly to the catabolic states observed in other chronic diseases, in which these processes significantly reduce quality of life and survival (⊃ Figure 11.1.7). Muscle wasting and malnutrition are associated with poorer outcomes also following HTx and LVAD implantation; pre-operative nutrition optimization is recommended.

Malignancy

Long-term complete recovery from any malignancy usually has no impact on the survival of advanced HF patients undergoing HTx

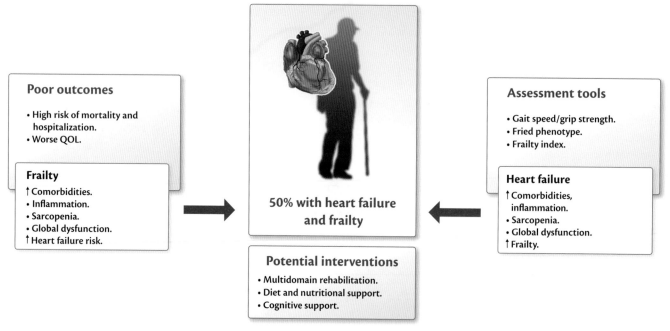

Figure 11.1.7 The inter-relationship between frailty and heart failure.
Frailty and heart failure share common pathological mechanisms, often coexist, and are associated with worse clinical and patient-oriented outcomes.
HF, heart failure; QoL, quality of life.
Source data from Pandey A, Kitzman D, Reeves G. Frailty Is Intertwined With Heart Failure: Mechanisms, Prevalence, Prognosis, Assessment, and Management. *JACC Heart Fail.* 2019 Dec;7(12):1001-1011. doi: 10.1016/j.jchf.2019.10.005.

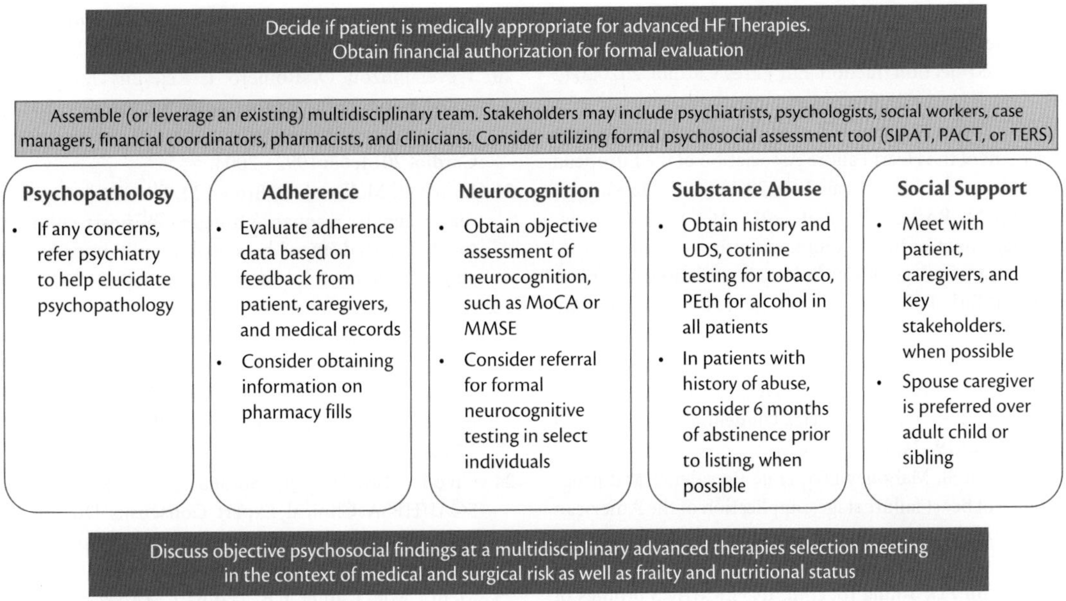

| Decide if patient is medically appropriate for advanced HF Therapies. Obtain financial authorization for formal evaluation |

Assemble (or leverage an existing) multidisciplinary team. Stakeholders may include psychiatrists, psychologists, social workers, case managers, financial coordinators, pharmacists, and clinicians. Consider utilizing formal psychosocial assessment tool (SIPAT, PACT, or TERS)

Psychopathology	Adherence	Neurocognition	Substance Abuse	Social Support
• If any concerns, refer psychiatry to help elucidate psychopathology	• Evaluate adherence data based on feedback from patient, caregivers, and medical records • Consider obtaining information on pharmacy fills	• Obtain objective assessment of neurocognition, such as MoCA or MMSE • Consider referral for formal neurocognitive testing in select individuals	• Obtain history and UDS, cotinine testing for tobacco, PEth for alcohol in all patients • In patients with history of abuse, consider 6 months of abstinence prior to listing, when possible	• Meet with patient, caregivers, and key stakeholders. when possible • Spouse caregiver is preferred over adult child or sibling

Discuss objective psychosocial findings at a multidisciplinary advanced therapies selection meeting in the context of medical and surgical risk as well as frailty and nutritional status

Figure 11.1.8 Stepwise approach to psychosocial assessment.
Stepwise approach to psychosocial assessment.
HF, heart failure; MMSE, mini-mental state evaluation; MoCA, Montreal cognitive assessment; PACT, Psychosocial assessment of candidates for transplantation; Peth, phosphatidylethanol; SIPAT, Stanford integrated psychosocial assessment for transplantation; TERS, transplant evaluation rating scale; UDS, urine drug screen.
Reproduced from Bui QM, Allen LA, LeMond L, Brambatti M, Adler E. Psychosocial Evaluation of Candidates for Heart Transplant and Ventricular Assist Devices: Beyond the Current Consensus. *Circ Heart Fail.* 2019 Jul;12(7):e006058. doi: 10.1161/CIRCHEARTFAILURE.119.006058 with permission from Wolters Kluwer.

or LVAD implantation. Patients suffering from any malignancy, or just recently recovering from one, should be carefully assessed on an individual basis to determine the probability of relapse post HTx due to chronic immunosuppression. Decisions in the cancer survivors requiring advanced HF therapy should be tailored to individual patients and involve multidisciplinary teams.

Social determinants of health

Social determinants of health (SDOH) are the conditions in which people are born, grow, educate, work, live, and age, as well as other factors affecting and shaping the daily life of the patients. It has been shown that patients with a greater number of negative SDOH fare worse. Although not yet studied in advanced HF patients, SDOH may influence the morbidity and mortality of these individuals and should play a significant role in choosing the most appropriate management strategy for those patients (➲ Figure 11.1.8).

Future directions

Despite the many advances outlined in this chapter for the accurate assessment of advanced heart failure, there is still much work that needs to be done. The ventricular assist device community has made great strides in developing a common set of data variables and definitions to be used internationally. Likewise, the heart transplant community has reached an important consensus on the grading of endomyocardial biopsies. These kind of data standards must be developed for the assessment of advanced heart failure. Risk scores should be established that can be universally validated and are applicable in general cardiology clinics as well as tertiary care centres. Predictive scores need to include

key social determinants of outcome that will allow a more diverse application of life-saving advanced therapies.

Conclusion

Enormous gaps exist in the correct and timely recognition of when patients with HF have reached the advanced stages of their disease. Often patients believed to have advanced HF are simply patients not receiving optimal guidelines-directed medical therapy. Frequently, patients are referred to specialized centres for consideration of advanced therapies, but these are subsequently avoided by the application of the appropriate medical therapy. Conversely, patients are commonly referred to specialized centres when their illness is associated with multi-organ failure which renders advanced therapies futile. Much has been learned since heart transplantation and mechanical circulatory support have become available. Progress has occurred in the recognition of key clinical features, in the utilization of various imaging techniques and in the development of scores for the risk stratification of potential candidates for advanced HF therapies. The optimal evaluation of advanced HF patients requires simultaneous consideration of multiple diagnostic modalities and the participation of multidisciplinary teams.

References

1. Groenewegen A, Rutten FH, Mosterd A, Hoes AW. Epidemiology of heart failure. Eur J Heart Fail. 2020;22(8):1342–1356.
2. Truby LK, Rogers JG. Advanced heart failure. JACC: Heart Failure. 2020;8(7):523–536.
3. Guglin M, Zucker MJ, Borlaug BA, *et al.* Evaluation for Heart Transplantation and LVAD Implantation: JACC Council Perspectives. J Am Coll Cardiol. 2020;75(12):1471–1487.

4. Corrà U, Magini A, Paolillo S, Frigerio M. Comparison among different multiparametric scores for risk stratification in heart failure patients with reduced ejection fraction. Eur J Prev Cardiol. 2020;27(2 suppl):12–18.

5. Crespo-Leiro MG, Metra M, Lund LH, et al. Advanced heart failure: a position statement of the Heart Failure Association of the European Society of Cardiology. Eur J Heart Fail,2018;20(11),1505–1535.

6. Yancy CW, Jessup M, Bozkurt B, et al.. 2013 ACCF/AHA guideline for the management of heart failure: executive summary: a report of the American College of Cardiology Foundation/American Heart Association Task Force on practice guidelines. Circulation. 2013;128(16):1810–52.

7. Fang JC, Ewald GA, Allen LA, et al. Heart Failure Society of America Guidelines Committee. Advanced (stage D) heart failure: a statement from the Heart Failure Society of America Guidelines Committee. .J Card Fail. 2015;21(6):519–34.

8. Ammar KA, Jacobsen SJ, Mahoney DW, et al. Prevalence and prognostic significance of heart failure stages: application of the American College of Cardiology/American Heart Association heart failure staging criteria in the community. Circulation. 2007;115(12):1563–70.

9. Stevenson LW, Pagani FD, Young JB, et al. INTERMACS profiles of advanced heart failure: the current picture. J Heart Lung Transplant 2009; 28:535–541.

10. Cooper LB, Mentz RJ, Stevens SR, et al. Hemodynamic Predictors of Heart Failure Morbidity and Mortality: Fluid or Flow? J Card Fail. 2016;22(3):182–9.

11. Brandon N, Mehra MR. "Flexo-dyspnea": a novel clinical observation in the heart failure syndrome. J Heart Lung Transplant. 2013; 32(8):844–5

12. Thibodeau JT, Turer AT, Gualano SK, et al. Characterization of a novel symptom of advanced heart failure: bendopnea. ACC Heart Fail. 2014 Feb;2(1):24–31.

13. Lala A, McNulty SE, Mentz RJ, et al. Relief and Recurrence of Congestion During and After Hospitalization for Acute Heart Failure: Insights From Diuretic Optimization Strategy Evaluation in Acute Decompensated Heart Failure (DOSE-AHF) and Cardiorenal Rescue Study in Acute Decompensated Heart Failure (CARESS-HF). Circ Heart Fail. 2015;8(4):741–8.

14. Cameli M, Loiacono F, Sparla S, et al. Systematic Left Ventricular Assist Device Implant Eligibility with Non-Invasive Assessment: The SIENA Protocol. J Cardiovasc Ultrasound 2017;25(2):39–46.

15. Taylor AJ, Cerqueira M, Hodgson JM, et al. ACCF/SCCT/ACR/ AHA/ASE/ASNC/NASCI/SCAI/SCMR 2010 appropriate use criteria for cardiac computed tomography. A report of the American College of Cardiology Foundation Appropriate Use Criteria Task Force, the Society of Cardiovascular Computed Tomography, the American College of Radiology, the American Heart Association, the American Society of Echocardiography, the American Society of Nuclear Cardiology, the North American Society for Cardiovascular Imaging, the Society for Cardiovascular Angiography and Interventions, and the Society for Cardiovascular Magnetic Resonance. J Am Coll Cardiol 2010; 56: 1864–1894.

16. Aziz W, Claridge S, Ntalas I, et al. Emerging role of cardiac computed tomography in heart failure. ESC Heart Fail. 2019 Oct;6(5):909–920.

17. Raman SV, Sahu A, Merchant AZ, Louis LB, Firstenberg MS, Sun B. Noninvasive assessment of left ventricular assist devices with cardiovascular computed tomography and impact on management. J Heart Lung Transplant 2010; 29: 79– 85.

18. Raman SV, Tran T, Simonetti OP, Sun B. Dynamic computed tomography to determine cardiac output in patients with left ventricular assist devices. J Thorac Cardiovasc Surg 2009; 137: 1213– 1217.

19. Lund LH, Edwards LB, Kucheryavaya AY, et al. The registry of the International Society for Heart and Lung Transplantation: thirty-first official adult heart transplant report–2014; focus theme: retransplantation. J Heart Lung Transplant 2014; 33: 996– 1008.

20. Wever-Pinzon O, Romero J, Kelesidis I, et al. Coronary computed tomography angiography for the detection of cardiac allograft vasculopathy: a meta-analysis of prospective trials. J Am Coll Cardiol 2014; 63: 1992– 2004.

21. Lum YH, McKenzie S, Brown M, Hamilton-Craig C. Impact of cardiac magnetic resonance imaging on heart failure patients referred to a tertiary advanced heart failure unit: improvements in diagnosis and management. Intern Med J. 2019;49(2):203–211.

22. Kim RJ, Wu E, Rafael A, et al. The use of contrast-enhanced magnetic resonance imaging to identify reversible myocardial dysfunction. N Engl J Med 2000; 343:1445–53.

23. Melero-Ferrer JL, López-Vilella R, Morillas-Climent H, et al. Novel imaging techniques for heart failure. Card Fail Rev 2016;2(1): 27–34.

24. Givertz MM, Fang JC, Sorajja P, et al. Executive Summary of the SCAI/HFSA Clinical Expert Consensus Document on the Use of Invasive Hemodynamics for the Diagnosis and Management of Cardiovascular Disease.J Card Fail. 2017;23(6):487–491.

25. Mehra MR, Canter CE, Hannan MA, et al. International Society for Heart Lung Transplantation (ISHLT) Infectious Diseases, Pediatric and Heart Failure and Transplantation Councils. The 2016 International Society for Heart Lung Transplantation listing criteria for heart transplantation: A 10-year update. J Heart Lung Transplant. 2016;35(1):1–23.

26. Costard-Jäckle A, Fowler MB. Influence of preoperative pulmonary artery pressure on mortality after heart transplantation: testing of potential reversibility of pulmonary hypertension with nitroprusside is useful in defining a high-risk group. J Am Coll Cardio. 1992;19(1):48–54.

27. Dupont M, Mullens W, Skouri HN, et al. Prognostic role of pulmonary arterial capacitance in advanced heart failure. Circ Heart Fail. 2012;5(6):778–85.

28. Wagner J, Agostoni P, Arena R, et al. The Role of Gas Exchange Variables in Cardiopulmonary Exercise Testing for Risk Stratification and Management of Heart Failure with Reduced Ejection Fraction, Am Heart J, 2018; 202:116–126,

29. Swank AM, Horton J, Fleg JL, et al. Modest increase in peak VO2 is related to better clinical outcomes in chronic heart failure patients: results from heart failure and a controlled trial to investigate outcomes of exercise training. Circ Heart Fail 2012; 5:579–585.

30. Mancini DM, Eisen H, Kussmaul W, Mull R, Edmunds LH Jr, Wilson JR. Value of peak exercise oxygen consumption for optimal timing of cardiac transplantation in ambulatory patients with heart failure. Circulation. 1991;83(3):778–86.

31. Guazzi M, Arena R, Halle M, Piepoli MF, Myers J, Lavie CJ. 2016 focused update: clinical recommendations for cardiopulmonary exercise testing data assessment in specific patient populations. Circulation 2016;133: e694–711.

32. Malhotra R, Bakken K, D'Elia E, Lewis GD. Cardiopulmonary Exercise Testing in Heart Failure. .JACC Heart Fail. 2016; 4(8):607–16.

33. Lund LH, Trochu JN, Meyns B, et al. Screening for heart transplantation and left ventricular assist system: results from the ScrEEning for advanced Heart Failure treatment (SEE-HF) study. Eur J Heart Fail. 2018;20(1):152–160.

34. Evans RS, Kfoury AG, Horne BD, et al. Clinical Decision Support to Efficiently Identify Patients Eligible for Advanced Heart Failure Therapies. J Card Fail. 2017;23(10):719–726.

35. Thorvaldsen T, Benson L, Ståhlberg M, Dahlström U, Edner M, Lund LH. Triage of patients with moderate to severe heart failure: who should be referred to a heart failure center? J Am Coll Cardiol. 2014;63(7):661–671.

36. Di Tanna GL, Wirtz H, Burrows KL, Globe G. Evaluating risk prediction models for adults with heart failure: A systematic literature review. PLoS One 2020;15(1): e0224135.

37. Aaronson KD, Schwartz JS, Chen TM, Wong KL, Goin JE, Mancini DM. Development and prospective validation of a clinical index to predict survival in ambulatory patients referred for cardiac transplant evaluation. Circulation. 1997;95(12):2660–7.

38. Levy WC, Mozaffarian D, Linker DT, et al. The Seattle Heart Failure Model: prediction of survival in heart failure. Circulation 2006;113(11):1424–33.

39. Pocock SJ, Ariti CA, McMurray JJV, et al. Meta-Analysis Global Group in Chronic Heart Failure. Predicting survival in heart failure: a risk score based on 39 372 patients from 30 studies. Eur Heart J 2013;34(19):1404–13.

40. Sartipy U, Dahlström U, Edner M, Lund LH. Predicting survival in heart failure: validation of the MAGGIC heart failure risk score in 51,043 patients from the Swedish heart failure registry. Eur J Heart Fail. 2014;16(2):173–9.

41. Pocock SJ, Ariti CA, McMurray JJV, et al. Predicting survival in heart failure: a risk score based on 39 372 patients from 30 studies. Eur Heart J 2013;34(19):1404–13.

42. Kato TS, Stevens GR, Jiangn J, et al. Risk stratification of ambulatory patients with advanced heart failure undergoing evaluation for heart transplantation. J Heart Lung Transplant. 2013 ;32(3): 333–40.

43. Abe S, Yoshihisa A, Takiguchi M, et al. Liver dysfunction assessed by model for end-stage liver disease excluding INR (MELD-XI) scoring system predicts adverse prognosis in heart failure. PLoS One. 2014;9(6): e100618.

44. Agostoni P, Corrà U, Cattadori G, et al. MECKI Score Research Group. Metabolic exercise test data combined with cardiac and kidney indexes, the MECKI score: a multiparametric approach to heart failure prognosis. Int J Cardiol. 2013;167(6):2710–8.

45. Agostoni P, Paolillo S, Mapelli M, et al. Multiparametric prognostic scores in chronic heart failure with reduced ejection fraction: a long-term comparison. Eur J Heart Fail. 2018;20(4):700–710.

CHAPTER 11.2

Advanced heart failure: management

Daniela Tomasoni, Marianna Adamo, and Marco Metra

Contents

Introduction

The prevalence of heart failure (HF) has increased and the number of patients who progress to an advanced stage of HF has grown in recent years.[1,2] This poses a challenge to clinicians, as such patients usually have severe symptoms, that is New York Heart Association (NYHA) class III or IV, poor quality of life, and high rates of hospitalizations despite being on optimal medical, surgical, and device therapies.[3,4] Prognostic stratification is crucial for the timely referral of patients with chronic HF to advanced care, to properly convey expectations to patients and families, and to plan treatment and follow-up strategies (➔ Figure 11.2.1).[1,3] Patients with advanced HF refractory to medical therapy and cardiac resynchronization therapy (CRT) and who do not have absolute contraindications should be referred for heart transplantation. Mechanical circulatory support should also be considered as bridge to transplant or destination therapy in selected patients.[1,3] The purpose of this chapter is to summarize the management of advanced HF patients, focusing on disease-modifying medical treatment, the management of congestion, including pharmacological therapy and renal replacement therapy, and the use of inotropes. Mechanical circulatory support, heart transplantation, palliative cares, and end-of-life management will be discussed in the following chapters.

Disease-modifying drugs

Guideline-directed medical treatment that has been demonstrated to improve CV outcome in patients with symptomatic HF with reduced ejection fraction (HFrEF) includes neurohormonal modulators and sodium glucose cotransporter type 2 (SGLT2) inhibitors.[1] Neurohormonal modulators include the angiotensin receptor neprylisin inhibitor (ARNI) sacubitril/valsartan, angiotensin converting enzyme inhibitors (ACEi) or angiotensin receptor blockers (ARB), beta-blockers, and mineralocorticoid receptor antagonists (MRA). The proportion of patients with advanced HF enrolled in landmark clinical trials that have led to the indication to these agents is widely variable. ➔ Table 11.2.1 reports pharmacological outcome trials in HF, highlighting results in subgroups of patients in NYHA class III or IV and with lower LVEF. Landmark trials with beta-blockers, ACEi, and MRA had a relatively high proportion of patients in NYHA class III or IV and/or with low LVEF with no interaction between these variables and treatment effect, supporting their use in advanced HF patients. On the other hand, in the Prospective Comparison of ARNI with ACEi to Determine Impact on Global Mortality and Morbidity in Heart Failure (PARADIGM-HF) trial, fewer than 1% of patients had a NYHA functional class IV.[5] Pre-specified subgroup analyses showed a significant interaction (p = 0.03) between NYHA class at randomization and the effect of treatment on the primary endpoint, with major benefits in the subgroup of patients with NYHA class I or II vs NYHA class III or

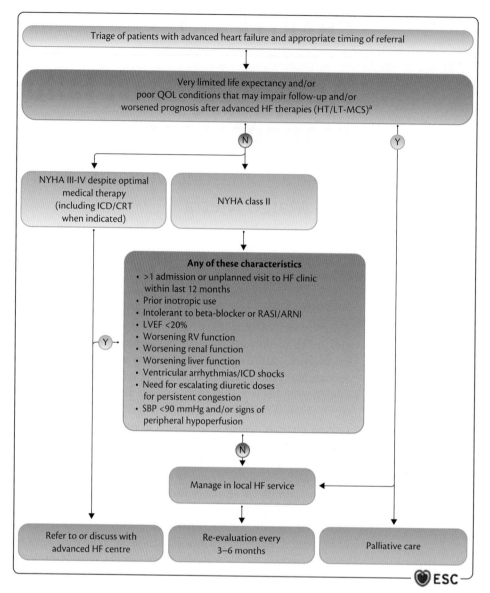

Figure 11.2.1 Triage of patients with advanced heart failure and appropriate timing of referral.

ARNI, angiotensin receptor-neprilysin inhibitor; CRT, cardiac resynchronization therapy; HF, heart failure; HT, heart transplantation; ICD, implantable cardioverter-defibrillator; LT-MCS, long-term mechanical circulatory support; LVEF, left ventricular ejection fraction; NYHA, New York Heart Association; RASi, renin-angiotensin system inhibitor; RV, right ventricular; SBP, systolic blood pressure; QOL, quality of life.

[a] Limited life expectancy may be due by major comorbidities such as cancer, dementia, end-stage organ dysfunction; other conditions that may impair follow-up or worsen post-treatment prognosis include frailty, irreversible cognitive dysfunction, psychiatric disorder, or psychosocial issues.

McDonagh TA, Metra M, Adamo M, et al; ESC Scientific Document Group. 2021 ESC Guidelines for the diagnosis and treatment of acute and chronic heart failure. *Eur Heart J.* 2021 Sep 21;42(36):3599-3726. doi: 10.1093/eurheartj/ehab368. © The European Society of Cardiology. Reprinted by permission of Oxford University Press.

IV. This interaction was not observed considering CV death. The rationale of the LIFE (LCZ696 in Hospitalized Advanced Heart Failure) study was to assess the feasibility, efficacy, and safety of such treatment in the most advanced phases of the disease.[6] This was a 24-week prospective, multicentre trial comparing the use of sacubitril/valsartan vs valsartan alone in patients with a LVEF <35%, recent NYHA class IV symptoms, and elevated N-terminal pro-brain natriuretic peptide (NT-proBNP) levels.[6] The study was prematurely stopped due to the Coronavirus 2019 (COVID-19) pandemic at the point when 335 patients had been randomized. No difference between sacubitril/valsartan and valsartan was shown in the primary endpoint of change from baseline in the area under the curve for NT-proBNP levels through 24 weeks. Sacubitril/valsartan did not improve the composite endpoint of number of days alive, out of hospital, and free from HF events and did not decrease the risk of death from CV causes or HF hospitalization, HF hospitalization, CV death, or all cause death, compared to valsartan.[7] The study was not, however, powered to detect changes in CV death and/or HF hospitalizations and results may have been influenced by the relatively small sample size and the relatively short study duration.

Thus, while only 25% of patients included in PARADIGM-HF were in NYHA class III-IV, the trial suggested a larger benefit of sacubitril/valsartan on the primary endpoint in the

Table 11.2.1 Pharmacological outcome trials investigating GDMT in HFrEF and including patients with NYHA III–IV

Study name (year)	Drug comparisons	Number of patients	Inclusion criteria	Characteristics of patients included			Effect of treatment on primary outcome
				Age (years)	NYHA	LVEF as %	
	ACEi						
CONSENSUS (1987)	enalapril vs placebo	253	NYHA IV; congestive HF, cardiomegaly on chest X-ray	71	IV (100%)	–	Enalapril reduced total mortality by 40% at 6 months (26% vs 44%, p = 0.002) and by 31% at 1 yr (52% vs 36%, p = 0.001)
SOLVD-T (1991)	enalapril vs placebo	2569	NYHA I–IV; LVEF ≤ 35%; chronic congestive HF	61	III–IV (32%)	25 6–22 (37%) 23–29 (32%)	Enalapril reduced total mortality by 16% (35% vs 40%, p = 0.004); consistent results in subgroups: NYHA I, II, III, IV, and LVEF 6–22%, 23–29%, 30–35% (p-value for interaction > 0.05)
ATLAS (1999)	high vs low dose lisinopril	3164	NYHA II–IV; LVEF ≤ 30%; if NYHA II, inclusion required treatment for HF in an emergency room or hospital within 6 months	63 ± 10	III–IV (84%)	23 ± 6	No difference in total mortality (43% vs 45%, p = 0.13); consistent results in subgroups: NYHA II, III, IV, and LVEF < 24 vs ≥ 24%
	ARB						
VALHeFT (2001)	valsartan vs placebo	5010	NYHA II–IV; LVEF ≤ 40%	63 ± 11	III–IV (38%)	27 ± 7 ≥ 27 (48%)	No difference in total mortality (19.7 vs 19.4, p = 0.80). Valsartan reduced the composite outcome of mortality and morbidity (cardiac arrest with resuscitation, HF hospitalization, and intravenous inotropic or vasodilator use for ≥ 4 hours by 13% (29% vs 32%, p = 0.009); consistent results in subgroups: NYHA III/IV vs II, and LVEF < 27% vs ≥27%
CHARM-Alternative (2003)	candesartan instead of ACEI vs placebo	2028	NYHA II–IV; LVEF ≤ 40%	67 ± 11	III–IV (52%)	30 ± 7	Candesartan reduced the composite outcome of cardiovascular death and HF hospitalization by 23% (33% vs 40%, p < 0.001)
HEAAL (2009)	High vs low dose losartan	3834	NYHA II–IV; LVEF ≤ 40%	66 (56–73)	III–IV (31%)	33 (28–37)	High dose losartan reduced the composite outcome of death or HF hospitalization by 10% (43% vs 46%, p = 0.03); consistent results in subgroups: NYHA III/IV vs I/II, and LVEF < 25%, 25–34%, and ≥ 35% (p-value for interaction > 0.05)
	ACEi/ARB						
ELITE I (1997)	losartan vs captopril	722	NYHA II–IV; LVEF ≤ 40%; chronic HF	73 ± 6	III–IV (35%)	30 ± 7	No difference in tolerability (persistent increase in creatinine) (11% vs 11%, p = 0.63)

(continued)

Table 11.2.1 Continued

Study name (year)	Drug comparisons	Number of patients	Inclusion criteria	Characteristics of patients included			Effect of treatment on primary outcome
				Age (years)	NYHA	LVEF as %	
ELITE II (2000)	losartan vs captopril	3152	NYHA II–IV; LVEF < 40%; chronic HF	71 ± 7	III–IV (48%)	31 ± 7 ≤ 25 (9%)	No difference in total mortality; consistent results in subgroups (18% vs 16%, p = 0.16): NYHA III/IV vs II, and LVEF ≤ 25 vs > 25%
CHARM-Added (2003)	candesartan + ACEI vs ACEI	2548	NYHA II–IV and LVEF ≤ 40%; if NYHA II, inclusion required hospitalization for cardiac reason within the last 6 months	64 ± 11	III–IV (76%)	28 ± 8	Candesartan + ACEI reduced the composite outcome of cardiovascular death and HF hospitalization by 15% (38% vs 42%, p = 0.01)
BB							
CIBIS-II (1999)	bisoprolol vs placebo	2647	NYHA III–IV; LVEF ≤ 35%; stable chronic HF	61 (24–80)	III–IV (100%)	28 ± 6	Bisoprolol reduced total mortality by 34% (12% vs 17%, p < 0.001); consistent results in subgroups: NYHA III vs IV
MERIT-HF References (1999)	metoprolol CR/XL vs placebo	3991	NYHA II–IV; LVEF ≤ 40%	64 ± 10	III–IV (59%)	28 ± 7	Metoprolol CR/XL reduced total mortality by 34% (7% vs 11%, p<0.001); consistent results in subgroups: NYHA II, III, IV, and LVEF lower vs middle + upper tertile
COMET (2003)	metoprolol vs carvedilol	3029	NYHA II–IV; LVEF ≤ 30%; chronic HF; previous admission for CV reason	62 ± 11	III–IV (52%)	26 ± 7 ≤ 25 (46%)	Carvedilol reduced mortality by 17% (34% vs 40%, p = 0.002); consistent results in subgroups; NYHA II, III, IV, and LVEF ≤ 25 vs > 25%
COPERNICUS (2001)	carvedilol vs placebo	2289	NYHA III–IV for ≥ 2 months; LVEF < 25%; clinically euvolaemic	63 ± 11	III–IV (100%)	20 ± 4	Carvedilol reduced total mortality by 35% (11% vs 17%, p < 0.001); consistent results in subgroups: LVEF < 20 vs ≥ 20%
SENIORS (2005)	nebivolol vs placebo	2128	HF confirmed as HF hospitalization in recent 12 months and/or LVEF ≤ 35% in recent 6 months	76 ± 5	III–IV (41%)	36 (13) ≤ 35 (64%)	Nebivolol reduced the composite outcome of total mortality and CV hospitalizations by 14% (31% vs 35%, p = 0.04); consistent results in subgroups; LVEF ≤ 35 vs > 35% (p-value for interaction > 0.05)
MRA							
RALES (1999)	spironolactone vs placebo	1663	NYHA III–IV; LVEF ≤ 35% within 6 months	65 ± 12	III–IV (100%)	25 ± 7	Spironolactone reduced total mortality by 30% (35% vs 46%, p < 0.001); consistent results in subgroups: NYHA III vs IV, LVEF < 26 vs ≥ 26%

Table 11.2.1 Continued

Study name (year)	Drug comparisons	Number of patients	Inclusion criteria	Characteristics of patients included			Effect of treatment on primary outcome
				Age (years)	NYHA	LVEF as %	
	ARNI						
PARADIGM-HF (2014)	sacubitril/valsartan vs enalapril	8399	NYHA II–IV; LVEF ≤ 40% (changed to ≤ 35% during the study); BNP ≥ 150 pg/ml or NT-proBNP ≥ 600 pg/ml (BNP ≥ 100 pg/ml or NT-proBNP ≥ 400 pg/ml if HF hospitalization within 12 months)	64 ± 11	III–IV (25%)	29 ± 6 ≤ 35 (89%)	Sacubitril/valsartan reduced the composite outcome of CV mortality and hospitalization for HF by 20% (22% vs 27%, p < 0.001); consistent results in subgroups: LVEF ≤ 35 vs > 35% (p-value for interaction > 0.05) whereas sacubitril/valsartan showed greater effect in NYHA I/II vs III/IV (p-value for interaction = 0.03)
LIFE (2021)	sacubitril/valsartan vs valsartan	335	NYHA IV in previous 3 months; LVEF ≤ 35% and ≤ 25% within 12 months; BNP ≥250 pg/ml or NT-proBNP ≥800 pg/ml; ≥1 additional objective finding of advanced HF	–	IV (100%)	–	Sacubitril/valasartan was not superior to valsartan with respect to lowering NT-proBNP levels (primary endpoint); HR for CV death or HF hospitalization 1.32 (0.86 –2.03)
	SGLT-2i						
DAPA-HF (2019)	dapagliflozin vs placebo	4744	NYHA II–IV; LVEF ≤ 40%; NT-proBNP > 600 pg/ml (> 400 pg/ml if HF hospitalization within 12 months, and > 900 pg/ml if atrial fibrillation/flutter at baseline)	66 ± 11	III–IV (32%)	31 ± 7 ≤ median (53%)	Dapagliflozin reduced the composite outcome of CV death or worsening HF by 26% (16% vs 21%, p<0.001); consistent results in subgroups LVEF < median vs > median (p-value for interaction > 0.05), whereas dapagliflozin showed greater effect in NYHA II vs III/IV (p-value for interaction < 0.05)
EMPEROR-reduced (2020)	empagliflozin vs placebo	3730	NYHA II–IV; LVEF < 40%; NT-proBNP > 600 pg/ml if LVEF < 30%, > 1000 pg/ml if LVEF 31–35%, and > 2500 pg/ml if LVEF 36–40%; if LVEF >30% then HF hospitalization within 12 months)	67 + 11	III–IV (25%)	27 + 6 <30 (73%)	Empagliflozin reduced the composite outcome of CV death or worsening HF by 25% (19% vs 25%, p < 0.001); consistent results in subgroups LVEF < 30 vs > 30%, whereas empagliflozin showed greater effect in NYHA II vs III/IV

Values are expressed as mean (± standard deviation), median (interquartile range), or number (percentage).

ACEI, angiotensin-converting enzyme inhibitor; ARB, angiotensin receptor blocker; ARNI, angiotensin receptor neprilysin inhibitor; BB, beta-blocker; BNP, brain natriuretic peptide; CR, controlled release; CV, cardiovascular; HF, heart failure; HR, hazard ratio; LV, left ventricle; LVEF, left ventricular ejection fraction; LVIDD, left ventricular internal diameter end diastole; MRA, mineralocorticoid receptor antagonist; NT-proBNP, N-terminal pro B-type natriuretic peptide; NYHA, New York Heart Association; SGLT-2i, sodium-glucose cotransporter-2 inhibitor XL, extended release; yrs, years.

patients with less severe HF,[5] and LIFE failed to show a benefit of sacubitril/valsartan over valsartan in patients with advanced HF.[6] However, although we have no evidence for ARNI versus ACEi or ARB, treatment with these drugs remains indicated in patients with advanced HF.[1] The same applies also to beta-blockers and MRA.[1]

Importantly, in clinical practice patients with advanced HF often cannot tolerate neurohormonal antagonists and their up-titration. This intolerance is related to features of the advanced stage of the HF, with frequent low cardiac output and hypotension, peripheral hypoperfusion, and end-organ worsening dysfunction, namely kidney dysfunction.[8] The use of suboptimal doses of neurohormonal modulators is associated with worse outcome and the presence of haemodynamic limitations to ACEi identifies patients with severe HF and with a very poor prognosis (mortality over 50% at 1 year).[9] Thus, intolerance to neurohormonal antagonists is a marker of advanced HF and a criterion to trigger referral to a specialized advanced HF centre (➲ Table 11.2.2).[1] In the simple mnemonic 'I NEED HELP', that was created for timely identification of patients requiring advanced HF therapies, 'P' refers to 'Prognostic medication' (e.g. inability to up-titrate or need to decrease/cease ACEi, beta-blockers, ARNIs, or MRAs) (➲ Table 11.2.3).[10] Most recently, Mehra et al. proposed a novel algorithm for the early identification of patients who need advanced therapies, the so-called rule of three which includes (1) repetitive hospitalizations for heart failure (e.g. ≥2 events in a year), (2) staircase diuretic requirements over time (e.g. an increase of oral loop diuretics therapy by 50% in the preceding 6 months) to maintain clinical stability, and (3i) intolerance to neurohormonal therapy with onset of cardiorenal perturbation (➲ Table 11.2.4).[11]

In the last years, two major trials have shown benefits of SGLT2 inhibitors on morbidity and mortality in patients with HFrEF.[12,13] Their effects were independent from HF severity, including NYHA class, and background therapy. They had mild to absent effects on blood pressure and, thus, may be better tolerated than ARNI/ACEi/ARB, and had favorable long-term effects on kidney function.[12,13] Favourable effects were also shown in trials with in-hospital initiation of SGLT2 inhibitors in patients with decompensated HF.[14–16] Thus, there are reasons to consider that SGLT2 inhibitors may be well tolerated and effective also in the patients with advanced HF and/or with a recent hospitalization for HF.[17,18]

Management of fluid overload

Diuretic therapy

Frequent hospitalizations caused by acute HF decompensation are a hallmark of advanced HF and are an ominous prognostic marker.[1,19] Diuretics are the mainstay of medical treatment of advanced HF both to treat and to prevent episodes of acute decompensation, and to improve symptoms caused by congestion. Their main mechanism of action is increased sodium and water excretion. However, they may cause electrolyte abnormalities and further neurohormonal activation. It is therefore recommended that diuretics are administered at the lowest doses that keep the patients free of congestion.[1,20,21]

Loop diuretics, particularly furosemide, is the mainstay of diuretic treatment.[1] To date, no large randomized studies have compared different loop diuretics, furosemide, bumetanide, and torsemide. The Torsemide Comparison with Furosemide for Management of Heart Failure (TRANSFORM-HF) trial randomized 2859 participants discharged after hospitalization for HF to torsemide or furosemide. Torsemide compared with furosemide

Table 11.2.2 Suggested clinical, laboratory, and echocardiographic criteria to trigger referral to a specialized heart failure or advanced heart failure unit

Clinical	Laboratory	Imaging	Risk score data
◆ ≥ 1 HF hospitalization in last year	◆ eGFR ≤ 45 mL/min	◆ LVEF ≤ 30%	◆ MAGGIC predicted survival ≤ 80% at 1 year
◆ NYHA class III–IV	◆ SCr ≥ 160 micromoles/L	◆ Large area of akinesis/dyskinesis or aneurysm	◆ SHFM predicted survival ≤ 80% at 1 year
◆ Intolerant of optimal dose of any GDMT HF drug	◆ Kþ ≥ 5.2 or < 3.5 mmol/L	◆ Moderate–severe mitral regurgitation	◆ MECKI predicted survival ≤ 80% at 1 year
◆ Increasing diuretic requirement	◆ Hyponatraemia	◆ RV dysfunction	
◆ SBP ≤ 90 mmHg	◆ Hb ≤ 120 g/L	◆ Systolic PA pressure ≥ 50 mmHg	
◆ Inability to perform CPET	◆ Persistently elevated high BNP/NT-proBNP, e.g. NTproBNP ≥ 1000 pg/mL	◆ Moderate-severe tricuspid regurgitation	
◆ 6MWT ≤ 300 m	◆ Abnormal liver function test	◆ Difficult to grade aortic stenosis	
◆ CRT non responder clinically	◆ Low albumin	◆ IVC dilated or without respiratory variation	
◆ Cachexia, unintentional weight loss			
◆ KCCQ decrease ≥ 5 units			

6MWT, 6-minute walk test; BNP, B-type natriuretic peptide; CPET, cardiopulmonary exercise test; CRT = cardiac resynchronization therapy; eGFR = estimated glomerular filtration rate; GDMT, guideline-directed medical therapy; Hb, haemoglobin; HF, heart failure; IVC, inferior vena cava; Kþ, potassium; KCCQ, Kansas City Cardiomyopathy Questionnaire; LVAD, left ventricular assist device; LVEF, left ventricular ejection fraction; MAGGIC, Meta-Analysis Global Group in Chronic Heart Failure; MECKI, Metabolic Exercise test data combined with Cardiac and Kidney Indexes; NT-proBNP, N-terminal pro-B-type natriuretic peptide; NYHA, New York Heart Association; PA, pulmonary artery; RV, right ventricular; SBP, systolic blood pressure; SCr, serum creatinine; SHFM, Seattle Heart Failure Model.

Moderate mitral regurgitation alone is not sufficient but is one factor suggesting risk of progression and should be considered together with other variables.

Note that this table reflects many clinically relevant but sometimes subjective and non-specific criteria. With these criteria, sensitivity has been prioritized over specificity, i.e. many criteria may be present in patients who do not need referral, but by considering these criteria in a comprehensive assessment, there is a lower risk that high-risk patients may be missed or referred too late. While cut-offs exist for transplantation listing or LVAD implantation, there are no data to support specific cut-offs for referral to a HF centre.

Source data from McDonagh TA, Metra M, Adamo M, et al; ESC Scientific Document Group. 2021 ESC Guidelines for the diagnosis and treatment of acute and chronic heart failure. *Eur Heart J.* 2021 Sep 21;42(36):3599-3726. doi: 10.1093/eurheartj/ehab368; and Crespo-Leiro MG, Metra M, Lund LH, et al. Advanced heart failure: a position statement of the Heart Failure Association of the European Society of Cardiology. *Eur J Heart Fail.* 2018 Nov;20(11):1505-1535. doi: 10.1002/ejhf.1236.

Table 11.2.3 The mnemonic 'I need help' for the early identification of patients who need advanced therapies

I NEED HELP		
I	Inotropes	Previous or ongoing need for inotropes
N	NYHA class/natriuretic peptide	Persisting NYHA class III or IV and/or persistently high BNP or NT-proBNP
E	End-organ dysfunction	Worsening renal or liver dysfunction in the setting of heart failure
E	Ejection fraction	Very low ejection fraction < 20%
D	Defibrillator shocks	Recurrent appropriate defibrillator shocks
H	Hospitalizations	More than 1 hospitalization with heart failure in the last 12 months
E	Oedema/escalating diuretics	Persisting fluid overload and/or increasing diuretic requirement
L	Low blood pressure	Consistently low BP with systolic <90 to 100 mmHg
P	Prognostic medication	Inability to up-titrate (or need to decrease/cease) ACEi, beta-blockers, ARNIs, or MRAs

ACEI, angiotensin-converting enzyme inhibitor; ARNI, angiotensin receptor neprilysin inhibitor; BP, blood pressure; BNP, brain natriuretic peptide; MRA, mineralocorticoid receptor antagonist; NT-proBNP, N-terminal pro B-type natriuretic peptide; NYHA, New York Heart Association.

Reproduced from Baumwol J. "I Need Help"-A mnemonic to aid timely referral in advanced heart failure. *J Heart Lung Transplant.* 2017 May;36(5):593-594. doi: 10.1016/j.healun.2017.02.010 with permission from Elsevier.

did not result in a significant difference in all-cause mortality over 12 months.[22] The mode of administration of furosemide, bolus versus continuous infusion, and its starting dose, low versus high, were not associated with significant differences in symptoms relief and outcomes in the Determining optimal dose and duration of diuretic treatment in people with acute HF (DOSE-AHF) Study.[23] A practical algorithm for the management of diuretic therapy in patients with acute HF was proposed by the Heart Failure Association (HFA) of the European Society of Cardiology and included in the recent HF ESC guidelines.[1,20] According to this

Table 11.2.4 The rule of three for the early identification of patients who need advanced therapies

The rule of three	
1	Repetitive hospitalizations for heart failure (e.g. ≥ 2 events in a year)
2	Staircase diuretic requirements over time (e.g. an increase of oral loop diuretics therapy by 50% in the preceding 6 months) to maintain clinical stability
3	Intolerance to neurohormonal therapy with onset of cardiorenal perturbation

Reproduced from Mehra MR, Gustafsson F. Left Ventricular Assist Devices at the Crossroad of Innovation in Advanced Heart Failure. *J Card Fail.* 2021 Nov;27(11):1291-1294. doi: 10.1016/j.cardfail.2021.06.003 with permission from Elsevier.

algorithm, intravenous loop diuretic treatment must be started at 1-2 times the daily oral loop diuretic with the dose then doubled if urinary sodium excretion remains less than 50–70 mEq/L and/or a urine output volume is less than 100–150 ml/h after 2 and 6 hours, respectively, from the start of i.v. diuretic administration. Further doubling of the loop diuretic dose or combination with a diuretic with a different site of action, e.g. a thiazide diuretic or metolazone or acetazolamide, must be considered when the diuretic response remains insufficient.[1,20]

Along with poor tolerance to neurohormonal modulators and frequent episodes of HF decompensation, loop diuretic resistance is another hallmark of advanced HF.[11] Diuretic resistance is a response to long-term loop diuretic use, leading to nephron remodeling, hypertrophy, and hyperfunction in different parts of the nephron and to increased renin secretion. Low gastrointestinal absorption of oral furosemide due to gut congestion may be another mechanism and is the basis of the efficacy of intravenous or alternative routes of administration.In the frequent case of diuretic resistance persisting after i.v. administration and dose increase, combination diuretic therapy is generally adopted (see earlier). However, concomitant administration of a thiazide diuretic or metolazone may lead to hyponatremia, hypokalemia, and worsen renal function.[24] Strategies of concomitant administration of acetazolamide or SGLT2 inhibitors, both acting on the proximal tubule, are currently tested in randomized trials.[20]

Vasopressin receptor antagonists (VRA) are aquaretic agents acting on the arginine vasopressin receptors and cause an increase in urine flow and the excretion of electrolyte-free water. The Efficacy of Vasopressin Antagonism in Heart Failure Outcome Study with Tolvaptan (EVEREST) trial failed to demonstrate positive long-term effects on outcomes when the selective V2 receptor antagonist tolvaptan was added to standard HF therapy in the acute setting.[25] Tolvaptan is currently indicated only in patients with severe hyponatraemia. As advanced stages of HF are characterized by inappropriately high levels of arginine vasopressin, leading to plasma expansion and dilutional hyponatraemia, the selective V_2-receptor antagonist tolvaptan may be considered as a further decongestive strategy.[3]

Lastly, high-dose furosemide has been combined with small-volume hypertonic saline solution infusion (150 mL of 1.4-4.6% NaCl) in patients with diuretic resistant decompensated acute HF and this has led to increased diuresis and natriuresis and was well tolerated. Larger randomized trials are required to confirm the safety and efficacy of this approach.[26,27]

Renal replacement therapy

Renal replacement therapy is reserved as a bail-out strategy to relieve congestion when medical treatment has failed.[1,28] Ultrafiltration removes plasma water across a semipermeable membrane using a machine-generated transmembrane pressure gradient.[20] Simplified ultrafiltration devices permit fluid removal in lower-acuity hospital settings. The effectiveness of ultrafiltration has been evaluated in relatively small randomized clinical trials with inconclusive results (➲ Table 11.2.5).[29–34] Relatively slow ultrafiltration rates, that is less than 250–500 mL/h with frequent

Table 11.2.5 Ultrafiltration clinical trials

Trial, year	N	Inclusion criteria	Study treatment	Results
RAPID-HF, 2005[31]	40	Hospitalized with HF, 2+ edema and ≥ 1 additional sign of congestion	UF vs usual medical care	Weight loss after 24 h was 2.5 kg vs 1.86 kg in the UF and usual care groups, respectively (p = 0.240)
UNLOAD, 2007[29]	200	Hospitalized with HF, ≥ 2 signs of fluid overload	UF vs intravenous diuretic	At 48 h, weight (5.0 ± 3.1 kg vs. 3.1 ± 3.5 kg; p = 0.001) and net fluid loss (4.6 vs. 3.3 l; p = 0.001) were greater in the ultrafiltration group. Dyspnea scores were similar (5.4 ± 1.1 vs. 5.2 ± 1.2); p = 0.588. HF rehospitalization at 90 days: 18% (UF) vs. 32% (standard care), p = 0.037
CARRESS-HF, 2012[30]	188	Hospitalized with HF, ≥2 signs of congestion, and recent worsened renal function (≥0.3 mg/dl sCr increase)	UF vs stepped pharmacologic therapy	Ultrafiltration was inferior to pharmacologic therapy with respect to the bivariate end point of the change in the serum creatinine level and body weight 96 hours after enrollment (P = 0.003) Higher rates of serious adverse events in the UF patients (72% vs. 57%, P = 0.03)
CUORE, 2014[32]	56	NYHA III or IV, ≥4 kg weight gain from peripheral fluid overload, over 2 months	UF vs standard medical care	Lower incidence of rehospitalizations for HF at 1 year in the UF group (HR 0.14, 95% CI 0.04-0.48; P = .002)
AVOID-HF, 2016[33]	224	Hospitalized with HF; ≥ 2 criteria for fluid overload; receiving daily oral loop diuretic agents	UF vs intravenous loop diuretics	Estimated days to first HF event were similar (62 vs 34 in UF and loop diuretics treatment, respectively (p = 0.106). UF patients had fewer HF and CV events, but more adverse events.
ULTRADISCO, 2011[34]	30	Hospitalized for HF, ≥ 2+ peripheral edema, ≥ 1 other criteria for volume overload	UF vs diuretics	UF group showed a greater improvement in haemodynamics

HF, heart failure; HR, hazard ratio; NYHA, New York Heart Association; sCr, serum creatinine; UF, ultrfiltration.
Reproduced from Costanzo MR, Ronco C, Abraham WT, et al. Extracorporeal Ultrafiltration for Fluid Overload in Heart Failure: Current Status and Prospects for Further Research. *J Am Coll Cardiol*. 2017 May 16;69(19):2428-2445. doi: 10.1016/j.jacc.2017.03.528 with permission from Elsevier.

adjustments based on haematocrit, body weight, and signs of congestion are warranted.[28] Renal replacement therapy is indicated for the treatment of metabolic complications of anuria/oliguria such as hyperkalaemia, acidosis, and uraemia. Futile treatment must be, however, avoided as much as possible considering the poor prognosis and the comorbidities of many of these patients.[3]

Peritoneal dialysis might be an at-home option for patients with advanced HF, cardiorenal syndrome, and refractory fluid overload.[35] Unlike haemodialysis that uses a semipermeable membrane and a machine-generated transmembrane pressure gradient, the peritoneum itself is used as a filter in peritoneal dialysis. Solute molecules can be exchanged between the dialysate (delivered to the peritoneal cavity through a catheter) and the blood. The osmotic pressure gradient between the hypertonic dialysate and the hypotonic peritoneal capillary blood allows removal of sodium and water. In earlier studies, conducted in patients with HF and chronic kidney disease, this strategy led to weight loss, a better NYHA classification, improvement in quality of life, and a reduction in HF hospitalizations.[36,37] It offers many advantages, including haemodynamic stability and less inflammation compared to haemodialysis. However, the majority of these studies lacked a control group, have short follow-up, and are not powered to detect effects on mortality. Further large, controlled, randomized studies are needed.

Intravenous vasoactive agents and inotropes

Inotropes are indicated in patients with advanced HF who have a severe impairment in systolic function with low cardiac output and signs of end-organ perfusion.[1,3] However, since they have not had favourable effects on outcome, with the only notable exceptions of digoxin and, more recently, omecamtiv mecarbil, their routine administration is not recommended (➲ Table 11.2.6).[1,3,38] Thus, inotropic support may be considered only as a bridge to transplant or to long-term MCS, or as palliative treatment for relief of symptoms in patients without other treatment options.[1] In a meta-analysis including 66 studies (13 randomized controlled trials and 53 observational studies), treatment with inotropes in advanced HF outpatients was associated with a greater improvement in NYHA functional class than in controls with no difference in mortality with intermittent inotropes versus controls (pooled risk ratio, 0.68; 95% confidence interval (CI), 0.40 to 1.17; p = 0.16; 9 trials).[39]

Digitalis glycosides

The effects of digoxin on outcomes were assessed in the Digoxin Investigators Group (DIG) trial.[40] In this study, 6800 patients in sinus rhythm and with a LV EF ≤45% were randomized to

Table 11.2.6 Results of major trials with inotropes

Drug	Classification/mechanism of action	Trials	Summary of results
Dobutamine[55]	Calcitrope/β-adrenergic receptor agonist	FIRST, meta-analysis	Increased mortality, worsened HF, myocardial infarction and cardiac arrest with dobutamine vs. epoprosteonol
Milrinone[56,57]	Calcitrope/Phosphodiesterase-3 inhibitor	PROMISE; OPTIME-CHF	Higher incidence of hypotension, arrhythmia and mortality with milrinone vs. placebo
Enoximone[58,59]	Calcitrope/Phosphodiesterase-3 inhibitor	Enoximone Multicenter Trial Group; ESSENTIAL trials	No difference in mortality with enoximone vs placebo
Levosimendan[48,49,51,60,61]	Calcitrope/Phosphodiesterase-3 inhibitor	LIDO; REVIVE I; REVIVE II; SURVIVE; PERSIST; LION-HEART	Reduced mortality with levosimendan vs dobutamine. Increased symptomatic relief, lower natriuretic peptide levels and lower HF hospitalizations; mixed results regarding mortality with Levosimendan vs. placebo
Omecamtiv mecarbil[52,53,54,62]	Myotrope /Direct myosin activator	COSMIC-HF; GALACTIC-HF	Increased cardiac output, positive cardiac remodelling and reduced composite endpoint of CV mortality or HF events with Omecamtiv Mecarbil vs. placebo (major benefits in severe HF)

COSMIC-HF, Chronic Oral Study of Myosin Activation to Increase Contractility in Heart Failure; ESSENTIAL, Studies of Oral Enoximone Therapy in Advanced HF; FIRST, Flolan International Randomized Survival Trial; GALACTIC-HF, Global Approach to Lowering Adverse Cardiac Outcomes Through Improving Contractility in Heart Failure; HF, heart failure; LIDO, Levosimendan Infusion versus DObutamine; LION-HEART, Intermittent Intravenous Levosimendan in Ambulatory Advanced Chronic Heart Failure Patients; OPTIME-CHF, Outcomes of a Prospective Trial of Intravenous Milrinone for Exacerbations of Chronic Heart Failure; PERSIST, Effects of peroral levosimendan in the prevention of further hospitalisations in patients with chronic heart failure; PROMISE, Prospective Randomized Milrinone Survival Evaluation; REVIVE (I, II), Randomized EValuation of Intravenous LeVosimendan Efficacy; SURVIVE, Survival of Patients With Acute Heart Failure in Need of Intravenous Inotropic Support.

placebo or digoxin (mean dose 0.25mg/day) and followed for an average of 37 months. Most of the patients were on ACEi and diuretics. CV mortality was unaffected. However, there was a trend to less mortality for worsening HF (risk ratio (RR), 0.88; 95% CI, 0.77 to 1.01; p = 0.06) and a reduction in HF hospitalizations (RR, 0.72; 95% CI, 0.66 to 0.79; p < 0.001) and CV hospitalizations (RR0.87; 95% CI, 0.81–0.93; p < 0.001), as well as in the combined end-points of all-cause death and HF hospitalizations and of HF deaths or hospitalizations, in the digoxin versus the placebo group.[40] Further analyses showed the importance of serum digoxin levels so that digoxin was associated with an improvement in all outcomes with serum digoxin levels of 0.5–0.9 ng/mL. Digitoxin is a potential alternative to digoxin and is currently being evaluated in a randomized placebo-controlled trial (ClinicalTrials.gov Identifier:NCT03783429).[1]

Vasopressors

Vasopressors (norepinephrine, epinephrine) may favor myocardial ischaemia and tachyarrhythmias and are therefore indicated only in cases of severe hypotension with end-organ hypoperfusion. Norepinephrine was associated with better outcomes, compared with epinephrine, in a randomized trial and a meta-analysis.[1] A combination of norepinephrine and an inotropic agents with peripheral vasodilating activity may be considered in patients with hypotension and low cardiac output.[1] Vasopressors should be used at the lowest dose that obtains the desired clinical goals and discontinued as soon as organ perfusion is restored and/or congestion is relieved.

Dopamine

When administered at low doses (0.5–3 μg/kg per minute), dopamine stimulates dopaminergic 1 and dopaminergic 2 receptors with splanchnic and renal vasodilation and an increase in renal blood flow. At higher doses (3-5 μg/kg per minute), dopamine binds to β1-receptors and increases norepinephrine release from sympathetic nerve terminals with an increase in cardiac contractility and heart rate. At higher doses (5–20 μg/kg per minute), α1-receptor-mediated vasoconstriction dominates with an increase in peripheral vascular resistance.[41] Given these pharmacodynamics properties the use of low-dose dopamine was proposed in acute HF patients at risk for acute renal failure to improve diuresis and renal blood flow. However, the renal-protective role of dopamine has not been demonstrated.[42] It was compared with norepinephrine as first-line vasopressor therapy in patients with shock and was associated with more arrhythmic events and a greater mortality in patients with cardiogenic shock but not in those with hypovolaemic or septic shock. Although the trial included 1679 patients, significance was seen only in a subgroup analysis of the 280 patients with cardiogenic shock among whom fewer than 10% had myocardial infarction.[43]

Dobutamine

Dobutamine is a β-adrenergic receptor agonist, with high affinity for β1 adrenoreceptors and milder effect on β2. It causes an increase in cardiac output and a decrease in pulmonary capillary wedge pressure (PCWP).[41] Its administration was associated with an increased risk of death, tachyarrhythmias, and myocardial ischaemia in retrospective analyses of trials and observational studies.[38,41,44,45] However, both continuous and intermittent dobutamine may provide symptomatic relief and improvement in quality of life in patients with advanced HF symptoms refractory to standard therapy.[39,46,47]

Phosphodiesterase inhibitors

Milrinone and enoximone are phosphodiesterase inhibitors, with both inotropic and vasodilator properties, which increase cardiac output and reduce systemic vascular resistance and PCWP. This vasodilatory activity may cause hypotension and further peripheral and coronary hypoperfusion in patients who are already hypotensive at baseline. Similarly to dobutamine, their administration has been associated with an increased risk of death or adverse events.[38,41,44,45] To avoid their hypotensive effects, combination with norepinephrine may be considered.[1]

Levosimendan

The intermittent infusion of levosimendan may be considered because of the long half-life of its active metabolite (OR-1896) so that the effects of a 12–24h infusion can last longer (up to weeks). Levosimendan is the prototype of calcium sensitizers, which enhance the sensitivity of the contractile apparatus, namely troponin C, to calcium. It also acts on adenosine triphosphate (ATP)-dependent K^+ channels, resulting in peripheral vasodilatation. Levosimendan may increase cardiac output and lower PCWP without increasing myocardial oxygen demand. In the REVIVE (Randomized Multicentre Evaluation of Intravenous Levosimendan Efficacy) I and II trials, levosimendan provided an improvement in signs and symptoms of HF and a larger decline in natriuretic peptide levels compared to placebo, but it was associated with more frequent hypotension and cardiac arrhythmias and a numerically higher risk of death. The relation between baseline systolic blood pressure and the risk of death was bidirectional with an increase in patients with low values at baseline and a reduction in those with higher values.[48] In the Survival of Patients With Acute Heart Failure in Need of Intravenous Inotropic Support (SURVIVE) study, 1327 patients hospitalized with acute decompensated HF and who required inotropic support were randomized to either levosimendan (loading of 12µg/kg for 10 minutes, followed by infusion of 0.1 µg/kg per minute for 50 minutes; and increased to 0.2 µg/kg per minute for 23 hours) or dobutamine (5 µg/kg per minute and increased up to 40 µg/kg per minute). Despite greater reduction in natriuretic peptide levels, all-cause mortality at 180 days was similar in the two groups.[49] The administration of relatively high doses of levosimendan starting with a bolus may explain the occurrence of adverse events.

Intermittent infusions of levosimendan have been tested in small randomized controlled trials with favorable effects on symptoms, NT-proBNP plasma levels and a tendency to improved outcomes.[50,51] This treatment may be considered as a bridge to MCS and/or cardiac transplantation or to improve symptoms when other options are not available. Concomitant administration of norepinephrine may counteract hypotension in patients who need acute treatment for cardiogenic shock.[1,3]

Omecamtiv mecarbil

Cardiac myosin activators act on cardiac myosin enhancing the transition of the actin–myosin complex from the weakly bound to the strongly bound configuration, thus increasing the number of myosin heads interacting with the actin filament. Increased actin–myosin interaction prolongs the duration of systole and, hence, increases stroke volume in the absence of any change in intracellular calcium concentrations.[38,44,45] For this reason, cardiac myosin activators were recently re-defined as myotropes, acting on the sarcomere through a calcium-independent mechanism, and so different from calcitropes, inotropes that act through increased intracellular cAMP and calcium concentrations.[38] In the phase 2 COSMIC-HF (Chronic Oral Study of Myosin Activation to Increase Contractility in Heart Failure) trial, 20 weeks of oral treatment with omecamtiv mecarbil, compared to placebo, increased LV systolic ejection time, stroke volume, and ejection fraction, decreased the left ventricular end-systolic and end-diastolic dimensions, with a concomitant reduction in heart rate.[52] More recently, the Global Approach to Lowering Adverse Cardiac Outcomes Through Improving Contractility in Heart Failure (GALACTIC-HF) trial demonstrated beneficial effects on CV outcome improving contractility in patients with HFrEF. This phase 3 trial enrolled 8256 patients with symptomatic chronic HF and LVEF ≤35% and randomized them to receive omecamtiv mecarbil (using pharmacokinetic-guided doses of 25 mg, 37.5 mg, or 50 mg twice daily) or placebo, in addition to standard HF therapy. Omecamtiv mecarbil reduced the composite endpoint of a HF event or death from CV causes compared to placebo (HR, 0.92; 95% CI, 0.86–0.99; p = 0.03).[53] Omecamtiv mecarbil was more effective in advanced HF patients. Indeed, benefits were greater in patients with the lowest LVEF and were consistent in the subgroup of patients with NYHA class III or IV. Amongst the pre-specified subgroups, LVEF was the strongest modifier of the treatment effect of omecamtiv mecarbil. Patients with baseline LVEF ≤ 22% (lowest quartile) had the greatest relative risk reduction for the composite endpoint (hazard ratio (HR), 0.83; 95% CI, 0.73–0.95), compared to patients with LVEF ≥33% (HR, 0.99; 95% CI, 0.84–1.16; interaction as LVEF by quartiles, p = 0.013). These findings are consistent with the drug's mechanism of selectively improving systolic function and presents a promising opportunity to improve the outcomes in patients with advanced HF.[54]

Key messages

- Advanced HF patients may benefit from contemporary guideline-directed HF drugs. However, intolerance to neurohormonal antagonists is a marker of advanced HF and identifies patients with a very poor prognosis, who need non-conventional therapies.
- Loop diuretics represent the first choice in order to achieve euvolaemia. Advanced HF patients often develop diuretic resistance due to nephron remodelling and cardiorenal syndrome, requiring increasing dosage of loop diuretics. In cases of persistent congestion, a single step-approach starting from combination

therapies is recommended. Renal replacement therapy represents a bail-out strategy.

♦ Inotropes improve haemodynamics and may prevent worsening end-organ function. However, many studies showed that they may worsen the prognosis. Thus, continuous inotropes may be considered only in patients with low cardiac output and evidence of organ hypoperfusion as a bridge to MCS or heart transplantation. Intermittent long-term use of inotropes may be used as palliative therapy for the relief of symptoms in patients without other treatment options.

♦ The novel drug omecamtiv mecarbil may represent a promising opportunity to improve prognosis of patients with advanced HFrEF.

References

1. McDonagh TA, Metra M, Adamo M, *et al.* 2021 ESC Guidelines for the diagnosis and treatment of acute and chronic heart failure. Eur Heart J. 2021;42(36):3599–726.

2. Dunlay SM, Roger VL, Killian JM, *et al.* Advanced heart failure epidemiology and outcomes: a population-based study. JACC Heart Fail. 2021;9(10):722–32.

3. Crespo-Leiro MG, Metra M, Lund LH, *et al.* Advanced heart failure: a position statement of the Heart Failure Association of the European Society of Cardiology. Eur J Heart Fail. 2018;20(11):1505–35.

4. Truby LK, Rogers JG. Advanced heart failure: epidemiology, diagnosis, and therapeutic approaches. JACC Heart Fail. 2020;8(7):523–36.

5. McMurray JJ, Packer M, Desai AS, *et al.* Angiotensin-neprilysin inhibition versus enalapril in heart failure. N Engl J Med. 2014;371(11):993–1004.

6. Mann DL, Greene SJ, Givertz MM, *et al.* Sacubitril/valsartan in advanced heart failure with reduced ejection fraction: rationale and design of the LIFE trial. JACC Heart Fail. 2020;8(10):789–99.

7. Mann DL, Givertz MM, Vader JM, *et al.* Effect of treatment with sacubitril/valsartan in patients with advanced heart failure and reduced ejection fraction: a randomized clinical Trial. JAMA Cardiol. 2022;7(1):17–25.

8. Mullens W, Damman K, Testani JM, *et al.* Evaluation of kidney function throughout the heart failure trajectory – a position statement from the Heart Failure Association of the European Society of Cardiology. Eur J Heart Fail. 2020;22(4):584–603.

9. Kittleson M, Hurwitz S, Shah MR, *et al.* Development of circulatory-renal limitations to angiotensin-converting enzyme inhibitors identifies patients with severe heart failure and early mortality. J Am Coll Cardiol. 2003;41(11):2029–35.

10. Baumwol J. 'I Need Help'–A mnemonic to aid timely referral in advanced heart failure. J Heart Lung Transplant. 2017;36(5):593–4.

11. Mehra MR, Gustafsson F. Left ventricular assist devices at the crossroad of innovation in advanced heart failure. J Card Fail. 2021;27(11):1291–4.

12. McMurray JJV, Solomon SD, Inzucchi SE, *et al.* Dapagliflozin in patients with heart failure and reduced ejection fraction. N Engl J Med. 2019;381(21):1995–2008.

13. Packer M, Anker SD, Butler J, *et al.* Cardiovascular and renal outcomes with empagliflozin in heart failure. N Engl J Med. 2020;383(15):1413–24.

14. Bhatt DL, Szarek M, Steg PG, *et al.* Sotagliflozin in patients with diabetes and recent worsening heart failure. N Engl J Med. 2021;384(2):117–28.

15. Damman K, Beusekamp JC, Boorsma EM, *et al.* Randomized, double-blind, placebo-controlled, multicentre pilot study on the effects of empagliflozin on clinical outcomes in patients with acute decompensated heart failure (EMPA-RESPONSE-AHF). Eur J Heart Fail. 2020;22(4):713–22.

16. Voors AA, Angermann CE, Teerlink JR, *et al.*. The SGLT2 inhibitor empagliflozin in patients hospitalized for acute heart failure. Nature Med. 2022; 28(3):568–74.

17. Tomasoni D, Fonarow GC, Adamo M, *et al.* Sodium-glucose co-transporter 2 inhibitors as an early, first line therapy in patients with heart failure and reduced ejection fraction. Eur J Heart Fail. 2022; 24(3):431–41.

18. Rao VN, Murray E, Butler J, *et al.* In-hospital initiation of sodium-glucose cotransporter-2 inhibitors for heart failure with reduced ejection fraction. J Am Coll Cardiol. 2021;78(20):2004–12.

19. Tomasoni D, Lombardi CM, Sbolli M, Cotter G, Metra M. Acute heart failure: More questions than answers. Prog Cardiovasc Dis. 2020;63(5):599–606.

20. Mullens W, Damman K, Harjola VP, *et al.* The use of diuretics in heart failure with congestion – a position statement from the Heart Failure Association of the European Society of Cardiology. Eur J Heart Fail. 2019;21(2):137–55.

21. Kapelios CJ, Laroche C, Crespo-Leiro MG, *et al.* Association between loop diuretic dose changes and outcomes in chronic heart failure: observations from the ESC-EORP Heart Failure Long-Term Registry. Eur J Heart Fail. 2020;22(8):1424–37.

22. Greene SJ, Velazquez EJ, Anstrom KJ, *et al.* Pragmatic design of randomized clinical trials for heart failure: rationale and design of the TRANSFORM-HF Trial. JACC Heart Fail. 2021;9(5):325–35.

23. Felker GM, Lee KL, Bull DA, *et al.* Diuretic strategies in patients with acute decompensated heart failure. N Engl J Med. 2011;364(9):797–805.

24. Brisco-Bacik MA, Ter Maaten JM, Houser SR, *et al.* Outcomes associated with a strategy of adjuvant metolazone or high-dose loop diuretics in acute decompensated heart failure: a propensity analysis. J Am Heart Assoc. 2018;7(18):e009149.

25. Konstam MA, Gheorghiade M, Burnett JC, Jr., *et al.* Effects of oral tolvaptan in patients hospitalized for worsening heart failure: the EVEREST outcome trial. JAMA. 2007;297(12):1319–31.

26. Licata G, Di Pasquale P, Parrinello G, *et al.* Effects of high-dose furosemide and small-volume hypertonic saline solution infusion in comparison with a high dose of furosemide as bolus in refractory congestive heart failure: long-term effects. Am Heart J. 2003;145(3):459–66.

27. Griffin M, Soufer A, Goljo E, *et al.* Real world use of hypertonic saline in refractory acute decompensated heart failure: A U.S. Center's Experience. JACC Heart Fail. 2020;8(3):199–208.

28. Costanzo MR, Ronco C, Abraham WT, *et al.* Extracorporeal ultrafiltration for fluid overload in heart failure: current status and prospects for further research. J Am Coll Cardiol. 2017;69(19):2428–45.

29. Costanzo MR, Guglin ME, Saltzberg MT, *et al.* Ultrafiltration versus intravenous diuretics for patients hospitalized for acute decompensated heart failure. J Am Coll Cardiol. 2007;49(6):675–83.

30. Bart BA, Goldsmith SR, Lee KL, *et al.* Ultrafiltration in decompensated heart failure with cardiorenal syndrome. N Engl J Med. 2012;367(24):2296–304.

31. Bart BA, Boyle A, Bank AJ, *et al.* Ultrafiltration versus usual care for hospitalized patients with heart failure: the Relief for Acutely Fluid-Overloaded Patients With Decompensated Congestive Heart Failure (RAPID-CHF) trial. J Am Coll Cardiol. 2005;46(11):2043–6.

32. Marenzi G, Muratori M, Cosentino ER, et al. Continuous ultrafiltration for congestive heart failure: the CUORE trial. J Card Fail. 2014;20(1):9–17.

33. Costanzo MR, Negoianu D, Jaski BE, et al. Aquapheresis versus intravenous diuretics and hospitalizations for heart failure. JACC Heart Fail. 2016;4(2):95–105.

34. Giglioli C, Landi D, Cecchi E, et al. Effects of ULTRAfiltration vs. DIureticS on clinical, biohumoral and haemodynamic variables in patients with deCOmpensated heart failure: the ULTRADISCO study. Eur J Heart Fail. 2011;13(3):337–46.

35. Grossekettler L, Schmack B, Meyer K, et al. Peritoneal dialysis as therapeutic option in heart failure patients. ESC Heart Fail. 2019;6(2):271–9.

36. Koch M, Haastert B, Kohnle M, et al. Peritoneal dialysis relieves clinical symptoms and is well tolerated in patients with refractory heart failure and chronic kidney disease. Eur J Heart Fail. 2012;14(5):530–9.

37. Nunez J, Gonzalez M, Minana G, et al. Continuous ambulatory peritoneal dialysis as a therapeutic alternative in patients with advanced congestive heart failure. Eur J Heart Fail. 2012;14(5):540–8.

38. Psotka MA, Gottlieb SS, Francis GS, et al. Cardiac calcitropes, myotropes, and mitotropes: JACC Review Topic of the Week. J Am Coll Cardiol. 2019;73(18):2345–53.

39. Nizamic T, Murad MH, Allen LA, et al. Ambulatory inotrope infusions in advanced heart failure: a systematic review and meta-analysis. JACC Heart Fail. 2018;6(9):757–67.

40. Digitalis Investigation Group. The effect of digoxin on mortality and morbidity in patients with heart failure. N Engl J Med. 1997;336(8):525–33.

41. Metra M, Bettari L, Carubelli V, Cas LD. Old and new intravenous inotropic agents in the treatment of advanced heart failure. Prog Cardiovasc Dis. 2011;54(2):97–106.

42. Chen HH, Anstrom KJ, Givertz MM, et al. Low-dose dopamine or low-dose nesiritide in acute heart failure with renal dysfunction: the ROSE acute heart failure randomized trial. JAMA. 2013;310(23):2533–43.

43. De Backer D, Biston P, Devriendt J, et al. Comparison of dopamine and norepinephrine in the treatment of shock. N Engl J Med. 2010;362(9):779–89.

44. Ahmad T, Miller PE, McCullough M, et al. Why has positive inotropy failed in chronic heart failure? Lessons from prior inotrope trials. Eur J Heart Fail. 2019;21(9):1064–78.

45. Maack C, Eschenhagen T, Hamdani N, et al. Treatments targeting inotropy. Eur Heart J. 2019;40(44):3626–44.

46. Martens P, Vercammen J, Ceyssens W, et al. Effects of intravenous home dobutamine in palliative end-stage heart failure on quality of life, heart failure hospitalization, and cost expenditure. ESC Heart Fail. 2018;5(4):562–9.

47. Chernomordik F, Freimark D, Arad M, et al. Quality of life and long-term mortality in patients with advanced chronic heart failure treated with intermittent low-dose intravenous inotropes in an outpatient setting. ESC Heart Fail. 2017;4(2):122–9.

48. Packer M, Colucci W, Fisher L, et al. Effect of levosimendan on the short-term clinical course of patients with acutely decompensated heart failure. JACC Heart Fail. 2013;1(2):103–11.

49. Mebazaa A, Nieminen MS, Packer M, et al. Levosimendan vs dobutamine for patients with acute decompensated heart failure: the SURVIVE Randomized Trial. JAMA. 2007;297(17):1883–91.

50. Oliva F, Comin-Colet J, Fedele F, et al. Repetitive levosimendan treatment in the management of advanced heart failure. Eur Heart J Suppl. 2018;20(Suppl I):I11–I20.

51. Comin-Colet J, Manito N, Segovia-Cubero J, et al. Efficacy and safety of intermittent intravenous outpatient administration of levosimendan in patients with advanced heart failure: the LION-HEART multicentre randomised trial. Eur J Heart Fail. 2018;20(7):1128–36.

52. Teerlink JR, Felker GM, McMurray JJ, et al. Chronic Oral Study of Myosin Activation to Increase Contractility in Heart Failure (COSMIC-HF): a phase 2, pharmacokinetic, randomised, placebo-controlled trial. Lancet. 2016;388(10062):2895–903.

53. Teerlink JR, Diaz R, Felker GM, et al. Cardiac myosin activation with omecamtiv mecarbil in systolic heart failure. N Engl J Med. 2021;384(2):105–16.

54. Teerlink JR, Diaz R, Felker GM, et al. Effect of ejection fraction on clinical outcomes in patients treated with omecamtiv mecarbil in GALACTIC-HF. J Am Coll Cardiol. 2021;78(2):97–108.

55. O'Connor CM, Gattis WA, Uretsky BF, et al. Continuous intravenous dobutamine is associated with an increased risk of death in patients with advanced heart failure: insights from the Flolan International Randomized Survival Trial (FIRST). Am Heart J. 1999;138:78–86.

56. Packer M, Carver JR, Rodeheffer RJ, et al. Effect of oral milrinone on mortality in severe chronic heart failure. The PROMISE Study Research Group. N Engl J Med. 1991;325:1468–75.

57. Cuffe MS, Califf RM, Adams KF Jr, et al. and Outcomes of a Prospective Trial of Intravenous Milrinone for Exacerbations of Chronic Heart Failure (OPTIME-CHF) Investigators. Short-term intravenous milrinone for acute exacerbation of chronic heart failure: a randomized controlled trial. JAMA. 2002; 287:1541–7.

58. Metra M, Eichhorn E, Abraham WT, et al., for the ESSENTIAL Investigators. Effects of low-dose oral enoximone administration on mortality, morbidity, and exercise capacity in patients with advanced heart failure: the randomized, double-blind, placebo-controlled, parallel group ESSENTIAL trials. Eur Heart J. 2009;30:3015–26.

59. Lowes BD, Shakar SF, Metra M, et al. Rationale and design of the enoximone clinical trials program. J Card Fail 2005;11:659–69.

60. Follath F, Cleland JG, Just H, et al. and Steering Committee and Investigators of the Levosimendan Infusion versus Dobutamine (LIDO) Study. Efficacy and safety of intravenous levosimendan compared with dobutamine in severe low-output heart failure (the LIDO study): a randomised double-blind trial. Lancet. 2002;360:196–202.

61. Nieminen MS, Cleland JG, Eha J, et al. Oral levosimendan in patients with severe chronic heart failure—the PERSIST study. Eur J Heart Fail. 2008;10:1246–54.

62. Felker GM, Solomon SD, Claggett B, et al. Assessment of omecamtiv mecarbil for the treatment of patients with severe heart failure: a post hoc analysis of data from the GALACTIC-HF randomized clinical trial. JAMA Cardiol. 2022;7:26.

CHAPTER 11.3

Mechanical circulatory support

Mandeep Mehra and Finn Gustafsson

Contents

Introduction

The history of mechanical circulatory support spans over five decades. Soon after development of the heart-lung machine, the idea of providing prolonged circulatory support to patients emerged. In 1963, Dr Liotta and Dr Cooley implanted the first artificial ventricle in a patient with post-cardiotomy cardiogenic shock. In 1967, the first intra-aortic balloon pump (IABP) was implanted by Dr Kantrowitz in New York.[1] In the 1970s, several groups were developing systems for mechanical circulatory support (MCS), but the next breakthroughs came in the following decade. In 1984, a report of the first total artificial heart intended for long-term use was published,[2] and in the same year an electrically driven pulsatile left ventricular (LV) assist device (Novacor™) was used in a patient. Since then multiple short- and long-term MCS devices have been developed and at present a spectrum of devices are available to choose from in order to meet the needs of patients in different clinical situations.

Current devices can be divided into *short-term* and *long-term* MCS and into *left ventricular-*, *right ventricular (RV)*, or *biventricular* devices. Some devices are implanted *percutaneously*, and some devices are implanted *surgically*. As experience with systems evolves overlapping use of systems occur in individual cases, for instance by prolonged use of devices intended for short term use. This chapter reviews devices for short term support as well as devices for durable assisted circulation.

Short-term devices

Short-term devices are used in a variety of clinical situations ranging from high risk percutaneous coronary intervention (PCI) in patients with normal ventricular function to acute decompensated heart failure, cardiogenic shock, and cardiac arrest. The systems have typically been developed for only a few days' use and they can be rapidly implanted percutaneously or with minimal surgical assistance. In recent years, several systems have been developed and tested for longer duration use (e.g. several weeks) (◆ Table 11.3.1).

Intra-aortic balloon pump

The intra-aortic balloon pump (IABP) (◆ Figure 11.3.1) is simple to place and relatively inexpensive. It is typically inserted via the femoral artery using the Seldinger technique but can also be placed by axillary access. The balloon is placed in the descending aorta and provides circulatory support by diastolic augmentation of the central arterial pressure, improving coronary and cerebral perfusion, as well as systolic unloading of the LV. Haemodynamically, the IABP leads to a decrease in pulmonary capillary wedge pressure and a small increase in cardiac output typically in the range of 0. 5 litres per minute. Inflation and deflation of the balloon is triggered by ECG (or the arterial pressure wave form in atrial fibrillation) and

Table 11.3.1 Devices used for short and intermediate MCS

Cardiac chamber support	Device	Implantation	Type
Left ventricle	IABP	Percutaneous	Pneumatic
	Impella 2.5, CP, 5.0, 5.5	Percutaneous	Microaxial
	TandemHeart	Percutaneous	Rotary
	Levitronix Centrimag, Medos	Sternotomy	Rotary
	Berlin Heart Excor	Sternotomy	Pneumatic
Right ventricle			
	Impella RP	Percutaneous	Microaxial
	ProtekDuo (with pump e.g. TandemHeart)	Percutaneous	Rotary
Left and right ventricle			
	VA-ECMO	Percutaneous/ Sternotomy	Rotary
	Bi-VAD (e.g. Levitronix Centrimag)	Sternotomy	Rotary
	Berlin Heart Excor	Sternotomy	Rotary

the degree of support can be adjusted by setting the ratio between augmented and not augmented cardiac cycles (1:1, 1:2). The main complication risk of the IABP is bleeding. Despite widespread use, there is no documentation from randomized clinical trials to support efficacy of IABP over medical therapy in cardiogenic shock. In the largest study, the randomized IABP-SHOCK-2 trial, IABP was compared 1:1 to medical therapy in more than 600 patients with cardiogenic shock related to acute myocardial infarction (AMI). The trial showed no difference between IABP and medical therapy alone on the primary endpoint which was mortality after 30 days.[3]

Percutaneous axial flow pumps (Impella)

Impellas are percutaneous, microaxial flow pumps which for left-sided support can provide flows of either 3.5 litres per minute (Impella CP) or approximately 5 litres per minute (Impella 5.0 or 5.5) (➲ Figure 11.3.2). Use of these devices has increased substantially over recent years.[4] The first generation Impella 2.5 has been abandoned in many centres in favour of the Impella CP. The Impella CP is placed in the catheterization laboratory under fluoroscopy via the right femoral artery, requiring a 14 F sheath. The tip of the Impella is advanced to the LV, leaving the pump inlet in the mid LV cavity and the outlet in the aorta just distal to the aortic valve. It is approved for a maximum of 14 days of support. Impella 5.0 and 5.5 can provide full LV support for most patients but require surgical cut down of the femoral or axillary artery to introduce and secure the 21 F sheath required. An axillary approach is generally preferred – the Impella 5.5 is specifically designed for that – because of greater mobility in awake patients and anticipated lower risk of vascular complications, especially in patients with peripheral vascular disease. Impella 2.5 and Impella CP are indicated for cardiogenic shock refractory to inotropic support or in high risk PCI and Impella 5.0/5.5 is indicated in cardiogenic shock typically with intended longer duration of support and targeting patients with very poor LV function and/or larger circulatory demands.

The left-sided Impellas increase cardiac output and decrease LV filling pressure (➲ Figure 11.3.3). Published observational studies have documented an increase in cardiac index of 18–42 % with Impella 2.5 and 50-83 % with Impella 5.05, which is considerably more than achieved with the IABP. However, clinical studies have yet to document benefits of Impella use on mortality in cardiogenic shock. In the ISAR-SHOCK trial (n = 25), patients in post MI cardiogenic shock were randomized to IABP or Impella 2.5 and while the early increase in cardiac index was greater in the Impella group, no difference between the devices was shown for mortality. In the IMPRESS trial, 48 patients were randomized

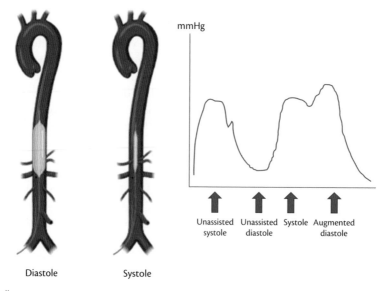

Diastole   Systole

Unassisted systole | Unassisted diastole | Systole | Augmented diastole

Figure 11.3.1 The intra-aortic balloon pump.

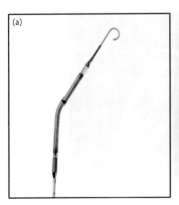
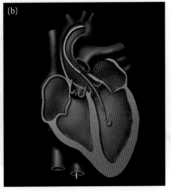
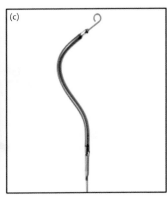

Figure 11.3.2 The Impella family.
Impella CP (a) placed in the LV (b). Impella RP (c), note the shape designed for placement of the tip in the pulmonary artery.

to IABP or Impella CP. The trial showed no difference in mortality but greater bleeding risk with the microaxial pump. A larger retrospective, propensity-matched study comparing patients in cardiogenic shock due to MI treated with Impella versus patients treated with an IABP from the IAPB-SHOCK-2 trial showed no difference in 30 day all-cause mortality but more complications in the Impella group.[6] In a recent, even larger propensity-matched analysis of outcome with Impella and IABP in cardiogenic shock complicating MI, a higher in-hospital mortality and higher risk of complications was found in patients treated with Impella.[7] The results of these studies have reduced the enthusiasm for use of microaxial pump support in cardiogenic shock in some centres, but it is important to emphasize that these studies were not randomized and suffer from confounding by indication. An adequately powered study comparing Impella CP with optimal medical therapy in cardiogenic shock associated with AMI is underway.[8]

TandemHeart

The TandemHeart consists of a left atrial cannula, a femoral artery cannula, and an extracorporeal rotary pump (⊙ Figure 11.3.4). The left atrial cannula typically is placed by central venous access and transseptal puncture. The TandemHeart can provide full support with flow rates up to 5 litres per minute and offers

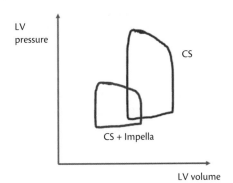

Figure 11.3.3 Left ventricular (LV) unloading in cardiogenic shock (CS) before and after Impella support. The pressure–volume curve is shifted down- and leftward and cardiac work is reduced.

effective decompression of the left atrium and consequently, the LV. The system can be connected to an oxygenator in case of hypoxia. One limitation of the system is the expertise required for transseptal puncture in the acute setting. In a randomized trial of 42 cardiogenic shock patients, the TandemHeart provided better LV unloading and greater cardiac output than an IABP, but there was no difference in survival.[9] Similar findings were reported in a slightly small study, which also documented higher risk of complications with the TandemHeart.[10]

Percutaneous RV support systems

Two percutaneous systems are available for RV support, the Impella RP (⊙ Figure 11.3.2) and the use of either a TandemHeart or CentiMag pump via a Protek Duo cannula system (⊙ Figure 11.3.5). These are used most often in patients with acute RV failure due to right ventricular MI, pulmonary embolism, or RV failure after heart transplantation or implantation of a durable left ventricular assist device (LVAD). The Impella RP is placed via a 21 F sheath in the femoral vein and advanced to the main pulmonary artery facilitated by the curved shape of the pump catheter (⊙ Figure 11.3.2). The pump inlet is the level of the inferior vena cava and right atrium and the outlet in the main pulmonary artery. The pump can deliver a maximum of 4–5 litres per minute and provides prompt RV unloading. Combination of the Impella RP with a left-sided Impella for biventricular support (so called Bi-Pella) has recently been reported.[11]

The Protek Duo system (29 or 31 F) consists of a double lumen catheter which can be placed via the right internal jugular vein and advanced through the right atrium and RV until the tip is placed in the main pulmonary artery. Blood flows into the outer channel through side holes on the catheter in the RA and the blood is subsequently pumped into the inner channel by means of a connected rotary pump. The inner channel exits in the main pulmonary artery. The Protek Duo cannula can be used with the TandemHeart rotary pump and an oxygenator can be connected in case of lung failure. Patient mobilization and ambulation with this system is possible. The largest published experience with this system reports on 27 patients and the one-year survival in this cohort was 81%.[12]

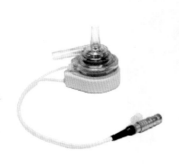

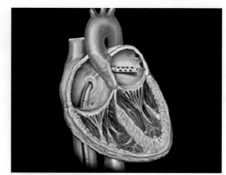

Figure 11.3.4 TandemHeart.

New systems

Several new short- and intermediate-term MCS systems are in development or testing. The NuPulseCV (iVAS) system is a portable IABP intended for longer-term use. The system is placed via the subclavian artery and has so far been shown to be feasible and improve quality of life and six-minute walking test in an observational study.[13] The Aortix pump is a rotary pump delivered via the femoral artery to the thoracic aorta which can deliver up to 5 litres flow per minute. It unloads the LV and improves perfusion of abdominal organs including the kidney. So far, human data have only been reported for high risk PCI patients, showing feasibility.[14]

Extracorporeal membrane oxygenation (ECMO)

The use of ECMO support has increased dramatically in recent years in part because of application in older patients.[15,16] ECMO can provide oxygenation in ventilator treatment refractory hypoxia in the form of veno-venous (VV)-ECMO. In this situation two venous cannulas (e.g. femoral and jugular) are inserted and connected to a rotary pump and an oxygenator. Recently, single vessel cannulation using double lumen catheters have been introduced (see earlier regarding the Protek Duo). Successful VV-ECMO requires adequate function of the left ventricle and is indicated in pulmonary – but not in cardiac – failure.

Veno-arterial (VA)-ECMO connects the venous circulation to the arterial circulation bypassing both the heart and the pulmonary circulation. VA-ECMO can be placed percutaneously or centrally, via sternotomy. The latter is the rule in post-cardiotomy

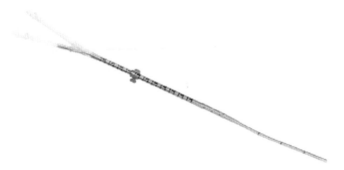

Figure 11.3.5 The Protek Duo cannula.

shock, typically when the patient cannot be weaned off cardiopulmonary bypass after cardiac surgery. The percutaneous approach is typically used in non-cardiotomy cardiogenic shock. Percutaneous VA-ECMO can be inserted in the catherization laboratory, the CCU, or even in the field, by mobile outreach ECMO teams. In percutaneous VA-ECMO, a venous cannula is typically placed via the femoral vein with the tip in the inferior vena cava or the RA and an arterial cannula is inserted in the femoral artery and advanced to the common iliac artery or the abdominal aorta. The drained venous blood is oxygenated in an oxygenator and pumped back into the arterial circulation at normal systemic pressures. VA-ECMO can deliver flows greater than 5 litres per minute and can consequently provide full circulatory support even in the setting of cardiac standstill (and lung failure). To avoid limb ischaemia in relation to the arterial cannulation, a short catheter (typically 5–10 F) is inserted in the superior femoral artery (i.e. distal to the arterial ECMO cannula) and connected to the arterial cannula by a Y-tube to provide distal perfusion of the leg. Alternative VA-ECMO cannulation possibilities include the axillary vein and artery allowing for patient mobilization.

Contraindications to VA-ECMO include advanced age and significant comorbidity. VA-ECMO is not useful in unrepaired aortic dissection or severe aortic regurgitation which will result in massive pulmonary oedema. ECMO should not be instituted in patients without potential for cardiac recovery if the patient is not a candidate for durable MCS or cardiac transplantation.

No large, randomized studies comparing VA-ECMO to medical therapy in cardiogenic shock are available. One small study showed no difference in mortality after 30 days, but the study was clearly underpowered. Several retrospective studies and meta-analyses of retrospective data have been published. In a meta-analysis including retrospective analysis of 235 patients with cardiogenic shock, VA-ECMO was associated with superior survival compared with IABP. Randomized studies of the use of VA-ECMO in cardiogenic shock are ongoing and will hopefully improve our understanding of the optimal use of this intervention.

VA-ECMO is a very powerful MCS system but also associated with significant risks. Bleeding is common both from cannulation sites and elsewhere (gastrointestinal, cerebral). A meta-analysis found major bleeding to occur in more than 40% of patients treated with ECMO.[17] Other important complications include stroke and infection. Even though the incidence of leg ischaemia is reduced substantially by use of a distal perfusion cannula, leg amputations still occur.

Two VA-ECMO specific complications deserve specific mentioning. The *Harlequin* or *North-South syndrome* may arise when there is significant lung failure combined with cardiac recovery, implying that a significant pulmonary perfusion occurs without adequate oxygenation resulting in systemic ejection of deoxygenated blood by the LV. The deoxygenated blood will supply the head and the upper extremities while oxygenated blood from the arterial ECMO cannula will supply the lower parts of the body. This leads to the skin colour difference indicated by the name and is associated with risk of cerebral and cardiac hypoxia. The problem can often be solved by moving from a peripheral to a central cannulation approach, by changing the configuration to add a venous cannula position to the superior vena cava by jugular access, or to add a third circuit, also referred to as VAV ECMO. VA-ECMO increases arterial blood pressure and afterload which may prevent effective emptying of the failing LV, in turn leading to pulmonary congestion. In severe cases, LV contractility, in the setting of increased afterload imposed by the VA-ECMO, is insufficient to open the aortic valve. This leads to risk of thrombosis of the LV cavity. The risks of pulmonary congestion and LV thrombosis must be mitigated by ensuring appropriate LV emptying. In some cases, inotropic therapy will be enough to unload the LV and the pulmonary circulation. However, high dose inotropic therapy is associated with increased myocardial oxygen consumption and even myocardial toxicity which could lead to lower chance of LV recovery and, hence, the possibility of ECMO weaning. Alternative approaches to LV and LA unloading are implantation of an IABP, an Impella (ECPELLA), or surgical or transvenous (and transseptal) insertion of an LA vent. An LA vent is a catheter connecting the LA to the ECMO venous drainage cannula which will prevent pressure increases in the LA exceeding those in the venous circulation. When used as an LV unloading strategy, an Impella or an IABP can be left in place as the ECMO support is weaned off, allowing for a two-step weaning process of MCS.

There are no randomized comparisons of the different strategies for LV unloading nor does agreement exist as to when unloading is necessary, but a meta-analysis of retrospective studies indicated a survival benefit of adding an IABP compared to ECMO without LV unloading.[18] Some authors advocate for instituting LV unloading in all ECMO runs prophylactically. As per experience, this is far from always necessary and LV unloading, both mechanical and pharmacological, carries its own risks of adverse events. However, a VA-ECMO circuit running without aortic valve opening is certain to result in pulmonary congestion and almost always requires intervention.

Short/intermediate term surgical LVADs/RVADs (extracorporeal circulatory pumps)

A variety of surgically implanted, extracorporeal circulatory support devices exist, such as the rotary Medos or the Levitronix CentriMag pumps or pulsatile pumps like the Berlin Heart Excor.

They are implanted through a sternotomy or left lateral thoracotomy and they can provide full circulatory support. Most often they are used in patients who cannot be weaned off cardiopulmonary bypass, that is after cardiac surgery, where access to the thoracic cavity is already available. They can be used to support left, right, or both ventricles. If biventricular support is needed two pumps are required. For right-heart failure, typically the RA and the pulmonary artery are cannulated. For left-sided support inflow is in either the LA or LV and outflow is in the aorta. The chest can be closed, and patients can be supported with these devices for months and even ambulate while on circulatory support.

Strategy for short term MCS in cardiogenic shock

Patients in cardiogenic shock failing to respond to inotropic support should be considered for MCS. Before initiating MCS, it is essential that potential contraindications are identified, and implantation in irreversible shock must be avoided as this will make MCS futile. It is important to consider the aim of MCS before implantation as this may affect the choice of MCS type. In principle there are three possible aims: (i) cardiac recovery and weaning of MCS, (ii) stabilization of the circulation and recovery of end-organ function enabling implantation of durable MCS (see later), or (iii) stabilization of the circulation and recovery of end-organ function enabling listing for urgent heart transplantation. The choice of device strategy depends on the clinical scenario, patient characteristics, and centre preference and experience (➲ Figure 11.3.6).

In patients with post-cardiotomy shock most often central cannulation is performed and short-intermediate type pumps, like the Levitronix Centrimag, are used. In case of isolated LV failure, LVAD configuration is used. When biventricular failure or intractable ventricular arrythmias are present, surgeons will often place the patient on VA-ECMO even if oxygenation is acceptable because of the ease of this approach in a clinically unstable situation, but biventricular assist devices with two rotary pumps can be inserted if oxygenation is adequate. VA-ECMO can subsequently be downgraded to extracorporeal LVAD support in the days following if RV function and oxygenation are acceptable. This permits a longer duration of support, allowing for greater possibility of recovery of end-organ function or chance of a donor heart offer if transplantation is the goal of the therapy. If the intended goal is durable LVAD, downscaling from VA-ECMO to extracorporeal LVAD allows for evaluation of RV function if this was questionable prior to instituting ECMO.

In the catheterization laboratory, percutaneous approaches are used but may require surgically assisted vascular access for instance for the Impella 5.5. Similar to the situation for surgical devices, the requirements for left-, right, or biventricular support must be evaluated. This decision often relies on the underlying diagnosis and echocardiography but may be assisted by invasive haemodynamic measurements (e.g. LV and RV filling pressures) if available. If arterial oxygenation cannot be achieved by oxygen supplementation or invasive ventilation, percutaneous VA-ECMO is the strategy of choice. There is little data to help decide between IABP, Impella, and TandemHeart for left sided support,

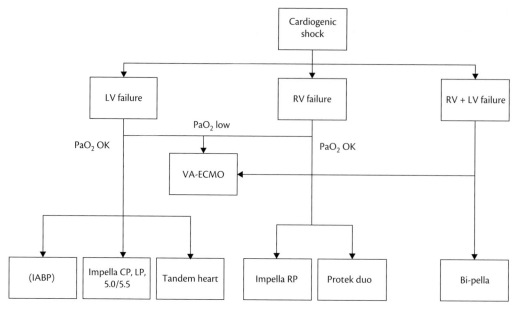

Figure 11.3.6 Flow diagram of strategy for short term mechanical circulatory support in cardiogenic shock.

but if cardiac output is severely reduced IABP may not be very effective and the use of Impella for this indication in the setting of acute MI has increased substantially in recent years. Ventricular septal rupture and papillary muscle rupture complicating AMI remain indications for IABP as a bridge to corrective surgery.

Durable assisted circulation

The late 1960s was a period of great ebullience. Humans reached the moon and the quest for a total artificial heart began in earnest. Shortly thereafter, it was realized that the technological challenges and compatibility coupled with challenges of durability required a shift to a lesser option, leading to the advent of the concept for supporting the left ventricle alone while leaving the right ventricle unsupported mechanically.[19] In the early concept phases, it was asserted that support targeting the left ventricle must necessarily replace its function with a similar pulsatile pump mechanism. As a result of this, the early generation left ventricular assist systems (LVAS) were bulky, heavy, required placement in the abdomen, and possessed displacement chambers and valves to allow for mimicking contractile function. A pivotal trial, REMATCH (Randomized Evaluation of Mechanical Assistance for the Treatment of Congestive Heart Failure), published in 2001, was the first study to reliably demonstrate that survival of transplant ineligible refractory, predominantly inotropic therapy supported heart failure is improved by implantation of a LVAS.[20] This study used an early generation pulsatile flow device and demonstrated a 48% reduction in risk of death at 1-year. However, the LVAS used, as previously discussed, was of limited durability and meaningful 'out of hospital' survival was prolonged by a short median duration of only 5 months. Complications encountered included strokes, multisystem organ failure, device failure, and infections which reduced enthusiasm for widespread adoption. As engineers persisted in refining this technology, the realization that support could be provided without pulsatile flow led to the development

of continuous flow left ventricular assist systems (CF-LVAS).[21] These turbo-pumps were smaller in profile, had fewer moving parts, did not require valves for ensuring optimal flow, and consequently were more durable. A landmark trial compared the older bulky pulsatile LVAS studied in REMATCH to a newer generation axial continuous flow LVAS, the HeartMate II (Abbott, USA), and demonstrated a marked improvement in short- and long-term survival, along with an improvement in functional capacity and meaningful quality of life prolongation.[22] This CF-LVAS required anchoring within an abdominal pump pocket. To facilitate a smaller design for a pump that could be implanted into the thoracic cavity without an abdominal pocket, a centrifugal CF-LVAS, the HeartWare HVAD (Medtronic, USA), was then introduced and demonstrated to be non-inferior in a randomized trial compared to the HeartMate II LVAS.[23] A greater incidence of strokes with this centrifugal pump was noted while the HeartMate II was plagued by an increased incidence of de-novo pump thrombosis requiring pump replacement. The HeartWare HVAD pump could be implanted via less-invasive surgical techniques that did not require a sternotomy and this LVAS was also suited for children and those adults with a smaller body surface area (⊃ Figure 11.3.7).[24] A newer centrifugal device, with a fully magnetically levitated system, the HeartMate 3 LVAS was subsequently introduced.[25–27] This device was engineered to specifically overcome problems of pump thrombosis by the creation of a frictionless motor, wider gaps to facilitate blood flow and minimize red blood cell destruction, and an intrinsic pulsatility algorithm engineered by asynchronous fixed speed changes of the rotor. The HeartMate 3 has quickly become the most used LVAS since it has been shown to nearly eliminate the complication of pump thrombosis, markedly reduce stroke rates, as well as demonstrate a decrease in bleeding complications.[26] This pump has been tested in the MOMENTUM 3 ((Multicenter Study of MagLev Technology in Patients Undergoing Mechanical Circulatory Support Therapy

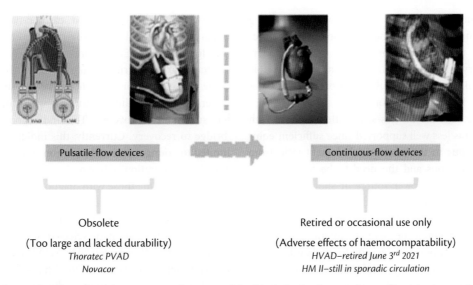

Pulsatile-flow devices

Continuous-flow devices

Obsolete

(Too large and lacked durability)
Thoratec PVAD
Novacor

Retired or occasional use only

(Adverse effects of haemocompatability)
HVAD—retired June 3rd 2021
HM II—still in sporadic circulation

Figure 11.3.7 The evolution of mechanical circulatory support. The nature of durable device development is one of introduction, application, experience, re-engineering, and obsolescence of older technology.

Reproduced from Mehra MR, Gustafsson F. Left Ventricular Assist Devices at the Crossroad of Innovation in Advanced Heart Failure. *J Card Fail*. 2021 Nov;27(11):1291–1294. doi: 10.1016/j.cardfail.2021.06.003 with permission from Elsevier.

with HeartMate 3) trial, which reported its results in 1028 patients randomly allocated to either the HeartMate 3 pump or the HeartMate II LVAS.[28] The fully magnetically levitated HeartMate 3 pump was associated with less frequent need for pump replacement than the HeartMate II device and was superior with respect to survival free of disabling stroke or reoperation to replace or remove a malfunctioning device. The need for pump replacement, occurrence of stroke of any severity, major bleeding, and gastrointestinal haemorrhage were lower in the centrifugal-flow pump group than in the axial-flow pump group. In real world experiences, this LVAS has been shown to not only be life prolonging when compared to the other devices, but to do so while reducing morbidity and cost of care (➲ Figure 11.3.8).[29,30] More recently, the HeartWare HVAD manufacturer discontinued its production and distribution, leaving the HeartMate 3 LVAS as the principal choice for adults and selected children and people with smaller body sizes.[31] While we now recognize the short-and intermediate-term durability of LVAS, with outcomes shown to

compare favourably with those achieved with heart transplantation, long-term durability beyond 7–10 years remains an open question.

Patient level indications

The patients in whom LVAS should be employed include those with severe persistent systolic heart failure symptoms who have failed to respond to optimal medical management. Commonly, these patients have marked functional limitation indicated by a peak oxygen consumption of < 12 mL/kg/min; or the patient is bound to continuous intravenous inotropic therapy owing to symptomatic hypotension, demonstrates worsening renal function, or persistent refractory congestion. Such a patient population with features of advanced heart failure may be identified using mnemonics such as 'I NEED HELP' or more simply by presence of three simple clinical features including: (i) recurrent hospitalizations for heart failure, (ii) inability to tolerate neurohormonal directed medical therapy, and (iii) increasing

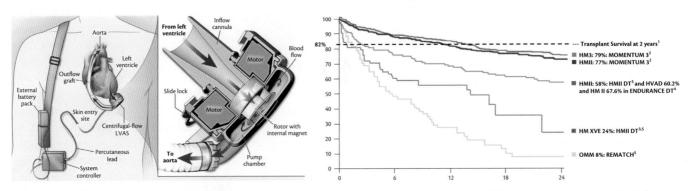

Figure 11.3.8 The HeartMate 3 left ventricular assist system and improvement in survival with durable pumps which now reaches similar survival with heart transplantation at 2 years.

Reproduced from Sidhu K, Lam PH, Mehra MR. Evolving trends in mechanical circulatory support: Clinical development of a fully magnetically levitated durable ventricular assist device. *Trends Cardiovasc Med*. 2020 May;30(4):223–229. doi: 10.1016/j.tcm.2019.05.013 with permission from Elsevier; and Mehra MR, Naka Y, Uriel N, et al; MOMENTUM 3 Investigators. A fully magnetically levitated circulatory pump for advanced heart failure. *N Engl J Med*. 2017 Feb;376(5):440–450. doi: 10.1056/NEJMoa1610426..

diuretic requirements to maintain stability with worsening cardiorenal syndrome.[31] Those patients who are no longer responding to cardiac resynchronization therapy or have moderately severe secondary mitral regurgitation (and are not amenable to percutaneous repair) may be particularly important candidates for consideration for LVAS implantation.[32]

Currently, the role of LVAS in 'less sick' patients (those with moderate symptoms) is less well supported since sufficient equipoise does not exist due to the adverse risk–benefit ratio from device-related complications and the need to be tethered to a driveline that connects to a power source. It should be recognized that although LVAS were initially designed for short-term support as a bridge to recovery or to cardiac transplantation, the most frequent use today entails permanent support for lifetime therapy ('destination therapy'). The decision to implant LVAS dichotomously as either a bridge to transplantation or for destination therapy is not always clear and, in several instances, these devices are used as a 'bridge to decision' (in those with potentially reversible underlying relative contraindications, such as renal insufficiency or pulmonary hypertension, who may become candidates for transplantation in the future). As such, terminology that creates gaps in patient selection ought to be avoided and we advocate a single indication in those patients that meet the threshold for consideration. Besides clinical features that point to the need for incremental cardiac support, outcomes are dependent on important factors including the state of disease in the right ventricle (dilation, elevated filling pressures, severity of tricuspid regurgitation, contractile insufficiency), non-cardiac

morbidity (cardiohepatic and cardiorenal syndrome), nutritional status (hypoalbuminemia), and overall condition (frailty) (➲ Figure 11.3.9).[33] Social support systems and care provider engagement are also critical features to ensuring a successful outcome. In selected circumstances, the decision to implant LVAS is performed with the intention to wean once cardiac function has sufficiently recovered. This indication is referred to as a 'bridge to recovery'. Currently, this indication is infrequent and limited to younger patients with non-ischaemic cardiomyopathy and shorter duration of having lived with heart failure. Such patients may include those with diagnoses including myocarditis or peripartum cardiomyopathy.

Society guidelines across the globe now provide endorsement for LVAD implantation in selected advanced heart failure patients. The recently released 2022 AHA/ACC/HFSA Guideline for the Management of Heart Failure[50] has suggested that in patients with NYHA class IV symptoms who are deemed to be dependent on continuous intravenous inotropes or temporary MCS, durable LVAD implantation is effective to improve functional status, quality of life, and survival (Class I: Strong recommendation based on high quality evidence). The Guideline also advocates such use in patients with advanced heart failure in NYHA IV symptoms who are yet to require inotropic therapy but do so with a moderate recommendation (Class 2A). It is important to note that these guidelines remain agnostic to the therapeutic intent of either bridge to transplantation or destination therapy. In some contrast, the 2021 ESC Guidelines for the diagnosis and treatment of acute and chronic heart failure[51] generally agree with the

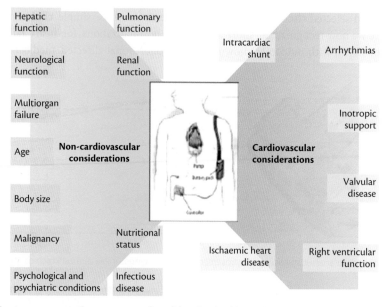

Figure 11.3.9 The complex evaluation parameters for assessment of candidacy for durable mechanical circulatory support.

patient severity indication as outlined above but provide separate categorization for therapeutic intent including bridging strategies to transplant, recovery or candidacy, or destination therapy. They also provide more specificity within the framework of severity of disease including use of the INTERMACS 1–4 profile, a LVEF < 25% and more than three hospitalizations for heart failure in the preceding year, a low cardiopulmonary exercise reserve, and evidence of haemodynamic aberrations with consequent end-organ dysfunction. These guidelines endorse such treatment using a 2A (moderate) level of recommendation.

Management of LVAS and their complications

Forward flow across LVAS circuits is critically dependent on management of systemic blood pressure. Continuous flow LVAS rely on pressure gradients between the left ventricular cavity and the aorta. Blood pressure is typically measured by using a Doppler ultrasound (which measures mean or opening blood pressure, which is less than the systolic blood pressure) since a peripheral pulse may not always be detectable. The ideal mean arterial blood pressure should be kept to < 90 mmHg and antihypertensive drug therapy prescribed using renin–angiotensin–aldosterone system (RAAS) drugs or other vasodilators.[34]

The blood flow path through current devices results in increased shear stress which is manifested in the form of low-grade haemolysis and the development of an acquired von Willebrand disease due to loss of high molecular weight multimers.[35,36] This haematological aberration has been associated with a risk of gastrointestinal bleeding, particularly resulting from arteriovenous malformations in the intestines. Therefore, a common complication encountered in patients is that of an anaemia, often due to iron deficiency. The administration of intravenous iron, while clinically utilized, has not been adequately tested in this population for effectiveness as well as safety. Gastrointestinal bleeding is a particularly vexing complication with significant recurrence risk once encountered. Therapy to abrogate this complication is not always successful, has been largely anecdotal, and includes several avenues of clinical intervention, for example, interventional endoscopic treatments or drugs, such octreotide, thalidomide, danazol, digoxin, and RAAS inhibitors.[37] Often reducing anticoagulation targets and eliminating antiplatelet therapy is required to treat this problem.

Other haemocompatibility-related adverse outcomes include neurological events (ischaemic and haemorrhagic strokes) and device-related thrombosis leading to pump malfunction. Antiplatelet therapy using aspirin in doses of 81–325 mg daily along with warfarin targeted to an INR of 2–3 is required for current LVAS to avoid the morbidity of haemocompatibility-related adverse events. On the one hand, this therapy protects against thrombotic complications while on the other, it predisposes the patient to bleeding complications. Strokes have been documented to occur with a frequency ranging from 10% with the HeartMate 3 LVAS to as much as 29% with the HeartWare HVAD device, by 2 years of treatment.[31] Optimal control of blood pressure is associated with improved rates of strokes, with some devices such as the HeartWare HVAD pump. Another cause of significant morbidity

is pump thrombosis requiring reoperation for device malfunction. This complication with the older devices was noted in 6–12% of LVAS implants, occurred early (in the first 6 months), and more commonly encountered with the HeartMate II device than with the HeartWare HVAD pump. The subclinical phase of LVAS thrombosis is characterized by increasing haemolysis and elevation in the device power. Progressively, inability to 'unload' the left ventricle is manifest leading to decompensated heart failure and possibly haemodynamic compromise. Lactate dehydrogenase is an excellent (although non-specific) biomarker of haemolysis and hence impending or established pump thrombosis. Patients who have suspected LVAD thrombosis and do not undergo LVAD exchange or cardiac transplantation have a 6-month mortality rate of 48%, inferring that medical therapy for VAD thrombosis may be inadequate (or cause harm in the case of thrombolytic use). Reoperation (pump exchange) carries a modest 6.5% perioperative mortality risk and a 65% 2-year survival following exchange. Fortunately, the HeartMate 3 LVAS is associated with pump thrombosis only rarely and generally due to ingestion-related thrombosis rather than de novo development of clots within the device. This observation has led investigators to study either modification of anticoagulation regimens or to consider elimination of antiplatelet therapy in the background, which has been the mainstay of such treatments since the inception of LVAS.[38,39]

The unsupported right ventricle in the presence of an optimally functioning LVAS often demonstrates worsening function and results in congestion requiring diuretic therapy. Despite a decrease in right-sided afterload with LVAS, increased device flow results in a greater right heart preload and induces mechanical dys-synchrony of the septum due its nature of trans-apical left ventricular unloading. This also decreases mechanical efficiency of torsion-related contractile function and uncovers right ventricular dilatation and maladaptation between the right ventricle and pulmonary circuit.[40] Cardiac arrhythmias are common, although less frequent with the HeartMate 3, but often require antiarrhythmic therapy since such events can trigger low flow through the device.[41] Whether cardiac resynchronization therapy or an implantable defibrillator are associated with benefits remains uncertain and emerging evidence points to a signal of potential harm in some cases, especially with cardiac resynchronization therapy. This may have important implications for replacement of device generators when nearing depletion.

Infection is common, often involving the driveline (the conduit connecting the device to the external controller and batteries) which occurs in 1 in 5 patients following LVAS implant.[42] Such an infection is treated with local internal exploration and requires long-term suppressive antibiotics unless the patient undergoes cardiac transplantation, or the device is exchanged. Infection and its inflammatory sequelae predispose to thrombosis and heighten the risk of neurological complications, leading to a worsening milieu in haemocompatibility. It has been noted that generalized infections, unrelated to the LVAS components itself are more often encountered in LVAS recipients. Whether this is due to an altered immunological milieu in such individuals remains a question for ongoing scientific inquiry.[43]

LVAS-facilitated myocardial recovery

LVAS support is associated with improvements to the shape and size of the left ventricle; however, normalization of ventricular geometry and recovery of function is noted in few highly selected individuals. Changes are seen as early as within the first month of mechanical unloading. Despite these observed changes, at a cellular level, abnormal gene expression changes associated with adverse remodeling persist.[44] For example, the expression of more than 3000 genes have been found to be modified in response to HF in a transcriptomic analysis of biopsies taken from patients with failing and non-failing hearts when compared to those with LVAD support. Mechanical unloading was associated with persistence of abnormal gene expression in 95% of dysregulated genes, and further dysregulation of genes in other pathways were noted.[45] The discoveries of transcriptional abnormalities observed through fluctuating patterns of microRNAs and long non-coding RNAs may open new avenues for gene discovery and potential novel therapeutic strategies in predicting recovery; however, this remains an open question for inquiry in the realm of predictive biomarker development. Importantly, the extra-cellular matrix composition and structure do not necessarily revert to a normal state and architecture with reverse remodeling. A few studies have shown that LVAD implantation is associated with decreased total collagen deposition while others yield conflicting results. One study demonstrated that extra-cellular matrix volume was initially increased in response to LVAD implantation, with subsequent volume reduction with longer support. Mechanical unloading with LVAD support does not seem to reverse levels of matrix metalloproteinases but when paired with neurohormonal directed therapy, improvements may be noted. Efforts to clinically recover patients with LVAS implants are associated with variable outcomes. In the recently reported RESTAGE study, 40 patients were enrolled from 6 centres who were an average age of 35 years old with non-ischaemic cardiomyopathy and heart failure symptoms of an average of 20 months duration. LVAD speed of the HeartMate II was optimized with an aggressive pharmacological regimen, and regular echocardiograms were performed at reduced LVAD speed to test underlying myocardial function.[46] Overall, half of these highly selected patients were explanted within 18 months and survival free from repeat LVAS implant or transplantation was 90% at 1-year and 77% at 2 years. While the promise of recovery is enticing, the prediction of recovery is difficult and applicable to a small population of candidates with severe advanced stage heart failure.

Total artificial heart

Those patients with severe right-sided heart failure or conditions that do not allow placement of an LVAS (restrictive cardiomyopathy, massive anterior MI with fragile myocardium in the early stages post-infarction, complex congenital heart disease) require consideration for biventricular support. In such patients, either a biventricular assist device approach (difficult to perform since it requires two separate pumps with distinct power sources) or a total artificial heart pump can be considered. The SynCardia total artificial heart is a pulsatile, implantable pump that consists of two polyurethane ventricles with pneumatically driven diaphragms, and four tilting disc valves.[47] This requires excision of the native ventricles and thus cannot be employed as a myocardial recovery strategy. This device operates on a steep physiological curve and has little adaptability to tolerate either systemic blood pressure changes or large shifts in blood volume. As the ventricles are excised, most patients exhibit a sharp decline in renal function due to the loss of natriuretic peptide expression by the myocardium, but this often recovers once alternate pathways for such natriuretic peptide expression are engaged or the renal system resets its needs for such adaptive hormonal availability. Severe haemolysis is common due to the presence of four mechanical valves and aberrant erythropoiesis is noted, leading to a severe anaemia. Newer artificial hearts using biocompatible surfaces are under development, such as the CARMAT pump, as well as those that use continuous flow technology.[48] These devices have yet to mature clinically to be advocated for routine use (➲ Figure 11.3.10).

Future directions

For short-term devices smaller and biocompatible pumps will facilitate easier percutaneous insertion and lead to fewer adverse events. Additionally, generation of firm evidence for either broad benefit of MCS in cardiogenic shock or clear definition of sub-populations where short term MCS is truly useful remains an unmet need which must be solved. These developments will not occur independently as safer and more efficient pumps may broaden the population where MCS will be indicated (➲ Figure 11.3.11).

Although durable LVAS are available worldwide, their use and indications vary from country to country, largely due to the individual and care provider burden, health care resource use and consequent high costs. Cost-effectiveness studies suggest improvement with the newer devices, yet some countries only allow use of this technology as a bridge to transplantation (e.g. UK), while awaiting more definitive long-term studies for lifetime use.[29,49] However, a recent cost-effectiveness analysis from the UK perspective has demonstrated that the use of destination therapy meets the threshold for cost implications considered as acceptable.[52] The use of LVAS in moderately symptomatic ambulatory patients with chronic systolic heart failure is still discouraged throughout the world, pending introduction of haemocompatible or biocompatible devices that are fully internalized without the need for an external driveline. Several novel device platforms are currently in pre-clinical phases and smaller pumps that provide more natural circulatory flow with fully internally powered systems are expected.

Summary and key messages

Several short- and intermediate-term pumps are available to assist the circulation in cardiogenic shock. The clinical profile of the patient is the main determinant of the optimal system with LV and RV function as well as pulmonary oxygenation being the most important factors. The use of percutaneous MCS including ECMO has increased dramatically in recent years, but firm

Emerging Technology for Biventricular Support

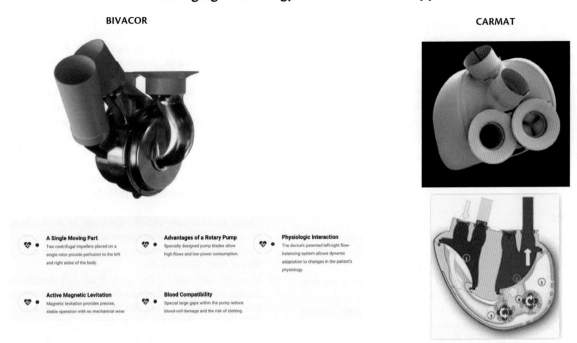

Figure 11.3.10 Total artificial hearts in evolution. The CARMAT and BIVACOR devices seek to provide more biocompatible and physiological smart pumping capability to replace physiological cardiac function with devices.
BIVACOR Source: https://bivacor.com

LVADs in Pre-clinical Phase Evaluation

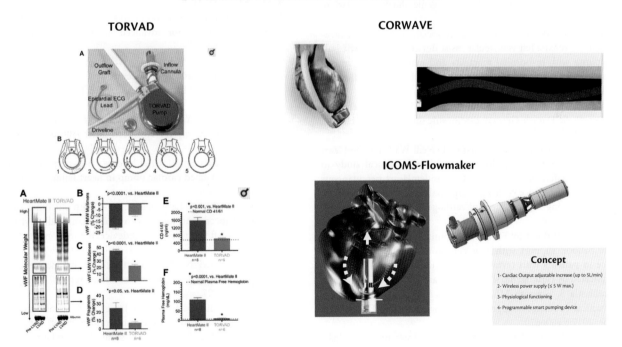

Figure 11.3.11 Left ventricular assist systems in evolution. The TORVAD, CORWAVE, and ICOMS devices are just a few different directions that the field is moving in to engineer more durable devices with novel mechanisms and flow characteristics.
TORVAD Source: Bartoli CR, Hennessy-Strahs S, Gohean J, et al, A Novel Toroidal-Flow Left Ventricular Assist Device Minimizes Blood Trauma: Implications of Improved Ventricular Assist Device Hemocompatibility. *Ann Thorac Surg.* 2019 Jun;107(6):1761-1767. CORWAVE Source: https://www.corwave.com/product/corwave-lvad/ICOMS Source: http://fineheart.fr/the-technologie

evidence for clinical benefit from large randomized trials is still awaited. Durable MCS has evolved considerably, and current, implantable, centrifugal devices are effective and reliable leading to improved survival, quality of life, and functional capacity with demonstration of excellent long-term survival.[53] They are indicated in advanced HF irrespective of whether the patient may be a candidate for transplantation or not and prediction of outcome at an individualized level is now possible.[54, 55] In some patients sufficient LV recovery allows for explant of the LVAS without recurrence of advanced HF. Patients with biventricular failure may be treated with a total artificial heart. Future LVAS development is expected to allow for implantation of less advanced HF patients.

References

1. Kantrowitz A, Tjonneland S, Freed PS, Phillips SJ, Butner AN, Sherman JL. Initial clinical experience with intraaortic balloon pumping in cardiogenic shock. JAMA. 1968;203:113–8.

2. DeVries WC, Anderson JL, Joyce LD, et al. Clinical use of the total artificial heart. N Engl J Med. 1984;310:273–8.

3. Thiele H, Zeymer U, Neumann F-J, et al. Intra-aortic balloon counterpulsation in acute myocardial infarction complicated by cardiogenic shock (IABP-SHOCK II): final 12 month results of a randomised, open-label trial. Lancet. 2013;382:1638–45.

4. Khera R, Cram P, Lu X, et al. Trends in the use of percutaneous ventricular assist devices: analysis of national inpatient sample data, 2007 through 2012. JAMA Intern Med. 2015;175:941–50.

5. van Dort DIM, Peij KRAH, Manintveld OC, et al. Haemodynamic efficacy of microaxial left ventricular assist device in cardiogenic shock: a systematic review and meta-analysis. Neth Heart J. 2020;28:179–89.

6. Schrage B, Ibrahim K, Loehn T, et al. Impella support for acute myocardial infarction complicated by cardiogenic shock. Circulation. 2019;139:1249–58.

7. Dhruva SS, Ross JS, Mortazavi BJ,et al. Association of use of an intravascular microaxial left ventricular assist device vs intra-aortic balloon pump with in-hospital mortality and major bleeding among patients with acute myocardial infarction complicated by cardiogenic shock. JAMA. 2020;323:734–45.

8. Udesen NJ, Moller JE, Lindholm MG,et al. Rationale and design of DanGer shock: Danish-German cardiogenic shock trial. Am Heart J. 2019;214:60–8.

9. Burkhoff D, Cohen H, Brunckhorst C, O'Neill WW, TandemHeart Investigators Group. A randomized multicenter clinical study to evaluate the safety and efficacy of the TandemHeart percutaneous ventricular assist device versus conventional therapy with intraaortic balloon pumping for treatment of cardiogenic shock. Am Heart J. 2006;152:469.e1–8.

10. Thiele H, Sick P, Boudriot E, et al. Randomized comparison of intra-aortic balloon support with a percutaneous left ventricular assist device in patients with revascularized acute myocardial infarction complicated by cardiogenic shock. Eur Heart J. 2005;26:1276–83.

11. Kuchibhotla S, Esposito ML, Breton C, et al. Acute biventricular mechanical circulatory support for cardiogenic shock. J Am Heart Assoc. 2017;6:e006670.

12. Salna M, Garan AR, Kirtane AJ, et al. Novel percutaneous duallumen cannula-based right ventricular assist device provides effective support for refractory right ventricular failure after left ventricular assist device implantation. Interact Cardiovasc Thorac Surg. 2020;30:499–506.

13. Uriel N, Jeevanandam V, Imamura T, et al. Clinical outcomes and quality of life with an ambulatory counterpulsation pump in advanced heart failure patients: results of the multicenter feasibility trial. Circ Heart Fail. 2020;13:e006666.

14. Vora AN, Schuyler Jones W, DeVore AD, Ebner A, Clifton W, Patel MR. First-in-human experience with Aortix intraaortic pump. Catheter Cardiovasc Interv. 2019;93:428–33.

15. Maxwell BG, Powers AJ, Sheikh AY, Lee PHU, Lobato RL, Wong JK. Resource use trends in extracorporeal membrane oxygenation in adults: an analysis of the Nationwide Inpatient Sample 1998–2009. J Thorac Cardiovasc Surg. 2014;148:416–421.e1.

16. Lorusso R, Gelsomino S, Parise O, et al. Venoarterial extracorporeal membrane oxygenation for refractory cardiogenic shock in elderly patients: trends in application and outcome from the Extracorporeal Life Support Organization (ELSO) Registry. Ann Thorac Surg. 2017;104:62–9.

17. Cheng R, Hachamovitch R, Kittleson M,et al. Complications of extracorporeal membrane oxygenation for treatment of cardiogenic shock and cardiac arrest: a meta-analysis of 1,866 adult patients. Ann Thorac Surg. 2014;97:610–6.

18. Russo JJ, Aleksova N, Pitcher I, et al. Left Ventricular unloading during extracorporeal membrane oxygenation in patients with cardiogenic shock. J Am Coll Cardiol. 2019;73:654–62.

19. Sidhu K, Lam PH, Mehra MR. Evolving trends in mechanical circulatory support: clinical development of a fully magnetically levitated durable ventricular assist device. Trends Cardiovasc Med. 2020;30:223–9.

20. Rose EA, Gelijns AC, Moskowitz AJ, et al. Longterm use of a left ventricular assist device for end-stage heart failure. N Engl J Med. 2001;345:1435–43.

21. Stewart GC, Mehra MR. A history of devices as an alternative to heart transplantation. Heart Fail Clin. 2014;10:S1–12.

22. Slaughter MS, Rogers JG, Milano CA, et al. Advanced heart failure treated with continuous-flow left ventricular assist device. N Engl J Med. 2009;361:2241–51.

23. Rogers JG, Pagani FD, Tatooles AJ,et al. Intrapericardial left ventricular assist device for advanced heart failure. N Engl J Med. 2017;376:451–60.

24. McGee E, Danter M, Strueber M,et al. Evaluation of a lateral thoracotomy implant approach for a centrifugal-flow left ventricular assist device: The LATERAL clinical trial. J Heart Lung Transplant. 2019;38:344–51.

25. Mehra MR, Naka Y, Uriel N, et al. A fully magnetically levitated circulatory pump for advanced heart failure. N Engl J Med. 2017;376:440–50.

26. Mehra MR, Goldstein DJ, Uriel N, et al. Two-year outcomes with a magnetically levitated cardiac pump in heart failure. N Engl J Med. 2018;378:1386–95.

27. Gustafsson F, Shaw S, Lavee J, et al. Six-month outcomes after treatment of advanced heart failure with a full magnetically levitated continuous flow left ventricular assist device: report from the ELEVATE registry. Eur Heart J. 2018;39:3454–60.

28. Mehra MR, Uriel N, Naka Y, et al. A fully magnetically levitated left ventricular assist device – final report. N Engl J Med. 2019;380:1618–27.

29. Pagani FD, Mehra MR, Cowger JA, et al. Clinical outcomes and healthcare expenditures in the real world with left ventricular assist devices – The CLEAR-LVAD study. J Heart Lung Transplant. 2021;40:323–33.

30. Pagani FD, Cantor R, Cowger J, et al. Concordance of treatment effect: an analysis of The Society of Thoracic Surgeons Intermacs database. Ann Thorac Surg. 2022; 113(4):1172–82.

31. Mehra MR, Gustafsson F. Left ventricular assist devices at the cross-road of innovation in advanced heart failure. J Card Fail. 2021; 27(11):1291–94.

32. Kanwar MK, Rajagopal K, Itoh A, *et al*. Impact of left ventricular assist device implantation on mitral regurgitation: An analysis from the MOMENTUM 3 trial. J Heart Lung Transplant. 2020;39:529–37.

33. Stewart GC, Givertz MM. Mechanical circulatory support for advanced heart failure: patients and technology in evolution. Circulation. 2012;125:1304–15.

34. Castagna F, Stohr EJ, Pinsino A, *et al*. The unique blood pressures and pulsatility of LVAD patients: current challenges and future opportunities. Curr Hypertens Rep. 2017;19:85.

35. Mehra MR. The burden of haemocompatibility with left ventricular assist systems: a complex weave. Eur Heart J. 2019;40:673–7.

36. Bansal A, Uriel N, Colombo PC, *et al*. Effects of a fully magnetically levitated centrifugal-flow or axial-flow left ventricular assist device on von Willebrand factor: A prospective multicenter clinical trial. J Heart Lung Transplant. 2019;38:806–16.

37. Kataria R, Jorde UP. Gastrointestinal bleeding during continuous-flow left ventricular assist device support: state of the field. Cardiol Rev. 2019;27:8–13.

38. Netuka I, Ivak P, Tučanova Z, *et al*. Evaluation of low-intensity anti-coagulation with a fully magnetically levitated centrifugal-flow circulatory pump-the MAGENTUM 1 study. J Heart Lung Transplant. 2018;37:579–86.

39. Mehra MR, Crandall DL, Gustafsson F, *et al*. Aspirin and left ventricular assist devices rationale and design for the International Randomized, Placebo-Controlled, Non-Inferiority ARIES HM3 trial. Eur J Heart Fail. 2021;23(7):1226–37.

40. Houston BA, Shah KB, Mehra MR, Tedford RJ. A new 'twist' on right heart failure with left ventricular assist systems. J Heart Lung Transplant. 2017;36:701–7.

41. Kumar A, Tandon V, O'Sullivan DM, Cronin E, Gluck J, Kluger J. ICD shocks in LVAD patients are not associated with increased subsequent mortality risk. J Interv Card Electrophysiol. 2019;56:341–8.

42. Patel CB, Blue L, Cagliostro B, *et al*. Left ventricular assist systems and infection-related outcomes: A comprehensive analysis of the MOMENTUM 3 trial. J Heart Lung Transplant. 2020;39:774–81.

43. Mehra MR, Woolley AE. Imaging the crevasse of left ventricular assist device infection. JACC Cardiovasc Imaging. 2020;13:1203–5.

44. Drakos SG, Mehra MR. Clinical myocardial recovery during long-term mechanical support in dvanced heart failure: Insights into moving the field forward. J Heart Lung Transplant. 2016;35:413–20.

45. Margulies KB, Matiwala S, Cornejo C, Olsen H, Craven WA, Bednarik D. Mixed messages: transcription patterns in failing and recovering human myocardium. Circ Res. 2005;96:592–9.

46. Birks EJ, Drakos SG, Patel SR, *et al*. Prospective multicenter study of myocardial recovery using left ventricular assist devices (RESTAGEHF (Remission from Stage D Heart Failure)): medium-term and primary end point results. Circulation. 2020;142:2016–28.

47. Copeland JG, Smith RG, Arabia FA, *et al*. Cardiac replacement with a total artificial heart as a bridge to transplantation. N Engl J Med. 2004;351:859–67.

48. Netuka I, Pya Y, Bekbossynova M, *et al*. Initial bridge to transplant experience with a bioprosthetic autoregulated artificial heart. J Heart Lung Transplant. 2020;39:1491–3.

49. Mehra MR, Salerno C, Cleveland JC, *et al*. Healthcare resource use and cost implications in the MOMENTUM 3 long-term outcome study. Circulation. 2018;138:1923–34.

50. Heidenreich PA, Bozkurt B, Aguilar D, *et al*. 2022 AHA/ACC/HFSA Guideline for the Management of Heart Failure: Executive Summary: A report of the American College of Cardiology/American Heart Association Joint Committee on Clinical Practice Guidelines. Circulation. 2022 145:e895–e1032.

51. McDonagh TA, Metra M, Adamo M, *et al*; ESC Scientific Document Group. 2021 ESC Guidelines for the diagnosis and treatment of acute and chronic heart failure: Developed by the Task Force for the diagnosis and treatment of acute and chronic heart failure of the European Society of Cardiology (ESC). With the special contribution of the Heart Failure Association (HFA) of the ESC. Eur J Heart Fail. 2022;24(1):4–131.

52. Lim HS, Shaw S, Carter AW, Jayawardana S, Mossialos E, Mehra MR. A clinical and cost-effectiveness analysis of the HeartMate 3 left ventricular assist device for transplant-ineligible patients: A United Kingdom perspective. J Heart Lung Transplant. 2022;41(2):174–186.

53. Mehra MR, Goldstein DJ, Cleveland JC, *et al*. Five-year outcomes in patients with fully magnetically levitated vs axial-flow left ventricular assist devices in the MOMENTUM 3 randomized trial. JAMA. 2022;328(12):1233–1242.

54. Mehra MR, Nayak A, Morris AA, *et al*. Prediction of survival after implantation of a fully magnetically levitated left ventricular assist device. JACC Heart Fail. 2022;10(12):948–959.

55. Mehra MR, Nayak A, Desai AS. Life-prolonging benefits of LVAD therapy in advanced heart failure: a clinician's action and communication Aid. JACC Heart Fail. 2023:S2213-1779(23)00249-4.

CHAPTER 11.4

Heart transplantation

Davor Miličić, Mandeep Mehra,
and Randall C Starling

Contents

Introduction

Advanced heart failure is a final phase of heart failure syndrome, where the patient becomes refractory to guideline-directed medical and device therapy.[1,2] For these patients heart transplantation is still considered the gold standard of treatment, if there are no contraindications.[1,2] Over time, post transplant survival rates have increased, and today reach about 90% after the first year, with median survival of 12.5 years.[3,4,5] In addition to survival, transplantation brings a significant improvement of functional status and quality of life in the majority of appropriately selected patients.[4,5]

As modern therapies enable more patients to survive milder or moderate forms of heart failure, the world is faced with a growing population of patients with advanced heart failure, which is inherently a progressive disorder. After a decline in heart transplant numbers between 1993 and 2004, recorded by the International Society for Heart and Lung Transplantation (ISHLT) Transplant Registry, numbers of heart transplantations have been increasing, and reached a peak in 2016, with a total of 5832 heart transplants at 346 centres, mostly in Europe and North America.[6] However, even in Europe and North America transplant rates are far below needs, while in the rest of the world the number of heart transplant procedures is extremely low. Therefore the majority of patients eligible for heart transplantation either die or are implanted with a ventricular assist device (VAD), as a potential bridge to transplant (BTT) or destination treatment (DT). In general, there is a huge, paradigmatic gap between what modern medicine can offer to treat advanced heart failure, and the reality, where we face increasing numbers of patients implanted with a VAD, as a temporary replacement or even alternative to transplantation in countries with low transplant rates or no heart transplant programme at all. Even in Europe, heart transplant rates significantly differ among countries, and are not always correlated with national GDP or health expenditures, but mostly reflect local organ donor rates (➲ Figure 11.4.1 and ➲ Figure 11.4.2).[7]

Referral and patient selection

Patients with suspected advanced heart failure should be referred to an advanced heart failure centre for further evaluation, and to define optimal management. Timely referral is mandatory for successful implementation of advanced, life-saving therapies – transplantation or/and mechanical circulatory support (MCS). A patient with 'single organ failure', that is without serious and irreversible multi-organ damage, especially of brain, lungs, liver, or kidneys, should be considered an optimal candidate for heart transplantation, in the absence of other contraindications. However, heart transplantation may be considered in a broad spectrum of patients with advanced heart failure, who do not have absolute contraindications. Because of the donor organ shortage, and

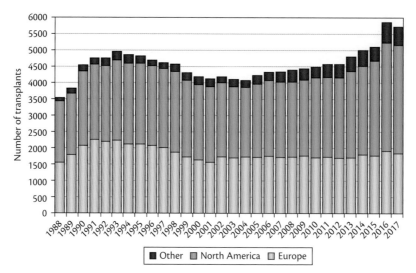

Figure 11.4.1 International Society for Heart and Lung Transplantation data on heart transplant numbers per year (1998–2017).
Reproduced from Khush KK, Cherikh WS, Chambers DC, et al; International Society for Heart and Lung Transplantation. The International Thoracic Organ Transplant Registry of the International Society for Heart and Lung Transplantation: Thirty-sixth adult heart transplantation report - 2019; focus theme: Donor and recipient size match. *J Heart Lung Transplant.* 2019 Oct;38(10):1056-1066. doi: 10.1016/j.healun.2019.08.004 with permission from Elsevier.

even if there are no absolute contraindications for heart transplantation, a durable left ventricular assist device (LVAD) can be implemented as a bridge to heart transplantation BTT. Nowadays there is a substantial number of patients (50% or more) on transplant lists who are already implanted with an LVAD as a durable BTT. For patients with severe biventrivcular or isolated right ventricular failure, biventricular mechanical support or isolated right ventricular support (RVAD) may be considered as a BTT. Those procedures require highly experienced centres, and therefore the rates of biventricular mechanical support or isolated RVAD support occur sporadically rather than routinely. In a case of absolute contraindications for heart transplantation, LVAD can be applied as a DT. In patients with contraindications to advanced therapies, the palliative approach remains the only therapeutic option. ➲ Box 11.4.1 lists indications and contraindications for heart transplantation.[1,2]

Diagnostic evaluation and patient phenotypes

Diagnostic evaluation of potential heart transplantation candidates should be performed in specialized centres by an expert team. Selection of such patients should aim to assure significant improvement in both life expectancy and quality of life. In addition, a patient's informed consent and clear motivation to be treated by heart transplatation is mandatory. In general, heart transplant candidates are patients with the end-stage heart disease not remediable by optimal evidence-based medical and device therapies.

The majority of patients being evaluated for heart transplantation are advanced heart failure patients with reduced ejection fraction (HFrEF), that is patients with dilated and hypocontractile myocardium of ischaemc or non-ischaemic etiology. Their candidacy for transplantation should include documented refractoriness to maximum tolerated doses of renin angiotensin aldosterone system inhibitors

(angiotensin-converting enzyme-inhibitors or sacubitril/valsartan or eventually angiotensin-receptor antagonists), beta-blockers and mineralocorticoid receptor antagonists (MRA), as well as refractoriness to cardioresynchronization therapy (CRT-P or CRT-D) if previously indicated and implanted according to guidelines. In addition, other less invasive methods to improve patients' status and prognosis should be checked, such as possibility of revascularization procedures, exceptionally palliative reconstructive surgery, or rehabilitation programmes.

A much smaller but significant proportion of patients with the advanced heart failure phenotypically present without heart dilatation and hypokinesia, and, if not responsive to approved therapies, could be also assessed for heart transplantation. That includes entities as hyertrophic cardiomyopathies, restrictive cardiomyopathies, arrhythmogenic right ventricle cardiomyopathy/dysplasia, and infiltrative cardiomyopathies.[3] That group of cardiomyopathies as potential indications for heart transplantation will be discussed later in this text, after general principles of pretransplant evaluation.

Functional capacity, prognosis, and haemodynamics

In general, diagnostic evaluation protocols consider patients with severe symptoms and/or signs of heart failure in a functional class NYHA IIIb or IV. The evaluation is based on three elements wich should be taken into account together with other relevant clinical data and/or comorbidities.[3]

1. Cardiopulmonary stress testing

Maximal test is defined as one with expiratory exchange ratio (RER) > 1.05 and reaching anaerobic treshold on optimal medical therapy. In a patient receiving a beta-blocker peak oxygen comsumption cut-off is defined as ≤ 12 ml/kg/min, and in a patient intolerant of a beta-blocker, a cut-off peak oxygen

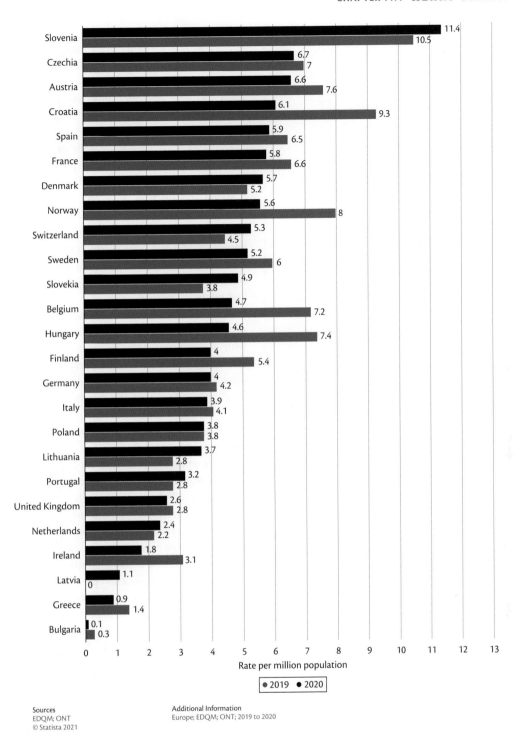

Figure 11.4.2 Rate of heart transplants per million population in Europe, 2019–2020.

consumption as a criterion for listing should be ml/kg/min.[3] In women and generally in patients < 50 years, ≤ 50% of predicted VO2 can be considered as additional criterion.[3]

2. Heart failure prognostic survival scores should be used in addition to cardiopulmonary stress testing in ambulatory patients.

An estimated 1-year survival calculated by the Seattle heart Failure Model of < 80% or the Heart Failure Survival Score in the medium- to high-risk range should be considered for listing in a context of cardiopulmonary stress testing and right-heart catheterization parameters.[3]

3. Diagnostic right-heart catheterization

Right heart catheterization (RHC) should be considered as mandatory for all adult candidates for heart transplantation, and should be repeated at least annually. The need for more frequent RHC should be individualized according to the severity of pulmonary hypertension, clinical stability of heart

Box 11.4.1 Indications and contraindications for heart transplantation

Indications

Advanced heart failure

No other therapeutivc option except for LVAD as BTT

Contraindications

Active infection except LVAD/driveline infection

Severe peripheral or cerebrovascular disease

Irreversible pulmonary hypertension despite pharmacological challenge

Malignancy (to be decided in collaboration with oncologist)

Irreversible liver dysfunction and/or cirrhosis

Irreversible renal dysfunction (e.g. creatinine clearence < 30 mL/min/1.73 m²)

Systemic disease with multi-organ involvement

Any other serious comorbidity with poor prognosis

BMI > 35 kg/m²

Current alcochol or drug abuse

Psychological instability incompatible with appropriate post-transplant magament

Social conditions or insufficient social support incompatible with compliant outpatient care

Source data from McDonagh TA, Metra M, Adamo M, et al; ESC Scientific Document Group. 2021 ESC Guidelines for the diagnosis and treatment of acute and chronic heart failure. *Eur Heart J*. 2021 Sep 21;42(36):3599-3726. doi: 10.1093/eurheartj/ehab368; and Crespo-Leiro MG, Metra M, Lund LH, *et al*. Advanced heart failure: a position statement of the Heart Failure Association of the European Society of Cardiology. *Eur J Heart Fail*. 2018 Nov;20(11):1505-1535. doi: 10.1002/ejhf.1236.

failure, and presence of MCS.[3] Frequency of RHC if more than once a year also depends on individual centre preferences/capabilities. Periodic RHC should in general not be performed in children.[3]

Irreversible pulmonary hypertension, transpulmonary gradient above the defined limit and/or elevated pulmonary vascular resistance (PVR) significantly increase risk of post transplantation right heart failure and mortality.[3] Cut-off limits of haemodynamic parameters are as follows[3]:

- PVR > 5 Wood Units or in children PVRI >6 Wood Units
- Transpulmonary pressure gradient > 16-20 mmHg
- Systolic pulmonary artery pressure > 60 mmHg in conjunction with any of the forementioned parameters
- PVR not reducible to < 2.5 Wood Units with a vasodilator, without a consequent fall of systolic blood pressure <85 mmHg.

Age and co-morbidities

Age: The upper age limit for eligibility for transplantation is generally accepted as 70 years. Some centres perform transplantation in patients over 70 years, using local specific donor and recipient criteria. Report of heart transplantation outcomes in carefully selected septuagenarians showed acceptable outcomes with fewer rejections but a higher mortality than in younger patients.[8]

Obesity: According to the reported evidence-based data, obesity within the body mass index (BMI) range < 35kg/m² is not associated with higher mortality rates after transplantation. However, BMI > 35 kg/m² is associated with higher post transplant morbitiy and mortality, and patients should be recommended to achieve their BMI < 35 kg/m² before being listed for heart transplantation.[9,10]

Diabetes with HbA1c > 7.5% or 58 mmol/l or end-organ damage, with an exception of non-proliferative retinopathy, is considered as a relative contraindication for heart transplantation.[3]

Renal dysfunction as a relative contraindication for heart transplantation should be defined as eGFR < 30 ml/min/1.73 m.[2,3] Renal diagnostic work up is mandatory to prove or exclude irreversibility of renal failure, which includes renal imaging by use of sonography and/or CT or MRI, estimation of proteinuria and renal arterial flow. Post-renal dysfunction should be evaluated and treated, if possible.

Peripheral and cerebrovascular disease not amenable to revascularization should be considered as major comorbidities with a significant negative impact on post-transplant survival and quality of life.[3] Serious peripheral arterial disease should limit eligibility for transplantation, as it substantially limits rehabilitation. Symptomatic cerebrovascular disease should be considered as a contraindication for heart transplantation, as it could be related to increased risk of post-transplant stroke and functional decline.[11]

Active systemic infection means a serious contraindication for transplantation, as it could seriously interfere with the clinical course in patients receiving high doses of immunosuppressive medications in the early post-transplant period.

Chronic persistent infections, such as HIV and hepatitis B and C, should be carefully evaluated and elaborated together with experienced HIV or hepatology specialists.

Exceptionally, stable HIV patients compliant with antiretroviral therapies and with no detectable HIV-RNA and CD4 counts > 200 cells/µl, and with no opportunistic infections could be considered for listing.[3] Data on carefully selected HIV patients receiving heart transplants showed similar short-term survival rates as in general post transplant population, but there is no data on their long-term survival.[13,14,15,16,17]

As well as donor organ shortage, another serious limitation for listing patients with HIV are numerous interactions between immunusupressive medications and antiretroviral drugs.[15,18]

Acute hepatitis B and C represent contraindications for heart transplantation.[3] Resolved hepatitis B or C infection in potential candidates for heart transplantation should receive hepatobiliar system imaging and liver biopsy, as cirrhosis and hepatocellular carcinoma represent absolute contraindications for transplantation. Serological and viral load testing and checking every 3 months and at the time of transplantation is mandatory. In chronic hepatitis C infection, HCV genotype should be determined.[3] In the light of new antiviral therapies the issue of heart transplantation in patients with controlled hepatitis B or C becomes a challenge, and long-term outcomes for those potential recipients are unknown.[12]

Malignancies: Active malignancy is an absolute contraindication for heart transplantation, with the exception of superficial skin basal or squamous cell carcinoma.[3] Patients in a complete remission for at least 5 years could be considered for transplantation in agreement with consultant oncologist. In the meantime, oncology patients with the advanced heart failure with a favourable prognosis regarding their malignant disease, could be supported with LVAD as a bridge to candidacy (BTC) or, if transplantation is contraindicated, to maintain with LVAD-support as a DT.[3]

Frailty is an evolving issue, particularly while assessing older potential heart recipients. There are several proposed modalities to assess frailty, from grip strength or gait speed to established questionnaires.[19,20,21] Frailty should become a matter of concern if three of the following symptoms are present: unintentional weight loss ≥ 10 pounds/ ≥ 5 kg within the past year, muscle loss, fatigue, slow walking speed, and low degree of physical activity.[3]

Psychosocial inadequacy could represent a temporary or definite contraindication for heart transplantation. Thus, a comprehensive psychosocial work-up is an essential part of the evaluation of potential transplant candidates. Compliance with recommended pharmacological therapies, regular follow-up, and lifestyle changes are essential for post transplant short- and long-term outcomes.[3] Active psychosis, intellectual disability, dementia, and/or inability to comply with instructions represent prohibiting elements for listing a patient for a heart transplant. Inadequate social conditions could also seriously limit candidacy for listing, if the heart team presumes serious difficulties in complying with a complex post transplant regimen.[3]

Tobacco, alcohol and other substance abuse: Active tobacco smoking and smoking during the 6 months prior to transplantation are associated with poorer outcomes, and therefore considered as a relative contraindication for listing.[3] In general, there is an evidence-based consensus of a deleterious effect of smoking history for post transplant outcomes. The largest, recent multicentre analysis on more than 32,000 patients revealed that cigarette smoking history in heart transplant recipients represents an independent risk for 1, 2, and 10-year mortality, and morbidity including higher risk of hospitalization for acute rejection and infection, increased risk of graft failure, and higher incidence of malignancies.[22] It has been also documented that cigarette smoking in a donor was associated with increased post transplant mortality.[22] Active alcohol and drugs abusers should also not be considered as heart transplant candidates.[3]

Special considerations

End-stage heart disease without inherent left ventricular dilatation and severely reduced systolic function: Among all myocardial phenotypes in patients under consideration for heart transplantation, there is proportionally small but important group of patients with the end-stage heart failure due to non-dilated and non-ischaemic cardiomyopathies, that is, hypertrophic, restrictive, infiltrative, and arrhythmogenic right ventricular cardiomyopathy/dysplasia (ARVC/D). These patients, if refractory to conventional medical and device therapies, would generally not be candidates for an LVAD, neither as a BTT, nor as a DT. Thus transplantion represents the only active treatment option in appropriately selected patients.[3]

Non-obstructive hypertrophic cardiomyopathy is a rare but serious disease, as time from diagnosis to the terminal heart failure has been reported as from 4 to 10 years, with worse predictable outcomes in younger patients and if already family members affected.[3,23,24] Severe heart failure refractory to conventional treatment can occur in patients with severe diastolic dysfunction and preserved systolic function, and these patients could substantially benefit from heart transplantation, as much as patients with more common indications for transplantation.[23,24] The other, more frequent scenario of advanced heart failure in hypertrophic cardiomyopathy is due to severe myocardial remodelling leading in the terminal phase to a phenotype resembling dilated cardiomyopathy: dilated and thinned, fibrotic and hypocontractile left ventricle with a combined systolic and diastolic dysfunction and symptoms and signs of severe heart failure.

ARVC/D is a genetically determined, rare disease, which could, as well as the right ventricle, affect the other myocardial territories.[25] It is usually complicated by serious and/or fatal ventricular arrhythmias, and rarely with the advanced heart failure.[26]

Left-ventricular non-compaction also represents a rare, genetically determined disease which could lead to the advanced heart failure and thus could be evaluated for heart transplantation.[27]

Restrictive and infiltrative cardiomyopathies are of a heterogeneous origin, but phenotypically characterized by stiff and thickened, not-dilated ventricles with preserved or mildly reduced ventricular contractility and dilated atria.[28] Defining aetiology is mandatory in the diagnostic work-up as, with the exception of idiopathic restrictive cardiomyopathy, some patients suffer from systemic disorders with predominant myocardial involovement, and usually need cause-targeted therapies, such as enzyme replacement in Anderson–Fabry disease,[29] immunosuppression in sarcoidosis and endomyocardial fibrosis, or disease-specific therapies in amyloid light-chain (AL) or transthyretin related (TTR) amyloidosis.

AL-amyloidosis in which amyloid derives from and indolent clone of plasma cells, can represent an indication for heart transplantation in a patient with seriously affected myocardium, and consecutive severe heart failure, which does not allow implementation disease-specific therapy.[30] Transplantation should be realized in experienced multidisciplinary centres, and autologous stemm cell transplantation performed as soon as possible after post heart transplantation recovery. Collaboration with haematologists is essential.[3,30]

TTR amyloidosis (ATTR) is a multi-organ infiltrative disease caused by depositions of TTR amyloid, which is produced predominantly in the liver. Thus liver transplantation can stop disease progression, and bring favourable outcomes in appropriately selected patients.[3,31] Cardiomyopathy caused by TTR amyloidosis is frequently misdiagnosed and underdiagnosed.[31] There are two types of TTR amyloidosis: hereditary (hATTR) and wild type (ATTRwt).

hATTR is an autosomal dominant inherited disorder, with variable penetration. Range of potential phenotypes coresponds with various genotypes, from polineuropathy to cardiomyopathy and mixed phenotype. Age at diagnosis varies according to certain genotype, and median life expectancy at time of diagnosis is 2–5 years.[31]

ATTRwt is the most common cause of amyloidosis-related cardiomyopathy, and causes 13–37% cases of heart failure with preserved ejection fraction (HFpEF).[3,31] Clinical presentation occurs more in older men, with a median survival at time of diagnosis 3–5 years.[31] Heart transplantation with or without combined liver transplantation is a viable treatment option with favourable outcomes in appropriately selected patients with TTR amyloid cardiomyopathy.[32,33]

Allocation of donor hearts

Organs are allocated according to legal regulations of each country, either per country or within countries associations, for example, EUROTRANSPLANT or Scandinavia Transplant. Principles of organs allocation are organ recipient-oriented and include blood group, body size, emergency status, and waiting time on a transplant list. Arbitary upper age limit for heart donation is 65 years. Absolute contraindications for heart donation are cardiac and non-cardiac disorders. Cardiac contraindication is a significant structural and/or functional myocardial, valvular, pericardial, or congential heart disease, clinically relevant arrhythmogenic substrate, complex coronary artery disease, or prior coronary artery by pass surgery. Non-cardiac absolute contraindications are sepsis or uncontrolled infections, and active malignant diseases.[3]

Donor evaluation

Every brain-dead patient should be considered as a potential multi-organ donor. Basic work-up of a potential heart donor consists of medical history and clinical examination, ECG, transthoracic echocardiography (TTE), bedside haemodynamics, and, in haemodynamically unstable patients Swan–Ganz catheterization, in order to optimize haemodynamic management of a potential donor. If TTE insite is insufficient due to a poor acoustic window, transoesophageal echocardiography (TEE) should be performed to acquire adequate information about donor heart structure and function. Coronary angiography is a part of a standard work-up in all potential donors from the age from 50 years upwards, but also in younger patients with cardiovascular risk factor(s). The rest of a work-up is standardized as for other organ donor evaluation, including virology/serology tests.[3]

Donor–recipient matching

Decision making about realization of heart transplantation should be done by experienced advanced heart failure cardiologist(s) and heart transplant surgeon(s), with the possibility of consulting other experts, for example, immunologists, anaesthesiologists. Independent transplant coordinators from national or transnational transplant organizations conduct initial matching and propose potential transplant candidate(s) to transplant centres chosen by predefined criteria. In the chosen centre, a heart transplant cardiologist in collaboration with a transplant surgeon designates the transplant recepient according to urgency status, waiting time, recipient's availability, and immunological and anthropometric compatibility with a donor.

ABO-incompatibility is an absolute contraindication for heart transplantation. Exceptionally, it can be considered in infants with immature immunological system, and only in experienced paediatric heart transplantation centres.[3,34]

Immunoincompatibility, that is high panel reactive antibody (PRA) is associated with a significantly reduced number of potential donors. It can be seen more often in multiparous women, patients supported by mechanical assist devices, patients who have received multiple blood transfusions, congenital heart disease patients surgically implanted with autologous homografts, and others. Patients waiting on transplant lists should be periodically checked for PRA in order to confirm their reactivity is below 20%.[35]

Human leucocyte antigen (HLA) matching for heart transplantation is in general not mandatory for approving heart transplantation. Despite some controversies about HLA-missmatch and its influence on post transplant complications, there is a general agreement that HLA-DR missmatch is associated with worse prognosis in transplant recipients.[36] A modern approach might move us forward towards precision medicine, and may include typing at serological split antigen levels by use of the Epitope Mismatch Algorithm to calculate the number of amino acid differences in antibody-verified HLA eplets, that is amino acid mismatch load (AAMM) with regard to HLA-DR and HLA-AB between donor and recipient.[37] Currently, HLA and in particular HLA-DSA (donor-specific antibodies) can be used as parameters for prediction of possible graft outcomes, rather than for recipient–donor matching.

Donor–recipient size matching is usually based on body weight and BMI. Traditionally it has been considered that > 20% discrepancy in body weight should be regarded as significant for heart transplantation. However, there are no clear data about significant correlations of body weight and size of the heart, except for extreme diferencies in body weight, as in body height and body surface area.[38] According to the ISHLT guidelines, the difference in BMI between donor and recipient should not be > 20%, and also that no transplantation should be done from a donor with body weight < 70% of the recipient.[38] However, it seems that the graft size and function is more important than the body weight, and that undersizing should not be a matter of serious concern in male-to-male, male-to-female, or female-to-female heart transplantation.[39] One of the novel paremeters for donor–recipient matching, still not in a ruotine use, is predicted heart mass (PHM), which can be calculated including weight, height, sex, and age.[39,40] In a case of the same height and weight of the donor and recipient, for opposite sexes the difference in PHM for male vs female is 19%.[40,41]

Sex donor–recipient difference could be associated with worse outcomes if the donor is a female, and the recipient is a male, but not vice versa. In practice, additional attention should be focused on male recipients receiving a heart from female donors, in particular regarding the graft quality.[3,39,40,41]

Mechanical circulatory support as a bridge to transplant

MCS is a very useful and often unavoidable treatment modality for a substantial proportion of patients on transplant lists, as the world is faced with increasing numbers of heart transplant candidates, and not enough donor hearts by far.

Currently at least of 50% of patients listed for heaart transplantation are bridged with MCS.[4]

Patients with cardiogenic shock (INTERMACS 1 and 2) could be bridged by use of paracorporeal circulatory support as a BTT or bridge to bridge. Despite some centres still using the intra-aortic balloon pump (IABP), state of the art temporary support is either extracorporeal membrane oxygenation (ECMO), which ensures both circulatory and respiratory support, or temporary continuous flow assist devices for supporting the left ventricle, or exceptionally the right ventricle or both ventricles (see ➲ Chapter 11.3).

Durable LVAD is an option for patients with indicators of predictable deterioration while waiting for a donor heart, such as repeated heart failure hospitalizations, a need for escalating dose of diuretics, inotrope dependence, intolerance of conventional medical therapy for heart failure, progression of functional incapability, or secondary deterioration of other organs function, particularly liver and kidney. Post transplant survival in patients previously implanted with continuous flow LVAD seems not to be significantly adversely affected in comparison with those only transplanted and previously not bridged with LVAD.[4]

Patients with a potential temporary contraindication for transplantation, such as high PVR or unresolved outcome of a malignant disease, should be also considered for implantable continuous flow LVAD.[1,2,3,4]

Obesity, uncontrolled diabetes mellitus, potentially reversible renal dysfunction, and alcohol, tobacco, and drug abuse could be indications for BTC with LVAD.[3]

If the aforementioned unfavourable haemodynamics and risk factors ameliorate during VAD support, then the patient can be considered for heart transplantation, otherwise VAD support should remain as the DT.

MCS may raise some unfavourable issues for transplantation, such as allosensitization. It is recommended to screen VAD patients for sensitization at various intervals and reconsider transplantation in patients with high PRAs. However, it has been stated recently that sensitization in the LVAD population may not be related to higher rejection rates or worse survival after transplantation, and thus the value of desensitization therapy remains questionable.[4]

Dynamic listing should be a part of listing strategies in ambulatory, non-inotrope-dependent patients. Those patients should be re-evaluated every 3–6 months after listing, including cardiopulmonary stress testing and heart failure survival prognostic scores, as well as their tolerance and responsiveness to the guideline-approved conventional medical and device therapies.[3]. That might imply de-listing a patient due to clinical and functional improvement, or re-listing of a previously de-listed patient due to deterioration.

Recipient work-up at the time of transplantation

Patients listed for heart transplantation should be regularly checked at 3–6 month intervals,[3] and contact maintained with the heart transplant centre in case of any relevant clinical or laboratory change. However, a careful but breif update at transplant admission time is mandatory to rule out potential new, clinically relevant problems. Routine haematology and biochemistry tests, and chest X-ray should be performed, and, if neccessary, any kind of additional diagnostics, for example, right heart catheterization. Heart transplant centres should be established within comprehensive, tertiary hospitals, enabling permanent provision of any necessary medical/surgical consultancy, diagnostics or therapy.

Donor heart explanation and preservation

The most used method of donor heart preservation is heart preservation in cardiac arrest followed by static cold storage in a crystalloid heart preservation solution. Acceptable level of such heart protection is < 6 hours.[42] To minimize graft dysfunction caused by ischaemia-reperfusion graft injury, preservation solutions have been developed to ameliorate ischaemia tolerance and reduce harm from graft ischwemia.[43] Recently various methods for beating heart warm preservation have been developed.[43] Apart from the ability to prolong out-of-body time between donor heart explantation and opening of the aortic clamp in the recipient patient, these systems offer more options for better donor organ diagnosis and management, including coronary angiography.[43]

Surgical aspects of heart transplantation

For years the prevailing surgical approach was the Shumway and Lower biatrial technique, whereby the recipient right atrium is anastomosed to the donor right atrium, the recipient left atrium to the donor left atrium, and the pulmonary artery and the aorta to the respective anatomic structures of the donor heart.[45] Biatrial technique results in abnormally enlarged atria and distorted atrial geometry, with a potential consequence of atrivetricular valves regurgitation, particulary tricuspid insufficiency. In addition, because of the proximity of the right atrial suture line to the sinus node, sinus node dysfunction can occur as a consequence of the sinus node injury.[46]

This method has been largely replaced by the bicaval technique, thereby avoiding annular distorsion of the donor tricuspid valve, and with less need for permanent pacemaker implantation, also with better haemodynamic results, and improved long-term post transplant survival.[44] The bicaval technique is therefore recommended as the method of choice as long as there is no caval vein anomaly. The bicaval approach preserves donor atria, combining the standard left atrial anastomosis with the bicaval anastomosis.[46,47]

Immediate post transplant management

After the surgical procedure, the newly transplanted patient is transferred from the operating room to the dedicated intensive care unit. Intensive postoperative management should be conducted by an experienced team, in order to prevent and treat postoperative complications, ensure appropriate haemodynamic status, and normal allograft function.

Immediate care should be focused on both recovery from the surgical procedure and innitial immunosuppressive strategies.[48]

Invasive haemodynamic monitoring and support is challenged by a threat of vasodilatory hypotension, right heart failure, and acute allograft dysfunction. It is critical to allow the ventricles and the sinus node to recover from ischaemic injury.[48]

Vasopressor and inotropic support should be carefully guided by assessing cardiac performance. The first step would be a gradient vasoconstrictor removal, and usually continuation with dobutamin and/or milrinone for at least 48 hours to allow the transplanted myoardium to recover from ischaemic injury.[49,50]

Most patients can be extubated and weaned from ventilator within the first 24 hours, and others should be extubated as soon as possible, to avoid the risk of ventilator-associated pneumonia. Antibiotics are given routinely, primarily to prevent operative site infection, for 24 hours or more. However, it seems that a preventative antibiotic regimen did not show clear evidencebased benefits in solid organs in the immediate post transplant period.[48]

For discussion of immunosuppressant induction, ➜ Immunosuppression, p. 724.'

Postoperative complications

Most relevant postoperative complications include vasodilatory hypotension, acute allograft dysfunction, renal failure, and post transplant arrhythmias.

Vasodilatory hypotension

Vasodilatory hypotension is a frequent complication after heart transplantation or any open heart surgery using cardiopulmonary bypass with membrane oxygenation. It can be, at least partially, explained by a systemic inflammatory response with consecutive vasodilatory cytokines release.[52] Alternatively vasodilatory hypotension could be baroreflex-mediated endogenous arginine vasopressin depletion.[53] It has been hypothesized that preoperative excessive vasopressin release in patients with severely decompensated heart failure could induce endogenous arginine vasopressin depletion, potentiated by an acute stress such as cardiopulmonary bypass.[54] Postoperative vasoplegia can be also mediated by preoperative use of vasodilatory drugs, either neurohormonal inhibitors for chronic heart failure treatment, or inodilators such as milrinone.[1] The mainstay treatment of postoperative vasodilation is norepinephrine, although there is a potential problem of catecholamine resistance as well as toxicity, if administered in higher

dosages. According to several underpowered trials testing vasopressin compared to norepinephrine in postcardiotomy surgery, and the most relevant, the VANCS trial,[50,] administration of vasopressin could be superior, particularly in regard to less serious complications, rather than mortality alone. However, it seems not be applicable for vasoplegia in septic shock.[51]

Acute graft dysfunction

Acute graft dysfunciton could be a very serious and fatal perioperative complication in heart transplant recipients, accounting for 30% of early post transplant deaths.[55] Among other reasons, it can be caused by unrecognized or neglected donor organ dysfunction, having in mind that myocardial inury to some extent occurs in all brain death organ donors, and in some cases could be prohibitive for organ harvesting.[56] Furthermore, acute graft dysfunction can be caused by prolonged ischaemic time, inappropriate organ preservation, and ischaemia–reperfusion injury.[57] Hyperacute graft rejection can occur as the most dramatic cause of graft dysfunction and death, in patients with pretransplant elevated PRA, that is previously formed antibodies to HLAs. Prospective HLA cross matching in those patients can be useful to prevent that complication.[3]

In order to start on-time treatment and stop progression of the acute graft failure, transplanted patients should be carefully monitored perioperatively, from intraoperative transesophageal monitoring of the heart function, to measuring pulmonary artery saturation and cardiac output in intensive care setting. ECG dynamics, such as ST-segment changes, QRS microvoltage, and arrhythmias, although non-specific for acute rejection, should raise awareness of its possiblility and initiate work up to define other potential causes, such as pericarditis/pericardial effusion or acute myocardial infarction.

Treatment of graft dysfunction begins with inodilators, such as dobutamine or milrinone, and more severe cases usually require various modalities of NCS, from ECMO and/or temporary VAD to durable VAD support. In patients without irreversible other organ damage, high-risk retransplantation may be considered as well.[57]

Right heart failure

Right heart failure is one of the most frequent post transplant complications, and could be caused be innapropriate graft preservation or reperfusion, ischaemic injury, and also by the allograft right ventricle afterload missmatch, as many heart transplant patients suffer from a certain grade of pretransplant pulmonary hypertension. Last but not least, donor–recipient missmatch, such as a smaller donor heart transplanted to a larger recipient can also result in right heart frailure.[57]

Elevated central venous pressure combined with a low cardiac output can be indicative of right heart failure, and thus a Swan–Ganz catheter might be used to continuously evaluate haemodynamics and tailor precise fluid management. Echo-guided right ventricular shape and function follow-up is also mandatory, often by use of the transoesophageal approach for an adequate right ventricle visualization.

Inotropes may be given sometimes for several weeks, and milrinone should be usually prefered over dobutamine, due to its vasodilatory effect within the pulmonary vascular bed.[57] Inhaled nitric oxide could be beneficial in patients with pulmonary hypertension and low cardiac output.[58]

Post transplant renal failure

Post transplant renal failure is a frequent complication occuring in up to 50% transplanted patients.[57] Preoperatively, many transplant candidates suffer from some either reversible or ireversible renal dysfunction. Perioperatively they often experience ischaemic kidney injury due to aortic crosss clamping or post operative hypotension, and also from nephrotoxic medications, for example, calcineurin inhibitors, antibiotics, etc. Although there are controversies regarding cut-off glomerulal filtration for listing a patient on a transplant list,[59] a need for haemodialysis in the immediate post transplant period, as well as a decrease in glomerulal filtration of more than 25% during the first post transplant year, have been found to be substantially associated with a worse survival in heart transplant recipients.[59] A significant preoperative congestion, followed by perioperative need for blood transfusions, increases the fluid overload, and could be a trigger for renal failure, and therefore has to be managed by loop diuretics or, if neccessary, temporary mechanical renal replacement.[57]

Post transplant rhythm disturbancies

Post transplant rhythm disturbances include bradycardia and taachyarrhythmias. As a transplanted heart is denervated, the usual postoperative sinus node frequency at rest is 90 or more per minute. The bicaval technique reduces the probability of sinus node dysfunction compared to the biatrial approach. However, epicardial pacing wires should remain until sinus node dysfunction is ruled out or recovered.[57] Among supraventricular arrhythmias, atrial fibrillation or flutter are the most common, and can be indicative of immune rejection, prior to other symptoms, or signs of myocardial dysfunction on echocardiography. Ventricular arhythmias occur less often, and can be rather associated with myocardial ischaemia or perioperative myocardial infarction, than with the graft rejection.[57]

Extended post transplantation management and follow-up

Surveillance, diagnosis, and classification of heart allograft rejection

Cardiac allograft rejection remains one of the major post transplant complications, despite advances in immunosuppressive medications resulting in gradually reduced rejection rates. It is also well known that over the course of the post transplant period, the risk of rejection decreases, in parallel with decreased intensity of immunosuppressive treatment. Clinical presentation of the rejection may be acute or chronic, and immune rejection mechanisms cellular, humoral, or mixed.

Endomyocardial biopsy (EMB) is still considered the gold standard for diagnosing and grading potential allograft rejection, enabling histopatological evaluation of the allograft tissue. It is performed either via the right jugular vein or femoral vein, using a percutaneous approach.[60]

There is no consensus regarding post transplantation EMB biopsy regimen and EMB scheduling protocols vary widely among transplant centres. A conservative aproach includes weekly EMB at the first month post transplantation, biweekly at the second month, monthly between the third and the sixth month, then every 3 months between month 7 and 12, every 3 months, between months 12 and 18, and every 6–12 months after the nineteenth month post transplantation.[57] In the era of efficient immunosuppressive protocols, non-invasive surveillance methods, including gene profiling, can help reduce significantly EMB frequency, especially after the first post transplant year. Thus routine surveillance EMB is tending to be replaced by symptom-triggered EMB.[62,63]

There was a diversity of rejection grading systems up to the 1980s, then in 1990, the ISHLT published a simple, universal rejection grading system, which was widely adopted, and enabled uniformity in rejection evaluation, easier communication among transplant centres, multicentre evaluation of transplant outcomes, and multicentre trials in the field. That classification served successfully over a decade, until in 2005, ISHLT published a revised Position Statement on this issue, to address new challenges and inconsistencies, and incorporate recent knowledge on antibody-mediated rejection (AMR) (⮀ Table 11.4.1). ⮀ Table 11.4.2 is taken from the 2005 ISHLT Position Statement and compares ISHLT rejection grading schemes 2005 vs 1990.[64]

Table 11.4.1 ISHLT AMR grading

Grade	Description
pAMR 0: Negative for pathologic AMR	Both histologic and immunopathologic studies are negative
pAMR 1 (H+): Histopathologic AMR alone	Histologic findings are present while immunopathologic findings are negative
pAMR 1 (I+): Immunopathologic AMR alone	Histologic findings are negative while immunopathologic findings are positive (CD68+ and/or C4d+)
pAMR 2: Pathologic AMR	Both histologic and immunopathologic findings are present
pAMR 3: Severe pathologic AMR	Interstitial haemorrhage, capillary fragmentation, mixed inflammatory infiltrates, endothelial cell pyknosis, and/or karyorrhexis, and marked oedema and immunopathologic findings are present

AMR, antibody mediated rejection.
Reproduced from Stewart S, Winters GL, Fishbein MC, *et al*. Revision of the 1990 working formulation for the standardization of nomenclature in the diagnosis of heart rejection. *J Heart Lung Transplant*. 2005 Nov;24(11):1710-20. doi: 10.1016/j.healun.2005.03.019 with permission from Elsevier.

Table 11.4.2 ISHLT standardized cardiac biopsy grading acute cellular rejection

2004		1990	
Grade 0 R*	**No rejection**	**Grade 0**	**No rejection**
Grade 1 R, mild	Interstitial and/or perivascular infiltrate With up to 1 focus of myocyte damage	Grade 1, mild A–Focal	Focal perivascualar and/or interstitial infiltrate without myocyte damge
		D–Diffuse	Diffuse infiltrate without myocyte damage
		Grade 2 moderate (focal)	Once focus of infiltrate with associated myocyte damge
Grade 2 R, moderate	Two or more foci of infiltrate with associated myocyte damage	Grade, moderate A–Focal	Multifocal infiltrate with myocyte damage Diffuse inlitrate with myocyte damage Diffuse, polymorphous infiltrate with extensive myocyte damage ± oedema, ± haemorrhage + vasculitis
Grade 3 R, sever	Diffuse infiltrate with multifocal myocyte damage ± oedema, ± haemorrhage ± vasculitis	B–Diffuse	Diffuse, polymorphous infiltrate with extensive myocyte damage ± oedmea, ± haemorrhage + vasculitis

*R denotes revised grade to avoid confusion with 1990 scheme.
Reproduced from Stewart S, Winters GL, Fishbein MC, *et al.* Revision of the 1990 working formulation for the standardization of nomenclature in the diagnosis of heart rejection. *J Heart Lung Transplant.* 2005 Nov;24(11):1710-20. doi: 10.1016/j.healun.2005.03.019 with permission from Elsevier.

Immunosuppression

Introduction of cyclosporine into clinical practice in the 1980s allowed solid organ transplantation to progress from anecdotal attempts to routine method for treating end-stage organ failure. In the meantime, development of potent immunosuppressive medications and combined immunosuppression protocols did not eliminate the threat of acute or chronic organ rejection as one of the major potential complications in patients with transplanted organs. Immune rejection can be T-cell mediated, that is cellular, and/or antibody mediated, that is humoral.

Therapeutic modulation of the immune response in transplant recipients consists of three main strategies: (1) induction, (2) maintenance, and (3) rejection therapy.

Glucocorticoids play an important role in induction therapy, in treating rejection episodes, and also are still used as part of maintanance immunosuppression in a certain proportion of transplanted patients. They inhibit the transcription factors activator protein-1 and nuclear factor kappa-B, which play important role in production of plethora of cytokines.[65] Glucocorticoids provide a general, non-specific immune supression, by limiting function and number of white blood cells, primarily depleting lymphocytes.[66]

Perioperatively, high-dose steroids are used parenterally, with a quick transition to an oral regimen, Due to numerous side-effects, the goal is to gradually de-escalate steroids over the first 6 months, and finally to withdraw them. However, for treating acute rejection, high-dose parenteral steroids remain the first therapeutic option.[66]

Most centres prescribe oral steroids after transplantation with biopsy guided tapering. By introduction of novel immunusuppressants, early steroid weaning, or even steroid avoidance remain sustainable options for a substantial proportion of transplanted patients, particularly in those who develop significant steroid-associated side-effects. However, although many patients may be completely weaned off steroids, it has been reported that about 60% of pateints take glucocorticoids permanently.[66]

Commonly used immunosuppressive agents in heart transplantation, and their most common side-effects are summarized in ➲ Table 11.4.3.

Induction therapy

Induction therapy includes a combination of polyclonal or monoclonal antibody medications together with a foundational immunosuppressive drugs. Current practice reflects heterogenous use of induction immunosuppressant protocols in various centres. Approximately 50% of patients undergoing heart transplantation receive immunnsuppressant induction with either polycloncal anti-thymocyte globulin (ATG) or a monoclonal, interleukin-2 receptor antibody – basiliximab or dacilizumab.[66]

Polyclonal ATG is available from two species: rabbit, following immunization with human thymocytes, and horse, following immunization with human T-cells. Application of ATG results in rapid depletion of recipient T-lymphocytes. It seems that rabbit ATG is more potent in decreasing circulating T-lymphocyte counts, with no difference in safety compared to horse-derived ATG, including risk of the posttransplant lymphoproliperative disorder (PTLD) or infections.[67]

Interleukin-2 receptor antagonists are directed to the apha-subunit of IL-2 receptor on activated T-cells, thus attenuating T-cell proliferation and allograft directed immune reaction.[68] Potential advantages of IL-2 receptor antagonists – basiliximab, and dacilizumab – are fewer PTLDs and infections, with continued effectiveness in reducing acute rejection.[68]

Monoclonal antithymocyte antibody – muromonab (OKT3) – is a murine antibody targeted towards T-cell CD-3+ receptor, which results in opsonization of T-cells and their removal by

Table 11.4.3 Commonly used immunosuppressive agents in heart transplantation. Quoted doses and levels vary between centers and individual patients according to required efficacy and adverse events

Agent	Doses/target levels	Common side effects**
Induction therapy		
Anti-thymocyte globulin	0.75 mg–1.5 mg/kg (3 days)	Thrombocytopenia, allergic reaction
Basiliximab	20 mg day 1 and 4	Allergic reaction
Maintenance therapy		
Calcineurin inhibitors		
Cyclosporine	Month 0–3: 200–300 µg/L* Month 3–12: 100–200 µg/L* >12 months: 80–120 µg/L*	Renal failure, tremor, hypertension, hyperlipidemia, diabetes, hirsutism, gingival hyperplasia
Tacrolimus	Month 0–3: 12–15 µg/L* Month 3–12: 10–12 µg/L* >12 months: 5–8 µg/L*	Renal failure, tremor, hypertension, hyperlipidemia, diabetes
Antiproliferative drugs		
Mycophenolate mofetil (MMF)	1.0–1.5 g bid	Leucopenia, diarrhoea
Azathioprine	50–150 mg od	Bone marrow suppression
Glucocorticoids		
Methylprednisolone	At transplant: 1–2 g iv	Diabetes, osteoporosis, hyperlipidemia, hypertension, cushingoid appearance, acne
Prednisolone	0.2 mg/kg tapering to 0.1 mg/kg or taper to 0	Diabetes, osteoporosis, hyperlipidemia, hypertension, cushingoid appearance, acne
Proliferation signal inhibitors		
Everolimus	3–8 µg/L	Diarrhea, bone marrow suppression, oedema, stomatitis, pneumonitis
Sirolimus	4–8 µg/L	Diarrhea, bone marrow suppression, oedema, stomatitis, pneumonitis

*When combined with MMF or azathioprine, ** All agents: infection, increased cancer risk; od: once daily; bid: twice daily.
Courtesy of F. Gustafsson.

circulating macrophages.[66] Because of potential side-effects, particularly 'cytokine release syndrome', such as headache, nausea, vomiting, fever, chest pain, or pulmonary oedema, as well as increased risk for PTLD, cytomegalovirus (CMV), or fungal infections, the use of muronomab has been practically abandoned.[69]

A meta-analysis of the available randomized trials in heart transplantation indicate that ATG is probably associated with a lower risk of biopsy-proven rejection compared with basiliximab, but no difference in mortality has been demonstrated.[68] Risks with both drugs include higher rates of infection.[68]

Induction therapy allows for delayed introduction of calcineurin inhibitors, which is an advantage in recipients with renal impairment. However, there is no clear evidence for use of induction therapy, but it remains in many centres either as a universal strategy, or implemented in high-risk patients, e.g. with preformed antibodies, positive retrospective crossmatch or renal dysfunction).[70]

Maintenance immunosuppressive therapy

Maintenance immunosuppressive therapy includes combination of foundational immunosuppressive medications. Beside glucocorticoids , discussed previously in this text, maintenance treatment includes combination of two of three classes of medications: Calcineurin inhibitors plus anti-metabilites, or proliferation signal inhibitors. Calcineurin inhibitors include cyclosporine A or tacrolimus. Anti-metabolites include mycophenalate mofetil, enteric coated mycophenolate sodium, and azathioprine. Proliferation signal inhibitors include sirolumus and everloimus.[66] For glucocorticoids, a preferable strategy should aim to deescalate dosages of steroid oral formulation over the first six months, and then to withdraw steroid from the maintenance therapy.[70] Some of the possible maintenance strategies are schematically presented in ◗ Figure 11.4.3.

Calcineurin inhibitors

Calcineurin inhibitors (CNIs) inhibit the phosphatase action of calcineurin, wihch is a crucial enzyme for the production of inflammatory cytokynes, including IL-2, thus inhibiting the expansion of CD4+ and CD8+ cells, and differentiation of CD4+ T cells.[71]

For many years, cyclosporine was the mainstay of maintanance immunosuppression, but today it has been replaced by tacrolimus

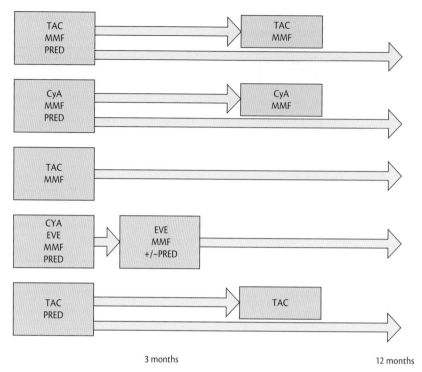

Figure 11.4.3 Immunosuppressive maintenance strategies.
Courtesy of F. Gustafsson.

(TAC) in most centres. Studies, including meta-analysis, have suggested that tacrolimus might slightly be more effective in preventing acute cellular rejection than cyclosporine.[72] The adverse event profiles for the two CNIs are quite similar, with renal dysfunction being of major clinical importance. Recent data from ISHLT show that at 1 year after heart transplant more than 90% of patients are treated with TAC. Studies have shown that patients may even be managed with TAC as monotherapy. Recently a once-daily formulation of TAC has been introduced, and while its use may be associated with higher adherence rates, no effect on outcome in allograft recipients has been demonstrated.[72]

Antiproliferative agents/cell cycle inhibitors

Azathioprine (AZA) was a part of original transplant protocols, but now has been almost completely replaced by mycophenolate mofetil (MMF), as MMF has demonstrated superior outcomes to AZA, especially with respect to development of allograft vasculopathy.[73] However, MMF is relatively often associated with gastrointestinal side-effects and leucopenia. AZA is mainly used in patients with intolerable gastrointestinal adverse reactions to MMF, particulary if enteric-coated formulation of MMF is not sufficient in reducing side–effects.[66]

AZA becomes an active metabolite which is converted into a purine analogue. When incorporated into nuclear DNA, that metabolite inhibits DNA synthesis and consequential T-and B-cells proliferation.[66] MMF is a non-competitive inhibitor of of inosine monophhosphate dehydrogenase, which is a key enzyme in guanine nucleotide production. MMF selectively blocks de novo guanine nucleotide production in proliferating lymphocytes, where the only pathway for purine synthesis is de novo.[66] MMF is a pro-drug which is being metabolized to mycophenolic acid.

Proliferation signal inhibitors/ mTOR inhibitors

Sirolimus (rapamycin) and everolimus are proliferation signal inhibitors (PSIs) that inhibit the enzyme kinase mammalian target of rapamycin (mTOR), which phosphorylates cell-cycle regulatory proteins involved in T-cell proliferation, and thus disrupts growth and differentiation of T- and B-lymphocytes and inhibits vascular smooth muscle cells proliferation.[66]

Everolimus is the most commonly used PSI in adult heart transplant recipients, as a substitute for either antiproliferative drugs or for CNIs. PSIs are associated with lower rates of allograft vasculopathy than AZA and MMF,[74] and if used, either with low doses of CNI, or, even more so, with MMF in the absence of CNIs (CNI-free regimen), improvement in renal function is obtained. Early introduction of a PSI-based CNI-free regimen is associated with the greatest improvement in renal function, but carries an increased risk of acute rejection.[75] Furthermore, PSIs are not tolerated by approximately 30% of patients, and for these reasons PSIs are rarely used as a primary strategy but often in patients who develop renal dysfunction with CNIs.

Candidates for being converted from MMF to PSI are patients with rejection from de novo donor-specific antibodies (DSA), as well as patients with CMV mismatch, or acquired CMV infection, or cardac allograft vasculopathy. In some malignancies, especially PSI or CNI-free regimen with PSI and MMF might be used, with low mainanance immunosuppressants doses.[76]

Rejection surveillance and treatment

There should be comprehensive rejection surveillance and treatment performed by assessing symptoms and clinical status, ECG, biomarkers, echocardiogram, and periodical endomyocardial biopsies, as the gold standard for diagnosing and grading allograft rejection. Signs and symptoms or heart failure can signal rejection, as well as arrhythmias, among which atrial fibrillation or flutter appear most frequently. Microvoltage in ECG can be associated with oedema of myocardium allograft walls and/or presence of pericardial effusion. Elevation of natriuretic peptides and/or cardiac troponin can also be a consequence of rejection.[57] Echocardiography can show reduced contractility, thickened myocardium due to oedematous walls, pericardial effusion, and/or dilation of myocardial chambers with atrioventricular valves relative insufficiency.

Endomyocardial biopsies (EMB) should be performed periodically according to defined schedules, especially immediately after heart transplantation and later on, usually up to 5 years or more if clinically relevant rejection was diagnosed in the previous post transplant follow-up.[57] The EMB should assess both cellular and humoral (AMR) according to the ISHLT criteria (➲ Box 11.4.1 and ➲ Table 11.4.4).[64] Occasionaly, rejection diagnosis can be supported by use of cardiac CT, positron emmsion tomography or MRI, where late gadolinium enhancement could be associated with rejection, but in general those methods should not be used as a replacement for EMB.

Mild, asymptomatic cellular rejection (ISHLT-1R) does not require treatment, but closer clinical surveillance. Asymptomatic moderate cellular rejection (ISHLT-2R) especially if later than 12 months after transplantation, may also not require specific treatment, but in most cases just a modification of a mantainance therapy, and closer surveillance, including clinical assessment, echocardiography evaluation, and follow up EMB.[77] Severe cellular rejection (ISHLT-3R) should be treated, regardless of symptoms.[77] Usual management of rejection should include a high dose of glucocrticoid, i.e. methylprednisolone 500 mg intravenously over 3 days, then in parallel with reduction of the high dosage, rabbit ATG could be added for its cytolytic T- and B-lymphocites activity.[57,77] Control EMB should be done usually from day 7 after starting rejection treatment.

In a case of suspected rejection, HLA antibodies should be checked, and if there are no HLA antibodies, non-HLA antibodies should be assessed in addition.

AMR can occur immediately after heart transplantation in a hyperacute form, or later, as acute or chronic. If AMR is suspected, EMB analysis should be expanded to include immunocytochemistry stains for complement split products, IgM, IgG, and IgA, and possibly antibody.[70,77] The goals of AMR treatment should be: (i) to disrupt injury of the allograft mediated by the humoral immune reaction, by use of intravenous corticosteroid and cytolytic medications (e.g. ATG); (ii) to remove circulating anti-HLA antibodies by use of (a) plasmapheresis, (b) intravenous immunoglobulin (IVIG can be applied 1 g/kg daily for 2 days up to the maximal total dosage of 140 g) and /or (c) immune apheresis

(immunoadsorption).[57,70,77] In a hyperacute AMR, besides intravenous corticosteroid and cytolytic medications, intravenous calcineurin inhibitor (cyclosporine A or TAC), and metabolic cycle inhibitor (MMF) may be considered.[77]

In a rejection presenting with cardiogenic shock, inotropes and vasopressors along with Swan–Ganz catheter haemodynamic monitoring should be titrated to achieve cardiac index > 2.0 L/min/m². As a bridge to recovery, acute MCS may be indicated.[57,76,77] In some cases retransplantation may also be considered, having in mind that in a case of a hyperacute AMR, survival after retransplantation is rather poor.[77]

Special considerations

Sensitization and desensitization

The exposure of the immune system to foreign HLA molecules results in anti-HLA antibody production and therefore sensitized patients. Most relevant risk factors for allosensitization are: blood product transfusions, multiparity, black ethnicity, viral infections, homograft or VAD implantation and retransplantation. [79,80]

Sensitization is traditionally measured with the panel-reactive antibody (PRA) testing, which is calculated by the percentage of positive reactions in the PRA assay, and is defined by a result ranging from 10 to 25%.[80] Currently, calculated PRA (cPRA) may be preferred. cPRA is derived from HLA frequencies among approximately 12,000 donors in the United States and it represents the percentage of actual organ donors who express one or more of the unacceptable HLAs as defined by the recipient anti-HLA antibodies.[81]

Desensitization is usually reserved for highly sensitized patients defined by a cPRA value ≥ 50–80% or by multiple positive crossmatches.[80] Desensitization treatments are aimed to counteract immune mechanisms responsible for sensitization. That includes removal of antibodies via plasmapheresis, immunoadsorption or total plasma exchange, inhibition of antibodies with use of intravenous immunoglobulin (IVIG), B cell depletion with rituximab, plasma cell depletion with bortezomib, or complement inhibition by use eculizumab and/or IVIG. Contemporary strategies usually include a combination of treatments targeting different of mechanisms, for example, plasmapheresis and/or IVIG and/or rituximab.[82–84] In the case of recurrent rejections, photopheresis could be considered as an add-on treatment.[78]

Donor specific anti-HLA antibodies (DSA) remain an issue in the early and late post-transplant period. Specifically de novo DSA development has an increased chance to occur over time, and DSA presence has been associated with worse prognosis.[85] It is also important to note that DSA developing de novo after the first post-transplant year has a worse prognosis.[86]

Cardiac allograft vasculopathy

Cardiac allograft vasculopathy (CAV) with a prevalence of 30% at 5 years and 50% at 10 years after heart transplantation has been identified as the main cause of mortality 3–10 years after transplantation.[87] Pathogenesis of CAV is related to repetitive endothelial damage caused by a combination of immunologic and non-immunologic mechanisms. Alloimunity in CAV includes HLA mismatch, DSA and/or episodes of acute cellular rejection and AMR.[88] Direct endothelial damage and inflammation stimulate proliferation of smooth muscle cells and deposition of the extracellular matrix, which leads to progressive vessel lumen narrowing. Cytomegalovirus, hepatitis C, and hepatitis B virus may increase the risk of CAV by both direct and immune-mediated injury.[88] Some non-immunological factors, such as dyslipidaemia, diabetes, hypertension, and smoking, enhance donor-transferred coronary atherosclerosis, and therefore should be appropriately modified and treated.[89] While obliterative intimal proliferation with diffuse distal vessel pruning reflects the CAV caused by immune-mediated mechanisms, focal and eccentric lesions in proximal segments of coronary arteries reflect predominant atherosclerotic aetiology.[88,89]

Serial screening for CAV is recommended since graft denervation masks angina symptoms, and allows silent progression of ischaemia until it causes complications with graft failure, myocardial dysfunction, arrhythmias, infarction, or sudden cardiac death. The gold standard for diagnosing CAV is coronary angiography. An increase in maximal intimal thickness of ≥ 0.5 mm during the first post transplant year on intravascular ultrasound is often used as a surrogate marker of rapidly progressive CAV.[90] When vascular changes are concentric and longitudinal, angiography may underestimate the severity of vascular changes, and only intravascular ultrasound or optical coherence tomography can diagnose graft vasculopathy in a patient with unexplained graft failure and no evidence of rejection. Dobutamine stress echocardiography is the best-validated non-invasive method, and may be used instead of angiography in heart recipients with significantly reduced renal function, or free of angiographically proven disease five years after transplantation.[91] In patients with poor acoustic window, stress myocardial perfusion scintigraphy is an alternative. In general, patients diagnosed with CAV should be regularly checked by echocardiography, and annually by coronary angiography.[90]

Despite evolving treatment approaches for CAV, focus should be on prevention and early detection, as already haemodynamically significant CAV can be treated only palliatively.

Besides better survival, the use of MMF, as opposed to AZA for immunosuppression, was associated with a trend toward a lower maximal intimal thickness.[92] mTOR inhibitors inhibit the proliferation of vascular fibroblast and smooth muscle cells, with a beneficial effect on graft vessels.[93] However, the use of everolimus and sirolimus is limited by side-effects, including increased risk of early post transplant infection and enhanced nephrotoxicity of CNIs, which may be alleviated by use of CNI-minimization immunosuppressive protocols. Besides CAV prevention, early introduction of everolimus in CNI-free protocols was shown to improve renal function, although at the expense of more frequent graft rejection.[94]

Statins are routinely prescribed for the majority of heart transplant recipients, aimed primarily to prevent CAV and atherosclerosis.

Once CAV is established, CNI replacement with sirolimus and continuation of MMF and steroid, or replacement of MMF with sirolimus and continuation of CNI and steroid may be useful.[93] Unlike in conventional coronary atherosclerosis, PCI in CAV has unsatisfactory long-term results. Due to high restenosis rates, control angiography is recommended 6 months after PCI. In selected patients, retransplantation remains as the curative option. There is no consensus on the role of prophylactic implantable cardioverter–defibrillators in patients with severe CAV.

Infections

Infections in heart recipients represent an important cause of morbidity and mortality. The risk of infections in allograft recipients depends on the intensity of immunosuppression, and on epidemiologic exposure of both donor and patient.

Donor selection process should include infection screening with respect to the risk of microbial transmission, such as hepatitis B and C, or HIV, and a stratification of future infection risk in order to tailor anitmicrobial prophylaxis in recipients (e.g. CMV serology).[70] Considering the COVID-19 pandemic, all donors and recipients should be screened for the presence of SARS-Cov-2, and if positive, not accepted for heart transplantation. On top of the standard vaccination protocol (see ISHLT Listing Critera for Heart Transplantation),[3] vaccination against COVID-19 should be performed in both transplant candidates and transplant recipients, as it has been shown as safe and effective.[95]

Many heart transplant centres give prophylactic peri-operative antibiotic therapy according to the specific hospital microbial flora to reduce early infection risk.

An obligatory part of pre-transplant patient work-up is a thorough evaluation of microbial exposure to prevent opportunistic infections in the post transplant period.

In heart allograft recipients, as in other solid organ recipients, post transplant infections are defined as early (within 1 month), intermediate (1–12 months), and late (> 12 months). Infections occurring within 1 month following heart transplantation are most commonly hospital-related and dependent on donor/recipient factors. Intermediate infections are mostly opportunistic, with decreasing risk by the end of the first post transplant year that correlates with routine reduction in immunosuppressive therapy, especially steroids. Antimicrobial prophylaxis is given for opportunistic infections, and usually prescribed during the first 3–12 post-transplantation months. Although the majority of late infections are by their nature community-acquired, it is important to be vigilant for late reactivation of opportunistic agents such as *Mycobacterium tuberculosis*, *Aspergillus* family fungi, or CMV, that may mimic non-infectious diseases.[70] Different centres suggest and use diverse post transplant follow-up protocols, that include particular antimicrobial drugs regimens.

A significant number of infections can be prevented by patient education, patient exposure reduction, reduction in immunosuppressive drug levels (e.g. steroid-free protocols), and vaccination.

COVID-19 outbreak brought COVID-19 infection as an important issue in allgoraft recipients. Recently a flow diagram of managment COVID-19 infection in heart transplant patients has been proposed (Figure 11.4.4).[96]

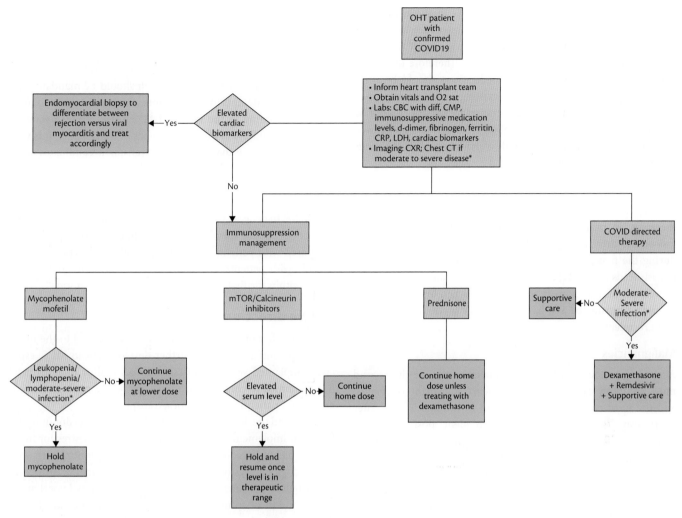

Figure 11.4.4 Flow diagram with suggested management in heart transplant patients affected with COVID-19.
Reproduced from Ballout JA, Ahmed T, Kolodziej AR. COVID-19 and Heart Transplant: A Case Series and Review of the Literature. *Transplant Proc.* 2021 May;53(4):1219-1223. doi: 10.1016/j.transproceed.2021.02.015 with permission from Elsevier.

Arterial hypertension

Arterial hypertension is a common comorbidity in heart transplant recipients and associated with worse outcome.[97] Denervation status of transplanted heart, water, and salt retention as a side-effect of glucocorticoid therapy, and vasoconstriction mediated by CNI, make heart transplant recipients prone to hypertension development. Everolimus-based regimens have shown a more favourable blood pressure profile over the first 1 to 3 years after heart transplantation.[98] Despite obligatory diet and lifestyle modification, majority of patients need antihypertensive medications for the appropriate blood pressure regulation. No class of antihypertensive drugs has been proven to be superior in heart transplant recipients, and usually patients need a combination of antihypertensives for hypertension management.[99] However, medications should be prescribed with caution, as dydiropropyridine calcium channel antagonists may be associated with increased circulating levels of cyclosporine, and renin-angiotensin-aldosterone antagonists may interfere with renal function.

Dyslipidaemia

The use of glucocorticoids, CNIs, and PSIs, such as everolimus or sirolimus, as well as other transplant-related medications, such as triazole angifungals, are associated with an elevated prevalence of dyslipidemia in heart transplant recipients. Statins are usually effective in reducing total cholesterol and low-density lipoprotein cholesterol.

However, it seems that the role of statins in management of heart transplant patients are far greater than lipid lowering, and therefore statins should be initiated very early after heart transplantation, irrespective of the lipid profile. According to the evidence from the pooled analysis, it has been suggested that statins improve survival, may prevent fatal rejection episodes, decrease the incidence of coronary vasculopathy, and even may decrease terminal cancer risk.[100]

Diabetes mellitus

Diabetes mellitus can adversely affect both graft and patient survival,[77] and is frequent in patients after heart transplantation, with a greater than 30% incidence of post transplant diabetes mellitus%.[101] High doses of glucocorticoids in the early post-operative phase and glucocorticoids in maintenance therapy, as well as calcineurin inhibitors, may predispose heart transplant recipients to new onset diabetes mellitus.[70] Therefore the use of diabetogenic immunosuppressive medications should be minimized in patients with either pre-existing or newly developed diabetes mellitus. Diabetes in post transplant patients should be controlled according to current diabetes management guidelines, although a less restrictive approach of HbA1c goal in the range 7.5–8.0% range has been proposed.[102]

Osteoporosis

Osteoporosis is a common side-effect of immunosuppressive therapies, in particular glucocorticoids. Bone mineral density loss occurs already early post transplant, and bone fractures peak during the first 2 years after heart transplantation.[102] As osteoporosis leads in general to an increased morbidity and mortality, prevention of osteoporosis with vitamin D and bisphosphonates should be considered and has proven to be useful in heart transplant recipients.[103]

Malignancies

According to the ISHLT Register, malignancies are the second most common cause of death in heart transplant recipients, and the most common cause of death in the first 5 years after heart transplantation.[6] The most frequent post transplant cancer risk factors are higher recipient age, male sex, smoking, pre-transplant malignancy, diabetes mellitus, more than one hospitalization for rejection during the first year after transplantation.[6,104] The Registry data from 2006-2011 show that within the first five post transplant years 12.4% of patients developed malignancy: 8.4% had a skin malignancy; 4.5% non-skin solid cancer; and 0.9% post transplant lymphoproliferative disorder (PTLD).[2] The most common post-transplant malignancy is non-melanoma skin cancer. Cumulative skin cancer incidence varies from 14.9% to 42%, being up to eight times higher than in general population. Any kind of solid organ cancer appeared in 2.9% in 1-year, 6.2% in 5-year, and 10.1% in 10 year survivors.[104] Lung cancer is the most frequent post-transplant solid organ cancer followed by prostate, colorectal, and breast cancers.[105] PTLD is a unique type of malignancy after organ transplantation. Risk of lymphomas is 20–30 times higher in children and young adults after heart transplant than in the non-transplant population. Most PTLD results from Epstein-Barr virus infection. Induction therapy with ATG is considered as a risk factor for PTLD. More recent studies demonstrate a lower risk of PTLD in using a cumulative reduced doses of ATG.[106] There is existing evidence that swithching from CNI to mTOR inhibitor might help reducing de novo malignancies. A single-centre cohort analysis with a mean follow-up of 10 years has shown a reduced incidence of de novo malignancies and PTLD in heart transplant patients who were converted to sirolimus with complete CNI withdrawal.[107] Furthermore, switching to mTOR containing immunosuppression after the initial diagnosis of malignancy has been shown to decrease mortality.[108]

Retransplantation

This should be reserved for highly selected patients with severe graft dysfunction and failure. As we are facing a far lower supply of donor hearts than is needed to meet demand, a rational approach in listing patients for retransplantation should be mandatory, to prevent futile attempts to save pateints with predictable poor outcomes. According to the ISHLT data, cardiac retransplantation represents about 3% of the total number of transplants.[6] It is very important to know that potential retransplant candidates carry very different post retransplantation mortality risk, and therefore each decision should be made by an experienced team, taking into account the individual risk profile for each potential retransplant candidate. In general, patients with chronic rejection and/or CAV have an acceptable survival prognosis after the retransplantation, compared with patients with primary graft dysfunction, and especially with patients with acute rejection or early graft failure, that is within the first year post original transplantation.[109-111]

Future directions

As the number of donors is far too small compared to the numbers of potential recipients, further development in MCS, especially implanted ventricular assist devices and/or total artificial heart is aimed to compensate a huge gap between allograft availability and patients in a need for a transplant.

To expand the donor pool, use of extended criteria donor hearts has been implemented in some transplantation centres for high-risk recipients. Extended criteria hearts include donor hearts with impared global systolic function and/or regional wall-motion abnormalities, coronary artery diseases, as well as hypertensive hearts, and those from donors with cardiovascular death (DCD). To minimize ischaemia-induced damage in DCD hearts, a methodology of ex vivo perfusion systems have been developed, with favourable short-term clinical outcomes.[112,113]

Conclusion

Despite all advances in drug and device therapies for heart failure, it is a progressive entity that may develop in to the advanced form, which is by definition refractory to conventional treatments. After the introduction of cyclosporine in the 1980s, heart transplantation, as for other solid organ allotransplantations, became a state-of-the-art therapy for the end-organ failure in appropriately selected patients. In the meantime, development of surveillance tools as well as advances in immunosuppressive regimens, and other evidence-based therapeutic procedures, established heart transplantation as the best treatment option for terminal myocardial disease, with a median survival of about 13.5 years and a very good quality of life for the majority of recipients, selected according to the current guidelines. However, the world is faced with a growing population affected by advanced heart failure, and, at the same time, far too few donor organs are available. Therefore, durable continuous flow (left) ventricular assist devices should be widely but carefully used, to safely bridge potential transplant recipients to the transplantation. For now, it seems unlikely that sophisticated implantable heart pumps, total artificial hearts, regenerative therapies, or genetically engineered xenotransplants will be able in the near future to replace cardiac allograft transplantation as the only real currative method for treating patients with terminal heart disease.

In conclusion, heart transplantation, despite the threat of the graft rejection and numorous potential non-immunologically driven complications, remains the golden therapeutic standard for all patients with advanced heart failure suitable for transplantation.

References

1. McDonagh TA, Metra M, Adamo M, et al. 2021 ESC Guidelines for the diagnosis and treatment of acute and chronic heart failure, European Heart Journal 2021;42(36):3638–44.

2. Crespo-Leiro MG, Metra M, Lund LH, et al. Advanced heart failure: a position statement of the Heart Failure Association of the European Society of Cardiology. Eur J Heart Fail 2018;20:1505–35.

3. Mehra MR, Canter CE, Hannan MM, et al. International Society for Heart Lung Transplantation (ISHLT), Infectious Diseases, Pediatric and Heart Failure and Transplantation Councils. The 2016 International Society for Heart Lung Transplantation listing criteria for heart transplantation: a 10-year update. J Heart Lung Transplant 2016; 35:1–23.

4. Khush KK, Cherikh WS, Chambers DC, et al. International Society for Heart and Lung Transplantation. The International Thoracic Organ Transplant Registry of the International Society for Heart and Lung Transplantation; Thirty-sixth adult heart transplantation report – 2019; focus theme: donor and recipient size match. J Heart Lung Transplant 2019;38(10):1056–66.

5. Lund LH, Edwards LN, Kucheryaya AY, et al. International Society for Heart and Lung Transplantation. The Registry of the International Society for Heart and Lung Transplantation. Thirtieth official adult heart transplant report – 2013; focus theme: age. J Heart Lung Transplant 2013;32:951–64.

6. Klush KK, Cherikh WS, Chambers DC, et al. The International Thoracic Organ Transplant Registry of the International Society for Heart and Lung Transplantation Report – 2018; focus theme: multiorgan transplantation. J Heart Lung Transplant 2018;37:1155–68.

7. Stuart C. Newsletter Transplant: International Figures on Donation and Transplantation 2020, pp 54–59. European Directorate for the Quality of Medicines & HealthCare Strasbourg.

8. Goldstein DJ, Bello R, Shin JJ, et al. Outcomes of cardiac transplantation in septuagenarians. J Heart Lung Transplant 2012; 31:679–85.

9. Weiss ES, Allen JG, Russel SDl Shah AS, Conte JV. Impact of recipient body mass index on organ allocation and mortality in orthotopic heart transplantation. J Heart Lung Transplant 2009;28:1150–7.

10. Russo MJ, Hong KN, Davies RR, et al. The effect of body mass index on survival following heart transplantation: do outcomes support consensus guidelines? Ann Surg 2010; 251:144–52.

11. Patlolla V, Mogulla V, DeNofrio D, Konstam MA, Krishnamani R. Outcomes in patients with symptomatic cerebrovascular disease undergoing heart transplantation. J Am Coll Cardiol 2011; 58:1036–41.

12. Sekar B, Newton PJ, Williams SG, Shaw SM. Should we consider patients with coexistent hepatitis B or C infection for orthotopic heart transplantation? J Transplant 2013;2013:748578.

13. Blumberg EA, Rogers CC, and the AST Infectious Diseases Community of Practice. Human immunodeficiency virus in solid organ transplantation. Am J Transplant. 2013;13:169–78.

14. Uriel, N, Nahumi N,Colombo PC, et al. Advanced heart failure in patients infected with human immunodeficiency virus: is there equal access to care? J Heart Lung Transplant 2014; 33:924–30.

15. Aguero F, Castel MA, Cocchi S, et al. An update on heart transplantation in human immunodeficiendy virus-infected patients. Am J Transplantation 2016;16:21–8.

16. Simps DB, Uriel N, Gonzales-Costello J, et al. Human immunodeficiency virus infection and left ventricular assist devices: a case series. J Heart Lung Transplant 2011;30:1060–4.

17. Castel MA, Perez-Villa F, Miro JM. Heart transplantation in HIV infected patients: more cases in Europe. J Heart. Lung Transplant 2011;30:1418.

18. Van Maarseveen EM, Rogers CC, Trofe-Clark J, van Zuilen AD, Mudrikovas T. Drug-naive interactions between antiretroviral and immunosuppressive agent sin HIV-infected patients after solid organ transplantation: a review. AIDS Patient Care STDS 2012; 26: 568–81.

19. Afilalo J, Mottillo S, Eisenberg MJ, et al. Addition of frailty and disability to cardiac surgery risk scores identifies elderly patients at high risk of mortality or major morbidity. Circ Cardiovasc Qual Outcomes 2012;5:222–8.

20. Khan H. Kalogeropoulos AP, Georgiopoulou VV, et al. Frailty and risk for heart failure in older adults; the health, aging and body somposition study. Am Heart J 2013; 166:887–94.

21. Afilalo. J, Eisenberg MJ, Morin JF, et al. Gait speed as incremental predictor of mortality and major morbidity in elderly patients undergoing cardiac surgery. J Am Coll Cardiol 2010; 56:1668–76.

22. Ohiomoba RO, Youmans QR, Akanyirige PW, et al. History of cigarette smoking and heart transplant outcomes. Int J Cardiol Heart Vasc. 2020;30:100599,

23. Biagini E, Spirito P, Leone O, et al. Heart transplantation in hypertrophic cardiomyopathy. Am J Cardiol 2008; 101:387–92,

24. Maron MS, Kalsmith. BM, Udelson JE, et al. Survival after cardiac transplantation in patients with hypertrophic cardiomyopathy. Circ Heart Fail 2010; 3:574–9,

25. Marcus FI, McKenna WJ, Sherill. D, et al. Diagnosisof arrhythmogenic right ventricular cardiomyopathy/dysplasia: proposed modification of the task force criteria. Circulation 2010; 121:1533–41,

26. Pinamonti B, Dragos AM, Pyxaras SA et al. Prognostic predictors in arrhythmogenic right ventricular cardiomyopathy: results from a 10-year registry. Eur Hear J 2011; 32:1105–13.

27. Ottaviani G, Segura AM, Rajapreyar IN, et al. Left ventricular nonconpaction cardiomyopathy in end-stage heart failure patients undergoing orthotopic heart transplantation. Cardiovasc Pathol 2016; 25(4):293–9.

28. Maron BJ, Towbin JA, Thiene G, et al. Contemporary definitions and classification of the cardiomyopathies: an American Heart Association scientific statement from the Council on Clinical Cardiology. Heart Failure and Transplantation Committee: Quality of Care and Outcomes Research and Functional Genomics and Translational Biology Interdisciplinary Working Groups: and Council on Epidemiology and Prevention. Circulation 2006; 113:1807–16.

29. Scaefer RM, Tylki-Szumanska A, Hilz MJ. Enzyme replacement therapy for Fabry disease: a systemic review of available evidence. Drugs 2009;69:2179–205.

30. Falk RH, Alexander KM, Liao R, Dorbala S. AL (Light-Chain) cardiac amyloidosis: a review of diagnosis and therapy. J Am Coll Cardiol 2016; 68:1323–41.

31. Rugberg FL, Grogan M, Hanna M, Kelly JW, Maurer MS. Transthyretin amyloid cardiomyopathy: JACC State-of-the-Art Review. J Am Coll Cardiol 2019; 11:73:2872–91.

32. Chen Q, Moriguchi J, Levine R, *et al.* Outcomes of heart transplantation in cardiac amyloidosis patients: a single center experience. Transplant Proc 2021; 53:329–334

33. Kirsten AV, Kreusser MM, Blum P, *et al.* Improved outcomes after heart transplantation for cardiac amyloidosis in the modern era. J Heart Lung Transplant 2018; 7:611–18.

34. West J, Pollock-Barziv SM, Diopchaud AI, *et al.* ABO-incompatible heart. Transplantation in infants. N Eng J Med 2021;344:793–800.

35. Chen JM, Edwards NM. Donor selection and management of the high-risk donor. In: Cardiac Transplantation, NM Edwards, JM Chen and Mazzeo PA, editors, Humana Press Inc. 2004, pp 19–36

36. Cacciatore F, Palmieri V, Amerelli C, Malello C, Napoli C. Further evidence of HLA DR matching in determining heart transplantation outcome. Transpl Int 2020; 33:1551–2.

37. Osoria Jaramillo E, Hasnoot GW, Kaider A, *et al.* Molecular level HLA mismatch is associated with rejection and worsened graft survival in heart transplant recipients – a retrospective study. Transpl Int 2020; 202;9:1078–88.

38. Chan BBK, Fleischer KJ, Bergin JD, *et al.* Weight is not an accurate criterion for adult cardiac transplant size matching. Ann Thorac Surg 1991;52:1230–6.

39. Oprzedkiewicz, A, Mado H, Szezurek W, *et al.* Donor-recipient matching in heart transplantation. The Open Cardiovascular Medicine Journal 2020;14:42–7.

40. Kransdorf EP, Kittleson MM, Bench LR, *et al.* Predicted heart mass is the optimal metric size for match in heart transplantation. J Heart Lung Transplant 2019;38:156–65.

41. Reed RM, Netzer G, Hunsicker L. *et al.* Cardiac size and sex-matching in heart transplantation: size matters in matters of seks and the heart. JACC Heart Fail 2014;2:73–83.

42. Ghodsizad A, Bordel V, Ungerer M, Karck M, Bekeredjian R, Ruhparwar A. Ex-vivo coronary angiography of a donor heart in the organ care system. Heart Surg Forum 2012; 15:161–3.

43. Li, Y, Guo S, Liu G, *et al.* Three preservation solutions for cold storage of cardiac allografts: A systematic review and meta-analysis. Artif Organs 2016; 40:489–96

44. Monteguado Vela M, Garcia Saez D, Simon AR. Current approaches in retrieval and heart preservation. Ann Cardiothor Surg 2018; 7:67–74.

45. Shumway NE, Lower R, Stofer RC. Transplantation of the heart. Adv Surg 1966;2:265–84.

46. Forni A, Faggian G, Luciani GB, *et al.* Reduced incidence of cardiac arrhythmias after orthotopic heart transplantation with direct bicaval anastomosis. Transplant Proc 1996;28:289–92.

47. Aziz TM, Burgess MI, El-Gamel A, *et al.* Orthotopic cardiac transplantation technique: survey of current practice. Ann Thorac Surg, 1999: 68; 1242–6 and Davies RR *et al.* Standard vs. bicaval techniques for orthotopic heart transplantation: An analysis from the United Network of Organ Sharing database. J Thorac Cardiovasc Surg 2010; 140: 700–8.

48. Siney PP. Posttransplant management. In Cardiac Transplantation: The Columbia University Medical Center/New York-Presbyterian Hospital Manual, Edwards NM, Chen JM, Mazzeo PA, editors; Humana Press, Totowa, New Jersey, 2004, pp 123–55.

49. Lisboa LA, de Amelda JP, Gerent AM, *et al.* Vasopressin versus norepinephrine in patients with vasoplegic shock after cardiac surgery. The VANCS randomized controlled trial. Anesthaesiology 2017; 126:85–93.

50. Hajjar LA, Vincent JL, Galas, FRBG, *et al.* Vasopressin versus norepinephrine in patients with vasoplegic shockafter cardiac surgery. The VANCS randomized controlled trial. Anesthesiology 2017;126:85–93.

51. Russel JA. Vassopressin, norepinephrine and vasodilatory shock after cardiac surgery: another VASST difference? Anesthesiology 2017;126:9–11.

52. Morales DLS, Gregg D, Helman DN, *et al.* Arginine vasopressin in the treatment of 50 patients with postcardiotomy vasodilatory shock. Ann Thorac Surg 2000;69:102–6.

53. Landry DW, Oliver JA. The pathogenesis of vasodilatory shock. N Engl J Med 2001;345:588–95.

54. Robertson GL. The regulation of vasopressin function in health and disease. Rec Prog Horm Res 1997;33:333–86.

55. Hosenpund JD, Bennet LE, Berkeley MK *et al.* The Registry of the International Society for Heart and Lung Transplantation: fifteenth official report – 1998. J Heart Lung Transplant 1998;17:656–8.

56. Hosenpund JD, Novick RJ, Breen TJ, at al. The Registry of the International Society for Heart and Lung Transplantation: twelfth official report –1995. J Heart Lung Transplant 1995;14:805–15.

57. Pinney SP. Posttransplant management. In: Cardiac Transplantation, Edwards NM, Chen JM, Mazzeo PA, editors. Humanna Press Inc 2004, pp 123–155

58. Ardehali A, Hughes K, Sadeghi A, *et al.* Inhaled nitric oxide for pulmonary hypertension after heart transplantation. Transplantation 2001; 72:638–41.

59. Kolsrund O, Karason K, Holmberg E *et al.* Renal function and outcome after heart transplantation. J Thorac Cardiovasc Surg 2018; 155:1593–604.

60. Murphy JM, Frantz R, Cooper L. Endomyocardial biopsy. In: Murphy J, Lloyd M, editors. Mayo Clinic Cardiology Concise Textbook. Minnesota: Rochester; 2007. p 1481

61. Stuart S, Winters GL, Fishbein C, *et al.* Revision of the 1990 working formulation of nomenclature in the diagnosis of heart rejection. ISHLT Consensus Report. J Heart Lung Transplant 2015; 24:1710–20.

62. Oh KT, Mustehsan MH, Goldstein DJ, Saeed O, Jorde UP. Patel SR. Protocol endomyocardial biopsy beyond 6 months – it is time to move on. Am J Transplant 2021;21:825–9.

63. Wu YL, Ye Q, Ho C. Cellular and functional imaging of cardiac transplant rejection, Curr Cardiovasc Imaging Rep 2011;4:50–62.

64. Stuart S, Winters GL, Fishbein C, *et al.* Revision of the 1990 working formulation of nomenclature in the diagnosis of heart rejection. ISHLT Consensus Report. J Heart Lung Transplant 2005; 24:1710–20.

65. Stehlik J, Edward LB, Kucheryavaya AY, *et al.* The Registry of the International Society for Heart and Lung Transplantation twenty-seventh official adult heart transplant report – 2010 J Heart Lung Transp 2010; 29:1089–103.

66. Lindenfeld J, Miller GG, Shakar SF, *et al.* Drug therapy in the heart transplant recipient: part II: immunosuppressive drugs. Circulation 2004;110:3858–65.

67. Beiras-Fernandez A, Thein A, Hammer C. Induction of immunosuppression with polyclonal antithymocyte globulins: an overview. Exp Clin Transplant 2003;1:79–84.

68. Møller CH, Gustafsson F, Gluud C, Steinbrüchel DA. Interleukin-2 receptor antagonists as induction therapy after heart transplantation: systematic review with meta-analysis of randomized trials. J Heart Lung Transplant 2008;27:835–42.

69. Opelz G, Henderson R. Incidence of non Hodkin lymphoma in kidney and heart transplant recipients. Lancet 1993;342:1514–16.

70. Jessup M, Acker M. Cardiac transplantation. In: Heart Failure, Mann DL editor, Elsevier, Saunders 2011; pp 787–801.

71. Urschel S, Altamirano-Diaz LA, West LJ. Immunosupression armamentarium in 2010: mechanistic and clinical considerations. Pediatr Clin North Am 2010;57:433–57.

72. Penninga L, Møller CH, Gustafsson F, Steinbrüchel DA, Gluud C. Tacrolimus versus cyclosporine as primary immunosuppression after heart transplantation: systematic review with meta-analyses and trial sequential analyses of randomised trials. Eur J Clin Pharmacol 2010;66:1177–87.

73. Eisen HJ, Kobashigawa J, Keogh A, *et al.* Three-year results of a randomized, double-blind, controlled trial of mycophenolate mofetil

versus azathioprine in cardiac transplant recipients. J Heart Lung Transplant 2005;24:517–25.

74. Eisen HJ, Kobashigawa J, Starling RC, et al. Everolimus versus mycophenolate mofetil in heart transplantation: a randomized, multicenter trial. Am J Transplant 2013;13:1203–16.

75. Andreassen AK, Andersson B, Gustafsson F, et al. Everolimus initiation and early calcineurin inhibitor withdrawal in heart transplant recipients: a randomized trial. Am J Transplant 2014;14:1828–38.

76. Chang DH, Young JC, Dilibero D, Patel JK, Kobashigawa JA. Heart transplant immunusupression strategies at Cedars-Sinai Medical Center. Int J Heart Fail 2021; 3:15–30.

77. Constanzo MR, Dipchand A, Starling R. et al. The International Society of Heart and Lung Transplantation Guidelines for the care of heart transplant recipients. J Heart Lung Transplant 2010; 29:914–56.

78. Kirklin JK, Brown RN, Huang ST et al. Rejection with hemodynamic compromise: objective evidence for eficacy photopheresis. J Heart Lung Transplant 2006; 25:283–8.

79. Al-Mohaissen MA, Virani SA. Allosensitization in heart transplantation: an overview. Can J Cardiol 2014;30(2):161–72.

80. Colvin MM, Cook JL, Chang PP, et al. Sensitization in heart transplantation: emerging knowledge: a scientific statement from the American Heart Association. Circulation 2019;139(12):e553–78.

81. Cecka JM. Calculated PRA (CPRA) – the new measure of sensitization for transplant candidates. Am J Transplant 2010;10:26–9.

82. Leech SH, Lopez-Cepero M, LeFor WM, et al. Management of the sensitized cardiac recipient: the use of plasmapheresis and intravenous immunoglobulin. Clin Transplant 2006;20(4):476–84.

83. Vo AA, Lukovsky M, Toyoda M, et al. Rituximab and intravenous immune globulin for desensitization during renal transplantation. N Engl J Med 2008;359(3):242–51.

84. Kobashigawa JA, Patel JK, Kittleson MM, et al. The long-term outcome of treated sensitized patients who undergo heart transplantation. Clin Transplant 2011;25(1):E61–7.

85. Smith JD, Banner NR, Hamour IM, et al. De novo donor HLA-specific antibodies after heart transplantation are an independent predictor of poor patient survival. Am J Transplant 2011;11(2):312–19.

86. Ho EK, Vlad G, Vasilescu ER, et al. Pre- and posttransplantation allosensitization in heart allograft recipients: major impact of de novo alloantibody production on allograft survival. Hum Immunol 2011;72(1):5–10.

87. Lund LH, Edwards LB, Dipchand AI, et al. The Registry of the International Society for Heart and Lung Transplantation: thirty-third adult heart transplant report – 2016; focus theme: primary diagnostic indications for transplant. J Heart Lung Transplant 2016;35:1158–69.

88. Patel CB, Holley CL. Cardiac allograft vasculopathy: a formidable foe. J Am Coll Cardiol 2019;74:52–53.

89. Nikolova AP, Kobashigawa JA. Cardiac allograft vasculopathy: the enduring enemy of cardiac transplantation. Transplantation 2019;103:1338–48.

90. Payne GA, Hage FG, Acharya D. Transplant allograft vasculopathy: role of multimodality imaging in surveillance and diagnosis. J Nucl Cardiol. 2016; 23:713–27.

91. Elkaryoni A, Abu-Sheasha G, Altibi AM, Hassan A, Ellakany K, Nanda NC. Diagnostic accuracy of dobutamine stress echocardiography in the detection of cardiac allograft vasculopathy in heart transplant recipients: A systematic review and meta-analysis study. Echocardiography 2019;36(3):528–36.

92. Kaczmarek I, Ertl B, Schmauss D, et al. Preventing cardiac allograft vasculopathy: long-term beneficial effects of mycophenolate mofetil. J Heart Lung Transplant. 2006;25(5):550–6.

93. Bellumkonda L, Patel J. Recent advances in the role of mammalian target of rapamycin inhibitors on cardiac allograft vasculopathy. Clin Transplant. 2020;34(1):e13769.

94. Schaffer SA, Ross HJ. Everolimus: efficacy and safety in cardiac transplantation. Expert Opin Drug Saf. 2010;9(5):843–54.

95. Aslam S, Goldstein DR, Vos R, et al. COVID-19 vaccination in our transplant recipients: The time is now. J Heart Lung Transplant. 2021;40(3):169–71.

96. Ballout JA, Ahmed T, Kolodziej AR. COVID-19 and Heart Transplant: A Case Series and Review of the Literature. Transplant Proc. 2021;53(4):1219–23.

97. Lund LH, Edwards LB, Kucheryavaya AY, et al. The Registry of the International Society for Heart and Lung Transplantation: thirty-first official adult heart transplant report – 2014; focus theme: retransplantation. J Heart Lung Transplant 2014;33:996–1008.

98. Andreassen AK, Broch K, Eiskjær H, et al. Blood pressure in de novo heart transplant recipients treated with everolimus compared with a cyclosporine-based regimen: results from the randomized SCHEDULE trial. Transplantation 2019;103:781–8.

99. Brozena SC, Johnson MR, Ventura H, et al. Effectiveness and safety of diltiazem or lisinopril in treatment of hypertension after heart transplantation: results of a prospective, randomized multicenter trail. J Am Coll Cardiol 1996;27:1707–12.

100. Vallakati A, Reddy S, Dunlap ME, Taylor DO. Impact of statin use after heart transplantation. A meta analysis. Circ Heart Fail 2016;9:e003265.

101. Zielińska K, Kukulski L, Wróbel M, Przybyłowski P, Zakliczyński M, Strojek K. Prevalence and risk factors of new-onset diabetes after transplantation (NODAT). Ann Transplant. 2020 Aug 25;25:e926556.

102. Wallia A, Illuri V, Molitch ME. Diabetes care after transplant: definitions, risk factors, and clinical management. Med Clin North Am 2016;100:535–50.

103. Leidig-Bruckner G, Hosch S, Dodidou P, Ritschel D, Conradt C, Klose C, et al. Frequency and predictors of osteoporotic fractures after cardiac or liver transplantation: a follow-up study. Lancet 2001;357:342–7.

104. Youn JC, Stehlik J, Wilk AR, , et al. Temporal trends of de novo malignancy development after heart transplantation. J Am Coll Cardiol. 2018;71(1):40–9.

105. Crespo-Leiro MG, Villa-Arranz A, Manito-Lorite N, et al. Lung cancer after heart transplantation: results from a large multicenter registry. Am J Transplant. 2011;11(5):1035–40.

106. Hertig A, Zuckermann A. Rabbit antithymocyte globulin induction and risk of post-transplant lymphoproliferative disease in adult and pediatric solid organ transplantation: an update. Transpl Immunol 2015;32(3):179–87.

107. Asleh R, Clavell AL, Pereira NL, et al. Incidence of malignancies in patients treated with sirolimus following heart transplantation. J Am Coll Cardiol. 201;73(21):2676–88.

108. Rivinius R, Helmschrott M, Ruhparwar A, et al. Analysis of malignancies in patients after heart transplantation with subsequent immunosuppressive therapy. Drug Des Devel Ther. 2014;9:93–102.

109. Miller RJH, Clarke BA, Howlett JG, et al. Outcomes in patients undergoing heart transplantation: a propensity matched cohort analysis of the UNOS Registry. J Heart Lung Transpl 2019;38:1067–74.

110. Radovancevic B, McGiffin DC, Kobashigawa JA, et al. Retransplantation in 7,290 primary transplant patients: a 10-year multi-institutional study. J Heart Lung Transplant 2003;22:862–8.

111. Tjang YS, Tenderich G, Hornik L, Körfer R. Cardiac retransplantation in adults: an evidence-based systematic review. Thorac Cardiovasc Surg. 2008;56(6):323–7.

112. Kim IC. Youn JC, Komashigawa JA. The past, present and future of heart transplantation. Korean Circ J 2018; 48:565–90.

113. Ardehalli A, Esmaillan F, Deng M, et al. Ex-vivo perfusion of donor hearts for human heart transplantation (PROCEED II): a prospective open-label, multicentre randomised non-inferiority trial. Lancet 2015; 385:2577–84.

CHAPTER 11.5

Palliative care in the heart failure trajectory

Tiny Jaarsma, Donna Fitzsimons,
Lisa Hjelmfors, Loreena Hill,
Ekaterini Lambrinou, and Anna Strömberg

Contents

Introduction

Palliation is an essential but often overlooked aspect of heart failure (HF) care that urgently requires implementation. As a result of advanced pharmaceutical, device, and surgical interventions, patients with HF have an improved longevity; however, this may come at a cost of greater symptom burden.[1] HF can have a major influence on the patient's emotional, physical, spiritual, and social well-being and patients with HF often have typical palliative care needs.[2]

The World Health Organization (WHO) defines palliative care as '*an approach that improves the quality of life of patients (adults and children) and their families who are facing problems associated with life-threatening illness. It prevents and relieves suffering through the early identification, correct assessment and treatment of pain and other problems, whether physical, psychosocial or spiritual.*'[3]

Palliative care aims to prevent and alleviate suffering through early detection, careful analysis, and treatment of physical, mental, social, and existential problems through collaboration across multi-professional specialties. Palliative care should be offered/available early in the disease trajectory along with life-prolonging treatment.

In this chapter, the relevance of palliative care in HF management is described. Furthermore, the importance of control and management of the most common HF symptoms are discussed. The chapter presents different organizational models of palliative care and argues for coordinated, interdisciplinary care, and it addresses ethical issues such as challenging conversations with difficult decisions, ethical issues related to implantation and deactivation of devices, and deprescribing medication. Finally, practical recommendations regarding how to communicate with the patient and family during the HF trajectory are provided.

Considering palliative care in the HF trajectory

The trajectory of HF is often unpredictable, which is why it is has been difficult to pinpoint a specific time when palliative care should be considered. However, palliative care (according to the WHO definition) is relevant and important to all patients with HF regardless of stage of their illness. Optimal symptom control and a systematical addressing of patients' and families' needs and preferences for treatment should be the focus of care.[4] In this way, palliative care can be offered in parallel with usual HF care throughout the whole illness trajectory.[4]

In the past two decades, there has been widespread discussion in the literature regarding the integration of palliative care within HF management and there is broad consensus that we should consider a palliative approach early within the patient journey.[6,7] In addition, we must abandon outdated notions that we *either* offer disease-modifying

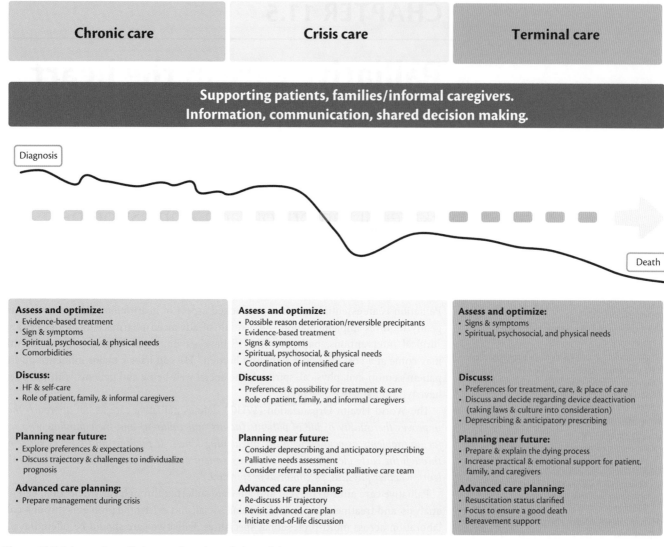

Figure 11.5.1 Integrating palliative care throughout the heart failure trajectory.
Reproduced from Hill L, Prager Geller T, Baruah R, et al. Integration of a palliative approach into heart failure care: a European Society of Cardiology Heart Failure Association position paper. Eur J Heart Fail. 2020 Dec;22(12):2327-2339. doi: 10.1002/ejhf.1994 with permission from John Wiley and Sons.

interventions, *or* palliative care – because evidence confirms that it is the combination of the two that have the potential to offer greatest benefit to patients and their families.[4,8] Indeed, it could be argued that all aspects of HF management are, in fact, palliative in nature, because the focus is on treating symptoms, rather than curing the disease. Thus, integrating palliative approaches into conventional HF management aimed at disease modification is a necessary and logical step (⊃ Figure 11.5.1). For patients with HF, it is assumed that basic palliative care needs can be managed by the patient's cardiologist, HF nurse, or general practitioner, while more complex palliative care needs should be managed by multidisciplinary specialist teams with specialist training in palliative care.[5,9] Palliative care interventions that are combined with HF management can improve patient outcomes and decrease costs and utilization.[10] The addition of palliative care to evidence-based HF care can improve quality of life, psychosocial (anxiety/depression), physical and spiritual well-being.[11]

The implementation of palliative care in HF care is conventionally based on prognostication or risk of death, whereas it should be initiated on recognition of the palliative care needs of the patient and family.

Organization of palliative care provision to HF patients

A variety of different models that integrate the provision of palliative care within a specialist HF services are available. An integrated approach is not widespread within clinical practice, and it is estimated that less than a quarter of European countries have designated palliative care units for people with advanced HF.[12] It is important to recognize the heterogeneity of HF service provision between different countries, and to appreciate the impact of different healthcare infrastructures on the continuity of patient care. Thus a worldwide 'one size fits all' approach is unlikely to be feasible and we need to consider the wider contextual issues

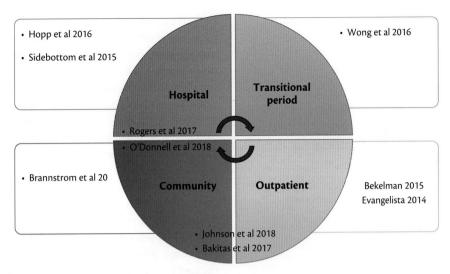

Figure 11.5.2 Studies illustrating setting of multidisciplinary care provision.

to determine the most appropriate model and affect meaningful change (➲ Figure 11.5.2).

Primary palliative care

Perhaps the most common model of integrated palliative care in the HF field is the concept of primary palliative care that emphasizes the role of the generalist HF team members, such as a HF nurse of doctor. This approach assumes that all clinicians are competent in providing basic palliative care interventions and is consistent with the belief that palliative care should be available for all patients and begin from the point of diagnosis in HF.[13] The core components of primary palliative care include symptom management, communication regarding the goals of care, advance care planning, and psychosocial care and care coordination.[14] The unpredictable disease trajectory in HF means that it is vitally important not to delay the initiation of supportive and palliative care discussions, and in that context a primary approach is advantageous, because it does not require specialist referral. Given the rising incidence of HF associated with the aging demographic, it has been asserted that primary palliative care is the most sustainable model to effectively and efficiently address the patients' needs.[15]

Many of the core components of palliative care such as symptom assessment and management, psychosocial support, and advance care planning are central to the provision of high-quality HF care, and so the integrated approach has the potential to produce a more feasible and cost effective management plan.

Specialist palliative care

A registry study that evaluated 31,060 deaths from heart disease concluded that only 10.6% of the patients with heart diseases died in a palliative care setting.[16] Furthermore, few patients and their families were aware of the possible symptoms that could occur during the illness trajectory and the imminence of death.[16] In a study from the United Kingdom, the worlds' largest primary care database was explored to find how many patients with HF were recognized as needing a palliative care approach. Of the patients with HF that were in the database, 7% (234/3122) were in a palliative care register compared to 48% (3669/7608) of cancer patients. Twenty-nine patients with HF were entered into the register just within a week of their death.[17]

Most of the studies that have evaluated models of integration focus on adding a specialist palliative care referral into an existing heart failure service. Several large-scale studies such as ENABLE CHF-PC,[18] PAL-HF,[11] and PREFER,[19] have tested innovative models of integrated care. A recent systematic review of the available evidence considered data from 23 different studies and found an improvement in patient reported outcomes (symptom burden, depression, functional status, quality of life), as well as resource use and costs of care.[20] However, it is also clear that where referral to specialist palliative care occurs, it is often late in the disease trajectory and patients' symptoms may be advanced.

It would seem that in terms of referral to Specialist Palliative Care, timing is everything for patients with advanced heart failure and their families, since many studies confirm that often we offer too little, too late.[21] The HFA guidance document sets out important triggers that may precipitate involvement of a specialist palliative care team.[15] It is very useful to reflect upon these critical opportunities, as key points when more specific expertise is valuable and if not already done, the concept of palliative care can be introduced to patients and their families (➲ Table 11.5.1).

Interdisciplinary approach

The concept of palliative care takes a holistic view of the patient and their family, therefore palliative care provision is not the sole terrain of one profession, rather it requires effective interdisciplinary working, communication and collaboration.[15,20]

Within the literature, there is a strong evidence base for nurse-led HF care, and specialist HF nurses play an important role in the delivery of effective HF care at the end of life. However, given the complexity of the biopsychosocial issues affecting people with advanced HF, the contribution of pharmacists, social workers, psychologists etc. is also vital. Data from qualitative studies suggest that dealing with such complexity is challenging for patients

Table 11.5.1 Possible triggers for the involvement of specialist palliative care for those with HF

Refractory or complex symptoms
When there is spiritual or existential distress
Recurrent HF admissions
Increasingly frequent appropriate ICD shocks
When considering ICD deactivation or non-replacement
Before LVAD implantation or transplant referral
When initiating palliative inotropic therapy
Declining functional status due to progressive HF or a comorbidity
If patients and/or informal carers/surrogates disagree on goals of care
If there is a request for assisted suicide

and caregivers in particular, with high levels of anxiety and uncertainty contributing to poor quality of life, widespread uncertainty, and inability to plan ahead.[22] Thus co-ordination across the care pathway is necessary because although these patients have high rates of repeat hospitalization, they will spend the majority of their time at home. In that context, the family doctor and community nursing team also play a significant role in helping to manage the complexity of symptoms and the unpredictable disease trajectory that typifies heart failure, even in the early stages.

Symptom management

Successful symptom management is one of the cornerstones of palliative care in patients with HF and it can improve the quality of life for both patients and their families during the HF trajectory.[15] A holistic palliative symptom management approach to patients with HF does not only address the physical aspect of symptoms, but also the psychological, social, and spiritual dimensions of suffering to achieve total symptom relief. In order to manage symptoms, successfully clinicians need to systematically assess symptoms using clinical skills and tools for patient reported symptoms, for example, the Edmonton Symptom Assessment Scale, Kansas City Cardiomyopathy Questionnaire, the Memorial Symptom Assessment Scale-Heart Failure.[23-26]

Symptom-monitoring is also an important component of self-care performed by the patients themselves or supported by their family caregivers.[27-29] To increase knowledge and skills related to symptom monitoring, patients with HF and their caregivers should be educated and supported to manage symptoms from diagnosis and throughout the HF trajectory, including information on frequency, how to assess intensity, rate, and duration of a symptoms. Telemonitoring may be a useful and effective tool to support both symptom monitoring and management in selected patients.[30]

The most common symptoms in HF are shortness of breath (breathlessness) and fatigue. Almost all patients in the more advanced stages of the condition have these symptoms. Breathlessness and fatigue can be unspecific and difficult to assess objectively but a visual analogue scale or numeric rating scale can be used, and patients can learn to monitor the different levels of breathlessness and fatigue and the impact it has on their daily life activities and exercise intolerance. Successful symptom management mainly relies on patients' (and/or their caregivers') ability to monitor and interpret symptoms and take appropriate actions to manage the symptoms.[28,29] Symptom management can include both self-care and medical treatment as shown in ⊃ Table 11.5.2.[31]

Symptom management in HF is complex and there are several challenges related to symptoms in patients with HF. Since most

Table 11.5.2 Overview of the clinical and self-care management of the most common heart failure symptoms

Symptoms	Medical treatment	Self-care
Breathlessness	Optimal medical therapy. Consider benzodiazepines for anxiety and opiates in end of life care Assess co-morbidities	Non-pharmacology: Sitting upright, hand-held fans, relaxation techniques, breathing exercises Pharmacology: Optimal HF medical therapy. Consider benzodiazepines for anxiety and opiates (morphine) Little benefit of supplementary oxygen in advanced HF alone
Oedema	Flexible diuretic intake Optimal medical heart failure therapy	Support stockings
Fatigue	Optimal medical heart failure therapy Assess co-morbidities	Exercise, physical activity, adequate nutrition
Thirst and xerostomia	Artificial saliva as gel or tablets	Intensified oral hygiene, rinse mouth frequently, free fluid intake, candies, chewing gum, suck ice cubes, or frozen fruit pieces
Pain	Assess cause of pain, e.g. cardiac, musculoskeletal, existential Use appropriate pain medication but avoid NSAIDs	Exercise, physical activity, relaxation techniques, breathing exercises
Nausea and/or poor appetite	Assess cause of nausea. Prescribe antiemetic drugs Replace medications that may cause nausea or other gastrointestinal problems	Dietary changes, avoid triggering smells, alternative or complementary medicine, e.g. acupressure, acupuncture
Anxiety/depression	SSRIs can be used safely and relatively well tolerated in HF but have limited evidence of efficacy	Psychoeducational support, exercise and psychological therapies, e.g. cognitive behavioral therapy

NSAIDs, non-steroidal anti-inflammatory drug; SSRIs, Selective serotonin reuptake inhibitors.

patients with HF have both cardiac and non-cardiac comorbidities causing end-organ damage, this may lead to a range of persistent, distressing and debilitating symptoms. Furthermore, several of the co-morbid conditions, that often occur simultaneously with HF, share a similar symptomatology, such as fatigue, shortness of breath and exercise intolerance. A deterioration of any of these symptoms in a person in addition suffering from more conditions, such as HF, chronic obstructive pulmonary disease (COPD), and renal failure can make it complicated to trace the cause of the deterioration. Additionally a high prevalence of cognitive impairment often occurs in combination with limited social support further complicating HF symptom monitoring and management.[32]

Recently frailty has been highlighted as an important clinical issue to assess in patients with HF. The Heart Failure Association has proposed a HF-specific definition of frailty including four domains: clinical (co-morbidities, weight loss, falls), psycho-cognitive (cognitive impairment, dementia, depression), functional (activities of daily living, Instrumental activities of daily living), low/non mobility, balance), and social (living alone, poor/no social support, institutionalization). Frailty is more common in persons with HF, compared to the general population within the same age span. There is much overlap between HF symptoms and components of frailty since the two syndromes mimic each other. Frail patients with HF are often more symptomatic, but frailty is not per se correlated linearly with HF disease severity.[33]

Due to the complexities already outlined, symptoms as experienced by patients may not always reflect an objective change in the HF condition.[28] However, in more advanced stages symptoms are more obvious and easier to detect and interpret for patients. Patients with the greatest needs of symptom management are those with characteristics of advanced HF as described in ➲ Table 11.5.3.

Table 11.5.3 'Need Help'—Characteristics of patients of advanced heart failure in great need of help with regard to symptom management

N	NYHA / Natriuretic peptides	Persisting NYHA class III or IV and/or high NT-proBNP
E	End-organ dysfunction	Worsening renal or liver dysfunction
E	Ejection fraction	Very low ejection fraction < 20%
D	Defibrillator shocks	Recurrent appropriate defibrillator shocks
H	Hospitalizations	> One hospitalization with heart failure in the last 12 months
E	Oedema	Persisting fluid overload and/or increasing diuretic requirement
L	Low blood pressure	Consistently low BP with systolic < 90 to 100 mmHg
P	Poor medication tolerance	Inability to up-titrate (or need to decrease/terminate) ACEI, beta-blockers, ARNIs, or MRAs

Source data from Crespo-Leiro, M.G., *et al.* Advanced heart failure: a position statement of the Heart Failure Association of the European Society of Cardiology. *Eur J Heart Fail*, 2018. 20(11): p. 1505–1535.

Ethical issues

Challenging conversations with difficult decisions

Contrary to belief, communication to inform advanced planning and future decision-making should ideally be undertaken when the patient's HF symptoms are stable and he/she has the ability to contribute to the conversation, rather than when death is imminent.[34] A patient's preference towards quality over quantity of life can change in accordance with symptoms and their treatment status. For example, hypothetically, members of the general public believed that if they had HF, 83% would prefer care focused on quality of life rather than on survival.[35] In reality, however evidence confirms that despite multiple symptoms, patients with HF remain reluctant to trade quality of life for increased length of life.[36,37] Professionals have a responsibility to respect patients' autonomy and encourage informed shared decision-making through-out the HF trajectory. Choices are complex, rather than black and white, for example option of either curative treatment or palliative care, but a balanced arrangement aligned to both patients' and healthcare professionals' expectations. Unrealistic treatment expectations can have detrimental consequences, leading to unnecessary anxiety, distress, and lack of much needed specialist support.[38] The communication and supportive relationship between the professional, patient, and informal caregiver may be thrown into disarray causing mistrust and confusion at a time when clarity and empathy are paramount.

The Integrated Palliative Care Outcome Scale is a patient-reported outcome measure that has been found to empower patients to become more engaged in the clinical consultation and to highlight their unmet needs.[39] Furthermore, a number of 'checklists' have been developed to encourage both patients and healthcare professionals to initiate difficult conversations, for example a 'question prompt list'.[40] Nevertheless, it is important to achieve this intricate balance between offering patients open, frank yet compassionate, personally connected conversations that acknowledge end-of-life, but yet do not remove hope for life before death.[41]

Ethical issues related to implantation of devices: ICD/CRT/LVAD

The implantation of implantable cardioverter defibrillator (ICD) or cardiac resynchronization device +/- ICD are perceived by many patients as life-saving.[42] Over the years the device may have discharged a successful shock, reinforcing this misconception. However, as HF progresses, the patient becomes more at risk of an arrhythmia and subsequent shock. As our society has a growing elderly population, with many experiencing at least one co-morbidity (e.g. renal disease or cancer), there is an increased likelihood of inappropriate or futile shock being delivered when death is imminent. This was most vividly portrayed in the study that interrogated 125 ICDs post death and concluded more than one third of patients had experienced a ventricular tachyarrhythmia within the last hour of life.[43]

International guidelines recommend that professionals discuss the option of ICD deactivation with the patient and family.[44,45] Deactivation is a simple non-invasive procedure whereby the shock function of the ICD is 'switched off'. At end of life there is an increased risk of the patient experiencing painful and futile shocks. Nevertheless, all too often the discussion and decision is left until death is imminent, placing additional anxiety on family members.

A number of studies have investigated the experience of a shock from the ICD and the subsequent cause of psychological distress with a negative impact on quality of life.[46,47] This may be acceptable while there is equipoise between acceptable quality of life and longevity; however, when the patient transitions into the last phase of life,[15] this argument may no longer be sustainable.

There is increasing awareness of the importance of informed choice concerning advanced HF therapies, such as ventricular assist devices (VAD) and the importance of inclusion of a palliative approach is recommended.[48] Patients in the advanced stages of HF, particularly those referred to or awaiting VAD or transplantation should receive a palliative care consultation before their intervention, to enable realistic treatment expectations and encourage family-centred discussions about provisions following their demise.

Deprescribing of evidence-based medications

The deprescribing of medications is not giving up hope, rather it is a proactive, individualized approach that requires a continuous revision of good prescribing principles and takes into consideration the context of goals of care, life expectancy, values, and preferences.[49] There are several reasons to de-prescribe, which may include risk of adverse drug event (increased with polypharmacy), limited benefit of evidence-based medications, and poor adherence to recommended treatment regimen. Professionals may encounter difficulties in discontinuing therapy due to robust prescribing guidelines, the dearth of deprescribing advice, adverse events recurrence after discontinuation, and patient's medication attachment (https://deprescribing.org). Many patients will have become familiar with their medication regimen and will have been informed at the time of initiation of the purposes of the medications. Any changes to this regimen will lead to unease and an awareness of declining health. Deprescribing requires professionals to be sensitive to potential issues and adopt an approach of good communication and information to ensure the patient and family members are committed and agree with changes made to medications.

A step-wise approach to deprescribing includes[49]:

1. A polypharmacy recognizing phase (appropriate indication, drug interaction)

2. Identifying futile treatment and adverse drug effects, and prioritizing the worse drug withdrawal

3. Withdrawal planning, communication to patient and caregiver, and process coordination

4. Monitoring withdrawal adverse drug events after gradual discontinuation

Communication with the patient and family during the HF trajectory

Patients with HF might not always be aware that their illness is life-limiting and often health-care professionals lack insight into their patients' future treatment preferences.[34] Explanations such as 'reluctance to dispel hope', 'uncertainty how and when to initiate conversations', and 'inadequate training' have been documented as reasons why this stalemate situation may occur.[50–52]

Recent position papers from both Palliative and HF Associations outlined a number of key recommendations that include the systematic review and addressing of patients' and family members' supportive needs and their preferences for care, as well as highlighting advance care planning and appropriate communication.[15,53]

Patients with HF prefer clear and honest and repeated opportunities to discuss these matters at a time when they are in a stable physical and/or cognitive state; they also prefer being able to process and respond to the information they receive.[52,54] Trust, empathy and hope are the core of patient centered communication.[3,46]

Both health professionals and patients enter an emotionally laden condition where they must confront and manage with issues about treatment, care, self-care, and the process of dying and at the same time issues beyond their health condition concerning patients' personal life. There can be uncertainties about life expectancy as well as treatment outcomes, and high-level communication skills are critical to each end-of-life decision-making discussion.[15,55] Bad news can be defined as any information viewed by a patient as negative to his/her current and future situation, which results in a cognitive or emotional deficit for a period of time after it is received.[56] Effective communication goes beyond what is said and what is done during an encounter with a patient. Moreover, what palliative care communication offers is the further ability to respond to rhetorical questions about life and death; the ability to know when to speak and when to say nothing; to provide the hand of comfort to the patient. It is much more than the giving of and asking for information.

Decision-making considers a constellation of physiological, psychosocial, and spiritual concerns, and their combined effect on the patient's medical treatment and quality of life at the end of life. This process includes the conversation in which healthcare professional gives the patient or their family bad news, and subsequent conversations related to treatment and care. Cultural and religious beliefs should also be considered to better ensure responsive healthcare practice.[57]

Timing of discussing the HF trajectory

Since HF is a condition with a fluctuating and unpredictable disease trajectory associated with a severe symptom burden and poor quality of life, it is important to initiate such conversations sooner, rather than later. Death from HF can be sudden, due to an ischaemic event or electric instability of the heart, or it can be slow, due to episodes of decompensation or progressive organ failure. It might be a challenge when to initiate a conversation about end of life. A screening tool that can be used to aid recognition if a patient is close to the end of life and to tailor advanced palliative care to HF patients is the 'surprise question': would you be surprised if this patient were to die within the next year?[15] If the answer to that surprise-question is 'no', a discussion concerning end-of-life care could be initiated by health care professionals, for example by introducing a communication tool to help the patient and the family pose questions that are important to them concerning future care.

If the HF trajectory is not adequately discussed, issues around end-of-life care tend to be addressed too late, possibly resulting in an unsatisfactory end-of-life care for both patients and their families.[22] Critical events such as the diagnosis of HF, perceptions of a change in clinical condition (e.g. experiences of frequent exacerbations), presentation of unrealistic expectations (e.g. patient with HF seeing treatments as curative), discussions about treatment complications or decisions (e.g. ICD implantation) or referral to palliative care may all act as prompts to start end-of-life discussions.[15,22]

The impact of early discussions can also extend to those close to patients prior to death, and into bereavement allowing them to prepare for death while also maintaining hope. Maintaining hope has been identified as extremely important to patients and relatives. Hope is not necessarily incompatible with knowledge of life-threatening disease or prognosis, and can mean more than simply survival.[58] Patients seem to maintain hope while also acknowledging their prognoses, whether they continue to hope: to live longer than expected; to enjoy a good quality of life; to achieve personal goals and self-manage themselves, or to have a peaceful death. An honest and clear communication provides and signposts clear opportunities for patients and relatives to discuss their preferences and concerns with the health care professional, including chances for them to be revisited and changed.[15,50]

Communication tools

Tools are available to support clinicians to communicate with patients with chronic and critical illness for example the BREAKS protocol[59] or the ABCDE protocol that help to prepare and structure a difficult conversation (➲ Table 11.5.4).[60] Other protocols include the SPIKES protocol in which setting up the consultation, assessing the patient's perception, and obtaining the patient's invitation are considered, and in giving information to the patient and addressing the patient's emotions with empathic responses are encouraged.[61]

Future directions

For several decades now the literature has been replete with assertions that patients with HF have sub-optimal care in the last stages of their illness. Palliative care should be considered throughout the HF trajectory meaning that palliative care should be offered/available early in the disease trajectory along with life-prolonging treatment. This means that heart failure teams must abandon the notion that they have to choose between disease-modifying interventions and palliative care, but need to combine the two approaches.

Table 11.5.4 ABCDE protocol for delivering bad news

A	**Advanced preparation**
	Review the patient's history, mentally rehearse, and emotionally prepare. Arrange for a support person if the patient desires. Determine what the patient knows about his or her illness.
B	**Build a therapeutic environment/relationship**
	Ensure adequate time and privacy. Provide seating for everyone. Maintain eye contact and sit close enough to touch the patient, if appropriate.
C	**Communicate well**
	Avoid medical jargon, and use plain language. Allow for silence, and move at the patient's pace.
D	**Deal with patient and family reactions**
	Address emotions as they arise. Actively listen, explore feelings, and express empathy.
E	**Encourage and validate emotions**
	Correct misinformation. Explore what the bad news means to the patient. Be cognizant of your emotions and those of your staff.

Source data from Rabow, M.W. and S.J. McPhee, Beyond breaking bad news: how to help patients who suffer. *West J Med*, 1999. 171(4):260–3.

Furthermore, optimal symptom control should be a main focus of HF management care and must be a vital part in education of professionals. Better assessment of palliative care needs supported by evidence-based validated PROMs is advised.[15]

The notion that palliative care can only be delivered by palliative care specialist should also be abandoned. HF management with a palliative care approach should be provided by all professionals. Where relevant, specialist palliative care should seriously be included in the multi-disciplinary team model with flexibility in regard to the optimal fit in different health-care systems available resources, and the spectrum of professional competences.[15]

Summary and key messages

- Palliative care should be a vital component of HF management ➲ Figure 11.5.3.
- Palliative care can be offered in parallel with usual HF care throughout the whole illness trajectory.
- The core components of primary palliative care include symptom management, communication regarding the goals of care, advance care planning, and psychosocial care and care co-ordination
- Successful symptom management is one of the cornerstones of palliative care in patients with HF, and it can improve the quality of life for both patients and their families during the HF trajectory.
- Optimal symptom control and a systematical addressing of patients' and families' needs and preferences for treatment should be the focus of care.
- Communication to inform advanced planning and future decision-making should ideally be undertaken when the patient's HF symptoms are stable and he/she has the ability to contribute to the conversation, rather than when death is imminent.

Supporting patients, families/informal caregivers

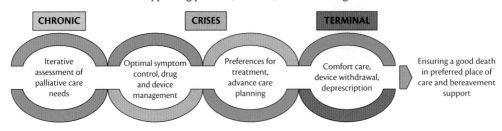

Information, communication, shared decision-making

Figure 11.5.3 Palliative care in heart failure.

References

1. Alpert, C.M., *et al.* Symptom burden in heart failure: assessment, impact on outcomes, and management. Heart Failure Review, 2017. **22**(1):25–39.

2. Olano-Lizarraga, M., *et al.et al.* The personal experience of living with chronic heart failure: a qualitative meta-synthesis of the literature. J Clin Nurs, 2016. **25**(17–18):2413–29.

3. Palliative care. 2020. https://www.who.int/news-room/fact-sheets/detail/palliative-care.

4. Chow, J. and H. Senderovich. It's time to talk: challenges in providing integrated palliative care in advanced congestive heart failure. A narrative review. Curr Cardiol Rev, 2018. **14**(2):128–37.

5. Remawi, B.N., *et al.* Palliative care needs-assessment and measurement tools used in patients with heart failure: a systematic mixed-studies review with narrative synthesis. Heart Fail Rev, 2021. **26**(1):137–55.

6. Jaarsma, T., *et al.* Palliative care in heart failure: a position statement from the palliative care workshop of the Heart Failure Association of the European Society of Cardiology. Eur J Heart Fail, 2009. **11**(5):433–43.

7. Fitzsimons, D., *et al.* The challenge of patients' unmet palliative care needs in the final stages of chronic illness. Palliat Med, 2007. **21**(4):313–22.

8. Lewin, W.H. and K.G. Schaefer. Integrating palliative care into routine care of patients with heart failure: models for clinical collaboration. Heart Fail Rev, 2017. **22**(5):517–24.

9. Quill, T.E. and A.P. Abernethy. Generalist plus specialist palliative care--creating a more sustainable model. N Engl J Med, 2013. **368**(13):1173–5.

10. Diop, M.S., *et al.* Palliative care interventions for patients with heart failure: a systematic review and meta-analysis. J Palliat Med, 2017. **20**(1):84–92.

11. Rogers, J.G., *et al.* Palliative care in heart failure: The PAL-HF randomized, controlled clinical trial. J Am Coll Cardiol, 2017. **70**(3):331–341.

12. Seferović, P.M., *et al.* The Heart Failure Association Atlas: rationale, objectives, and methods. Eur J Heart Fail, 2020. **22**(4):638–45.

13. Kavalieratos, D., *et al.* Palliative care in heart failure: rationale, evidence, and future priorities. J Am Coll Cardiol, 2017. **70**(15):1919–30.

14. Gelfman, L.P., *et al.* The state of the science on integrating palliative care in heart failure. Journal of Palliative Medicine, 2017. **20**(6):592–603.

15. Hill, L., *et al.* Integration of a palliative approach into heart failure care: a European Society of Cardiology Heart Failure Association position paper. Eur J Heart Fail, 2020. **22**(12):2327–39.

16. Brännström, M., *et al.* Unequal care for dying patients in Sweden: a comparative registry study of deaths from heart disease and cancer. Eur J Cardiovasc Nurs, 2012. **11**(4):454–9.

17. Gadoud, A., *et al.* Palliative care among heart failure patients in primary care: a comparison to cancer patients using English family practice data. PLoS One, 2014. **9**(11):e113188.

18. Bakitas, M.A., *et al.* Effect of an early palliative care telehealth intervention vs usual care on patients with heart failure: the ENABLE CHF-PC randomized clinical trial. JAMA Intern Med, 2020. **180**(9):1203–13.

19. Brännström, M. and K. Boman. Effects of person-centred and integrated chronic heart failure and palliative home care. PREFER: a randomized controlled study. Eur J Heart Fail, 2014. **16**(10):1142–1151.

20. Datla, S., *et al.* Multi-disciplinary palliative care is effective in people with symptomatic heart failure: A systematic review and narrative synthesis. Palliat Med, 2019. **33**(8):1003–16.

21. McIlfatrick, S., *et al.* 'The importance of planning for the future': Burden and unmet needs of caregivers' in advanced heart failure: A mixed methods study. Palliat Med, 2018. **32**(4):881–90.

22. Fitzsimons, D., *et al.* Inadequate communication exacerbates the support needs of current and bereaved caregivers in advanced heart failure and impedes shared decision-making. J Cardiovasc Nurs, 2019. **34**(1):11–19.

23. Bruera, E., *et al.* The Edmonton Symptom Assessment System (ESAS): a simple method for the assessment of palliative care patients. J Palliat Care, 1991. **7**(2):6–9.

24. Zambroski, C.H., *et al.* Impact of symptom prevalence and symptom burden on quality of life in patients with heart failure. Eur J Cardiovasc Nurs, 2005. **4**(3):198–206.

25. Green, C.P., *et al.* Development and evaluation of the Kansas City Cardiomyopathy Questionnaire: a new health status measure for heart failure. J Am Coll Cardiol, 2000. **35**(5):1245–55.

26. Spertus, J.A. and P.G. Jones. Development and Validation of a Short Version of the Kansas City Cardiomyopathy Questionnaire. Circ Cardiovasc Qual Outcomes, 2015. **8**(5):469–76.

27. Jaarsma, T., *et al.* Factors related to self-care in heart failure patients according to the middle-range theory of self-care of chronic illness: a literature update. Curr Heart Fail Rep, 2017. **14**(2):71–77.

28. Riegel, B., *et al.* Integrating symptoms into the middle-range theory of self-care of chronic illness. ANS Adv Nurs Sci, 2019. **42**(3):206–15.

29. Riegel, B., T. Jaarsma, and A. Strömberg. A middle-range theory of self-care of chronic illness. ANS Adv Nurs Sci, 2012. **35**(3):194–204.

30. Jaarsma, T., *et al.* Self-care of heart failure patients: practical management recommendations from the Heart Failure Association of the European Society of Cardiology. Eur J Heart Fail, 2021.;**23**(1):157–74.

31. McDonagh, T.A., *et al.* 2021 ESC Guidelines for the diagnosis and treatment of acute and chronic heart failure. Eur Heart J, 2021. **42**(36):3599–726.

32. Crespo-Leiro, M.G., *et al.* Advanced heart failure: a position statement of the Heart Failure Association of the European Society of Cardiology. Eur J Heart Fail, 2018. **20**(11):1505–35.

33. Vitale, C., *et al.* Heart Failure Association/European Society of Cardiology position paper on frailty in patients with heart failure. Eur J Heart Fail, 2019. **21**(11):1299–1305.

34. Hill, L., *et al.* End of life decision making in patients with an implantable cardioverter defibrillator (ICD): exploring the reality. European Journal of Cardiovascular Nursing, 2014. **13**(supplement 1):S9.

35. Lainscak, M., *et al.* General public awareness of heart failure: results of questionnaire survey during Heart Failure Awareness Day 2011. Arch Med Sci, 2014. **10**:355–360.

36. Stevenson, L.W., *et al.* Changing preferences for survival after hospitalisation with advanced heart failure. Journal of American College of cardiology, 2008. **52**:1702–8.

37. Lokker, M.E., *et al.* The prevalence and associated distress of physical and psychological symptoms in patients with advanced heart failure attending a South African medical center. Journal of Cardiovascular Nursing, 2016. **31**(4):313–22.

38. Campbell, R.T., *et al.* Which patients with heart failure should receive specialist palliative care? Eur J Heart Fail, 2018. **20**(9):1338–47.

39. Kane, P.M., *et al.* Understanding how a palliative-specific patient-reported outcome intervention works to facilitate patient-centred care in advanced heart failure: A qualitative study. Palliative Medicine, 2018. **32**(1):143–55.

40. Hjelmfors, L., *et al.* Using co-design to develop an intervention to improve communication about the heart failure trajectory and end-of-life care. BMC Palliative care, 2018. **17**(1):85.

41. Molzahn, A.E., *et al.* Life and priorities before death: A narrative inquiry of uncertainty and end of life in people with heart failure and their family members. Eur J Cardiovasc Nurs, 2020. **19**(7):629–37.

42. Hill, L., *et al.* Patients' perception of implantable cardioverter defibrillator deactivation at the end of life. Palliat Med 2015;**29**(4):310–23.

43. Westerdahl, A.K., *et al.* Implantable cardioverter-defibrillator therapy before death high risk for painful shocks at the end of life. Circulation, 2014. **129**:422–9.

44. Padeletti, L., *et al.* EHRA Expert Consensus Statement on the management of cardiovascular implantable electronic devices in patients nearing end of life or requesting withdrawal of therapy. Europace, 2010. **12**(10):1480–9.

45. Lampert, R., *et al.* HRS Expert Consensus Statement on the Management of Cardiovascular Implantable Electronic Devices (CIEDs) in patients nearing end of life or requesting withdrawal of therapy. Heart Rhythm, 2010. **7**(7):1008–26.

46. Irvine, J., *et al.* Quality of life in the Canadian Implantable Defibrillator study (CIDS) Am.Heart J., 2002. **144**:282–9.

47. Habibović, M., *et al.* Posttraumatic stress and anxiety in patients with an implantable cardioverter defibrillator: Trajectories and vulnerability factors. Pacing Clin Electrophysiol., 2017. **40**(7):817–23.

48. Verdoorn, B.P., *et al.* Palliative medicine and preparedness planning for patients receiving left ventricular assist device as destination therapy-challenges to measuring impact and change in institutional culture. J Pain Symptom Manage, 2017. **54**(2):231–6.

49. Scott, I.A., *et al.* Reducing inappropriate polypharmacy: the process of deprescribing. Jama Intern Med, 2015. **175**(5):827–34.

50. Barclay, S., *et al.* End-of-life care conversations with heart failure patients: a systematic literature review and narrative synthesis. Br J Gen Pract, 2011. **61**:e49–e62.

51. De Vleminck, A., *et al.* Barriers to advance care planning in cancer, heart failure and dementia patients: a focus group study on general practitioners' views and experiences. PLoS One, 2014. **9**(1):e84905.

52. Hjelmfors, L., *et al.* Communicating prognosis and end of life care to heart failure patients: A survey of heart failure nurses' perspectives Eur J Cardiovasc Nurs, 2014. **13**(2):152–61.

53. Sobanski, P.Z., *et al.* Palliative care for people living with heart failure: European Association for Palliative Care Task Force expert position statement. Cardiovasc Res, 2020. **116**(1):12–27.

54. Kelemen, A.M., G. Ruiz, and H. Groninger. Choosing words wisely in communication with patients with heart failure and families. Am J Cardiol, 2016. **117**(11):1779–82.

55. Berkey, F.J., J.P. Wiedemer, and N.D. Vithalani. Delivering bad or life-altering news. Am Fam Physician, 2018. **98**(2):99–104.

56. Fallowfield, L. and V. Jenkins. Communicating sad, bad, and difficult news in medicine. Lancet, 2004. **363**(9405):312–9.

57. Cain, C.L., *et al.* Culture and palliative care: preferences, communication, meaning, and mutual decision making. J Pain Symptom Manage, 2018. **55**(5):1408–19.

58. Brighton, L.J. and K. Bristowe. Communication in palliative care: talking about the end of life, before the end of life. Postgrad Med J, 2016. **92**(1090):466–70.

59. Narayanan, V., B. Bista, and C. Koshy. 'BREAKS' protocol for breaking bad news. Indian J Palliat Care, 2010. **16**(2):61–5.

60. Rabow, M.W. and S.J. McPhee. Beyond breaking bad news: how to help patients who suffer. West J Med, 1999. **171**(4):260–3.

61. Baile, W.F., *et al.* SPIKES-A six-step protocol for delivering bad news: application to the patient with cancer. Oncologist, 2000. **5**(4):302–11.

SECTION 12

Comorbidities and clinical conditions

CHAPTER 12.1

Clinical aspects of chronic kidney disease in heart failure

Pieter Martens and
Hans-Peter Brunner-La Rocca

Contents

Introduction

Both acutely and chronically, heart failure can cause kidney failure and kidney failure can cause heart failure. In addition, underlying pathologies or pre-existing comorbidities can result in simultaneous heart failure (HF) and kidney failure. These conditions are summarized by the term cardiorenal syndrome, and can be classified into five different groups. In individual patients, however, it can be difficult to determine if the kidneys or the heart is the (initial) trigger for the cardiorenal syndrome. Importantly, both the heart and the kidney are heavily intertwined, can worsen each other's prognosis, and potentially lead to under-utilization of disease modifying therapies.[1] Moreover, the concomitant presence of HF and chronic kidney disease (CKD) seems to accelerate the progression of both conditions. Chapter 5.7 mainly focuses on the renal consequences of heart failure (i.e. cardiorenal syndrome types 1 and 2), while this chapter covers the effects of renal failure on the heart (cardiorenal syndrome types 3 and 4).[2] This includes both diagnosis and management. In addition, this chapter provides definitions of CKD, the prognostic relevance of CKD in heart failure, assessment of kidney function, the implications of CKD on symptoms and management of heart failure as well as the management of end-stage renal failure in relation to heart failure.

Definition of CKD

In efforts to harmonize the definition of CKD, a previous consensus statement advises defining kidney function and CKD according to the Kidney Disease Improving Global Outcomes (KDIGO) classification (⊃ Figure 12.1.1), which is based on objective measurement of specific kidney measures such as a decrease in glomerular filtration rate (GFR), and the presence of evidence of kidney damage, being most often detected by albuminuria (or abnormal urine sediment, histologic or structural abnormalities).[3] While CKD is often used interchangeably for an estimated (e)GFR<60mL/min/1.73m^2, it needs to be pointed out that patients with an eGFR>60mL/min/1.73m^2 can also have CKD if albuminuria or other markers of kidney damage are present. An additional element of the definition of CKD relates to the chronicity of the findings. By definition, CKD implies the presence of kidney damage (low eGFR or albuminuria) over a time period of more than 3 months.

Prevalence of CKD in relation to heart failure

The worldwide prevalence of CKD is estimated to be 697.5 million people (9.1% of the entire population).[4] In heart failure patients, the prevalence of CKD is much higher, affecting around 55% of patients, with a similar high prevalence in both heart failure

Definition of CKD-stage according to the 2012 KDIGO guidelines, with colours indicating risk to progression of CKD and guide to intensity of follow-up				Albuminuria: description and range		
				A1	**A2**	**A3**
				Normal to mild increase	Moderately increased	Severely increased
				<30mg/g <30mg/mmol	30–300mg/g 3–30mg/mmol	>300mg/g >30mg/mmol
GFR–categories (ml/min/1.73m²)	G1	Normal or high	≥90			
	G2	Mildly decreased	60–89			
	G3a	Mild to moderate decreased	45–59			
	G3b	Moderate to severely decreased	30–44			
	G4	Severely decreased	15–29			
	G5	Kidney failure	<15			

Figure 12.1.1 Classification of chronic kidney disease according to Kidney Disease Improving Global Outcomes (KDIGO).
Source data from Kellum JA, Lameire N; KDIGO AKI Guideline Work Group. Diagnosis, evaluation, and management of acute kidney injury: a KDIGO summary (Part 1). *Crit Care.* 2013 Feb 4;17(1):204. doi: 10.1186/cc11454.

with preserved (HFpEF) and reduced ejection fraction (HFrEF).[5] This high prevalence is not surprising as both conditions accelerate each other and cluster in older patients with certain co-morbidities such as hypertension, obesity, diabetes, or other cardiovascular risk factors. Additionally, patients with CKD and heart failure might respond differently to classic treatments, as the perceived risk associated with therapies (e.g. slight decrease in eGFR) might lead to suboptimal use of disease modifying therapies.[1] De novo heart failure in CKD is estimated to occur with an incidence of around 17% to 21% per year. The severity of CKD (reflected in ➲ Figure 12.1.1) also determines the risk for heart failure. Indeed, as CKD severity increases so does the prevalence of heart failure. It is estimated that 44% of patients on haemodialysis suffer from heart failure (➲ Figure 12.1.2).[6]

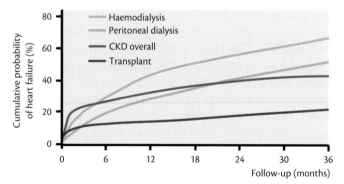

Figure 12.1.2 Prevalence of de novo heart failure in patients with chronic kidney disease (CKD).
Source data from Collins AJ, Foley R, Herzog C, et al. Excerpts from the United States Renal Data System 2007 annual data report. *Am J Kidney Dis.* 2008 Jan;51(1 Suppl 1):S1-320. doi: 10.1053/j.ajkd.2007.11.001.

Prognostic value of CKD in heart failure

GFR is a strong predictor of clinical outcomes in heart failure patients, illustrated by the observation that GFR is more closely related to outcome than left ventricular ejection fraction (LVEF).[7] A large meta-analysis, encompassing over one million patients with chronic heart failure, illustrated that CKD (defined as GFR <60mL/min/1.73m²) is associated with a doubling in risk of all-cause mortality.[5] GFR is the net result of the total number of functioning nephrons, the ultrafiltration coefficient (K_f), and the net Starling forces (P_{UF}) across the glomerular capillaries (the latter being determined by the hydrostatic and oncotic forces in the capillaries versus the Bowman space), as reflected in ➲ Figure 12.1.3. Importantly, GFR deterioration is especially of prognostic relevance if it reflects permanent loss of functioning nephrons. As such, one needs to understand the pathophysiologic mechanism behind GFR changes to understand the impact on clinical outcome. Indeed, an increase in serum creatinine (often termed worsening renal function or WRF) in the setting of acute HF is not always associated with adverse clinical outcome.[8-10] This is explained by the unique position of the kidney in the altered haemodynamics in HF. Congestion in heart failure affects the renal blood flow and subsequently the net Starling forces (P_{UF}) across the glomerular membrane, thus reflecting a haemodynamic alteration rather than a permanent loss in functioning nephrons.[11-13] No study has ever documented that WRF in acute heart failure or chronic heart failure is associated with a loss in functioning nephrons. Importantly, relief of congestion in acute HF is associated with better outcomes despite a temporary decrease in GFR.[14] Yet, therapies used to alleviate congestion in acute heart failure also influence glomerular haemodynamics.[15] For instance, the macula densa is lined with the NKCC receptor (which is also inhibited by loop diuretics) to assess chloride

$$GFR = N \times L_P \times S \times (P_{GC} - P_B - \pi_{GC})$$

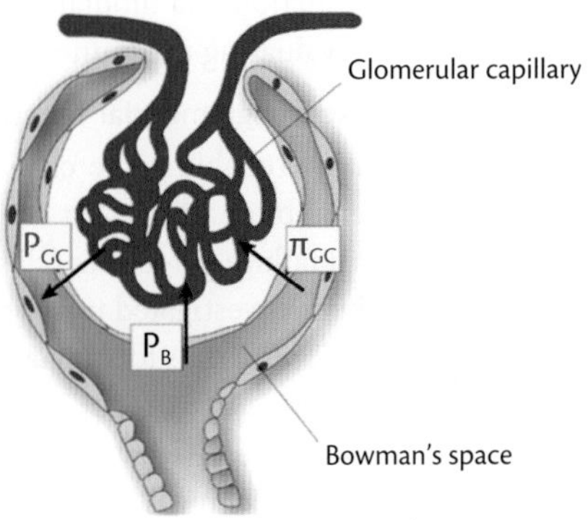

N	= Number of functional nephrons
L_P	= Hydraulic conductivity glomerular capillary
S	= Filtration area
P_{GC}	= Hydrostatic pressure glomerular capillary
P_B	= Hydrostatic pressure Bowman's space
π_{GC}	= Colloid osmotic pressure glomerular capillary

Figure 12.1.3 Determination of glomerular filtration rate.
The oncotic pressure in the Bowman's space is negligible and not reflected in this figure.
Courtesy of Frederik Verbrugge.

content in the ultrafiltrate.[16] Therefore, treatment with loop diuretics can cause a decrease in GFR as they might induce more renin release. However, as loop diuretics also relieve congestion, this drop in GFR is not necessarily indicative of poor prognosis[17,18] and decongestion may even increase GFR. Numerous studies in acute heart failure have documented that effective decongestion (good diuretic response and relief of congestion) is associated with an improved prognosis, even if creatinine increases.[17,19] As such, a position paper from the cardiorenal working group of the Heart Failure Association (HFA) has proposed evaluating creatinine changes during decongestion in light of the decongestive effectiveness, something that was also recognized in the 2021 ESC heart failure guidelines.[1,20]

In the setting of chronic heart failure, an *unprovoked* decrease in the GFR is often clinically relevant as it mostly reflects a permanent loss of functioning nephrons (most often driven by intraglomerular hypertension or chronic hypoperfusion-related damage).[21] Progressive nephron loss results in an accelerated decline of GFR over time leading to the premature development of end-stage renal disease or experiencing a major adverse renal event.[5] This is such a common finding in heart failure that adverse renal events are becoming frequent secondary endpoints in randomized controlled trials (RCTs) of novel heart failure drugs. Additionally, CKD is associated with the highest population attributable risk (how much the development of a certain endpoint is related to a certain risk factor) to develop heart failure related mortality.[22] In healthy individuals, the average annual decline in eGFR has been shown to be 0.6–1mL/min/1.73m^2 per year after the age of 30–50.[23] In comparison in the GISSI-HF trial, patients with chronic heart failure experienced a decline in the slope of GFR of around 2.57 mL/min/1.73m^2 per year.[24] Importantly, heart failure itself remained independently associated with a more pronounced decline in GFR over time after adjustment for other well-known risk factors associated with progression towards end stage kidney disease.[24] Not surprisingly, assessment of GFR slopes is becoming a frequent trial endpoint in RCTs, serving as a proxy for the development of end-stage renal disease.[25,26] However, one needs to interpret changes in GFR

carefully, because in clinical practice GFR changes are often provoked. For instance SGLT2- and renin-angiotensin-aldosterone system (RAAS) inhibitors reduce intra-glomerular pressures, resulting in a haemodynamic-related drop in GFR.[25–31] However, this drop in GFR is not reflective of progressive nephron loss. In contrast, the sustained reduction in intra-glomerular pressures is associated with attenuation of the loss of nephrons over time, because it limits the intra-glomerular hypertension occurring in heart failure (or frequent co-morbid conditions such as diabetes and obesity).[32,33] As such, the early part of the eGFR slope in heart failure patients receiving guideline-directed medical therapies is obscured by the glomerular haemodynamic effect of these agents and these agents (SGLT2-I and RAASi) lead to a reduction in major adverse renal events.

Evaluation of the kidney in patients with heart failure

In clinical practice, renal function evaluation should almost always be a part of every encounter cardiologists have with their heart failure patients as most have CKD. ● Figure 12.1.1 outlines the need for frequent kidney function evaluation and the simultaneous evaluation of cardiac and kidney function during in- and outpatient visits as a consequence. Such simultaneous kidney evaluation: (1) aids in a better understanding of the underlying cardiorenal physiology, (2) improves initiation, adaptation, or continuation of evidence-based heart failure therapies, (3) results in better stratification of patients at risk of adverse outcome, and (4) identifies the presence of systemic diseases (e.g. light chain amyloidosis) or coexistence of independent renal disease (e.g. renal artery stenosis during RAAS titration). Importantly, kidney function is more than just the assessment of glomerular filtration. Indeed, as congestion is key in heart failure patients, understanding the role of regulators of the volume status in heart failure is paramount; however, this latter is more a reflection of the kidney's tubular function than its glomerular function. A wide variety of laboratory and imaging techniques are available to help the clinician differentiate between functional and structural renal derangements in heart failure. Importantly, the interpretation of renal function depends on the setting in which the patient is presenting (acute heart failure vs chronic heart failure).

Biomarkers

To be of clinical utility, biomarkers need to be studied in the clinical context of heart failure, and able to guide changes in patient care on top of currently existing alternatives. As such, a renal biomarker detecting acute kidney injury in nephrology cannot just be extrapolated to a situation of heart failure. ⊃ Table 12.1.1 provides an overview of the potential prognostic, diagnostic, and clinical utility of blood and urinary biomarkers studied in heart failure. Aside from glomerular filtration, renal function also encompasses renal secretion and absorption. All these processes are altered in HF as they are influenced by intra- and extrarenal haemodynamics and neurohormonal activation.[34–36] Therefore,

we try to make a differentiation in blood biomarker information of glomerular function and tubular function and the role of urine biomarkers in evaluating the kidney.

Plasma biomarkers of glomerular function

Plasma creatinine (enabling the calculation of eGFR) and urea are the only renal biomarkers that currently are strongly recommended in heart failure guidelines (class I), although their clinical value has not been investigated in appropriate clinical trials (level of evidence C).[20] Numerous formulae exist to estimate GFR based on serum creatinine, cystatin C or a combination of both (⊃ Table 12.1.2).[37] While formulae exist using both serum creatinine and serum cystatin C, in clinical practice estimation based on solely serum creatinine probably suffices, with the CKD-EPI formula being most commonly used in clinical practice Plasma levels of urea are not only related to glomerular filtration but also relate to tubular urea reabsorption and thus neurohormonal activation

Table 12.1.1 Overview of laboratory and urinary renal biomarkers in heart failure

	Marker	Prognostically relevant	Diagnostic for WRF	Therapeutically relevant
BLOOD BIOMARKER	**Glomerular function**			
	Creatinine	++	++	++
	Cystatin C	+	+	?
	Urea	+++	?	++
	SuPAR	+	?	?
	Pro-enkephalin	+	?	?
	Tubular function			
	NGAL	++	−	?
	H-FABP	+	?	?
	β2-microglubulin	+	?	?
URINE BIOMARKER	**Glomerular function and integrity**			
	Creatinine	+	?	+
	Albumin	+++	?	++
	Tubular function/injury			
	NGAL	++	+	?
	KIM-1	+	+	?
	NAG	+	+	?
	Cystatin C	+	+	?
	β2-microglubulin	+	+	?
	NPs	+	?	?
	L/H-FABP	+	?	?
	IGFBP7	?	+	?
	TIMP2	?	+	?
	Diuretic efficiency (natriuresis / mg diuretic)	+++	+/?	++

WRF, worsening of renal function; SuPAR, soluble urokinase plasminogen activator receptor, NGAL, neutrophil gelatinase-associated lipocalin, H-FABP, Heart-type fatty acid binding protein, KIM-1, kidney injury molecule 1, NAG, N-acetyl-β-glucosaminidase, NPs, natriuretic peptides, L-FABP, liver fatty acid binding protein IGFBP7, insulin-like growth factor binding protein 7, TIMP2, tissue inhibitor of metalloproteinases 2.
Source data from Mullens W, Damman K, Testani JM, et al. Evaluation of kidney function throughout the heart failure trajectory - a position statement from the Heart Failure Association of the European Society of Cardiology. *Eur J Heart Fail.* 2020 Apr;22(4):584-603. doi: 10.1002/ejhf.1697.

Table 12.1.2 Limitations of markers and formulas for estimation of GFR

Marker/ formula	Limitation
Serum creatinine	◆ Variability in creatinine production across individuals ◆ Dependency on muscle mass ◆ Tubular secretion leading to overestimation of glomerular function ◆ Variability of the extent of tubular secretion between individuals ◆ Extra-renal clearance of creatinine ◆ Tubular reabsorption in case of low tubular flow ◆ Late marker of AKI ◆ Assumption of unchanged volume of distribution ◆ Exponential relationship with eGFR
Serum cystatin C	◆ Increased levels in case of inflammation ◆ Increased levels with thyroid dysfunction ◆ More expensive than serum creatinine ◆ Not always readily available in every laboratory ◆ Assumption of unchanged volume of distribution ◆ Absolute values difficult to interpret due to limited clinical experience
Cockcroft and Gault $$\frac{(140 - age) \times weight}{72 \times sCr} \times (0.85 \text{ if female})$$	◆ Formula with lowest accuracy to estimate GFR in comparison to gold standard measurement ◆ Based on creatinine thus sensitive to limitation related to serum creatinine
MDRD $175 \times sCr^{-1.154} \times Age^{-0.203} \times (0.742 \text{ if female})$	◆ Better than Cockcroft-Gault but worse than CKD-EPI$_{creat}$ for estimation GFR in comparison to gold standard measurement ◆ Poorly calibrated in GFR>60mL/min/1.73m² ◆ Worse in predicting outcome in HF in comparison to Cockcrof-Gault ◆ Based on creatinine thus sensitive to limitation related to serum creatinine
CKD-EPI$_{creat}$ $A \times (sCr/B)^C \times 0.993^{age} \times (1.159 \text{ if African American})$ With A,B,C being dependent on the gender and serum creatinine value	◆ Worse in predicting outcome in HF in comparison to Cockcrof-Gault ◆ Poorly calibrated in GFR > 90mL/min/1.73m² ◆ Based on creatinine thus sensitive to limitation related to serum creatinine
CKD-EPI$_{cys}$ $133 \times (sCys/0.8)^A \times 0.996^{age} \times B$ With A and B being dependent on the gender and serum cystatine C value	◆ Based on cystatin C thus sensitive to limitation related to cystatin C
CKD-EPI$_{creat-cys}$ $A \times (sCr)^{BC} \times (sCys/0.8)^D \times 0.995^{age} \times (1.08 \text{ if African American})$ With A,B,C being dependent on the gender and serum cystatine C and the serum creatinine value	◆ Based on creatinine thus sensitive to limitation related to serum creatinine ◆ Based on cystatin C thus sensitive to limitation related to cystatin C

Source data from Mullens W, Damman K, Testani JM, et al. Evaluation of kidney function throughout the heart failure trajectory - a position statement from the Heart Failure Association of the European Society of Cardiology. *Eur J Heart Fail.* 2020 Apr;22(4):584-603. doi: 10.1002/ejhf.1697.

in heart failure.[37] Proximal nephron sodium and water reabsorption results in solvent drag leading to more urea reabsorption. In addition, collecting ducts reabsorb urea under situations of vasopressin stimulation.[38] Therefore, it is not surprising that urea is a powerful predictor of outcomes. Other plasma biomarkers have been investigated to give information about glomerular function, but their precise role in heart failure management remain undefined (➲ Table 12.1.1).[39]

Plasma biomarkers of tubular function

On a daily basis, the healthy kidneys filter 180 L of ultra-filtrate containing 1.5 kg of NaCl. However, significantly less than 1% of this NaCl and only a tiny fraction of other solutes are excreted into the urine, which illustrates that small derangements in tubular function might have a substantial impact on volume and electrolyte homeostasis.[40] As the renal tubules consume the most oxygen in the kidney, they are sensitive to hypoxia, which is often present in HF when both renal arterial and venous flow are impeded. Currently there is no consensus on how to assess tubular function, resulting in a large number of investigated biomarkers (➲ Table 12.1.1).[41] Most of these markers can be found in the urine as they are produced or leak out of the tubular cells, while some can also be found in the plasma and are sometimes (partly) filtered or secreted and appear in urine as well. The large majority of plasma tubular injury biomarkers have been investigated in the research setting, and many of these assays are not clinically available for bedside use. The most extensively studied plasma tubular injury biomarker is neutrophil gelatinase-associated lipocalin (NGAL).[42] In the AKINESIS trial (Acute Kidney Injury N-gal Evaluation of Symptomatic heart failure Study), plasma

NGAL was not superior to plasma creatinine in predicting WRF or adverse in hospital outcome in patients with AHF.[43] Therefore plasma biomarkers reflecting tubular function have a limited role in heart failure as yet.

Urine biomarkers and diuretic response

As one of the main tasks of the renal tubules is to regulate sodium and volume status, which is particularly hampered in heart failure, a more precise assessment of the tubular function might be the evaluation of urine itself.[3] Urine is easily sampled and readily available in clinical practice. Due to its direct relation to the nephron, it is exquisitely useful for the evaluation of renal function. Numerous biomarkers can be measured in the urine including markers of glomerular function (e.g. urinary creatinine), glomerular integrity, and podocyte function (e.g. albuminuria) and urinary markers of tubular function and injury (e.g. urinary tubular injury markers, urinary sediment analysis, urinary electrolytes) as reflected in ⮕ Table 12.1.1. Most importantly, urine electrolyte concentrations and urinary volume can be used as a functional test to determine the tubular function, which might be of particular interest in heart failure. Indeed, heart failure is characterized by a very early loss in natriuretic responsiveness, which contributes to development of diuretic resistance and ongoing congestion.[44] Numerous studies in AHF have suggested that a good diuretic response is associated with better outcome. More recently, the 2021 ESC heart failure guidelines stipulate measuring diuretic response (urinary spot sodium sample and urinary volume) after diuretic administration in AHF.[20]

Renal imaging

Renal ultrasonography allows the measurement of kidney size (and abnormalities), which could be indicative of the chronicity of the disease. A sudden decline in renal function warrants imaging to rule out a urinary tract obstruction. Furthermore, renal artery evaluation should be considered in specific situations, such as severe decline in eGFR following initiation of a RAAS-blocker. Detailed echocardiography allows the assessment of cardiac filling pressures non-invasively.[45,46] However, in the process towards developing haemodynamic congestion, metrics of renal venous flow might become disrupted before metrics indicative of cardiac filling pressures (e.g. e′, E/e′, E/A-ratio, systolic pulmonary artery pressure).[47] Renal ultrasonography allows the clinician to assess such renal venous flow patterns, which can be measured at the bedside using an abdominal broad-band 2.5–5 MHz echo-probe. A continuous venous flow-pattern is associated with low renal venous pressures, while increased venous pressures are associated with a discontinuous renal venous flow signal.[48] Examples of different possible measurements are illustrated in ⮕ Figure 12.1.4. Interestingly, a discontinuous renal venous flow in a response to volume expansion is associated with a reduced diuretic response independent of the underlying GFR.[47] Although additional confirmation studies are warranted, renal venous flow pattern assessment might help to guide decongestive therapy.

Clinical features of CKD in heart failure

Chronic kidney disease hardly causes any symptoms unless CKD is at an advanced stage. In addition, these symptoms are rather non-specific, such as fatigue, loss of appetite, or sleeping problems. Mild to moderate CKD cannot be detected clinically and requires blood sampling for diagnosis and to determine renal function (for details, see earlier). Despite this, patients with significant CKD may be more susceptible to fluid retention and electrolyte disturbances. For example, worsening renal function may increase the risk of fluid retention and, as a consequence, cardiac decompensation. In addition, CKD-related hyperkalaemia may limit the use of evidence-based therapy for HF. Also, the response to diuretic therapy may be reduced in advanced CKD, where isolated thiazide treatment is less effective and the required dose of loop diuretics is often higher. Thus, changes in response to diuretic therapy might indicate deterioration of renal function or increased neurohumoral stimulation of both.

Therapeutic approach to CKD

Heart failure therapies and their impact on progression of kidney dysfunction

Observational data indicate that the proportion of patients using either a beta-blocker, ACE-I/ARB/ARNI, or MRA decreases with increasing severity of renal dysfunction.[49] Additionally, the proportion of patients taking all three of these agents is only 15% if patients have an eGFR in the range 45–60 mL/min/1.73m² and only 5% if eGFR is in the range 30–45 mL/min/1.73m².[49] Yet, many classes of different guideline-directed medical therapies (GDMT) can safely be initiated in patients with lower GFR. ⮕ Table 12.1.3 shows the range of eGFR in which medical therapy can be initiated and the expected effect on eGFR, both acutely and chronically. While some agents lead to an acute drop in eGFR after initiation (⮕ Table 12.1.3), these acute changes are most often only transient and not accompanied with persistent renal damage. Additionally, the reno-protective effect of ACE-I and ARB are well known in patients with CKD. Furthermore, in heart failure specifically, the classes of ARNI and SGLT2i have been shown to reduce the annual decline in eGFR slope (most pronounced for SGLT2i). None of the RCTs with the agents shown in ⮕ Table 12.1.3 found any statistical interaction between the presence of CKD and the treatment effect on the primary endpoint. Therefore, in terms of relative risk reduction, these agents are equally effective in patients with CKD. Because patients with CKD actually are at the highest baseline risk to develop cardiovascular death or heart failure hospitalization, the absolute risk reduction effect is even more pronounced in HF patients with CKD.

Therapeutic consideration in chronic kidney disease

As indicated above, CKD shares many similarities with chronic heart failure, including chronic low-grade inflammation, and hence, the two conditions may share common treatment strategies. This is nicely demonstrated by the positive effects of SGLT2-inhibition in heart failure and in CKD independently of other conditions. Also, the impact of associated conditions shows

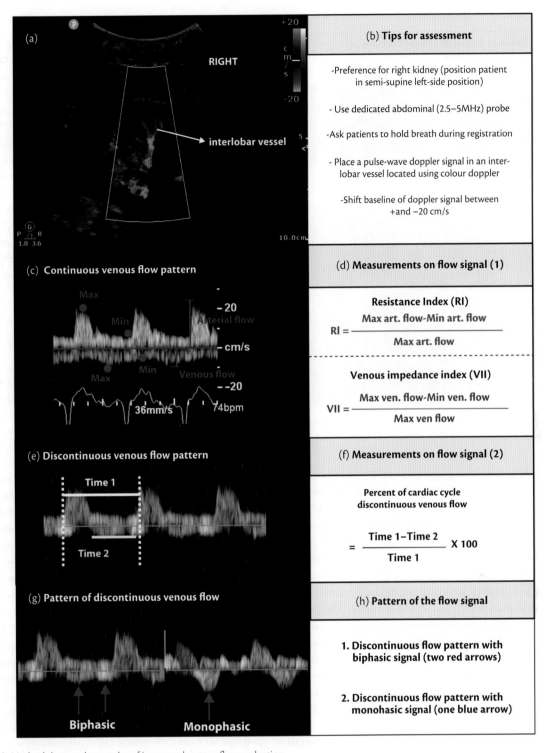

Figure 12.1.4 Methodology and examples of intra-renal venous flow evaluation.
Source data from Mullens W, Damman K, Testani JM, et al. Evaluation of kidney function throughout the heart failure trajectory - a position statement from the Heart Failure Association of the European Society of Cardiology. *Eur J Heart Fail.* 2020 Apr;22(4):584–603. doi: 10.1002/ejhf.1697.

significant overlap. An important example is iron deficiency, which is highly prevalent in both CKD and chronic heart failure. Not surprisingly, the risk of iron deficiency increases in the presence of both diseases, depending on the severity of each of them. The value of intravenous iron therapy has been established in patients with HFrEF, although supporting studies were of small to medium size

only and with limited follow-up.[20] Subgroup analysis suggests that the beneficial effect may be particularly present in HFrEF patients with CKD. Intravenous iron supplementation might even improve renal function. In contrast, the evidence of iron supplementation in isolated CKD is poor and limited to end-stage CKD only. Still, a recent study suggests that more aggressive iron replacement is

Table 12.1.3 Initiation of HF drugs in relation to baseline CKD-status

Drug	Evidence according to baseline eGFR enrolment criteria				Acute drop GFR	Impact on GFR slope in HF trial	CKD treatment interaction	Treatment effect with CKD
	ESRD	15–30	30–60	>60				
ACE-I/ARB	Moderate evidence if dialysis, weak evidence if not on dialysis				Yes	No (beneficial effect of around 1-2mL/min/1.73m² per year in CKD trials)	No	Relative benefit: ~ Absolute benefit: ↑
Beta-blockers					No	No	Yes (potentially higher RRR in MERIT-HF but some conflicting results)	Relative benefit: ~ Absolute benefit: ↑
MRA					Yes	No	No	Relative benefit: ~ Absolute benefit: ↑
ARNI					Yes	Yes (around 0.5 mL/min/ 1.73 m² per year)	No	Relative benefit: ~ Absolute benefit: ↑
SGLT2-i		>20			Yes	Yes (around 1-2 mL/min/ 1.73 m² per year)	No	Relative benefit: ~ Absolute benefit: ↑
Ivabradine					No	No	No	Relative benefit: ~ Absolute benefit: ↑
Vericiguat					No	No	No	Relative benefit: ~ Absolute benefit: ↑
Omecamtiv mecarbil					No	No	No	Relative benefit: ~ Absolute benefit: ↑

Key: Dark grey = strong evidence, mid-grey = moderate evidence, light grey = no data,
CKD, chronic kidney disease (eGFR < 60 mL/min), GFR, glomerular filtration rate. RRR, relative risk reduction. Drug abbreviations as in main text.

associated with fewer cardiovascular events.[50] Effects of isolated treatment of iron deficiency in CKD are, however, unknown as studies on iron replacement included erythropoiesis-stimulating agent use for treatment of CKD related anaemia, which is standard in CKD. In contrast, erythropoiesis-stimulating agent use is not indicated in chronic heart failure and mild to moderate anaemia as it did not improve outcome but increased the risk of thrombo-embolic events, as long as there is no other indication for its use.[51] Anaemia related to (end-stage) CKD could be such an indication, although the effect of erythropoiesis-stimulating agent has not been specifically investigated in CKD patients having heart failure.

Another important aspect is that CKD may limit heart failure therapy. This does not only apply to end-stage CKD, as discussed below. In particular, hyperkalaemia may limit the use of inhibitors of RAAS including ARNI.[20] Potassium-binding drugs (patiromer and sodium zirconium cyclosilicate; others with more side-effects) have been introduced, which may allow initiation or up-titration of RAAS-inhibition even in patients susceptible to hyperkalaemia. Smaller studies in patients with CKD and heart failure showed that the use of such potassium-binding agents is safe and well tolerated (mainly patiromer). Although patho-physiologically convincing, the approach of using evidence-based therapy in combination with potassium-binding agents to enable this therapy has not yet been proven to improve clinical outcomes as compared to the use of less RAAS-inhibition only. Accordingly, recent guidelines do not make clear recommendations about their use.[20] An outcome study using patiromer has been conducted

(NCT03888066), although the COVID pandemic required a reduction in the number of included patients and the adjustment of the primary end point, significantly limiting the value of this study.[52] With the use of patiromer, which was well tolerated, average serum potassium was lower, and the number of patients with serum potassium of >5.5 mmol/L significantly decreased from 19.4% to 13.9%, despite higher concurrent use of MRA and RAAS. However, there was no effect at all on number of hospitalizations or mortality.[52]

Heart failure and end-stage kidney disease

Evidence for all drugs in patients with eGFR <30 mL/min/1.73m² is very limited (⊃ Table 12.1.3), but does not suggest that drugs improving outcome and diuretics cause harm to the kidneys.[53] Obviously, patients with end-stage kidney disease and heart failure are still in need of medical therapy. Still, it must be emphasized that very close monitoring of renal function and electrolytes is crucial in these patients. As discussed above, the ability of the kidneys to adapt is extremely limited in end-stage kidney disease and even small changes in cardiac function may cause (further) deterioration of renal function, severe electrolyte disturbances (particularly hyperkalaemia), and fluid retention. In addition, some drugs are renally cleared (e.g. most ACE-inhibitors) and dosage must be adjusted accordingly or alternatives used that are not cleared exclusively by the kidneys (e.g. most ARBs, fosinopril).

Obviously, dialysis may be applied if required by the level of renal function. Whether peritoneal dialysis is safer compared to haemodialysis in patients with heart failure due to less direct effect on haemodynamics is a matter of debate and the evidence is rather limited. Still, theoretical considerations favour peritoneal dialysis as no high-flow arteriovenous shunt is required, infection risk may be lower, and it may help to better correct hyponatraemia.[54] If peritoneal dialysis also impacts outcome in patients with end-stage kidney disease not yet fulfilling the criteria for dialysis but with significant difficulties to achieve a sufficient fluid balance has only been studied in very small studies and is presently reserved for very selected patients.[55]

Future directions

Although the strong link between the kidney and the heart is beyond doubt, a better understanding is required as to how and by which mechanisms the two organs impact each other. Only with improved understanding can specific therapies be developed to prevent the negative impact of the failing of one organ on the other, beyond the treatment of (common) underlying risk factors and diseases. This is particularly true for CKD, where no specific therapy is available and treatment is mainly directed to reduce underlying risk factors such as hypertension. In addition, the impact of renal replacement therapy for decongestion in chronic heart failure patients on clinical outcomes needs to be properly investigated. This particularly applies in patients with advanced (i.e. eGFR <30 mL/min/1.73m^2) but not yet end-stage CKD with insufficient response to diuretic therapy in the chronic setting.

Most importantly, there is an urgent need for testing of standard medical therapies in patients with eGFR <20(–30) mL/min/1.73m^2, where proper evidence is lacking. In clinical practice, a significant proportion of patients belong to this category. They have a high absolute risk, but what their treatment should be is unknown. In fact, major HF guidelines recommend not to initiate standard GDMT in these patients, which in clinical practice is not only not possible but most likely also not appropriate.[20] Clinical studies are needed to investigate if GDMT regarding both efficacy and safety is similar (apart from considering changed pharmacokinetics) in these patients compared to those with better renal function.

Conclusion

The kidney and the heart are heavily intertwined and can alter each other's prognosis. Limited physiological reserve underscores the importance of close monitoring in the setting of CKD. CKD worsens the prognosis of patients with HF. Yet GDMT works equally well in patients with CKD, underscoring the importance of adequate implementation of life saving therapies.

Summary and key messages

- GFR is determined by the number of glomeruli, Starling forces, and the ultrafiltration coefficient, with the number of glomeruli carrying important prognostic meaning.
- While dose reductions of some neurohormonal blockers might be needed in CKD, neurohormonal blockers remain grossly underused.
- The prevalence of heart failure in patients on haemodialysis is as high as 44%.
- CKD doubles the risk for all-cause mortality (being a far stronger predictor of outcome than LVEF).
- In acute heart failure, the assessment of renal tubular function through measuring urine output and urinary sodium content after loop diuretic administration is advised by ESC HF guidelines.
- Higher all-cause mortality risk in CKD with maintained relative risk reductions by GDMT results in larger absolute risk reductions with GDMT.
- Misinterpretation of eGFR changes often results in inappropriate discontinuation of GDMT.
- A drop in eGFR after initiation of ACE-I/ARB/ARNI/MRA/SGLT2i does not alter the treatment benefits of these agents.

References

1. Mullens W, Damman K, Testani JM, et al. Evaluation of kidney function throughout the heart failure trajectory - a position statement from the Heart Failure Association of the European Society of Cardiology. Eur J Heart Fail 2020;22(4):584–603.
2. Ronco C, Haapio M, House AA, Anavekar N, Bellomo R. Cardiorenal syndrome. J Am Coll Cardiol 2008 ;52(19):1527–39.
3. Levey AS, Eckardt KU, Dorman NM, et al. Nomenclature for kidney function and disease-executive summary and glossary from a Kidney Disease: Improving Global Outcomes (KDIGO) consensus conference. Eur Heart J 2020;41(48):4592–8.
4. GBD Chronic Kidney Disease Collaboration. Global, regional, and national burden of chronic kidney disease, 1990–2017: a systematic analysis for the Global Burden of Disease Study 2017. Lancet 2020;395(10225):709–33.
5. Damman K, Valente MA, Voors AA, O'Connor CM, van Veldhuisen DJ, Hillege HL. Renal impairment, worsening renal function, and outcome in patients with heart failure: an updated meta-analysis. Eur Heart J 2014;35(7):455–69.
6. Collins AJ, Foley R, Herzog C, et al. Excerpts from the United States Renal Data System 2007 annual data report. Am J Kidney Dis 2008;51(1 Suppl 1):S1–320.
7. Hillege HL, Girbes AR, de Kam PJ, et al. Renal function, neurohormonal activation, and survival in patients with chronic heart failure. Circulation 2000;102(2):203–10.
8. Damman K, Navis G, Voors AA, et al. Worsening renal function and prognosis in heart failure: systematic review and meta-analysis. J Card Fail 2007;13(8):599–608.
9. Smith GL, Lichtman JH, Bracken MB, et al. Renal impairment and outcomes in heart failure: systematic review and meta-analysis. J Am Coll Cardiol 2006;47(10):1987–96.
10. Harjola VP, Mullens W, Banaszewski M, et al. Organ dysfunction, injury and failure in acute heart failure: from pathophysiology to diagnosis and management. A review on behalf of the Acute Heart Failure Committee of the Heart Failure Association (HFA) of the European Society of Cardiology (ESC). Eur J Heart Fail 2017;19(7):821–36.
11. Matthews JC, Koelling TM, Pagani FD, Aaronson KD. The right ventricular failure risk score a pre-operative tool for assessing the risk of right ventricular failure in left ventricular assist device candidates. J Am Coll Cardiol 2008;51(22):2163–72.
12. Mullens W, Abrahams Z, Francis GS, et al. Importance of venous congestion for worsening of renal function in advanced decompensated heart failure. J Am Coll Cardiol 2009;53(7):589–96.
13. Mullens W, Nijst P. Cardiac output and renal dysfunction: definitely more than impaired flow. J Am Coll Cardiol 2016;67(19):2209–12.

14. Metra M, Davison B, Bettari L, *et al.* Is worsening renal function an ominous prognostic sign in patients with acute heart failure? The role of congestion and its interaction with renal function. Circ Heart Fail 2012;5(1):54–62.

15. Trivedi H, Dresser T, Aggarwal K. Acute effect of furosemide on glomerular filtration rate in diastolic dysfunction. Ren Fail 2007;29(8):985–9.

16. Wilcox CS, Welch WJ, Murad F, *et al.* Nitric oxide synthase in macula densa regulates glomerular capillary pressure. Proc Natl Acad Sci USA 1992;89(24):11993–7.

17. Testani JM, Chen J, McCauley BD, Kimmel SE, Shannon RP. Potential effects of aggressive decongestion during the treatment of decompensated heart failure on renal function and survival. Circulation 2010;122(3):265–72.

18. Testani JM, Brisco MA, Chen J, McCauley BD, Parikh CR, Tang WH. Timing of hemoconcentration during treatment of acute decompensated heart failure and subsequent survival: importance of sustained decongestion. J Am Coll Cardiol 2013;62(6):516–24.

19. Verbrugge FH, Duchenne J, Bertrand PB, Dupont M, Tang WH, Mullens W. Uptitration of renin-angiotensin system blocker and beta-blocker therapy in patients hospitalized for heart failure with reduced versus preserved left ventricular ejection fractions. Am J Cardiol 2013;112(12):1913–20.

20. McDonagh TA, Metra M, Adamo M, *et al.* 2021 ESC Guidelines for the diagnosis and treatment of acute and chronic heart failure. Eur Heart J 2021;42(36):3599–726.

21. Denic A, Mathew J, Lerman LO, *et al.* Single-nephron glomerular filtration rate in healthy adults. N Engl J Med 2017;376(24):2349–57.

22. van Deursen VM, Urso R, Laroche C, *et al.* Co-morbidities in patients with heart failure: an analysis of the European Heart Failure Pilot Survey. Eur J Heart Fail 2014;16(1):103–11.

23. Halbesma N, Brantsma AH, Bakker SJ, *et al.* Gender differences in predictors of the decline of renal function in the general population. Kidney Int 2008;74(4):505–12.

24. Damman K, Masson S, Lucci D, *et al.* Progression of renal impairment and chronic kidney disease in chronic heart failure: An analysis from GISSI-HF. J Card Fail 2017;23(1):2–9.

25. Packer M, Anker SD, Butler J, *et al.* Cardiovascular and renal outcomes with empagliflozin in heart failure. N Engl J Med 2020;383(15):1413–24.

26. Wanner C, Inzucchi SE, Lachin JM, *et al.* Empagliflozin and progression of kidney disease in type 2 diabetes. N Engl J Med 2016;375(4):323–34.

27. Effects of enalapril on mortality in severe congestive heart failure. Results of the Cooperative North Scandinavian Enalapril Survival Study (CONSENSUS). N Engl J Med 1987;316(23):1429–35.

28. McMurray JJ, Packer M, Desai AS, *et al.* Angiotensin-neprilysin inhibition versus enalapril in heart failure. N Engl J Med 2014;371(11):993–1004.

29. McMurray JJ, Krum H, Abraham WT, *et al.* Aliskiren, enalapril, or aliskiren and enalapril in heart failure. N Engl J Med 2016;374(16):1521–32.

30. McMurray JJV, Solomon SD, Inzucchi SE, *et al.* Dapagliflozin in patients with heart failure and reduced ejection fraction. N Engl J Med 2019;381(21):1995–2008.

31. Rossignol P, Cleland JG, Bhandari S, *et al.* Determinants and consequences of renal function variations with aldosterone blocker therapy in heart failure patients after myocardial infarction: insights from the Eplerenone Post-Acute Myocardial Infarction Heart Failure Efficacy and Survival Study. Circulation 2012;125(2):271–9.

32. Mullens W, Martens P. Exploiting the natriuretic peptide pathway to preserve glomerular filtration in heart failure. JACC Heart Fail 2018;6(6):499–502.

33. Mullens W, Martens P. Empagliflozin and renal sodium handling: an intriguing smart osmotic diuretic. Eur J Heart Fail 2021;23(1):79–82.

34. Cody RJ, Ljungman S, Covit AB, *et al.* Regulation of glomerular filtration rate in chronic congestive heart failure patients. Kidney Int 1988 Sep;34(3):361–7.

35. Cody RJ, Torre S, Clark M, Pondolfino K. Age-related hemodynamic, renal, and hormonal differences among patients with congestive heart failure. Arch Intern Med 1989;149(5):1023–8.

36. Packer M, Lee WH, Kessler PD. Preservation of glomerular filtration rate in human heart failure by activation of the renin-angiotensin system. Circulation 1986;74(4):766–74.

37. Schrier RW. Blood urea nitrogen and serum creatinine: not married in heart failure. Circ Heart Fail 2008;1(1):2–5.

38. Kazory A. Emergence of blood urea nitrogen as a biomarker of neurohormonal activation in heart failure. Am J Cardiol 2010;106(5):694–700.

39. Hayek SS, Sever S, Ko YA, *et al.* Soluble urokinase receptor and chronic kidney disease. N Engl J Med 2015;373(20):1916–25.

40. Verbrugge FH, Dupont M, Steels P, *et al.* The kidney in congestive heart failure: 'are natriuresis, sodium, and diuretics really the good, the bad and the ugly?' Eur J Heart Fail 2014;16(2):133–42.

41. van Veldhuisen DJ, Ruilope LM, Maisel AS, Damman K. Biomarkers of renal injury and function: diagnostic, prognostic and therapeutic implications in heart failure. Eur Heart J 2016;37(33):2577–85.

42. Schmidt-Ott KM, Mori K, Li JY, *et al.* Dual action of neutrophil gelatinase-associated lipocalin. J Am Soc Nephrol 2007;18(2):407–13.

43. Maisel AS, Wettersten N, van Veldhuisen DJ, *et al.* Neutrophil gelatinase-associated lipocalin for acute kidney injury during acute heart failure hospitalizations: The AKINESIS study. J Am Coll Cardiol 2016;68(13):1420–31.

44. McKie PM, Schirger JA, Costello-Boerrigter LC, *et al.* Impaired natriuretic and renal endocrine response to acute volume expansion in pre-clinical systolic and diastolic dysfunction. J Am Coll Cardiol 2011;58(20):2095–103.

45. Nagueh SF. Non-invasive assessment of left ventricular filling pressure. Eur J Heart Fail 2018;20(1):38–48.

46. Mullens W, Borowski AG, Curtin RJ, Thomas JD, Tang WH. Tissue Doppler imaging in the estimation of intracardiac filling pressure in decompensated patients with advanced systolic heart failure. Circulation 2009;119(1):62–70.

47. Nijst P, Martens P, Dupont M, Tang WHW, Mullens W. Intrarenal flow alterations during transition from euvolemia to intravascular volume expansion in heart failure patients. JACC Heart Fail 2017;5(9):672–81.

48. Iida N, Seo Y, Sai S, *et al.* Clinical implications of intrarenal hemodynamic evaluation by doppler ultrasonography in heart failure. JACC Heart Fail 2016;4(8):674–82.

49. Patel RB, Fonarow GC, Greene SJ, *et al.* Kidney function and outcomes in patients hospitalized with heart failure. J Am Coll Cardiol 2021;78(4):330–43.

50. Macdougall IC, White C, Anker SD, *et al.* Intravenous iron in patients undergoing maintenance hemodialysis. N Engl J Med 2019;380(5):447–58.

51. Swedberg K, Young JB, Anand IS, *et al.* Treatment of anemia with darbepoetin alfa in systolic heart failure. N Engl J Med 2013;368(13):1210–9.

52. Butler J, Anker SD, Lund LH, *et al.* Patiromer for the management of hyperkalemia in heart failure with reduced ejection fraction: the DIAMOND trial. Eur Heart J 2022; 43(41):4362–73.

53. Jankowski J, Floege J, Fliser D, Bohm M, Marx N. Cardiovascular disease in chronic kidney disease: Pathophysiological insights and therapeutic options. Circulation 2021;143(11):1157–72.

54. Albakr RB, Bargman JM. A comparison of hemodialysis and peritoneal dialysis in patients with cardiovascular disease. Cardiol Clin 2021;39(3):447–53.

55. Cnossen TT, Kooman JP, Krepel HP, *et al.* Prospective study on clinical effects of renal replacement therapy in treatment-resistant congestive heart failure. Nephrol Dial Transplant 2012;27(7):2794–9.

56. Kellum JA, Lameire N. Diagnosis, evaluation, and management of acute kidney injury: a KDIGO summary (Part 1). Crit Care 2013;17(1):204.

CHAPTER 12.2

Dyskalaemia in heart failure

João Pedro Ferreira, Kevin Damman, Wilfried Mullens, and Javed Butler

Contents

Introduction

Potassium (K^+) is the most abundant cation in humans; 98% of K^+ is located intracellularly ($\approx$140 mEq/L) and 2% is located extracellularly ($\approx$3.8–5.0 mEq/L). Potassium is essential for normal cellular function and alterations in K^+ regulation can lead to neuro-muscular, gastrointestinal and cardiac abnormalities.[1] The potassium content and distribution among the body compartments both depend on a complex interplay of multiple factors including renal and gastrointestinal function, diet, medications and supplements, neuro-hormonal status, and acid base balance.[2] Derangements in any of these may result in disruption of K^+ homeostasis, leading to abnormal K^+ concentrations. Under normal conditions, the kidneys are responsible for up to 90–95% of K^+ elimination, with the colon being responsible for the remainder. In the setting of chronic renal impairment, colonic K^+ excretion may increase by three-fold.[3] Furthermore, the cellular sodium–potassium-ATPase pump (stimulated by aldosterone, catecholamines, and insulin) preserves a high intracellular potassium concentration in the advent of an adverse concentration gradient. The resting transmembrane potential difference depends on intracellular and extracellular potassium concentrations. Because cardiac repolarization relies on potassium influx, hypokalaemia lengthens the action potential and increases QT dispersion.[4] Hyperkalaemia leads to a shortening of the repolarization time which may lead to QT interval shortening.[4] Both hypo- and hyperkalaemia may be life-threatening conditions by increasing the risk of ventricular arrhythmia and sudden cardiac death.[5]

Dyskalaemia (i.e. both hypokalaemia and hyperkalaemia) in heart failure (HF) is common because of HF itself and its commonly related comorbidities, and because of the medications used to treat HF and these comorbidities. Dyskalaemia in HF has important prognostic implications.[6,7] Critical comorbidities include chronic kidney disease (CKD), diabetes, frailty, and ageing. Relevant drugs include loop and/or thiazide diuretics, mineralocorticoid receptor antagonists (MRAs), angiotensin converting enzyme inhibitors (ACEi), angiotensin receptor blockers (ARBs), angiotensin-neprilysin inhibitors (ARNi), and beta-blockers[8, 9]. All of these treatments may cause K^+ alterations, resulting in either hypokalaemia or hyperkalaemia; K^+ changes can impact clinical outcomes directly and also by limiting the use of guideline-recommended medical therapy. Heart failure patients are often multi-morbid and poly-medicated, further complicating K^+ concentrations and management.

In HF, as in other conditions, e.g. myocardial infarction, hypertension, kidney disease, or in the general population,[10–14] the relationship between K^+ concentrations and adverse outcomes appears to be U-shaped, where both low- and high K^+ levels are associated with adverse outcomes,[15–17] although it remains unclear to what extent dyskalaemia is a risk factor itself vs a risk marker representing the patient's overall clinical status, other comorbidities, and/or use or non-use of HF medications. While moderate to severe hyperkalaemia has been the focus of acute clinical care, observational data suggest that hypokalaemia is, at least, as detrimental.[10] These data have clinical and research implications; hypokalaemia-associated risk in HF has not been the focus of as much research, and overall, the safe serum K[+] zone is not well established.

While literature is emerging concerning the epidemiology, pathophysiology, outcomes, and acute management of moderate to severe hyperkalaemia, practical guidance on chronic management and guideline-derived comorbidity optimization in a broader group of patients with dyskalaemia remains poorly described. This chapter aims to provide such guidance.

Measuring circulating potassium levels

Interpretation of circulating K[+] values and, consequently, the assessment of the risk of dyskalaemia, depends on the quality and nature of measurement. Blood levels of K[+] can be measured either in serum or plasma. Serum measurements require clotting before analysis whereas plasma levels can be measured immediately. K[+] is continuously released from cells during clotting; therefore, serum values are generally higher, by 0.1–0.4 mmol/L, and the difference is greater at higher absolute values (i.e. at low K[+] the difference is closer to 0.1 and at high K[+] the difference is closer to 0.4).[18] Therefore, hyperkalaemia may result from haemolysis subsequent to erroneous blood sample handling and/or long waiting periods before the analysis is performed.[19] This 'pseudo-hyperkalaemia' can be misleading and result in incorrect interpretation and patient management. Thus, it is important to confirm the diagnosis of hyperkalaemia before instituting medical management, except in life-threatening emergencies.

The literature regarding dyskalaemia and cardiovascular disease discussed herein is limited by the fact that serum vs plasma measurements are often not known or reported, or they are mixed together.

Hypokalaemia
Incidence and causes

Hypokalaemia, defined by a serum K[+] ≤3.5 mmol/L, is associated with adverse events; although the associated risk may vary by the level of hypokalaemia and by its correction or not. Potassium levels in the lower third of the normal range (K[+] 3.5–4.0 mmol/L) may even be associated with a higher risk compared to the range of 4–5, and often occur frequently in patients with HF, even in the context of ACEi/ARB and MRA treatment,[20,21] The most frequent cause of hypokalaemia is the use of diuretics, especially during periods of (aggressive) decongestion, either during an episode of hospitalisation for HF or in the outpatient setting. Also, excessive neurohormonal activation or diuresis with intravascular volume depletion results in excessive aldosterone production, which induces sodium and water reabsorption with concomitant K+ excretion.[22] Advanced HF with malnutrition and cachexia may also cause hypokalaemia. Hypokalaemia-associated risks include potentially life-threatening ventricular arrhythmias, particularly in the context of preexisting structural cardiac abnormalities, associated electrolyte disturbances (such as hypomagnesaemia), ischaemic substrate and/or and reduced EF,[23,24]

Prognostic implications
Observational studies

Observational studies suggest that hypokalaemia is associated with excess morbidity and mortality in HF. The lower the K[+] levels the higher the risk, starting at K[+] levels below approximately 4.0 mmol/L, but the risk increases steeply with K[+] levels below 3.5 mmol/L. A K[+] <3.5 mmol/L is infrequently observed (<5%) but has been consistent and independently associated with poor outcomes,[6,7,21,25–29] The associations of K[+] levels with the outcomes and the main patient features are detailed in ➲ Table 12.2.1.

Table 12.2.1 Serum potassium levels and outcomes in observational studies adjusted for potential confounders

Study / K[+] level (mmol/L)	<3.5	3.5–4.0	4.1–5.0	5.1–5.5	>5.5
Aldahl M. et al (2017)	3.2 (2.4–4.1)	1.6 (1.3–2.0)	Ref. (1)	1.6 (1.3–2.0)	3.3 (2.6–4.2)
Nunez J. *el al* (2018)	2.4 (1.4–3.9)	1.1 (0.8–1.4) [§]	Ref. (1)	1.5 (1.0–2.0) [§]	2.5 (1.5–3.5) [§]
Linde C. *et al* (2019) [§§]	2.0 (1.5–2.5)	1.3 (1.1–1.5)	Ref. (1)	1.3 (1.1–1.5)	1.5 (1.3–1.8) *
Hoss S. *et al* (2016)	2.3 (1.6–3.4)	1.2 (0.9–1.6)	Ref. (1)	0.8 (0.6–1.2)	0.9 (0.5–1.4)
Matsushita K. *et al* (2019)	1.6 (1.5–1.7)	1.1 (1.0–1.2) [§]	Ref. (1)	1.1 (1.0–1.2) [§]	1.7 (1.5–1.9)
Desai AS. *et al* (2018)	1.6 (1.1–2.1)	1.3 (1.2–1.6) [§]	Ref. (1)	1.3 (1.1–1.7) [§]	1.7 (1.2–2.5)
Cooper L. *et al* (2020) [§]	2.0 (1.0–3.0)	1.5 (1.2–1.8)	Ref. (1)	1.0 (0.9–1.3)	1.0 (0.8–1.4)

[§] Estimates derived from continuous 'spline' curves.

[§§] Estimates derived from forest plots.

* The relative risk for patients with K[+] between 5.5 and 6.0 mmol/L was 1.5 (1.3–1.8), and for K[+] > 6.0 mmol/L was 3.0 (2.0–4.0). Patients with K[+] > 5.5 mmol/L had higher odds for renin–angiotensin–aldosterone system inhibitor discontinuation.

** K[+] levels > 6.0 mmol/L are more likely to have a causal association with worse outcomes; levels between 5.5 and 6.0 mmol/L were not consistently associated with worse prognosis and even when they are the associations are not overwhelmingly strong to exclude another explanation.

The adjustment variables varied across studies, but systematically included age, sex, renal function, co-morbid conditions, such as diabetes, hypertension, and atrial fibrillation, and measures of disease severity such as NYHA class.

Reproduced from Ferreira JP, Butler J, Rossignol P, et al. Abnormalities of Potassium in Heart Failure: JACC State-of-the-Art Review. *J Am Coll Cardiol.* 2020 Jun 9;75(22):2836–2850. doi: 10.1016/j.jacc.2020.04.021 with permission from Elsevier.

The studies that report the associations by left ventricular ejection fraction (LVEF) suggest that the association of hypokalaemia with outcomes is similar regardless of the LVEF,[7,21] even though the risk of ventricular arrhythmias is greater with lower EF.

Clinical trials

Secondary analyses of clinical trials also support such associations regardless of EF, i.e. the associations are similar in HF with reduced ejection fraction (HFrEF) and HF with preserved ejection fraction (HFpEF) and will be discussed together. In the TOPCAT trial of spironolactone treatment for patients with HFpEF, hypokalaemia (<3.5 mmol/L) was associated with a 1.6-fold increase in the relative risk of death.[30.] Spironolactone treatment reduced the risk of incident hypokalemia.[30] In the EMPHASIS-HF trial of eplerenone treatment in patients with HFrEF, patients with K^+ levels < 4.0 mmol/L at baseline had an increased risk of HF rehospitalization or cardiovascular death if taking placebo (hazard ration (HR) (95% CI) = 1.37 (1.05–1.79), p = 0.02), but no such risk if taking eplerenone (HR (95% CI) = 0.87 (0.62–1.23), p = 0.44); p for interaction = 0.04.[31] In the RALES (Randomized Aldactone Evaluation Study) in patients with severe HFrEF, hypokalaemia (<3.5 mmol/L) was also associated with an increased risk of death. Patients taking spironolactone experienced 10% less hypokalaemia episodes at the <3.5 mmol/L and 20% less at the <4 mmol/L cut-off marks.

In the PARADIGM-HF trial evaluating angiotensin–neprilysin inhibition versus enalapril in heart failure trial in HFrEF patients, 3% or fewer of the patients had investigator-reported hypokalaemia.[32] A secondary analysis of the PARADIGM-HF trial focusing on serum potassium showed that, compared with normokalaemia, both hypokalaemia (<3.5 mmol/L) and hyperkalaemia (>5.5 mmol/L) were associated with a higher risk for cardiovascular death. However, potassium abnormalities were similarly associated with sudden death and pump failure death, as well as non-cardiovascular death and heart failure hospitalization, findings that suggest that potassium abnormalities may mainly be markers rather than mediators of an increased risk of death.[33] In PARAGON-HF (angiotensin–neprilysin inhibition in HFpEF) trial in patients with HFpEF fewer than 5% had investigator-reported hypokalaemia,[34] and similar findings to those described for PARADIGM-HF were found in PARAGON-HF, whereby potassium abnormalities may mainly be markers rather than mediators of risk of death.

It is likely that potassium abnormalities can be direct causes of fatal arrhythmias and death at extreme values (e.g. <3 and >6 mmol/L), but that the commonly observed associations at milder potassium values represent a marker of disease severity and not a direct cause of death. In any case, maintaining a potassium level between 3.5 and 5.5 mmol/L seems desirable.

In summary, clinically relevant hypokalaemia (<3.5 mmol/L) is not very common, but it is independently associated with a higher event rate. Aldosterone antagonists lessen the risk for hypokalaemia and part of their therapeutic effect may be explained by reducing this risk. While the observational data are consistent across many studies, the proportion of outcomes that may be directly attributed to hypokalaemia vs hypokalaemia being a marker for a sicker patient population (i.e. reverse causation) is uncertain. The fact that hypokalaemia is associated with mortality even after extensive adjustment, and that risk is ameliorated when hypokalaemia is corrected, suggests that hypokalaemia is a strong risk marker and a potential cause of death at extreme values.[25] Considering the link between structural heart disease and the risk for arrhythmia in the presence of hypokalaemia, avoiding hypokalaemia in HF patients seems prudent (➔ Figure 12.2.2).

Management

Maintaining serum potassium concentrations in the normal range should be a therapeutic goal and attaining a potassium concentration of at least 4.0 mmol/L seems desirable.[17]

Thiazide-type diuretics are a major cause of hypokalaemia, and if thiazides are necessary for lowering blood pressure or to achieve adequate decongestion, the lowest possible dose should be used.[35] Loop diuretics may cause less hypokalaemia than thiazides with the average potassium fall after the usual doses of furosemide (≈0.3 mmol/L) being less than after the usual doses of thiazides (≈0.6 mmol/L); moreover, contrary to thiazides the potassium fall with loop diuretics is little influenced by the dose or duration of treatment.[36,37] However, in sicker patients, with higher degrees of renin-angiotensin-aldosterone system (RAAS) activation as well as higher doses of loop diuretics, the risk of hypokalaemia may still be considerable. A more effective strategy may be to up-titrate ACEi or ARB if possible and to use MRAs as soon as possible. A potassium-rich diet may be followed in selected patients, but care should be given in patients on RAAS inhibitor therapy who may be at simultaneous risk of hyperkalaemia.[38] Despite these efforts, in patients with persistent hypokalaemia, oral potassium supplements may be used to increase K^+ levels, but only after ACEi/ARB and MRA initiation and up-titration has been tried (➔ Table 12.2.2 and ➔ Figure 12.2.1).

Monitoring

In the presence of hypokalaemia below 3.5 mmol/L and after initiation of MRA therapy, frequent K^+ and renal function monitoring is recommended. It is appropriate to measure K^+ and creatinine in the first week after hypokalaemia detection and/or MRA initiation, with one additional measurement per month for the next 3 months (i.e. 4 measures in total) or until potassium levels are in the normal range.[39] If the K^+ levels are below 3 mmol/L an in-hospital treatment with telemetry (or other facility where close surveillance is possible) is desirable due to the high risk of fatal events. Another common clinical scenario is the patient with HFrEF (and thus at risk of ventricular arrhythmias) admitted with volume overload and appropriately treated with high dose diuretics, where K^+ falls dramatically and may put patients at risk of arrhythmias. These patients may benefit from an early introduction of MRAs (not only as a diuretic adjuvant but also as a means to balance K^+) and might need several K^+ measurements per 24-hour period and continuous telemetry, particularly in the absence of an implantable cardioverter defibrillator. A synthesis

Table 12.2.2 Management of dyskalaemia

Serum K$^+$ (mmol/L)	Therapeutic recommendations (providing renal function is stable and eGFR > 30 ml/min/1.73m^2 and blood pressure is stable and systolic BP >100 mmHg)

<3.5	1. If associated with 'de novo' ECG alterations: in-hospital admission
	2. If no ECG alterations:
	   2.1. Stop thiazides (if diuretics are necessary for congestion relief, prefer loop diuretics)
	   2.2. Stop potassium binders
	   2.3. Initiate MRA
	   2.4. If already on MRA, then increase dose
	3. Increase ACEi/ARBs/ARNi dose to guideline-recommended targets
	4. Monitor K$^+$ and creatinine at 1 week, 1 month, 2 months, and 3 months
	   4.1. Until K$^+$ is in the 'normal' range
	   4.2. Adapt MRA dose if necessary (see also ➔ Table 12.2.3)
	5. Initiate a potassium supplement if none of the above steps works

3.5–3.9	1. Stop thiazides (prefer loop diuretics for congestion relief)
	2. Stop potassium binders
	3. Initiate MRA (or increase dose, if already taking one)
	4. Increase ACEi/ARBs/ARNi dose to guideline-recommended targets
	5. Monitor K$^+$ and creatinine at 1 week, 1 month, 2 months, and 3 months
	   4.1. Until K$^+$ is in the 'normal' range
	   4.2. Adapt MRA dose if necessary (see also ➔ Table 12.2.3)

4.0–5.0	1. Patient is in the target zone 2. Initiate or maintain RAASi and MRA dose
5.1–5.5	1. Individualize management based on patient risk and reliability of medical compliance and follow up 2. ACEi/ARBs, ARNi and MRA may be maintained (see also ➔ Table 12.2.3) 3. Monitor K$^+$ and creatinine closely 4. Eliminate K$^+$ supplements and NSAIDs, and decrease K$^+$ rich foods (whenever possible) 5. If reliable clinical follow-up and serum potassium assessment is doubtful, may consider potassium binder preferably over compromising RAASi therapy

5.6–6.0	1. Perform ECG and if 'de novo' ECG alterations: in-hospital admission
	2. Assess the possibility of hemolysis and repeat sample, if necessary
	3. Initiate a diuretic or increase its dose (if necessary)
	4. Eliminate K$^+$ supplements and NSAIDs, and decrease K$^+$ rich foods (whenever possible)
	5. Reassess K$^+$ levels after 1 week; if K$^+$ levels still high:
	   5.1. and on maximal tolerated/guideline-recommend RAASi dose, consider a K$^+$ binder (do not stop RAASi but may decrease the dose up to 50% of the guideline recommended dose)
	   5.2. if RAASi dose <50% of guideline recommendation, consider a K$^+$ binder and RAASi up-titration
	6. Monitor K$^+$ and creatinine at 1 week, 1 month, 2 months, and 3 months
	   5.1. Until K+ is in the 'normal' range
	   5.2. Adapt ACEi/ARB, ARNi and MRA dose if necessary (see also ➔ Table 12.2.3)

> 6.0	1. If associated with 'de novo' ECG alterations: in-hospital admission
	2. If no ECG alterations:
	   2.1. Assess the possibility of haemolysis and repeat sample, if necessary
	   2.2. Initiate a diuretic or increase its dose (if necessary)
	   2.3. Eliminate K+ supplements and NSAIDs, and decrease K+ rich foods (whenever possible)
	   2.4. Initiate a K$^+$ binder
	3. Reassess K+ levels after 1 week; if K+ levels still high:
	   3.1. Reduce MRA/ACEi/ARB/ARNI dose by 50% of the guideline-recommended dose (but do not decrease below 50%) and maintain K$^+$ binder or initiate one if not yet started; repeat the K$^+$ assessment after 1 week and if K$^+$ still > 6.0 mmol/L stop the MRA maintaining the K$^+$ binder
	   3.2. When K+ levels < 6.0 mmol/L, reintroduce the MRA maintaining the K$^+$ binder and see the above panel
	4. Monitor K+ and creatinine at 1 week, 1 month, 2 months, and 3 months
	   4.1. Until K$^+$ is in the 'normal' range
	   4.2. Adapt RAASi dose to guideline-recommended targets

MRA, mineralocorticoid receptor antagonist; ACEi/ARB, angiotensin converting enzyme inhibitor/angiotensin receptor blocker; RAASi, renin-angiotensin aldosterone inhibitor; eGFR, estimated glomerular filtration rate; BP, blood pressure.

Reproduced from Ferreira JP, Butler J, Rossignol P, et al. Abnormalities of Potassium in Heart Failure: JACC State-of-the-Art Review. *J Am Coll Cardiol.* 2020 Jun 9;75(22):2836-2850. doi: 10.1016/j.jacc.2020.04.021 with permission from Elsevier.

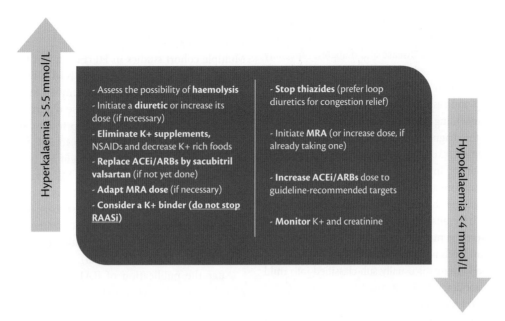

Figure 12.2.1 Management of hyperkalaemia and hypokalaemia.
ACEi/ARBs, angiotensin converting enzyme inhibitors/angiotensin receptor blockers; MRA, mineralocorticoid receptor antagonist; RAASi, renin-angiotensin-aldosterone system inhibitors.
Reproduced from Ferreira JP, Butler J, Rossignol P, et al. Abnormalities of Potassium in Heart Failure: JACC State-of-the-Art Review. *J Am Coll Cardiol.* 2020 Jun 9;75(22):2836-2850. doi: 10.1016/j.jacc.2020.04.021 with permission from Elsevier.

of the management of potassium disturbances is provided in ➲ Table 12.2.2 and ➲ Figure 12.2.1.

Hyperkalaemia

Incidence and causes

Hyperkalaemia in HF is often associated with the use of RAASi (ACEi/ARBs/MRAs) including the use of ARNi sacubitril-valsartan, and also with patient factors including older age, diabetes, and CKD, that is the patients who most benefit from RAASi. The occurrence of hyperkalaemia often limits RAASi use and/or leads to dose reductions and discontinuations, thereby reducing their potential benefits.

Hyperkalaemia is a major concern for clinicians, particularly in association with the use of MRAs.[40] The fear of hyperkalaemia and the related underuse of RAASi therapy is understandable, as

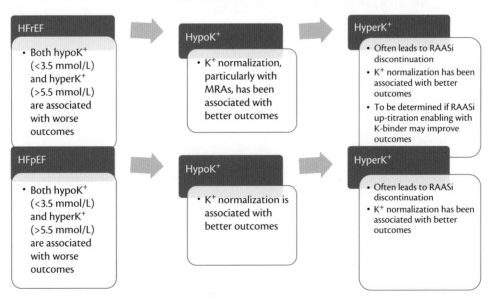

Figure 12.2.2 Outcome associations of dyskalaemia in HFrEF and HFpEF.
HFrEF, heart failure with reduced ejection fraction; HFpEF, heart failure with preserved ejection fraction; MRA, mineralocorticoid receptor antagonist; RAASi, renin-angiotensin-aldosterone system inhibitors.
Reproduced from Ferreira JP, Butler J, Rossignol P, et al. Abnormalities of Potassium in Heart Failure: JACC State-of-the-Art Review. *J Am Coll Cardiol.* 2020 Jun 9;75(22):2836-2850. doi: 10.1016/j.jacc.2020.04.021 with permission from Elsevier.

a sizable proportion of HF patients develop moderate to severe hyperkalaemia with RAASi therapy, a risk which is compounded in the presence of comorbid renal disease and diabetes, especially in the elderly.[41] It should be noted, however, that hyperkalaemia may result from haemolysis resulting in 'pseudo-hyperkalaemia' that can be misleading and result in incorrect interpretation and patient management, including RAASi discontinuation. Thus, it is important to confirm the diagnosis of hyperkalaemia before instituting medical management, except in life-threatening emergencies.

In a large, contemporary, international HF population, it was found that hyperkalaemia, impaired kidney function, and hypotension were the main causes for the non-prescription or underdosing of RAASi,[42] and in a large analysis of the Swedish HF Registry, CKD and older age were the major reasons for MRA non-use, independent of potassium levels and other confounders.[43]

The severity of hyperkalaemia is usually sub-classified into mild (> 5.0– < 5.5 mmol/L), moderate (5.5–6.0 mmol/L), and severe (> 6.0 mmol/L). The threshold risk for the development of hyperkalaemia-associated arrhythmic emergencies and death varies widely between patients.[23] It is often stated that the rapidity of change rather than the absolute K^+ level leads to rhythm disturbances. However, data are not conclusive and this assertion can be questioned based on observational associations showing that even mild hyperkalaemia is associated with worse outcomes. Because the risk of arrhythmia for a given potassium level varies between patients, an ECG should be obtained in both hyper- and hypokalaemia to detect precursors to arrhythmia, even though the sensitivity of ECG to detect hyperkalaemia associated rhythm disturbances is poor.[44,45]

Prognostic impact

Observational studies

Multiple cohort studies in HFrEF suggest that while ACEi/ARB use in routine clinical practice is relatively good (≥ 80%), MRA use remains low, ranging from only 30 to 60%. Hyperkalaemia is mentioned by surveys or in case report forms as a reason for not prescribing ACEi/ARBs in up to 10% of cases, whereas for MRAs this proportion can go up to 35%.[42,43,46] For ACEi/ARBs and beta-blockers the clinical benefit has been shown to be dose-dependent[47,48]; optimal dosing of MRA for outcome benefit has not been tested but data derived from the EMPHASIS-HF renal function stratified analysis, suggest that (at least for eplerenone) MRA doses should be adapted according to the patients' renal function, with lower doses provided to patients with impaired renal function[49] (⊘ Table 12.2.3).

After the publication of RALES, the use of spironolactone rose dramatically in Canada and the rates of hyperkalaemia also rose over a similar time-frame. Some authors related these findings to an overall increase in morbidity and mortality rates.[50] This unnerved many clinicians and may have contributed to poor MRA use. However, less publicized was a similar study from Scotland, where a similarly dramatic increase in the use of spironolactone after RALES was not associated with an increase in hyperkalaemia (or CKD), and the hospital admissions for hyperkalaemia and outpatient hyperkalaemia events actually fell.[51] These differences may be due to different potassium monitoring strategies (usual potassium monitoring in Ontario, Canada vs close monitoring in Tayside, Scotland), different

Table 12.2.3 Spironolactone and eplerenone dose adjustment proposal

Serum K^+ (mmol/L)	Dose adjustment (providing renal function is stable and eGFR >30 mL/min/1.73m² and blood pressure is stable and systolic BP >100 mmHg)
	Baseline: ⌐ eGFR ≥ 50 mL/min/1.73m² → spironolactone dose = 25 mg/d or eplerenone 50 mg/d ⌐ eGFR 30–49 mL/min/1.73m² → spironolactone dose = 25 mg every other day or eplerenone 25 mg/d
< 4.0	Increase dose: If spironolactone dose = 25 mg/d →increase to 50 mg/d or if eplerenone dose = 50 mg/d → increase to 100 mg/d If spironolactone dose = 25 mg every other day →increase to 25 mg/d or if eplerenone dose =25 mg/d →increase to 50 mg/d
4.0–5.4	No adjustment recommended
5.5–5.9	Decrease dose: If spironolactone dose = 50 mg/d →decrease to 25 mg/d or if eplerenone dose = 100 mg/d →decrease to 50 mg/d If spironolactone dose =25 mg/d →decrease to 25 mg very other day or if eplerenone dose =50 mg/d →decrease to 25 mg/d If spironolactone dose =25 mg every other day →interrupt treatment and reassess K^+ within 1 week or if eplerenone dose =25 mg/d →interrupt treatment and reassess K^+ within 1 week
≥ 6.0	Stop MRA treatment and reassess K^+ levels after 1 week When K^+ levels <6.0 mmol/L, initiate a K^+ binder and reintroduce MRA
	Stop MRA treatment at any case if eGFR ≤ 30 mL/min/1.73m² and reintroduce upon clinical decision i.e. upon renal function improvement and K^+ stabilization.

MRA, mineralocorticoid receptor antagonist; eGFR, estimated glomerular filtration rate; BP, blood pressure.

Reproduced from Ferreira JP, Butler J, Rossignol P, et al. Abnormalities of Potassium in Heart Failure: JACC State-of-the-Art Review. *J Am Coll Cardiol*. 2020 Jun 9;75(22):2836-2850. doi: 10.1016/j.jacc.2020.04.021 with permission from Elsevier.

populations (older patients in Ontario, Canada, who were treated with ACE inhibitors, regardless of whether or not they had previously been hospitalized for HF vs patients who had a hospital admission for HF in Tayside, Scotland) and the age of the patients, much older in the Canadian report compared with the Scottish (79 vs 73 yrs). Importantly, the hyperkalaemia-associated increased risk in HF may be largely due to avoiding RAASi in prevalent hyperkalaemia or stopping RAASi therapy once the patient's potassium starts to rise (i.e. hyperkalaemia may be a risk marker for sub-optimal RAASi use rather than a risk factor in itself).[52] This possibility has now been explored in several analyses. In the BIOSTAT-CHF study, specifically designed to evaluate factors associated with RAASi up-titration, hyperkalaemia was not an independent risk factor for worse outcomes but was an independent risk factor for lower sub-optimal ACEi/ARB doses.[53] In the Swedish HF registry, both hypo- and hyperkalaemia were associated with increased mortality, short- and long-term, with the familiar U-shaped relationship previously described.[21] After adjustment hypokalaemia remained independently associated with both short- and long-term mortality. In contrast, hyperkalaemia was independently associated with only short-term, but not long-term mortality, suggesting that in the longer term, hyperkalaemia is a risk marker for other confounders, such as suboptimal RAASi use.[54] In a recent observational study including patients initiating MRA therapy, the occurrence of hyperkalaemia led to MRA discontinuation in 47% and dose reduction in 10% of patients. Once MRA was discontinued, over 75% of the patients were not restarted on MRAs during the subsequent year.[55]

Finally, in the large ESC-HF-LT Registry, and in concordance with the previous reports, hyper- and hypokalaemia were both associated with worse outcomes. However, after adjusting for discontinuation of a RAASi (ACEI/ARB or MRA), hyperkalaemia was no longer associated with an increased risk.[56] These findings suggest that hyperkalaemia may be a risk factor for RAASi underuse and discontinuation which mediates the association with worse outcomes.[54] Together, these findings suggest that hyperkalaemia leads to RAASi underuse and permanent discontinuation which increase the risk of adverse outcomes, beyond its potential proarrhythmogenic properties.[52,54] As the associations of K[+] levels with outcomes are U-shaped, in most of the studies referenced above, hyperkalaemia was also associated with increased mortality risk. Potassium levels above 5.5 mmol/L and especially 6.0 mmol/L have been consistently associated with poor outcomes. The strength of the associations for K[+] > 6.0 mmol/L is similar to those observed for K[+] < 3.5 mmol/L, and correction of hyperkalaemia is also associated with mitigation of its associated risk.[6,7,21,26–28] The detailed prognostic associations and main patient characteristics are summarized in ❥ Table 12.2.1.

Clinical trials

The prognostic implications of hyperkalaemia in clinical trials appear similar to those found in observational studies and are also similar across the spectrum of ejection fraction, therefore HFrEF and HFpEF will be discussed together. For example, in a post-hoc analysis of the TOPCAT trial in patients with HFpEF, K[+] levels >5.5 mmol/L were associated with a 1.7-fold increase in the relative risk of death.[30] In a post-hoc analysis from the RALES trial in patients with severe HFrEF, hyperkalaemia (> 5.5 mmol/L) was associated with increased risk of death.[57] The benefit with spironolactone was seen even when K[+] levels reached 6.0 mmol/L. Similar findings were reported from the EMPHASIS-HF trial in patients with mildly symptomatic HFrEF, where eplerenone retained its survival benefits without interaction with the baseline K[+] levels.[58] In the PARADIGM-HF trial in patients with HFrEF trial fewer than 18% of the patients had K[+] levels > 5.5 mmol/L throughout the follow-up with no differences between the sacubitril/valsartan and enalapril groups. Potassium levels > 6.0 mmol/L occurred in 4% of the patients treated with sacubitril/valsartan and in 6% of the patients treated with enalapril, a difference that was statistically significant.[32] Moreover, in patients taking an MRA the hyperkalaemia risk was attenuated by sacubitril/valsartan.[59]

In the PIONEER-HF trial in patients with acute HF, the hyperkalaemia rates were similar to PARADIGM-HF and were not statistically different between groups.[60] In the PARAGON-HF trial in HFpEF, fewer than 16% of the patients had K[+] levels > 5.5 mmol/L throughout the follow-up. Potassium levels > 6.0 mmol/L occurred in 3% of the patients treated with sacubitril/valsartan and in 4% of the patients treated with valsartan.[34] Moreover, in patients taking an MRA, the hyperkalaemia risk was similar in the sacubitril/valsartan and the valsartan groups. Even with normokalaemia, CKD is associated with sub-optimal use of RAASi. In the RALES, EMPHASIS-HF, and PARADIGM trials, there was no significant interaction between the treatment effect and baseline creatinine levels or CKD status (defined as eGFR < 60 mL/min/1.73m[2]). HF trials have mainly excluded patients with eGFR <30 mL/min/1.73m[2], but two large observational studies suggest that RAASi drugs may be as effective in the elderly and in patients with eGFR < 30 mL/min/1.73m[2], often excluded from trials.[61,62]

As also described in the hypokalaemia section, in the PARADIGM-HF and PARAGON-HF trials, both hypo- and hyperkalaemia were associated with an increased risk of cardiovascular death but also with non-cardiovascular death, suggesting that the majority of 'mild' potassium abnormalities (at least as low as 3 and as high as 6 mmol/L) may be markers of underlying disease severity, rather than a mediator of cardiovascular death.[33]

In summary, potassium levels persistently above 6.0 mmol/L are strongly associated with higher mortality rates in HF, but importantly, hyperkalaemia is also a marker for poor RAASi use. When hyperkalaemia reverts to normal, the associated risk is reduced but poor RAASi use persists, illustrating that even sporadic and non-recurring episodes of hyperkalaemia may have long-term consequences. MRAs increase the risk of hyperkalaemia but their benefit in HFrEF is likely seen throughout the potassium spectrum until the K[+] levels reach 6.0 mmol/L. In chronic HFrEF, sacubitril/valsartan likely reduces the risk of hyperkalaemia, as compared to enalapril, especially in the context of concomitant MRA use (❥ Figure 12.2.2).

Management

A synthesis of the management of potassium disturbances is provided in ➲ Table 12.2.2 and Figure 12.2.1. A detailed history of diet, use of supplements, salt substitutes, and concomitant medications that may contribute to hyperkalaemia should be performed. Restriction of dietary potassium to <2.4 g/d is recommended in patients with stage 3 (eGFR <60 mL/min per 1.73 m²) or higher CKD.[63] When sodium restriction is advised, the use of salt substitutes including potassium may expose these patients to a risk of hyperkalaemia. Although patients are often educated to avoid commonly recognized high-potassium foods, many such foods may remain unrecognized by patients and clinicians. Furthermore, it is increasingly clear that patients receive lay information that potassium-rich foods are also often promoted as being healthy foods, so patients receive conflicting messages. Thus, education by a dietician is recommended. This common-sense recommendation, although embedded in nephrology practice, is frequently overlooked by general physicians and (HF) cardiologists. Therapy with RAASi and ARNIs should be started at a low dose and titrated to the maximum tolerated evidence-based dose up to a K⁺ level of 5.5 mmol/L.

Current guidelines recommend that patients with hyperkalaemia should be started on a low K⁺ diet and be initiated on a non-K⁺ sparing diuretic or to increase the diuretic dose if already on a diuretic.[63–65] However, this may lead to volume depletion, a worsening in renal function, and to a stimulation of the RAAS.[66] K⁺ supplements should be discontinued, and drugs that may compromise renal function and increase K⁺ levels, such as NSAIDs, should also be stopped.

Recommendations exist on when to reduce the dose or stop RAASi and ARNIs.[8] In general, it is recommended not to stop RAASi or ARNis when the K+ levels are between 5.0 and 5.5 mmol/L,[67] unless patient follow-up is unreliable in which case the clinician may choose to lower the dose, trying not to decrease below 50% of the guideline-recommended dose. If a short-term cessation of RAASi or ARNi is deemed necessary, this should be kept to the shortest time possible, and RAASi or ARNi should be reintroduced as soon as possible while monitoring K+ levels.[8, 68] Potassium binders (see also later) may be used to facilitate continuation of RAASi therapy. If K+ levels are between 5.5 and 6.0 mmol/L, it is recommended to reduce MRAs or ACEi/ARB, or ARNi dose by 50% and recheck the serum potassium in 5–7 days until it has returned to baseline. If serum potassium does not return to baseline in the short term, long-term compromise of MRAs, ACEi/ARB, or ARNi is not recommended and the use of potassium binders for RAASi enablement should be strongly considered[1] (➲ Table 12.2.2 and ➲ Figure 12.2.1). The dyskalaemia associated-risk and the potential benefits of its prompt correction are depicted in ➲ Figure 12.2.3.

Monitoring

As per guidelines for ACEi/ARB use,[6,68] it is recommended that blood chemistry, including serum creatinine and serum potassium are checked 1–2 weeks after initiation, 1–2 weeks after final dose titration, and every 4 months thereafter. The same recommendation is reasonable also for ARNis. For MRA use, checks should be performed at 1 and 4 weeks after starting/increasing dose and at 8 and 12 weeks; 6, 9, and 12 months, and 4-monthly thereafter. After an episode of hyperkalaemia, it is recommended that blood chemistry, including serum creatinine and serum potassium, should be monitored frequently and serially until potassium and creatinine have plateaued. Proposed guidance on

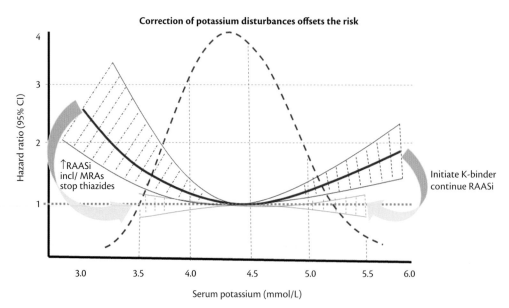

Figure 12.2.3. Association of serum potassium with all-cause death and the benefits of a prompt correction of dyskalemia.
Legend: RAASi, renin-angiotensin aldosterone inhibitor; MRA, mineralocorticoid receptor antagonist; ↑, increase.
Reproduced from Ferreira JP, Butler J, Rossignol P, et al. Abnormalities of Potassium in Heart Failure: JACC State-of-the-Art Review. *J Am Coll Cardiol*. 2020 Jun 9;75(22):2836-2850. doi: 10.1016/j.jacc.2020.04.021 with permission from Elsevier.

MRA-dose adjustments is provided in → Table 12.2.3. However, the rates of appropriate monitoring are very low in clinical practice and a rise in potassium level represents a frequent cause for RAASi dose reduction or discontinuation; actions that may deprive HF patients of therapy proven to improve outcomes.[39,57,69] Indeed, in a study of HF from the Swedish HF registry, and in one of new MRA users in the Stockholm CREAtinine Measurements (SCREAM) health-care utilization cohort, in treated patients RAASi drugs were often stopped over time, and in untreated patients or patients where RAASi was stopped, these were rarely re-started.[21,70] More intense monitoring, using potential future devices for self-monitoring or point-of-care monitoring and disease management programmes, including specialist HF nurse assistance with education of the patient, and follow-up (in person or by telephone) may help optimize safer use of RAASi and merits further investigation.[71] The use of deep-learning models for the screening of potassium abnormalities with ECGs could also be considered as a possibility, after prospective validation.[72]

Potassium binders

The recent availability of safe and tolerable gastrointestinal potassium binders allows for chronic management of hyperkalaemia and may enable RAASi therapy optimization.[73–76] Sodium and calcium polystyrene sulfonate (SPS or CPS) are widely available cation exchange resins that remove potassium via the gastrointestinal tract; these compounds have been around for many years, yet neither SPS nor CPS have been tested in adequately powered randomized trials to assess their safety, tolerability, and efficacy in the long term.[77,78] In the short term, these compounds have poor tolerability, an unstable onset of action, and an unpredictable magnitude of potassium lowering.[79,80] The use of SPS may be associated with volume expansion, since SPS exchanges potassium for sodium. Some reports have also evidenced a potentially increased colonic necrosis risk, although with very low absolute rates and potential for confounding.[81]

Two new agents, patiromer and sodium zirconium cyclosilicate (SZC), also act to remove potassium by exchanging cations (calcium for patiromer, and sodium and hydrogen for SZC) for potassium in the gastrointestinal tract thus increasing its faecal excretion.[79,82,83] The Food and Drug Administration and European Medicines Agency regulatory agencies have both approved patiromer and SZC for the treatment of hyperkalaemia in patients receiving RAASi. Once patients' manifest potassium levels in the hyperkalaemic range, many see their RAASi therapy reduced or discontinued but the use of potassium binders help facilitates preservation of RAASi use and dosing.[84,85] For example, in the PEARL-HF (evaluation of the efficacy and safety of RLY5016, a polymeric potassium binder, in a double-blind, placebo-controlled study in patients with chronic heart failure) trial,[84] 105 patients with HF and a history of hyperkalaemia resulting in discontinuation of a RAASi or CKD, were randomized to patiromer or placebo for 4 weeks. At the end of treatment, patiromer had significantly lowered serum K+ levels and reduced hyperkalaemia (7.3% in patiromer vs 24.5% in placebo) and

enabled a higher proportion of patients on spironolactone 50 mg/day (91% in patiromer vs 74% in placebo).

Notwithstanding, hypokalaemia (K+ < 3.5 mmol/L) occurred in 6% of patients taking patiromer vs 0% of the patients taking placebo (p = 0.094). Additionally, hypomagnesaemia occurred in 24% of the patients taking patiromer vs 2% taking the placebo (p = 0.001). In patients with resistant hypertension and CKD, patiromer also enabled more patients to continue treatment with spironolactone with less hyperkalaemia.[85] The HARMONIZE (Hyperkalaemia Randomized Intervention Multidose ZS-9 Maintenance) trial[74] studied the effects of SZC on serum potassium levels; 87 patients in the trial had documented HF with baseline K+ > 5.0 mmol/L. Among these, 93% achieved the target potassium level of 3.5–5 mmol/L within 48 h of receiving open-label SZC without adjusting RAASi doses. Oedema was reported in 2.4% of the placebo group and up to 14.3% with the highest dose of SZC (15 g daily; no increased oedema risk was seen in patients treated with the lowest dose of 5 g daily).[86] Together, these findings support the potential use of K-binders to enable RAASi up-titration.[75] Practical guidance for the use of these binders in HF is proposed in → Table 12.2.4.

Whether the use of potassium binders enabling optimal RAASi therapy may improve outcomes is under investigation. For example, the DIAMOND (Patiromer for the Management

Table 12.2.4 Proposal for potassium binder use

Serum K+ (mmol/L)	K-binder use
< 5.5	Maintain guideline-recommended treatment Do not stop K-binder if the patient is taking one Consider initiating K-binder between 5.0–5.5 mmol/L if reliable patient follow-up is a concern and therefore consideration is given to compromising RAASi dosing
5.5–5.9	Adapt MRA dose as suggested in → Table 12.2.3 Do not reduce ACEi/ARB/ARNi Re-assess K+ levels after 1 week; if K+ levels still high add K-binder, preferably those with long term enablement data, i.e. patiromer or SZC ♦ Reassess K+ levels after 1 week (a ≈1 mmol/L K+ decrease could be expected) ♦ If K+ <5.5 mmol/L increase MRA dose and maintain K-binder for 1 additional week, then continue routine follow-up ♦ If K+ 5.5-5.9 mmol/L do not increase MRA and maintain/uptitrate K-binder for 1 additional week reassessing K+ afterwards
≥ 6.0	Adapt MRA dose as suggested in → Table 12.2.4 Reduce ACEi/ARB/ARNi in 50% Re-assess K+ levels after 1 week; if K+ levels still high add a K-binder similar to as recommended for potassium levels 5.5-5.9 mmol/L

RAASi, renin-angiotensin aldosterone system inhibitor; MRA, mineralocorticoid receptor antagonist; ACEi/ARB/ARNi, angiotensin converting enzyme inhibitor/angiotensin receptor blocker/angiotensin receptor neprilysin inhibitor.
Reproduced from Ferreira JP, Butler J, Rossignol P, et al. Abnormalities of Potassium in Heart Failure: JACC State-of-the-Art Review. J Am Coll Cardiol. 2020 Jun 9;75(22):2836-2850. doi: 10.1016/j.jacc.2020.04.021 with permission from Elsevier.

of Hyperkalemia in Subjects Receiving RAASi Medications for the Treatment of Heart Failure; ClinicalTrials.gov Identifier: NCT03888066) study will evaluate the potential of patiromer to improve outcomes by enabling HF patients, with or without CKD, to be treated with RAASi therapy in accordance with HF treatment guidelines. The PRIORITIZE-HF (Potassium Reduction Initiative to Optimize RAAS Inhibition Therapy With Sodium Zirconium Cyclosilicate in Heart Failure; ClinicalTrials.gov Identifier: NCT03532009) study will evaluate whether SZC may enable target-dose RAASi up-titration if HF patients.

Gaps in evidence and future directions

A better estimation of the dietary K^+, implementation of K^+ dietary counselling in HF disease management programmes, and their impact on maintenance of optimal blood K^+ levels and outcomes in HF patients requires further investigation to better guide dietary recommendations in HF patients with dyskalaemia.

Potassium monitoring strategy recommendations are currently based on algorithms used in RAASi trials, but which are not being implemented in current practice. New strategies to help embed these recommendations in HF management programmes should be investigated, including using new point-of-care self-measurements remote monitoring technologies.

Whether the use of K-binders may maximize the use of RAASi in HF patients is being investigated in the PRIORITIZE-HF trial. But further research is required to ascertain whether RAASi up-titration enabled by K-binders can improve patients' outcomes. The ongoing DIAMOND study is designed to address this issue.

K-binders may be used to study the potential benefit of RAASi in populations not studied in the past due to the risk of hyperkalaemia, such as patients with eGFR < 30 mL/min/1.73 m^2. Also, K-binders may enable investigating the benefit of higher doses MRA therapy.

Hypokalaemia is common in HF and little is known about the best approach to identify and correct it. Future research should target hypokalaemia; for example, using pragmatic algorithms with MRA dose adjustments, and/or algorithms using potassium supplements, based on K^+ levels.

The potential impact of potassium disturbances on sudden cardiac death has been rarely reported in the literature; given the pro-arrhythmogenic risk of both hypo- and hyperkalaemia a better understanding of the associations and mechanisms by which potassium may increase the risk for sudden death is warranted.

Hypomagnesaemia has been underreported in HF studies and little is known about its prognostic impact and further research is also required in this field.

The sodium-glucose co-transporter 2 inhibitors (SGLT2i), dapagliflozin and empagliflozin, have recently been shown to reduce morbidity and mortality in patients with heart failure and reduced ejection fraction, with and without diabetes in the DAPA-HF (Dapagliflozin in Patients with Heart Failure and Reduced Ejection Fraction) and EMPEROR-Reduced (Cardiovascular and Renal Outcomes with Empagliflozin in Heart Failure) trials.[87–89] No excessive hyper- of hypokalaemia adverse events with SGLT2i were found in these trials; however, the effect of these drugs on serum potassium requires further study and subsequent secondary analyses will certainly report these findings.

Conclusion

Dyskalaemia can be life-threatening if not corrected, either directly or indirectly by impacting provision of optimal medical therapy. Serum potassium below 3.5–4.0 mmol/L may portend a similar death risk as potassium above 5.5–6.0 mmol/L. Based on current observational data, it seems prudent to keep the serum potassium concentration between 4.0 and 5.0 mmol/L. More research and education about dyskalaemia may help increase awareness about the issue and thus improve clinical practice, including: (1) identifying patients at risk, (2) preventing dyskalaemia with available 'life-style' changes, including dietary changes (although this may not be sustainable on the long-run and may deprive patients of healthy food), (3) monitoring serum potassium, at least as per guidelines, and maybe more intensively in patients who experienced dyskalaemia episodes, (4) treating emerging rise of potassium with dose adjustments of drugs likely to increase serum potassium, and/or using potassium binders, and (5) enabling optimal medical therapy in selected patients with potassium binders without compromising life-saving medications. Worsening chronic comorbidities are rarely attributed to hyperkalaemia in the setting of sub-optimal RAASi therapy even when the two are related. However, novel potassium binders might provide a potential opportunity to not compromise on long-term optimal medical therapy of patients with chronic cardiovascular and renal diseases in whom RAASi therapy is known to be beneficial. This hypothesis is currently under investigation.

References

1. Palmer BF. Managing hyperkalemia caused by inhibitors of the renin-angiotensin-aldosterone system. *N Engl J Med*. 2004;351(6):585–92. doi:10.1056/NEJMra035279
2. Palmer BF. Regulation of potassium homeostasis. *Clin J Am Soc Nephrol*. 2015;10(6):1050–60. doi:10.2215/cjn.08580813
3. Mathialahan T, Maclennan KA, Sandle LN, Verbeke C, Sandle GI. Enhanced large intestinal potassium permeability in end-stage renal disease. *J Pathol*.;206(1):46–51. doi:10.1002/path.1750
4. Fisch C, Knoebel SB, Feigenbaum H, Greenspan K. Potassium and the monophasic action potential, electrocardiogram, conduction and arrhythmias. *Prog Cardiovasc Dis*. 1966;8(5):387–418. doi:10.1016/s0033-0620(66)80029-4
5. Macdonald JE, Struthers AD. What is the optimal serum potassium level in cardiovascular patients? *J Am Coll Cardiol*. 2004;43(2):155–61. doi:10.1016/j.jacc.2003.06.021
6. Aldahl M, Jensen AC, Davidsen L, *et al*. Associations of serum potassium levels with mortality in chronic heart failure patients. *Eur Heart J*. 2017;38(38):2890–6. doi:10.1093/eurheartj/ehx460
7. Nunez J, Bayes-Genis A, Zannad F, *et al*. Long-term potassium monitoring and dynamics in heart failure and risk of mortality. *Circulation*. 2018;137(13):1320–30. doi:10.1161/circulationaha.117.030576
8. Ponikowski P, Voors AA, Anker SD, *et al*. 2016 ESC Guidelines for the diagnosis and treatment of acute and chronic heart failure: The Task Force for the diagnosis and treatment of acute and chronic heart failure of the European Society of Cardiology (ESC). Developed with the special contribution of the Heart Failure Association (HFA) of the ESC. *Eur J Heart Fail*. 2016; 2016;37(27):2129–200. doi:10.1002/ejhf.592

9. Yancy CW, Jessup M, Bozkurt B, et al. 2016 ACC/AHA/HFSA Focused Update on New Pharmacological Therapy for Heart Failure: An Update of the 2013 ACCF/AHA Guideline for the Management of Heart Failure: A Report of the American College of Cardiology/American Heart Association Task Force on Clinical Practice Guidelines and the Heart Failure Society of America. J Am Coll Cardiol. 2016;68(13):1476–88. doi:10.1016/j.jacc.2016.05.011

10. Collins AJ, Pitt B, Reaven N, et al. Association of serum potassium with all-cause mortality in patients with and without heart failure, chronic kidney disease, and/or diabetes. Am J Nephrol. 2017;46(3):213–221. doi:10.1159/000479802

11. Krogager ML, Torp-Pedersen C, Mortensen RN, et al. Short-term mortality risk of serum potassium levels in hypertension: a retrospective analysis of nationwide registry data. Eur Heart J. 2017; 2017;38(2):104–112. doi:10.1093/eurheartj/ehw129

12. Goyal A, Spertus JA, Gosch K, et al. Serum potassium levels and mortality in acute myocardial infarction. JAMA. 2012;307(2):157–64. doi:10.1001/jama.2011.1967

13. Pitt B, Rossignol P. Serum potassium in patients with chronic heart failure: once we make a U-turn where should we go? Eur Heart J. 2017;38(38):2897–9. doi:10.1093/eurheartj/ehx537

14. Kovesdy CP, Matsushita K, Sang Y, et al. Serum potassium and adverse outcomes across the range of kidney function: a CKD Prognosis Consortium meta-analysis. Eur Heart J. 2018; 2018;39(17):1535–42. doi:10.1093/eurheartj/ehy100

15. Hayes J, Kalantar-Zadeh K, Lu JL, Turban S, Anderson JE, Kovesdy CP. Association of hypo- and hyperkalemia with disease progression and mortality in males with chronic kidney disease: the role of race. Nephron Clin Pract. 2012;120(1):c8–16. doi:10.1159/000329511

16. Shiyovich A, Gilutz H, Plakht Y. Potassium Fluctuations are associated with inhospital mortality from acute myocardial infarction. Soroka Acute Myocardial Infarction II (SAMI-II) Project. Angiology. 2018;69(8):709–17. doi:10.1177/0003319717740004

17. Kovesdy CP, Appel LJ, Grams ME, et al. Potassium homeostasis in health and disease: A scientific workshop cosponsored by the National Kidney Foundation and the American Society of Hypertension. J Am Soc Hypertens. 2017;11(12):783–800. doi:10.1016/j.jash.2017.09.011

18. Cooper LB, Savarese G, Carrero JJ, et al. Clinical and research implications of serum versus plasma potassium measurements. Eur J Heart Fail. 2019;21(4):536–7. doi:10.1002/ejhf.1371

19. Meng QH, Wagar EA. Pseudohyperkalemia: A new twist on an old phenomenon. Crit Rev Clin Lab Sci. 2015;52(2):45–55. doi:10.3109/10408363.2014.966898

20. Bielecka-Dabrowa A, Mikhailidis DP, Jones L, Rysz J, Aronow WS, Banach M. The meaning of hypokalemia in heart failure. Int J Cardiol. 2012;158(1):12–7. doi:10.1016/j.ijcard.2011.06.121

21. Savarese G, Xu H, Trevisan M, et al. Incidence, predictors, and outcome associations of dyskalemia in heart failure with preserved, mid-range, and reduced ejection fraction. JACC Heart Fail. 2019;7(1):65–76. doi:10.1016/j.jchf.2018.10.003

22. Weber KT. Aldosterone in congestive heart failure. N Engl J Med. 2001;345(23):1689–97. doi:10.1056/NEJMra000050

23. Gettes LS. Electrolyte abnormalities underlying lethal and ventricular arrhythmias. Circulation. 1992;85(1 Suppl):I70–6.

24. Spencer AP. Digoxin in heart failure. Crit Care Nurs Clin North Am. 2003;15(4):447–52.

25. Cooper LB, Benson L, Mentz RJ, et al. Association between potassium level and outcomes in heart failure with reduced ejection fraction: a cohort study from the Swedish Heart Failure Registry. Eur J Heart Fail. 2020; 2020;22(8):1390–8. doi:10.1002/ejhf.1757

26. Linde C, Qin L, Bakhai A, et al. Serum potassium and clinical outcomes in heart failure patients: results of risk calculations in 21 334

patients in the UK. ESC Heart Fail. 2019;6(2):280–90. doi:10.1002/ehf2.12402

27. Hoss S, Elizur Y, Luria D, Keren A, Lotan C, Gotsman I. Serum potassium levels and outcome in patients with chronic heart failure. Am J Cardiol. 2016;118(12):1868–74. doi:10.1016/j.amjcard.2016.08.078

28. Matsushita K, Sang Y, Yang C, et al. Dyskalemia, its patterns, and prognosis among patients with incident heart failure: A nationwide study of US veterans. PLoS One. 2019;14(8):e0219899. doi:10.1371/journal.pone.0219899

29. Basnet S, Dhital R, Tharu B, Ghimire S, Poudel DR, Donato A. Influence of abnormal potassium levels on mortality among hospitalized heart failure patients in the US: data from National Inpatient Sample. J Community Hosp Intern Med Perspect. 2019;9(2):103–7. doi:10.1080/20009666.2019.1593778

30. Desai AS, Liu J, Pfeffer MA, et al. Incident hyperkalemia, hypokalemia, and clinical outcomes during spironolactone treatment of heart failure with preserved ejection fraction: Analysis of the TOPCAT Trial. J Card Fail. 2018;24(5):313–20. doi:10.1016/j.cardfail.2018.03.002

31. Rossignol P, Girerd N, Bakris G, et al. Impact of eplerenone on cardiovascular outcomes in heart failure patients with hypokalaemia. Eur J Heart Fail. 2017;19(6):792–9. doi:10.1002/ejhf.688

32. McMurray JJ, Packer M, Desai AS, et al. Angiotensin-neprilysin inhibition versus enalapril in heart failure. N Engl J Med. Sep 11 2014;371(11):993–1004. doi:10.1056/NEJMoa1409077

33. Ferreira JP, Mogensen UM, Jhund PS, et al. Serum potassium in the PARADIGM-HF trial. Eur J Heart Fail. 2020; 22(11):2056–64. doi:10.1002/ejhf.1987

34. Solomon SD, McMurray JJV, Anand IS, et al. Angiotensin-neprilysin inhibition in heart failure with preserved ejection fraction. N Engl J Med. 2019;381(17):1609–20. doi:10.1056/NEJMoa1908655

35. Felker GM, Ellison DH, Mullens W, Cox ZL, Testani JM. Diuretic therapy for patients with heart failure: JACC state-of-the-art review. J Am Coll Cardiol. 2020;75(10):1178–95. doi:10.1016/j.jacc.2019.12.059

36. Morgan DB, Davidson C. Hypokalaemia and diuretics: an analysis of publications. Br Med J. 1980;280(6218):905–8. doi:10.1136/bmj.280.6218.905

37. Tannen RL. Diuretic-induced hypokalemia. Kidney Int. 1985;28(6):988–1000. doi:10.1038/ki.1985.229

38. Cohn JN, Kowey PR, Whelton PK, Prisant LM. New guidelines for potassium replacement in clinical practice: a contemporary review by the National Council on Potassium in Clinical Practice. Arch Intern Med. 2000;160(16):2429–36. doi:10.1001/archinte.160.16.2429

39. Cooper LB, Hammill BG, Peterson ED, et al. Consistency of laboratory monitoring during initiation of mineralocorticoid receptor antagonist therapy in patients with heart failure. JAMA 2015;314(18):1973–5. doi:10.1001/jama.2015.11904

40. Ko DT, Juurlink DN, Mamdani MM, et al. Appropriateness of spironolactone prescribing in heart failure patients: a population-based study. J Card Fail. 2006;12(3):205–10. doi:10.1016/j.cardfail.2006.01.003

41. Chang AR, Sang Y, Leddy J, et al. Antihypertensive Medications and the Prevalence of Hyperkalemia in a Large Health System. Hypertension. 2016;67(6):1181–8. doi:10.1161/hypertensionaha.116.07363

42. Maggioni AP, Anker SD, Dahlstrom U, et al. Are hospitalized or ambulatory patients with heart failure treated in accordance with European Society of Cardiology guidelines? Evidence from 12,440 patients of the ESC Heart Failure Long-Term Registry. Eur J Heart Fail. 2013;15(10):1173–84. doi:10.1093/eurjhf/hft134

43. Savarese G, Carrero JJ, Pitt B, et al. Factors associated with underuse of mineralocorticoid receptor antagonists in heart failure with reduced ejection fraction: an analysis of 11 215 patients from the Swedish Heart Failure Registry. Eur J Heart Fail. 2018;20(9):1326–34. doi:10.1002/ejhf.1182

44. Rossignol P, Legrand M, Kosiborod M, et al. Emergency management of severe hyperkalemia: Guideline for best practice and opportunities for the future. *Pharmacol Res*. 2016;113(Pt A):585–91. doi:10.1016/j.phrs.2016.09.039

45. Depret F, Peacock WF, Liu KD, Rafique Z, Rossignol P, Legrand M. Management of hyperkalemia in the acutely ill patient. *Ann Intensive Care*. 2019;9(1):32. doi:10.1186/s13613-019-0509-8

46. Komajda M, Anker SD, Cowie MR, et al. Physicians' adherence to guideline-recommended medications in heart failure with reduced ejection fraction: data from the QUALIFY global survey. *Eur J Heart Fail*. 2016;18(5):514–22. doi:10.1002/ejhf.510

47. Konstam MA, Neaton JD, Dickstein K, et al. Effects of high-dose versus low-dose losartan on clinical outcomes in patients with heart failure (HEAAL study): a randomised, double-blind trial. *Lancet*. 2009;374(9704):1840–8. doi:10.1016/s0140-6736(09)61913-9

48. Packer M, Poole-Wilson PA, Armstrong PW, et al. Comparative effects of low and high doses of the angiotensin-converting enzyme inhibitor, lisinopril, on morbidity and mortality in chronic heart failure. ATLAS Study Group. *Circulation*. 1999;100(23):2312–8.

49. Ferreira JP, Abreu P, McMurray JJV, et al. Renal function stratified dose comparisons of eplerenone versus placebo in the EMPHASIS-HF trial. *Eur J Heart Fail*.;21(3):345–51. doi:10.1002/ejhf.1400

50. Juurlink DN, Mamdani MM, Lee DS, et al. Rates of hyperkalemia after publication of the Randomized Aldactone Evaluation Study. *N Engl J Med*. 2004;351(6):543–51. doi:10.1056/NEJMoa040135

51. Wei L, Struthers AD, Fahey T, Watson AD, Macdonald TM. Spironolactone use and renal toxicity: population based longitudinal analysis. *BMJ*. 2010;340:c1768. doi:10.1136/bmj.c1768

52. Epstein M, Reaven NL, Funk SE, McGaughey KJ, Oestreicher N, Knispel J. Evaluation of the treatment gap between clinical guidelines and the utilization of renin-angiotensin-aldosterone system inhibitors. *Am J Manag Care*. 2015;21(11 Suppl):S212–20.

53. Beusekamp JC, Tromp J, van der Wal HH, et al. Potassium and the use of renin-angiotensin-aldosterone system inhibitors in heart failure with reduced ejection fraction: data from BIOSTAT-CHF. *Eur J Heart Fail*. 2018;20(5):923–30. doi:10.1002/ejhf.1079

54. Lund LH, Pitt B. Is hyperkalaemia in heart failure a risk factor or a risk marker? Implications for renin-angiotensin-aldosterone system inhibitor use. *Eur J Heart Fail*. 2018;20(5):931–32. doi:10.1002/ejhf.1175

55. Trevisan M, de Deco P, Xu H, et al. Incidence, predictors and clinical management of hyperkalaemia in new users of mineralocorticoid receptor antagonists. *Eur J Heart Fail*. 2018;20(8):1217–26. doi:10.1002/ejhf.1199

56. Rossignol P, Lainscak M, Crespo-Leiro M, Laroche C, Piepoli M, al e. Unravelling the interplay between hyperkalaemia, renin-angiotensin-aldosterone inhibitor use and clinical outcomes. Data from 9 222 chronic heart failure patients of the ESC HFA EORP Heart Failure Long-Term Registry. Eur J Heart Fail. 2020;22(8):1378–89.

57. Vardeny O, Claggett B, Anand I, et al. Incidence, predictors, and outcomes related to hypo- and hyperkalemia in patients with severe heart failure treated with a mineralocorticoid receptor antagonist. *Circ Heart Fail*. 2014;7(4):573–9. doi:10.1161/circheartfailure.114.001104

58. Rossignol P, Dobre D, McMurray JJ, et al. Incidence, determinants, and prognostic significance of hyperkalemia and worsening renal function in patients with heart failure receiving the mineralocorticoid receptor antagonist eplerenone or placebo in addition to optimal medical therapy: results from the Eplerenone in Mild Patients Hospitalization and Survival Study in Heart Failure (EMPHASIS-HF). *Circ Heart Fail*. 2014;7(1):51–8. doi:10.1161/circheartfailure.113.000792

59. Desai AS, Vardeny O, Claggett B, et al. Reduced risk of hyperkalemia during treatment of heart failure with mineralocorticoid receptor antagonists by use of sacubitril/valsartan compared with enalapril: a secondary analysis of the PARADIGM-HF Trial. *JAMA Cardiol*. 2017;2(1):79–85. doi:10.1001/jamacardio.2016.4733

60. Velazquez EJ, Morrow DA, DeVore AD, et al. Angiotensin-neprilysin inhibition in acute decompensated heart failure. *N Engl J Med*. 2019;380(6):539–48. doi:10.1056/NEJMoa1812851

61. Edner M, Benson L, Dahlstrom U, Lund LH. Association between renin-angiotensin system antagonist use and mortality in heart failure with severe renal insufficiency: a prospective propensity score-matched cohort study. *Eur Heart J*. Sep 7 2015;36(34):2318–26. doi:10.1093/eurheartj/ehv268

62. Savarese G, Dahlstrom U, Vasko P, Pitt B, Lund LH. Association between renin-angiotensin system inhibitor use and mortality/morbidity in elderly patients with heart failure with reduced ejection fraction: a prospective propensity score-matched cohort study. *Eur Heart J*. 2018;39(48):4257–65. doi:10.1093/eurheartj/ehy621

63. K/DOQI clinical practice guidelines on hypertension and antihypertensive agents in chronic kidney disease. *Am J Kidney Dis*. 2004;43(5 Suppl 1):S1–290.

64. Rosano GMC, Tamargo J, Kjeldsen KP, et al. Expert consensus document on the management of hyperkalaemia in patients with cardiovascular disease treated with renin angiotensin aldosterone system inhibitors: coordinated by the Working Group on Cardiovascular Pharmacotherapy of the European Society of Cardiology. *Eur Heart J Cardiovasc Pharmacother*. 2018;4(3):180–8. doi:10.1093/ehjcvp/pvy015

65. Andrassy KM. Comments on 'KDIGO 2012 Clinical Practice Guideline for the Evaluation and Management of Chronic Kidney Disease'. *Kidney Int*. 2013; 84(3):622–3.

66. Zannad F, Rossignol P. Cardiorenal syndrome revisited. *Circulation*. 2018;138(9):929–44. doi:10.1161/circulationaha.117.028814

67. Bakris GL, Pitt B, Weir MR, et al. Effect of patiromer on serum potassium level in patients with hyperkalemia and diabetic kidney disease: The AMETHYST-DN Randomized Clinical Trial. *JAMA*. 2015;314(2):151–61. doi:10.1001/jama.2015.7446

68. Yancy CW, Jessup M, Bozkurt B, et al. 2013 ACCF/AHA guideline for the management of heart failure: executive summary: a report of the American College of Cardiology Foundation/American Heart Association Task Force on practice guidelines. *Circulation*. 2013;128(16):1810–52. doi:10.1161/CIR.0b013e31829e8807

69. Ferreira JP, Rossignol P, Machu JL, et al. Mineralocorticoid receptor antagonist pattern of use in heart failure with reduced ejection fraction: findings from BIOSTAT-CHF. *Eur J Heart Fail*. 2017;19(10):1284–93. doi:10.1002/ejhf.900

70. Thorvaldsen T, Benson L, Dahlstrom U, Edner M, Lund LH. Use of evidence-based therapy and survival in heart failure in Sweden 2003–2012. *Eur J Heart Fail*. 2016;18(5):503–11. doi:10.1002/ejhf.496

71. Rossignol P, Coats AJ, Chioncel O, Spoletini I, Rosano G. Renal function, electrolytes, and congestion monitoring in heart failure. *Eur Heart J Suppl*. 2019;21(Suppl M):M25–31. doi:10.1093/eurheartj/suz220

72. Galloway CD, Valys AV, Shreibati JB, et al. Development and validation of a deep-learning model to screen for hyperkalemia from the electrocardiogram. *JAMA Cardiol*. 2019;4(5):428–436. doi:10.1001/jamacardio.2019.0640

73. Kosiborod M, Rasmussen HS, Lavin P, et al. Effect of sodium zirconium cyclosilicate on potassium lowering for 28 days among outpatients with hyperkalemia: the HARMONIZE randomized clinical trial. *JAMA*. 2014;312(21):2223–33. doi:10.1001/jama.2014.15688

74. Anker SD, Kosiborod M, Zannad F, et al. Maintenance of serum potassium with sodium zirconium cyclosilicate (ZS-9) in heart failure patients: results from a phase 3 randomized, double-blind, placebo-controlled trial. *Eur J Heart Fail*. 2015;17(10):1050–6. doi:10.1002/ejhf.300

75. Zannad F, Ferreira JP, Pitt B. Potassium binders for the prevention of hyperkalaemia in heart failure patients: implementation issues and future developments. *Eur Heart J Suppl.* 2019;21(Suppl A):A55–60. doi:10.1093/eurheartj/suy034

76. Weir MR, Bakris GL, Bushinsky DA, *et al.* Patiromer in patients with kidney disease and hyperkalemia receiving RAAS inhibitors. *N Engl J Med.* 15 2015;372(3):211–21. doi:10.1056/NEJMoa1410853

77. Lepage L, Dufour AC, Doiron J, *et al.* Randomized clinical trial of sodium polystyrene sulfonate for the treatment of mild hyperkalemia in CKD. *Clin J Am Soc Nephrol.* 2015;10(12):2136–42. doi:10.2215/cjn.03640415

78. Bianchi S, Regolisti G. Pivotal clinical trials, meta-analyses and current guidelines in the treatment of hyperkalemia. *Nephrol Dial Transplant.* 2019;34(Supplement_3):iii51–iii61. doi:10.1093/ndt/gfz213

79. Pitt B, Bakris GL. New potassium binders for the treatment of hyperkalemia: current data and opportunities for the future. *Hypertension.* 2015;66(4):731–8. doi:10.1161/hypertensionaha.115.04889

80. Zannad F, Rossignol P, Stough WG, *et al.* New approaches to hyperkalemia in patients with indications for renin angiotensin aldosterone inhibitors: Considerations for trial design and regulatory approval. *Int J Cardiol.* 2016;216:46–51. doi:10.1016/j.ijcard.2016.04.127

81. Pitt B, Rossignol P. Potassium lowering agents: Recommendations for physician and patient education, treatment reappraisal, and serial monitoring of potassium in patients with chronic hyperkalemia. *Pharmacol Res.* 2017;118:2–4. doi:10.1016/j.phrs.2016.07.032

82. Tamargo J, Caballero R, Delpon E. New drugs for the treatment of hyperkalemia in patients treated with renin-angiotensin-aldosterone system inhibitors – hype or hope? *Discov Med.* 2014;18(100):249–54.

83. Spinowitz BS, Fishbane S, Pergola PE, *et al.* Sodium zirconium cyclosilicate among individuals with hyperkalemia: a 12-month phase 3 study. *Clin J Am Soc Nephrol.* 7 2019;14(6):798–809. doi:10.2215/cjn.12651018

84. Pitt B, Anker SD, Bushinsky DA, Kitzman DW, Zannad F, Huang IZ. Evaluation of the efficacy and safety of RLY5016, a polymeric potassium binder, in a double-blind, placebo-controlled study in patients with chronic heart failure (the PEARL-HF) trial. *Eur Heart J.* 2011;32(7):820–8. doi:10.1093/eurheartj/ehq502

85. Agarwal R, Rossignol P, Romero A, *et al.* Patiromer versus placebo to enable spironolactone use in patients with resistant hypertension and chronic kidney disease (AMBER): a phase 2, randomised, double-blind, placebo-controlled trial. *Lancet.* 2019;394(10208):1540–50. doi:10.1016/s0140-6736(19)32135-x

86. Zannad F, Hsu BG, Maeda Y, *et al.* Efficacy and safety of sodium zirconium cyclosilicate for hyperkalaemia: the randomized, placebo-controlled HARMONIZE-Global study. *ESC Heart Fail.* 2020; 7(1):54–64.doi:10.1002/ehf2.12561

87. McMurray JJV, Solomon SD, Inzucchi SE, *et al.* Dapagliflozin in Patients with Heart Failure and Reduced Ejection Fraction. *N Engl J Med.* 2019; 381(21):1995–2008 doi:10.1056/NEJMoa1911303

88. Packer M, Anker SD, Butler J, *et al.* Cardiovascular and Renal Outcomes with Empagliflozin in Heart Failure. *N Engl J Med.* 2020;383(15):1413–24 doi:10.1056/NEJMoa2022190

89. Zannad F, Ferreira JP, Pocock SJ, *et al.* SGLT2 inhibitors in patients with heart failure with reduced ejection fraction: a meta-analysis of the EMPEROR-Reduced and DAPA-HF trials. *Lancet.* Aug 28 2020; 396(10254):819–29doi:10.1016/s0140-6736(20)31824-9

CHAPTER 12.3

Chronic lung disease

Josep Masip, Karina Portillo, and Mattia Arrigo

Contents

Introduction

The heart and the lung are essential organs that have close structural and functional interactions. Left-sided heart failure (HF) is associated with pulmonary congestion affecting lung function during episodes of acute decompensation and producing permanent lung parenchymal changes in chronic states. Conversely, lung diseases have an impact on the heart, predominantly affecting the right ventricle (RV), causing changes that may further precipitate or contribute to the development of HF. In addition, the main manifestations of HF are related to lung congestion or pulmonary hypertension (PH). Therefore, lung diseases and HF are common entities with a reciprocal relationship. Chronic lung diseases (CLD), in particular chronic obstructive pulmonary disease (COPD), are prevalent in up to one-third of patients with HF because both conditions share several risk factors (e.g. age, smoking) and have mutual detrimental effects on clinical course and survival.[1,2] This chapter addresses the impact that CLD have on the heart, preceding HF, as well as the impact that HF can have on the lung in both acute and chronic settings.

Impact of lung diseases on the heart

The involvement of the heart in lung diseases is a frequent finding, and RV alterations have been described even in early stages of chronic respiratory diseases.[3,4] PH is one of the most relevant complications of lung diseases, especially in COPD and diffuse interstitial lung diseases (ILD).[5] This PH due to lung diseases, which is allocated to Group 3 of the World Symposium on Pulmonary Hypertension (WSPH) clinical classification, and PH due to left heart disease (WSPH Group 2) are considered the most frequent forms of PH.[6] On the other hand, although cardiac abnormalities in these diseases have been mainly associated with the RV, several studies have reported that the left ventricle (LV) may also be affected.[7]

In CLD, the evaluation of cardiac chambers and the estimation of systolic pulmonary artery pressure (PAP) by echocardiography (ECHO) are complicated by the frequency of suboptimal quality images. Right-heart catheterization, as the gold standard for diagnosing PH, is not routinely recommended in the evaluation of lung diseases. Therefore, these drawbacks have generated several methodological limitations in studies that analyse the coexistence of respiratory and cardiovascular (CV) diseases, as well as in the real-world clinical practice. To overcome these limitations it is recommended to combine different ECHO parameters with advanced imaging techniques such as magnetic resonance image (MRI), computed tomography scanning (CT), nuclear scintigraphy, or positron emission tomography.

Chronic obstructive pulmonary disease

COPD and CV disease are major causes of death worldwide. Together they are responsible for approximately 60% of all tobacco-related deaths. CV disease is highly prevalent in patients with COPD and is an important cause of mortality in this population. The cardiac abnormality most related to COPD has traditionally been considered to be RV dysfunction, but many recent publications have also reported pathological LV changes in the autopsied hearts of COPD patients.[8] At present, due to advances in imaging techniques, various ventricular abnormalities have been demonstrated in these patients.

Pathophysiology of cardiac alterations in COPD

The pathophysiology of the development of ventricular alterations in COPD involves multifactorial processes. Several studies have shown that CV events are more common in patients with COPD compared to smokers without COPD.[9] However, whether this is simply due to the higher prevalence of traditional CV risk factors (systemic hypertension, diabetes mellitus, reduced physical activity, and dyslipidaemia) in COPD patients, or whether there is a particular pathophysiological connection, is still widely debated. While some authors propose systemic inflammation as the aetiological pathway, recent studies indicate that sustained systemic inflammation occurs in only a proportion of patients with COPD. Thus, the association between RV and LV impairment in COPD is much more complex, and may involve other factors: biological (deterioration in forced expiratory volume in 1 second (FEV1), emphysema, hyperinflation), neurohumoral (excess sympathetic activity), and genetic background (polymorphisms of the metalloproteinases, telomere shortening etc.).[3,7,10,11]

Ventricular interdependence describes the phenomenon in which both RV pressure and volume overload cause the interventricular septum to shift toward the LV, modifying its geometry ('D-shape'). Dilatation of the RV also increases the constrictive effect of the pericardium, all of which can result in a reduction in the distensibility and filling of the LV. This mechanism may explain why a preserved ejection fraction (EF) can be observed in the LV, despite a sub-optimal filling phase.

RV alterations in COPD

Necropsy studies have revealed RV hypertrophy in up to 40% of COPD patients.[10] In clinical practice, adequate evaluation of the RV is essential, since its dysfunction is related to poorer oxygen supply to the tissues, lower exercise tolerance, and as an independent prognostic factor in these patients.[11] The guidelines of the European Society of Cardiology and the European Respiratory Society (ESC/ERS) have proposed that ECHO evaluation is indicated in all patients with symptoms of greater severity than the underlying pulmonary disease may suggest.[6] Several non-invasive ECHO parameters of elevated PAP and RV dysfunction have been proposed, with different cut-off values.[12] Some authors found that the RV end-diastolic diameter index and the RV wall thickness were increased in COPD patients compared to a control group.[13] These parameters together with the end-diastolic filling rate are independent predictors of exercise capacity and mortality.[14]

RV index of myocardial performance (RIMP) evaluated by tissue Doppler imaging, with a cut off of 0.43, has been recognized as being able to identify remodelling of the RV in COPD patients without PH.[12] Free wall RV longitudinal strain (fwRVLS) of the basal portion with a cut-off <−23% has also been associated with an early impairment of RV function.[12,13]

RV morphological changes and right atrial (RA) dilation are associated with a decrease in exercise tolerance in COPD patients with mild to moderate disease, independently of the degree of the airflow severity.[14] This clinical outcome highlights the need to include assessment of RA in the ECHO report when evaluating pulmonary diseases.[12,15]

Other imaging techniques such 3D ECHO, speckle tracking ECHO, and MRI are used to describe RV changes in COPD patients with normoxaemia or mild hypoxeamia. The RV-EF during exercise measured by nuclear techniques has been described as a strong predictor of mortality in patients who are candidates for lung transplantation.

Pulmonary hypertension in COPD (WSPH 3)

PH is a relevant complication in the natural history of patients with COPD, since its presence is associated with shorter survival, an increased risk of exacerbations, and greater use of health care resources.[11] The actual prevalence of PH in COPD remains uncertain and varies widely according to the targeted population, the definition applied, and the diagnostic approach used to identify PH. According to updated classifications, PH is defined as a mean PAP greater than 20 mmHg, which is the upper normal limit shown in healthy subjects, with a pulmonary vascular resistance (PVR) greater than 2 Wood Units.[16]

In COPD, most haemodynamic studies have been performed in patients with advanced disease in whom PH is expected to occur more frequently, with a prevalence of PH ranging from 23% to 91%.[17] However, the prevalence of PH in milder disease is lower. Some reports have shown that up to 70% of patients might have abnormal mean PAP during exercise, which is associated with decreased cardiac output.[17,18]

The rate of PH progression in COPD is normally slow (an increase of <1 mmHg per year) and the degree of PH in COPD is usually of mild-to-moderate magnitude.[6,11] However, a subgroup of patients (1–5% according to published series) may develop severe pre-capillary PH and present with specific clinical features including moderate airway obstruction with deterioration of gas exchange and low carbon monoxide diffusion capacity (DLCO).[17] It is important to identify these patients with predominant vascular involvement since they represent a clinically distinct vascular phenotype of poor prognosis in the scope of COPD population.[16,17,18,19]

The left ventricle in COPD
Left ventricular hypertrophy

Ventriculography and autopsy studies in patients with chronic bronchitis and emphysema often show LV hypertrophy and increased ventricular mass.[8] Anderson et al.[20] using ECHO, reported a prevalence of LV hypertrophy of 21.4% in men and

43.2% in women with normoxaemic COPD and no underlying PH; the LV mass was significantly greater than that of controls.

Diastolic ventricular dysfunction

Various studies in COPD patients have described a higher rate of LV diastolic dysfunction compared to age-matched controls, even in those without CV risk factors.[7] Its prevalence also varies considerably, reaching 90% in some series of COPD patients with severe airflow limitation.[8] The most frequently described pattern is one of slow relaxation, which is characterized by reduced E and increased A waves, with an E:A ratio < 1.[12]

Systolic left ventricular dysfunction

The reported prevalence of systolic LV dysfunction in patients with stable COPD in different series in non-selected populations ranges from 8 to 25%,[21,22] and varies widely depending on the presence of CV risk factors (0–16% in COPD patients without these risk factors).[7]

Heart failure

HF may remain unnoticed in patients with COPD, since both entities have similar signs and symptoms that frequently overlap. Natriuretic peptides are crucial for the correct diagnosis.

The prevalence of HF in patients with COPD in different series ranges from 7% to 31%.[22,23] Rutten et al.[24] reported a prevalence of HF around 20% in a cohort of patients with stable COPD. During a 4-year follow-up period, mortality among patients diagnosed of HF was higher, regardless of other factors such as age, sex, history of ischaemic heart disease, or systemic hypertension. Therefore, incident HF is a significant and independent predictor of all-cause mortality and it appears to be independent of LVEF.[9]

Idiopathic pulmonary fibrosis and diffuse parenchymal lung disease

More than 200 entities have been described under the term of ILD. Among them, idiopathic pulmonary fibrosis (IPF) has recently generated special interest due to the emerging therapies for its management.

IPF is particularly associated with the development of PH and RV dysfunction. The presence of PH is associated with a worse prognosis.[5,25]

The prevalence of PH in IPF may vary depending upon the population evaluated and the mean PAP cut-off criteria used. Studies with right-heart catheterization have indicated that the prevalence of PH in IPF ranges between 31% and 46%.[25] Although IPF patients with early and moderate disease tend to have less frequent PH, the ARTEMIS-IPF trial that included patients with non-severe IPF with a mean forced vital capacity (FVC) of 68% of predicted, showed that the prevalence of PH at baseline was 10%.[26] In line with this observation, a lower contractile reserve of the RV, evaluated by stress ECHO, has been described in early stages of the disease.[27]

Combined pulmonary fibrosis and emphysema (CPFE) is a syndrome characterized by the coexistence of emphysema in the upper lobes and pulmonary fibrosis, predominantly in the lower lobes, associated with a distinctive functional profile. Spirometric values appear to be practically unchanged, contrasting with a severe reduction in DLCO, hypoxaemia, and oxygen desaturation on exertion. These patients are particularly prone to develop severe PH.[28] The PH prevalence in CFPE has been observed as being between 47% and 90%, much higher than in COPD or IPF alone.[6,29] In most published series, the diagnosis of PH was established by a transthoracic ECHO, with a criterion of a tricuspid regurgitation velocity >2.8 m/s. The study by Cottin et al.[28] demonstrated that PH played a critical role in the prognosis of these patients. The 5-year probability of survival was 25% in patients with PH diagnosed by ECHO compared with 75% in those with no signs of PH at the time of diagnosis. The mean survival time in this series was 6.1 years, dropping to 3.9 years in those patients with associated PH.

Pathophysiology of cardiac alterations in interstitial lung diseases

There are many mechanisms that have been shown to play a role in the development of RV changes and PH in fibrotic lung disease in genetically susceptible individuals. RV damage is considered to be due to the increase of PVR secondary to hypoxic vasoconstriction and the progressive rearrangement and fibrotic distortion of alveolar parenchyma. Many diverse mediators including endothelin 1 (ET-1), transforming growth factor-β, prostaglandin-E2, bone morphogenetic protein receptor type 2, adenosine signalling, hyaluronan, and IL-6, can lead to an imbalance in endothelium-derived vasodilator factors shifting the balance towards fixed obliteration and narrowing of pulmonary vessels.[30]

Lung alterations in heart failure

Pathophysiology of lung alterations in acute heart failure

In acute heart failure (AHF) syndromes the lungs are commonly affected by pulmonary congestion secondary to LV and left atrial (LA) alterations. The dysfunction in the left heart chambers may be triggered by different insults, such as myocardial ischaemia or necrosis, arrhythmia, cardiomyopathy, and valvular, pericardial, or systemic diseases.

Whatever the cause, the process is triggered by an increase in the LA pressures transmitted backwards to the pulmonary veins and the capillary bed. This rise of the hydrostatic pressure in the pulmonary microcirculation unbalances the Starling forces in the capillaries, increasing the transit of fluid to the interstitial space (➲ Figure 12.3.1), resulting in interstitial and peri-bronchovascular oedema.

The excess of fluid in the interstitium is usually drained by the lymphatic system, but when the oedema surpasses the capacity of the lymphatic system to drain the fluid and keep pleural pressure low, the fluid moves across the visceral pleura creating pleural effusions, and also reaching the air spaces, causing alveolar oedema.[31]

The extent of interstitial and alveolar oedema is related to the degree, duration, and rate of the increase in the hydrostatic capillary pressure. The oncotic pressure usually does not play a significant role, but three additional factors may impact the progression of oedema. One is the frequently observed disruption in

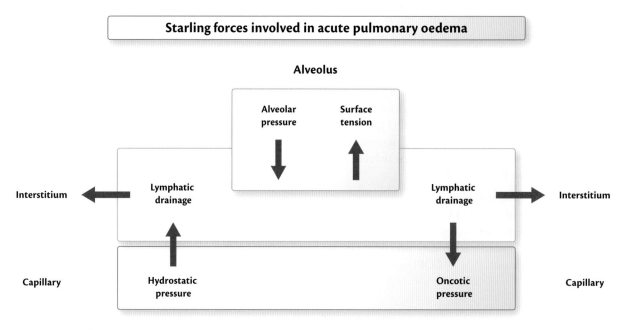

Figure 12.3.1 Scheme of the Starling forces involved in the alveolar-capillary units. Oncotic pressure, lymphatic drainage and intra-alveolar pressure are forces against oedema formation.

the anatomic configuration of the capillary–alveolar membrane, provoking what is called 'alveolar–capillaries membrane stress failure'.[32] Another is the alveolar fluid reabsorption capacity[33] which depends on the active transport of sodium and chloride across the alveolar epithelial barrier (primarily in alveolar epithelial type I and type II cells by means of the Na^+/K^+-ATPase), whereas water follows passively through aquaporins, which are water channels predominantly on alveolar epithelial type I cells.[34] Finally, the interstitium plays an important role in Na^+ and fluid homeostasis. Total body Na^+ levels are increased in HF. A large part of the Na^+ is distributed in the interstitium of different tissues as free cations bound to negatively charged biopolymers, glycosaminoglycan (GAG) networks.[35] These GAG networks function as Na^+ buffers and play an important role in fluid homeostasis and endothelial function. Long-term Na^+ overload and neurohumoral up-regulation cause dysfunction of interstitial GAG networks, resulting in increased vascular resistance and permeability, as well as fluid accumulation in the interstitium and oedema.[35]

Classically, the alveolar fluid in patients with AHF has low protein content and may be clearly differentiated from cases of non-cardiogenic pulmonary oedema, typically seen in sepsis, in which there is a direct inflammatory injury of the capillary membrane permeability, allowing the transition of large amounts of proteins. However, this differentiation is often not so clear after alveolar–capillaries membrane stress failure, where increased levels in plasma surfactant, elevated C-reactive protein levels, and tumour necrosis factor (TNF)-α, are suggestive of acute membrane alterations with pulmonary parenchymal inflammation, which may be observed several days after the resolution of the hydrostatic pressure rise. The membrane alterations in AHF are usually reversible, but in cases of severe injury or after repeated episodes of

decompensation, there is an incomplete remodelling leading to permanent lung alterations (➲ Figure 12.3.2).

The translation of these alterations of the microcirculation into clinical scenarios may produce different phenotypes, ranging from mild AHF decompensations with minimal lung alterations, to severe acute pulmonary oedema (APO) or cardiogenic shock (CS), where acute lung injury and severe acute respiratory failure may be present. In a continuum of increasing pulmonary congestion, APO is the clinical scenario where the alveolar flooding provokes progressive acute respiratory failure that may lead to death in minutes or hours, unless therapeutic intervention is applied quickly.

Dyspnoea is the most common symptom of AHF and is related to several disorders: interstitial and alveolar oedema, even mild, increases the stiffness of the lung, reducing its compliance; peribronchial oedema causes obstruction to the air-flow; the flooded alveoli have a shunt effect and ventilation–perfusion mismatch, leading to hypoxaemia, which aggravates dyspnoea. However, acute respiratory failure defined by hypoxaemia, with or without hypercapnia, is seen in slightly more than half of the patients with AHF, comprising those with APO, cardiogenic shock, and some with acute decompensated HF. Cases with severe APO mainly show hypoxaemia and acidosis, predominantly of respiratory origin with hypercapnia, whereas in cases of cardiogenic shock, acidosis is predominantly metabolic (lactic acidosis). Hypercapnia may be explained by decreased alveolar ventilation secondary to alveolar inundation, respiratory muscle fatigue, long elapsed time from the onset of symptoms, and the presence of COPD or previous respiratory disorders.

The impact in the lungs has been seen even in patients with acute cardiac conditions with apparently no signs of HF. In a

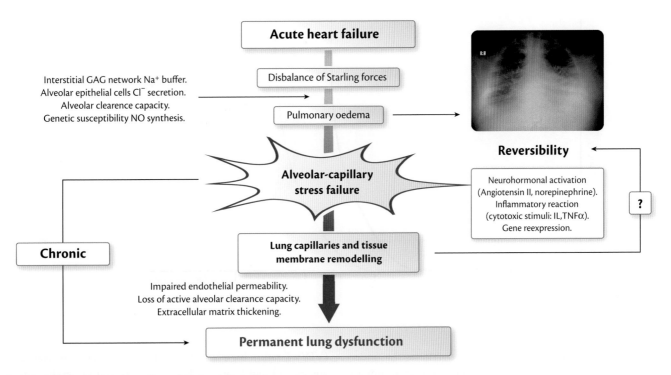

Figure 12.3.2 Pathophysiology of lung alterations in heart failure.
Acute decompensations may result in alveolar-capillary stress failure which is often reversible. In severe cases or after repeated failures, there is a remodelling process that leads to permanent lung dysfunction.
GAG: glycosaminoglycan; NO: Nitric oxide; TNF: Tumor necrosis factor: IL: Interleukin

series of 220 patients with acute myocardial infarction (AMI), we found some degree of hypoxaemia measured by oxygen saturation, in nearly 50%.[36] Hypoxaemia was mainly related to age and the presence of AHF, which was diagnosed in nearly 30% of the patients. Some authors have suggested that an alteration in alveolar–capillary membrane gas conductance (DM) may contribute to an abnormal gas exchange in patients with AMI. Guazzi et al. described patients with AMI in stable condition, with left ventricular ejection fraction (LVEF) > 50% and pulmonary capillary wedge pressure (PCWP) < 16 mmHg, who showed 30% less DM than controls.[37] When patients presented with AHF, these authors found that gas diffusion, measured by DLCO was preserved in the initial stages, probably because the increment in the volume of blood in the capillaries, compensated the decrease of membrane conductance.

Lung alterations in chronic HF

After capillary stress failure, there is impairment in diffusion and DM, not compensated by the increase in capillary volume. When remodelling produces irreversible alterations, gas diffusion and membrane conductance further deteriorates, probably because of fluid accumulation or fibrotic processes, while capillary volume decreases, most likely as a consequence of an increased vascular resistance, micro embolism, local thrombosis, increased intrapulmonary shunt, and low blood flow.[38]

Chronic HF patients have higher thresholds for triggering pulmonary oedema than 'de novo' HF patients, and tolerate higher levels of elevated capillary pressure[39] (➲ Figure 12.3.3).

Although the increase in hydrostatic pressure in the capillaries is the main trigger for developing pulmonary oedema, as has been mentioned before, other factors such as sodium, chloride, nitric oxide (NO), and the interstitium, may influence the process. More than half of chronic HF patients have an altered alveolar fluid clearance capacity, with anomalous transport of chloride and sodium, which may play an important role in the genesis of pulmonary oedema.[33] In addition, individual genetic susceptibility with defective NO synthesis, a mechanism that seems essential in the development of high-altitude pulmonary oedema (HAPE), may contribute to trigger oedema formation in some patients.[40] In subjects prone to HAPE, this genetic NO alteration leads to an exaggerated hypoxic pulmonary hypertension through an impaired vasodilation and non-homogeneous hypoxic pulmonary vasoconstriction, which leaves some capillaries not protected, exposed to regional overperfusion, and oedema. In patients with HF, the rise in LA pressure increases endothelial NO synthase activity, altering chloride secretion and decreasing Na+ absorption in the membrane, affecting the alveolar clearance rate.[34]

The remodelling process of capillaries and small arteries shows endothelial dysfunction, proliferation of myofibroblasts, fibrosis, and extracellular matrix deposition. These changes may be mediated by neurohormonal activation (angiotensin II, norepinephrine), inflammatory reaction (cytotoxic stimuli, IL, TNFα), and gene re-expression.[32] The alveolar gas diffusion becomes impaired because the path from air to blood is increased (thickening of extracellular matrix), and there is a loss of the fine balance of molecular mechanisms involved in fluid reabsorption and

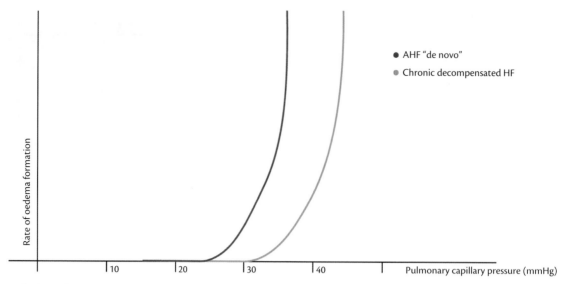

Figure 12.3.3 The level of pulmonary capillary pressure to trigger pulmonary oedema is higher in patients with chronic heart failure (HF) than in AHF (acute heart failure).

clearance.[41] The impairment in gas transfer reflects the underlying lung tissue damage and has independent prognostic impact, playing a role in the pathogenesis of the exercise limitation and ventilatory abnormalities observed in these patients.

The ventilatory response to exercise in patients with chronic HF is greater than normal, with high ventilatory output (➲ Figure 12.3.4). The more severe the HF, the greater the tachypnoea and the smaller the tidal volume (VT) at a given exercise expired volume per unit time.[42] The magnitude of the ventilatory response is inversely related to the arterial partial CO_2 pressure ($PaCO_2$) and directly related to the CO_2 production and dead space volume/tidal volume ratio (VD/VT). Increased dead space ventilation

(VD/VT ratio), high VA/Q (ventilation/perfusion mismatching), augmented ventilatory needs due to increased CO_2 production, alteration in lung mechanics, reduced lung diffusion, and overactive reflexes from metabolic, baro, or chemo-receptors, are possible explanations for the hyperventilation seen in these patients.[43]

Peak oxygen consumption (peak-VO_2) may reflect better than New York Heart Association (NYHA) class the functional limitations of these patients. As HF advances, peak-VO_2 declines. In addition, there is a progressive decrease of resting FEV_1, FVC, DLCO, DM, and capillary volume, in parallel to the severity of HF and the fall in the peak-VO_2.[44] Therefore, patients with chronic HF have a restrictive ventilatory pattern. The increased intrathoracic

Physiologic response to exercise in normal subjects and in patients with chronic HF

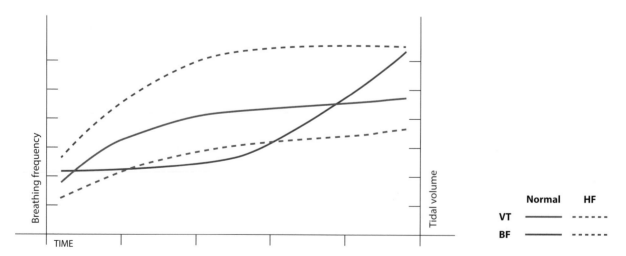

Figure 12.3.4 Scheme of the physiologic response to exercise of normal subjects and patients with chronic heart failure (HF). In normal subjects, breathing frequency increases mainly at the end of the exercise while tidal volume increases earlier. In HF patients there is higher breathing frequency at the onset and shows an early significant increase. Indeed, tidal volume (VT) in HF patients is lower than in normal subjects, and experiences mild increase during the exercise. Solid lines are normal subjects. Dashed lines are patients with chronic HF. Red line is breathing frequency and blue line tidal volume (VT).

fluid content, progressive fibrosis, and the place occupied by an enlarged heart may account for these alterations. FEV$_1$ and FVC are inversely associated with risk of future coronary heart disease and CV events in older community-dwelling adults and may add to CV risk stratification in the elderly.

In addition to altered ventilatory response to exercise, chronic HF patients have other ventilatory and sleep-related breathing disorders such as Cheyne–Stokes respiration, obstructive sleep apnoea, and central sleep apnoea.

Pulmonary hypertension

Chronic pulmonary venous congestion is often associated with an increase in PVR and the transpulmonary pressure gradient. This PH, classified as the WSPG group 2, is frequently called 'reactive' because it may reverse in hours or days with vasodilators. The endothelium plays a central role in the local control of vascular tone through the regulated release of NO and ET-1.[45] The dysfunction of the endothelial cells dysregulates this system, leading to vasoconstriction and remodelling of the arterial wall, with abnormalities of elastic fibres, intimal fibrosis, smooth muscle cell proliferation. and medial hypertrophy, which result in vascular stiffness and PH. This secondary PH attributable to structural remodelling from chronic LV failure is often referred as 'fixed' because it is not rapidly responsive.

The PAP further depends on the performance of the RV. High pulmonary pressures may be achieved by the RV if PH develops slowly, allowing the RV remodelling and adaptation (mainly hypertrophy). Conversely, in cases of RV failure, PAP may be relatively low despite a marked elevation of the PVR.

PH is seen in patients with both HF with reduced (HFrEF), and preserved ejection fraction (HFpEF) showing similar manifestations, but different pathophysiology with pulsatile and resistive loading.[46] In HFrEF haemodynamic drivers for PH are LV dilatation with eccentric remodelling, secondary dynamic mitral regurgitation (MR), and LA enlargement. In HFpEF, concentric remodelling with increased LV diastolic stiffness, atrial functional MR, and a stiff LA are the major driving forces. Vascular stress failure and remodelling similarly affect veins, capillaries, and small arteries. Patients with HFpEF and metabolic syndrome may have metabolic injury in addition to that induced by pressure (⮞ Figure 12.3.5). Independently of the LVEF, the occurrence of PH in patients with HF worsens the prognosis.

Diagnostic approach to lung dysfunction in HF

As previously mentioned, chronic pulmonary dysfunction and HF may share similar clinical presentations and have reciprocal detrimental effects on disease progression. Chronic pulmonary congestion may alter alveolar physiology and gas exchange, and severe long-standing lung disease might cause pre-capillary PH, which can result in RV dysfunction (*cor pulmonale*), worsening systemic congestion and organ dysfunction.[47] Furthermore, concerns related to possible adverse effects of specific treatment for one disease may lead to significant undertreatment of the other disease, with a negative impact on symptoms control and survival.[48] However, mislabelling is common and it is estimated that up to one third of patients with HF are treated as COPD patients and vice versa.[49]

Given the significant overlap in symptoms and signs, such as shortness of breath, fatigue, decreased functional capacity, the distinction of both syndromes based solely on the clinical examination is challenging.[49] For example, pulmonary auscultation might reveal wheezing indicating airflow limitation and bronchial

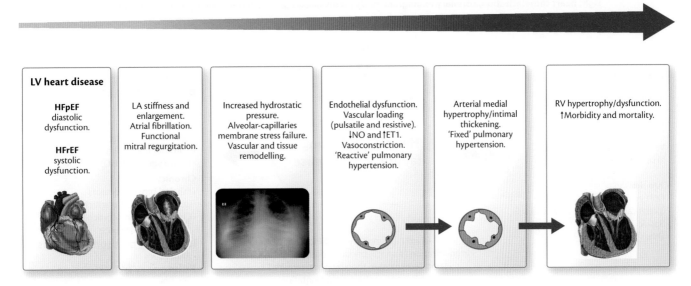

Figure 12.3.5 Sequence of events and reactions in chronic heart failure patients from cardiac remodeling in preclinical phases, to pulmonary hypertension and right ventricle failure.

ET$_1$: Endotelin-1; HFpEF: Heart failure with preserved ejection fraction; HFrEF: Heart failure with reduced ejection fraction; LA: left atrium; LV: Left ventricle; NO: Nitric oxide; RV: Right ventricle.

hyperresponsiveness both in acutely exacerbated COPD and in acute HF (*asthma cardiale*).[50,51] Pulmonary imaging (i.e. computed tomography) is of high value to describe acute and chronic morphologic alterations of lung parenchyma (e.g. inflammatory infiltrates, emphysema, interstitial patterns), but is frequently not appropriate in acute settings to distinguish COPD exacerbations from acute HF and to guide therapeutic decisions (e.g. diuretics, corticosteroids, antibiotic treatment). The value of lung ultrasound (LUS) in patients with chronic lung disease is controversial, since B-lines might arise from pulmonary congestion but also other conditions such as fibrosis. Hence, diagnosing COPD in a patient with HF, or HF in a patient with COPD, requires clinical awareness, understanding of the overlaps, and testing for both diseases (➲ Figure 12.3.6). Normal circulating natriuretic peptides in patients with COPD virtually rule out the coexistence of HF while elevated levels require further investigations (e.g. ECHO) to confirm the presence of a structural heart disease and estimate the consequences of pulmonary disease on the heart (mainly PH and RV dysfunction).

Pulmonary function tests, mainly spirometry, are mandatory to diagnose chronic respiratory diseases in HF patients and the mainstay for the diagnosis of COPD is evidence of an irreversible pulmonary obstruction on spirometry. According to the Global Initiative for Chronic Obstructive Lung Disease (GOLD) criteria, COPD is confirmed by an FEV1/FVC ratio of 0.70 or less after challenge with a short-acting bronchodilator. COPD is further classified according to the proportion of the measured FEV1 to the predicted value and the frequency of exacerbations in different stages (I–IV) and risk classes (A–D).[52] Of note, the FEV1/FVC

ratio is unaffected by HF, at least when the patient is euvolemic, while both FEV1 and FVC are reduced similarly by up to 20% from baseline.[53] As such, it is evident that severity of obstructive lung disease in a COPD patient is overestimated in the presence of acute HF. This is also true for diffusion capacity since gas exchange is limited by fluid accumulation in the alveolar–capillary membrane. Conversely, bronchospasms and nocturnal attacks of dyspnoea and coughing are frequently observed in patients with HF but without COPD. These alterations resolve with haemodynamic stabilization and decongestion. Therefore, spirometry should be performed in a euvolemic condition and restrictive patterns are frequently observed in chronic HF patients. Spiroergometry is of great value to differentiate cardiac, pulmonary, and metabolic/muscular components of limited exercise capacity and provides valuable information for prognosis and future treatment decisions.

Finally, acute pulmonary disease (e.g. pneumonia, exacerbated COPD) and HF have a strong interrelationship[8,54]: (i) acute HF might mimic pulmonary disease (e.g. butterfly pneumonia in APO or right upper lobe pneumonia in acute mitral valve dysfunction), (ii) acute pulmonary infections are one of the most common precipitating factors for acute HF and, (iii) chronic HF is an important risk factor for pulmonary diseases, in particular pneumonia. Acute HF precipitated by infections, and in particular by pulmonary infections, is associated with higher mortality at 3 and 12 months.[54,55] Of note, the risk of death peaks 3–4 weeks after disease onset and might result from the interplay between intrinsic physiology and clinician behaviour. Indeed, there are complex interactions between infection and a combination of

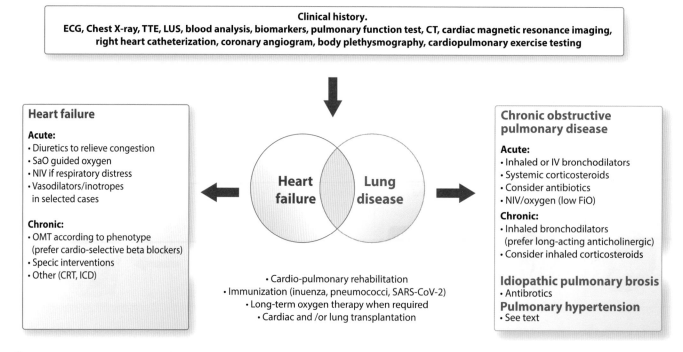

Figure 12.3.6 Diagnostic approach (upper part) and main therapies for patients with heart failure (left) and chronic lung diseases (right).
CRT cardiac resynchronization therapy, CT computed tomography; ECG: electrocardiogram; ICS: Inhaled corticosteroids; ICD implantable cardioverter-defibrillator, LUS: lung ultrasound, OMT optimal medical therapy, NIV non-invasive ventilation, TTE transthoracic ultrasound.

endothelial dysfunction, plaque instability, activated coagulation, volume overload, inflammatory and ischaemic myocardial injury, and arrhythmia, which may lead to death.[56] However, the relative neglect of the implied acute pulmonary disease by clinicians focused on the heart might lead to potentially suboptimal management and adverse outcomes.

Besides COPD, ILD, in particular IPF, may mimic the signs and symptoms of HF, especially if PH has developed. The differential characteristics of these three entities are presented in ⮕ Table 12.3.1. PH may be suspected in cases of greater reduction of DLCO (< 30%), of the 6-min walking distance, often with oxygen desaturation to below 85% or impaired heart-rate recovery after exertion.[57]

Formal cardiopulmonary exercise testing (CPET) can be very helpful in differentiating between HF and chronic lung disease. In HF, there is a commonly seen pattern of increased ventilatory responses to exercise but very rarely in the chronic HF patient does significant hypoxaemia occur. Rather there is a hyperventilatory pattern with relative hypocapnia. In contrast in predominantly lung disease patients, there is frequently a pattern of earlier hypoxaemia and CO_2 retention. Such observations may help in the differentiation of the relative contributions to exercise limitation in a patient with both heart and lung disease.

Therapeutic implications of chronic lung diseases in patients with heart failure

Patients with relevant comorbidities are frequently excluded from clinical trials, therefore evidence-based recommendations on the optimal treatment in patients with concomitant HF and severe pulmonary disease are limited.

Disease-modifying therapy for HF, including angiotensin-converting enzyme (ACE)-inhibitors, angiotensin-receptor blockers (ARB), mineralocorticoid receptor antagonists (MRA), angiotensin receptor/neprilysin inhibitors (ARNi), and sodium-glucose cotransporter 2 inhibitors (SGLT2i) displays similar tolerability and efficacy regarding the reduction of CV mortality and HF readmissions irrespective of the presence of COPD[58,59] Therefore, these drugs should be prescribed to HF patients, according to the LVEF, as recommended by the 2021 ESC Guidelines for the treatment of HF.

Beta-blockers (BB) are largely underused and underdosed in patients with obstructive lung disease (i.e. COPD and asthma)

Table 12.3.1 Main differential features of patients with HF, COPD, or IPF

	Chronic HF	COPD	IPF
Prevalence	High	High	Rare
Background	AF? Heart disease	Tobacco +++/ pollutants Chronic cough Sputum production	Tobacco Environmental exposure Genetic factors
Age (mean)	~ 75	~ 70	~ 65
Dyspnoea characteristics	Orthopnoea	Long expiration time	On exertion
Inspection	Peripheral oedema?	Barrel chest?	Finger clubbing (~50%)
Auscultation	Coarse crackles	Low heart sounds Decreased breath sounds Rhonchi and wheezing	Velcro-crackles
Chest X-ray	Cardiomegaly Interstitial-alveolar oedema Pleural effusions?	Flat diaphragm ↑ Retrosternal air space Horizontal ribs	Interstitial pattern
Pulmonary function test	FVC↓ FEV$_1$↓ DLCO↓	Airflow limitation FEV$_1$/FVC <70 FEV$_1$ ↓↓ *DLCO ↓↓	FVC↓↓ FEV$_1$/FVC ↑↑ DLCO ↓↓↓
ECG	Abnormal	–	–
Natriuretic peptides	Elevated	**	**
Blood gases	-	***Hypercapnia??	Hypoxemia
ECHO	LV systolic and/or diastolic dysfunction Mild PH?	Mild–moderate PH?	Mild–moderate PH?
Main chronic treatment	Diuretics/vasodilators	Bronchodilators Corticosteroids LTOT	Antifibrotic therapy LTOT

* If emphysema or PH coexist; ** Mildly elevated in advanced stages; *** Exacerbations or advanced stages
COPD: Chronic obstructive pulmonary disease; IPF: Idiopathic pulmonary fibrosis; FVC: Forced vital capacity; FEV-1: Forced expiratory volume in 1 second; DLCO: Diffusing capacity for carbon monoxide; ECG: Electrocardiogram; ECHO: Echocardiogram; PH: pulmonary hypertension; LTOT: Long-term oxygen therapy

because of concerns of adverse effects on pulmonary obstruction and outcome.[60] While many patients with pulmonary obstruction have been excluded from the large clinical trials testing BB for HFrEF, several meta-analyses and propensity-matched cohorts found a maintained prognostic benefit of the use of BB in HFrEF patients.[61] The reduction in clinical events related to HF surpasses the minimal reduction in FEV1 induced by BB, in particular when using beta1-selective agents such as bisoprolol, metoprolol succinate, or nebivolol. Observational studies have suggested even a decrease in mortality and frequency of acute exacerbations in COPD patients without HF treated with BB, but these data could not be confirmed in a recent controlled study and remain controversial.[62,63] The contraindication to BB in patients with asthma derives from older series and may be considered – in patients with well-controlled disease – as only a relative contraindication. In clinical practice, starting with low doses of beta1-selective agents under close monitoring for signs of airway obstruction may allow the initiation of BB in HFrEF. In BB-intolerant patients in sinus rhythm, ivabradine might be considered. It is our strong opinion, that patients with clear indication for a beta-blocking agent should not be withheld from such treatment, provided they present with a stable respiratory condition.

On the other hand, the treatment of the underlying pulmonary disease might be affected by the presence of HF. Inhaled bronchodilators, anticholinergic agents, and steroids are the most frequently used therapeutic agents for COPD and asthma. Observational studies have reported an association between inhaled beta2-agonists and increased mortality and hospitalization in patients with coexisting pulmonary disease and HF,[64] but these data have never been confirmed by dedicated randomized trials and remain controversial. In this context, caution should be exercised before restricting the use of inhaled beta2-agonists in COPD patients with concomitant HF. Nevertheless, long-acting anticholinergic drugs might represent a better first-line choice in this context, since these drugs showed good efficacy for the treatment of COPD.

Treatment with inhaled corticosteroids for COPD appears to be safe in patients with HF. Conversely, courses of systemic corticosteroids used to treat COPD or asthma exacerbations can induce sodium and water retention, possibly contributing to acute HF.

There is some concern with the interaction of the antifibrotics with proven efficacy in IPF (pirfenidone and nintedanib), in patients with high-risk of bleeding, because they inhibit the receptors for platelet-derived growth factor and vascular endothelial growth factor. Therefore, their use should be cautious in HF patients under anticoagulant or anti-aggregant therapy, although the pivotal trials that excluded patients with high-risk of bleeding, the most frequent bleeding was epistaxis, not reporting a higher rate of major bleedings.[58]

Oxygen non-invasive ventilation

Although non-invasive ventilation is indicated in COPD exacerbations and APO, as first line therapy,[65] positive pressure ventilation may aggravate RV dysfunction in patients with PH. In addition, it should be considered that weaning from mechanical ventilation is often difficult in intubated patients with CLD.

In patients with PH Group 3 with hypoxaemia, the correction of alveolar hypoxia with long-term oxygen seems to be the preferred therapeutic measure to reduce PH.[6] Long-term oxygen treatment improves life expectancy, which might be related to its retardation of PH development.

Treatment for PH

Regarding the treatment of PH, pulmonary vasodilators, such as calcium channel blockers, endothelin receptor antagonists, phosphodiesterase-5 inhibitors, and prostacyclin analogues, commonly used in the treatment of patients with pulmonary arterial hypertension (those with PH from WSHP Group 1), have been tested in patients with PH-WSHP 3 with inconclusive results, and to date, are not recommended. In COPD patients with PH, some meta-analyses, including sildenafil or bosentan, showed improvements in haemodynamics but the effect on exercise capacity was inconsistent.[66,67] Nevertheless, the subset of patients with PH that is disproportionately severe to their COPD may derive the most benefit from pulmonary arterial hypertension -specific treatment in improving exercise capacity, haemodynamics, and probably survival.[67,68] A recent large-scale trial has demonstrated that inhaled treprostinil was associated with improved outcomes in the PH-ILD population.[68]

Future directions

Although HF and CLD are the most prevalent chronic diseases, currently accounting for the largest proportion of hospital admissions, there are some emergent aspects that may give a hoping light for the future. From one side, prevention will be crucial. Healthier diet and lifestyle habits, with a decrease in pollution and reduced tobacco use, will have an enormous impact in the prevention of ischaemic CV disease, and hence, HF and CLD burden. Another important aspect will be early detection. By individual genetic and epigenetic information (proteomics, metabolomics, genomics), wide proliferation of biomarkers, big data implementation, together with the improvement in image and advanced digital technologies, these illnesses may be detected early, allowing a prompt personalized approach. Finally, new integrated treatments will be developed combining regenerative medicine based on cellular engineering and gene therapy, with improved monitoring through telemedicine and personal devices. The conjunction of these scenarios will have a great impact in the control of CLD and HF.

Summary and key messages

HF and CLD are frequently associated. One third of the patients with HF have CLD and conversely, nearly 20% of the CLD have HF.[24] The most prevalent diseases are COPD and ILD (pulmonary fibrosis). In the genesis of COPD, tobacco and pollution play a major role, and airflow limitation ($\downarrow$ FEV$_1$) is the main alteration, whereas decreased $\downarrow$FVC and impaired diffusion (DLCO) are key in ILD, showing hypoxemia, initially on exertion.

CLD have an impact on the heart, primarily by the development of PH, but biological, inflammatory, neurohormonal, and genetic factors also play an important role.

In COPD patients, PH usually progresses slowly and is usually seen in the late course of the disease, but it is often detectable earlier on exertion. Some COPD patients may present a 'vascular phenotype' characterized by a severe PH and gas exchange deterioration, in relation to the degree of the illness.

IPF has gained relevance within the scope of ILD, after the development of some effective antifibrotic therapies, which may be used in patients with HF. Patients with IPF tend to develop PH, but specific treatments used in pulmonary arterial hypertension (WSPH Group 1) have not been shown to be effective and are not recommended. Long-term oxygen therapy is indicated in hypoxaemic patients with CLD and PH.

The LV may also be affected in CLD by different mechanisms. Conversely, pulmonary congestion secondary to LV failure may provoke permanent lung alterations after the remodelling of capillary stress failure.

Decreased FVC and FEV_1, with restrictive pattern, and impaired DLCO and DM are commonly observed in patients with chronic HF.

Echocardiography, by assessing PAP, RA structure, and RV function, as well as pulmonary function tests, are crucial for the identification of HF and CLD.

Standard therapies for HF and COPD are commonly indicated, with the preference for anticholinergic inhalators and cardioselective BB. Cardiopulmonary rehabilitation, vaccination, or cardiac/lung transplant in very advanced stages are alternative therapeutic measures that should be considered in both entities.

References

1. Fonarow GC, Stough WG, Abraham WT, et al. Characteristics, treatments, and outcomes of patients with preserved systolic function hospitalized for heart failure: a report from the OPTIMIZE-HF Registry. J Am Coll Cardiol 2007; 50: 768–77.

2. Muñoz-Ferrera A, Rodriguez-Ponsa L, Garcia-Olivé I, et al. Airflow limitation in patients with heart failure: Prevalence and associated factors. Med Clin (Barc) 2019;153: 191–5.

3. Santos S, Peinado VI, Ramírez J, et al. Characterization of pulmonary vascular remodelling in smokers and patients with mild COPD. Eur Respir J 2002;19: 632–8.

4. D'Andrea A, Stanziola A, Di Palma E, et al. Right ventricular structure and function in idiopathic pulmonary fibrosis with or without pulmonary hypertension. Echocardiography 2016;33: 57–65.

5. Harder EM, Waxman AB. Clinical trials in group 3 pulmonary hypertension. Curr Opin Pulm Med. 2020;26: 391–6.

6. Humbert M, Kovacs G, Hoeper MM, et al. ESC/ERS Scientific Document Group. 2022 ESC/ERS Guidelines for the diagnosis and treatment of pulmonary hypertension. Eur Heart J 2022;43:3618–731.

7. Portillo K, Abad-Capa J, Ruiz-Manzano J. Chronic obstructive pulmonary disease and left ventricle. Arch Bronconeumol 2015;51: 227–34.

8. Kohama A, Tanouchi J, Hori M, Kitabatake A, Kamada T. Pathologic involvement of the left ventricle in chronic cor pulmonale. Chest 1990;98: 794–800.

9. Singh D, Agusti A, Anzueto A, et al. Global Strategy for the Diagnosis, Management, and Prevention of Chronic Obstructive Lung Disease: the GOLD science committee report 2019. Eur Respir J 2019;53: 1900164.

10. Weitzenblum E, Chaouat A, Kessler R. Pulmonary hypertension in chronic obstructive pulmonary disease. Pneumonol Alergol Pol 2013;81: 390–8

11. Barberà JA, Peinado VI, Santos S. Pulmonary hypertension in chronic obstructive pulmonary disease. Eur Respir J 2003;21: 892–905.

12. Mandoli GE, De Carli G, Pastore MC, et al. Right cardiac involvement in lung diseases: a multimodality approach from diagnosis to prognostication. J Intern Med 2021;289: 440–9.

13. Hilde JM, Skjørten I, Grøtta OJ, et al. Right ventricular dysfunction and remodeling in chronic obstructive pulmonary disease without pulmonary hypertension. J Am Coll Cardiol 2013;62: 1103–11.

14. Cuttica MJ, Shah SJ, Rosenberg SR, et al. Right heart structural changes are independently associated with exercise capacity in non-severe COPD. PLoS One 2011;6: e29069.

15. Li Y, Wang Y, Zhai Z, Guo X, Yang Y, Lu X. Real-time three-dimensional echocardiography to assess right ventricle function in patients with pulmonary hypertension. PLoS One 2015;10: e0129557.

16. Simonneau G, Montani D, Celermajer DS, et al. Haemodynamic definitions and updated clinical classification of pulmonary hypertension. Eur Respir J. 2019;53: 1801913.

17. Portillo K, Torralba Y, Blanco I, et al. Pulmonary hemodynamic profile in chronic obstructive pulmonary disease. Int J Chron Obstruct Pulmon Dis 2015;10: 1313–20.

18. Hilde JM, Skjørten I, Hansteen V, et al. Haemodynamic responses to exercise in patients with COPD Eur Respir J 2013;41:1031–41.

19. Kovacs G, Agusti A, Barberà JA, et al. Pulmonary vascular involvement in chronic obstructive pulmonary disease. Is there a pulmonary vascular phenotype? Am J Respir Crit Care Med 2018;198: 1000–1011.

20. Anderson WJ, Lipworth BJ, Rekhraj S, Struthers AD, George J. Left ventricular hypertrophy in COPD without hypoxemia: the elephant in the room? Chest 2013;143: 91–97.

21. Macchia A, Rodriguez Moncalvo JJ, Kleinert M, et al. Unrecognised ventricular dysfunction in COPD. Eur Respir J 2012;39: 51–8.

22. Freixa X, Portillo K, Paré C, et al.. Echocardiographic abnormalities in patients with COPD at their first hospital admission. Eur Respir J 2013;41: 784–91.

23. Boudestein LC, Rutten FH, Cramer MJ, Lammers JW, Hoes AW. The impact of concurrent heart failure on prognosis in patients with chronic obstructive pulmonary disease. Eur J Heart Fail 2009;11: 1182–8.

24. Rutten FH, Cramer MJ, Lammers JW, Grobbee DE, Hoes AW. Heart failure and chronic obstructive pulmonary disease: An ignored combination? Eur J Heart Fail 2006;8: 706–11.

25. Collum SD, Amione-Guerra J, Cruz-Solbes AS, et al. Pulmonary hypertension associated with idiopathic pulmonary fibrosis: current and future perspectives. Can Respir J 2017;2017:1430350.

26. Raghu G, Behr J, Brown KK, et al. Treatment of idiopathic pulmonary fibrosis with ambrisentan: a parallel, randomized trial. Ann Intern Med 2013;158: 641–9.

27. D'Andrea A, Stanziola A, D'Alto M, et al. Right ventricular strain: An independent predictor of survival in idiopathic pulmonary fibrosis. Int J Cardiol 2016;222: 908–10.

28. Cottin V, Nunes H, Brillet PY, et al. Combined pulmonary fibrosis and emphysema: a distinct underrecognised entity. Eur Respir J 2005;26: 586–93.

29. Portillo K, Morera J. Combined pulmonary fibrosis and emphysema syndrome: a new phenotype within the spectrum of smoking-related interstitial lung disease. Pulm Med 2012;2012: 867870.

30. Farkas L, Gauldie J, Voelkel NF, Kolb M. Pulmonary hypertension and idiopathic pulmonary fibrosis: a tale of angiogenesis, apoptosis, and growth factors. Am J Respir Cell Mol Biol 2011;45: 1–15.

31. Ware L, Matthay, M. Acute pulmonary edema. N Engl J Med 2005;353: 2788–96..

32. Guazzi M. Alveolar-capillary membrane dysfunction in heart failure. evidence of a pathophysiologic role. Chest 2003; 124:1090–1102.

33. Verghese GM, Ware LB, Matthay BA, Matthay MA. Alveolar epithelial fluid transport and the resolution of clinically severe hydrostatic pulmonary edema. J Appl Physiol 1999;87: 1301–12.

34. Londino JD, Matalon S. Chloride secretion across adult alveolar epithelial cells contributes to cardiogenic edema. PNAS 2013; 110: 10055–6.

35. Nijst P, Verbrugge FH, Grieten L, et al. The pathophysiological role of interstitial sodium in heart failure. J Am Coll Cardiol 2015;65: 378–88.

36. Masip J, Gayà M, Páez J, et al. Pulse oximetry in the diagnosis of acute heart failure. Rev Esp Cardiol (Engl Ed) 2012;65: 879–84.

37. Guazzi M. Alveolar gas diffusion abnormalities in heart failure. J Card Fail 2008; 14: 695–702.

38. Guazzi M, Phillips SA, Arena R, CJ. Lavie CJ. Endothelial dysfunction and lung capillary injury in cardiovascular diseases. Prog Cardiovasc Dis 2015; 57:454–2.

39. Clark AL, Cleland JG. Causes and treatment of oedema in patients with heart failure. Nat Rev Cardiol 2013;10: 156–70.

40. Scherrer U, Rexhaj E, Jayet PY, Allemann Y, Sartori C. New insights in the pathogenesis of high-altitude pulmonary edema. Prog Cardiovasc Dis 2010;52: 485–92.

41. Agostoni P, Bussotti M, Cattadori G, et al. Gas diffusion and alveolar-capillary unit in chronic heart failure. Eur Heart J 2006;27: 2538–43.

42. Agoston P, Cattadori G, Bussottia M, Apostolo A. Cardiopulmonary interaction in heart failure. Pulm Pharmacol Therap 20 2007: 130–4.

43. Clark AL, Davies C, Francis DP, Coats AS. Ventilatory capacity and exercise tolerance in patients with chronic stable heart failure. Eur J Heart Fail 2000; 2:47–51.

44. Guazzi M, Reina G, Tumminello G, Guazzi MD. Exercise ventilation inefficiency and cardiovascular mortality in heart failure: the critical independent prognostic value of the arterial CO_2 partial pressure. Eur Heart J 2005;26: 472–80.

45. Moraes DL, Colucci WS, Givertz MM. Secondary pulmonary hypertension in chronic heart failure the role of the endothelium in pathophysiology and management. Circulation. 2000;102:1718–23.

46. Guazzi M, Ghio S, Adir Y. Pulmonary hypertension in HFpEF and HFrEF. J Am Coll Cardiol 2020;76: 1102–11.

47. Arrigo M, Huber LC, Winnik S, et al. Right ventricular failure: pathophysiology, diagnosis and treatment. Card Fail Rev 2019; 5: 140–6.

48. Canepa M, Franssen FME, Olschewski H, et al. Diagnostic and therapeutic gaps in patients with heart failure and chronic obstructive pulmonary disease. JACC Heart Fail 2019; 7: 823–33..

49. Caroci Ade S, Lareau SC. Descriptors of dyspnea by patients with chronic obstructive pulmonary disease versus congestive heart failure. Heart Lung 2004; 33: 102–10.

50. Petermann W, Barth J, Entzian P. Heart failure and airway obstruction. Int J Cardiol 1987; 17: 207–9..

51. Cabanes LR, Weber SN, Matran R, et al. Bronchial hyperresponsiveness to methacholine in patients with impaired left ventricular function. N Engl J Med 1989; 320(20): 1317–22..

52. Global strategy for prevention, diagnosis and treatment of chronic obstructive pulmonary disease (2021 report). https://goldcopd.org/2023-gold-report-2/

53. Guder G, Rutten FH, Brenner S, et al. The impact of heart failure on the classification of COPD severity. J Card Fail 2012; 18: 637–44.

54. Arrigo M, Tolppanen H, Sadoune M, et al. Effect of precipitating factors of acute heart failure on readmission and long-term mortality. ESC Heart Fail 2016; 3: 115–21..

55. Arrigo M, Gayat E, Parenica J, et al. Precipitating factors and 90-day outcome of acute heart failure: a report from the intercontinental GREAT registry. Eur J Heart Fail 2017;19: 201–8.

56. Corrales-Medina VF, Musher DM, Shachkina S, Chirinos JA. Acute pneumonia and the cardiovascular system. Lancet 2013;381: 496–505..

57. Cleemput JV, Sonaglioni A, Wuyts WA, Bengus M, Stauffer JL, Harari S. Idiopathic pulmonary fibrosis for cardiologists: differential diagnosis, cardiovascular comorbidities, and patient management. Adv Ther 2019: 36: 298–317.

58. Dewan P, Docherty KF, Bengtsson O, et al. Effects of dapagliflozin in heart failure with reduced ejection fraction and chronic obstructive pulmonary disease: an analysis of DAPA-HF. Eur J Heart Fail 2021; 23: 632–43.

59. Ehteshami-Afshar S, Mooney L, Dewan P, et al. Clinical characteristics and outcomes of patients with heart failure with reduced ejection fraction and chronic obstructive pulmonary disease: insights from PARADIGM-HF. J Am Heart Assoc 2021; 10: e019238..

60. Huber LC, Arrigo M. Betablocker und Asthma bronchiale: Ja oder Nein? Cardiovasc Med 2016; 19: 256–60.

61. Sin DD, McAlister FA. The effects of beta-blockers on morbidity and mortality in a population-based cohort of 11,942 elderly patients with heart failure. Am J Med 2002; 113: 650–6..

62. Rutten FH, Zuithoff NPA, Hak E, Grobbee DE, Hoes AW. β-blockers may reduce mortality and risk of exacerbations in patients with chronic obstructive pulmonary disease. Arch Intern Med 2010;170: 880.

63. Dransfield MT, Voelker H, Bhatt SP, et al. Metoprolol for the prevention of acute exacerbations of COPD. N Engl J Med 2019; 381: 2304–14.

64. Hawkins NM, Wang D, Petrie MC, et al. Baseline characteristics and outcomes of patients with heart failure receiving bronchodilators in the CHARM programme. Eur J Heart Fail 2010; 12: 557–65.

65. Masip J, Peacock WF, Price S, et al. Indications and practical approach to noninvasive ventilation in acute heart failure. Eur Heart J 2018; 39:17–25.

66. Seeger W, Adir Y, Barberà JA, et al. Pulmonary hypertension in chronic lung diseases. J Am Coll Cardiol 2013;62 (25 Suppl):D109–16..

67. Harder EM, Waxman AB. Clinical trials in group 3 pulmonary hypertension. Curr Opin Pulm Med 2020;26: 391–6.

68. Waxman A, Restrepo-Jaramillo R, Thenappan T, et al. Inhaled treprostinil in pulmonary hypertension due to interstitial lung disease. N Engl J Med 2021;384:325–3.4

CHAPTER 12.4

Ventilatory abnormalities and sleep disordered breathing

Piergiuseppe Agostoni, Elisabetta Salvioni, Maria Rosa Costanzo, and Andrew JS Coats

Contents

Introduction

In chronic heart failure, both the pattern and neural control of ventilation are frequently altered at rest and during exercise, as well as during the day and during sleep. This is associated with mechanical respiratory abnormalities, inefficient ventilation, and anomalous respiratory patterns. Several symptoms reported by heart failure patients, such as dyspnoea, fatigue, exercise limitation, and poor quality sleep, are linked to ventilation. Moreover abnormalities of respiration have a strong prognostic power in chronic heart failure and are as a result candidate targets for therapy. Among the principal abnormalities, both alveolar capillary membrane diffusion[1] and the minute ventilation/carbon dioxide production (VE/VCO$_2$) slope during exercise [2] have a recognized prognostic role, while the alveolar capillary membrane mechanics of ventilation, and the chemoreflex responses are specific targets of therapy. Similarly, sleep disorders and daytime oscillatory breathing both play a pivotal prognostic role and are possible therapeutic targets.

In normoxic conditions, regulation of ventilation is described by the following equation:

$$VE = 863 \times VCO_2/[PaCO_2 \times (1 - VD/VT)]$$

where VCO$_2$ is the amount of expired CO$_2$ output, PaCO$_2$ is the CO$_2$ set point in the systemic arterial blood regulated by the chemo and metabo-receptors (also known as ergoreceptors), and V_D/V_T (ratio of dead-space ventilation (V_D) to tidal ventilation (V_T)) represents the mechanical efficiency of ventilation due to ventilation/perfusion mismatch and alveolar capillary membrane abnormalities. According to Wasserman *et al.* in heart failure VCO$_2$, PaCO$_2$, and V_D/V_T account of 47%, 8%, and 45% of the increased of ventilation during exercise.[3] The present chapter starts from the basic physiology of ventilatory abnormalities to review abnormalities of ventilatory patterns during day and night.

Spirometric abnormalities in heart failure

In chronic heart failure, standard spirometry can be normal or can show a restrictive pattern. This pattern of alveolar volume reduction is due to the combined effects of intrathoracic fluid increase and cardiomegaly, both of which utilize part of the intrathoracic space otherwise available for ventilation. These abnormalities can be partially corrected by better control of lung fluid such as by intensified diuretic therapy. Abnormalities in the alveolar capillary membrane are also seen in chronic heart failure and are characterized by a reduction of both components of diffusion capacity: membrane diffusion and capillary volume. Mechanical and diffusion abnormalities increase as the severity of heart failure increases. During physical activity in normal subjects, lung diffusion increases, due to recruitment of more effectively operating pulmonary vessels, but this is not the case in patients with severe heart failure in whom exercise leads to a worsening of gas exchange, which persists even after activity has ceased. Alveolar capillary membrane diffusion is usually now measured by one of two tracers, carbon monoxide (CO) or nitric oxide (NO). The former is representative of membrane diffusion and capillary volume, the latter of the membrane diffusion alone, given that the resistance of haemoglobin to NO is negligible. The study of both diffusion components and of the capillary volume is possible through the classic three-step Roughton and Forster method or by the single-step double tracer method, which is based on the simultaneous analysis of diffusing capacity of the lungs for carbon monoxide (DLCO) and diffusing capacity of the lungs for nitric oxide (DLNO). In contrast, the Roughton and Forster method is based on the competition between CO and oxygen for haemoglobin, so that it is measured by using three manoeuvres with a standard CO dose mixed with three different oxygen inhalation fractions, specifically 20%, 40%, and 60%. Lung diffusion is variably influenced by heart failure treatment, being unaffected by dialysis or diuretic treatment, but positively affected by angiotensin-converting enzyme (ACE) inhibitors, but not by angiotensin receptor blockers (ARB), or mineralocorticoid receptor antagonists (MRA) and negatively affected by β_1-β_2 receptor blockers. This is due to the anatomical changes which the alveolar capillary membrane undergoes and specifically to the increase in its cellular, protein, and connective and fibrotic tissue components and to the regulatory action of bradykinin and alveolar β_2 receptors on gas exchange.[4,5]

Ventilation during exercise

Ventilation during exercise progressively increases for a given VO$_2$ (oxygen consumption) as a consequence of inefficiency of ventilation. In severe heart failure, ventilation can be double that found in normal subjects at the same level of VO$_2$. In heart failure, respiratory rate increases early while the tidal volume increase is blunted (➡ Figures 12.4.1 and ➡ 12.4.2) leading to the so-called shallow breathing pattern.

The shallow breathing pattern is highly inefficient, being associated with an increase of dead space ventilation, reduction of end tidal CO$_2$ pressure, and increase in the PCO$_2$ (partial pressure of carbon dioxide) arterial to end-tidal gradient. From a physiological point of view, instead of the physiological reduction of end-tidal lung volumes during exercise, the presence of expiratory flow limitation pushes functional residual capacity toward higher volumes leading to an increase in the intrathoracic pressure swings (➡ Figure 12.4.3).[6]

This inefficiency of ventilation is analysed by the relationship between ventilation and VCO$_2$, which can be reported as the VE/VCO$_2$ ratio, and is usually measured at the anaerobic threshold or as the lowest recorded value, or as the slope of the VE vs VCO$_2$ relationship. Regardless of how it is measured, the VE/VCO$_2$ has a strong and independent prognostic power in heart failure. Of note, since the VE/VCO$_2$ is higher in females and it increases with age, it should be normalized and presented as a percentage of a predicted value.[7]

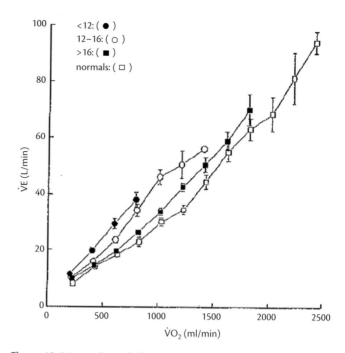

Figure 12.4.1 Ventilation (VE) as a function of oxygen uptake VO$_2$ for each patient group and the control group.

Reproduced from Wasserman K, Zhang YY, Gitt A, Belardinelli R, Koike A, Lubarsky L, Agostoni PG. Lung function and exercise gas exchange in chronic heart failure. *Circulation*. 1997 Oct 7;96(7):2221-7. doi: 10.1161/01.cir.96.7.2221. with permission from Wolters Kluwer

Cheyne–Stokes respiration and exercise oscillatory ventilation

On top of the ventilatory abnormalities described above, a peculiar ventilatory pattern characterized by regular oscillations of tidal volume has been described following the pioneering work of John Cheyne and William Stokes. Specifically, Cheyne–Stokes respiration is characterized by progressive tidal volume reductions down to complete apnoea followed by a progressive increase in tidal volumes. Cheyne–Stokes respiration has been described in several diseases including neurological, cardiologic, and respiratory conditions, as well as at high altitude. A variant of Cheyne–Stokes respiration is present during exercise in severe heart failure patients and it is characterized by hyperpnoea followed by hypopnea. This behaviour is named exercise oscillatory ventilation (EOV) or periodic breathing (PB). Several definitions of EOV have been proposed. Indeed, EOV is determined by the combined characteristics of the ventilatory pattern (amplitude, cycle length, and/or oscillatory time), according to definitions of Ben-Dov,[8] Corrà,[9] Kremser,[10] Leite,[11] and Sun.[12] ➡ Figure 12.4.4 shows the EOV-positive ventilatory pattern and the synthesis of the EOV definitions and illustrates the minimum of oscillatory cycles or duration recommended for each definition.

Specifically, the definition of EOV proposed by Ben Dov et al. requires at least two consecutive cyclic fluctuations with an amplitude ≥ 25% of the average ventilation during the cycle, and a cycle length between 30 and 60 seconds; Kremser et al.'s definition requires the presence of oscillation > 66% of the total exercise time with an average amplitude of the oscillation > 15% of ventilation

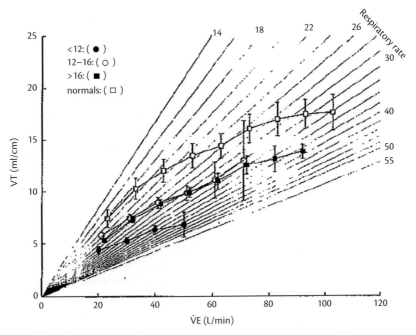

Figure 12.4.2 Tidal volume (VT) normalized to height as a function of exercise ventilation (VE) for normal subjects and the three groups of heart failure patients included in the study.

Reproduced from Wasserman K, Zhang YY, Gitt A, Belardinelli R, Koike A, Lubarsky L, Agostoni PG. Lung function and exercise gas exchange in chronic heart failure. *Circulation*. 1997 Oct 7;96(7):2221-7. doi: 10.1161/01.cir.96.7.2221. with permission from Wolters Kluwer.

at rest; Leite et al.'s definition requires at least three consecutive cyclic fluctuations of ventilation with an amplitude ≥ 5L/min; Sun et al.'s definition, like Leite et al.'s, requires at least three consecutive cyclic fluctuations of ventilation but with an amplitude > 30% of the average ventilation. Finally, Corrà et al.'s EOV definition requires an oscillation of ventilation for at least 60% of exercise time with an amplitude of oscillation > 15% of the average ventilation at rest. According to the American Heart Association, the EOV definition of Corrà et al. is the most reliable. Regardless of its definition, EOV can last for the entire exercise period or can end before exercise finishes. The reasons behind this phenomenon are unknown, although reduction of transit time, that is, the time needed to convey the blood gas signal from the alveoli to the chemoreceptor, seems to play a major role. Of note, in patients being treated with a left ventricular assist device (LVAD), an increase in LVAD output reduces and even cancels EOV.[13] Moreover, Schmid et al.[13a] reported that in 50% of patients with EOV ending during exercise the VO₂–work relationship slope increases, showing that EOV increases the work of breathing.

Depending on the definition applied, the prevalence of EOV varies as shown by Ingle et al.[14] Regardless of the definition, EOV is more frequently observed in patients with severe heart failure and it has a strong prognostic power.[15,16] Specifically, Cornelis et al.[17] found a four-fold greater risk of adverse cardiovascular events in heart failure EOV-positive patients compared to their counterparts without EOV. In an analysis of the Metabolic Exercise test data combined with Cardiac and Kidney Indexes (MECKI) score data set, Rovai et al.[18] found that EOV is associated with lower survival of heart failure patients with reduced or mid-range left ventricular ejection fraction in a 2-year follow-up, regardless of

age and sex (➲ Figure 12.4.5). Of note, the time frame of the cardiovascular risk increase between reduced and mid-range ejection fraction patients was different and delayed by 18 months in mid-range patients (➲ Figure 12.4.6).

EOV is also a target of treatment. Indeed, it can be cancelled when a further respiratory stimulus is applied, such as an external dead volume or when breathing with a hypercapnic air mixture.[19,20] Similarly, acetazolamide treatment reduces EOV.[19] However, EOV reduction, or even disappearance, obtained via added dead space or with acetazolamide treatment, was associated with a reduction in exercise performance.[19] In contrast, when severe heart failure is treated as with levosimendan, EOV disappearance is associated with exercise performance improvement.

Sleep breathing disorders

The study of ventilation during sleep has a pivotal role in the analysis of respiratory abnormalities in heart failure. There are two major forms of sleep-related breathing abnormalities seen in heart failure: central sleep apnoea (CSA) and obstructive sleep apnoea (OSA); a combination of the two can also be observed, the so-called mixed sleep apnoea. CSA is characterized by the absence of respiratory movements due to fluctuation of the central respiratory drive. CSA occurs when PaCO₂ falls below the apnoeic threshold, followed by hyperpnoea when PaCO₂ rises again. A similar phenomenon has been observed at high altitude, particularly in the male sex, and it is prevented by acetazolamide.[21] OSA derives from the collapse of the pharynx and upper airways leading to thoracic movements without effective air flow. The reported cause of OSA in heart failure is a shift of fluid from the legs and abdomen to central structures, including the upper airways

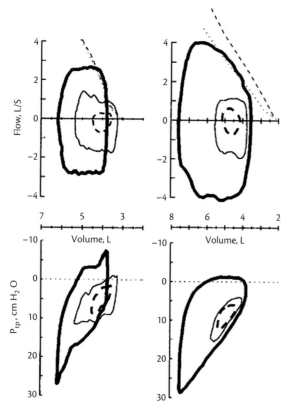

Figure 12.4.3 Composite tidal flow–volume and transpulmonary pressure (Ptp)–volume loops at rest (dashed lines), at 40% of maximal ventilation (thin solid lines), and at maximum exercise (thick solid lines) in typical chronic heart failure (left) and normal (right) subjects. The 2 oblique lines on flow-volume loops are partial forced expiratory flows recorded at rest (dotted line) and at maximum exercise (dashed line). Total lung capacity is at the interception of x- and y-axes on the flow–volume loops. Chronic heart failure subject: at rest, EFR, i.e. the difference in flow between near end tidal expiration and forced flow at the same absolute volume, is much less than in the normal individual because of the lower functional residual capacity (FRC). At the beginning of exercise, FRC decreases and Ptp (PtpFRC) becomes slightly negative. Tidal expiratory flow near FRC encroaches on forced expiratory flow, thus suggesting initial occurrence of expiratory flow limitation (EFL). Then, FRC tends to increase above resting value at the end of exercise whereas PtpFRC becomes more negative. The increase in PtpFRC is not associated with increase in flow, thus suggesting further EFL. Forced expiratory flow at maximum exercise (dashed oblique line) is similar to resting conditions (dotted oblique line), which is consistent with lack of bronchodilatation. Normal subject: FRC decreases early during exercise and remains low through the end of exercise. PtpFRC becomes slightly negative over the second half of tidal expiration. EFL would have likely occurred at maximum exercise if forced expiratory flow had not increased.
Reproduced from Agostoni P, Pellegrino R, Conca C, Rodarte JR, Brusasco V. Exercise hyperpnea in chronic heart failure: relationships to lung stiffness and expiratory flow limitation. *J Appl Physiol* (1985). 2002 Apr;92(4):1409-16. doi: 10.1152/japplphysiol.00724.2001 with permission from American Physiological Society.

when the patient lies down to rest. In heart failure patients treated with LVADs, an increase of cardiac output is associated with a relevant reduction of CSAs but an increase of OSAs.[22] Mixed apnoea starts as a CSA episode and ends with OSA if airway collapse ensues. ◑ Figure 12.4.7 reports an example of OSA, CSA, mixed apnoea, and hypopnoea. Cheyne–Stokes respiration is a type of periodic breathing characterized by hyperpnea followed by hypopnoea or apnoea due to CSA (◑ Figure 12.4.8). It

is classically more regularly oscillating (with a periodicity of between 30 and 120 seconds) compared to irregularly spaced non-Cheyne–Stokes forms of apnoeic CSA.

Ventilation during sleep can be measured by different technologies at different levels, starting from the simple transcutaneous haemoglobin oxygen saturation and heart rate monitoring (type IV). The gold standard for sleep disease evaluation is overnight full polysomnography, which requires simultaneous and continuous monitoring of electroencephalogram, eye movements, electromyogram of the chin, ECG, body position, haemoglobin oxygen saturation, and oronasal flow as well as direct video view of patients during sleep (type I). However, type I polysomnography requires patients to be hospitalized, is extremely expensive, and does not allow recording of sleeping patterns in the place where the patient is more comfortable, for example, in their home. Type II polysomnography is similar to full polysomnography but without video recording, being continuous monitoring of physiological parameters performed outside the hospital. In contrast to type I, type II does not require the presence of a technician and can performed using portable devices. Type III is like type II but without electroencephalogram signals. At present, a type III recording is also obtainable by use of a wearable transducer based on the simultaneous recordings of at least three thoracic movements.[23] In such a case, apnoea is defined as the absence of movement (central apnoea) or as the presence of contrasting movements whose sum is equal to zero (obstructive apnoea). Information on the quality of sleep can also be obtained in patients fitted with pacemakers by intrathoracic impendence changes during sleep. The most well-known parameter to assess ventilation during sleep is the apnoea-hypopnoea index (AHI), the number of episodes per hour.

The diagnosis of sleep apnoea in heart failure requires at least type III monitoring to identify OSA and CSA and to quantify AHI. A diagnosis of OSA is made with an AHI > 15 or > 5 and concomitant presence of sleeplessness, non-restorative sleep, fatigue, insomnia, and gasping or snoring. CSA is diagnosed when central apnoeas are predominant. The severity of sleep disorders is commonly defined by AHI frequency as light (AHI between 5 and 14 events per hour), moderate (AHI between 15 and 29), and severe in case of AHI >30.

OSA can be observed even in healthy individuals with a greater prevalence in the male sex, while CSA is rarely reported.[24] Many diseases are associated with OSA and CSA (◑ Box 12.4.1). Of note, CSA and OSA can both be frequently observed in heart failure patients and particularly in those with severe heart failure, where CSA begins to be the dominant form. Consequently, the frequency of sleep disorders varies in different reports from 28% to 82% of cases.[25] Sleep disorders have been associated with a worsened heart failure prognosis. Hanly et al.[26] reported a mortality of 86% in heart failure patients with Cheyne–Stokes respiration vs 56% in patients without this type of respiratory pattern. Moreover, Cheyne–Stokes respiration is observed combined with exercise-induced oscillatory ventilation.[27–30] Indeed, the presence of sleep disorders, regardless OSA or CSA pattern, is associated with transient episodes of hypoxia which can lead to arrhythmias

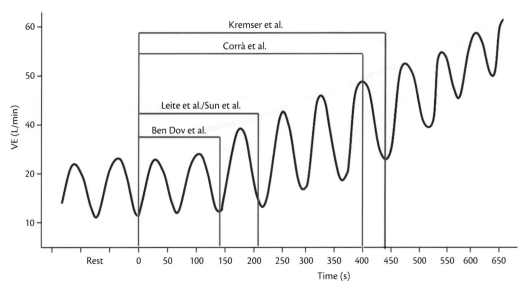

Figure 12.4.4 EOV-positive ventilatory pattern.
CPET, cardiorespiratory exercise test; EOV, exercise oscillatory ventilation; VE, minute ventilation; SD, standard deviation. *Visible oscillation in three or more CPET parameters.

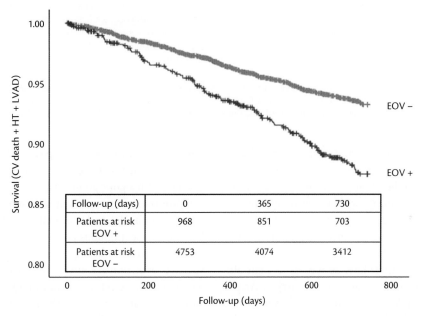

Figure 12.4.5 Survival and presence of exercise oscillatory ventilation (EOV) in the total population. Kaplan–Meier survival curves of study endpoint (cardiovascular (CV) death, urgent heart transplant (HT), or left ventricular assist device (LVAD) implantation) according to the presence or absence of EOV (EOV+ and EOV−) in the entire study population at 2-year follow-up (p = 0.000; χ2 = 34.0).

Reproduced from Rovai S, Corrà U, Piepoli M, Vignati C, Salvioni E, Bonomi A, Mattavelli I, Arcari L, Scardovi AB, Perrone Filardi P, Lagioia R, Paolillo S, Magrì D, Limongelli G, Metra M, Senni M, Scrutinio D, Raimondo R, Emdin M, Lombardi C, Cattadori G, et al; MECKI Score Research Group (see Appendix 1). Exercise oscillatory ventilation and prognosis in heart failure patients with reduced and mid-range ejection fraction. *Eur J Heart Fail*. 2019 Dec;21(12):1586-1595. doi: 10.1002/ejhf.1595 with permission from John Wiley and Sons.

including atrial fibrillation as well as fatal arrhythmias, as shown by the increased nocturnal discharge rate of implantable defibrillators.[31] Transient hypoxia is also associated with myocardial perfusion abnormalities, leading to sympathetic stimulation and myocardial ischaemia, both possible causes of myocyte apoptosis and necrosis, adrenoreceptor down regulation, and desensitization. Accordingly, polysomnography is suggested in cases of paroxysmal or recurrent atrial fibrillation, refractory hypertension,

unanticipated pulmonary hypertension with and without right ventricular failure, malignant arrhythmias, or obesity.[25]

Some pathophysiological aspects can help differentiate OSA from CSA. First of all, OSA is associated with negative intrathoracic pressures developing due to the respiratory muscles being stimulated and contracting against a closed airway. These muscles are not active in the apnoeic phases in CSA, and hence intrathoracic pressures do not fall. Secondly, heart failure CSA

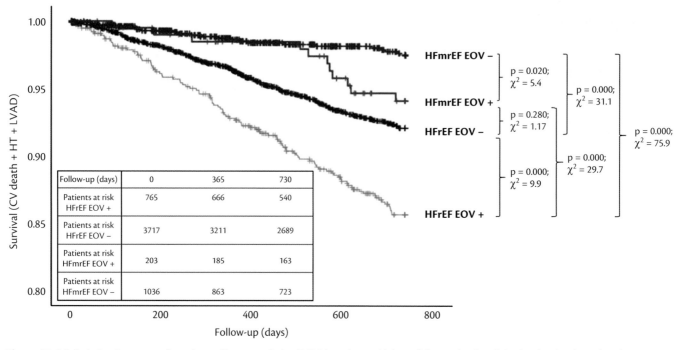

Figure 12.4.6 Surival and presence of exercise oscillatory ventilation (EOV) in patients with heart failure and reduced ejection fraction (HFrEF) and in patients with heart failure and mid-range ejection fraction (HFmrEF). Kaplan–Meier survival curves of study endpoint (cardiovascular (CV) death, urgent heart transplant (HT), or left ventricular assist device (LVAD) implantation) stratified according to the presence or absence of EOV (EOV+ and EOV−) in patients with HFrEF and in patients with HFmrEF. Comparison between groups (HFmrEF EOV− vs HFmrEF EOV+: p = 0.020, χ2 = 5.4; HFmrEF EOV− vs HFrEF EOV−: p = 0.000, χ2 = 31.1; HFmrEF EOV− vs. HFrEF EOV+: p = 0.000, χ2 = 75.9; HFmrEF EOV+ vs HFrEF EOV−: p = 0.280, χ2 = 1.17; HFmrEF EOV+ vs. HFrEF EOV+: p = 0.000, χ2 = 29.7; HFrEF EOV− vs. HFrEF EOV+: p = 0.000, χ2 = 9.9).

Reproduced from Rovai S, Corrà U, Piepoli M, Vignati C, Salvioni E, Bonomi A, Mattavelli I, Arcari L, Scardovi AB, Perrone Filardi P, Lagioia R, Paolillo S, Magrì D, Limongelli G, Metra M, Senni M, Scrutinio D, Raimondo R, Emdin M, Lombardi C, Cattadori G, et al; MECKI Score Research Group (see Appendix 1). Exercise oscillatory ventilation and prognosis in heart failure patients with reduced and mid-range ejection fraction. *Eur J Heart Fail.* 2019 Dec;21(12):1586-1595. doi: 10.1002/ejhf.1595 with permission from John Wiley and Sons.

patients have a greater sympathetic stimulation, as shown by the high urinary and plasma norepinephrine levels.[32] Thirdly, CSA is sometimes associated with heart rate oscillations, an event not observed with OSA. The combined oscillation of ventilation and heart rate has likely a further negative prognostic effect. Fourthly, CSA can be observed in severe heart failure patients during daytime in awake subjects which is not the case for OSA.[33]

In patients with severe heart failure, as well as at high altitude as described at the end of the nineteenth century by Angelo Mosso at Capanna Regina Margherita on top of Monte Rosa (4600 mt, Italian-Swiss Alps), Cheyne–Stokes respiration has also been found during daytime. This event is, however, rarer than

night-time Cheyne–Stokes respiration likely due to a higher sympathetic activity. Again, daytime Cheyne–Stokes ventilation is associated with a poor prognosis.

Optimization of heart failure treatment is the first-line treatment for both OSA and CSA in these patients. Severe OSA should be treated by continuous positive airway pressure (CPAP) which, in addition to clinical improvements in sleep quality, may be associated with positive effects on cardiac function (increases in left ventricular ejection fraction) and reductions of blood pressure, heart rate, and sympathetic tone.[34–36] A positive effect of OSA treatment by CPAP on heart failure mortality has been suggested, but no randomized double-blind studies are at present

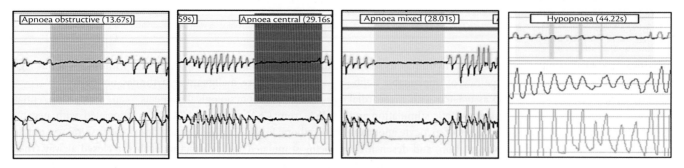

Figure 12.4.7 Example of obstructive sleep apnoea, central sleep apnoea, mixed apnoea, and hypopnoea.

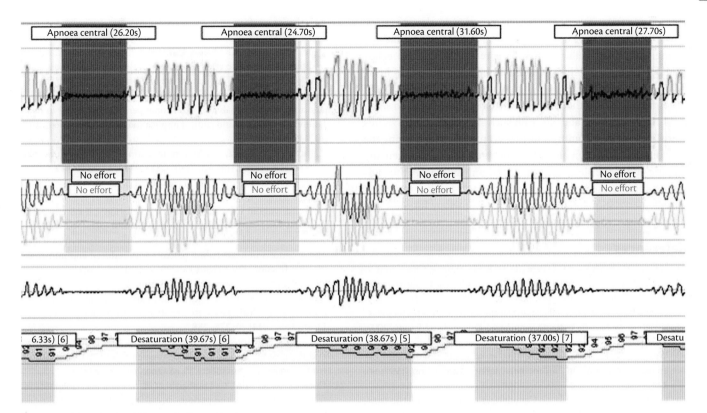

Figure 12.4.8 Example of Cheyne–Stokes respiration.

Box 12.4.1 Clinical characteristics of obstructive and central apnoea

Disease associated with obstructive sleep apnoea

- Unexplained daytime somnolence
- Abnormal sleep noises (gasping, choking, loud apnoeas) with respiratory effort witnessed by bed partners
- Fatigue
- Resistant arterial hypertension
- Cardiac rhythm abnormalities
- Obesity/high waist and neck circumference
- Narrow oropharynx
- Heart failure symptoms, in particular peripheral oedema

Disease associated with central sleep apnoea

- Less commonly daytime somnolence
- Repetitive sleep apnoeas without abnormal noises, and without respiratory effort
- Poor quality of sleep
- Possible association with periodic breathing during exercise
- Cardiac rhythm abnormalities
- Heart failure symptoms, in particular peripheral oedema

Source data from Parati, G., C. Lombardi, F. Castagna, P. Mattaliano, P.P. Filardi, P. Agostoni, *et al.* Heart failure and sleep disorders. *Nat Rev Cardiol*, 2016;13:389–403.

available.[37,38] The SAVE trial, the largest trial (2717 patients) of CPAP in OSA patients with cardiovascular disease (but excluding those with NYHA (New York Heart Association) class III or IV heart failure), reported no improvement in the primary composite end point of death from cardiovascular causes, myocardial infarction, stroke, or hospitalization for unstable angina, heart failure, or transient ischemic attack after a mean follow-up of 3.7 years. The trial reported 17.0% events in the treatment group vs 15.4% in the control group, hazard ratio with CPAP, 1.10; 95% confidence interval, 0.91 to 1.32; p = 0.34). CPAP did, however, significantly reduce snoring and daytime sleepiness and improved health-related quality of life and mood.[39]

Pharmacological treatment of CSA has been suggested using acetazolamide and theophylline. The rationale for CSA and EOV treatment with acetazolamide is strong, but the long-term effects are unclear.[19,25] In particular, acetazolamide may be also useful in severe heart failure, not only for CSA treatment but also when a combined diuretic treatment is needed. In contrast, the arrhythmogenic action of theophylline precludes its use in heart failure, although a reduction of CSA has been reported.[40] The SERVE-HF trial used positive pressure airway masks to treat heart failure with reduced ejection fraction (HFrEF) patients with CSA, and this led to an excess in cardiovascular mortality so this form of therapy is contra-indicated in this setting.[41] An alternative of an implantable phrenic nerve stimulation device has been shown to improve sleep quality and to reduce central apnoeas and the AHI in patients with CSA.[42] In a subset of these patients with heart failure (n = 96), improvements were reported in sleep metrics, Epworth Sleepiness Scale, patient global assessment Minnesota Living with Heart Failure Questionnaire (MLHFQ), and echocardiographic parameters. In addition the 6-month rate of heart failure hospitalization was 4.7% in treatment patients and 17.0% in control patients, although the trials to date have been too small to prove or disprove any effect on such major outcomes.[43] Thus guidelines advise including a formal sleep study to determine the type of sleep apnoea in any HFrEF patient prior to commencing therapy and if the sleep apnoea is predominantly CSA they advise against the use of positive pressure airway masks but suggest phrenic nerve stimulation as an alternative therapy for these patients to improve symptoms.

References

1. Guazzi, M., J. Myers, M.A. Peberdy, D. Bensimhon, P. Chase, and R. Arena. Exercise oscillatory breathing in diastolic heart failure: prevalence and prognostic insights. Eur Heart J, 2008; 29: 2751–2759.

2. Arena, R., J. Myers, J. Abella, et al. Development of a ventilatory classification system in patients with heart failure. Circulation, 2007; 115: 2410–2417.

3. Wasserman, K., Y.Y. Zhang, A. Gitt, et al. Lung function and exercise gas exchange in chronic heart failure. Circulation, 1997; 96: 2221–2227.

4. Contini, M., A. Apostolo, G. Cattadori, et al. Multiparametric comparison of CARvedilol, vs. NEbivolol, vs. BIsoprolol in moderate heart failure: the CARNEBI trial. Int J Cardiol, 2013; 168: 2134–2140.

5. Mutlu, G.M. and J.I. Sznajder. Mechanisms of pulmonary edema clearance. Am J Physiol Lung Cell Mol Physiol, 2005; 289: L685–695.

6. Agostoni, P., R. Pellegrino, C. Conca, J.R. Rodarte, and V. Brusasco. Exercise hyperpnea in chronic heart failure: relationships to lung stiffness and expiratory flow limitation. J Appl Physiol (1985), 2002; 92: 1409–1416.

7. Salvioni, E., U. Corra, M. Piepoli, et al. Gender and age normalization and ventilation efficiency during exercise in heart failure with reduced ejection fraction. ESC Heart Fail, 2020; 7: 371–380.

8. Ben-Dov, I., K.E. Sietsema, R. Casaburi, and K. Wasserman. Evidence that circulatory oscillations accompany ventilatory oscillations during exercise in patients with heart failure. Am Rev Respir Dis, 1992; 145: 776–781.

9. Corrà, U., A. Giordano, E. Bosimini, et al. Oscillatory ventilation during exercise in patients with chronic heart failure: Clinical correlates and prognostic implications. Chest, 2002; 121: 1572–1580.

10. Kremser, C.B., M.F. O'Toole, and A.R. Leff. Oscillatory hyperventilation in severe congestive heart failure secondary to idiopathic dilated cardiomyopathy or to ischemic cardiomyopathy. Am J Cardiol, 1987; 59: 900–905.

11. Leite, J.J., A.J. Mansur, H.F.G. De Freitas, et al. Periodic breathing during incremental exercise predicts mortality in patients with chronic heart failure evaluated for cardiac transplantation. J Am Coll Cardiol, 2003; 41: 2175–2181.

12. Sun, X.G., J.E. Hansen, J.F. Beshai, and K. Wasserman. Oscillatory breathing and exercise gas exchange abnormalities prognosticate early mortality and morbidity in heart failure. J Am Coll Cardiol, 2010; 55: 1814–1823.

13. Vignati, C., A. Apostolo, G. Cattadori, et al. Lvad pump speed increase is associated with increased peak exercise cardiac output and vo2, postponed anaerobic threshold and improved ventilatory efficiency. Int J Cardiol, 2017; 230: 28–32.

13a. Schmid, J.P., A. Apostolo, L. Antonioli, G. Cattadori, M. Zurek, M. Contini, P. Agostoni. Influence of exertional oscillatory ventilation on exercise performance in heart failure. Eur J Cardiovasc Prev Rehabil. 2008; 15: 688–692.

14. Ingle, L., A. Isted, K.K. Witte, J.G. Cleland, and A.L. Clark. Impact of different diagnostic criteria on the prevalence and prognostic significance of exertional oscillatory ventilation in patients with chronic heart failure. Eur J Cardiovasc Prev Rehabil, 2009; 16: 451–456.

15. Agostoni, P. and E. Salvioni. Exertional periodic breathing in heart failure: Mechanisms and clinical implications. Clin Chest Med, 2019; 40: 449–457.

16. Agostoni, P., U. Corra, and M. Emdin. Periodic breathing during incremental exercise. Ann Am Thorac Soc, 2017; 14: S116–S122.

17. Cornelis, J., J. Taeymans, W. Hens, P. Beckers, C. Vrints, and D. Vissers. Prognostic respiratory parameters in heart failure patients with and without exercise oscillatory ventilation – a systematic review and descriptive meta-analysis. Int J Cardiol, 2015; 182: 476–486.

18. Rovai, S., U. Corra, M. Piepoli, et al. Exercise oscillatory ventilation and prognosis in heart failure patients with reduced and mid-range ejection fraction. Eur J Heart Fail, 2019; 21: 1586–1595.

19. Apostolo, A., P. Agostoni, M. Contini, L. Antonioli, and E.R. Swenson. Acetazolamide and inhaled carbon dioxide reduce periodic breathing during exercise in patients with chronic heart failure. J Card Fail, 2014; 20: 278–288.

20. Gargiulo, P., A. Apostolo, P. Perrone-Filardi, S. Sciomer, P. Palange, and P. Agostoni. A non invasive estimate of dead space ventilation from exercise measurements. PLoS One, 2014; 9: e87395.

21. Caravita, S., A. Faini, C. Lombardi, et al. Sex and acetazolamide effects on chemoreflex and periodic breathing during sleep at altitude. Chest, 2015; 147: 120–131.

22. Apostolo, A., S. Paolillo, M. Contini, et al. Comprehensive effects of left ventricular assist device speed changes on alveolar gas exchange, sleep ventilatory pattern, and exercise performance. J Heart Lung Transplant, 2018; 37: 1361–1371.

23. Contini, M., A. Sarmento, P. Gugliandolo, et al. Validation of a new wearable device for type 3 sleep test without flowmeter. PLoS One, 2021; 16: e0249470.

24. Levy, P., M. Kohler, W.T. McNicholas, et al. Obstructive sleep apnoea syndrome. Nat Rev Dis Primers, 2015; 1: 15015.

25. Parati, G., C. Lombardi, F. Castagna, et al. Heart failure and sleep disorders. Nat Rev Cardiol, 2016; 13: 389–403.

26. Hanly, P.J. and N.S. Zuberi-Khokhar. Increased mortality associated with Cheyne–Stokes respiration in patients with congestive heart failure. Am J Respir Crit Care Med, 1996; 153: 272–276.

27. Oldenburg, O., B. Lamp, L. Faber, H. Teschler, D. Horstkotte, and V. Topfer. Sleep-disordered breathing in patients with symptomatic heart failure: a contemporary study of prevalence in and characteristics of 700 patients. Eur J Heart Fail, 2007; 9: 251–257.

28. Corra, U., M. Pistono, A. Mezzani, et al. Sleep and exertional periodic breathing in chronic heart failure: prognostic importance and interdependence. Circulation, 2006; 113: 44–50.

29. Meguro, K., H. Adachi, S. Oshima, K. Taniguchi, and R. Nagai. Exercise tolerance, exercise hyperpnea and central chemosensitivity to carbon dioxide in sleep apnea syndrome in heart failure patients. Circ J, 2005; 69: 695–699.

30. Lanfranchi, P.A., A. Braghiroli, E. Bosimini, et al. Prognostic value of nocturnal Cheyne–Stokes respiration in chronic heart failure. Circulation, 1999; 99: 1435–1440.

31. Bitter, T., N. Westerheide, C. Prinz, et al. Cheyne-Stokes respiration and obstructive sleep apnoea are independent risk factors for malignant ventricular arrhythmias requiring appropriate cardioverter-defibrillator therapies in patients with congestive heart failure. Eur Heart J, 2011; 32: 61–74.

32. Naughton, M.T., D.C. Benard, P.P. Liu, R. Rutherford, F. Rankin, and T.D. Bradley. Effects of nasal CPAP on sympathetic activity in

patients with heart failure and central sleep apnea. Am J Respir Crit Care Med, 1995; 152: 473–479.

33. Brack, T., I. Thuer, C.F. Clarenbach, *et al.* Daytime Cheyne–Stokes respiration in ambulatory patients with severe congestive heart failure is associated with increased mortality. Chest, 2007; 132: 1463–1471.

34. Franklin, K.A., J.B. Nilsson, C. Sahlin, and U. Naslund. Sleep apnoea and nocturnal angina. Lancet, 1995; 345: 1085–1087.

35. Kaneko, Y., J.S. Floras, K. Usui, *et al.* Cardiovascular effects of continuous positive airway pressure in patients with heart failure and obstructive sleep apnea. N Engl J Med, 2003; 348: 1233–1241.

36. Mansfield, D.R., N.C. Gollogly, D.M. Kaye, M. Richardson, P. Bergin, and M.T. Naughton. Controlled trial of continuous positive airway pressure in obstructive sleep apnea and heart failure. Am J Respir Crit Care Med, 2004; 169: 361–366.

37. Wang, H., J.D. Parker, G.E. Newton, *et al.* Influence of obstructive sleep apnea on mortality in patients with heart failure. J Am Coll Cardiol, 2007; 49: 1625–1631.

38. Kasai, T., K. Narui, T. Dohi, *et al.* Prognosis of patients with heart failure and obstructive sleep apnea treated with continuous positive airway pressure. Chest, 2008; 133: 690–696.

39. R.D. McEvoy, N.A. Antic, E. Heeley, et al. CPAP for prevention of cardiovascular events in obstructive sleep apnea. N Engl J Med, 2016; 375: 919–931.

40. Javaheri, S., T.J. Parker, L. Wexler, J.D. Liming, P. Lindower, and G.A. Roselle. Effect of theophylline on sleep-disordered breathing in heart failure. N Engl J Med, 1996; 335: 562–567.

41. Cowie, M.R., H. Woehrle, K. Wegscheider, *et al.* Adaptive servo-ventilation for central sleep apnea in systolic heart failure. N Engl J Med, 2015; 373: 1095–1105.

42. Costanzo, M.R., P. Ponikowski, S. Javaheri, et al. Transvenous neurostimulation for central sleep apnoea: a randomised controlled trial. Lancet, 2016; 388: 974–982.

43. Costanzo, M.R., P. Ponikowski, A. Coats *et al.* Phrenic nerve stimulation to treat patients with central sleep apnoea and heart failure. Eur J Heart Fail 2018; 20: 1746–1754.

CHAPTER 12.5

Pulmonary hypertension associated with left heart disease

Irene M Lang and Stephan Rosenkranz

Introduction

The commonest cause of pulmonary hypertension (PH) is left heart disease (LHD). Significant advances have occurred over the past five years in the area of pre-capillary pulmonary hypertension (PAH) with positive findings in genetics, proteomics and metabolomics, but the understanding of PH-LHD has remained poor. PH in heart failure with preserved ejection fraction (PH-HFpEF) represents the most complex situation because it is usually misdiagnosed as Group 1 PH and treated as Group 1 PH. In a large cohort referred for invasive haemodynamic assessment, PH-HFpEF was very common (46.1% of the population in[1]). The discussion of PH-LHD is important within this ESC textbook because PH is an important prognostic indicator of heart failure (⮕ Figure 12.5.1).

PH-LHD is the consequence of a 1:1 upstream transmission of elevated left atrial pressure, labeled as 'isolated post-capillary PH' (Ipc-PH). In 13% of cases with PH-LHD an increase in mean pulmonary arterial pressure (mPAP) occurs that is disproportional to left atrial pressure due to an additional contribution of pulmonary vascular disease, with decreased right ventricular–pulmonary vascular coupling and increased mortality, and these cases are labeled as combined post- and pre-capillary PH (Cpc-PH).[3] Patients with 'pre-capillary' pulmonary disease can be identified by an elevated diastolic pulmonary vascular pressure gradient (DPG) $\geq$ 7 mmHg. At present, the prognostic relevance of DPG has been confirmed in some reports,[3] but has also been refuted by others,[4] and so has been the classification by the 2015 ESC/ERS guidelines in: (1) 'isolated post-capillary PH' (Ipc-PH; DPG < 7mmHg and/or pulmonary vascular resistance (PVR) < 3WU) and (2) 'combined post- and pre-capillary PH' (Cpc-PH; DPG $\geq$ 7mmHg and/or PVR $\geq$ 3WU).[5] A recent analysis of a very large dataset concluded that elevated transpulmonary gradient (TPG), PVR, and DPG are all associated with mortality and cardiac hospitalizations.[1] Taken together, existing data suggest that patients with an elevated DPG (roughly 16% of the population[6]) harbour a particularly severe pulmonary vascular disease component,[6] that involves the arterial vascular bed beyond venous and intermediate vessel changes,[7] while the majority of cases of PH-LHD is classified as Ipc-PH-type, and may be regarded as a comorbidity of LHD ⮕ Figure 12.5.2.[8] The 2022 definition of PH-LHD is shown in ⮕ Table 12.5.1.

Prevalence and definition

Prevalence of PH-LHD

Globally, PH is the most common cause of right heart failure, with a prevalence estimate of 1%, increasing up to 10% in individuals aged >65 years.[9] In 65–80% of cases PH is due to left heart disease, including myocardial disease, coronary disease, valve disease, and pericardial disease. For example, in a series of patients with aortic valve

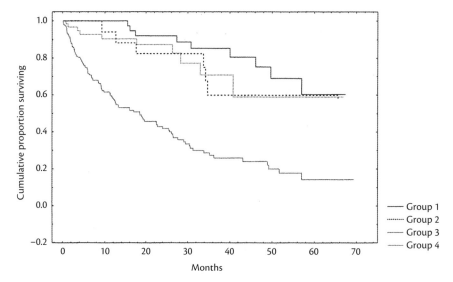

Figure 12.5.1 Survival rates without urgent heart transplantation in patients grouped according to the coupling between mean pulmonary arterial pressure (PAP) and right ventricular ejection fraction (RVEF). Group 1 = normal PAP/preserved RVEF (n = 73); group 2 = normal PAP/low RVEF (n = 68); group 3 = high PAP/preserved RVEF (n = 21); and group 4 = high PAP/low RVEF (n = 215).
Reproduced from Ghio S, Gavazzi A, Campana C, Inserra C, Klersy C, Sebastiani R, Arbustini E, Recusani F, Tavazzi L. Independent and additive prognostic value of right ventricular systolic function and pulmonary artery pressure in patients with chronic heart failure. *J Am Coll Cardiol.* 2001 Jan;37(1):183-8. doi: 10.1016/s0735-1097(00)01102-5 with permission Elsevier.

stenosis, a common LHD in the older population, mPAP ≥ 25 mmHg was found in 239 (48%) patients. Of those, 64 patients (13%) had Cpc-PH, 144 (28%) had Ipc-PH, and 31 patients (6%) had pre-capillary PH.[10] In heart failure with reduced ejection fraction (HFrEF), the prevalence of PH as assessed by right heart catherization was reported to be between 40 and 75%.[11,12] In heart failure with preserved ejection fraction (HFpEF), studies utilizing either echocardiography or invasive assessments with right heart catherization indicate a PH prevalence between 36 and 83%.[13–15] However, while PH is common in HFpEF, the condition is multi-faceted.[16–19] To identify distinct phenotypic subgroups in a cohort of individuals with HFpEF unsupervised clustering analysis has recently resulted in three phenogroups based on criteria in which PH was not included.[20]

Definition and classification of PH-LHD

PH-LHD denotes pulmonary hypertension due to left heart disease, meaning that PH occurs as a consequence of LHD. In the new guidelines of PH, PH-LHD was defined as: (1) post capillary PH when mPAP ≥ 20 mmHg and pulmonary arterial wedge pressure (PAWP) > 15 mmHg; and if (1) applies, then (2) Ipc-PH, when PVR < 2 Wood Units (WU); and (3) Cpc-PH when PVR

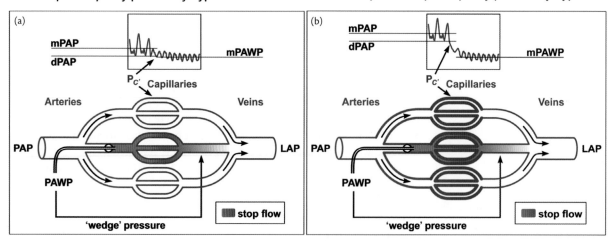

Figure 12.5.2 Schematic representation of the pulmonary circulation with corresponding pressure decay curves that arise from inflation of the Swan-Ganz balloon, in (a) isolated post-capillary pulmonary hypertension (Ipc-PH) and (b) combined post- and precapillary pulmonary hypertension (Cpc-PH). In Ipc-PH there is no significant pressure difference between mean pulmonary arterial pressure (mPAP) and pulmonary arterial wedge pressure (PAWP). In contrast, in Cpc-PH there is a pressure difference between mPAP and PAWP due to an additional component of pulmonary vascular disease at the level of the capillary bed, both on the arterial and the venous side.

Table 12.5.1 Haemodynamic definitions of pulmonary hypertension: 2022 ESC-ERS Guidelines on the diagnosis and treatment of pulmonary hypertension

Classification	Characteristics	Clinical groups
Pre-capillary PH	mPAP > 20 mmHg PAWP ≤ 15 mmHg PVR ≥ 3WU	1,3,4 and 5
Isolated post-capillary PH (Ipc-PH)	mPAP > 20 mmHg PAWP > 15mmHg PVR < 3WU	2 and 5
Combined pre- and post-capillary PH (Cpc-PH)	mPAP > 20 mmHg PAWP > 15 mmHg PVR ≥ 3WU	2 and 5

Reproduced from Simonneau G, Montani D, Celermajer DS, et al. Haemodynamic definitions and updated clinical classification of pulmonary hypertension. Eur Respir J. 2019 Jan 24;53(1):1801913. doi: 10.1183/13993003.01913-2018 with permission from European Respiratory Society.

≥ 2 WU (➲ Table 12.5.1). Still, major unanswered questions are whether DPG can be substituted by PVR, and whether Cpc-PH and idiopathic pulmonary arterial hypertension (iPAH) with comorbidities are distinct entities. Cpc-PH occurs in fewer than 20% of cases with PH-LHD, and is usually accompanied by other conditions, such as low DLCO,[21] valve disease, or other comorbidities.[6] The best way to describe the pre-capillary component of post-capillary PH remains controversial: none of the haemodynamic variables proposed to describe PH-LHD are free from limitations. Future studies may employ other physical measures, e.g. pulmonary waveform analyses or right ventricular flow dynamics to discriminate pulmonary vascular disease in the context of LHD. In addition, the disease history needs to be taken into account. For example, if a patient with diagnosed iPAH survives many years on modern treatments and acquires aortic valve stenosis, amyloidosis, or coronary artery disease, adding a component of left heart disease to the haemodynamic readout, then *PAH with comorbidities* may be diagnosed. In contrast to this concept, nowadays, these patients and patients with Cpc-PH are referred to by some as '*PAH with comorbidities*', or '*atypical PAH*'. In the new PH Guidelines, the definition of PH-LHD has been revised as PH associated with LHD, thus including PH-LHD, and PH occurring together with LHD.

Diagnosis

Non-invasive diagnosis

Algorithms have been devised to non-invasively and safely rule out pre-capillary PH and diagnose post-capillary PH without invasive right heart catheterization because this is a major unmet need in a majority of patients who are referred today for diagnostic investigation to a heart failure or PH clinic. According to a decision tree that followed the echocardiographic estimate of a pulmonary artery systolic pressure of > 36mmHg, patients were stratified by the presence or absence of an electrocardiographic right ventricular strain pattern and serum N-terminal brain natriuretic peptide (NT-proBNP) levels below and above 80 pg/

mL 100% sensitivity for pre-capillary PH was achieved, with only one false positive case per five patients.[22] Furthermore, a simple echocardiographic score for diagnosing precapillary versus postcapillary PH was proposed, including the ability to discriminate between Ipc-PH and Cpc-PH. This score[23] is based on seven points (2 for E/e' ratio ≤ 10, 2 for a dilated non-collapsible inferior vena cava, 1 for a left ventricular eccentricity index ≥ 1.2, 1 for a right-to-left heart chamber dimension ratio > 1, and 1 for the right ventricle forming the heart apex) and was applied in 230 consecutive patients referred for evaluation of pulmonary hypertension. The data suggest that the score behaves less well for Cpc-PH than for Ipc-PH (AUC 73% vs 85% for Ipc-PH). In summary, while the differentiation between pre- and postcapillary PH is facilitated by modern echocardiography and other imaging[24] providing subtle measures of left ventricular dysfunction and pulmonary hypertension, invasive right heart catheterization is still unavoidable today to differentiate Cpc-PH from Ipc-PH. Particularly in the presence of risk factors for Cpc-PH, or very poor right ventricular function by echocardiography invasive assessment is clinically indicated and needs to be performed.

The diagnostic dilemma of PH-LHD

A major diagnostic dilemma is to differentiate PH-LHD from '*PAH with comorbidities*'. The term 'PAH with comorbidities' was introduced at the time of the AMBITION trial, when naive patients with PAH were enrolled in a trial testing the efficacy and safety of upfront combination drug treatment against upfront monotherapy.[25] Although inclusion haemodynamic thresholds were set according to the PH guidelines definition at mPAP ≥ 25 mmHg, PVR ≥ 240 dyn·sec/cm⁵, and PAWP or left ventricular end-diastolic pressure (LVEDP) ≤ 15 mmHg, demographics of a significant proportion of enrolled patients were those of PH-LHD, including characteristic comorbidities such as diabetes, hypertension, coronary artery disease, and obesity.[26–29] Consequently, the study leadership introduced revised criteria as per a subsequent amendment to select for patients with a more precapillary phenotype. The steering committee introduced new thresholds such as mPAP ≥ 25 mmHg, PVR ≥ 300 dyn·sec/cm⁵, PAWP or LVEDP ≤12 mmHg if PVR was ≥ 300 to < 500 dyn·sec/cm⁵ or PAWP or LVEDP ≤ 15 mm Hg if PVR was ≥ 500 dyn·sec/cm⁵. Since then it has become evident that demographics of patients with PAH have changed over recent decades, with more elderly and comorbid patients found to have '*PAH with comorbidities*'. Whether this entity is separate and new, or a variant of PH-LHD (CpC-PH subtype) is unknown. Opitz et al. compared clinical phenotypes of iPAH, 'PAH with comorbidities', which these authors called atypical PH, and PH-HFpEF and found similarities, an observation which tempted them to conclude that pre-capillary, combined post- and pre-capillary PH, and post-capillary pulmonary hypertension comprised a pathophysiological continuum.[30] However, differential treatment responses and diverging prognoses speak against this concept. Recently, the authors of the Comparative, Prospective Registry of Newly Initiated Therapies for Pulmonary Hypertension (COMPERA) performed a cluster analysis of 841 patients with an IPAH diagnosis based on age, sex, diffusion capacity of the lung for carbon monoxide (DLCO; < 45% vs ≥ 45% predicted), smoking status, and presence of comorbidities (obesity, hypertension, coronary heart disease, diabetes mellitus), and identified Cluster 1 (n = 106; 12.6%): median age 45 years, 76% females, no comorbidities, mostly never smokers, DLCO ≥ 45%; Cluster 2 (n = 301; 35.8%): median age 75 years, 98% females, frequent comorbidities, no smoking history, DLCO mostly ≥ 45%; and Cluster 3 (n = 434; 51.6%): median age 72 years, 72% males, frequent comorbidities, history of smoking, and low DLCO. Patients in Cluster 1 had a better response to PAH treatment than patients in the two other clusters. One of the main shortfalls of the COMPERA phenomapping analysis is that there was no corelab for haemodynamic phenotyping, only selected comorbidities were collected, and the timing of the occurrence of comorbidities (from the start versus during the course of confirmed precapillary pulmonary hypertension) are unknown.[31] Haemodynamic phenotyping remains at the centre of diagnosis, and right heart catheterization has been embraced by the new heart failure guidelines for heart failure types that are commonly accompanied by pulmonary hypertension, such as constrictive and restrictive disease, congenital heart disease, and high output heart failure, as well as selected cases with HFpPEF.[32]

Haemodynamic variables to dissect pulmonary hypertension due to left heart disease subsets: with or without pulmonary vascular disease

Best practice suggests that right heart catherization should be performed in a stable clinical condition with no prior diuresis or fluid supplements (→ Table 12.5.2). Proper levelling at the mid-chest and 'zero-ing' the transducer to atmospheric pressure are requested. Patients should be positioned supine with legs flat, and pressures recorded during no-breath-hold-spontaneous-breathing. All measurements, including thermodilution cardiac outputs or cardiac output estimates by the direct Fick should be repeated in triplicate to obtain values within a 10% agreement.

PAWP is the primary key haemodynamic measurement for the diagnosis of post-capillary disease and is assessed as stop–flow pressure with the balloon inflated in the pulmonary artery at end-diastole closely reflecting LVEDP or LA pressure. In the absence of mitral stenosis, PAWP measured at end-diastole (i.e. typically as the mean of the A-wave or alternatively, a QRS-gated approach) more closely approximates LVEDP. By contrast, mean PAWP (averaged throughout the cardiac cycle) in the presence of large V waves (mitral regurgitation or non-compliant left atrium) will be higher than end-diastolic PAWP and will overestimate LVEDP. PAWP is clearly different from capillary pressure that may be estimated by pulmonary artery occlusion waveform analysis.[33] PAWP measurements are used instead of capillary pressure values to differentiate pre- from post-capillary disease states. While current definitions are based on a PAWP > 15 mmHg measured at end-expiration, analyses of large patient-based datasets suggest that PAWP > 12 mmHg may be a more appropriate threshold,[34] including confirmatory data from waveform analysis. The presence of large V waves signifies the presence of LHD.

TPG is calculated by subtracting mean pulmonary arterial wedge pressure (mPAWP) from mPAP, and diastolic gradient (DPG) as the difference between diastolic pulmonary arterial pressure minus PAWP.[6,35,36] PVR is calculated as TPG/cardiac output.[3,4] DPG was used in the 1970s in combination with PAWP, cardiac output (or arterio-venous oxygen content difference) and systemic blood pressure measurements for the differential diagnosis of cardiac and pulmonary causes of acute respiratory failure.[37] Recently, in a large haemodynamic database of stable patients with more than 10 years of follow-up it was found that elevated DPG ≥ 7 mmHg was associated with more advanced pulmonary vascular remodelling and consequently, with prognosis.[6] Disparity in the association of DPG with outcomes in different databases that were subsequently published (→ Table 12.5.2) may be associated with sources of error in retrospectively recorded pressures, errors in PAWP (underwedging or overwedging, excessive V waves), errors in diastolic pulmonary arterial pressure due to high frequency noise, catheter whip (with underestimation of PA diastolic pressure) as well as excessive respiratory variation and/or inadequate calibration; these errors may result in false negative values limiting clinical utility. Another factor accounting for the divergent experience with DPG as a correlate of pulmonary vascular disease[6,12,38–45,46] is the variability of patient populations studied with regards to heart failure aetiology, disease characteristics, the contribution of acute heart failure, disease duration, age, sex, treatment era, and contemporary practices during which the data were collected.

PVR is a commonly used measure to describe the pulmonary vascular bed in haemodynamic terms. In the new haemodynamic definitions and updated clinical classification of pulmonary hypertension,[47] a PVR > 2 WU was introduced as an additional criterion for the definition of pre-capillary,[48] and post-capillary PH,[49] and that definition was also taken up in the most recent guidelines for adult congenital heart disease where it appears particularly useful. PVR > 2 WU as a prognostic cut-off has been based on scientific evidence derived from heart failure populations.[11] Most recent data from the large US Veterans Affairs healthcare system catheterization database (2007–2012)[50] that had supported the mPAP threshold of 20 mmHg suggest that the effective PVR threshold may be as low as 2.2 WU in specific subsets.[51] These data illustrate that disease-specific cut-offs may emerge when more prospective large databases are analysed. In the preoperative evaluation of heart transplant recipients, PVR ≥3 WU remained associated with a significant increase in hazard for 30-day mortality after cardiac transplantation, even in the presence of low mPAP.[52]

Pulmonary vascular compliance is the stroke volume, measured in mL, needed to elevate PA pressure by 1 mmHg and is calculated as stroke volume divided by the difference between systolic and diastolic pulmonary arterial pressure (also called pulse pressure). Pulmonary arterial compliance calculated by that formula is usually greatly overestimated, but unfortunately not in a systematic fashion, with more severe overestimation in more severe disease states.

Table 12.5.2 Haemodynamic variables to define the pulmonary vascular component of PH-LHD

Parameter	TPG	DPG	PVR	PAC	Pulmonary wave forms	High fidelity pressure volume–loops
Measurement	mPAP-PAWP	dPAP-PAWP	(mPAP-PAWP)/CO	SV/(sPAP-dPAP)	% upstream resistance	Ees/Ea
Strength of physiological background	-/+	+++	+++	+	+++	+++++
Dependent on quality of PAWP recording	++	+++	+	-	-	-
Information	Describes the pressure gradient across the lungs	Describes the degree of pulmonary vascular disease	Describes the resistance across the lungs	Describes the volume needed to elevate PA pressure by 1 mmHg, and is a measure of distensibility (capacity of all arteries and arterioles to accumulate blood in systole and release it in diastole)	Describes capillary pressure, and define the steepness of the pressure decay between the PA and PAWP	Informs about RV contractility, PA elastance and coupling
Specific limitations	Included in PVR Limited relevance	Highly dependent on quality of PAWP Small number	Interdependent numerator and denominator	Small number non-linearly overestimating PAC	Technically demanding	Technical learning curve, preload reduction necessary, by separate 8F access
Marker of disease	+	++	++	–/+	–/+	+
Marker of prognosis	–/+	++	++	++	++	++++
Clinical usefulness	++	+++	+++	-	-/+	–

Conductance catheterization measures pressures and volumes simultaneously, allowing after calibration of volumes and stop–flow to assess right ventricle (RV) contractility as end-systolic elastance (Ees) and arterial elastance (Ea) or RV afterload and their ratio, Ees/Ea which describes RV–PA coupling. While the main readout of pressure volume loops is RV contractility, RV chamber stiffness can be read from the end-diastolic pressure–volume relationship of multi-beat pressure–volume loops with preload reduction. The arterial part describes RV afterload which is pulmonary vascular disease.

Using capillary pressure estimates PVR can be partitioned into larger arterial (upstream, Rup) and small arterial plus venous (downstream, Rds) components. In healthy subjects, PVR follows an almost equal distribution across the pulmonary circulation with ~60% Rup and ~40% Rds.[53] In iPAH, there is a similar PVR partitioning pattern, yet with significant elevation of mPAP and Pc', which is increased as arteriolar pulmonary vascular remodelling extends to the capillary–venous compartment. The discrepancy between the pulmonary artery occlusion waveform analysis estimates of capillary pressure is greatest in the presence of pulmonary vascular disease, and the magnitude of discordance is proportional to the severity of the disease. When partitioning of small vessel resistance is used for estimation of capillary pressure, the only parameter that is able to discriminate low upstream resistance of less than 60% without performing waveform analysis is DPG ≥ 7mmHg.

All these measures have been implicated as prognostic markers in PH-LHD, with variable importance, possibly depending on the nature and size of cohorts that were studied.[54] More recently, pulmonary effective arterial elastance (Ea), calculated as ratio of mPAP to SV in mmHg/mL, was introduced as a measure of total right ventricular afterload and prognosis of PH-LHD.[55] ⦿ Table 12.5.1 provides a summary of currently used parameters and techniques to assess the pulmonary vascular component of RV afterload, including coupling as the overall measure of energy transfer between the RV and the pulmonary vascular bed.

Isolated post-capillary and combined pre and post-capillary pulmonary hypertension – are they clinical phenotypes?

The prevalence of Cpc-PH is less than 20% of the total heart failure population.[3] There is no predilection for males or females, and most patients are elderly (60 plus years) and in New York Heart Association (NYHA) functional class III at presentation. While stable ischaemic heart disease, atrial fibrillation, and body mass index are similar, arterial hypertension tends to be more common in Ipc-PH. In Cpc-PH associated with diastolic heart failure, mild valvular heart disease and interstitial lung disease are more common. In Cpc-PH due to systolic heart failure, milder degrees of chronic obstructive pulmonary disease appear to aggravate pulmonary vascular disease. Other comorbidities of PH-LHD include a low DLCO,[21] as well as sleep apnoea,[56] which occurs in approximately 50% of all heart failure patients, and has consequences such as intermittent hypoxaemia, arousal, and intra-thoracic pressure swings leading to neurohormonal stimulation, oxidative stress, and inflammation. While sleep apnoea is a cause of PH in 10% of cases, severe PH due solely to obstructive sleep apnoea is rare. Prospective screening needs to be performed to couple sleep apnoea with a particular haemodynamic heart failure phenotype. Taken together, Ipc-PH and Cpc-PH clearly represent clinical phenotypes, but differential diagnosis is not possible based on the clinical presentation alone. Furthermore, several large datasets have confirmed the prognostic value of the differentiation between Ipc-PH and Cpc-PH. Gerges et al. and other investigators have described the dismal prognosis of Cpc-PH, which is similarly poor as that of iPAH.[57]

The 2018 WHO writing group[49] has proposed to approach the diagnosis of PH-LHD in three steps: (1) identification of a clinical phenotype taking into account all comorbid conditions to establish the characteristics of Group 2 PH; (2) assessment of a pre-test probability to identify which patients deserve an invasive evaluation; (3) haemodynamic characterization, which could include provocative testing (e.g. exercise or fluid loading) in selected cases in whom classification is difficult despite the invasive assessment at rest.

Management of PH-LHD

Drug treatment of PH-LHD

A collective progress in pulmonary vascular and heart failure medicine reinforces the critical importance of accurate haemodynamic assessment. The proper distinction between PAH and PH-LHD, and the distinction between Ipc-PH and Cpc-PH may be challenging, yet it has direct therapeutic consequences. Except for a single study,[58] randomized controlled trials have failed to show evidence that PAH-specific therapy benefits PH-LHD.[59][60] Furthermore, notwithstanding that the presence of pulmonary vascular disease may justify the use of drugs approved for PAH, the single trial that was designed to target Cpc-PH delivered a signal of harm.[61] Another signal of harm came from a randomized study of sildenafil in valvular heart disease PH.[62] These data lend support to the concept of keeping drugs that are approved for the treatment of PAH away from patients with PH-LHD. For the management of PH-LHD it remains important to decide whether PH is the comorbidity of LHD,[8] or LHD is the comorbidity of PAH.[25] In the majority of patients, PH is the comorbidity of LHD and treatment of underlying left heart disease remains the best choice.

Systemic light chain amyloidosis (AL) with cardiac involvement is the most common form of cardiac amyloidosis. The severity of heart disease dictates the prognosis in AL amyloidosis. Advances in chemotherapy and immunotherapy that suppress light chain production have improved outcomes. These recent improvements in survival rates have enabled therapies such as implanted cardiac defibrillators and heart transplantation that were previously not indicated for patients with advanced AL cardiomyopathy. For transthyretin amyloidosis (ATTR), the second most common form of amyloidosis with cardiac involvement, there is also significant progress in treatment. In cardiac TTR amyloidosis, parameters of RV size and function correlated well with symptom severity.[63] Therapies that stabilize transthyretin, such as tafamidis, have been successful. Tafamidis inhibits non-mutant TTR amyloidogenesis in a dose-dependent manner and stabilizes the two most clinically significant amyloidogenic mutants with similar efficacy.[64] A phase III trial of 441 patients with wild-type and hereditary ATTR cardiac amyloidosis tested tafamidis against placebo.[65] The pooled tafamidis arms (80 mg and 20 mg doses) showed a reduction in all-cause mortality (HR 0.70, 95% CI 0.51–0.96) and cardiovascular hospitalization (HR 0.68, 95% CI 0.56–0.81). Information on the regression of PH has not been published, but significant improvement in the 6-min walk test and quality of life occurred and a smaller increase in proBNP at months 12 and 30, and tafamidis was well tolerated. Treatment of wild-type and hereditary ATTR cardiac amyloidosis with tafamidis is labelled as a class I guidelines recommendation.[32]

Similar success was made in the treatment of hypertrophic cardiomyopathy, another common cause for PH-LHD[66]: in the EXPLORER-HCM trial, a phase 3, randomized, double-blind, placebo-controlled mutlicentre trial, patients with hypertrophic cardiomyopathy with a left ventricular outflow tract gradient of 50 mmHg or greater and NYHA class II–III symptoms were treated with placebo or mavacamten and experienced improved exercise capacity, less left ventricular outflow tract obstruction, NYHA functional class, and health status under treatment with mavacamten.[67]

Management of tricuspid regurgitation

PH is frequently associated with RV and right atrial (RA) dilatation and functional tricuspid regurgitation (TR),[68] which serves to make the diagnosis of PH[5] on the one hand, but is a driver of heart failure progression. In left heart disease, functional TR can result from multiple mechanisms including dilation of the tricuspid valve annulus, RV and RA remodelling, increased RV pressures, and atrial fibrillation.[69] Furthermore, presence of a pacemaker and defibrillator lead, reduced tricuspid annulus plane systolic excursion (TAPSE), and tricuspid annulus dilation are independently associated with development of significant TR.[70] Primary TR caused by an anatomical abnormality of the tricuspid valve apparatus is far rarer. Moderate or severe TR is associated with an increased mortality risk, and in isolated TR an effective regurgitant orifice ≥ 40 mm^2 was shown to be prognostically relevant.[71] Recently, the burden of TR and its impact on mortality have become more and more evident, particularly in HFpEF.[72] More interest has focused on the tricuspid valve in recent years following the advent of percutaneous tricuspid valve repair.[73] In isolated severe TR, there is preliminary evidence for clinical improvement after successful transcatheter treatment with the edge-to-edge MitraClip technique, including improved NYHA functional class and an increase of the 6-min walking distance.[73] In both surgical and interventional approaches to treat TR, high mortality rates have been reported, and patient selection is crucial. It is important to bear in mind that reducing TR in situations of increased RV afterload may lead to RV failure, or not correct the underlying uncoupling of the RA from the inferior vena cava.[74] In many instances, medical/electric cardioversion or atrial fibrillation ablation may be more effective than structural intervention at the tricuspid valve.

Future directions

Pathophysiology of PH-LHD remains a research topic. Because fluid overload appears as one of the disease characteristics, the understanding of the role of SGLT-2 inhibitors to specifically treat PH-LHD is a goal to be achieved in the near future. Furthermore, novel imaging to understand involvement of the pulmonary vasculature (arterioles, capillaries, veins) will impact disease classification in the future, as not all PH-LHD is the same. Finally, mechanical support of the right ventricle has been refined over the past years, with the concept to attenuate the spiral of vascular injury to the lung by lowering pulse pressure.[75]

Summary and key messages

- The commonest cause of pulmonary hypertension (PH) is left heart disease (LHD).

- LHD may occur in PH (PH is the first and the leading diagnosis):
  - as a consequence of ageing of diagnosed PAH, e.g. coronary artery disease, or degenerative mitral or aortic valve disease.
  - as a consequence of corrective heart surgery, e.g. in PH due to congenital heart disease.
  - as a comorbidity, e.g. of CTEPH.

- PH may occur in LHD (LHD is the first and the leading diagnosis):
  - as a consequence of severe chronic heart failure (all types, particularly HFmrEF and HFpEF).
  - as a consequence of comorbidities such as lung disease, malignancy, chemotherapy, and other treatments including surgeries, renal impairment, and genetic disorders.
  - as a consequence of concurrent causes of PH such as congenital heart disease, connective tissue disease, or hemolytic anemia.

- Haemodynamic phenotyping, including provocation with exercise and fluid loading remains at the centre of diagnosis.

- Precise aetiologic assessment is very important for treatment.

Sources of funding

This manuscript was supported by FWF SFB-F54 'Cellular Mediators Linking Inflammation and Thrombosis' and WWTF LCS 18-090.

Disclosures

IML has relationships with drug companies including AOPOrphan Pharmaceuticals, Actelion, MSD, Neutrolis, Ferrer, and United Therapeutics. Relationships include being an investigator in trials, consultancy services, research grants, and membership of scientific advisory boards.

References

1. Vanderpool RR, Saul M, Nouraie M, Gladwin MT and Simon MA. association between hemodynamic markers of pulmonary hypertension and outcomes in heart failure with preserved ejection fraction. *JAMA Cardiology*. 2018;3:298–306.

2. Ghio S, Gavazzi A, Campana C, et al. Independent and additive prognostic value of right ventricular systolic function and pulmonary artery pressure in patients with chronic heart failure. *Journal of the American College of Cardiology*. 2001;37:183–8.

3. Gerges M, Gerges C, Pistritto AM, Lang MB, Trip P, Jakowitsch J, Binder T and Lang IM. Pulmonary hypertension in heart failure. Epidemiology, right ventricular function, and survival. *American Journal of Respiratory and Critical Care Medicine*. 2015;192:1234–46.

4. Tedford RJ, Beaty CA, Mathai SC, et al. Prognostic value of the pre-transplant diastolic pulmonary artery pressure-to-pulmonary capillary wedge pressure gradient in cardiac transplant recipients with pulmonary hypertension. *Journal of Heart and Lung Transplantation* 2014;33:289–97.

5. Galie N, Humbert M, Vachiery JL, et al. 2015 ESC/ERS Guidelines for the diagnosis and treatment of pulmonary hypertension: The Joint Task Force for the Diagnosis and Treatment of Pulmonary Hypertension of the European Society of Cardiology (ESC) and the European Respiratory Society (ERS): Endorsed by: Association for European Paediatric and Congenital Cardiology (AEPC), International Society for Heart and Lung Transplantation (ISHLT). *European Heart Journal*. 2016;37:67–119.

6. Gerges C, Gerges M, Lang MB, Zhang Y, Jakowitsch J, Probst P, Maurer G and Lang IM. Diastolic pulmonary vascular pressure gradient: a predictor of prognosis in 'out-of-proportion' pulmonary hypertension. *Chest*. 2013;143:758–66.

7. Fayyaz AU, Edwards WD, Maleszewski JJ et al. Global pulmonary vascular remodeling in pulmonary hypertension associated with heart failure and preserved or reduced ejection fraction. *Circulation*. 2018;137:1796–810.

8. Tichelbäcker T, Dumitrescu D, Gerhardt F, et al. Pulmonary hypertension and valvular heart disease. *Herz*. 2019;44:491–501.

9. Hoeper MM, Humbert M, Souza R, et al. A global view of pulmonary hypertension. *Lancet Respiratory Medicine*. 2016;4:306–22.

10. Weber L, Rickli H, Haager PK, et al. Haemodynamic mechanisms and long-term prognostic impact of pulmonary hypertension in patients with severe aortic stenosis undergoing valve replacement. *European Journal of Heart Failure*. 2019;21:172–81.

11. Miller WL, Grill DE and Borlaug BA. Clinical features, hemodynamics, and outcomes of pulmonary hypertension due to chronic heart failure with reduced ejection fraction: pulmonary hypertension and heart failure. *JACC Heart Failure*. 2013;1:290–9.

12. Tampakakis E, Leary PJ, Selby VN, et al. The diastolic pulmonary gradient does not predict survival in patients with pulmonary hypertension due to left heart disease. *JACC Heart Failure*. 2015;3:9–16.

13. Lam CS, Roger VL, Rodeheffer RJ, Borlaug BA, Enders FT and Redfield MM. Pulmonary hypertension in heart failure with preserved ejection fraction: a community-based study. *Journal of the American College of Cardiology*. 2009;53:1119–26.

14. Leung CC, Moondra V, Catherwood E and Andrus BW. Prevalence and risk factors of pulmonary hypertension in patients with elevated pulmonary venous pressure and preserved ejection fraction. *American Journal of Cardiology*. 2010;106:284–6.

15. Shah AM, Shah SJ, Anand IS, *et al.* Cardiac structure and function in heart failure with preserved ejection fraction: baseline findings from the echocardiographic study of the Treatment of Preserved Cardiac Function Heart Failure with an aldosterone antagonist trial. *Circulation. Heart Failure.*. 2014;7:104–15.

16. Pieske B, Tschöpe C, de Boer RA, *et al.* How to diagnose heart failure with preserved ejection fraction: the HFA-PEFF diagnostic algorithm: a consensus recommendation from the Heart Failure Association (HFA) of the European Society of Cardiology (ESC). *European Heart Journal.* 2019;40:3297–317.

17. Barandiarán Aizpurua A, Sanders-van Wijk S, Brunner-La Rocca HP, *et al.* Validation of the HFA-PEFF score for the diagnosis of heart failure with preserved ejection fraction. *European Journal of Heart Failure.* 2020;22:413–21.

18. Reddy YNV, Carter RE, Obokata M, Redfield MM and Borlaug BA. A simple, evidence-based approach to help guide diagnosis of heart failure with preserved ejection fraction. *Circulation.* 2018;138:861–70.

19. Hwang IC, Cho GY, Choi HM, *et al.* H2FPEF score reflects the left atrial strain and predicts prognosis in patients with heart failure with preserved ejection fraction. *Journal of Cardiac Failure.* 2021;27:198–207.

20. Segar MW, Patel KV, Ayers C, *et al.* Phenomapping of patients with heart failure with preserved ejection fraction using machine learning-based unsupervised cluster analysis. *European Journal of Heart Failure.* 2020;22:148–58.

21. Hoeper MM, Meyer K, Rademacher J, Fuge J, Welte T and Olsson KM. Diffusion capacity and mortality in patients with pulmonary hypertension due to heart failure with preserved ejection fraction. *JACC Heart Failure.* 2016;4:441–9.

22. Bonderman D, Wexberg P, Martischnig AM, Heinzl H, Lang MB, Sadushi R, Skoro-Sajer N and Lang IM. A noninvasive algorithm to exclude pre-capillary pulmonary hypertension. *European Respiratory Journal.* 2011;37:1096–103.

23. D'Alto M, Romeo E, Argiento P, *et al.* A simple echocardiographic score for the diagnosis of pulmonary vascular disease in heart failure. *Journal of Cardiovascular Medicine (Hagerstown).* 2017;18:237–43.

24. Hur DJ and Sugeng L. Non-invasive multimodality cardiovascular imaging of the right heart and pulmonary circulation in pulmonary hypertension. *Frontiers in Cardiovascular Medicine.* 2019;6:24.

25. Galiè N, Barberà JA, Frost AE, *et al.* Initial use of ambrisentan plus tadalafil in pulmonary arterial hypertension. *New England Journal of Medicine.* 2015;373:834–44.

26. Ling Y, Johnson MK, Kiely DG, *et al.* Changing demographics, epidemiology, and survival of incident pulmonary arterial hypertension: results from the pulmonary hypertension registry of the United Kingdom and Ireland. *American Journal of Respiratory and Critical Care Medicine.* 2012;186:790–6.

27. Frost AE, Badesch DB, Barst RJ, *et al.* The changing picture of patients with pulmonary arterial hypertension in the United States: how REVEAL differs from historic and non-US Contemporary Registries. *Chest.* 2011;139:128–37.

28. Hoeper MM, Huscher D, Ghofrani HA, *et al.* Elderly patients diagnosed with idiopathic pulmonary arterial hypertension: results from the COMPERA registry. *International Journal of Cardiology.* 2013;168:871–80.

29. Rådegran G, Kjellström B, Ekmehag B, *et al.* Characteristics and survival of adult Swedish PAH and CTEPH patients 2000–2014. *Scandinavian Cardiovascular Journal.* 2016;50:243–50.

30. Opitz CF, Hoeper MM, Gibbs JS, *et al.*. Pre-capillary, combined, and post-capillary pulmonary hypertension: a pathophysiological continuum. *Journal of the American College of Cardiology.* 2016;68:368–78.

31. Hoeper MM, Pausch C, Grünig E, *et al.* Idiopathic pulmonary arterial hypertension phenotypes determined by cluster analysis from the COMPERA registry. *Journal of Heart and Lung Transplantation.* 2020;39:1435–44.

32. McDonagh TA, Metra M, Adamo M, *et al.* 2021 ESC Guidelines for the diagnosis and treatment of acute and chronic heart failure. *European Heart Journal.* 2021;42:3599–726.

33. Gerges C, Gerges M, Fesler P, *et al.* In-depth haemodynamic phenotyping of pulmonary hypertension due to left heart disease. *European Respiratory Journal.* 2018;51(5):1800067.

34. Gerges C, Gerges M, Skoro-Sajer N, *et al.* Hemodynamic thresholds for precapillary pulmonary hypertension. *Chest.* 2016;149:1061–73.

35. Harvey RM, Enson Y and Ferrer MI. A reconsideration of the origins of pulmonary hypertension. *Chest.* 1971;59:82–94.

36. Naeije R, Vachiery JL, Yerly P and Vanderpool R. The transpulmonary pressure gradient for the diagnosis of pulmonary vascular disease. *European Respiratory Journal.* 2013;41:217–23.

37. Stevens PM. Assessment of acute respiratory failure: cardiac versus pulmonary causes. *Chest.* 1975;67:1–2.

38. Al-Naamani N, Preston IR, Paulus JK, Hill NS and Roberts KE. Pulmonary arterial capacitance is an important predictor of mortality in heart failure with a preserved ejection fraction. *JACC Heart Failure.* 2015;3:467–74.

39. Howard C, Rangajhavala K and Safdar Z. Pulmonary artery diastolic pressure gradient as an indicator of severity of illness in patients with pulmonary hypertension related to left-sided heart disease. *Therapeutic Advances in Respiratory Disease.* 2015;9:35–41.

40. O'Sullivan CJ, Wenaweser P, Ceylan O, *et al.* Effect of pulmonary hypertension hemodynamic presentation on clinical outcomes in patients with severe symptomatic aortic valve stenosis undergoing transcatheter aortic valve implantation: insights from the new proposed pulmonary hypertension classification. *Circulation Cardiovascular Interventions.* 2015;8:e002358.

41. Brunner NW, Yue SF, Stub D, *et al.* The prognostic importance of the diastolic pulmonary gradient, transpulmonary gradient, and pulmonary vascular resistance in patients undergoing transcatheter aortic valve replacement. *Catheterization and Cardiovascular Interventionss.* 2017;90:1185–91.

42. Mazimba S, Mejia-Lopez E, Black G, *et al.* Diastolic pulmonary gradient predicts outcomes in group 1 pulmonary hypertension (analysis of the NIH primary pulmonary hypertension registry). *Respiratory Medicine.* 2016;119:81–6.

43. Nagy AI, Venkateshvaran A, Merkely B, Lund LH and Manouras A. Determinants and prognostic implications of the negative diastolic pulmonary pressure gradient in patients with pulmonary hypertension due to left heart disease. *European Journal of Heart Failure.* 2017;19:88–97.

44. Adir Y, Guazzi M, Offer A, Temporelli PL, Cannito A and Ghio S. Pulmonary hemodynamics in heart failure patients with reduced or preserved ejection fraction and pulmonary hypertension: Similarities and disparities. *American Heart Journal.* 2017;192:120–7.

45. Palazzini M, Dardi F, Manes A, *et al.* Pulmonary hypertension due to left heart disease: analysis of survival according to the haemodynamic classification of the 2015 ESC/ERS guidelines and insights for future changes. *European Journal of Heart Failure.* 2018;20(2):248–55.

46. Ciftci O, Unal EN, Dellaloglu Z, *et al.* Relationship between preoperative diastolic transpulmonary gradient with pulmonary vascular resistance and 1-year and overall mortality rates among patients undergoing cardiac transplant. *Experimental and Clinical Transplantation* 2019;17:231–235.

47. Simonneau G, Montani D, Celermajer DS, Denton CP, Gatzoulis MA, Krowka M, Williams PG and Souza R. Haemodynamic

definitions and updated clinical classification of pulmonary hypertension. *European Respiratory Journal*. 2019;53(1):1801913.

48. Simonneau G, Gatzoulis MA, Adatia I, *et al*. Updated clinical classification of pulmonary hypertension. *Journal of the American College of Cardiology*. 2013;62:D34–41.

49. Vachiery JL, Tedford RJ, Rosenkranz S, *et al*. Pulmonary hypertension due to left heart disease. *European Respiratory Journal*. 2019;53(1):1801897.

50. Maron BA, Hess E, Maddox TM, *et al*. Association of borderline pulmonary hypertension with mortality and hospitalization in a large patient cohort: insights from the veterans affairs clinical assessment, reporting, and tracking program. *Circulation*. 2016;133:1240–8.

51. Maron BA, Brittan EL, Hess E, *et al*. Pulmonary vascular resistance and clinical outcomes in patients with pulmonary hypertension: a retrospective cohort study. *Lancet Respiratory Medicine*. 2020;8:873–84.

52. Crawford TC, Leary PJ, Fraser CD, 3rd, *et al*. Impact of the new pulmonary hypertension definition on heart transplant outcomes: expanding the hemodynamic risk profile. *Chest*. 2020;157:151–61.

53. Maggiorini M, Melot C, Pierre S, *et al*. High-altitude pulmonary edema is initially caused by an increase in capillary pressure. *Circulation*. 2001;103:2078–83.

54. Caravita S, Faini A, Carolino D'Araujo S *et al*. Clinical phenotypes and outcomes of pulmonary hypertension due to left heart disease: Role of the pre-capillary component. *PloS one*. 2018;13:e0199164.

55. Tampakakis E, Shah SJ, Borlaug BA, *et al*. Pulmonary effective arterial elastance as a measure of right ventricular afterload and its prognostic value in pulmonary hypertension due to left heart disease. *Circulation. Heart Failure*. 2018;11:e004436.

56. Javaheri S, Javaheri S and Javaheri A. Sleep apnea, heart failure, and pulmonary hypertension. *Current Heart Failure Reports*. 2013;10:315–20.

57. Naeije R, Gerges M, Vachiery JL, Caravita S, Gerges C and Lang IM. Hemodynamic phenotyping of pulmonary hypertension in left heart failure. *Circulation. Heart Failure*. 2017;10(9):e004082.

58. Guazzi M, Vicenzi M, Arena R and Guazzi MD. Pulmonary hypertension in heart failure with preserved ejection fraction: a target of phosphodiesterase-5 inhibition in a 1-year study. *Circulation*. 2011;124:164–74.

59. Bonderman D, Ghio S, Felix SB, *et al*. Riociguat for patients with pulmonary hypertension caused by systolic left ventricular dysfunction: a phase IIb double-blind, randomized, placebo-controlled, dose-ranging hemodynamic study. *Circulation*. 2013;128:502–11.

60. Hoendermis ES, Liu LC, Hummel YM, *et al*. Effects of sildenafil on invasive haemodynamics and exercise capacity in heart failure patients with preserved ejection fraction and pulmonary hypertension: a randomized controlled trial. *European Heart Journal*. 2015;36:2565–73.

61. Vachiery JL, Delcroix M, Al-Hiti H, Efficace M, Hutyra M, Lack G, Papadakis K and Rubin LJ. Macitentan in pulmonary hypertension due to left ventricular dysfunction. *The European Respiratory Journal*. 2018;51 (2):1701886.

62. Bermejo J, Yotti R, Garcia-Orta R, *et al*.Sildenafil for improving outcomes in patients with corrected valvular heart disease and persistent pulmonary hypertension: a multicenter, double-blind, randomized clinical trial. *European Heart Journal*. 2018;39:1255–64.

63. Binder C, Duca F, Stelzer PD, *et al*. Mechanisms of heart failure in transthyretin vs. light chain amyloidosis. *European Heart Journal Cardiovascular Imaging*. 2019;20:512–24.

64. Bulawa CE, Connelly S, Devit M, *et al*. Tafamidis, a potent and selective transthyretin kinetic stabilizer that inhibits the amyloid cascade. *Proceedings of the National Academy of Sciences of the USA*. 2012;109:9629–34.

65. Maurer MS, Schwartz JH, Gundapaneni B, *et al*. Tafamidis treatment for patients with transthyretin amyloid cardiomyopathy. *New England Journal of Medicine*. 2018;379:1007–16.

66. Musumeci MB, Mastromarino V, Casenghi M, *et al*. Pulmonary hypertension and clinical correlates in hypertrophic cardiomyopathy. *International Journal of Cardiology*. 2017;248:326–32.

67. Olivotto I, Oreziak A, Barriales-Villa R, *et al*. Mavacamten for treatment of symptomatic obstructive hypertrophic cardiomyopathy (EXPLORER-HCM): a randomised, double-blind, placebo-controlled, phase 3 trial. *Lancet*. 2020;396:759–69.

68. Mentias A, Patel K, Patel H, *et al*. Effect of pulmonary vascular pressures on long-term outcome in patients with primary mitral regurgitation. *Journal of the American College of Cardiology*. 2016;67:2952–61.

69. Prihadi EA, Delgado V, Leon MB, Enriquez-Sarano M, Topilsky Y and Bax JJ. Morphologic types of tricuspid regurgitation: characteristics and prognostic implications. *JACC Cardiovasc Imaging*. 2019;12:491–99.

70. Prihadi EA, van der Bijl P, Gursoy E, *et al*. Development of significant tricuspid regurgitation over time and prognostic implications: new insights into natural history. *European Heart Journal*. 2018;39:3574–81.

71. Topilsky Y, Nkomo VT, Vatury O, *et al*. Clinical outcome of isolated tricuspid regurgitation. *JACC Cardiovascular Imaging*. 2014;7:1185–94.

72. Borlaug BA, Kane GC, Melenovsky V and Olson TP. Abnormal right ventricular-pulmonary artery coupling with exercise in heart failure with preserved ejection fraction. *European Heart Journal*. 2016;37:3293–302.

73. Nickenig G, Kowalski M, Hausleiter J, *et al*. Transcatheter treatment of severe tricuspid regurgitation with the edge-to-edge MitraClip technique. *Circulation*. 2017;135:1802–14.

74. Marcus JT, Westerhof BE, Groeneveldt JA, Bogaard HJ, de Man FS and Vonk Noordegraaf A. Vena cava backflow and right ventricular stiffness in pulmonary arterial hypertension. *European Respiratory Journal*. 2019;54:1900625.

75. Gerges C, Vollmers K, Pritzker MR, Gainor J, Scandurra J, Weir EK and Lang IM. Pulmonary artery endovascular device compensates for loss of vascular compliance in pulmonary arterial hypertension. *Journal of the American College of Cardiology*. 2020;76:2284–6.

CHAPTER 12.6

Ventricular arrhythmias and sudden death in heart failure

Alessandro Trancuccio, Alessia Chiara Latini, Carlo Arnò, Deni Kukavica, Andrea Mazzanti, and Silvia G Priori

Contents

The impact of ventricular arrhythmias and sudden death in heart failure

Ventricular arrhythmias (VAs) are highly prevalent in patients with chronic heart failure (HF),[1] and range from isolated premature ventricular complexes to more severe arrhythmias, such as non-sustained or sustained ventricular tachycardia (VTns and VTs, respectively) and, lastly, to ventricular fibrillation.[2] The clinical relevance of VAs, which may cause sudden cardiac death (SCD), is related to the fact that they represent an important competing cause of death in patients with HF.

Importantly, SCD has been deemed to account for approximately 50% of all deaths in HF,[3] but SCD rates have been declining over time.[4] A recent meta-analysis by Shen et al.[4] analyzed data from all the randomized clinical trials (RCTs) enrolling more than 1000 patients that were conducted from 1995 to 2014, including only patients without an implantable cardioverter-defibrillator (ICD), to evaluate the impact of the increasing use of evidence-based pharmacotherapies able to reduce incidence of SCD in HF. Interestingly, the authors demonstrated that the SCD rates have declined by 44% over the past 20 years (⮞ Figure 12.6.1).

Accordingly, while the first trials conducted in the late 1990s[5,6] reported annual rates of SCD around 6% per annum, more recent studies have found rates of approximately 3%.[7,8] It is important to highlight that data deriving from RCTs may not be representative of 'real-world clinical practice' because trial patients are selected by stringent criteria that often exclude older individuals and patients with co-morbidities. Furthermore, in clinical trials compliance to the therapeutic regimen is strictly controlled. It is therefore important to highlight that the trend supporting the reduction of the incidence of SCD has been also confirmed in real-world studies.[9] Although the rates of SCD have significantly reduced over the years, recent data from the PARADIGM-HF trial estimate the cumulative incidence in patients with HF to be 8.8% at three years.[4] Additionally, another important concept that emerged from the aforementioned meta-analysis by Shen et al.[4] is that the proportion of deaths attributable to SCD remained substantially unvaried during

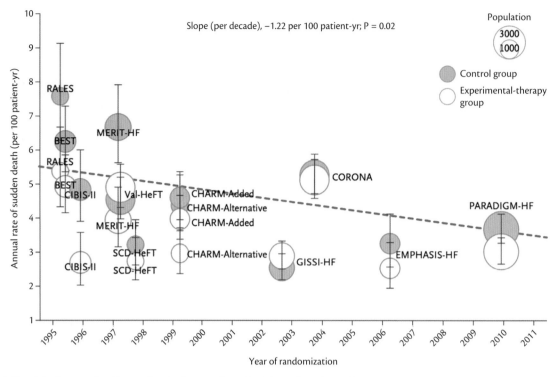

Figure 12.6.1 Trends in the rate of sudden cardiac death across the main trials conducted over the past 20 years.

the last 20 years, with SCD accounting for around 40% of the total number of deaths of these patients. This finding is consistent with the fact that current pharmacological therapy (beta-blockers (BBs), ACE-inhibitors (ACE-I), and mineralocorticoid receptor antagonists (MRA)) seems equally effective in reducing mortality due to arrythmias and due to worsening of HF.

In patients with HF the overall risk of death is given by a combined risk of SCD and a risk of dying from other causes, cardiovascular or otherwise. The contribution of SCD as a competing cause of death in patients with HF is variable and depends on the stage of the disease. In patients with mild to moderate HF (New York Heart Association (NYHA) functional class II and III), SCD is the cause of death in 50–60% of cases, while in the end-stage (NYHA IV) patients are more likely to die from pump failure, with SCD being the cause of death in only 20 to 30% of the cases.[10] Additionally, the proportion of deaths attributable to SCD is age-dependent, it competes with other causes of death, both cardiovascular and non-cardiovascular (e.g. cancer, metabolic diseases, etc.). As shall be discussed later, the concept of competitive risk has relevant implications for the management and prognosis of patients with HF.

Aetiology and pathogenesis of ventricular arrhythmias in heart failure

HF is a complex clinical syndrome resulting from several causes, often coexisting and interacting in a single patient (➲ Figure 12.6.2). It has been traditionally classified in post-ischaemic and non-ischaemic forms, with the former being the most studied by virtue of the high frequency of coronary artery disease in the

general population. However, this classification is reductive, and it disregards some important aspects.

First, the prevalence of the different causes of HF varies among different geographical areas, with myocardial infarction (MI) being the leading cause in higher-income countries, in contrast to lower-income countries, in which hypertensive heart disease, rheumatic heart disease, and myocarditis prevail.[11,12] Of note, other aetiologies, which are rare in Europe, are worthy of mention for their high arrhythmic potential (e.g. Chagas disease in South America).[11]

Secondly, the grouping of all other causes under the umbrella term of 'non-ischaemic HF' clusters together an extremely heterogeneous spectrum of diseases. An important proof of this concept is the growing awareness of the role of inherited cardiomyopathies in HF. In fact, the increasing use of genetic analysis in clinical practice has shed light on familial cardiomyopathies as an important but underestimated cause of HF, in patients who are usually younger than those suffering from ischaemic heart disease. This is not only relevant for classification purposes but has crucial implications for the management of patients. As discussed more in detail in the section regarding risk stratification, several forms of cardiomyopathies are associated with an increased risk of SCD,[2] such as those secondary to mutations in the following genes: *LMNA, FLNC, PLN, RBM20,* and *DSP*.[13]

These important differences notwithstanding, in the following section the general mechanisms that have been implicated in arrhythmogenesis of VAs in HF are dissected. We will inspect the arrhythmogenic mechanisms of VAs at three different levels[14] (➲ Figure 12.6.3):

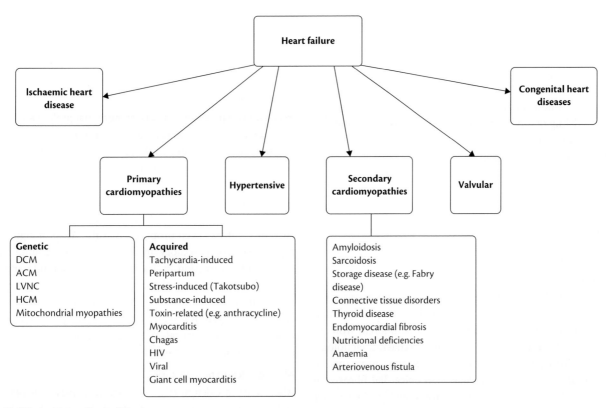

Figure 12.6.2 Aetiology of heart failure.
Source data from Ziaeian B, Fonarow GC. Epidemiology and aetiology of heart failure. *Nat Rev Cardiol.* 2016 Jun;13(6):368–78.

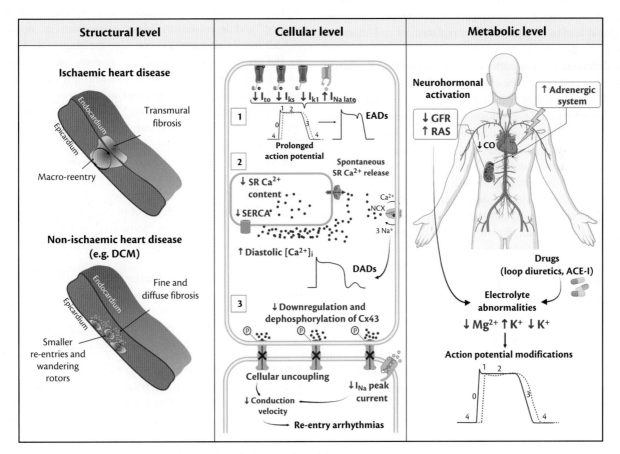

Figure 12.6.3 Arrhythmogenic mechanisms of ventricular arrhythmias in heart failure.

1. Structural level:
   a. Replacement and interstitial fibrosis
   b. Left ventricle (LV) geometric remodeling and myocardial stretch
2. Cellular level (remodeling of the electrophysiological properties of the cardiomyocyte):
   a. Remodeling of ion channels and prolongation of action potential duration
   b. Altered Ca^{2+} homeostasis
   c. Intercellular uncoupling (reduced connexin 43)
3. Metabolic level:
   a. Neurohormonal activation
   b. Electrolyte abnormalities.

Structural abnormalities

Replacement and interstitial fibrosis

The presence of fibrosis constitutes an anatomic substrate for the genesis of re-entrant VAs. However, it should be emphasized that the replacement fibrosis secondary to a MI is different from fibrosis found in patients with HF of non-ischaemic aetiology. Compared with post-MI, in which the ischaemic wavefront of necrosis results in more endocardial than epicardial fibrosis, in HF of non-ischaemic aetiology, the fibrosis tends to be smaller and less confluent, with less endocardial involvement and with reduced transmural extension[15,16] (➲ Figure 12.6.3). Additionally, chronic pressure overload secondary to valvular heart disease or hypertension, as well as a consequence of hypertrophic cardiomyopathy may lead to the coexistence of replacement and interstitial fibrosis.[16]

The differences in the pattern of fibrosis result in the generation of different types of re-entry. Seminal studies conducted in the 1990s demonstrated that in MI the presence of post-infarct replacement fibrosis (i.e. confluent scar) determines sites of conduction block and anisotropic conduction leading to macro-reentrant VT.[17,18] On the other hand, finer replacement fibrosis (typical of HF related to dilated cardiomyopathy (DCM)) tends to be associated with smaller circuits and with wandering rotors.[19] Lastly, *in silico* studies support the hypothesis of microreentries as the sole arrhythmogenic mechanism associated with diffuse interstitial fibrosis.[20] These differences have important clinical implications in terms of suitability for ablative procedures, as discussed in the section regarding the clinical management.

Geometric remodeling and myocardial stretch

In addition to the development of fibrosis, other structural abnormalities such as LV geometric remodeling and myocardial stretch are implicated in the arrhythmogenesis of HF. Volume and pressure overload, or a combination of both, cause different LV geometric adaptations (eccentric hypertrophy and concentric hypertrophy, respectively), which can contribute to the arrhythmogenic *milieu*[21,22] In fact, it is very well recognized that cardiac hypertrophy is an important pro-arrhythmogenic factor,[23] and it has been demonstrated in animal models of HF that both increased preload and afterload (i.e. increased myocardial stretch)

can promote the development of VAs.[24] Additionally, myocardial stretch has been demonstrated to induce afterdepolarizations,[25] which can cause triggered activity, which in turn may act as a trigger for VAs.

Cellular remodeling

Ion channel remodeling and action potential prolongation

A growing body of evidence deriving both from animal models[26] and from studies on human tissue[27,28] has shown that HF is characterized by alterations in ionic currents that determine a prolongation of the cardiac action potential (AP). These alterations include both a reduction in the outward potassium currents Ito,[27,29,30] IKs,[29–31] and IK1,[27,32] and an increase in the late sodium current.[33,34] It has been proposed that the AP-prolonging effects represent a compensatory mechanism, which counterbalances the loss of contraction by increasing the amplitude and/or the duration of the Ca^{2+}-transient.[19] The resultant prolongation of the AP can promote the onset of early afterdepolarizations,[35,36] which can be the trigger for re-entry arrhythmias, especially when combined with an anatomical substrate predisposing to a critical degree of conduction slowing.[19,37]

Altered calcium homeostasis

Alterations in calcium (Ca^{2+}) homeostasis play a pivotal role in arrhythmogenesis in patients with HF. In particular, it has been demonstrated that cardiomyocytes from patients with HF are characterized by increased diastolic cytoplasmic Ca^{2+} concentration (i.e. 'Ca^{2+} overload'),[38] decreased sarcoplasmic reticulum Ca^{2+} content[38] and decreased sarcoplasmic reticulum Ca^{2+} uptake.[39,40]

Additionally, alterations in Na^+/Ca^{2+} exchanger (NCX), crucial for the maintenance of normal Ca^{2+} homeostasis, have been reported, but their role in HF remains unclear. Although not consistently, most studies in different animal models of different forms of HF have found increased NCX expression at the mRNA and protein level.[41–43] Importantly, these findings were later confirmed in a study on explanted human hearts, where Schillinger and colleagues[44] found increased protein levels of NCX by 56%, and patients with complex VAs (VTns or VTs) had significantly higher levels of NCX than patients without them. Lastly, in a recent study on a porcine model of post-MI HF, the inward NCX current (i.e. Ca^{2+} efflux) was increased during the plateau phase of action potential, consistently with an increased functional role of NCX in HF.[34]

According to the classical arrhythmogenic theories, the combination of all the aforementioned Ca^{2+} handling abnormalities may promote the occurrence of spontaneous Ca^{2+} release from the sarcoplasmic reticulum, which can ultimately lead to NCX-mediated delayed afterdepolarizations and triggered arrhythmias.[19]

Altered intercellular coupling

Gap junctions mediate electrical coupling between cardiac myocytes, forming the cell-to-cell pathways for an orderly spread of the wave of electrical excitation responsible for synchronous contraction.[45]

Interestingly, both downregulation[46–48] and dephosphorylation[47] of connexin-43 (Cx43), a major gap junctional protein, have been described as a general feature of HF. In support of this, samples collected from human explanted hearts showed reduction of Cx43, and redistribution to other regions of the cardiomyocyte distant from their physiologic localization at the intercalated disc.[48] Different studies have proposed a link between Cx43 expression and reduced sodium current amplitude in ventricular[49,50] and atrial cardiomyocytes,[51] while super-resolution fluorescence localization microscopy in murine adult cardiomyocytes demonstrated that the NaV1.5 channels that conduct the inward sodium current, localization at the intercalated disks is Cx43-dependent.[52] Therefore, it is not surprising to observe a reduction of the peak sodium current density in HF cardiomyocytes.[33]

The role of these alterations in cell-to-cell communication in HF is pivotal in the arrhythmogenesis, since intercellular uncoupling, combined with a reduction of peak sodium current, results in slowed conduction, thereby increasing the susceptibility of the failing heart to re-entrant arrhythmias.[45]

Metabolic abnormalities

Neurohormonal activation

The decreased cardiac output in HF results in a series of maladaptive compensatory mechanisms which can contribute to arrhythmogenesis. These include the activation of the adrenergic nervous system and the renin-angiotensin system (RAS).

It is well established that neurohumoral activation may influence the substrate in the failing heart and may represent a trigger for lethal VA. Both experimental evidence[53] and clinical studies[5,54] have demonstrated a clear association between adrenergic system and RAS activation and SCD. In 2000, Cao and colleagues demonstrated in ventricular biopsy and autopsy specimens a correlation between VAs and increased density of sympathetic nerves in patients with HF, suggesting that abnormally increased post-injury sympathetic nerve density may contribute to the occurrence of ventricular tachyarrhythmias and SCD.[55] With regards to RAS activation, it has been observed that transgenic overexpression of angiotensin-converting enzyme-related carboxypeptidase (ACE2) in mice induced connexin dysregulation, and presumably gap junction remodeling, resulting in profound electrophysiological disturbances and an increased rate of SCD.[56]

Electrolyte abnormalities

Other metabolic alterations involved in the arrhythmogenesis of HF include electrolyte imbalance, especially alterations of serum levels of potassium and magnesium. Both hypokalaemia and hyperkalaemia can potentiate the already elevated risk of arrhythmias in patients with HF.[57,58] Hypokalaemia can result from the adaptive activation of RAS or can be secondary to the use of loop diuretics, while hyperkalaemia is usually due to the use of RAS inhibitors. Additionally, patients with chronic HF frequently have clinically relevant abnormalities of the serum magnesium, which has been associated a high prevalence of VAs and an increased risk of SCD.[59]

Risk stratification

As previously highlighted, SCD is a major cause of death in HF patients,[60] and hence an appropriate arrhythmic risk stratification

is mandatory. At the same time, in the post-DANISH trial world risk stratification represents a challenging issue for the physician. There are factors which have been extensively explored and proved to be strongly associated with SCD, such as a reduced LVEF and a higher NYHA functional class.[61] However, other factors may be considered and could represent future opportunities to provide a more accurate definition of the SCD risk in these patients. Among these promising new risk stratification approaches, it is important to mention the emerging role of cardiac magnetic resonance imaging and genetic analysis, as well as the identification of novel serum and electrophysiological markers.

Moreover, it should be kept in mind that patients with HF present with a wide range of comorbidities and, consequently, there are competing risks contributing to overall mortality, both cardiovascular (e.g. non-tachyarrhythmic events such as bradyarrhythmias; non-shockable rhythms; and vascular accidents) and non-cardiovascular (e.g. cancer, metabolic diseases, etc.), which ought to be considered in the occurrence of SCD, making risk stratification in these patients even more difficult.[62]

LVEF and NYHA class

An LVEF ≤ 35% in patients with a NYHA II or III functional class is a well-established predictor of SCD, and it still represents, according to the current ESC guidelines, the main indication for ICD use in primary prevention of SCD.[61] However, some studies showed that the rate of appropriate ICD shocks in these patients may be overestimated,[63,64] proving that risk stratification needs to be refined. It should be considered that solid data in support of the use of LVEF ≤ 35% derive from studies like MADIT I, MADIT II, and SCD-HeFT that were published between 1996 and 2005,[65–67] and that the pharmacological treatment has changed remarkably since then. It would be reasonable to re-evaluate whether the currently used threshold for EF would still confirm the same predictive value in the patients of today. Unfortunately, the Class I recommendations for the use of the ICD[68] have become an obstacle to the organization of a novel trial because randomizing patients to an ICD arm or to a no-ICD arm would deprive those the subjects randomized to the no-ICD treatment of a Class I recommended therapy (the ICD), thus constituting a legal and ethical obstacle.

Serum biomarkers

The identification of serum biomarkers that are indicators of patients at higher risk for SCD could provide other helpful and non-invasive methods to improve risk stratification in HF.

Serum B-type natriuretic peptide (BNP) or its precursor N-terminal prohormone of brain natriuretic peptide (NT-pro-BNP) could be useful prognostic tools, since higher values of these peptides have been demonstrated to be associated with an elevated risk of VAs and SCD, both in HF with reduced[69] and preserved LVEF.[70]

Similarly, to BNP and NT-pro-BNP, also higher levels of cardiac troponin T have been linked to a higher risk of VAs and SCD in patients with left ventricular dysfunction of both ischaemic and non-ischaemic aetiology.[71]

Recently, circulating microRNAs (miRNAs), which are involved in the biochemical pathways underlying pathological processes such as fibrosis, apoptosis, and inflammation, have been associated for the first time with a higher risk of SCD in patients with HF.[72]

Imaging markers

Imaging techniques such as transthoracic echocardiography and contrast-enhanced cardiac magnetic resonance imaging could be useful for early recognition of patients at higher risk of SCD.

Enlargement of both LV and left atrium in patients with DCM has been associated with a higher risk of SCD and/or major VAs.[73] Speckle-tracking echocardiography could be another useful tool for these patients, since arrhythmic events have been shown to be associated with lower values of LV global longitudinal strain and a higher mechanical dispersion of the LV.[74]

Cardiac magnetic resonance imaging allows both the assessment of the function and the morphology of the myocardium. Tissue characterization allows the assessment of replacement fibrosis using late gadolinium enhancement. A recent prospective multi-centre study on 1,508 patients with non-ischaemic DCM identified midwall late gadolinium enhancement in more than three wall segments as an independent predictor of both overall mortality (HR: 2.077, 95% CI: 1.211–3.562, P = 0.008) and major adverse arrhythmic events (HR: 1.693, 95% CI: 1.084–2.644; P = 0.021).[75]

All these parameters could be of great interest since they may help identify patients with a normal LVEF but who are still at high risk of experiencing potentially fatal VA.

Electrophysiological markers

Several ECG parameters, including QRS duration, fragmented ECG complexes, signal-averaged ECG, microvolt T wave alternans and heart rate variability, have been proposed as prognostic indicators of VAs and SCD in HF, both in ischaemic and non-ischaemic aetiologies.[76–82] However, the positive predictive accuracy of these parameters is still insufficient to allow them to be used as a risk-stratification tool.[76]

Studies mainly conducted on patients with ischaemic HF, which evaluated the role of invasive electrophysiological testing to stratify the risk of SCD, have yielded conflicting results.[76,83–85] Importantly, in the MADIT II study, the inducibility of VAs during the electrophysiological study was associated with an increased risk of VT but not of VF.[85] It should be highlighted that the discrepancies observed between the studies can be related to the differences in patient selection and stimulation protocols. A well-known concept is that the more aggressive the stimulation protocol, the less specific is the result in the case of inducibility. Lastly, in patients with non-ischaemic HF, inducible VTs during programmed ventricular stimulation identified a subgroup of patients at higher risk for an SCD surrogate, defined either as appropriate ICD shock or as documented SCD.[86]

Genetics

Patients with HF of non-ischaemic aetiology are frequently affected by primitive forms of cardiomyopathy,[11] such as DCM and arrhythmogenic cardiomyopathy (ACM), two forms of cardiomyopathy frequently overlapping with each other and typically caused by genetic mutations in genes encoding for structural proteins of the cardiomyocyte.[87]

The genetic background in these cases is of great help, and it has been extensively demonstrated how certain specific genetic mutations expose patients with familial forms of cardiomyopathy to a much higher risk of developing fatal VA. For instance, mutations in Lamin A/C (*LMNA*)[88,89] and filamin C (*FLNC*)[90] genes, especially if non-missense, are associated with a particularly high risk of major VAs. Other than the aforementioned, desmosomal gene mutations are also causative of particularly arrhythmogenic phenotypes, independently from the residual LVEF.[13] Among desmosomal gene mutations, truncating mutations in the desmoplakin (*DSP*) gene lead to a particularly arrhythmogenic phenotype, compared to plakophilin-2 (*PKP2*), the most commonly found gene in ACM.[91,92] Lastly, other noteworthy gene mutations associated with highly arrhythmogenic forms of DCM/ACM are found in genes such as phospholamban (*PLN*, particularly the founder mutation p.Arg14del)[93] or RNA-binding motif protein 20 (*RBM20*).[94]

Recognition of specific genetic profiles linked to a higher arrhythmic burden is critical and could represent a further step towards precision medicine in the field of HF. In clinical practice, this would translate into consideration of primary prevention of SCD for patients who do not still show an overt LV dysfunction but who are nonetheless at risk of fatal VAs based on the sole presence of specific genetic mutations.

Myocardial sympathetic innervation

Another risk factor which has been associated with a major risk of life-threatening VAs in patients with ischaemic HF is an incremented inhomogeneity in myocardial sympathetic innervation, estimated by the extent of sympathetic denervation in the heart with PET imaging. Interestingly, the amount of denervated myocardium is associated with a higher risk of VAs independently from other parameters, such as LVEF or the extent of the infarcted area.[95]

Therapeutic approach

The therapeutic approach to prevent ventricular arrhythmias and SCD in patients with HF is complicated by the multifactorial mechanisms that may generate rhythm disturbances. As described in the previous section, the aetiology of the ventricular dysfunction as well as the patient-specific clinical characteristics, including comorbidities, concomitant therapies, and life expectancy may determine the prevailing arrhythmogenic mechanisms and therefore the most successful treatment. This section will illustrate the different therapeutic strategies available to date, including both pharmacological therapies, ablation procedures, and the implantable defibrillator.

Pharmacological treatment

Optimal pharmacological therapy for HF: BBs, ACE-I, and MRAs

Current guidelines recommend the use of optimal pharmacological therapy with BBs, ACE-I (or, when intolerant, angiotensin receptor blockers (ARBs)), and mineralocorticoid receptor antagonists (MRAs) titrated to the maximum tolerated dose, in all patients with HF and systolic dysfunction to reduce SCD and total mortality (Class I, level A indication).[68,96]

BBs constitute the cornerstone of pharmacological treatment for patients with HF and reduced ejection fraction. Several trials demonstrated their efficacy in reducing the risk of SCD, estimating the risk reduction at 40%, and overall mortality, estimating it at approximately 35%, in cohorts recruiting both ischaemic and non-ischaemic HF patients.[10,54,97–101]

At variance with BBs, beneficial effects of ACE-I on mortality seem to be related more to a slowing of HF progression than a specific reduction of SCD.[102,103] However, ACE-I occasionally causes worsening of renal function, hyperkalaemia, symptomatic hypotension, cough, and, rarely, angioedema. Therefore, ACE-i should only be used in patients with adequate renal function (estimated GFR (eGFR) ≥30 mL/min/1.73 m^2) and a normal serum potassium.[104]

It has been demonstrated that addition of MRAs reduce mortality and rates of SCD in patients with HF treated with ACE-Is and BBs.[68] Pitt and colleagues demonstrated in 1999 that spironolactone reduced the risk of SCD by 29% in an RCT involving patients with both ischaemic and non-ischaemic HF.[5] The same group, in 2003, demonstrated that also eplerenone, a selective aldosterone blocker, titrated to a maximum of 50 mg per day reduced the rate of SCD by 21% in patients with LV dysfunction after MI. MRAs can cause hyperkalaemia and worsening renal function, which were uncommon in the RCTs, but may occur more frequently in common clinical practice, especially in elderly and comorbid patients. Both should be used in patients with adequate renal function and a normal serum potassium.[104]

Angiotensin receptor neprilysin inhibitor (sacubitril/valsartan)

McMurray and colleagues[8] demonstrated the superiority of sacubitril/valsartan over enalapril in reducing the overall mortality in HF patients with elevated plasma BNP levels (BNP ≥ 150 pg/mL or NT-proBNP ≥ 600 pg/mL or, if they had been hospitalized for HF within the previous 12 months, BNP ≥ 100 pg/mL or NT-proBNP ≥ 400 pg/mL), and eGFR ≥ 30 mL/min/1.73 m^2 of body surface area, who were able to tolerate separate treatments periods with enalapril (10 mg twice a day) and sacubitril/valsartan (97/103 mg twice a day) during a run-in period. In the PARADIGM-HF trial, Desai and colleagues[105] examined the effect of sacubitril/valsartan on the mode of death, demonstrating that the 20% reduction in cardiovascular death was attributable primarily to reductions in the incidence of both SCD (HR: 0.80, 95% CI: 0.68–0.94, P: 0.008) and death due to progressive HF.

Amiodarone

The use of amiodarone in patients with HF is controversial. It has been proven that amiodarone does not have a favourable effect on survival,[67,68,106] and additionally, its chronic use is profoundly limited by the presence of numerous end-organ toxicities leading to thyroid, lung, and liver disease. The randomized double-blind placebo-controlled European Myocardial Infarct Amiodarone Trial (EMIAT)[107] enrolled 1486 survivors of MI with LVEF ≤ 40%, demonstrating that amiodarone did not reduce the risk of all-cause mortality and cardiac mortality compared to placebo, while there was a 35% risk reduction in arrhythmic deaths. Similarly, a meta-analysis conducted on 15 RCTs revealed that the use of amiodarone in patients with HF was neutral with respect to all-cause mortality, but it reduced by 26% the incidence of SCD, independently of dosage, aetiology of HF, and concomitant use of BBs.[108] In the light of the aforementioned, there is no evidence for the systematic prophylactic use of amiodarone in all patients with depressed LV function, but amiodarone may be reasonably used in optimally treated HF patients with previous VTs who are not eligible for an ICD or in HF patients treated with an ICD and symptomatic VAs or recurrent shocks.[2]

With regards to amiodarone, its use in the context of Chagas disease merits a special mention. In fact, there is some evidence that amiodarone has a specific anti-*T. cruzi* activity, disrupting parasites' Ca^{2+} homeostasis and blocking ergosterol biosynthesis.[109] A recent meta-analysis showed that amiodarone is effective in reducing VA in patients with Chagas disease, but this analysis did not identify sufficient data regarding its effect on SCD reduction.[110]

Class I anti-arrhythmic drugs

In 1991, a seminal study designed to test the hypothesis that suppression of ventricular ectopies after a MI would result in reducing post-ischaemic SCD (CAST trial) showed that the use of class I anti-arrhythmic drugs (AADs) was paradoxically associated with an increased risk of arrhythmic death.[111] It is thought that the pro-arrhythmic properties of these drugs, which are blockers of the sodium channel, in the context of HF are related to their effect on slowing of conduction velocity, which might facilitate the onset of re-entry arrhythmias. As a consequence of this game-changing finding, class I AADs are contraindicated in patients with HF.[68,96] Two possible exceptions to this indication are represented by quinidine and mexiletine, which have been used alone or in conjunction with other class III AADs to achieve arrhythmia suppression in patients with HF, albeit this indication has never been formally evaluated in the context of RCTs.[1]

Diuretics and digoxin

Diuretics and digoxin are still used by many patients with HF, but they do not reduce rates of all-cause mortality or SCD,[68] and provide only symptomatic relief.

Device therapy

Implantable cardioverter defibrillator in secondary prevention of SCD

An ICD is recommended to reduce the risk of SCD and all-cause mortality in patients with HF who have recovered from a VA causing haemodynamic instability, and who are expected to survive for > 1 year with good functional status.[96] This recommendation is supported by the data that ICD implantation reduces by 28% the risk of death, due to a 50% reduction in SCD risk.[112]

Implantable cardioverter defibrillator in primary prevention of SCD

The current risk stratification scheme for the prediction of life-threatening VAs in patients with HF is based mainly on the degree of systolic dysfunction of the LV, with LVEF < 35% set as the high-risk threshold for SCD, based on the results of RCTs. Current guidelines recommend the use of an ICD in patients with symptomatic HF (NYHA class II–III) and LVEF ≤ 35% after ≥ 3 months of optimal medical therapy who are expected to survive for at least 1 year with good functional status, with a class I level A indication in patient with ischaemic aetiology and class I level B indication in patients with non-ischaemic aetiology.[68] While there are more data to support the use of ICDs in ischaemic HF, in patients with non-ischaemic aetiologies reduction in all-cause mortality and arrhythmic mortality is supported as well (➲ Table 12.6.1).

The recent DANISH trial[119] conducted on 1,116 patients with symptomatic non-ischaemic HF (LVEF≤35%) demonstrated that prophylactic ICD implantation was associated with a significant reduction of SCD, but it was not associated with a significant reduction in the long-term overall mortality. However, it is remarkable that the subgroup analyses in the DANISH trial revealed that age was the only factor showing a significant interaction with the treatment (ICD or not ICD). Indeed, the rate of death from any cause was significantly lower among patients younger than 68 years than among patients 68 years of age or older (HR: 0.64, 95% CI: 0.45–0.90, P = 0.01). Put together, these data highlight the pressing need to consider the competitive risks of death when managing patients with HF. Therefore, when evaluating the role of the ICD in reducing the overall mortality, it must be considered that the greater the competitive risk of dying suddenly, the greater the utility of ICD. In other words, it is not a mere question of establishing whether the ICD itself would be effective or not, but rather of identifying the patients in which the competitive risk of dying suddenly is greater than other causes of death, and who could hence benefit the most from the implant.

A recent meta-analysis (➲ Figure 12.6.4) collected all available RCTs comparing the role of ICD in primary prevention of SCD. Although ICD therapy was associated with a statistically significant reduction in SCD in all three groups studied (i.e. patients with acute MI, ischaemic HF, non-ischaemic HF), the effects on overall mortality were consistently different. Two RCTs[114,115] did not demonstrate a beneficial role of ICD implanted within 40 days after an MI in reducing the overall mortality and, accordingly, an ICD is contraindicated in this time period. In a meta-analysis of 11 trials, the authors demonstrated a significant and quantitatively reproducible reduction in death from any cause in patients with HF and reduced ejection fraction resulting from both ischaemic and non-ischaemic disease (HR 0.76), thus providing strong support for the role of ICD implant primary prevention of SCD also in patients with non-ischaemic aetiologies.[121]

However, when dealing with patients with non-ischaemic HF, the underlying cause of the disease needs to be considered in the therapeutic choice, particularly in the case of inherited cardiomyopathies. Both DCM and ACM can progress to HF, sometimes with overlapping phenotypes between the two. In particular, the growing use of genetic analysis in clinical practice in the last decade has brought increasingly strong evidence about the existence of subgroups of patients with inherited cardiomyopathies who are at higher risk of SCD. Although genotype–phenotype correlations in the literature are still scarce, the emerging issue is that the use of LVEF ≤ 35% as the only risk marker for patients with cardiomyopathy-related HF is not sufficient to assist the physicians in selecting the patients most likely to benefit from an ICD implantation in primary prevention of SCD. Consequently, current guidelines suggest the use of LVEF < 45% as the threshold for ICD implantation in patients with mutations in *LMNA*, *FNLC*, and *PLN*.[68,122] Moreover, as a general concept, patients with inherited cardiomyopathies should be referred to highly specialized tertiary centers and undergo there an evaluation specifically tailored on their phenotype and risk factors.

Cardiac resynchronization therapy

Two RCTs (COMPANION, CARE-HF)[120,123] randomized patients with moderate to severe symptomatic HF (NYHA class III or IV) and QRS duration ≥ 120 ms to either optimal medical therapy or optimal medical therapy plus cardiac resynchronization therapy (CRT). The COMPANION trial[120] demonstrated that CRT-pacemaker (CRT-P) and CRT-defibrillator (CRT-D) reduced the all-cause mortality by 24% and 36%, respectively, but only CRT-D reduced the rate of SCD. The CARE-HF trial[123] demonstrated that CRT-P reduced both the overall mortality by 40% and the risk of SCD by 46%. Other two RCTs[124,125] enrolled patients with mild or moderate symptoms and showed that CRT-D was superior to ICD alone in reducing the overall mortality. Importantly, different meta-analyses[126,127] conducted on these RCTs revealed that CRT was beneficial only in patients with left bundle branch block, and not in patients with other types of conduction defects. Accordingly, current guidelines recommend CRT for patients with HF and LVEF ≤ 35% who have a life expectancy with good functional status of > 1 year if they are in sinus rhythm and have a markedly prolonged QRS duration (≥ 130 ms) and an ECG that shows left bundle branch block, irrespective of symptom severity.

Catheter ablation

Although ICDs effectively terminate life-threatening VAs, they do not prevent arrhythmia recurrence. For the purpose of prevention of arrhythmic recurrence, catheter ablation is used in patients with recurrent ICD shocks due to sustained VT.[68] Nonetheless, the available evidence does not support a benefit of VT catheter ablation to reduce mortality, as confirmed also by a recent meta-analysis.[128] Therefore, it is important to highlight that catheter ablation cannot be considered as an alternative to ICD implantation.

As previously highlighted, in patients with ischaemic HF, scar-mediated macro-re-entry is the common pathophysiological mechanism and catheter ablation targets the isthmus of slow conduction (critical isthmus) within VT re-entry circuit. Several studies have evaluated the role of catheter ablation in the treatment of VTs, in different populations: (1) patients with recurrent ICD shocks, (2) patients with a first episode of VT, and (3) patients with electrical storms.

Table 12.6.1 Randomized clinical trials conducted in primary prevention of SCD in patients with HF, divided by ischaemic or non-ischaemic aetiology.

Heart failure with ischaemic heart disease

Colonna1	Author, Year	Randomized (N)	Study groups	Follow-up (months)	Inclusion criteria	Exclusion criteria	Primary Endpoint	HR (95% CI)	Reference
CABG-Patch	Bigger, 1997	900	ICD vs SMT	32	Undergoing CABG, abnormal ECG	Sustained VT or VF	Overall mortality	1.07 (0.81–1.42)	113
MADIT-I	Moss, 1996	196	ICD vs SMT	27	NYHA 1-3, MI, NSVT	CA, syncopal VT	Overall mortality	0.46 (0.26–0.82)	65
MADIT-II	Moss, 2002	1232	ICD vs SMT	20	NYHA 1-3, MI	MI within 1 month	Overall mortality	0.69 (0.51–0.93)	66
DINAMIT	Hohnloser, 2004	674	ICD vs SMT	30	Recent MI	NYHA 4	Overall mortality	1.08 (0.76–1.55)	114
IRIS	Steinbeck, 2009	898	ICD vs SMT	37	Recent MI	NYHA 4, VA before or ≥ 48 h after	Overall mortality	1.04 (0.81–1.35)	115

Heart failure without ischaemic heart disease

Colonna1	Author, year	Randomized (N)	Study groups	Follow-up (months)	Inclusion criteria	Exclusion criteria	Primary endpoint	HR (95% CI)	Reference
CAT	Bänsch, 2002	104	ICD vs SMT	66	NYHA 2-3, recent DCM diagnosis	Valvular, HCM or restrictive, prior MI	Overall mortality	0.80 (0.39–0.64)	116
AMIOVIRT	Strickberger, 2003	103	ICD vs SMT	24	NYHA 1-3, asymptomatic	Syncope	Overall mortality	0.87 (0.32–2.42)	117
DEFINITE	Kadish, 2004	458	ICD vs SMT	29	Symptomatic DCM, ambient arrhythmias	NYHA 4, familial cardiomyopathy	Overall mortality	0.65 (0.40–1.06)	118
DANISH	Køber, 2016	1116	ICD vs SMT	67.6	NYHA 2-4, raised NT-proBNP	-	Overall mortality	0.87 (0.68–1.12)	119

Heart failure with both ischaemic and non-ischaemic heart disease

Colonna1	Author, year	Randomized (N)	Study groups	Follow-up (months)	Inclusion criteria	Exclusion criteria	Primary endpoint	HR (95% CI)	Reference
COMPANION	Bristow, 2004	1520	CRT-D vs SMT	15.8	NYHA 3-4, recent HF hospitalization	-	Death from or hospitalization for HF	0.80 (0.68–0.85)	120
SCD-HeFT	Bardy, 2005	1676	ICD vs SMT	45.5	NYHA 2-3, OMT	-	Overall mortality	0.77 (0.62–0.96)	67

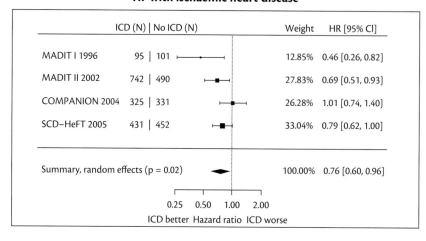

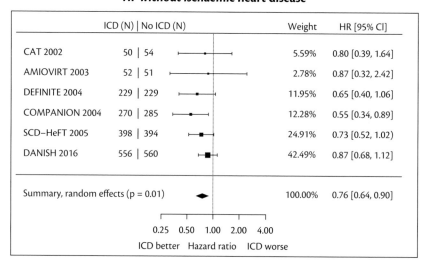

Figure 12.6.4 Implantable cardioverter defibrillators for primary prevention of death in left ventricular dysfunction with and without ischaemic heart disease: a meta-analysis of 8567 patients in 11 trials.

Reproduced from Shun-Shin MJ, Zheng SL, Cole GD, Howard JP, Whinnett ZI, Francis DP. Implantable cardioverter defibrillators for primary prevention of death in left ventricular dysfunction with and without ischaemic heart disease: a meta-analysis of 8567 patients in the 11 trials. *Eur Heart J.* 2017 Jun 7;38(22):1738-1746. doi: 10.1093/eurheartj/ehx028 with permission from Oxford University Press.

The most extensively studied population is that of patients with ischaemic HF who experienced multiple ICD interventions. In the Cooled RF trial (2000) the elimination of all inducible VTs was achieved in 41% of patients and the rate of recurrence during 243 ± 153 days of follow-up was 46%.[129] The Multicenter Thermocool Ventricular Tachycardia Ablation Trial (2008) showed that catheter ablation abolished all inducible VTs in 49% of patients and freedom from recurrent VT at 6-month follow-up was achieved for 53% of patients.[130] The EURO-VT multicentre study (2009) assessed the efficacy and safety of electro-anatomical mapping in combination with irrigated ablation technology for ablation of recurrent VT after MI.[131] Ablation was acutely successful in 81% of patients, and 49% of patients experienced VT recurrence after a mean follow-up of 12 ± 3 months. The Post-Approval THERMOCOOL VT Trial (2016)[132] showed that 62% of patients were free from sustained VT recurrences at 6-month follow-up, with 41.3% of patients reported being free of any VT at the 3-year mark. The recent multicentre, randomized VANISH trial[133] enrolled 259 patients with ischaemic cardiomyopathy and an ICD who continued to experience VT despite the use of AADs to compare the strategies of escalating anti-arrhythmic therapy versus catheter ablation. Notably, there was a significant reduction of the composite primary outcome (i.e., death, VT storm, or appropriate ICD shock) among patients undergoing catheter ablation than among those receiving an escalation in AAD therapy (HR: 0.72, 95% CI: 0.53–0.98, P = 0.04). Consequently, according to the recent HRS/EHRA/APHRS/LAHRS expert consensus statement,[134] in patients with ischaemic HF who experience recurrent monomorphic VT despite chronic amiodarone therapy, catheter ablation is recommended in preference to escalating AAD therapy. Catheter ablation is also recommended in patients with recurrent symptomatic monomorphic VT despite AAD therapy, or when AAD therapy is contraindicated or not tolerated.[134]

Other studies focused on the role of catheter ablation in patients who experienced their first episode of VT. In 2007, Reddy et al.[135] conducted a RCT in which ablation was performed with the use of a substrate-based approach in which the myocardial scar is mapped and ablated while the heart remains predominantly in sinus rhythm (i.e. without the need for VT induction). Interestingly, the authors observed a significant reduction of ICD therapy from 33% in the control group to 12% in the ablation group. The VTACH trial (2010)[136] evaluated the role of prophylactic VT ablation before ICD implantation in patients with previous MI, reduced ejection fraction, and haemodynamically stable VT. Although catheter ablation did not affect mortality, the rate of survival free from recurrent VT over 2 years was higher in the ablation group (47%) compared with the control arm (29%). The CALYPSO pilot study found an increased time to first VT recurrence with ablation versus AADs,[137] but on the other hand, the Substrate Modification Study (SMS) failed to meet its primary endpoint of time to first VT/VF recurrence.[138] However, in the SMS study catheter ablation reduced the total number of ICD interventions.[138] Therefore, in patients with ischaemic heart disease and an ICD who experience a first episode of monomorphic VT, catheter ablation may be considered (Class IIb indication) to reduce the risk of recurrent VT or ICD therapies.[134]

Several studies evaluated the application of catheter ablation in patients with ICDs and with electrical storm, demonstrating that catheter ablation can terminate potentially life-threatening electrical storms with high acute success rate, but with a significant mortality.[139-141] Therefore, in patients with ischaemic heart disease and VT storm refractory to AAD therapy, catheter ablation is currently recommended.[134]

While the role of catheter ablation has been well elucidated in patients with myocardial infarction and scar, the different structural substrate between patients with ischaemic or non-ischaemic HF profoundly influences the outcome of the ablation procedure. In fact, areas of scar in non-ischaemic cardiomyopathy (e.g. DCM, ACM) tend to be smaller and more often located in the mid-myocardium or epicardial layers[142] as compared to patients with ischaemic HF, and therefore, patients with VT related to post-myocardial scar tend to have a better outcome following catheter ablation than patients with VT due to non-ischaemic cardiomyopathy.[15,142] Another intrinsic limit of ablative procedures in patients with non-ischaemic cardiomyopathy is the progressive nature of the disease, which renders them non-resolutive in the long run. Nonetheless, several studies have shown good results of ablation in patients with non-ischaemic aetiology, with VT-free survival ranging from 40% to 70% at 1 year post catheter ablation.[143-147] Given the presence of epicardial substrate and VT circuits that cannot be successfully ablated from the endocardium, in patients with non-ischaemic cardiomyopathy epicardial mapping and catheter ablation can significantly reduce VT recurrence.[148] However, due to an increased risk of complications or late adhesions preventing future pericardial access, current guidelines state that epicardial ablation may be reserved to first-line endocardial approach failures, except when ECG or imaging suggests a predominant epicardial substrate.[134]

Conclusions

The clinical relevance of VAs in HF is related to the fact that they are a frequent cause of SCD, which, in turn, accounts for almost half of the deaths of these patients.

When dealing with VAs and SCD in HF, the issue is complex and multifaceted, since HF is not a unitary clinical entity, but it rather represents the evolution of many heterogeneous cardiac conditions. Consequently, the arrhythmogenic mechanisms leading to VAs and SCD in HF are equally varied, involving several abnormalities at different levels: structural, metabolic, and cellular. In addition, associated comorbidities are a common feature of patients with HF and may have substantial influence on arrhythmias, their complications, treatment, prognosis, and mortality of patients with HF.

Therefore, the clinical management of these patients is arduous, and synergistic combinations are often required to reach the goal of a personalized therapy. Current pharmacological therapies are effective in reducing the risk of life-threatening VAs but do not abolish it and therefore SCD still remains a major cause of death in patients affected by HF.

A difficult challenge for the clinician is to identify subjects who are at the highest risk of dying suddenly and who may benefit most from ICD implantation. The only risk factor which has been consistently and independently associated with SCD is represented by the reduction of LVEF. It is clear, however, that a single parameter cannot be the only guide for prevention of SCD and more refined risk stratification strategies are urgently needed.

References

1. Santangeli P, Rame JE, Birati EY, Marchlinski FE. Management of ventricular arrhythmias in patients with advanced heart failure. *J Am Coll Cardiol.* 2017;69:1842–1860.
2. Lip GYH, Heinzel FR, Gaita F, *et al.* European Heart Rhythm Association/Heart Failure Association joint consensus document on arrhythmias in heart failure, endorsed by the Heart Rhythm Society and the Asia Pacific Heart Rhythm Society. *Eur J Heart Fail.* 2015;17:848–874.
3. Kannel WB, Plehn JF, Cupples LA. Cardiac failure and sudden death in the Framingham Study. *Am Heart J.* 1988;115:869–875.
4. Shen L, Jhund PS, Petrie MC, *et al.* Declining risk of sudden death in heart failure. *N Engl J Med.* 2017;377:41–51.
5. Pitt B, Zannad F, Remme WJ, Cody R, *et al.* The effect of spironolactone on morbidity and mortality in patients with severe heart failure. Randomized Aldactone Evaluation Study Investigators. *N Engl J Med.* 1999;341:709–717.
6. Eichhorn EJ, Domanski MJ, Krause-Steinrauf H, Bristow MR, Lavori PW. A trial of the beta-blocker bucindolol in patients with advanced chronic heart failure. *N Engl J Med.* 2001;344:1659–1667.
7. Zannad F, McMurray JJ V, Krum H, *et al.* Eplerenone in patients with systolic heart failure and mild symptoms. *N Engl J Med.* 2011;364:11–21.
8. McMurray JJ V, Packer M, Desai AS, *et al.* Angiotensin-neprilysin inhibition versus enalapril in heart failure. *N Engl J Med.* 2014;371:993–1004.
9. Cubbon RM, Gale CP, Kearney LC, *et al.* Changing characteristics and mode of death associated with chronic heart failure caused by left ventricular systolic dysfunction: a study across therapeutic eras. *Circ Heart Fail.* 2011;4:396–403.

10. Effect of metoprolol CR/XL in chronic heart failure: Metoprolol CR/XL Randomised Intervention Trial in Congestive Heart Failure (MERIT-HF). *Lancet*. 1999;353:2001–2007.

11. Ziaeian B, Fonarow GC. Epidemiology and aetiology of heart failure. *Nat Rev Cardiol*. 2016;13:368–378.

12. Roger VL. Epidemiology of heart failure. *Circ Res*. 2013;113:646–659.

13. Gigli M, Merlo M, Graw SL, et al. Genetic risk of arrhythmic phenotypes in patients with dilated cardiomyopathy. *J Am Coll Cardiol*. 2019;74:1480–1490.

14. Masarone D, Limongelli G, Rubino M, et al. Management of arrhythmias in heart failure. *J Cardiovasc Dev Dis*. 2017;4.(1):3

15. Nakahara S, Tung R, Ramirez RJ, et al. Characterization of the arrhythmogenic substrate in ischemic and nonischemic cardiomyopathy implications for catheter ablation of hemodynamically unstable ventricular tachycardia. *J Am Coll Cardiol*. 2010;55:2355–2365.

16. Eijgenraam TR, Silljé HHW, de Boer RA. Current understanding of fibrosis in genetic cardiomyopathies. *Trends Cardiovasc Med*. 2020;30:353–361.

17. Pogwizd SM, Hoyt RH, Saffitz JE, Corr PB, Cox JL, Cain ME. Reentrant and focal mechanisms underlying ventricular tachycardia in the human heart. *Circulation*. 1992;86:1872–1887.

18. Stevenson WG, Khan H, Sager P, et al. Identification of reentry circuit sites during catheter mapping and radiofrequency ablation of ventricular tachycardia late after myocardial infarction. *Circulation*. 1993;88:1647–1670.

19. Coronel R, Wilders R, Verkerk AO, Wiegerinck RF, Benoist D, Bernus O. Electrophysiological changes in heart failure and their implications for arrhythmogenesis. *Biochim Biophys Acta*. 2013;1832:2432–2441.

20. Balaban G, Costa CM, Porter B, et al. 3D electrophysiological modeling of interstitial fibrosis networks and their role in ventricular arrhythmias in non-ischemic cardiomyopathy. *IEEE Trans Biomed Eng*. 2020;67:3125–3133.

21. Konstam MA, Kramer DG, Patel AR, Maron MS, Udelson JE. Left ventricular remodeling in heart failure: current concepts in clinical significance and assessment. *JACC Cardiovasc Imaging*. 2011;4:98–108.

22. Verma A, Meris A, Skali H, et al. Prognostic implications of left ventricular mass and geometry following myocardial infarction: the VALIANT (VALsartan In Acute myocardial iNfarcTion) Echocardiographic Study. *JACC Cardiovasc Imaging*. 2008;1:582–591.

23. Aronow WS, Epstein S, Schwartz KS, Koenigsberg M. Correlation of complex ventricular arrhythmias detected by ambulatory electrocardiographic monitoring with echocardiographic left ventricular hypertrophy in persons older than 62 years in a long-term health care facility. *Am J Cardiol*. 1987;60:730–732.

24. Zabel M, Koller BS, Sachs F, Franz MR. Stretch-induced voltage changes in the isolated beating heart: importance of the timing of stretch and implications for stretch-activated ion channels. *Cardiovasc Res*. 1996;32:120–130.

25. Franz MR. Mechano-electrical feedback. Cardiovasc. Res. 2000;45:263–266.

26. Aiba T, Tomaselli G. Electrical remodeling in dyssynchrony and resynchronization. *J Cardiovasc Transl Res*. 2012;5:170–179.

27. Beuckelmann DJ, Näbauer M, Erdmann E. Alterations of K+ currents in isolated human ventricular myocytes from patients with terminal heart failure. *Circ Res*. 1993;73:379–385.

28. Vermeulen JT, McGuire MA, Opthof T, et al.Triggered activity and automaticity in ventricular trabeculae of failing human and rabbit hearts. *Cardiovasc Res*. 1994;28:1547–1554.

29. Tsuji Y, Opthof T, Kamiya K, et al. Pacing-induced heart failure causes a reduction of delayed rectifier potassium currents along with decreases in calcium and transient outward currents in rabbit ventricle. *Cardiovasc Res*. 2000;48:300–309.

30. Li G-R, Lau C-P, Ducharme A, Tardif J-C, Nattel S. Transmural action potential and ionic current remodeling in ventricles of failing canine hearts. *Am J Physiol Heart Circ Physiol*. 2002;283:H1031–41.

31. Tsuji Y, Zicha S, Qi X-Y, Kodama I, Nattel S. Potassium channel subunit remodeling in rabbits exposed to long-term bradycardia or tachycardia: discrete arrhythmogenic consequences related to differential delayed-rectifier changes. *Circulation*. 2006;113:345–355.

32. Pogwizd SM, Schlotthauer K, Li L, Yuan W, Bers DM. Arrhythmogenesis and contractile dysfunction in heart failure: Roles of sodium-calcium exchange, inward rectifier potassium current, and residual beta-adrenergic responsiveness. *Circ Res*. 2001;88:1159–1167.

33. Valdivia CR, Chu WW, Pu J, et al. Increased late sodium current in myocytes from a canine heart failure model and from failing human heart. *J Mol Cell Cardiol*. 2005;38:475–483.

34. Hegyi B, Bossuyt J, Griffiths LG, et al. Complex electrophysiological remodeling in postinfarction ischemic heart failure. *Proc Natl Acad Sci U S A*. 2018;115:E3036–E3044.

35. Nattel S, Maguy A, Le Bouter S, Yeh Y-H. Arrhythmogenic ionchannel remodeling in the heart: heart failure, myocardial infarction, and atrial fibrillation. *Physiol Rev*. 2007;87:425–456.

36. Weiss JN, Garfinkel A, Karagueuzian HS, Chen P-S, Qu Z. Early afterdepolarizations and cardiac arrhythmias. *Heart Rhythm*. 2010;7:1891–1899.

37. Michael G, Xiao L, Qi X-Y, Dobrev D, Nattel S. Remodelling of cardiac repolarization: how homeostatic responses can lead to arrhythmogenesis. *Cardiovasc Res*. 2009;81:491–499.

38. Baartscheer A, Schumacher CA, Belterman CNW, Coronel R, Fiolet JWT. SR calcium handling and calcium after-transients in a rabbit model of heart failure. *Cardiovasc Res*. 2003;58:99–108.

39. Zarain-Herzberg A, Afzal N, Elimban V, Dhalla NS. Decreased expression of cardiac sarcoplasmic reticulum Ca(2+)-pump ATPase in congestive heart failure due to myocardial infarction. *Mol Cell Biochem*. 1996;163–164:285–290.

40. Arai M, Alpert NR, MacLennan DH, Barton P, Periasamy M. Alterations in sarcoplasmic reticulum gene expression in human heart failure. A possible mechanism for alterations in systolic and diastolic properties of the failing myocardium. *Circ Res*. 1993;72:463–469.

41. Yoshiyama M, Takeuchi K, Hanatani A, et al. Differences in expression of sarcoplasmic reticulum Ca2+-ATPase and Na+-Ca2+ exchanger genes between adjacent and remote noninfarcted myocardium after myocardial infarction. *J Mol Cell Cardiol*. 1997;29:255–264.

42. Winslow RL, Rice J, Jafri S, Marbán E, O'Rourke B. Mechanisms of altered excitation-contraction coupling in canine tachycardiainduced heart failure, II: model studies. *Circ Res*. 1999;84:571–586.

43. Wang Z, Nolan B, Kutschke W, Hill JA. Na+-Ca2+ exchanger remodeling in pressure overload cardiac hypertrophy. *J Biol Chem*. 2001;276:17706–17711.

44. Schillinger W, Schneider H, Minami K, Ferrari R, Hasenfuss G. Importance of sympathetic activation for the expression of Na+-Ca2+ exchanger in end-stage failing human myocardium. *Eur Heart J*. 2002;23:1118–1124.

45. Severs NJ, Bruce AF, Dupont E, Rothery S. Remodelling of gap junctions and connexin expression in diseased myocardium. *Cardiovasc Res*. 2008;80:9–19.

46. Wiegerinck RF, van Veen TAB, Belterman CN, et al. Transmural dispersion of refractoriness and conduction velocity is associated with heterogeneously reduced connexin43 in a rabbit model of heart failure. *Hear Rhythm*. 2008;5:1178–1185.

47. Ai X, Pogwizd SM. Connexin 43 downregulation and dephosphorylation in nonischemic heart failure is associated with enhanced colocalized protein phosphatase type 2A. *Circ Res.* 2005;96:54–63.

48. Kostin S, Rieger M, Dammer S, et al. Gap junction remodeling and altered connexin43 expression in the failing human heart. *Mol Cell Biochem.* 2003;242:135–144.

49. Danik SB, Rosner G, Lader J, Gutstein DE, Fishman GI, Morley GE. Electrical remodeling contributes to complex tachyarrhythmias in connexin43-deficient mouse hearts. *FASEB J Off Publ Fed Am Soc Exp Biol.* 2008;22:1204–1212.

50. Jansen JA, Noorman M, Musa H, et al. Reduced heterogeneous expression of Cx43 results in decreased Nav1.5 expression and reduced sodium current that accounts for arrhythmia vulnerability in conditional Cx43 knockout mice. *Heart Rhythm.* 2012;9:600–607.

51. Desplantez T, McCain ML, Beauchamp P, et al. Connexin43 ablation in foetal atrial myocytes decreases electrical coupling, partner connexins, and sodium current. *Cardiovasc Res.* 2012;94:58–65.

52. Agullo-Pascual E, Lin X, Leo-Macias A, et al. Super-resolution imaging reveals that loss of the C-terminus of connexin43 limits microtubule plus-end capture and NaV1.5 localization at the intercalated disc. *Cardiovasc Res.* 2014;104:371–381.

53. Yamada C, Kuwahara K, Yamazaki M, et al. The renin-angiotensin system promotes arrhythmogenic substrates and lethal arrhythmias in mice with non-ischaemic cardiomyopathy. *Cardiovasc Res.* 2016;109:162–173.

54. The Cardiac Insufficiency Bisoprolol Study II (CIBIS-II): a randomised trial. *Lancet.* 1999;353:9–13.

55. Cao JM, Fishbein MC, Han JB, et al. Relationship between regional cardiac hyperinnervation and ventricular arrhythmia. *Circulation.* 2000;101:1960–1969.

56. Donoghue M, Wakimoto H, Maguire CT, et al. Heart block, ventricular tachycardia, and sudden death in ACE2 transgenic mice with downregulated connexins. *J Mol Cell Cardiol.* 2003;35:1043–1053.

57. Nolan J, Batin PD, Andrews R, Lindsay SJ, et al. Prospective study of heart rate variability and mortality in chronic heart failure: results of the United Kingdom heart failure evaluation and assessment of risk trial (UK-heart). *Circulation.* 1998;98:1510–1516.

58. Sarwar CMS, Papadimitriou L, Pitt B, et al. Hyperkalemia in Heart Failure. *J Am Coll Cardiol.* 2016;68:1575–1589.

59. Gottlieb SS, Baruch L, Kukin ML, Bernstein JL, Fisher ML, Packer M. Prognostic importance of the serum magnesium concentration in patients with congestive heart failure. *J Am Coll Cardiol.* 1990;16:827–831.

60. Alvarez CK, Cronin E, Baker WL, Kluger J. Heart failure as a substrate and trigger for ventricular tachycardia. *J Interv Card Electrophysiol..* 2019;56:229–247.

61. Priori SG, Blomström-Lundqvist C, Mazzanti A, et al. 2015 ESC Guidelines for the management of patients with ventricular arrhythmias and the prevention of sudden cardiac death: The Task Force for the Management of Patients with Ventricular Arrhythmias and the Prevention of Sudden Cardiac Death of the European Society of Cardiology (ESC) Endorsed by: Association for European Paediatric and Congenital Cardiology (AEPC). *Europace* 2015;17:1601–1687.

62. Packer M. Nonarrhythmic sudden cardiac death in chronic heart failure – a preventable event? *JAMA Cardiol.* 2019;4:721–722.

63. Chen C-Y, Stevenson LW, Stewart GC, et al. Real world effectiveness of primary implantable cardioverter defibrillators implanted during hospital admissions for exacerbation of heart failure or other acute co-morbidities: cohort study of older patients with heart failure. *BMJ.* 2015;351:h3529.

64. Sabbag A, Suleiman M, Laish-Farkash A, et al. Contemporary rates of appropriate shock therapy in patients who receive implantable device therapy in a real-world setting: From the Israeli ICD Registry. *Heart Rhythm.* 2015;12:2426–2433.

65. Moss AJ, Hall WJ, Cannom DS, et al. Improved survival with an implanted defibrillator in patients with coronary disease at high risk for ventricular arrhythmia. Multicenter Automatic Defibrillator Implantation Trial Investigators. *N Engl J Med.* 1996;335:1933–1940.

66. Moss AJ, Zareba W, Hall WJ, et al. Prophylactic implantation of a defibrillator in patients with myocardial infarction and reduced ejection fraction. *N Engl J Med.* 2002;346:877–883.

67. Bardy GH, Lee KL, Mark DB, et al. Amiodarone or an implantable cardioverter-defibrillator for congestive heart failure. *N Engl J Med.* 2005;352:225–237.

68. Priori SG, Blomström-Lundqvist C, Mazzanti A, et al. 2015 ESC Guidelines for the management of patients with ventricular arrhythmias and the prevention of sudden cardiac death – Web Addenda.. *Europace.* 2015;17:1601–1687.

69. Levine YC, Rosenberg MA, Mittleman M, et al. B-type natriuretic peptide is a major predictor of ventricular tachyarrhythmias. *Heart Rhythm.* 2014;11:1109–1116.

70. Adabag S, Langsetmo L. Sudden cardiac death risk prediction in heart failure with preserved ejection fraction. *Heart Rhythm.* 2020;17:358–364.

71. Nakamura H, Niwano S, Fukaya H, et al. Cardiac troponin T as a predictor of cardiac death in patients with left ventricular dysfunction. *J Arrhythm.* 2017;33:463–468.

72. Silverman MG, Yeri A, Moorthy MV, et al. Circulating miRNAs and risk of sudden death in patients with coronary heart disease. *JACC Clin Electrophysiol.* 2020;6:70–79.

73. Stolfo D, Ceschia N, Zecchin M, et al. Arrhythmic risk stratification in patients with idiopathic dilated cardiomyopathy. *Am J Cardiol.* 2018;121:1601–1609.

74. Haugaa KH, Goebel B, Dahlslett T, et al. Risk assessment of ventricular arrhythmias in patients with nonischemic dilated cardiomyopathy by strain echocardiography. *J Am Soc Echocardiogr Off Publ Am Soc Echocardiogr.* 2012;25:667–673.

75. Guaricci AI, Masci PG, Muscogiuri G, et al. CarDiac magnEtic Resonance for prophylactic Implantable-cardioVerter defibrillAtor ThErapy in Non-Ischaemic dilated CardioMyopathy: an international Registry.. 2021; *Europace* 2021;23:1072–1083.

76. Goldenberg I, Huang DT, Nielsen JC. The role of implantable cardioverter-defibrillators and sudden cardiac death prevention: indications, device selection, and outcome. *Eur Heart J.* 2020;41:2003–2011.

77. Hartikainen JE, Malik M, Staunton A, Poloniecki J, Camm AJ. Distinction between arrhythmic and nonarrhythmic death after acute myocardial infarction based on heart rate variability, signal-averaged electrocardiogram, ventricular arrhythmias and left ventricular ejection fraction. *J Am Coll Cardiol.* 1996;28:296–304.

78. Bailey JJ, Berson AS, Handelsman H, Hodges M. Utility of current risk stratification tests for predicting major arrhythmic events after myocardial infarction. *J Am Coll Cardiol.* 2001;38:1902–1911.

79. Huikuri H V, Raatikainen MJP, Moerch-Joergensen R, et al. Prediction of fatal or near-fatal cardiac arrhythmia events in patients with depressed left ventricular function after an acute myocardial infarction. *Eur Heart J.* 2009;30:689–698.

80. Hombach V, Merkle N, Torzewski J, et al. Electrocardiographic and cardiac magnetic resonance imaging parameters as predictors of a worse outcome in patients with idiopathic dilated cardiomyopathy. *Eur Heart J.* 2009;30:2011–2018.

81. Kitamura H, Ohnishi Y, Okajima K, et al. Onset heart rate of microvolt-level T-wave alternans provides clinical and prognostic value in nonischemic dilated cardiomyopathy. *J Am Coll Cardiol.* 2002;39:295–300.

82. Salerno-Uriarte JA, De Ferrari GM, Klersy C, et al. Prognostic value of T-wave alternans in patients with heart failure due to nonischemic cardiomyopathy: results of the ALPHA Study. J Am Coll Cardiol. 2007;50:1896–1904.

83. Bourke JP, Richards DA, Ross DL, McGuire MA, Uther JB. Does the induction of ventricular flutter or fibrillation at electrophysiologic testing after myocardial infarction have any prognostic significance? Am J Cardiol. 1995;75:431–435.

84. Roy D, Marchand E, Théroux P, Waters DD, Pelletier GB, Bourassa MG. Programmed ventricular stimulation in survivors of an acute myocardial infarction. Circulation. 1985;72:487–494.

85. Daubert JP, Zareba W, Hall WJ et al. Predictive value of ventricular arrhythmia inducibility for subsequent ventricular tachycardia or ventricular fibrillation in Multicenter Automatic Defibrillator Implantation Trial (MADIT) II patients. J Am Coll Cardiol. 2006;47:98–107.

86. Gatzoulis KA, Vouliotis A-I, Tsiachris D, et al. Primary prevention of sudden cardiac death in a nonischemic dilated cardiomyopathy population: reappraisal of the role of programmed ventricular stimulation. Circ Arrhythm Electrophysiol. 2013;6:504–512.

87. McNally EM, Mestroni L. Dilated cardiomyopathy: genetic determinants and mechanisms. Circ Res. 2017;121:731–748.

88. van Berlo JH, de Voogt WG, van der Kooi AJ, et al. Meta-analysis of clinical characteristics of 299 carriers of LMNA gene mutations: do lamin A/C mutations portend a high risk of sudden death? J Mol Med (Berl). 2005;83:79–83.

89. van Rijsingen IAW, Arbustini E, Elliott PM, et al. Risk factors for malignant ventricular arrhythmias in lamin a/c mutation carriers a European cohort study. J Am Coll Cardiol. 2012;59:493–500.

90. Ortiz-Genga MF, Cuenca S, Dal Ferro M, et al. Truncating FLNC mutations are associated with high-risk dilated and arrhythmogenic cardiomyopathies. J Am Coll Cardiol. 2016;68:2440–2451.

91. López-Ayala JM, Gómez-Milanés I, Sánchez Muñoz JJ, et al. Desmoplakin truncations and arrhythmogenic left ventricular cardiomyopathy: characterizing a phenotype. Europace. 2014;16:1838–1846. . 2014;16:1838–1846.

92. Smith ED, Lakdawala NK, Papoutsidakis N, et al. Desmoplakin cardiomyopathy, a fibrotic and inflammatory form of cardiomyopathy distinct from typical dilated or arrhythmogenic right ventricular cardiomyopathy. Circulation. 2020;141:1872–1884.

93. van der Zwaag PA, van Rijsingen IAW, Asimaki A, et al. Phospholamban R14del mutation in patients diagnosed with dilated cardiomyopathy or arrhythmogenic right ventricular cardiomyopathy: evidence supporting the concept of arrhythmogenic cardiomyopathy. Eur J Heart Fail. 2012;14:1199–1207.

94. van den Hoogenhof MMG, Beqqali A, Amin AS, et al. RBM20 mutations induce an arrhythmogenic dilated cardiomyopathy related to disturbed calcium handling. Circulation. 2018;138:1330–1342.

95. Fallavollita JA, Heavey BM, Luisi AJJ, et al. Regional myocardial sympathetic denervation predicts the risk of sudden cardiac arrest in ischemic cardiomyopathy. J Am Coll Cardiol. 2014;63:141–149.

96. Ponikowski P, Voors AA, Anker SD, et al. 2016 ESC Guidelines for the diagnosis and treatment of acute and chronic heart failure: The Task Force for the diagnosis and treatment of acute and chronic heart failure of the European Society of Cardiology (ESC) Developed with the special contribution of the Heart Failure Association (HFA) of the ESC. Eur Heart J. 2016;37:2129–2200.

97. Hjalmarson A, Goldstein S, Fagerberg B, et al. Effects of controlled-release metoprolol on total mortality, hospitalizations, and well-being in patients with heart failure: the Metoprolol CR/XL Randomized Intervention Trial in congestive heart failure (MERIT-HF). JAMA. 2000;283:1295–1302.

98. Packer M, Coats AJ, Fowler MB, et al.. Effect of carvedilol on survival in severe chronic heart failure. N Engl J Med. 2001;344:1651–1658.

99. Packer M, Bristow MR, Cohn JN, et al. The effect of carvedilol on morbidity and mortality in patients with chronic heart failure. U.S. Carvedilol Heart Failure Study Group. N Engl J Med. 1996;334:1349–1355.

100. Packer M, Fowler MB, Roecker EB, et al. Effect of carvedilol on the morbidity of patients with severe chronic heart failure: results of the carvedilol prospective randomized cumulative survival (COPERNICUS) study. Circulation. 2002;106:2194–2199.

101. Flather MD, Shibata MC, Coats AJS, et al.. Randomized trial to determine the effect of nebivolol on mortality and cardiovascular hospital admission in elderly patients with heart failure (SENIORS). Eur Heart J. 2005;26:215–225.

102. CONSENSUS Trial Study Group. Effects of enalapril on mortality in severe congestive heart failure. Results of the Cooperative North Scandinavian Enalapril Survival Study (CONSENSUS). N Engl J Med. 1987;316:1429–1435.

103. Garg R, Yusuf S. Overview of randomized trials of angiotensin-converting enzyme inhibitors on mortality and morbidity in patients with heart failure. JAMA. 1995;273:1450–1456.

104. McMurray JJ V, Adamopoulos S, Anker SD, et al. ESC Guidelines for the diagnosis and treatment of acute and chronic heart failure 2012: The Task Force for the Diagnosis and Treatment of Acute and Chronic Heart Failure 2012 of the European Society of Cardiology. Developed in collaboration with the Heart Failure Association (HFA) of the ESC. Eur Heart J. 2012;33:1787–1847.

105. Desai AS, McMurray JJ V, Packer M, et al. Effect of the angiotensin-receptor-neprilysin inhibitor LCZ696 compared with enalapril on mode of death in heart failure patients. Eur Heart J. 2015;36:1990–1997.

106. Singh SN, Fletcher RD, Fisher SG, et al. Amiodarone in patients with congestive heart failure and asymptomatic ventricular arrhythmia. Survival trial of antiarrhythmic therapy in congestive heart failure. N Engl J Med. 1995;333:77–82.

107. Julian DG, Camm AJ, Frangin G, et al. Randomised trial of effect of amiodarone on mortality in patients with left-ventricular dysfunction after recent myocardial infarction: EMIAT. European Myocardial Infarct Amiodarone Trial Investigators. Lancet. 1997;349:667–674.

108. Piccini JP, Berger JS, O'Connor CM. Amiodarone for the prevention of sudden cardiac death: a meta-analysis of randomized controlled trials. Eur Heart J. 2009;30:1245–1253.

109. Benaim G, Sanders JM, Garcia-Marchán Y, et al. Amiodarone has intrinsic anti-Trypanosoma cruzi activity and acts synergistically with posaconazole. J Med Chem. 2006;49:892–899.

110. Stein C, Migliavaca CB, Colpani V, et al.. Amiodarone for arrhythmia in patients with Chagas disease: A systematic review and individual patient data meta-analysis. PLoS Negl Trop Dis. 2018;12:e0006742.

111. Echt DS, Liebson PR, Mitchell LB, et al. Mortality and morbidity in patients receiving encainide, flecainide, or placebo. The Cardiac Arrhythmia Suppression Trial. N Engl J Med. 1991;324:781–788.

112. Connolly SJ, Hallstrom AP, Cappato R, et al. Meta-analysis of the implantable cardioverter defibrillator secondary prevention trials. AVID, CASH and CIDS studies. Antiarrhythmics vs Implantable Defibrillator study. Cardiac Arrest Study Hamburg . Canadian Implantable Defibrillator Study. Eur Heart J. 2000;21:2071–2078.

113. Bigger JTJ. Prophylactic use of implanted cardiac defibrillators in patients at high risk for ventricular arrhythmias after coronary-artery bypass graft surgery. Coronary Artery Bypass Graft (CABG) Patch Trial Investigators. N Engl J Med. 1997;337:1569–1575.

114. Hohnloser SH, Kuck KH, Dorian P, et al. Prophylactic use of an implantable cardioverter-defibrillator after acute myocardial infarction. N Engl J Med. 2004;351:2481–2488.

115. Steinbeck G, Andresen D, Seidl K, et al. Defibrillator implantation early after myocardial infarction. N Engl J Med. 2009;361:1427–1436.

116. Bänsch D, Antz M, Boczor S, et al. Primary prevention of sudden cardiac death in idiopathic dilated cardiomyopathy: the Cardiomyopathy Trial (CAT). *Circulation*. 2002;105:1453–1458.

117. Strickberger SA, Hummel JD, Bartlett TG, et al. Amiodarone versus implantable cardioverter-defibrillator:randomized trial in patients with nonischemic dilated cardiomyopathy and asymptomatic nonsustained ventricular tachycardia—AMIOVIRT. *J Am Coll Cardiol*. 2003;41:1707–1712.

118. Kadish A, Dyer A, Daubert JP, et al. Prophylactic defibrillator implantation in patients with nonischemic dilated cardiomyopathy. *N Engl J Med*. 2004;350:2151–2158.

119. Køber L, Thune JJ, Nielsen JC, et al. Defibrillator implantation in patients with nonischemic systolic heart failure. *N Engl J Med*. 2016;375:1221–1230.

120. Bristow MR, Saxon LA, Boehmer J, et al. Cardiac-resynchronization therapy with or without an implantable defibrillator in advanced chronic heart failure. *N Engl J Med*. 2004;350:2140–2150.

121. Shun-Shin MJ, Zheng SL, Cole GD, Howard JP, Whinnett ZI, Francis DP. Implantable cardioverter defibrillators for primary prevention of death in left ventricular dysfunction with and without ischaemic heart disease: a meta-analysis of 8567 patients in the 11 trials. *Eur Heart J*. 2017;38:1738–1746.

122. Towbin JA, McKenna WJ, Abrams DJ, et al. 2019 HRS expert consensus statement on evaluation, risk stratification, and management of arrhythmogenic cardiomyopathy. *Heart Rhythm*. 2019;16:e301–e372.

123. Cleland JGF, Daubert J-C, Erdmann E, et al. The effect of cardiac resynchronization on morbidity and mortality in heart failure. *N Engl J Med*. 2005;352:1539–1549.

124. Moss AJ, Hall WJ, Cannom DS, et al. Cardiac-resynchronization therapy for the prevention of heart-failure events. *N Engl J Med*. 2009;361:1329–1338.

125. Tang ASL, Wells GA, Talajic M, et al. Cardiac-resynchronization therapy for mild-to-moderate heart failure. *N Engl J Med*. 2010;363:2385–2395.

126. Sipahi I, Chou JC, Hyden M, Rowland DY, Simon DI, Fang JC. Effect of QRS morphology on clinical event reduction with cardiac resynchronization therapy: meta-analysis of randomized controlled trials. *Am Heart J*. 2012;163:260–7.e3.

127. Cunnington C, Kwok CS, Satchithananda DK, et al. Cardiac resynchronisation therapy is not associated with a reduction in mortality or heart failure hospitalisation in patients with non-left bundle branch block QRS morphology: meta-analysis of randomised controlled trials. *Heart*. 2015;101:1456–1462.

128. Martinez BK, Baker WL, Konopka A, et al. Systematic review and meta-analysis of catheter ablation of ventricular tachycardia in ischemic heart disease. *Heart Rhythm*. 2020;17:e206–e219.

129. Calkins H, Epstein A, Packer D, et al. Catheter ablation of ventricular tachycardia in patients with structural heart disease using cooled radiofrequency energy: results of a prospective multicenter study. *J Am Coll Cardiol*. 2000;35:1905–1914.

130. Stevenson WG, Wilber DJ, Natale A, et al. Irrigated radiofrequency catheter ablation guided by electroanatomic mapping for recurrent ventricular tachycardia after myocardial infarction: the multicenter thermocool ventricular tachycardia ablation trial. *Circulation*. 2008;118:2773–2782.

131. Tanner H, Hindricks G, Volkmer M, et al.. Catheter ablation of recurrent scar-related ventricular tachycardia using electroanatomical mapping and irrigated ablation technology: results of the prospective multicenter Euro-VT-study. *J Cardiovasc Electrophysiol*. 2010;21:47–53.

132. Marchlinski FE, Haffajee CI, Beshai JF, et al. Long-term success of irrigated radiofrequency catheter ablation of sustained ventricular tachycardia: Post-approval THERMOCOOL VT Trial. *J Am Coll Cardiol*. 2016;67:674–683.

133. Sapp JL, Wells GA, Parkash R, et al. Ventricular tachycardia ablation versus escalation of antiarrhythmic drugs. *N Engl J Med*. 2016;375:111–121.

134. Cronin EM, Bogun FM, Maury P, et al. 2019 HRS/EHRA/APHRS/LAHRS expert consensus statement on catheter ablation of ventricular arrhythmias.. *Europace*. 2019;21:1143–1144.

135. Reddy VY, Reynolds MR, Neuzil P, et al. Prophylactic catheter ablation for the prevention of defibrillator therapy. *N Engl J Med*. 2007;357:2657–2665.

136. Kuck K-H, Schaumann A, Eckardt L, et al. Catheter ablation of stable ventricular tachycardia before defibrillator implantation in patients with coronary heart disease (VTACH): a multicentre randomised controlled trial. *Lancet*. 2010;375:31–40.

137. Al-Khatib SM, Daubert JP, Anstrom KJ, et al. Catheter ablation for ventricular tachycardia in patients with an implantable cardioverter defibrillator (CALYPSO) pilot trial. *J Cardiovasc Electrophysiol*. 2015;26:151–157.

138. Kuck K-H, Tilz RR, Deneke T, et al. Impact of substrate modification by catheter ablation on implantable cardioverter-defibrillator interventions in patients with unstable ventricular arrhythmias and coronary artery disease: results from the multicenter randomized controlled SMS ((Substrate Modification Study). *Circ Arrhythm Electrophysiol*. 2017;10.e004422

139. Carbucicchio C, Santamaria M, Trevisi N, et al. Catheter ablation for the treatment of electrical storm in patients with implantable cardioverter-defibrillators: short- and long-term outcomes in a prospective single-center study. *Circulation*. 2008;117:462–469.

140. Deneke T, Shin D, Lawo T, et al. Catheter ablation of electrical storm in a collaborative hospital network. *Am J Cardiol*. 2011;108:233–239.

141. Muser D, Liang JJ, Pathak RK, et al. Long-term outcomes of catheter ablation of electrical storm in nonischemic dilated cardiomyopathy compared with ischemic cardiomyopathy. *JACC Clin Electrophysiol*. 2017;3:767–778.

142. Mathuria N, Tung R, Shivkumar K. Advances in ablation of ventricular tachycardia in nonischemic cardiomyopathy. *Curr Cardiol Rep*. 2012;14:577–583.

143. Proietti R, Essebag V, Beardsall J, et al. Substrate-guided ablation of haemodynamically tolerated and untolerated ventricular tachycardia in patients with structural heart disease: effect of cardiomyopathy type and acute success on long-term outcome.. *Europace*. 2015;17:461–467.

144. Muser D, Santangeli P, Castro SA, et al. Long-term outcome after catheter ablation of ventricular tachycardia in patients with nonischemic dilated cardiomyopathy. *Circ Arrhythm Electrophysiol*. 2016;9:e004328.

145. Dinov B, Fiedler L, Schönbauer R, et al. Outcomes in catheter ablation of ventricular tachycardia in dilated nonischemic cardiomyopathy compared with ischemic cardiomyopathy: results from the Prospective Heart Centre of Leipzig VT (HELP-VT) Study. *Circulation*. 2014;129:728–736.

146. Tokuda M, Tedrow UB, Kojodjojo P, et al. Catheter ablation of ventricular tachycardia in nonischemic heart disease. *Circ Arrhythm Electrophysiol*. 2012;5:992–1000.

147. Tung R, Vaseghi M, Frankel DS, et al. Freedom from recurrent ventricular tachycardia after catheter ablation is associated with improved survival in patients with structural heart disease: An International VT Ablation Center Collaborative Group study. *Heart Rhythm*. 2015;12:1997–2007.

148. Cano O, Hutchinson M, Lin D, et al. Electroanatomic substrate and ablation outcome for suspected epicardial ventricular tachycardia in left ventricular nonischemic cardiomyopathy. *J Am Coll Cardiol*. 2009;54:799–808.

CHAPTER 12.7

Management of atrial fibrillation in heart failure

Andreas Metzner, Laura Rottner,
Ruben Schleberger, Fabian Moser, and
Paulus Kirchhof

Contents

Introduction

Heart failure and atrial fibrillation are two of the epidemics in cardiovascular medicine and their incidences are expected to further rise in the future.[1] Their prevalence in the USA is projected to increase to >770,000 newly diagnosed patients with heart failure in 2040,[2] and from 3.3 million in 2020 to >5.1 millions of patients with atrial fibrillation in 2040.[3,4] Approximately one in three patients with heart failure has atrial fibrillation, and vice versa.[5–7] One explanation is that both entities share identical risk factors. Arterial hypertension, diabetes mellitus, obesity, smoking, sleep apnoea, kidney disease, coronary artery disease, and valvular heart disease are conditions that may cause or contribute to both heart failure and atrial fibrillation.[8] In addition, all inherited cardiomyopathies have a high incidence of concomitant atrial fibrillation, thus reflecting shared genetic causes and shared genomic traits.[9]

Heart failure and atrial fibrillation also sustain and aggravate each other. Heart failure may lead to left atrial enlargement, increasing left atrial pressure and functional mitral regurgitation, thus increasing the risk for atrial fibrillation. Atrial fibrillation reduces cardiac output and can even lead to tachycardia-mediated cardiomyopathy.[10] Some degree of tachycardiomyopathy can be detected in 20–30% of patients suffering from atrial fibrillation.[10] Patients with prevalent atrial fibrillation have a significantly higher risk for additional development for both, heart failure with preserved or reduced ejection fraction.[11] Patients with heart failure also have a significantly higher risk of developing atrial fibrillation compared to patients without heart failure. It is more likely that atrial fibrillation antedates rather than follows heart failure. It was also shown that new onset atrial fibrillation in patients with heart failure and reduced or preserved ejection fraction significantly increases mortality when compared to patients with new onset of atrial fibrillation and without heart failure.[11] These numbers and interrelations also demonstrate the highly relevant socioeconomic impact as well as present and future challenges for medical systems.

Regarding treatment of atrial fibrillation in the setting of heart failure important trials were performed and published over recent years and improved our understanding of interactions of both conditions and, at the same time, challenged previous treatment recommendations. Studies such as the Ablation Versus Amiodarone for Treatment of Persistent Atrial Fibrillation in Patients With Congestive Heart Failure and an Implanted Device: Results From the AATAC Multicenter Randomized Trial[12] or the Catheter Ablation of Atrial Fibrillation with Heart Failure[13] trial randomized patients with atrial fibrillation and concomitant heart failure with reduced ejection fraction into antiarrhythmic drug-based and interventional ablation arms. While the first study defined recurrence of atrial fibrillation as the primary endpoint, the latter study defined a composite endpoint of death from any cause or worsening heart failure as the primary endpoint. Both studies found significant benefits for ablation of atrial fibrillation demonstrating the rising

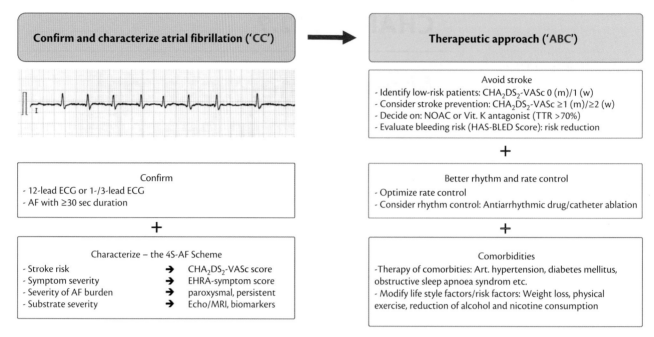

Figure 12.7.1 The CC to ABC algorithm of the 2020 ESC atrial fibrillation guidelines.
Based on more recent data, 'B' may refer to 'Better rhythm and rate control' in patients with atrial fibrillation and heart failure. The emphasis on rhythm control is emerging based on new evidence.
AF, atrial fibrillation; Art., arterial; ECG, electrocardiogram; f, female; m, male; MRI, magnetic resonance imaging; NOAC, direct oral anticoagulant; TTR, time in therapeutic range.

importance of interventional treatment strategies. More recently, the EAST–AFNET 4 trial showed that systematic rhythm control therapy, given to all patients irrespective of LV function (800/2789 patients in that trial had heart failure), improves outcomes in patients with recently diagnosed atrial fibrillation compared to usual care.[7,14] These favourable outcomes with regard to reduction of cardiovascular outcomes have been confirmed for the main cohort of the EAST-AFNET 4 trial and in several subgroup analyses.[14a,14b] The effectiveness of early rhythm control is mediated by the presence of sinus rhythm at 12 months in the EAST-AFNET 4 trial.[14c] A recently published substudy of the CABANA trial suggests that atrial fibrillation ablation may have better outcomes than rhythm control using antiarrhythmic drugs in patients with heart failure.[15] The sub-analysis of patients with atrial fibrillation and heart failure randomized in the EAST—AFNET 4 trial also underpins that systematic initiation of rhythm control therapy improves outcomes in patients with atrial fibrillation and heart failure across the spectrum of left ventricular functions.[35]

This chapter proposes a contemporary approach to the management of patients with atrial fibrillation and heart failure.

Diagnostic approach to atrial fibrillation

The symptoms of atrial fibrillation and heart failure often overlap and the two diseases often occur together. Screening for atrial fibrillation should thus be part of the work-up of all patients with heart failure, and work-up for heart failure is necessary in all patients with atrial fibrillation.

Diagnostic algorithm

The current ESC atrial fibrillation guidelines contain the 'CC to ABC pathway' that offers guidance for the diagnostic and

therapeutic approach to atrial fibrillation (CC: *Confirm and characterise*, ABC: *Avoid stroke/anticoagulation; better symptom control; cardiovascular risk factors and concomitant diseases*; ⊃ Figure 12.7.1).[16] Confirmation and characterization of atrial fibrillation are mainly based on widely available diagnostic tools and clinical scores. For in-depth information about the underlying conditions and the myocardial substrate, especially in the context of heart failure, more specialized imaging tools like cardiac magnetic resonance imaging and laboratory markers might be necessary.

Screening

Although screening for atrial fibrillation is technically feasible using several different technical tools (e.g. Holter ECG and blood pressure monitors, implantable loop recorders, wrist bands, smart watches, and phones), data on screening benefit and optimal strategy are scarce. The guidelines recommend opportunistic screening in a population > 65 years (IB) and consideration of systematic screening in patients at high risk (e.g. > 75 years, IIaB). Based on the recently published STROKESTOP outcomes study, population-based ECG screening could prevent strokes in the long term.[16a]

Confirmation of diagnosis

To establish the diagnosis of atrial fibrillation, ECG documentation (> 30 seconds) is required. Implanted devices can detect atrial high-rate episodes which might represent subclinical atrial fibrillation and require confirmation by conventional ECG. In addition, the ECG provides valuable information on the type of heart failure, e.g. showing bundle branch block, signs of ischaemia, and/or of cardiomyopathies. The latter are of particular relevance in patients with atrial fibrillation and heart failure as all inherited cardiomyopathies can present with atrial fibrillation.

Characterization of atrial fibrillation

The guidelines contain the mnemonic '4S-AF-Scheme' (*stroke risk*; *symptoms*; *severity of burden*; *substrate*) for a comprehensive characterization of atrial fibrillation. The keywords can be addressed using the CHA_2DS_2-VASc Score for stroke risk and the EHRA symptom score for symptom evaluation. For assessment of the substrate severity (e.g. atrial enlargement, dysfunction, and fibrosis), imaging technics like echocardiography and cardiac magnetic resonance imaging or biomarkers are helpful.

Echocardiography

Transthoracic echocardiography is the most useful, widely available tool in patients with suspected heart failure to establish the diagnosis and it provides immediate information on chamber volumes, ventricular systolic and diastolic function, wall thickness, valve function, and pulmonary hypertension. Differentiation of patients with heart failure based on left ventricular ejection fraction, usually measured using echocardiography, is important in establishing the diagnosis and in determining appropriate treatment.

The diagnosis of heart failure with preserved ejection fraction is more challenging than the diagnosis of heart failure with reduced ejection fraction. Left ventricular diastolic dysfunction is thought to be the underlying pathophysiological abnormality in patients with heart failure with preserved ejection fraction, thus its assessment plays an important role in diagnosis. Although echocardiography is at present the only imaging technique that can allow for the diagnosis of diastolic dysfunction, no single echocardiography variable is sufficiently accurate to be used in isolation to make a diagnosis of left ventricular diastolic dysfunction. Therefore, a comprehensive echocardiography examination incorporating all relevant two-dimensional and Doppler data is recommended.

In patients with atrial fibrillation transthoracic echocardiography is essential in the assessment of structural and functional changes (i.e. left atrial size, valvular abnormalities) and to guide treatment.

Cardiac magnetic resonance imaging

Magnetic resonance imaging is the gold standard for evaluation of cardiac morphology and measurements of volume, mass, and cardiac function. It is the best modality for patients with non-diagnostic echocardiographic studies, to visualize the right heart, and is the method of choice in patients with congenital heart disease.[17] Magnetic resonance imaging also allows characterization of myocardial structure using late gadolinium enhancement along with T1 mapping. It thereby allows differentiation between ischaemic and non-ischaemic origins of heart failure. In addition, it is useful to identify the presence of myocarditis and to diagnose specific cardiomyopathies, such as infiltrative processes or left ventricular non-compaction.

Patients with heart failure with reduced ejection fraction and atrial fibrillation without late gadolinium enhancement exhibited significantly greater improvement in systolic function after restoration of sinus rhythm. Further stratification with magnetic resonance imaging may identify patients who benefit from the restoration of sinus rhythm and certain therapies, such as catheter ablation.[18] Although imaging of the ventricular myocardium is well

established, there are important limitations related to the spatial resolution of the thin atrial myocardium. Assessment of left atrial fibrosis with late gadolinium enhancement has been described but only rarely applied and reproduced in clinical practice.[19] Further clinical limitations include lower availability and higher costs compared with echocardiography as well as safety issues in patients with certain implanted pacemakers or defibrillators.

Biomarkers

Natriuretic peptides, in particular B-type natriuretic peptide and its pro-hormone fragment, are markers of cardiac load and stress, including end-diastolic left ventricular pressure as they are released from cardiomyocytes in response to stretch. Elevated natriuretic peptides help establish an initial working diagnosis and to identify those who require further cardiac investigation. Patients with normal plasma concentrations are unlikely to have heart failure (high negative predictive value). Therefore, the use of natriuretic peptides is recommended for ruling-out heart failure, but not to establish the diagnosis.

Their plasma concentrations are elevated in patients with atrial fibrillation as well. Furthermore, natriuretic peptides provide prognostic information in patients with atrial fibrillation.[20,20a] Circulating biomarkers provide quantifiable measures of clinical or subclinical disease states in patients with atrial fibrillation and enable prediction of atrial fibrillation when long-term monitoring or even an ECG is not feasible.[21] Furthermore, biomarkers (e.g. troponin, natriuretic peptides, growth differentiation factor 15, von Willebrand factor, or bone morphogenic protein-10) can help to estimate prognosis and assess risk once atrial fibrillation has been diagnosed. Clinical scores including biomarkers (e.g. the ABC-stroke risk score considering age, previous stroke/transient ischaemic attack, high-sensitivity troponin T, and N-terminal-prohormone B-type natriuretic peptide) can improve stroke risk prediction significantly over clinical scores.[22]

Specific aspects in patients with atrial fibrillation and heart failure

The diagnostic evaluation of patients presenting with atrial fibrillation and heart failure with preserved ejection fraction can be particularly challenging. It might be unclear which condition is predominantly responsible for the symptoms. In those cases, a stepwise approach has been suggested by the 7th AFNET/EHRA consensus conference (➲ Figure 12.7.2).[23] The first overtly presenting condition may stratify patients with primary and secondary causes, possibly enabling differential therapy. It has been proposed to observe the initial response to diuretics and a 'diagnostic cardioversion'. This information can define the further management pathway including a potentially more aggressive rhythm control management. Those who respond well to diuretics may have heart failure with preserved ejection fraction as their predominant condition, while in those who respond well to cardioversion, atrial fibrillation may be the main driver of symptoms. The patients with predominant heart failure with preserved ejection fraction might potentially benefit more from identification and treatment of underlying risk factors. Patients predominantly suffering from atrial fibrillation may benefit from

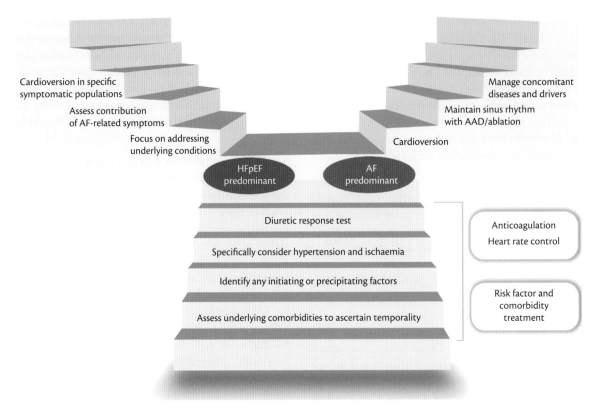

Figure 12.7.2 Acute management of patients presenting with atrial fibrillation and heart failure with preserved ejection fraction.
This proposal for a sequence of acute interventions is based on expert consensus from the 7th AFNET/EHRA consensus conference. This approach is expected to improve patient wellbeing and reduce incidence of adverse events. The lower staircase is a common to both management of heart failure with preserved ejection fraction and atrial fibrillation, the upper staircases illustrate separate management priorities. The approach may be adjusted in patients with early atrial fibrillation.
AAD, antiarrhythmic drugs; AF, atrial fibrillation; HFpEF, heart failure with preserved ejection fraction.

antiarrhythmic drugs, cardioversion, or ablation to improve symptoms, disease substrate, and possibly even prognosis.

Tachymyopathy

Some patients with persistent atrial fibrillation and otherwise unexplained left ventricular systolic dysfunction suffer from an arrhythmia-mediated cardiomyopathy, sometimes even despite adequate ventricular rate control. The left ventricular dysfunction is partially or even completely reversible in these patients. Frequently the clinical history cannot determine the temporal relationship of the two conditions. The restoration of sinus rhythm, and especially rhythm control therapy using catheter ablation, can lead to considerable improvements in left ventricular ejection fraction, cardiac remodelling, and functional capacity.[18] Of note, systematic rhythm control therapy and symptom-restricted rhythm control therapy have similar long-term effects on left ventricular function in patients with recently diagnosed atrial fibrillation and heart failure, while systematic rhythm control improves outcomes.[35] Coronary angiography is recommended in patients with heart failure and intermediate to high pre-test probability of coronary artery disease in the presence of probable ischaemia in non-invasive stress test. Coronary angiography is also recommended in patients with a history of symptomatic ventricular arrhythmia or aborted cardiac arrest. In patients with a low pre-test probability, the use of computed tomography is reasonable to determine whether an obstructive coronary artery disease is present.[17]

Therapeutic approach to atrial fibrillation

Treatment algorithm of the ESC atrial fibrillation guidelines 2020

The Atrial Fibrillation Better Care (ABC) approach is part of the ESC guidelines as a recommendation for structured atrial fibrillation treatment.[24] The acronym stands for Avoid stroke/anticoagulation, Better symptom control and Cardiovascular risk factors and concomitant diseases (⊃ Figure 12.7.1). The approach has recently been evaluated in a post-hoc analysis of the AFFIRM trial and achieved an improved outcome with less major adverse events in patients with multiple comorbidities.[25]

1. Acute atrial fibrillation therapy

The ABC approach can generally be applied in the acute and long-term care of patients with atrial fibrillation. In case of rapid ventricular response with haemodynamic instability, emergency electrical cardioversion might be necessary.[16] Anticoagulation should be started as soon as possible and underlying heart failure as well as precipitating factors should be treated according to the respective guidelines.

2. Anticoagulation/avoid stroke

The CHA$_2$DS$_2$-VASc score offers a compromise between practicability and accuracy making it an essential tool for stroke-risk assessment, stroke prevention, and anticoagulation management. In individuals with CHA$_2$DS$_2$-VASc score 2 (male) or 3 (female), oral anticoagulation is recommended. Frequent re-evaluations are important, as unknown risk factors may come to light during the time after first diagnosis of atrial fibrillation. The HAS-BLED score should be applied in all patients before the beginning of anticoagulation to determine the bleeding risk, but it is generally recommended to modify risk factors and intensify surveillance instead of withholding anticoagulation. Direct oral anticoagulants (apixaban, dabigatran, edoxaban, rivaroxaban) remain the preferred treatment. Dose reduction apart from evidence-based recommendations should be avoided.

3. Rhythm and rate control therapy

Rate control should be applied in every patient. The target heart rate is <110 beats per minute, based on results of the RACE, RACE II, and AFFIRM trials.[26–28] While betablockers are the standard agent to achieve rate control, the small, randomized RATE-AF trial showed that low-dose digoxin improves symptoms and potentially lowers pro-BNP better in patients with permanent atrial fibrillation and symptoms of heart failure.[29] Long-term rhythm control therapy has traditionally been applied in patients still being symptomatic under rate control. The clinical benefits of rhythm control therapy, delivered as early rhythm control or as catheter ablation, are discussed in detail below with special consideration of patients with atrial fibrillation and heart failure. These recent results suggest that systematic rhythm control therapy is the emerging default therapy in patients with recently diagnosed atrial fibrillation and heart failure. The patients' preference regarding medical or interventional rhythm control is a central concept in the current atrial fibrillation guidelines. While medical therapy with agents like flecainide, propafenone, and others has a Class IA recommendation, catheter ablation is an alternative treatment option (Class IIaB recommendation for paroxysmal atrial fibrillation, Class IIbC recommendation for persistent atrial fibrillation without high risk of recurrence). Flecainide and propafenone are agents suitable for patients without structural heart disease, whereas amiodarone and dronedarone can be used in individuals with known cardiac conditions. In individuals with paroxysmal or persistent atrial fibrillation, who have previously had an unsuccessful medical therapy or who cannot tolerate medical therapy, catheter ablation is the treatment of choice (class IA recommendation) in the guidelines.

4. Cardiovascular risk factors and concomitant diseases

The occurrence of atrial fibrillation is often promoted by lifestyle factors and cardiovascular comorbidities. For patients with atrial fibrillation and heart failure with reduced ejection fraction, meticulous use of disease-modifying therapies is needed. Rhythm control therapy may be needed to disrupt the vicious circle of atrial fibrillation-induced atrial damage. The RACE III trial was able to demonstrate that treatment of risk factors and cardiovascular comorbidities stabilizes sinus rhythm in patients with heart failure, but even a comprehensive, integrat care approach can only prevent a small part of the atrial fibrillation recurrence as shown during long-term follow-up.[30,31]

Early rhythm control: The emerging treatment standard for patients with AF and heart failure

The results of the recently published EAST-AFNET 4 trial indicate that an early start for rhythm control therapy reduces cardiovascular events in comparison to standard therapy according to the guidelines.[7] In total 2789 patients with atrial fibrillation diagnosed within a year prior to randomization were randomized in 135 European centres. The intervention consisted of antiarrhythmic medication or catheter ablation, and cardioversion when needed, while patients in the control group received rate control therapy at baseline with additional rhythm therapy in case of persisting symptoms. The EARLY-AF and the STOP-AF First trials were published a few months later and demonstrated that an interventional approach using cryoballoon ablation as the first-line therapy was superior to antiarrhythmic drug treatment regarding atrial fibrillation recurrence rates with an equal safety profile.[32,33] Early intervention by catheter ablation may achieve additional benefits for patients with heart failure with reduced ejection fraction as a meta-analysis of 26 studies including 1838 heart failure patients has demonstrated. Recurrence rates were lower when ablation was performed earlier after first diagnosis of atrial fibrillation or heart failure.[34] A recently published heart failure sub-analysis of the EAST-AFNET 4 trial, including patients with heart failure with preserved and reduced ejection fraction, has reported a clinical benefit for individuals randomized to early rhythm control.[35] The safety of early rhythm control therapy has since been confirmed in the UK Biobank and in several large healthcare data sets.[35a,35b,35c] Thus, early rhythm control therapy should be an integral part of the management in patients with heart failure and atrial fibrillation.

Antiarrhythmic medication or catheter ablation

Antiarrhythmic drug treatment doubles the number of patients maintaining sinus rhythm, with amiodarone being the most effective antiarrhythmic agent. Still, especially amiodarone comes along with several potentially severe side-effects. Catheter ablation is more effective in maintaining sinus rhythm than antiarrhythmic drugs. The CABANA trial, which was published in 2019 compared medical and interventional rhythm control therapy and found no difference in the primary endpoint, which comprised death, disabling stroke, serious bleeding, and cardiac arrest.[36] Both groups had an improvement of life quality, with a greater effect in the ablation group. This was confirmed by the CAPTAF trial from 2019.[37] The complication rates of antiarrhythmic drug therapy and interventional rhythm control are in general similar. The heart failure sub-analysis of the CABANA trial suggests a clinical benefit of atrial fibrillation ablation compared to antiarrhythmic drug therapy, suggesting that atrial fibrillation ablation could be preferred to antiarrhythmic drug therapy where both options exist.[15]

Specific aspects of atrial fibrillation treatment in patients with heart failure

Atrial fibrillation and heart failure are often linked, and both are associated with high morbidity and mortality. To improve outcome in heart failure patients, several studies have evaluated drug-based or interventional approaches of atrial fibrillation treatment.

Amiodarone is the only drug recommended for rhythm control in patients with acute heart failure. Dronedarone, while associated with reduced mortality in one study, had higher rates of heart failure, stroke, and death in patients with permanent atrial fibrillation in the PALLAS trial.[38,39] In the AATAC trial patients with persistent atrial fibrillation and congestive heart failure were randomized to catheter ablation or drug therapy with amiodarone.[12] The primary outcome (recurrence of atrial fibrillation) was significantly reduced in the catheter ablation group, as were the secondary outcomes of mortality and hospitalization. The results were confirmed in a meta-analysis published in 2018 by Turagam et al., which included several randomized controlled studies.[40] In contrast to the general atrial fibrillation patient collective, patients with heart failure seem to benefit from ablation not only regarding their symptom status, but also regarding mortality, left ventricular function, and exercise capacity. The main driver of the aforementioned meta-analysis is the CASTLE-AF study which is the largest randomized controlled trial to show a reduction in the composite endpoint of all-cause mortality and hospitalization for heart failure.[13] These results have been repeated in recent heart failure sub-analyses of the CABANA trial and the EAST-AFNET4 trial: while the initial analysis of CABANA showed no difference regarding mortality in patients with atrial fibrillation comparing catheter ablation and medical therapy,[36] the sub-analysis focused on patients with clinically diagnosed heart failure showed a reduction of the primary endpoint consisting of death, disabling stroke, serious bleeding, or cardiac arrest.[15] Rillig et al. furthermore demonstrated a reduction of the primary endpoint (mortality, stroke, hospitalization for worsening heart failure or acute coronary syndrome) after randomization to early rhythm control therapy in their sub-analysis of the EAST-AFNET 4 trial including patients with heart failure.[35] In summary, rhythm control therapy emerges as the default therapy for all patients with atrial fibrillation and heart failure, irrespective of their left ventricular function. Atrial fibrillation ablation seems to be more effective and may be preferred where available. Considering patient preferences, antiarrhythmic drug therapy is a safe alternative that also reduces cardiovascular outcomes in the long term.

Optimal patient selection for catheter ablation in patients with atrial fibrillation and concomitant heart failure

The aforementioned studies provide substantial evidence showing that patients with atrial fibrillation and heart failure should receive rhythm control therapy, potentially with a preference to atrial fibrillation ablation. Nevertheless, they included heterogeneous patient cohorts and variable ablation strategies. Further selection among patients with atrial fibrillation and heart failure might thus be important to balance procedure related complication risks and potential benefit of rhythm control. Additional interventional studies are especially warranted to test the beneficial effect of rhythm control therapy in patients with atrial fibrillation and heart failure with preserved or only mildly reduced ejection fraction.

The role of patient characteristics, type of atrial fibrillation and atrial fibrillation burden

Freedom from recurrent atrial fibrillation may not be the most relevant therapeutic target for rhythm control therapy. Prevention of atrial fibrillation progression to chronic forms could be clinically more useful.[41] A post hoc analysis of the CASTLE-AF study demonstrated that atrial fibrillation recurrence (determined by an episode > 30 seconds) was not associated to the primary endpoint, whereas an atrial fibrillation burden of 6% or less predicted freedom from the primary endpoint, compared to those with atrial fibrillation burden > 6%.[42]

Upcoming trials, such as RAFT-AF (Randomized Ablation-based atrial Fibrillation rhythm control versus rate control Trial in patients with heart failure and high burden Atrial Fibrillation), will provide additional information on the effect of atrial fibrillation burden on post-ablation outcome in patients with atrial fibrillation and heart failure.[43] In their seventh EHRA/AFNET 4 Consensus Statement, Fabritz et al. offer a recurrence-risk-based therapy selection (➲ Figure 12.7.3): patients at low risk of recurrence are offered initial therapy with antiarrhythmic drugs, patients at higher risk of recurrence would benefit from atrial fibrillation ablation, and those at highest risk of recurrent atrial fibrillation might benefit from initial combination therapy with ablation and antiarrhythmic drugs.[23]

Traditionally, the electrophysiology community has sought to treat the 'ideal patient' with the highest likelihood of acute and long-term procedural success, i.e. a younger patient with recent-onset heart failure, recent-onset atrial fibrillation, fast ventricular rates, idiopathic cardiomyopathy, absence of ventricular late gadolinium enhancement, lower ejection fraction, minimal to moderate left atrial enlargement (<55 mm), left atrial fibrosis < 10%, and no or only few comorbidities.[44] The recent data clearly suggest that rhythm control therapy should be offered to all patients with recently diagnosed atrial fibrillation, and especially those with atrial fibrillation and heart failure. This paradigm shift from the 'ideal patient' to the 'high-risk patient' will take time to implement but has the potential to prevent many atrial fibrillation-related complications. Risk-based selection of rhythm control therapy and using rhythm control to reduce cardiovascular risk are the emerging concepts that should guide rhythm control therapy in patients with atrial fibrillation, and especially those with atrial fibrillation and heart failure.

The impact of underlying type of cardiomyopathy and structural heart disease

There is only sparse data on whether the underlying type of cardiomyopathy plays a role for the improvement of left ventricular ejection fraction during rhythm control therapy. Previous studies found that left ventricular improvement after catheter ablation was more pronounced in patients suffering from tachycardia-mediated cardiomyopathy or dilated cardiomyopathy than in those with ischaemic cardiomyopathy.[10,45] These findings are in line with data from a large, international, multicentre registry. The authors reported that the increase in left ventricular ejection fraction was the highest in patients suffering from dilated cardiomyopathy, and furthermore, that the likelihood of the composite endpoint (stroke or death) was significantly reduced in patients with tachycardia-mediated cardiomyopathy compared with other types of cardiomyopathies.[46]

Apart from ablation efficacy, procedural safety might deserve special attention in patients with heart failure. A multicentre

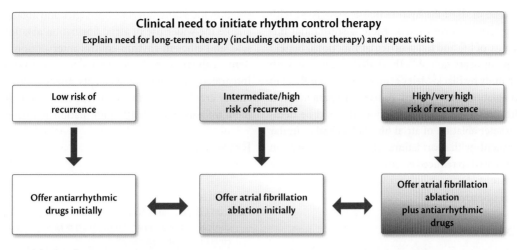

Figure 12.7.3 Suggested rhythm therapy management tree.
This proposal for a recurrence-risk-based therapy selection is based on the expert consensus from the 7th AFNET/EHRA consensus conference. AAD, antiarrhythmic drugs; AF, atrial fibrillation.

study focusing on the periprocedural risk for complications during catheter ablation in patients with different types of cardiomyopathies showed that catheter ablation is associated with a low-to-moderate incidence of major complications in this patient population. Interestingly, hypertensive cardiomyopathy was an independent predictor for complications, in particular thromboembolic events.[47] Therefore, prevention of these events by optimizing patient selection and adjunct or uninterrupted anticoagulation might be essential to enhance patient outcomes.

Young patients with atrial fibrillation and heart failure with reduced ejection fraction, and those with abnormal morphology or structure of the right or left ventricle, should undergo workup for inherited cardiomyopathies.

The impact of left atrial and left ventricular fibrosis

Local voltage abnormalities are used as a surrogate for diseased cardiac tissue. Extensive left atrial tissue fibrosis has been used to predict a less beneficial outcome after atrial fibrillation ablation.[48] Additional ablation strategies targeting low-voltage areas have been developed to improve clinical outcomes of atrial fibrillation ablation.[49] However, long-term success rates are lower in patients with heart failure compared to patients without underlying cardiac condition[46] and controversies still exist regarding an optimal ablation strategy in this special patient cohort.

The impact of atrial fibrillation ablation on biventricular pacing during cardiac resynchronization therapy

Cardiac resynchronization therapy has evolved as a standard treatment in heart failure patients with stable sinus rhythm, impaired systolic left ventricular function, and left bundle branch block.[16] Data on cardiac resynchronization therapy in patients with heart failure and concomitant atrial fibrillation is sparse since most trials for cardiac resynchronization therapy excluded patients with atrial fibrillation. The therapeutic effect of resynchronization has been shown to be lower in patients with atrial arrhythmias compared to patients with stable sinus rhythm due to impaired biventricular pacing delivery in irregular atrio-ventricular electrical conduction,

resulting in fusion and pseudo-fusion beats.[50] To maintain sinus rhythm in this setting, treatment options range from rate control to rhythm control with antiarrhythmic drugs or catheter ablation as well as AV-nodal ablation.

Previous randomized trials, such as CASTLE-AF or the AATAC focusing on clinical outcome after atrial fibrillation ablation in heart failure patients, included patients with resynchronization therapy. Detailed outcomes have not yet been reported.[12,13] Nevertheless, Fink et al. were able to show, that pulmonary vein isolation improved biventricular capture, left ventricular ejection fraction, and functional NYHA class.[51] On the other hand, AV-nodal ablation has been investigated and proved to increase exercise capacity, left ventricular ejection fraction, and reverse remodelling in patients with resynchronization therapy and atrial fibrillation.[52,53] A possible disadvantage of AV-nodal ablation might be the loss of atrial contraction, which is seen after restoration of stable sinus rhythm. The PABA-CHF (Pulmonary Vein Antrum Isolation vs. AV-nodal Ablation with Bi-Ventricular Pacing for Congestive Heart Failure) trial addressed this issue and reported that catheter ablation resulted in 88% atrial fibrillation-free survival and an absolute increase in left ventricular ejection fraction by 8% at six months of follow-up compared with no relevant change in left ventricular ejection fraction (–1%) in the pace-and-ablate group ($P < 0.001$). In addition, functional capacity and quality of life significantly improved in patients randomized to atrial fibrillation ablation.[54]

Results of catheter ablation in patients with heart failure with or without reduced ejection fraction

Although most studies on patients suffering from atrial fibrillation and heart failure included individuals with reduced ejection fraction only, there are also data showing beneficial effects of catheter ablation for patients with heart failure with mid-range or preserved ejection fraction. Cha et al. analysed a prospective cohort of patients with systolic dysfunction, isolated diastolic dysfunctionor preserved ventricular function, who underwent radiofrequency-ablation for atrial fibrillation. The authors found that although an ablative approach for atrial fibrillation in patients with systolic or diastolic dysfunction is associated with an increased long-term recurrence risk, there is substantial improvement of quality of life and left ventricular functional benefit regardless the type of heart failure.[55] These data are in line with results of a larger study by Black-Meier et al. assessing the effect of atrial fibrillation ablation on long-term outcome in patients with heart failure with preserved ejection fraction. It could be demonstrated that catheter ablation of atrial fibrillation had a similar effectiveness in patients with heart failure with preserved ejection fraction when compared to reduced ejection fraction, irrespective of presence of systolic dysfunction and without differences regarding functional improvements.[56]

Future perspectives

An integrative treatment approach to atrial fibrillation and heart failure is important for further reduction of the disease burden. Systematic rhythm control therapy emerges as a default part of the management of patients with atrial fibrillation and heart failure. Local availability of therapy options, patient choice, and the estimated risk of recurrent atrial fibrillation can help to guide the choice of rhythm control, either atrial fibrillation ablation or antiarrhythmic drug therapy. The management of atrial fibrillation needs to be integrated into optimal medical heart failure therapy. To improve quality of life both of atrial fibrillation and of heart failure symptoms, an integrated care model which provides patient-centered care is essential. This model should involve access to all specialist treatment options, reducing concomitant risk factors, early life style education programmes, to achieve consistent delivery of these best individual treatments and treatment choices to all patients with heart failure and atrial fibrillation. These options might be accompanied by technical progress in artificial intelligence models in continuous health parameter acquisition. In the future these integrated patient care measures might help to stop atrial fibrillation and heart failure progression at an early stage, ideally before the first symptoms and hospital admission or complication occur.

Summary and key messages

Heart failure and atrial fibrillation are increasingly prevalent and associated with high morbidity and mortality. Each condition markedly enhances the risk associated with the other, leading to coexistence of atrial fibrillation and heart failure in many patients. Treatment and research therefore need to consider both entities and their interaction.

The current ESC atrial fibrillation guidelines contain the 'CC to ABC pathway' that offers guidance for the diagnostic and therapeutic approach to atrial fibrillation (CC: Confirm and characterize, ABC: Avoid stroke/anticoagulation; better symptom control; cardiovascular risk factors and concomitant diseases).[16] The results of the EAST-AFNET 4 trial and earlier studies evaluating rhythm control therapy in patients with atrial fibrillation and reduced ejection fraction encourage the systematic use of rhythm control as part of the default treatment in patients with atrial fibrillation and heart failure. Recent advances in catheter ablation including novel technologies and ablative strategies may enable the wider use of atrial fibrillation ablation as an effective, safe, and efficient rhythm control intervention, especially in patients with atrial fibrillation and reduced left ventricular function. Integrated management concepts and consideration of patient choice are important factors influencing the best choice of treatment for patients with atrial fibrillation and heart failure.

References

1. Braunwald E. Cardiovascular medicine at the turn of the millennium: triumphs, concerns, and opportunities. N Engl J Med, 1997; 337:1360–1369.
2. Lam CSP, Donal E, Kraigher-Krainer E, Vasan RS. Epidemiology and clinical course of heart failure with preserved ejection fraction. Eur J Heart Fail 2011; 13:18–28.
3. Go AS, Hylek EM, Phillips KA, et al. Prevalence of diagnosed atrial fibrillation in adults: national implications for rhythm management and stroke prevention: the AnTicoagulation and Risk Factors in Atrial Fibrillation (ATRIA) Study. JAMA 2001; 285:2370–2375.
4. Kornej J, Börschel CS, Benjamin EJ, Schnabel RB. Epidemiology of atrial fibrillation in the 21st century: novel methods and new insights. Circ Res 2020; 127:4–20.
5. Kotecha D, Piccini JP. Atrial fibrillation in heart failure: what should we do? Eur Heart J 2015; 36:3250–3257.
6. Chua W, Purmah Y, Cardoso VR, et al. Data-driven discovery and validation of circulating blood-based biomarkers associated with prevalent atrial fibrillation. Eur Heart J 2019; 40:1268–1276.
7. Kirchhof P, Camm AJ, Goette A, et al. Early rhythm-control therapy in patients with atrial fibrillation. N Engl J Med 2020; 383:1305–1316.
8. Trulock KM, Narayan SM, Piccini JP. Rhythm control in heart failure patients with atrial fibrillation: contemporary challenges including the role of ablation. J Am Coll Cardiol 2014; 64:710–721.
9. Lubitz SA, Yin X, Lin HJ, et al. Genetic risk prediction of atrial fibrillation. Circulation 2017; 135:1311–1320.
10. Verma A, Kalman JM, Callans DJ. Treatment of patients with atrial fibrillation and heart failure with reduced ejection fraction. Circulation 2017; 135:1547–1563.
11. Santhanakrishnan R, Wang N, Larson MG, et al. Atrial fibrillation begets heart failure and vice versa: temporal associations and differences in preserved versus reduced ejection fraction. Circulation 2016; 133:484–492.
12. Di Biase L, Mohanty P, Mohanty S, et al. Ablation versus amiodarone for treatment of persistent atrial fibrillation in patients with congestive heart failure and an implanted device: results from the AATAC multicenter randomized trial. Circulation 2016; 133:1637–1644.
13. Marrouche NF, Brachmann J, Andresen D, et al. Catheter ablation for atrial fibrillation with heart failure. N Engl J Med 2018; 378:417–427.
14. Metzner A, Suling A, Brandes A, et al. Anticoagulation, therapy of concomitant conditions, and early rhythm control therapy: a detailed analysis of treatment patterns in the EAST-AFNET 4 trial. Europace 2022; 24(4):552–64.
14a. Rillig A, Borof K, Breithardt G, et al. Early rhythm control in patients with atrial fibrillation and high comorbidity burden. Circulation 2022; 146(11):836–47.
14b. Willems S, Borof K, Brandes A, et al. Systematic, early rhythm control strategy for atrial fibrillation in patients with or without symptoms: the EAST-AFNET 4 trial. Eur Heart J 2022; 43(12):1219–30.
14c. Eckardt L, Sehner S, Suling A, et al. Attaining sinus rhythm mediates improved outcome with early rhythm control therapy of atrial fibrillation: the EAST-AFNET 4 trial. Eur Heart J 2022; 43(40):4127–44.

15. Packer DL, Piccini JP, Monahan KH, et al. Ablation versus drug therapy for atrial fibrillation in heart failure: results from the CABANA Trial. Circulation 2021; 143:1377–1390.

16. Hindricks G, Potpara T, Dagres N, et al. 2020 ESC Guidelines for the diagnosis and management of atrial fibrillation developed in collaboration with the European Association of Cardio-Thoracic Surgery (EACTS). Eur Heart J 2020; 42(5):373–498.

16a.Svennberg E, Friberg L, Frykman V, et al. Clinical outcomes in systematic screening for atrial fibrillation (STROKESTOP): a multicentre, parallel group, unmasked, randomised controlled trial. Lancet 2021; 398(10310):1498–506.

17. Ponikowski P, Voors AA, Anker SD, et al. 2016 ESC Guidelines for the diagnosis and treatment of acute and chronic heart failure: The Task Force for the diagnosis and treatment of acute and chronic heart failure of the European Society of Cardiology (ESC) developed with the special contribution of the Heart Failure Association (HFA) of the ESC. Eur Heart J 2016; 37:2129–2200.

18. Willems S, Meyer C, de Bono J, et al. Cabins, castles, and constant hearts: rhythm control therapy in patients with atrial fibrillation. Eur Heart J. 2019;40:3793–9c

19. Oakes RS, Badger TJ, Kholmovski EG, et al. Detection and quantification of left atrial structural remodeling with delayed-enhancement magnetic resonance imaging in patients with atrial fibrillation. Circulation 2009; 119:1758–1767.

20. Schrage B, Geelhoed B, Niiranen TJ, et al. Comparison of cardiovascular risk factors in european population cohorts for predicting atrial fibrillation and heart failure, their subsequent onset, and death. J Am Heart Assoc 2020; 9:e015218.

20a.Brady P, Chua W, Nehaj F, et al. Interactions between atrial fibrillation and natriuretic peptide in predicting heart failure hospitalization or cardiovascular death. J Am Heart Assoc 2022; 11:e022833.

21. Freedman B, Camm J, Calkins H, et al. Screening for atrial fibrillation: A report of the AF-SCREEN International Collaboration. Circulation 2017; 135:1851–1867.

22. Hijazi Z, Lindbäck J, Alexander JH, et al. The ABC (age, biomarkers, clinical history) stroke risk score: a biomarker-based risk score for predicting stroke in atrial fibrillation. Eur Heart J 2016; 37:1582–1590.

23. Fabritz L, Crijns HJGM, Guasch E, et al. Dynamic risk assessment to improve quality of care in patients with atrial fibrillation: the 7th AFNET/EHRA Consensus Conference. Europace; 2021; 23(3):329–344.

24. Lip GYH. The ABC pathway: an integrated approach to improve AF management. Nat Rev Cardiol 2017; 14:627–628.

25. Proietti M, Romiti GF, Olshansky B, Lane DA, Lip GYH. Comprehensive management with the ABC (Atrial Fibrillation Better Care) pathway in clinically complex patients with atrial fibrillation: a post hoc ancillary analysis from the AFFIRM trial. J Am Heart Assoc 2020; 9:e014932.

26. Wyse DG, Waldo AL, DiMarco JP, et al. A comparison of rate control and rhythm control in patients with atrial fibrillation. N Engl J Med 2002; 347:1825–1833.

27. Van Gelder IC, Hagens VE, Bosker HA, et al. A comparison of rate control and rhythm control in patients with recurrent persistent atrial fibrillation. N Engl J Med 2002; 347:1834–1840.

28. Van Gelder IC, Healey JS, Crijns HJGM, et al. Duration of device-detected subclinical atrial fibrillation and occurrence of stroke in ASSERT. Eur Heart J 2017; 38:1339–1344.

29. Kotecha D, Bunting KV, Gill SK, et al. Effect of digoxin vs bisoprolol for heart rate control in atrial fibrillation on patient-reported quality of life: the RATE-AF randomized clinical trial. JAMA 2020; 324:2497–2508.

30. Rienstra M, Hobbelt AH, Alings M, et al. Targeted therapy of underlying conditions improves sinus rhythm maintenance in patients with persistent atrial fibrillation: results of the RACE 3 trial. Eur Heart J 2018; 39:2987–2996.

31. Rienstra M. Targeted therapy of underlying conditions in patients with persistent atrial fibrillation and mild to moderate stable heart failure: long-term outcome of the RACE 3 Trial. Data presented at EHRA Congress 2021.

32. Wazni OM, Dandamudi G, Sood N, et al.. Cryoballoon ablation as initial therapy for atrial fibrillation. N Engl J Med 2020; 384(4):316–324.

33. Andrade JG, Wells GA, Deyell MW, et al. Cryoablation or drug therapy for initial treatment of atrial fibrillation. N Engl J Med 2020; 384(4):305–315.

34. Anselmino M, Matta M, D'Ascenzo F, et al. Catheter ablation of atrial fibrillation in patients with left ventricular systolic dysfunction: a systematic review and meta-analysis. Circ Arrhythm Electrophysiol 2014; 7:1011–1018.

35. Rillig A, Magnussen C, Ozga A-K, et al. Early Rhythm Control Therapy in Patients with Atrial Fibrillation and Heart Failure. Circulation 2021;144:845–858.

35a.Gottschalk S, Kany S, Konig HH, et al. Cost-effectiveness of early rhythm control vs. usual care in atrial fibrillation care: an analysis based on data from the EAST-AFNET 4 trial. Europace 2023; 25(5):euad051.

35b.Dickow J, Kany S, Roth Cardoso V, et al. Outcomes of early rhythm control therapy in patients with atrial fibrillation and a high comorbidity burden in large real-world cohorts. Circ Arrhythm Electrophysiol 2023; 16(5):e011585.

35c.Kim D, Yang PS, You SC, et al. Early rhythm control therapy for atrial fibrillation in low-risk patients: A nationwide propensity score-weighted study. Ann Intern Med 2022; 175(10):1356–65.

36. Packer DL, Mark DB, Robb RA, et al. Effect of catheter ablation vs antiarrhythmic drug therapy on mortality, stroke, bleeding, and cardiac arrest among patients with atrial fibrillation: The CABANA randomized clinical trial. JAMA 2019; 321:1261–1274.

37. Blomström-Lundqvist C, Gizurarson S, Schwieler J, et al. Effect of catheter ablation vs antiarrhythmic medication on quality of life in patients with atrial fibrillation: The CAPTAF randomized clinical trial. JAMA 2019; 321:1059–1068.

38. Hohnloser SH, Crijns HJGM, van Eickels M, et al. Effect of dronedarone on cardiovascular events in atrial fibrillation. N Engl J Med 2009; 360:668–678.

39. Connolly SJ, Camm AJ, Halperin JL, et al. Dronedarone in high-risk permanent atrial fibrillation. N Engl J Med 2011; 365:2268–2276.

40. Turagam MK, Garg J, Whang W, et al. Catheter ablation of atrial fibrillation in patients with heart failure: a meta-analysis of randomized controlled trials. Ann Intern Med 2019; 170:41–50.

41. Kuck K-H, Merkely B, Zahn R, et al. Catheter ablation versus best medical therapy in patients with persistent atrial fibrillation and congestive heart failure: the Randomized AMICA trial. Circ Arrhythm Electrophysiol 2019; 12(12):e007731.

42. Brachmann J, Sohns C, Andresen D, et al. Atrial fibrillation burden and clinical outcomes in heart failure: The CASTLE-AF trial. JACC Clin Electrophysiol 2021; 7:594–603.

43. Parkash R, Wells G, Rouleau J, et al. A randomized ablation-based atrial fibrillation rhythm control versus rate control trial in patients with heart failure and high burden atrial fibrillation: The RAFT-AF trial rationale and design. Am Heart J 2021; 234:90–100.

44. Link MS, Haïssaguerre M, Natale A. Ablation of atrial fibrillation: patient selection, periprocedural anticoagulation, techniques, and preventive measures after ablation. Circulation 2016; 134:339–352.

45. Prabhu S, Ling L-H, Ullah W, et al. The impact of known heart disease on long-term outcomes of catheter ablation in patients with atrial

fibrillation and left ventricular systolic dysfunction: a multicenter international study. J Cardiovasc Electrophysiol 2016; 27:281–289.

46. Ullah W, Ling L-H, Prabhu S, et al. Catheter ablation of atrial fibrillation in patients with heart failure: impact of maintaining sinus rhythm on heart failure status and long-term rates of stroke and death. Europace 2016; 18:679–686.

47. Hoffmann BA, Kuck K-H, Andresen D, et al. Impact of structural heart disease on the acute complication rate in atrial fibrillation ablation: results from the German Ablation Registry. J Cardiovasc Electrophysiol 2014; 25:242–249.

48. Marrouche NF, Wilber D, Hindricks G, et al. Association of atrial tissue fibrosis identified by delayed enhancement MRI and atrial fibrillation catheter ablation: the DECAAF study. JAMA 2014; 311:498–506.

49. Jadidi AS, Lehrmann H, Keyl C, et al. Ablation of persistent atrial fibrillation targeting low-voltage areas with selective activation characteristics. Circ Arrhythm Electrophysiol 2016; 9:e002962.

50. Kalscheur MM, Saxon LA, Lee BK, et al. Outcomes of cardiac resynchronization therapy in patients with intermittent atrial fibrillation or atrial flutter in the COMPANION trial. Heart Rhythm 2017; 14:858–865.

51. Fink T, Rexha E, Schlüter M, et al. Positive impact of pulmonary vein isolation on biventricular pacing in nonresponders to cardiac resynchronization therapy. Heart Rhythm 2019; 16:416–423.

52. Doshi RN, Daoud EG, Fellows C, et al. Left ventricular-based cardiac stimulation post AV nodal ablation evaluation (the PAVE study). J Cardiovasc Electrophysiol 2005; 16:1160–1165.

53. Gasparini M, Auricchio A, Regoli F, et al. Four-year efficacy of cardiac resynchronization therapy on exercise tolerance and disease progression: the importance of performing atrioventricular junction ablation in patients with atrial fibrillation. J Am Coll Cardiol 2006; 48:734–743.

54. Khan MN, Jaïs P, Cummings J, et al. Pulmonary-vein isolation for atrial fibrillation in patients with heart failure. N Engl J Med 2008; 359:1778–1785.

55. Cha Y-M, Wokhlu A, Asirvatham SJ, et al. Success of ablation for atrial fibrillation in isolated left ventricular diastolic dysfunction: a comparison to systolic dysfunction and normal ventricular function. Circ Arrhythm Electrophysiol 2011; 4:724–732.

56. Black-Maier E, Ren X, Steinberg BA, et al. Catheter ablation of atrial fibrillation in patients with heart failure and preserved ejection fraction. Heart Rhythm 2018; 15:651–657.

CHAPTER 12.8

Diabetes, prediabetes, and heart failure

Giuseppe Rosano, Javed Butler,
Petar M Seferović, Jelena Seferović, and
Francesco Cosentino

Contents

Introduction

There is a strong association between type 2 diabetes mellitus (T2DM) and heart failure (HF). T2DM and prediabetes, have been associated with an increased likelihood of developing HF in the general population. Patients with a history of HF have a greater propensity for new-onset T2DM, whilst known T2DM and prediabetes aggravate the risks of complications and mortality in individuals with HF. Recent advances in pharmacological treatment, in particular the introduction of sodium-glucose cotransporter-2 (SGLT2) inhibitors, have significantly advanced the possibilities to prevent the occurrence of HF in patients with T2DM. Likewise, considerable progress has been made in the treatment of HF with concomitant T2DM. There are now possibilities to hold up the progression of T2DM in the setting of HF with reduced ejection fraction (HFrEF), as well as to prevent hospitalizations and reduce mortality with the available therapies. This chapter summarizes the epidemiology, pathophysiology, and prevention of HF in T2DM and provides an overview of contemporary treatment options for HF and T2DM.

Epidemiology

It is presently estimated that there are 64 million people with HF[1] and 537 million adults with T2DM worldwide.[2] In Europe alone, the prevalence of HF is estimated at 14 million patients[3], and that of T2DM at 61 million people.[2] Of note, the prevalence of both conditions is expected to rise, due to the ageing population and the mounting burden of risk factors.

Risk of HF in patients with T2DM

Observational data indicate that T2DM is a strong independent risk factor for developing HF in the general population. According to the First NHANES study (National Health and Nutrition Examination Survey), T2DM was associated with an 85% greater adjusted risk of developing HF in the general population of individuals without previous HF over 19 years of follow-up.[4] More recently, a population-based study of 1.9 million individuals without know cardiovascular disorders demonstrated that HF was one the most common first presentations of cardiovascular disease, developing in 14.4% of patients with T2DM over 5.5 years of follow-up.[5] The occurrence of HF was more frequent than that of myocardial infarction or stroke, with an adjusted hazard ratio of 1.56 compared to the individuals without T2DM.[5] The risk of HF increases even with milder forms of dysglycaemia (i.e. prediabetes) as demonstrated in the ARIC (Atherosclerosis Risk in Communities) study, where the respective adjusted hazard ratios of individuals with glycosylated haemoglobin A1c (HbA1c) 5.5–6.0% and 6.0–6.4% were 16% and 40% higher compared to the reference group.[6] Poor glycaemic control is yet another risk factor for incident HF in patients with T2DM, as each 1% increase in HbA1c conferred an 8% increased risk of incident HF in a cohort of almost 50,000 patients with T2DM.[7] T2DM is also a risk factor for HF in individuals with asymptomatic left ventricular (LV) dysfunction (i.e. pre-HF according to the universal definition of HF), which bears important implications for the prevention.[8,9] It is important to note that unrecognized pre-HF and HF may be frequent in patients with T2DM, particularly in the elderly. A cohort study of 581 patients with T2DM using a comprehensive diagnostic approach and the European Society of Cardiology (ESC) criteria, indicated that the prevalence of unknown HF was 27.7%, with HFpEF being the more common phenotype than HFrEF (22.9% vs 4.8%).[10] A high prevalence of pre-HF was also suggested, in the form of LV systolic (25.8%) and LV diastolic (25.1%) dysfunction.[10]

The prevalence of HF among the general population of patients with T2DM is approximately 12%, and increases with the age and accompanying comorbidities, especially coronary artery disease and chronic kidney disease.[11] In the recent cardiovascular outcome trials of patients with T2DM and established cardiovascular disorders or with multiple risk factors, the prevalence of known HF ranged between 10% and 28%, albeit data on the clinical type of HF were not well characterized in those studies (➲ Tables 12.8.1–12.8.3).

Risk of T2DM in patients with HF

Epidemiological data indicate that the prevalence of T2DM in patients with HF is between 12% and 30%, which is significantly higher compared with individuals without HF (➲ Figure 12.8.1).

The prevalence of T2DM was even higher in clinical trials of HF, where the presence of T2DM was more scrupulously ascertained compared to observational studies. Indeed, both trials of HFrEF, and those of HF with preserved ejection fraction (HFpEF), reported the prevalence of known T2DM between ~15% and more than 40%.[12-18] According to the clinical trial and registry data, T2DM is present in ~40% of patients admitted to hospitals with acute HF, regardless of LV ejection fraction.[19-21] The awareness of T2DM seems to be poor among patients with HF as suggested by the pooled data from the CHARM (Candesartan in Heart failure Assessment of Reduction in Mortality and morbidity) Programme where prediabetes was present in 20–22%, and undiagnosed T2DM in 22% and 26% of patients with HFpEF and HFrEF, respectively.[22]

There appears to be a significant global and regional variation in the prevalence of T2DM in patients with HF. According to the ESC Heart Failure Long-Term Registry, the reported prevalence of T2DM in patients with chronic HFpEF and HFrEF in Europe was 29% and 32%, respectively.[23] However, more recent data suggest considerable regional heterogeneity of comorbid T2DM in individuals with HF across Europe, with the highest prevalence in the Mediterranean region (47%), followed by western and eastern Europe (37% and 33%, respectively).[24] Regional heterogeneity was also observed in the Americas, with the prevalence of T2DM being lower in Central/South America (31%) compared with the United States (45% and 42% for HFpEF and HFrEF,

respectively).[21,24] The prevalence of T2DM in HF appears to be particularly high in the Asia-Pacific region, where concomitant T2DM was reported as 44–57%.[25,26] On the other hand, a considerably lower prevalence of T2DM was reported in patients with HF in Sub-Saharan Africa (11.4%).[27] The reasons for the observed heterogeneity are currently speculative and likely reflect differences in diagnostic accuracy, as well as biological factors, including diversities in population age and gender structure, the aetiology of HF, and the prevailing risk factors.

Clinical presentation, complications, and outcomes in patients with HF and T2DM

A vast body of evidence indicates that concomitant T2DM and HF impart a more serious clinical presentation, greater risk of complications, and worse prognosis compared to either condition alone.

In patients hospitalized for acute HF, most observational data suggest higher risk of mortality associated with T2DM. In the ALARM-HF registry (4953 patients with acute HF from six European countries, Mexico, and Australia), in-hospital mortality rates were significantly higher in patients with T2DM compared to those without T2DM (11.7 vs 9.8%, p = 0.01), particularly among the elderly, with acute coronary syndrome, with lower LV ejection fraction, and in those not receiving disease-modifying therapies.[28] In the ESC Heart Failure Long-Term registry, among 6926 patients admitted to hospitals for acute HF, the presence of T2DM was an independent predictor of higher short-term (all-cause in-hospital mortality hazard ratio, 1.77) and long-term mortality rates (1-year all-cause mortality hazard ratio 1.16), as well as a higher risk of readmission for worsening HF (hazard ration 1.32).[29] However, in a Korean registry (5625 patients with acute HF patients) and in the Get With the Guidelines registry in the United States (n = 364,480 acute HF patients), the presence of T2DM was not independently associated with higher in-hospital mortality, but the association with adverse prognosis became apparent with a longer follow-up.[21,30] Clinical trial data confirm these observations. In the EVEREST trial (Efficacy of Vasopressin Antagonism in Heart Failure Outcome Study with Tolvaptan), in 4133 patients hospitalized with acute HF, the presence of T2DM was associated with a higher risk of cardiovascular death after 9.9 months of follow-up.[19]

In patients with chronic HF, observational and clinical trial data suggest that T2DM is associated with adverse prognosis, with the size effect varying depending on outcome, the studied populations and, to some extent, on the variables used to control the association. In the ESC Heart Failure Long-Term registry, enrolling 9428 outpatients with chronic HF, the presence of T2DM was associated with a 28% higher adjusted risk for 1-year all-cause mortality, a 28% higher cardiovascular mortality and a 37% higher adjusted risk for HF hospitalizations.[31] Similar results were shown in other registries of patients with chronic HF,[32] regardless of the aetiology of HF (ischaemic vs non-ischaemic).[33] Clinical trials of patients with chronic HFrEF and HFpEF support these observations (➲ Figure 12.8.2).

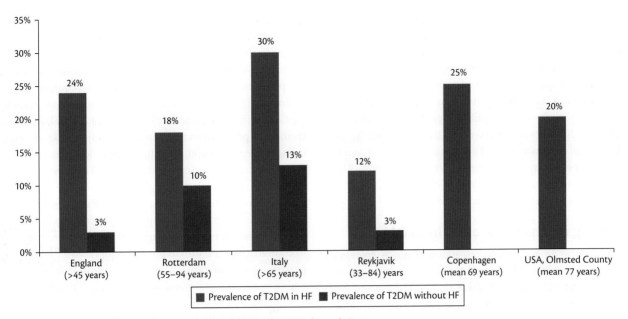

Figure 12.8.1 Prevalence of T2DM in patients with heart failure in the general population.
Reproduced from Pfeffer MA, Swedberg K, Granger CB, et al; CHARM Investigators and Committees. Effects of candesartan on mortality and morbidity in patients with chronic heart failure: the CHARM-Overall programme. *Lancet*. 2003 Sep 6;362(9386):759-66. doi: 10.1016/s0140-6736(03)14282-1 with permission from Elsevier.

A meta-analysis of 31 registries and 12 clinical trials with 381,725 patients with acute and chronic HF demonstrated that T2DM is an independent predictor of adverse long-term outcomes, including all-cause death (random-effects hazard ratio, 1.28), cardiovascular death (random-effects hazard ratio, 1.34) and HF hospitalizations (random-effects hazard ratio 1.35). In addition to known T2DM, pre-diabetes and unrecognized T2DM also confer an increased risk of adverse clinical outcomes

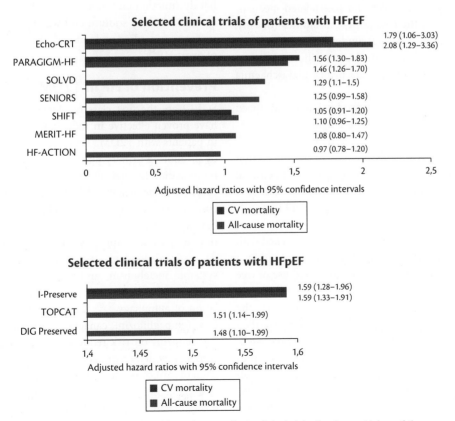

Figure 12.8.2 The association of T2DM and all-cause and cardiovascular mortality in clinical trials of patients with heart failure.
Reproduced from Pfeffer MA, Swedberg K, Granger CB, et al; CHARM Investigators and Committees. Effects of candesartan on mortality and morbidity in patients with chronic heart failure: the CHARM-Overall programme. *Lancet*. 2003 Sep 6;362(9386):759-66. doi: 10.1016/s0140-6736(03)14282-1 with permission from Elsevier.

(albeit lower than known T2DM), both in patents with HFrEF and HFpEF.[22,34]

Not only does T2DM adversely affect morbidity and mortality in HF, but it also has unfavourable impact on symptoms, functional status, and quality of life, and increases the risk of complications, such as vascular events (myocardial infarction and stroke).[35,36] In patients with HFpEF, the presence of T2DM was associated with increased markers of inflammation, fibrosis, and endothelial dysfunction, and echocardiographic evidence of greater LV hypertrophy, and elevated filling pressures.[14,37] These patients also had more comorbidities (hypertension, renal dysfunction, obesity) and more pronounced congestion.[14,15,38]

Underlying mechanisms of HF in T2DM

Despite long-standing scientific research and much epidemiological evidence linking T2DM with HF, the mechanisms responsible for the development of HF in T2DM have not been fully elucidated.[39] Among the most important and well understood contributors to HF in T2DM are myocardial ischaemia and infarction.[40] Indeed, hyperglycaemia, hyperinsulinaemia, and proatherogenic dyslipidaemia in T2DM are associated with accelerated atherosclerosis, extensive epicardial coronary artery disease, and microvascular endothelial dysfunction. HF that develops in this setting of myocardial ischaemia and infarction usually takes the phenotype of HFrEF.[40,41] However, HF in T2DM can occur in the absence of significant coronary artery stenosis, and most commonly manifests as HFpEF.[40,41] In this setting, it was postulated that several complex and interrelated mechanisms, in combination with the effect of comorbidities (obesity, hypertension chronic kidney disease), underlie the pathophysiology of HF. These mechanisms may also contribute to the severity of HF in patients with concomitant myocardial ischaemia and vice versa.

Hyperglycaemia leads to excessive production of advanced glycated end-products (AGEs), which were associated with increased myocardial interstitial fibrosis, reduced LV compliance[42,43] and the development of diastolic dysfunction.[44] The interaction between AGEs and the vascular vessel wall leads to endothelial dysfunction, increased vascular permeability, leukocyte adhesion, activation of fibroblastsand promotion of vascular wall remodelling, which results in increased vascular stiffening.[45]

Hyperinsulinaemia and insulin resistance were associated with profound changes in myocardial metabolism, characterized by a shift away from glucose utilization towards increased use of free fatty acids.[46,47] The metabolic shift is produced by impaired glucose uptake into the cardiomyocytes, and simultaneous increase in the availability of free fatty acids, triglycerides, and non-esterified fatty acids abundantly produced by the liver. Since the uptake of free fatty acids is not insulin-dependent, they become the preferred metabolic fuel for the myocardial energy production, at an expense of increased myocardial oxygen consumption, fragmentation of cellular mitochondrial network, and greater production of free oxygen species. Mitochondrial dysfunction and augmentation of oxidative stress directly contribute to the cardiac contractile

dysfunction in T2DM.[48] In addition, increased uptake of non-esterified fatty acids, which are not a substrate for beta-oxidation, results in their accumulation in the cardiomyocytes and perturbation in several cellular signalling processes, which is referred to as lipotoxicity.[49,50] Cardiac magnetic resonance imaging was used to document that impaired insulin signalling is associated with a significant increase in cardiac lipid content.[49] This leads to the activation of proinflammatory and profibrotic cytokines, excessive collagen deposition, and cardiomyocyte loss due to apoptosis, with a resultant increase in myocardial wall stiffness and impaired diastolic function. Diastolic dysfunction is further aggravated by the alteration in the expression and phosphorylation of titin protein in the cardiomyocytes. Impaired insulin signalling is responsible for a switch towards the more 'stiffer' titin isoform,[51] which, in combination with titin hypo-phosphorylation,[52] leads to higher passive myocardial tension and impaired diastolic relaxation. In addition, inflammation and oxidative stress in T2DM foster the development of microvascular endothelial dysfunction.[53] Lower bioavailability of nitric oxide in the myocardium, hampers titin phosphorylation and results in the activation of signalling pathways responsible for cardiomyocyte hypertrophy.

Collectively, the pathological processes in T2DM portend the occurrence of myocardial contractile dysfunction, LV remodelling, and diastolic dysfunction, and the resulting HF phenotype depends on the prevailing pathophysiological mechanism. In addition, extra-cardiac abnormalities associated with T2DM, such as obesity, impaired vascular stiffness, systemic endothelial dysfunction, autonomic nervous system perturbations and excessive kidney sodium and water retention, contribute to an increase in cardiac preload and afterload and the development of overt HF.[54,55]

Prevention of HF in T2DM

SGLT2 are the first class of glucose-lowering medications that have proven effective in reducing the risk of HF-related events in patients with T2DM. They exert their glucose-lowering effect by promoting urinary glucose excretion and have an additional modest diuretic, natriuretic, and uricosuric effects.[56] However, cardiovascular benefits of SGLT2 inhibitors extend beyond glucose lowering and include several postulated mechanisms, which have not yet been conclusively proven. These include a reduction in plasma volume without neurohormonal activation, a decrease in blood pressure, favourable impact on cardiac and systemic metabolism, anti-inflammatory effects, improvement in endothelial function, increased erythropoiesis, and modulation of autophagy.[57-60] The favourable effect of SGLT2 inhibitors (empagliflozin, canagliflozin, dapagliflozin, ertugliflozin, sotagliflozin) on risk reduction in HF hospitalization has been consistently demonstrated in patients with T2DM across a spectrum of cardiovascular risk and regardless of earlier HF history [61-64] (➲ Table 12.8.1). Furthermore, SGLT2 inhibitors (canagliflozin, dapagliflozin and sotagliflozin) have also proven beneficial in reducing HF hospitalizations in patients with diabetic nephropathy[65] or chronic kidney disease[66,67] (➲ Table 12.8.1).

Table 12.8.1 Effect of SGLT2 inhibitors on risk reduction in CV outcomes and HF hospitalization

Medication	Trial	Patients, n	Patient characteristics	HbA$_{1c}$ (mean)	History of HF	Follow-up (mean or median)	Primary outcome, (HR, 95% CI)	HF hospitalization (HR, 95% CI)
Empagliflozin	EMPA-REG OUTCOME[61]	7,020	T2DM and Established CVD	8.1%	10%	3.1 years	Death from CV causes, nonfatal MI, or nonfatal stroke: 0.86 (0.74–0.99); p = 0.04 for superiority	0.65 (0.50–0.85)
Canagliflozin	CANVAS Program[62]	10,142	T2DM and Established CVD (66%); CV risk factors (34%)	8.2%	14%	3.2 years	Death from CV causes, nonfatal MI, or nonfatal stroke: 0.86 (0.75–0.97); p = 0.02 for superiority	0.67 (0.52–0.87)
Canagliflozin	CREDENCE[65]	4,401	T2DM and Albuminuric chronic kidney disease	8.3%	~15%	2.62 years	End-stage kidney disease, doubling of serum creatinine level, or death from renal or CV causes: 0.70 (0.59–0.82); p = 0.00001	0.61 (0.47–0.80)
Dapagliflozin	DECLARE TIMI-58[63]	17,160	T2DM and Established CVD (41%); CV risk factors (59%)	8.3%	10%	4.2 years	Death from CV causes, nonfatal MI, or nonfatal stroke*: 0.93 (0.84–1.03); p = 0.17 CV death or HF hospitalization*. 0.83 (0.73–0.95); p = 0.005)	0.73 (0.61–0.88)*
Dapagliflozin	DAPA-CKD[66]	4,094	Chronic kidney disease and T2DM ~67%	---	~11%	2.4 years	Sustained decline in the eGFR ≥ 50%, end-stage kidney disease, or death from renal or CV causes: 0.61; (0.51–0.72); p < 0.001	0.71 (0.55–0.92)**
Ertugliflozin	VERTIS-CV[64]	8246	T2DM and Established CVD	8.2%	~24%	3.5 years	Death from CV causes, nonfatal MI, or nonfatal stroke 0.97 (0.85–1.11); p < 0.001 for noninferiority	0.70 (0.54–0.90)
Sotagliflozin	SCORED[67]	10,584	T2DM and Chronic kidney disease and established CV risk factors	8.3%	31%	1.3 years	Total no. of deaths from CV causes, HF hospitalizations and urgent visits for HF 0.74 (0.63–0.88); p<0.001	0.67 (0.55–0.82)

*Coprimary efficacy outcomes.

** Composite of death from cardiovascular causes or hospitalization for heart failure.

CI, confidence interval; CV, cardiovascular; CVD, cardiovascular disease; HbA1c, glycosylated haemoglobin A1c; HF, heart failure; HR, hazard ratio.

A meta-analysis of six cardiovascular and kidney outcome trials in patients with T2DM confirmed a 22% lower risk of cardiovascular death or HF hospitalization, as well as a lower risk of cardiovascular and kidney events with SGLT2 inhibitors.[68] Therefore, 2021 European Society of Cardiology guidelines for the management of acute and chronic HF and expert consensus documents recommend the use of SGLT2 inhibitors in individuals with T2DM to prevent hospitalizations for HF, major cardiovascular events, end-stage renal dysfunction, and cardiovascular death.[69,70]

Treatment of HF in patients with T2DM

Current evidence suggests that the use of disease-modifying HF medications and devices provides similar beneficial effects in patients with T2DM compared with those without T2DM.

A meta-analysis of six pivotal randomized trials of angiotensin-converting enzyme (ACE) inhibitors (enalapril, captopril, zofenopril, trandolapril) in HFrEF has demonstrated that a random effect pooled estimate of risk reduction in all-cause mortality was similar in patients with T2DM (risk reduction, 0.84) and in those without T2DM (risk reduction, 0.85).[71] Likewise, subgroup analyses of key clinical trials with angiotensin receptors blockers (ARBs) in HFrEF did not show evidence of heterogeneity in treatment effects with respect to T2DM status.[72–74] More recently, a subgroup analysis of the PARADIGM-HF trial (Prospective Comparison of ARNI With an ACE-Inhibitor to Determine Impact on Global Mortality and Morbidity in Heart Failure) demonstrated consistent treatment benefits with sacubitril/valsartan vs enalapril in patients with HFrEF, across a range of HbA1c levels and regardless of T2DM status.[36] In addition to their beneficial effects on cardiovascular outcomes, clinical trial data suggest that the use of ACE inhibitors and ARBs reduces the risk of incident T2DM in patients with HFrEF.[75,76] Likewise, in the PARADIGM-HF trial sacubitril/valsartan was associated with a greater improvement in glycaemic control compared with enalapril, as well as a greater reduction in the requirement for the initiation of insulin or glucose-lowering drugs.[77]

A meta-analysis of pivotal clinical trials with beta-blockers (bisoprolol, carvedilol, and metoprolol-succinate) in HFrEF provided pooled estimates of risk reduction in all-cause mortality of 0.65 in patients without T2DM and of 0.77 in patients with T2DM.[71] Although the relative risk reduction may have been less for patients with T2DM, because of their greater total risk of adverse outcomes, the absolute risk reduction was likely equal to or greater than in patients without T2DM.[71] Mineralocorticoid receptor antagonists have demonstrated consistent efficacy and safety in HFrEF, irrespectively of T2DM status,[78,79] even in patients at high risk of hyperkalaemia or worsening renal function.[80] Finally, ivabradine was shown to provide a similar risk reduction in cardiovascular mortality or HF hospitalization in patients with and without T2DM.[81]

Considering the beneficial effects of implantable cardioverter defibrillator (ICD), a prespecified sub-analysis of the MADIT-II trial (Multicenter Automatic Defibrillator Implantation Trial II)

suggested consistent reduction in mortality in patients with and without T2DM[82]. However, a *post hoc* sub-analysis of the SCD-HeFT trial (Sudden Cardiac Death in Heart Failure Trial) indicated that the benefit of ICD may be attenuated in individuals with T2DM, which may be a consequence of a higher all-cause increased mortality risk attributed by T2DM.[83] In addition, in clinical trials of cardiac resynchronization therapy (CRT), the overall benefit of CRT was not influenced by T2DM status.[84,85]

The most recent advance in the treatment of HF in patients with and without T2DM has come with SGLT2 inhibitors. In patients with HFrEF (LV ejection fraction ≤40%), both dapagliflozin and empagliflozin have been proven effective in improving cardiovascular outcomes with a similar effectiveness in patients with and without T2DM. In the DAPA-HF trial (Dapagliflozin in Patients with Heart Failure and Reduced Ejection Fraction), there was a 26% risk reduction in the primary composite outcome of cardiovascular mortality or HF hospitalization with dapagliflozin vs placebo and both components of the primary outcome were significantly reduced.[86] Dapagliflozin treatment also led to a 32% lower risk of new onset T2DM.[87] In the EMPEROR-Reduced, empagliflozin reduced the combined primary endpoint of cardiovascular death or HF hospitalization by 25%. Although, there was no significant reduction in cardiovascular mortality in EMPEROR-Reduced, a meta-analysis of both trials indicated a significant reduction in mortality with SGLT2 inhibition, without evidence of heterogeneity between treatments. Further clinical data have extended the evidence for the role of SGLT2 inhibitors in the treatment to HFpEF and acute HF. The SOLOIST-WHF trial (Sotagliflozin in Patients with Diabetes and Recent Worsening Heart Failure) demonstrated that in diabetic patients with a recent HF hospitalization sotagliflozin compared with placebo reduced the risk of the total number of cardiovascular deaths, hospitalizations, and urgent visits for HF treatment by 33%.[88] Similar benefits were observed with sotagliflozin in patients with LV ejection fraction <.50% and ≥.50%.[88] The EMPEROR-Preserved trial (Empagliflozin in Heart Failure with a Preserved Ejection Fraction) demonstrated a significant improvement in cardiovascular outcomes with the use of empagliflozin in patients with HFpEF (LV ejection fraction >40%).[89] Compared with placebo, the risk of cardiovascular death or HF hospitalization was reduced by 21% with empagliflozin, which was primarily driven by a significant risk reduction in HF hospitalization.[89] The treatment effects were consistent regardless of baseline LV ejection fraction and T2DM status. Most recently, in the EMPULSE trial (Empagliflozin in Patients Hospitalized for Acute Heart Failure) including patients hospitalized for acute HF (regardless of left ventricular ejection fraction), those patients treated with empagliflozin were 36% more likely to experience a clinical benefit (a composite of death, number of HF events, time to first HF event, and change in Kansas City Cardiomyopathy Questionnaire—Total Symptom Score from baseline to 90 days) compared with placebo. There was no evidence for treatment interaction in patients with and without T2DM.[90]

Advanced HF in patients with T2DM

Individuals with T2DM constitute a significant fraction of patients with advanced HF requiring long-term mechanical circulatory support (MCS) or heart transplantation. In two cohort studies of consecutive patients receiving long-term patients receiving MCS, T2DM was reported in ~40%.[91,92] Those patients had a higher prevalence of ischaemic HF aetiology and MCS was more often selected as destination therapy.[91,92] The presence of T2DM was associated with increased risk of long-term all-cause mortality and non-fatal complications.[91,92] Preoperative glycaemic control was not associated with outcomes, but following MCS implantation, a significant improvement in glycaemic control was observed.[92]

In patients with advanced HF, uncontrolled T2DM (i.e. HbA1c >7.5%) and T2DM-related end-organ damage, except for non-proliferative retinopathy, are relative contraindications for heart transplantation.[93] In selected patients with uncontrolled T2DM, MCS may be considered as a bridge to candidacy.[93] According to the US United Network of Organ Sharing database, concomitant T2DM is present in 18.1% of adult heart transplant recipients.[94] Median survival following heart transplantation was similar in patients with uncomplicated T2DM (9.3 years) and those without T2DM (10.1 years), but when stratified by disease severity, heart transplant recipients with more severe T2DM (i.e. one of more T2DM-related complications) had significantly worse survival compared to individuals without T2DM.[94] Although acute rejection and the incidence of transplant coronary artery disease were similar in patients with and without T2DM, the risk of renal failure and severe infections was higher in patients with T2DM and inversely related to the number of T2DM-related complications.[94] There is also a risk of worsening glycaemic control with the use of immunosuppressive agents.

Glycaemic targets and the choice of glucose-lowering medications in patients with HF and T2DM

Although intensive glycaemic control provides long-term benefits in the prevention of microvascular complications (retinopathy, nephropathy, and peripheral neuropathy), it was not proven effective in reducing the risk of HF or cardiovascular mortality in patients with T2DM. A meta-analysis of eight clinical trials, with a total of 37,229 patients with T2DM, did not show a significant difference in the risk of HF between intensive glycaemic control and standard of care treatment.[95] Observational data suggest that in patients with HF receiving glucose-lowering medications, the association between glycaemic control (i.e. HgA1c levels) and mortality appears to be U-shaped,[96] with the lowest mortality risk associated with modest glycaemic control (i.e. HbA1c levels 7.0–7.9%).

More recently, a focus has been put on cardiovascular outcomes and the associated risk of HF with several glucose-lowering medications (dipeptidyl peptidase-4 (DPP4) inhibitors, glucagon like peptide-1 receptor agonists (GLP-1 RA), and SGLT2 inhibitors).

DPP-4 inhibitors demonstrated non-inferiority compared with placebo with respect to cardiovascular outcomes, but a concern has been raised about a significantly higher risk of HF hospitalizations with saxagliptin,[97] a non-significant increase in HF risk with alogliptin[98] (Table 12.8.2), as well as a non-significant increase in mortality with vildagliptin in a small trial of patients with T2DM and HFrEF.[99]

GLP-1 RA proved to be effective in reducing cardiovascular outcomes and likely have a neutral effect on the risk of HF in the general population of patients with T2DM (Table 12.8.3). However, in two small, randomized trials of patients with HFrEF, the use of liraglutide led to more adverse CV events compared with placebo,[100,101] which raised a safety issue for patients with HF.

Although SGLT2 inhibitors had a varied effect on cardiovascular outcomes depending on the study medication and patient characteristics, all SGLT2 inhibitors have proven effective in reducing the risk of HF hospitalization in their respective trials, regardless of CV risk burden or a history of HF (Table 12.8.1).

Possible risks and recommendations on the use of DPP4 inhibitors, GLP-1 RA, SGLT2 inhibitors and other glucose lowering medications for the treatment of T2DM in patients with HF are summarized in Table 12.8.4.4.

Table 12.8.2 Risk of HF hospitalization associated with the use of PDD4 inhibitors compared with placebo in the pivotal cardiovascular outcome trials

Medication	Trial	Patients, n	Patient characteristics	HbA$_{ic}$ (mean)	History of HF	Follow-up (mean or median)	HF hospitalization (HR, 95% CI)a	P-value
Saxagliptin	SAVOR-TIMI 53[97,104]*	16,492	Established CVD; multiple CV risk factors	8.0%	2105 (13%)	2.1 years	1.27 (1.07–1.51)	0.007
Alogliptin	EXAMINE[98]	5380	Recent acute coronary syndrome	8.0%	1533 (28%)	1.5 years	1.07 (0.79–1.46)	0.66
Sitagliptin	TECOS[105]	14,671	Established CVD	7.2%	2643 (18%)	3 years	1.00 (0.83–1.20)	0.98
Linagliptin	CARMELINA[106]	6991	High CV and renal risk	7.9%	1876 (27%)	2.2 years	0.90 (0.74–1.08)	0.26

CI, confidence interval; CV, cardiovascular; CVD, cardiovascular disease; HbA$_1$, glycated haemoglobin; HF, heart failure; HR, hazard ratio. *Treatment vs. placebo.

Seferović PM, Coats AJS, Ponikowski P, et al. European Society of Cardiology/Heart Failure Association position paper on the role and safety of new glucose-lowering drugs in patients with heart failure. Eur J Heart Fail. 2020 Feb;22(2):196-213. doi: 10.1002/ejhf.1673. (C) European Society of Cardiology reproduced by Oxford University Press.

Table 12.8.3 Risk of HF hospitalization associated with the use of GLP1 RA inhibitors compared with placebo in the pivotal cardiovascular outcome trials.

Medication	Trial	Patients, n	Patient characteristics	HbA₁c (mean)	History of HF	Follow-up (mean or median)	HF hospitalization (HR, 95% CI)*	P-value
Lixisenatide	ELIXA	6068	Recent acute coronary syndrome	~7.7%	1358 (22%)	2.1 years	0.96 (0.75–1.23)	0.75
Liraglutide	LEADER	9340	Age > 50 years and established CVD Age > 60 years and CV risk factors	8.7%	1667 (18%)	3.8 years	0.87 (0.73–1.05)	0.14
Semaglutide (subcutaneous)	SUSTAIN-6	3297	Age > 50 years and established CVD Age ≥ 60 years and CV risk factors	8.7%	777 (24%)	2.1 years	1.11 (0.77–1.61)	0.57
Semaglutide (oral)	PIONEER 6'	3183	Age > 50 years and established CVD; Age ≥ 60 years and CV risk factors	8.2%	388 (12%)	1.3 years	0.86 (0.48–1.55)	-
Exenatide	EXSCEL	14,752	Established CVD (73%) CV risk factors (37%)	8.0%	2389 (16%)	3.2 years	0.94 (0.78–1.13)	-
Albiglutide	Harmony Outcome	9463	Established CVD	~8.7%	1922 (20%)	1.5 years	0.85 (0.70–1.04)†	0.11
Dulaglutide	REWIND	9901	Established CVD (31.5%) CV risk factors (68.5%)	~7.3%	853 (8.6%)	5.4 years	0.93 (0.77–1.12) ‡	0.46

CI, confidence interval; CV, cardiovascular; CVD, cardiovascular disease; HbA₁c, glycated haemoglobin; HF, heart failure; HR, hazard ratio.

*Treatment vs placebo; †A composite of CV death or HF hospitalization.

‡HF hospitalization or urgent HF visit.

Seferović PM, Coats AJS, Ponikowski P, et al. European Society of Cardiology/Heart Failure Association position paper on the role and safety of new glucose-lowering drugs in patients with heart failure. *Eur J Heart Fail*. 2020 Feb;22(2):196-213. doi: 10.1002/ejhf.1673. (C) European Society of Cardiology reproduced by Oxford University Press.

Table 12.8.4 Risks, precautions, and recommendations for the use of glucose-lowering medications in accordance with the 2021 ESC Guidelines for the diagnosis and treatment of acute and chronic heart failure

Medication	Risks and cautions	Recommendations for use
DPP4 inhibitors	Increase risk of HF hospitalization with saxagliptin.	Not recommended to reduce cardiovascular events in patients with HF
GLP-1 RA	May be associated with increased risk of adverse events in HFrEF (liraglutide)	Not recommended to prevent HF events in patients with HF
SGLT2 inhibitors	Consistently lower risk of HF hospitalization	Recommended to prevent hospitalizations for HF, major cardiovascular events, end-stage renal dysfunction, and cardiovascular death
Metformin	Increased risk of lactic acidosis in patients with eGFR <30 mL/min/1.73m^2 or hepatic impairment	Generally safe to be used in patients with HF except in patients with renal and liver impairment
Sulfonylurea drugs	The risk of HF exacerbation may be increased Increased risk of hypoglycaemia	They are not a preferred treatment in patients with HF and, if needed, patients should be monitored for evidence of worsening of HF
Thiazolidinediones	Documented higher risk of HF hospitalization	Contraindicated in patients with HF
Insulin	May be associated with fluid retention and weight gain Increased risk of hypoglycaemia The higher risk of HF exacerbation may be increased	Insulin therapy is indicated in patients with type 1 diabetes and for the control of hyperglycaemia in some patients with T2DM with monitoring of signs of worsening HF

DPP4, dipeptidyl peptidase-4; eGFR, estimated glomerular filtration rate; GLP1-RA, glucagon like peptide-1 receptor agonists; HF, heart failure; SGLT2, sodium-glucose cotransporter 2; T2DM, type 2 diabetes mellitus.
Source data from McDonagh TA, Metra M, Adamo M, et al; ESC Scientific Document Group. 2021 ESC Guidelines for the diagnosis and treatment of acute and chronic heart failure. *Eur Heart J.* 2021 Sep 21;42(36):3599-3726. doi: 10.1093/eurheartj/ehab368

Lifestyle modifications and multidisciplinary approach

Patients with T2DM and HF often face the burden of physical inactivity, poor dietary habits, and obesity. Clinical trial evidence suggests that exercise training is safe in patients with HFrEF and T2DM and associated with greater improvement in exercise capacity compared with standard care, despite worse baseline functional status and lesser adherence.[102] Promoting healthy lifestyle changes, improving dietary habits, smoking cessation, and maintenance of heathy body weight may be beneficial in patients with HF and T2DM. Furthermore, education of patients and family members and empowerment for self-care are important treatment goals. Given the complexity of disease management, particularly in patients with multiple glucose-lowering agents, comorbidities (e.g. chronic kidney disease), poor health status, frailty, and/or cognitive impairment, there is a requirement for a multidisciplinary approach including a collaboration between multiple specialists (cardiologists/HF specialist, endocrinologists/diabetologists, nephrologists, primary care physicians, pharmacists, trained nurses, and many others).[103]

Future directions

Although a significant progress has occurred in the understanding of the bidirectional relationship between T2DM and HF, the mechanisms underlying this relationship remain insufficiently elucidated. Advancing knowledge of the fundamental mechanisms is critical for the development of novel targeted treatment options and an informed approach to use of the existing drugs and their impact on disease progression. Given the growing burden of both of T2DM and HF, it is of great significance to develop effective strategies for the prevention of HF in patients with T2DM, as exemplified by the promising results with SGLT2 inhibitors. On the other hand, more attention needs to be focused on the recognition of pre-diabetes and undiagnosed diabetes in patients with HF in order to mitigate their adverse prognostic impact. Also, there is a need to develop evidence-based multidisciplinary team care of patients with HF and T2DM to provide the more comprehensive management and support.

References

1. Groenewegen A, Rutten FH, Mosterd A, Hoes AW. Epidemiology of heart failure. Eur J Heart Fail. 2020;22(8):1342–56.
2. Federation ID. IDF Diabetes Atlas, 10th edn. Brussels, Belgium: International Diabetes Federation. 2021.
3. Seferović PM, Vardas P, Jankowska EA, Maggioni AP, Timmis A, Milinković I, et al. The Heart Failure Association Atlas: Heart Failure Epidemiology and Management Statistics 2019. Eur J Heart Fail. 2021;23(6):906–14.
4. He J, Ogden LG, Bazzano LA, Vupputuri S, Loria C, Whelton PK. Risk factors for congestive heart failure in US men and women: NHANES I epidemiologic follow-up study. Arch Intern Med. 2001;161(7):996–1002.
5. Shah AD, Langenberg C, Rapsomaniki E, Denaxas S, Pujades-Rodriguez M, Gale CP, et al. Type 2 diabetes and incidence of cardiovascular diseases: a cohort study in 1·9 million people. Lancet Diabetes Endocrinol. 2015;3(2):105–13.
6. Matsushita K, Blecker S, Pazin-Filho A, Bertoni A, Chang PP, Coresh J, et al. The association of hemoglobin a1c with incident heart failure among people without diabetes: the atherosclerosis risk in communities study. Diabetes. 2010;59(8):2020–6.
7. Iribarren C, Karter AJ, Go AS, Ferrara A, Liu JY, Sidney S, et al. Glycemic control and heart failure among adult patients with diabetes. Circulation. 2001;103(22):2668–73.
8. Shindler DM, Kostis JB, Yusuf S, Quinones MA, Pitt B, Stewart D, et al. Diabetes mellitus, a predictor of morbidity and mortality in the Studies of Left Ventricular Dysfunction (SOLVD) Trials and Registry. Am J Cardiol. 1996;77(11):1017–20.

9. Bozkurt B, Coats AJS, Tsutsui H, Abdelhamid CM, Adamopoulos S, Albert N, et al. Universal definition and classification of heart failure: a report of the Heart Failure Society of America, Heart Failure Association of the European Society of Cardiology, Japanese Heart Failure Society and Writing Committee of the Universal Definition of Heart Failure: Endorsed by the Canadian Heart Failure Society, Heart Failure Association of India, Cardiac Society of Australia and New Zealand, and Chinese Heart Failure Association. Eur J Heart Fail. 2021;23(3):352–80.

10. Boonman-de Winter LJ, Rutten FH, Cramer MJ, Landman MJ, Liem AH, Rutten GE, et al. High prevalence of previously unknown heart failure and left ventricular dysfunction in patients with type 2 diabetes. Diabetologia. 2012;55(8):2154–62.

11. Nichols GA, Hillier TA, Erbey JR, Brown JB. Congestive heart failure in type 2 diabetes: prevalence, incidence, and risk factors. Diabetes Care. 2001;24(9):1614–19.

12. Pfeffer MA, Swedberg K, Granger CB, Held P, McMurray JJ, Michelson EL, et al. Effects of candesartan on mortality and morbidity in patients with chronic heart failure: the CHARM-Overall programme. Lancet. 2003;362(9386):759–66.

13. Pitt B, Pfeffer MA, Assmann SF, Boineau R, Anand IS, Claggett B, et al. Spironolactone for heart failure with preserved ejection fraction. N Engl J Med. 2014;370(15):1383–92.

14. Kristensen SL, Mogensen UM, Jhund PS, Petrie MC, Preiss D, Win S, et al. Clinical and echocardiographic characteristics and cardiovascular outcomes according to diabetes status in patients with heart failure and preserved ejection fraction: A report from the I-Preserve trial (Irbesartan in Heart Failure With Preserved Ejection Fraction). Circulation. 2017;135(8):724–35.

15. Solomon SD, McMurray JJV, Anand IS, Ge J, Lam CSP, Maggioni AP, et al. Angiotensin–neprilysin inhibition in heart failure with preserved ejection fraction. N Engl J Med. 2019;381(17):1609–20.

16. McMurray JJ, Packer M, Desai AS, Gong J, Lefkowitz MP, Rizkala AR, et al. Angiotensin-neprilysin inhibition versus enalapril in heart failure. N Engl J Med. 2014;371(11):993–1004.

17. McMurray JJ, Ostergren J, Swedberg K, Granger CB, Held P, Michelson EL, et al. Effects of candesartan in patients with chronic heart failure and reduced left-ventricular systolic function taking angiotensin-converting-enzyme inhibitors: the CHARM-Added trial. Lancet. 2003;362(9386):767–71.

18. Yusuf S, Pitt B, Davis CE, Hood WB, Cohn JN. Effect of enalapril on survival in patients with reduced left ventricular ejection fractions and congestive heart failure. N Engl J Med. 1991;325(5):293–302.

19. Sarma S, Mentz RJ, Kwasny MJ, Fought AJ, Huffman M, Subacius H, et al. Association between diabetes mellitus and post-discharge outcomes in patients hospitalized with heart failure: findings from the EVEREST trial. Eur J Heart Fail. 2013;15(2):194–202.

20. Packer M, O'Connor C, McMurray JJV, Wittes J, Abraham WT, Anker SD, et al. Effect of ularitide on cardiovascular mortality in acute heart failure. N Engl J Med. 2017;376(20):1956–64.

21. Echouffo-Tcheugui JB, Xu H, DeVore AD, Schulte PJ, Butler J, Yancy CW, et al. Temporal trends and factors associated with diabetes mellitus among patients hospitalized with heart failure: Findings from Get With The Guidelines-Heart Failure registry. Amer Heart J. 2016;182:9–20.

22. Kristensen SL, Jhund PS, Lee MMY, Køber L, Solomon SD, Granger CB, et al. Prevalence of prediabetes and undiagnosed diabetes in patients with HFpEF and HFrEF and associated clinical outcomes. Cardiovasc Drugs Ther. 2017;31(5–6):545–9.

23. Chioncel O, Lainscak M, Seferovic PM, Anker SD, Crespo-Leiro MG, Harjola VP, et al. Epidemiology and one-year outcomes in patients with chronic heart failure and preserved, mid-range and reduced ejection fraction: an analysis of the ESC Heart Failure Long-Term Registry. Eur J Heart Fail. 2017;19(12):1574–85.

24. Tromp J, Bamadhaj S, Cleland JGF, Angermann CE, Dahlstrom U, Ouwerkerk W, et al. Post-discharge prognosis of patients admitted to hospital for heart failure by world region, and national level of income and income disparity (REPORT-HF): a cohort study. Lancet Glob Health. 2020;8(3):e411–22.

25. Tromp J, Claggett BL, Liu J, Jackson AM, Jhund PS, Køber L, et al. Global differences in heart failure with preserved ejection fraction: The PARAGON-HF trial. Circ Heart Fail. 2021;14(4):e007901.

26. Bank IEM, Gijsberts CM, Teng TK, Benson L, Sim D, Yeo PSD, et al. Prevalence and Clinical Significance of Diabetes in Asian Versus White Patients With Heart Failure. JACC Heart Fail. 2017;5(1):14–24.

27. Damasceno A, Mayosi BM, Sani M, Ogah OS, Mondo C, Ojji D, et al. the causes, treatment, and outcome of acute heart failure in 1006 Africans from 9 countries: results of the Sub-Saharan Africa survey of heart failure. Archives of Internal Medicine. 2012;172(18):1386–94.

28. Parissis JT, Ikonomidis I, Rafouli-Stergiou P, Mebazaa A, Delgado J, Farmakis D, et al. Clinical characteristics and predictors of in-hospital mortality in acute heart failure with preserved left ventricular ejection fraction. Am J Cardiol. 2011;107(1):79–84.

29. Targher G, Dauriz M, Laroche C, Temporelli PL, Hassanein M, Seferovic PM, et al. In-hospital and 1-year mortality associated with diabetes in patients with acute heart failure: results from the ESC-HFA Heart Failure Long-Term Registry. Eur J Heart Fail. 2017;19(1):54–65.

30. Kong MG, Jang SY, Jang J, Cho H-J, Lee S, Lee SE, et al. Impact of diabetes mellitus on mortality in patients with acute heart failure: a prospective cohort study. Cardiovasc Diabetol. 2020;19(1):49.

31. Dauriz M, Targher G, Laroche C, Temporelli PL, Ferrari R, Anker S, et al. Association between diabetes and 1-year adverse clinical outcomes in a multinational cohort of ambulatory patients with chronic heart failure: results from the ESC-HFA Heart Failure Long-Term Registry. Diabetes Care. 2017;40(5):671–8.

32. Johansson I, Edner M, Dahlström U, Näsman P, Rydén L, Norhammar A. Is the prognosis in patients with diabetes and heart failure a matter of unsatisfactory management? An observational study from the Swedish Heart Failure Registry. Eur J Heart Fail. 2014;16(4):409–18.

33. Cubbon RM, Adams B, Rajwani A, Mercer BN, Patel PA, Gherardi G, et al. Diabetes mellitus is associated with adverse prognosis in chronic heart failure of ischaemic and non-ischaemic aetiology. Diab Vasc Dis Res. 2013;10(4):330–6.

34. Pavlović A, Polovina M, Ristić A, Seferović JP, Veljić I, Simeunović D, et al. Long-term mortality is increased in patients with undetected prediabetes and type-2 diabetes hospitalized for worsening heart failure and reduced ejection fraction. Eur J Prev Cardiol. 2019;26(1):72–82.

35. MacDonald MR, Petrie MC, Varyani F, Ostergren J, Michelson EL, Young JB, et al. Impact of diabetes on outcomes in patients with low and preserved ejection fraction heart failure: an analysis of the Candesartan in Heart failure: Assessment of Reduction in Mortality and morbidity (CHARM) programme. Eur Heart J. 2008;29(11):1377–85.

36. Kristensen SL, Preiss D, Jhund PS, Squire I, Cardoso JS, Merkely B, et al. Risk related to pre-diabetes mellitus and diabetes mellitus in heart failure with reduced ejection fraction: insights from prospective comparison of ARNI with ACEI to determine impact on global mortality and morbidity in heart failure trial. Circ Heart Fail. 2016;9: e002560.

37. Lindman BR, Dávila-Román VG, Mann DL, McNulty S, Semigran MJ, Lewis GD, et al. Cardiovascular phenotype in HFpEF patients with or without diabetes: a RELAX trial ancillary study. J Am Coll Cardiol. 2014;64(6):541–9.

38. Jackson AM, Rørth R, Liu J, Kristensen SL, Anand IS, Claggett BL, et al. Diabetes and pre-diabetes in patients with heart failure and preserved ejection fraction. Eur J Heart Fail. 2022;24:497–509.

39. Seferović PM, Paulus WJ. Clinical diabetic cardiomyopathy: a two-faced disease with restrictive and dilated phenotypes. Eur Heart J. 2015;36(27):1718–27.

40. Marwick TH, Ritchie R, Shaw JE, Kaye D. Implications of underlying mechanisms for the recognition and management of diabetic cardiomyopathy. J Am Coll Cardiol. 2018;71(3):339–51.

41. Polovina M, Lund LH, Đikić D, Petrović-Đorđević I, Krljanac G, Milinković I, et al. Type 2 diabetes increases the long-term risk of heart failure and mortality in patients with atrial fibrillation. Eur J Heart Fail. 2020;22(1):113–25.

42. Goh SY, Cooper ME. Clinical review: The role of advanced glycation end products in progression and complications of diabetes. J Clin Endocrinol Metab. 2008;93(4):1143–52.

43. Hegab Z, Gibbons S, Neyses L, Mamas MA. Role of advanced glycation end products in cardiovascular disease. World J Cardiol. 2012;4(4):90–102.

44. Huynh K, Bernardo BC, McMullen JR, Ritchie RH. Diabetic cardiomyopathy: mechanisms and new treatment strategies targeting antioxidant signaling pathways. Pharmacol Ther. 2014;142(3):375–415.

45. Basta G, Schmidt AM, De Caterina R. Advanced glycation end products and vascular inflammation: implications for accelerated atherosclerosis in diabetes. Cardiovasc Res. 2004;63(4):582–92.

46. Amaral N, Okonko DO. Metabolic abnormalities of the heart in type II diabetes. Diab Vasc Dis Res. 2015;12(4):239–48.

47. Bayeva M, Sawicki KT, Ardehali H. Taking diabetes to heart–deregulation of myocardial lipid metabolism in diabetic cardiomyopathy. J Am Heart Assoc. 2013;2(6):e000433.

48. Montaigne D, Marechal X, Coisne A, Debry N, Modine T, Fayad G, et al. Myocardial contractile dysfunction is associated with impaired mitochondrial function and dynamics in type 2 diabetic but not in obese patients. Circulation. 2014;130(7):554–64.

49. McGavock JM, Lingvay I, Zib I, Tillery T, Salas N, Unger R, et al. Cardiac steatosis in diabetes mellitus: a 1H-magnetic resonance spectroscopy study. Circulation. 2007;116(10):1170–5.

50. Poornima IG, Parikh P, Shannon RP. Diabetic cardiomyopathy: the search for a unifying hypothesis. Circ Res. 2006;98(5):596–605.

51. Krüger M, Babicz K, von Frieling-Salewsky M, Linke WA. Insulin signaling regulates cardiac titin properties in heart development and diabetic cardiomyopathy. J Mol Cell Cardiol. 2010;48(5):910–6.

52. Hopf AE, Andresen C, Kötter S, Isić M, Ulrich K, Sahin S, et al. Diabetes-induced cardiomyocyte passive stiffening is caused by impaired insulin-dependent titin modification and can be modulated by neuregulin-1. Circ Res. 2018;123(3):342–55.

53. Tabit CE, Chung WB, Hamburg NM, Vita JA. Endothelial dysfunction in diabetes mellitus: molecular mechanisms and clinical implications. Rev Endocr Metab Disord. 2010;11(1):61–74.

54. Heerspink HJ, Perkins BA, Fitchett DH, Husain M, Cherney DZ. Sodium glucose cotransporter 2 inhibitors in the treatment of diabetes mellitus: cardiovascular and kidney effects, potential mechanisms, and clinical applications. Circulation. 2016;134(10):752–72.

55. Obokata M, Reddy YNV, Pislaru SV, Melenovsky V, Borlaug BA. Evidence supporting the existence of a distinct obese phenotype of heart failure with preserved ejection fraction. Circulation. 2017;136(1):6–19.

56. Lambers Heerspink HJ, de Zeeuw D, Wie L, Leslie B, List J. Dapagliflozin a glucose-regulating drug with diuretic properties in subjects with type 2 diabetes. Diabetes Obes Metab. 2013;15(9):853–62.

57. Inzucchi SE, Zinman B, Fitchett D, Wanner C, Ferrannini E, Schumacher M, et al. How does empagliflozin reduce cardiovascular mortality? insights from a mediation analysis of the EMPA-REG OUTCOME trial. Diabetes Care. 2018;41(2):356–63.

58. Filippatos TD, Liontos A, Papakitsou I, Elisaf MS. SGLT2 inhibitors and cardioprotection: a matter of debate and multiple hypotheses. Postgrad Med. 2019;131(2):82–8.

59. Oelze M, Kröller-Schön S, Welschof P, Jansen T, Hausding M, Mikhed Y, et al. The sodium-glucose co-transporter 2 inhibitor empagliflozin improves diabetes-induced vascular dysfunction in the streptozotocin diabetes rat model by interfering with oxidative stress and glucotoxicity. PLoS One. 2014;9(11):e112394.

60. Palmiero G, Cesaro A, Vetrano E, Pafundi PC, Galiero R, Caturano A, et al. Impact of SGLT2 Inhibitors on Heart Failure: From Pathophysiology to Clinical Effects. Int J Mol Sci. 2021;22(11):5863.

61. Zinman B, Wanner C, Lachin JM, Fitchett D, Bluhmki E, Hantel S, et al. Empagliflozin, cardiovascular outcomes, and mortality in type 2 diabetes. N Engl J Med.. 2015;373(22):2117–28.

62. Neal B, Perkovic V, Mahaffey KW, de Zeeuw D, Fulcher G, Erondu N, et al. Canagliflozin and cardiovascular and renal events in type 2 diabetes. N Engl J Med. 2017;377(7):644–57.

63. Wiviott SD, Raz I, Bonaca MP, Mosenzon O, Kato ET, Cahn A, et al. Dapagliflozin and cardiovascular outcomes in type 2 diabetes. N Engl J Med. 2019;380(4):347–57.

64. Cannon CP, Pratley R, Dagogo-Jack S, Mancuso J, Huyck S, Masiukiewicz U, et al. Cardiovascular outcomes with ertugliflozin in type 2 diabetes. N Engl J Med. 2020;383(15):1425–35.

65. Perkovic V, Jardine MJ, Neal B, Bompoint S, Heerspink HJL, Charytan DM, et al. Canagliflozin and renal outcomes in type 2 diabetes and nephropathy. N Engl J Med. 2019;380(24):2295–306.

66. Heerspink HJL, Stefánsson BV, Correa-Rotter R, Chertow GM, Greene T, Hou FF, et al. Dapagliflozin in patients with chronic kidney disease. N Engl J Med. 2020;383(15):1436–46.

67. Bhatt DL, Szarek M, Pitt B, Cannon CP, Leiter LA, McGuire DK, et al. Sotagliflozin in patients with diabetes and chronic kidney disease. N Engl J Med. 2020;384(2):129–39.

68. McGuire DK, Shih WJ, Cosentino F, Charbonnel B, Cherney DZI, Dagogo-Jack S, et al. Association of SGLT2 inhibitors with cardiovascular and kidney outcomes in patients with type 2 diabetes: a meta-analysis. JAMA Cardiology. 2021;6(2):148–58.

69. McDonagh TA, Metra M, Adamo M, Gardner RS, Baumbach A, Böhm M, et al. 2021 ESC Guidelines for the diagnosis and treatment of acute and chronic heart failure. Eur Heart J. 2021;42(36):3599–726.

70. Seferović PM, Fragasso G, Petrie M, Mullens W, Ferrari R, Thum T, et al. Heart Failure Association of the European Society of Cardiology update on sodium-glucose co-transporter 2 inhibitors in heart failure. Eur J Heart Fail. 2020;22(11):1984–6.

71. Shekelle PG, Rich MW, Morton SC, Atkinson CS, Tu W, Maglione M, et al. Efficacy of angiotensin-converting enzyme inhibitors and beta-blockers in the management of left ventricular systolic dysfunction according to race, gender, and diabetic status: a meta-analysis of major clinical trials. J Am Coll Cardiol. 2003;41(9):1529–38.

72. MacDonald MR, Petrie MC, Varyani F, Östergren J, Michelson EL, Young JB, et al. Impact of diabetes on outcomes in patients with low and preserved ejection fraction heart failure: An analysis of the Candesartan in Heart failure: Assessment of Reduction in Mortality and morbidity (CHARM) programme. Eur Heart J. 2008;29(11):1377–85.

73. Cohn JN, Tognoni G. A randomized trial of the angiotensin-receptor blocker valsartan in chronic heart failure. N Engl J Med. 2001;345(23):1667–75.

74. Konstam MA, Neaton JD, Dickstein K, Drexler H, Komajda M, Martinez FA, et al. Effects of high-dose versus low-dose losartan on clinical outcomes in patients with heart failure (HEAAL study): a randomised, double-blind trial. Lancet. 2009;374(9704):1840–8.

75. Yusuf S, Ostergren JB, Gerstein HC, Pfeffer MA, Swedberg K, Granger CB, et al. Effects of candesartan on the development of a new diagnosis of diabetes mellitus in patients with heart failure. Circulation. 2005;112(1):48–53.

76. Vermes E, Ducharme A, Bourassa MG, Lessard M, White M, Tardif JC. Enalapril reduces the incidence of diabetes in patients with

chronic heart failure: insight from the Studies Of Left Ventricular Dysfunction (SOLVD). Circulation. 2003;107(9):1291–6.

77. Seferovic JP, Claggett B, Seidelmann SB, Seely EW, Packer M, Zile MR, et al. Effect of sacubitril/valsartan versus enalapril on glycaemic control in patients with heart failure and diabetes: a post-hoc analysis from the PARADIGM-HF trial. Lancet Diabetes Endocrinol. 2017;5(5):333–40.

78. Pitt B, Zannad F, Remme WJ, Cody R, Castaigne A, Perez A, et al. The effect of spironolactone on morbidity and mortality in patients with severe heart failure. Randomized Aldactone Evaluation Study Investigators. N Engl J Med. 1999;341(10):709–17.

79. Zannad F, McMurray JJ, Krum H, van Veldhuisen DJ, Swedberg K, Shi H, et al. Eplerenone in patients with systolic heart failure and mild symptoms. N Engl J Med. 2011;364(1):11–21.

80. Eschalier R, McMurray JJ, Swedberg K, van Veldhuisen DJ, Krum H, Pocock SJ, et al. Safety and efficacy of eplerenone in patients at high risk for hyperkalemia and/or worsening renal function: analyses of the EMPHASIS-HF study subgroups (Eplerenone in Mild Patients Hospitalization And SurvIval Study in Heart Failure). J Am Coll Cardiol. 2013;62(17):1585–93.

81. Komajda M, Tavazzi L, Francq BG, Böhm M, Borer JS, Ford I, et al. Efficacy and safety of ivabradine in patients with chronic systolic heart failure and diabetes: an analysis from the SHIFT trial. Eur J Heart Fail. 2015;17(12):1294–301.

82. Wittenberg SM, Cook JR, Hall WJ, McNitt S, Zareba W, Moss AJ. Comparison of efficacy of implanted cardioverter-defibrillator in patients with versus without diabetes mellitus. Am J Cardiol. 2005;96(3):417–9.

83. Bardy GH, Lee KL, Mark DB, Poole JE, Packer DL, Boineau R, et al. Amiodarone or an implantable cardioverter-defibrillator for congestive heart failure. N Engl J Med. 2005;352(3):225–37.

84. Ghali JK, Boehmer J, Feldman AM, Saxon LA, Demarco T, Carson P, et al. Influence of diabetes on cardiac resynchronization therapy with or without defibrillator in patients with advanced heart failure. J Card Fail. 2007;13(9):769–73.

85. Moss AJ, Hall WJ, Cannom DS, Klein H, Brown MW, Daubert JP, et al. Cardiac-resynchronization therapy for the prevention of heart-failure events. N Engl J Med. 2009;361(14):1329–38.

86. McMurray JJV, Solomon SD, Inzucchi SE, Køber L, Kosiborod MN, Martinez FA, et al. Dapagliflozin in patients with heart failure and reduced ejection fraction. N Engl J Med. 2019;381(21):1995–2008.

87. Inzucchi SE, Docherty KF, Køber L, Kosiborod MN, Martinez FA, Ponikowski P, et al. Dapagliflozin and the incidence of type 2 diabetes in patients with heart failure and reduced ejection fraction: an exploratory analysis from DAPA-HF. Diabetes Care. 2021;44(2):586–94.

88. Bhatt DL, Szarek M, Steg PG, Cannon CP, Leiter LA, McGuire DK, et al. Sotagliflozin in patients with diabetes and recent worsening heart failure. N Engl J Med. 2020;384(2):117–28.

89. Anker SD, Butler J, Filippatos G, Ferreira JP, Bocchi E, Böhm M, et al. Empagliflozin in heart failure with a preserved ejection fraction N Engl J Med. 2021;85(16):1451–1461.

90. Voors AA, Angermann CE, Teerlink JR, Collins SP, Kosiborod M, Biegus J, et al. The SGLT2 inhibitor empagliflozin in patients hospitalized for acute heart failure: a multinational randomized trial. Nature Medicine. 2022;28(3):568–74.

91. Vest AR, Mistak SM, Hachamovitch R, Mountis MM, Moazami N, Young JB. Outcomes for patients with diabetes after continuous-flow left ventricular assist device implantation. J Card Fail. 2016;22(10):789–96.

92. Asleh R, Briasoulis A, Schettle SD, Tchantchaleishvili V, Pereira NL, Edwards BS, et al. Impact of diabetes mellitus on outcomes in

patients supported with left ventricular assist devices. Circ Heart Fail. 2017;10(11):e004213.

93. Mehra MR, Canter CE, Hannan MM, Semigran MJ, Uber PA, Baran DA, et al. The 2016 International Society for Heart Lung Transplantation listing criteria for heart transplantation: A 10-year update. J Heart Lung Transplant. 2016;35(1):1–23.

94. Russo MJ, Chen JM, Hong KN, Stewart AS, Ascheim DD, Argenziano M, et al. Survival after heart transplantation is not diminished among recipients with uncomplicated diabetes mellitus. Circulation. 2006;114(21):2280–7.

95. Castagno D, Baird-Gunning J, Jhund PS, Biondi-Zoccai G, MacDonald MR, Petrie MC, et al. Intensive glycemic control has no impact on the risk of heart failure in type 2 diabetic patients: evidence from a 37,229 patient meta-analysis. Am Heart J. 2011;162(5):938–48.e2.

96. Lawson CA, Jones PW, Teece L, Dunbar SB, Seferovic PM, Khunti K, et al. association between type 2 diabetes and all-cause hospitalization and mortality in the uk general heart failure population: stratification by diabetic glycemic control and medication intensification. JACC Heart Fail. 2018;6(1):18–26.

97. Scirica BM, Braunwald E, Raz I, Cavender MA, Morrow DA, Jarolim P, et al. Heart failure, saxagliptin, and diabetes mellitus: observations from the SAVOR-TIMI 53 randomized trial. Circulation. 2014;130(18):1579–88.

98. Zannad F, Cannon CP, Cushman WC, Bakris GL, Menon V, Perez AT, et al. Heart failure and mortality outcomes in patients with type 2 diabetes taking alogliptin versus placebo in EXAMINE: a multicentre, randomised, double-blind trial. Lancet. 2015;385(9982):2067–76.

99. McMurray JJV, Ponikowski P, Bolli GB, Lukashevich V, Kozlovski P, Kothny W, et al. Effects of vildagliptin on ventricular function in patients with type 2 diabetes mellitus and heart failure: a randomized placebo-controlled trial. JACC Heart Fail. 2018;6(1):8–17.

100. Jorsal A, Kistorp C, Holmager P, Tougaard RS, Nielsen R, Hänselmann A, et al. Effect of liraglutide, a glucagon-like peptide-1 analogue, on left ventricular function in stable chronic heart failure patients with and without diabetes (LIVE)-a multicentre, double-blind, randomised, placebo-controlled trial. Eur J Heart Fail. 2017;19(1):69–77.

101. Margulies KB, Hernandez AF, Redfield MM, Givertz MM, Oliveira GH, Cole R, et al. Effects of liraglutide on clinical stability among patients with advanced heart failure and reduced ejection fraction: a randomized clinical trial. JAMA. 2016;316(5):500–8.

102. Banks AZ, Mentz RJ, Stebbins A, Mikus CR, Schulte PJ, Fleg JL, et al. Response to exercise training and outcomes in patients with heart failure and diabetes mellitus: insights from the HF-ACTION trial. J Card Fail. 2016;22(7):485–91.

103. Seferović PM, Coats AJS, Ponikowski P, Filippatos G, Huelsmann M, Jhund PS, et al. European Society of Cardiology/Heart Failure Association position paper on the role and safety of new glucose-lowering drugs in patients with heart failure. Eur J Heart Fail. 2020;22(2):196–213.

104. Scirica BM, Bhatt DL, Braunwald E, Steg PG, Davidson J, Hirshberg B, et al.; SAVOR-TIMI 53 Steering Committee and Investigators. Saxagliptin and cardiovascular outcomes in patients with type 2 diabetes mellitus. N Engl J Med. 2013;369:1317–1326.

105. Green JB, Bethel MA, Armstrong PW, Buse JB, Engel SS, Garg J, et al.; TECOS Study Group. Effect of sitagliptin on cardiovascular outcomes in type 2 diabetes. N Engl J Med.2015;373:232–242.

106. Rosenstock J, Perkovic V, Johansen OE, Cooper ME, Kahn SE, Marx N, et al.; CARMELINA Investigators. Effect of inagliptin vs placebo on major cardiovascular events in adults with type 2 diabetes and high cardiovascular and renal risk: the CARMELINA randomized clinical trial. JAMA. 2019;321:69–79.

CHAPTER 12.9

Heart failure in systemic immune-mediated diseases

Giacomo De Luca, Luca Moroni, Alessandro Tomelleri, Renzo Marcolongo, Lorenzo Dagna, Alida LP Caforio, and Marco Matucci-Cerinic

Contents

Introduction

Patients with systemic rheumatic diseases have an increased risk of developing cardiovascular complications.[1] These include vascular damage with accelerated atherosclerosis, myocardial and pericardial involvement, valvular abnormalities, arrhythmia, and heart failure (HF). The high risk of cardiovascular pathology is primarily due to chronic inflammation and autoimmunity.[1]

The prevalence of HF is high since it represents the final result of various pathogenic mechanisms, related to a chronic proinflammatory state. Increased concentration of inflammatory cytokines (IL-1b, IL-6, TNF-a) correlates with the NYHA functional class in HF patients, acts as a direct cardiodepressant factor in patients with sepsis, and is directly involved in myocardial inflammation and fibrosis, leading to cardiac dysfunction.[2]

Here we summarize the prevalence, pathogenic mechanisms, clinical features, and management of HF in the most common systemic rheumatic diseases.

Systemic sclerosis

Systemic sclerosis (SSc) is a rare connective tissue disease characterized by early inflammation, aberrant activation of the immune system, and diffuse vascular damage, eventually leading to fibrosis of skin and internal organs, including the heart.[3]

Cardiac involvement in SSc is often unrecognized. Depending on the diagnostic technique, contemporary reviews suggest a clinical incidence of cardiac involvement in 15–35% of patients with SSc.[4] Autopsy studies documented widespread inflammatory, fibrotic, and vasculopathic myocardial abnormalities in up to 80% of SSc patients, including those without 'ante-mortem' cardiac symptoms.[4]

Even though often clinically silent, cardiac involvement is a major determinant of mortality in SSc. It is classified into a 'direct' or 'primary' heart disease, and an 'indirect' or 'secondary' to other organs' involvement (i.e. pulmonary arterial hypertension (PAH), scleroderma renal crisis). Primary heart involvement includes myocarditis, cardiac fibrosis, arrhythmias and conduction system abnormalities, pericardial disease, and both systolic and diastolic HF.[3,4]

Left ventricular systolic dysfunction

Overt congestive HF occurs in more advanced disease, but systolic dysfunction (SD) is often clinically occult. Systolic or diastolic dysfunction (DD) may occur early in SSc heart disease, years before becoming clinically evident. Left ventricular (LV) SD, defined by reduced LV ejection fraction (LVEF) at echocardiography, is uncommon in SSc and it is not a sensitive marker of cardiac loss of function. Segmental or exercise-induced dysfunction are more prevalent.[4,5] Male sex, age, digital ulcerations, myositis, and lack of treatment with calcium-channel blockers emerged as independent factors associated with LV dysfunction, suggesting that markers of SSc severity, as well as markers of microvascular lesions, are associated with reduced LVEF.[5]

Both myocardial fibrosis and myocardial inflammation could be associated with LV dysfunction. Myocarditis is increasingly reported and represents an important mechanism of myocardial damage, preceeding the devolopment of fibrosis.[6,7] At endomyocardial biopsy (EMB), the degree of myocardial inflammation and fibrosis has been associated with a poor outcome.[6]

Even in the absence of a reduced LVEF, SSc patients with EMB-proven myocarditis tend to present more frequently with HF and a higher NYHA class compared to patients with other forms of myocarditis. These clinical features are paralleled by a higher degree of myocardial fibrosis, possibly related to the worse cardiac prognosis.[7]

An early recognition of myocardial damage and a prompt therapeutic intervention are of cardinal importance to improve patients' outcome. The diagnosic approach should include a comprehensive clinical and laboratoristic assessment, an accurate echocardiographic evaluation, cardiac magnetic resonance (CMR) imaging, nuclear imaging, and, in selected cases, EMB.

Cardiac enzymes (high-sensitive cardiac troponin (hs-cTn) and NT-proBNP) may be useful screening biomarkers of early cardiac damage and may improve patients' risk stratification.[8]

Echocardiography is a fundamental tool for the non-invasive and routinely assessment of LV systolic function in SSc patients. However, traditional echocardiographic parameters are ineffective in detecting an early subclinical systolic impairment. Speckle tracking echocardiography (STE) is a reproducible technique used to assess myocardial deformation at both segmental and global levels, which can be used to evaluate both global and regional LV and RV systolic function. The STE-derived global longitudinal strain and global circumferential strain are significantly impaired in SSc, even in the absence of significant impairment of the LVEF.[9] Thus, global longitudinal strain might become a low-cost, non-invasive and reliable tool to detect early cardiac involvement and SD in SSc-patients.

CMR can non-invasively detect both focal and diffuse myocardial fibrosis as well as myocardial oedema in SSc-patients. The study of myocardial tissue using the novel mapping techniques further improves the CMR sensibility to detect a subclinical heart involvement before the occurrence of clinically evident heart disease. Using CMR, impaired LV and RV systolic dysfunction can be detected in approximately 20% of SSc-patients (➲ Figure 12.9.1a–d).

There are no long-term outcome studies of the treatment of LV-SD associated with SSc. Traditional therapy for HF is implemented, including diuretics, angiotensin-converting enzyme (ACE) inhibitors (or angiotensinreceptor blockers (ARBs)), and aldosterone antagonists. Calcium-channel blockers are widely adopted in SSc for Raynaud's phenomenon, and are useful in preventing LV dysfunction.[5]

Recently, it has been debated whether immunosuppression may be useful to treat LV systolic dysfunction related to myocarditis in SSc. A recent European Society of Cardiology position paper recommends performing EMB including search for possible infectious agents by PCR on EMB tissue to differentiate immune-mediated (infection-negative) myocarditis from infectious forms; only the former may be candidates to

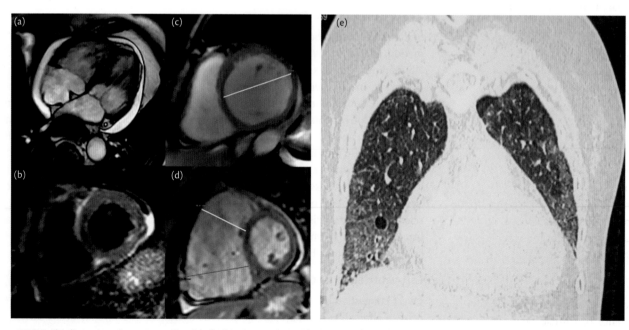

Figure 12.9.1 Cardiac magnetic resonance imaging findings in a patient with systemic sclerosis heart involvement: (a) pericardial effusion; (b) myocardial oedema; (c) left ventricular dilation; (d) right ventricular dilation; (e) chest X-ray showing cardiomegaly with massive right ventricular enlargement in a patient with SSc.

immunosuppression.[10] Immunosuppressive therapy improved symptoms and normalized cardiac enzymes in the majority of studies and case-reports on SSc myocarditis.[6,7,10] The efficacy of rituximab and intravenous immunoglobulins has been only anecdotally reported in SSc myocarditis with HF.[10] The increased risk of renal crisis in SSc patients treated with high-dose steroids and the potential cardiotoxicity of cyclophosphamide should be taken into account when designing the therapeutic strategy.

Emerging evidence supports the use of anti-cytokine agents to curb myocardial inflammation, preventing cardiac dysfunction and the progression to fibrosis.[2,11] IL-1/IL-6-mediated inflammation, indeed, lead to apoptosis of cardiomyocytes, loss of contractile tissue, fibrosis, and cardiomyopathy, and directly causes impaired contractile function, clinically characterized by HF.[11] IL-1 and IL-6 inhibition may have a remarkable therapeutic potential in systolic HF related to myocarditis.

Therapies to reduce the burden of established myocardial fibrosis, are still lacking and eagerly awaited.

Diastolic dysfunction and HFpEF

Although SD in SSc is uncommon, the awareness of DD has significantly grown in non-systolic HF. In SSc, LV-DD is a common finding in up to 44% of cases at baseline evaluation, it increases during follow-up, and can predict a poor prognosis,[12] thus emphasizing the need for its prompt recognition. The high frequency of DD in SSc could be explained by the underlying myocardial fibrosis, together with the subtle myocardial inflammation and vascular damage that jointly represent the substrates for the development of LV-DD.

Even patients with PAH present a high prevalence of DD, associated with worse haemodynamics and outcome.[12] Thus, it remains highly contentious whether the commonly detected DD is truly a manifestation of primary SSc heart disease or whether it secondary to other cardiac pathologies: DD is regarded as the precursor of HF with preserved ejection fraction (HFpEF), which has equal morbidity and mortality as HF with reduced EF (HFrEF). HFpEF is more difficult to disclose than HFrEF, as patients show normal ejection fraction and levels of natriuretic peptides are significantly lower.

Targeted therapies for DD and HFpEF are based on ACE-inhibitors, ARBs, diuretics, and beta blockers.[12]

Pulmonary arterial hypertension and right heart failure

Right HF (RHF) in SSc may result from PAH or pulmonary hypertension (PH) secondary to lung or heart disease. PAH is a severe complication which affects up to 12–14% of all SSc patients during the disease course, particularly those with limited subset and anti-centromere (or, rarely, anti-Th/To) antibodies, and has a 50% mortality rate within 3 years from diagnosis.[13] Compared with the idiopathic form of PAH, patients with SSc-PAH have a three-fold increased risk of death and may receive a diagnosis late in the course of disease because of its insidious onset and the high prevalence of cardiac, musculoskeletal, and pulmonary parenchymal comorbidities.[13] The continuous screening of SSc-patients using algorithms (such as DETECT) through the study of clinical variables, pulmonary function tests, immunological, biological, electrocardiographic and echocardiographic parameters, is essential to identify asymptomatic PAH patients eligible for effective vasoactive therapies.[13]

Once PAH is diagnosed, the capacity of the RV to function under the increased load determines both severity of symptoms and survival (⊛ Figure 12.9.1e). Signs and symptoms of RHF by history, echocardiogram, and right heart catheterization (RHC) are associated with a significantly increased risk of death.[13]

However, the indices that usually reflect advanced RV failure are still crude; novel tools for timely assessment of the presence and extent of subclinical RHF are needed. Recently, the tricuspid annular plane systolic excursion (TAPSE) emerged as a robust PAH outcome measure in SSc.[14]

The diagnosis, clinical management and treatment of SSc-PAH rely on the guidelines of the European Society of Cardiology for PH.[15]

Inflammatory myositis and antisynthetase syndrome

Polymyositis (PM) and dermatomyositis (DM) are rare idiopathic inflammatory myopathies that affect the heart with tachyarrhythmia, conduction disturbances, myocarditis, and HF.[16]

Older autopsy studies revealed cardiac abnormalities in up to 40% of PM/DM patients. A detailed cardiologic assessment of 32 patients with DM/PM revealed cardiac symptoms in only two individuals but conduction disturbances in more than 50% and LV diastolic dysfunction in 42% of the cases studied by echocardiography.[16]

Cardiac involvement was reported in 9.3% of 162 cases with idiopathic inflammatory myopathy followed-up for 5 years, but it might have been under-diagnosed due to the study retrospective design.[17] Interstitial lung disease is one of the most common extramuscular manifestations found in up to 5–30% of the cases, leading to PH and RHF.[16]

Antisynthetase syndrome (AS) is characterized by autoimmune myopathy, interstitial lung disease, cutaneous involvement, arthritis, fever, and the presence of myositis-specific autoantibodies (directed against tRNA-synthetases). The prevalence of myocarditis in AS is reported in up to 42% of patients; it is not linked to autoantibody specificity and associated with an active myositis.[18] Cardiac MRI can reveal late hypersignals in T1-images, and immunosuppressive therapy led to recovery in the majority of patients, while 25% developed a chronic HF in a French retrospective study.[18]

PH secondary to severe ILD or left heart disease is another serious complication and a cause of RHF and death in patients with PM, DM, and AS.[16–18]

Systemic lupus erythematotus, Sjogren syndrome, mixed connective tissue disease and antiphospholipid syndrome

Systemic lupus erythematosus (SLE) disease burden includes higher risk of cardiovascular events, including a prevalence of HF between 1% and 10% and an increased risk of HF hospitalizations.[19]

A recent meta-analysis attributes to primary Sjogren syndrome (pSS) an increased likelihood of HF in comparison to the general population.[20]

In SLE and pSS, cardiovascular (CV) factors are over-represented.[21,22] However, aberrant host immune responses and chronic inflammation, that may lead to accelerated atherosclerosis and primary CV events, are the most likely aetiologic factors.[19] Beyond inflammatory mediators, circulating anti-Ro/La antibodies and antiphospholipid antibodies may contribute to subclinical atherosclerosis, since they are more frequently found in patients with myocardial infarction (MI) associated with SLE, pSS, and antiphospholipid syndrome (APS).[21-23]

Smouldering diffuse myocardial dysfunction, possibly contributing to the excess of HF in SLE and APS population has been demonstrated in CMR studies.[19-23]

Patients with SLE and APS, moreover, display significantly worse LV diastolic parameters as compared to sex and age-matched controls, significantly correlating with disease activity and disease duration.[24] LV-DD is the most frequently observed cardiac substrate for HF in SLE patients regardless of SLE-specific cardiac involvement,[25] whereas HFrEF is prominent in myocarditis, MI and, rarely, in medication-induced cardiotoxicity leading to dilated cardiomyopathy. RV-DD also occurs in subjects with primary APS and stands for a primary process independent of concomitant valvular disease or SD.

Pericardial involvement is the most frequent cause of symptomatic cardiac disease in SLE and pericardial effusion is observed in over 50% of patients in the disease course. However, large effusions leading to cardiac tamponade or constrictive pericarditis are rare and thus its impact on the risk of HF is limited.[19]

The prevalence of myocarditis in SLE is estimated at 8–57%,[22,26] while it is exceptional in pSS. SLE myocarditis is associated with disease activity and can lead to global hypokinesis, conduction abnormalities, dilated cardiomyopathy, and HF.[10,26] Valvular disease occurs in 11–60% of patients in SLE and/or APS as verrucous thrombotic non-bacterial (Libman–Sacks) endocarditis, but significant valvular dysfunction leading to HF is rare[22,24] (< 6% of cases).

Congenital heart block may develop in fetuses of Ro/SSA autoantibody-positive women. Later in life, individuals with congenital heart block show a significantly increased risk of cardiovascular comorbidity with cardiomyopathy and HF.[27]

The impact of PAH related to SLE, APS, and pSS on HF development is limited: in SLE and APS, PAH has a widely variable prevalence, possibly associated to *in-situ* macro- or microthromboses/embolism, while pSS represents the cause of only 1% of CTDs-related PAH.[19-23]

Anaemia and chronic kidney disease in SLE patients are also a shared risk factor for HF, but data on their influence on HF risk are lacking. Finally, glucocorticoids and other immunosuppressive therapies of these conditions may modify the risk of HF in this population: immunomodulating treatment, indeed, can improve CV profile through reduction of inflammatory activity.[19-23] However, cardiotoxicity from medication (glucocorticoids, cyclophosphamide, and hydroxychloroquine) is also reported.[19,28]

Mixed connective tissue disease is a overlap disease with features of SSc, SLE, PM/DM, and rheumatoid arthritis (RA). Cardiac findings are comparable to those described in the diseases that constitute the overlap syndrome.

Large-vessel vasculitides

Large-vessel vasculitides are chronic inflammatory diseases affecting the aorta and its main branches. Two are the main diseases composing the spectrum of large-vessel vasculitides: giant cell arteritis (GCA) and Takayasu arteritis (TAK).[29]

GCA (or Horton's disease) is diagnosed in patients older than 50 years old, and TAK in women below 40 years of age.[29]

GCA patients are at increased risk of developing cardiovascular disease, eventually evolving towards overt HF. GCA carries an intrinsic risk of causing aortic aneurysms of the ascending aorta,[30,31] increasing over the disease course and more frequently detected in patients who display signs of aortic inflammation at disease onset, but can potentially arise in all GCA patients, even in those with apparently good control of the disease. The subsequent development of HF is related to aortic insufficiency.[32] Current international guidelines recommend a periodic screening of GCA patients with transthoracic echocardiogram and chest X-ray to monitor ascending aorta aneurysms formation.[33]

GCA patients are at increased risk of suffering from coronary artery disease and MI,[34,35] especially at early stages. Systemic inflammation and long-term steroid use could represent the trigger factors for MI in GCA patients.[36] Anecdotal reports described myocarditis as a cause of HF in GCA patients.[37]

Coronary involvement in TAK is reported in around 30% of patients, and it is likely underestimated since coronary arteries are not commonly evaluated in the diagnostic workup of TAK, unless symptomatic. Coronary arteries, however, are among the vessels potentially involved in TAK patients.[38] According to a cohort study evaluating hospital records of women who accessed the Emergency Department over 8 consecutive years, among patients aged < 40 who had ischaemic heart disease, 10% were eventually diagnosed with TAK.[39]

TAK patients can also develop ascending aorta aneurysms and aortic insufficiency.[40] In addition, in a non-negligible fraction of patients, the disease involves the pulmonary artery, causing PH and RHF.[41] When the inflammatory process affects renal arteries, TAK patients are at high risk of developing arterial hypertension, which can contribute to HF.[42] Lastly, albeit rarely, cases of myocarditis have also been described in patients with TAK.[43]

Antineutrophil cytoplasmic antibody (ANCA)-associated vasculitides

The antineutrophil cytoplasmic antibody (ANCA)-associated vasculitides (AAV) are a group of rare autoimmune diseases characterized by inflammatory cell infiltration causing necrosis of small and medium-sized vessels affecting various organs, including the heart. Cardiac involvement is associated with poor prognosis and high mortality.[10,44]

The AAV comprise: granulomatosis with polyangiitis, microscopic polyangiitis, and eosinophilic granulomatosis with polyangiitis.[29]

AAV patients are at increased risk of developing HF because of different potential causal factors: primary cardiac involvement may manifest as myocarditis, pericarditis, valvular heart disease, and coronary vessels arteritis.[10,45] Renal and pulmonary involvement can contribute to the development of acute and chronic HF.[45] Finally, the detrimental effects of systemic inflammation contribute to the burden of cardiovascular disease, including HF, and can be reduced by immunosuppressive therapy.[45]

Rheumatoid arthritis, ankylosing spondylitis, and psoriatic arthritis

RA is a chronic, systemic, inflammatory, disorder that primarily involves synovial joints, but other organs and tissues may also be affected, including the heart.[46] Various forms of heart disease can be seen in RA patients: pericardial and myocardial disease,[10] HF,[10] valvular disease, coronary artery disease, and arrythmias.

Compared to the general population, subjects with RA have a higher risk of cardiovascular disease (CVD) and HF, resulting in premature morbidity and mortality. Indeed, RA is an independent risk factor for accelerated CVD.[46] The burden of CVD in RA patients is mainly related to systemic inflammation and disease activity.[46] The incidence HF (mainly non-ischaemic HF and both HFrEF and HFpEF) is increased up to two-fold, independently from of other cardiovascular risk factors; it increases rapidly during the disease course and represents an important contributor to increased mortality in RA. The relative risk of ischaemic HF develops more slowly over time.[47,48]

Glucocorticoids and nonsteroidal anti-inflammatory drugs (NSAIDs) may also impact on the HF incidence. Inflammation is indeed the major CV risk factor. Besides accelerated atherosclerosis, pro-inflammatory cytokines and mediators are involved in multiple mechanisms of cardiac damage: endothelial dysfunction and vessel abnormalities, insulin-resistance, changes in lipid levels, oxidative stress, reduction of cardiac contractility and HF.[49]

In RA, higher C-reactive protein is associated with greater HF risk, methotrexate is associated with ≈25% lower HF risk, supporting the notion that curbing systemic inflammation and achieving RA disease control are essential to reduce the burden of HF in these patients.[49]

Spondyloarthritis comprises a family of disorders, including ankylosing spondylitis, nonradiographic axial spondyloarthritis and forms of arthritis associated with psoriasis (PsA) and with inflammatory bowel diseases. These conditions primarily affect joints and the axial skeleton and are associated with increased cardiovascular morbidity and mortality. The increased CV risk has been attributed to systemic inflammation and increased prevalence of traditional CV risk factors, especially in PsA.[50] Metabolic syndrome, diabetes mellitus, and atherosclerosis, indeed, occur more commonly in patients with PsA than in the general population, and are related to disease severity.

HF, however, is not only associated with the known cardiac risk factors, such as hypertension and diabetes, but also with the burden of inflammation related to the skin and joint disease, since patients with more active arthritis and psoriasis as well as those with higher levels of inflammatory blood markers, are at higher risk of HF. This notion highlights the importance of controlling inflammation in patients with psoriasis and PsA to potentially reduce the risk of future HF.

Aortic valve involvement could be an additional cause of HF in patients with AS.[46,50]

Future directions

Patients with many systemic rheumatic diseases have an increased risk of developing heart failure and other cardiovascular complications. The high risk of HF seems to be primarily related to chronic inflammation and disease activity. Thus, disease control and dampening of systemic inflammation are crucial to reduce the CVDburden in rheumatic patients. Similarly, a systematic evaluation of the CV risk and of the cardiac manifestations should be adopted for an early identification of patients at higher risk and to allow a prompt therapeutic intervention. In this view, close collaboration between cardiologists and rheumatologist is crucial.

While therapeutic strategies to curb systemic inflammation are available in the vast majority of rheumatic diseases, current treatments are not specifically targeted to mechanisms of heart damage and should be combined with traditional cardiologic therapy and treatment of cardiovascular risk factors.

A detailed comprehension of pathogenic mechanisms of HF could pave the way to targeted therapeutic approaches.

Key messages

- Patients with systemic rheumatic diseases present a high cardiovascular risk.
- Heart failure could represent a frequent and underecognized complication of many systemic rheumatic disease, and is associated with a poor prognosis.
- Chronic systemic inflammation represents the major mechanism leading to heart failure in patients with systemic immune-mediated diseases.
- Myocardial inflammation, myocardial fibrosis, vascular and valvular disease, accelerated atherosclerosis, pharmacological intervention, and higher burden of traditional cardiovascular risk factors also contribute to the occurrence of heart failure in patients with rheumatic diseases.
- Disease control and dampening of systemic inflammation are crucial to reduce the cardiovascular disease burden in rheumatic patients.
- A systematic evaluation of the cardiovascular risk profile and of the cardiac manifestations is needed for an early identification of patients at higher risk and to allow a prompt therapeutic intervention.
- Close collaboration between cardiologists and rheumatologists is crucial to reduce the burden of heart failure and cardiovascular disease in patients with rheumatic diseases.

References

1. Prasad M, Hermann J, Gabriel SE, et al. Cardiorheumatology. cardiac involvement in systemic rheumatic disease. *Nat Rev Cardiol.* 2015;12(3):168–176. doi:10.1038/nrcardio.2014.206

2. De Luca G, Cavalli G, Campochiaro C, Tresoldi M, Dagna L. Myocarditis: An interleukin-1-mediated disease? *Front Immunol.* 2018;9:1335. doi:10.3389/fimmu.2018.01335

3. Denton CP, Khanna D. Systemic sclerosis. *Lancet.* 2017;390(10103):1685–1699. doi:10.1016/S0140-6736(17)30933-9

4. Champion HC. The heart in scleroderma. *Rheum Dis Clin North Am.* 2008;34(1):181–190. doi:10.1016/j.rdc.2007.12.002

5. Allanore Y, Meune C, Vonk MC, et al. Prevalence and factors associated with left ventricular dysfunction in the EULAR Scleroderma Trial and Research group (EUSTAR) database of patients with systemic sclerosis. *Ann Rheum Dis.* 2010;69(1):218–221. doi:10.1136/ard.2008.103382

6. Mueller KAL, Mueller II, Eppler D, et al. Clinical and histopathological features of patients with systemic sclerosis undergoing endomyocardial biopsy. Assassi S, ed. *PLoS One.* 2015;10(5):e0126707. doi:10.1371/journal.pone.0126707

7. De Luca G, Campochiaro C, De Santis M, et al. Systemic sclerosis myocarditis has unique clinical, histological and prognostic features: a comparative histological analysis. *Rheumatology.* 2020;59(9):2523–2533. doi:10.1093/rheumatology/kez658

8. Bosello S, De Luca G, Berardi G, et al. Cardiac troponin T and NT-proBNP as diagnostic and prognostic biomarkers of primary cardiac involvement and disease severity in systemic sclerosis: A prospective study. *Eur J Intern Med.* 2019;60:46–53. doi:10.1016/j.ejim.2018.10.013

9. Guerra F, Stronati G, Fischietti C, et al. Global longitudinal strain measured by speckle tracking identifies subclinical heart involvement in patients with systemic sclerosis. *Eur J Prev Cardiol.* 2018;25(15):1598–1606. doi:10.1177/2047487318786315

10. Caforio ALP, Adler Y, Agostini C, Allanore Y, Anastasakis A, Arad M, et al. Diagnosis and management of myocardial involvement in systemic immune-mediated diseases: a position statement of the European Society of Cardiology Working Group on Myocardial and Pericardial Disease. Eur Heart J. 2017;38(35):2649–2662. doi:10.1093/eurheartj/ehx321. PMID: 28655210

11. De Luca G, Cavalli G, Campochiaro C, et al. Interleukin-1 and systemic sclerosis: getting to the heart of cardiac involvement. *Front Immunol.* 2021;12:819. doi:10.3389/fimmu.2021.653950

12. Tennøe AH, Murbræch K, Andreassen JC, et al. Systolic dysfunction in systemic sclerosis: prevalence and prognostic implications. *ACR Open Rheumatol.* 2019;1(4):258–266. doi:10.1002/acr2.1037

13. Bruni C, De Luca G, Lazzaroni MG, et al. Screening for pulmonary arterial hypertension in systemic sclerosis: A systematic literature review. *Eur J Intern Med.* 2020;78:17–25. doi:10.1016/j.ejim.2020.05.042.

14. Forfia PR, Fisher MR, Mathai SC, et al. Tricuspid annular displacement predicts survival in pulmonary hypertension. *Am J Respir Crit Care Med.* 2006;174(9):1034–1041. doi:10.1164/rccm.200604-547OC

15. Galiè N, Chairperson E, Humbert M, et al. 2015 ESC/ERS Guidelines for the diagnosis and treatment of pulmonary hypertension. *Eur Heart J.* 2015;46:903–975. doi:10.1183/13993003.01177-2015

16. Gonzalez-Lopez L, Gamez-Nava JI, Sanchez L, et al. Cardiac manifestations in dermato-polymyositis. *Clin Exp Rheumatol.* 1996;14(4):373–379. Accessed June 20, 2021. https://europepmc.org/article/med/8871835

17. Dankó K, Ponyi A, Constantin T, Borgulya G, Szegedi G. Long-term survival of patients with idiopathic inflammatory myopathies according to clinical features: a longitudinal study of 162 cases. *Medicine (Baltimore).* 2004;83(1):35–42. doi:10.1097/01.md.0000109755.65914.5e

18. Dieval C, Deligny C, Meyer A, et al. Myocarditis in patients with antisynthetase syndrome: Prevalence, presentation, and outcomes. *Medicine (Baltimore)..* 2015;94(26):e78. doi:10.1097/MD.0000000000000798

19. Dhakal BP, Kim CH, Al-Kindi SG, Oliveira GH. Heart failure in systemic lupus erythematosus. *Trends Cardiovasc Med.* 2018;28(3):187–197. doi:10.1016/j.tcm.2017.08.015

20. Beltai A, Barnetche T, Daien C, et al. Cardiovascular morbidity and mortality in primary sjögren's syndrome: a systematic review and meta-analysis. *Arthritis Care Res (Hoboken).* 2020;72(1):131–139. doi:10.1002/acr.23821

21. Bruce IN, Urowitz MB, Gladman DD, Ibañez D, Steiner G. Risk factors for coronary heart disease in women with systemic lupus erythematosus: The Toronto Risk Factor Study. *Arthritis Rheum.* 2003;48(11):3159–3167. doi:10.1002/art.11296

22. Bartoloni E, Baldini C, Schillaci G, et al. Cardiovascular disease risk burden in primary Sjögren's syndrome: results of a population-based multicentre cohort study. *J Intern Med.* 2015;278(2):185–192. doi:10.1111/joim.12346

23. Kolitz T, Shiber S, Sharabi I, Winder A, Zandman-Goddard G. Cardiac manifestations of antiphospholipid syndrome with focus on its primary form. *Front Immunol.* 2019;10(MAY):941. doi:10.3389/fimmu.2019.00941

24. Paran D, Caspi D, Levartovsky D, et al. Cardiac dysfunction in patients with systemic lupus erythematosus and antiphospholipid syndrome. *Ann Rheum Dis.* 2007;66(4):506–510. doi:10.1136/ard.2005.044073

25. Mavrogeni S, Koutsogeorgopoulou L, Dimitroulas T, Markousis-Mavrogenis G, Kolovou G. Complementary role of cardiovascular imaging and laboratory indices in early detection of cardiovascular disease in systemic lupus erythematosus. *Lupus.* 2017;26(3):227–236. doi:10.1177/0961203316671810

26. Comarmond C, Cacoub P. Myocarditis in auto-immune or auto-inflammatory diseases. *Autoimmun Rev.* 2017;16(8):811–816. doi:10.1016/j.autrev.2017.05.021

27. Mofors J, Eliasson H, Ambrosi A, et al. Comorbidity and long-term outcome in patients with congenital heart block and their siblings exposed to Ro/SSA autoantibodies in utero. *Ann Rheum Dis.* 2019;78(5):696–703. doi:10.1136/annrheumdis-2018-214406

28. Zhao H, Wald J, Palmer M, Han Y. Hydroxychloroquine-induced cardiomyopathy and heart failure in twins. *J Thorac Dis.* 2018;10(1):E70–E73. doi:10.21037/jtd.2017.12.66

29. Jennette JC, Falk RJ, Bacon PA, et al. 2012 Revised International Chapel Hill Consensus Conference Nomenclature of Vasculitides. *Arthritis Rheum.* 2013;65(1):1–11. doi:10.1002/art.37715

30. Amiri N, De Vera M, Choi HK, Sayre EC, Avina-Zubieta JA. Increased risk of cardiovascular disease in giant cell arteritis: A general population-based study. *Rheumatol (United Kingdom).* 2016;55(1):33–40. doi:10.1093/rheumatology/kev262

31. Jud P, Verheyen N, Dejaco C, et al. Prevalence and prognostic factors for aortic dilatation in giant cell arteritis – a longitudinal study. *Semin Arthritis Rheum.* 2021;51(4):911–918. doi:10.1016/j.semarthrit.2020.11.003

32. Bekeredjian R, Grayburn PA. Valvular heart disease: Aortic regurgitation. *Circulation.* 2005;112(1):125–134. doi:10.1161/CIRCULATIONAHA.104.488825

33. Marie I, Proux A, Duhaut P, et al. Long-term follow-up of aortic involvement in giant cell Arteritis: A series of 48 patients. *Medicine (Baltimore).* 2009;88(3):182–192. doi:10.1097/MD.0b013e3181a68ae2

34. Li L, Neogi T, Jick S. Giant cell arteritis and vascular disease-risk factors and outcomes: A cohort study using UK Clinical Practice Research Datalink. *Rheumatol (United Kingdom).* 2017;56(5):753–762. doi:10.1093/rheumatology/kew482

35. Udayakumar PD, Chandran AK, Crowson CS, Warrington KJ, Matteson EL. Cardiovascular risk and acute coronary syndrome in giant cell arteritis: A population-based retrospective cohort study. *Arthritis Care Res.* 2015;67(3):396–402. doi:10.1002/acr.22416

36. Greigert H, Zeller M, Putot A, et al. Myocardial infarction during giant cell arteritis: A cohort study. *Eur J Intern Med.* 2021;89:30–38. doi:10.1016/j.ejim.2021.02.001

37. Kushnir A, Restaino SW, Yuzefpolskaya M. Giant cell arteritis as a cause of myocarditis and atrial fibrillation. *Circ Hear Fail.* 2016;9(2):e002778. doi:10.1161/CIRCHEARTFAILURE.115.002778

38. Rav-Acha M, Plot L, Peled N, Amital H. Coronary involvement in Takayasu's arteritis. *Autoimmun Rev.* 2007;6(8):566–571. doi:10.1016/j.autrev.2007.04.001

39. Cavalli G, Tomelleri A, Di Napoli D, Baldissera E, Dagna L. Prevalence of Takayasu arteritis in young women with acute ischemic heart disease. *Int J Cardiol.* 2018;252:21–23. doi:10.1016/j.ijcard.2017.10.067

40. Yang KQ, Meng X, Zhang Y, et al. Aortic aneurysm in Takayasu arteritis. *Am J Med Sci.* 2017;354(6):539–547. doi:10.1016/j.amjms.2017.08.018

41. Yang J, Peng M, Shi J, Zheng W, Yu X. Pulmonary artery involvement in Takayasu's arteritis: Diagnosis before pulmonary hypertension. *BMC Pulm Med.* 2019;19(1):1–9. doi:10.1186/s12890--019-0983-7

42. Hong S, Ghang B, Kim YG, Lee CK, Yoo B. Longterm outcomes of renal artery involvement in Takayasu arteritis. *J Rheumatol.* 2017;44(4):466–472. doi:10.3899/jrheum.160974

43. Kotake T, Sueyoshi E, Sakamoto I, Izumida S. Myocarditis associated with Takayasu arteritis. *Eur Heart J.* 2015;36(38):2564. doi:10.1093/eurheartj/ehv169

44. Guillevin L, Pagnoux C, Seror R, Mahr A, Mouthon L, Toumelin P Le. The five-factor score revisited: Assessment of prognoses of systemic necrotizing vasculitides based on the french vasculitis study group (FVSG) cohort. *Medicine (Baltimore).* 2011;90(1):19–27. doi:10.1097/MD.0b013e318205a4c6

45. Soulaidopoulos S, Madenidou A-V, Daoussis D, et al. Cardiovascular Disease in the Systemic Vasculitides. *Curr Vasc Pharmacol.* 2020;18(5):463–472.doi:10.2174/1570161118666200130093432

46. Agca R, Heslinga SC, Rollefstad S, et al. EULAR recommendations for cardiovascular disease risk management in patients with rheumatoid arthritis and other forms of inflammatory joint disorders: 2015/2016 update. *Ann Rheum Dis.* 2016;76(1):17–28. doi:10.1136/annrheumdis-2016-209775

47. Ferreira MB, Fonseca T, Costa R, et al. Prevalence, risk factors and proteomic bioprofiles associated with heart failure in rheumatoid arthritis: The RA-HF study. *Eur J Intern Med.* 2021;85:41–49. doi:10.1016/j.ejim.2020.11.002

48. Mantel Ä, Holmqvist M, Andersson DC, Lund LH, Askling J. Association between rheumatoid arthritis and risk of ischemic and nonischemic heart failure. *J Am Coll Cardiol.* 2017;69(10):1275–1285. doi:10.1016/j.jacc.2016.12.033

49. Taylor PC, Atzeni F, Balsa A, Gossec L, Müller-Ladner U, Pope J. The key comorbidities in patients with rheumatoid arthritis: a narrative review. *J Clin Med.* 2021;10(3):509. doi:10.3390/jcm10030509

50. Buleu F, Sirbu E, Caraba A, Dragan S. heart involvement in inflammatory rheumatic diseases: a systematic literature review. *Medicina (B Aires).* 2019;55(6):249. doi:10.3390/medicina55060249

CHAPTER 12.10

Liver and gut dysfunction

Yuri Lopatin and Gianluigi Savarese

Introduction

Although gastrointestinal symptoms are common and have been well described in patients with heart failure (HF), the interaction between the heart, the liver, and the gut has only recently become a subject of close attention. The major reason for such scrutiny is related not only to the prognostic significance of liver and gut dysfunction in HF, but also to the contribution of such dysfunction to disease progression, which can potentially be modified by existing or future interventions. Taking into account the bidirectional nature of the relationships between the heart, the liver, and the gastrointestinal system, the hypotheses of the heart–liver axis and heart–gut axis in HF have been put forward. Moreover, it was proposed to consider these complex relationships in the context of the special cardio-hepatic and cardio-intestinal syndromes in HF.[1,2]

The heart–liver axis

Heart failure often provokes liver damage, which is described with the terms 'congestive hepatopathy' (CH) or 'acute cardiogenic liver injury' (ACLI).[3–6] Other terms used previously to refer to the latter include ischaemic hepatitis, hypoxic hepatitis, and shock liver. CH is the chronic congestion of the liver parenchyma induced by impaired hepatic venous outflow secondary to a right-sided cardiac failure, which eventually leads to the organ damage. ACLI refers to the necrosis of hepatocytes within the liver parenchyma provoked by a sudden and significant drop in hepatic perfusion from a systemic circulatory failure (⊃ Figure 12.10.1).

CH is a more common cause of liver dysfunction in HF compared to acute changes in hepatic perfusion. Its prevalence ranges from 15% to 65%, depending on the definition and the type of liver function abnormality.[7] In HF, the elevated central venous pressure transmits to the hepatic veins without any attenuation because of the lack of valves in the latter. Increased hepatic venous pressure causes sinusoidal congestion, dilation of sinusoidal fenestrae, and exudation of protein and fluid into the space of Disse, which impairs the diffusion of oxygen and nutrients to hepatocytes. Excess fluid in the space of Disse is drained into the hepatic lymphatics, but in the case of excessive lymph formation this may lead to the development of ascites with a high protein concentration, which distinguishes cardiac ascites from other types.[2] Prolonged congestion results in progressive hepatocyte atrophy and necrosis within zone 3 of the hepatic acinus (centrilobular parenchyma located adjacent to central hepatic veins), perisinusoidal and perivenular deposition of fibrotic tissue, and, if untreated, bridging fibrosis between the central veins, and, eventually, cirrhosis.[8]

The prevalence of ACLI in acute HF is estimated at 20–30%[9] and is associated with a significant risk of in-hospital death.[6] The ACLI is usually attributed to acute coronary

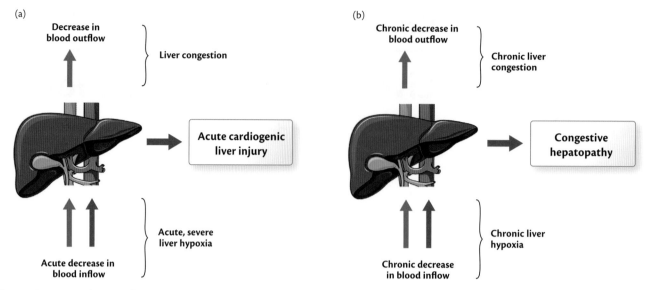

Figure 12.10.1 Mechanisms of liver injury in heart failure.

(a) Acute cardiogenic liver injury usually develops following severe liver hypoxia in the setting of liver congestion (i.e. cardiogenic shock). (b) Congestive hepatopathy results from chronic liver congestion associated with chronic liver hypoxia (i.e. chronic severe congestive heart failure).

Reproduced from Xanthopoulos A, Starling RC, Kitai T, Triposkiadis F. Heart failure and liver disease: cardiohepatic interactions. *JACC Heart Fail.* 2019 Feb;7(2):87–97. doi: 10.1016/j.jchf.2018.10.007 with permission from Elsevier.

events, sustained cardiac arrhythmias, or transient severe hypotension. However, the acute decline in hepatic perfusion is not the only cause of ACLI. ACLI and CH often coexist in HF patients and exacerbate one another. Passive liver congestion may predispose hepatocytes to a greater hypoxic injury resulting from hypotension.[10] The histological feature of ACLI is centriolobular necrosis, which may expand to mid-zonal hepatocytes (zone 2 of the hepatic acinus), especially in the case of prolonged ischaemia. The depletion of the compensatory mechanisms preventing ischaemic damage, such as adenosine-triggering hepatic artery vasodilation in response to a decrease in portal blood flow and an increase of oxygen diffusion into hepatocytes in response to hypoxia, also contribute to liver damage.[11,12]

Clinical manifestations and diagnosis of liver dysfunction in HF

Liver dysfunction in HF may be asymptomatic for a long time and is usually identified through abnormalities detected by routine biochemical tests.[13]

The clinical presentation of CH is dominated rather by symptoms and signs of right-sided HF than by those of liver involvement. When symptomatic, patients may present a mild and dull right upper quadrant pain, nausea, loss of appetite, and weight loss. Depending on the severity and duration of the congestion, physical examination reveals jaundice, hepatomegaly, hepatojugular reflux, pulsatile liver, ascites, and splenomegaly. In HF patients the loss of liver pulsatility over time suggests the progression of CH to cardiac cirrhosis.[3,14]

The common laboratory abnormalities in CH are elevated serum cholestasis markers, including mild hyperbilirubinaemia with a predominantly unconjugated fraction, alkaline phosphatase, and gamma-glutamyl transferase.[15] The degree of cholestasis is related to the severity of both the elevation of right atrial pressure and tricuspid regurgitation.[7,16] A mild increase in the alanine aminotransferase (ALT) and aspartate aminotransferase (AST) levels, the prothrombin time, as well as a mild decrease in the albumin level are also seen in patients with CH.[17] It was shown that among conventional tests of liver function the total bilirubin is the strongest predictor of outcomes in HF patients.[17,18]

The clinical manifestations of ACLI vary from asymptomatic cases to conditions resembling acute viral hepatitis with symptoms of nausea, vomiting, weakness, apathy, anorexia, right upper quadrant pain, and in few cases, mental confusion, flapping tremor, oliguria, jaundice, and even hepatic coma.[3,19] The onset of symptoms is preceded by a latency period of 2 to 24 hours after the acute event.

Typical laboratory findings in ACLI include rapid, transient rises in AST, ALT, and lactate dehydrogenase (LDH) levels to 10–20 times the upper limit of normal values, and even up to 2000-fold increases.[20] The ratio of serum ALT to LDH below 1.5 early in the course of liver injury is generally considered as a pathognomonic sign of ACLI.[12] The peak of AST is seen earlier and at higher levels than the peak of ALT. A progressive increase in the bilirubin level is usually observed but is seldom severe. An early and sharp deterioration in renal function and prolongation of the prothrombin time may also support the presence of ACLI. Following the restoration of haemodynamic stability, these laboratory abnormalities generally return to normal within 7 to 10 days.[15] Importantly, the abnormal liver function tests have an unfavorable impact on mortality in patients with acute HF.[20,21]

Imaging tests play an important role in the assessment of liver dysfunction in HF.[22] Abdominal ultrasound findings include hepatomegaly, an irregular and nodular liver, dilation of inferior vena cava and hepatic veins and a loss of the normal triphasic hepatic venous waveform. Computed tomography and magnetic resonance imaging help to better identify the morphological characteristics of the liver and to reveal abnormal kinetics of intravenous contrast enhancement including retrograde hepatic venous opacification during the early phase of intravenous contrast material injection and a predominantly peripheral heterogeneous pattern of hepatic enhancement due to stagnant blood flow. To estimate the liver parenchymal stiffness, both ultrasound and magnetic resonance elastography are applied; however, these methods cannot reliably distinguish the contributing components of congestion and fibrosis to the liver stiffness. Liver biopsy may be used to differentiate between parenchymal congestion and fibrosis, although this method is not often applied for this purpose.

In any case, the confirmation of liver dysfunction in HF patients should be based on a careful evaluation of the history of the disease, clinical manifestation, biochemical profile, and results of imaging tests, and, of course, on exclusion of other causes of liver damage. Regarding the latter, the potential presence of systemic diseases, such as amyloidosis or haemochromatosis, simultaneously resulting in HF and liver disease should be taken into consideration.

Prognosis and treatment of liver dysfunction in HF

The prognosis of HF patients with a liver dysfunction is generally determined by the underlying cardiac disease. In addition to abnormal liver function tests, clinical risk scores, such as the Model for End Stage Liver Disease (MELD) and the Model for End Stage Liver Disease Excluding INR (international normalized ratio; MELD-XI), are helpful for the prognostication of outcomes in HF.[23,24] However, they rather predict cardiac- but not liver-related mortality.[13] Importantly, MELD and MELD-XI scores may predict morbidity and mortality in patients undergoing heart transplantation (HT) or left ventricular assist device (LVAD) implantation.[25-27]

Treatment of CH consists of the management of the underlying cardiac disease. At the moment, there are no specific therapies for CH.[13] Diuretics are beneficial for the elimination of hepatic congestion, but require caution to avoid precipitating hepatic ischaemia. Early manifestations of CH can be reversed by the improvement of systemic and liver haemodynamics. Moreover, improvements of liver function were seen even in patients with advanced HF following the HT and the LVAD implantation.[28,29] However, if CH is suspected, potential candidates for HT should be carefully examined for the presence of cardiac cirrhosis, which is a contraindication for HT.[2,13] Liver dysfunction can alter the pharmacokinetics and pharmacodynamics of HF medications; however, there are no clear recommendations for modifying drug dosages in CH yet.[5,13]

The management of ACLI is based on a timely identification and removal of the precipitating cause. When needed, oxygen and ventilator support, inotropes, vasopressors, myocardial revascularization procedures, and mechanical circulatory support should be used in patients with ACLI. There are limited data

on the ability of N-acetylcysteine to reduce hepatic damage in ACLI by improving the microcirculation of the liver.[15]

The heart–gut axis

The heart–gut axis hypothesis in HF is nowadays a topic of intensive investigation and is supported by relevant evidence. In HF, decreased cardiac output and venous congestion directly affect the gut, leading to increased sympathetic vasoconstriction, intestinal mucosal ischaemia, hypoxia, bowel wall oedema, altered mucosal barrier with leakage of endotoxins, microbial components and metabolites (e.g. lypopolysaccharides), and juxtamucosal bacterial overgrowth.[30-33] It is currently estimated that 3000–5000 microbial species are located in the gut.[34,35] Among bacterial product levels increased in patients with HF, trimethylamine N-oxide (TMAO) and lipopolysaccharides (LPS) seem to play a major role. TMAO is the metabolite deriving from the bacterial digestion of dietary choline, phosphatidylcholine, and carnitine, which are present, for example, in red meat.[36] LPS is a component of Gram-negative bacteria outer membranes. These molecules are involved in systemic inflammation,[37-40] endothelial dysfunction,[41] adverse remodeling, and fibrosis,[42-46] which are key mechanisms in HF (➲ Figure 12.10.2). TMAO levels have been identified to have a prognostic role in HF, with high TMAO levels independently associated with more symptomatic and advanced HF, higher long-term mortality risk and significantly contributing to patient risk stratification for in-hospital mortality for acute HF.[42,47–51] Similarly, concentrations of LPS are higher in patients with more severe HF,[52] and decrease after recompensation[32] and following intensified diuretic treatment.[39]

In HF patients it has also been shown that changes in gut microbiota composition (dysbiosis), that is, a significantly decreased diversity of the intestinal microbiome, is paralleled by an enrichment of potential pathogenic bacteria such as *Shigella*, *Salmonella*, *Yersinia entercolitica*, and *Candida* species, and by a reduction in species producing short-chain fatty acids (SCFAs), which might be affected by changes in fluid balance, bowel congestion and ischaemia, and dysmotility, characterizing HF status.[53-56] SCFAs provide energy for intestinal epithelial cells, have an immune regulatory function by acting on the NF-kB pathway, and facilitate tight junctions supporting intestinal wall integrity, which is altered in HF.[57] Notably, supplements of SCFAs given to SCFA-depleted mice have been shown to exert antihypertrophic and antifibrotic effects, as well as a repair capacity after myocardial infarction.[58,59] Additionally, a decrease in bacterial richness, a lower Firmicutes/Bacteroidetes ratio and an increase in small intestinal bacterial overgrowth have been associated with worse outcomes.[60,61]

The gut as a new therapeutic target in HF

The interaction between the gut and the heart in HF has put a spotlight on gut dysfunction as a potential target for HF treatments.

In a murine genetic model of dilated cardiomyopathy, neither fibres, which are a substrate for fermentation that produces SCFA, nor supplementation with the SCFA acetate could attenuate cardiac

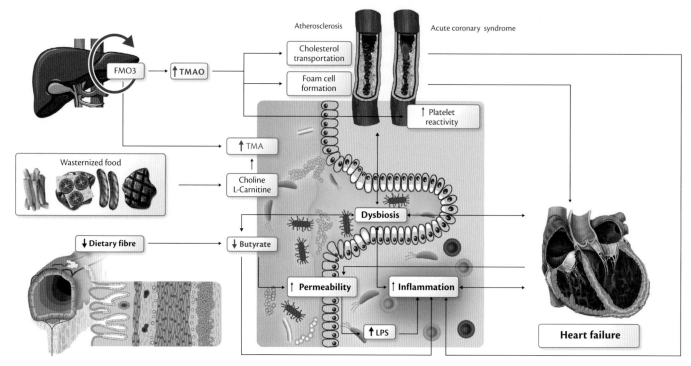

Figure 12.10.2 Diet–gut-heart interactions: proposed mechanisms.

Interactions between diet and the gut microbiome could contribute to atherosclerosis, acute coronary syndromes, and heart failure through common and separate mechanisms. Westernized food rich in red meat promotes bacterial production of TMA, which is oxidized in the liver to the pro-athero-genic metabolite, TMAO. TMAO may contribute to atherosclerosis by interference with cholesterol transportation, foam cell formation and platelet aggregation, the latter playing a potential role in acute coronary syndromes. Reduced dietary fibre is associated with reduced bacterial production of the short chain fatty acid butyrate, which has immune modulatory effects in the gut mucosa, and also serves as the main energy substrate for colonocytes. Reduction of butyrate levels in the gut could promote local inflammation, aggravate dysbiosis and contribute to impaired gut barrier function, the latter resulting in leakage of bacterial toxins such as LPS, further fuelling local and systemic inflammation.

FMO3; flavin-containing monooxygenase 3, LPS; lipopolysaccharide, TMA; trimetylamine, TMAO; trimethylamine-N-oxide.

Reproduced from Trøseid M, Andersen GØ, Broch K, Hov JR. The gut microbiome in coronary artery disease and heart failure: Current knowledge and future directions. *EBioMedicine.* 2020 Feb;52:102649. doi: 10.1016/j.ebiom.2020.102649 with permission from Elsevier.

remodelling or cardiomyocyte apoptosis, suggesting that increasing SCFA production cannot override a strong genetic contribution to the development of HF.[62] However, withdrawal of TMAO from the diet and inhibiting gut microbial conversion of choline to TMAO with a choline trimethylamine lyase inhibitor has shown beneficial effects on ventricular remodeling and cardiac function in a different murine model of HF (transverse aortic constriction).[45]

In a randomized controlled trial, treatment with probiotics reduced levels of TMAO, transforming growth factor beta (TGF-β), and C-reactive protein (CRP), without any effect on ejection fraction in 44 subjects with myocardial infarction who underwent coronary intervention.[63]

Surprisingly, TMAO levels have not been shown to be affected by HF guideline-recommended therapies.[51] This might suggest that therapeutic intervention targeting gut dysfunction in HF might be potentially additive to current HF treatments. The probiotic *Lactobacillus rhamnosus* GR-1 attenuated left ventricular hypertrophy, atrial natriuretic peptide expression, systolic and diastolic cardiac function in rat models of sustained coronary artery occlusion.[64] The ongoing GutHeart randomized controlled trial (phase II) is currently testing the hypothesis that targeting gut microbiota might be beneficial in HF, by randomizing 150 patients with stable HF and left ventricular ejection fraction < 40% to receive 1:1:1 the antibiotic rifamixin, the probiotic yeast

Sacchraromyces boulardii, or no treatment to assess differences in ejection fraction after 3 months of treatment.[65]

Finally, faecal microbiota transplantation, that is delivery of faecal matter from a healthy donor into the gastrointestinal tract of a patient by endoscopy, also represents a therapy with great potential, which is currently mainly investigated for the treatment of metabolic syndrome.[66]

Summary

There is a growing body of evidence on the involvement of the liver and the gut in the pathogenesis of HF. Nevertheless, gaps in knowledge on the burden of liver and gut dysfunction in HF, on validated biomarkers confirming their presence and predicting clinical outcomes, and, most important, on effective treatment strategies still exist. With all the evidence demonstrating the fundamental role of guideline-directed HF management in such patients, the search for new therapeutic modalities to remove liver and gut dysfunction should be a subject of further investigation.

References

1. Laribi S, Mebazaa A. Cardiohepatic syndrome: liver injury in decompensated heart failure. Curr Heart Fail Rep. 2014;11(3):236–40.
2. Sundaram V, Fang JC. Gastrointestinal and liver issues in heart failure. Circulation. 2016;133(17):1696–703.

3. Møller S, Bernardi M. Interactions of the heart and the liver. Eur Heart J. 2013;34(36):2804–11.

4. Samsky MD, Patel CB, DeWald TA, Smith DA, Felker GM, Rogers JG, et al. Cardiohepatic interactions in heart failure: an overview and clinical implications. J Am Coll Cardiol. 2013; 61(24):2397–05.

5. Pendyal A., Gelow JM. Cardiohepatic interactions: implications for management in advanced heart failure. Heart Fail Clin. 2016;12(3):349–61.

6. Tapper EB, Sengupta N, Bonder A. The incidence and outcomes of ischemic hepatitis: a systematic review with meta-analysis. Am J Med. 2015;128(12):1314–21.

7. van Deursen VM, Damman K, Hillege HL, van Beek AP, van Veldhuisen DJ, Voors AA. Abnormal liver function in relation to hemodynamic profile in heart failure patients. J Card Fail. 2010;16(10):84–90.

8. Dai DF, Swanson PE, Krieger EV, Liou IW, Carithers RL, Yeh MM. Congestive hepatic fibrosis score: a novel histologic assessment of clinical severity. Mod Pathol. 2014;27(12):1552–8.

9. Harjola V-P, Mullen, W, Banaszewsk, M, Bauersachs J, Rocca H-PB-L, Chioncel O, et al. Organ dysfunction, injury and failure in acute heart failure: From pathophysiology to diagnosis and management. A review on behalf of the Acute Heart Failure Committee of the Heart Failure Association (HFA) of the European Society of Cardiology (ESC). Eur J Heart Fail. 2017;19(7):821–36.

10. Birrer R, Takuda Y, Takara T. Hypoxic hepatopathy: pathophysiology and prognosis. Intern Med. 2007;46:1063–70.

11. De La Monte SM, Arcidi JM, Moore GW, Hutchins GM. Midzonal necrosis as a pattern of hepatocellular injury after shock. Gastroenterology. 1984;86(4):627–31.

12. Xanthopoulos A, Starling RC, Kitai T, Triposkiadis F. Heart failure and liver disease: cardiohepatic interactions. JACC Heart Fail. 2019;7(2):87–97.

13. Fortea JI, Puente Á, Cuadrado A, Huelin P, Pellón R, González Sánchez FJ, et al. Congestive hepatopathy. Int J Mol Sci. 2020;21(24):9420.

14. Kavoliuniene A, Vaitiekiene A, Cesnaite G. Congestive hepatopathy and hypoxic hepatitis in heart failure: a cardiologist's point of view. Int J Cardiol. 2013;166(3):554–8.

15. Ford RM, Book W, Spivey JR. Liver disease related to the heart. Transplant Rev (Orlando). 2015;29(1):33–7.

16. Lau GT, Tan HC, Kritharides L. Type of liver dysfunction in heart failure and its relation to the severity of tricuspid regurgitation. Am J Cardiol. 2002;90(12):1405–9.

17. Allen LA, Felker GM, Pocock S, McMurray JJV, Pfeffer MA, Swedberg K, et al. Liver function abnormalities and outcome in patients with chronic heart failure: data from the Candesartan in Heart Failure: Assessment of Reduction in Mortality and Morbidity (CHARM) program. Eur J Heart Fail. 2009;11(2):170–7.

18. Suzuki K, Claggett B, Minamisawa M, Packer M, Zile MR, Rouleau J, et al. Liver function and prognosis, and influence of sacubitril/valsartan in patients with heart failure with reduced ejection fraction. Eur J Heart Fail. 2020;22(9):1662–71.

19. Fouad YM, Yehia R. Hepato-cardiac disorders. World J Hepatol. 2014;6(1):41–54.

20. Çaglı K, Fatma Basar FN, Tok D, Turak O, Basar Ö. How to interpret liver function tests in heart failure patients? Turk J Gastroenterol. 2015;26(3):197–203.

21. Biegus J, Hillege HL, Postmus D, Valente MA, Bloomfield DM, Cleland JG, et al. Abnormal liver function tests in acute heart failure: relationship with clinical characteristics and outcome in the PROTECT study. Eur J Heart Fail. 2016;18(7):830–9.

22. Wells ML, Venkatesh SK. Congestive hepatopathy. Abdom Radiol. 2018;43(8):2037–51.

23. Kim MS, Kato TS, Farr M, Wu C, Givens RC, Collado E, et al. Hepatic dysfunction in ambulatory patients with heart failure: application of the MELD scoring system for outcome prediction. J Am Coll Cardiol. 2013;61(22):2253–61.

24. Abe S, Yoshihisa A, Takiguchi M, Shimizu T, Nakamura Y, Yamauchi H, et al. Liver dysfunction assessed by model for end-stage liver disease excluding INR (MELD-XI) scoring system predicts adverse prognosis in heart failure. PLoS One. 2014;9(6):e100618

25. Chokshi A, Cheema FH, Schaefle KJ, Jiang J, Collado E, Shahzad K, et al. Hepatic dysfunction and survival after orthotopic heart transplantation: application of the MELD scoring system for outcome prediction. J Heart Lung Transplant. 2012;31:591–600.

26. Deo SV, Al-Kindi SG, Altarabsheh SE, Hang D, Kumar S, Ginwalla MB, et al. Model for end-stage liver disease excluding international normalized ratio (MELD-XI) score predicts heart transplant outcomes: evidence from the registry of the United Network for Organ Sharing. J Heart Lung Transplant. 2016;35:222–7.

27. Yang JA, Kato TS, Shulman BP, Takayama H, Farr M, Jorde UP, et al. Liver dysfunction as a predictor of outcomes in patients with advanced heart failure requiring ventricular assist device support: use of the Model of End-stage Liver Disease (MELD) and MELD eXcluding INR (MELD-XI) scoring system. J Heart Lung Transplant. 2012;31:601–10.

28. Dichtl W, Vogel W, Dunst KM, Grander W, Alber HF, Frick M, et al. Cardiac hepatopathy before and after heart transplantation. Transpl Int. 2005;18:697–702.

29. Russell SD, Rogers JG, Milano CA, Dyke DB, Pagani FD, Aranda JM, et al. HeartMate II Clinical Investigators. Renal and hepatic function improve in advanced heart failure patients during continuous-flow support with the HeartMate II left ventricular assist device. Circulation. 2009;120:2352–7.

30. Sandek A, Swidsinski A, Schroedl W, Watson A, Valentova M, Herrmann R, et al. Intestinal blood flow in patients with chronic heart failure: a link with bacterial growth, gastrointestinal symptoms, and cachexia. J Am Coll Cardiol. 2014;64(11):1092–102.

31. Krack A, Richartz BM, Gastmann A, Greim K, Lotze U, Anker SD, et al. Studies on intragastric PCO2 at rest and during exercise as a marker of intestinal perfusion in patients with chronic heart failure. Eur J Heart Fail. 2004;6(4):403–7.

32. Sandek A, Bjarnason I, Volk HD, Crane R, Meddings JB, Niebauer J, et al. Studies on bacterial endotoxin and intestinal absorption function in patients with chronic heart failure. Int J Cardiol. 2012;157(1):80–5.

33. Sandek A, Bauditz J, Swidsinski A, Buhner S, Weber-Eibel J, von Haehling S, et al. Altered intestinal function in patients with chronic heart failure. J Am Coll Cardiol. 2007;50(16):1561–9.

34. Almeida A, Mitchell AL, Boland M, Forster SC, Gloor GB, Tarkowska A, et al. A new genomic blueprint of the human gut microbiota. Nature. 2019;568(7753):499–504.

35. Pasolli E, Asnicar F, Manara S, Zolfo M, Karcher N, Armanini F, et al. Extensive unexplored human microbiome diversity revealed by over 150,000 genomes from metagenomes spanning age, geography, and lifestyle. Cell. 2019;176(3):649–62 e20.

36. Koeth RA, Wang Z, Levison BS, Buffa JA, Org E, Sheehy BT, et al. Intestinal microbiota metabolism of L-carnitine, a nutrient in red meat, promotes atherosclerosis. Nat Med. 2013;19(5):576–85.

37. Gnauck A, Lentle RG, Kruger MC. The characteristics and function of bacterial lipopolysaccharides and their endotoxic potential in humans. Int Rev Immunol. 2016;35(3):189–218.

38. Charalambous BM, Stephens RC, Feavers IM, Montgomery HE. Role of bacterial endotoxin in chronic heart failure: the gut of the matter. Shock. 2007;28(1):15–23.

39. Niebauer J, Volk HD, Kemp M, Dominguez M, Schumann RR, Rauchhaus M, et al. Endotoxin and immune activation in chronic heart failure: a prospective cohort study. Lancet. 1999;353(9167):1838–42.

40. Medzhitov R, Preston-Hurlburt P, Janeway CA, Jr. A human homologue of the *Drosophila* Toll protein signals activation of adaptive immunity. Nature. 1997;388(6640):394–7.

41. McGarrity S, Anuforo O, Halldorsson H, Bergmann A, Halldorsson S, Palsson S, et al. Metabolic systems analysis of LPS induced endothelial dysfunction applied to sepsis patient stratification. Sci Rep. 2018;8(1):6811.

42. Organ CL, Otsuka H, Bhushan S, Wang Z, Bradley J, Trivedi R, et al. Choline diet and its gut microbe-derived metabolite, trimethylamine N-oxide, exacerbate pressure overload-induced heart failure. Circ Heart Fail. 2016;9(1):e002314.

43. Tang WH, Wang Z, Kennedy DJ, Wu Y, Buffa JA, Agatisa-Boyle B, et al. Gut microbiota-dependent trimethylamine N-oxide (TMAO) pathway contributes to both development of renal insufficiency and mortality risk in chronic kidney disease. Circ Res. 2015;116(3):448–55.

44. Shuai W, Wen J, Li X, Wang D, Li Y, Xiang J. High-choline diet exacerbates cardiac dysfunction, fibrosis, and inflammation in a mouse model of heart failure with preserved ejection fraction. J Card Fail. 2020;26(8):694–702.

45. Organ CL, Li Z, Sharp TE, 3rd, Polhemus DJ, Gupta N, Goodchild TT, et al. Nonlethal inhibition of gut microbial trimethylamine n-oxide production improves cardiac function and remodeling in a murine model of heart failure. J Am Heart Assoc. 2020;9(10):e016223.

46. Felisbino MB, McKinsey TA. Epigenetics in cardiac fibrosis: emphasis on inflammation and fibroblast activation. JACC Basic Transl Sci. 2018;3(5):704–15.

47. Tang WH, Wang Z, Fan Y, Levison B, Hazen JE, Donahue LM, et al. Prognostic value of elevated levels of intestinal microbe-generated metabolite trimethylamine-N-oxide in patients with heart failure: refining the gut hypothesis. J Am Coll Cardiol. 2014;64(18):1908–14.

48. Suzuki T, Heaney LM, Bhandari SS, Jones DJ, Ng LL. Trimethylamine N-oxide and prognosis in acute heart failure. Heart. 2016;102(11):841–8.

49. Troseid M, Ueland T, Hov JR, Svardal A, Gregersen I, Dahl CP, et al. Microbiota-dependent metabolite trimethylamine-N-oxide is associated with disease severity and survival of patients with chronic heart failure. J Intern Med. 2015;277(6):717–26.

50. Yuzefpolskaya M, Bohn B, Nasiri M, Zuver AM, Onat DD, Royzman EA, et al. Gut microbiota, endotoxemia, inflammation, and oxidative stress in patients with heart failure, left ventricular assist device, and transplant. J Heart Lung Transplant. 2020;39(9):880–90.

51. Suzuki T, Yazaki Y, Voors AA, Jones DJL, Chan DCS, Anker SD, et al. Association with outcomes and response to treatment of trimethylamine N-oxide in heart failure: results from BIOSTAT-CHF. Eur J Heart Fail. 2019;21(7):877–86.

52. Ebner N, Foldes G, Schomburg L, Renko K, Springer J, Jankowska EA, et al. Lipopolysaccharide responsiveness is an independent predictor of death in patients with chronic heart failure. J Mol Cell Cardiol. 2015;87:48–53.

53. Luedde M, Winkler T, Heinsen FA, Ruhlemann MC, Spehlmann ME, Bajrovic A, et al. Heart failure is associated with depletion of core intestinal microbiota. ESC Heart Fail. 2017;4(3):282–90.

54. Pasini E, Aquilani R, Testa C, Baiardi P, Angioletti S, Boschi F, et al. Pathogenic gut flora in patients with chronic heart failure. JACC Heart Fail. 2016;4(3):220–7.

55. Kummen M, Mayerhofer CCK, Vestad B, Broch K, Awoyemi A, Storm-Larsen C, et al. Gut microbiota signature in heart failure defined from profiling of 2 independent cohorts. J Am Coll Cardiol. 2018;71(10):1184–6.

56. Cui X, Ye L, Li J, Jin L, Wang W, Li S, et al. Metagenomic and metabolomic analyses unveil dysbiosis of gut microbiota in chronic heart failure patients. Sci Rep. 2018;8(1):635.

57. Peng L, Li ZR, Green RS, Holzman IR, Lin J. Butyrate enhances the intestinal barrier by facilitating tight junction assembly via activation of AMP-activated protein kinase in Caco-2 cell monolayers. J Nutr. 2009;139(9):1619–25.

58. Kaye DM, Shihata WA, Jama HA, Tsyganov K, Ziemann M, Kiriazis H, et al. Deficiency of prebiotic fiber and insufficient signaling through gut metabolite-sensing receptors leads to cardiovascular disease. Circulation. 2020;141(17):1393–403.

59. Tang TWH, Chen HC, Chen CY, Yen CYT, Lin CJ, Prajnamitra RP, et al. Loss of gut microbiota alters immune system composition and cripples postinfarction cardiac repair. Circulation. 2019;139(5):647–59.

60. Mayerhofer CCK, Kummen M, Holm K, Broch K, Awoyemi A, Vestad B, et al. Low fibre intake is associated with gut microbiota alterations in chronic heart failure. ESC Heart Fail. 2020;7(2):456–66.

61. Mollar A, Villanueva MP, E NU, Carratal AA, Mora F, Bayes-GenIs A, et al. Hydrogen- and methane-based breath testing and outcomes in patients with heart failure. J Card Fail. 2019;25(5):319–27.

62. Jama HA, Fiedler A, Tsyganov K, Nelson E, Horlock D, Nakai ME, et al. Manipulation of the gut microbiota by the use of prebiotic fibre does not override a genetic predisposition to heart failure. Sci Rep. 2020;10(1):17919.

63. Moludi J, Saiedi S, Ebrahimi B, Alizadeh M, Khajebishak Y, Ghadimi SS. Probiotics supplementation on cardiac remodeling following myocardial infarction: a single-center double-blind clinical study. J Cardiovasc Transl Res. 2021;14(2):299–307.

64. Gan XT, Ettinger G, Huang CX, Burton JP, Haist JV, Rajapurohitam V, et al. Probiotic administration attenuates myocardial hypertrophy and heart failure after myocardial infarction in the rat. Circ Heart Fail. 2014;7(3):491–9.

65. Mayerhofer CCK, Awoyemi AO, Moscavitch SD, Lappegard KT, Hov JR, Aukrust P, et al. Design of the GutHeart-targeting gut microbiota to treat heart failure-trial: a Phase II, randomized clinical trial. ESC Heart Fail. 2018;5(5):977–84.

66. Marotz CA, Zarrinpar A. Treating obesity and metabolic syndrome with fecal microbiota transplantation. Yale J Biol Med. 2016;89(3):383–388.

CHAPTER 12.11

Iron deficiency in heart failure

Ewa A Jankowska, Stefan D Anker, and Piotr Ponikowski

Contents

Iron deficiency as a global health problem

Iron deficiency (ID) is the most prevalent nutritional deficiency worldwide,[1,2] being particularly common in women, children, and the elderly. It is also common in those with chronic diseases and in individuals with low economic status.[1,2] Iron deficiency anaemia (IDA) currently affects 1.2 billion people, whereas ID without anaemia is at least twice as common.[1,2] ID is associated with numerous unfavourable consequences, seen globally at the population level, for example, higher healthcare costs, poor pregnancy outcomes, reduced school performance, decreased productivity, high morbidity, and mortality.[1-5] ID ranks as the thirteenth leading risk factor for global disability adjusted life-years (DALYs).[3] IDA is responsible for a significant proportion of years lived with disability (YLDs) due to communicable, maternal, neonatal, and nutritional disorders, accounting for 5.5% of all YLDs.[4] The economic burden imposed by ID/IDA is substantial, including the very substantial cost consequences of ID/IDA-related decreased productivity.[5]

Iron deficiency leads to defective energy metabolism

Iron is critically needed for the optimal functioning of both haematopoietic and non-haematopoietic cells. Iron, despite being perceived as mainly serving a critical factor for erythropoiesis, thrombopoiesis, and immune responses, is also present in all living cells where it plays important roles in multiple metabolic pathways[6-8] (➲ Figure 12.11.1). Classical teaching is that the consequences of ID may include IDA, immunodeficiency, thrombocytosis, and coagulopathy. However, it has been recently acknowledged that being a component of respiratory chain proteins in mitochondria and other enzymes crucial for energetic reactions, iron is also critical for the maintenance of optimal cellular energy metabolism.[6-11] Hence, it is not surprising that iron is particularly relevant for tissues with high energy demands, such as myocardium, kidneys, and skeletal muscles, as well as those with high mitogenic activity such as haematopoietic cells of all lines[7,9-11] (➲ Figure 12.11.2). Therefore, ID itself should be distinguished from IDA. Although untreated ID can result in anaemia as a consequence of being more advanced and long-lasting, ID itself reveals several highly relevant unfavourable effects in humans, including patients with heart failure (HF) even in the absence of anaemia.

Pathophysiological concepts of iron deficiency in heart failure

The cause of the high prevalence of ID in HF remains imperfectly understood. Taking into account that fact that iron is not actively excreted from the body, the pathogenesis of ID in HF might be thought to be associated with reduced iron intake, abnormal iron loss, and/or abnormal iron distribution to those body compartments where it is not available for metabolic processes. There are limited data to support the concept that

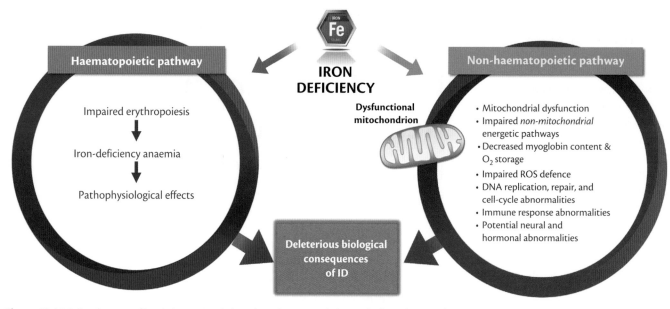

Figure 12.11.1 Involvement of iron in haematopoietic and non-haematopoietic metabolic pathways in humans.

inadequate dietary iron intake and/or low gastrointestinal iron bioavailability in instrumental in the ID that so frequently accompanies HF. Theoretically, low gastrointestinal iron bioavailability may be a consequence of intestinal interstitial oedema, the use of drugs lowering gastric pH (e.g. omeprazole or H2 receptor-antagonists), or the ingestion of food containing calcium, tannins, phosphates, or antiacids.[12–14] Iron loss in HF may also occur in the course of incidental gastrointestinal disorders (peptic ulcer, gastritis, duodenitis, colitis, diverticulitis) as well as menstrual blood loss, and blood loss from the urinary tract and other sources. It should be noted, however, that despite the plausibility of these pathomechanisms their relative contributions to the development of ID in patients with HF remain uncertain.

Some experts have hypothesized that the pathomechanisms triggering ID in the course of HF are similar to those seen in patients with chronic kidney disease (CKD). Patients with CKD demonstrate predominantly functional ID. This type of ID is driven principally by inflammation, which in turn stimulates the hepatic production of hepcidin. Hepcidin acts systemically to trigger mechanisms that shift iron into reticuloendothelial cells, where it remains trapped and is unavailable for widespread metabolic needs.[7,15–17] Importantly, however, there is little or no evidence that inflammation is a major trigger for ID in patients with HF, and this concept still remains equivocal and disputable. Importantly, patients with HF both in the chronic[18,19] and acute settings[20] demonstrate extremely low (not high!) circulating hepcidin levels, which suggests that ID seen in the course HF is associated with predominantly depleted iron stores rather than inflammation-triggered iron redistribution.

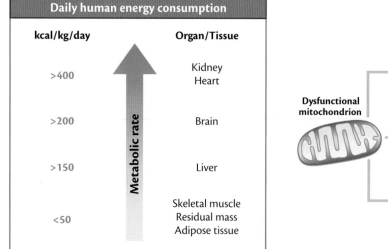

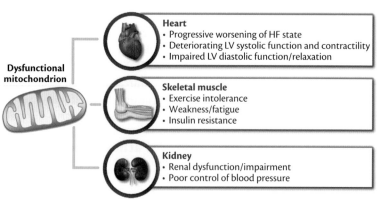

Figure 12.11.2 Mitochondrial dysfunction due to iron deficiency impairs functioning of organs characterised by high daily energy consumption.

Definition of iron deficiency in heart failure

According to haematological standards, bone marrow aspiration with the assessment of iron stores remains the 'gold standard' method to diagnose ID.[8,21,22] The invasive nature and limitations on the availability of this procedure makes it impractical to be used in routine clinical practice, particularly outside specialist haematology units. Importantly, the assessment of iron stores in bone marrow provides insight mainly into the iron status of erythropoietic processes. A biomarker-based approach seems to be more suitable for a diagnosis of ID in patients with HF. Instead specific peripheral blood biomarkers which reflect stored and utilized iron pools (described below) are recommended for the assessment of iron status in patients with HF.

Circulating ferritin is a reliable surrogate of iron stored in the body, predominantly in hepatocytes and reticuloendothelial cells. As a rule, the lower the serum ferritin, the more depleted are body iron stores. In the general population, absolute ID can be diagnosed when serum ferritin is at a level <30 ng/mL or by some accounts when serum ferritin is <12–15 ng/mL.[8,22–24] However, the fact that ferritin belongs is an acute phase protein and its production is increased during inflammation means that the ferritin level alone is insufficient to accurately rule ID in or out.[22,25] Therefore, in clinical conditions accompanied by inflammation (such as both CKD and HF), the interpretation of circulating ferritin is not straightforward; its level reflects iron stores, but only after the correcting the measured level for the effect of ongoing inflammation, an effect that is very difficult to quantify. Therefore, the definition of ID in most common use in HF research and clinical practice is a pragmatic one that considers higher cut-off values for serum ferritin ,such as <100 ng/mL or even higher, between 100–299 ng/mL, if they are accompanied by a low TSAT (<20%). Transferrin saturation (TSAT) reflects the pool of utilized iron that is available for use by metabolizing cells. TSAT is the percentage of transferrin which binds iron and is calculated as a ratio of serum iron and TIBC × 100% (TIBC, total iron binding capacity by transferrin).[7,8,22,25]

According to both the 2016 and 2021 ESC guidelines on HF,[26,27] the following definition of ID is recommended to be applied in patients with HF: serum ferritin <100 ng/mL, or serum ferritin 100–299 ng/mL with TSAT (<20%). This definition has been used in several trials of intravenous iron supplementation in patients with HF,[28–30] which have shown beneficial clinical effect, thereby demonstrating the ability of this pragmatic definition to identify individuals who likely will benefit from this therapy. Importantly the ESC guidelines emphasize the need to screen all patients with HF for the presence of ID utilizing serum ferritin and TSAT as the screening tools, irrespective of haemoglobin level, left ventricular ejection fraction (LVEF), and kidney function, in order to detect a potentially treatable co-morbidity.[26,27]

There have been attempts to propose alternative definitions of ID in patients with HF, either by utilizing novel iron biomarkers (e.g. hepcidin, soluble transferrin receptor (sTfR))[19,20] or by using standard biomarkers (ferritin, TSAT, iron) in different ways (L,M). A new pathophysiological definition of ID is based on the combined assessment of low serum hepcidin (reflecting depleted iron stores more accurately than ferritin) and high sTfR (reflecting depleted intracellular iron) has recently been proposed.[19,20] TfR is the membrane entrance pathway for iron import into all cells; it is upregulated when intracellular metabolic needs for iron are not met in order to facilitate the iron entrance to the cells and is later shed in excess to the circulation.[8,23] Although low hepcidin, high sTfR, low serum ferritin, low TSAT, and low serum iron have proven their prognostic value in patients with HF,[19,20,31–33] their utility as diagnostic tools applied in therapeutic algorithms have not been yet been adequately tested.

Prevalence and clinical consequences of iron deficiency in heart failure

ID is a non-cardiovascular co-morbidity prevalent across the whole spectrum of HF. When applying the aforementioned definition of ID (serum ferritin <100 ng/mL, or serum ferritin 100–299 ng/mL with TSAT (<20%), the prevalence of ID in patients with HF ranges between 35% and 83%, being particularly prevalent in patients after an episode of acute HF (72–83%). Moreover, the following features identify patients with HF who are more likely to be iron deficient: female sex, advanced NYHA class, anaemia, high plasma N-terminal pro-B-type natriuretic peptide (NT-pro-BNP), and high serum high-sensitivity C-reactive protein (hsCRP).[19,20,34–49]

In observational studies in patients with HF, ID (regardless of concomitant anaemia) has been associated with impaired aerobic performance (expressed by lower peak oxygen consumption), higher ventilatory response to exercise (VE-VCO$_2$ slope), reduced submaximal exercise capacity (expressed by the shorter 6-minute walking test distance), and poor health related quality of life (➲ Figure 12.11.3).[34,38,43,50–54] Iron deficient non-anaemic patients with HF have much worse exercise capacity and poorer quality of life compared to anaemic patients without ID.[38,43,51]

In cohort studies in patients with HF, ID (regardless of concomitant anaemia) has independently predicted the risk of all-cause death, cardiovascular death, combined death, or nonfatal cardiovascular events (HF hospitalization, acute coronary syndrome, severe arrhythmia, stroke), combined death, or heart transplantation (➲ Figure 12.11.3).[34,20,35–37,40,41,55]

Oral iron supplementation in heart failure

There is evidence that oral iron supplementation is not effective in iron-deficient patients with HF. In the IRONOUT trial, 16-week oral iron supplementation administered in iron deficient patients with HF did not result in significant change in serum ferritin, TSAT, or peak oxygen consumption.[56] Therefore, such therapy cannot be currently recommended.

Intravenous iron supplementation in heart failure

There is now a large and growing body of evidence that intravenous iron supplementation is effective and safe in iron-deficient patients with HF.

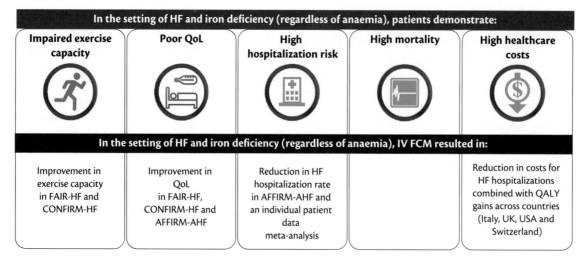

Figure 12.11.3 Clinical consquences of iron deficiency in patients with heart failure, and the effects of intravenous supplementation in this patient cohort.

It is worthy of note that previously used parenteral iron preparations were not free of toxicity, being associated with a high level of clinically relevant adverse events when administered as an iron oxyhydroxide complex. These preparations could induce oxidative stress and were associated with multiple adverse events including hypotension, nausea, vomiting, abdominal and lower back pain, peripheral oedema, and a metallic taste.[57–59] These side-effects have been largely circumvented by the introduction of compounds containing iron in a core surrounded by a carbohydrate shell, thereby eliminating the vast majority of adverse reactions, including allergic ones.[60] Up to now, five new parental formulations have been tested in patients with HF: iron sucrose, iron dextran, iron isomaltose, and ferric gluconate have been administered to groups of 136, 40, 20, and 13 patients, respectively.[61–71] The vast majority of evidence on safety and efficacy of intravenous iron supplementation in patients with HF comes from studies with ferric carboxymaltose (FCM).[28–30] These are reviewed below.

In the FAIR-HF trial, intravenous FCM administered in iron-deficient patients with HF and LVEF < 45% improved self-reported patient global assessment at week 24 and NYHA class at week 24 (primary endpoints) as well as increasing the distance of a 6-minute walk test and improving quality of life.[28,72] The improvement in aforementioned characteristics was seen in both anaemic and non-anaemic patients, even though the clinical improvement in non-anaemic patients was not accompanied by an increase in haemoglobin level.[72,73]

In the CONFIRM-HF trial, intravenous FCM administered in iron-deficient patients with HF and LVEF < 45% increased the distance of a 6-minute walking test at week 24 (primary endpoint) and this treatment effect was sustained to week 52.[29] Throughout the study, an improvement in NYHA class, patient global assessment, and quality of life in patients treated with intravenous FCM was also demonstrated. Treatment with FCM was associated with a reduction in the risk of hospitalizations for worsening HF at week 52 (secondary endpoint).[29]

In the AFFIRM-AHF trial, intravenous FCM administered to iron-deficient patients with HF and left ventricular ejection fraction ≤ 50% who had stabilized after an episode of acute HF resulted in a trend towards a reduction in total HF hospitalizations and cardiovascular death at week 52 (p = 0.059) (primary endpoint). It was also associated with a nominally significant reduction in total HF hospitalizations without an evident effect on cardiovascular mortality during the 52-week follow-up.[30] There was also a clinically meaningful improvement in quality of life seen as early as 4 weeks after treatment initiation and lasting up to week 24.[74] Cost-effectiveness analysis of the AFFIRM-AHF trial has confirmed that intravenous iron supplementation with FCM in iron-deficient patients after an episode of acute HF is dominant in the UK, USA, and Switzerland, and is highly cost-effective in Italy.[75]

Evidence coming from clinical trials has been supported by the results of two meta-analyses.[76,77] The meta-analysis of Jankowska et al.[83] included five trials in iron deficient patients with HF and LVEF ≤ 45%. It has been shown that in this patient cohort intravenous iron therapy as compared to placebo reduces the risk of combined all-cause death or cardiovascular hospitalization, the risk of combined cardiovascular death or HF hospitalization, and the risk of HF hospitalization, but without an effect on either all-cause or cardiovascular mortality.[76] Moreover, this intervention resulted in an improvement in exercise capacity (an increase in 6-minute walking test distance), an alleviation of HF symptoms (a reduction in NYHA class), and an improvement in quality of life and self-reported patient global assessment.[83] The individual patient data meta-analysis of Anker et al.[77] included data extracted from four trials comparing FCM with placebo in iron-deficient patients with HF and LVEF ≤ 45%. Compared with those taking placebo, patients on FCM had lower rates of recurrent cardiovascular hospitalizations and cardiovascular death, lower rates of recurrent HF hospitalizations and cardiovascular death, and lower rates of recurrent cardiovascular hospitalizations and all-cause death.[77] Time-to-first-event analyses showed similar findings, with somewhat attenuated treatment effects.[77]

Recommendations for iron deficiency complicating HF

The results of the FAIR-HF,[28,72] CONFIRM-HF,[29] and AFFIRM-AHF,[30,74] trials along with a meta-analysis[76] have established the basis for the ESC recommendation that intravenous iron supplementation with FCM should be considered in symptomatic patients with LVEF < 45% and ID (defined as above) in order to alleviate HF symptoms, improve exercise capacity, and quality of life.[27]

The major results of the AFFIRM-AHF trial[30] have led the foundations for the recommendation that intravenous iron supplementation with FCM should be considered in symptomatic HF patients recently hospitalized for HF and with LVEF < 50% and ID (defined as above) in order to reduce the risk of HF hospitalization.[27]

Practical advice on the diagnosis and treatment of ID in patients with HF are provided in ⊃ Table 12.11.1.

Table 12.11.1 Practical advice on diagnosis and treatment of ID in patients with HF

All patients with HF, regardless of haemoglobin level, kidney function and LVEF, are recommended to be screened periodically for ID using serum ferritin and TSAT
Screening for ID can be performed at any time during the course of HF, also during hospitalization for HF worsening
Diagnosis of ID in patients with HF is based on the following criteria: serum ferritin <100 ng/mL, or serum ferritin 100–299 ng/mL with TSAT < 20%
Patients with HF who do not have ID at baseline should be rechecked regarding their iron status every 12 months afterwards
Oral iron supplementation is not effective in iron deficient patients with HF and cannot be recommended
Intravenous iron supplementation with FCM should be considered in symptomatic patients with LVEF < 45% and ID in order to alleviate HF symptoms, improve exercise capacity, and quality of life
Intravenous iron supplementation with FCM should be considered in symptomatic HF patients recently hospitalized for HF and with LVEF < 50% and ID in order to reduce the risk of HF hospitalization
Following the dosing regime from the CONFIRM-HF[29] and AFFIRM-AHF trials,[30] intravenous FCM is administered according to a fixed scheme based on the subject's body weight and haemoglobin level at baseline and administered at weeks 0 and 6 (the total dose is between 0.5–2.0 g of FCM, and if the calculated dose exceeds 1 g, the dose remaining above 1 g is administered at week 6)
If ID is diagnosed in a hospitalized patient after an episode of acute HF, the first dose should be administered already in hospital before discharge
Intravenous iron supplementation with FCM can be administered in patients with HF in the outpatient setting
There is no need to perform any anti-allergic tests before intravenous FCM administration
Intravenous iron supplementation should not be administered in patients with HF if haemoglobin level exceeds 15 g/dL
Intravenous iron supplementation can be administered in patients with HF, regardless of kidney function, blood pressure, and heart rate
Patients with HF who have received the calculated dose of intravenous FCM should be rechecked regarding their iron status after 3–6 months

Future perspectives

Although ID is highly prevalent in HF, it origin still remains unknown. The ongoing clinical trials are expected to provide evidence on the effect of this therapy on long-term cardiovascular mortality in iron-deficient patients with HF (FAIR-HF2 (NCT03036462), IRONMAN (NCT02642562), HEART-FID (NCT03037931)) as well as on exercise capacity and quality of life in iron-deficient patients with HF with preserved ejection fraction (FAIR-HFpEF (NCT03074591)).

Anaemia without iron deficiency in heart failure

Anaemia (haemoglobin <12 g/dL in women and <13 g/dL in men) is common in all forms of HF, and is associated with worse clinical status and a higher risk of poor clinical outcomes. Simlar to ID, anaemia may have multiple causes in HF; as well as ID, these include chronic blood loss, relative erythropoietin deficiency secondary to CKD, haemodilution, and inflammation. Yet in the absence of ID, no specific therapy to correct anaemia has been proven to provide reliable clinical benefits, other than transfusion to correct severe anaemia such as that caused by acute or severe blood loss. Other causes of anaemia, beyond blood loss and ID, should be sought as specific therapies may be available for deficiency, including vitamin B12 or folate deficiencies or haemoglobinopathies. The 2021 ESC guidelines for HF specifically state that 'Treatment of anaemia in HF with erythropoietin stimulating agents is not recommended in the absence of other indications for this therapy.' This is because of the risk of adverse events and lack of efficacy seen in trials of this therapy for anaemia in patients with HF.

References

1. Al-Naseem A, Sallam A, Choudhury S, Thachil J. Iron deficiency without anaemia: a diagnosis that matters. Clin Med (Lond). 2021;21:107–13.
2. Zimmermann MB, Hurrell RF.Nutritional iron deficiency. Lancet. 2007;370:511–20.
3. Murray CJ, Lopez AD. Measuring the global burden of disease. N Engl J Med. 2013;369:448–57.
4. Vos T, Flaxman AD, Naghavi M, Lozano R, Michaud C, Ezzati M, et al. Years lived with disability (YLDs) for 1160 sequelae of 289 diseases and injuries 1990–2010: a systematic analysis for the Global Burden of Disease Study 2010. Lancet. 2012;380:2163–96.
5. Hunt JM. Reversing productivity losses from iron deficiency: the economic case. J Nutr. 2002;132(4 Suppl):794S–801S.
6. Andrews NC. Disorders of iron metabolism. N Engl J Med 1999;341:1986–95.
7. Jankowska EA, Von Haehling S, Anker SD, MacDougall IC, Ponikowski P. Iron deficiency and heart failure: Diagnostic dilemmas and therapeutic perspectives. Eur Heart J 2013;34:816–26.
8. Goodnough LT, Nemeth E, Ganz T. Detection, evaluation, and management of iron-restricted erythropoiesis. Blood 2010;116:4754–61.
9. Paul BT, Manz DH, Torti FM, Torti SV. Mitochondria and Iron: current questions. Expert Rev Hematol. 2017;10:65–79. Erratum in: Expert Rev Hematol. 2017;10:275.
10. Boyman L, Karbowski M, Lederer WJ. Regulation of mitochondrial ATP production: Ca2+ signaling and quality control. Trends Mol Med. 2020;26:21–39.

11. Brown DA, Perry JB, Allen ME, Sabbah HN, Stauffer BL, Shaikh SR, et al. Expert consensus document: Mitochondrial function as a therapeutic target in heart failure. Nat Rev Cardiol. 2017;14:238–50.

12. Hughes CM, Woodside J V, McGartland C, Roberts MJ, Nicholls DP, McKeown PP. Nutritional intake and oxidative stress in chronic heart failure. Nutr Metab Cardiovasc Dis. 2012;22:376–82.

13. Lourenço BH, Vieira LP, Macedo A, Nakasato M, Marucci M de FN, Bocchi EA. Nutritional status and adequacy of energy and nutrient intakes among heart failure patients. Arq Bras Cardiol. 2009;93:541–48.

14. Hallberg L, Hulthén L. Prediction of dietary iron absorption: An algorithm for calculating absorption and bioavailability of dietary iron. Am J Clin Nutr. 2000;71:1147–60.

15. Ueda N, Takasawa K. Impact of inflammation on ferritin, hepcidin and the management of iron deficiency anemia in chronic kidney disease. Nutrients. 2018;10:1173.

16. Wish JB, Aronoff GR, Bacon BR, Brugnara C, Eckardt KU, Ganz T, et al. Positive iron balance in chronic kidney disease: how much is too much and how to tell? Am J Nephrol. 2018;47:72–83.

17. Macdougall IC, Malyszko J, Hider RC, Bansal SS. Current status of the measurement of blood hepcidin levels in chronic kidney disease. Clin J Am Soc Nephrol. 2010;5(9):1681–9.

18. Weber CS, Beck-Da-Silva L, Goldraich LA, Biolo A, Clausell N. Anemia in heart failure: Association of hepcidin levels to iron deficiency in stable outpatients. Acta Haematol. 2013;129:55–61.

19. Jankowska EA, Malyszko J, Ardehali H, Koc-Zorawska E, Banasiak W, von Haehling S, et al. Iron status in patients with chronic heart failure. Eur Heart J. 2013;34:827–34.

20. Jankowska EA, Kasztura M, Sokolski M, Bronisz M, Nawrocka S, Kowska-Florek WO, et al. Iron deficiency defined as depleted iron stores accompanied by unmet cellular iron requirements identifies patients at the highest risk of death after an episode of acute heart failure. Eur Heart J. 2014;35:2468–76.

21. Gale E, Torrance J, Bothwell T. The quantitative estimation of total iron stores in human bone marrow. J Clin Invest. 1963;42:1076–.82.

22. Pasricha S-RS, Flecknoe-Brown SC, Allen KJ, Gibson PR, McMahon LP, Olynyk JK, , et al. Diagnosis and management of iron deficiency anaemia: a clinical update. Med J Aust. 2010;193:525–32.

23. Koulaouzidis A, Said E, Cottier R, Saeed AA. Soluble transferrin receptors and iron deficiency, a step beyond ferritin. A systematic review. J Gastrointestin Liver Dis. 2009;18:345–52.

24. Ali MA, Luxton AW, Walker WH. Serum ferritin concentration and bone marrow iron stores: a prospective study. Can Med Assoc J. 1978;118:945–46.

25. Wish JB. Assessing iron status: beyond serum ferritin and transferrin saturation. Clin J Am Soc Nephrol. 2006;1:S4–8.

26. Ponikowski P, Voors AA, Anker SD, Bueno H, Cleland JGF, Coats AJS, et al. 2016 ESC Guidelines for the diagnosis and treatment of acute and chronic heart failure: The Task Force for the diagnosis and treatment of acute and chronic heart failure of the European Society of Cardiology (ESC)Developed with the special contribution of the Heart Failure Association (HFA) of the ESC. Eur Heart J. 2016;37(27):2129–200. Erratum in: Eur Heart J. 2018;39:860.

27. McDonagh TA, Metra M, Adamo M, Gardner RS, Baumbach A, Böhm M, et al. 2021 ESC Guidelines for the diagnosis and treatment of acute and chronic heart failure. Eur Heart J. 2021;42:3599–726. Erratum in: Eur Heart J. 2021 Dec 21;42(48):4901.

28. Anker SD, Comin Colet J, Filippatos G, Willenheimer R, Dickstein K, Drexler H, et al. Ferric carboxymaltose in patients with heart failure and iron deficiency. N Engl J Med. 2009;361:2436–48.

29. Ponikowski P, van Veldhuisen DJ, Comin-Colet J, Ertl G, Komajda M, Mareev V, et al.. Beneficial effects of long-term intravenous iron therapy with ferric carboxymaltose in patients with symptomatic heart failure and iron deficiency. Eur Heart J. 2015;36:657–68.

30. Ponikowski P, Kirwan BA, Anker SD, McDonagh T, Dorobantu M, Drozdz J, et al. Ferric carboxymaltose for iron deficiency at discharge after acute heart failure: a multicentre, double-blind, randomised, controlled trial. Lancet. 2020;396:1895–904.

31. Grote Beverborg N, van der Wal HH, Klip IT, Anker SD, Cleland J, Dickstein K, et al. Differences in clinical profile and outcomes of low iron storage vs defective iron utilization in patients with heart failure: results from the DEFINE-HF and BIOSTAT-CHF studies. JAMA Cardiol. 2019;4:696–701.

32. Cleland JG, Zhang J, Pellicori P, Dicken B, Dierckx R, Shoaib A, Wong K, et al. Prevalence and outcomes of anemia and hematinic deficiencies in patients with chronic heart failure. JAMA Cardiol. 2016;1:539–47.

33. Sierpinski R, Josiak K, Suchocki T, Wojtas-Polc K, Mazur G, Butrym A, et al. High soluble transferrin receptor in patients with heart failure: a measure of iron deficiency and a strong predictor of mortality. Eur J Heart Fail. 2021;23(6):919–32. Erratum in: Eur J Heart Fail. 2022 Mar;24(3):591.

34. Okonko DO, Mandal AKJ, Missouris CG, Poole-Wilson PA. Disordered iron homeostasis in chronic heart failure: Prevalence, predictors, and relation to anemia, exercise capacity, and survival. J Am Coll Cardiol. 2011;58:1241–51.

35. Jankowska EA, Rozentryt P, Witkowska A, Nowak J, Hartmann O, Ponikowska B, et al. Iron deficiency: An ominous sign in patients with systolic chronic heart failure. Eur Heart J. 2010;31:1872–80.

36. Parikh A, Natarajan S, Lipsitz SR, Katz SD. Iron deficiency in community-dwelling US adults with self-reported heart failure in the National Health and Nutrition Examination Survey III: Prevalence and associations with anemia and inflammation. Circ Hear Fail 2011;4:599–606.

37. Klip IT, Comin-Colet J, Voors AA, Ponikowski P, Enjuanes C, Banasiak W, et al. Iron deficiency in chronic heart failure: An international pooled analysis. Am Heart J. 2013;165:575–82.e3.

38. Comín-Colet J, Enjuanes C, González G, Torrens A, Cladellas M, Meroño O, et al. Iron deficiency is a key determinant of health-related quality of life in patients with chronic heart failure regardless of anaemia status. Eur J Heart Fail 2013;15:1164–72.

39. Kasner M, Aleksandrov AS, Westermann D, Lassner D, Gross M, Von Haehling S, et al. Functional iron deficiency and diastolic function in heart failure with preserved ejection fraction. Int J Cardiol. 2013;168:4652–7.

40. Rangel I, Gonçalves A, de Sousa C, Leite S, Campelo M, Martins E, et al. Iron deficiency status irrespective of anemia: a predictor of unfavorable outcome in chronic heart failure patients. Cardiology. 2014;128:320–6.

41. Yeo TJ, Yeo PSD, Ching-Chiew Wong R, Ong HY, Leong KTG, Jaufeerally F, et al. Iron deficiency in a multi-ethnic Asian population with and without heart failure: prevalence, clinical correlates, functional significance and prognosis. Eur J Heart Fail. 2014;16:1125–32.

42. Schou M, Bosselmann H, Gaborit F, Iversen K, Goetze JP, Soletomas G, et al. Iron de fi ciency: Prevalence and relation to cardiovascular biomarkers in heart failure outpatients. Int J Cardiol. 2015;195:143–8.

43. Ebner N, Jankowska EA, Ponikowski P, Lainscak M, Elsner S, Sliziuk V, et al. The impact of iron deficiency and anaemia on exercise capacity and outcomes in patients with chronic heart failure. Results from the Studies Investigating Co-morbidities Aggravating Heart Failure. Int J Cardiol. 2016;205:6–12.

44. Núñez J, Domínguez E, Ramón JM, Núñez E, Sanchis J, Santas E, et al.. Iron deficiency and functional capacity in patients with advanced heart failure with preserved ejection fraction. Int J Cardiol. 2016;207:365–7.

45. Cohen-Solal A, Damy T, Terbah M, Kerebel S, Baguet JP, Hanon O, et al.. High prevalence of iron deficiency in patients with acute decompensated heart failure. Eur J Heart Fail. 2014;16:984–91.

46. de Silva R, Rigby AS, Witte KKA, Nikitin NP, Tin L, Goode K, et al. Anemia, renal dysfunction, and their interaction in patients with chronic heart failure. Am J Cardiol. 2006;98:391–8.

47. von Haehling S, Gremmler U, Krumm M, Mibach F, Schön N, Taggeselle J, et al. Prevalence and clinical impact of iron deficiency and anaemia among outpatients with chronic heart failure: The PrEP Registry. Clin Res Cardiol. 2017;106:436–43.

48. Wienbergen H, Pfister O, Hochadel M, Michel S, Bruder O, Remppis BA, et al.. Usefulness of iron deficiency correction in management of patients with heart failure [from the Registry Analysis of Iron Deficiency-Heart Failure (RAID-HF) Registry]. Am J Cardiol. 2016;118:1875–80.

49. Van Aelst LNL, Abraham M, Sadoune M, Lefebvre T, Manivet P, Logeart D, et al. Iron status and inflammatory biomarkers in patients with acutely decompensated heart failure: early in-hospital phase and 30-day follow-up. Eur J Heart Fail. 2017;19:1075–76.

50. Jankowska EA, Rozentryt P, Witkowska A, Nowak J, Hartmann O, Ponikowska B, et al. Iron deficiency predicts impaired exercise capacity in patients with systolic chronic heart failure. J Card Fail. 2011;17:899–906.

51. Enjuanes C, Klip IT, Bruguera J, Cladellas M, Ponikowski P, Banasiak W, et al. Iron deficiency and health-related quality of life in chronic heart failure: Results from a multicenter European study. Int J Cardiol. 2014;174:268–75.

52. Martens P, Nijst P, Verbrugge FH, Smeets K, Dupont M, Mullens W. Impact of iron deficiency on exercise capacity and outcome in heart failure with reduced, mid-range and preserved ejection fraction. Acta Cardiol. 2018;73:115–23.

53. Alcaide-Aldeano A, Garay A, Alcoberro L, Jiménez-Marrero S, Yun S, Tajes M, et al. Iron deficiency: impact on functional capacity and quality of life in heart failure with preserved ejection fraction. J Clin Med. 2020;9:1199.

54. Bekfani T, Pellicori P, Morris D, Ebner N, Valentova M, Sandek A, et al.Iron deficiency in patients with heart failure with preserved ejection fraction and its association with reduced exercise capacity, muscle strength and quality of life. Clin Res Cardiol. 2019;108:203–11.

55. Aung N, Ling HZ, Cheng AS, Aggarwal S, Flint J, Mendonca M, et al. Expansion of the red cell distribution width and evolving iron deficiency as predictors of poor outcome in chronic heart failure. Int J Cardiol; 2013;168:1997–2002.

56. Lewis GD, Malhotra R, Hernandez AF, McNulty SE, Smith A, Felker GM, et al. Effect of oral iron repletion on exercise capacity in patients with heart failure with reduced ejection fraction and iron deficiency: The IRONOUT HF randomized clinical trial. JAMA. 2017;317(19):1958–66. Erratum in: JAMA. 2017;317(23):2453.

57. Heath CW, Strauss MB, Castle WB. Quantitative aspects of iron deficiency in hypochromic anemia: (the parenteral administration of iron). J Clin Invest. 1932;11:1293–312.

58. Goetsch AT, Moore C V, Minnich V. Observations on the effect of massive doses of iron given intravenously to patients with hypochromic anemia. J Lab Clin Med. 1946;31:466.

59. Evans RW, Rafique R, Zarea A, Rapisarda C, Cammack R, Evans PJ, et al. Nature of non-transferrin-bound iron: studies on iron citrate complexes and thalassemic sera. J Biol Inorg Chem; 2007;13:57–74.

60. Macdougall IC. Evolution of iv iron compounds over the last century. J Ren Care 2009;35 Suppl 2:8–13.

61. Bolger AP, Bartlett FR, Penston HS, O'Leary J, Pollock N, Kaprielian R, Chapman CM. Intravenous iron alone for the treatment of anemia in patients with chronic heart failure. J Am Coll Cardiol 2006;48:1225–7.

62. Toblli JE, Lombraña A, Duarte P, Di Gennaro F. Intravenous iron reduces NT-pro-brain natriuretic peptide in anemic patients with chronic heart failure and renal insufficiency. J Am Coll Cardiol 2007;50:1657–65.

63. Okonko DO, Grzeslo A, Witkowski T, Mandal AKJ, Slater RM, Roughton M, et al. Effect of intravenous iron sucrose on exercise tolerance in anemic and nonanemic patients with symptomatic chronic heart failure and iron deficiency. J Am Coll Cardiol. 2008;51:103–12.

64. Usmanov RI, Zueva EB, Silverberg DS, Shaked M. Intravenous iron without erythropoietin for the treatment of iron deficiency anemia in patients with moderate to severe congestive heart failure and chronic kidney insufficiency. J Nephrol. 2008;21:236–42.

65. Terrovitis J V., Kaldara E, Ntalianis A, Sventzouri S, Kapelios C, Barbarousi D, et al. Intravenous iron alone is equally effective with the combination of iron and erythropoietin for the treatment of iron-deficiency anemia in advanced heart failure. J Am Coll Cardiol. 2012;60:2255–6.

66. Beck-Da-Silva L, Piardi D, Soder S, Rohde LE, Pereira-Barretto AC, De Albuquerque D, et al. IRON-HF study: A randomized trial to assess the effects of iron in heart failure patients with anemia. Int J Cardiol. 2013;168:3439–442.

67. Toblli JE, Di Gennaro F, Rivas C. Changes in echocardiographic parameters in iron deficiency patients with heart failure and chronic kidney disease treated with intravenous iron. Hear Lung Circ.2015;24:686–95.

68. Gaber R, Kotb NA, Ghazy M, Nagy HM, Salama M, Elhendy A. Tissue doppler and strain rate imaging detect improvement of myocardial function in iron deficient patients with congestive heart failure after iron replacement therapy. Echocardiography. 2012;29:13–18.

69. Kaminsky BM, Pogue KT, Hanigan S, Koelling TM, Dorsch MP. Effects of total dose infusion of iron intravenously in patients with acute heart failure and anemia (Hemoglobin < 13 g/dl). Am J Cardiol. 2016;117:1942–6.

70. Hildebrandt PR, Bruun NE, Nielsen OW, Pantev E, Shiva F, Videbæk L, et al. Effects of administration of iron isomaltoside 1000 in patients with chronic heart failure. A pilot study. Transfus Altern Transfus Med.2010;11:131–7.

71. Reed BN, Blair EA, Thudium EM, Waters SB, Sueta CA, Jensen BC, Rodgers JE. Effects of an accelerated intravenous iron regimen in hospitalized patients with advanced heart failure and iron deficiency. Pharmacotherapy 2015;35:64–71.

72. Comin-Colet J, Lainscak M, Dickstein K, Filippatos GS, Johnson P, Lüscher TF, et al. The effect of intravenous ferric carboxymaltose on health-related quality of life in patients with chronic heart failure and iron deficiency: a subanalysis of the FAIR-HF study. Eur Heart J. 2013;34:30–8.

73. Filippatos G, Farmakis D, Colet JC, Dickstein K, Lüscher TF, Willenheimer R, et al. Intravenous ferric carboxymaltose in iron-Deficient chronic heart failure patients with and without anaemia: A subanalysis of the FAIR-HF trial. Eur J Heart Fail. 2013;15:1267–6.

74. Jankowska EA, Kirwan BA, Kosiborod M, Butler J, Anker SD, McDonagh T, et al. The effect of intravenous ferric carboxymaltose on health-related quality of life in iron-deficient patients with acute heart failure: the results of the AFFIRM-AHF study. Eur Heart J. 2021;42:3011–20.

75. McEwan P, Ponikowski P, Davis JA, Rosano G, Coats AJS, Dorigotti F, et al. Ferric carboxymaltose for the treatment of iron deficiency in heart failure: a multinational cost-effectiveness analysis utilising AFFIRM-AHF. Eur J Heart Fail. 2021;23:1687–97.

76. Jankowska EA, Tkaczyszyn M, Suchocki T, Drozd M, von Haehling S, Doehner W, et al. Effects of intravenous iron therapy in iron-deficient patients with systolic heart failure: a meta-analysis of randomized controlled trials. Eur J Heart Fail. 2016;18:786–95.

77. Anker SD, Kirwan BA, van Veldhuisen DJ, Filippatos G, Comin-Colet J, Ruschitzka F, et al. Effects of ferric carboxymaltose on hospitalisations and mortality rates in iron-deficient heart failure patients: an individual patient data meta-analysis. Eur J Heart Fail. 2018;20:125–33.

CHAPTER 12.12

Cognitive impairment and depression

Wolfram Doehner, Cristiana Vitale, and Mehmet Birhan Yilmaz

Contents

Introduction

Heart failure (HF), being particularly common in the elderly, is commonly presenting as a syndrome associated with multi-organ dysfunction and many co-morbidities. Co-morbidities can complicate the diagnosis of HF, can worsen symptomatic status and disease progression, and can make treatment more difficult and more expensive. Of these HF-related co-morbidities brain disorders are some of the most prevalent and the most difficult to manage.[1] The elderly HF patient with patterns of increasing comorbidities poses a complex challenge for modern health care systems. Foremost to account for these challenges are higher brain function disorders, namely cognitive decline and/or dementia and depression which make patient self-care and treatment compliance more difficult and which add dramatically to the cost of health care provision for the HF itself. With the ageing of developed societies, more patients with HF present with these multiple co-morbidities thus HF emerging as the most frequent reason for hospitalization.

The heart and the brain are commonly subject to similar disease processes and pathophysiological mechanisms, and a disorder in each can mutually affect the other. The heart and the brain are both subject to the structural and functional decline of ageing, including tissue atrophy,[2] fibrosis, ischaemia, infarction, macro and micro vascular dysfunction, and tissue inflammation (➔ Figure 12.12.1).[3] Neurological co-morbidities including stroke, depression, cognitive decline, and autonomic dysfunction (beside cardiac and vascular regulation) have received little commentary in recent HF guidelines[4] despite being common, clinically relevant, and difficult to manage.[5] Therapeutic strategies in this setting, therefore remain largely empirical. The haemodynamic effects of the HF on higher cerebral function are still poorly understood,[6] but should not be underestimated.[7]

Dementia in heart failure

Heart failure is an independent risk factor for cognitive decline with an estimated prevalence for cognitive decline between 25% and 75%[8,9] and a 60% increased risk of dementia.[10] Unfortunately, many cases are not recognized.[11] When present it carries a loss of independence, a significantly impaired quality of life, and a worse prognosis.[12] In HF many aspects of higher cerebral function can be impaired, including cognition, attention, memory, language, psychomotor function, and visuo-spatial acuity.[13,14] Although the precise pathophysiological processes involved are not fully understood, poor perfusion, micro-embolic events, and other ischaemic syndromes may play a role, along with possible effects of disruptions of the blood–brain barrier, cerebral inflammation, and endothelial- and neurovascular unit dysfunction. Early detection of cognitive decline is always challenging and the study of subtle differences in brain function in HF is in its infancy, with many questions remaining unanswered. Clinical features associated with cognitive

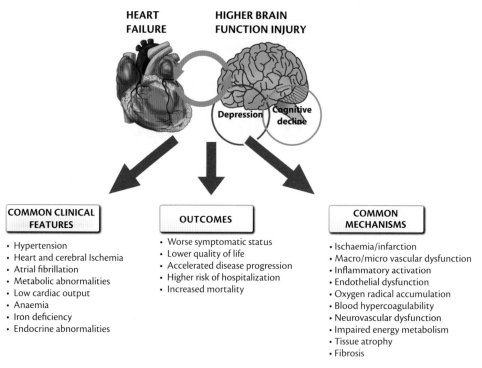

Figure 12.12.1 Shared features between heart failure, cognitive impairment, and depression.

decline and dementia include hypertension as a risk factor for both, stroke, atrial fibrillation (AF), metabolic abnormalities, low cardiac output, depression, anaemia, iron deficiency, and endocrine abnormalities.[15,16] Cognitive impairment in HF can have a variety of clinical manifestations from mild memory problems through to dementia requiring permanent nursing home care or equivalent, and have been reported both in HFrEF and HFpEF.[17] Cognitive impairment can have a stealthy onset or it can develop acutely, associated with delirium typically during an episode of acute haemodynamic decompensation.[18] Delirium can occur during episodes of acute decompensation of HF and is associated with increased mortality and length of hospital stay. The mechanisms underlying the association between acute delirium and HF remain poorly understood.

Mechanisms of cognitive decline in heart failure

Fundamental mechanisms of declining cerebral function in heart failure include sudden (and repeated) vascular injury (stroke), chronic impaired cerebral perfusion (low flow HF), and cardiovascular risk factors affecting cerebral perfusion.

Stroke in patients with heart failure

Stroke, in particular multiple mini strokes or events of silent cerebral ischaemia, are a common cause of disability, cognitive decline, and dementia in HF, as in the general population.[19,20] In patients with HF, however, strokes are more likely because HF is prone to blood hypercoagulability, endothelial dysfunction, inflammatory activation, and malfunctioning of cerebral autoregulation along with a higher incidence of AF. HF is prevalent in ca. 10% of all strokes,[21,22] and when they occur subsequent re-strokes and death are more likely to follow.[23,24] Silent brain infarctions are also very

common in HF (two- to four-fold higher prevalence than in the non HF population of similar age) and may be responsible for a progressive deterioration of cognitive function. In the Framingham Study, HF lead to a 4.1, for men and 2.8, for women, greater risk of stroke compared to those without HF.[25] AF as a common comorbidity in HF further increases the risk of stroke, as does an ischaemic aetiology of the HF. Other co-morbidities, including peripheral arterial disease, hypertension, valvular heart disease, diabetes, chronic kidney disease (CKD), can further increase the risk of stroke. Dementia can be delayed or prevented if strokes can be prevented or treated very early, to limit cerebral tissue loss. Oral anticoagulants are indicated in HF patients with AF but the balance of benefit and risk in patients with HFrEF with maintained sinus rhythm is less clear. The ESC 2021 guidelines[4] state that there is no data to support a routine strategy of anticoagulation in patients with HF patients who are in sinus rhythm without the presence or history of AF. The recently published COMMANDER-HF trial did not report a benefit of oral anticoagulation with rivaroxaban to improve the composite primary endpoint of death, myocardial infarction, or stroke. However, a reduction of the endpoint component stroke alone was observed in this trial (HF 0.66, 95% CI 0.47–0.95).[26] Early thrombolytic treatment of an ischaemic stroke within the first 4.5 hours after symptom onset and even beyond this point in selected patients can improve outcomes, although an increased bleeding risk after thrombolysis in HF should be taken into consideration.[27] Another therapeutic option in acute ischaemic stroke is mechanical thrombectomy.

Impaired cerebral perfusion

Low cardiac output may account for reduced cerebral perfusion although cerebrovascular auto-regulation is capable of maintaining perfusion pressure over a wide range of vascular pressure. Physiological cerebrovascular auto-regulation is active both globally and regionally in response to functional cerebral activity and local oxygen demands. The vascular variability is locally controlled by pericytes, perivascular cells with contractile capacity at the capillary level.[28] This vascular autoregulation is impaired in HF. The resulting hypoperfusion seen with both acute or chronic HF may cause or worsen cognitive decline in HF. Low blood pressure (<139 mmHg) was observed to relate to reduced cognitive function in HF patients.[29] However, it is unclear if the low blood pressure is directly related to cognitive impairment (vial reduced perfusion pressure) or indirectly as a function of more severe HF. Further HF-related pathophysiological mechanisms, such as inflammatory activation, oxygen radical accumulation, endothelium dysfunction, and impaired energy metabolism, may contribute to impaired cerebral perfusion and hence to progressing cognitive decline. Impaired tissue perfusion is particularly present in episodes of acute decompensated HF and a temporary severe cognitive impairment up to significant delirium is a complication in acute HF associated with increased mortality.[30] After haemodynamic stabilization, cognitive impairment may recover up to or below the level prior to the acute event.[31]

Diagnostic and therapeutic concepts of dementia in heart failure

Cognitive disorders in HF may range from barely recognizable mild cognitive impairment to progressive and debilitating dementia, to significant but temporary delirium related to acutely decompensated HF.

Cognitive decline via impairment of perception, learning, memory, problem solving, and social communication contributes to progressive loss of functional independence and quality of life, worsening of adherence to therapy, to symptomatic HF progression, prolonged in-hospital stay, and increased mortality. Self-care in HF is a cognitively demanding process requiring adherence to several non-pharmacological interventions and medications. Hence, even mild cognitive impairment can potentially result in impaired self-care, which may incorrectly be attributed to poor motivation or poor treatment compliance and account for delayed engagement to seek assistance from disease management programmes.[32]

Therefore, early recognition of the cognitive impairment in HF represents the most important initial step for establishing effective concepts to prevent further cognitive decline.

Diagnosis and monitoring cognitive function in heart failure

Multiple validated questionnaires exist to screen for, and to an extent, grade cognitive impairment. These include the Mini Mental Status Examination (MMSE) and the Montreal Cognitive Assessment (MoCA). Both scores were suggested for use in the previous ESC guidelines on diagnosis and treatment of HF but this message was lost in the current ESC Guidelines.[4]

The MMSE has been used to screen for cognitive deficits, but it is not very sensitive in detecting mild cognitive impairment

(MCI). The MoCA is considered to be more sensitive to subtle changes.[33] These screening tools can be helpful in differentiating acute from chronic cognitive decline in HF. The questionnaires detect the clinically measurable cognitive decline, whereas the pathophysiological structural antecedents may be present but functionally unrecognized months or years earlier. For example cerebral atrophy, white matter hyperintensities,[34] loss of grey matter,[35] and silent cerebral infarcts[36] are frequent findings in cerebral imaging in HF patients with and without cognitive dysfunction.[37] Those imaging findings may help to recognize the risk of and search for signs of cognitive impairment.

MCI is the mildest form of cognitive decline and may remain undetected in many cases. It is advisable to address cognitive implications of HF in patient education as in family and relatives education in order to ensure awareness and early recognition of mild symptoms. Establishing comprehensive concepts to target cognitive decline together with sufficient monitoring concepts on self-care, treatment adherence, and symptom progression may improve quality of life and prognosis of the patients. Screening for cognitive impairment should be considered in elderly patients with HF when admitted with acute HF or upon casually reported deficits by the patients or relatives. Screening and review should also be regularly performed in the outpatient settings. Primary care can often pick up early milder changes, perhaps being reported by carers and family members.

Management of cognitive decline in heart failure

Very little is said in most HF guidelines concerning the management of cognitive decline, dementia, or delirium. Further research is clearly needed to investigate preventive and interventional strategies to improve outcomes, especially self-care. It is important to recognize the presence or progression of cognitive impairment and not to dismiss it as poor motivation or compliance. Depression is also a frequent accompaniment of HF and the overlap or combination with cognitive decline adds further complexity to both diagnostics and treatment. Early recognition of cognitive deficits require engagement of support facilities and engagement in disease management programmes to assist in self-care and to maintain an adequate treatment regimen.

Treatments of heart failure affecting cognitive function

Angiotensin converting enzyme inhibitors and angiotensin receptor blockers, beta blockers and mineralocorticoid receptor antagonists

Angiotensin converting enzyme inhibitors and angiotensin receptor blockers have been shown to improve cognitive function in both hypertension and HF.[38,39] Beta-blockers worsen dizziness and hypotension in HF which is a theoretical risk for worsening cognitive function in fragile elderly HF patients. Sacubitril/valsartan in the PARADIGM-HF trial, whilst reducing mortality and morbidity, was associated with more hypotension compared to patients randomized to enalapril, and there is an as yet unresolved concern about its potential to promote Alzheimer's disease[40] via inhibition of neprilysin-mediated degradation of β-amyloid (Aβ) and the potential accumulation of Aβ in the brain. However, analyses of PARADIGM did not find any increased risk of dementia or Alzheimer's.[41] The mineralocorticoid receptor antagonist spironolactone was shown to improve some domains of cognitive impairments in animal studies and has been tested in schizophrenia patients in SPIRO-TREAT trial.[42]

Sodium glucose co-transporter-2 inhibitors

Sodium glucose co-transporter (SGLT-2) inhibitors, as the latest improvement in therapy for HF irrespective of the EF, showed neuroprotective properties, cerebral infarct-limiting properties by improving brain microvasculature and potentially other pathways, and seem to be good candidates for improving cognitive dysfunction of HF.[43]

Devices

Biventricular pacing has repeatedly been reported to improve cognitive function likely via improved haemodynamic capacity[44] as has been shown for heart transplantation. In turn, devices used to treat HF such as left ventricular assist devices (LVAD) carry an increased risk of embolic stroke, bleeding, and thrombotic complications.[45] Of note, cognitive impairment remains as a significant risk factor for stroke and death following LVAD implantation.[46] Changes in systemic immune state, platelet function. and acquired von Willebrand syndrome may potentially lead to cerebral infarction and haemorrhage. Other devices such as veno-arterial extracorporeal membrane oxygenation (VA-ECMO) are similarly thought to lead to an increased risk of thrombosis, bleeding, and neurological events.

Depression in chronic heart failure

Depression is an important comorbidity in HF patients, with major depression affecting up to 30% of patients and many patients having depressive symptoms. The prevalence of depression is higher in women and increases with age and advanced New York Heart Association classes (class III, IV).[47] In patients with HF, depression has a negative impact on their psychosocial and functional status and it is associated with poorer compliance to guideline-directed medical therapy, lower self-care, poor quality of life, greater morbidity and mortality, increased hospitalization, and higher health care costs. [48]

Adverse effects of depression on HF are supposedly mediated by shared pathophysiological mechanisms, including dysregulation of the autonomic system, inflammation, procoagulant state, increased activity of the hypothalamic–pituitary–adrenal axis, arrhythmias, and social factors but also by lower treatment compliance, and lower self-care. There is conflicting evidence that cardiovascular medications, such as beta-blockers and mineralocorticoid receptor antagonists, may be associated with depression. However, the use of hydrophilic beta-blockers is associated with a lower risk of central neurological symptoms, as they do not significantly cross the blood/brain barrier.

Diagnosing depression in heart failure

Despite the relevant negative impact of depression in HF, this condition remains frequently under-diagnosed. Depression can be easily overlooked in the routine care of HF patients because symptoms of the two conditions overlap, thus being misinterpreted both by physicians and patients themselves. Current ESC guidelines on HF recommend to screen HF patients for depression only upon clinical suspicion of depression.[4] It is advisable to address the potential for depressive mood shifts in patient education, as in family and relatives education, in order to ensure awareness and early recognition of the respective symptoms. Establishing comprehensive care concepts to address depressive changes may benefit treatment adherence, self-care, and may improve quality of life and prognosis of the patients.

Given the overlap between cardiac and psychological symptoms, an accurate diagnosis of major depression in HF patients can be challenging. Screening tools for early detection of mood changes (such as the Patient Health Questionnaire-2 and -9, Beck Depression Inventory, and Geriatric Depression Scale) are not routinely used in clinical practice in HF. Furthermore, it is unclear whether different, more specific, diagnostic instruments (questionnaires and structured interview) should be used in patients with HF compared to those commonly used.

Therapeutic concepts on depression in heart failure

Although remission from depression may improve cardiovascular outcomes, successful intervention strategies specific for the setting of HF have not been demonstrated. Adequate depression treatment includes non-pharmacological and pharmacological therapies. Short-term exercise training and cognitive behavioural therapy (CBT) are safe and have shown beneficial effects on depressive symptoms, but their sustainability in long-term clinical practice is unknown.[49]

Antidepressant agents may safely be used in HF patients, but monoamine oxidase inhibitors and tricyclic antidepressants are usually avoided due to their unfavourable effects on blood pressure and pro-arrhythmic potential, respectively.[50] Notably, many of the commonly utilized antidepressants (such as citalopram, escitalopram, fluoxetine, and venlafaxine) may prolong the QT interval. Therefore their used should be carefully weighted and monitored in HF patients. Selective serotonin reuptake inhibitors (SSRIs) appear to be safe and are commonly used in HF. The results of two major randomized trials (SADHART-CHF and MOOD-HF) did, however, not show superiority over placebo in reducing depressive symptoms in patients with HF in the short- and long-term. [51,52] Transcranial magnetic stimulation for the treatment of depression is contraindicated in HF patients with pacemakers and implanted devices.

The combination of CBT with a SSRI is currently regarded the preferred management of depression in patients with HF patients. However, a multidisciplinary approach for comprehensive patient care, also involving patient education, could be the key to an effective management of depression in HF patients. More research is warranted to develop novel and safer treatments targeted at depression in patients with HF.

Future directions

Further work is needed to address gaps in the evidence and to raise awareness of cognitive functional decline and depression in patients with HF. Unfortunately, in the current guidelines, reduced information on cognitive function and depression as comorbidities in HF has been noted compared to the previous guidelines. Tools to assess dynamic cognitive decline in the course of HF need to be evaluated for widespread and easy clinical applicability in HF patients. Further studies are warranted to establish if a specific antidepressant therapy regimen may be superior for application in HF. More likely, however, multimodal treatment approaches may be most effective to prevent or slow down the decline in cognitive function and depressive disorder. Consequently, future work needs to evaluate improved concepts of comprehensive care that includes multiple parties involved in patient care (e.g. patients, families, primary medical and social services or specialized services) as well as optimized medical, physical, and rehabilitation treatments. Novel innovative treatment concepts, such as remote and telemedical care, specialized HF nurse programmes, rehabilitation or exercise programmes, and comprehensive disease management concepts, need to be evaluated for efficacy, applicability, and cost effectiveness. Importantly, improving awareness among both patient, relatives and health care providers is required for early detection and therapy. Hence, beside novel research efforts, further education and advocating are required to advance therapeutic success of these comorbidities on HF.

Summary and key messages

Cognitive impairment and depression are common comorbidities and complications in HF with pronounced prevalence in the elderly patient population. These functional brain disorders have been proven to worsen the symptomatic status, decrease quality of life, contribute to disease progression, and increase mortality of the patients. Despite this significant impact on HF morbidity and mortality, cognitive function and depression remain poorly addressed in current diagnostic and treatment guidelines for HF and are often overlooked in clinical evaluation of ambulatory or hospitalized patients. Early recognition, patient education, and diagnostic workup are most important to raise awareness for this complication for patients, their social networks, attending physicians, and health care structures. Establishing multifaceted care concepts to target cognitive impairment and depression within comprehensive HF care models may substantially slow down progression of brain functional decline and support improved treatment adherence, quality of life, symptomatic status, and prognosis of the patients.

References

1. Scherbakov N, Doehner W. Heart-brain interactions in heart failure. Card Fail Rev. 2018;4:87–91.
2. Kohara K, Okada Y, Ochi M, Ohara M, Nagai T, Tabara Y, Igase M. Muscle mass decline, arterial stiffness, white matter hyperintensity, and cognitive impairment: Japan Shimanami Health Promoting Program study. J Cachexia Sarcopenia Muscle. 2017;8(4):557–566.
3. Doehner W, Ural D, Haeusler KG, Čelutkienė J, Bestetti R, Cavusoglu Y, et al. Heart and brain interaction in patients with heart failure: overview and proposal for a taxonomy A position paper from the Study Group on Heart and Brain Interaction of the Heart Failure Association Eur J Heart Fail. 2018;20(2):199–215.
4. McDonagh TA, Metra M, Adamo M, Gardner RS, Baumbach A, Böhm M, et al. 2021 ESC Guidelines for the diagnosis and treatment of acute and chronic heart failure. Eur Heart J. 2021;42:3599–3726. Erratum in: Eur Heart J 2021;42(48):4901.
5. van Bilsen M, Patel HC, Bauersachs J, Böhm M, Borggrefe M, Brutsaert D, et al. The autonomic nervous system as a therapeutic target in heart failure: a scientific position statement from the Translational Research Committee of the Heart Failure Association of the European Society of Cardiology. Eur J Heart Fail. 2017;19:1361–1378.
6. Roy B, Woo MA, Wang DJJ, Fonarow GC, Harper RM, Kumar R. Reduced regional cerebral blood flow in patients with heart failure. Eur J Heart Fail. 2017;19:1294–130.2
7. Erkelens CD, van der Wal HH, de Jong BM, Elting JW, Renken R, Gerritsen M, et al. Dynamics of cerebral blood flow in patients with mild non-ischaemic heart failure Eur J Heart Fail. 2017;19:261–268.
8. Hajduk AM, Lemon SC, McManus DD, Lessard DM, Gurwitz JH, Spencer FA, et al. Cognitive impairment and self-care in heart failure. Clin Epidemiol. 2013;5:407–416.
9. Ampadu J, Morley JE Heart failure and cognitive dysfunction. Int J Cardiol. 2015;178:12–23
10. Wolters FJ, Segufa RA, Darweesh SKL, Bos D, Ikram MA, Sabayan B, et al. Coronary heart disease, heart failure, and the risk of dementia: A systematic review and meta-analysis. Alzheimers Dement. 2018;14:1493–1504.
11. Hanon O, Vidal JS, de Groote P, Galinier M, Isnard R, Logeart D, et al. Prevalence of memory disorders in ambulatory patients aged C70 years with chronic heart failure (from the EFICARE Study). Am J Cardiol. 2014;113:1205–1210.
12. Zuccala G, Pedone C, Cesari M, Onder G, Pahor M, Marzetti E, et al. The effects of cognitive impairment on mortality among hospitalized patients with heart failure. Am J Med. 2003;115:97–103.
13. Pressler SJ, Subramanian U, Kareken D, Perkins SM, Graduz-Pizlo I, Sauve MJ, et al. Cognitive deficits in chronic heart failure. Nurs Res. 2010;59:127–139.
14. Alwerdt J, Edwards JD, Athilingam P, O'Connor ML, Valdes EG. Longitudinal differences in cognitive functioning among older adults with and without heart failure. J Aging Health. 2013;25:1358–1377.
15. Alosco ML, Brickman AM, Spitznagel MB, et al The independent association of hypertension with cognitive function among older adults with heart failure. J Neurol Sci. 2012;323:216–220.
16. Jankowska EA, Biel B, Majda J, Szklarska A, Lopuszanska M, Medras M, et al Anabolic deficiency in men with chronic heart failure: prevalence and detrimental impact on survival Circulation 2006;114:1829–1837.
17. Čelutkienė J, Vaitkevičius A, Jakštienė S, Jatužis D. Expert opinion-cognitive decline in heart failure: more attention is needed. Card Fail Rev. 2016; 2(2):106–109.
18. Alagiakrishnan K, Mah D, Ahmed A, Ezekowitz J. Cognitive decline in heart failure. Heart Fail Rev. 2016;21:661–673.
19. Townsend N, Wilson L, Bhatnagar P, Wickramasinghe K, Rayner M, Nichols M. Cardiovascular disease in Europe: epidemiological update 2016. Eur Heart J. 2016;37:3232–3245.
20. Feigin VL, Mensah GA, Norrving B, Murray CJ, Roth GA; GBD 2013 Stroke Panel Experts Group. Atlas of the Global Burden of Stroke (1990–2013): The GBD 2013 study. Neuroepidemiology. 2015; 45(3):230–236.

21. Hebert K, Kaif M, Tamariz L, Gogichaishvili I, Nozadze N, Delgado MC, Arcement LM. Prevalence of stroke in systolic heart failure. J Card Fail. 2011;17:76–81.

22. Kristensen SL, Jhund PS, Køber L, McKelvie RS, Zile MR, Anand IS, et al. Relative importance of history of heart failure hospitalization and N-terminal pro–B-type natriuretic peptide level as predictors of outcomes in patients with heart failure and preserved ejection fraction. JACC Heart Fai.l 2015;3:478–486.

23. Haeusler KG, Laufs U, Endres M. Chronic heart failure and ischemic stroke. Stroke. 2011;42:2977–2982.

24. Katsanos AH, Parissis J, Frogoudaki A, Vrettou AR, Ikonomidis I, Paraskevaidis I, et al. Heart failure and the risk of ischemic stroke recurrence: A systematic review and meta-analysis. J Neurol Sci. 2016;362:182–187.

25. Kannel WB, Wolf PA, Verter J. Manifestations of coronary disease predisposing to stroke The Framingham study. JAMA. 1983;250:2942–2446.

26. Zannad F, Anker SD, Byra WM, Cleland JGF, Fu M, Gheorghiade M, et al. Rivaroxaban in patients with heart failure, sinus rhythm, and coronary disease N Engl J Med. 2018;379:1332–1342.

27. Whiteley WN, Slot KB, Fernandes P, Sandercock P, Wardlaw J. Risk factors for intracranial hemorrhage in acute ischemic stroke patients treated with recombinant tissue plasminogen activator: a systematic review and meta-analysis of 55 studies. Stroke. 2012;43:2904–2909.

28. Dalkara T, Alarcon-Martinez L. Cerebral microvascular pericytes and neurogliovascular signaling in health and disease. Brain Res. 2015;1623:3–17.

29. Zuccalà G, Onder G, Pedone C, Carosella L, Pahor M, Bernabei R, et al. Hypotension and cognitive impairment: selective association in patients with heart failure. Neurology. 2001,11;57:1986–1992.

30. Harjola VP, Mullens W, Banaszewski M, Bauersachs J, Brunner-La Rocca HP, et al. Organ dysfunction, injury and failure in acute heart failure: from pathophysiology to diagnosis and management A review on behalf of the Acute Heart Failure Committee of the Heart Failure Association (HFA) of the European Society of Cardiology (ESC). Eur J Heart Fail. 2017;19:821–836.

31. Kindermann I, Fischer D, Karbach J, Link A, Walenta K, Barth C, et al. Cognitive function in patients with decompensated heart failure: the Cognitive Impairment in Heart Failure (CogImpair-HF) study. Eur J Heart Fail. 2012;14:404–413.

32. Lovell J, Pham T, Noaman SQ, Davis MC, Johnson M, Ibrahim JE. Self-management of heart failure in dementia and cognitive impairment: a systematic review. BMC Cardiovasc Disord. 2019;19:99.

33. Cameron J, Worrall-Carter L, Page K, Stewart S, Ski CF. Screening for mild cognitive impairment in patients with heart failure: Montreal cognitive assessment versus mini mental state exam. Eur J Cardiovasc Nurs. 2013; 12:252–260.

34. Jefferson AL, Tate DF, Poppas A, Brickman AM, Paul RH, Gunstad J, et al. Lower cardiac output is associated with greater white matter hyperintensities in older adults with cardiovascular disease. J Am Geriatr Soc. 2007;55:1044–1048.

35. Almeida OP, Garrido GJ, Etherton-Beer C, Lautenschlager NT, Arnolda L, Alfonso H, Flicker L. Brain and mood changes over 2 years in healthy controls and adults with heart failure and ischaemic heart disease. Congest Heart Fail. 2013;19: E29–E34.

36. Cogswell RJ, Norby FL, Gottesman RF, Chen LY, Solomon S, Shah A, Alonso A. High prevalence of subclinical cerebral infarction in patients with heart failure with preserved ejection fraction. Eur J Heart Fail. 2017;19:1303–1309.

37. Suzuki H, Matsumoto Y, Ota H, Sugimura K, Takahashi J, Ito K, et al. Structural brain abnormalities and cardiac dysfunction in patients with chronic heart failure. Eur J Heart Fail. 2018;20:936–938.

38. Zuccala G, Onder G, Marzetti E, et al. Use of ACE-inhibitors and variations in cognitive performance among patients with heart failure. Eur Heart J. 2005; 26, 226–233.

39. Böhm M, Kindermann I. Does angiotensin-converting-enzyme inhibitor therapy improve cognitive function in heart failure patients? Nat Clin Pract Cardiovasc Med. 2005;2:448–44.9

40. Alessio G, Lombardi F. Neprilysin inhibition for heart failure. N Engl J Med. 2014, 371: 2335–2337.

41. Cannon JA, Shen L, Jhund PS, Kristensen SL, Køber L, Chen F, et al. Dementia-related adverse events in PARADIGM-HF and other trials in heart failure with reduced ejection fraction. Eur J Heart Fail. 2017;19:129–137.

42. Wehr MC, Hinrichs W, Brzózka MM, Unterbarnscheidt T, Herholt A, Wintgens JP, et al. Spironolactone is an antagonist of NRG1-ERBB4 signaling and schizophrenia-relevant endophenotypes in mice. EMBO Mol Med. 2017;9:1448–1462.

43. Wiciński M, Wódkiewicz E, Górski K, Walczak M, Malinowski B. Perspective of SGLT2 inhibition in treatment of conditions connected to neuronal loss: focus on Alzheimer's Disease and ischemia-related brain injury. Pharmaceuticals (Basel). 2020;13:379.

44. Duncker D, Friedel K, König T, Schreyer H, Lüsebrink U, Duncker M, et al. Cardiac resynchronization therapy improves psycho-cognitive performance in patients with heart failure. Europace. 2015;17:1415–1421.

45. McIlvennan CK, Magid KH, Ambardekar AV, Thompson JS, Matlock DD, Allen LA. Clinical outcomes after continuous-flow LVED; a systematic review. Cir Heart Fail. 2014;7: 1003–1013.

46. Pavol MA, Boehme AK, Willey JZ, Festa JR, Lazar RM, Nakagawa S, et al. Predicting post-LVAD outcome: Is there a role for cognition? Int J Artif Organs. 2021;44:237–242.

47. Rutledge T, Reis VA, Link SE, Greenberg BH, Mills PJ. Depression in heart failure: a meta analytic review of prevalence, intervention effects, and associations with clinical outcomes. J Am Coll Cardiol. 2006;48:1527–1537.

48. Ramos S, Prata J, Bettencourt P, Gonçalves FR, Coelho R. Depression predicts mortality and hospitalization in heart failure: a six-years follow-up study. J Affect Disord 2016;201:162–170.

49. Jeyanantham K, Kotecha D, Thanki D, Dekker R, Lane DA. Effects of cognitive behavioural therapy for depression in heart failure patients: a systematic review and meta-analysis. Heart Fail Rev 2017;22:731–741.

50. Fernandez A, Bang SE, Srivathsan K, Vieweg WV Cardiovascular side effects of newer antidepressants. Anadolu Kardiyol Derg 2007;7:305–309.

51. O'Connor CM, Jiang W, Kuchibhatlla M, Sliva SG, Cuffe MS, Callwood DD, et al. Safety and efficacy of sertraline for depression in patients with heart failure: results of the SADHART-CHF (Setraline Against Depression and Heart Disease in Chronic Heart Failure) trial. J Am Coll Cardiol. 2010;56:692–699.

52. Angermann CE, Gelbrich G, Störk S, Gunold H, Edelmann F, Wachter R, et al. Effect of escitalopram on all-cause mortality and hospitalization in patients with heart failure and depression: the MOOD-HF randomized clinical trial. JAMA. 2016;315:2683–2693.

CHAPTER 12.13

Cancer and heart failure

Dimitrios Farmakis*, Alexander Lyon*,
Rudolf de Boer, and Yuri Belenkov

Contents

Introduction

Cancer is increasing in prevalence as a comorbidity affecting heart failure (HF) patients. This has been attributed to several factors:[1–3]

1 shared risk factors, such as ageing, smoking, obesity;

2 increasing survival of HF patients who can live to develop cancer;

3 frequent use of cross-sectional imaging and contact with healthcare professionals that results in increased cancer detection;

4 common prescription of anticoagulation and/or antiplatelet agents unmasking cancer due to the detection of bleeding or iron deficiency;

5 emerging evidence that HF itself may *per se* increase the risk of new cancer development or progression.

The impact of the diagnosis of cancer in a HF patient, and vice versa, depends upon a variety of factors (➲ Figure 12.13.1). From a cardiological perspective, the severity of the HF syndrome, the treatments required, and the prognosis of the patient may all influence the selection of cancer treatments that can be administered safely.[1] From an oncological perspective, the specific type of cancer, its stage, the prognosis, and, importantly, the cardiovascular (CV) safety of available treatment options will all determine the final choice of cancer treatments.[4]

An essential and fundamental component in the management of patients is the effective communication among the oncology team, the HF team, and, ideally, the cardio-oncology team to discuss the impact of HF on cancer management, and vice versa in order to minimize risks but also to improve survival and other clinical outcomes.[4]

Treating cancer in patients with heart failure

The risk of cardiotoxicity

Systemic anticancer therapies may cause CV toxicity of different forms.[5] As a result, the balance between their anti-tumour activity and CV side effects should be carefully assessed by a multi-disciplinary team of specialists before administering them to patients with known HF.[5] The risk of cardiotoxicity is associated with a constellation of risk factors (➲ Figure 12.13.2). Drugs, such as anthracyclines, 5-fluourouracil, and capecitabine, the human epidermal growth factor receptor 2 (HER2) targeting antibody trastuzumab, or tyrosine kinase inhibitors (TKIs) targeting vascular endothelial

---

* DF and AL have contributed equally and share the lead author role.

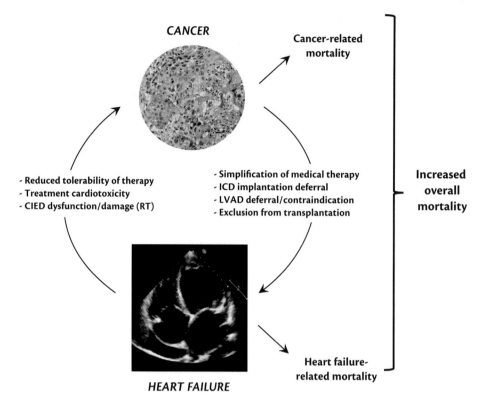

Figure 12.13.1 Cancer and heart failure carry an independent risk of mortality, but also potentially hinder the treatment of one another, with the result being a further increase in mortality. Diagnosis of cancer worsens the prognosis of a patient with pre-existing heart failure, and each condition carries an independent risk of mortality and potentially hinders treatment of the other one. ICD: implantable cardioverter defibrillator; LVAD: left ventricular assist device; CIED: cardiac implantable electronic device; RT: radiotherapy.

Reproduced from Ameri P, Canepa M, Anker MS, et al; Heart Failure Association Cardio-Oncology Study Group of the European Society of Cardiology. Cancer diagnosis in patients with heart failure: epidemiology, clinical implications and gaps in knowledge. *Eur J Heart Fail.* 2018 May;20(5):879–887. doi: 10.1002/ejhf.1165 with permission from John Wiley and Sons.

growth factor (VEGF)-directed, may cause or aggravate left ventricle (LV) systolic or diastolic dysfunction and may precipitate myocardial ischaemia or arrhythmia by a variety of mechanisms.[6,7] Hence their use in patients with pre-existing HF must be extremely cautious. Other oncological therapies may increase the risk of vascular events that could have a secondary impact on HF. These include gonadotropin-releasing hormone (GnRH) agonists and anti-androgens, used to treat locally advanced and metastatic prostate cancer, VEGF TKI for various solid tumours, and BCR-ABL TKI for chronic myeloid leukaemia.[8] In addition,

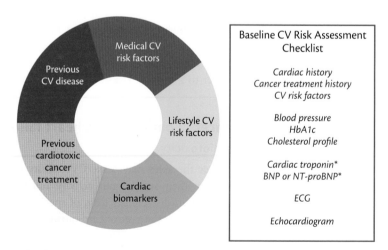

Figure 12.13.2 Risk factors associated with an increased risk of cardiotoxicity in patients with cancer scheduled to receive potentially cardiotoxic anticancer regimens and main modalities used for baseline risk stratification.

Reproduced from Lyon AR, Dent S, Stanway S, et al. Baseline cardiovascular risk assessment in cancer patients scheduled to receive cardiotoxic cancer therapies: a position statement and new risk assessment tools from the Cardio-Oncology Study Group of the Heart Failure Association of the European Society of Cardiology in collaboration with the International Cardio-Oncology Society. *Eur J Heart Fail.* 2020 Nov;22(11):1945–1960. doi: 10.1002/ejhf.1920 with permission from John Wiley and Sons.

many systemic anti-neoplastic drugs, both cardiotoxic and non-cardiotoxic, are frequently administered with large amounts of concomitant intravenous fluid to minimize nephrotoxicity; care should therefore be given in patients with pre-existing HF who are prone to fluid retention.[5]

Cytotoxic chemotherapy

Cytotoxic chemotherapy is indicated for a range of solid tumours and bone marrow malignancies. Anthracyclines, including doxorubicin, epirubicin, daunorubicin, and idarubicin, are well known to cause myocardial dysfunction, either via a direct myocyte toxic injury or functional toxicity without injury, or indirectly via increased risk of atrial tachyarrhythmias.[9] The risk of anthracycline-induced cardiotoxicity depends upon a number of variables including demographics, CV risk factors and disease and prior cardiotoxic therapies (⊃ Figure 12.13.3).[5] The risk also depends upon the severity of HF as indicated by symptoms, LV size and function (baseline left ventricular ejection fraction (LVEF)), natriuretic peptide level, tolerance of and response to guideline-targeted doses of HF medication, and HF aetiology. Genetic background is also crucial as the risk of cardiotoxicity is higher in patients with mutations associated with cardiomyopathy.[10]

⊃ Figure 12.13.3 depicts the Heart Failure-International Cardio-Oncology Society (HFA-ICOS) baseline risk assessment proforma for cancer patients scheduled to receive anthracycline chemotherapy, and ⊃ Figure 12.13.4 shows the cardiac monitoring plan during therapy with anthracycline-based regimens.[4,11] HF per se places patients at very high risk for anthracycline-related cardiotoxicity and therefore alternative non-anthracycline regimens should be considered, while if they are started on an anthracycline-based regimen, they should be followed with echocardiography and cardiac biomarkers every two cycles during chemotherapy and at 3 and 12 months post-treatment.

Besides causing cardiotoxicity, cytotoxic chemotherapy may also destabilize HF patients, particularly their fluid balance and diuretic requirements. For example, platinum-based chemotherapies require co-administration of relatively large fluid volumes to reduce nephrotoxicity. Amending infusion protocols to minimize fluid volume, increase the duration of the infusion time, and co-administration of additional loop diuretic doses is advisable. In contrast, many cytotoxic chemotherapy regimens cause severe nausea, vomiting, and/or diarrhoea which can cause dehydration and diuretic doses, and sometimes doses of RAASi need to be temporarily reduced or interrupted to reduce the risk of acute kidney injury, but should be restarted when the patient's fluid balance has stabilized.

Electrolyte imbalance, particularly hypokalaemia and hypomagnesaemia, are common following cytotoxic chemotherapies and increase the risk of QTc prolongation and both atrial and ventricular arrhythmias.[5] Replacement to maintain normal levels is recommended, and ECGs monitoring is required to assess QTc interval given it is frequently increased in patients with HF at baseline. Avoidance of QTc prolonging drugs, such as anti-emetics and antibiotics with QTc prolonging potential, which are also frequently used in cancer patients is important.[5]

Targeted therapies

Targeted cancer therapies are currently used to treat a wide range of malignancies, including solid tumours and haematological malignancies. Targeted therapies have been associated with a wide range of CV toxicities, including asymptomatic LV dysfunction, HF, arterial hypertension, thromboembolic events, myocardial ischaemia, QT prolongation, and arrhythmias.[5]

According to HFA-ICOS baseline CV risk assessment proformas,[12] a history of HF places patients at high or very high risk for cardiotoxicity also during treatment with targeted anticancer agents. These agents include HER2-targeted therapies (e.g. trastuzumab, pertuzumab, lapatinib), VEGF inhibitors (e.g., bevacizumab, sunitinib, pazopanib, sorafenib), multi-targeted TK/BCR-ABL inhibitors (e.g. ponatinib, nilotinib, dasatinib), proteasome inhibitors (e.g. carfilzomib, bortezomib), and RAF/MEK inhibitors (e.g. dabrafenib/trametinib).[4] In addition, patients with baseline HF are also at high risk for cardiotoxicity during treatment with immune checkpoint inhibitors (e.g. ipilimumab, nivolumab, pembrolizumab, azetolizumab, avelumab).[13]

Radiation therapy

The prevalence of pericardial disease due to radiation and chemotherapy is unknown because there are no large multicentre studies or registries for radiation-induced CV disease.[14] In most cases, pericardial disease may develop in parallel with myocardial damage when using radiotherapy together with anthracyclines, immune checkpoint inhibitors, or more rarely after methotrexate, bleomycin, or bone marrow transplantation.[13,15] Acute pericarditis during radiotherapy is usually observed in patients with Hodgkin's lymphoma, breast cancer, and lung cancer.[16] Most commonly, acute pericarditis resolves spontaneously without any treatment. However, in up to 20% of patients after high-dose radiotherapy administration, occurrence of chronic exudative and/or constrictive pericarditis are described.[17,18] Delayed effects of radiotherapy can occur in the period from 6 months to 15 years and includes both acute pericarditis and chronic pericardial effusion (usually asymptomatic), with an absolute cumulative incidence of 2–5%.[19] Transthoracic echocardiography is the imaging method of choice for suspected pericardial disease due to chemo-radiotherapy. Cardiac CT and MRI, especially with late gadolinium enhancement, can be useful, particularity for detecting calcifications, infiltrative lesions, and masses.[5]

Treatment of pericardial diseases due to chemo-radiotherapy does not differ from that recommended for other aetiologies. The prescription of non-steroid anti-inflammatory drugs can sometimes be contra-indicated if there are haemostatic disorders due to cancer treatment. Acute radiation-induced pericarditis requires colchicine therapy, and ICI-induced pericarditis requires both colchicine and steroids.[20] Pericardiocentesis is recommended in the cases with significant pericardial effusion and cardiac tamponade.

Baseline evaluation and management

Baseline CV risk stratification of cancer patients scheduled to receive potentially cardiotoxic anticancer regimens is based on

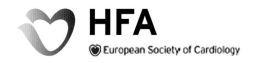 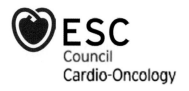 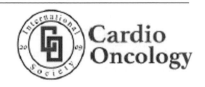

BASELINE CARDIO-ONCOLOGY RISK ASSESSMENT

ANTHRACYCLINE CHEMOTHERAPY

Risk Factor	Risk Factor Present	Score	Level of Evidence
Previous cardiovascular disease			
Heart failure or cardiomyopathy		VERY HIGH	B
Severe valvular heart disease		HIGH	C
Myocardial infarction or previous coronary revascularisation (PCI or CABG)		HIGH	C
Stable angina		HIGH	C
Baseline LVEF <50%		HIGH	B
Baseline LVEF 50–54%		MEDIUM^2	C
Cardiac Biomarkers (where available)			
Elevated baseline troponin*		MEDIUM^1	C
Elevated baseline BNP or NT-proBNP*		MEDIUM^1	C
Demographic and cardiovascular risk factors			
Age ≥80 years		HIGH	B
Age 65–79 years		MEDIUM^2	B
Hypertension ⌀		MEDIUM^1	B
Diabetes mellitus ✦		MEDIUM^1	C
Chronic kidney disease ⊀		MEDIUM^1	C
Previous cardiotoxic cancer treatment			
Previous anthracycline exposure		HIGH	B
Previous radiotherapy to left chest or mediastinum		HIGH	C
Previous non-anthracycline-based chemotherapy		MEDIUM^1	C
Lifestyle risk factors			
Current smoker or significant smoking history		MEDIUM^1	C
Obesity (BMI >30)		MEDIUM^1	C
RISK LEVEL			

LEGEND
BMI = Body mass index
BNP = Brain natriuretic peptide
CABG = Coronary artery bypass graft
LVEF = Left ventricular ejection fraction
NT-proBNP = N-terminal pro-brain natriuretic peptide
* Elevated above the upper limit of normal for local laboratory reference range
⌀ Systolic blood pressure (BP) >140 mmHg or diastolic BP >90 mmHg, or on treatment
✦ HbA1c >7.0% or >53 mmol/mol or on treatment
⊀ Estimated glomerular filtration rate <60 ml/min/1.73m^2

LOW RISK = no risk factor OR one MEDIUM1 RF
MEDIUM RISK = MEDIUM RFs with a total of 2–4 points
HIGH RISK = MEDIUM RFs with a total of ≥5 points OR any HIGH RF
VERY HIGH RISK = any VERY HIGH RF

Figure 12.13.3 HFA-ICOS Baseline risk assessment proforma for cancer patients scheduled to receive anthracycline chemotherapy.
Reproduced from Lyon AR, Dent S, Stanway S, et al. Baseline cardiovascular risk assessment in cancer patients scheduled to receive cardiotoxic cancer therapies: a position statement and new risk assessment tools from the Cardio-Oncology Study Group of the Heart Failure Association of the European Society of Cardiology in collaboration with the International Cardio-Oncology Society. *Eur J Heart Fail.* 2020 Nov;22(11):1945–1960. doi: 10.1002/ejhf.1920 with permission from John Wiley and Sons.

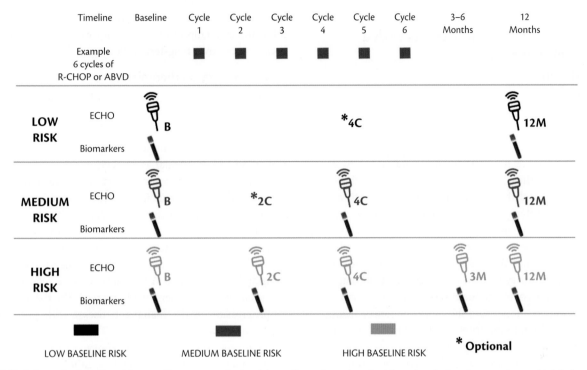

Figure 12.13.4 Example of cardiotoxicity surveillance protocol using echocardiography and cardiac biomarkers for lymphoma patients scheduled to receive 6 cycles of ABVD or R-CHOP chemotherapy. Heart failure patients will be in the High Risk group with increased monitoring.

Reproduced from Čelutkienė J, Pudil R, López-Fernández T, et al. Role of cardiovascular imaging in cancer patients receiving cardiotoxic therapies: a position statement on behalf of the Heart Failure Association (HFA), the European Association of Cardiovascular Imaging (EACVI) and the Cardio-Oncology Council of the European Society of Cardiology (ESC). *Eur J Heart Fail.* 2020 Sep;22(9):1504–1524. doi: 10.1002/ejhf.1957 with John Wiley and Sons.

history, clinical evaluation, ECG, cardiac imaging and cardiac biomarkers (➲ Figure 12.13.2).[4] The Heart Failure Association (HFA) in collaboration with ICOS has developed a series of structured baseline risk assessment proformas to stratify the risk of cardiotoxicity associated with specific anticancer regimens.[4] There are six different risk proformas for corresponding anticancer drug classes, including:

1 anthracyclines,

2 HER2 targeted therapies,

3 VEGF inhibitors,

4 multi-targeted kinase inhibitors including BCR-ABL TKIs,

5 proteasome inhibitors/immunomodulatory drugs, and

6 androgen deprivation therapies.[4]

The level of cardiotoxicity risk determined by these proformas guides subsequent patient management as well as the form and frequency of cardiac monitoring, if needed, in the course of anticancer treatment. Patients with increased risk of cardiotoxicity associated with planned anticancer regimens should ideally be referred for cardio-oncology consultation before starting cancer treatment. Appropriate guidance is provided by the corresponding HFA position papers.[4,11,21]

In general, a history of HF places patients with a new cancer diagnosis at high or very high risk of cardiotoxicity from a broad range of anticancer agents.[4] For this reason, HF patients are generally excluded from clinical trials in the field of oncology and therefore evidence on the efficacy and safety of many anticancer agents in HF is very limited. As a result, patients with HF who are being diagnosed with cancer should be referred for cardiology assessment, preferably by a cardio-oncology specialist, before the initiation of any anticancer therapy.[4]

The initial management of patients with HF and a new cancer diagnosis before the onset of cancer treatment requires:

1 meticulous assessment of HF status, including clinical review, ECG, echocardiogram, and measurement of baseline cardiac biomarkers (troponin, natriuretic peptides);

2 optimization of HF therapy, increasing renin-angiotensin-aldosterone inhibitors and betablocker doses to guideline-targeted doses as tolerated;

3 careful selection of anticancer regimen, weighing the risks and benefits of cardiotoxic versus non-cardiotoxic treatments upon cancer and HF prognosis;

4 development of a cardiac monitoring plan during cancer treatment;

5 patient education regarding monitoring body weight, blood pressure, and heart rate at home.

The above should ideally be guided by a multidisciplinary team of oncology, HF, and cardio-oncology specialists.

Treating heart failure in patients with a new cancer diagnosis

Medical therapies

When a HF patient is newly diagnosed with cancer, the evidence-based HF medication should ideally continue according to guideline recommendations.[22] However, temporary dose reduction or even interruption of HF medications may be required when patients' performance health status deteriorates due to cancer or its treatment.[1] Thus, cancer patients, particularly those with advanced cancer and those being actively treated with chemotherapy, often develop hypotension, volume depletion, electrolyte disturbances, or renal function worsening due to vomiting, diarrhoea or other side-effects of cancer or its therapy.[1] In addition, new tachyarrhythmias resulting from electrolyte disturbances, stress, pulmonary emboli, or infection may decompensate a HF patient in the context of the effects of the cancer or its treatment. Infections resulting from the cancer or cancer treatments may be an indication to interrupt sodium-glucose cotransporter type 2 inhibitors (SGLT2i) temporarily (sick days rule) and resume once the infection has cleared. Furthermore, as cancer or its therapy may cause thrombocytopaenia, the risk–benefit balance for anticoagulation and/or antiplatelets should be reviewed, with potential interruption until bleeding risk has been minimized or corrected, taking under consideration both cancer and cardiac prognosis.[23] Advice on home monitoring of weight and blood pressure is necessary along with periodic monitoring of renal function, electrolytes, and blood count, and frequent revision of HF medications.

Device therapies

HF patients with advanced or metastatic cancer may represent a contraindication to eligibility for device therapy depending upon the prognosis of the cancer. An implantable cardioverter-defibrillator (ICD) may be withheld if predicted life expectancy is less than 1 year for either cardiac or oncological reasons.[22] Decisions regarding eligibility for an ICD should be kept under constant review as patients can show substantial responses to modern targeted anti-cancer therapies that may prolong cancer-progression-free survival and may merit ICDs if the competing risk of sudden cardiac death is high.

Cardiac implantable electronic devices (pacemakers, cardiac resynchronization therapy (CRT)-P, cardiac resynchronization therapy-D) are commonly used in patients with HF and reduced LV ejection fraction (HFrEF), and therefore may be present in a HF patient with a new cancer diagnosis. In these patients, clinical surveillance should include interrogation of the cardiac implantable electronic devices (CIED) before and after radiotherapy, because of the possibility of CIED dysfunction or damage caused by the radiation.[24,25] Direct CIED irradiation with high-energy (more than 10 MV) or neutron-producing beams should be avoided, and the estimated cumulative dose to the CIED should be limited. ECG monitoring should be available during radiotherapy sessions for pacing-dependent patients.[24] Cardiac imaging (echocardiography, cardiac CT, MRI) may be required following irradiation to the chest, for example, in lymphoma or breast cancer, over long-term follow-up.[26]

Advanced surgical therapies

Patients with active malignancy or a history of recently treated cancer who develop HF may not be clinically suitable for the full range of available therapeutic options for HF and this is particularly true for advanced surgical therapies, including cardiac transplantation and ventricular assist devices.[1]

Active cancer is a contraindication for cardiac transplantation and the same is true for patients with a history of recently treated cancer (within the last 5 years), with the exception of non-melanoma skin cancer.[22] Patients with well-controlled or low-grade malignancy (e.g. prostate cancer) should be reviewed on a case-by-case basis by the heart transplantation multidisciplinary team. An additional issue related to cardiac transplantation in patients with cancer is the risk of recurrence or progression of the malignant disease with post-transplant immunosuppression.[27]

Long-term mechanical circulatory support (MCS) with implantable ventricular assist devices, either as a bridge to transplantation or as destination therapy, is also contraindicated in patients with cancer and a poor prognosis, as defined by a life expectancy of less than 2 years.[28] In the INTERMACS Registry, among patients who received a ventricular assist device, those with a history of cancer had worse outcomes that those without.[28] However, according to the International Society for Heart and Lung Transplantation guidelines, patients with a history of treated cancer who are in long-term remission or are considered free of disease may be candidates for MCS as bridge to transplantation (class I, level of evidence C), while those with a life-expectancy greater than 2 years may also be candidates for MCS as destination therapy.[29]

Given the ongoing advances in anticancer therapies and the continuous improvement in prognosis provided by new and emerging modalities, decision making in patients with cancer and HF in need for advanced surgical therapies should be guided by a multidisciplinary team including oncology, HF, CV surgery, and cardio-oncology specialists.

Exercise rehabilitation

Impairment of cardiorespiratory fitness (CRF) is a strong predictor of patient outcomes during and following cancer treatment. It has been shown that low CRF is associated with poor quality of life, increased morbidity, worse CV risk factor profile, and is an independent predictor of all-cause, cancer-related, and CV disease (CVD)-related mortality in cancer survivors.[30,31] A study in a cohort of 1632 cancer survivors (mean, 7 years post treatment) showed that the risk of CVD-related mortality decreased by 14% per 1 metabolic equivalent (MET) (3.5 mLO2/kg/min) increase in CRF, suggesting that CRF may an intervention target in cancer survivors.[31]

Exercise must be regarded as a potent multi-targeted approach that addresses multiple mechanisms of CV toxicity, including CRF impairment, CV injury, and CV risk factors.[32] CPET-guided exercise facilitates development of training programmes that are individualized to a person's fitness level and targeted to specific mechanisms of injury, and that systematically progress to optimize physiologic adaptation.[33] Current evidence demonstrates that supervised exercise therapies (including high-intensity interval training) is safe and well tolerated,[34] attenuates cardiotoxicity risk and improves CRF.

Heart failure and cancer drug–drug interactions

May anticancer drugs have multiple interactions with medications taken by patients with prevalent HF or CVD in general. It is important to consult with pharmacists and be aware of drug–drug interactions, particularly for cancer patients receiving TKIs, many of which have interactions involving cytochrome CYP3A4 or p-glycoprotein-mediated metabolism. Statins, angiotensin receptor–neprilysin inhibitors (ARNI), angiotensin-converting enzyme inhibitors (ACEi), angiotensin receptor blocker (ARBs), and SGLT2 inhibitors must be reviewed to ensure compatibility. Caution must also be taken in patients on cancer drugs which prolong QTc interval given many HF patients have prolonged QTc, and to avoid cardiac QTc prolonging drugs such as amiodarone. Furthermore, direct oral anticoagulants (DOAC) that are often prescribed in HF patients due to concomitant atrial fibrillation should also be used with extreme caution in patients being actively treated with anticancer agents. All DOAC should be avoided when anticancer regimens include strong inducers or inhibitors of p-glycoprotein such as doxorubicin, vinblastine, imatinib, or vandetanib.[35] In addition, DOAC and particularly apixaban and rivaroxaban and apixaban should be used cautiously with anticancer agents that are substrates for CYP3A4.[35]

Cancer causing cardiac cachexia and heart failure

Advanced cancer is often followed by progressive muscle wasting, leading to weight loss and cachexia. It seems that this process does not spare the heart either, as cancer has been associated with myocardial atrophy and energy depletion, a condition termed cardiac cachexia.[36,37] Implicated mechanisms include the release of pro-inflammatory cytokines by cancer cells, followed by dysregulation of several pathways including Akt/mammalian target of rapamycin (mTOR), AMP-activated protein kinase (AMPK), peroxisome proliferator-activated receptor gamma (PPAR-γ) coactivator 1α, and nuclear factor-κB (NF-κB) that in turn promote protein catabolism, reduction in oxidative defences, and impaired oxidative metabolism.[36] It has been postulated that exercise training may attenuate these processes, reducing potentially cancer-associated cardiac cachexia.[36]

The development of HF in patients with cancer results from the interaction of three main factors, the cardiotoxic effects of anticancer therapy, the CV background of the patient, and the effects of the cancer itself (➲ Figure 12.13.5).[9] Many anticancer therapies cause LV dysfunction and HF, including anthracyclines, targeted therapies such as HER2-targeted agents, VEGF inhibitors, multi-targeted TKI, and RAF/MEK inhibitors, proteasome inhibitors, and immune checkpoint inhibitors.[12] In addition, anticancer therapies may cause HF indirectly, through other forms of CV toxicity that may in turn lead to the development or exacerbation of HF, including arterial hypertension, myocardial ischaemia, thromboembolic events, arrhythmias, and myocarditis.[5] Patients' pre-existing CVD and risk factors, along with genetic predisposition, increase the susceptibility to cardiotoxicity. Finally, cancer may affect the heart directly through the invasion of cardiac tissues and mostly indirectly through secretion of metabolic by products and toxic factors, induction of cardiac cachexia, autonomic nervous system imbalance, and others (➲ Figure 12.13.5).[3]

Increased risk of cancer in heart failure patients

Over recent years, there has been a growing interest towards pathogenetic mechanisms that may link heart failure and cancer in a reciprocal manner (➲ Figure 12.13.6) following an increasing awareness that CVD in general, and HF in particular, are associated with an increased risk of cancer.[3] Epidemiological studies have described a higher incidence of cancer in patients with prevalent HF, including malignant lymphoma, colorectal cancer, breast cancer, and urogenital cancer.[38-45] The reasons for this intriguing phenomenon have been discussed in more detail in recent years.[46-48] First, there may be observational and ascertainment bias, as patients with prevalent CVD often undergo more blood and radiological examinations, that may prompt early diagnosis of cancer. Furthermore, patients with prevalent CVD frequently use anticoagulants, which may trigger tumours and polyps to bleed and become detected. However, the excess in cancer diagnoses is relatively stable over time which does not support this explanation. Another explanation is the effect of shared mechanisms that induce pathophysiological changes in the heart and other organs and also have an effect on tumour initiation and/or growth.[3] For instance, CVD is characterized by chronic, low-grade inflammation, and this has been linked to cancer formation as well. In the CANTOS trial, which evaluated the effects of the anti-inflammatory IL-1 antibody canakinumab on coronary artery disease, canakinumab prevented coronary events and HF,[49] but quite strikingly, it also dose-dependently prevented incident lung cancer,[50] providing evidence for a shared pathophysiology.

Another hypothesis is that a damaged heart secretes factors that may promote tumour growth. In a mouse model of precancerous colorectal polyps, the presence of post-myocardial infarction HF, independent from haemodynamic factors, caused the polyps to grow.[51] They identified several circulating factors, most notably

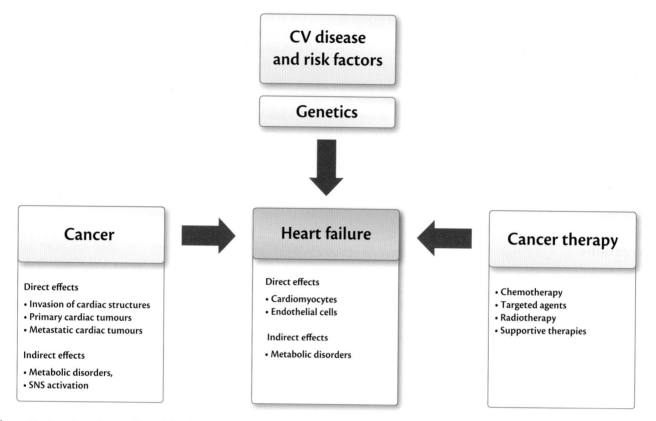

Figure 12.13.5 Determinants of heart failure in patients with cancer.
CV, cardiovascular; SNS, sympathetic nervous system.
Reproduced from Farmakis D, Mantzourani M, Filippatos G. Anthracycline-induced cardiomyopathy: secrets and lies. *Eur J Heart Fail*. 2018 May;20(5):907–909. doi: 10.1002/ejhf.1172 with permission from John Wiley and Sons.

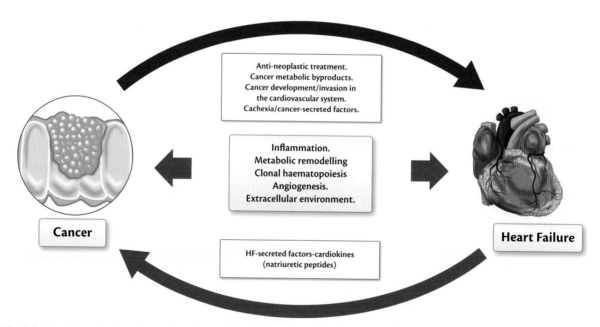

Figure 12.13.6 Potential mechanisms for a reciprocal relationship between heart failure and cancer CV, cardiovascular; HF, heart failure.
Reproduced from de Boer RA, Hulot JS, Tocchetti CG, et al. Common mechanistic pathways in cancer and heart failure. A scientific roadmap on behalf of the Translational Research Committee of the Heart Failure Association (HFA) of the European Society of Cardiology (ESC). *Eur J Heart Fail*. 2020 Dec;22(12):2272–2289. doi: 10.1002/ejhf.2029 with permission from John Wiley and Sons.

serpinA3, that were produced by failing hearts and elevated in plasma of human patients with HF. This has been validated by independent groups. Another study showed that extracellular matrix proteins may play a role in HF-derived cancer growth,[42] especially periostin. It has been reported that changes in the immune system induced by myocardial infarction accelerated breast cancer growth, adding immunological phenomena to the reverse cardio-oncology hypothesis. The connection between HF and cancer, however, is likely dependent on the aetiology of HF, the model, and the type of cancer: In a murine model of renal cancer, post-myocardial infarction HF did not accelerate tumour growth.[52]

The different aspects of the connection between CV disease and HF on one hand, and incident cancer of the other hand have been summarized.[3,46] It even has been proposed that, in parallel to the heart–kidney axis, cancer and CVD are also interconnected at various levels.[53] In this regard, it is interesting to realize that CV risk may be predicted by tumour markers,[54] while cancer risk can accurately be predicted by CV risk.[55] Future research should identify the pathways that are most notably implicated and, since these are phenomena that go across different organ systems and medical specialties, they will require development of relevant experimental models[55] and trans-disciplinary networks.

Summary and key messages

The diagnosis of cancer in a HF patient introduces multiple complexities for both HF and cancer management. Close communication among the HF, oncology, and cardio-oncology teams is important to optimize HF and cancer treatments in order to minimize risks and achieve the best outcomes for both conditions. HF medication should ideally be optimized to help reduce the risk of decompensation during the cancer treatment. Avoiding cardiotoxic cancer therapies and large intravenous fluid volumes is important where possible. Baseline optimization of HF medication and close monitoring during cardiotoxic cancer treatments is recommended given that HF patients have a high risk of cardiotoxicity. Following the ESC 2021 HF and ESC 2022 Cardio-Oncology guidelines[56] will help minimize the risk of CV complications for HF patients during oncology treatment. The choice of advanced HF therapies, including implantable devices, such as cardiac resynchronization therapy, ICDs, and LVADs, depends on cancer type, stage, and prognosis, and requires multidisciplinary team discussion regarding short- and long-term prognosis. Careful attention to potential drug–drug interactions between HF and cancer drugs is important, particularly regarding QT prolongation drugs and anticoagulants. Fluid balance and management can frequently be disrupted by the impact of the cancer and/or its treatments and patient education and monitoring fluid intake and weight is important.

Future directions

Prospective trials are required in multiple areas of this field. The implementation and refinement of the baseline risk assessment approach and its impact upon adherence to cancer treatment,

cancer outcomes, and CV disease and HF prevention need to be studied. The efficacy of cardioactive drugs and other interventions suggested for the primary prevention cancer therapy-related cardiotoxicity remains to be proven. The optimal treatment of HF caused by cancer treatment also requires trials, and in particular the impact of novel HF therapies including sacubitril/valsartan and SGLT2i. Pharmacogenomic studies regarding drug–drug interactions, and the impact of cardiomyopathy-related gene mutations are areas where genetics can impact this field. Digital technologies, including AI algorithms to improve risk prediction, are areas of future research. Finally, the potential reverse pathogenetic relationship between HF and cancer, with HF causing cancer is currently an attractive field of research.

References

1. Ameri P, Canepa M, Anker MS, Belenkov Y, Bergler-Klein J, Cohen-Solal A, et al. . Cancer diagnosis in patients with heart failure: epidemiology, clinical implications and gaps in knowledge. *Eur J Heart Fail* 2018;**20**:879–887.
2. Farmakis D, Stafylas P, Giamouzis G, Maniadakis N, Parissis J. The medical and socioeconomic burden of heart failure: A comparative delineation with cancer. *Int J Cardiol* 2016;**203**:279–281.
3. Boer RA de, Hulot J-S, Tocchetti CG, Aboumsallem JP, Ameri P, Anker SD, et al. Common mechanistic pathways in cancer and heart failure. A scientific roadmap on behalf of the Translational Research Committee of the Heart Failure Association (HFA) of the European Society of Cardiology (ESC). *Eur J Heart Fail* 2020;**22**:2272–2289.
4. Lyon AR, Dent S, Stanway S, Earl H, Brezden-Masley C, Cohen-Solal A, et al. Baseline cardiovascular risk assessment in cancer patients scheduled to receive cardiotoxic cancer therapies: a position statement and new risk assessment tools from the Cardio-Oncology Study Group of the Heart Failure Association of the European Society of Cardiology in collaboration with the International Cardio-Oncology Society. *Eur J Heart Fail* 2020;**22**:1945–1960.
5. Zamorano JL, Lancellotti P, Rodriguez Muñoz D, Aboyans V, Asteggiano R, Galderisi M, et al. 2016 ESC Position Paper on cancer treatments and cardiovascular toxicity developed under the auspices of the ESC Committee for Practice Guidelines: The Task Force for cancer treatments and cardiovascular toxicity of the European Society of Cardiology (ESC). *Eur Heart J* 2016;**37**:2768–2801.
6. Mercurio V, Pirozzi F, Lazzarini E, Marone G, Rizzo P, Agnetti G, et al. Models of heart failure based on the cardiotoxicity of anticancer drugs. *J Card Fail* 2016;**22**:449–458.
7. Di Lisi D, Madonna R, Zito C, Bronte E, Badalamenti G, Parrella P, et al. Anticancer therapy-induced vascular toxicity: VEGF inhibition and beyond. *Int J Cardiol* 2017;**227**:11–17.
8. Kirichenko YY, Ilgisonis IS, Belenkov YN, Privalova EV, Naymann YI, Lyamin AM, et al. [The effect of chemotherapy on endothelial function and microcirculation in patients with gastric cancer]. *Kardiologiia* 2020;**60**:89–95.
9. Farmakis D, Mantzourani M, Filippatos G. Anthracycline-induced cardiomyopathy: secrets and lies. *Eur J Heart Fail* 2018;**20**:907–909.
10. Garcia-Pavia P, Kim Y, Restrepo-Cordoba MA, Lunde IG, Wakimoto H, Smith AM, et al. Genetic variants associated with cancer therapy-induced cardiomyopathy. *Circulation* 2019;**140**:31–41.
11. Čelutkienė J, Pudil R, López-Fernández T, Grapsa J, Nihoyannopoulos P, Bergler-Klein J, et al. Role of cardiovascular imaging in cancer patients receiving cardiotoxic therapies: a position statement on behalf of the Heart Failure Association (HFA), the European Association of Cardiovascular Imaging (EACVI) and the Cardio-Oncology

Council of the European Society of Cardiology (ESC). *Eur J Heart Fail* 2020;**22**:1504–1524.

12. Zhang L, Reynolds KL, Lyon AR, Palaskas N, Neilan TG. The evolving immunotherapy landscape and the epidemiology, diagnosis, and management of cardiotoxicity: JACC: CardioOncology Primer. *JACC CardioOncology* 2021;**3**:35–47.

13. Ball S, Ghosh RK, Wongsaengsak S, Bandyopadhyay D, Ghosh GC, Aronow WS, et al. Cardiovascular toxicities of immune checkpoint inhibitors: JACC Review Topic of the Week. *J Am Coll Cardiol* 2019;**74**:1714–1727.

14. Ghosh AK, Crake T, Manisty C, Westwood M. Pericardial disease in cancer patients. *Curr Treat Options Cardiovasc Med* 2018;**20**:60.

15. Cazin B, Gorin NC, Laporte JP, Gallet B, Douay L, Lopez M, Najman A, et al. Cardiac complications after bone marrow transplantation. A report on a series of 63 consecutive transplantations. *Cancer* 1986;**57**:2061–2069.

16. Armanious MA, Mohammadi H, Khodor S, Oliver DE, Johnstone PA, Fradley MG. Cardiovascular effects of radiation therapy. *Curr Probl Cancer* 2018;**42**:433–442.

17. Gagliardi G, Constine LS, Moiseenko V, Correa C, Pierce LJ, Allen AM, Marks LB. Radiation dose-volume effects in the heart. *Int J Radiat Oncol Biol Phys* 2010;**76**:S77–85.

18. Adler Y, Charron P, Imazio M, Badano L, Barón-Esquivias G, Bogaert J, et al. 2015 ESC Guidelines for the diagnosis and management of pericardial diseases: The Task Force for the Diagnosis and Management of Pericardial Diseases of the European Society of Cardiology (ESC) Endorsed by: The European Association for Cardio-Thoracic Surgery (EACTS). *Eur Heart J* 2015;**36**:2921–2964.

19. Applefeld MM, Wiernik PH. Cardiac disease after radiation therapy for Hodgkin's disease: analysis of 48 patients. *Am J Cardiol* 1983;**51**:1679–1681.

20. Chiabrando JG, Bonaventura A, Vecchié A, Wohlford GF, Mauro AG, Jordan JH, et al. Management of acute and recurrent pericarditis: JACC State-of-the-Art Review. *J Am Coll Cardiol* 2020;**75**:76–92.

21. Pudil R, Mueller C, Čelutkienė J, Henriksen PA, Lenihan D, Dent S, et al. Role of serum biomarkers in cancer patients receiving cardiotoxic cancer therapies: a position statement from the Cardio-Oncology Study Group of the Heart Failure Association and the Cardio-Oncology Council of the European Society of Cardiology. *Eur J Heart Fail* 2020;**22**:1966–1983.

22. McDonagh TA, Metra M, Adamo M, Gardner RS, Baumbach A, Böhm M, et al. 2021 ESC Guidelines for the diagnosis and treatment of acute and chronic heart failure. *Eur Heart J* 2021;**42**:3599–3726.

23. Farmakis D. Anticoagulation for atrial fibrillation in active cancer: what the cardiologists think. *Eur J Prev Cardiol* 2021;**28**:608–610.

24. Viganego F, Singh R, Fradley MG. Arrhythmias and other electrophysiology issues in cancer patients receiving chemotherapy or radiation. *Curr Cardiol Rep* 2016;**18**:52.

25. Fradley MG, Lefebvre B, Carver J, Cheung JW, Feigenberg SJ, Lampert R, et al. How to manage patients with cardiac implantable electronic devices undergoing radiation therapy. *JACC CardioOncology* 2021;**3**:447–451.

26. Lancellotti P, Nkomo VT, Badano LP, Bergler J, Bogaert J, Davin L, et al. Expert Consensus for multi-modality imaging evaluation of cardiovascular complications of radiotherapy in adults: A report from the European association of cardiovascular imaging and the American society of echocardiography. *J Am Soc Echocardiogr* 2013;**26**:1013–1032.

27. Sigurdardottir V, Bjortuft O, Eiskjær H, Ekmehag B, Gude E, Gustafsson F, et al. Long-term follow-up of lung and heart transplant recipients with pre-transplant malignancies. *J Heart Lung Transplant* 2012;**31**:1276–1280.

28. Arnold SV, Jones PG, Allen LA, Cohen DJ, Fendler TJ, Holtz JE, et al.. Frequency of poor outcome (death or poor quality of life) after left ventricular assist device for destination therapy: results from the INTERMACS registry. *Circ Heart Fail* 2016;**9**:e002800.

29. Feldman D, Pamboukian SV, Teuteberg JJ, Birks E, Lietz K, Moore SA, et al. The 2013 International Society for Heart and Lung Transplantation Guidelines for mechanical circulatory support: executive summary. *J Heart Lung Transplant* 2013;**32**:157–187.

30. Fardman A, Banschick GD, Rabia R, Percik R, Fourey D, Segev S, et al. Cardiorespiratory fitness and survival following cancer diagnosis. *Eur J Prev Cardiol* 2021: 2021;28(11):1242–1249.

31. Groarke JD, Payne DL, Claggett B, Mehra MR, Gong J, Caron J, et al.Association of post-diagnosis cardiorespiratory fitness with cause-specific mortality in cancer. *Eur Heart J Qual Care Clin Outcomes* 2020;**6**:315–322.

32. Scott JM, Nilsen TS, Gupta D, Jones LW. Exercise therapy and cardiovascular toxicity in cancer. *Circulation* 2018;**137**:1176–1191.

33. Sasso JP, Eves ND, Christensen JF, Koelwyn GJ, Scott J, Jones LW. A framework for prescription in exercise-oncology research. *J Cachexia Sarcopenia Muscle* 2015;**6**:115–124.

34. Wallen MP, Hennessy D, Brown S, Evans L, Rawstorn JC, Wong Shee A, Hall A. High-intensity interval training improves cardiorespiratory fitness in cancer patients and survivors: A meta-analysis. *Eur J Cancer Care (Engl)* 2020;**29**:e13267.

35. Steffel J, Collins R, Antz M, Cornu P, Desteghe L, Haeusler KG, et al. 2021 European Heart Rhythm Association practical guide on the use of non-vitamin k antagonist oral anticoagulants in patients with atrial fibrillation. *EP Europace* 2021;**23**:1612–1676.

36. Belloum Y, Rannou-Bekono F, Favier FB. Cancer-induced cardiac cachexia: pathogenesis and impact of physical activity (review). *Oncol Rep* 2017;**37**:2543–2552.

37. Anker MS, Sanz AP, Zamorano JL, Mehra MR, Butler J, Riess H, et al. Advanced cancer is also a heart failure syndrome: a hypothesis. *J Cachexia Sarcopenia Muscle* 2021;**12**:533–537.

38. Banke A, Schou M, Videbaek L, Møller JE, Torp-Pedersen C, Gustafsson F, et al.Incidence of cancer in patients with chronic heart failure: a long-term follow-up study. *Eur J Heart Fail* 2016;**18**:260–266.

39. Hasin T, Gerber Y, Weston SA, Jiang R, Killian JM, Manemann SM, et al.Heart failure after myocardial infarction is associated with increased risk of cancer. *J Am Coll Cardiol* 2016;**68**:265–271.

40. Berton G, Cordiano R, Cavuto F, Bagato F, Segafredo B, Pasquinucci M. Neoplastic disease after acute coronary syndrome: incidence, duration, and features: the ABC-4* Study on Heart Disease. *J Cardiovasc Med (Hagerstown)* 2018;**19**:546–553.

41. Selvaraj S, Bhatt DL, Claggett B, Djoussé L, Shah SJ, Chen J, et al. Lack of association between heart failure and incident cancer. *J Am Coll Cardiol* 2018;**71**:1501–1510.

42. Avraham S, Abu-Sharki S, Shofti R, Haas T, Korin B, Kalfon R, et al. Early cardiac remodeling promotes tumor growth and metastasis. *Circulation* 2020;**142**:670–683.

43. Koelwyn GJ, Newman AAC, Afonso MS, Solingen C van, Corr EM, Brown EJ, et al. Myocardial infarction accelerates breast cancer via innate immune reprogramming. *Nat Med* 2020;**26**:1452–1458.

44. Boer RA de, Meijers WC, Meer P van der, Veldhuisen DJ van. Cancer and heart disease: associations and relations. *Eur J Heart Fail* 2019;**21**:1515–1525.

45. Tini G, Bertero E, Signori A, Sormani MP, Maack C, De Boer RA, et al. Cancer mortality in trials of heart failure with reduced ejection fraction: a systematic review and meta-analysis. *J Am Heart Assoc* 2020;**9**:e016309.

46. Aboumsallem JP, Moslehi J, Boer RA de. Reverse cardio-oncology: cancer development in patients with cardiovascular disease. *J Am Heart Assoc* 2020;**9**:e013754.

47. Wit S de, Boer RA de. From studying heart disease and cancer simultaneously to reverse cardio-oncology. *Circulation* 2021;**144**:93–95.

48. Koelwyn GJ, Aboumsallem JP, Moore KJ, Boer RA de. Reverse cardio-oncology: Exploring the effects of cardiovascular disease on cancer pathogenesis. *J Mol Cell Cardiol* 2021;**163**:1–8.

49. Ridker PM, Everett BM, Thuren T, MacFadyen JG, Chang WH, Ballantyne C, et al.Antiinflammatory therapy with canakinumab for atherosclerotic disease. *N Engl J Med* 2017;**377**:1119–1131.

50. Ridker PM, MacFadyen JG, Thuren T, Everett BM, Libby P, Glynn RJ, CANTOS Trial Group. Effect of interleukin-1β inhibition with canakinumab on incident lung cancer in patients with atherosclerosis: exploratory results from a randomised, double-blind, placebo-controlled trial. *Lancet* 2017;**390**:1833–1842.

51. Meijers WC, Maglione M, Bakker SJL, Oberhuber R, Kieneker LM, Jong S de, et al.Heart failure stimulates tumor growth by circulating factors. *Circulation* 2018;**138**:678–691.

52. Shi C, Aboumsallem JP, Wit S de, Schouten EM, Bracun V, Meijers WC, et al. Evaluation of renal cancer progression in a mouse model of heart failure. *Cancer Commun Lond Engl* 2021;**41**:796–799.

53. Boer RA de, Aboumsallem JP, Bracun V, Leedy D, Cheng R, Patel S, et al.A new classification of cardio-oncology syndromes. *Cardiooncol ogy* 2021;**7**:24.

54. Shi C, Wal HH van der, Silljé HHW, Dokter MM, Berg F van den, Huizinga L, et al. Tumour biomarkers: association with heart failure outcomes. *J Intern Med* 2020;**288**:207–218.

55. Lau ES, Paniagua SM, Liu E, Jovani M, Li SX, Takvorian K, Suthahar N, et al. Cardiovascular risk factors are associated with future cancer. *JACC CardioOncology* 2021;**3**:48–58.

56. Lyon AR, Lopez-Fernandez T, Couch LS, *et al.*; ESC Scientific Document Group. 2022 ESC Guidelines on cardio-oncology developed in collaboration with the European Hematology Association (EHA), the European Society for Therapeutic Radiology and Oncology (ESTRO) and the International Cardio-Oncology Society (IC-OS). *Eur Heart J* 2022;**43**:4229–361.

CHAPTER 12.14

Pregnancy and heart failure

Johann Bauersachs, Denise Hilfiker-Kleiner, and Karen Sliwa

Contents

Introduction

The number of women with cardiovascular disease who become pregnant is increasing due to preexisting cardiac disease, such as congenital heart disease and/or increasing maternal age, and comorbidities, such as hypertension, diabetes, cancer, and autoimmune disorders. Maternal heart disease is present in 1% to 4% of pregnancies and accounts for up to 15% of maternal deaths. The ESC Registry Of Pregnancy And Cardiac disease (ROPAC) reports a mortality of 0.6%, and heart failure occurrence in 11% of pregnancies complicated by maternal heart disease.[1]

Pre-conception counselling and knowledge regarding timely (but also appropriate) referral to specialized care is, therefore, of utmost importance to ensure optimal maternal and foetal outcome. There is a need to distinguish patients with a potential risk of developing heart failure, such as women with a history of cardiotoxic therapies (e.g. for malignant conditions) but without heart failure before pregnancy, from those women who already have symptoms and signs of heart failure, as care must be tailored according to those different scenarios needing specific advice and risk stratification.

Women with a known diagnosis of left ventricular (LV) dysfunction due to a cardiomyopathy or presenting with (de novo) heart failure during pregnancy will usually require continuation of medical therapy which may adversely affect the foetus. Accurate information on the foetal effects of medication is important to weigh the advantages of treating the mother against the possible long-lasting negative effects on the child. However, clear guidelines/directions on how to counsel these patients before, during or after pregnancy are limited.

This chapter refers to recently published papers,[2,3] and will fill important gaps in knowledge and is, therefore, a much-needed reference for all physicians dealing with women at risk or presenting with signs of heart failure.

Physiology of the cardiovascular system during pregnancy and the peripartum phase

Physiological changes during pregnancy are substantial, with increases in basal oxygen consumption, blood volume, and red cell mass. Haemodynamic changes in the maternal circulation already start in the first trimester, including profound systemic vasodilation with a drop in blood pressure.[4] Venous compliance and blood volume are increased, as well as renal plasma flow and glomerular filtration rate. Activation of the renin-angiotensin-aldosterone system in pregnancy maintains blood pressure and helps retain salt and water as maternal systemic and renal arterial dilation creates an 'underfilled' cardiovascular system.[5]

Cardiac output rises by about 50% by the mid-third trimester, and stroke volume and heart rate increase over the course of pregnancy. In response to the 'volume overload' signal in pregnancy, and the increase in cardiac stroke work, the maternal heart undergoes physiological (eccentric) hypertrophy associated with increased capillarization. In late pregnancy LV global strain is significantly decreased, with a slight reduction of LV ejection fraction (LVEF). An additional marked change in cardiac function occurs during labour and delivery, with the maximum cardiac output related to increased heart rate and preload caused by the uterine contractions, increased circulating catecholamines, and autotransfusion of 300–500 mL blood from the uterus into the maternal circulation.[4] Most morphological and functional changes in pregnancy reverse postpartum to the pre-pregnancy status.

Endocrine and systemic alterations in pregnancy include major changes in hormones (oestrogen, progesterone, and prolactin), which also impact on the cardiovascular system to support the growing foetus and counteract pregnancy stresses. In this regard, oestrogen, progesterone, and relaxin promote vascular relaxation.[6] Importantly, in normal uncomplicated pregnancy, the risk for thrombosis is 4- to 10-fold higher and maximal around term as the factors VII, X, VIII, fibrinogen, and von Willebrand factor rise throughout gestation.[7]

Thrombotic risk and physiological pregnancy-induced changes in the cardiovascular system can be negatively affected by comorbidities, such as maternal obesity and gestational diabetes mellitus, and impact on the cardiovascular system in pregnancy, increasing the risk for complications, such as hypertension and preeclampsia.[5] Delaying pregnancy to older age may increase the risk of cardiovascular disease in both women and their children. However, the (patho-) physiological mechanisms are not fully understood.

Pathophysiology of heart failure during pregnancy and the peripartum period

Hypertensive disorders in pregnancy include preeclampsia and HELLP-syndrome and affect up to 8% of pregnant women worldwide.[8] Pregnancies complicated by preeclampsia or HELLP are a leading cause for premature delivery, with high risk for maternal, foetal, and neonatal morbidity and mortality.

Preeclampsia de novo, or superimposed on chronic hypertension, is defined as blood pressure >140/90 mmHg and at least one of the following criteria: proteinuria, other maternal organ dysfunction, or uteroplacental dysfunction with foetal growth restriction. HELLP syndrome is defined as reduction of platelet count below 100,000/dL, and an elevation of liver transaminases. Preeclampsia and its more severe form, HELLP, result from a mismatch between uteroplacental supply (with impaired placenta due to ischaemic and/or oxidative stress damage) and foetal demands, leading to systemic inflammatory maternal and foetal manifestations.

Pathomechanisms of preeclampsia include impaired trophoblast invasion and incomplete spiral artery remodelling, leading to placental ischaemia and increased serum levels of soluble fms-like tyrosine kinase-1.[8] Tumor necrosis factor α, interleukins, oxidized lipid products, and asymmetric dimethylarginine may also contribute to the pathophysiology of preeclampsia and HELLP, in part by promoting endothelial dysfunction. Levels of the N-terminal 16 kDa fragment (16-kDa prolactin) directly correlate with adverse outcome in preeclampsia and HELLP syndrome. In women with preeclampsia, increased afterload leads to adverse concentric LV remodelling associated with increased wall thickness, diastolic dysfunction, left atrial enlargement, and increased LV and RV filling pressures.[8] Together with increased vascular resistance, these changes also precipitate pulmonary oedema in some patients with preeclampsia, which is aggravated by increased vascular permeability and volume overload.

Delivery is the main cure for severe preeclampsia and HELLP syndrome and symptoms then resolve quickly. However, patients with preeclampsia or HELLP may continue to have a higher risk for cardiovascular complications, and LV remodelling and diastolic dysfunction can persist up to 12 months after delivery.[9] Therefore, it is suggested to also monitor blood pressure, urine albumin level, fasting glucose, and lipids in the postpartum period of women with preeclampsia and HELLP syndrome, and implement treatment according to the ESC guidelines.[10]

Peripartum cardiomyopathy

Possible pathomechanisms leading to peripartum cardiomyopathy (PPCM) are provided in a comprehensive and detailed overview by Ricke-Hoch et al.[11] Among these are inflammation and autoimmune reactions with elevated levels of various circulating cytokines.

Genetic background and alterations also seem to contribute to PPCM, as African ancestry is a risk factor for PPCM.[5] However, the recently published international data from the EuroObservational Research programme on PPCM clearly demonstrated that PPCM is a global disease, with women from the Middle East having a particularly poor rate of cardiac recovery.[12] In some PPCM patients, familial clustering and histories of cardiomyopathies have also been reported, as well as some known genetic variants.[13] In addition, mutations in genes of the DNA damage repair pathway were found, suggesting that impaired repair systems in the maternal heart after pregnancy may also increase the risk for PPCM.[14] Experimental evidence suggests impairment in catecholamines and the cAMP-PKA signaling as potential pathomechanisms initiating and driving PPCM. Moreover, the β1-adrenoceptor agonist dobutamine in PPCM patients with cardiogenic shock was associated with adverse cardiac outcome.[15]

Many of the pathomechanisms in PPCM converge on a common pathway which involves unbalanced oxidative stress and the generation of the anti-angiogenic 16-kDa prolactin.[5] Central roles for protection of the maternal heart from oxidative stress have been associated with major signalling pathways, including the signal transducer and activator of transcription 3 and peroxisome proliferator-activated receptor γ coactivator 1α. In experimental PPCM in mice, cardiac knockout of these factors ultimately results in PPCM.[5, 11] The hormone prolactin, periodically released from the pituitary gland during nursing, appears to be a major player. Prolactin rises during pregnancy and is specifically high postpartum. Driven by enhanced oxidative stress in PPCM prolactin undergoes proteolytic cleavage to the shorter 16-kDa prolactin that induces endothelial and myocardial damage and dysfunction. Blocking prolactin with the dopamin D2 receptor agonist bromocriptine has emerged as a potential disease specific therapy for PPCM and been added to the ESC guidelines on cardiac disease in pregacy as a possible therapeutic option.[10]

Cardiovascular risk during pregnancy in female cancer survivors

Heart failure and cancer are epidemiologically associated, share common risk factors, and pathophysiological pathways, and may promote the onset of the respective other disease.[16] Malignant diseases may directly induce cardiac dysfunction, whereas several anti-tumour therapies display acute and/or late cardiotoxicity associated with heart failure. Common risk factors, cardiotoxic treatment, genetic variants (associated with cardiomyopathies and/or cancer) increase the risk for subsequent heart failure. The multi-hit hypothesis linking cancer, cardiotoxic treatments, and heart failure recognizes increased cardiac stress imposed by pregnancy as an important factor for heart failure development during pregnancy, even in apparently healthy cancer survivors.[3,17]

More and more female cancer survivors following curative treatment of a malignancy in childhood or young adulthood reach child-bearing age and require counselling and preventive/adjunctive treatment before/during pregnancy. Survivors of curative paediatric cancer treatment, including anthracycline chemotherapy, and/or radiation to the chest, display a dose-related several-fold increased risk of heart failure development at long-term follow-up,[18] and lifelong surveillance for cardiomyopathy/heart failure is recommended in cancer survivors.[19]

Pregnancy-related cardiovascular complications, predominantly heart failure, are more frequent in survivors of cardiotoxic cancer therapies, especially when cardiomyopathy is present before pregnancy. In a small cohort of cancer survivors, the incidence of heart failure during pregnancy was 0% in women without, but 31% in patients with a previous diagnosis of cardiomyopathy.[20] In another small study of cancer survivors, 15% of the non-pregnant control group, but 28% of the pregnant women, developed a new cardiomyopathy. Higher cumulative anthracycline dose and younger age at treatment were associated with higher incidence of heart failure development.[21] In a large retrospective study in cancer survivors, the majority of women were diagnosed with cardiomyopathy, either prior to pregnancy or later than five months after pregnancy,[22] and only 0.3% developed a new pregnancy-associated cardiomyopathy.

Risk factors for pregnancy-induced heart failure in female cancer survivors include[3]:

◆ LVEF < 50% pre-pregnancy (higher risk if LVEF < 40% pre-pregnancy)
◆ Previous anthracycline chemotherapy (higher risk in women who received a total cumulative doxorubicin dose ≥ 250 mg/m^2 or equivalent)

◆ Previous chest radiation therapy (higher risk if total cumulative chest radiation dose ≥35 Gy)
◆ Cancer diagnosis and treatment at young age (<10 years)
◆ Time from cancer treatment to pregnancy >15 years.

While the absolute risk of pregnancy-induced heart failure in cancer survivors appears to be rather low, the risk is higher in cancer survivors who received anthracycline chemotherapy or chest radiation. Unfortunately, in many countries survivors of childhood cancer are still not thoroughly followed over decades after curative treatment, and chemotherapy-associated cardiomyopathy is not diagnosed before pregnancy.

All female cancer survivors who received anthracycline or chest radiation are recommended to have their obstetric care delivered by a multidisciplinary pregnancy heart team, including an obstetrician and a cardiologist, should have a personalized surveillance plan to monitor cardiovascular health during their pregnancy, and should be reviewed with clinical history, examination, and echocardiography to assess LV function at the end of the first trimester of all pregnancies.[3]

Cardiovascular risk in women receiving chemotherapy during pregnancy

Although chemotherapy is only occasionally required during pregnancy, these women are at higher risk, even in the absence of known heart failure, and appropriate risk assessment before starting chemotherapy, cardiac monitoring during chemotherapy, and delivery involving the pregnancy heart team is recommended, in collaboration with a cardio-oncology team.[23] New malignancies during pregnancy include breast cancer and Hodgkin's lymphoma where anthracycline chemotherapy is indicated.

As many novel antineoplastic agents, such as immune checkpoints inhibitors, are developed every year with new and often unexpected cardiovascular side-effects, an infrastructure is needed that enables fast and intense interaction between cardiologists, oncologists, and gynaecologists to best serve the needs of these women suffering from cancer and requiring chemotherapy during pregnancy.

Counselling before pregnancy in patients at risk for or with pre-existing chronic heart failure

In women with adult congenital heart disease (ACHD) pre-pregnancy counselling, including genetic counselling, is essential.[24] Although many patients with ACHD or acquired heart disease tolerate pregnancy well, it is necessary to identify those at higher risk. In general, risk stratification must be done before entering a pregnancy and adequate contraception is essential in patients in whom pregnancy is considered to pose a high risk.

According to the modified (m) WHO classification, an intermediate increased risk of maternal mortality or moderate-to-severe increase in morbidity (mWHO II–III) occurs in patients with, for example, mild LV impairment (EF > 45%), hypertrophic cardiomyopathy, mild mitral stenosis, moderate aortic stenosis,

Table 12.14.1 Congenital heart disease with high (mWHO class III) and extremely high risk (mWHO class IV) for pregnancy according to modified (m) WHO classification

Significantly increased risk of maternal mortality or severe morbidity (mWHO class III) (cardiac event rate 19–27%)	Extremely high risk of maternal mortality or severe morbidity (mWHO class IV)* (cardiac event rate 40–100%)
Unrepaired cyanotic heart disease	Pulmonary arterial hypertension
Moderate LV impairment (EF 30–45%)	Severe LV impairment (EF <30% or NYHA class III–IV)
Systemic RV with good or mildly decreased ventricular function	Systemic RV with moderate or severely decreased ventricular function
Fontan circulation. If the patient is otherwise well and the cardiac condition uncomplicated	Fontan with any complication
Severe asymptomatic AS	Severe symptomatic AS
Moderate mitral stenosis	Severe mitral stenosis
Moderate aortic dilatation (40–45 mm in Marfan syndrome or other HTAD; 45–50 mm in BAV, 20–25 mm/m² in Turner syndrome)	Severe aortic dilatation (>45 mm in Marfan syndrome or other HTAD; >50 mm in BAV, >25 mm/m² in Turner syndrome)
Mechanical valve	Severe (re-)coarctation

AS, aortic stenosis; ASI, aortic size index; BAV, bicuspid aortic valve; CHD, congenital heart defect; EF, ejection fraction; HTAD, heritable thoracic aortic disease; LV, left ventricle/ventricular; mWHO, modified World Health Organization; NYHA, New York Heart Association; RV, right ventricle/ventricular; TOF, tetralogy of Fallot. *Pregnancy should definitely be avoided in women with these conditions.

Baumgartner H, De Backer J, Babu-Narayan SV, et al; ESC Scientific Document Group. 2020 ESC Guidelines for the management of adult congenital heart disease. *Eur Heart J.* 2021 Feb 11;42(6):563-645. doi: 10.1093/eurheartj/ehaa554. © European Society of Cardiology. Reprinted by Oxford University Press.

or atrioventricular septal defect. These patients can become pregnant but should be followed bi-monthly during pregnancy.

mWHO class III includes patients with a significantly increased risk of maternal mortality or severe morbidity (estimated maternal cardiac event rate of 19–27%). Patients classified as mWHO III (➲ Table 12.14.1) include those with moderate LV impairment (EF 30–45%), previous PPCM without any residual LV impairment, any kind of mechanical valve, systemic right ventricle with good or mildly decreased ventricular function, uncomplicated Fontan circulation, unrepaired cyanotic heart disease, other complex heart disease, moderate mitral stenosis, or severe asymptomatic aortic stenosis. These patients require expert counselling by a pregnancy heart team at an expert centre and monthly or bi-monthly follow-up during pregnancy.

Pregnancy should definitely be avoided in patients classified as mWHO class IV (➲ Table 12.14.1), and if pregnancy occurs, termination should be discussed, as they are at extremely high risk (40–100%) of maternal mortality or severe morbidity. mWHO IV includes patients with pulmonary arterial hypertension (PAH), severe LV dysfunction (LVEF <30%, NYHA class III–IV), previous PPCM with any residual LV impairment, systemic right ventricles with moderately or severely decreased function, Fontan patients with any previous complication, severe symptomatic aortic stenosis, severe mitral stenosis, or (re)coarctation.[10,24]

In patients with known chronic heart failure, standard drugs such as angiotensin-converting enzyme (ACE)-inhibitors, angiotensin receptor blocker (ARB), angiotensin receptor–neprilysin inhibitors (ARNI), mineralocorticoid receptor antagonists (MRAs), ivabradine, and SGLT-2 inhibitors are contraindicated during pregnancy as they are associated with a high risk of foetal adverse events in all trimesters (➲ Table 12.14.2).[2] They should be stopped prior to conception, with close clinical and echocardiographic monitoring. If the ejection fraction falls, further discussion should occur reconsidering the safety of pregnancy.

A specific group of patients in need for counselling pre-pregnancy are all female cancer survivors. Recommendations for the management of pregnancy in female cancer survivors include[3]:

◆ All female cancer survivors who are at high risk of pregnancy-induced cardiovascular complications should have their obstetric care delivered by a multidisciplinary team specialized in the care of high-risk pregnancies: the pregnancy heart team.

◆ All female cancer survivors who received anthracycline or chest radiation should be counselled about the potential cardiovascular risks associated with pregnancy, and prior to all planned pregnancies are recommended to have a cardiology review including resting echocardiography and risk assessment.

Managing pregnancies in patients with chronic heart failure

In the large ROPAC database of pregnancies in patients with known heart disease the prevalence of heart failure was 10.6%.[1] In these patients the risk for cardiovascular events and death, as well as preterm labour and delivery, are elevated. Furthermore, foetal and neonatal deaths are increased. Patients with known heart failure thus need specialized care, both before (➲ Counselling before pregnancy in patients at risk for or with pre-existing chronic heart failure, p. 885) and during pregnancy; successful pregnancy can be achieved under the care of an experienced 'pregnancy heart team'.[3, 10]

Concentrations of natriuretic peptides are quantitative plasma biomarkers of the presence and severity of haemodynamic cardiac stress and heart failure.[25] As the severity of heart failure is a strong predictor of cardiac complications in women during and after pregnancy, quantifying heart failure severity using natriuretic peptide measurements may facilitate the detection of patients at high-risk for cardiac complications.[26]

Management of heart failure should follow established guidelines,[27] and pre-pregnancy management must include

Table 12.14.2 Risks and safety of medications during pregnancy and lactation

Drug class	Use in pregnancy Summary	Use in lactation Summary	Drugs with lactation safety data	Relative infant dose from breast milk	Infant monitoring
ACEI	Avoid (*contraindicated*) – teratogenic	Use with caution (*limited data*). Clinically insignificant levels of captopril and enalapril found in breast milk	Enalapril (most data) Captopril	0.02–0.2%	Observe for oedema, hypotension, weight gain, lethargy, pallor, and poor feeding, especially pre-term infants and those under 2 months
ARB	Avoid (*contraindicated*) –fetotoxic	Avoid (*no published data*) and/or consider ACEI instead (better established safety profile)	–	–	–
Beta-blocker	Use with caution (*limited data*). Beta-blockers can cause intrauterine growth restriction. If used near delivery, newborn infant should be closely monitored for 24–48 h for signs and symptoms of beta-blockade, such as hypotension and bradycardia, regardless of breastfeeding	Use with caution (*limited data*). Metoprolol is present in small levels in breast milk, with some transfer into infant serum; No adverse reactions in breastfed infants have been observed. No detectable levels of bisoprolol were also found in breast milk in a single case study	Metoprolol (most data) Bisoprolol	1.4%	Observe for signs or symptoms of beta-blockade, such as hypotension and bradycardia
MRA	Avoid (*not recommended*) –feminization of rat fetus and limited data in humans	Use with caution (*limited data*). All diuretics may theoretically suppress milk supply and mothers should be monitored for this. Clinically insignificant levels of canrenone (spironolactone active metabolite) found in breast milk. Single case report of no harm with breastfeeding and spironolactone	Spironolactone	2–4.3% [exrapolated from canrenone (spironolactone active metabolite) data]	Observe for fluid loss, dehydration, feeding/weight gain and lethargy
Loop diuretic	Use with caution (*limited data*). Potential reduction in placental blood flow but use is often unavoidable	Use with caution (*no data*). All diuretics may theoretically suppress milk supply and mothers should be monitored for this. High protein binding and short half-life should limit passage into breast milk	–	–	Observe for fluid loss, dehydration, feeding/weight gain and lethargy

(continued)

Table 12.14.2 Continued

Drug class	Use in pregnancy	Use in lactation	Drugs with lactation safety data	Relative infant dose from breast milk	Infant monitoring
	Summary	**Summary**			
Thiazide diuretic	Use with caution (*limited data*). Potential reduction in placental blood flow but use is often unavoidable	Use with caution (*limited data.*) All diuretics may theoretically suppress milk supply and patients on high doses may need to monitor this. Small levels of hydrochlorothiazide were found in breast milk and were undetectable in infant serum in a single case study	Hydrochlorothiazide	1.68%	Observe for fluid loss, dehydration, feeding/weight gain and lethargy
ARNI	Avoid (*contraindicated*) – ARBs are known to be fetotoxic	Avoid (*no published data*), consider different feeding method for infant in discussion with mother or consider ACEI instead (*better established safety profile*)	–	–	–
Ivabradine	Avoid (*conraindicated*) – teratogenic	Avoid (*no published data*) or consider different feeding method for infant in discussion with mother	–	–	–
Cardiac glycoside	Use with extreme caution only (limited data). ESC guidelines for the management of cardiovascular disease during pregnancy suggest to allow digoxin in atrial fibrillation if needed	Use with caution (*limited data*). Small levels of digoxin in breast milk, undetectable levels in infant serum (other than in very high doses) and no observed adverse effects in the nursing infants	Digoxin	2.7–2.8%	No special requirement
Vasodilators	Use with caution (*limited data*)	Use with caution (*limited data*). Small levels of hydralazine in breast milk and infant serum and no observed adverse effects in the nursing infants	Hydralazine	1.2%	No special requirements
Nitrates	Use with caution (*limited data*)	Use with caution (*no data*)	–	–	Observe for drowsiness, lethargy, poor feeding, flushing and weight gain
VKA	First trimester – avoid (contraindicated). Significant risk to foetus. Foetal/infant death or abnormalities in 37% of cases following first trimester exposure. Consider LMVH instead	Use with caution (*limited data*). No detectable levels of warfarin in breast milk (at usual therapeutic doses), no warfarin activity in breastfed infants and no observed adverse effects in the nursing infants	Warfarin	–	No special requirements

Drug	Pregnancy	Breastfeeding			
VKA	Second/third trimester – use with extreme caution (*limited data*), only in cases with compelling indication(s). Foetal/infant death or abnormalities in 16% of cases following second trimester exposure and 27% in third trimester exposure. Risk to foetus is dose-dependent, with doses >5 mg/day related to worse outcomes. Consider LMVH as potential alternative after assessing individual thrombotic risk profile of the mother and dose of VKA needed and indication(s) for anticoagulation. Good communication and joint decision making with the patient are vital				
NOAC	Avoid (*Contraindicated*)	Avoid. Small levels of rivaroxaban in breast milk in a single case study		1.34%	–
Unfractionated heparin	Use with caution (*limited data*)	Use with caution (*limited data*). Due to very high molecular weight, it would not be expected to be present in breast milk. Also likely to be rapidly destroyed in infant gastric contents		–	No special requirements
LMWH	Use with caution (*limited data*)	Use with caution (*limited data*). Little or no levels detectable in breast milk. Oral adsorption unlikely. No anti-Xa activity observed in breastfed infants	Dalteparin, Enoxaparin	–	No special requirements
Synthetic pentasaccharide (fondaparinux)	Avoid (*limited data*) unless allergy or adverse reaction to LMWH	Avoid (*no published data*) and/or consider LMWH instead (*better established safety profile*)		–	

ACEI, angiotensin-converting enzyme inhibitor; ARB, angiotensin receptor blocker; ARNI, angiotensin receptor-neprilysin inhibitor; ESC, Europen Society of Cardiology; LWMH, low molecular weight heparin; MRA, mineralocorticoid receptor antagonist; NOAC, non-vitamin K antagonist oral anticoagulant; VKA, vitamin K antagonist.

Sources used to compile this table are available in the online supplement to Bauersachs J, et al. *Eur J Heart Fail.* 2019 Jul;21(7):827–843.

Reproduced from Bauersachs J, König T, van der Meer P, et al. Pathophysiology, diagnosis and management of peripartum cardiomyopathy: a position statement from the Heart Failure Association of the European Society of Cardiology Study Group on peripartum cardiomyopathy. *Eur J Heart Fail.* 2019 Jul;21(7):827–843. doi: 10.1002/ejhf.1493 with permission from John Wiley and Sons.

modification of existing heart failure medications to avoid teratogenicity and minimize harm to the foetus (➲ Figure 12.14.1). If drugs that are contraindicated during pregnancy, such as ACE-inhibitors, ARB, ARNI, MRA, or SGLT2 inhibitors have been inadvertently taken during the first trimester, they should be stopped, and the patient monitored closely (maternal echocardiography and foetal ultrasound). Beta-blockers are considered to be safe in pregnancy although they may be associated with foetal growth restriction and hypoglycaemia. Beta-1 selective drugs, such as metoprolol and bisoprolol, are preferred,

as they are associated with fewer effects on foetal growth, uterine relaxation, and peripheral vasodilation. Carvedilol may also be used as heart failure therapy. Loop and thiazide diuretics can be continued, if necessary, for the treatment of pulmonary congestion.[2,10]

Sub-pulmonary ventricular failure may also occur, especially in patients with PAH. Bed rest and fluid balance with diuretics and inotropes could be used. In cases of PAH, targeted therapy with phosphodiesterase-5 inhibitors or prostaglandins may be considered.[28,29]

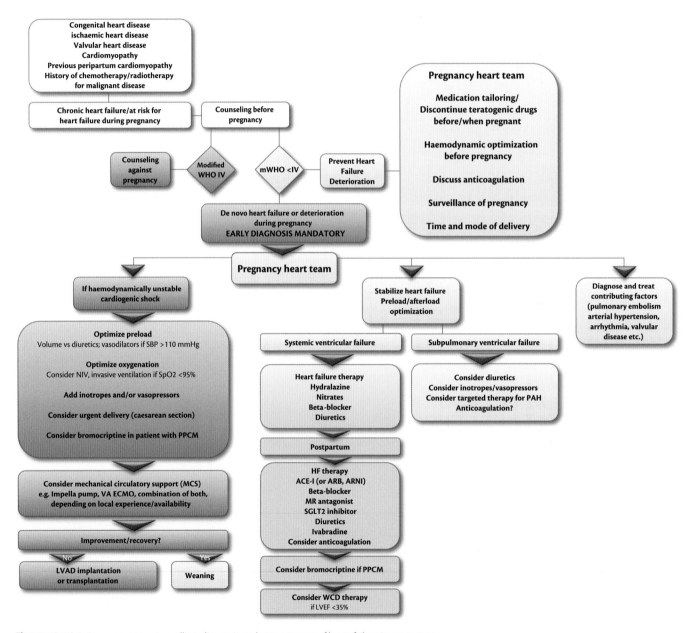

Figure 12.14.1 Pre-pregnancy counselling, diagnosis, and management of heart failure in pregnancy.

ACE-I, angiotensin-converting enzyme inhibitor; HF, heart failure; ARB, angiotensin receptor blocker; ARNI, angiotensin receptor–neprilysin inhibitor; LVAD, left ventricular assist device; MR, mineralocorticoid receptor; PAH, pulmonary arterial hypertension; PPCM, peripartum cardiomyopathy; SBP, systolic blood pressure; sodium–glucose cotransporter; SpO2, blood oxygen saturation; VA ECMO, veno-arterial extracorporeal membrane oxygenation; WCD, wearable cardioverter-defibrillator.

Source data from Sliwa K, van der Meer P, Petrie MC, et al. Risk stratification and management of women with cardiomyopathy/heart failure planning pregnancy or presenting during/after pregnancy: a position statement from the Heart Failure Association of the European Society of Cardiology Study Group on Peripartum Cardiomyopathy. *Eur J Heart Fail.* 2021 Apr;23(4):527–540. doi: 10.1002/ejhf.2133.

Iron deficiency, a common comorbidity in patients with heart failure, triggers heart failure worsening, circulatory decompensation, and is associated with higher mortality.[30] Also, in pregnant women, iron deficiency (both with and without anaemia) is highly prevalent with unfavourable consequences on the health status of the foetus and the mother. Iron deficiency compromises erythropoiesis, but also triggers coagulopathy and thromboembolic events, and impairs foetal and maternal cardio(myocyte) function by compromising energy metabolism.[31] In patients with chronic heart failure, intravenous iron supplementation improved symptoms.[32]

Diagnosis and management of de novo and acute heart failure during pregnancy or postpartum

Distinguishing symptoms and signs of normal pregnancy from heart failure demands careful clinical assessment and investigation which makes the diagnosis of de novo heart failure during pregnancy challenging. A high level of suspicion ensures that the diagnosis is not missed in patients without known heart failure. Quite often, heart failure symptoms such as dyspnoea develop in patients with pregnancy-associated hypertension/eclampsia. This form of hypertensive heart failure with preserved LVEF responds well to application of diuretics and lowering of blood pressure.[8]

If acute heart failure (AHF) develops in a pregnant patient, either with or without previously known heart failure, immediate referral to an ICU and assessment of heart failure severity and foetal status are crucial. Urgent echocardiography is recommended to detect left and/or right heart failure, valvular abnormalities, etc. To ensure rapid diagnosis, decision-making, and therapy, a prespecified interdisciplinary task force and management algorithm are recommended (➡ Figure 12.14.1).[2,10] Multidisciplinary care includes cardiologists, intensivists, obstetricians, neonatologists, anaesthetists, and cardiac surgeons. Timely diagnosis and treatment are crucial. A recommended treatment algorithm for patients with AHF is given in ➡ Figure 12.14.2.[3]

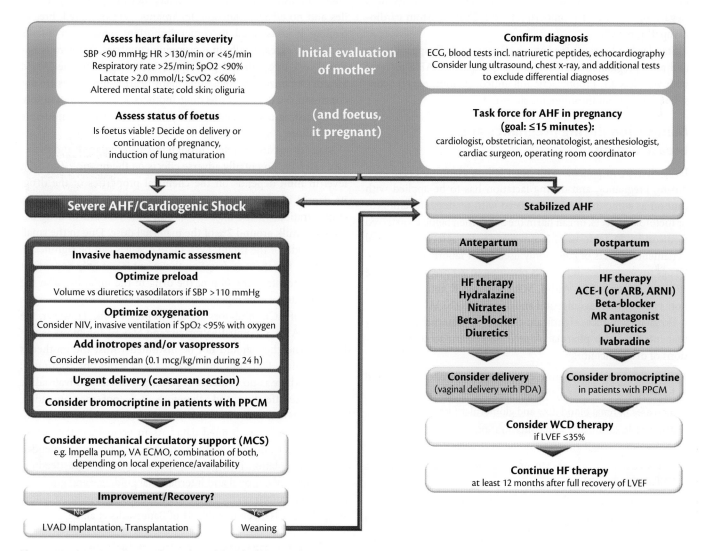

Figure 12.14.2 Management of acute heart failure (HF) during/after pregnancy: rapid interdisciplinary workup and treatment of the mother and foetus. ACE-I, angiotensin-converting enzyme inhibitor; AHF, acute heart failure; ARB, angiotensin receptor blocker; ARNI, angiotensin receptor–neprilysin inhibitor; ECG, electrocardiogram; HR, heart rate; LVAD, left ventricular assist device; LVEF, left ventricular ejection fraction; MR, mineralocorticoid receptor; NIV, non-invasive ventilation; PDA, peridural anaesthesia; PPCM, peripartum cardiomyopathy; SBP, systolic blood pressure; ScvO2, central venous oxygen saturation; SpO2, blood oxygen saturation; VA ECMO, veno-arterial extracorporeal membrane oxygenation; WCD, wearable cardioverter-defibrillator.

A patient in cardiogenic shock or severe AHF requiring inotropes or vasopressors should be transferred early to a tertiary centre capable of providing mechanical circulatory support (MCS) and ventricular assist devices (VADs).[33,34] Urgent delivery by Caesarean section (irrespective of gestation) should be considered with MCS available. PPCM patients seem to be especially sensitive to the toxic effects of beta-adrenergic agonists, which should be avoided whenever possible; the calcium sensitizer levosimendan may be an alternative.[15]

In patients with stabilized or subacute AHF, management goals are similar to AHF in non-pregnant patients, but foetotoxic agents (ACE inhibitors, ARB, ARNI, MRA) must be avoided.[2,3,27] Loop diuretics should be used in patients with symptoms or signs of congestion, despite concerns about placental blood flow. Nitrates appear safe in pregnancy. After stabilization, initiation and uptitration of beta-blockers should be performed with caution. If high resting heart rate persists in the presence of beta-blockade, or intolerance thereof, treatment with ivabradine may be initiated in patients who are not pregnant or breastfeeding. Regarding the use of bromocriptine, see ⊃ Peripartum cardiomyopathy, p. 893.

Standard indications for anticoagulation in AHF apply during and after pregnancy.[10] In pregnant or postpartum AHF patients with very low EF, prophylactic full anticoagulation may be considered to prevent thromboembolic events.

Medication during pregnancy and breastfeeding

Drug therapy in patients with heart failure planning pregnancy, during pregnancy, and during lactation has to be applied with caution as some drugs are associated with teratogenic, embryo- or foetotoxic effects, or can harm the baby when being transferred to the milk. ⊃ Table 12.14.2, summarizes the safety or potential detrimental effects of commonly used heart failure medications. Drugs to be avoided in patients planning to get pregnant include ACE inhibitors, ARBs, ARNI, MRA, vitamin K antagonists, and non-vitamin K antagonist oral anticoagulants (NOAC).

Pregnancy induces significant changes in maternal physiology that interfere with pharmacokinetic and pharmacodynamic actions of drugs including:

- increases in plasma volume, cardiac output, stroke volume, and heart rate
- increases in renal blood flow and glomerular filtration rate
- decrease in serum albumin concentration
- increases in coagulation factors and fibrinogen
- increased activity of liver cytochrome P450 enzymes, for example, CYP2D6 and CYP3A4
- delayed gastric emptying, nausea and vomiting.

The increase in maternal intravascular and extravascular fluid volumes during pregnancy with a decrease in albumin and altered binding of alpha-1-acid glycoprotein affects drug distribution. This leads to an increase of the unbound drug fraction affecting the bio-availability of drugs that have a high protein binding.[35]

Serum concentrations of total drug in pregnant women underestimate the concentrations of free drug. A greater fluctuation in the unbound drug concentration occurring during the dosing interval may potentiate the pharmacodynamic effects at peak or reduce therapeutic effect at trough. More frequent dosing is advisable with an adjustment according to the pharmacodynamic effect observed for cardiovascular drugs with direct effect on physiological parameters, such as heart rate or blood pressure. Thus, given the altered pharmacokinetic of most drugs observed during pregnancy, the dosage of cardiovascular drugs should be titrated according to their pharmacodynamic effect on the mother and the foetus (e.g. heart rate, blood pressure, INR, aPTT).[10]

Breastfeeding in patients with heart failure is controversial. In patients with severe heart failure preventing lactation may be considered due to the high metabolic demands of lactation and breastfeeding (class IIb recommendation[10]). Stopping lactation enables safe treatment with all established heart failure drugs. Although in a collective of PPCM patients in South Africa where breastfeeding was terminated, normal growth percentiles and no adverse outcome for infants were observed, breastfeeding is considered to confer important benefits to infants and mothers, especially in developing countries. Numerous national and international guidelines, including from the World Health Organization, advise that many heart failure drugs are not contraindicated in breastfeeding mothers if used with caution. Breastfeeding is tolerated by many women with mild–moderate heart failure.

Many drugs are excreted through the maternal milk and therefore can have potentially adverse effects on the infant.[36] The drug level in milk depends on the chemical properties of the drug, its degree of plasma protein binding, and the maternal serum concentration. In the majority of cases the amount of drug excreted in milk around 2% of the maternal dose. Due to the small body weight of the infant, even these dosages can be significant. Therefore, the effect of drugs on the infant is not only dependent on the percentage fraction of the drug in the milk, but also the daily amount of milk ingested by the infant and the infant's weight.

Levels of ACE inhibitors are low in breast milk. However, the safety of ARB, sacubitril/valsartan, and SGLT2 inhibitors is unknown, and they should not be instituted whilst the mother is breastfeeding. Diuretics and beta blockers should be continued; however, there is no evidence regarding the safety of ivabradine during breastfeeding and, therefore, it is not recommended. Digoxin, MRA, and Vitamin K antagonists should be used with caution as there are limited data.[2] As in pregnancy, the risk of NOAC is not known, and they are therefore not recommended for anticoagulation post-partum if the mother is breastfeeding. A summary of national and international guidance and guideline recommendations on the safety of breastfeeding and heart failure drug therapy is given in Table S1 of Bauersachs et al.[2]

Delivery in patients with heart failure

The safe delivery of a woman with heart failure is a challenge requiring the input of a multidisciplinary team to achieve the best outcome. In terms of timing the delivery, considerations include the gestational age at presentation, whether there is a reversible underlying reason for heart failure, and the response to medical measures.[3] At least prophylactic anticoagulation should be considered, and in some patients with, for example, persisting atrial fibrillation or intracardiac thrombus, therapeutic anticoagulation needs to be instituted. Delivery should be considered, ideally from 32 weeks, when foetal survival without disability is expected, or earlier, including termination of pregnancy, when the response to medical therapy is suboptimal, the precipitating problem is irreversible, and/or there is a significant risk to the life or long-term health of the woman of continuing the pregnancy.

In patients with acute and/or severe heart failure often delivery will be by Caesarean section, as advised by the ESC guidelines,[10] and only occasionally vaginal delivery may be possible. Clearly these patients should be cared for in tertiary centres with an established pregnancy heart team and the availability of MCS. The delivery plan has to be made by the pregnancy heart team including obstetricians, neonatologists, cardiologists, anaesthetists, and cardiac surgeons (in case MCS is necessary). Close attention to fluid balance is key, in conditions of hypovolaemia secondary to blood loss and vasodilation.

If vaginal delivery is attempted, effective pain relief is essential and an instrumental delivery, without prior maternal effort, is likely to be the safest approach.[3] Vaginal delivery is associated with less blood loss and lower risk of infection, venous thrombosis, and embolism, and should be advised for most women with mild-moderate heart failure. Careful use of uterotonics, avoiding agents like ergometrine and carboprost, and the early or even prophylactic use of mechanical approaches, including brace suture and balloon compression, for the management or prevention of post-partum haemorrhage are advised. Once delivery is achieved and after the immediate peripartum period, an important consideration is effective contraception.

Adult congenital heart disease and right heart failure

In the large prospective ROPAC registry, ACHD is the most prevalent diagnosis (58%).[1] The majority of ACHD patients tolerate pregnancy well with a mortality rate of 0.2%. However, due to the heterogeneity of this group, the type and complexity of CHD needs to be considered.[10,24] While heart failure rate was 7% for the total ACHD group and 13% in patients with complex CHD, it was 5% and 6% for simple and moderate defects. The vast majority of these patients had their condition treated at a very young age. Maternal mortality complicates pregnancy in 0.1% of women with corrected CHD and in 0.7% with uncorrected CHD. Pre-pregnancy counselling (➲ Counselling before pregnancy, p. 885) and the optimization of cardiac status prior to pregnancy may account for the relatively good outcomes.[1]

Pregnancy must be avoided in patients classified as mWHO class IV (➲ Table 12.14.1) including patients with PAH, severe LV dysfunction, and Fontan patients with any previous complication. Patients in mWHO class III, such as those with LVEF 30–45%,

systemic right ventricle with good or mildly decreased ventricular function, uncomplicated Fontan circulation, unrepaired cyanotic heart disease, or other complex heart disease, require expert counselling by a pregnancy heart team at an expert centre and monthly or bimonthly follow-up during pregnancy.

Although, in general, the patients with regurgitant lesions often tolerate pregnancy well, severe valve regurgitation can cause heart failure. Regarding occurrence of clinically overt heart failure, in the ROPAC registry, there was a peak around the end of the second trimester (typically women with a shunt lesion) and in the first days after delivery (women with diminished LVEF). Treatment of heart failure is essentially the same as outside pregnancy, respecting contraindications to embryo-/fetotoxic drugs. In patients with a systemic right ventricle (transposition of the great arteries with a Senning/Mustard procedure or congenitally corrected transposition of the great arteries patients), there is no evidence that medication such as ACE-inhibitors are effective. Early delivery is advised when heart failure cannot be stabilized with bedrest and medication.

Specific cardiomyopathies

Cardiomyopathies are a heterogeneous group of heart muscle diseases with structural and functional abnormalities, including PPCM, hypertrophic cardiomyopathy (HCM), dilated cardiomyopathy (DCM), and restrictive cardiomyopathy (RCM), as well as left ventricular non-compaction, arrhythmogenic right ventricular cardiomyopathy (ARVC) and Takotsubo syndrome. The epidemiology and management of cardiomyopathies and heart failure during/after pregnancy has been reviewed recently.[3,37]

Peripartum cardiomyopathy

PPCM presents with heart failure with reduced LVEF (< 45%) in previously cardiac-healthy women towards the end of pregnancy, or in the months following delivery. PPCM has major geographical variations in incidence (1–100 in 10,000 live births).[2] In two-thirds of patients the diagnosis of PPCM is made post-delivery, and patients are usually only diagnosed when they have severe symptoms,[38] raising the possibility that those with less severe presentation may go undiagnosed. A high index of suspicion is encouraged from midwives, obstetricians, and general practitioners to not miss the diagnosis in patients with mild–moderate symptoms. Investigations for possible PPCM should include an electrocardiogram, as well as natriuretic peptide determination or/and echocardiography. No specific biomarkers for PPCM are established to date, thus the differentiation from other cardiomyopathies is not easily possible.[2] Important differential diagnoses include pulmonary embolism, myocardial infarction, hypertensive heart disease during pregnancy, and pre-existing heart disease.

PPCM is associated with a mortality rate of around 6% at 6 months but has a good chance of myocardial recovery (around 50%; recovery occurring up to 3 years after diagnosis).[12] As for all patients with heart failure during/after pregnancy, a management plan should be formulated taking into account the wellbeing of the mother and baby. Drug therapy pre-delivery follows the general rules outlined above. If PPCM is diagnosed post-delivery, there are several key aspects of management. Therapy should include drugs that are safe during lactation (if the woman is breast-feeding).[2] In women who are not breastfeeding medical therapy should reflect conventional guideline-directed heart failure therapy. As pro-coagulant activity is increased during and early after pregnancy, and a high rate of thrombo-embolic events have been observed in the EURObservational Research Programme (EORP) PPCM worldwide registry (7% in the first 30 days after delivery),[12] initial treatment with low molecular weight heparin or oral anticoagulation, at least in prophylactic dose, should be considered if there is not an indication for therapeutic anticoagulation due to other reasons.

The 2018 ESC Guidelines for the management of cardiovascular diseases during pregnancy[10] has added a recommendation regarding the use of bromocriptine in PPCM (class IIB). Bromocriptine (2.5 mg once daily) for 1 week may be considered in uncomplicated cases, whereas prolonged treatment (2.5 mg twice daily for 2 weeks, then 2.5 mg once daily for 6 weeks) may be considered in patients with EF < 25% and/or cardiogenic shock.[2,39] Bromocriptine treatment must always be accompanied by anticoagulation in at least prophylactic dosages.

As many patients with PPCM have a good chance for recovery, or at least marked improvement of LVEF with guideline-directed heart failure drug therapy, cardiac resynchronization therapy and implantable cardioverter defibrillators for primary prevention should be avoided during the first 6–12 months. Prior to discharge, counselling should include advice about contraception and the risk of subsequent pregnancies.[40] When and whether to stop heart failure drug therapy after LV recovery is uncertain. While some experts advocate indefinite treatment, cautious tapering of medication after complete and sustained LV recovery may be feasible.[2]

The risk of subsequent pregnancies depends upon whether LV ejection fraction has recovered (usually defined as >50–55%).[40] For PPCM patients with recovered EF that is sustained after tapering of RAAS blockers, during a subsequent pregnancy the rate of death is <1% and a risk of recurrent heart failure is around 10%. These patients need close follow-up during a subsequent pregnancy by an expert heart team. For those who have not recovered, the risk is substantially higher (risk of death around 10%, and recurrent heart failure 25–50%), thus subsequent pregnancy is not recommended in patients with prior PPCM without LV recovery.[40]

Hypertrophic cardiomyopathy

The observed incidence of HCM in pregnancy is < 1:1000; echocardiography is crucial for diagnosis. Maternal mortality is low (0.5%), and complications or worsening of symptoms occur in 29% of cases.[10,41] Foetal mortality is comparable to the general population; however, the risk of premature birth is increased (26%). Risk is higher in women who are symptomatic before pregnancy or exhibit diastolic dysfunction, severe LV outflow

tract obstruction (LVOTO), or arrhythmia.[3] Symptoms and medication before pregnancy are also risk factors for maternal cardiac events.

Most women with HCM are mWHO class II (only slightly increased risk of maternal mortality/morbidity) and should be assessed during each trimester. Those in class III (e.g. with moderate LV impairment) should be assessed monthly or bi-monthly. A recent randomized study on the effectiveness of implanted cardiac rhythm recorders for detecting arrhythmias in pregnant women with structural heart disease suggests that these devices could be considered in HCM to facilitate early detection of arrythmia or re-assurance of the mother and avoiding harmful medication.[42] Beta-blockers should be continued if they are already being taken, and effects on the foetus may require monitoring by the gynaecologist. Beta-blockers should be started when new symptoms occur, for rate control in atrial fibrillation, and to suppress ventricular arrhythmias. Cardioversion should be considered for poorly tolerated persistent atrial fibrillation. Therapeutic anticoagulation is recommended for those with paroxysmal or persistent arrhythmias.

In patients with stiff ventricles and LVOTO, hypovolaemia may be poorly tolerated. Patients' risk for sudden cardiac death, especially in those with a past history or a family history of sudden death, should be re-assessed and need close surveillance with prompt investigation if they develop palpitations or presyncope. When indicated, a device should be implanted.

Low-risk cases may proceed with vaginal delivery. Caesarean section should be considered in patients with severe LV outflow tract obstruction, pre-term labour while on oral anticoagulation, or severe heart failure. However, in the ROPAC study, only 5% of patients required emergency Caesarean section.[41] During delivery, monitoring of heart rate and rhythm should be considered in patients with a high risk of developing arrhythmias.

Restrictive cardiomyopathy

RCM is characterized by ventricular wall stiffness caused by abnormalities intrinsic to the myocardium, or to the endomyocardial layer.[43] LV hypertrophy associated with myocardial stiffness predominates in infiltrative and storage diseases, with accumulation of the pathological material in the myocardium and variable interstitial and/or replacement fibrosis. Classic features of RCM are severe diastolic dysfunction, markedly elevated filling pressures with atrial enlargement, and a predisposition to atrial fibrillation. Patients with RCM may have low blood pressure and suffer from orthostatic hypotension and hypoperfusion if volume is depleted. Endomyocardial fibrosis is the leading cause of RCM in tropical regions, while amyloid cardiomyopathy is the most common cause of the infiltrative form. In some patients, specific therapies should be considered after the aetiology of RCM has been established. There are only a few reports on patients diagnosed with RCM during pregnancy.[37] Care for these patients needs to focus on treatment of heart failure with preserved ejection fraction and potential rhythm disturbances, especially atrial fibrillation.

Arrhythmogenic right ventricular cardiomyopathy

ARVC is a rare, inheritable, chronic, and progressive cardio-myopathy characterized by loss of cardiomyocytes, followed by fibrofatty replacement in the right ventricle, associated with arrhythmia and RV failure. Its prevalence is 0.02–0.05%, but it is one of the leading causes of sudden cardiac death in young women.[37] For women who have not had an ICD implant before pregnancy, ARVC severity score is highly predictive for the occurrence of ventricular arrhythmias, and echocardiographic and signal-averaged ECGs are markers of ventricular arrhythmias.[44] As ventricular arrhythmia and disease progression in ARVC are worsened by vigorous exercise, pregnancy-associated haemo-dynamic stress may, theoretically, lead to disease progression. However, in a recently published large cross-sectional cohort study,pregnancy did not affect cardiac structure or function in ARVC, supporting previous reports of well-tolerated pregnancies in this patient group.[45]

Moreover, serious cardiac symptoms did not worsen during pregnancy, number of pregnancies was not associated with arrhythmic events, and higher number of pregnancies was not associated with worse outcome in women with ARVC. Thus, the long-term effect of pregnancy is well tolerated, and pregnancy appears relatively safe in women with ARVC.[3] Nevertheless, ARVC patients should be referred to an experienced centre for structured follow-up from early pregnancy until after delivery.

Left ventricular non-compaction cardiomyopathy

Left ventricular non-compaction (LVNC) is a rare, inherited heart disease characterized by hypertrabeculation of the myocardium with deep intertrabecular recesses, and an increased risk of thromboembolic events. A subset of patients develop LV dysfunction and heart failure. During normal pregnancy, there is a transient increase in LV trabeculation which occurs in one-quarter of women. Also, in patients with PPCM, reversible increases in LV trabeculation have been observed. This makes diagnosis of LVNC during pregnancy challenging.[46]

Pregnancy in LVNC is often complicated by heart failure and arrhythmias, but no deaths during pregnancy have been reported.[47] There is no specific treatment, but anticoagulation is recommended for patients with LVNC and a history of thrombo-embolic events, atrial fibrillation, intracardiac thrombi, or impaired LV function.[37]

Takotsubo syndrome

Takotsubo syndrome (TTS) is an acute and usually reversible heart failure syndrome with initial presentation similar to acute coronary syndrome.[48,49] Often triggered by emotional stress, and much more common in women than in men, classical TTS is characterized by reversible LV dysfunction with extensive apical cardiac akinesia. However, other transient wall motion abnormalities of the LV have also been described. Cardiac function recovers almost entirely within a few days/weeks if the patient survives the acute phase. However, life-threatening complications such as cardiogenic shock, ventricular rupture, and ventricular fibrillation occur in more than 10%.[49] The pathophysiology of TTS is not well understood, and clinical management is not based on clear evidence. Most of the reported TTS cases in pregnant women occurred after Caesarean delivery, but TTS has also been reported in women during pregnancy, or after a spontaneous abortion. Similar to non-pregnant patients with TTS, recovery was observed between 4 days and 3 months.[37]

The European task force position statement suggests classifying TTS into lower- and higher-risk categories,[48] and recommend considering an ACE inhibitor/ARNI and a beta-blocker in the higher-risk groups. However, given that ACE inhibitors/ARNI are contraindicated in pregnancy, and evidence for beta-blockers is not established in TTS, these agents should not be used during pregnancy. In severe cases with life-threatening haemodynamic instability MCS should be considered. In the rare event of an LV thrombus, anticoagulation is mandatory, whereas routine anticoagulation for dyskinesis without thrombus is not recommended.

Dilated cardiomyopathy

DCM includes acquired and inherited conditions characterized by LV dilatation and systolic dysfunction in the absence of significant abnormalities in loading conditions or coronary artery disease. Causes include pathogenic gene variants in 20–35%, and/or acquired triggers including prior viral infection, immune-mediated, and drug-induced LV dysfunction.[43] More than 50 gene mutations seem to be associated with DCM, but the genetic contribution of 12 of them have recently been re-enforced.[3,50] DCM and PPCM may share a genetic predisposition,[13] as, in a minority of PPCM patients, DCM gene variants can be detected. However, PPCM and DCM are considered distinct disease entities. The differentiation sometimes may be challenging, especially when the patient presents in the last trimester of pregnancy. In general, DCM is a pre-existing cardiomyopathy known before pregnancy, but may also become clinically apparent during the course of pregnancy. Women carrying pathogenic mutations associated with DCM, but without previous disease manifestation, are at elevated risk during pregnancy as the cardiovascular stress during pregnancy may present a second hit.[5,17]

Patients with pre-existing DCM receiving current disease-modifying medication may show substantial/complete recovery of LV systolic function.[43] However, pregnancy is often poorly tolerated in women with DCM, and significant deterioration in LV function (depending on the residual severity of LV dysfunction) may occur.[1] Predictors of maternal mortality include the degree of symptoms (approximately 7% for NYHA class III or IV) and EF < 40%.[1,37] Patients with LVEF < 30%, and/or NYHA class III/IV, belong to mWHO class IV and should be counselled against pregnancy. In patients with LVEF > 30%/NYHA class I–II, drugs contraindicated during pregnancy need to be tapered cautiously and LV function checked thereafter to detect significant deterioration that may preclude pregnancy. All patients with DCM who are pregnant require close joint cardiac and obstetric care by the pregnancy heart team, since there is a high risk of heart failure deterioration, maternal mortality, and foetal loss.

Standard indications for anticoagulation in DCM include intracardiac thrombi and atrial fibrillation; as anticoagulant agent mainly low molecular weight heparin is used, but vitamin K antagonists may be taken in the second and third trimester.[10]

A new diagnosis of DCM carries potential implications for the patient, but her relatives may potentially require clinical screening of family members and referral to experts in cardiovascular genetics. For all patients with DCM and/or carrying DCM mutations, careful pre-pregnancy evaluation, risk-stratification, and counselling is mandated before a future pregnancy is considered.

Cardiac transplantation – LV assist devices

Patients, and their foetus, are at elevated risk during pregnancy after heart transplantation.[3] There are case reports of successful conception and delivery in patients after heart transplantation, and also in patients with long-term VADs. Multidisciplinary care is mandatory, preferably coordinated by the transplant centre.[51]

Pre-conception counselling includes the risks to the mother and the foetus, including graft rejection, graft dysfunction, infection, and teratogenicity of immunosuppressive agents.[3] Some centres recommend paternal HLA testing prior to conception as the risk of autograft rejection is high if the donated heart and father have the same HLA antigen, and the recipient develops donor-specific antibodies.[52] As children of mothers with CHD as the reason for heart transplantation have up to 10% risk of congenital disease in the foetus, this risk should also be considered in pre-conception counselling and early foetal screening is indicated. Pregnancy should be avoided for at least one year after transplantation as the risk of spontaneous abortion is 10–20%. Successful pregnancy is most likely when graft function is normal with no signs of rejection. Where clinically indicated, standard investigations up to and including endomyocardial biopsy should be undertaken prior to pregnancy. In patients at high risk of rejection and/or with poor baseline graft function, pregnancy should be strongly discouraged until these risks can be reduced.[3]

The most common maternal complication during pregnancy is hypertension which may result in foetal growth restriction and preterm delivery. Thromboembolic events are also frequent in cardiac transplant recipients and clinical suspicion should remain high.

All drugs including immunosuppression, need to be reviewed prior to conception, with cessation/substitution of teratogenic drugs, and close monitoring of drug levels (especially if drug metabolism can be altered by pregnancy, for example, for cyclosporine). Careful monitoring is necessary in case of hyperemesis gravidarum with poor absorption of immunosuppressive medication. As all immunosuppressive medications enter the foetal circulation, the management of immunosuppression in the pregnant post-transplant recipient should be conducted by dedicated experts. Furthermore, all immunosuppressive agents are excreted into breast milk with unknown long-term effects. Thus, breast-feeding is not recommended.

Future directions

Patients with previously known or newly developing cardiomyopathy/heart failure during or after pregnancy are a highly complex and diverse patient group, with often markedly elevated risk for adverse maternal and foetal outcomes. Most of the care provided is based on clinical experience, but not on firm evidence. Clinical registries such as the ROPAC registry have provided data on these patients, but much more research is needed to get firm ground for pre-pregnancy counselling, as well as for management during pregnancy and thereafter.

Summary and key messages

Patients with pre-existing heart failure or developing heart failure during pregnancy are at elevated (sometimes at very high) risk for adverse outcomes, including death of the mother and the child. Pre-pregnancy counselling is crucial of women with pre-existing heart failure, or at risk of developing heart failure during pregnancy. All women with a history of chemo-/radiotherapy for malignant diseases need specific pre-pregnancy assessment and counselling. Management of pregnancy and the postpartum period for women with a previously known cardiomyopathy/heart failure, or developing heart failure during pregnancy/postpartum, requires expert care in a multi-disciplinary pregnancy heart team.

Conflicts of interest

JB reports honoraria for lectures and/or consulting: Novartis, BMS, Pfizer, Vifor, Bayer, Servier, Daichii Sankyo, CVRx, MSD, Boehringer Ingelheim, AstraZeneca, Abiomed, Abbott, Medtronic, Cardior; Research support: Zoll, CVRx, Vifor, Abiomed. DH and KS report no conflict of interests.

References

1. Roos-Hesselink J, Baris L, Johnson M, De Backer J, Otto C, Marelli A, et al. Pregnancy outcomes in women with cardiovascular disease: evolving trends over 10 years in the ESC Registry Of Pregnancy And Cardiac disease (ROPAC). European Heart Journal. 2019;40(47):3848–55.
2. Bauersachs J, Konig T, van der Meer P, Petrie MC, Hilfiker-Kleiner D, Mbakwem A, et al. Pathophysiology, diagnosis and management of peripartum cardiomyopathy: a position statement from the Heart Failure Association of the European Society of Cardiology Study Group on peripartum cardiomyopathy. European Journal of Heart Failure. 2019;21(7):827–43.
3. Sliwa K, van der Meer P, Petrie MC, Frougadi A, Johnson MR, Hilfiker-Kleiner D, et al. Risk stratification and management of women with cardiomyopathy/heart failure planning pregnancy or presenting during/after pregnancy: a position statement from the Heart Failure Association of the European Society of Cardiology Study Group on Peripartum Cardiomyopathy. European Journal of Heart Failure. 2021, 23(4):527–40.
4. Chung E, Leinwand LA. Pregnancy as a cardiac stress model. Cardiovascular research. Cardiovasc Res 2014;101(4):561–70.

5. Hilfiker-Kleiner D, Haghikia A, Nonhoff J, Bauersachs J. Peripartum cardiomyopathy: current management and future perspectives. European Heart Journal. 2015;36(18):1090–7.

6. Sanghavi M, Rutherford JD. Cardiovascular physiology of pregnancy. Circulation. 2014;130(12):1003–8.

7. Brenner B. Haemostatic changes in pregnancy. Thromb Res. 2004;114(5–6):409–14.

8. Ives CW, Sinkey R, Rajapreyar I, Tita ATN, Oparil S. Preeclampsia-pathophysiology and clinical presentations: JACC State-of-the-Art Review. Journal of the American College of Cardiology. 2020;76(14):1690–702.

9. Beale AL, Meyer P, Marwick TH, Lam CSP, Kaye DM. Sex differences in cardiovascular pathophysiology: why women are overrepresented in heart failure with preserved ejection fraction. Circulation. 2018;138(2):198–205.

10. Regitz-Zagrosek V, Roos-Hesselink JW, Bauersachs J, Blomstrom-Lundqvist C, Cifkova R, De Bonis M, et al. 2018 ESC Guidelines for the management of cardiovascular diseases during pregnancy. European Heart Journal. 2018;39(34):3165–241.

11. Ricke-Hoch M, Hoes MF, Pfeffer TJ, Schlothauer S, Nonhoff J, Haidari S, et al. In peripartum cardiomyopathy plasminogen activator inhibitor-1 is a potential new biomarker with controversial roles. Cardiovascular Research. 2020;116(11):1875–86.

12. Sliwa K, Petrie MC, van der Meer P, Mebazaa A, Hilfiker-Kleiner D, Jackson AM, et al. Clinical presentation, management, and 6-month outcomes in women with peripartum cardiomyopathy: an ESC EORP registry. European Heart Journal. 2020;41(39):3787–97.

13. Ware JS, Li J, Mazaika E, Yasso CM, DeSouza T, Cappola TP, et al. Shared genetic predisposition in peripartum and dilated cardiomyopathies. New Engl J Med. 2016;374(3):233–41.

14. Pfeffer T, Schlothauer S, Pietzsch S, Schaufelberger M, Aubert B, Ricke-Hoch M, et al. Increased cancer prevalence in peripartum cardiomyopathy. JACC CardioOncology. 2019;1:196–205.

15. Stapel B, Kohlhaas M, Ricke-Hoch M, Haghikia A, Erschow S, Knuuti J, et al. Low STAT3 expression sensitizes to toxic effects of beta-adrenergic receptor stimulation in peripartum cardiomyopathy. European Heart Journal. 2017;38(5):349–61.

16. de Boer RA, Hulot JS, Tocchetti CG, Aboumsallem JP, Ameri P, Anker SD, et al. Common mechanistic pathways in cancer and heart failure. A scientific roadmap on behalf of the Translational Research Committee of the Heart Failure Association (HFA) of the European Society of Cardiology (ESC). European Journal of Heart Failure. 2020;22(12):2272–89..

17. Pfeffer TJ, Pietzsch S, Hilfiker-Kleiner D. Common genetic predisposition for heart failure and cancer. Herz. 2020;45(7):632–6.

18. Fidler MM, Reulen RC, Henson K, Kelly J, Cutter D, Levitt GA, et al. Population-based long-term cardiac-specific mortality among 34 489 five-year survivors of childhood cancer in Great Britain. Circulation. 2017;135(10):951–63.

19. Armenian SH, Hudson MM, Mulder RL, Chen MH, Constine LS, Dwyer M, et al. Recommendations for cardiomyopathy surveillance for survivors of childhood cancer: a report from the International Late Effects of Childhood Cancer Guideline Harmonization Group. Lancet Oncology. 2015;16(3):e123–36.

20. Liu S, Aghel N, Belford L, Silversides CK, Nolan M, Amir E, et al. Cardiac outcomes in pregnant women with treated cancer. Journal of the American College of Cardiology. 2018;72(17):2087–9.

21. Thompson KA, Hildebrandt MA, Ater JL. Cardiac outcomes with pregnancy after cardiotoxic therapy for childhood cancer. Journal of the American College of Cardiology. 2017;69(5):594–5.

22. Hines MR, Mulrooney DA, Hudson MM, Ness KK, Green DM, Howard SC, et al. Pregnancy-associated cardiomyopathy in survivors of childhood cancer. J Cancer Surviv. 2016;10(1):113–21.

23. Lyon AR, Dent S, Stanway S, Earl H, Brezden-Masley C, Cohen-Solal A, et al. Baseline cardiovascular risk assessment in cancer patients scheduled to receive cardiotoxic cancer therapies: a Position Statement and new risk assessment tools from the Cardio-Oncology Study Group of the Heart Failure Association of the European Society of Cardiology in collaboration with the International Cardio-Oncology Society. European Journal of Heart Failure. 2020;22:1945–60.

24. Baumgartner H, De Backer J, Babu-Narayan SV, Budts W, Chessa M, Diller GP, et al. 2020 ESC Guidelines for the management of adult congenital heart disease. European Heart Journal. 2021; 42(6):563–645.25. Mueller C, McDonald K, de Boer RA, Maisel A, Cleland JGF, Kozhuharov N, et al. Heart Failure Association of the European Society of Cardiology practical guidance on the use of natriuretic peptide concentrations. European Journal of Heart Failure. 2019;21(6):715–31.

26. Resnik JL, Hong C, Resnik R, Kazanegra R, Beede J, Bhalla V, et al. Evaluation of B-type natriuretic peptide (BNP) levels in normal and preeclamptic women. American Journal of Obstetrics And gynecology. 2005;193(2):450–4.

27. McDonagh TA, Metra M, Adamo M, Gardner RS, Baumbach A, Böhm M, et al. 2021 ESC Guidelines for the diagnosis and treatment of acute and chronic heart failure: The Task Force for the diagnosis and treatment of acute and chronic heart failure of the European Society of Cardiology (ESC). Developed with the special contribution of the Heart Failure Association (HFA) of the ESC. European Heart Journal. 2021;42(36):3599–726.

28. Bassily-Marcus AM, Yuan C, Oropello J, Manasia A, Kohli-Seth R, Benjamin E. Pulmonary hypertension in pregnancy: critical care management. Pulmonary Medicine. 2012;2012:709407.

29. Zengin E, Sinning C, Schrage B, Mueller GC, Klose H, Sachweh J, et al. Right heart failure in pregnant women with cyanotic congenital heart disease--The good, the bad and the ugly. International Journal of Cardiology. 2016;202:773–5.

30. Jankowska EA, Kasztura M, Sokolski M, Bronisz M, Nawrocka S, Oleskowska-Florek W, et al. Iron deficiency defined as depleted iron stores accompanied by unmet cellular iron requirements identifies patients at the highest risk of death after an episode of acute heart failure. European Heart Journal. 2014;35(36):2468–76.

31. Georgieff MK, Krebs NF, Cusick SE. The benefits and risks of iron supplementation in pregnancy and childhood. Annu Rev Nutr. 2019;39:121–46.

32. Anker SD, Comin Colet J, Filippatos G, Willenheimer R, Dickstein K, Drexler H, et al. Ferric carboxymaltose in patients with heart failure and iron deficiency. New England Journal of Medicine. 2009;361(25):2436–48.

33. Chioncel O, Parissis J, Mebazaa A, Thiele H, Desch S, Bauersachs J, et al. Epidemiology, pathophysiology and contemporary management of cardiogenic shock - a position statement from the Heart Failure Association of the European Society of Cardiology. European Journal of Heart Failure. 2020;22(8):1315–41.

34. Bauersachs J, Arrigo M, Hilfiker-Kleiner D, Veltmann C, Coats AJ, Crespo-Leiro MG, et al. Current management of patients with severe acute peripartum cardiomyopathy: practical guidance from the Heart Failure Association of the European Society of Cardiology Study Group on peripartum cardiomyopathy. European Journal of Heart Failure. 2016;18(9):1096–105.

35. Loebstein R, Lalkin A, Koren G. Pharmacokinetic changes during pregnancy and their clinical relevance. Clinical Pharmacokinetics. 1997;33(5):328–43.

36. Ito S. Mother and child: medication use in pregnancy and lactation. Clinical Pharmacology and Therapeutics. 2016;100(1):8–11.

37. Schaufelberger M. Cardiomyopathy and pregnancy. Heart. 2019;105(20):1543–51.

38. Sliwa K, Mebazaa A, Hilfiker-Kleiner D, Petrie MC, Maggioni AP, Laroche C, et al. Clinical characteristics of patients from the worldwide registry on peripartum cardiomyopathy (PPCM): EURObservational Research Programme in conjunction with the Heart Failure Association of the European Society of Cardiology Study Group on PPCM. European Journal of Heart Failure. 2017;19(9):1131–41.

39. Hilfiker-Kleiner D, Haghikia A, Berliner D, Vogel-Claussen J, Schwab J, Franke A, et al. Bromocriptine for the treatment of peripartum cardiomyopathy: a multicentre randomized study. European Heart Journal. 2017;38(35):2671–9.

40. Sliwa K, Petrie MC, Hilfiker-Kleiner D, Mebazaa A, Jackson A, Johnson MR, et al. Long-term prognosis, subsequent pregnancy, contraception and overall management of peripartum cardiomyopathy: practical guidance paper from the Heart Failure Association of the European Society of Cardiology Study Group on Peripartum Cardiomyopathy. European Journal of Heart Failure. 2018;20(6):951–62.

41. Goland S, van Hagen IM, Elbaz-Greener G, Elkayam U, Shotan A, Merz WM, et al. Pregnancy in women with hypertrophic cardiomyopathy: data from the European Society of Cardiology initiated Registry of Pregnancy and Cardiac disease (ROPAC). European Heart Journal. 2017;38(35):2683–90.

42. Sliwa K, Azibani F, Johnson MR, Viljoen C, Baard J, Osman A, et al. Effectiveness of implanted cardiac rhythm recorders with electrocardiographic monitoring for detecting arrhythmias in pregnant women with symptomatic arrhythmia and/or structural heart disease: a randomized clinical trial. JAMA cardiology. 2020;5(4):458–63.

43. Seferovic PM, Polovina M, Bauersachs J, Arad M, Gal TB, Lund LH, et al. Heart failure in cardiomyopathies: a position paper from the Heart Failure Association of the European Society of Cardiology. European Journal of Heart Failure. 2019;21(5):553–76.

44. Calkins H, Corrado D, Marcus F. Risk Stratification in Arrhythmogenic Right Ventricular Cardiomyopathy. Circulation. 2017;136(21):2068–82.

45. Castrini AI, Lie OH, Leren IS, Estensen ME, Stokke MK, Klaeboe LG, et al. Number of pregnancies and subsequent phenotype in a cross-sectional cohort of women with arrhythmogenic cardiomyopathy. European Heart Journal Cardiovascular Imaging. 2019;20(2):192–8.

46. Gati S, Papadakis M, Papamichael ND, Zaidi A, Sheikh N, Reed M, et al. Reversible de novo left ventricular trabeculations in pregnant women: implications for the diagnosis of left ventricular noncompaction in low-risk populations. Circulation. 2014;130(6):475–83.

47. Ueda Y, Kamiya CA, Nakanishi A, Horiuchi C, Miyoshi T, Hazama R, et al. Cardiomyopathy phenotypes and pregnancy outcomes with left ventricular noncompaction cardiomyopathy. Int Heart J. 2018;59(4):862–7.

48. Lyon AR, Bossone E, Schneider B, Sechtem U, Citro R, Underwood SR, et al. Current state of knowledge on Takotsubo syndrome: a Position Statement from the Taskforce on Takotsubo Syndrome of the Heart Failure Association of the European Society of Cardiology. European Journal of Heart Failure. 2016;18(1):8–27.

49. Napp LC, Bauersachs J. Takotsubo syndrome: between evidence, myths, and misunderstandings. Herz. 2020;45(3):252–66.

50. Mazzarotto F, Tayal U, Buchan RJ, Midwinter W, Wilk A, Whiffin N, et al. Reevaluating the genetic contribution of monogenic dilated cardiomyopathy. Circulation. 2020;141(5):387–98.

51. Costanzo MR, Dipchand A, Starling R, Anderson A, Chan M, Desai S, et al. The International Society of Heart and Lung Transplantation Guidelines for the care of heart transplant recipients. Journal of Heart and Lung Transplantation 2010;29(8):914–56.

52. O'Boyle PJ, Smith JD, Danskine AJ, Lyster HS, Burke MM, Banner NR. De novo HLA sensitization and antibody mediated rejection following pregnancy in a heart transplant recipient. Am J Transplant. 2010;10(1):180–3.

CHAPTER 12.15

Frailty in heart failure

Ewa A Jankowska, Cristiana Vitale,
and Dong-Ju Choi

Contents

Heart failure, ageing, and multimorbidity

Heart failure (HF) is recognized as a cardiogeriatric syndrome.[1,2] There is a strong relationship between HF and ageing. Elderly people have a higher incidence and prevalence of HF; they usually have advanced heart disease, more severe symptoms, poorer quality of life, and worse clinical outcomes with a particularly high burden of HF hospitalization and associated health care costs.[1,2]

Although new pharmacotherapies, invasive procedures, and devices, which have been demonstrated to improve clinical status and outcomes, have been implemented in patients with HF, quality of life and prognosis of older patients with HF remain poor, which is also due to a suboptimal implementation of these therapies in elderly subjects.

HF is a complex clinical syndrome with the contribution of several pathomechanisms, such as neuro-hormonal activation, inflammation, insulin resistance, catabolic/anabolic imbalance, quantitative and qualitative malnutrition, immobility, sarcopenia, and skeletal dysfunction. These abnormalities are particularly exaggerated in elderly individuals with HF, and, on the other hand, independently of HF, they also contribute to the pathological process of ageing and the development of frailty.

Moreover, HF is a prime example of a clinical entity that is accompanied by multiple cardiovascular (CV) and non-CV diseases.[3,4] Comorbidities contribute in different ways to the progression of HF, the pathological process of ageing, and the development of frailty.

Concept of frailty

Frailty is not just a simple reflection of the ageing process. Ageing itself predisposes to frailty, but is not a synonym for frailty. Similarly, multimorbidity predisposes to frailty, but is not a synonym for frailty. There is a heterogeneity in the rate of age-related decline in the functioning of particular systems and organs as well as the development of particular comorbidities. Therefore, the biological age is much more important than the chronological one, and frailty is related to pathological (accelerated) ageing. It needs to be acknowledged that frailty is a distinct biological syndrome that underlies its heterogeneity. Frailty syndrome is the consequence of an exaggerated decline in functional reserves of multiple systems and organs leading to the accumulation of deficits in numerous functions of an organism, which together finally translate into poor global functioning and unfavourable survival.[5,6,7,8]

Pathophysiological concepts underlying frailty in heart failure

There are mutual and bidirectional relationships between frailty and HF.[5] Multisystem dysfunction, being a central feature of frailty syndrome, is accompanied by the systemic nature of HF. Frailty and HF share several pathophysiological mechanisms and

Box 12.15.1 Shared pathophysiological mechanisms between frailty and heart failure syndromes

Skeletal dysfunction and sarcopenia (reduced muscle mass)

Concomitant reduction in fat and bone mass

Catabolic/anabolic imbalance

Deficiency in gonadal and adrenal androgens (e.g. testosterone, DHEAS)

Abnormalities in thyroid functioning

Quantitative and qualitative malnutrition

Inadequate exercise activity

Low cholesterol and low albumin levels

Deficiencies of vitamins and micronutrients (e.g. vitamin D, B12, folic acid, iron)

Electrolyte imbalance (e.g. hyponatremia)

Insulin resistance

Mitochondrial dysfunction, energy depletion, not optimal energy metabolism

Tissue hypoxia and hypoperfusion

Inflammation and inadequate immune response

Cellular apoptosis ad necrosis

Neurohormonal activation

Autonomic imbalance

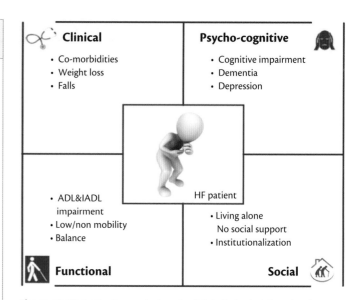

Figure 12.15.1 The four main domains (clinical, physical–functional, cognitive–psychological, and social) contributing to the Heart Failure Frailty Score (HFFS).
ADL, activities of daily living; HF, heart failure; IADL, instrumental activities of daily living.

accelerate mutually the progression of coexisting syndromes (Box 12.15.1).[5,7,8] These pathomechanisms become particularly exaggerated during haemodynamic decompensation, hence recurrent HF hospitalizations accelerate the progression of frailty and pathological process of ageing. Comorbidities prevalent in older patients with HF additionally contribute to these abnormalities.[5,7,8]

Definition of frailty in heart failure

There are two major approaches regarding the assessment of frailty: one is based on the phenotype features (e.g. the Fried phenotype model) and the other is based on the cumulative number of deficits (e.g. the deficit index Rockwood model).[5,6,7,8] According to the Fried frailty phenotype model, a decline in physiological reserves is reflected by the following phenotype features (abnormalities): weight loss, weakness, poor endurance, slowness, and low physical activity level. Pre-frailty and frailty are confirmed by the presence of 1–2 and 3–5 out of five phenotype features, respectively.[9,10] The two major limitations of this approach in the context of HF patients are a significant overlap between thephenotype features and HF symptoms,[10,] and the omission of other deficits that are common and relevant in patients with HF (e.g. comorbidities, cognitive dysfunction, social status).[11] According to the deficit index Rockwood model, frailty status is an accumulation of health deficits across multiple domains, and the deficit index uses a multidisciplinary list of variables covering information on signs, symptoms, comorbidity burden, laboratory results, and everyday activities.[9,12,13] There are some limitations of this approach in the context of HF patients: a complex and numerous list of items contributing to this index, a lack of standardization, and a lack of weighting of deficits.[9,12,13]

Currently, there is no consensus on how best to define frailty in HF.[5,6,7,8] Several frailty tools have been developed, and many of them are complex and not suitable for everyday clinical practice. Until now, none of them has been dedicated for patients with HF. Therefore, the HFA has set up an initiative to establish the definition of frailty in HF, and accordingly to derive and validate a specific diagnostic tool, the Heart Failure Frailty Score (HFFS).[14]

According to the HFA experts, in patients with HF, frailty is defined as a multidimensional dynamic state, independent of age, that makes the individual with HF more vulnerable to the effect of stressors.[14] The experts believe that a holistic approach is more reliable than the physical approach in recognizing those patients with HF who are also frail. This new diagnostic tool includes four domains – (clinical, physical–functional, cognitive–psychological, and social) – as the main determinants of frailty in HF patients (➲ Figure 12.15.1).[14] Indeed, these four domains have been identified by Gorodeski et al.[15] as the key factors affecting health outcomes in elderly patients with HF. However, Gorodeski et al.[15] include frailty as an element of the physical domain, whereas according to the HFA all four domains should be incorporated as determinants of the proposed new HF frailty score as they well reflect the holistic approach of the HFA score.

Prevalence of frailty in heart failure and clinical consequences

Frailty is prevalent in patients with HF. Its prevalence depends on the applied criteria for frailty and the character of the population under investigation. Frailty defined using the Fried frailty phenotype is reported in 20–50% of outpatients with HF.[16,17,18] Frailty is much more common in patients with HFpEF than in those with HFrEF (60–90%), which may be associated with older age and a higher number of comorbidities.[18,19] Frailty is particularly common in patients with acute HF (60–70%) and in those with advanced HF (50–65%).[20,21]

Frailty in patients with HF translates into worse functional status, poorer quality of life,[22,23] increased disability and dependence on others, along with an increased risk of recurrent CV and non-CV hospitalizations, including HF hospitalizations and high mortality.[17,19,24,25]

Management of frailty in heart failure

Frailty in patients with HF requires special attention, as frail patients are more susceptible to adverse events during the administration of life-saving therapies. On the other hand, it has been shown that advanced HF therapies, such as left ventricular assist device and heart transplantation, reduce the frailty burden in patients with severe HF.[26]

Taking into consideration the domain management approach proposed by Gorodeski et al.[15] and the frailty concept in HF, incorporating deficits in several domains,[14] it seems reasonable to implement therapies that target deficits in medical, physical function, emotion and cognition, and social environmental domains as well as to screen and treat comorbidities optimally. In particular, systemic interventions (e.g. exercise training, nutritional support, cognitive activation) are presumed to bring several benefits and improve patient-oriented outcomes in frail patients with HF. There is no doubt that skeletal dysfunction and sarcopenia contribute to the progression of frailty in patients with HF, hence it is not surprising that supervised exercise training can improve exercise capacity and quality of life in patients with HF.[27,28,29] However, these studies included limited numbers of frail subjects and did not tackle the directly functional limitations that are common in elderly subjects. Taking into consideration that malnourishment and nutritional deficiencies are common and have a multiple origin in frail patients with HF, nutritional support seems to be justified here. One may consider the general nutritional supplementation with increased caloric intake on the one hand and also more targeted therapies on the other. For example, it has been shown in a meta-analysis, that multi-nutrient and protein supplementation improve physical function in frail subjects.[30] Moreover, individualized nutritional counselling reduces mortality and HF readmission rates in malnourished patients with HF.[31]

Perspectives and conclusions

Frailty is a multidimensional, multisystem syndrome that is highly prevalent in older patients with HF and contributes to poor functional status and worse clinical outcomes. The integration of routine frailty screening into outpatient and inpatient clinical practice can identify older patients with HF and frailty, enhance risk stratification, and facilitate novel management strategies to improve outcomes and reduce the burden of frailty in this high-risk, vulnerable population. The assessment of frailty should constitute an element of routine clinical assessment in order to better describe overall clinical status and prognosis in patients with HF as well as adjust therapeutic strategies. The new Heart Failure Frailty Score specifically designed for patients with HF is under development.

A comprehensive therapeutic approach should be implemented to target deficits in the aforementioned frailty domains in frail patients with HF (e.g. multidisciplinary programmes, exercise training, nutritional support, cognitive stimulation, social support, drugs improving the function of skeletal muscles). There should be investigations in frail patients with HF of the role of exercise training, exercise-related interventions to improve functional limitations, nutritional intervention designed specifically for particular patients (e.g. high energy and protein diet for cachectic subjects, specific supplementation of vitamins, and micronutrients for specific deficiencies, such as iron deficiency, vitamin B12 deficiency) as well as interventions stimulating cognitive function, improving memory, concentration, and other mental capabilities. Particularly in frail individuals, the selection of therapeutic strategies should be designed according to the priorities discussed with patients themselves and their care givers. Interventions improving quality of life and preventing disability and dependence on others should be prioritized.

References

1. Alghamdi F, Chan M. Management of heart failure in the elderly. Curr Opin Cardiol. 2017 Mar;32(2):217–223. doi: 10.1097/HCO.0000000000000375. PMID: 28059840.

2. Osmanska J, Jhund PS. Contemporary Management of Heart Failure in the Elderly. Drugs Aging. 2019 Feb;36(2):137–146. doi: 10.1007/s40266-018-0625-4. PMID: 30535931.

3. Triposkiadis F, Giamouzis G, Parissis J, Starling RC, Boudoulas H, Skoularigis J, et al. Reframing the association and significance of co-morbidities in heart failure. Eur J Heart Fail. 2016 Jul;18(7):744–58. doi: 10.1002/ejhf.600. Epub 2016 Jun 30. PMID: 27358242.

4. Mentz RJ, Kelly JP, von Lueder TG, Voors AA, Lam CS, Cowie MR, et al. Noncardiac comorbidities in heart failure with reduced versus preserved ejection fraction. J Am Coll Cardiol. 2014 Dec 2;64(21):2281–93. doi: 10.1016/j.jacc.2014.08.036. Epub 2014 Nov 24. PMID: 25456761; PMCID: PMC4254505.

5. Pandey A, Kitzman D, Reeves G. Frailty Is Intertwined With Heart Failure: Mechanisms, Prevalence, Prognosis, Assessment, and Management. JACC Heart Fail. 2019 Dec;7(12):1001–1011. doi: 10.1016/j.jchf.2019.10.005. PMID: 31779921; PMCID: PMC7098068.

6. Uchmanowicz I, Łoboz-Rudnicka M, Szeląg P, Jankowska-Polańska B, Łoboz-Grudzień K. Frailty in heart failure. Curr Heart Fail Rep. 2014 Sep;11(3):266–73. doi: 10.1007/s11897-014-0198-4. PMID: 24733407.

7. Uchmanowicz I, Nessler J, Gobbens R, Gackowski A, Kurpas D, Straburzynska-Migaj E, et al. Coexisting Frailty With Heart Failure. Front Physiol. 2019 Jul 3;10:791. doi: 10.3389/fphys.2019.00791. PMID: 31333480; PMCID: PMC6616269.

8. Wleklik M, Uchmanowicz I, Jankowska EA, Vitale C, Lisiak M, Drozd M, et al. Multidimensional Approach to Frailty. Front Psychol. 2020 Mar 25;11:564. doi: 10.3389/fpsyg.2020.00564. PMID: 32273868; PMCID: PMC7115252.

9. Fried LP, Tangen CM, Walston J, Newman AB, Hirsch C, Gottdiener J, et al. Cardiovascular Health Study Collaborative Research Group. Frailty in older adults: evidence for a phenotype. J Gerontol A Biol Sci Med Sci. 2001 Mar;56(3):M146–56. doi: 10.1093/gerona/56.3.m146. PMID: 11253156.

10. Bandeen-Roche K, Xue QL, Ferrucci L, Walston J, Guralnik JM, Chaves P, et al. Phenotype of frailty: characterization in the women's health and aging studies. J Gerontol A Biol Sci Med Sci. 2006 Mar;61(3):262–6. doi: 10.1093/gerona/61.3.262. PMID: 16567375.

11. Dodson JA, Truong TT, Towle VR, Kerins G, Chaudhry SI. Cognitive impairment in older adults with heart failure: prevalence, documentation, and impact on outcomes. Am J Med. 2013 Feb;126(2):120–6. doi: 10.1016/j.amjmed.2012.05.029. Erratum in: Am J Med. 2013 Jun;126(6):e25. PMID: 23331439; PMCID: PMC3553506.

12. Rockwood K, Song X, MacKnight C, Bergman H, Hogan DB, McDowell I, Mitnitski A. A global clinical measure of fitness and frailty in elderly people. CMAJ. 2005 Aug 30;173(5):489–95. doi: 10.1503/cmaj.050051. PMID: 16129869; PMCID: PMC1188185.

13. Searle SD, Mitnitski A, Gahbauer EA, Gill TM, Rockwood K. A standard procedure for creating a frailty index. BMC Geriatr. 2008 Sep 30;8:24. doi: 10.1186/1471-2318-8-24. PMID: 18826625; PMCID: PMC2573877.

14. Vitale C, Jankowska E, Hill L, Piepoli M, Doehner W, Anker SD, et al. Heart Failure Association/European Society of Cardiology position paper on frailty in patients with heart failure. Eur J Heart Fail. 2019 Nov;21(11):1299–1305. doi: 10.1002/ejhf.1611. Epub 2019 Oct 23. PMID: 31646718.

15. Gorodeski EZ, Goyal P, Hummel SL, Krishnaswami A, Goodlin SJ, Hart LL, et al. Geriatric Cardiology Section Leadership Council, American College of Cardiology. Domain Management Approach to Heart Failure in the Geriatric Patient: Present and Future. J Am Coll Cardiol. 2018 May 1;71(17):1921–1936. doi: 10.1016/j.jacc.2018.02.059. PMID: 29699619; PMCID: PMC7304050.

16. McDonagh J, Martin L, Ferguson C, Jha SR, Macdonald PS, Davidson PM, Newton PJ. Frailty assessment instruments in heart failure: A systematic review. Eur J Cardiovasc Nurs. 2018 Jan;17(1):23–35. doi: 10.1177/1474515117708888. Epub 2017 May 4. PMID: 28471241.

17. Yang X, Lupón J, Vidán MT, Ferguson C, Gastelurrutia P, Newton PJ, et al. Impact of Frailty on Mortality and Hospitalization in Chronic Heart Failure: A Systematic Review and Meta-Analysis. J Am Heart Assoc. 2018 Dec 4;7(23):e008251. doi: 10.1161/JAHA.117.008251. PMID: 30571603; PMCID: PMC6405567.

18. Sze S, Pellicori P, Zhang J, Weston J, Clark AL. Identification of Frailty in Chronic Heart Failure. JACC Heart Fail. 2019 Apr;7(4):291–302. doi: 10.1016/j.jchf.2018.11.017. Epub 2019 Feb 6. PMID: 30738977.

19. Sanders NA, Supiano MA, Lewis EF, Liu J, Claggett B, Pfeffer MA, et al. The frailty syndrome and outcomes in the TOPCAT trial. Eur J Heart Fail. 2018 Nov;20(11):1570–1577. doi: 10.1002/ejhf.1308. Epub 2018 Sep 18. PMID: 30225878.

20. Madan SA, Fida N, Barman P, Sims D, Shin J, Verghese J, et al. Frailty Assessment in Advanced Heart Failure. J Card Fail. 2016 Oct;22(10):840–4. doi: 10.1016/j.cardfail.2016.02.003. Epub 2016 Feb 13. PMID: 26883168.

21. Joyce E. Frailty in Advanced Heart Failure. Heart Fail Clin. 2016 Jul;12(3):363–74. doi: 10.1016/j.hfc.2016.03.006. PMID: 27371513.

22. Denfeld QE, Winters-Stone K, Mudd JO, Hiatt SO, Lee CS. Identifying a Relationship Between Physical Frailty and Heart Failure Symptoms. J Cardiovasc Nurs. 2018 Jan/Feb;33(1):E1–E7. doi: 10.1097/JCN.0000000000000408. PMID: 28353543; PMCID: PMC5617768.

23. Denfeld QE, Winters-Stone K, Mudd JO, Gelow JM, Kurdi S, Lee CS. The prevalence of frailty in heart failure: A systematic review and meta-analysis. Int J Cardiol. 2017 Jun 1;236:283–289. doi: 10.1016/j.ijcard.2017.01.153. Epub 2017 Feb 10. PMID: 28215466; PMCID: PMC5392144.

24. Volpato S, Cavalieri M, Guerra G, Sioulis F, Ranzini M, Maraldi C, et al. Performance-based functional assessment in older hospitalized patients: feasibility and clinical correlates. J Gerontol A Biol Sci Med Sci. 2008 Dec;63(12):1393–8. doi: 10.1093/gerona/63.12.1393. PMID: 19126854; PMCID: PMC6138871.

25. Vidán MT, Blaya-Novakova V, Sánchez E, Ortiz J, Serra-Rexach JA, Bueno H. Prevalence and prognostic impact of frailty and its components in non-dependent elderly patients with heart failure. Eur J Heart Fail. 2016 Jul;18(7):869–75. doi: 10.1002/ejhf.518. Epub 2016 Apr 12. PMID: 27072307.

26. Maurer MS, Horn E, Reyentovich A, Dickson VV, Pinney S, Goldwater D, et al. Can a Left Ventricular Assist Device in Individuals with Advanced Systolic Heart Failure Improve or Reverse Frailty? J Am Geriatr Soc. 2017 Nov;65(11):2383–2390. doi: 10.1111/jgs.15124. Epub 2017 Sep 21. PMID: 28940248; PMCID: PMC5681378.

27. Flynn KE, Piña IL, Whellan DJ, Lin L, Blumenthal JA, Ellis SJ, et al; HF-ACTION Investigators. Effects of exercise training on health status in patients with chronic heart failure: HF-ACTION randomized controlled trial. JAMA. 2009 Apr 8;301(14):1451–9. doi: 10.1001/jama.2009.457. Erratum in: JAMA. 2009 Dec 2;302(21):2322. PMID: 19351942; PMCID: PMC2690699.

28. O'Connor CM, Whellan DJ, Lee KL, Keteyian SJ, Cooper LS, Ellis SJ, et al.; HF-ACTION Investigators. Efficacy and safety of exercise training in patients with chronic heart failure: HF-ACTION randomized controlled trial. JAMA. 2009 Apr 8;301(14):1439–50. doi: 10.1001/jama.2009.454. PMID: 19351941; PMCID: PMC2916661.

29. Pandey A, Parashar A, Kumbhani D, Agarwal S, Garg J, Kitzman D, et al. Exercise training in patients with heart failure and preserved ejection fraction: meta-analysis of randomized control trials. Circ Heart Fail. 2015 Jan;8(1):33–40. doi: 10.1161/CIRCHEARTFAILURE.114.001615. Epub 2014 Nov 16. PMID: 25399909; PMCID: PMC4792111.

30. Veronese N, Stubbs B, Punzi L, Soysal P, Incalzi RA, Saller A, Maggi S. Effect of nutritional supplementations on physical performance and muscle strength parameters in older people: A systematic review and meta-analysis. Ageing Res Rev. 2019 May;51:48–54. doi: 10.1016/j.arr.2019.02.005. Epub 2019 Feb 28. PMID: 30826500.

31. Bonilla-Palomas JL, Gámez-López AL, Castillo-Domínguez JC, Moreno-Conde M, López Ibáñez MC, Alhambra Expósito R, et al. Nutritional Intervention in Malnourished Hospitalized Patients with Heart Failure. Arch Med Res. 2016 Oct;47(7):535–540. doi: 10.1016/j.arcmed.2016.11.005. PMID: 28262195.

SECTION 13

Self-care and patient education

CHAPTER 13.1

Self-care and patient education

Tiny Jaarsma, Loreena Hill,
Ekaterini Lambrinou, Anna Strömberg,
and Tina Hansen

Contents

Introduction

The successful delivery of modern health care requires the active involvement of patients and caregivers. Heart failure (HF) management programmes emphasize the role of self-care to improve patient outcomes and prevent HF deterioration and exacerbations. Effective communication and information by the multidisciplinary team across all care settings promote involvement. When there is a greater emphasis on self-care, the ability to participate in daily tasks requires knowledge as well as interpretation, skills, and action. Patient education and self-care support is the responsibility of all health-care providers taking care of patients with HF, and within the HF team the roles and responsibilities should be clearly defined. There are several approaches to education of patients and caregivers. This chapter discusses these approaches and presents some resources that can be used in education of patients and their family members or other informal caregivers.

Self-care in patients with heart failure

Self-care is essential in the long-term management of HF. Self-care is defined as the process of maintaining health through health-promoting practices and managing illness and is performed in both healthy and ill states.[1] Self-care is an overarching concept based on three key concepts: self-care maintenance, self-care monitoring, and self-care management (➲ Figure 13.1.1).[2]

- Self-care maintenance includes behaviours used by patients to preserve health, to maintain physical and emotional stability, or to improve well-being. These may be health-promoting behaviours (e.g. smoking cessation, preparing healthy food, physical activity, coping with stress) or illness-related behaviours (e.g. taking medication as prescribed).

- Self-care monitoring is the process of observing oneself for changes in signs and symptoms, for example by checking body weight, or monitoring symptoms or heart rate. The goal of self-care monitoring is recognition that a change has occurred. The monitoring of symptoms is effective when the person or an informal caregiver is able to both recognize and interpret the sign or symptom. In other words, only checking for changes in symptoms or signs without interpreting the meaning or significance of the change is not sufficient.

- Self-care management is the response to occurring signs and symptoms. Self-care management involves an evaluation of changes in physical and emotional signs and symptoms to determine if action is needed. These changes may be due to illness, treatment, or the environment (e.g. changing diuretic dose in response to symptoms).

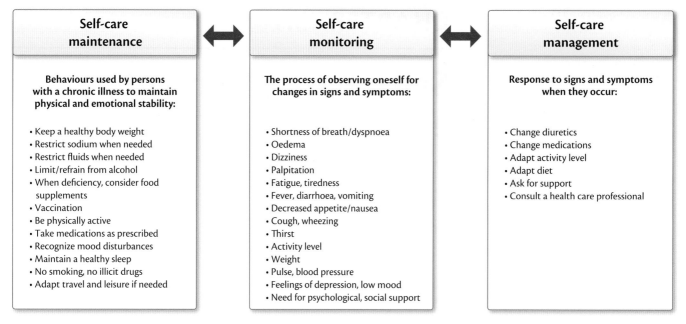

Figure 13.1.1 Patient self-maintenance, monitoring and management.

For patients with HF, it might be necessary to regulate and adapt self-care during the course of the disease, for example in times of deterioration, if comorbidities occur, or in case of specific advanced treatment. Self-care is found to be important in influencing outcomes in patients with HF; those who report more effective self-care have a better quality of life, and lower mortality and hospital readmission compared to those who report poor self-care.[3] Education and support are essential to enhance self-care behaviour that aims to improve HF-related outcomes.[4,5]

Having support from a family member or informal carer is very important for patients with HF. Family caregivers have been found to be crucial for supporting and improving patient self-care. On the other hand, there is an increasing awareness that caregiving could affect the caregiver's health negatively and cause a physical and financial burden as well as psychosocial distress.[6]

Education on self-care for patients and their caregivers

Recent guidelines and position papers recommend that all health-care professionals within the patient's multidisciplinary team should have a role in the education of patients and their caregivers as part of their vital remit in care provision.[3,7,8] For many health-care professionals, patient education relates to verbal dialogue, perhaps with information repeated on a number of occasions or reinforced by a written booklet or handout. However, this may not always ensure adequate comprehension and understanding. It is often assumed that patients and family members, when provided with the necessary knowledge, are motivated to become actively involved and improve their self-care behaviour, including adherence with pharmacological and non-pharmacological treatment.[9] This may work in the initial days after discharge, but for continued adherence supportive interventions can ensure patients

and informal caregivers continue to remain engaged. Indeed, studies that evaluated patient discharge education when combined with a support programme, have found positive benefits. A meta-analysis noted that comprehensive discharge planning (including one-on-one teaching sessions, discharge protocols, and home care coordination) combined with post-discharge support resulted in a 25% relative reduction in hospital readmissions over 3–12 months after discharge.[10]

Additional strategies have been implemented to complement the information provided by professionals.

Health literacy can be defined as 'the degree to which individuals have the capacity to obtain, process, and understand basic health information and services needed to make appropriate health decisions'.[11] A recent systematic review stated that the level of health literacy was found to be low in patients with HF. Further inadequate health literacy has been found to be associated with lower quality of life and survival and higher health-care utilization.[12]

New approaches and techniques need to be considered and tools and resources need to be tailored to the patient and caregivers. Successful improvement of the level of health literacy in chronic conditions may be achieved with a combination of several strategies, and structured education and information contributing to shared decision making.[13]

A recent scientific statement from American Heart Association highlighted that there have only been a handful of intervention trials evaluating support to caregivers. The studies included a large majority of female family caregivers and the educational intervention and skill training were mainly delivered face-to-face.[6]

Techniques and approaches

One technique, for example 'Teach-back', is recognized as a best practice strategy[14] to improve disease-specific knowledge, and understanding, treatment adherence and self-efficacy leading to reduced hospital readmissions.[15,16] Consultations whereby information is provided to the patient and informal caregiver should employ such a technique. Existing literature indicates that the most important time to provide HF patients with relevant information and ensure understanding is pre-discharge.[17]

A successful approach to elicit behaviour change is that of motivational interviewing.[18] Defined as 'a person-centred counselling style for addressing the common problem of ambivalence about change', its benefit in comparison to informational sessions within HF management is becoming increasingly well evidenced.[19] For self-care interventions to be effective, there must be a supportive relationship with the professional, an individualized approach, efforts to promote self-efficacy, practical information, and ongoing support from informal caregivers.[20] Unsurprisingly, the incorporation of motivational interviewing within a randomized control trial to improve self-care management, found positive results particularly regarding the inclusion of caregivers to improve patients' self-care management.[19] In a systematic review published in 2020, eight randomized control trials involving 758 patients, found motivational interviewing was better than simple advice-giving. This systematic review concluded that these interventions had the potential to improve the immediate risk of hospital readmission as well as long-term outcomes through better medication adherence and self-care behaviours.

It is important both the patient and caregiver feel they can initiate questions during consultations. The 'ASK ME 3' (http://www.ihi.org/resources/Pages/Tools/Ask-Me-3-Good-Questions-for-Your-Good-Health.aspx) is an online educational programme to encourage patients to ask questions about their condition to promote healthy lifestyle. Driven by patient autonomy, the education of patients and informal caregivers will promote shared health-care decision-making, alongside an agreed management plan, which will have greater likelihood of success.

Tools and resources

Patients might prefer a multi-model style of learning including e-health,[21] ranging from more 'basic/traditional' material to more innovative ones. Resources include hard copy education with printed education materials (brochures, flyers, leaflets), teaching sessions, telemedicine, and digital health (websites and video education) telephone interventions, interactive voice response reminder systems, gaming, and computer-aided learning application.[21,22]

Brochures, flyers, and leaflets

Printed education materials, consisting mostly of booklets, allow patients to have easy access to information over time.[4] Using printed material with verbal instructions, either personally or in groups, can enhance self-care behaviours.

Websites and video education

The internet has become a powerful, accessible resource for many patients to use for their own medical management and comprehension.[8] It is also a practical method as patients can replay the videos whenever they desire or go back to read the information again.[18] The Heart Failure Matters website (www.heartfailurematters.org) provides practical information from diagnosis, medications, lifestyle recommendations to palliative care, that patients and informal caregivers can readily access. It has a number of communication prompts and tools to enable patients to ask questions on topics they are uncertain about.

Adding images related to the words can contribute to involvement of the learner's mind and his/her active learning. Video education may enhance retention of health information. The visual absorption of information increases patients' confidence by showing actual persons living with HF, modelling healthy behaviours and, at the same time, demonstrating that healthy behaviours are achievable. Using visual role modelling to demonstrate self-care behaviours seems to stimulate learning and health literacy and to improve clinical outcomes in chronic diseases including heart failure.[23]

Internet access has opened up a plethora of resources to use as education materials, but the writing style and language of most medically relevant articles favour a small percentage of the general public and, at the same time, not all e-health materials have been assessed for the quality of the information provided (e.g. DISCERN and CUA quality rating tool).[24,25]

Gaming

Historical strategies to educating patients is moving from a written or verbal format to a more digital format, facilitated by smartphones, apps, and innovative software.[26] With the current advances in technology, more innovative ways are possible to educate and develop patients' skills to enable successful self-care behaviour. Studies are using artificial intelligence to engage the patient to learn through 'gaming' or provision of information through avatar type interactions.[27]

Other technologies used in self-care education

Technology that can support HF self-care range from invasive devices that monitor lung impedance and pulmonary artery pressure to mobile applications that track HF symptoms, blood pressure, heart rate and rhythm, and adherence to medications. The digital solutions rarely target support to caregivers in their role and life situation, despite the impact they have on a daily basis to support self-care so this is an area in need of further development.

Special considerations

Special attention is warranted in particular to those patients showing poor adherence to medical therapy or unpredictable self-care pattern.[28,29] This may indicate some degree of cognitive impairment, with older patients with more severe HF found to have poorer executive functioning. In addition, the more severe the HF, it was associated with poorer total recall memory, poorer visuospatial recall ability, psychomotor slowing, and poorer executive function.[30] The provision of information and re-checking comprehension may not be sufficient if the patient is aware of what he/she needs to undertake but is physically, socially, or psychologically challenged to do so.

With advanced technology, many professionals become caught up in the jargon, using complex terminology to explain pending investigations or technology. During the Covid pandemic, as we have learnt how to use digital technology more effectively within the clinical environment, such technology may be simply extended to provide a visual overview of, for example, the catheterization room or the device clinic. This reinforces the importance of learning not just through words but images, pictures, and real-life scenarios. Once again the valuable role of family members and informal caregivers cannot be underestimated and should be included, as much as possible, in information-giving sessions.[31]

When using technology, consideration of patients' perceived electronic health (eHealth) literacy skills or digital health literacy skills is crucial for improving the delivery of health information, and instruments to assess eHealth literacy scale can be used.[32]

Future directions

Adequate patient self-care is essential in the effective management of HF. Patient education allows patients to understand what is beneficial and to help to make decisions about their self-care jointly with their health-care professionals. Education to improve self-care should be tailored to the individual patient and based on, where available, scientific evidence or expert opinion. A personalized and tailored approach to self-care support is needed. This includes using a range of teaching and educational techniques and optimal use of communication skills and where relevant technological support and tools. Training in communication skills should be structurally integrated in education of health-care professionals and educational seminars.

Summary and key messages

Optimal self-care improves patient outcomes and can prevent deterioration and exacerbations. With a greater emphasis on self-care, the ability to participate in daily life requires knowledge as well as interpretation, skills, and action. New patient teaching strategies are needed to support the development of tactical and situational skills, foster coherence, and use trusted resources. As HF management programmes develop, including coaching interventions that target skill-building tactics, such as role-playing in specific situations, may be one option.[33] Gone are the days when education relies on verbal and written information alone. Patients with HF as well as their caregivers require tailored information that is delivered in a format and engaging way that they can understand and which will lead to positive behaviour changes.

References

1. Riegel, B., T. Jaarsma, and A. Stromberg. A middle-range theory of self-care of chronic illness. ANS Adv Nurs Sci, 2012. 35(3): 194–204.
2. Riegel, B., et al. Integrating symptoms into the middle-range theory of self-care of chronic illness. ANS Adv Nurs Sci, 2019;42(3):206–15.
3. Jaarsma, T., et al. Self-care of heart failure patients: practical management recommendations from the Heart Failure Association of the European Society of Cardiology. Eur J Heart Fail, 2021;23(1):157–74.
4. Veroff, D.R., et al. Improving self-care for heart failure for seniors: the impact of video and written education and decision aids. Popul Health Manag, 2012. 15(1): 37–45.
5. McDonagh, T.A., et al. 2021 ESC Guidelines for the diagnosis and treatment of acute and chronic heart failure. Eur Heart J, 2021. 42(36): 3599–726.
6. Kitko, L., et al. Family caregiving for individuals with heart failure: a scientific statement from the American Heart Association. Circulation, 2020. 141(22): e864–e878.
7. Rasmusson, K., M. Flattery, and L.S. Baas. American Association of Heart Failure Nurses position paper on educating patients with heart failure. Heart Lung, 2015. 44(2): 173–7.
8. Ponikowski, P., et al. 2016 ESC guidelines for the diagnosis and treatment of acute and chronic heart failure. The task force for the diagnosis and treatment of acute and chronic heart failure of the European Society of Cardiology. 2016. 37(27):2129–200.
9. Strömberg, A. The crucial role of patient education in heart failure. Eur J Heart Fail, 2005. 7(3):363–9.
10. Phillips, C.O., et al. Comprehensive discharge planning with postdischarge support for older patients with congestive heart failure: a meta-analysis. JAMA, 2004. 291(11): 1358–67.
11. Nielsen-Bohlman L, Panzer AM, Kindig, DA. Health Literacy: A Prescription to End Confusion. 2004, Washington, DC: The National Academies Press.
12. Fabbri, M., et al. Health literacy and outcomes among patients with heart failure: a systematic review and meta-analysis. JACC Heart Fail, 2020. 8(6):451–60.
13. Kher, A., S. Johnson, and R. Griffith. Readability assessment of online patient education material on congestive heart failure. Adv Prev Med, 2017. 2017: 9780317.
14. Anderson, K.M., S. Leister, and R. De Rego. The 5Ts for teach back: an operational definition for teach-back training. Health Lit Res Pract, 2020. 4(2): e94–103.
15. Ha Dinh, T.T., et al. The effectiveness of the teach-back method on adherence and self-management in health education for people with chronic disease: a systematic review. JBI Database System Rev Implement Rep, 2016. 14(1): p. 210–47.
16. Peter, D., et al. Reducing readmissions using teach-back: enhancing patient and family education. J Nurs Adm, 2015. 45(1): 35–42.
17. Mebazaa, A., et al. Recommendations on pre-hospital & early hospital management of acute heart failure: a consensus paper from the Heart Failure Association of the European Society of Cardiology, the European Society of Emergency Medicine and the Society of Academic Emergency Medicine. Eur J Heart Fail, 2015. 17(6): 544–58.
18. Miller W, R.S. Motivational interviewing: helping people change 3rd Edition ed. 2013, New York: Guilford Press.
19. Vellone, E., et al. Motivational interviewing to improve self-care in heart failure patients (MOTIVATE-HF): a randomized controlled trial. ESC Heart Fail, 2020. 7(3):1309–18.
20. Clark, A.M., et al. A systematic review of the main mechanisms of heart failure disease management interventions Heart, 2016. 9:707–711.
21. Boyde, M. and R. Peters. Education material for heart failure patients: what works and what does not? Curr Heart Fail Rep, 2014. 11(3):314–20.
22. Austin, L.S., C.O. Landis, and K.H. Hanger, Jr. Extending the continuum of care in congestive heart failure: an interactive technology self-management solution. J Nurs Adm, 2012. 42(9):442–6.
23. Reid, K.R.Y., et al. Using video education to improve outcomes in heart failure. Heart Lung, 2019. 48(5): 386–94.

24. Cajita, M.I., et al. Quality and health literacy demand of online heart failure information. J Cardiovasc Nurs, 2017. 32(2):156–64.

25. Klompstra, L., et al. A clinical tool (CUE-tool) for health care professionals to assess the usability and quality of the content of medical information websites: Electronic Delphi Study. J Med Internet Res, 2021. 23(2):e22668.

26. Topol, E.J., S.R. Steinhubl, and A. Torkamani. Digital medical tools and sensors. JAMA, 2015. 313(4): 353–4.

27. Barrett, M., et al. Artificial intelligence supported patient self-care in chronic heart failure: a paradigm shift from reactive to predictive, preventive and personalised care. EPMA J, 2019. 10(4):445–64.

28. Hawkins, L.A., et al. Cognitive impairment and medication adherence in outpatients with heart failure. Heart & Lung, 2012. 41(6): 572–82.

29. Davis, K.K., et al. Targeted intervention improves knowledge but not self-care or readmissions in heart failure patients with mild cognitive impairment. . Eur J Heart Fail, 2012. 14(9):1041–9.

30. Pressler, S.J., et al. Cognitive deficits in chronic heart failure. Nurs Res, 2010. 59(2):127–39.

31. Doherty, L.C., D. Fitzsimons, and S.J. McIlfatrick. Carers' needs in advanced heart failure: A systematic narrative review. Eur J Cardiovasc Nurs, 2016. 15(4):03–12.

32. Lin, C.Y., et al. Psychometric Evaluation of the Persian eHealth Literacy Scale (eHEALS) among elder Iranians with heart failure. Eval Health Prof, 2020. 43(4): 222–9.

33. Dickson, V.V. and B. Riegel. Are we teaching what patients need to know? Building skills in heart failure self-care. Heart Lung, 2009. 38(3): 253–61.

SECTION 14

Multidisciplinary approach to heart failure management

CHAPTER 14.1

Multidisciplinary approach to heart failure management

Loreena Hill, Friedrich Koehler, Tiny Jaarsma, Marija Polovina, Katherine McCreary, and Andrew JS Coats

Contents

Rationale and introduction

Evidence over the last three decades has shown that a collaborative team approach involving interdisciplinary healthcare professionals can improve the outcome of patients with heart failure (HF), as well as reduce healthcare costs.[1-3] This involves contribution from a HF specialist, be that cardiologist or physician, as well as a HF nurse, general practitioner and an allied professional, such as a pharmacist, physiotherapist, or psychologist. Management of the patient, from diagnosis to death, should be coordinated and documented in a management plan that can be initiated within primary care or the acute hospital setting. The predominant purpose of the multidisciplinary disease team (MDT) approach is to ensure patients undergo appropriate investigations, receive an accurate diagnosis, and are guided through the initiation and titration of evidence-based medications, tailored education, and follow-up, all depending on individual needs.[4] The emphasis is on a seamless patient-centred approach and care planning, from diagnosis to death.[5]

For many years the precise benefits of an MDT management programme remained debated, accounting for the diversity in roles and delivery (i.e. setting) of different programmes. Some studies reported no or limited benefits on primary endpoints, such as reduced hospital admissions or mortality in ambulatory patients with HF.[6] However, other studies reported benefits in terms of improved quality of life and medication compliance,[7,8] reflecting the possible impact of the diverse nature of different MDT programmes. An individual patient data meta-analysis of 20 studies, including 5624 patients, concluded that self-management interventions in HF patients improved outcomes despite heterogeneity in the intensity, content, and personnel who delivered the intervention.[9] The American study by Rich et al.[3] randomized 156 patients to receive patient education on diet and available social services, a medication review, and an intense follow-up post-discharge versus usual care. The intervention was delivered by a variety of professionals, including a nurse, dietician, physician, and social services representative. The results showed that this MDT strategy was associated with improved medication compliance during the first 30 days ($p = 0.003$). Within the UK, a home-based MDT intervention was designed by Stewart et al.[7] and delivered to patients (n = 200) discharged after an acute hospital admission. The intervention composed of remedial counselling, advice to improve treatment adherence, a simple exercise regimen, symptom monitoring, such as weighing and titration of diuretic, and beta-blocker therapy. The intervention was facilitated by a nurse, physician, and cardiologist. Results from this randomized control trial (RCT) reported a 40% reduction in unplanned readmissions ($p = 0.03$) at 6 months, with reduced days in hospital ($p = 0.02$) and a trend towards improved survival ($p = 0.098$).

It is evident across many countries that there is considerable diversity in the delivery of MDT for HF care. Recent evidence from the Heart Failure Association (HFA) Atlas project found that the diagnosis and management of patients varied according to resource allocation, depending importantly on whether the country is a high-income European Society of Cardiology (ESC) member country or a middle-income country. Furthermore, the median number of hospitals with dedicated HF centres was 1.16 per million people, ranging from < 0.10 in the Russian Federation and Ukraine to >7 in Norway and Italy.[10] As a result, depending on resources and healthcare setting, the ability to request initial investigations, including blood tests (B-type natriuretic peptide (BNP)), echocardiogram, and electrocardiogram may differ between MDT programmes. Additional investigations may be warranted to determine the aetiology of the HF diagnosis, these being mainly carried out within a hospital or advanced HF setting.

In 2017, van Spall et al.[11] published a meta-analysis of 53 RCTs and concluded that both nurse home-visits and disease management clinics for HF reduced all-cause mortality compared to usual care, with nurse home-visits being the most effective. This was supported by a Cochrane review in 2020,[12] which reported on 47 RCTs and found that case management MDT interventions potentially reduced all-cause mortality and readmissions, unlike clinic-based interventions. As many services are transitioning into the community, due to the intense demand for hospital beds, what should the components of a 21st century MDT approach look like?

A multidisciplinary approach to HF diagnosis and management has been endorsed by many professional organizations, including the HFA of the ESC. The HFA has proposed to enhance development and implementation of the MDT approach into existing healthcare systems of the HFA-accredited Quality of Care Centres. This will provide a platform for standardizing and coordinating multidisciplinary management of HF across all levels of care (community, specialized, and advanced).[13]

Current models in practice

Professional clinical guidelines for HF recommend a multidisciplinary HF management programme throughout the HF trajectory; from onset, through critical events, periods of apparent stability, and its terminal stages.[1,4,14] Conceptually, disease management should include key elements, such as a coordinated system of care, delivery system support, support for patient

---

Box 14.1.1 Core characteristics of a MDT HF programme

- Patient or person-centred approach.
- Employs a multidisciplinary team of medical, nursing, and allied professionals.
- Targets high-risk symptomatic patients and has a proactive approach towards prevention.
- Competent and professionally educated staff.
- Patient and carer engagement in the condition and its management.

---

self-care, identification of at-risk populations, continual feedback loop between patient and care provider, measures of clinical and other outcomes, and the goal of improving overall health.[14] Different parts are not designated to one or two members of the MDT team, but rather it is the responsibility of each member to ensure the patient has a clear plan of management. Nevertheless, HF management programmes continue to vary significantly, with different service models, including a clinic-based approach (in primary, secondary, or tertiary care), a home-based programme, case management, or a hybrid of these. Components and services within each model may also differ, for example some primary care services incorporate tele-monitoring. Importantly, no service model has been shown to be consistently superior to others.[11]

Characteristics and components of a heart failure management programme

Clinical trials have included complex, bundled interventions, making it difficult to determine the efficiency and effectiveness of each specific component. Despite this we can summarize the following characteristics (➲ Box 14.1.1) and components (➲ Box 14.1.2) as being commonly recommended.

Box 14.1.2 Components of an effective multidisciplinary programme

- Optimized medical and device treatment.
- Adequate patient education, with emphasis on self-care including patient involvement in symptom monitoring (see also ➲ Chapter 13.1).
- Provision of psychosocial support to patients and family caregivers.
- Follow-up after discharge (regular clinic and/or home-based visits; possibly telephone support or telemonitoring).
- Easy access to health care (in-person or telephone contact) and facilitated access to care during episodes of decompensation.
- Assessment of (and appropriate intervention in response to) an unexplained change in weight, nutritional status, functional status, quality of life, sleep problems, psychosocial problems, or other findings (e.g. laboratory values).
- Access to advanced treatment options and palliative care.

Team members

The differing inputs from HF practitioners and healthcare experts within the allied professions varies with the nature and complexity of healthcare organization, patient diagnosis, and condition, and locally available resources. For example, the patient with HF with reduced ejection fraction (HFrEF) requires intensive medication review, while the patient with HF with preserved ejection fraction (HFpEF) may benefit more from management of causative factors of his/her comorbidities (e.g. weight, diet). Allied professionals active within the HF MDT include pharmacists, dieticians, physiotherapists, psychologists, primary care providers, occupational therapists, and social workers. They work collaboratively within the team to achieve the patient's holistic needs.[15,16] This list is not comprehensive and team members may vary according to the needs of the specific patient (➲ Figure 14.1.1). In Anglo-Saxon and Scandinavian countries, a HF-nurse frequently cares for the out-patient follow-up of HF-patients. In contrast, in countries in Central and Eastern Europe as well as Mediterranean countries a general practitioner-based healthcare system is more common. Essentially, it is not a matter of who provides the best care for HF patients, but rather how patients can best receive integrated care. Each healthcare professional should collaborate with each other to ensure person-centred care that fits the individual patient's situation, as well as each local healthcare system. A clear description of roles and responsibilities, alongside due emphasis on good communication is warranted to ensure avoidance of fragmented care.[17]

In ➲ Figure 14.1.2a, a model with the HF clinic in the centre is depicted, a model that is often used to describe the coordinating role of a HF service. However, a more patient-centred approach is suggested, in which patients and their caregivers are the foci and important part of the team.

Each member of the MDT makes a valued contribution towards improving the quality of life for patients with HF and their family members throughout the disease trajectory. The coordination of care requires an interlocuter who, as shown in ➲ Figure 14.1.2b, may be the case manager or HF nurse. This role would be to ensure that the patient receives the essential components of the MDT intervention, identifying and negotiating any barriers to care delivery.

The characteristics and components of the MDT intervention should be evident, irrespective of its delivery setting. Nevertheless, at certain points of the illness trajectory certain components of the MDT intervention take precedence over others. The following will discuss the role of the MDT in three scenarios: community setting, during hospitalization, and post-discharge management.

Delivery of the MDT within a community setting (diagnosis)

The diagnosis of HF is established on the basis of current or prior symptoms or signs of HF (dyspnoea, exercise intolerance, evidence of fluid overload) and objective evidence of cardiac dysfunction, as the cause of symptoms.[1] There is no single test for HF, and the diagnosis relies on the clinical judgement of the specialist. There is a paucity of data about the characteristics of patients with symptoms of HF living in the community, but available reports suggest that they tend to be older and have a high burden of comorbidities and frailty at the time of presentation.[18–20] The diagnosis of HF may be missed in those patients, especially if presenting with atypical symptoms and/or without signs of fluid overload, which may have serious prognostic implications.[21]

Although the organization of healthcare services varies across different countries, community-based healthcare professionals (general practitioners, family physicians, primary care specialists, geriatricians, and allied professionals) can play an important part in the diagnosis and management of patients suspected of having HF. Community-based physicians should proactively search for signs and symptoms suggestive of HF, particularly among individuals with multiple risk factors or a history of cardiovascular disease, and perform essential diagnostic work-up using electrocardiography, chest radiography, laboratory assessment, and natriuretic peptide testing, if available.[1] Through collaboration with a specialist services, patients with abnormal findings can be rapidly referred for an echocardiographic examination and

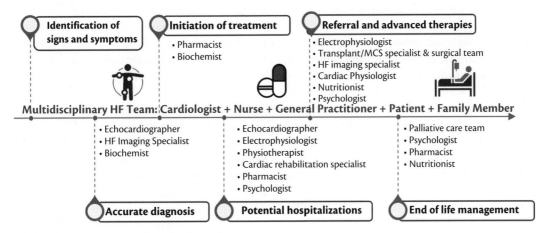

Figure 14.1.1 Multidisciplinary HF team: coordinated and complimentary care.
This is not an exclusive list of allied professionals, but dependent on patient need and available resources.

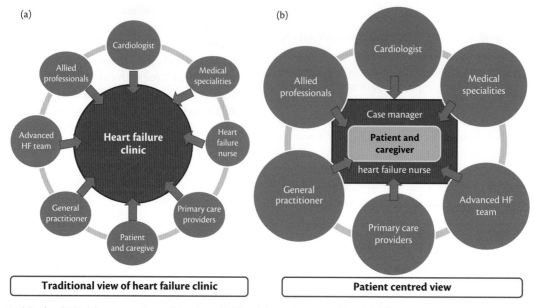

Figure 14.1.2   Models of multidisciplinary care: the traditional model (a) and the patient-centred model (b).
Source data from Annema C, Luttik ML, Jaarsma T. Reasons for readmission in heart failure: Perspectives of patients, caregivers, cardiologists, and heart failure nurses. *Heart Lung.* 2009 Sep-Oct;38(5):427–34. doi: 10.1016/j.hrtlng.2008.12.002.

a HF specialist review, to confirm the diagnosis, provide aetiological assessment, and initiate pharmaceutical therapies in accordance with current HF guidelines. The utility of a collaborative community-based assessment coupled with BNP testing as a strategy for an early identification and treatment of individuals at high risk of developing HF (n = 1374) was evaluated in the STOP-HF trial.[22] Participants were randomly assigned to a BNP-guided cooperative management between a general practitioner and a cardiologist or alternatively to a control group whereby they received routine care. In the intervention group, patients with a BNP level ≥ 50 pg/mL were referred for echocardiography and a review by a cardiologist, who developed a future management plan. The study reported a significant reduction in the primary endpoint of left ventricular dysfunction with or without HF in the intervention group (odds ratio, 0.55; 95% confidence interval, 0.37–0.82; p = 0.003), likely due to a facilitated introduction of disease-modifying therapies (i.e. angiotensin-converting enzyme inhibitors) and a greater utilization of diagnostic procedures.

Patient follow-up should also be coordinated between community-based practitioners and secondary or tertiary level specialists, to ensure treatment optimization and adherence, monitoring of HF decompensation or symptom deterioration, and provision of protocols for a timely referral to higher levels of care. As the number of patients with HF increases and healthcare resources come under increasing strain, there is an increasing focus on incorporating new ways of working by the team to manage this complex group of patients.

Telemedicine/virtual outreach

Telemedicine represents one facet of electronic health (e-Health) in cardiology. The underlying clinical evidence for, and the clinical feasibility of, telemedicine for the care of patients suffering

cardiovascular disorders are well understood within the HF world. Three landmark studies (IN-TIME, CHAMPION, TIM-HF2) have found superiority in terms of mortality and morbidity in patients with remote patient management in contrast to patients without telemedicine.[23–25] Thus it represents an innovative supplement to the 'traditional' care given in out-patient clinics and hospitals with direct face-to-face contact. In telemedicine home measurement devices can be used for daily transfer of vital parameters from the patient's home to the HF-professionals, to provide daily indirect contact between patients and their MDT.

Telemedicine for HF is currently in a transition from clinical trial settings into real-world clinical practice. In contrast to drugs or medical devices, which directly influence the pathogenesis of HF, telemedicine represents an element within a comprehensive MD care programme. Healthcare systems therefore play a fundamental role in the implementation of telemedicine into routine practice. Depending on the model of MDT care provision telemedical supervision for HF patients may be also provided directly by the GP, resulting in different professional groups using the same technology. While HF-nurses (tele-)monitor patients themselves, most GPs only care for one or two HF-patients eligible for HF telemonitoring. Therefore, large telemedical centres (TMC) have been established, especially in GP-based healthcare systems, to provide telemedical services for entire regions (e.g. an area with four million inhabitants).

A regional TMC is usually situated in a third level HF-centre and is staffed with HF-specialists and HF-nurses, who review incoming vital parameters of 500–1000 HF-patients. If any transferred vital parameters fall below pre-specified thresholds, the TMC will contact the patient's GP to modify therapy as needed. In the case of an emergency, the TMC staff can admit the patient to the next available emergency room. Some TMCs even provide a 24/7 service, which can play a vital role in the telemonitoring of patients with left ventricular assist devices (LVAD).[26]

Novel technologies utilizing artificial intelligence within TMCs, such as decision support systems are under investigation to increase the capacities of an individual TMC.[27] This would resolve the issue of upscaling, which appears to be the predominant issue when trying to transfer randomized controlled trial settings into HF-care daily practices.

In addition to the technological hurdles of remotely monitoring large cohorts of HF-patients, the reimbursement of tele-monitoring in HF-patients is a relevant concern. For example, in December 2020 a new regulation was passed in Germany, regarding the reimbursement of tele-monitoring for HF-patients with reduced ejection fraction, < 40%.[28] This new regulation allows primary care physicians (GP and/or cardiologist) to decide whether a HF-patient requires a 24/7 tele-monitoring or whether tele-monitoring during office hours would suffice. Such regulations help in the acceptance and implementation of tele-medical services, which are vital in improving patient's prognosis and quality of life.

During hospitalization (implantable devices/surgical interventions)

Over a 20-year period (1998–2019), the age-adjusted rates of first hospitalization within the UK increased by 28% for both all-cause and HF admissions, and by 42% for non-cardiovascular admissions.[29] This increase has been particularly noticeable within the female population and in patients with comorbidities, such as diabetes or renal disease.[30] On admission, patients require accurate assessment and triage to ensure they are managed in the most appropriate clinical setting. There is increased evidence to indicate that patients admitted with HF have an improved survival, for up to one year, when they are treated and followed up within specialist cardiac units.[31,32] This may be accounted for by the fact that patients managed by a specialist MDT are increasingly more likely to undergo diagnostic investigations such as cardiac magnetic imaging, referral for device or surgical interventions and have evidence-based medications prescribed.[33]

Device therapy is increasingly important in the management of life-threatening arrhythmia and clinical HF. In its broader application, encompassing acute haemodynamic support for patients with cardiogenic shock (i.e. intra-aortic balloon pump: IABP), short term haemodynamic support along with IABP with ventricular assist devices, and chronic haemodynamic support using mechanical circulatory support (MCS) devices for destination therapy or a bridge to cardiac transplantation. Research throughout the evolution of advanced therapies has unanimously concluded that successful outcomes rely on robust patient selection, which can be conducted in the acute hospitalization setting or the outpatient setting.

For selected patients, implantable cardioverter defibrillators (ICDs) can improve mortality benefit by treating lethal ventricular arrhythmias and in certain eligible patient groups, cardiac resynchronization therapy reduces morbidity and mortality.[34] In recent years, there has been increasing interest in the clinical implications of frailty in patients with cardiovascular disease in general, HF being no exception, with frailty scoring providing valuable information on prognosis. Recent clinical guidelines stress that patients with serious comorbidities who are unlikely to survive substantially more than one year with good quality of life are unlikely to obtain substantial benefit from an implantable cardioverter defibrillator.[4] However, assessment in clinical practice remains a challenge, and consensus is lacking on the best tool to use.[35] What is clear is that a collaborative approach from primary care physicians, nurses, physiotherapist, and electrophysiologist, is an integral first step in ensuring appropriate patient selection and individualized decision-making, particularly regarding defibrillator therapy.[36]

When considering both in-patient and out-patient device implantation consultations, patient counselling and education are vital to ensure shared decision-making and ongoing patient compliance. Information and education should include details on the immediate implantation phase, and consider long-term implications on driving, incidence and dealing with inappropriate therapies, lead failure, and device deactivation. As with any educational process, it should be multi-staged, beginning at pre-implantation and continuing through-out post implantation management.[37] The depth of information may be tailored according to the patient's need with respect for indication for the device, cognitive ability, psychological coping and his/her preference. Chava et al. reviewed length of hospital stay and readmission rates following the implementation of MDT HF rounds. The MDT within the study included a cardiologist, case manager, pharmacist, social worker, and a nutritionist. Results were promising showing reduced length of stay from 5.7 days to 5 days, and 30-day readmissions decreased from 27.6% to 17.22% (p-value 0.026).[38]

One of the key challenges is coordination and communication across team members. A number of methods have been developed to improve the transition of care for the patient while in hospital, as well as from hospital to home. Cowie et al.[39] reported preliminary findings on the 'Optimize heart failure program', an initiative implemented in 45 countries, with the purpose of improving outcomes post-discharge. Using pre- and post-discharge checklists, as well as a printed and smartphone application ('My HF Passport'), positive results in terms of optimization of pharmacological therapy have been achieved.

Cardiac physiologists play a vital role in patient device management, particularly with regards to device optimization and home monitoring. To date, remote monitoring via pacing devices has been disappointing and studies have failed to demonstrate an improved prognosis.[40,41] Limited data from a dedicated implantable pulmonary artery device (CardioMEMS) in selected patients is encouraging,[25] although more convincing results from larger trial are desired. In overwhelmed healthcare settings, it is possible that with growing device monitoring capabilities, the resulting huge data burden could easily overwhelm services. Collaborative working with electrophysiologists, HF specialists, and cardiac physiologists is essential to identify patients who would benefit from remote monitoring.

Although no studies have reported on the impact of a multidisciplinary approach on the survival of patients with MCS or cardiac transplant, a team approach is required to ensure all practical, physical, psychological, and social consequences of LVAD implantation are addressed.[42] Robust pre-assessment in this patient group includes assessment of the risk of anesthesia as well as psychological status, nutritional status, and pulmonary function, all aided by appropriate cardiac imaging. In addition, it may be necessary to include a palliative MDT approach to ensure the patient has an understanding of prognosis and expectations of treatment, while in-hospital and at home.[43] During the immediate post-operative stage, patient care will be shared between the intensivists/critical care doctors, surgeons, intensive care nurses, and cardiologists. On discharge, care should be coordinated by the cardiologist, HF nurse, MCS device or transplant coordinator, and be supported by a team of allied professionals including nutritionist, physiotherapist, psychologist and social worker as well as the patient's GP. The GP is an integral member of the team, regularly communicating with the patient and family members, as well as providing day-to-day care including blood tests, medication adherence and organizing important community services, as required.

At the vulnerable post-discharge phase (drug titration, education)

A survey carried out in 2018–2019 found over 16,000 consultant physicians are currently employed within the UK, of which 10.4% are cardiologists.[44] This proportion of cardiologists is similar to that in most ESC countries and may actually in some countries be exceeded by a factor of 2–10.[45] For cardiologists, the main role is the efficient diagnosis of HF, accurate identification of aetiology, and reversible/ irreversible contributing factors for decompensation, with initiation of appropriate evidence-based therapies in accordance with patient and country-specific needs. Within clinical guidelines, all patients with suspected HF are recommended to have an echocardiogram;[4] however, only 66% of patients within the EuroHeart failure survey programme had this completed.[46] Unfortunately, this investigation remains on a downward trend with the recent 2020/2021 UK audit revealing only 86% of patients with suspected HF had an echocardiogram compared to 92% in 2014/2015. Certainly this is only one investigation, required for diagnosis, with others including blood investigations (including BNP), and electrocardiogram.

Cardiologists, working alongside the HF nurses, can achieve optimization of medications more efficiently and for patients who are not responding to optimal treatment, identify those eligible for device and surgical interventions. Surgical interventions can range from revascularization to potential implantation of an MCS (e.g. LVAD). Once optimized on appropriate drug and device therapies, and symptomatically stable, patients with HF may be discharged for continued long-term follow-up with their primary care team, under the guidance of their GP. Good collaboration and a creation of a seamless service across primary and secondary care will ensure that should the patient's symptoms deteriorate,

clear pathways are in place for timely re-referral and re-review at the specialist centre.

The vital role of the nurse in the pre- discharge and transition to out-patient care delivery of patients with HF has been highlighted within position papers and clinical guidelines.[16,47] Over the past two decades nurses have contributed to the management of patients with HF, particularly those recently admitted due to a decompensation of their condition.[3] Traditionally their focus was on patient education and optimization of evidence-based medications, such as beta-blockers and renin–angiotensin–aldosterone system inhibitors according to agreed protocols.[48,49] Due to the increasing number of patients diagnosed with HF, their crucial role has complemented and in some instances taken on the responsibilities of other members of the HF MDT team. Many nurses act as 'interlocutor', improving communication with the patient and relevant family members, between primary and secondary care, and across specialisms. This is becoming increasing relevant due to the advancing age of our HF population and the complexity of their health status. Education on their HF condition and monitoring of symptoms, advising on relevant lifestyle changes that may be necessary, and discussing treatment expectations and prognosis, all aim to empower the patient to be self-caring.[50] Further enhancement of the role of the HF nurse has been the emergence of non-medical prescribing within the UK. Many HF nurses can now independently initiate, titrate, and optimize evidence-based therapies.

Within at least seven European countries, some degree of prescribing by nurses has become established. Within the UK, nurses who have completed a recognized prescribing course can act as autonomous practitioners, completing a clinical examination before issuing the relevant prescription and advising on follow-up.[51] This has positively impacted patient satisfaction and the speed at which important guideline directed medications can be titrated. In addition in 2016, the HFA published the Heart Failure Nurse curriculum, providing guidance on the essential knowledge, skills, and behaviours required of the nurse managing patients across different care settings.[52] The important role nurses play has been recognized by their inclusion by the HFA in healthcare settings wishing for recognition as a 'centre of excellence' in the provision of HF care.[13]

Patient benefit from the optimization of their medications has inspired the developing role of not only the HF nurses but also pharmacists. As an essential allied professional, they are playing more of an increased contributory role in the MDT as they support the optimization of evidence-based medications.[53] Essentially noted within a primary care setting, the role of the pharmacist with the HF team within the hospital setting is increasing. Within the increasing complexity of the HF population, who often present with a range of comorbidities and polypharmacy, the pharmacist can play a crucial role in medication reconciliation, observation of essential drug interactions, and optimization prior to discharge.

The early integration of a palliative care approach into the management of the patient with HF has been recommended within a recent HFA position statement and expert guidelines.[4,54] As the patient nears end of life and symptoms become more distressing, input from specialist palliative care professionals would be appropriate. This may be either in an advisory capacity or direct management, depending on symptoms and patient's wishes. The cardiologist may have to initiate the difficult conversation that no further treatment options are available or lead the discussion and shared decision to deactivate an implantable device. This can only be successfully achieved through an empathetic relationship, built up over time with the patient and family members, as well as awareness and knowledge of their expectations.

The complexity of HF is underscored by its frequent association with multiple comorbidities. Depending on which comorbidities and their severity, patients will require tailored care coordinated by the HF MDT, with input from a number of specialists.

Collaboration with specialists

Multimorbidity, defined as the co-existence of two or more chronic conditions, is highly prevalent in HF.[55,56] The reported prevalence of multimorbidity has increased over the past two decades, with the average number of comorbidities being higher in patients with HFpEF than in those with HFrEF, in both women (5.53 vs 4.94; p < 0.0001) and men (5.20 vs 4.82; p < 0.0001).[57] The rising burden of comorbidities is of concern given that they may precipitate cardiac decompensation and increase the risk of both non-fatal complications and mortality.[57,58]

In order to achieve a holistic approach that would allow patient-tailored provision of disease-modifying therapies for HF and the appropriate management of comorbidities, collaboration between multiple specialists is often required. However, this approach may inadvertently increase the risk of conflicting medical advice, polypharmacy, poor adherence, and adverse drug interactions. Therefore, a multispecialist team should have established means of communication and cooperation in a joint effort to provide safe and rationalized therapeutic interventions.

Diabetes and endocrine disorders

The management of diabetes in HF should address several treatment goals, which may be more challenging than in the general population. These goals include: (i) glycaemic control (i.e. maintaining glycosylated haemoglobin A1c ~7.0%), whilst avoiding hypoglycaemia, which may have detrimental consequences in HF; (ii) control of cardiovascular risk factors and lifestyle modification, whilst taking into account limited ability to exercise, and (iii) screening and prevention of micro- and macrovascular complications.

Sodium-glucose cotransporter-2 (SGLT2) inhibitors have been proven effective in reducing the risk of HF hospitalizations in individuals with diabetes, and the combined risk of HF hospitalization or cardiovascular mortality in patients with HFrEF, with or without diabetes. Their addition as one of the four pillars of HF management confirmed this importance.[4] Therefore, SGLT2 inhibitors should be the preferred treatment of type 2 diabetes in patients with HF.[59] However, patients with diabetes frequently require more than one oral glucose-lowering medication and/or insulin for glycaemic control, and insulin is a mandatory treatment of type 1 diabetes mellitus. The more complex therapeutic regimens (i.e. two or more glucose-lowering medications/insulin) may aggravate the risk of hypoglycaemia. Moreover, several antidiabetic drugs (e.g. thiazolidinediones, saxagliptin) have been associated with a greater risk of worsening HF. Therefore, a MDT approach, comprising of HF specialist, a diabetologist/endocrinologist, a nutritionist, and an HF nurse should be involved in all patients with HF requiring the more complex management of diabetes.[60] The risk of hypoglycaemia and other complications (diabetic ketoacidosis, infections) may be exacerbated in emergencies and critical conditions (e.g. trauma, sepsis, worsening renal function), where successful management hinges on multispecialist care. Even in diabetic patients principally managed by the cardiologist, a periodic consultation with a diabetologist/endocrinologist should be considered to optimize strategies for long-term prevention of micro- and macrovascular complications.[60]

Besides diabetes, an endocrinologist should be involved in the diagnosis and management of endocrine disorders known to cause or exacerbate HF, including thyroid dysfunction (in particular, thyrotoxicosis), growth hormone excess (acromegaly), hypopituitarism, pheochromocytoma, and Cushing syndrome.

Chronic kidney disease

Chronic kidney disease (CKD) imposes difficulties for the management of HF due to frequently encountered diuretic resistance, electrolyte abnormalities, adverse drug reactions, concomitant cardiovascular comorbidities, anaemia, and secondary hyperparathyroidism. The management of HF patients with CKD should be a shared responsibility between HF specialist team and nephrologist, with a focus on the provision of HF therapies with proven cardio-renal benefits (i.e. angiotensin converting enzyme inhibitors or angiotensin receptor blockers or sacubitril/valsartan, SGLT2 inhibitors), management of hyperkalaemia, cardiovascular risk reduction, and the treatment of anaemia and hyperparathyroidism. In particular, institution of renal replacement therapy should be considered in patients with acute/advanced HF, refractory volume overload and end-stage kidney disease.[1] Also, in patients on dialysis, a close cross-specialist collaboration is needed to optimize the dialysis schedule and volume of ultrafiltration for the maintenance of volume control and prevention of hypotension.

Future directions

Patients often have existing comorbidites, adding complexity to their HF management and requiring input from a range of disciplines across specialisms. A MDT approach, consisting of a HF specialist (cardiology/nurse), general practitioner and allied professionals has been proven to be beneficial. Further research is required into the specific content, intensity, and delivery; however, the model is often dictated by country-specific and healthcare resources.

Extending the remit of the team to include other specialisms, such as endocrinology, requires clear lines of communication and coordination. The HFA-accredited Quality of Care Centres aims to foster standardized and coordinated multidisciplinary management of patients with HF across community, specialized, and advanced centres.

Summary and key messages

♦ All patients should receive care that is coordinated and delivered by a team of expert multidisciplinary and multispecialism professionals.

♦ Clear lines of communication and documentation are needed to ensure seamless continuity of care irrespective of the patient's place of care (i.e. community, specialist and advanced).

♦ Early involvement of professionals is required to compliment and support the HF MDT, according to the individual needs of the patient.

♦ A central member of the team should be identified to coordinate the team approach and ensure services and resources are accessed throughout the patient's illness.

References

1. Ponikowski P, Voors AA, Anker SD, Bueno H, Cleland JGH, Coats AJS, et al. 2016 ESC guidelines for the diagnosis and treatment of acute and chronic heart failure. The task force for the diagnosis and treatment of acute and chronic heart failure of the European Society of Cardiology2016; Eur Heart J. 2016;37(27):2129–200

2. Yancy CW, Jessup M, Bozkurt B, Butler J, Casey DE, Drazner MH, et al. 2013 ACCF/AHA Guideline for the Management of Heart Failure A Report of the American College of Cardiology Foundation/American Heart Association Task Force on Practice Guidelines Developed in Collaboration With the American College of Chest Physicians, Heart Rhythm Society and International Society for Heart and Lung Transplantation Endorsed by the American Association of Cardiovascular and Pulmonary Rehabilitation. Circulation. 2013;128:e240–327.

3. Rich MW, Gray DB, Beckham V, Wittenberg C, Luther P. Effect of a multidisciplinary intervention on medication compliance in elderly patients with congestive heart failure. Am J Med. 1996;101(3):270–6.

4. McDonagh TA, Metra M, Adamo M, Gardner RS, Baumbach A, Böhm M, et al. 2021 ESC Guidelines for the diagnosis and treatment of acute and chronic heart failure. Eur Heart J. 2021;42(36):3599–726.

5. Hill L. Producing an effective care plan in advanced heart failure. Eur Heart J Suppl. 2019;21(Suppl M):M61–3.

6. Jaarsma T, van der Wal MH, Lesman-Leegte I, Luttik ML, Hogenhuis J, Veeger NJ, et al. Effect of moderate or intensive disease management program on outcome in patients with heart failure: Coordinating Study Evaluating Outcomes of Advising and Counseling in Heart Failure (COACH). Arch Intern Med. 2008;168(3):316–24.

7. Stewart S, Marley JE, Horowitz JD. Effects of a multidisciplinary, home-based intervention on unplanned readmissions and survival among patients with chronic congestive heart failure: a randomised controlled study. Lancet. 1999;354(9184):1077–83.

8. McMurray JJ, Stewart S. Nurse led, multidisciplinary intervention in chronic heart failure. Heart. 1998;80(5):430–1.

9. Jonkman NH, Westland H, Groenwold RH, Agren S, Atienza F, Blue L, et al. Do self-management interventions work in patients with heart failure? an individual patient data meta-analysis. Circulation. 2016;133(12):1189–98.

10. Seferović PM, Vardas P, Jankowska EA, Maggioni AP, Timmis A, Milinković I, et al. The Heart Failure Association Atlas: Heart Failure Epidemiology and Management Statistics 2019. Eur J Heart Fail. 2021;23(6):906–14.

11. Van Spall HGC, Rahman T, Mytton O, Ramasundarahettige C, Ibrahim Q, Kabali C, et al. Comparative effectiveness of transitional care services in patients discharged from the hospital with heart failure: a systematic review and network meta-analysis. Eur J Heart Fail. 2017;19:1427–43.

12. Takeda A, Martin N, Taylor RS, Taylor SJ. Disease management interventions for heart failure. Cochrane Database Syst Rev. 2019;1(1):Cd002752.

13. Seferović PM, Piepoli MF, Lopatin Y, Jankowska E, Polovina M, Anguita-Sanchez M, et al. Heart Failure Association of the European Society of Cardiology Quality of Care Centres Programme: design and accreditation document. Eur J Heart Fail. 2020;22(5):763–74.

14. Krumholz HM, Currie PM, Riegel B, Phillips CO, Peterson ED, Smith R, et al. A taxonomy for disease management: a scientific statement from the American Heart Association Disease Management Taxonomy Writing Group. Circulation. 2006;114(13):1432–45.

15. Morton G, Masters J, Cowburn PJ. Multidisciplinary team approach to heart failure management. Heart. 2018;104(16):1376–82.

16. McDonagh TA, Blue L, Clark AL, Dahlström U, Ekman I, Lainscak M, et al. European Society of Cardiology Heart Failure Association Standards for delivering heart failure care. Eur J Heart Fail. 2011;13(3):235–41.

17. Hendriks JM, Jaarsma T. The multidisciplinary team approach in cardiovascular care. Eur J Cardiovasc Nurs. 2020; 20(2): 91–2.

18. Senni M, Tribouilloy CM, Rodeheffer RJ, Jacobsen SJ, Evans JM, Bailey KR, et al. Congestive heart failure in the community: a study of all incident cases in Olmsted County, Minnesota, in 1991. Circulation. 1998;98(21):2282–9.

19. Chen HH, Lainchbury JG, Senni M, Bailey KR, Redfield MM. Diastolic heart failure in the community: clinical profile, natural history, therapy, and impact of proposed diagnostic criteria. J Cardia Fail. 2002;8(5):279–87.

20. Altimir S, Lupón J, González B, Prats M, Parajón T, Urrutia A, et al. Sex and age differences in fragility in a heart failure population. Eur J Heart Fail. 2005;7(5):798–802.

21. Akosah KO, Moncher K, Schaper A, Havlik P, Devine S. Chronic heart failure in the community: missed diagnosis and missed opportunities. J Card Fail. 2001;7(3):232–8.

22. Ledwidge M, Gallagher J, Conlon C, Tallon E, O'Connell E, Dawkins I, et al. Natriuretic peptide-based screening and collaborative care for heart failure: the STOP-HF randomized trial. JAMA. 2013;310(1):66–74.

23. Hindricks G, Taborsky M, Glikson M, Heinrich U, Schumacher B, Katz A, et al. Implant-based multiparameter telemonitoring of patients with heart failure (IN-TIME): a randomised controlled trial. Lancet. 2014;384(9943):583–90.

24. Koehler F, Koehler K, Deckwart O, Prescher S, Wegscheider K, Kirwan BA, et al. Efficacy of telemedical interventional management in patients with heart failure (TIM-HF2): a randomised, controlled, parallel-group, unmasked trial. Lancet. 2018;392(10152):1047–57.

25. Abraham WT, Adamson PB, Bourge RC, Aaron MF, Costanzo MR, Stevenson LW, et al. Wireless pulmonary artery haemodynamic monitoring in chronic heart failure: a randomised controlled trial. Lancet. 2011;377(9766):658–66.

26. 5GmedCamp. 5GMedCamp 2021 [Available from: https://www.5gmedcamp.de/.

27. Meyer A, Zverinski D, Pfahringer B, Kempfert J, Kuehne T, Sündermann SH, et al. Machine learning for real-time prediction of complications in critical care: a retrospective study. Lancet Respir Med. 2018;6(12):905–14.

28. Beschluss des Gemeinsamen Bundesausschusses über eine Änderung der Richtlinie Methoden vertragsärztliche Versorgung: Telemonitoring bei Herzinsuffizienz. 2020.

29. Lawson CA, Zaccardi F, Squire I, Ling S, Davies MJ, Lam CSP, et al. 20-year trends in cause-specific heart failure outcomes by sex, socioeconomic status, and place of diagnosis: a population-based study. Lancet Public Health. 2019;4(8):e406–20.

30. Mosterd A, Hoes AW. Clinical epidemiology of heart failure. Heart. 2007;93(9):1137–46.

31. National Institute for cardiovascular Outcomes (NICOR) BSoHF, Barts Health NHS Trust, The Healthcare Quality Improvement partnership (HQIP). National Cardiac Audit Programme: National Heart Failure Audit (NHFA), 2021 summary report 2021. 14 October 2021.

32. Boom NK, Lee DS, Tu JV. Comparison of processes of care and clinical outcomes for patients newly hospitalized for heart failure attended by different physician specialists. Am Heart J. 2012;163(2):252–9.

33. Cowie MR, Anker SD, Cleland JGF, Felker GM, Filippatos G, Jaarsma T, et al. Improving care for patients with acute heart failure: before, during and after hospitalization. ESC Heart Fail. 2014;1(2):110–45.

34. Cleland JG, Abraham WT, Linde C, Gold MR, Young JB, Claude Daubert J, et al. An individual patient meta-analysis of five randomized trials assessing the effects of cardiac resynchronization therapy on morbidity and mortality in patients with symptomatic heart failure. Eur Heart J. 2013;34(46):3547–56.

35. Hoogendijk EO, Afilalo J, Ensrud KE, Kowal P, Onder G, Fried LP. Frailty: implications for clinical practice and public health. Lancet. 2019;394(10206):1365–75.

36. Turner G, Clegg A. Best practice guidelines for the management of frailty: a British Geriatrics Society, Age UK and Royal College of General Practitioners report. Age Ageing. 2014;43(6):744–7.

37. Hill LM, McIlfatrick S, Taylor B, Dixon L, Fitzsimons D. Implantable cardioverter defibrillator (ICD) functionality: patient and family information for advanced decision-making. BMJ Support Palliat Care. 2022;12(e2):e219–25.

38. Chava R, Karki N, Ketlogetswe K, Ayala T. Multidisciplinary rounds in prevention of 30-day readmissions and decreasing length of stay in heart failure patients: A community hospital based retrospective study. Medicine (Baltimore). 2019;98(27):e16233.

39. Cowie MR, Lopatin YM, Saldarriaga C, Fonseca C, Sim D, Magaña JA, et al. The Optimize Heart Failure Care Program: Initial lessons from global implementation. Int J Cardiol. 2017;236:340–4.

40. Boriani G, Da Costa A, Quesada A, Ricci RP, Favale S, Boscolo G, et al. Effects of remote monitoring on clinical outcomes and use of healthcare resources in heart failure patients with biventricular defibrillators: results of the MORE-CARE multicentre randomized controlled trial. Eur J Heart Fail. 2017;19(3):416–25.

41. Lindenfeld J, Zile MR, Desai AS, Bhatt K, Ducharme A, Horstmanshof D, et al. Haemodynamic-guided management of heart failure (GUIDE-HF): a randomised controlled trial. Lancet. 2021;398(10304):991–1001.

42. Ben Gal T, Ben Avraham B, Milicic D, Crespo-Leiro MG, Coats AJS, Rosano G, et al. Guidance on the management of left ventricular assist device (LVAD) supported patients for the non-LVAD specialist healthcare provider: executive summary. Eur J Heart Fail. 2021;23(10):1597–609.

43. O'Donnell AE, Schaefer KG, Stevenson LW, DeVoe K, Walsh K, Mehra MR, et al. Social worker-aided palliative care intervention in high-risk patients with heart failure (SWAP-HF): a pilot randomized clinical trial. JAMA Cardiol. 2018;3(6):516–9.

44. Royal College of Physicians RcoPoE, Royal College of Physicians and Surgeons of Scotland Focus on Physicians: Census of consultant physicians and higher speciality training 2018, Medical Workforce Unit 2018.

45. Seferovic PM, Stoerk S, Filippatos G, Mareev V, Kavoliuniene A, Ristic AD, et al. Organization of heart failure management in European Society of Cardiology member countries: survey of the Heart Failure Association of the European Society of Cardiology in collaboration with the Heart Failure National Societies/Working Groups. Eur J Heart Fail. 2013;15(9):947–59.

46. Cleland JG, Swedberg K, Follath F, Komajda M, Cohen-Solal A, Aguilar JC, et al. The EuroHeart Failure survey programme – a survey on the quality of care among patients with heart failure in Europe. Part 1: patient characteristics and diagnosis. Eur Heart J. 2003;24(5):442–63.

47. Mebazaa A, Yilmaz MB, Levy P, Ponikowski P, Peacock WF, Laribi S, et al. Recommendations on pre-hospital & early hospital management of acute heart failure: a consensus paper from the Heart Failure Association of the European Society of Cardiology, the European Society of Emergency Medicine and the Society of Academic Emergency Medicine. Eur J Heart Fail. 2015;17(6):544–58.

48. Güder G, Störk S, Gelbrich G, Brenner S, Deubner N, Morbach C, et al. Nurse-coordinated collaborative disease management improves the quality of guideline-recommended heart failure therapy, patient-reported outcomes, and left ventricular remodelling. Eur J Heart Fail. 2015;17(4):442–52.

49. Boyde M, Turner C, Thompson DR, Stewart S. Educational interventions for patients with heart failure: a systematic review of randomized controlled trials. J Cardiovasc Nurs. 2011;26(4):E27–35.

50. Jaarsma T, Hill L, Bayes-Genis A, La Rocca HB, Castiello T, Čelutkienė J, et al. Self-care of heart failure patients: practical management recommendations from the Heart Failure Association of the European Society of Cardiology. Eur J Heart Fail. 2021;23(1):157–74.

51. Kroezen M, van Dijk L, Groenewegen PP, Francke AL. Nurse prescribing of medicines in Western European and Anglo-Saxon countries: a systematic review of the literature. BMC Health Serv Res. 2011;11:127.

52. Riley JP, Astin F, Crespo-Leiro MG, Deaton CM, Kienhorst J, Lambrinou E, et al. Heart Failure Association of the European Society of Cardiology heart failure nurse curriculum. Eur J Heart Fail. 2016;18(7):736–43.

53. Dempsey J, Gillis C, Sibicky S, Matta L, MacRae C, Kirshenbaum J, et al. Evaluation of a transitional care pharmacist intervention in a high-risk cardiovascular patient population. Am J Health Syst Pharm. 2018;75(17 Supplement 3):S63–s71.

54. Hill L, Prager Geller T, Baruah R, Beattie JM, Boyne J, de Stoutz N, et al. Integration of a palliative approach into heart failure care: a European Society of Cardiology Heart Failure Association position paper. Eur J Heart Fail. 2020; 22(12):2327–39

55. Khan MS, Samman Tahhan A, Vaduganathan M, Greene SJ, Alrohaibani A, Anker SD, et al. Trends in prevalence of comorbidities in heart failure clinical trials. Eur J Heart Fail. 2020;22(6):1032–42.

56. Chamberlain AM, St Sauver JL, Gerber Y, Manemann SM, Boyd CM, Dunlay SM, et al. Multimorbidity in heart failure: a community perspective. Am J Med. 2015;128(1):38–45.

57. Pandey A, Vaduganathan M, Arora S, Qamar A, Mentz RJ, Shah SJ, et al. Temporal trends in prevalence and prognostic implications of comorbidities among patients with acute decompensated heart failure: The ARIC Study Community Surveillance. Circulation. 2020;142(3):230–43.

58. Braunstein JB, Anderson GF, Gerstenblith G, Weller W, Niefeld M, Herbert R, et al. Non cardiac comorbidity increases prevenatble hospitalisations and mortaility among Medicare beneficiaries with chronic heart failure. J Am Coll Cardiol. 2003;42(7): 1226–33.

59. Cosentino F, Grant PJ, Aboyans V, Bailey CJ, Ceriello A, Delgado V, et al. 2019 ESC Guidelines on diabetes, pre-diabetes, and cardiovascular diseases developed in collaboration with the EASD. Eur Heart J. 2020;41(2):255–323.

60. Seferović PM, Coats AJS, Ponikowski P, Filippatos G, Huelsmann M, Jhund PS, et al. European Society of Cardiology/Heart Failure Association position paper on the role and safety of new glucose-lowering drugs in patients with heart failure. Eur J Heart Fail. 2020;22(2):196–213.

SECTION 15

Clinical trial design and interpretation

CHAPTER 15.1

Clinical trial design and interpretation

Gianluigi Savarese, Marija Polovina, and Gerasimos Filippatos

Contents

Introduction

Evidence-based medicine (EBM) has been ranked as one of the 15 most important milestones in modern medicine. David Sackett (McMaster University, Hamilton, Canada) introduced the concept of EBM in the 1980s as the application of the best available research to clinical care, which requires the integration of evidence with clinical expertise and patient values.[1] The implementation of the concept of EBM has led to the development of grading of evidence to support decision-making in clinical practice, as reported in the international medical guidelines[2] (◯ Figure 15.1.1).

Randomized controlled trials (RCT) represent a large proportion of high-quality EBM and are the gold standard to test treatment benefit in medicine.[3]

The aim of this chapter is to provide an overview on the key aspects involved in clinical trial design, to guide a structured critical appraisal of RCTs performed in the field of heart failure (HF).

Equipoise

The concept of equipoise represents the central ethical principle for RCTs and supports the rationale for conducting a trial that would test efficacy and/or safety of a novel treatment against placebo, only if there is substantial uncertainty regarding benefit related with specific treatment. If there is evidence that a beneficial treatment/treatment standard in a specific setting exists, it is unethical not to compare the investigational intervention to the standard of care.[4]

RCT phases

Potential new treatments are tested in a sequential manner though phase I–IV trials. Phase I/II and III/IV trials can also be quite common.[5] Phase I trials usually aim to explore potential toxic effects and tolerance issues in ~20–100 healthy volunteers or people with the disease/condition over several months. In phase II, the aim is to assess whether the treatment shows efficacy, in general in terms of surrogate outcomes, while considering different doses/timing combinations and monitoring for side-effects.[6] They usually enroll up to several hundred patients with the disease of interest and last up to ~2 years. In phase III up to 3000 patients with the disease of interest are enrolled and the purpose is to investigate efficacy, in most of cases in terms of hard outcomes (mortality/morbidity), and monitoring adverse reaction. These studies last up to ~4 years. In phase IV several thousand patients are enrolled to obtain long-term data on morbidity and safety (post-marketing studies).

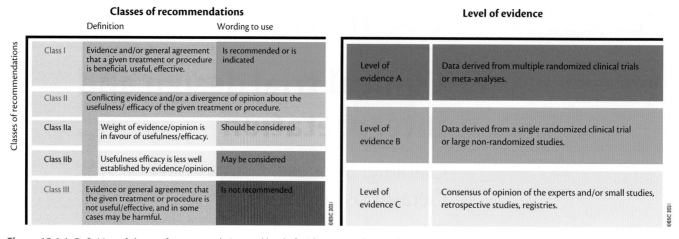

Figure 15.1.1 Definition of classes of recommendations and level of evidence according to the 2021 ESC Guidelines on Heart Failure. McDonagh TA, Metra M, Adamo M, et al; ESC Scientific Document Group. 2021 ESC Guidelines for the diagnosis and treatment of acute and chronic heart failure. *Eur Heart J*. 2021 Sep 21;42(36):3599-3726. doi: 10.1093/eurheartj/ehab368. © European Cardiology Society. Reprinted with permission from Oxford Unviersity Press.

Randomization

The term randomization refers to the procedure of allocating patients by chance to the study arms receiving different treatments. It ensures that each patient has the same chance of receiving any investigated intervention, for example, the treatment under investigation or the control, which leads to comparable patient characteristics across the study arms except for the intervention that each arm receives.[7] Randomization is the only procedure that allows an unbiased evaluation of treatment efficacy, free of confounding from any known and unknown, measured and unmeasured confounder.[8] In contrast to RCTs, in observational studies it is possible to use statistical methods to adjust for known and measured confounders, but it is not possible to adjust for unknown or unmeasured (i.e. variables not collected in the database) confounders. Therefore, a role for residual confounding cannot be ruled out with this study design, which leads to the inability of observational studies to assess efficacy, whereas only associations between exposures and outcomes can be evaluated.[9] For example in the RALES and EMPHASIS trials randomizing patients with HF and reduced ejection fraction (HFrEF), both spironolactone and eplerenone reduced mortality and morbidity.[10,11] In a registry-based study considering patients receiving vs non-receiving spironolactone, the population on treatment had more severe HF and comorbidity burden compared with those who were not treated, reflecting the 2016 European Society of Cardiology Guidelines recommendation of initiating mineralocorticoid receptor antagonists whether patients were still symptomatic and had an EF ≤ 35% despite the therapy with an angiotensin converting enzyme inhibitor (ACEi) or a beta-blocker.[12,13] After extensive adjustments using a propensity score matching design, there was no association between use of spironolactone and survival, which was explained by residual confounding, indication bias or a potential lower benefit associated with spironolactone outside the clinical trial setting.[13]

Several types of randomization techniques can be considered for RCT design.[7] Simple randomization is based on a single sequence of random assignments. It can be achieved by flipping a coin and considering heads for treatments and tails for controls, by throwing a dice and considering even numbers for the treatments and odd numbers for controls, or computer-generated random numbers and applying similar rules. Ad-hoc software exists for random allocation of patients in clinical studies. Although this randomization technique is likely to be successful in providing comparable populations and equal number of patients across the study arms whether the sample size is large (n > 100), it might fail in these purposes if the sample overall size is small, or during interim analyses when the enrollment has not been completed.[14]

By using permuted block randomization, patients are randomized to a treatment or a control within blocks containing predefined randomly assigned treatment assignments.[15] This method allows a balance in sample size in the treated vs. control groups to be maintained over time. The block size is usually defined as a multiple of the number of treatment arms, for example, if the trial has two arms, the block size might contain four, six, or eight patients, etc. Smaller blocks allow the desired sample size to be more easily preserved across the study groups. If blocks of six patients are chosen, e.g. ABAABBA where A is the study treatment and B is the control, meaning that patient 1 will receive the treatment, patient 2 will receive the control, patient 3 the treatment, etc, the same sample size in both arms will be ensured every six enrolled patients, although treated and control patients might not be comparable for some covariates within the block. Guaranteeing balanced sample sizes across the study groups maximizes statistical power and reduces risk of bias.[15]

Stratified randomization aims to guarantee that specific patient characteristics which are prognostically relevant and can influence treatment response are equally distributed across the trial arms, which is particularly relevant for small trials (n < 100) where the risk of enrolling non-comparable study groups is higher.[16] Covariates of interest for stratifications need to be identified before the study begins. Whether the researcher is for example interested to stratify by sex and age < or ≥ 65 years, there will be four strata. Randomization to treatment vs control is separately performed within each stratum, usually using a permute block randomization approach. Stratified randomization has been shown to prevent type I errors and improve power for small trials (< 400 patients) only when the covariates involved in the stratification process have large prognostic effect. Stratified randomization facilitates interim analyses which might consider small sample sizes. Additionally, it is particularly relevant for subgroup analyses, when some subgroups are particularly small and, in combination with block randomization, to guarantee that treatment assignments within subgroups is balanced, that is each subgroup becomes a small individual trial.[16] One example for a RCT using stratified permuted block randomization is the EMPEROR-Reduced, testing the efficacy of empagliflozin vs placebo in patients with HFrEF, which used a computer pseudo-random number generator to produce the blocks, and stratification was performed according to geographical regions (North America, Latin America, Europe, Asia, other), diabetes status at the screening, estimated glomerular filtration rate < vs ≥ 60 mL/min/1.73m^2 at the screening.[17] A stratified randomization approach with permuted blocks has been used in the DAPA-HF where stratification was performed by diabetes status at the screening.[18] Stratifying by diabetes in these trials, allowed to properly assess sodium-glucose co-transporter-2 (SGLT2i) inhibitors in patients with and without diabetes.

Blinding or masking

Blinding procedures are often adopted in RCTs to avoid a certain number of biases that might arise if the patient, the investigator, the outcome assessors, and data analysts know the treatment allocation. In a single-blinded trial the patient is usually blinded; in a double-blinded trial both the patient and the investigator are usually blinded; in a triple-blinded trial the patient, the investigator, and outcome assessor are blinded; in a quadruple-blinded trial also the data analyst might be blinded. Blinding the patient avoids the possibility that patients' favourable expectations or apprehension might lead to change their behaviours, such as seeking additional adjunct interventions or leaving the trial, or that patients might subjectively report outcome measures based on treatment allocation. Blinding the investigator prevents physicians to transfer their expectations regarding the study interventions to the patients, to provide different care based on the treatment allocation, for example, additional care whether being randomized to placebo is perceived as a missed chance of receiving a beneficial treatment, to differently withdraw study participants from the trial, and to be influenced on whether and how reporting potential clinical events to outcome assessors. Blinding the outcome assessors ensure an impartial evaluation of the outcomes. Blinding the data analyst until the completion of the analyses avoids a conscious or unconscious selection of specific statistical methods or

selective reporting of outcome measures.[19] Blinding is not always possible since it depends on the type of intervention under investigation, and if it is not used, an RCT is defined as open-label trial. However, when it is not feasible to blind patients and investigators, blinding the outcome assessor remains a useful option, that is, prospective, randomized, open-label, blinded-endpoint evaluation RCTs (PROBE). A PROBE design is preferred in those settings where blinding is difficult to achieve, for instance when the use of the study intervention is laboratory-guided, when side-effects of the study intervention makes the treatment easily recognizable, such as in trials on devices. Indeed, in the GUIDE-IT trial randomizing patients with HFrEF to either usual care or a strategy adjusting therapy aiming to achieve a target NTproBNP <1000 pg/mL with primary outcome being the composite of cardiovascular mortality and HF hospitalization, although patients were not blinded and masking investigators was not feasible due to the tested intervention, the adjudication committee was blinded to the treatment assignment to minimize the risk of bias.[20] In the MADIT-CRT trial aiming to assess whether cardiac resynchronization therapy (CRT) reduced mortality or HF events in HF patients with mild symptoms, EF ≤ 30% and a QRS ≥ 130 ms, both patients and investigators were not blinded, but the end point adjudication committee was blinded.[21] Pros of a PROBE design vs a double-blinded approach are the lower costs, enhanced patient compliance, and the greater similarity of the trial setting to the real-world clinical practice. However, cons are the potential presence of an investigator bias – the reporting bias – since the investigator might be influenced in the choice of reporting a clinical event to the outcome assessor based on the patient's treatment allocation.[22]

There are different techniques to mask a comparator. The most frequent approach is to produce a placebo which seems completely the same as the treatment, for example, shape, colour, absence of specific marks, same packaging components. Over-encapsulation might be considered, that is, placing products into an opaque capsule which avoids identifying the contents. When comparing two active drugs which might have very different appearance, the double-dummy method can be considered, that is, the patient receiving treatment A will receive a placebo for treatment B which appears exactly as treatment B, and the patient receiving treatment B will receive a placebo for treatment A which appears exactly as treatment A. This will lead to each patient receiving two pills. In the FAIR-HF trial ferric carboxymaltose was tested against placebo with self-reported patient global assessment and New York Heart Association (NYHA) function class at week 24 as primary outcomes. Ferric carboxymaltose solution is dark brown and therefore easily distinguishable from the placebo which was 0.9% saline solution. In order to blind at least one study investigator, unblinded study personnel were required for preparation and administration of study treatments and for ensuring that patients could not observe the actual received treatment. To ensure that the blinded investigator remained blinded, post-treatment iron biomarkers analyses were sent only to the unblinded personnel who were responsible for acting in case of severe anemia or elevated iron parameters.[23]

Selection criteria

Patients included in clinical trials should closely reflect the population that the intervention is intended for. Ideally, broad selection criteria and appropriate representation of specific groups of patients (e.g. females, elderly, ethnic minorities) should allow the trial results to be generalizable to the population. Earlier clinical trials of patients with HF were criticized for under-representation of women, older patients, and those of other ethnicities/races apart from white people.[24] This has been largely improved in the more recent trials, however, there remains the question about the generalizability of trial results due to the narrow eligibility criteria. Investigators often opt for an 'enrichment' of the trial population for patients with characteristic that make them more likely to experience cardiovascular endpoints of interest (e.g. elevated levels of natriuretic peptides can be used to identify patients with greater risk of cardiovascular compared with non-cardiovascular events).[25] This provides a relatively homogeneous trial population which should allow for the more precise estimates of the treatment effect but limits the generalizability. Patients are usually excluded from trials based on the lack of equipoise, most frequently when the expected risk is considered to outweigh the potential benefits (e.g. individuals with severe renal or hepatic impairment).[26] Furthermore, excluding patients who are more likely to be lost to follow-up, or those whose outcomes might be 'censored' by competing events (e.g. older or sicker individuals) is a common strategy to prevent bias from non-random loss of subjects at different stages of the trial.[26] However, all these factors may limit the generalizability of trial results to the real-world patients. For example, an analysis of the eligibility for sacubitril/valsartan of outpatients with HF from a contemporary national registry in Sweden has demonstrated that only 32% of the registry patients would be eligible for sacubitril/valsartan based on strict ('literal') application of the PARADIGM-HF trial inclusion/exclusion criteria.[27] However, with a more 'pragmatic' interpretation of the PARADIGM-HF eligibility criteria (i.e. use of selected inclusion/exclusion criteria deemed most likely to influence the likelihood of patients receiving sacubitril/valsartan in real-world settings) a total of 63% of the registry patients would be considered eligible for the drug.[27] The most important unmet inclusion criteria in the real-world patients were related to the severity of HF status (i.e. lack of elevated natriuretic peptide levels or NYHA class II–IV), whereas major exclusion criteria limiting eligibility were hypotension and renal dysfunction.[27]

Outcomes

An outcome (also called an event or endpoint) is a variable that is being monitored and recorded during a trial to objectively document the impact of a given intervention (or exposure) on the health of the study population.[28] There are four types of outcome:

1 **Primary outcome** is defined by the ClinicalTrials.gov as 'the outcome measure(s) of the greatest importance specified in the protocol, usually the one(s) used in the power calculation'. It is the variable most relevant to answer the research question and ideally it should be patient centred (e.g. hospitalization, mortality, quality of life). The primary outcome needs to be pre-specified before the start of the trial to avoid false-positive and false-negative errors. False-positive errors may arise from the statistical testing of many outcomes resulting in a situation where statistical test is significant by chance and the conclusion is not true in the population. False-negative error (i.e. a situation where the intervention is truly effective but the trial failed to identify a statistically significant effect because the sample size was too small) can be prevented through the estimation of the sample size necessary for an adequately powered study.[29] To do so, the investigators need to specify what a clinically meaningful difference in the primary outcome between the two treatment arms (e.g. intervention arm vs placebo or an active control) would be. This information, or an estimate of the effect size based on previous research (e.g. a pilot study), can enable calculation of the appropriate sample size to detect the pre-determined clinically significant difference to a certain degree of power.[30]

2 **Secondary outcome** is defined by the ClinicalTrials.gov as 'an outcome measure that is of lesser importance than a primary outcome but is a part of a pre-specified analysis plan for evaluating the effects of the intervention(s) under investigation'. There may be more than one secondary outcome; however, the investigators need to choose only the most relevant ones to reduce the risk of false-positive errors deriving from testing multiple outcomes. Also, because the sample size is calculated for the primary outcome, statistical testing of secondary outcomes may yield false-negative results.

3 **Other pre-specified outcome measures** (i.e. exploratory outcomes) are defined by the ClinicalTrials.gov as 'any other measurements (excluding post-hoc measures), that will be used to evaluate the intervention(s)'. These include exploratory endpoints.

4 **Post-hoc outcomes** include outcomes specified after the trial has started. Post-hoc analyses need to be interpreted with caution, and unless confirmed prospectively or in different datasets, they should be considered as preliminary.

In addition, surrogate outcomes and composite outcomes are frequently used in clinical trials of patients with HF, sometimes as primary outcome measures.

Surrogate outcomes might represent biomarkers or other measures, for example, NYHA class, left ventricular ejection fraction or parameters related to functional capacity, that can be used as a substitute for a hard clinical outcome, for example, mortality, because of their strong correlation. For example, changes in concentrations of natriuretic peptides have been used as a marker of disease progression in HF. Surrogate outcomes tend to occur before clinical outcomes and their use can reduce the sample size, duration, and cost of a trial, but there is a risk of an overestimation of the treatment effect in the clinical sense. For example, the PARAMOUNT trial assessed the efficacy of sacubitril/

valsartan compared with valsartan on the change in N-terminal pro-B type natriuretic peptide (NT-proBNP) concentration at 12 weeks (primary outcome) in patients with HF with preserved ejection fraction (HFpEF).[31] The results demonstrated a significant reduction in NT-proBNP with sacubitril/valsartan vs valsartan, which set the expectations that similar clinical benefit could be demonstrated in a prospective randomized trial. However, the PARAGON-HF trial, which assessed the efficacy of sacubitril/valsartan compared with valsartan for risk reduction in cardiovascular mortality and total (first and recurrent) hospitalizations for HF, failed to demonstrate a significant difference between the two study arms.[32]

Composite outcome is made up of several variables, and usually includes clinical outcomes of interest for disease progression (e.g. hospitalization for HF) and fatal events (e.g. cardiovascular or all-cause death). The use of a composite outcome has the advantage of increasing the power of the trial when each of the primary outcome components is rare, or when there is a risk of competitive events (e.g. patients who die cannot have a hospitalization for HF). It also reduces the duration and costs of a trial. The most common way to analyse a composite endpoint is by assessing the time to the first occurring event with the standard Cox proportional hazards analysis. However, there is a need for a cautious interpretation, because if the intervention is proven effective in reducing the primary composite outcome, it does not necessarily mean that it reduces the risk of its components. For example, in the EMPEROR-Preserved trial, there was a significant 21% risk reduction in the primary outcome composed of cardiovascular mortality or hospitalization for HF with empagliflozin vs placebo, which was primarily driven by a 27% risk reduction in HF hospitalizations, whereas there was no significant reduction in cardiovascular mortality.[33] Furthermore, the use of a time-to-the-first event analysis neglects the fact that an individual can experience more than one non-fatal event. Alternatively, a composite endpoint can be analysed by models for recurrent events (e.g. regression models based on count data or Cox-based models including those of Andersen and Gill, Prentice, Williams and Peterson or, Wei, Lin and Weissfeld).[34] However, when using these more complex analyses, it must be taken into the account that for each event there exist separate processes that may be correlated or not, and that treatment effects may be different depending on the type and timing of an event. After the occurrence of an event, the risk for a subsequent event may change (e.g. the risk of death may increase following HF hospitalization), and this may also depend on the timing of the previous event. Also, the occurrence of the first event may modify the relative treatment effect for a subsequent event. Therefore, depending on the type of events included in the composite outcome, a careful selection of a recurrent events analysis is required to provide interpretable and meaningful results in the clinical context.[34]

A different approach to the analysis of composite outcomes is the use of win ratio.[35] The win ratio takes in the account the relative priorities of the components (by creating a clinically relevant hierarchical order of event analysis) and allows the components to be analysed as separate types of outcomes.[36] The order of analysis provides that the clinically most relevant outcomes are analysed first, whilst less important outcomes are tested only if more relevant ones have been accounted for. Inclusion of multiple components increases the study power (because more patients potentially had an 'event') and allows for the less relevant outcomes to be considered as a part of the primary outcome (e.g. treatment effect on quality of life and functional status). To perform this analysis patients in the intervention arm and the control group are arranged into matched pairs based on their risk profiles. If, for example, the composite outcome is made up of cardiovascular mortality and HF hospitalization, cardiovascular mortality is the first event to be analysed (because it is clinically more relevant). For each matched pair, the patient in the intervention arm is labelled a 'winner' or a 'loser' depending on who had experienced cardiovascular mortality first (if cardiovascular mortality occurred first in the control group patient, intervention group patient is labelled a 'winner').[35] If none of the patients in the matched pair have died, then they are labelled a 'winner' or a 'loser' depending on who had HF hospitalization first. If none of the composite component events has occurred, then they are considered tied. The win ratio is calculated as the total number of winners divided by the total numbers of losers.[35] When win ratio analysis was compared to the Cox proportional hazard analysis by reanalysing several clinical trials, the results were reassuringly similar with only minor differences in treatment effect size and p-values.[37] The win ratio analysis was recently used in the EMPULSE trial of empagliflozin in patients hospitalized for acute HF.[38]

Superiority vs non-inferiority RCTs

All the large pharmacological and device RCTs in HF have been designed to test the superiority of a treatment vs standard care (➲ Figure 15.1.2). The null hypothesis is that the treatment and control have the same efficacy and therefore the aim is to reject such a hypothesis and show that the treatment significantly reduces the risk of the primary outcome.[39]

Other trials might test non-inferiority or equivalence. Non-inferiority trials aim to demonstrate that treatments are equal in terms of treatment effect, that is a new treatment is not unacceptably worse than an established active control. In particular, in order to demonstrate non-inferiority, the lower bound of the confidence interval of the treatment effect difference between the new intervention and the active control has to be higher than a pre-specified non-inferiority margin.[39] Significance level is usually set as one-sided p-value of 0.025. The non-inferior margin can consist of an absolute difference or a risk ratio, and since it can have great influence on the trial outcome, the rational for its choice and whether it is based on absolute or relative scale must be clearly stated a priori. Both clinical and statistical considerations explain the choice of a specific non-inferiority margin.[40] Although the new treatment might be 'only' non-inferior to the gold standard therapy, a better safety profile, lower costs, or better manageability might lead the new treatment to become the preferred one. In equivalence trials, the aim is to demonstrate that the new treatment is non-inferior and non-superior compared to

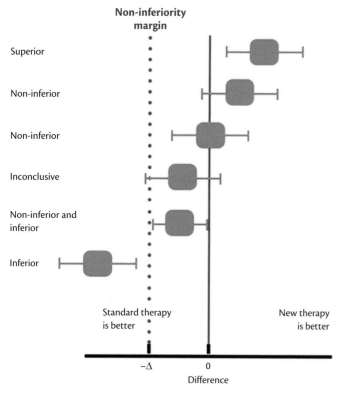

Figure 15.1.2 Superiority vs non-inferiority randomized controlled trials. Reproduced from Head SJ, Kaul S, Bogers AJ, Kappetein AP. Non-inferiority study design: lessons to be learned from cardiovascular trials. *Eur Heart J.* 2012 Jun;33(11):1318-24. doi: 10.1093/eurheartj/ehs099 with permission from Oxford University Press.

the gold standard, and therefore two margins are considered rather than only the non-inferiority one, and the significance level is set as a two-sided p value of 0.05.[40]

Different potential trial designs in HF

The parallel arm design is the most commonly used study design in HF trials. At the time of randomization patients are allocated to the treatment or control (e.g. placebo) arm, and then followed-up over time.

A crossover design is less frequently used in HF trials: two or more treatments are consecutively administered to each study participant. Advantage of this study design is the removal of between-subject differences since within-patient comparisons are analysed, that is, each study participant is the control of himself/herself due to the fact that he/she receives both the treatment and the control during different phases of the study. This leads to greater biological homogeneity and the need of a smaller sample size compared with parallel arm designs. One key assumption for this study design is that the treatment effect is temporary and disappears before the next study drugs is initiated, that is, there is no carry-over effect. Therefore, a washout period might be needed before starting the next treatment. A crossover design is not appropriate if the primary outcome is irreversible, for example, mortality.[41] One example for crossover trial design in HF is the NEAT-HFpEF trial.[42] Patients with HFpEF were randomized to

a 6-week dose-escalation regimen of isosorbide mononitrate (30, 60, 120 mg once daily) or placebo, with crossover to the other group for 6 weeks. Patients could be first assigned to 6 weeks of placebo and then switch to isosorbide mononitrate or vice versa. Primary outcome was the daily activity level. The same patient was compared with him/herself during the different treatment periods.[42]

A factor design is used to investigate two or more independent interventions in the same RCT.[43,44] In a 2 × 2 factorial design patients are randomized to treatment A or placebo A, and then patients receiving both treatment A or placebo A are also randomized to treatment B or placebo B. As a consequence, there will be four trial arms, that is, treatment A + treatment B; treatment A + placebo B; placebo A + treatment B, placebo A + placebo B. Benefits of this trial design includes the improved efficiency, that is less need of resources and smaller sample size compared with conducting two trials to investigate two research questions. Cons are linked with the assumption that the two investigated treatments do not interact, and if they do, estimates might be not precise and biased. An example of 2 × 2 factorial design in HF is the DANHEART trial, randomizing 1500 HFrEF patients to hydralazine-isosorbide dinitrate or placebo (H-HeFT) and to metformin or placebo (Met-HeFT).[45]

An adaptive design allows modification of the design during the conduct of the study based on the accumulating data to maximize statistical efficiency and improve outcome/reduce risk in trial participants.[46,47] For example, response-adaptive randomization allows to modify randomization ratio (e.g. from 1:1 to 2:1, 3:1) in favour of the treatment arm if the accumulating evidence shows that the treatment might be beneficial. Other features of adaptive RCTs include group sequential stopping, sample size re-estimation, which might be also used to repower non-inferiority trials to show superiority during an interim analysis, and enrichment strategies (e.g. biomarkers-based) (➲ Figure 15.1.3).[47] Since the adaptive approach is based on an evaluation of the treatment effect in posterior probabilities, Bayesian statistical approaches are usually adopted. In an adaptive platform RCT multiple treatments, for example—four to five different drugs, can be tested in parallell vs a control/placebo and at multiple pre-specified interim analyses withdrawn or continuation might be decided based on signals of futility or efficacy, respectively.[46]

Registry-based RCTs (RRCT) aim to improve trial efficiency by reducing complexity and costs through using registries for several elements involved in the conductance of a RCT.[48] Automated procedures can be implemented in a registry to automatically identify patients fulfilling the selection criteria to enter the RCT, that is, screening, which favour minimally selected consecutive enrollment. Since patients' data are already available within the registry, whether a patient is randomized, further data collection through complex case report forms might not be needed. In a RRCT, a registry can also be used for ascertaining the occurrence of a key trial endpoint, for example, mortality, without need of adjudication. A RRCT is the ideal environment to efficiently and effectively perform in a randomized setting an open-label assessment of

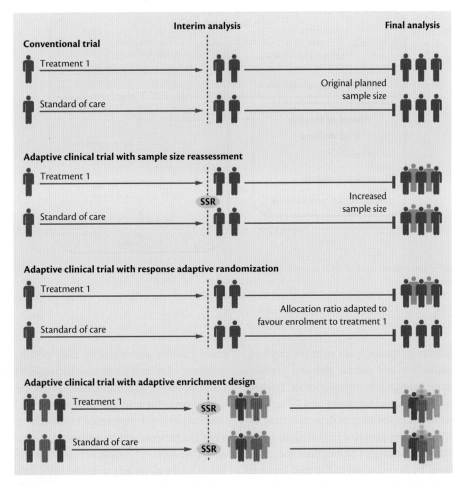

Figure 15.1.3 Adaptive trial design.
SSR, sample size reassessment.
Source: Thorlund K, Haggstrom J, Park JJ, Mills EJ. Key design considerations for adaptive clinical trials: a primer for clinicians. *BMJ*. 2018 Mar 8;360:k698. doi: 10.1136/bmj.k698. PMID: 29519932; PMCID: PMC5842365.Creative Commons CC-BY-NC 4.0 (https://creativecommons.org/licenses/by-nc/4.0/).

an already available treatment, when an extensive monitoring for safety issues is not required and the outcomes is univocally defined. Conversely, in a setting where a comprehensive safety assessment is required, blinding is preferred, many patient characteristics need to be collected, and formal adjudication of clinical events is required, some but not all the functionalities of a RRCT could be implemented.[48] An example of RRCT in HF is the SPIRRIT-HFpEF trial planning to randomize 3200 patients with HF and EF ≥ 40% 1:1 to open label spironolactone or eplerenone in addition to usual care vs usual care alone. Primary outcome is a composite of cardiovascular death and total HF hospitalizations. For the sites enrolling in Sweden, prospective and retrospective screening is performed though the Swedish HF registry. Randomization is executed after the signature of the informed consent through a module integrated within the registry. Patient baseline characteristics are obtained through the Swedish HF registry and exported to the trial case report form, which also includes information on laboratory values and treatment decisions collected during the follow-up. SPIRRIT-HFpEF has a PROBE design, and therefore although endpoint data are collected through the linkage of the Swedish HF registry with the National Patient Registry and the

Cause of Death Registry, formal adjudication by a blinded adjudication committee is then required[49] (➲ Figure 15.1.4).

Key approaches to the analysis of RCT data: intention-to-treat vs per-protocol analysis

In an RCT, after randomization patients might deviate from the trial protocol, for example, discontinue the treatment, being lost to follow-up, etc. Although it might seem attractive to exclude these patients from the statistical analyses to ensure integrity, this would lead to several issues: (1) violation of the randomization: removal of a study participant from one arm might lead to unbalanced study arms in terms of patient characteristics; (2) selection bias: patients with more severe disease might be more likely to experience adverse events and discontinue the study treatment, which might lead to a selective exclusion of sicker patients and unbalanced study arms; (3) reduction of the sample size; (4) deviation from daily clinical practice, where even if patients are prescribed with a treatment they might actively not take it, and therefore the benefits observed in a RCT would exaggerate what later is observed in clinical practice.[50] Therefore, the main scope of conducting an intention-to-treat (ITT) analysis of RCT data,

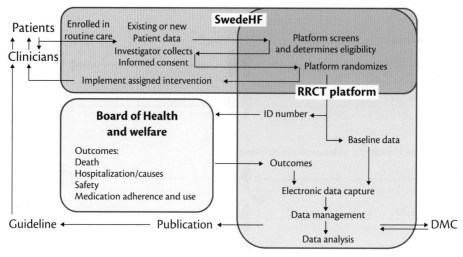

Figure 15.1.4 SPIRRIT-HFpEF registry-based randomized controlled trial platform (RRCT).
DMC, data monitoring committee.
Reproduced from Lund LH, Oldgren J, James S. Registry-Based Pragmatic Trials in Heart Failure: Current Experience and Future Directions. *Curr Heart Fail Rep.*
2017 Apr;14(2):59-70. doi: 10.1007/s11897-017-0325-0 with permission from Springer.

that is, including the patients in the analyses as at the random-ization, preserves randomization and sample size and prevents biases. This is the preferred approach in superiority RCT where demonstrating efficacy is the aim, and adopting an ITT analysis is more conservative, that is, the probability of demonstrating su-periority is less compared with a per-protocol (PP) analysis where patients received the treatment strategies throughout the entire follow-up period as defined by the protocol of the trial (optimal conditions). In equivalence and non-inferiority RCTs, a PP ana-lysis might be more conservative since ITT might tend to attenuate between-arms differences, which might make the demonstration of non-inferiority/equivalence more likely.[39] Therefore, for non-inferiority/equivalence trials both ITT and PP might be more similar in importance.[39] Overall, ITT remains the gold standard for main RCT analysis and use of PP as supporting sensitivity analysis is recommended, in particular in non-inferiority trials. PP analyses might provide important hypothesis-generating re-sults, suggesting treatment effects when adequate strategies for improving patients' compliance are implemented.[50] They might be also particularly relevant for safety analyses, where it is rele-vant to know whether the study participant is or not on treatment. The term modified intention-to-treat is quite widely used to de-scribe an analysis that excluded those participants who did not receive a defined minimum amount of the intervention.[51]

Subgroup and post-hoc analyses of RCTs

A subgroup analysis is defined as the assessment of the treatment effect for a specific outcome in subgroups of patients defined ac-cording to specific baseline characteristics.[52] Subgroup analysis are defined 'pre-specified' when planned at the time of the trial design in terms of considered patient characteristics, and statistical methods used include test for interaction. Pre-specification prevents the possibility of publishing only subgroups providing significant re-sults and therefore pre-specified subgroups analyses are considered

more credible and valuable than post-hoc analyses.[52,53] The as-sessment of several subgroups increases the chance of type I error (false positive), and multiplicity might be addressed with formal adjustments for multiple comparisons.[54] Whether stratified ran-domization is not performed to consider specific patient strata, for example, patients with vs without diabetes in EMPEROR-Reduced and DAPA-HF,[17,18] treatment and control groups might not be balanced for all patient characteristics within the different strata of patients. Additionally, lack of a statistically significant interaction might be explained by the lack of statistical power rather than by the lack of heterogeneity in treatment effect, and therefore whether or not inferential subgroup analysis is the objective, stratified ran-domization, subgroup size, and power must be adequately con-sidered at the time of trial design.[54] Subgroup analyses showing no heterogeneity in the context of a positive RCT might be supportive but still considered in light of what reported above, for example underpower.[54] In neutral trials, exploratory subgroup analyses can be at best considered hypothesis generating. For example, in the PARAGON-HF trial, sacubitril/valsartan significantly reduced the primary outcome (cardiovascular death or total HF hospitaliza-tions) in patients with lower ejection fraction and in women but not in the overall trial population.[55] This finding, affected by all the above-mentioned limitations of subgroup analyses and coming from an overall neutral trial, can only be considered hypothesis generating. Clinical plausibility and confirmation of findings iden-tified through subgroup analysis in subsequent ad-hoc designed RCTs are always needed.

Summary and key messages

♦ RCTs represent the gold standard to test treatment benefit in medicine.

♦ Randomization is the only procedure that allows an unbiased evaluation of treatment efficacy, allowing for controlling for any known and unknown, measured and unmeasured confounder.

- Observational studies allow adjustments for known and measured confounders, but not for unknown or unmeasured confounders.
- Blinding procedures represent a further strategy to reduce risk of bias in RCTs.
- Selection criteria in RCTs aim to include population that the intervention is intended for.
- Broad selection criteria increase generalizability of RCTs findings but might increase the risk of competing events. Specific selection criteria aim to enrich the trial population for the occurrence of cardiovascular endpoints of interest and reduce the risk of competing events.
- ITT analysis is the gold standard for main RCT analysis and using PP as supporting sensitivity analysis is recommended, in particular in non-inferiority trials.
- Subgroup analyses are defined 'pre-specified' when planned at the time of the trial design. Pre-specification prevents a selective reporting of results, and therefore pre-specified subgroups analyses are considered more credible and valuable than post-hoc analyses.
- Novel and more dynamic trial design might make possible running more, more effective, and cheaper randomized controlled trials in the heart failure field.

References

1. Evidence-Based Medicine Working G. Evidence-based medicine. A new approach to teaching the practice of medicine. JAMA. 1992;268(17):2420–5.
2. McDonagh TA, Metra M, Adamo M, Gardner RS, Baumbach A, Bohm M, et al. 2021 ESC Guidelines for the diagnosis and treatment of acute and chronic heart failure. Eur Heart J. 2021;42(36):3599–726.
3. Pearce W, Raman S, Turner A. Randomised trials in context: practical problems and social aspects of evidence-based medicine and policy. Trials. 2015;16:394.
4. Freedman B. Equipoise and the ethics of clinical research. N Engl J Med. 1987;317(3):141–5.
5. Stanley K. Design of randomized controlled trials. Circulation. 2007;115(9):1164–9.
6. Hare JM, Bolli R, Cooke JP, Gordon DJ, Henry TD, Perin EC, et al. Phase II clinical research design in cardiology: learning the right lessons too well: observations and recommendations from the Cardiovascular Cell Therapy Research Network (CCTRN). Circulation. 2013;127(15):1630–5.
7. Pocock SJ. Allocation of patients to treatment in clinical trials. Biometrics. 1979;35(1):183–97.
8. Akobeng AK. Understanding randomised controlled trials. Arch Dis Child. 2005;90(8):840–4.
9. Norgaard M, Ehrenstein V, Vandenbroucke JP. Confounding in observational studies based on large health care databases: problems and potential solutions - a primer for the clinician. Clin Epidemiol. 2017;9:185–93.
10. Pitt B, Zannad F, Remme WJ, Cody R, Castaigne A, Perez A, et al. The effect of spironolactone on morbidity and mortality in patients with severe heart failure. Randomized Aldactone Evaluation Study Investigators. N Engl J Med. 1999;341(10):709–17.
11. Zannad F, McMurray JJ, Krum H, van Veldhuisen DJ, Swedberg K, Shi H, et al. Eplerenone in patients with systolic heart failure and mild symptoms. N Engl J Med. 2011;364(1):11–21.
12. Ponikowski P, Voors AA, Anker SD, Bueno H, Cleland JG, Coats AJ, et al. 2016 ESC Guidelines for the diagnosis and treatment of acute and chronic heart failure: The Task Force for the diagnosis and treatment of acute and chronic heart failure of the European Society of Cardiology (ESC). Developed with the special contribution of the Heart Failure Association (HFA) of the ESC. Eur J Heart Fail. 2016;18(8):891–975.
13. Lund LH, Svennblad B, Melhus H, Hallberg P, Dahlstrom U, Edner M. Association of spironolactone use with all-cause mortality in heart failure: a propensity scored cohort study. Circ Heart Fail. 2013;6(2):174–83.
14. Roberts C, Torgerson D. Randomisation methods in controlled trials. BMJ. 1998;317(7168):1301.
15. Broglio K, Randomization in clinical trials: permuted blocks and stratification. JAMA. 2018;319(21):2223–4.
16. Kernan WN, Viscoli CM, Makuch RW, Brass LM, Horwitz RI. Stratified randomization for clinical trials. J Clin Epidemiol. 1999;52(1):19–26.
17. Packer M, Butler J, Filippatos GS, Jamal W, Salsali A, Schnee J, et al. Evaluation of the effect of sodium-glucose co-transporter 2 inhibition with empagliflozin on morbidity and mortality of patients with chronic heart failure and a reduced ejection fraction: rationale for and design of the EMPEROR-Reduced trial. Eur J Heart Fail. 2019;21(10):1270–8.
18. McMurray JJV, DeMets DL, Inzucchi SE, Kober L, Kosiborod MN, Langkilde AM, et al. A trial to evaluate the effect of the sodium-glucose co-transporter 2 inhibitor dapagliflozin on morbidity and mortality in patients with heart failure and reduced left ventricular ejection fraction (DAPA-HF). Eur J Heart Fail. 2019;21(5):665–75.
19. Schulz KF, Grimes DA. Blinding in randomised trials: hiding who got what. Lancet. 2002;359(9307):696–700.
20. Felker GM, Ahmad T, Anstrom KJ, Adams KF, Cooper LS, Ezekowitz JA, et al. Rationale and design of the GUIDE-IT study: Guiding Evidence Based Therapy Using Biomarker Intensified Treatment in Heart Failure. JACC Heart Fail. 2014;2(5):457–65.
21. Moss AJ, Brown MW, Cannom DS, Daubert JP, Estes M, Foster E, et al. Multicenter automatic defibrillator implantation trial-cardiac resynchronization therapy (MADIT-CRT): design and clinical protocol. Ann Noninvasive Electrocardiol. 2005;10(4 Suppl):34–43.
22. Kohro T, Yamazaki T. Cardiovascular clinical trials in Japan and controversies regarding prospective randomized open-label blinded end-point design. Hypertens Res. 2009;32(2):109–14.
23. Anker SD, Colet JC, Filippatos G, Willenheimer R, Dickstein K, Drexler H, et al. Rationale and design of Ferinject assessment in patients with IRon deficiency and chronic Heart Failure (FAIR-HF) study: a randomized, placebo-controlled study of intravenous iron supplementation in patients with and without anaemia. Eur J Heart Fail. 2009;11(11):1084–91.
24. Heiat A, Gross CP, Krumholz HM. Representation of the elderly, women, and minorities in heart failure clinical trials. Arch Intern Med. 2002;162(15):1682–8.
25. Savarese G, Orsini N, Hage C, Vedin O, Cosentino F, Rosano GMC, et al. Utilizing NT-proBNP for eligibility and enrichment in trials in HFpEF, HFmrEF, and HFrEF. JACC: Heart Failure. 2018;6(3):246–56.
26. Britton A, McKee M, Black N, McPherson K, Sanderson C, Bain C. Threats to applicability of randomised trials: exclusions and selective participation. J Health Serv Res Policy. 1999;4(2):112–21.
27. Savarese G, Hage C, Benson L, Schrage B, Thorvaldsen T, Lundberg A, et al. Eligibility for sacubitril/valsartan in heart failure across the ejection fraction spectrum: real-world data from the Swedish Heart Failure Registry. J Intern Med. 2021;289(3):369–84.
28. Ferreira JC, Patino CM. Types of outcomes in clinical research. J Bras Pneumol. 2017;43(1):5.

29. Andrade C. The primary outcome measure and its importance in clinical trials. J Clin Psychiatry. 2015;76(10):e1320–3.

30. Kendall JM. Designing a research project: randomised controlled trials and their principles. Emerg Med J. 2003;20(2):164–8.

31. Solomon SD, Zile M, Pieske B, Voors A, Shah A, Kraigher-Krainer E, et al. The angiotensin receptor neprilysin inhibitor LCZ696 in heart failure with preserved ejection fraction: a phase 2 double-blind randomised controlled trial. Lancet. 2012;380(9851):1387–95.

32. Solomon SD, McMurray JJV, Anand IS, Ge J, Lam CSP, Maggioni AP, et al. Angiotensin-neprilysin inhibition in heart failure with preserved ejection fraction. New Eng J Med. 2019;381(17):1609–20.

33. Anker SD, Butler J, Filippatos G, Ferreira JP, Bocchi E, Böhm M, et al. Empagliflozin in heart failure with a preserved ejection fraction. New Eng J Med. 2021;385(16):1451–61.

34. Ozga A-K, Kieser M, Rauch G. A systematic comparison of recurrent event models for application to composite endpoints. BMC Med Res Method. 2018;18(1):2.

35. Pocock SJ, Ariti CA, Collier TJ, Wang D. The win ratio: a new approach to the analysis of composite endpoints in clinical trials based on clinical priorities. Eur Heart J. 2012;33(2):176–82.

36. Redfors B, Gregson J, Crowley A, McAndrew T, Ben-Yehuda O, Stone GW, et al. The win ratio approach for composite endpoints: practical guidance based on previous experience. Eur Heart J. 2020;41(46):4391–9.

37. Ferreira JP, Jhund PS, Duarte K, Claggett BL, Solomon SD, Pocock S, et al. Use of the win ratio in cardiovascular trials. JACC: Heart Failure. 2020;8(6):441–50.

38. Voors AA, Angermann CE, Teerlink JR, Collins SP, Kosiborod M, Biegus J, et al. The SGLT2 inhibitor empagliflozin in patients hospitalized for acute heart failure: a multinational randomized trial. Nature Med. 2022;28(3):568–74.

39. Head SJ, Kaul S, Bogers AJ, Kappetein AP. Non-inferiority study design: lessons to be learned from cardiovascular trials. Eur Heart J. 2012;33(11):1318–24.

40. Macaya F, Ryan N, Salinas P, Pocock SJ. Challenges in the design and interpretation of noninferiority trials: insights from recent stent trials. J Am Coll Cardiol. 2017;70(7):894–903.

41. Li T, Yu T, Hawkins BS, Dickersin K. Design, analysis, and reporting of crossover trials for inclusion in a meta-analysis. PLoS One. 2015;10(8):e0133023.

42. Redfield MM, Anstrom KJ, Levine JA, Koepp GA, Borlaug BA, Chen HH, et al. Isosorbide mononitrate in heart failure with preserved ejection fraction. N Engl J Med. 2015;373(24):2314–24.

43. Jaki T, Vasileiou D. Factorial versus multi-arm multi-stage designs for clinical trials with multiple treatments. Stat Med. 2017;36(4):563–80.

44. Lubsen J, Pocock SJ. Factorial trials in cardiology: pros and cons. Eur Heart J. 1994;15(5):585–8.

45. Wiggers H, Kober L, Gislason G, Schou M, Poulsen MK, Vraa S, et al. The DANish randomized, double-blind, placebo controlled trial in patients with chronic HEART failure (DANHEART): A 2 × 2 factorial trial of hydralazine-isosorbide dinitrate in patients with chronic heart failure (H-HeFT) and metformin in patients with chronic heart failure and diabetes or prediabetes (Met-HeFT). Am Heart J. 2021;231:137–46.

46. Lawler PR, Hochman JS, Zarychanski R. What are adaptive platform clinical trials and what role may they have in cardiovascular medicine? Circulation. 2022;145(9):629–32.

47. Bhatt DL, Mehta C. Adaptive designs for clinical trials. N Engl J Med. 2016;375(1):65–74.

48. James S, Rao SV, Granger CB. Registry-based randomized clinical trials--a new clinical trial paradigm. Nat Rev Cardiol. 2015;12(5):312–6.

49. Lund LH, Oldgren J, James S. Registry-based pragmatic trials in heart failure: current experience and future directions. Curr Heart Fail Rep. 2017;14(2):59–70.

50. Tripepi G, Chesnaye NC, Dekker FW, Zoccali C, Jager KJ. Intention to treat and per protocol analysis in clinical trials. Nephrology (Carlton). 2020;25(7):513–7.

51. Schulz KF, Altman DG, Moher D, Group C. CONSORT 2010 statement: updated guidelines for reporting parallel group randomised trials. PLoS medicine. 2010;7(3):e1000251.

52. Wang R, Lagakos SW, Ware JH, Hunter DJ, Drazen JM. Statistics in medicine--reporting of subgroup analyses in clinical trials. N Engl J Med. 2007;357(21):2189–94.

53. Schuhlen H. Pre-specified vs. post-hoc subgroup analyses: are we wiser before or after a trial has been performed? Eur Heart J. 2014;35(31):2055–7.

54. Drexel H, Pocock SJ, Lewis BS, Saely CH, Kaski JC, Rosano GMC, et al. Subgroup analyses in randomized clinical trials: Value and limitations Review #3 on important aspects of randomized clinical trials in cardiovascular pharmacotherapy. Eur Heart J Cardiovasc Pharmacother. 2021:302–10.

55. Solomon SD, McMurray JJV, Anand IS, Ge J, Lam CSP, Maggioni AP, et al. Angiotensin-Neprilysin Inhibition in Heart Failure with Preserved Ejection Fraction. N Engl J Med. 2019;381(17):1609–20.

SECTION 16

Digital health in heart failure

CHAPTER 16.1

Digital health in heart failure

Arvind Singhal and Martin R Cowie

Introduction

Digital health technologies are emerging as some of the most powerful disrupters to how healthcare is delivered in the twenty-first century, and cardiologists have been at the forefront of this transformation. Heart failure (HF) physicians have been using some basic digital technologies for decades, such as telephone consultations and electronic health records, but digital technologies have so far had limited impact on how HF care was delivered. The conventional model of HF outpatient care, with scheduled face-to-face visits often many months apart, was largely unchanged for decades. The COVID-19 pandemic and the related social-distancing measures and health service demands accelerated implementation of digital technologies, with teleconsultation rapidly becoming the default option in many institutions, and with remote monitoring being used where this was possible. This chapter discusses the application of digital health in heart failure, including teleconsultation, remote monitoring, wearable devices, Apps, and electronic health records, along with the opportunities and barriers that need to be addressed to optimize the impact of these technologies on the outcome and experience of patient care, and workload for healthcare professionals and organizations.

What is digital health?

Digital health is defined by the World Health Organization (WHO) as *'a broad umbrella term encompassing e-Health, as well as emerging areas, such as the use of advanced computing sciences in 'Big Data', genomics and artificial intelligence'*, whereas e-Health is *'the use of information and communications technology in support of health and health-related fields'.*[1] ➲ Table 16.1.1 outlines key definitions in digital health, and ➲ Figure 16.1.1 illustrates the domains of digital health and e-health.

Digital health interventions increasingly underpin all healthcare activity, but healthcare settings are at different levels of digital maturity. The smartphone has been a key driver for digital transformation, even in resource-poor settings where they provide an opportunity to deliver care and advice to traditionally poorly served areas. The smartphone today is a portable, powerful personal computer and communications device. Smartphone penetration ranges from 80% of adults in high income countries such as USA, UK, France and Germany, to 60% in China, and 37% in India,[2] but smartphone usage in lower income countries is growing rapidly.

As technologies evolve and begin to demonstrate clinical and cost-effectiveness, healthcare organizations are increasingly being asked to assess how and where digital health may improve or support clinical and organizational practice. A report into digital

Table 16.1.1 Definitions

Term	Definition
Digital health	A broad umbrella term encompassing eHealth (which includes mHealth), as well as emerging areas, such as the use of advanced computing sciences in 'big data', genomics and artificial intelligence
e-Health	The use of information and communications technology in support of health and health-related field
m-Health	Medical and public health practice supported by mobile devices
Telehealth	Delivery of health care services, where patients and providers are separated by distance (often used interchangeably with telemedicine)
Teleconsultation	The use of information and communications technology to consult with patients or other providers separated by distance
Remote monitoring	A subset of telehealth that facilitates patient monitoring as well as the timely transfer of patient-generated data from patient to care team and back to the patient (often used interchangeably with telemonitoring)
Wearable	A non-invasive sensor that is worn i.e. a device that is externally applied to the body, measures a signal and collects these data which can then be transmitted and/or stored for further analysis and decision-making

transformation in healthcare before the COVID-19 pandemic, led by the cardiologist Eric Topol, was commissioned by the UK Secretary of State for Health to help identify key opportunities for digital health.[3] The areas he predicted to demonstrate the largest short-term impact included telemedicine, smartphone applications (Apps), and sensors and wearables for remote diagnostic purposes. Other digital technologies, such as artificial intelligence, big data, and robotics, are likely to play an increasing role (particularly in image interpretation and predictive analytics) over a longer period of time.

Teleconsultation

Teleconsultation (consultation with patients or other healthcare professionals separated by distance using information and communications technology) had been encouraged by healthcare systems as a solution to overburdened outpatient departments before the COVID-19 pandemic,[4] but its usage in hospital outpatient services was exceptional until recently. A report on telemedicine by the Organisation for Economic Co-operation and Development (OECD) found that the number of teleconsultations represented just 0.1–0.2% of all face-to-face consultations in OECD countries,[5] with a lack of clear reimbursement mechanisms cited as the most frequent barrier to adopting telemedicine services. Video consultations have been generally well received in primary care,[6,7] but have so far had limited evaluation in HF specialist care.

A small study in HF patients found video consultations to be broadly acceptable for patients chosen by their clinician as being appropriate for video consultation, but challenges included establishing a good connection, communication difficulties due to latency and connection degradation, and difficulty in conducting examinations (see ⮩ Table 16.1.2 for suggestions on how to address these issues).[8] Another study explored 'virtual' physical examinations via video consultation in HF patients in more detail: video consultations conducted by HF nurses were complemented by remote physiological measurements from home sphygmomanometers and oxygen saturation probes. Although in all patients some form of examination was accomplished, the clinical team found significant challenges in performing an examination for HF via video consultations, with particular difficulties in communicating examination instructions (such as feeling for leg oedema) and ensuring patients or carers conducted the examination whilst simultaneously making it visible to the clinician.[9]

In March 2020 as the COVID-19 pandemic swept across the world, many health care organizations rapidly moved to teleconsultation for routine outpatient appointments to minimize the risk of COVID-19

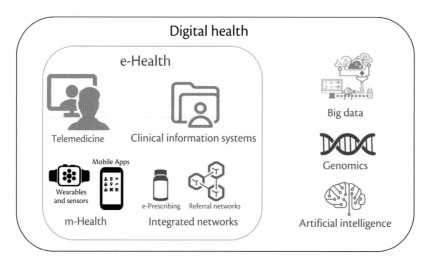

Figure 16.1.1 Domains of digital health and e-Health.

Table 16.1.2 Challenges to conducting video consultations for HF patients, and suggested solutions

Challenges	Possible solution
Difficulty using video consultation platform	◆ Careful selection of platform ◆ Clear instructions sent in advance
Awkward start to consultation	◆ Clear introduction, check audio and visual feed, establish rapport and explain what to expect
Privacy concerns	◆ Use of secure, encrypted platform ◆ Ensure consultation takes place in private place on both sides ◆ Participants clarify if anyone else is present in consultation out of view
Disruption in audio/video feed	◆ Test hardware and platform before consultation ◆ Ensure fast internet connection on both sides ◆ Telephone as backup ◆ Summarize key points of conversation at the end and check understanding
Latency resulting in conversational overlap	◆ Turn-taking in conversation ◆ Invite patient to continue if accidental interruption
Difficulty in conducting examinations	◆ Clear instructions and acknowledgement of limitations

transmission to patients and staff. To incentivize this, reimbursement mechanisms were amended in several healthcare systems; in the USA, for example, temporary measures allowed telehealth services to be billed as if they were in-person services for patients enrolled in Medicare or Medicaid, resulting in more than a 2000-fold increase in telemedicine consultations between January and June 2020.[10] Similarly, in France where reimbursement of telehealth technologies was made available before the COVID-19 pandemic, the number of physicians providing teleconsultations rose from 3000 in February 2020 to 56,000 in April 2020.[11] The extent to which enthusiasm for teleconsultation will remain after the COVID-19 pandemic will be determined by clinician and patient experience during this widespread rollout, and reimbursement, but teleconsultation is likely to play a larger role in the routine management in HF outpatient care than before the pandemic.

Remote monitoring for decompensation of HF

In addition to teleconsultation, telemedicine also includes remote monitoring (RM, also termed telemonitoring), which is the use of telecommunication technologies to monitor patient status at a distance. ➲ Figure 16.1.2 illustrates the principles behind RM in HF care, and ➲ Table 16.1.3 lists key randomized controlled trials (RCTs) in RM.

HF decompensation is a critical event with high mortality; European registry data show that hospitalization carries a 24% risk of death within 1 year.[12] Early signs of decompensation are unlikely to coincide with a routine outpatient clinic appointment, and patients tend to seek professional advice only when their symptoms are advanced.[13] Identifying when patients may be deteriorating at a point when intervention may re-stabilize the syndrome without the need for hospitalization has obvious attractions. Motivated patients have long been encouraged to self-monitor symptoms, weight, and other physiological variables, such as blood pressure; however, many HF patients lack the requisite knowledge, equipment (such as scales and automatic sphygmomanometers), or confidence for effective self-care. Access to clinical advice, often through an HF nurse telephone service, is therefore critical to ensure patients are supported in their journey of self-care.

Structured telephone support

Structured telephone support (STS) offers a basic level of RM; patients are called by a member of the HF team to discuss symptoms, drug therapy, and compliance with lifestyle measures. They may be asked to provide measurements, for example weight and blood pressure or pulse rate. STS has been deployed in various forms in different healthcare settings with mixed results. a 2015 meta-analysis reported a marginal mortality benefit (risk ratio 0.87 for all-cause mortality; 95% CI, 0.77–0.98) and reduction in HF hospitalizations (risk ratio, 0.85; 95% CI 0.77–0.93) but no effect on all-cause hospitalizations.[14] Given that telephone calls are primarily initiated by healthcare professionals at pre-set, protocol-driven times, they are often unable to detect more rapid changes in clinical status. STS is relatively labour-intensive, and costs vary according to the intensity of monitoring: a 2013 health technology assessment projected costs between £31.60 and £235 (€35–€265) per patient per year in the UK.[15]

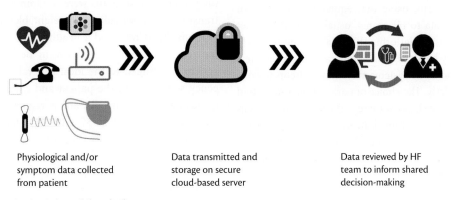

Physiological and/or symptom data collected from patient   Data transmitted and storage on secure cloud-based server   Data reviewed by HF team to inform shared decision-making

Figure 16.1.2 Remote monitoring in heart failure (HF).

Table 16.1.3 Key randomized controlled trials in remote monitoring of HF

Study	Patient population	Intervention	Endpoints	Results
Non-invasive remote monitoring				
Tele-HF (Chaudhry 2010)[67]	1653 patients with recent HF hospitalization	Interactive telephone system	All-cause death or hospitalization	No significant difference between groups
TIM-HF (Koehler 2011)[68]	710 HF patients NYHA II or III with LVEF ≤ 35% and history of HF decompensation within previous 2 years or LVEF ≤ 25%	Telemonitoring system collecting ECG, blood pressure and body weight data, connected to 24/7 call centre	All-cause death Composite of cardiovascular death and hospitalization	No significant difference between groups
BEAT HF (Ong 2016)[69]	1437 patients with recent HF hospitalization	Health coaching telephone calls and telemonitoring collecting blood pressure, heart rate, weight, and symptom data	All-cause hospitalization	No significant difference between groups
TIM-HF2 (Koehler 2018)[16]	1571 HF patients with NYHA II or III and history of HF hospitalization within previous 12 months, without depression	Telemonitoring system collecting ECG, blood pressure, body weight, oxygen saturation and health status questionnaire data, connected to 24/7 call centre	Percentage of days lost to unplanned cardiovascular hospitalization or all-cause death	Primary outcome 4.88% in RM group vs 6.64% in control group (p = 0.046)
CIED based remote monitoring				
DOT-HF (Van Veldhuisen 2011)[20]	335 HFrEF (LVEF ≤35%) patients with ICD or CRT and HF hospitalization within previous 12 months	Audible patient alert from device for reduced thoracic impedance	Composite of All-cause mortality and HF hospitalization	Increased HF hospitalization in intervention group: hazard ratio 1.79 (1.08–2.95, p = 0.022)
IN-TIME (Hindricks 2014)[22]	664 HFrEF (LVEF ≤35%) patients with NYHA II-III with ICD or CRT without permanent AF	Device RM collecting multiparameter data transmitted daily and reviewed by healthcare professionals	Composite score of all-cause death, HF hospitalization, change in NYHA class and change in self-assessment	Primary outcome reduced in intervention group (worsening score 18.9% in intervention vs 27.2% in control, p = 0.013)
REM-HF (Morgan 2017)[21]	1650 HF patients with ICD or CRT	Device RM collecting multiparameter data transmitted weekly and reviewed by healthcare professionals	Death from any cause or unplanned cardiovascular hospitalization	No significant difference between groups
Implantable haemodynamic monitor				
CHAMPION (Abraham 2011)[24]	550 HF patients with NYHA III and HF hospitalization within previous 12 months	Daily remote pulmonary artery pressure monitoring reviewed by healthcare professionals	Rate of HF hospitalization at 6 months	Primary outcome reduced in intervention group: hazard ratio 0.63 (0.52–0.77, p < 0.0001)

AF, atrial fibrillation, CIED, cardiac implantable electronic devices , CRT, cardiac resynchronization therapy, ECG, electrocardiography, HF, heart failure, HFrEF, heart failure with reduced ejection fraction, ICD, implantable cardioverter–defibrillator, LVEF, left ventricular ejection fraction, NYHA, New York Heart Association, RM, remote monitoring.

Non-invasive remote monitoring systems

A less labour-intensive and more automated type of RM is a non-invasive 'standalone' system, using the regular transmission of selected physiological data to HF teams, usually via an internet connection to a web-based platform. The data may be regularly reviewed, or teams may be alerted when a parameter is outside a pre-specified range, and some systems may allow patients to contact their HF team directly. The choice of parameters transmitted varies between different systems as there is no clear consensus as to which data are most useful, though heart rate, blood pressure, oxygen saturations, and weight are the most frequent features.

The evidence base for standalone telemonitoring systems is mixed, with RCTs failing to show consistent benefit. The largest positive RCT of telemonitoring is the TIM-HF2 study in which 1571 German HF patients with New York Heart Association (NYHA) class II–III symptoms and an HF hospitalization in the preceding 12 months were randomized to a wireless system, transmitting daily readings of weight, blood pressure, oxygen saturations, heart rate, and a health status questionnaire to a centralized 24/7 monitoring centre in Berlin, or usual care.[16] The system was linked to the local general practitioners, the emergency services, and the patient and carers. The composite outcome of all-cause mortality and percentage days hospitalized was reduced (risk ratio, 0.8; 95% CI, 0.65–1.00), though crucially this study excluded patients with depression, or NYHA class I or IV symptoms.

A Cochrane meta-analysis of 18 randomized telemonitoring trials showed a mortality benefit (risk ratio, 0.80 for all-cause mortality; 95% CI, 0.68–0.94) and reduction in HF-related hospitalizations (risk ratio, 0.71; 95%, CI 0.68–0.83);[14] however, the heterogeneity of interventions, health service structures, patients studied, and definitions of 'usual care' has made it difficult to make specific recommendations based on these data. However, the most recent HF guidelines of the European Society of Cardiology make a Class 2B, Level B 'may be considered' recommendation for the use of non-invasive home telemonitoring for patients with HF in order to reduce the risk of recurrent cardiovascular and HF hospitalization, and cardiovascular mortality (➲ Box 16.1.1).[17] During the COVID-19 pandemic remote monitoring of chronic conditions was recommended by many organizations, such as the Centre for Disease Controls and Prevention in the USA, in order to maintain continuity of care in the absence of face-to-face contact.[18] The European Society of Cardiology (ESC) guideline discusses the cessation of face-to-face consultations during the pandemic, highlighting some of the advantages of home telemonitoring, including maintenance of quality of care, facilitating rapid access to care when needed, reduced patient travel costs, and minimizing the frequency of face-to-face clinic visits.[17] Importantly, the guideline mentions that where social distancing is important, and with the rising importance of the 'green' agenda, home telemonitoring only needs to show non-inferiority (rather than superiority) to usual care to be recommended as an appropriate means of supporting care.[17]

Invasive remote monitoring through implantable devices

Invasive options for remote monitoring come in two main forms: cardiac implantable electronic devices (CIEDs), such as implantable cardioverter defibrillators with algorithms for detecting decompensation, and implantable haemodynamic monitors.

Some modern CIEDs come equipped with 'diagnostic' capabilities by collecting physiological data, such as intrathoracic impedance, heart rate variability, patient activity, and intensity of heart sounds. Intrathoracic impedance correlates negatively with pulmonary fluid content; increasing pulmonary oedema results in a fall in intrathoracic impedance.[19] Impedance measurements were therefore an obvious target for remote monitoring in CIEDs, but one randomized trial of device-based impedance alerts resulted in a 79% increase in HF hospitalization.[20] This may have resulted from the anxiety triggered by an audible alert from the device, alongside the low specificity of alerts when using impedance alone as a trigger.

Multiparameter monitoring, where several physiological variables are incorporated into alerts, has been developed to improve the sensitivity and specificity of decompensation alerts. Two large RCTs have assessed the impact on outcomes with differing results. The REM-HF study randomized 1650 patients with HF and a CIED to routine remote multi-parametric monitoring or usual care at nine English hospitals. Over an average follow-up of 2.8 years, RM failed to show an improvement over usual care in terms of death or hospitalization.[21] The IN-TIME study tested CIED monitoring using measures of tachyarrhythmia, suboptimal biventricular pacing, increased ventricular ectopy, and decreased patient activity, randomizing 664 patients to RM or usual care.[22] Patients in the RM group had a reduction in the primary endpoint of death, HF hospitalization, change in NYHA class, and change in patient self-assessment (odds ratio, 0.63; 95% CI, 0.43–0.90), though much of this benefit may have been principally realized in patients with atrial fibrillation. A promising multiparameter algorithm is the HeartLogic™ score. In the MultiSENSE study, a multiparameter algorithm combined data from heart sounds, respiration, thoracic impedance, heart rate, and activity to produce a personalized 'score' (the HeartLogic™ score); this algorithm was tested on 400 patients with CIEDs and HF and a score above the determined threshold had a 70% sensitivity and 86% specificity for predicting HF decompensation, with a median lead time of 34 days before decompensation.[23] Using this score to guide therapy is under evaluation in a RCT in the USA (NCT03237858).

Box 16.1.1 Guidelines on Remote Monitoring (RM) for HF events

European Society of Cardiology – 2021 ESC guidelines for the diagnosis and treatment of acute and chronic heart failure[17]

Recommendations for exercise, multidisciplinary management and monitoring of patients with heart failure

'Monitoring of pulmonary artery pressures using a wireless implantable haemodynamic monitoring system (CardioMems) may be considered in symptomatic patients with HF in order to improve clinical outcomes (Class IIb, level B.)

Non-invasive home telemonitoring may be considered for patients with HF in order to reduce the risk of recurrent cardiovascular and HF hospitalisation, and cardiovascular death (Class IIb, level B.)'

American College of Cardiology Foundation/American Heart Association – 2013 ACCF/AHA Guideline for the Management of Heart Failure[33]

Systems of care to promote care coordination for patients with chronic HF

'The quality of evidence is mixed for specific components of HF clinical management interventions, such as home-based care, disease management, and remote telemonitoring programs.'

'Overall, very few specific interventions have been consistently identified and successfully applied in clinical practice.'

American Heart Association – Using Remote Patient Monitoring Technologies for Better Cardiovascular Disease Outcomes (2019)[71]

Heart failure

'Although recent systematic reviews and meta analyses have shown a positive effect on HF-related admissions and mortality rates and all-cause mortality rates, the bulk of the literature consists of low-quality and inconsistent evidence about the beneficial effect [of remote monitoring].'

HF, heart failure; HFrEF, heart failure with reduced ejection fraction; LVEF, left ventricular ejection fraction, IN-TIME, INfluence of Home Monitoring on The clinical Management of heart failurE patients with impaired left ventricular function.

Implantable haemodynamic monitors

Implantable haemodynamic monitors have shown more promise at preventing HF hospitalization. Pulmonary artery pressure (PAP) increases in response to increasing intracardiac pressure or fluid volume, with rises in pressure typically preceding symptoms by some weeks. A randomized trial of an implanted wireless pulmonary artery pressure monitor (the CardioMEMS™ device) showed that remote daily PAP monitoring, and titration of medications in response to changes in pressure, reduced subsequent HF hospitalization by 33% in NYHA class III patients who had been admitted for HF in the previous year (hazard ratio, 0.57; 95% CI, 0.55–0.80).[24] Patients with heart failure with preserved ejection fraction (HFpEF) as well as heart failure with reduced ejection fraction (HFrEF) were included in the study, and data from NYHA Class III patients in Germany, The Netherlands, UK, and Ireland confirm this benefit,[25,26] The GUIDE HF study examined the impact in a broader spectrum of patients, including those with milder symptoms,[27] but was complicated by a dramatic reduction in HF hospitalization risk during COVID-19 lockdowns. In February 2022, the US Food & Drug Administration extended the approval for the use of CardioMEMS™ in HF patients in NYHA Class II with either an HF hospitalization in the previous year and/ or elevated natriuretic peptides. Cost-effectiveness may be more of a challenge to prove in the European setting, where the cost of hospitalization is substantially lower than in the USA; however, in England the National Institute for Health and Care Excellence recently approved its use in 'routine' specialist practice on the basis of the available evidence.[28] Pulmonary artery diastolic pressure is often used as a surrogate for left atrial pressure, but it is possible to directly measure left atrial pressure with wireless implantable devices. In 2016, the LAPTOP-HF randomized trial studied the use of a haemodynamic monitoring system collecting data from the left atrium (NCT01121107), but the trial was stopped early because of concern regarding the risk of implanting the left atrial pressure sensor across the inter-atrial septum. Following that setback, a newer left atrial pressure monitoring device is currently being studied for safety and efficacy (NCT03775161).

Wearables

The direct-to-consumer health technology industry, now worth billions of dollars annually, continues to grow year-on-year. Nearly 20% of Americans now report using fitness monitors to track their health statistics.[29] A key difference between remote monitoring systems and wearables is who pays; RM systems are generally 'prescribed' by clinicians and reimbursed or paid for by healthcare systems or insurance companies, but wearable devices such as activity monitors, heart rate monitors, and 'smart' watches are largely marketed directly to (and paid for by) consumers as tools for 'health and lifestyle maintenance'. As such, the incentives for development differ, with wearable technologies focusing little on proving clinical and cost-effectiveness, and more on user experience. Despite this, some wearable devices are becoming increasingly accurate and sophisticated in what they can measure.

We define a wearable device as a non-invasive sensor that is worn (i.e. a device that is externally applied to the body), measures a signal, and collects these data, which can then be transmitted and/or stored for further analysis and decision-making.[30] The continuous monitoring of physiological signals from a wearable device could, in theory, allow a more personalized and empowered experience for the person living with HF. Currently only limited data are available to guide their use in HF patients; commercial wearables tend to target younger, more technologically familiar consumers, whereas the average age of an HF patient is around 80 years in high income countries. Even where they have a smartphone, they may not use it as such, relying only on the ability to make and receive telephone calls. ➲ Figure 16.1.3 illustrates wearable technologies that may be used in HF, alongside implantable device and RM technologies currently in use. The current ESC HF guideline states that it is uncertain whether wearable technology for measuring heart rate or rhythm, and lung congestion, offer added benefits to conventional home telemonitoring.[17]

Activity monitors

Most wearable devices incorporate an activity monitor, which is usually an accelerometer measuring movement at the level of the device (usually the wrist). The movement data are then converted into estimates of physical activity by an algorithm; the exact mechanism of device and algorithm varies between manufacturers. A study validating the accuracy of 10 commercially available activity monitors found that most devices had very high accuracy estimating step count in laboratory conditions (i.e. walking on a treadmill), with half of the devices having < 1% error deviation.[31] The accuracy of monitors, however, is greatly influenced by the type of movement detected, with wrist-worn devices typically undercounting steps at low ambulation speeds and overcounting steps during sedentary activity (such as playing cards) in older adults,[32] which is particularly relevant for HF patients.

Exercise and rehabilitation

Exercise training in HF improves exercise capacity and quality of life, reduces the risk of hospitalization, and is a Class I recommendation in both the ESC and American College of Cardiology (ACC)–American Heart Association (AHA) guidelines for HF.[17,33] Activity monitors could potentially help with patient adherence and delivering exercise training at home to widen participation. A sub-study of the Teledi@log clinical trial found that cardiac rehabilitation participants (20% of whom had HF) increased their mean step count from a baseline of 5899 steps per day to 7890 steps per day after 1 year of telephone-based cardiac rehabilitation with Fitbit™ activity monitors.[34]

Functional classification and prognostication

Functional classification using NYHA class is subjective, and there is significant variation in assessment by healthcare professionals. Six-minute walk tests are cumbersome and rarely performed outside clinical trials, and formal cardiopulmonary exercise testing is expensive, time consuming, and has limited availability. Activity monitors could provide an objective measure of functional status

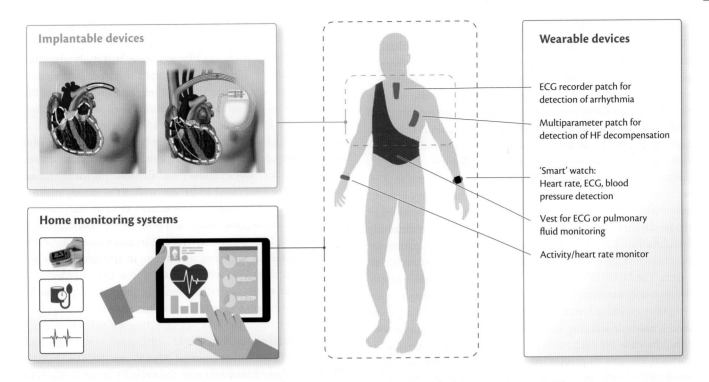

Figure 16.1.3 Wearables used in the monitoring of heart failure (HF) alongside implantable devices and remote monitoring systems. ECG, electrocardiogram.

based on an individual's usual activity patterns. Low step counts are associated with more severe symptoms and poorer prognosis. A study of 50 HF patients measured step counts over two weeks using activity monitors; mean step counts were significantly different between physician-assessed NYHA classes, although there was some overlap in activity levels between class II and III participants.[35] A prospective cohort study of 170 Japanese HF patients found that low step count (< 4889 steps per day), measured via a waist-worn monitor, was the strongest independent predictor of mortality over a median follow-up of 3.7 years, beating even VO_{2MAX} measured by exercise testing.[36] Currently no evidence or guidance exists as to whether these data can be used to guide decision-making or treatment.

Heart rate monitors

Many wrist-worn wearables are also able to measure heart rate using photoplethysmography (PPG). PPG works by illuminating a capillary bed with a light emitting diode and then measuring the pulsatile change in light absorption.[37] PPG-based heart rate measurement is very sensitive to artefact; thus, the type of activity being performed greatly influences its accuracy. A study of the accuracy of PPG wristbands in healthy volunteers found that during treadmill exercise the 95% limits of agreement with ECG were more than +/- 20 bpm for each of the four devices tested. A study specifically in HF patients found that Fitbit[TM] and Apple[TM] Watch devices consistently underestimated heart rate during exercise, particularly during dynamic heart rate change.[38] Thus, PPG-based heart rate monitoring may be best suited to measure resting or average heart rates in HF patients. They could theoretically be used, for example, to titrate negatively chronotropic HF

medications, such as β-blockers, though such use has not been studied in clinical trials.

Heart rate variability (HRV), which is a measure of the variation in the R–R interval, has been studied as a biomarker of several pathologies including HF. A reduction in HRV is associated with increased sympathetic nervous system activity and more advanced HF.[39] Intervals between pulse waves are closely related to R–R intervals, so PPG could be used to estimate HRV.[40] A validation study found that whilst PPG-derived pulse rate variability correlated well with HRV in healthy subjects at rest, the performance was significantly worse after exercise or in patients with pre-existing cardiovascular disease.[41] An American study aims to recruit 40 patients with HF to validate the Apple[TM] Watch's HRV algorithm against 24-hour Holter monitoring and correlate with patient health status (NCT04510779).

Blood pressure control

Blood pressure is an important measurement in HF; hypertension is a modifiable risk factor for HF and ischaemic heart disease, and hypotension result from the disease, or treatment with disease-modifying therapy or diuretics. Automatic oscillometric blood pressure cuffs have been in use for several years, but many now are able to connect with smartphones via Bluetooth® allowing easier recording of trends. Miniaturized oscillometric sphygmomanometers can now be incorporated into wristwatches. A smartwatch-integrated sphygmomanometer (Omron[TM] HeartGuide) showed excellent correlation with manual measurement across a range of blood pressures; the mean differences were -0.9 +/- 6.8 mmHg for systolic blood pressure and –1.1 +/- 5.5 mmHg for diastolic pressure, meeting American National Standards Institute criteria.[42]

Wearables for detection of HF decompensation

Wearable devices may also be able to act as non-invasive alternatives to remote monitoring systems for detection of HF decompensation (see above section on remote monitoring). Dielectric sensing (applying a low-power electromagnetic impulse across a tissue) is a non-invasive method of estimating pulmonary fluid content, similar to thoracic impedance. The Remote Dielectric Sensing (ReDS™) system is a wearable vest being studied for HF monitoring. In an observational study of 50 HF patients, ReDS™-directed titration of medical therapy was associated with an 87% reduction in hospitalization compared with the 90 days prior to enrolment, and a subsequent 79% increase in hospitalizations in the 90 days following removal of the vest.[43] The vest is currently being evaluated in a clinical trial (NCT03586336). Multiparameter patch sensors have also shown promise for the detection of HF events. The LINK-HF study investigated the use of a patch sensor continuously measuring ECG signals, thoracic impedance, body temperature, and accelerometry in 100 HF patients. Using these data, a machine learning algorithm was used to create a personalized baseline for each patient. Following this, a prognostic algorithm was able to predict impending decompensation with a sensitivity of 88% and a specificity of 86% a median of 6.5 days before the HF event.[44] Whether such alerts can provide a window for intervention to prevent HF hospitalization needs to be investigated further. Finally, multiple electrodes embedded in textiles could allow for extraction of data similar to those used by implanted device-based algorithms such as HeartLogic™, including heart rate, heart rate variability, respiratory rate, and thoracic impedance; a 'smart textile' vest measuring these parameters to predict HF decompensation is being studied in an ongoing trial (NCT03719079).

Arrhythmia detection in HF

Atrial fibrillation (AF) is common in HF, and the presence of AF has therapeutic implications, such as the need for decision making regarding oral anticoagulation and rate or rhythm control. Methods of AF detection have advanced beyond a simple 24-hour Holter monitor, and now a variety of options are available. For patients with paroxysmal symptoms, a patient-activated electrocardiogram (ECG) recorder such as the Kardia™ mobile device can provide symptom-ECG correlation; these devices are now regularly used in many high-income countries, and some reimbursement bodies, including the National Health Service (NHS) in England have provided a framework for reimbursement, allowing clinicians to 'prescribe' them.

For asymptomatic patients in whom there is a high clinical suspicion of AF, screening can involve either irregular pulse detection or ECG detection. ECG detection is the gold-standard, and options include Holter monitors which are typically worn for 24–48 hours, patch recorders which can record up to 2 weeks of data, wearable vests which can record up to 4 weeks of data, and finally implantable loop recorders which can last up to 2–3 years. Irregular pulse detection can be used in opportunistic screening, but requires confirmation with an ECG. PPG algorithms can detect irregular pulses, but cannot differentiate between AF and other causes.

The Apple Heart Study was a large-scale cohort study where the Apple™ Watch PPG algorithm was used to screen participants for AF. Patients who had an irregular pulse notification from the algorithm (0.5% of total study population) were asked to participate in a teleconsultation, and those who agreed were sent a 2-week ECG patch recorder. Thirty-four per cent of patients who sent back the patch had a confirmed episode of AF during the recording period; 77% of irregular pulse alerts during simultaneous recording were confirmed to be AF, with atrial ectopy making up most of the remainder.[45] Much like AF detected through implantable devices, however, it is still uncertain how these data can be best used. Further research is required into the utility of this approach in HF patients, and whether an intervention following opportunistic screening with a smart watch can improve outcomes such as stroke or death. A recently announced 'pragmatic' randomized trial aims to enrol 150,000 patients with an Apple™ Watch to investigate the effect of detecting AF through the device on all-cause mortality, stroke, anticoagulation usage, and health resource utilization amongst other things (NCT04276441). PPG-based algorithms could also theoretically generate alerts to other paroxysmal tachycardias;[46] feasibly a similar approach of ECG patch testing following a sudden tachycardia alert could be studied for the detection of ventricular tachycardia in heart failure patients, which could provide more data for decisions regarding defibrillator therapy. Further research is needed in this area, and currently no PPG-based technologies are licensed outside AF detection.

Apps

The growing demand for education and self-management has led to a proliferation of healthcare Apps over the past decade; in 2017 it was estimated that 325,000 health Apps were available on smartphones.[47] The scale of this booming market makes it challenging to regulate and for clinicians to know which apps to recommend. Language and local regulatory differences have so far prevented an international consensus on assessing healthcare Apps, leading local organizations to adopt their own assessment approach; the Catalan government, for example, created a public library of accredited health Apps with the Fundación TIC Salud Social (ICT Social Health Foundation).

One example of the use of healthcare Apps is remote access to healthcare information and services. Estonia's 'e-Health record' is an example of a nationwide system whereby patients and emergency services are able to remotely access summary health data via an 'e-Patient portal'. Other countries are similarly following suit; the UK NHS has recently launched the NHS App which allows patients to access their summary medical record (including test results) and book appointments, with further functionality such as repeat prescriptions planned in the near future. Patient education is a key factor in improving health outcomes, particularly in cardiovascular disease, with improvements in diet, exercise, smoking cessation, and medication compliance helping to optimize the outcome of care and lifestyle choices. Health literacy, which is the ability of patients to understand and use written healthcare information, is poor in Europe; in a study across eight European countries, 47% of participants had low or inadequate health literacy, rising to 61% for those with more than one long-term illness.[48] Sufficient knowledge for adequate self-care in HF patients is similarly lacking.[49] Despite this, a recent review identified only 10 Apps specifically designed for HF patients on Google Play and Apple App stores,[50] none of which have been evaluated in an RCT setting. Four of these were produced by scientific societies (including the American Heart Association). This may be because commercial demand for HF-specific Apps is currently low given the elderly demographic of HF patients, but as patients become more digitally engaged (smartphone penetration increases each year, even in the elderly population) Apps may prove more popular. An App-based HF disease management programme, with remote monitoring, drug titration decision support, and patient education, has been developed and evaluated in Canada.[51]

Electronic health records

Electronic health records (EHRs) are a key component of digital health. Different EHRs offer varying levels of functionality, from basic 'read-only' access to clinical notes, to real-time display of clinical signs and observations and electronic prescribing. There is no unified approach to EHRs across Europe; even within a single country, individual healthcare organizations typically must procure their own software and are at varying levels of digital maturity. Uptake of EHRs in primary care has been far ahead of hospital-based systems; a survey of primary care doctors across Europe found that 96% routinely use EHRs,[52] whereas hospitals have been slower to adopt and usually use different systems that do not integrate easily with primary care. Interoperability between systems is therefore a key challenge; data cannot easily be transferred from one system to another, the coding used may differ, and much of the information may not be easily searchable.

Across Europe, there is also the issue of language differences, and patients may have healthcare interactions across international borders. The European Union's (EU) 'eHealth Digital Service Infrastructure' (eHDSI) aims to allow cross-border sharing of EHRs, electronic prescription and dispensation of medications by 2021 in 22 EU countries. Ninety per cent of EU citizens expect to be able to access their own health data,[53] but the ability to do this is currently limited, and consequently there is a political drive in the EU to ensure better access of citizens to their own health data, within the constraints of digital security and confidentiality.

Whilst patients and politicians are enthusiastic for EHRs, they have so far had a mixed reception from clinicians: a survey of US primary care physicians reported that although 63% believed EHRs have generally led to improved care, 74% reported that using an EHR increased their workload, and 68% stated that EHRs took valuable time away from patient care.[54] A time and motion study from the US showed that 49% of clinician time was spent on EHRs and administration.[55] This may be because EHRs are often procured on the basis of their administrative functionality, such as for billing, rather than on clinician user experience.

Fears of over-reliance on technology may also contribute to scepticism of EHRs, as system failures can bring organizations to a halt. In 2017, the UK NHS was struck by a cyberattack, resulting in near-total computer blackouts in infected trusts; one acute trust, the second largest in the UK, was estimated to have lost £4.8 million (€5.5 million) from lost activity and IT costs[56] during the attack. Cybersecurity and backup protocols are therefore of the utmost importance to ensure confidence in EHRs.

Data from remote monitoring devices and wearables can complement data already in many EHRs, such as blood and imaging results. EHRs are vital for synthesizing these different data streams to assist clinical decision making and patient-clinician interactions (❯ Figure 16.1.2). Interoperability between these IT systems is therefore crucial, but difficult to achieve without clear, mandated Application Programming Interface (API) standards; this requires international co-ordination and regulation. Without automatic integration with EHRs, gathering patient data generates extra work for clinicians or administrative staff, and adds potential for error. Accurately recording all data that can influence a clinical decision is vital from both a clinical and medicolegal point of view.

Some EHRs allow embedding of algorithms which can be used as decision aids. An example of basic algorithms is the use of alerts when a certain parameter or threshold is met, such as an alert for acute kidney injury (AKI). Unfortunately, many decision aids are embedded based on assumptions as opposed to RCT data. A recent large RCT of over 6000 patients found that EHR-based AKI alerts made no difference overall to the primary endpoint of progression of AKI, receipt of dialysis, or death, but analysis of non-teaching hospitals found the primary endpoint higher with the intervention (relative risk, 1.49; 95% CI, 1.12–1.98; p = 0.006), driven by increased mortality.[57] More refined algorithms with greater predictive power may be produced by machine learning, but they must also demonstrate an ability to improve clinical outcomes.

Barriers to the implementation of digital health

The EU e-Health action plan 2012–2020[58] identified several barriers to widespread implementation of digital health technologies including:

- lack of awareness of, and confidence in e-Health solutions among patients, citizens and healthcare professionals
- lack of interoperability between e-Health solutions
- limited large-scale evidence of the cost-effectiveness of e-Health tools and services
- lack of legal clarity for health and wellbeing mobile applications and the lack of transparency regarding the utilization of data collected by such applications
- inadequate or fragmented legal frameworks including the lack of reimbursement schemes for e-Health services
- high start-up costs involved in setting up e-Health systems
- regional differences in accessing ICT services, limited access in deprived areas.

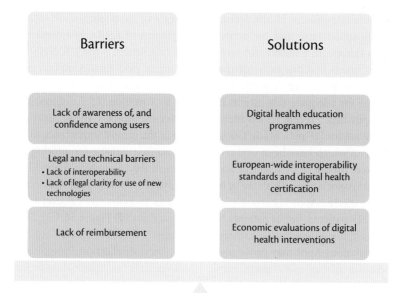

Figure 16.1.4 Barriers and solutions to deployment of digital health interventions.

⮕ Figure 16.1.4 suggests some broad solutions to tackling these issues, proposed by the ESC e-Cardiology working group.[59] A crucial barrier to overcome, however, is the 'digital divide'.

The digital divide

The digital divide refers to the growing gap between individuals and groups who are able to benefit from digital technologies, and those who are not. It also tends to follows the 'inverse care law', where those who are most in need of healthcare services have least access to them;[60] older age, low health literacy, and low socioeconomic status are factors associated with low uptake of new technologies, as well as poor health status.[59] Digital literacy, which is the ability to use information and communication technologies to find, evaluate, create, and communicate information[61] must be addressed to ensure greater uptake in target groups. Patient education programmes are therefore essential to tackle the notion that digital interventions are inferior, and to ensure patients can easily access the intervention. Co-design of products with patients is essential for wide uptake and to ensure products are fit for target audiences, and financial support from healthcare systems or insurers may be necessary to help purchase technology and access to high speed internet for patients with low disposable incomes.

Time as a resource

Co-design of products with healthcare professionals is also necessary to ensure they achieve their desired benefits. Reimagined workflows must be more efficient and technologies should be designed to save time, for example by automating tasks to free up healthcare workers to focus on patient contact, diagnosis and education; the Topol report describes this as 'the gift of time',[3] but digital health has yet to convincingly deliver on this promise. RM systems in HF, for example, have been reported to increase workload by some clinicians, and a survey of three European countries found that attitudes to RM were less positive if healthcare professionals were older and identified as having less computer experience.[62] A report into digital transformation of healthcare in Europe by Deloitte identified that the three most commonly encountered challenges to implementing new digital technologies were bureaucracy in healthcare, cost of technology, and finding the right technologies.[63] It is important to align stakeholders' interests in picking the right technology; healthcare professionals' time is a valuable resource which needs to be factored into health economic decisions. EHRs, as described above, are an important example of where promised efficiency benefits have often not been realized.

Regulatory issues

Medical device regulation

A key issue determining how digital technologies are regulated is their stated purpose. If a technology is intended for use for diagnosis, prevention, monitoring, or treatment of disease it is classified as a medical device, and must therefore meet the appropriate legislative standards. In the USA medical devices are regulated by the Food and Drug Administration, whilst in the EU the legislative framework is provided by the EU Medical Devices Regulation. Approval across the EU is provided by member state national regulatory bodies which can provide a 'CE mark' (Conformité Européenne) if the technology proves safety and effectiveness. In general, if the device might provide data that would influence medical decision-making, it must conform to these higher standards, but if it only makes claims to support health and lifestyle decision-making, it may be able to access the consumer market provided it is safe, functions as it claims to function, and does not make claims that cannot be supported. Many manufacturers, particularly in the wearables market, are careful to avoid making definite medical claims and instead market their products for fitness, health, and 'wellness'. This passes legal liability on to the physician if they choose to use it to inform medical decision making.

Data governance

Remote monitoring, wearable devices, and machine algorithms generate lots of patient-level data; a key issue is who 'owns' and can legally access and/or process these data. As more data are collected on individuals the 'digital fingerprint' becomes more likely to be identifiable even if anonymized. In the USA, medical information is regulated by the Health Insurance Portability and Accountability Act (HIPAA), but the focus of this regulation is on insurance companies rather than technology companies which are not currently covered. In the EU, the General Data Processing Regulation (GDPR) is much stricter and mandates a Data Protection Impact Assessment for all technologies that process personal data. Though many technology companies may be tempted to store user data outside of the EU to avoid this, the GDPR also regulates international transfers of personal data of EU citizens.[64]

Integration into healthcare system

Regulatory approval is only one step towards adoption of new technologies, which must also demonstrate clinical and organizational value before being integrated into healthcare systems. These measures judged by a variety of bodies, depending on the healthcare system and key payers. Systems with nationalized healthcare services or state-based insurance models often use national health technology assessment bodies to judge whether a technology should be reimbursed where the payer is the state. The evidence frameworks for evaluation of digital technologies is in rapid evolution; an example of its use in practice is the NICE evidence standards framework for digital technologies, outlining the goals new technologies must meet in order to meet criteria for approval.[65] The Zio™ patch was approved in this way for the diagnosis of suspected arrhythmia.

Evaluating technologies marketed directly at consumers, such as many wearable devices, is more complex and evolving. From the healthcare professional perspective, data from such devices are increasingly being 'offered' to clinicians by patients (for example, data from a wrist-worn heart rate monitor), and it can be difficult for that clinician to assess the likely validity of the data, or to incorporate the data into the electronic medical record, and to robustly document how the data has influenced decision-making. The uncertainty, extra workload, and concern regarding legal liability may lead the healthcare professional to ignore the data, leading to the patient feeling disempowered or, at best, rather distanced from the decision-making processes. Incentivizing digital technologies by remuneration for the clinician or the health system is likely to lead to more rapid adoption, as has been seen with a variety of home telemonitoring systems for HF in France after the 'ETAPES' government initiative was rolled out, and the German government recently published similar draft legislation.

Future scope

EHRs are essential for the synthesis and recording of different data streams, but a growing concern is of 'information overload'; more data than ever are being generated and recorded in patient records, but information is 'filed' in a traditional way, and as such retrieving and summarizing medical histories can be challenging and time-consuming. One solution is Natural Language Processing, whereby machine learning algorithms scan through records and extract relevant diagnoses and summarize medical histories in plain language, though such algorithms are yet to be formally evaluated. Self-management of HF based on certain parameters may become feasible as simple biomarkers and early interventions are validated. A recent RCT demonstrated self-management of blood pressure using an automated digital intervention providing feedback to patients resulted in a greater blood pressure reduction compared with the control group.[66] Continuous blood glucose monitors such as Freestyle Libre™ have revolutionized self-care in type I diabetes mellitus; extending this model to HF, patients may be educated to self-titrate diuretics based on pulmonary pressure readings if this shown to be effective, for example.

Conclusions

Digital health interventions have increased the range of possible interactions between the person living with HF and their healthcare team. Technologies and healthcare systems are at different levels of digital maturity, and HF patients and their clinical advisors have a wide range of digital literacy. The intervention must be tailored to the ability of the patient (and clinical team) to engage with the technology, and the needs of the HF patient. ➔ Figure 16.1.5 provides an example of a 'digital menu' for HF patients. Technologies such as CIEDs require minimal input from the patient whilst implantable haemodynamic monitors simply require the patient to interact with the transmitter ('pillow') daily, and thus are suitable for most patients when clinically indicated. On the other hand, teleconsultation, wearable

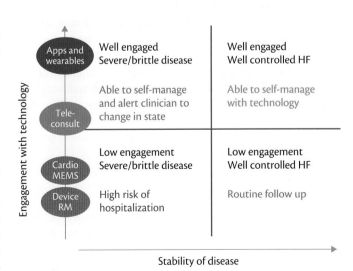

Figure 16.1.5 The 'digital menu' for managing heart failure (HF).

devices and Apps generally require more technological famil-iarity and may be best suited to well-engaged patients who are able to self-manage to a degree. As HF patients become more fa-miliar with technology and markers of HF status become more robust, patients may become more 'activated' to take on more responsibility for their self-care. This 'democratization' of health data should aim to put the patient at the centre of digital health and decision-making.

Summary and key messages

◆ Digital health involves the use of information and communi-cation technology in health-related fields, and includes remote consultation and monitoring, but also wearable devices, Apps, and electronic health records.

◆ The COVID-19 pandemic accelerated the implantation of several digital technologies, most notably teleconsultation, as a result of social distancing rules and health service pressures.

◆ Teleconsultation involves consulting patients or healthcare pro-fessionals at a distance. Limited evidence suggests it is an ac-ceptable alternative to face-to-face consultation for amenable patients, but virtual physical examination can be challenging in HF patients.

◆ Remote monitoring of HF status has been part of HF man-agement for several years, though few technologies have demonstrated convincing reductions in hospitalization or mortality. The use of implantable pulmonary artery pressure monitors to guide HF therapy has shown a significant re-duction in HF hospitalization for NYHA III patients with a recent hospitalization. Machine learning algorithms using data from CIEDs and wearable patch sensors have shown good predictive value for HF hospitalization and are being investigated as tools to assist decision-making and action to prevent hospitalization.

◆ Wearable devices are being increasingly used by patients for 'health and lifestyle' and can measure physiological parameters with increasing accuracy. Activity, heart rate, pulse irregularity, and blood pressure may be measured, but it is unknown whether data from wearables can be used to better guide HF management. Smartphone Apps may be useful for patient education and to support self-care and rehabilitation, but have not yet been widely evaluated.

◆ Several barriers exist to the implantation of digital interventions including lack of confidence among users, legal, technical, and regulatory barriers, and reimbursement. Addressing these bar-riers requires a collaborative approach between all stakeholders (patients, healthcare workers, technology companies, govern-ments, and regulators).

Conflicts of interest

Dr Singhal's salary is funded by a fellowship from Abbott. Prof Cowie has provided consultancy advice to Medtronic, Abbott, Boston Scientific, We-Health, AstraZeneca and Bayer related to digital health, and has received research funds to his institution from Bayer, Boston Scientific, Medtronic and Abbott.

References

1. WHO guideline. Recommendations on digital interventions for health system strengthening. World Health Organization. 2019. Available from: https://www.who.int/publications/i/item/9789241550505 https://www.who.int/reproductivehealth/publications/digital-interventions-health-system-strengthening/en/. Accessed 19 June 2023.

2. Newzoo Global Mobile Market Report 2019. Available from: https://newzoo.com/insights/trend-reports/newzoo-global-mobile-market-report-2019-light-version. Accessed 25 January 2021.

3. Topol E. The Topol Review – Preparing the healthcare workforce to deliver the digital future. NHS Health Education England. 2019. Available from: https://topol.hee.nhs.uk. Accessed 25 January 2021.

4. Royal College of Physicians. Outpatients: The Future – Adding value through sustainability. 2018. Available from: https://www.rcplondon.ac.uk/projects/outputs/outpatients-future-adding-value-through-sustainability. Accessed 25 January 2021.

5. Oliveira Hashiguchi T. Bringing health care to the patient: An over-view of the use of telemedicine in OECD countries. OECD Health Working Papers, 2020, No. 116, OECD Publishing, Paris. doi: 10.1787/8e56ede7-en.

6. Thiyagarajan A, Grant C, Griffiths F, et al. Exploring patients' and clinicians' experiences of video consultations in primary care: a sys-tematic scoping review. BJGP open. 2020;4(1):bjgpopen20X101020 doi: 10.3399/bjgpopen20X101020. PMID: 32184212.

7. Donaghy E, Atherton H, Hammersley V, et al. Acceptability, bene-fits, and challenges of video consulting: a qualitative study in pri-mary care. Br J Gen Pract. 2019;69(686):e586–e594. doi: 10.3399/bjgp19X704141. PMID: 31160368.

8. Shaw SE, Seuren LM, Wherton J, et al. Video consultations between patients and clinicians in diabetes, cancer, and heart failure ser-vices: linguistic ethnographic study of video-mediated interaction. J Med Internet Res 2020;22(5):e18378. doi: 10.2196/18378. PMID: 32391799.

9. Seuren LM, Wherton J, Greenhalgh T, et al. Physical examinations via video for patients with heart failure: qualitative study using conversation analysis. J Med Internet Res. 2020;22(2):e16694. doi: 10.2196/16694. PMID: 32130133.

10. Patel SY, Mehrotra A, Huskamp HA, et al. Trends in outpatient care delivery and telemedicine during the COVID-19 pandemic in the US. JAMA Intern Med. 2021;181(3):388–391.

11. Richardson E, Aissat D, Williams GA, Fahy N. Keeping what works: Remote consultations during the Covid-19 pandemic. Eurohealth 2020; 26(2):73–76.

12. Crespo-Leiro MG, Anker SD, Maggioni AP, et al. European Society of Cardiology Heart Failure Long-Term Registry (ESC-HF-LT): 1-year follow-up outcomes and differences across regions. Eur J Heart Fail. 2016;18(6):613–25. doi: 10.1002/ejhf.566. PMID: 27324686.

13. Schiff GD, Fung S, Speroff T. Decompensated heart failure: symp-toms, patterns of onset and contributing factors. Am J Med 2003; 114: 625–30. doi: 10.1016/s0002–9343(03)00132–3. PMID: 12798449.

14. Inglis SC, Clark RA, Dierckx R et al. Structured telephone sup-port or non-invasive telemonitoring for patients with heart failure. Cochrane Database Syst Rev 2015; (10): CD007228. doi: 10.1002/14651858.CD007228.pub3. PMID: 26517969.

15. Pandor A, Thokala P, Gomersall T, et al. Home telemonitoring or structured telephone support programmes after recent discharge in patients with heart failure: systematic review and economic evalu-ation. Health Technol Assess. 2013;17(32):1–207, v-vi. doi: 10.3310/hta17320. PMID: 23927840.

16. Koehler F, Koehler K, Deckward O, et al. Efficacy of telemedical inter-ventional management in patients with heart failure (TIM-HF2):

a randomised, controlled, parallel-group, unmasked trial. Lancet. 2018;392(10152):1047–1057. doi: 10.1016/S0140–6736(18)31880–4. PMID: 30153985.

17. McDonagh TA, Metra M, Adamo M, Gardner RS, Baumbach A, Böhm M, et al; ESC Scientific Document Group. 2021 ESC Guidelines for the diagnosis and treatment of acute and chronic heart failure: Developed by the Task Force for the diagnosis and treatment of acute and chronic heart failure of the European Society of Cardiology (ESC). With the special contribution of the Heart Failure Association (HFA) of the ESC. Eur J Heart Fail. 2022;24(1):4–131. doi: 10.1002/ejhf.2333. PMID: 35083827.

18. Using Telehealth to Expand Access to Essential Health Services during the COVID-19 Pandemic. Centre for Disease Control and Prevention. 2019. Available from: https://www.cdc.gov/coronavirus/2019-ncov/hcp/telehealth.html. Accessed 25 January 2021.

19. Abraham WT. Intrathoracic impedance monitoring for early detection of impending heart failure decompensation. Congest Heart Fail. 2007;13(2):113–5. doi: 10.1111/j.1527–5299.2007.06255.x. PMID: 17392616.

20. Van Veldhuisen DJ, Braunschweig F, Conraads V, et al. Intrathoracic impedance monitoring, audible patient alerts, and outcome in patients with heart failure. Circulation. 2011;124(16):1719–26. doi: 10.1161/CIRCULATIONAHA.111.043042. PMID: 21931078.

21. Morgan JM, Kitt S, Gill J, et al. Remote management of heart failure using implantable electronic devices. Eur Heart J. 2017;38(30):2352–60. doi: 10.1093/eurheartj/ehx227. PMID: 28575235.

22. Hindricks G, Taborsky M, Glikson M, et al. Implant-based multiparameter telemonitoring of patients with heart failure (IN-TIME): a randomised controlled trial. Lancet 2014; 384:583–90. PMID: 25131977.

23. Boehmer JP, Hariharan R, Devecchi FG, et al. A multisensor algorithm predicts heart failure events in patients with implanted devices: results from the MultiSENSE Study. JACC Heart Fail. 2017;5(3):216–25. doi: 10.1016/j.jchf.2016.12.011. PMID: 28254128.

24. Abraham WT, Stevenson LW, Bourge RC, et al. Sustained efficacy of pulmonary artery pressure to guide adjustment of chronic heart failure therapy: Complete follow-up results from the CHAMPION randomised trial. Lancet. 2016;387(10017):453–61. doi: 10.1016/S0140–6736(15)00723–0. PMID: 26560249.

25. Angermann CE, Assmus B, Anker SD, et al. Pulmonary artery pressure-guided therapy in ambulatory patients with symptomatic heart failure: the CardioMEMS European Monitoring Study for Heart Failure (MEMS-HF). Eur J Heart Fail. 2021; 22(10):1891–1901. doi: 10.1002/ejhf.1943. PMID: 32592227.

26. Cowie MR, Flett A, Cowburn P, Foley P, Chandrasekaran B, Loke I, et al. Real-world evidence in a national health service: results of the UK CardioMEMS HF System Post-Market Study. ESC Heart Fail. 2022; 9: 48–56. doi: 10.1002/ehf2.13748.

27. Lindenfeld J, Zile MR, Desai AS, Bhatt K, Ducharme A, Horstmanshof D, et al. Haemodynamic-guided management of heart failure (GUIDE-HF): a randomised controlled trial. Lancet. 2021; 398: 991–1001. doi: 10.1016/S0140–6736(21)01754–2..

28. Percutaneous implantation of pulmonary artery pressure sensors for monitoring treatment of chronic heart failure. Interventional Procedure guidance IPG 711. 2021. Available at https://www.nice.org.uk/guidance/IPG711/chapter/1-Recommendations (accessed 5 March 2022)

29. Gallup Poll Social Series: Health and Healthcare. Available from: https://news.gallup.com/poll/269096/one-five-adults-health-apps-wearable-trackers.aspx. Published November 2019. Accessed 25 January 2021.

30. Singhal A, Cowie MR. The Role of wearables in heart failure. Curr Heart Fail Rep. 2020;17(4):125–132. doi: 10.1007/s11897–020–00467-x. PMID: 32494944.

31. Kooiman TJM, Dontje ML, Sprenger SR, et al. Reliability and validity of ten consumer activity trackers. BMC Sports Sci Med Rehabil. 2015;7:24. doi: 10.1186/s13102–015-0018–5. PMID: 26464801.

32. Tedesco S, Sica M, Ancillao A, Timmons S, Barton J, O'Flynn B. Accuracy of consumer-level and research-grade activity trackers in ambulatory settings in older adults. PLoS One. 2019; 14: e0216891. doi: 10.1371/journal.pone.0216891. PMID: 31112585; PMCID: PMC6529154.

33. Yancy CW, Jessup M, Bozkurt B, et al. 2013 ACCF/AHA guideline for the management of heart failure. Circulation. 2013;128(16):e240–327.

34. Thorup C, Hansen J, Grønkjær M, et al. Cardiac patients' walking activity determined by a step counter in cardiac telerehabilitation: data from the intervention arm of a randomized controlled trial. J Med Internet Res. 2016;18(4):e69. doi: 10.2196/jmir.5191. PMID: 27044310.

35. Baril JF, Bromberg S, Moayedi Y, Taati B, Manlhiot C, Ross HJ, et al. Use of free-living step count monitoring for heart failure functional classification: Validation study. J Med Internet Res. 2019;21(5):e12122.

36. Izawa KP, Watanabe S, Oka K, et al. Usefulness of step counts to predict mortality in Japanese patients with heart failure. Am J Cardiol. 2013;111(12):1767–71. doi: 10.1016/j.amjcard.2013.02.034. PMID: 23540653.

37. Allen J. Photoplethysmography and its application in clinical physiological measurement. Physiol Meas. 2007;28(3):R1–39. doi: 10.1088/0967–3334/28/3/R01. PMID: 17322588.

38. Moayedi Y, Abdulmajeed R, Duero Posada J, et al. Assessing the use of wrist-worn devices in patients with heart failure: feasibility study. JMIR Cardio. 2017;1(2):e8. doi: 10.2196/cardio.8301. PMID: 31758789.

39. Lombardi F. Clinical implications of present physiological understanding of HRV components. Card Electrophysiol Rev. 2002;6(3):245–9. doi: 10.1023/a:1016329008921. PMID: 12114846.

40. Elgendi M. On the analysis of fingertip photoplethysmogram signals. Curr Cardiol Rev. 2012;8(1):14–25. doi: 10.2174/157340312801215782. PMID: 22845812.

41. Pinheiro N, Couceiro R, Henriques J, et al. Can PPG be used for HRV analysis? 2016 Annu Int Conf IEEE Eng Med Biol Soc.2016: 2945–2949. doi: 10.1109/EMBC.2016.7591347. PMID: 28268930.

42. Kuwabara M, Harada K, Hishiki Y, Kario K. Validation of two watch-type wearable blood pressure monitors according to the ANSI/AAMI/ISO81060-2:2013 guidelines: Omron HEM-6410T-ZM and HEM-6410T-ZL. J Clin Hypertens (Greenwich). 2019;21(6):853–58. doi: 10.1111/jch.13499. PMID: 30803128.

43. Amir O, Ben-Gal T, Weinstein JM, et al. Evaluation of remote dielectric sensing (ReDS) technology-guided therapy for decreasing heart failure re-hospitalizations. Int J Cardiol. 2017;240:279–84. doi: 10.1016/j.ijcard.2017.02.120. Epub 2017 Mar 3. PMID: 28341372.

44. Stehlik J, Schmalfuss C, Bozkurt B, et al. Continuous wearable monitoring analytics predict heart failure hospitalization: the LINK-HF multicenter study. Circ Heart Fail. 2020 Mar;13(3):e006513. doi: 10.1161/CIRCHEARTFAILURE.119.006513. PMID: 32093506.

45. Perez M V., Mahaffey KW, Hedlin H, et al. Large-scale assessment of a smartwatch to identify atrial fibrillation. N Engl J Med. 2019;381(20):1909–17. doi: 10.1056/NEJMoa1901183. PMID: 31722151.

46. Ip JE. Wearable devices for cardiac rhythm diagnosis and management. JAMA. 20199;321(4):337–8. doi: 10.1001/jama.2018.20437. PMID: 30633301.

47. Device Software Functions Including Mobile Medical Applications. U.S. Food & Drug Administration. Available from: https://www.fda.gov/medical-devices/digital-health-center-excellence/device-softw

are-functions-including-mobile-medical-applications. Accessed 25 January 2021.

48. Sørensen K, Pelikan JM, Röthlin F, et al; HLS-EU Consortium. Health literacy in Europe: comparative results of the European health literacy survey (HLS-EU). Eur J Public Health. 2015;25(6):1053–8. doi: 10.1093/eurpub/ckv043. Epub 2015 Apr 5. PMID: 25843827.

49. Clark AM, Freydberg CN, McAlister FA, et al. Patient and informal caregivers' knowledge of heart failure: necessary but insufficient for effective self-care. Eur J Heart Fail 2009; 11: 617–21. doi: 10.1093/eurjhf/hfp058. PMID: 19414477.

50. Mortara A, Vaira L, Palmieri V, et al. Would you prescribe mobile health apps for heart failure self-care? An integrated review of commercially available mobile technology for heart failure patients. Card Fail Rev. 2020;6:e13. doi: 10.15420/cfr.2019.11. PMID: 32537246.

51. Ware P, Ross HJ, Cafazzo JA, Boodoo C, Munnery M, Seto E. Outcomes of a heart failure telemonitoring program implemented as the standard of care in an outpatient heart function clinic: pretest-posttest pragmatic study. J Med Internet Res. 2020; 22: e16538. doi: 10.2196/16538. PMID: 32027309; PMCID: PMC7055875.

52. Benchmarking deployment of eHealth among general practitioners. European Commission, Directorate-General for Communications Networks, Content and Technology. 2018. https://op.europa.eu/en/publication-detail/-/publication/d1286ce7-5c05-11e9-9c52-01aa75ed71a1/language-en /. Accessed 19 June 2023.

53. European Commission. Shaping Europe's digital future. 2018. Available from: https://ec.europa.eu/digital-single-market/en/news/infographic-digital-health-and-care-eu. Accessed 25 January 2021

54. The Harris Poll. How doctors feel about electronic health records: national physician poll. 2018. Available from: https://med.stanford.edu/content/dam/sm/ehr/documents/EHR-Poll-Presentation.pdf. Accessed 25 January 2021

55. Sinsky C, Colligan L, Li L, et al. Allocation of physician time in ambulatory practice: a time and motion study in 4 specialties. Ann Intern Med. 2016;165(11):753–60. doi: 10.7326/M16-0961. Epub 2016 Sep 6. PMID: 27595430.

56. Ghafur S, Kristensen S, Honeyford K, Martin G, Darzi A, Aylin P. A retrospective impact analysis of the WannaCry cyberattack on the NHS. NPJ Digit Med. 2019;2:98. doi: 10.1038/s41746-019-0161-6. PMID: 31602404; PMCID: PMC6775064.

57. Wilson FP, Martin M, Yamamoto Y, et al. Electronic health record alerts for acute kidney injury: multicenter, randomized clinical trial. BMJ. 2021;372:m4786. doi: 10.1136/bmj.m4786. PMID: 33461986.

58. European Commission. eHealth Action Plan 2012–2020: Innovative healthcare for the 21st century. 2012. Available from: https://health.ec.europa.eu/publications/ehealth-action-plan-2012-2020. Accessed 23 June 2023.

59. Frederix I, Caiani EG, Dendale P, et al. ESC e-Cardiology Working Group Position Paper: Overcoming challenges in digital health implementation in cardiovascular medicine. Eur J Prev Cardiol. 2019;26(11):1166–77. doi: 10.1177/2047487319832394. Epub 2019 Mar 27. PMID: 30917695.

60. Tudor Hart J. The inverse care law. Lancet. 1971; 297(7696), 405–412.

61. Museum and Library Services Act of 2010. US Pub. L. 111–340. 2010. Available from: https://www.congress.gov/bill/111th-congress/senate-bill/3984/text. Accessed 19 June 2023.

62. Lycholip E, Aamodt IT, Lie I, et al. Young and computer-literate healthcare professionals have the greatest expectations for heart failure telemonitoring. Eur Heart J- Digit Health, 2020;1 (1): 6–7. https://doi.org/10.1093/ehjdh/ztaa001

63. Shaping the future of European Healthcare. Deloitte. 2020. Shaping the future of European Healthcare. Deloitte. 2020. Available from https://www2.deloitte.com/content/dam/Deloitte/uk/Documents/life-sciences-health-care/deloitte-uk-shaping-the-future-of-european-healthcare.pdf. Accessed 19 June 2023.

64. Nielsen JC, Kautzner J, Casado-Arroyo R, et al. Remote monitoring of cardiac implanted electronic devices: legal requirements and ethical principles - ESC Regulatory Affairs Committee/EHRA joint task force report. Europace. 2020;22(11):1742–58. doi: 10.1093/europace/euaa168. PMID: 32725140.

65. NICE. Evidence Standards Framework. 2018. Available from https://www.nice.org.uk/about/what-we-do/our-programmes/evidence-standards-framework-for-digital-health-technologies. Accessed 4 Feb, 2021.

66. McManus RJ, Little P, Stuart B, et al. HOME BP investigators. Home and Online Management and Evaluation of Blood Pressure (HOME BP) using a digital intervention in poorly controlled hypertension: randomised controlled trial. BMJ. 2021;372:m4858. doi: 10.1136/bmj.m4858. PMID: 33468518.

67. Chaudhry SI, Mattera JA, Curtis JP, et al. Telemonitoring in patients with heart failure. N Engl J Med. 2010;363(24):2301–9. doi: 10.1056/NEJMoa1010029. Epub 2010 Nov 16. PMID: 21080835.

68. Koehler F, Winkler S, Schieber M, et al. Impact of remote telemedical management on mortality and hospitalizations in ambulatory patients with chronic heart failure: the telemedical interventional monitoring in heart failure study. Circulation. 2011;3;123(17):1873–80. doi: 10.1161/CIRCULATIONAHA.111.018473. Epub 2011 Mar 28. PMID: 21444883.

69. Ong MK, Romano PS, Edgington S, et al. Better Effectiveness After Transition–Heart Failure (BEAT-HF) Research Group. Effectiveness of remote patient monitoring after discharge of hospitalized patients with heart failure: the Better Effectiveness After Transition – Heart Failure (BEAT-HF) randomized clinical trial. JAMA Intern Med. 2016;176(3):310–8. doi: 10.1001/jamainternmed.2015.7712. PMID: 26857383.

70. American Heart Association. Using Remote Patient Monitoring Technologies for Better Cardiovascular Disease Outcomes: Guidance. 2019. Available from https://www.heart.org/-/media/files/about-us/policy-research/policy-positions/clinical-care/remote-patient-monitoring-guidance-2019.pdf?la=en. Accessed 25 January 2021.

SECTION 17

Big data in heart failure

CHAPTER 17.1

Big data in heart failure

Mamas A Mamas and Dipak Kotecha

Contents

Introduction

Big data has been characterized as large complex sets of rapidly growing data from disparate sources that require advanced techniques to store and analyse the information.[1] The rapid adoption of digital health systems across the fields of medicine has led to the exponential growth of such big data resources either from internal sources (e.g. electronic health record, apps and wearable technologies, imaging, genomics, clinical registries, administrative data), or external sources (e.g. web and social media sites, or biometric data).[2] Big data offers unprecedented opportunities to study population health, basic science, and the effects of medical care at scale.[3] Longitudinal data collected at the individual patient and population level consists of many natural experiments, including the natural history of disease amongst different clinical phenogroups, the efficacy of therapeutic interventions, and the potential for adverse outcomes or complications, and real-world clinical outcomes in patient groups not routinely recruited into randomized controlled trials, through which we can explore real-world evidence synthesis. In clinical settings, such information is captured by apps and wearable technology, electronic health records (EHRs), different imaging modalities which are recorded routinely as part of medical care and frequently form an essential part of care delivery. This data can be utilized through artificial intelligence to inform care delivery in patients with heart failure (HF), leveraging computer science to deal with the complexities of the multimorbid management of HF, help identify distinct clinical phenogroups, and facilitate a personalized HF patient centric approach. This chapter will overview how data derived from the electronic health record, wearable apps and technologies, and different imaging modalities can be leveraged through artificial intelligence and machine learning to aid delivery of healthcare and guide therapeutic strategies in patients with HF.

Electronic health records

Electronic healthcare records (EHR) are generated through the systematic collection of longitudinal patient and population level data during the routine delivery of healthcare that is electronically stored in a digital format.[4] EHRs contain demographic, administrative, claims (medical and pharmacy), procedural data, clinical history, and patient-centered (e.g. quality-of-life instruments, patient reported outcome measures, and caregiver assessments) data. The nature of the EHR varies according to healthcare system and country and may reflect single components of care, such as primary care, secondary care, disease, or procedure specific registries (e.g. HF or cardiac implantable electronic device registries) or may be integrated across more healthcare providers and institutions to more broadly represent hospital-wide or inter-hospital national systems. The EHR is dynamic, changing with each patient interaction with a healthcare provider, and may evolve reflecting changes in technology, coding, or healthcare practices.

EHR include both administrative datasets or disease specific datasets that provide important information at the population and hospital level around treatments and outcomes of important conditions such as HF. HF-specific national registries have been developed to capture condition-relevant data of patients admitted with a principal diagnosis of HF. The purpose of such registries is to improve the management of patients with HF by activity analysis, clinical quality assurance, clinical improvement work, and research, aiming for reduced mortality and morbidity and increased quality of life in patients with HF. These registries serve an important role for clinical audit and benchmarking of services.

There are several examples of national HF registries such as the US Get With The Guidelines HF registry (GWTG-HF) that was launched by the American Heart Association for performance improvement; this national registry enrols patients if they are admitted with worsening HF or develop HF symptoms during a hospitalization for which HF is the primary discharge diagnosis.[5] Other examples of national registries include the national HF audit (NHFA) of the UK that was established in 2007 to monitor and improve the quality of care of patients admitted to hospital with a diagnosis of principal HF, capturing data on their clinical presentation, characteristics, investigations, specialist input, management, and outcomes in the real world,[6] and the Swedish Heart Failure Registry (SwedeHF; www.SwedeHF.se). EHR from different countries can be combined to form international registries such as the EUROHEART programme, a rolling programme of cardiovascular surveys among the member nations of the European Society of Cardiology (ESC). One such survey of this programme, the EuroHeart Failure survey was initiated to describe the quality of hospital care, diagnostics, and therapeutics, for patients with suspected or confirmed HF in ESC member countries. The quality of management will be judged against the recommendations contained in the ESC guidelines on diagnosis and treatment of HF and highlight differences amongst European member states.[7]

Patient interactions with the secondary care hospital system may be captured through routine administrative data, such as the National Inpatient Sample (NIS), which is the largest all-payer inpatient health care database in the United States, developed by the Healthcare Cost and Utilization Project (HCUP) and sponsored by the Agency for Healthcare Research and Quality (AHRQ)[8] or Hospital Episode Statistics (HES) that captures hospital activity data collected as part of management, planning and reimbursement of NHS hospitals in England.[8] Finally, EHR used for HF research may be derived from the primary care healthcare records, for example, in the UK the Clinical Practice Research Datalink (CPRD) is a database of anonymized electronic, primary health records. In January 2017, the CPRD held data on nearly 17 million active and historical patients registered with 714 general practices across the UK. It contains longitudinal information on diagnoses, referrals, tests, and therapy records and can be linked to HES and mortality data.[9] These systems have now been adapted to run nationwide, data-driven, innovative randomized controlled trials such as DaRe2THINK.[10]

There are both advantages and disadvantages (➲ Figure 17.1.1) to the different EHR available for research purposes, and the

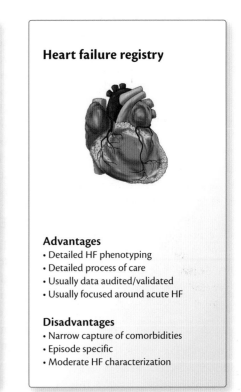

Primary care/Community

Advantages
• Complete capture of comorbidities
• Longitudinal (from cradle to grave)
• Focused around chronic HF

Disadvantages
• Poor HF characterization
• Non cardiology diagnosis
• Poor capture of inpatient care

Administrative/Hospital

Advantages
• Fuller capture of all comorbidities
• Capture of all primary/secondary admissions of pts with HF
• Focused around acute HF

Disadvantages
• Not longitudinal
• Episode specific
• Moderate HF characterization

Heart failure registry

Advantages
• Detailed HF phenotyping
• Detailed process of care
• Usually data audited/validated
• Usually focused around acute HF

Disadvantages
• Narrow capture of comorbidities
• Episode specific
• Moderate HF characterization

Figure 17.1.1. Advantages and disadvantages of different sources of electronic healthcare data of patients with heart failure (HF).

choice of EHR will depend on the nature of the research question. HF national registries are often focused around acute HF admissions and will provide granular data around the HF phenotype, in-hospital processes of care, drug therapies, and clinical outcomes. Such registries provide useful insight into processes of care around acute HF and can be used to answer research questions around this arena and for benchmarking. Nevertheless, many such registries are limited in that they do not provide longitudinal data and any data captured is limited to the single admission episode. Furthermore, whilst national HF registries capture a broad range of cardiovascular comorbid conditions, they do not capture data around other important comorbid conditions such as cancer, frailty, etc, that are commonly encountered in patients with HF and are known to be important determinants of prognosis and receipt of treatment. Importantly, HF registries do not capture hospital episodes of HF patients admitted with a different principal diagnosis and so cannot provide a true measure of HF burden to the wider health economy. Administrative datasets will often have national coverage, or national coverage relevant to the payer (e.g. Medicare or Medicaid) and capture data on all-cause admissions and may contain data from hundreds of millions hospital admissions. They will capture a broader range of comorbid conditions and will capture all hospital events that patients with HF may experience. Analogous to many of the HF national registries highlighted above, many of the administrative datasets do not capture longitudinal data and are limited to capturing information around medical treatments/outcomes during the index hospital event. Furthermore, administrative data does not contain the granularity of HF registries around the aetiology of HF, will lack detail around pharmacotherapy, left ventricular function, or biochemistry such as renal function or B-type natriuretic peptide. Whilst administrative datasets capture a broader range of comorbid conditions than HF registries, they will not capture the whole past medical history of the patient and will only capture important comorbid conditions thought relevant to the principal diagnosis. Finally primary care EHR, whilst providing the most granular data around a patient's past medical history and represents a complete record of a patient's interactions with primary care. The EHR is longitudinal and will contain prescription data and interactions with other healthcare providers such as social care that are often not captured in other administrative EHR. Whilst administrative EHR and HF registries capture data around hospitalization with a principal diagnosis of HF, they will not capture data around the longer-term trajectories and outcomes of stable patients with HF in the community that are not hospitalized. It is important to consider both the advantages and disadvantages of each data source when considering the use of EHR for HF research. A resource is now available by the ESC for researchers to examine worldwide and contemporary real-world data sources for HF.[11] The ESC and BigData@Heart, in collaboration with international stakeholders such as regulators, payers, patient representatives, and both academic and industry researchers have co-created a more transparent, socially licensed approach to research using coded healthcare data (CoDe-EHR; www.escardio.org/bigdata).

Electronic health records in research

EHR have been used widely in HF research, for observational studies, safety surveillance, clinical research to facilitate feasibility assessments and patient recruitment, registry based randomized controlled trials, and regulatory purposes such as safety surveillance of new technologies (➲ Figure 17.1.2).

Randomized controlled trials (RCTs) are considered the gold standard for evidence evaluation. However, they are often limited to recruitment of patients without significant comorbidities which is particularly relevant in conditions such as HF that is characterized by multimorbid elderly patients, and therefore HF patients recruited into RCTs are often not reflective of those encountered in everyday clinical practice. Increasingly it is recognized that observational research through the utility of EHR may be complementary to RCTs or provide insights where RCTs may not exist or in patient groups not recruited into RCTs. EHR can also be used to capture rare events or complications of treatments and are used by regulatory bodies for safety surveillance of new technologies.

EHR can provide insights into the real-world outcomes and disease trajectories of HF patients in the community, providing important data around prognosis[12,13] and its relationship with sex, ethnicity, and social deprivation[13,14] and can be used to investigate the natural history and progression of HF in the outpatients setting.[15] HF is recognized as a multimorbid state, and primary care EHR can capture important comorbidities such as diabetes, chronic obstructive pulmonary disease, or renal dysfunction and can be used to study how longitudinal changes in such comorbid conditions impact on HF prognosis.[16-18] EHR derived from primary care and community settings can provide important data that have been used to develop risk scores that predict incident HF[19] or validate risk scores in the community setting that have been developed to estimate the likelihood that heart failure with preserved ejection fraction (HFpEF) is present among patients with unexplained dyspnoea (H2FPEF and HFA-PEFF risk scores)[20] which can be embedded in the EHR and prospectively applied.

Administrative datasets can be used to describe the impact of important comorbidities on HF outcomes that are often not captured by HF specific national registries, such as frailty[21] and cancer,[22] and the large sample size of such cohorts, often in the millions, allows for the study of important, but less prevalent, comorbid conditions.

RCTs in HF are known to under-recruit women and ethnic minorities relative to disease distribution,[23] and administrative datasets have been used to highlight disparities in the risk of developing HF, its treatments and outcomes based on sex and race[24-26] that inform policy makers around social inequalities in the provision of healthcare at a societal level. Data derived from administrative datasets also allow the assessment of policy and its impact on patients with HF. For example, hospital-based financial incentives may exacerbate healthcare disparities, particularly if they penalize institutions that disproportionately serve minority patients or reward hospitals that avoid minority patients, and data assessing the impact of Medicare's Hospital Readmissions

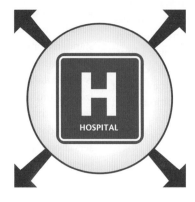

Observational studies

- Epidemiology
- Disease trajectories
- Outcomes in specific patient groups
- Treatment efficacy
- Prognosis/risk models
- Evidence implementation
- Guideline adherence
- Capture complications/rare events

Clinical research

- Registry randomized controlled trials
- Source data to populate eCRF
- Feasibility assessment
- Patient recruitment
- Endpoint or severe adverse effects ascertainment

Safety surveillance

- Post-marketing safety surveillance
- Active surveillance

Regulatory

- New market authorization
- Pharmacovigilance

Figure 17.1.2. Electronic healthcare records in research.
RCT, randomized controlled trial; SAE, serious adverse event. eCRF, electronic case report form.

Reduction Program (HRRP) has suggested that racial disparities may have widened substantially after the implementation of the HRRP in the United States.[27] Administrative datasets may also allow the study of indirect surrogate markers of quality of care, such as unplanned 30-day readmissions that are important for the wider health economy, particularly given that many healthcare institutions face financial penalties unplanned 30-day readmissions. Data derived from RCTs are often derived from lower risk patient groups and may under-estimate the healthcare and financial burden of readmissions, particularly given that the most common cause of unplanned readmissions following an acute HF event are not related to HF.[28,29] Administrative datasets provide important information to policy makers and clinicians around the causes, predictor costs, and outcomes associated with unplanned readmissions.[28,30]

National HF specific registries are often used as the basis of national audit, in which data derived from EHR are used to study differences in process of care across hospitals and differences in outcomes and are used to benchmark services at the individual hospital level that underpin many national reporting programmes. National HF registries provide insight into the epidemiology of HF, particularly around processes of care and their associated clinical outcomes. As an example, the UK national HF audit has shown three-fold differences in practices around referral to cardiology services post discharge amongst UK hospitals which is associated with a 20–30% decreased mortality at 30 days and 1-year.[31] National HF audits also provide important granular data around how extrinsic factors, such as changes in service delivery, introduction of new technologies, or pharmacotherapy,

may impact on HF admissions nationally. The importance of this has been shown recently, where national HF specific registries have been crucial in highlighting the impact of COVID-19 on HF services nationally.[6] National HF registries overcome the weakness of many RCTs that are underpowered to study temporal changes in patient characteristics or outcomes of important groups of patients with HF: for example it would not be feasible to study temporal trends in 7000 patients with dilated cardiomyopathy over a decade which can easily be studied in national HF registries such as in Sweden.[32]

Whilst RCTs can study the efficacy of pharmacotherapy and devices in patients with HF, they do not provide information on how such evidence-based therapy is implemented in the real world, and whether prescribing patterns impact on clinical outcomes. Data derived from HF specific registries enable the study of evaluate the association of HF hospitalization (HFH) with guideline-directed medical therapy prescribing patterns among patients in the real world[33] and provide insight into groups at greatest risk from inequalities in evidence-based therapies. Many of the commonly used risk stratification tools for predicting survival in patients with HF are derived from HF cohort studies also including data from RCTs, for example the Meta-analysis Global Group in Chronic Heart Failure (MAGGIC) that has developed a prognostic model in HF patients[34] and then validated it in the Swedish HF registry[35] and ESC HF long-term registry.[36] Whilst such prognosis models may be useful in the risk stratification of patients for the purposes of benchmarking or highlighting at-risk patient groups to clinicians, they can also be used as a research tool to assess the efficacy of treatments in RCTs at different levels of predefined risk.[37] Finally, national registries can be used to embed RCTs, in which a web-based module to randomize patients can be embedded into the existing infrastructure of the national registry enabling randomization at point of entry into the database. Patient demographics, medical history, concomitant medications, procedural/therapeutic intervention details, and index hospitalization clinical outcomes routinely coded into the registry's data collection form using standardized data elements are electronically captured without study site coordinator effort. Outcome data can be captured through the national registry or linkage of the registry to national mortality/hospital admission data. Whilst the concept of a trial design using a national registry as the basis for continuous enrolment and randomization of all-comers is potentially limited by the lack of formal central adjudication of clinical events, its advantages include that trials run in this manner cost 10% of conventional RCTs and allow for more rapid patient recruitment and larger trials. Examples of trials using this methodology include the TASTE trial,[38] IFR-SWEDEHEART trial[39] from the Swedish SCAAR registry, and SAFE-PCI from the US CathPCI registry.[40]

Apps and wearable technology

The rapid advance in technology available to every person has fuelled the development of new approaches that are applicable and potentially advantageous to healthcare and the goal of improving patient outcomes.[41,42] Consider that in the year 2000 consumers were able to purchase a desktop computer with a central processor speed of 500 Mhz, memory capacity of 128 megabytes, display resolution of 1024 × 768 and storage of 30 gigabytes. Just 20 years on, mobile phones (with a lower price tag) can provide central processing with 8 cores (each running at 2730 Mhz), 16,000 megabytes of memory, a display at 3200 × 1440 and storage 17 times higher (512 gigabytes). The digital transformation has led to profound societal changes, particularly with online websites and app development. Over 150 billion apps are download each year globally, and this is expected to rise beyond 150 billion annually within the next few years.[43]

In the context of HF, studies on apps have mainly focused on weight and symptom assessment, in addition to medication management and activity tracking/encouragement. Unfortunately, although large numbers of patients are using mobile health (mHealth) applications in the real world, scientific appraisal has been limited. In an integrative review,[44] a literature search from 2008 to 2017 identified 18 articles that tested mobile app or tablet-based mobile interventions in HF, of which seven were RCTs, only two of which had a sample size of 100 or more,[45,46] and four were pilot RCTs. Although there was considerable variability in quality of data, 8 of the 18 studies showed a trend or a significant reduction in re-hospitalization, highlighting the potential for benefit with HF apps. There is also an opportunity to better educate patients with HF on their condition and management, and the professional societies have taken on this important task with website content and apps,[47] including www.heartfailure matters.org.

Wearable technology has also rapidly evolved over recent years. Conventional physiological markers (e.g. the 6-minute walk test in HF) provide time-limited information and are subject to many personal and environmental factors. They are also challenging to perform and interpret in an ageing population with multimorbidity, which can interact with mobility and quality of life.[48] Conversely, wearables provide dynamic information, across greater periods of time, and in the patient's own home environment. The breadth of available wearable devices encompasses not only body location (from headbands to sensors embedded in clothing), but also type of information (from accelerometers to electrocardiograms).[49] In HF, wearables have application in patients with pre- or early HF (e.g. risk factor monitoring, such as obesity and hypertension), can contribute to understanding the response to therapy (e.g. heart rate and fluid status), and even add to prognostic and advanced HF care (oxygen saturation and atrial fibrillation detection). However, similar to the situation with mobile apps, scientific knowledge and rigour is only just evolving, restricting the clinical application of such devices. In a comprehensive review of wearables in HF, DeVore and colleagues identified a limited number of observational and small randomized studies evaluating wearables in HF, albeit with some promising signs of potential benefit for patient care (⮕Table 17.1.1).[50] Assessment of fluid volume status and the potential for reducing readmissions has also been demonstrated using electromagnetic signals obtained from a vest[51] and chest vibrations from a sternal patch.[52] Future innovations that have direct application to HF include more widespread use of smart sensors, smart mirrors, and connected smart-home devices, and not to forget, intelligent toilet seats![53]

The purpose for wearable devices is also broad in the published literature; we propose these can defined into four emerging groups:

1 Tele-rehab: measures of activity, for example an RCT of 64 hospitalized patients using a wrist monitor,[54] and 149 patients after cardiac surgery using an ankle monitor.[55]

2 Surrogate outcomes: using activity as a surrogate for clinical performance, such a trial of nitrates in 110 patients with HFpEF, where accelerometer data from a belt were used as the primary outcome.[56]

3 Dual purpose: wearables used as both the intervention and outcome, for example a step counter in 200 patients with HF and diabetes to provide feedback to patients as well as determine the primary outcome.[57]

4 Facilitation of evidence: for example, using an ingestible sensor connected to a cutaneous patch to monitor adherence to therapy.[58]

Regardless of the purpose, wearable devices still have considerable limitations and poor data on validation in clinical practice. Issues of data privacy, data protection and social licence need to be more openly discussed if patients are to accept these technologies in their daily lives. Further, the rapid development of consumer devices (mass produced, relatively cheap with a

Table 17.1.1 Studies of wearable devices in HF from a literature review (1995–2018)

First author, year	Device	Design	HF patients (no.)	Primary outcome	Main findings
Cook 2013[55]	Fitbit-One (San Francisco, CA)	Observational	22	Steps/day, length of stay, discharge disposition	Wireless monitoring of mobility after major surgery was feasible and practical
Thorup 2016[71]	Fitbit Zip (San Francisco, CA)	Randomized control trial (subset)	13	Pedometer	Cardiac telerehabilitation at a call centre can support walking activity using commercial pedometers
Redfield 2015[56]	Kersh activity monitor (Richardson, TX) Kionix Accelerometer (Ithaca, NY, subsidiary of ROHM, Inc Japan)	Randomized control trial	110	Daily activity level	During all dose regimens, activity in the isosorbide mononitrate group was lower than that in the placebo group
Dontje 2014[72]	SenseWear® Pro3 Armband (BodyMedia, Inc., Pittsburgh, PA)	Observational	68	Steps/day; METs	Daily physical activity in HF patients is considerable
Athilingam 2016[73]	Zephyr BioHarness and/or BioPatch (Medtronic, Dublin, Ireland)	Observational	25	Confidence in use of device	Patients reported moderate self-confidence in using HeartMapp
Chan 2016[74]	AliveCor, (San Francisco, CA)	Observational	97	AF detection	Community screening for AF with smartphone-based wireless single-lead ECG was feasible and it identified a significant proportion of citizens with newly diagnosed AF

AF, atrial fibrillation; ECG, electrocardiogram; HF, heart failure; METs, metabolic equivalents.
Reproduced from DeVore AD, Wosik J, Hernandez AF. The Future of Wearables in Heart Failure Patients. *JACC Heart Fail*. 2019 Nov;7(11):922-932. doi: 10.1016/j.jchf.2019.08.008 with permission from John Wiley and Sons.

'black-box' mentality) should be segregated from traditional medical devices (high grade, expensive, and regulated). This is reflected by the stance the regulators such as the US Food and Drug Administration, European Medicines Agency and the UK Medicines and Healthcare products Regulatory Agency have taken on the value of different types of wearables suitable for therapeutic approvals.

Artificial intelligence

The expansion of Big Data in the cardiovascular arena through the growth of heterogeneous collections of EHR datasets, data derived from wearables and apps, and imaging from patients with cardiovascular disease has lent itself to the use of state-of-the-art analysis using artificial intelligence (AI). AI consists of the development of computerized systems – analytical platforms that can perform tasks and undertake analyses that typically require human intelligence. The field of AI includes machine learning (ML), that provides computer systems the ability to learn and improve performance from experience without being explicitly programmed to do so. ML can be categorized into supervised and unsupervised learning, where supervised learning describes a computer algorithm trained on input data that has been labelled for a particular output. For example, the recognition of a tumour on a CT chest. The model is trained until it can detect the underlying patterns and relationships between the input data and the output labels, that is, it is trained until it can detect the tumour in the training data and then it can be applied for classification

or prediction of new (untaught) input. Supervised learning techniques have been used extensively in medical image analysis, and the availability of large amounts of training data with labels (e.g. whether there is a tumour in the CT chest example above) has been crucial in the success of these endeavours.[59] In contrast, unsupervised ML does not used labelled data points (e.g. whether a CT chest has a tumour), but rather aims to identify unknown natural structure or patterns present within a set of data points and has been used to identify previously unrecognized phenogroups within a clinical condition such as HF.[60]

Deep learning (DL) is a branch of ML that uses neural networks with multiple layers to progressively extract higher-level features from the raw data input. For example, in imaging processing, lower layers may identify edges whereas deeper layers may extract more granular facial features, such as the shape and colour of the eyes. DL algorithms perform a task repeatedly, each time optimizing it each time to improve the outcome and can be applied to supervised or unsupervised ML.

ML has been applied extensively to the field of HF and has proven to be effective in highlighting how such computer algorithms when applied to big data may advance our understanding of a heterogenous condition that is defined by a clinical phenotype but, in reality, represents disparate pathophysiological processes and clinical phenotypes under an umbrella term, currently only stratified by the ejection fraction of the left ventricle. Unsupervised ML was applied to data derived from the Patient-Centered Care Transitions in HF (PACT-HF) trial that separated patients according to different comorbidity profiles or phenogroups, each of which included patients across the LVEF spectrum. The classification of patients by clinical phenogroups and independent of LVEF resulted in greater separation of clusters and better association with clinical outcomes at 6 and 12 months than classification based on LVEF categories.[60] Such approaches may be particularly useful in identifying phenogroups in HF with preserved LV function (HFpEF) which clinically is characterized by a number of different phenotypes, where future intervention trials can be targeted.

ML may also be useful to select subgroups of patients who are likely to respond to HF therapies in clinical trials, particularly within traditional categories that have been difficult to demonstrate treatment efficacy in. Unsupervised ML algorithms have been successfully applied to clinical and echocardiographic data derived from the Multicenter Automatic Defibrillator Implantation Trial with Cardiac Resynchronization Therapy (MADIT-CRT) to identify two phenogroups that were associated with a substantially better treatment effect of CRT-D on the primary outcome (hazard ratio (HR), 0.35; 95% confidence interval (CI), 0.19–0.64; P = 0.0005, and HR, 0.36; 95% CI, 0.19–0.68; P = 0.001) than observed in the other groups (interaction P = 0.02).[61] Other studies have reported that unsupervised ML algorithms applied to ECG and echo images can optimize identification of CRT responders,[62] or can be used to predict outcomes in patients that have received CRT devices.[63] Using a series of interconnected AI algorithms on data from landmark placebo-controlled trials, the card*AI*c group were able identify and validate clusters of HFrEF patients according to the benefit they received from beta-blocker therapy.[64] This included a subgroup of patients with both HFrEF and AF who were younger, heavier, and more likely to have non-ischaemic cardiomyopathy than average, and who also demonstrated a significant reduction in mortality (odds ratio 0.57, 0.35–0.93; P = 0.023) distinct from most other patients with AF.[65]

Machine learning has been widely applied to disparate sources of data including EHR, imaging, and biochemistry leading to the development of prognosis models that outperform traditional models developed using classical statistical techniques. ML based algorithms have been used to develop models to predict outcomes for HF patients in the intensive care unit,[66] post cardiac transplant,[67] or general HF population.[68] Prognosis tools are not only useful in predicting outcomes in patients with established heart failure, but also important identifying those patients with cardiovascular risk factors that have the greatest risk of developing HF. Using data derived from four community cohorts (ARIC (Atherosclerosis Risk in Communities), DHS (Dallas Heart Study), JHS (Jackson Heart Study), and MESA (Multi-Ethnic Study of Atherosclerosis)) with adjudicated HF events, ML approaches that included 39 candidate variables across demographic, anthropometric, medical history, laboratory, and electrocardiographic domains contributed to the development of race-specific models for prediction of 10-year risk of heart failure in the community[69] with superior performance compared to established HF models. Such HF risk prediction models can identify high-risk individuals who are most likely to benefit from effective preventive therapies. These strategies may include lifestyle interventions to promote weight loss, intensive blood pressure control, and initiation of pharmacotherapies such as sodium-glucose cotransporter-2 inhibitors among individuals with type 2 diabetes.[70]

Future directions

Currently data from EHR from patients with HF is captured in silos, with isolated information/data captured from dedicated HF registries, primary care, and administrative sources with no cross linkage across data sources. It is difficult to track healthcare resource utilization of a patient with HF, particularly when healthcare events may not always relate to their HF but rather to comorbid conditions. This limits the potential to capture granular phenotype data, or to study their longitudinal trajectory across healthcare systems. Work is beginning to focus on linkage across different datasets captured from the individual patients at different points in their journey across healthcare systems, but importantly to integrate imaging and biological data for a greater systems-wide approach. With the advent of AI and machine learning approaches, real-time data capture will allow for dynamic modelling, with the performance of models updated/recalibrated with each additional datapoint. It remains to be seen whether integration of such risk scores into routine practice to guide treatment decisions will impact meaningfully on clinical outcomes in patients with HF. Similarly, while machine learning has identified phenogroups in HF that may respond to therapies, such as CRT devices, it is yet to be demonstrated that utilizing these machine learning algorithms improves clinical outcomes compared to standard practice. With the ability of AI derived tools to analyse disparate multi-modal sources of data, future work should focus how such prognosis models developed from such machine learning approaches should be implemented into clinical pathways, with consideration around the potential design of services that can deliver real-time changes in management, perhaps through e-health solutions such as apps. This will require seamless integration of parallel patient-facing systems across different healthcare providers which represents an important challenge for the future. Regardless of the purpose of these emerging data analytics and how they will integrate into e-health solutions, there are still considerable limitations and poor data on validation of such technologies in clinical practice. Issues of data privacy, data protection, and social licence need to be more openly discussed if patients are to accept these data driven solutions in their daily lives.

Key messages

- Big data represents a disparate, rapidly growing, source of information (datapoints) created during the routine delivery of healthcare to patients with HF. Currently this information is captured in silos, with little integration across different data sources and poor linkage to longitudinal outcomes. There is little data quality control or audit as to the reliability of such data.

- Big data offers unprecedented opportunities to leverage the growing field of artificial intelligence, and in particular machine learning to better understand the HF phenotype and different longitudinal trajectories in different patient groups and to begin to gain inroads into the delivery of personalized medicine to this complex group of patients.

- mHealth applications will change how HF care is delivered in healthcare systems of the future, with wearables central to this. Emerging areas include Tele-rehab: measures of activity; Surrogate outcomes: using activity as a surrogate for clinical performance; Dual purpose: wearables used as both the intervention and outcome; and Facilitation of evidence: measures of adherence.

- Regardless of the purpose, mhealth solutions still have considerable limitations and poor data on validation in clinical practice. Issues of data privacy, data protection, and social licence need to be more openly discussed if patients are to accept these technologies in their daily lives.

Disclosures

Prof. Kotecha reports grants from the National Institute for Health Research (NIHR CDF-2015-08-074; NIHR HTA-130280), the British Heart Foundation (PG/17/55/33087 and AA/18/2/34218), EU/EFPIA Innovative Medicines Initiative (BigData@Heart 116074), the European Society of Cardiology in collaboration with Boehringer Ingelheim/BMS-Pfizer Alliance/Bayer/Daiichi Sankyo/Boston Scientific (STEEER-AF NCT04396418), Amomed Pharma and IRCCS San Raffaele/Menarini (Beta-blockers in Heart Failure Collaborative Group NCT0083244); in addition personal fees from Bayer (Advisory Board), AtriCure (Speaker fees), Amomed (Advisory Board), Protherics Medicines Development (Advisory Board) and Myokardia (Advisory Board).

References

1. Raghupathi W, Raghupathi V. Big data analytics in healthcare: promise and potential. Health Inf Sci Syst 2014;**2**:3.

2. Wagle AA, Isakadze N, Nasir K, Martin SS. Strengthening the learning health system in cardiovascular disease prevention: time to leverage big data and digital solutions. Curr Atheroscler Rep 2021;**23**(5):19.

3. Martin GP, Mamas MA. Importance of quality control in 'big data': implications for statistical inference of electronic health records in clinical cardiology. Cardiovasc Res 2019;**115**(6):e63–e65.

4. Cowie MR, Blomster JI, Curtis LH, Duclaux S, Ford I, Fritz F, et al. Electronic health records to facilitate clinical research. *Clinical Res Cardiol.* 2017;**106**(1):1–9.

5. Smaha LA, American Heart A. The American Heart Association Get With The Guidelines program. Amer Heart J 2004;**148**(5 Suppl):S46–8.

6. Shoaib A, Van Spall HGC, Wu J, Cleland JGF, McDonagh TA, Rashid M, et al. Substantial decline in hospital admissions for heart failure accompanied by increased community mortality during COVID-19 pandemic. Eur Heart J Qual Care Clin Outcomes 2021;**7**(4): 378–387.

7. Cleland JG, Swedberg K, Cohen-Solal A, Cosin-Aguilar J, Dietz R, Follath F, et al. The Euro Heart Failure Survey of the EUROHEART survey programme. A survey on the quality of care among patients with heart failure in Europe. The Study Group on Diagnosis of the Working Group on Heart Failure of the European Society of Cardiology. The Medicines Evaluation Group Centre for Health Economics University of York. Eur J Heart Fail 2000;**2**(2):123–32.

8. Hines A, Stranges E, Andrews RM. Trends in hospital risk-adjusted mortality for select diagnoses by patient subgroups, 2000–2007: Statistical Brief #98. In. *Healthcare Cost and Utilization Project (HCUP) Statistical Briefs.* Rockville (MD); 2010.

9. Zghebi SS, Mamas MA, Ashcroft DM, Salisbury C, Mallen CD, Chew-Graham CA, et al. Development and validation of the DIabetes Severity SCOre (DISSCO) in 139 626 individuals with type 2 diabetes: a retrospective cohort study. BMJ Open Diabetes Res Care 2020;**8**(1):e000962

10. Kotecha D, Shukla D, Clinical Practice Research Datalink. Preventing stroke, premature death and cognitive decline in a broader community of patients with atrial fibrillation using healthcare data for pragmatic research: A randomised controlled trial (DaRe2THINK). Sponsor: University of Birmingham; Funder: National Institute for Health Research 2021; EudraCT 2020–005774–10; ClinicalTrials.gov NCT04700826; www.birmingham.ac.uk/dare2think

11. Studer R, Sartini C, Suzart-Woischnik K, Agrawal R, Natani H, Gill S, et al. Identification and mapping real-world data sources for heart failure, acute coronary syndrome, and atrial fibrillation. Cardiology 2022;**147**(1):98–106.:

12. Mamas MA, Sperrin M, Watson MC, Coutts A, Wilde K, Burton C, et al. Do patients have worse outcomes in heart failure than in cancer? A primary care-based cohort study with 10-year follow-up in Scotland. Eur J Heart Fail 2017;**19**(9):1095–1104.

13. Lawson CA, Zaccardi F, Squire I, Okhai H, Davies M, Huang W, et al. Risk factors for heart failure: 20-year population-based trends by sex, socioeconomic status, and ethnicity. Circ Heart Fail 2020;**13**(2):e006472.

14. Kubicki DM, Xu M, Akwo EA, Dixon D, Munoz D, Blot WJ, et al. Race and sex differences in modifiable risk factors and incident heart failure. JACC Heart Fail 2020;**8**(2):122–130.

15. Iorio A, Rea F, Barbati G, Scagnetto A, Peruzzi E, Garavaglia A, et al. HF progression among outpatients with HF in a community setting. Int J Cardio.2019;**277**:140–146.

16. Lawson CA, Testani JM, Mamas M, Damman K, Jones PW, Teece L, Kadam UT. Chronic kidney disease, worsening renal function and outcomes in a heart failure community setting: A UK national study. Int J Cardio. 2018;**267**:120–127.

17. Lawson CA, Mamas MA, Jones PW, Teece L, McCann G, Khunti K, Kadam UT. Association of medication intensity and stages of airflow limitation with the risk of hospitalization or death in patients with heart failure and chronic obstructive pulmonary disease. JAMA Netw Open 2018;**1**(8):e185489.

18. Lawson CA, Jones PW, Teece L, Dunbar SB, Seferovic PM, Khunti K, et al. Association between type 2 diabetes and all-cause hospitalization and mortality in the uk general heart failure population: stratification by diabetic glycemic control and medication intensification. JACC Heart Fail 2018;**6**(1):18–26.

19. Suthahar N, Lau ES, Blaha MJ, Paniagua SM, Larson MG, Psaty BM, et al. Sex-specific associations of cardiovascular risk factors and biomarkers with incident heart failure. J Amer Coll Cardiol 2020;**76**(12):1455–1465.

20. Selvaraj S, Myhre PL, Vaduganathan M, Claggett BL, Matsushita K, Kitzman DW, et al. Application of diagnostic algorithms for heart failure with preserved ejection fraction to the community. JACC Heart Fail 2020;**8**(8):640–653.

21. Kwok CS, Zieroth S, Van Spall HGC, Helliwell T, Clarson L, Mohamed M, et al. The Hospital Frailty Risk Score and its association with in-hospital mortality, cost, length of stay and discharge location in patients with heart failure short running title: Frailty and outcomes in heart failure. Int J Cardio 2020;**300**:184–190.

22. Tuzovic M, Yang EH, Sevag Packard RR, Ganz PA, Fonarow GC, Ziaeian B. National outcomes in hospitalized patients with cancer and comorbid heart failure. J Card Fail 2019;**25**(7):516–521.

23. Whitelaw S, Sullivan K, Eliya Y, Alruwayeh M, Thabane L, Yancy CW, et al. Trial characteristics associated with under-enrolment of females in randomized controlled trials of heart failure with reduced ejection fraction: a systematic review. Eur J Heart Fail 2021;**23**(1):15–24.

24. Downing NS, Wang C, Gupta A, Wang Y, Nuti SV, Ross JS, et al. Association of racial and socioeconomic disparities with outcomes among patients hospitalized with acute myocardial infarction, heart failure, and pneumonia: an analysis of within- and between-hospital variation. JAMA Netw Open 2018;**1**(5):e182044.

25. Mohamed MO, Volgman AS, Contractor T, Sharma PS, Kwok CS, Rashid M, et al. Trends of sex differences in outcomes of cardiac electronic device implantations in the United States. Can J Cardiol 2020;**36**(1):69–78.

26. Akwo EA, Kabagambe EK, Harrell FE, Jr., Blot WJ, Bachmann JM, Wang TJ, et al. Neighborhood deprivation predicts heart failure risk in a low-income population of blacks and whites in the southeastern United States. Circ Cardiovasc Qual Outcomes 2018;**11**(1):e004052.

27. Chaiyachati KH, Qi M, Werner RM. Changes to racial disparities in readmission rates after medicare's hospital readmissions reduction program within safety-net and non-safety-net hospitals. JAMA Netw Open 2018;**1**(7):e184154.

28. Kwok CS, Seferovic PM, Van Spall HG, Helliwell T, Clarson L, Lawson C, et al. Early unplanned readmissions after admission to hospital with heart failure. Am J Cardiol 2019;**124**(5):736–745.

29. Kwok CS, Amin AP, Shah B, Kinnaird T, Alkutshan R, Balghith M, et al. Cost of coronary syndrome treated with percutaneous coronary intervention and 30-day unplanned readmission in the United States.Catheter Cardiovasc Interv 2021;**97**(1):80–93.

30. Martin GP, Kwok CS, Van Spall HGC, Volgman AS, Michos E, Parwani P, et al. Readmission and processes of care across weekend and weekday hospitalisation for acute myocardial infarction, heart failure or stroke: an observational study of the National Readmission Database. BMJ Open 2019;**9**(8):e029667.

31. Emdin CA, Hsiao AJ, Kiran A, Conrad N, Salimi-Khorshidi G, Woodward M, et al. Referral for specialist follow-up and its association with post-discharge mortality among patients with systolic heart failure (from the National Heart Failure Audit for England and Wales). Am J Cardiol 2017;**119**(3):440–444.

32. Sjoland H, Silverdal J, Bollano E, Pivodic A, Dahlstrom U, Fu M. Temporal trends in outcome and patient characteristics in dilated cardiomyopathy, data from the Swedish Heart Failure Registry 2003–2015. BMC Cardiovasc Disord 2021;**21**(1):307.

33. Srivastava PK, DeVore AD, Hellkamp AS, Thomas L, Albert NM, Butler J, et al. Heart failure hospitalization and guideline-directed prescribing patterns among heart failure with reduced ejection fraction patients. JACC Heart Fail 2021;**9**(1):28–38.

34. Pocock SJ, Ariti CA, McMurray JJ, Maggioni A, Kober L, Squire IB, et al. Meta-Analysis Global Group in Chronic Heart F. Predicting survival in heart failure: a risk score based on 39 372 patients from 30 studies. Eur Heart J 2013;**34**(19):1404–13.

35. Sartipy U, Dahlstrom U, Edner M, Lund LH. Predicting survival in heart failure: validation of the MAGGIC heart failure risk score in 51,043 patients from the Swedish heart failure registry. Eur J Heart Fail 2014;**16**(2):173–9.

36. Canepa M, Fonseca C, Chioncel O, Laroche C, Crespo-Leiro MG, Coats AJS, et al. Investigators EHLTR. Performance of prognostic risk scores in chronic heart failure patients enrolled in the European Society of Cardiology Heart Failure Long-Term Registry. JACC Heart Fail 2018;**6**(6):452–62.

37. Simpson J, Jhund PS, Silva Cardoso J, Martinez F, Mosterd A, Ramires F, et al., Investigators P-H, Committees. Comparing LCZ696 with enalapril according to baseline risk using the MAGGIC and EMPHASIS-HF risk scores: an analysis of mortality and morbidity in PARADIGM-HF. J Am Coll Cardiol 2015;**66**(19):2059–71.

38. Frobert O, Lagerqvist B, Gudnason T, Thuesen L, Svensson R, Olivecrona GK, James SK. Thrombus aspiration in ST-Elevation myocardial infarction in Scandinavia (TASTE trial). A multicenter, prospective, randomized, controlled clinical registry trial based on the Swedish angiography and angioplasty registry (SCAAR) platform. Study design and rationale. Am Heart J 2010;**160**(6):1042–8.

39. Gotberg M, Christiansen EH, Gudmundsdottir IJ, Sandhall L, Danielewicz M, Jakobsen L, et al., i FRSI. Instantaneous wave-free ratio versus fractional flow reserve to guide PCI. New Engl J Med 2017;**376**(19):1813–23.

40. Hess CN, Rao SV, Kong DF, Aberle LH, Anstrom KJ, Gibson CM, et al. Embedding a randomized clinical trial into an ongoing registry infrastructure: unique opportunities for efficiency in design of the Study of Access site For Enhancement of Percutaneous Coronary Intervention for Women (SAFE-PCI for Women). Am Heart J 2013;**166**(3):421–8.

41. Kotecha D, Chua WWL, Fabritz L, Hendriks J, Casadei B, Schotten U, et al. European Society of Cardiology Atrial Fibrillation Guidelines Taskforce, CATCH ME Consortium, European Heart Rhythm Association. European Society of Cardiology smartphone and tablet applications for patients with atrial fibrillation and their health care providers. Europace 2018;**20**(2):225–33.

42. Rossello X, Stanbury M, Beeri R, Kirchhof P, Casadei B, Kotecha D. Digital learning and the future cardiologist. Eur Heart J 2019;**40**(6):499–501.

43. SensorTower. Global app downloads by year and App downloads forecast growth. sensortowercom 2020.

44. Athilingam P, Jenkins B. Mobile phone apps to support heart failure self-care management: integrative review. JMIR Cardio 2018;**2**(1):e10057.

45. Scherr D, Kastner P, Kollmann A, Hallas A, Auer J, Krappinger H, et al. Effect of home-based telemonitoring using mobile phone technology on the outcome of heart failure patients after an episode of acute decompensation: randomized controlled trial. J Med Internet Res 2009;**11**(3):e34.

46. Seto E, Leonard KJ, Cafazzo JA, Barnsley J, Masino C, Ross HJ. Mobile phone-based telemonitoring for heart failure management: a randomized controlled trial. J Med Internet Res 2012;**14**(1):e31.

47. Ahmed N, Ahmed S, Grapsa J. Apps and online platforms for patients with heart failure. Card Fail Rev 2020;**6**:e14.

48. Jones J, Stanbury M, Haynes S, Bunting KV, Lobban T, Camm AJ, et al. Importance and Assessment of Quality of Life in Symptomatic Permanent Atrial Fibrillation: Patient Focus Groups from the RATE-AF Trial. Cardiology 2020;**145**(10):666–75.

49. Piwek L, Ellis DA, Andrews S, Joinson A. The rise of consumer health wearables: promises and barriers. PLoS Med 2016;**13**(2):e1001953.

50. DeVore AD, Wosik J, Hernandez AF. The future of wearables in heart failure patients. JACC Heart Fail 2019;**7**(11):922–32.

51. Amir O, Ben-Gal T, Weinstein JM, Schliamser J, Burkhoff D, Abbo A, Abraham WT. Evaluation of remote dielectric sensing (ReDS) technology-guided therapy for decreasing heart failure rehospitalizations. Int J Cardiol 2017;**240**:279–84.

52. Inan OT, Baran Pouyan M, Javaid AQ, Dowling S, Etemadi M, Dorier A, et al. Novel wearable seismocardiography and machine learning algorithms can assess clinical status of heart failure patients. Circ Heart Fail 2018;**11**(1):e004313.

53. Conn NJ, Schwarz KQ, Borkholder DA. In-home cardiovascular monitoring system for heart failure: comparative study. JMIR Mhealth Uhealth 2019;**7**(1):e12419.

54. Thorup C, Hansen J, Grønkjær M, Andreasen JJ, Nielsen G, Sørensen EE, Dinesen BI. Cardiac patients' walking activity determined by

a step counter in cardiac telerehabilitation: data from the intervention arm of a randomized controlled trial. *J Med Internet Res* 2016;**18**(4):e69.

55. Cook DJ, Thompson JE, Prinsen SK, Dearani JA, Deschamps C. Functional recovery in the elderly after major surgery: assessment of mobility recovery using wireless technology. Ann Thorac Surg 2013;**96**(3):1057–61.

56. Redfield MM, Anstrom KJ, Levine JA, Koepp GA, Borlaug BA, Chen HH, et al. Isosorbide mononitrate in heart failure with preserved ejection fraction. N Engl J Med 2015;**373**(24):2314–24.

57. Sharma A, Mentz RJ, Granger BB, Heitner JF, Cooper LB, Banerjee D, et al. Utilizing mobile technologies to improve physical activity and medication adherence in patients with heart failure and diabetes mellitus: Rationale and design of the TARGET-HF-DM Trial. Am Heart J 2019;**211**:22–33.

58. Thompson D, Mackay T, Matthews M, Edwards J, Peters NS, Connolly SB. Direct adherence measurement using an ingestible sensor compared with self-reporting in high-risk cardiovascular disease patients who knew they were being measured: a prospective intervention. JMIR Mhealth Uhealth 2017;**5**(6):e76.

59. de Bruijne M. Machine learning approaches in medical image analysis: From detection to diagnosis. Med Image Anal 2016;**33**:94–7.

60. Gevaert AB, Tibebu S, Mamas MA, Ravindra NG, Lee SF, Ahmad T, et al. Clinical phenogroups are more effective than left ventricular ejection fraction categories in stratifying heart failure outcomes. ESC Heart Fail 2021; 10.1002/ehf2.13344.

61. Cikes M, Sanchez-Martinez S, Claggett B, Duchateau N, Piella G, Butakoff C, et al. Machine learning-based phenogrouping in heart failure to identify responders to cardiac resynchronization therapy. Eur J of Heart Fail 2019;**21**(1):74–85.

62. Lei J, Wang YG, Bhatta L, Ahmed J, Fan D, Wang J, Liu K. Ventricular geometry-regularized QRSd predicts cardiac resynchronization therapy response: machine learning from crosstalk between electrocardiography and echocardiography. Int J Cardiovasc Imaging 2019;**35**(7):1221–9.

63. Cai C, Tafti AP, Ngufor C, Zhang P, Xiao P, Dai M, et al. Using ensemble of ensemble machine learning methods to predict outcomes of cardiac resynchronization. J Cardiovasc Electrophysiol 2021; 10.1111/jce.15171.

64. Karwath A, Bunting KV, Gill SK, Tica O, Pendleton S, Aziz F, et al. Redefining beta-blocker response in heart failure patients with sinus rhythm and atrial fibrillation: a machine learning cluster analysis. Lancet 2021; **398**(10309):1427–35.

65. Kotecha D, Holmes J, Krum H, Altman DG, Manzano L, Cleland JG, et al. Beta-Blockers in Heart Failure Collaborative Group. Efficacy of beta blockers in patients with heart failure plus atrial fibrillation: an individual-patient data meta-analysis. Lancet 2014;**384**(9961):2235–43.

66. Li F, Xin H, Zhang J, Fu M, Zhou J, Lian Z. Prediction model of in-hospital mortality in intensive care unit patients with heart failure: machine learning-based, retrospective analysis of the MIMIC-III database. BMJ Open 2021;**11**(7):e044779.

67. Zhou Y, Chen S, Rao Z, Yang D, Liu X, Dong N, Li F. Prediction of 1-year mortality after heart transplantation using machine learning approaches: A single-center study from China. Int J Cardiol 2021; **339**:21–7.

68. Negassa A, Ahmed S, Zolty R, Patel SR. Prediction model using machine learning for mortality in patients with heart failure. Am J Cardiol 2021;**153**:86–93.

69. Segar MW, Jaeger BC, Patel KV, Nambi V, Ndumele CE, Correa A, et al. Development and validation of machine learning-based race-specific models to predict 10-year risk of heart failure: a multicohort analysis. Circulation 2021;**143**(24):2370–83.

70. Zelniker TA, Wiviott SD, Raz I, Im K, Goodrich EL, Bonaca MP, et al. SGLT2 inhibitors for primary and secondary prevention of cardiovascular and renal outcomes in type 2 diabetes: a systematic review and meta-analysis of cardiovascular outcome trials. Lancet 2019;**393**(10166):31–9.

71. Thorup C, Hansen J, Gronkjaer M, Andreasen JJ, Nielsen G, Sorensen EE, Dinesen BI. Cardiac patients' walking activity determined by a step counter in cardiac telerehabilitation: data from the intervention arm of a randomized controlled trial. J Med Internet Res 2016;**18**(4):e69.

72. Dontje ML, van der Wal MH, Stolk RP, Brugemann J, Jaarsma T, Wijtvliet PE, et al. Daily physical activity in stable heart failure patients. J Cardiovasc nurs 2014;**29**(3):218–26.

73. Athilingam P, Labrador MA, Remo EF, Mack L, San Juan AB, Elliott AF. Features and usability assessment of a patient-centered mobile application (HeartMapp) for self-management of heart failure. Appl Nurs Res 2016;**32**:156–63.

74. Chan NY, Choy CC. Screening for atrial fibrillation in 13 122 Hong Kong citizens with smartphone electrocardiogram. Heart (British Cardiac Society) 2017;**103**(1):24–31.

SECTION 18

Telemedicine and remote monitoring

CHAPTER 18.1

Telemedicine and remote monitoring in heart failure

Tarek Bekfani, Friedrich Koehler, and
William T Abraham

Contents

Introduction

Efforts to decrease mortality, reduce hospitalization rates, and improve the quality of life (QoL) of patients with HF have been modestly successful over the last decades. However, in spite of the introduction of many effective pharmacological and device therapies,[1] HF readmission rates remain high and represent a significant social and financial burden.[2] For example, the one-month readmission rate as a key indicator of hospital performance currently remains high at approximately 25%.[3] Consequently, the focus of HF disease management has shifted from managing episodes of decompensation requiring hospitalization, a reactive approach to HF care, to achieving and maintaining an euvolemic state in order to keep patients out of the hospital, a more proactive approach.[4,5,6]

In this regard, understanding the pathophysiology of HF and the development of HF decompensation is imperative. As a response to reduced cardiac output, the human body attempts to maintain an effective mean arterial pressure through a series of compensatory mechanisms. Over-activation of the sympathetic nervous system and renin-angiotensin-aldosterone system are among the earliest pathophysiological responses along with an increased metabolic rate driven by an active inflammatory process.[7,8] These changes in haemodynamics and neurohormones lead to the retention of salt and water by the kidneys, resulting in extracellular fluid volume excess. Paired with a decreased vascular compliance due to vasoconstriction, these changes produce increased cardiac filling pressures and increased interstitial pulmonary fluid, often referred to as haemodynamic and clinical congestion, respectively.[9]

Clinicians are used to intervening at a later stage in the development of decompensation, that is, when patients are overtly symptomatic or gain weight (phase C or D, ⮕ Figure 18.1.1). However, based on monitoring of physiological variables that change early, meaningful clinical intervention might be more effective at an earlier phase (phase A or B) prior to worsening symptoms or weight gain to control decompensation and reduce the risk of HF hospitalization. It is estimated that the earliest detectable changes in physiological measurements occur 10–20 days prior to an onset of worsening symptoms.[10]

Consequently, new technologies such as telemedicine (also known as remote monitoring (RM) or remote patient monitoring) are urgently required to match these unmet needs in patients with HF.

The importance of RM became even more crucial during the global COVID-19 pandemic, where social distancing was recommended and the number of in-person patient-physician contacts dramatically declined.[11]

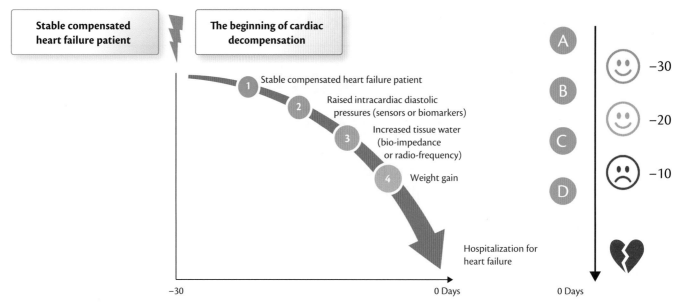

Figure 18.1.1 The phases of decompensated heart failure. Currently, action tends to be taken when patients are in phase C. Ideally, clinicians should react earlier when patients are still in phases A or B. RM offers different possibilities in this regard.

Source data from Adamson PB. Pathophysiology of the transition from chronic compensated and acute decompensated heart failure: new insights from continuous monitoring devices. Curr Heart Fail Rep. 2009 Dec;6(4):287-92. doi: 10.1007/s11897-009-0039-z.

Although the need and utility of RM appears intuitive, evidence to support the clinical benefit has been mixed and inconsistent. The following paragraphs will discuss the suggested criteria for successful RM in HF, the history of clinical trials in the field of RM, recent landmark trials and technologies in RM and fluid management, as well as the principles and structure of RM centres.

Criteria for successful remote monitoring of fluid management in heart failure

Based on reviewing the evidence and the tested technologies in clinical trials in the field of RM in HF, at least six characteristics of RM technologies seem to be important prerequisites for success (⊃ Figure 18.1.2).[5]

1 Appropriateness: sensors must measure the underlying pathophysiology contributing to worsening HF symptoms and clinical events (e.g. hospitalizations). Increases in intracardiac and pulmonary artery pressures and in lung fluid content seem to be among the earliest physiological changes and the proximate cause of worsening HF.[10] Thus, measurement of haemodynamic and/or pulmonary congestion may provide the best target and greatest opportunity for proactive intervention and avoidance of hospitalizations.

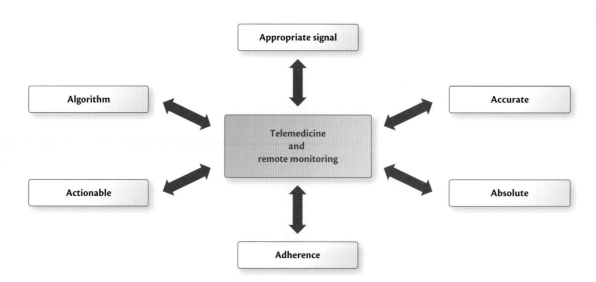

Figure 18.1.2 The six prerequisites for developing successful RM technologies in HF.

2 Accuracy: sensors must be accurate, providing measurements that have been validated against gold standards such as the Swan–Ganz catheter in the case of haemodynamic pressure sensors or chest computed tomography in the case lung fluid content sensors.

3 Absolute values: these values rather than relative ones seem to be more helpful. For example, in the case of lung fluid content assessment, it is not sufficient to know when the lungs are relatively wetter or dryer. Rather, it is imperative to know when the lungs are normally dry and, conversely, to know quantitatively the amount of abnormal fluid when wet in order to guide therapy. The relativistic nature of impedance-based technologies measuring lung fluid content may explain the failure to date of most trans-thoracic and intra-thoracic impedance assessment tools in HF management.

4 Actionability: The information gathered should be understood clearly to ascertain the appropriate response. In the case of implantable haemodynamic monitors, we understand the meaning of intracardiac and pulmonary artery pressures, and we know what to do with this information. In the case of relative changes in thoracic impedance, we do not.

5 Algorithm: an algorithm is required to support clinicians in making and implementing the right clinical decision depending on the information gained from the RM technology. The aim should be adjusting medical therapies when abnormal values are recorded.

6 Adherence: adherence of both patients and clinicians to effective RM technologies is essential to achieving the goal of keeping patients well and out of the hospital. For example, new technologies should be user friendly. Additionally, focusing on patient education and engagement with RM technologies, such as leveraging smart phone technology and the principles of social media engagement, could be supportive in achieving a high level of patient adherence.

Heart failure remote monitoring clinical trials

The effectiveness of RM to improve life expectancy, QoL, and to reduce HF re-hospitalizations has been demonstrated in several trials,[12-14] but not in others.[15-17] The outcomes of such studies are, in large part, related to the RM approach or technology used. In a recent Cochrane review, both non-invasive RM and structured telephone support have been shown to offer statistically and clinically meaningful benefits to patients with HF by reducing all-cause mortality and HF-related hospitalizations.[18] A meta-analysis of five trials evaluating the impact of haemodynamic-guided HF management in patients with symptomatic HF showed that haemodynamic-guided HF management using permanently implanted sensors and frequent filling pressure evaluation is superior to traditional clinical management strategies in reducing long-term HF hospitalization risk (38% relative risk reduction) in symptomatic patients.[19] On this background, some of the most recent and upcoming trials and technologies are summarized below as well as the evidence supporting RM in patients with HF (➲ Table 18.1.1).

Implantable electronic devices

One device, one parameter approach

CardioMEMS Heart Sensor Allows Monitoring of Pressure to Improve Outcomes in NYHA Class III Heart Failure Patients (CHAMPION trial)

The CHAMPION trial, published in 2011, investigated the utility of wireless pulmonary artery haemodynamic monitoring in chronic HF in reducing HF-hospitalization.[14] CardioMEMS™ is a small sensor placed in the pulmonary artery. Readings can be taken (usually once daily) of the pulmonary artery pressure (systolic, diastolic, and mean pressure). Patients were randomly assigned to management with the wireless implantable haemodynamic monitoring system (treatment group) or to a control group for at least 6 months. The trial showed a reduction in hospitalization for patients who were managed with this wireless implantable haemodynamic monitoring system. Information about pulmonary arterial pressure in addition to clinical signs and symptoms resulted in improved HF management, versus a standard of care approach alone.[13,20] The implantation of this wireless HF monitoring system in a real-world setting in patients with HF and New York Heart Association (NYHA) class III symptoms resulted in 80% reduction in HF admissions and 69% reduction in all-cause admissions, the latter largely due to the decrease in HF events.[14] The aim of the Hemodynamic Guided Management of Heart Failure (GUIDE-HF) clinical trial (NCT03387813) was to test the effectiveness of the CardioMEMS™ HF System in HF patients for whom there has been so far no indication for the use of this system, but who are at risk for future HF events or mortality (e.g. NYHA II or NYHA IV). Between March 2018 and December 2019, 1022 patients were enrolled, with 1000 patients implanted successfully, and follow-up was completed on 8 January 2021. There were 253 primary endpoint events (0.563 per patient-year) among 497 patients in the haemodynamic-guided management group (treatment group) and 289 (0.640 per patient-year) in 503 patients in the control group (hazard ratio, 0.88; 95% confidence interval, 0.74–1.05; p = 0.16). A pre-specified COVID-19 sensitivity analysis using a time-dependent variable to compare events before COVID-19 and during the pandemic suggested a treatment interaction ($p_{interaction}$ = 0.11) due to a change in the primary endpoint event rate during the pandemic phase of the trial, warranting a pre-COVID-19 impact analysis. In the pre-COVID-19 impact analysis, there were 177 primary events (0.553 per patient-year) in the intervention group and 224 events (0.682 per patient-year) in the control group (hazard ratio, 0.81; 95% CI, 0.66–1.00; p = 0.049). The authors concluded that haemodynamic-guided management of HF did not result in a lower composite endpoint rate of mortality and total heart failure events compared with the control group in the overall study analysis. However, a pre-specified pre-COVID-19 impact analysis indicated a benefit of haemodynamic-guided management on the primary outcome in the pre-COVID-19 period, primarily driven by a lower HF hospitalization rate compared with the control group.[21] This significant reduction in HF hospitalizations with pulmonary artery pressure-guided HF management was nearly identical to that seen in the CHAMPION trial, providing further support to the effectiveness

Table 18.1.1 Overview of recent and future studies in RM in patients with HF

	Number of patients	Recruitment status	Patients selection	Method	Primary outcomes measures
SMILE-HF	268	Terminated 2017	Patients with current hospitalization for ADHF, regardless of the LVEF	ReDS	The rate of recurrent events of HF readmissions
MANAGE-HF	2700	Completion estimated in January 2025	Implanted ICD/CRTD NYHA II-III	HeartLogic™	All-cause mortality. HF-hospitalization
PREEMPT-HF	3750	Study completion anticipated in January 2026	Documented HF ICD/CRTD with HeartLogic	HeartLogic™	To evaluate the association of HeartLogic sensors with 30-day HF readmission
TRIAGE-HF	100	Completed 2013–2015	Non-randomized, all subjects who have been implanted with an ICD or CRT-D for at least 3 months	Heart Failure Risk Status (HFRS) derived from implanted CRT-D or ICD devices with wireless telemetry to CareLink	HFRS performance characterization from baseline until a subject completes 8 months of follow-up. The clinical signs and symptoms of worsening HF that are associated with an Heart Failure Risk Status triggered by an OptiVol alert
MONITOR-HF	348	Completed 2019–2022	HF-patients with NYHA Class III who have experienced a HF-hospitalization within the past 12 months	CardioMEMS™	The mean difference in the KCCQ overall summary score at 12 months
CardioMEMS HF System OUS post Market Study	800	Recruiting (2016–2023)	HF-patients with NYHA Class III who have experienced a HF-hospitalization within the past 12 months.	CardioMEMS™	Freedom from device/system related complications. Freedom from pressure sensor failure. Annualized HF hospitalization rate at 1 year compared to the HF hospitalization rate in the year prior to enrolment
SIRONA-HF	15	Completed 2017–2019	NYHA Class III	Cordella™	Safety freedom form adverse events. Efficacy: Accuracy
PROACTIVE-HF	900	Completion estimated in May 2024	NYHA Class III	Cordella™	Prespecified safety and effectiveness endpoints to prove a smiliar risk/benefit profile to the CardioMEMS system
VECTOR-HF	30	Completed 2019–2022	NYHA III, ambulatory IV	V-LAP™	Safety: Device/system related complication. Performance accuracy
REM-HF	1650	Completed (2011–2014)	NYHA II-IV and implanted cardiac device (ICD, CRTD/P)	ICD, CRTD/P devices were used from multiple manufacturers (Medtronic, Boston Scientific, St. Jude Medical): Bi-ventricular pacing %, Nocturnal HR, Thoracic impedance only in Medtronic and some St. Jude medical devices. activity levels, AT/AF burden, ventricular arrhythmias, therapy from device, heart rate variability, lead integrity, device programming. V–V interval at time of D/L	Death or hospitalization from cardiovascular causes

Table 18.1.1 Continued

	Number of patients	Recruitment status	Patients selection	Method	Primary outcomes measures
IN-TIME	716	Completed (2007–2013)	NYHA II–III LVEF < 35% and ICD, CRTD/P	ICD, CRTD/P (BIOTRONIK GmBH, Germany)	A composite clinical score consisting of all-cause death, HF hospitalization, change in NYHA class, and change in patient global self-assessment
NANOSENSE	500	Completion estimated December 2021	At least 150 HF-patients. The patient is either hospitalized with a primary diagnosis of acute or was discharged with a primary diagnosis of AHF within 2 weeks prior to enrolment -NYHA Class II-IV at time of enrolment.	SimpleSENSE	To develop and validate a multi-parameter algorithm for the detection of HF prior to a HF event

AHF, acute heart failure; AF, atrial fibrillation; AT, atrial tachycardia; CRTD/P, cardiac resynchronization therapy defibrillator/pacemaker; HF, heart failure; HFRS, heart failure risk status; HR, heart rate; ICD, implantable cardioverter defibrillator; LVEF, left ventricular ejection fraction; NYHA, New York Heart Association.

of this approach. Of note, however, there was no improvement seen in the NYHA Class IV patients whose HF may have been too advanced to benefit from this RM approach. Recently, a further randomized clinical trial (MONITOR-HF) (NTR7673) that was conducted in Europe (Netherlands) proved that haemodynamic monitoring using CardioMEMS™ improves QoL, measured using Kansas City Cardiomyopathy Questionnaire (KCCQ), and reduces heart failure hospitalization in this group of patients. In total 348 patients with HF and NYHA Class III were enrolled between 2019 and 2022 in 25 centres in the Netherlands. The primary endpoint was the mean difference in the KCCQ overall summary score at 12 months. The secondary efficacy endpoint was the total number of heart failure hospitalizations (first and recurrent) and urgent unplanned visits with the need for intravenous diuretics during follow-up. Both the primary and the above-mentioned secondary endpoints were met.[22]

There are few published data on RM with CardioMEMS™ for patients with left ventricular assist devices (LVAD). In a retrospective analysis of 436 patients who had received a CardioMEMS™ device, 108 of whom also received an LVAD,[23] the mean pulmonary artery (PA) pressure at the time of CardioMEMS™ implantation was higher (p < 0.001) in the group that subsequently received an LVAD. Mean PA pressures decreased after LVAD-implantation and remained stable for 1 year. The authors concluded that monitoring PA-pressure may help with decision-making regarding the timing of LVAD-implantation and in the monitoring of these patients.

Implantable pulmonary artery pressure measurement (Cordella™)

Cordella™ is a pulmonary artery pressure sensor and provides comprehensive data on the health status of the patient at home. The data gathered can be then shared with health care providers for further evaluation and management. The Cordella Sensor integrates PA-pressure data into the Cordella system to proactively deliver the information necessary to improve patient care between office visits.

The SIRONA trial (Evaluating the Safety and Efficacy of the Cordella™ Heart Failure System NYHA Class III HF Patients) (NCT03375710) is a prospective, multi-centre, open-label, single-arm clinical trial. The primary safety endpoint was freedom from adverse events associated with the use of Cordella HF system through 30 days post-implant. The primary efficacy endpoint was the accuracy of Cordella Sensor PA pressure measurements relative to standard-of-care fluid-filled catheter pressure measurements obtained by standard right heart catheterization at 90 days post-sensor implant. The primary results of the first-in-human SIRONA-study are promising.[24] A further Prospective, Multi-Center, SingleArm Clinical Trial Evaluating the Safety and Efficacy of the Cordella™ Pulmonary Artery Sensor System in New York Heart Association (NYHA) Class III Heart Failure Patients (PROACTIVE-HF Trial) has completed enrollment with results expected in early 2024 (NCT04089059).

Left atrial haemodynamic monitoring system

An alternative to pulmonary arterial pressure monitoring is direct left atrial pressure monitoring.[25] Direct left atrial pressure monitoring has theoretical advantages in certain HF sub-populations, such as those patients with secondary or mixed pulmonary hypertension, where the PA pressure may not reflect the left atrial pressure, and in HF patients with secondary mitral regurgitation, where the left atrial pressure waveform may inform on dynamic or progressive changes in the secondary mitral regurgitation severity. A first-generation left atrial pressure monitoring system provided strong proof-of-concept for the approach.[26] The ongoing Left Atrium Monitoring systEm for Patients With Chronic sysTOlic & Diastolic Congestive heaRt Failure trial (VECTOR-HF, NCT03775161) studies the safety and reliability of the V-LAP™ device in patients with HF irrespective of LVEF. V-LAP is a wireless, battery-free microcomputer, placed directly across the interatrial septum. The first device was implanted in February 2019 and enrolment of the planned 30 patients was completed in December 2021, in six European centres across Germany, Israel,

Italy, and England. Presentation of preliminary results support the future potential for the use of this system, and additional studies are planned.

Multiparameter algorithms in implanted devices

One of the longest established methods of RM is using cardiac implantable electronic devices (CIEDs) to measure cardiopulmonary variables such as thoracic impedance (surrogate of lung fluid content), heart rate and heart rate variability, and patient activity level.[27] To date, studies have demonstrated the utility of such devices for predicting risk of future HF events; however, how to best use this information and to keep patients out of the hospital is still under investigation. Ongoing efforts and novel technologies seek to improve detection algorithms and utility of CIEDs in HF RM.

HeartLogic™ algorithm

The HeartLogic algorithm was developed using data from the MultiSENSE study (Multisensor Chronic Evaluation in Ambulatory Heart Failure Patients). The following sensor measurements were incorporated: heart sounds (S1, S3), lung impedance, respiratory rate and volume, activity, and night-time heart rate. The changes in sensor parameters were weighted and aggregated based on a risk determination, resulting in a single composite index to alert clinicians when a patient's HF is worsening.

HeartLogic was found to augment baseline N-terminal pro-B-type natriuretic peptide (NT-proBNP) assessment. Furthermore, a retrospective analysis indicated that the HeartLogic algorithm might be useful to detect gradual worsening of HF and to stratify risk of HF decompensation.[28,29] Two studies seek to provide further evidence for clinical benefit:

1 Multiple Cardiac Sensors for the Management of Heart Failure (MANAGE-HF) is a multi-centre, global, prospective, open label, multi-phase trial intended to evaluate the clinical efficacy of the HeartLogic HF diagnostic feature (NCT03237858). Phase II of the MANAGE-HF trial assessed the clinical integration and safety of RM of HF patients with implanted cardiac resynchronization therapy-D (CRT-D) or implantable cardioverter defibrillators (ICD) that contain the HeartLogic feature against patients with RM but without HeartLogic alerts. Two hundred patients with symptomatic HF (NYHA II-III) and left ventricular ejection fraction < 35% were enrolled. Further criteria for recruitment were hospitalization as a result of HF decompensation in the last 12 months or unexpected visit in the last 90 days due to HF worsening or an elevated natriuretic peptide concentration. During the period of follow-up there were 585 alerts. In 74% of these cases, HF-medications were adjusted. Optimizing HF-therapy within 2 weeks of alert resulted in faster recovery of HeartLogic scores. NT-proBNP decreased during the period of 12 months of follow-up. The authors concluded that monitoring using HeartLogic diagnostic is safe and might optimize the management of HF.

2 PREEMPT-HF-trial (Precision Event Monitoring for Patients with Heart Failure using HeartLogic) (NCT03579641) completed recruitment. The primary outcome is the association

of HeartLogic sensors with 30-day HF re-admission. Subjects were followed for about 12 months after baseline to observe the occurrence of clinical events. These are defined as follows: hospitalization (any cause), hospitalization due to HF, HF-readmission 30-days after discharge, and HF-outpatient visit where unscheduled intravenous diuretics are prescribed in a setting that does not involve patient admission (emergency department, outpatient clinic). The results are not yet published.

Heart failure risk status (HFRS) generated by cardiac implantable electronic devices (TRIAGE-HF)

HF-risk status (HFRS) generated by cardiac implanted electronic devices was investigated in 100 patients with HF in three Canadian centres for up to 8 weeks (TRIAGE-HF) (NCT 01798797). Measurements included impedance/OptiVol (Medtronic, MN, USA), patient activity, night heart rate, heart rate variability, percentage CRT pacing, atrial tachycardia/atrial fibrillation, and episodes of untreated and device-treated arrhythmia. Patients with a high HFRS score were contacted by telephone to assess symptoms, and compliance with prescribed therapies, nutrition, and exercise. Clinician-assessed and HFRS-calculated risk were compared at study baseline and exit. Twenty-four high HFRS episodes were observed. Measurements associated with an increased risk of HF hospitalization included OptiVol index (n = 20), followed by low patient activity (n = 18) and elevated night heart rate (n = 12). High HFRS was associated with symptoms of worsening HF in 63% of cases (n = 15) increasing to 83% of cases (n = 20) when non-compliance with pharmacological therapies and lifestyle was considered. The authors concluded that HFRS might be a useful tool for RM of HF.[30]

Intrathoracic impedance monitoring, audible patient alerts, and outcome in patients with heart failure (DOT-HF) trial

This trial studied 335 patients with chronic HF who had undergone implantation of an implantable cardioverter-defibrillator alone (18%) or with cardiac resynchronization therapy (82%). All devices featured a monitoring tool to track changes in intrathoracic impedance (OptiVol) and other diagnostic parameters. Patients were randomized to have information available to physicians and patients as an audible alert in case of preset threshold crossings (access arm) or not (control arm). The primary endpoint was a composite of all-cause mortality and HF hospitalizations. During 14.9 ± 5.4 months, this occurred in 48 patients (29%) in the access arm and in 33 patients (20%) in the control arm (p = 0.063; hazard ratio, 1.52; 95% confidence interval, 0.97–2.37). This was due mainly to more HF hospitalizations (hazard ratio, 1.79; 95% confidence interval, 1.08–2.95; p = 0.022), whereas the number of deaths was comparable (19 vs 15; p = 0.54). The number of outpatient visits was higher in the access arm (250 versus 84; p < 0.0001), with relatively more signs of HF among control patients during outpatient visits. Although the trial was terminated as a result of slow enrolment, a post hoc futility analysis indicated that a positive result would have been unlikely. The authors concluded that use of an implantable diagnostic tool to measure intrathoracic impedance with an audible patient alert did not improve outcome and increased heart failure hospitalizations and outpatient visits in heart failure patients.[31]

Fluid status monitoring wirelessly: Rationale and design of the OptiLink HF Study (Optimization of Heart Failure Management using OptiVol Fluid Status Monitoring and CareLink)

Patients recently implanted with an ICD with or without CRT were eligible if one of three conditions was met: prior HF hospitalization, recent diuretic treatment, or recent brain natriuretic peptide increase. Eligible patients were randomized (1:1) to have fluid status alerts automatically transmitted as inaudible text message alerts to the responsible physician or to receive standard care (no alerts). In the intervention arm, following a telemedicine alert, a protocol-specified algorithm with remote review of device data and telephone contact was prescribed to assess symptoms and initiate treatment. The primary endpoint was a composite of all-cause death and cardiovascular hospitalization, and 1002 patients were followed for an average of 1.9 years. The primary endpoint occurred in 227 patients (45.0%) in the intervention arm and 239 patients (48.1%) in the control arm (hazard ratio, 0.87; 95% confidence interval, 0.72–1.04; p = 0.13). There were 59 (11.7%) deaths in the intervention arm and 63 (12.7%) in the control arm (hazard ratio, 0.89; 95% confidence interval, 0.62–1.28; p = 0.52). Twenty-four per cent of alerts were not transmitted and 30% were followed by a medical intervention. In conclusion, among ICD patients with advanced HF, fluid status telemedicine alerts did not significantly improve outcomes. Adherence to treatment protocols by physicians and patients might be challenge for further developments in the telemedicine field.[32]

Remote Management of Heart Failure using implantable electronic devices (REM-HF)

REM-HF is the largest prospective and randomized clinical trial conducted on RM with implanted devices. In this trial, 1650 patients with HF who had an ICD were randomized to active weekly review of RM data or usual care across nine UK hospitals, with an average follow-up of 2.8 years. The primary outcome of death or hospitalization from cardiovascular causes was the same in the RM group (42.4%) and the control group (40.8%) of patients (p = 0.87), despite considerable extra activity being triggered by the remotely collected data.[33] In this study ICD, CRTD/P devices were used from multiple manufacturers (Medtronic, Boston Scientific, St. Jude Medical). Bi-ventricular pacing percentage, nocturnal heart rate, thoracic impedance only in Medtronic and some St. Jude medical devices, activity levels, atrial tachycardia/atrial fibrillation burden, ventricular arrhythmias, therapy from device, heart rate variability, lead integrity, and device programming were documented.

The influence of home monitoring on the clinical management of HF patients with impaired left ventricular function (IN-TIME)

The IN-TIME study was a prospective randomized trial that analysed the benefit on clinical outcomes of RM of implanted devices (Biotronik). In this study, 716 patients were recruited, and 664 patients were finally randomized to multiparameter RM in addition to standard of care or standard of care alone. At a set time every day (typically 03.00 a.m.) or on detection of tachyarrhythmia (atrial or ventricular), the devices transmitted cumulative and last-saved diagnostic data in 24 hours such as CRT-stimulation < 80%, pacing, impedance, or sensing safety issues. A small portable patient device received the data and relayed them automatically over mobile telephone links to the Biotronik Home Monitoring Service Center (Berlin, Germany). The primary end point was a composite clinical score. This included all-cause death, HF hospitalization, change in NYHA class, and change in patient global self-assessment. The composite clinical score was better in the RM population. Improvement in composite outcome mainly resulted from a lower death rate in the RM group (estimated 1-year mortality 2.7% versus 6.8% (HR 0.37; 95% CI 0.16–0.83, p = 0.012).[34]

While there is no clear explanation for the difference in the results between REM-HF and IN-TIME, the results could be attributed to the weekly RM in REM-HF compared with the daily review and intervention in IN-TIME.

Non-invasive-monitoring

Non-invasive monitoring for HF spans cardiac and extra-cardiac variables in an attempt to detect signs of cardiac decompensation.

The authors of the Trans-European Network-Home-Care Management System (TEN-HMS) trial investigated whether home telemonitoring (HTM) (weight, blood pressure, heart rate and rhythm with automated devices linked to a cardiology centre) improves outcomes compared to nurse telephone support (NTS) and usual care for patients with HF who are at high risk of hospitalization or death. Patients were randomly assigned to HTM, NTS, or usual care in a 2:2:1 ratio. The trial enrolled 426 patients. The primary endpoint was days lost as a result of death or hospitalization with NTS vs HTM at 240 days. There was no statistically significant difference between the two groups. The number of admissions and mortality were similar among patients randomly assigned to NTS or HTM, but the mean duration of admissions was reduced by 6 days with HTM. Patients randomly assigned to receive usual care had higher one-year mortality (45%) than patients assigned to receive NTS (27%) or HTM (29%) (p = 0.032).[15] In a sub-analysis of the TEN-HMS, the investigators tested the possibility of predicting hospitalization due to worsening heart failure using daily weight measurement. They concluded that many episodes of worsening heart failure are not necessarily associated with weight gain and therefore RM focused primarily on weight changes may not have great value for HF management.[35]

The effectiveness of RM after discharge of hospitalized patients with HF was investigated in the Better Effectiveness After Transition–Heart Failure (BEAT-HF) trial, a clinical randomized trial conducted in six centres in California, USA. The follow-up period was on average 180 days. Centralized registered nurses conducted RM reviews (daily blood pressure, heart rate, symptoms, and weight), protocolized actions, and telephone calls. The trial enrolled 1437 patients. The primary outcome was readmission for any cause within 180 days after discharge. Secondary outcomes were all-cause readmission within 30 days, all-cause mortality at 30 and 180 days, and QoL at 30 and 180 days. At the end, there was no reduction in 180-day readmissions among patients hospitalized for HF, in whom combined health coaching telephone calls and RM were performed.[16] Patient adherence was a major limitation in this trial, given that only about 60% of patients were adherent for more than half of the time in the first 30 days.

The Telemedical Interventional Management in Heart Failure II (TIM-HF-2) a randomized, controlled, multicentre trial (NCT 01878630) is a positive trial for non-invasive telemonitoring. Eligible patients with HF with reduced and preserved ejection fraction were randomized (1:1) to either RM + usual care or to usual care only. Patients were followed for 12 months. Patients in the intervention group used a set of multiple non-invasive devices on a daily basis. A telemedical centre staffed with HF-nurses and HF-specialists operated 24/7. The staff could, if needed immediately act remotely with changes in medication or with admission to emergency departments.

The primary outcome was the percentage of days lost due to unplanned cardiovascular hospitalizations or all-cause death during a one year follow-up. This endpoint focused on the impact of RM from the patient's perspective. The main secondary outcomes were all-cause mortality and cardiovascular mortality. The investigators found that patients assigned to RM had fewer lost days compared with patients assigned to usual care. The all-cause mortality was significantly lower in the RM-group, but there was no significant difference in cardiovascular mortality between the two groups.[12]

The sub-study of TIM-HF-2 investigated whether the biomarkers mid-regional pro-adrenomedullin (MR-proADM) and NT-proBNP could be used to identify low-risk patients unlikely to benefit from RM, thereby allowing more efficient allocation of the intervention. Both biomarkers were strongly associated with events. The primary endpoint of lost days increased from 1.0% (1.4%) in the lowest to 17.3% (17.6%) in the highest quintile of NT-proBNP (MR-proADM). The authors showed that Biomarker guidance in the RM would have saved about 150 working hours in a telemedical centre/year per 100 patients of the eligible population.[36]

Daily weight measurements

This is the easiest way to control euvolaemic status in patients with HF and it is still recommended by HF-specialists and ESC-HF guidelines.[37] However, daily weight change has low sensitivity for predicting HF hospitalization.

Lung fluid volume and lung impedance measurement

Some studies have focused on non-invasive lung impedance-guided treatment in patients with HF (Impedance HF-trial) and showed reduced mortality and reduced hospitalization rates due to acute HF (AHF).[38] In addition, the extent of change in pulmonary fluid content using lung-impedance based therapy during HF-hospitalization has been shown to be strongly predictive of HF readmission and event-free survival.[39]

Remote Dielectric Sensing (ReDS™) is an example of a non-invasive technology used in the field of RM that contains clinical algorithms and performs an absolute measurement of lung fluid volume by using a focused electromagnetic RADAR beam through the right lung. Normal lung measures 20–35% lung fluid content (default target range). The measurement can be done without any skin contact in up to 45 seconds. Uriel et al. showed strong correlations between ReDS™ and invasive haemodynamic

measurements using the pulmonary artery wedge pressure (PAWP).[40] In this study, receiver operating characteristic analysis of the ability to identify a PAWP ≥18 mm Hg resulted in a ReDS cutoff value of 34%, with an area under the curve of 0.85, a sensitivity of 90.7%, and a specificity of 77.1%. Overall, ReDS <34% carries a high negative predictive value of 94.9% for an elevated PAWP.

In the Evaluation Study of Remote Dielectric Sensing (ReDS) Technology-Guided Therapy for Decreasing Heart Failure Re-Hospitalizations, the investigators concluded that ReDS-guided management has the potential to reduce HF readmissions in AHF patients recently discharged from the hospital.[41] The results of SMILE-HF trial were presented at the HFSA 2019.[42] The study recruited 268 patients from 43 centres across the USA. The pre-specified endpoint of per-protocol changes in HF readmission were reduced in the ReDS™ treatment guided HF management arm (HR 0.52, 95% CI [0.31–0.87], p = 0.01), which equates to a 48% readmissions reduction.

Non-invasive intracardiac pressure monitoring

A novel method of intracardiac pressure monitoring (ICPM) uses a non-invasive portable ultrasound-based measurement system. The new system is based on image time series processing estimating the changes of the oscillating traceable regions via the introduction of the new ultrasound generalized M-mode and the notion of the derived image. The non-invasive system requires an initial calibration with simultaneous invasive pressure measurements, yet efforts are underway to eliminate this step using machine learning technology. The system has been successfully tested in animals (sheep).[43] Human validation trials were performed on 32 patients and a multicentre multinational study is pending. The intended in-home use will require the self-use of a portable ultrasound system by patients.

Voice signal recognition

Maor at al. enrolled 10,583 patients in Israel in their study. Patients were registered to a call centre for patients who had chronic conditions including congestive heart failure (CHF) between 2013 and 2018. A total of 223 acoustic features were extracted from 20 s of speech for each patient. A biomarker was developed based on a training cohort of non-CHF patients (n = 8316). The biomarker was tested on a mutually exclusive CHF study cohort (n = 2267) and was evaluated as a continuous and ordinal (4 quartiles) variable. Median age of the CHF study population was 77 (interquartile range 68–83) and 63% were men. During a median follow-up of 20 months (interquartile range 9–34), 824 (36%) patients died. Kaplan–Meier survival analysis showed higher cumulative probability of death with increasing quartiles (23%, 29%, 38%, and 54%; p < 0.001). The model consistently demonstrated an independent association of the biomarker with hospitalizations during follow-up (p < 0.001). The authors concluded that non-invasive vocal biomarker is associated with adverse outcome among CHF patients, suggesting a possible role for voice analysis in telemedicine and CHF patient care.[44] Perspectival, wearable medical devices or smartphones could have the potential to be effective in RM of patients with HF.

HF-diagnostics using wearable devices and technologies

There is currently a heightened focus on wearable monitoring technology both for detecting atrial fibrillation and for preventing hospitalization due to decompensated HF by observing early changes occurring before overt AHF takes place.[45,46]

Wearable health devices are part of digital and mobile health and represent potential instruments to improve HF care and outcomes. DeVore et al described this topic nicely in a recently published review article.[47] Available data are currently limited to observational studies or small clinical randomized trials. Wearables are being integrated into HF trials as an intervention to assess outcomes. This may include lifestyle, pharmacological, device, and mHealth interventions.[48] Future wearables for HF may be applied externally and include skin patches, watches, and contact lenses, and may monitor lactate or electrolytes.[49] In many cases, wearable devices employ a multi-sensor approach to emulate the risk predictive approach demonstrated using CIEDs.

The LINK-HF trial (NCT03037710) was a 'Multisensor Non-invasive Remote Monitoring for Prediction of Heart Failure Exacerbation'. LINK-HF examined the performance of a personalized analytical platform using continuous data streams to predict re-hospitalization after HF admission. Monitoring was performed up to 3 months using a disposable multisensor patch placed on the chest that recorded physiological data. Data were uploaded continuously via smartphone to a cloud analytics platform. Machine learning was used to design a prognostic algorithm to detect HF exacerbation. Altogether, 100 subjects aged 68.4 ± 10.2 years (98% male) were enrolled. The algorithm detected precursors of HF hospitalization with 76% to 88% sensitivity and 85% specificity. Median time between initial alert and readmission was 6.5 (4.2–13.7) days.[50] In conclusion LINK-HF trial showed that multivariate physiological telemetry from a wearable sensor can provide accurate early detection of impending re-hospitalization with a predictive accuracy comparable to implanted devices. The clinical efficacy and generalizability of this low-cost non-invasive approach to re-hospitalization mitigation should be further tested.

The Nanowear Wearable Heart Failure Management System Multiple Sensor Algorithm Development and Validation Trial is a multi-centre prospective, non-randomized, observational study (NCT03719079). The aim is to enroll up to 500 subjects in order to collect data which includes at least 150 HF hospitalizations in participating subjects. The trial was expected to be completed in December 2021, but has not yet been published. The study device is the Wearable Congestive Heart Failure Management System (WCHFS, also known as SimpleSENSE).

The observational multi-centre study titled 'Evaluating Mobile Health Tool Use for Capturing Patient-Centered Outcomes Measures in HF Patients' (NCT04191356) will evaluate the feasibility of a novel mobile health monitoring platform. The trial has stopped recruiting. Actual enrolment is 67 patients (April 2023). It was planned to enrol 170 patients with HF. The platform was supposed to capture patient-centered outcomes measures for 8 weeks. The primary outcome is the correlation between physiology and accelerometer data collected from Everion and Apple Watch (i.e. heart rate, single lead ECG report) with 6-minute walk test, laboratory (i.e. eGFR, troponin, creatinine, NT-proBNP) results, and QoL measured using Kansas City Cardiomyopathy Questionnaire (KCCQ)-12 and the 5-level and 5-dimensions European quality of life (EQ-5D-5L) questionnaire. Estimated study completion was July 2023.

These small feasibility studies may improve understanding of the technology but do not address the core issue of whether what can be done should be done. Only randomized controlled trials will help determine the clinical and financial effectiveness of RM.

More studies and evidence are required before a routine integration of these new technologies in the daily routine work-up or screening of patients with HF would become feasible. Furthermore, there are currently no RCTs evaluating the reliability and validity of the data measured by wearables and smartphones. In addition, the increasing number of apps and devices makes it difficult to assess their strengths and weaknesses. Data protection and data processing security issues have to be re-assessed for each new application.

The future will show if wearable technologies will prove themselves to be an effective means in the field of RM and the management of patients with HF. How wearable technologies can complement implanted technology and in what instances they can replace the more invasive technology have yet to be determined.[51]

Principles and structure of remote monitoring systems

Two patterns of RM (telecardiology) can be observed in patients with HF: (1) physician-to-physician RM, which enables an exchange of diagnostic information between different medical providers themselves, and (2) physician-to-patient RM, which allows a direct connection between doctors and patients in their homes.

Physician-to-physician RM

The telemedical information and communication technology (ICT) enabling exchange between physicians is mostly based on a telemedical transfer of image data such as echocardiographic findings of rare diseases (e.g. in adults with congenital heart defects or in cardiomyopathies in the context of cardiac involvement in systemic diseases, such as Fabry's disease). This telemedical use is usually combined with a video conference and time-shifted to the clinical examination of the patient. Certain diagnostics can also be performed by family doctors or HF-nurses as point-of-care diagnostics for focused questions. Therefore, this method is particularly suitable for screening and follow-up for HF patients in rural areas with sparsely medical care providers.

Physician-to-patient RM

This scenario describes a connection between cardiologists and patients themselves in their homes using telemedical measurement devices and other ICT infrastructure. This care concept is an addition to the existing outpatient care provided by a general practitioner and cardiologist.

The principles of the physician-to-patient relationship are similar to usual HF outpatient care except for the lack of direct physical contact in the telemedicine modality. All other characteristics, such as the provision of personal medical care, the medical standards, and confidentiality are basics in telemedical HF care.

Telemedicine in HF is indeed rapidly evolving[6] and both described scenarios are in use. A further example of the physician-to-physician approach is exchanging findings of HF patients, who are currently on vacation (e.g. on cruise ships), between medical service providers on board and a telemedicine centre (TMC).

However, the direct communication between patient and TMC is more common (physician-to-patient). The patient measures daily vital signs at home according to a defined measuring plan, such as blood pressure, heart rate and weight, or for example, uses ultrasound ICPM and transmits the measurements to the TMC. In this way, cardiac decompensation can be detected early, and further deterioration may be prevented by adjusting the HF-medications (➲ Figure 18.1.3).

Finally, physician-directed, patient self-management approaches are under investigation in RM for HF. In fact, such an approach has been used in HF for many years, as physicians have advised patients to take on their own a higher diuretic dose in response to rapid weight gain. Moreover, this variation of the physician-to-patient approach was tested in the HOMEOSTASIS trial,[26] where it was shown to be feasible, safe, and potentially effective to allow patients to adjust diuretic doses on their own according to a physician-prescribed algorithm, based on the changes in the directly measured left atrial pressure. This approach is analogous to the long-ago established approach to diabetes management using home glucometers.

Current questions and future outlook

Several questions remain open, however, and need to be answered: Which patients should be monitored? It seems to be reasonable to apply the RM primarily to symptomatic patients (NYHA II-III), who suffered from cardiac decompensation in spite of optimal medical therapy. The best timeframe to start RM would be pre-discharge or shortly after that.[19] The chance of these patients to decompensate again is much higher than those with stable HF and the heightened risk might justify the costs resulting from applying RM in this group of patients. In addition, the method of RM is still to be chosen. For example, devices with multiple sensors might be superior to single sensor method. Furthermore, telemonitoring with CIEDs provides diagnostic information about early markers regarding the onset of pulmonary congestion, for example, elevated left ventricular end diastolic pressure (LVEDP) or elevated left atrial pressure (LAP), decreased intrathoracic impedance, changes in pulmonary artery pressure (PAP), and arrhythmias. However, non-invasive devices like scales and blood pressure monitors have a 'late' sensitivity compared to implanted telemonitoring devices. To compensate for this systematic deficit of non-invasive devices, transferred vital parameters should be reviewed daily, which may require a 24/7 telemedical service. On the other hand, some advantages of non-invasive devices could be the low costs associated with these procedures and the absence of inherent safety concerns of implantable devices. To answer this question of which modality could be better, invasive vs. non-invasive monitoring, there is currently an RCT running in Germany to evaluate the benefits of PAP measurement vs. non-invasive telemedical intervention (PASSPORT-HF: NCT04398654).

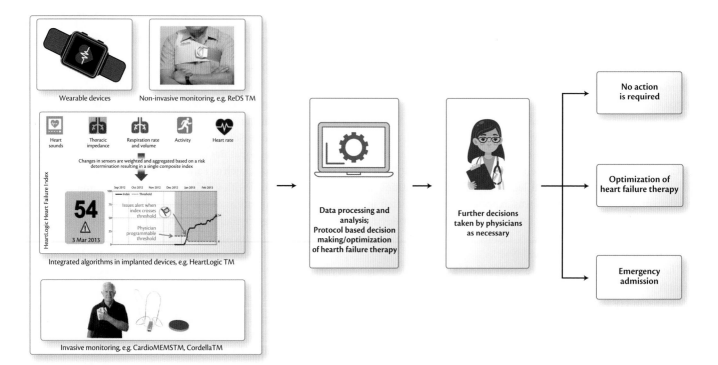

Figure 18.1.3 Different RM options (wearables, non-invasive devices like ReDS™, integrated algorithms in implanted cardiac devices such as HeartLogic™). The resulting data will be transferred to medical centres and be reviewed frequently by medical personnel (physicians, trained nurses, etc.). Accordingly, decisions can be made to modify medical therapy or to organize admission of the patient. Alternatively, no action may be required, assuring a stable condition of heart failure patients.

A further challenging step for the RM concept is the translation from study conditions to usual care in a 'real-world' setting. Currently, the TMC capacity is about 500 HF patients. For example, in Germany with approximately 200,000 patients meeting the TIM-HF2 inclusion criteria more than 200 TMCs would be necessary. Technological innovations like artificial intelligence are needed for upscaling this concept. Also, the use of a clinical decision support system in the TMC to support medical staff in their daily medical workflow is required.

Moreover, new sensor technologies are under investigation, for example, artificial intelligence-based voice analysis for the diagnosis of cardiac decompensation.[44]

Further issues should address responsibility for reviewing the transmitted data and the frequency of data transmission and review. Data should be transmitted securely to a medical centre. It is expected that medical personnel will receive a large volume of data that needs to be processed and analysed. Approving and paying for the additional costs resulting from RM is still an open question. In the USA, the Centers for Medicare and Medicaid Services have established programmes, such as the Chronic Care Management and Remote Patient Monitoring programmes, to support the applications of systems utilizing RM technologies in complex patients with chronic disease syndromes like HF. Moreover, an analysis based on the CHAMPION trial suggested that monitoring using the CardioMEMS™ device was cost-effective from a US-payer perspective, with the incremental cost to deliver one additional quality-adjusted life-year of approximately $30,000 in the USA.[52] Recent analysis performed by national researchers and health insurance companies in Germany showed that the additional non-invasive telemedical interventional management in patients with HF was cost-effective compared to standard care alone, since such intervention was associated with overall cost savings and superior clinical effectiveness.[53] A further aspect might be related to the different health systems worldwide. For example, the TIM-HF2 care model might be not easily applicable to other health care systems. The main issues to be considered are patient adherence and the required availability of medical teams (24-hour availability). Unanswered questions in the field of RM are summarized in ⊃ Figure 18.1.4. Additional clinical investigations will help to confirm and extend the existing evidence presented above and to answer some of the raised questions.

Summary and key messages

Development of objective means of monitoring fluid status with associated treatment algorithms to reduce hospitalizations has emerged as a priority in the care of HF patients.

RM is a promising way to monitor and manage patients with HF. RM could be performed non-invasively, through wearable devices, or by using developed algorithms integrated in ICDs or invasively through continuous measuring of the pulmonary artery or left atrial pressure. RM has been shown to improve the management and outcomes in patients with HF, but results do not apply to all technologies in all settings. Upcoming devices and technologies are being currently evaluated. Early results are promising. Questions regarding patient selection, timing of initiation and duration, and the most appropriate RM technology for each patient remain open. However, current evidence suggests that the most beneficial HF patient group are patients at high risk, recently hospitalized due to HF in functional class II or III. For the majority of stable HF patients there is no evidence for a beneficial effect of RM. Further larger, randomized studies are required to refine our current knowledge and optimize patient care.

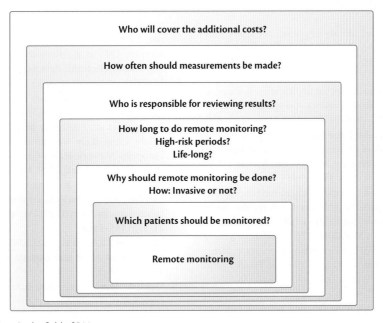

Figure 18.1.4 Unresolved questions in the field of RM.

References

1. Rosano, G.M.C., et al., Patient profiling in heart failure for tailoring medical therapy. A consensus document of the Heart Failure Association of the European Society of Cardiology. Eur J Heart Fail, 2021. **23**(6):872–81.

2. Epstein, A.M., A.K. Jha, and E.J. Orav, The relationship between hospital admission rates and rehospitalizations. N Engl J Med, 2011. **365**(24):2287–95.

3. van Oeffelen, A.A., et al., Prognosis after a first hospitalisation for acute myocardial infarction and congestive heart failure by country of birth. Heart, 2014. **100**(18):1436–43.

4. Dickinson, M.G., et al., Remote monitoring of patients with heart failure: a White Paper from the Heart Failure Society of America Scientific Statements Committee. J Card Fail, 2018. **24**(10): 682–94.

5. Abraham, W.T., et al., Patient monitoring across the spectrum of heart failure disease management 10 years after the CHAMPION trial. ESC Heart Fail, 2021. **8**(5):3472–82.

6. Brahmbhatt, D.H. and M.R. Cowie, Remote management of heart failure: an overview of telemonitoring technologies. Card Fail Rev, 2019. **5**(2):86–92.

7. Schrier, R.W. and W.T. Abraham, Hormones and hemodynamics in heart failure. N Engl J Med, 1999. **341**(8):577–85.

8. Bekfani, T., et al., A current and future outlook on upcoming technologies in remote monitoring of patients with heart failure. Eur J Heart Fail, 2021. **23**(1):175–85.

9. Kaye, D.M., et al., Adverse consequences of high sympathetic nervous activity in the failing human heart. J Am Coll Cardiol, 1995. **26**(5): 1257–63.

10. Adamson, P.B., Pathophysiology of the transition from chronic compensated and acute decompensated heart failure: new insights from continuous monitoring devices. Curr Heart Fail Rep, 2009. **6**(4): 287–92.

11. Cleland, J.G.F., et al., Caring for people with heart failure and many other medical problems through and beyond the COVID-19 pandemic: the advantages of universal access to home telemonitoring. Eur J Heart Fail, 2020. **22**(6):995–8.

12. Koehler, F., et al., Efficacy of telemedical interventional management in patients with heart failure (TIM-HF2): a randomised, controlled, parallel-group, unmasked trial. Lancet, 2018. **392**(10152): 1047–57.

13. Abraham, W.T., et al., Sustained efficacy of pulmonary artery pressure to guide adjustment of chronic heart failure therapy: complete follow-up results from the CHAMPION randomised trial. Lancet, 2016. **387**(10017):453–61.

14. Assaad, M., et al., CardioMems(R) device implantation reduces repeat hospitalizations in heart failure patients: A single center experience. JRSM Cardiovasc Dis, 2019. **8**:2048004019833290.

15. Cleland, J.G., et al., Noninvasive home telemonitoring for patients with heart failure at high risk of recurrent admission and death: the Trans-European Network-Home-Care Management System (TEN-HMS) study. J Am Coll Cardiol, 2005. **45**(10):1654–64.

16. Ong, M.K., et al., Effectiveness of remote patient monitoring after discharge of hospitalized patients with heart failure: the Better Effectiveness After Transition—Heart Failure (BEAT-HF) randomized clinical trial. JAMA Intern Med, 2016. **176**(3):310–8.

17. Qian, F., et al., Racial differences in heart failure outcomes: evidence from the Tele-HF Trial (Telemonitoring to Improve Heart Failure Outcomes). JACC Heart Fail, 2015. **3**(7):531–8.

18. Inglis, S.C., et al., Structured telephone support or non-invasive telemonitoring for patients with heart failure. Cochrane Database Syst Rev, 2015(10):CD007228.

19. Adamson, P.B., et al., Remote haemodynamic-guided care for patients with chronic heart failure: a meta-analysis of completed trials. Eur J Heart Fail, 2017. **19**(3):426–33.

20. Adamson, P.B., et al., CHAMPION trial rationale and design: the long-term safety and clinical efficacy of a wireless pulmonary artery pressure monitoring system. J Card Fail, 2011. **17**(1):3–10.

21. Lindenfeld, J., et al., Haemodynamic-guided management of heart failure (GUIDE-HF): a randomised controlled trial. Lancet, 2021. **398**(10304):991–1001.

22. Brugts, J.J., et al. Remote haemodynamic monitoring of pulmonary artery pressures in patients with chronic heart failure (MONITOR-HF): a randomised clinical trial. Lancet, 2023;401(10394):2113–23.

23. Kilic, A., et al., Changes in pulmonary artery pressure before and after left ventricular assist device implantation in patients utilizing remote haemodynamic monitoring. ESC Heart Fail, 2019. **6**(1): 138–45.

24. Mullens, W., et al., Digital health care solution for proactive heart failure management with the Cordella Heart Failure System: results of the SIRONA first-in-human study. Eur J Heart Fail, 2020; **22**(10):1912–19.

25. Di Mario, C., et al., A novel implantable left atrial pressure sensor in two heart failure patients. EuroIntervention, 2020; **16**(5):432–3.

26. Ritzema, J., et al., Physician-directed patient self-management of left atrial pressure in advanced chronic heart failure. Circulation, 2010; **121**(9):1086–95.

27. Hawkins, N.M., et al., Predicting heart failure decompensation using cardiac implantable electronic devices: a review of practices and challenges. Eur J Heart Fail, 2016. **18**(8):977–86.

28. Boehmer, J.P., et al., A Multisensor Algorithm Predicts Heart Failure Events in Patients With Implanted Devices: Results From the MultiSENSE Study. JACC Heart Fail, 2017. **5**(3):216–25.

29. Capucci, A., et al., Preliminary experience with the multisensor HeartLogic algorithm for heart failure monitoring: a retrospective case series report. ESC Heart Fail, 2019. **6**(2):308–18.

30. Virani, S.A., et al., Prospective evaluation of integrated device diagnostics for heart failure management: results of the TRIAGE-HF study. ESC Heart Fail, 201; **5**(5):809–17.

31. van Veldhuisen, D.J., et al., Intrathoracic impedance monitoring, audible patient alerts, and outcome in patients with heart failure. Circulation, 2011. **124**(16):1719–26.

32. Bohm, M., et al., Fluid status telemedicine alerts for heart failure: a randomized controlled trial. Eur Heart J, 2016. **37**(41):3154–63.

33. Morgan, J.M., et al., Remote management of heart failure using implantable electronic devices. Eur Heart J, 2017. **38**(30): 2352–60.

34. Hindricks, G., et al., Implant-based multiparameter telemonitoring of patients with heart failure (IN-TIME): a randomised controlled trial. Lancet, 2014;. **384**(9943):583–90.

35. Zhang, J., et al., Predicting hospitalization due to worsening heart failure using daily weight measurement: analysis of the Trans-European Network-Home-Care Management System (TEN-HMS) study. Eur J Heart Fail, 2009. **11**(4):420–7.

36. Mockel, M., et al., Biomarker guidance allows a more personalized allocation of patients for remote patient management in heart failure: results from the TIM-HF2 trial. Eur J Heart Fail, 2019. **21**(11):1445–1458.

37. McDonagh, T.A., et al., 2021 ESC Guidelines for the diagnosis and treatment of acute and chronic heart failure. Eur Heart J, 2021. **42**(36):3599–3726.

38. Shochat, M.K., et al., Non-Invasive Lung IMPEDANCE-Guided Preemptive Treatment in Chronic Heart Failure Patients: A Randomized Controlled Trial (IMPEDANCE-HF Trial). J Card Fail, 2016. **22**(9):713–22.

39. Kleiner Shochat, M., et al., Prediction of readmissions and mortality in patients with heart failure: lessons from the IMPEDANCE-HF extended trial. ESC Heart Fail, 2018. **5**(5):788–799.

40. Uriel, N., et al., Relationship between noninvasive assessment of lung fluid volume and invasively measured cardiac hemodynamics. J Am Heart Assoc, 2018. **7**(22):e009175.

41. Amir, O., et al., Evaluation of remote dielectric sensing (ReDS) technology-guided therapy for decreasing heart failure re-hospitalizations. Int J Cardiol, 2017. **240**:279–284.

42. Abraham, W.T., et al., Primary results of the Sensible Medical Innovations Lung Fluid Status Monitor Allows Reducing Readmission Rate of Heart Failure Patients (SMILE) trial. J Card Fail, 2019. **25**(11):938.

43. Brenner, A., A system and method for non-invasive measurement of cardiovascular blood pressure. Biomed J Sci&Tech Res, 2018;**7**(2):5758–60.

44. Maor, E., et al., Vocal biomarker is associated with hospitalization and mortality among heart failure patients. J Am Heart Assoc, 2020.;**9**(7):e013359.

45. Seshadri, D.R., et al., Accuracy of Apple Watch for detection of atrial fibrillation. Circulation, 2020. **141**(8):702–3.

46. Shah, A.J., et al., Detecting heart failure using wearables: a pilot study. Physiol Meas, 2020. *41*(4):1–7.

47. DeVore, A.D., J. Wosik, and A.F. Hernandez, The future of wearables in heart failure patients. JACC Heart Fail, 2019. **7**(11):922–32.

48. Allida, S., et al., mHealth education interventions in heart failure. Cochrane Database Syst Rev, 2020; **7**:CD011845.

49. Imani, S., et al., A wearable chemical-electrophysiological hybrid biosensing system for real-time health and fitness monitoring. Nat Commun, 2016. 7:11650.

50. Stehlik, J., et al., Continuous Wearable Monitoring Analytics Predict Heart Failure Hospitalization: The LINK-HF Multicenter Study. Circ Heart Fail, 2020. **13**(3):e006513.

51. Bonato, P., Advances in wearable technology and its medical applications. Conf Proc IEEE Eng Med Biol Soc, 2010. **2010**:2021–4.

52. Martinson, M., et al., Pulmonary artery pressure-guided heart failure management: US cost-effectiveness analyses using the results of the CHAMPION clinical trial. Eur J Heart Fail, 2017. **19**(5):652–60.

53. Sydow, H., et al., Cost-effectiveness of noninvasive telemedical interventional management in patients with heart failure: health economic analysis of the TIM-HF2 trial. Clin Res Cardiol, 2022.111(11):1231–44.

Index

For the benefit of digital users, indexed terms that span two pages (e.g., 52–53) may, on occasion, appear on only one of those pages.

Note: 'f ','t', and 'b' before page numbers indicate figures, tables, and boxes.